Kuerer's
BREAST SURGICAL ONCOLOGY

Kuerer's
BREAST SURGICAL ONCOLOGY

Editor

Henry M. Kuerer, MD, PhD, FACS

Professor, Department of Surgical Oncology
Director, Breast Surgical Oncology Training Program
University of Texas MD Anderson Cancer Center
Houston, Texas

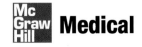

New York   Chicago   San Francisco   Lisbon   London   Madrid   Mexico City
Milan   New Delhi   San Juan   Seoul   Singapore   Sydney   Toronto

Kuerer's Breast Surgical Oncology

Copyright © 2010 by The McGraw-Hill Companies, Inc. All rights reserved. Printed in China. Except as permitted under the United States Copyright Act of 1976, no part of this publication may be reproduced or distributed in any form or by any means, or stored in a data base or retrieval system without the prior written permission of the publisher.

1 2 3 4 5 6 7 8 9 0 CTP/CTP 12 11 10 9

Set ISBN 978-0-07-160176-4; MHID 0-07-160176-7
Book ISBN 978-0-07-160178-8; MHID 0-07-160178-3
DVD ISBN 978-0-07-160179-5; MHID 0-07-160179-1

This book was set in Adobe Garamond by Glyph International.
The editors were Marsha S. Gelber and Peter J. Boyle.
The production supervisor was Catherine H. Saggese.
Art management was by Armen Ovsepyan.
Project management was provided by Deepti Narwat Agarwal, Glyph International.
The designer was Janice Bielawa.
The cover designer was Mary McKeon.
China Translation & Printing Services, Ltd., was printer and binder.

This book was printed on acid-free paper.

Library of Congress Cataloging-in-Publication Data

Kuerer's breast surgical oncology / [edited by] Henry Mark Kuerer.
       p. ; cm.
  Includes bibliographical references and index.
    ISBN-13: 978-0-07-160176-4 (set)
    ISBN-10: 0-07-160176-7 (set)
    ISBN-13: 978-0-07-160178-8 (book : alk. paper)
    ISBN-10: 0-07-160178-3 (book : alk. paper)   1. Breast–Cancer–Surgery.   I. Kuerer, Henry Mark.
  II. Title: Breast surgical oncology.
    [DNLM: 1. Breast Neoplasms–surgery. WP 870 K96 2010]
    RD539.8.K84 2010
    616.99'449059–dc22

                                      2009041007

McGraw-Hill books are available at special quantity discounts to use as premiums and sales promotions, or for use in corporate training programs. To contact a representative please e-mail us at bulksales@mcgraw-hill.com

DEDICATION

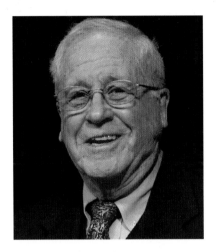

Bernard Fisher, MD

To Bernard Fisher, "father" of the field of breast surgical oncology and internationally renowned clinical cancer researcher, in honor of his lifetime achievements in advancing clinical science and his unwavering dedication to improving survival and quality of life for women with breast cancer.

The carefully designed clinical trials conducted by Dr. Fisher and his colleagues have improved our understanding of tumor metastases, advanced the field of breast cancer prevention, and improved our treatment of breast cancer by establishing the suitability of less radical surgical management and defining the roles of adjuvant and neoadjuvant therapy.

CONTENTS

SECTION 1

ETIOLOGY, ASSESSING RISK, INITIAL EVALUATION, AND MANAGEMENT

Thomas B. Julian, David Euhus, Irene L. Wapnir

SECTION 2

PATHOLOGY OF THE BREAST AND CLINICAL MANAGEMENT

Savitri Krishnamurthy, Rache M. Simmons

SECTION 3

IMAGING

Pat W. Whitworth, Terri-Ann Gizienski

SECTION 4

LANDMARK CLINICAL TRIALS IN BREAST SURGICAL ONCOLOGY

Eleftherios P. Mamounas

SECTION 5

OPERATIVE MANAGEMENT

Anthony Lucci, Tari King

SECTION 6

PLASTIC AND BREAST RECONSTRUCTION

Steven J. Kronowitz

SECTION 7

SYSTEMIC THERAPY OF BREAST CANCER
Lisa Carey, David W. Ollila

SECTION 8

RADIATION
Bruce G. Haffty

SECTION 9

FOLLOW-UP AND COMPLICATIONS FOLLOWING DIAGNOSIS AND THERAPY

Tara Breslin, Mehra Golshan

SECTION EDITORS

Tara M. Breslin, MD, MS
Assistant Professor of Surgery, University of Michigan, Ann Arbor, Michigan
Section 9

Lisa Carey, MD
Associate Professor, Department of Medicine, University of North Carolina, Lineberger Comprehensive Cancer Center
Section 7

David Euhus, MD
Professor, Surgery, University of Texas Southwestern Medical Center, Dallas, Texas
Section 1, Chapter 9

Terri-Ann Gizienski, MD
Mammography Department, UPMC Passavant, Pittsburgh, Pennsylvania
Section 3

Mehra Golshan, MD
Director of Breast Surgical Services, Brigham and Women's Hospital, Dana Farber Cancer Institute, Harvard Medical School, Boston, Massachusetts
Section 9

Bruce G. Haffty, MD
Professor and Chairman, Department of Radiation Oncology, Cancer Institute of New Jersey, Robert Wood Johnson Medical School, University of Medicine and Dentistry of New Jersey, New Brunswick, New Jersey
Section 8, Chapters 93, 96

Thomas B. Julian, MD
Associate Professor, Department of Human Oncology, Drexel University College of Medicine; Cancer Center, Allegheny General Hospital, Philadelphia, Pennsylvania
Section 1, Introduction, Chapter 42

Tari King, MD
Associate Professor, Department of Surgery, Weill Medical College of Cornell University; Jeanne A. Petrek Junior Faculty Chair, Memorial Sloan-Kettering Cancer Center, New York, New York
Section 5

Savitri Krishnamurthy, MD
Professor, Department of Pathology, Cytopathology Section, University of Texas MD Anderson Cancer Center, Houston, Texas
Section 2, Chapters 13, 24

Steven J. Kronowitz, MD
Associate Professor, Department of Plastic Surgery, University of Texas MD Anderson Cancer Center, Houston, Texas
Section 6, Chapter 75

Anthony Lucci, MD
Associate Professor, University of Texas MD Anderson Cancer Center, Houston, Texas
Section 5, Video 8

Eleftherios P. Mamounas, MD
Professor, Department of Surgery, Northeastern Ohio Universities College of Medicine, Rootstown, Ohio
Section 4, Chapter 42

David W. Ollila, MD
Associate Professor of Surgery, Department of Surgery, University of North Carolina, Chapel Hill, Chapel Hill, North Carolina
Section 7, Chapter 89

Rache M. Simmons, MD
Anne K. and Edwin C. Weiskopf Professor of Surgical Oncology, Medical Director of Clinical Research, Joan and Sanford Weill Medical College of Cornell University, Iris Cantor Women's Health Center, New York Presbyterian Hospital, New York, New York
Section 2, Introduction, Chapters 19, 67

Irene L. Wapnir, MD
Associate Professor of Surgery, Stanford University School of Medicine, Stanford, California
Section 1, Introduction

Pat W. Whitworth, MD
Clinical Associate Professor, Surgery, Vanderbilt University Medical Center, Nashville, Tennessee
Section 3, Chapters 33, 60

CONTRIBUTORS

Jeffrey Abrams, MD
Associate Director, Cancer Therapy Evaluation Program, Division of Cancer Treatment and Diagnosis, National Cancer Institute, Bethesda, Maryland
Chapter 41

Prachi Agarwala, MD
House Officer, Psychiatry, University of Michigan, Ann Arbor, Michigan
Chapter 100

Gretchen M. Ahrendt, MD
Director of Breast Surgical Services, Magee-Women's Hospital, University of Pittsburgh Medical Center, Pittsburgh, Pennsylvania
Introduction

Amy K. Alderman, MD
Assistant Professor, Department of Surgery, University of Michigan, Ann Arbor, Michigan
Chapter 73

Alison L. Allan, PhD
Oncology Scientist and Assistant Professor, Departments of Oncology and Anatomy and Cell Biology; Schulich School of Medicine, University of Western Ontario, London, Ontario, Canada
Chapter 3

Keith Amos, MD
Assistant Professor, Surgery, University of North Carolina School of Medicine, Chapel Hill, North Carolina
Chapter 83

Stewart Anderson, PhD
Professor, Biostatistics, University of Pittsburgh Graduate School of Public Health, Pittsburgh, Pennsylvania
Chapter 37

Eleni Andreopoulou, MD
Assistant Professor, Breast Medical Oncology, University of Texas MD Anderson Cancer Center, Houston, Texas
Chapter 36

Nimmi Arora, MD
Resident, Surgery, New York-Presbyterian Hospital, Weill Cornell Medical College, New York, New York
Chapter 19

Juhi Asad, DO
Attending, Breast Surgery, Colorado Surgical Service, Wheat Ridge, Colorado
Chapter 16

Werner P. Audretsch, MD
Director Interdisciplinary Breast Center, Breast Surgery, Sana Kliniken–Düsseldorf, Düsseldorf, Germany
Introduction

Gildy V. Babiera, MD
Associate Professor, Department of Surgical Oncology, University of Texas MD Anderson Cancer Center, Houston, Texas
Chapters 72, 90

Walter Baile, MD
Professor, Behavioral Science, University of Texas MD Anderson Cancer Center, Houston, Texas
Chapter 14

Bettina Ballardini, MD
Assistant, Breast Unit, Fondazione Maugeri Pavia and Universite degli Studi di Perugia, Scuola di Specializzazione in Chirurgia Generale, Pavia, Perugia, Italy
Chapter 61

Violetta Barbashina, MD
Assistant Attending Pathologist, Department of Pathology, Memorial Sloan-Kettering Cancer Center, New York, New York
Chapter 15

Harry Bartelink, MD, PhD
Professor, Radiotherapy Department, Netherlands Cancer Institute, Amsterdam, Netherlands
Chapter 45

Zainab Basir, MD
Associate Professor, Pathology, Medical College of Wisconsin, Milwaukee, Wisconsin
Chapter 23

Elisabeth K. Beahm, MD
Professor, Department of Plastic Surgery, University of Texas MD Anderson Cancer Center, Houston, Texas
Chapter 68

Isabelle Bedrosian, MD
Assistant Professor, Surgical Oncology, University of Texas MD Anderson Cancer Center, Houston, Texas
Chapter 65

Susan K. Boolbol, MD
Assistant Professor, Department of Surgery, Albert Einstein College of Medicine, New York, New York
Introduction; Chapter 16

Elin Borgen, MD, PhD
Department of Pathology, University of Oslo, Norwegian Radium Hospital, Oslo, Norway
Chapter 27

Judy C. Boughey, MD
Assistant Professor, Department of Surgery, Mayo Clinic, Rochester, Minnesota
Chapters 11, 44, 66

Stephan Braun, MD, PhD

Department of Gynecology, University Hospital of Obstetrics and Gynecology, Innsbruck Medical University, Innsbruck, Austria
Chapter 27

Edi Brogi, MD, PhD

Associate Professor of Clinical Pathology and Laboratory Medicine, Pathology and Laboratory Medicine, Weill Medical College of Cornell University; Memorial Sloan-Kettering Cancer Center, New York, New York
Chapter 15

Alexandra Shaye Brown, MD

Assistant Professor, Pathology and Laboratory Medicine, University of Mississippi Medical Center, Jackson, Mississippi
Chapter 54

Ervin B. Brown, MD

Associate Professor, Department of Surgical Oncology, University of Texas MD Anderson Cancer Center, Houston, Texas
Chapter 71

Horst Buerger, MD, PhD

Institute of Pathology Paderborn, Paderborn, Germany
Chapter 1

Grant W. Carlson, MD

Wadley R. Glenn Professor, Surgery, Emory University, Atlanta, Georgia
Chapter 74

Luigi Cataliotti, MD

University of Florence, Florence, Italy
Introduction

Anees B. Chagpar, MD

Associate Professor, Surgery, University of Louisville, Louisville, Kentucky
Chapter 69

C. Denise Ching, MD,

Fellow, Surgical Oncology, University of Texas, MD Anderson Cancer Center, Houston, Texas
Chapter 13

Marie-Rose Christiaens, MD, PhD

University Hospital Leuven, Gasthuisberg Campus, Leuven, Belgium
Introduction

Hiram S. Cody, MD

Professor of Clinical Surgery, Weill Medical College of Cornell University; Memorial Sloan-Kettering Cancer Center, New York, New York
Chapter 70

Beth Collins, MD

Resident/Fellow, Plastic and Reconstructive Surgery, Emory University, Atlanta, Georgia
Chapter 80

Christopher E. Comstock, MD

Professor of Clinical Radiology, Radiology, University of California San Diego School of Medicine, La Jolla, California
Chapter 5

Joseph P. Costantino, MD

Professor, Biostatistical Center, National Surgical Adjuvant Breast and Bowel Project, University of Pittsburgh Graduate School of Public Health, Pittsburgh, Pennsylvania
Chapter 37

Peter Cordeiro, MD

Professor, Surgery, Weill Medical College of Cornell University; Memorial Sloan-Kettering Cancer Center, New York, New York
Chapter 79

Massimo Cristofanilli, MD

Department of Breast Medical Oncology, University of Texas MD Anderson Cancer Center, Houston, Texas
Chapter 90

Walter M. Cronin, MPH

Associate Director, Biostatistical Center, National Surgical Adjuvant Breast and Bowel Project, Pittsburgh, Pennsylvania
Chapter 38

Brian J. Czerniecki, MD

Associate Professor, Harrison Department of Surgery Research, University of Pennsylvania, Philadelphia, Pennsylvania
Introduction, Chapter 91

E. Claire Dees, MD

Associate Professor, Medicine, University of North Carolina, Lineberger Comprehensive Cancer Center, Chapel Hill, North Carolina
Chapter 88

Amy C. Degnim, MD

Mayo Clinic, Rochester, Minnesota
Introduction, Chapter 11

Emmanuel Delay, MD, PhD

Department of Plastic and Reconstructive Surgery, Centre Léon Bérard, Lyon, France
Chapter 78

Andrea Denicoff, RN, MS, ANP

Cancer Therapy Evaluation Program, Division of Cancer Treatment and Diagnosis, National Cancer Institute, Bethesda, Maryland
Chapter 41

Jill R. Dietz, MD

Staff Surgeon, Women's Health Institute, Cleveland Clinic, Cleveland, Ohio
Introduction

James Dignam, PhD

Associate Professor, Department of Health Studies, University of Chicago, Chicago, Illinois
Chapter 4

J. Michael Dixon, MD

Professor of Surgery, Edinburgh Breast Unit, Western General Hospital, Edinburgh, Scotland, United Kingdom
Chapter 84

Laura Dominici, MD

Fellow, Breast Surgical Oncology, University of Texas MD Anderson Cancer Center, Houston, Texas
Chapter 14

Stephen B. Edge, MD
Professor of Surgery and Oncology, Department of Surgical
    Oncology, Roswell Park Cancer Institute and the University at
    Buffalo, Buffalo, New York
Chapter 13

Mahmoud B. El-Tamer, MD
Associate Professor, Breast Surgery, Columbia Presbyterian Medical
    Center, New York, New York
Introduction, Chapter 21

Laura J. Esserman, MD, MBA
Director, Carol Franc Buck Breast Care Center, Associate Director,
    Helen Diller Family Comprehensive Cancer Center, University of
    California—San Francisco, San Francisco, California
Chapter 6

Regina M. Fearmonti, MD
Resident, Plastic, Reconstructive, Craniomaxillofacial and Oral
    Surgery, Duke University, Durham, North Carolina
Chapter 68

Andrew H. Fenton, MD
Associate Professor, Department of Surgery, Northeastern Ohio
    Universities College of Medicine, Rootstown, Ohio
Introduction

Helio Rubens De Oliveira Filho, MD
Clinical Fellow, Breast Surgery, Senology Division, European
    Institute of Oncology, Milan, Italy
Chapter 55

Richard E. Fine, MD
Associate Clinical Professor, Department of Surgery, University of
    Tennessee, Chattanooga Unit, Chattanooga, Tennessee
Chapter 56

Bernard Fisher, MD
Distinguished Service Professor, Department of Surgery,
    University of Pittsburgh, Magee-Women's Hospital, Pittsburgh,
    Pennsylvania
Chapter 42

Bruno D. Fornage, MD
Professor of Radiology and Surgical Oncology, Diagnostic Radiology,
    University of Texas MD Anderson Cancer Center, Houston, Texas
Chapter 34

Prudence A. Francis, MD
Head, Breast Medical Oncology, Department of Medical Oncology,
    Peter MacCallum Cancer Centre, Melbourne, Australia
Chapter 86

Luke M. Funk, MD
Resident, General Surgery, Department of Surgery, Brigham and
    Women's Hospital, Boston, Massachusetts
Chapter 99

Colin M. Furnival, PhD, FRACS
Director, Centre for Breast Health, Royal Brisbane and Women's
    Hospital, Herston, Brisbane, Queensland, Australia
Chapter 17

Sheryl G. A. Gabram-Mendola, MD, MBA
Professor of Surgery, Emory University, Winship Cancer Institute,
    Director, AVON Comprehensive Breast Center at Grady,
    Atlanta, Georgia
Introduction

Jennifer R. Garreau, MD
Surgical Oncology Fellow, Surgical Oncology, John Wayne Cancer
    Institute, Santa Monica, California
Chapter 62

Charles E. Geyer, MD
National Surgical Adjuvant Breast and Bowel Project, Allegheny
    General Hospital, Pittsburgh, Pennsylvania
Chapter 42

Armando E. Giuliano, MD
Chief of Science and Medicine, Breast and Endocrine Department,
    John Wayne Cancer Institute, Santa Monica, California
Introduction, Chapters 26, 62

Michael Gnant, MD
Professor of Surgery, Department of Surgery, Medical University of
    Vienna, Vienna, Austria
Chapter 47

Viviana Negrón González, MD
Breast Surgical Oncology Fellow, Surgical Oncology, University of
    Texas MD Anderson Cancer Center, Houston, Texas
Chapter 90

Farzin Goravanchi, DO
Associate Professor, Anesthesiology and Pain Medicine, University of
    Texas MD Anderson Cancer Center, Houston, Texas
Chapter 52, Video 3

Robert J. Goulet Jr, MD
Indiana University, Indianapolis, Indiana
Chapter 59

Sharad Goyal, MD
Instructor, Department of Radiation Oncology, Cancer Institute of
    New Jersey, Robert Wood Johnson Medical School, University of
    Medicine and Dentistry of New Jersey, New Brunswick,
    New Jersey
Chapter 95

Ian Grady, MD
Assistant Professor, Family Medicine, University of California—Davis,
    Davis, California
Chapter 28

Caprice C. Greenberg, MD, MPH
Division of Breast Surgical Oncology, Brigham and Women's
    Hospital, Boston, Massachusetts
Chapter 99

Jennifer J. Griggs, MD, MPH
Associate Professor, Department of Medicine, Division of
    Hematology/Oncology, University of Michigan, Ann Arbor,
    Michigan
Chapter 98

Alicia Growney, MD
Clinical Lecturer, Surgery, University of Michigan, Ann Arbor,
    Michigan
Chapter 98

Moustapha Hamdi, MD
Professor, Department of Plastic and Reconstruction Surgery, Gent
    University Hospital, Gent, Belgium
Chapter 77

Nora M. Hansen, MD
Associate Professor of Surgery, Department of Surgery, Feinberg School of Medicine, Northwestern University, Chicago, Illinois
Introduction

Pat Hansen, MD
Director of Women's Imaging, MD Imaging, Attending Physician, Mercy Medical Center, University of California–Davis, Davis, California
Chapter 28

Jay K. Harness, MD
Clinical Professor of Surgery, Department of Surgery, University of California–Irvine, Orange, California
Chapter 30

Dennis R. Holmes, MD
Director, USC Breast Fellowship Program, University of Southern California, Norris Comprehensive Cancer Center, Los Angeles, California
Introduction

Kathleen C. Horst, MD
Assistant Professor, Department of Radiation Oncology, Stanford University Medical Center, Stanford, California
Chapter 97

Janet K. Horton, MD
Assistant Professor, Department of Radiation Oncology, Duke University, Durham, North Carolina
Chapter 88

Kevin Hughes, MD
Associate Professor, Department of Surgical Oncology, Harvard Medical School, Massachusetts General Hospital, Boston, Massachusetts
Chapter 50

Kelly K. Hunt, MD
Professor, Chief Surgical Breast Section, Department of Surgical Oncology, University of Texas MD Anderson Cancer Center, Houston, Texas
Chapter 44

Dezheng Huo, PhD, MD
Assistant Professor, Department of Health Studies, University of Chicago, Chicago, Illinois
Chapter 4

E. Shelley Hwang, MD, MPH
Chief, Division of Breast Surgical Oncology, Associate Professor, Department of Surgery, University of California–San Francisco, San Francisco, California
Chapter 6

Rosa Hwang, MD
Assistant Professor, Department of Surgical Oncology, University of Texas MD Anderson Cancer Center, Houston, Texas
Video 11

William Irvin, Jr, MD
Hematology/Oncology Fellow, Internal Medicine, University of North Carolina, Chapel Hill, North Carolina
Chapter 83

Raimund Jakesz, MD
Professor, Department of Surgery, Vienna Medical School, Vienna General Hospital, Vienna, Austria
Introduction, Chapter 47

Ronald C. Jones, MD
Chief, Department of Surgery, Baylor University Medical Center, Dallas, Texas
Introduction

Meredith Kato, MD
Research Fellow, Department of Surgery, Weill Medical College of Cornell University, New York, New York
Chapter 67

Manfred Kaufmann, MD
Klinik für Geburtshilfe und Gynäkologie, Frankfurt, Germany
Introduction

Thomas J. Kearney, MD
Associate Professor, Department of Surgery, Cancer Institute of New Jersey, Robert Wood Johnson Medical School, University of Medicine and Dentistry of New Jersey, New Brunswick, New Jersey
Introduction

Nazanin Khakpour, MD
Assistant Professor, Assistant Member, Department of Oncological Sciences and Surgery, Department of Women's Oncology, Moffitt Cancer Center, University of South Florida, Tampa, Florida
Introduction

Atif J. Khan, MD
Assistant Professor, Department of Radiation Oncology, Cancer Institute of New Jersey, Robert Wood Johnson Medical School, University of Medicine and Dentistry of New Jersey, Piscataway, New Jersey
Chapter 96

Kandice E. Kilbride, MD
Clinical Lecturer, Division of Surgical Oncology, University of Michigan, Ann Arbor, Michigan
Chapter 103

Julian Kim, MD
Professor and Chief, Division of Surgical Oncology, Case Western Reserve University, Cleveland, Ohio
Chapter 58, Video 12

Nancy Klauber-DeMore, MD
Associate Professor, Surgery, University of North Carolina at Chapel Hill, Chapel Hill, North Carolina
Chapter 88

Celina G. Kleer, MD
Harold Oberman Collegiate Professor and Associate Professor, Pathology, University of Michigan, Ann Arbor, Michigan
Chapter 22

Amanda L. Kong, MD
Assistant Professor, General Surgery, Medical College of Wisconsin, Milwaukee, Wisconsin
Chapter 54, Videos 4, 5

Ian E. Krop, MD, PhD
Dana-Farber Cancer Institute, Boston, Massachusetts
Chapter 87

Henry M. Kuerer, MD, PhD, FACS
Professor, Department of Surgical Oncology, Director, Breast Surgical Oncology Training Program, University of Texas MD Anderson Cancer Center, Houston, Texas
Introduction, Video 9

Arno Kuijper, MD, PhD
Department of Pathology, University Medical Center Utrecht, Utrecht, Netherlands
Chapter 1

Scott H. Kurtzman, MD
Professor, Department of Surgery, University of Connecticut School of Medicine; Waterbury Hospital, Farmington, Connecticut
Introduction

Michael D. Lagios, MD
Clinical Associate Professor, Department of Pathology, Stanford University Medical Center, Stanford, California
Chapter 18

Sunil R. Lakhani, MD
Professor, Molecular and Cellular Pathology, School of Medicine, University of Queensland, Herston, Brisbane, Queensland, Australia
Chapter 17

Christine Laronga, MD
Associate Member and Chief, Comprehensive Breast Program, Department of Women's Oncology, H. Lee Moffitt Cancer Center, Tampa, Florida
Chapter 12

Rakhshanda Layeequr-Rahman, MD
Associate Professor, Surgical Oncology, Department of Surgery, Texas Tech University Health Sciences Center, Amarillo, Texas
Introduction

H. Carisa Le-Petross, MD
Associate Professor, Breast Section, Diagnostic Radiology, University of Texas MD Anderson Cancer Center, Houston, Texas
Videos 1, 2

A. Marilyn Leitch, MD
Professor, Department of Surgery, University of Texas Southwestern Medical Center, Dallas, Texas
Chapter 64

Arthur Lerner, MD
White Plains Hospital Center, Valhalla, New York
Chapter 29

Jaime Lewis, MD
Resident, Department of Surgery, University of Cincinnati College of Medicine, Cincinnati, Ohio
Chapter 60

Jennifer Ligibel, MD
Instructor, Medicine, Harvard Medical School, Dana-Farber Cancer Institute, Boston, Massachusetts
Chapter 105

Jennifer D. Lorek, MD
Assistant Professor, Department of Pathology, Medical College of Wisconsin, Milwaukee, Wisconsin
Chapter 23

Albert Losken, MD
Assistant Professor, Department of Plastic and Reconstructive Surgery, Emory University, Atlanta, Georgia
Chapter 76

Susan M. Love, MD
Clinical Professor, Department of Surgery, David Geffen School of Medicine, University of California—Los Angeles, Los Angeles, California
Chapter 59

Helen Mabry, MD
Breast Care and Imaging Center, Orange, California
Chapter 26

E. Jane Macaskill, MBChB, MRCSEd
Specialist Registrar, Department of Surgery, Ninewells Hospital, University of Dundee, Dundee, Angus, United Kingdom
Chapter 84

Deborah J. MacDonald, PhD, APNG
Assistant Professor, Clinical Cancer Genetics, City of Hope Comprehensive Cancer Center, Duarte, California
Chapter 7

R. Douglas Macmillan, MD
Oncoplastic Breast Surgeon, Department of Surgery, Nottingham Breast Institute, City Hospital, Nottingham
Introduction

Aurora Madrigal, RN
Research Nurse, Breast Medical Oncology, University of Texas MD Anderson Cancer Center, Houston, Texas
Chapter 39

Julie A. Margenthaler, MD
Assistant Professor of Surgery, Department of Surgery, Washington University School of Medicine, St. Louis, Missouri
Introduction

Alice Matura, RN, MS
Director, Department of Surgical Oncology Protocol Research, University of Texas MD Anderson Cancer Center, Houston, Texas
Chapter 39

Colleen McCarthy, MD, FRCS
Assistant Associate Professor, Plastic and Reconstructive Service, Department of Surgery, Memorial Sloan-Kettering Cancer Center, New York, New York
Chapter 79

Beryl McCormick, MD
Attending and Member, Memorial Hospital, Radiation Oncology, Memorial Sloan-Kettering Cancer Center, New York, New York
Chapter 51

John McCraw, MD
Professor, Department of Surgery, University of Mississippi Medical Center, Jackson, Mississippi
Chapter 80

David R. McCready, MD, FRCSC
Professor, Gattuso Chair in Breast Surgical Oncology, Department of Surgery, University of Toronto, Toronto, Ontario, Canada
Chapter 20

Susan McKenney, RN
Associate Professor, Department of Surgery, University of North Carolina, Chapel Hill, North Carolina
Chapter 89

Sarah McLaughlin, MD
Assistant Professor of Surgery, Department of General Surgery,
    Mayo Clinic, Jacksonville, Florida
Chapter 70

Philip Meijnen, MD, PhD
Radiation Oncologist in Training, Department of Radiation
    Oncology, The Netherlands Cancer Institute, Antoni van
    Leeuwenhoek Hospital, Amsterdam, Netherlands
Chapter 45

Jane E. Méndez, MD
Assistant Professor of Surgery, Department of Surgery, Surgical
    Oncology Division, Boston University School of Medicine,
    Boston, Massachusetts
Chapter 72

Funda Meric-Bernstam, MD
Associate Professor, Department of Surgical Oncology, University of
    Texas MD Anderson Cancer Center, Houston, Texas
Chapter 85

Naomi Miller, MD
Staff Pathologist, Department of Pathology, University Health
    Network, Assistant Professor, Department of Laboratory
    Medicine and Pathobiology, University of Toronto, Toronto,
    Ontario, Canada
Chapter 20

Elizabeth A. Mittendorf, MD
Assistant Professor, Department of Surgical Oncology, University of
    Texas MD Anderson Cancer Center, Houston, Texas
Chapter 91

Leslie Montgomery, MD
Associate Professor, Department of Surgery, Memorial Sloan
    Kettering Cancer Center, New York, New York
Introduction, Chapter 53

Simonetta Monti, MD
Senior Assistant, Senology Division, European Institute of Oncology,
    Milan, Italy
Chapter 55, Video 7

Meena S. Moran, MD
Assistant Professor, Department of Therapeutic Radiology,
    Yale University School of Medicine, New Haven, Connecticut
Chapter 94

Elizabeth Morris, MD
Associate Attending Radiologist, Radiology, Memorial Sloan-
    Kettering Cancer Center, New York, New York
Chapter 35

Mary Morrogh, MD
Fellow, Department of Surgery, Breast Service, Memorial Sloan-
    Kettering Cancer Center, New York, New York
Chapter 61

Monica Morrow, MD
Chief, Breast Service; Anne Burnett Windfohr Chair of Clinical
    Oncology; Professor of Surgery, Weill Medical College of Cornell
    University, Memorial Sloan-Kettering Cancer Center, New York,
    New York
Introduction

P. K. Morrow, MD
Assistant Professor, Department of Breast Medical Oncology,
    University of Texas MD Anderson Cancer Center, Houston,
    Texas
Chapter 82

Maurice Y. Nahabedian, MD
Associate Professor, Plastic Surgery, Georgetown University,
    Washington, DC
Chapter 81

Venkat Narra, PhD
Associate Professor, Radiation Oncology, Cancer Institute of
    New Jersey, Robert Wood Johnson Medical School, University of
    Medicine and Dentistry of New Jersey, New Brunswick,
    New Jersey
Chapter 93

Bjørn Naume, MD, PhD
Department of Oncology, Norwegian Radium Hospital, National
    Hospital, University of Oslo, Oslo, Norway
Chapter 27

Heather B. Neuman, MD
Fellow, Surgery, Memorial Sloan-Kettering Cancer Center,
    New York, New York
Chapter 63

Lisa Newman, MD, MPH
University of Michigan Health System, Ann Arbor, Michigan
Introduction, Chapter 102

Steve Norton, CLT, CDT
Clinical Instructor, Lymphedema Therapy, Norton School of
    Lymphatic Therapy, Matawan, New Jersey
Chapter 104

Scott Oates, MD
Associate Professor, Department of Plastic Surgery, University of
    Texas MD Anderson Cancer Center, Houston, Texas
Video 11

Julia L. Oh, MD
Department of Radiation Oncology, University of Texas MD
    Anderson Cancer Center, Houston, Texas
Chapter 90

Niall J. O'Higgins, MCh, FRCS
Emeritus Professor of Surgery, University College Dublin, Ireland,
    Professor and Chairman, Department of Surgery, Royal College
    of Surgeons in Ireland-Medical University of Bahrain, Kingdom
    of Bahrain
Introduction

Haydee Ojeda-Fournier, MD
Assistant Clinical Professor, Department of Radiology, Moores
    Cancer Center, University of California—San Diego, La Jolla,
    California
Chapter 5

Michael P. Osborne, MD
Director of Breast Programs, Continuum Cancer Centers of
    New York, Beth Israel Medical Center, New York, New York
Chapter 16

Nicholas Osborne, MD
Resident, General Surgery; Robert Wood Johnson Clinical Scholar, Department of Surgery, University of Michigan, Ann Arbor, Michigan
Chapter 102

Soonmyung Paik, MD
Director, Division of Pathology, National Surgical Adjuvant Breast and Bowel Project Foundation, Pittsburgh, Pennsylvania
Chapter 40

Christoph Papp, MD
Ash Clinic, Salzburg, Austria
Chapter 80

Ronald Parris, MD
Assistant Professor, Anesthesiology and Pain Medicine, University of Texas MD Anderson Cancer Center, Houston, Texas
Chapter 52

Ann H. Partridge, MD, MPH
Assistant Professor, Department of Medicine, Dana-Farber Cancer Institute, Harvard Medical School, Boston, Massachusetts
Chapter 101

Helen A. Pass, MD
Assistant Professor of Clinical Surgery, Department of Surgery, Columbia University College of Physicians and Surgeons, New York, New York
Introduction

Ketan Patel, MD
Resident Physician, Department of Plastic Surgery, Georgetown University Hospital, Washington, DC
Chapter 81

Florentia Peintinger, MD
Associate Professor, Department of Gynecology, General Hospital Leoben, Leoben, Austria
Introduction

George E. Peoples, MD
Department of Surgery, Brooke Army Medical Center, Fort Sam Houston, Texas
Chapter 91

Barbara Persons, MD
Assistant Professor, Department of Surgery, Division of Plastic and Reconstructive Surgery, University of Mississippi Medical Center, Jackson, Mississippi
Chapter 80

Benjamin Pocock, MD
Clinical Instructor, Department of Breast Surgery, Columbia Presbyterian Medical Center, New York, New York
Chapter 21

Elisa Port, MD
Assistant Attending Surgeon and Assistant Professor, Surgery, Weill Medical College of Cornell University; Memorial Sloan-Kettering Cancer Center, New York, New York
Chapter 35

Richard M. Rainsbury, MD
Surgical Director, Oncoplastic Breast Surgery, Royal Hampshire County Hospital, Winchester, Hampshire, United Kingdom
Introduction

Roshni Rao, MD
Assistant Professor, Department of Surgery, Division of Surgical Oncology, University of Texas Southwestern Medical Center, Dallas, Texas
Chapter 64, Video 10

Lea Regolo, MD
Assistant, Department of Senology, Fondazione Maugeri, Pavia, Italy
Chapter 61

Michelle B. Riba, MD, MS
Clinical Professor and Associate Chair for Integrated Medical and Psychiatric Services, Department of Psychiatry, University of Michigan, Ann Arbor, Michigan
Chapter 100

Geoffrey Robb, MD
Professor and Chair, Department of Plastic Surgery, University of Texas MD Anderson Cancer Center, Houston, Texas
Video 6

Linda Robinson, MS, CGC
Supervising Genetic Counselor, Simmons Cancer Center, UT Southwestern Medical Center, Dallas, Texas
Chapter 8

Julia Rodriguez-Fernandez, MD
Senology Division, European Institute of Oncology, Milan, Italy
Chapter 55

Kari M. Rosenkranz, MD
Assistant Professor, Department of Surgery, Dartmouth Hitchcock Medical Center, Lebanon, New Hampshire
Chapter 66

Isabel T. Rubio, MD
Active Staff, Coordinator of Breast Surgical Oncology, Breast Surgical Oncology, Hospital Universitario Vall d'Hebron, Barcelona, Spain
Introduction

Kathryn J. Ruddy, MD
Medical Oncology and Hematology Fellow, Breast Oncology, Harvard Medical School, Dana-Farber Cancer Institute, Boston, Massachusetts
Chapter 101

Hope S. Rugo, MD
Clinical Professor of Medicine, Director, Breast Oncology Clinical Trials Program, Helen Diller Family Comprehensive Cancer Center, University of California San Francisco, San Francisco, California
Chapter 92

Emiel Rutgers, MD, PhD
Head, Department of Surgery, Netherlands Cancer Institute, Antoni van Leeuwenhoek Hospital, Amsterdam, Netherlands
Chapter 45

Michael S. Sabel, MD
Associate Professor, Department of Surgery, University of Michigan, Ann Arbor, Michigan
Chapter 22

Virgilio Sacchini, MD
Department of Surgery, Breast Service, Memorial Sloan-Kettering Cancer Center, New York, New York
Chapter 61

Sebastian F. Schoppmann, MD
Associate Professor, Department of Surgery, Medical University of
    Vienna, Vienna, Austria
Chapter 47

Gordon F. Schwartz, MD, MBA
Jefferson Medical College, Philadelphia, Pennsylvania
Introduction

Lisa M. Sclafani, MD
Associate Professor of Clinical Surgery, Weill Medical College of
    Cornell University; Memorial Sloan-Kettering Cancer Center,
    New York, New York,
Introduction, Chapter 57

Roger Sergel
ABC News, Needham, Massachusetts
Introduction

Elin R. Sigurdson, MD, PhD
Senior Member, Department of Surgical Oncology, Fox Chase
    Cancer Center, Philadelphia, Pennsylvania
Introduction

Melvin J. Silverstein, MD
Director, Breast Program, Hoag Memorial Hospital Presbyterian,
    Newport Beach, California, Clinical Professor of Surgery,
    Keck School of Medicine, University of Southern California,
    Los Angeles, California
Introduction, Chapter 18

S. Eva Singletary, MD
Professor, Department of Surgical Oncology, University of Texas
    MD Anderson Cancer Center, Houston, Texas
Chapters 13, 72

Chanel E. Smart, MD
Postdoctoral Research Scientist, Centre for Clinical Research,
    University of Queensland, Herston, Brisbane, Queensland,
    Australia
Chapter 17

Barbara L. Smith, MD, PhD
Division of Surgical Oncology, Department of Surgery,
    Massachusetts General Hospital, Boston, Massachusetts
Chapter 50

Howard Snider, MD
Medical Director, Alabama Breast Center, Montgomery, Alabama
Chapter 31A

Lawrence J. Solin, MD
Radiation Oncology, Albert Einstein Medical Center, Thomas
    Jefferson University, Philadelphia, Pennsylvania
Chapter 49

Atilla Soran, MD, MPH
Clinical Professor of Surgery, Department of Surgical Oncology,
    Magee-Women's Hospital, University of Pittsburgh, Pittsburgh,
    Pennsylvania
Chapter 10

April Spencer, MD
Breast Surgical Oncology Fellow, Department of Surgical Oncology,
    University of Texas MD Anderson Cancer Center, Houston,
    Texas
Chapter 71

Rand Stack, MD
St. Luke's-Roosevelt Hospital, New York, New York
Chapter 29

Edgar D. Staren, MD, PhD, MBA
Senior Vice President for Clinical Affairs and Chief Medical Officer,
    Cancer Treatment Centers of America, Zion, Illinois
Chapter 31B

Tanya W. Stephens, MD
Assistant Professor, Diagnostic Imaging, University of Texas MD
    Anderson Cancer Center, Houston, Texas
Chapter 36

Filip Stillaert, MD
Department of Plastic and Reconstructive Surgery, University
    Hospital Gent, Gent, Belgium
Chapter 77

Marieke Straver, MD
Department of Surgical Oncology, Netherlands Cancer Institute,
    Antoni van Leeuwenhoek Hospital, Amsterdam, Netherlands
Chapter 45

Rachel Streu, MD
Resident, Research Fellow, Department of Surgery, Section of Plastic
    Surgery, St. Joseph Mercy Hospital and University of Michigan
    Health System, Ann Arbor, Michigan
Chapter 73

W. Fraser Symmans, MD
Professor, Pathology, University of Texas MD Anderson Cancer
    Center, Houston, Texas
Chapter 25

Lorraine Tafra, MD
Breast Center for Anne Arundel Medical Center, Annapolis,
    Maryland
Introduction

Richard Theriault, DO, MBA
Professor, Breast Medical Oncology, University of Texas MD
    Anderson Cancer Center, Houston, Texas
Chapter 82

Karl Thomanek, MD
Department of Surgery, Medical University of Vienna, Vienna,
    Austria
Chapter 47

Sara M. Tolaney, MD, MPH
Instructor, Breast Oncology, Dana-Farber Cancer Institute, Boston,
    Massachusetts
Chapter 87

Sharon Tollin, ARNP
Lifetime Cancer Screening and Prevention Center, H. Lee Moffitt
    Cancer Center, Tampa, Florida
Chapter 12

Edward L. Trimble, MD
Head, Gynecologic Cancer Therapeutics, Division of Cancer
    Treatment and Diagnosis, National Cancer Institute, Bethesda,
    Maryland
Chapter 41

Theodore N. Tsangaris, MD

Associate Professor of Surgery, Chief of Breast Surgery, Director, Johns Hopkins Comprehensive Breast Center, Johns Hopkins University, Baltimore, Maryland

Chapter 59

Kiran Turaga, MD

Fellow in Surgical Oncology, Surgical Oncology, H. Lee Moffitt Cancer Center, Tampa, Florida

Chapter 12

Roderick R. Turner, MD

Adjunct Member, Department of Pathology, John Wayne Cancer Institute, Santa Monica, California

Chapter 26

Christopher B. Umbricht, MD, PhD

Assistant Professor, Surgery, Oncology and Pathology, Johns Hopkins University School of Medicine, Baltimore, Maryland

Chapter 2

Michael Untch, MD

Professor, Head of the Clinic, Clinic for Gynecology and Obstetrics, Gynecologic Oncology, Head of Breast Cancer Center, HELIOS Klinikum Berlin-Buch, Berlin, Germany

Chapter 48

Jayant S. Vaidya, PhD, MBBS

Senior Lecturer and Consultant Surgeon, Division of Surgery and Interventional Science, University College London, London, United Kingdom

Chapter 46

Elsken van der Wall, MD, PhD

Professor of Internal Medicine, Division of Internal Medicine and Dermatology, University Medical Center Utrecht, Utrecht, Netherlands

Chapter 1

Paul J. van Diest, MD, PhD

Professor, Department of Pathology, University Medical Center Utrecht, Utrecht, Netherlands

Chapter 1

Kimberly J. Van Zee, MD

Professor, Surgery, Weill Medical College of Cornell University; Memorial Sloan-Kettering Cancer Center, New York, New York

Chapter 63

Umberto Veronesi, MD

Professor, Scientific Directorate, Istituto Europeo di Oncologia, Milan, Italy

Chapter 43

Victor Vogel, MD

Professor, Medicine and Epidemiology, Magee-Women's Hospital, University of Pittsburgh, Pittsburgh, Pennsylvania

Chapter 10

Gunter von Minckwitz, MD, PhD

Managing Director, German Breast Group, Neu-Isenburg, Germany

Chapter 48

Karl von Smitten, MD, PhD

Associate Professor, Department of Gastrointestinal and General Surgery, Helsinki University Central Hospital, Helsinki, Finland

Introduction

Amanda J. Wheeler, MD

Assistant in Surgery, Division of Surgical Oncology, Department of Surgery, Massachusetts General Hospital, Boston, Massachusetts

Chapter 50

Eric B. Whitacre, MD

Breast Center of Southern Arizona, Tucson, Arizona

Chapter 32

Julia White, MD

Professor, Radiation Oncology, Medical College of Wisconsin, Milwaukee, Wisconsin

Chapter 51

D. Lawrence Wickerham, MD

Associate Chairman, National Surgical Adjuvant Breast and Bowel Project (NSABP), Pittsburgh, Pennsylvania

Chapter 42

Lisa Wiechmann, MD, MPH

Memorial Sloan-Kettering Cancer Center, New York, New York

Chapter 61

Edwin G. Wilkins, MD, MS

University of Michigan Medical Center, Taubman Health Care Center, Ann Arbor, Michigan

Chapter 73

Norman Wolmark, MD

Department of Surgical Oncology, Allegheny General Hospital, Pittsburgh, Pennsylvania

Chapter 42

Tina W. F. Yen, MD

Assistant Professor, Surgery, Medical College of Wisconsin, Milwaukee, Wisconsin

Chapter 23

Greg Yothers, PhD

Research Assistant Professor, Biostatistical Center, National Surgical Adjuvant Breast and Bowel Project, University of Pittsburgh, Graduate School of Public Health, Pittsburgh, Pennsylvania

Chapter 37

Bruce L. Youngson, MD

Assistant Professor, Department of Laboratory Medicine and Pathobiology, University of Toronto, Toronto, Ontario, Canada

Chapter 20

Ning J. Yue, PhD

Professor, Radiation Oncology, Cancer Institute of New Jersey, Robert Wood Johnson Medical School, University of Medicine and Dentistry of New Jersey, New Brunswick, New Jersey

Chapter 93

Vittorio Zanini, MD

Head, Unit of Senology and Oncoplastic Surgery, Fondazione Salvatore Maugeri, Pavia, Italy

Chapter 61

Victor Zannis, MD

Medical Director, Breast Care Center of the Southwest, Phoenix, Arizona

Chapter 95

Stefano Zurrida, MD

Associate Professor, Department of Senology, Istituto Europeo di Oncologia, Universite di Milano, Milan, Italy

Chapter 43

FOREWORD

A Look Forward from the Past

It is an honor to have *Kuerer's Breast Surgical Oncology* dedicated to me. When I began my surgical career nearly 60 years ago, surgery was the only treatment for breast cancer. There were no oncologists, and surgeons were generalists. Few operated exclusively on cancer patients, and still fewer limited their practices to women with breast cancer. The drama of medicine occurred in the operating theater, and surgeons devoted their efforts to developing the technical proficiency needed to perform feats of skill and daring, as it was the technical nuances of a surgical procedure rather than the characteristics of a tumor and its host that were believed to be responsible for patient survival.

The concepts that governed surgery for more than three quarters of the twentieth century were formulated by William S. Halsted, the Johns Hopkins University surgeon whose name was associated with the operation that he first described in 1891, the Halsted radical mastectomy. It was Halsted's contention that breast cancer was a local-regional disease that spread along lymphatic pathways by contiguous extension and that it could be cured only by surgeons more broadly interpreting what constituted the "region" and, consequently, conducting more expansive operations. During that era, I was trained to perform radical breast cancer operations according to the "rules" of Halsted. Should I have failed to comply with that dictum, I could have been excommunicated from the practice of surgery.

As a surgeon, I was concerned that, despite the increase in the magnitude of the operations being performed, there seemed to be little reduction in mortality. During that part of my career, I was also conducting laboratory research in liver regeneration and transplantation biology. Because of the scientific gestalt that I had acquired as a result of my efforts, I became sensitive to the fact that there was a lack of information available about the biological nature of the cancers that surgeons were treating. Thus, because it seemed to me that the benefits and failures of cancer surgery were more likely related to tumor biology than to technical proficiency, in the late 1950s I embarked on more than two decades of laboratory and clinical research related to the phenomenon of tumor metastasis. The findings from my investigations showed that (1) contrary to the prevailing thesis, the blood and lymphatic vascular systems were so interrelated that neither could be considered an independent route of tumor cell dissemination; (2) regional lymph nodes were not barriers to the dissemination of tumor cells, as had been proposed in the late nineteenth century; and (3) host factors were important in the development of metastases. I also found that dormant metastatic tumor cells did exist and that perturbation of the host by a variety of means could cause them to proliferate.

Those and other discoveries led me to formulate, in 1968, a hypothesis whose precepts were antithetical to Halsted's. Biological rather than anatomic or mechanistic in concept, my alternative hypothesis held that operative breast cancer was likely to be a systemic disease before its diagnosis, that it involved a complex spectrum of host–tumor interrelations, and that variations in local-regional surgery would be unlikely to substantially affect survival.

In 1957, I was one of a few surgeons who were founding members of the National Surgical Adjuvant Breast Project (NSABP). After serving on that group's executive committee, I became the group chairman in 1967. Fortunately, at that time I was also a member of the National Cancer Institute (NCI) Breast Cancer Task Force. Thus, when the latter group agreed with me that there should be a randomized clinical trial conducted to evaluate the relative merits of several surgical approaches for treating breast cancer, I was able to use the resources of the NSABP to conduct a study to test this hypothesis.

Begun in 1971, that trial compared the outcome of women treated with the conventional Halstedian operation with that of women in two other groups who had received less extensive breast-removal surgery. The women in one of the latter two groups were also treated with postoperative breast irradiation. During the next 25 years, the findings from that study showed that survival in the three groups was not significantly different. With support from the earlier findings from that trial, there was justification for me to initiate another trial in 1976 to further ascertain whether breast-conserving surgery in the form of lumpectomy, with or without the administration of breast radiation therapy, was as effective as mastectomy. As in the first study, results from the second trial failed to show, through 20 years of follow-up, a survival difference among the groups. The findings from both of those trials provided support for the alternative hypothesis. For the first time in the history of cancer surgery, there was a biological basis for a particular operative procedure, that is, lumpectomy. After the report of results from my studies, a radical change occurred in the surgical treatment of primary breast cancer. A new paradigm began to dictate the management of that disease, and strict Halstedian concepts were relegated to history.

At the same time that progress was occurring in the surgical arena, the era of systemic therapy was also beginning. In my hypothesis, I had also proposed that only with the use of systemic therapy after breast cancer surgery could further improvement in survival be achieved. In 1971, on the basis of new kinetic and biological principles, I designed and implemented a seminal clinical trial to determine the value of postoperative systemic adjuvant chemotherapy. The results from that study were the first to demonstrate that such therapy could favorably alter the outcome of women who had primary operable breast cancer.

Before leaving the chairmanship of the NSABP in 1994, I had conducted 20 randomized clinical trials involving women with invasive and noninvasive breast cancers. Those studies demonstrated the worth, or lack thereof, of chemotherapy and/or tamoxifen for reducing disease-free survival and improving survival in various cohorts of women with biologically heterogeneous breast tumors. The findings from those studies gave rise to a second treatment paradigm, one that governed the use of systemic adjuvant therapy. When I observed that the use of systemic therapy also reduced the incidence of local-regional tumor recurrence after surgery, I concluded that the surgical and systemic therapy paradigms had converged so that the treatment of breast cancer began to be governed by a single, unified paradigm.

In late 1972, I began to conduct additional clinical trials to evaluate a number of other hypotheses. Influenced by findings from my laboratory investigations, I initiated the first clinical trial to evaluate the worth of preoperative chemotherapy. Results from that study showed that patients who had been judged to need a mastectomy could, after receiving systemic therapy, undergo a lumpectomy. Perplexed that women with invasive cancer were being treated with breast-conserving surgery while those who had noninvasive cancer were undergoing mastectomy, I conducted several studies, the findings from which showed that lumpectomy followed by radiation therapy and tamoxifen could replace mastectomy for the treatment of appropriate patients with either intraductal or lobular carcinoma in situ. Finally, having found that tamoxifen decreased the incidence of contralateral breast cancer, I hypothesized that, in healthy women at increased risk, that drug could prevent breast cancer. Consequently, I initiated the first prevention trial in the United States to test that thesis. The results from that study demonstrated that the incidence of both invasive and noninvasive cancers was dramatically reduced; those findings have important biological and clinical implications that require further exploration.

In addition to progress made during the twentieth century relative to obtaining a better understanding of the biology of breast cancer and improvement in its treatment, detection, and prevention, another frequently overlooked accomplishment occurred: a change in the process of therapeutic decision making. Nonscientific approaches, such as anecdotalism, opinion, and inductivism, in deciding how to treat a patient were replaced by the use of information obtained from well-designed clinical trials. Nevertheless, prestigious medical journals continue to publish manuscripts in which anecdotal information is used to support biases. Such a practice is a disservice to physicians and their patients. Equally egregious is the plethora of advice about breast cancer that is being presented almost daily in the lay press and in other media outlets before credible data exist to prove its value. These actions not only connote a rejection of the scientific process but also create confusion in medical practice. Additionally, several recent innovations whose worth has not yet been sufficiently evaluated threaten to overturn some of the advances that have been made during the past few decades.

One of these changes relates to the use of modalities that have been developed as a consequence of research in engineering. The use of laser, cryo-, electro-, endoscopic, and robotic "surgery," as well as ultrasound, radiowaves, and stereotactic radiation is gaining acceptance in surgical practice as a consequence of a plethora of anecdotal reports about the effectiveness of these innovations. However, there is a need for information about such critical end points as distant disease-free survival and survival before the worth of these modalities can be determined. The assimilation of some of these innovations into surgical practice should not occur as a consequence of anecdotalism. Moreover, because such methodologies are used to eliminate localized tumors, and because cancer is apt to be a systemic disease, obtaining such information via the conduct of randomized clinical trials is obligatory. In many respects, the current era of engineered medicine is reminiscent of the Halstedian era in that it is currently based upon technological rather than biological principles.

Another significant circumstance that has occurred as a result of technological ingenuity is that which threatens the use of breast-conserving surgery. As a result of the evolution of magnetic resonance imaging (MRI) and other modalities, previously unidentified aberrations in the breast that are not associated with the primary lesion are now being detected. That circumstance, which has attracted considerable attention in both the media and in the medical literature, has led to a revival of the notion that breast-conserving surgery cannot be justified as long as there is the possibility that a single abnormal cell remains. As a consequence, an increasing number of mastectomies are being performed in women who are candidates for lumpectomy. Only when sufficient data are obtained about the biological and clinical significance of occult breast lesions that are being found by MRI can a meaningful decision be made about the propriety of the resurgence in the performance of mastectomies. The finding of additional lesions in the breast, the increasing information being obtained about circulating tumor cells, and recognition of the existence of dormant tumor cells all support my original thesis that breast cancer at the time of diagnosis can be a systemic disease and further indicate that frequent surgical procedures alone are inadequate to treat that disease in some cases.

Finally, the current description of the history of breast cancer surgery from my perspective serves as a prologue to the future of such surgery. It is fatuous to attempt to predict what will comprise that future. Because, however, it has been the findings obtained from laboratory and clinical research that have been responsible for the major changes related to breast cancer surgery during the past 30 years, it is likely that continuing efforts aimed at obtaining a better understanding of the biological nature of cancer will be responsible for progress in the future. It is the findings from research in molecular biology and genetics that are most likely to dictate the future status of cancer treatment and, ultimately, the fate of surgery. Cancer surgery as has been and as is currently being performed will almost certainly be replaced by other modalities that have resulted from scientific investigation. That process need not be viewed negatively by surgeons but should, rather, be embraced as an indication that progress has been made in the treatment of breast and other cancers.

Bernard Fisher, MD

PREFACE

The fields of oncology, general surgery, and surgical oncology have merged and evolved into the new specialty of breast surgical oncology. The intention of this textbook is to endow practitioners who treat breast diseases with cutting-edge, evidence-based information along with the clinical nuances related to the field of breast surgical oncology in order to help set current and future global standards of best practice. Toward this end, *Kuerer's Breast Surgical Oncology* provides a comprehensive dissemination of the highest level of knowledge in breast surgical oncology, leading-edge advancements in the multidisciplinary care of patients, an all-inclusive assessment and celebration of the major accomplishments made thus far in the field, and focused descriptions of the next wave of molecular and clinical studies needed to move the field forward over the next several years.

The textbook has several unique features: (1) complete integration of the relevant pathology of the disease entity with clinical management; (2) an atlas on breast ultrasound imaging and biopsy techniques; (3) special chapters on the influence of the media and Internet on breast cancer care and the funding of breast cancer research; (4) a separate section on the landmark trials that have shaped the field; (5) a major section of the textbook devoted to operative management; and (6) throughout the text, details regarding currently open and accruing clinical trials and future critical questions that need to be answered to move our field forward.

I am personally indebted to the contributing authors and section editors of this first edition. They represent an incredible mix of the current thought leaders in breast cancer from around the nation and world and our next wave of the most creative clinical scholars who have already begun to make their impact in the field.

Finally, it is my desire that the *Kuerer's Breast Surgical Oncology* provides you with insight and fresh ideas in the interest of our patients and their families. A bright future is anticipated for generations of women when breast cancer no longer imparts a threat to well-being or life. May the future begin with this present moment.

Henry M. Kuerer, MD, PhD, FACS

ACKNOWLEDGMENTS

This book began as a result of my own family experience. My mother, Cynthia Louise Kuerer, developed breast cancer when I was in high school. Very early on, I realized that breast cancer hits home, hitting women in the prime of their lives and impacting every facet of the lives that they touch. My mother was a fighter; after all, she had much to live for. Eventually, though, she lost her battle to ovarian cancer. When my mother was diagnosed, it became obvious how important it was to seek out experts and the latest and best treatments. Her multidisciplinary teams of clinicians listened to her and were compassionate, smart, and exceptional clinical scientists—just the role models any aspiring cancer surgeon could have hoped to have.

I am indebted to my chairman, Raphael E. Pollock, MD, PhD, FACS, for his unwavering leadership, mentorship, availability, and support, which allowed this book to come to fruition. I am also grateful to my colleagues and friends at MD Anderson who have fostered this program and continually provided exceptional guidance—in particular, S. Eva Singletary, MD, FACS, Kelly K. Hunt, MD, FACS, and Gabriel N. Hortobagyi, MD, FACP.

I am especially grateful to our group of world-class section editors and contributing authors.

Special thanks also to the superb editorial/art/production team headed by Marsha Gelber at McGraw-Hill, including Peter Boyle, Deepti Narwat, Catherine Delphia, Catherine Saggese, and Priscilla Beer, without whose tireless efforts this book could not have been published.

Finally, I am thankful for the enormous amount of hard work undertaken by my program coordinator, Monica Gonzalez, and our department's publication coordinator, Storm Weaver, to make this publication a great success.

Henry M. Kuerer, MD, PhD, FACS

Multidisciplinary Training for Breast Surgical Oncology

Henry M. Kuerer, Helen A. Pass, Rache Simmons, Scott H. Kurtzman, Luigi Cataliotti, Lisa A. Newman, Lisa M. Sclafani, Melvin J. Silverstein, Lorraine Tafra, Werner P. Audretsch, Ronald C. Jones, Manfred Kaufmann, R. Douglas Macmillan, Susan K. Boolbol, Gordon F. Schwartz, Thomas J. Kearney, Isabel T. Rubio, Jill R. Dietz, Niall J. O'Higgins, Richard M. Rainsbury, Mahmoud B. El-Tamer, Sheryl G.A. Gabram-Mendola, Marie-Rose Christiaens, Thomas B. Julian, Raimund Jakesz, Nazanin Khakpour, Florentia Peintinger, Amy C. Degnim, Leslie L. Montgomery, Nora M. Hansen, Irene L. Wapnir, Rakhshanda Layeequr-Rahman, Andrew H. Fenton, Elin R. Sigurdson, Karl von Smitten, Brian J. Czerniecki, Gretchen M. Ahrendt, Dennis R. Holmes, Julie A. Margenthaler, Armando E. Giuliano, and Monica Morrow

The past 20 years have seen an explosion in knowledge regarding the pathogenesis and treatment of breast cancer, and a natural outgrowth of this phenomenon is the emergence of multidisciplinary breast cancer subspecialties, including breast surgical oncology.[1-4]

A breast surgical oncologist is an oncologist who, although trained to utilize surgery as the primary mode of therapy, recognizes the essential need for multidisciplinary treatment for breast cancer as well. Thus, breast surgical oncologists must learn a broad range of skills beyond surgical skills. Breast surgical oncologists not only are aware of the results of the randomized clinical trials that have shaped our field, but also understand the need for such trials in establishing new treatment paradigms and understand the basic components of the design of such trials. With breast surgery, as with all surgery, the most critical component in delivering care is recognizing which patients do not need or will not benefit from therapy. In this regard, breast surgical oncologists must be highly trained in the differential diagnosis of benign breast entities, appreciate absolute and relative risk, understand genetic counseling and testing and identify resources available for genetic counseling and testing, and have a keen understanding of molecular diagnostics and therapeutics. Breast surgical oncologists must be able to keep up with technological advances in the field, such as image-guided breast interventions.

With the profusion of health information available on the Internet and from advocacy groups, patients, and their families have become increasingly savvy and are demanding specialized surgeons with focused practices in breast care. There are many paths to becoming an excellent breast surgical oncologist. In the past, the most common pathway in the United States was a 5-year general surgery residency. Another common pathway has been "on-the-job training": gradually increasing the numbers of patients with breast disease in one's practice over the course of a long career. Many of the current leaders in breast surgical oncology followed this path and were instrumental in developing the field of breast surgical oncology. More recently, the development of the field of surgical oncology and the establishment of general surgical oncology fellowships have added additional paths toward gaining breast surgical oncology experience.

This chapter discusses current breast surgical oncology fellowship training options in the United States and Europe, the role of breast surgical oncology within the multidisciplinary breast center model of care, the importance of work–life balance in maintaining career satisfaction and avoiding burnout, and the importance of mentorship.

CURRENT BREAST SURGICAL ONCOLOGY FELLOWSHIP TRAINING IN THE UNITED STATES

About a decade ago, breast specialists in Europe and the United States recognized the need to provide additional training to physicians who wanted to specialize in the care of patients with breast disease and developed breast fellowship programs. The leadership of breast cancer funding and advocacy groups and specialty societies in the United States recognized the need for comprehensive multidisciplinary training to enable surgeons to become proficient breast surgical oncologists, funded some of these programs, and developed premier structured and accredited interdisciplinary breast surgical oncology fellowship training programs. Leaders within the American Society of Breast Surgeons, the Society of Surgical Oncology, the American Society of Breast Disease, and Susan G. Komen for the Cure developed the curriculum for fellowship training, agreed upon appropriate outcome measures, and established guidelines for trainee assessment and fellowship program certification.

The general educational objectives of breast surgical oncology fellowship training are described in Table 1.[5] In brief, dedicated time in breast surgery, medical oncology, radiation oncology, pathology, breast imaging, and plastic and reconstructive surgery is required to provide the fellow with an in-depth understanding of each of these disciplines. The specific amount of time needed on each rotation varies among training programs. The requirement for exposure to multiple disciplines can be satisfied by block rotations or through integration of multiple specialty experiences during the week or month. Normal interactions with other specialties that occur as a part of breast surgical practice (eg, discussing a patient's film with the radiologist, reviewing slides in a multidisciplinary conference) do not satisfy this requirement.

The care of breast diseases is a rapidly changing field with new and important discoveries and treatment options emerging very frequently. Therefore the design of breast fellowship training recognizes the need for the specialist to be able to understand, critically analyze, and participate in research. Fellows are therefore also required to participate in relevant clinical research activities, such as the design of clinical protocols, the recruitment of patients to clinical trials, or participation in or observation of institutional review board or research review committee activities. Each fellow should initiate or participate in an investigative project and should be sufficiently familiar with statistical methods to properly evaluate research results. Scholarly activity is also expected, such as giving presentations at national meetings, delivering lectures, and authoring peer-reviewed publications.

Clinical experience alone is considered insufficient education in the breast fellowship training. Fellows participate in regularly scheduled didactic programs, including conferences, lectures, debate series, and journal clubs. They are also expected to present relevant literature at multidisciplinary case conferences. In smaller programs these educational requirements may also be satisfied in part by attendance at educational courses such as the School of Breast Oncology or other comprehensive, multidisciplinary Continuing Medical Education meetings. The didactic experience includes not only clinical breast problems but also translational science, clinical research, and ethical problems.

Some breast fellowship programs accept nonsurgeons as well as general surgeons. As an example, a 1-year fellowship program could include a 6-month rotation in the fellow's area of specialty (for example, a surgeon would spend 6 full months on a surgery rotation or a medical oncologist might spend only 1 month on a surgical rotation), as well as 2- to 4-week rotations in other areas, including Clinical Cancer Prevention, Genetics, Medical Oncology, Pathology, Plastic and Reconstructive Surgery, Radiation Oncology, Diagnostic Imaging, Surgery, and Community Service/Patient Advocacy and Research. Fellows could also spend time enhancing skills in counseling and in dealing with quality-of-life issues and end-of-life issues. In some of the current training programs, trainees interested in additional 1- or 2-year laboratory-based cancer research training may also elect to apply for a National Cancer Institute-supported research fellowship.

In order to ensure the highest-quality training programs, the learning objectives are rigorous. It is expected that not all objectives will be attained by all programs, and thus the adequacy of training is assessed globally rather than on the basis of any single learning objective. The Society of Surgical Oncology (SSO), together with representatives from the American Society of Breast Surgeons (ASBrS) and the American Society of Breast Disease (ASBD), visits and extensively reviews and approves breast fellowship training programs on an ongoing basis. Each fall the Society of Surgical Oncology administers and conducts a Matching Program to match qualified candidates with positions in approved training programs. To date, 32 standing breast fellowship programs have confirmed that they meet the criteria outlined in the guidelines and have agreed to be inspected within the next 3 years. Once a program successfully passes an inspection, it is considered an official "Society of Surgical Oncology–approved training program."

The Society of Surgical Oncology administers and conducts a Matching Program to match qualified candidates with positions in approved training programs. The prerequisites that make candidates eligible for enrollment in one of these programs are by and large uniform, with some exceptions. All candidates are generally required to have completed their graduate training from one of the Association of American Medical Colleges Liaison Committee on Medical Education listed medical schools followed by a general surgery residency program. Some programs accept applications from graduates of obstetrics/gynecology residency training programs and some also train candidates from nonsurgical residencies including medical oncology, radiology, and pathology. Candidates from nonsurgical residencies are not expected to do surgical procedures but receive additional multidisciplinary breast training relevant to their respective fields. Not all but some programs also entertain candidates from international residency programs as well. Any fellow who completes his or her fellowship in one of the approved programs will receive a joint certificate from the SSO, ASBD, and ASBrS. Information regarding breast fellowship training, eligibility, and the matching process can be obtained at the Society of Surgical Oncology website (*www.surgonc.org*).

TABLE 1 Current Interdisciplinary Breast Surgical Oncology Fellowship Training Curriculum Guidelines and General Learning Objectives

Breast Imaging
At the completion of the training period, the fellow should be able to
- Understand the techniques of diagnostic mammography, as well as the BI-RADS nomenclature and recommendations for additional views, and identify mammographic characteristics of benign and malignant disease.
- Demonstrate experience in performing breast sonography and distinguish between normal breast sonographic anatomy and sonographic characteristics of simple cysts, complex cysts, well-circumscribed probably benign masses, and solid masses of suspicious nature.
- Demonstrate experience in performing image-guided breast biopsy techniques.
- Demonstrate experience in selecting image-guided breast intervention procedures, including but not limited to ductograms, image-guided (ie, ultrasound, stereotactic, MRI, and others) fine-needle aspiration, and core biopsies.
- Discuss the evolving breast imaging technologies.
- Evaluate the present indications for and possible future applications of MRI in the management of malignant and benign breast disease.
- Select, recommend, and interpret the techniques of breast lymphoscintigraphy.
- Discuss the complexities, advantages, and disadvantages of breast screening trials in women in different age groups.

Breast Surgery
At the completion of the training period, the fellow should be able to
- Evaluate and manage common benign and malignant breast conditions.
- Assess the indications and contraindications for and demonstrate experience in performing and interpreting the results of common in-office procedures, including but not limited to breast sonography (see "Breast Imaging" earlier in the table), cyst aspiration, bone marrow biopsy, fine-needle aspiration, percutaneous core biopsy with and without image guidance, and skin punch biopsy.
- Assess the indications for techniques to optimize cosmetic outcome, minimize surgical trauma, and achieve best oncologic outcome for cancer operations for all major breast procedures, including but not limited to breast biopsy; wire localization biopsy; duct excision; lumpectomy; simple mastectomy; and modified radical mastectomy with or without skin sparing, chest wall resection, axillary lymph node dissection, and sentinel lymph node mapping. The fellow must demonstrate proficiency in the performance of these procedures.
- Demonstrate experience in interdisciplinary evaluation and presurgical treatment planning with multiple disciplines, including but not limited to radiology, plastic and reconstructive surgery, medical oncology, radiation oncology, medical oncology, and pathology.
- Identify the indications for and techniques of palliative surgical procedures for locoregional relapse as well as metastatic foci.
- Evaluate and manage arm lymphedema as a side effect of breast cancer treatment.
- Explain evolving surgical technologies such as percutaneous ablation, core vacuum resection, focused ultrasonography, ductal lavage, and ductoscopy.

Community Service and Outreach
The fellow should
- Identify and contact local patient advocacy organizations and participate in relevant activities.
- Identify ways to provide public service to the community.
- Promote the best standard of breast care and screening.

Genetics
At the completion of the training period, the fellow should be able to
- Identify patients at high risk for developing breast cancer, including those with risk factors such as pathologic, familial, and genetic factors and previous cancer-inducing therapies—eg, childhood radiation therapy.
- Discuss the epidemiologic evidence regarding the effect of environmental factors (broadly defined as nutrition, lifestyle, pollutants, chemicals, socioeconomic status, etc) on high-risk patients.
- Advise patients regarding estimations of risk by contemporary models and options for risk reduction through screening, medication, and surgery.
- Review the available clinical trials for breast cancer risk reduction and facilitate patient participation in such trials.
- Advise patients regarding indications, usefulness, costs, complications, and privacy issues of genetic testing.
- Take a detailed family pedigree and history.
- Interpret the various pathology findings as they influence risk.

(Continued)

TABLE 1 Current Interdisciplinary Breast Surgical Oncology Fellowship Training Curriculum Guidelines and General Learning Objectives (*Continued*)

- Describe and evaluate options for breast-conserving therapy in patients in whom an inherited susceptibility to breast cancer is suspected.
- Identify resources available for genetic counseling and testing.

Medical Oncology
At the completion of the training period, the fellow should be able to
- Assess the indications and contraindications for adjuvant systemic chemotherapy and hormonal therapies.
- Describe the mechanism of action, risks, and benefits of existing and developing targeted therapies and the indications for such therapies.
- Describe the prominent molecular pathways in the development and progression of breast cancer.
- Describe the most commonly prescribed chemotherapy and hormonal agents and their associated acute and chronic toxic effects.
- Identify and manage toxic effects of prescribed agents.
- Identify indications, techniques, and interdisciplinary coordination required for neoadjuvant and "sandwich" chemotherapy.
- Demonstrate proficiency in the interdisciplinary management of recurrent and metastatic disease, including palliative care.
- Balance the use, benefits, side effects, and costs of systemic chemotherapy and hormonal agents in patients with metastatic disease.
- Manage patient and family needs for psychosocial support, psychosocial intervention, hospice, and crisis management.

Pathology
At the completion of the training period, the fellow should be able to
- Explain and evaluate the benign and malignant pathological aspects of breast disease.
- Understand optimal techniques for marking, processing, and assessing pathology specimens.
- Identify special pathology issues pertinent to the treatment of breast cancer.
- Explain and evaluate immunohistochemical stains, cytology, and tumor markers and other indicators of prognosis and their relevance to treatment.
- Discuss evolving pathology technology.
- Stage breast cancer clinically and pathologically.

Plastic and Reconstructive Surgery
At the completion of the training period, the fellow should be able to demonstrate an understanding of reconstructive and surgical procedures such as
- Tissue expander, implant, and a variety of flap reconstruction techniques for immediate or delayed reconstruction after mastectomy.
- Oncoplastic techniques of breast conservation.
- General breast plastic procedures, such as augmentation and reduction, as they relate to total care of women with benign and malignant breast disease.
The fellow should also be able to explain and evaluate the planning and timing of adjuvant therapies in relation to plastic and reconstructive surgery.

Psycho-oncology
At the completion of the training period, the fellow should be able to
- Recognize changing needs for social support systems for patients and their families throughout diagnosis, treatment, transition to surveillance, and relapse.
- Recognize cultural diversity and the different needs of patients and their families from different cultural backgrounds with regard to illness and treatment.
- Exhibit a sensitive and culturally appropriate style of communicating with patients and their families.
- Explain and discuss all aspects of patient treatment and care with the patient in lay terms.
- Recognize patients at psychosocial high risk and identify resources for referral.
- Participate in existing support groups.
- Discuss complementary therapies/integrated care.

Radiation Oncology
At the completion of the training period, the fellow should be able to
- Describe the processes the patient experiences while undergoing breast radiation therapy, including simulation, treatment planning, treatment delivery, and acute and chronic effects of therapy.

TABLE 1 Current Interdisciplinary Breast Surgical Oncology Fellowship Training Curriculum Guidelines and General Learning Objectives (*Continued*)

- Assess the indications and contraindications for and complications of
  - Post-breast conservation radiation therapy in both DCIS and invasive carcinomas.
  - Postmastectomy radiation therapy.
  - Radiation therapy for management of chest wall recurrences.
  - Inclusion or exclusion of supraclavicular or internal mammary fields.
- Describe the common DCIS scoring systems and issues pertaining to the use of radiation therapy for DCIS.
- Describe and apply the considerations in combining systemic and radiation therapy.
- Describe and apply interdisciplinary management of recurrent disease.
- Identify the indications for and techniques of palliative radiation therapy procedures for locoregional relapse as well as metastatic foci.
- Assess the impact of radiation therapy on various surgical options for reconstruction.
- Discuss the evolving technologies of more localized radiation techniques.

Academic Research
At the completion of the training period, the fellow should be able to participate in
- Clinical trials development and patient enrollment.
- Prospective and retrospective clinical research.
- Enrollment of patients in available national protocols.
- The conduct and critical review of research studies.
- The preparation of manuscripts suitable for publication in lay or professional journals.

BI-RADS, Breast Imaging Reporting and Data System; DCIS, ductal carcinoma in situ; MRI, magnetic resonance imaging.

INITIAL EVALUATION OF BREAST FELLOWSHIP PROGRAMS IN THE UNITED STATES

After the second group of breast fellows had graduated from the combined SSO, ASBD, and ASBrS multidisciplinary program, the Training Committee of the American Society of Breast Disease undertook a survey to allow the graduated fellows from 2005 and 2006 to comment and assess their fellowship training as it pertained to their current practices. The results of this survey were presented by Dr Lisa Sclafani at a special session of the ASBD annual meeting in April 2007. Thirty of 43 fellows queried responded to the questionnaires. The results were enlightening.

In their current positions following breast fellowship training, two-thirds of respondents were practicing only breast surgery and only 8% stated that their practice was made up of less than 50% breast surgery. The respondents were working hard with 73% working more than 50 hours per week and 54% working more than 60 hours per week. The majority (90%) of respondents was found to be spending most of their time in clinical practice, but almost 60% were involved in teaching and over 80% had participated in academic publications or presentations at national meetings since their fellowship began. Ninety-three percent had given lectures to the public and 65% volunteered in a community-based breast cancer organization.

In their assessments, graduates were asked about deficiencies and successes in their training. The most common success stated was the ability to understand the multiple disciplines involved in treating breast cancer and the multidisciplinary nature of decision-making for these complex patients. Deficiencies noted included training in performance of image-guided biopsies and complex oncoplastic techniques. These areas are currently being addressed by the Training Committee. Overall, the queried fellows felt well prepared from their fellowship training to enter the practice of breast cancer treatment in a multidisciplinary setting.

CURRENT BREAST SURGICAL ONCOLOGY FELLOWSHIP TRAINING IN EUROPE

The European Society of Breast Cancer Specialists (EUSOMA) has established that diagnosis and treatment of breast diseases, and in particular breast cancer, are approached in widely different ways across Europe. Two particularly important aims of EUSOMA are to improve and standardize the level of patient care throughout Europe and to foster training, including multidisciplinary postgraduate training, in breast disease at the national and international levels.

EUSOMA has developed and published standards of training in breast cancer—which may be used for accreditation of specialists in Breast Radiology, Breast Diagnostic Radiography, Breast Care Nursing, Breast Surgery, Breast Pathology, Breast Medical Oncology, Breast Radiotherapy, and Breast Medical Physics—with the ultimate goal of increasing the standard of breast care available to all women across Europe.[6]

In Europe, candidates for accreditation in Breast Surgery must hold a current license to practice as a general surgeon, plastic surgeon, or gynecologist. At the completion of a 1-year training program (or 3 years for plastic surgery–trained fellows), breast surgery trainees are expected to have an advanced knowledge of the general principles involved in prevention and genetics, breast imaging and diagnosis, pathology, radiation therapy relating to breast cancer, and the use of systemic therapies for breast cancer in the preoperative and adjuvant setting and for advanced disease. Trainees are expected to attend breast clinics and see patients together with breast surgeons and radiologists specializing in breast diseases to gain clinical expertise in benign breast disease and primary breast cancer both in the clinic and in the operating theater. It is also expected that trainees spend time evaluating patients for radiation therapy and systemic therapy along with radiation oncologists and medical oncologists and gain experience with palliative care. Specific guidelines for breast surgery training in Europe are summarized in Table 2.

Trainees should understand which surgical procedures to recommend to each patient and should be clear about the protocols on which these recommendations are based (eg, they must know the criteria by which tumors are judged suitable or unsuitable for breast-conserving surgery). They should have performed such operations during their training.

Trainees should also gain experience with immediate or delayed reconstructive surgery after partial or total mastectomy (performed either by oncoplastic breast surgeons or by breast surgeons together with plastic surgeons). Trainees should also work on units where the plastic surgeon has a particular interest in breast disease, has a link to a designated breast unit, and supports the breast surgeon with techniques of tumor-specific immediate reconstruction. Alternatively, they should work with a dedicated oncoplastic breast surgeon. In the United Kingdom, 9 specific fellowships dedicated to oncoplastic surgery designed for senior breast oncology or plastic surgery trainees were started. Multidisciplinary training in breast surgery in the United Kingdom has been extended to include the acquisition of a broad range of oncoplastic skills.[7] This development is the product of an interface training initiative supported by general and plastic surgeons. This development began in 1996 with the inclusion of breast reconstruction in the curriculum for general surgeons with an interest in breast disease. Senior trainees from a background of general or plastic surgery can apply for a fellowship year, working in one of the 9 large multidisciplinary oncoplastic training centers in England. These fellowships provide concentrated training in all aspects of diagnosis, resection, reconstruction, and clinical management.

Trainees are required to attend regular, preferably weekly, multidisciplinary meetings where specialized breast surgeons, radiation oncologists, clinical oncologists, pathologists, and radiologists plan surgery and postsurgical treatments. Trainees are also expected to gain experience with using standardized

---

TABLE 2 Training Guidelines for Breast Surgery in Europe[*]

By the End of Training, Trainees Must Have
- Attended at least 40 diagnostic clinics and have been declared suitable by the trainer for seeing and advising patients by themselves.
- Assisted at 10 and personally performed 20 operations on benign lesions.
- Assisted at 10 and personally performed 15 axillary node sampling procedures (this includes sentinel lymph node biopsy).
- Assisted at 10 and personally performed 10 breast-conserving procedures.
- Assisted at 10 and personally performed 10 total mastectomies.
- Assisted at 10 and personally performed 5 skin-sparing mastectomies.
- Assisted at 10 and personally performed 10 full axillary clearances.
- Observed or assisted at 10 immediate and delayed total breast reconstructions using both implants and autologous tissue.
- Observed or assisted at 10 and personally performed 5 breast remodelling procedures after breast-conserving surgery (oncoplastic surgery).
- Attended at least 10 clinics with the radiation (clinical) oncologist at which decisions on adjuvant systemic therapy are made.
- Attended at least 10 follow-up clinics at which the side effects of surgery and radiation can be assessed.
- Attended at least 10 clinics at which women with advanced disease (both locally advanced and metastatic disease) are seen.
- Attended a regular, preferably weekly, pre- and post-surgical multidisciplinary case management meeting.
- Attended at least one genetic/family history clinic, in which women at risk are advised.

[*]Candidates must keep a log, signed by their trainer, of the operations they have attended as an assistant and the operations they have carried out, supervised or unsupervised, and also of the clinics they have attended and the multidisciplinary meetings they have attended.
Adapted and reproduced, with permission, from Cataliotti L, De Wolf C, Holland R, et al. Guidelines on the standards for the training of specialised health professionals dealing with breast cancer. Eur J Cancer. 2007;43:660-675.

data collection systems such as the EUSOMA Audit System on Breast Cancer Diagnosis and Treatment or an equivalent; to be able to critique the breast literature; and to have some knowledge of the ongoing research in breast cancer.

The qualification of a candidate to be a Specialist in Breast Surgery is assessed through a multiple-choice examination that tests the candidate's knowledge of the general principles of breast disease management (as detailed earlier in this section) together with a discussion of some clinical cases.

BREAST SURGICAL ONCOLOGY WITHIN THE MULTIDISCIPLINARY BREAST CENTER MODEL

Given increasing demand for breast surgical oncology services and a constant or diminishing supply of breast surgical oncologists, it should be possible for breast surgical oncologists to maintain an appropriate level of remuneration. However, for general surgeons or surgical oncologists whose practice has only a small percentage of patients with breast disease, this may not be possible. This is a complex problem because patients are now more likely to ask for breast specialists, but operating a practice with many breast patients may not be realistic because of a practice's geographical location or other constraints; therefore surgeons in those locations need to treat other diseases in order to maintain a practice. If a breast practice relies on procedures as the sole source of revenue, an acceptable level of income may be feasible only with a very large breast-focused practice due to the relatively low reimbursement fees for the amount of time required with these patients.

Multidisciplinary care has become the mainstay in the treatment of breast cancer patients. Decision-making has become increasingly complex and nuanced. Treatment plans are generally a joint decision between the patient and her surgeon, and thus the surgeon must be familiar with all aspects of the patient's treatment plan, to help and guide the patient in discussing treatment options. The complexities of these decisions are often poorly appreciated by the house staff, by other faculty within departments, and administrators. It is important for academic centers to highlight the education needed by residents, and raise the visibility of the Multidisciplinary Breast Cancer Team within the center through academic pursuits, including publications and presentations nationally, as well as in their own center.

Modern visionary academic and private entities have now come to understand that the best and most advanced breast-focused practices utilize a multidisciplinary approach to breast care including a team of experts in breast-specific surgical oncology, genetic counseling, physical medicine and rehabilitation, radiology, medical oncology, pathology, reconstructive surgery, and radiation therapy. At the institutional level, the current remuneration for the essential multidisciplinary and highest-quality care of a patient with breast cancer is sufficient to support all components of care and still leave revenue for continued program development, education, and research activities provided that there are a certain minimum number of patients treated annually. Many academic and private facilities operate on the principle that individual departments caring for patients with breast cancer must earn sufficient revenue to cover their expenses. When organizations instead implement the vision of multiple departments working in concert to care for breast cancer patients, it becomes clear that this is not only an economically successful model but also the only currently financially tolerable method of delivering excellence in breast care. Today, graduates of breast surgical oncology training programs are commanding appropriately high salaries as essential and critical members of multidisciplinary treatment teams.

IMPACT OF TRAINING ON THE NATIONAL ACCREDITATION PROGRAM FOR BREAST CENTERS

The general public often not only seeks out individuals with experience in the surgical treatment of breast cancer but also desires to be seen in a breast center that has the entire spectrum of specialized breast care services in an organized and central system. Breast centers are quite heterogeneous with respect to the overall quality and active involvement of essential multidisciplinary team members across the United States, and the American College of Surgeons, which has a long and distinguished history of accrediting cancer and trauma programs in the United States, recently undertook an effort to organize an accreditation program for breast centers. They recognized, from the onset, that breast cancer is a multidisciplinary disease and that an organizing committee should include all appropriate parties. A formal governing board of the National Accreditation Program for Breast Centers (NAPBC) was organized and conducted its first meeting in May 2006. The organizations represented on the board are listed in Table 3.

TABLE 3 Member Organizations of the National Accreditation Program for Breast Centers

American Board of Surgery
American Cancer Society
American College of Surgeons
American Society of Breast Disease
American Society of Breast Surgeons
American Society of Clinical Oncology
American Society for Therapeutic Radiology and Oncology
Association of Cancer Executives
Association of Oncology Social Work
College of American Pathologists
The Joint Commission
National Cancer Institute
National Cancer Registrars Association
National Consortium of Breast Centers
Oncology Nursing Society
Society of Surgical Oncology
Members-at-Large

The NAPBC has the following mission statement:

The National Accreditation Program for Breast Centers represents a consortium of national, professional organizations dedicated to the improvement of the quality of care and monitoring of outcomes of patients with diseases of the breast.

In order to fulfill this mission, the following objectives were agreed upon:

- Develop by consensus the criteria for breast centers and a survey process to monitor compliance.
- Strengthen the scientific basis for improving quality care.
- Establish a National Breast Disease Database to report patterns of care and effect quality improvement.
- Reduce the morbidity and mortality of breast cancer by improving screening mammography and advocating for increased access to and participation in clinical trials.

Many of the standards for Commission on Cancer approval are applicable to the NAPBC. For those breast centers that are also Commission on Cancer centers, there will be consolidation of Commission on Cancer approval and NAPBC site visits. It is possible that there will be consolidation of Commission on Cancer approval and NAPBC accreditation. The 20% to 30% of breast centers not associated with a Commission on Cancer-approved cancer program would be independently eligible for NAPBC survey and accreditation. Since the vast majority of the 1430 breast centers are in the community setting, accreditation by the NAPBC ensures patients that they can receive high-quality care close to home. The NAPBC is working toward site-visiting the more than 500 breast centers in the United States that have currently expressed interest in accreditation.

BREAST UNIT ACCREDITATION IN EUROPE

In Europe, the process of accreditation of breast units has cautiously started. The whole process consist of an initial certification (the center meets the recommendations of the EUSOMA guidelines) followed by full certification (and recertification) after 5 years depending on audit and performance indicators collected during those 5 years. The centers that fulfill the requirements are made public on the Internet at *www.senonetwork.org*.[8,9]

MAINTAINING WELLNESS AND LIFE BALANCE AS A BREAST SURGICAL ONCOLOGIST

There are few professions that by nature require the professional to deal with life-and-death situations on a daily basis. There are similarly few professions that have a profound daily impact on both the professional and his or her patients. Surgical oncology is one such profession. These attributes of surgical oncology, along with the rigors of training for this profession, attract individuals of a particular character and determination. One's career should provide meaning and a means of supporting one's life and loved ones, and it should be a source of daily enjoyment. Finding the right balance between family, loved

ones, outside interests that give one pleasure, and promoting one's career efforts is complex, and the balance often changes as one's career develops and flourishes. The traits that define the committed breast surgical oncologist also place him or her at risk for work-related stress and "burnout," a syndrome of emotional exhaustion and depersonalization that leads to decreased effectiveness at work. To maintain wellness and balance, surgical oncologists must schedule and include activities outside of work that give them pleasure, plan time with loved ones and friends, exercise daily, and get adequate rest and sleep to prevent the cycle of burnout and symptoms of depression (Table 4).

A recent survey of surgeons from the Society of Surgical Oncology found that more than 50% of respondents worked more than 60 hours per week and 24% performed more than 10 surgical cases per week.[10] Among the respondents, 72% were academic surgical oncologists, and 26% devoted at least 25% of their time to research.[10] Seventy-nine percent stated that they would become a surgical oncologist again given the choice. However, overall, 28% of respondents had burnout. Burnout was significantly more common among respondents age 50 years or younger and women. This is concerning because individuals experiencing burnout may be at risk for leaving the profession. Factors associated with a higher risk of burnout on multivariate analysis were devoting less than 25% of time to research, having lower physical quality of life, and being age 50 years or younger. Burnout was associated with lower satisfaction with career choice. Although surgical oncologists indicated a high level of career satisfaction, nearly one-third experienced burnout. The information in this study about factors

---

TABLE 4 Methods for Breast Surgical Oncologists to Maintain Career Satisfaction and Personal Wellness

Maintaining Career Satisfaction
Utilize the power of mentorship
Engage in clinical or translational research
Make time for work-related travel

Maintaining Personal Wellness
Relationships
    Protect time to spend with significant others
Spiritual practices
    Nurture spiritual aspects of self and cultivate interests
    that are personally joyous and emotionally satisfying
Attitudes
    Find meaning in work and personal endeavors
    Intentionally focus on aspects of your life that are
    emotionally positive and that you are grateful for
Physical and mental well-being
    Get proper exercise, sleep, nutrition, and medical care,
    and seek professional counseling when needed
    Consciously strive to maintain balance between work
    and personal life

associated with burnout should prompt increased efforts by program directors and surgeons to promote personal health and retain the best surgeons in the field.

A number of studies have explored the potential causes of physician burnout. Some have suggested that commitment to patients, attention to detail, and recognizing the responsibility associated with patients' trust—the very traits that define a good breast surgeon—also place physicians at greater risk for burnout. A mentality that puts personal life on hold during medical school, residency, and fellowship training in turn appears to foster a mentality of delayed gratification that many physicians carry with them into practice. The outcome of this mentality is that many physicians who were "hoping to reclaim" their personal life after completing fellowship find themselves delaying this task ever further into the future (eg, until after establishing their practice or until after becoming an associate professor). This can lead many physicians to put their personal life on hold right up to the time of their retirement. These observations suggest that the roots of surgeon burnout may have their origin early in the training process. Current medical students, residents, and fellows are the future of breast surgical oncology. Toward this end, we are obligated to design systematic interventions to help future breast surgeons both recognize and prevent burnout so that they can maintain resilience through the course of their career. In this regard, the critical importance of positive mentorship cannot be underestimated for mid and later level clinicians and faculty, but early on for our medical students and trainees.

THE CRITICAL IMPORTANCE OF MENTORSHIP

There have been no great individual success stories without mentorship. The field of breast surgery is in need of more and more creative individuals to provide and improve the care of our current and future generations of patients. With this in mind, it should be our goal for our trainees to rise to heights far above those who train them. The role of mentorship in surgery was recently highlighted by Dr Eva Singletary—Professor of Surgery at M.D. Anderson—in her Society of Surgical Oncology Presidential Address.[11] For those embarking on a career, it is helpful to find mentors early on and utilize their support abundantly. One way to do this is to keep one's eyes, ears, and all of the senses open. In this way, role models will rapidly identify themselves. In a career, one will have multiple role models as they develop. The beauty of the mentorship relationship is that often a mentor can simultaneously serve as a mentor and also be mentored by another individual. The receipt of mentorship is not limited to any particular point in one's career, and mentees (the ones who receive the mentorship) can concurrently or consecutively utilize a broad network of mentors to develop different kinds of expertise. The fact is, there is some innate ability required to be a great mentor or accept mentorship, but most of the skills involved can be taught and utilized successfully by mentors and trainees now and in the future. The essential rules on how to be the best mentor and mentee are highlighted in Tables 5 and 6, and should provide an excellent framework for maximizing professional goals and personal success.

TABLE 5 Being the Best Possible Mentor

What Mentors Do	What Mentors Do Not Do
Listen: function as a sounding board for problems and ideas; provide wise counsel	*Protect from experience:* do not assume the role of the problem solver for mentees
Support and facilitate: provide networking experience; share knowledge of the system; offer assistance where needed	*Threaten:* do not use threats or coercion to mold the professional lives of mentees
Teach by example: serve as a model for adhering to the highest values in every area of life	*Take credit:* do not assume credit for work the mentee has done, eg, writing their papers or applications
Encourage and motivate: help mentees to consistently move beyond their comfort zone	*Take over:* do not do what mentees should be doing themselves, eg, writing their papers or applications
Promote independence: give mentees every opportunity to learn by experience	*Force:* do not attempt to force mentees in one direction
Promote balance: serve as a model for balance between professional and personal needs and obligations	*Use undue influence:* do not use a sense of obligation to influence mentees' professional decisions
Rejoice in the success of their mentees: recognize that students may rise to greater levels than those who trained them	*Lose critical oversight:* do not allow friendship to shade over to favoritism
Convey joy: the joy that they find in their work is apparent to all around them	*Condemn:* do not convey to mentees that honest mistakes are career-altering disasters

Adapted and reproduced, with permission, from Singletary SE. Mentoring surgeons for the 21st century. Ann Surg Oncol. 2005;12:848-860.

TABLE 6 Maximizing Your Success with Mentorship

What Mentees Do	What Mentees Do Not Do
Take the initiative: recognize the need for mentoring and seek it out	*Avoid difficulties:* do not expect mentors to solve all their problems for them
Avoid perfectionism: accept that they will make mistakes, and learn from them	*Sidestep work:* do not expect mentors to do work that they should be doing themselves
Maintain balance: preserve time for family and friends	*Stay in their comfort zone:* do not shy away from new learning experiences
Work hard: be prepared to give their best	*Take advantage:* do not use friendship with a mentor as a tool to avoid work or escape consequences of their own activities
Support their peers: exchange personal and professional support with fellow trainees	*Bottle it up:* do not avoid talking about problems, anxieties, or grief because it makes them seem less than perfect
Take responsibility for the long-term results of patient care: accept that their job does not begin and end in the operating room	*Avoid total commitment:* recognize that their traineeship is a once-in-a lifetime opportunity
Welcome experience: be enthusiastic about pursuing the widest range of professional experience	*Let their egos get in the way:* recognize that everyone (faculty, residents, other trainees, nurses, and patients) has something to teach them
Seek counseling: solicit advice or counseling if they experience problems with depression, substance abuse, or burnout	*Work joylessly:* do not become so caught up in the rigors of training that they fail to experience the joy that should come from working in a field they love

Adapted and reproduced, with permission, from Singletary SE. Mentoring surgeons for the 21st Century. Ann Surg Oncol. 2005;12:848-860.

FUTURE DIRECTIONS: BREAST SURGICAL ONCOLOGY TRAINING IN THE FUTURE

In breast surgical oncology, as in several other highly focused disciplines and specialized areas of training within surgery, board eligibility and certification should be theoretically possible after a specified period of general surgery training of 3 or so years, and 2 to 3 years of focused breast-specific training that would include participation in research activities. The benefits and potential drawbacks of this breast surgical oncology fellowship training approach will be hotly debated over the next few years. The potential benefits include raising the standard of breast care and the outcome of women who develop breast cancer; potential drawbacks include requiring trainees to select an ultimate career field before having received enough exposure to this and other surgically based disciplines. Many surgeons with focused breast surgery practices feel they are better equipped physicians because of having had the full general surgery residency; however, this remains a theoretical perceived but unproven benefit. There are ongoing active discussions within the American Board of Surgery and the American College of Surgeons regarding possible future surgical specialty certification or recertification in the area of surgical oncology.[12] This is a very complex issue that will no doubt require a great deal of consideration before such a change would be implemented.

SUMMARY

The subspecialty of breast surgical oncology has emerged as a result of the recent explosion in knowledge regarding the pathogenesis and treatment of breast cancer as well as the growing complexity of the management of the breast cancer patient. Leaders of breast cancer funding and advocacy groups and specialty societies in the United States and Europe have recognized the need for comprehensive multidisciplinary training in breast surgical oncology, and they have developed standards for breast surgical oncology fellowship training programs. In brief, these programs require fellows to spend dedicated time in breast surgery, medical oncology, radiation oncology, pathology, breast imaging, and plastic and reconstructive surgery to acquire in-depth knowledge of these disciplines. Fellows are also required to receive training in genetics and psycho-oncology and to participate in relevant clinical research activities and community service and outreach. In the United States, the Society of Surgical Oncology, together with the American Society of Breast Surgeons and the American Society of Breast Disease, review and approve breast fellowship training programs and administer a matching program to link qualified candidates with positions in the training programs. A parallel effort in Europe is being led by the European Society of Breast Cancer Specialists, which has developed and published standards of training in breast cancer that are used for accreditation of specialists in breast radiology, breast diagnostic radiography, breast care nursing, breast surgery, breast pathology, breast medical oncology, breast radiotherapy, and breast medical physics—with the ultimate goal of increasing the standard of breast care available to all women across Europe. To maintain wellness and balance, breast surgical oncologists must schedule activities outside of work that give them pleasure, plan time with loved ones and friends, exercise daily, and get adequate rest and sleep to prevent the cycle of burnout and symptoms of depression. For those embarking on a career in breast surgical oncology, it is important to find mentors early on and abundantly utilize their support.

REFERENCES

1. Stitzenberg KB, Sheldon GF. Progressive specialization within general surgery: adding to the complexity of workforce planning. *J Am Coll Surg.* 2005;201:925-932.
2. Quinn McGlothin TD. Breast surgery as a specialized practice. *Am J Surg.* 2005;190:264-268.
3. Skinner KA, Helsper JT, Deapen D, et al. Breast cancer: do specialists make a difference? *Ann Surg Oncol.* 2003;10:606-615.
4. Morrow M. Organ-based subspecialization in surgical oncology: fragmentation as a path to progress? *J Surg Oncol.* 2007;96:1-2.
5. SSO requirements for breast fellowship. http://www.surgonc.org/default .aspx?id=66. Accessed October 5, 2008.
6. Cataliotti L, De Wolf C, Holland R, et al. Guidelines on the standards for the training of specialised health professionals dealing with breast cancer. *Eur J Cancer.* 2007;43:660-675.
7. Association of Breast Surgery at BASO, Association of Breast Surgery at BAPRAS, Trainee Interface Group in Breast Surgery. Oncoplastic breast surgery: a guide to good practice. *Eur J Surg Oncol.* 2007;33(suppl 1):S1-S23.
8. Blamey RW, Cataliotti L. EUSOMA accreditation of breast units. *Eur J Cancer.* 2006;42:1331-1337.
9. http://www.senonetwork.org. Accessed January 11, 2009.
10. Kuerer HM, Eberlein TJ, Pollock RE, et al. Career satisfaction, practice patterns and burnout among surgical oncologists: report on the quality of life of members of the Society of Surgical Oncology. *Ann Surg Oncol.* 2007;14:3029-3053.
11. Singletary SE. Mentoring surgeons for the 21st century. *Ann Surg Oncol.* 2005;12:848-860.
12. Pollock RE. Board certification in surgical oncology: does it make sense? *J Surg Oncol.* 2008;98:1-2.

The Influence of the News Media and the Internet on Breast Cancer Patient Care and Research

Roger Sergel

Any doctor involved with breast cancer is perhaps more likely than specialists in other fields to be faced with the opportunity to talk to the press. As medical specialties go, breast cancer is among the top in generating news. For at least 4 decades, breast cancer has generated interest both for advances in the field and human stories. This chapter seeks to explore some of the issues in breast cancer that received the greatest news coverage. It also attempts to critically examine how the press handled different stories and to offer some guidance on how doctors should and should not respond to the media and to the new world of Internet news. More than ever, doctors who treat breast cancer will be faced with patients who bring with them information from a wide range of sources. It is important for doctors to better understand how these media outlets approach their field.

THE DEVELOPMENT OF "BREAST CANCER" AS A "HOT" STORY

On March 17, 1999, 3 trials comparing high-dose chemotherapy with autologous bone marrow transplant (HDC/ABMT) and standard chemotherapy were presented at the annual meeting of the American Society of Clinical Oncology.[1] The 3 trials showed no difference in overall survival between the 2 treatments.

On November 30, 1995, the *New England Journal of Medicine* reported on the reanalysis and results after 12 years of follow-up in a randomized clinical trial comparing total mastectomy with lumpectomy with or without irradiation in the treatment of breast cancer by Fisher and associates.[2] The study found that "lumpectomy followed by breast irradiation is appropriate therapy for women with either negative or positive axillary nodes and breast tumors 4 cm or less in diameter."

On August 6, 2002, the largest study ever to look for environmental links to breast cancer, involving 1000 women from Long Island, found that the data, "based on the largest number of samples analyzed to date among primarily white women, do not support the hypothesis that organochlorines increase breast cancer risk among Long Island women."[3]

Each of these studies provided an important turning point in the news coverage of these issues that ultimately turned out to be wrong. The media in each case created an impression that the story was different.

In the case of a controversial HDC/ABMT treatment, the media had done numerous stories suggesting that HDC/ABMT was the last hope for women with breast cancer, and that health plans that denied the treatment were more interested in profits than women's lives. In the case of scientific misconduct, the public heard suggestions in news reports that the National Surgical Breast and Bowel Project (NSABP) studies, which concluded that lumpectomy was as effective as modified radical mastectomy, might have the results called into question because of scientific misconduct involving patients entered into the trial by one Dr Roger Poisson. And in the example of the environmental role in breast cancer risk, patient advocates and politicians regularly made their case through the media that the breast cancer rate was significantly higher among Long Island women and that studies were needed to prove that environmental factors were responsible.

These stories, which unfolded in the 1990s, involved complex issues that were in sharp contrast to the simpler themes for breast cancer coverage in 1970s. Much of the reporting in the 1970s sought to simply get the public talking about breast cancer. Efforts to increase public awareness received a significant boost September 24, 1974, when First Lady Betty Ford had surgery to remove her right breast after a lump was detected. Mrs Ford not only openly discussed her cancer but went on to become an advocate for increased public understanding of breast cancer. Mrs Ford said, "So many thousands of women in the world have breast cancer, I felt I had to share my experience with them so they would take precautions for themselves."[4] The media worked closely with the American Cancer Society in informing the public about early detection. Commenting on the skepticism at that time about mammography, Dr Len Lichtenfeld with the American Cancer Society said he believes the press exposure was "responsible for getting mammography on the map."[5]

Throughout the 1970s breast cancer began to grow as a "hot" story. Joann Rodgers, former National Science Reporter for Hearst Newspapers, said that during that time there were a lot of women coming into journalism and medical beats were often given to them. Rodgers, Director of Media Relations at Johns Hopkins Medical Institutions, said "editors were pounding on you to cover the story."[6] She recalls one incident where a local American Cancer Society in Maryland was pushing for a story about breast self-exam. Rodgers said she told the ACS people that the story was not news. "They went to my editor and I was ordered to write the story," Rodgers said.

PATIENT ADVOCACY

The increased press interest was coming at a time when patient advocates were urging women to become equal partners in the decision-making process about treatments that were affecting their bodies and lives. There were also major changes taking place in how organized medicine approached breast cancer, as detailed in *The Politics of Breast Cancer* by Mareen Hogan Casamayou.[7]

"Enlightened" physicians began to encourage the formation of breast cancer support groups, with hospital and breast care centers. Many oncology nurses took up the cudgel of patient advocacy, doing what they could to meet the informational needs of women whose doctors displayed traditional paternalistic behavior. At the same time the American Cancer Society had its Reach to Recovery Program, in which former breast cancer patients would visit the bedside of a woman after her mastectomy and offer emotional support and certain accoutrements (such as a prosthesis) for physical recovery. In addition, the National Cancer Institute began its own national hotline, 1-800-4-CANCER, in the mid-1970s.

IMPORTANT BREAST CANCER RESEARCH ADVANCES

During this period, there were important research advances:

- 1973: Metastatic breast cancer was shown to be moderately sensitive to a single chemotherapy agent.
- 1974: The FDA approved the first drug specifically for breast cancer.
- 1974: A study found mastectomy provided no benefit over lumpectomy.

However, as years have passed, the media have had to move beyond being a cheerleader for public awareness and into more difficult areas of interpreting research advances, understanding and explaining the patient advocacy movement, presenting allegations of scientific misconduct, and responsibly reporting on celebrities who can use the media as a platform to convey misleading information.

NEWS COVERAGE OF CELEBRITIES

When an editor brings a story about breast cancer to the attention of a reporter, the first suggestion the editor is going to make is "Find a patient." Breast cancer coverage has been defined by the personal story. For a reporter, focusing on the patient gives a human dimension to the story.

In many cases this may involve people the public admires. In fact, Marissa Weiss of breastcancer.org got 150 celebrities to record definitions of terms, because she felt the public would be more interested in hearing complicated medical language explained by a celebrity. Dr Larry Wickerham, chairman of the NSABP, said that following the announcement by actress Christina Applegate that she had undergone a bilateral mastectomy, his institution experienced what he described as the "Applegate effect," where more women inquired about bilateral mastectomy.[8]

The impact of celebrities is not just anecdotal. In Australia, it was announced on May 17, 2005 that singer Kylie Minogue had breast cancer. In a study published in *Medicine and the Media* in September 2005, researchers from Sydney found that subsequently there was a "20-fold increase in news coverage of breast cancer" and a 40% increase in bookings for screenings in the 2 weeks following the disclosure. According to the study there was an additional "101% increase in on-screened women in the eligible age-group 40 to 69 years."[9] However, there is also evidence that suggests that celebrity exposure may impact understanding but not bring about significant changes in behavior. A 1989 study on the impact of media coverage of Nancy Reagan's experience on breast cancer screening did find a significant increase in "knowledge of lifetime risk of breast cancer."[10] However, only 6% to 8% of the women surveyed were influenced to contact a health professional, and 1.5% to 2% were influenced to have their first mammogram.[10]

But celebrity coverage can also produce outcomes that many researchers find troubling. In April 2000, actress, author, and businesswoman Suzanne Somers met with Dr Melvin Silverstein, Director of the University of Southern California Norris Lee Breast Center, following a mammogram. In an extensive account, *People* magazine details what followed.[11] Silverstein told Somers her mammogram looked fine but suggested that she might want to have an ultrasound. Somers said that a 2.4-cm tumor was detected in her right breast. Somers had a lumpectomy followed by radiation.

At the time of her treatment, Somers' books had focused more on her life and approaches to diet and weight loss. *People* reported Somers had been taking plant-based estrogen for 3 years, for menopause. But Somers, who would later turn her belief in bioidentical hormones into several books, did not heed Silverstein's advice to stop taking the hormones. Instead, a year later on CNN's "Larry King Live" she revealed that she had been treated for breast cancer and had decided to continue taking the hormones, to forego chemotherapy, and to treat herself with injections of mistletoe extract called Iscador.

This news set off a firestorm in the press. And it raised some fundamental questions about how the press should handle such information. How extensively should the story be covered? Should Somers be given a forum for her medical views? If the medical community believes her views are wrong, how should the media provide coverage? Are there opportunities, even if Somers' views are highly controversial, to use the story for greater public understanding of breast cancer treatments? What responsibility does the broadcast press have if they decide to put her on the air?

The first question was quickly answered by the press. Somers' approach to her treatment was widely covered in both the print and broadcast press. Somers was a celebrity, and the press felt her comments were news. Magazines such as *People* told the personal story of Somers, which included details of her initial diagnosis and her conversations with her surgeon, Dr Mel Silverstein; how she dealt with the stories about her liposuction, which she said was done because the radiation treatments created swelling where her breast met her back; and her reasons for refusing chemotherapy. But *People* also provided an interview with Barie Cassileth, who ran the complementary medicine program at Memorial Sloan Kettering Cancer Center.[12] Cassileth cited 2 studies that found "the 5-year survival rate for patients using Iscador was no better than for the control group." She said: "What they are saying is that Iscador has no value in the treatment of cancer." The Cassileth interview was what is called a "sidebar" article, which goes with the main article. The question can legitimately be asked whether such views belonged in the main article, where far more people would have read it.

But some in the media not only believe Somers' opinions were news but they used the story to explore issues raised by the controversy. WABC-TV New York's medical editor, Dr Jay Adlersburg, called the Somers episode an "opportunity to do a story on alternative and sometimes wacky treatments that people use in the face of more evidence-based treatments."[13] An article in *Newsday* in May 2001 provided some background on the treatment Somers had chosen.[14] It said "although it is unclear from clinical trials whether it's actually effective mistletoe is not considered such a wacky treatment in Europe. In fact in Germany it is the most widely used oncological drug according to a study in the May/June issue of the *Journal of Alternative Therapies*." And CNN, whose 1-hour broadcast of Somers on "Larry King Live" had triggered extensive press coverage, provided a report from their medical correspondent Elizabeth Cohen that looked at a study from Holland that showed "skin cancer metastasized to the brain in 19 percent of the patients who took mistletoe but in only 7 percent of the patients who didn't take it."[15]

But some in the medical press and the research community believe the Somers story should not have been covered. A *Buffalo News* article of May 2001 described Dr Stephen Edge, chief of breast surgery at Roswell Park, as "livid."[16] Dr Edge was angry about the effect Somers' statements would have on other women, particularly concerning her choice of unproven rather than proven therapy. "If Suzanne Somers stops 100 women from taking Tamoxifen 10 of those women are going to die because of it, and that's not right. Celebrities with these diseases need to take their status seriously." Peggy Peck, executive editor of *MedPage Today*, a Web site aimed primarily at physicians, said "responsible press should not report such claims. Chemotherapy has been shown to save lives but there is no evidence to back this [Somers] claim."[17] Dr Marie Savard, a women's health specialist and medical contributor to ABC News, believes the broadcast press has "an obligation to either footnote each statement of such extreme nature or provide a concurrent expert."[18]

When Somers provided her views originally on "Larry King," during the questioning King did press Somers on how the medical community strongly opposed her views, but he did not press her to provide the evidence for her decision. Few of the stories attempted to pin Somers down on her responsibility as a celebrity and how she could separate the effect of saying she believed in something from her celebrity status. But following her disclosures about her approach to treatment, Somers upped the ante on the controversy by coming out with 3 books that touted the use of bioidentical hormones. She also included her views of Iscador and chemotherapy. This meant her views on breast cancer therapy were no longer just news, they might impact the sales of her books.

So it is unusual to see a celebrity pinned down about his or her health views and the impact on the public. A September 2008 broadcast on *Nightline* provided a rare case of broadcast journalism doing some very tough questioning about Somers' ability to separate what she did from her public message.[19] ABC News correspondent Lisa Fletcher did a report on Somers that ended with her pressing Somers. While Fletcher's questions focused on Somers' views on bioidentical hormones, Somers' answers seem likely to reflect her general view of her role in the media spotlight, including her use of Iscador instead of chemotherapy.

> FLETCHER: You are accused of making yourself a human guinea pig.
> SOMERS: So I think I will be watched till the day I die in a sense because I have been chosen to be the face of this.
> FLETCHER: But then how do you take that, which is an unknown and recommend that to other women in good conscience. Not knowing what the outcome is?
> SOMERS: I never give advice. I say, this is the way I've gone. If you want to have what I have go that way. Read up about it. Read my books.

And later in the interview:

> FLETCHER: But are there peer-reviewed scientific studies that say that that's right and that it is safe?
> SOMERS: Well, do you want to wait until all these studies are in?
> FLETCHER: I don't want to be a human lab rat.
> SOMERS: Well, then that's the choice you make.

Fletcher concluded her report by saying, "All the controversy and criticism it seems has only made Somers more resolved to spread her message, no matter the cost."

The Somers story presented journalistic challenges but it was basically a simple story to report. However, in the 1990s, reporters faced one of the most difficult stories about breast cancer in the past 25 years: HDC with ABMT.

HOW THE MEDIA REPORTED ON THE HIGH-DOSE CHEMOTHERAPY/AUTOLOGOUS BONE MARROW TRANSPLANT CONTROVERSY

In February 1990, this author and ABC News Medical Dr Tim Johnson did a report on *20/20* about HDC.[20] The story discussed the effectiveness of chemotherapy, the side effects, and how they could be managed. The story then took a turn into the issue of chemotherapy dosing. Dr Johnson said: "When chemotherapy was first introduced the theory often was the less the better. More recently that thinking has changed and in 1985 one of the country's leading cancer experts, then head of the National Cancer Institute, charged that some doctors were misusing chemotherapy by giving doses that were too low."

That narration was followed by a sound bite from Dr Vincent DeVita, then at Memorial Sloan Kettering, who said "there are clearly people who are losing their lives because they are not getting adequate chemotherapy." The story introduced others who were concerned about underdosing, including Dr Irwin Krakoff at M.D. Anderson, who used the phrase "killing with kindness"; and Dr William Hrynuik with the University of California, San Diego and an advocate of HDC. At the end of the report we noted that HDC with bone marrow transplant for breast cancer was relatively new, and many insurance companies would not pay for it because they thought it was experimental. And we then introduced Dr Craig Henderson, then at Dana Farber Cancer Institute, who said that he saw no evidence yet that bone marrow transplants prolong lives. Our story set the HDC/ABMT debate in the context of the underdosing issue. Prior to our story there had been major research developments, which included

- 1984: Paper by Hrynuik and Bush that maintained a relationship existed between dose rate in metastatic disease and average dose of chemotherapy.
- 1986: Hrynuik study that extended the dose–response rate theory to stage II patients.
- 1988: Article where Henderson and Dan Hayes challenged the dose–response theory.
- 1988: Dr Bill Peters, then at Duke Medical Center, report on the phase 2 results of HDC/ABMT.
- 1989: Founding of Response Technology, the company that set up centers for treating patients with stem cells and HDC.[21]

So the stage was set for the rise of HDC/ABMT that took place in the early 1990s. This story also began to unfold at a time when the issue of HMOs was getting more press attention. Stories were appearing about HMOs overruling doctors and denying care. As is often the case, the media tended to focus on only one villain, because it is an easier story to tell. Little press attention was paid to the employers, who often provided the HMOs with the economic guidelines that lead to the coverage decisions. The press framed the story as a battle between HMOs and women with breast cancer. And many of the stories focused primarily on women with recurrence of breast cancer, with coverage that was characterized with emotionally charged words. Phrases such as "only hope," "keep her alive," and "best chance to survive" were repeatedly linked to those patients

seeking HDC/ABMT. It was not just the reporters who used strong words in their stories. In many cases quotes from doctors conveyed a sense that this was proven therapy. For example, a 1993 *Austin American Statesman* newspaper article quoted Dr Richard Champlin of M.D. Anderson: "About 20 percent or more have survived 5 years and we believe some of these patients will be cured."[22] And in a 1996 story in the *Los Angeles Times*, a woman seeking HDC/ABMT says she was told by Dr Roy Jones at the University of Colorado that the procedure offered "as much as a 20% to 30% chance of an outright cure."[23]

There was also a general lack of discussion of side effects and mortality in many stories. And when the issue of cost was raised it was usually in the context of how the patient could not afford the high cost of the treatment, if the insurance company would not provide coverage. But many critics believe that the biggest failing in the coverage of HDC/ABMT was the press not explaining that this was an unproven treatment, which had never been studied in randomized clinical trials. Dr Larry Norton, Deputy Physician-in-Chief for Breast Cancer Programs at Memorial Sloan Kettering and past president of American Society of Clinical Oncology (ASCO), says the press was not willing to explain how science works. In reference to HDC/ABMT, Norton said, "If they (the public) don't understand the scientific method they are not going to understand what we are talking about." Norton said, "we tried repeatedly to get the message out that this was not established therapy and the press wouldn't listen."[24] Norton said the press found (and still finds) the process of explaining clinical trials too complicated.

Some doctors go even further, saying that the press coverage had a role in the length of time it took to enroll patients and get answers from the trials. Dr Wickerham says that "women and their families were reluctant to go into trials where there was a 50/50 chance of getting standard treatment."[25] Dr Susan Love, clinical professor of surgery at UCLA and author of *Dr Susan Love's Breast Cancer Book*, calls the press coverage of HDC/ABMT a "terrible travesty" that was "handled badly" by the media.[26] Love believes the media had a responsibility not to repeat what everybody was saying. "Their job should be the muckrakers and to say the emperor has no clothes," Love said.

But there are those, both within the press and without, who take a different view. Joann Rodgers of Johns Hopkins thinks it would have been difficult for the media on its own to sort through the science. Rodgers says, "How would you even pose the question to physicians who were jumping on the bandwagon?…Do you want to make the argument that science writers not put on TV anything that is not peer reviewed?"[27] And Dr George Sledge, codirector of the Breast Cancer Research Program at the Indiana University Simon Cancer Center, is also sympathetic to the position of the press. "I've never blamed the press for its handling of the BMT thing," he says. "When distinguished professors at Harvard and Duke tell you something works you tend to believe it—not just you guys but also a large number of physicians."[28]

In the highly researched 2007 book *False Hope*, authors Richard Rettig, Peter Jacobson, Cynthia Farquhar, and Wade Aubrey explored the controversy in great detail. The authors said responsibility for what went wrong included members of the medical profession, lawyers, judges, juries, federal health administrators, and the news media, which "played a critical role in promoting HDC/ABMT to breast cancer patients and persuading legislators to force insurers to pay for the procedure."[21] The authors reviewed hundreds of newspaper articles and dozens of television stories and concluded that the stories convinced readers and viewers that "first, HDC made sense; if a little chemotherapy could cure early cancers then obviously higher doses were needed for more advanced cancers. Second HDC was an advanced breast cancer patient's only hope. Third, the only thing standing between a patient and the potential cure was money which insurers did not want to spend."[21]

False Hope suggests reporters got the story wrong because of the "culture of journalism." The authors say the media have a history of embracing new treatments put forward by charismatic doctors holding prestigious positions in the medical establishment. The book says reporters "accepted without question reports from institutions like ASCO and Duke University, as well as doctors publicizing the treatment." And further, the authors say reporters were attracted to the stories because "hope sells" and "medical reporters had gotten used to being the bearer of good news and their employers knew from sales figures that while readers were keenly interested in health information, they preferred stories that offered a sense of hope."

The authors believe the media failed to cast a critical eye the way political reporters do with politicians. But *False Hope* goes even further by charging the media with a bias due to economic interests. "As the media have grown increasingly dependent on advertising by drug companies they have also become increasingly reluctant to run stories attacking the pharmaceutical industry." The remedy offered by *False Hope* is for journalism schools to start "teaching students to question the motives of doctors and hospitals and to 'follow the money' as investigative reporters like to say."

There are many in the press and research community who believe the media did not make clear the lack of definitive studies and relied too heavily on several leading experts. However, the suggestion in *False Hope* of a bias due to financial ties is questionable. ABC News does have a large number of pharmaceutical ads on many of its news programs, but the author has never had any experience of having this financial relationship on the sales side intrude into the editorial independence in the medical reporting at ABC News. Although it would be difficult to prove, the way that the press covers medical stories, which we follow every day, does not seem to this author to suggest drug company influence. What is more, at the time of our reporting on this topic, Dr Timothy Johnson and this author had no information regarding which companies made the drugs being used for the treatment of these patients.

REPORTING OF SCIENTIFIC MISCONDUCT IN THE NSABP STUDIES

It is hard to imagine, from a public relations and news coverage perspective, how things could have gone any worse for the leadership of the NSABP in 1994. Multiple developments created a news coverage story line that cast the prestigious NSABP's research and its cofounder and scientific director, Dr Bernard Fisher, in an extremely negative light. Here is what happened:

1. A news story broke suddenly for which the NSABP was not prepared.
2. Dr Fisher's name became associated with words in news stories describing fraudulent activities of a researcher working on NSABP studies.
3. The subject was of interest to a powerful congressman (Congressman John Dingell) who could drive news coverage by his ability to hold public hearings and pick witnesses.
4. This problem upset the most powerful government agency (National Cancer Institute) in cancer, and reflected poorly on its director.
5. Editors of the most powerful medical journal (New England Journal of Medicine) felt the credibility of what they published had been called into question.
6. An extensive explanation of what happened was not given publically on Capitol Hill until much later.

This public relations nightmare was created by a series of events that may provide lessons about how the press responds to such stories, and what potential important lessons can be learned from a story of this nature.

Any public relations person will advise that when there is very negative news being reported, it is necessary to get out front with your story. There appears to be no indication that the NSABP was prepared for the story on March 13, 1994, by John Crewdson of the *Chicago Tribune*.[29] Crewdson, in a Sunday story, detailed how Dr Roger Poisson had falsified data on patients involved in the NSABP lumpectomy versus mastectomy study. The first problem is that the story broke on a Sunday. Weekends are a bad time to deal with a news story. Reporters can not access as many sources on the weekend, so what happens is that the original story will drive the coverage. When reporters can reach other sources, sometimes they will take a different approach to a story. For example, 2 key elements to the story in retrospect are numerous other studies supported the conclusions of the NSABP lumpectomy versus mastectomy study, and the 100 patients whose records had been altered were spread out over multiple studies. But with the Crewdson story setting the tone, news organizations on Sunday followed what the *Tribune* reported. The author first saw the details of this story in a wire report that summarized the Crewdson article. Once the wire framed the story with Crewdson's information, then television and radio news organizations, at both the network and local level, reported the story as Crewdson did. The "100 cases," for example, were repeatedly referred to.

The CBS News story that day said:

> But an investigation by the U.S. National Cancer Institute has now revealed that Dr Richard Poisson and his assistants, who collaborated in the studies, falsified or fabricated the results of research carried out on some 100 cancer patients treated at Montreal's Saint Luc Hospital.[30]

ABC News said that here were "documented 111 separate instances in which the falsified data was submitted."[31] And news stories used words that would frame the story. Not only was "fraud" used repeatedly but the story was viewed as so unsettling that stronger words appeared. The ABC News correspondent Karen Burnes said that the *Tribune* story "reveals a chilling case of greed and ego which superseded all else, including the treatment of women." Dr Bernard Fisher, who was regarded worldwide as one of the most important figures in breast cancer research, had a brief sound bite on the CBS story saying "there was no evidence that the results were affected by what was done." And the ABC story had a sound bite from a Sloan Kettering physician who said "we need to reassure our patients that there are other trials that still say that this is safe." But those messages would be lost in the sea of "fraud," "scientific misconduct," and "ego."

By the next day, as people read the story and heard the story on television and radio, a new angle emerged. Once a story such as this has 24 hours under its belt, it begins to pick up a momentum of its own. No one is going to change the story line and get reporters to start questioning whether the results were affected or get them to emphasize that some of the data of one doctor out of 5000 is not going to change the statistical validity of a study. Reporters next began to hear from breast cancer patients and patient advocacy groups, who reacted to the story as it was framed on Sunday. So reporters began to focus on an additional story line that would add momentum to the outrage over the revelations; CBS News anchor Paula Zahn interviewed Dr Maureen Cavanah of Boston University Medical Center on the morning after the story broke:

ZAHN: But you must concede that there are women out there in this country, on the basis of this study, who went in and had lumpectomies and not radical mastectomies and those that are now being told they should line up for lumpectomies. How should they feel about this morning? Even though you're saying the science should still stand, shouldn't they be concerned about what message this sends?[32]

Now the story line was: "Danger! These data are going to call into question whether women who have lumpectomies will die sooner than if they had a mastectomy." This story line suggested that the scientific fraud was going to result in potential earlier deaths of women who had received lumpectomy compared to women who received mastectomy. It was an absurd suggestion, but it provides a critical lesson in the importance of trying to do everything possible to take back control of a story. Or at least try to turn the story.

The NSABP and Dr Fisher were not only facing an out-of-control story, building momentum, but other researchers and the government officials were providing reporters with sound bites that added to the negative impression of how the NSABP had handled the discovery of scientific misconduct. On NPR's "All Things Considered" the day after the story was published, reporter Noah Adams had a sound bite from an official of the Office of Research Integrity (ORI):

DOROTHY MCFARLANE, Investigator: We found in a review of over 1500 cases entered by Dr Poisson between 1977 and 1990, that in 100 of these cases there was data that had been falsified or fabricated.[33]

Dr Janet Osuch, in a "MacNeil-Lehrer NewsHour" story on PBS on March 30, 1994, did not mention Dr Fisher by name, but clearly laid blame at his feet for not sharing the information about Poisson's data with other researchers in NSABP.[34] Osuch said, "I feel very betrayed, very betrayed. I think that an issue of scientific misconduct is a very serious issue. I feel that the NSABP failed to disclose to the membership, and I hold them accountable for that."

And then the *New England Journal of Medicine* editors, who were upset that Fisher had not informed them of the fraudulent data, added to criticism for the delay in correcting the data. In a commentary titled "Setting the Record Straight in the Breast Cancer Trials" the *Journal* said "there is no excuse for the 4 year delay between the first indication of misconduct in 1999 and the publication of the reanalysis which we hope will take place in 1994."[35] By the time Dr Fisher appeared before the Dingell committee in April 1994, most would have considered that he personally had little chance of turning the story even slightly.

There may be a temptation for physicians and researchers to look at this episode and blame the news media. But the quotes above provide evidence that there were many people who personally expressed that they were upset with Dr Fisher, and this had an impact on how the story was being framed. The story is classic example of how it is nearly impossible to turn a big story, once it heads in a certain direction. The process can be called unfair, or press bias, or the press love of sensationalism. There are plenty of people who believe Dr Fisher was not treated fairly. And there were news reports that made that case.

One of the best was a series by the *Pittsburgh Post Gazette* reporter McKenzie Carpenter, which painted a very different picture of Fisher. She told about the "renegade" who had challenged the radical mastectomy and believed, contrary to prevailing thinking, that cancer spread through the blood and lymph vessels. She told how Dr Fisher took over the NSABP and began selling his idea of randomized comparative trials between radical and simple mastectomy. Carpenter described how Fisher brought 500 institutions and 5000 physicians into NSABP studies.

Carpenter also went through the data and again painted a very different picture. She described the falsifications by Dr Poisson as "small changes in the dates that determined whether women met the deadline by enrolling in the studies."[36] The story also provided an explanation of how Dr Fisher had planned to get the word out about the falsified data. She described his plan as a "careful deliberate approach—the way Fisher had always done things." As for not informing the *New England Journal of Medicine*, the story quoted Fisher as saying that the NSABP had concluded there was no change in the outcome. "When you get no change in the results," Fisher said, "you don't call up the *New England Journal of Medicine* and say 'Guess what? Nothing happened.'"[36]

Carpenter provided details about how Fisher felt about the Dingell hearing. "For Fisher it was a total unmitigated disaster, the low point of his life." And Carpenter also went through point by point the accusations by Dingell, and concluded, "It was a dramatic drilling. But it wasn't true." And the final installment of the series ended with the reporter's conclusions:

In the case of Dr Bernard Fisher, the facts are these. He never was accused of falsifying information. The fraud committed by Poisson on 99 patient records has not changed the basic outcome of the studies he directed at NSABP. There is no evidence of systematic fraud in the other medical centers Fisher oversaw.[36]

Perhaps Dr Fisher, speaking at ASCO in 1993, before the story broke, said it best:

> Politics, personalities, process, publicity, media coverage, fiscal concerns and other secondary considerations must not be permitted to take on a life of their own and like a cancer, destroy our true mission.

The mission goes on, but that "life of their own" is the legacy of this story. On a positive note, the government's investigation and in part the widespread media coverage surrounding the scientific misconduct in the NSABP clinical trials brought to light the essential need for checks and balances and continuous auditing of trials for source documentation that are now considered routine and generally required for all clinical trials performed in the United States and around the world. And Dr Fisher was personally cleared of all charges of scientific misconduct.

THE BREAST CANCER IN LONG ISLAND STORY

Another example of misleading reporting, also based on statistics, emerged in Long Island during the 1980s. Dan Fagin, a reporter for *Newsday* who covered the story for over a decade, laid out the following timeline in a 2002 story. In July 1983, New York State said the breast cancer rate in Nassau County was 30% higher than the national average.[37] Six months later, Nassau politicians commissioned the state health department to do an $800,000 study of the county's breast cancer rate. Three years later the study concluded that risk factors such as being Jewish, having children late in life, and eating a high-fat diet were the main reasons for the higher rate.[37] Advocacy groups responded that such an explanation was "blaming the victim," and pressed for more studies. The groups were convinced that environmental factors were a major reason for the higher rate. In 1990 the state health department found that areas with contaminated water wells and hazardous waste sites did not have higher breast cancer rates.[37] Undeterred, a month later a group was formed called 1 in 9, or the Long Island Breast Cancer Action Committee. Throughout this time, the story was being widely covered by the local press.

The Long Island group became part of the national advocacy efforts for breast cancer in Washington in the early 1990s, and with the help of some powerful political allies, including Senator Alfonse D'Amato, the Long Island groups pushed for passage of a bill that included money to fund environmental studies of Long Island's breast cancer rates. The National Cancer Institute was charged with developing a plan and came up with proposals for 12 studies that would ultimately cost around $30 million.[37] What Fagin describes as the "cornerstone" of this research was an $8 million study comparing environmental exposure of women with breast cancer to those who did not have cancer. From 1994 to 2002, a series of studies and cancer maps provided no strong evidence of the environmental link. And in 2002 the cornerstone study found no evidence that pollution is an important cause of breast cancer in Long Island women.[37]

The Long Island story is instructive for a number of reasons. Fagin, who is now director of the NYU Science, Health and Environmental Reporting Program, says that during the time

that the NCI-funded studies were going on, there were data showing that breast cancer rates in affluent suburbs in other parts of the country were high, including in Chicago and San Francisco. "But by that time the train had left the station." Fagin, whose coverage was consistently balanced and thoughtful, said reporting by other press was generally "shallow." The national press also eventually picked up on the story. As was true with the NSABP story, this is another case where the reporting of science gets politicized. In this case it was done by advocacy groups and politicians. But perhaps even more important is how the Long Island breast cancer story provided a hint of what was to come from combining advocacy groups with politicians who are seeking to pressure science to provide the answers they want.

A popular movement that suspects that mercury in vaccines causes autism has taken the Long Island story a step further. Not only have they combined patient advocacy with political support, but they have added celebrity spokespeople. Some elements of this movement bitterly attack scientists for refusing to agree with their views. They believe the Centers for Disease Control and Prevention, the World Health Organization, and the Institute of Medicine have all come up with the "wrong" answer by failing to find a link between vaccines and autism. And they are not a state movement but a national movement. Some use the Internet to ridicule reporters who present stories in what they believe are a biased way. Their congressional supporters have called members of the press to Washington to explain their reporting on autism, which the congressmen and these autism groups believe is not accurate.

This growing willingness of advocacy groups and their political supporters to ignore scientific evidence presents serious challenges for the press. And the increasingly hostile tactics, using the Internet as a bludgeon, are a new challenge for reporters who cover this story and researchers who could get in their sights if they end up on the "wrong side" of a scientific issue. Suddenly, what is communicated in any form, be it e-mail response or story, could end up widely distributed on the Internet among many people who believe that the press is allied with scientists in keeping the "true" environmental risks from the public.

GUIDANCE FOR DEALING WITH THE PRESS

For some doctors, the e-mail message or call from the media may be dreaded. For others it may be welcomed. From the beginning of the communication until the story airs, there is a great deal of information about the process that is important for the doctor to understand. First is the news organization. Doctors will want to know the news organization the reporter represents. And this is getting increasingly complicated with the growth of the Internet. Doctors can get calls from reporters working for unfamiliar Web sites. One advantage of the Internet is that information about such sites is easily accessed. Simply by going to the site and clicking on "about us" it is possible for a doctor to get a sense of the Web site.

If the reporter is from a recognized newspaper or news organization, it is a good idea to find out whether or not the reporter is a medical specialist or a general reporter. These are questions that doctors at institutions with public relations departments can get answered before speaking to the reporter. Even an office assistant or other gatekeeper can answer these questions for doctors who are not represented by someone in public affairs. How a doctor approaches an interview may be quite different if a reporter is a medical specialist, who can be expected to have some general understanding of the clinical trial process. A general assignment reporter may or may not have any idea of how medical studies are done.

Major national news organizations now have multiple "platforms" providing news. ABC News, for example, has its major daily weekday programs, a newsmagazine (*20/20*), weekend broadcasts, overnight and early-morning news broadcasts, video news service to ABC affiliates, ABC Radio, and digital outlets (ABCNews.com and ABC News NOW). Other network news organizations and cable news have multiple programs and digital outlets. Audiences for these platforms may vary significantly, from major programs whose audiences are counted in the multi-millions to individual digital stories whose readers may be in the hundreds. Doctors may want their PR to triage the specific platform for a national news organization to get a sense of the size of the audience. There is generally going to be a big difference between the number of viewers watching a story on the network evening newscasts and the number reading a story on a national news outlet's Web site.

Web site traffic will vary dramatically depending upon whether a story appears on the home page. A reporter will not know in advance whether or not that is the case. But a doctor looking for a story on the Internet where he or she is quoted who finds the story on the home page should know that a lot more people will be reading the story than if the story only was included in the Web site's health section. There is the possibility of linkage to a major Web site with high traffic volume. Even though a story appears in a health section of a Web site, if it gets linked as the lead story on Google Health or the Drudge Report, then all bets are off on traffic.

It is also worth noting that there is often an inverse relationship between length of time on air and size of audience. As you go down in time you generally go up in audience. A 12-second sound bite in a 90-second piece on an evening network newscast may be seen by over 8 million people. Or a doctor may be invited to participate in a 1-hour webcast. Unless there is something extraordinary about the webcast, chances are the audience is going to be very small. There are obvious exceptions, such as 4-minute interviews on morning national news programs or lengthy interviews on nationally syndicated radio programs.

It is also reasonable to establish before an interview whether the reporter is working on a news story with a deadline or on a feature. If a reporter is on deadline, the doctor needs to decide whether it is possible to do the interview prior to the deadline. Reporters will seek multiple sources and usually have a backup source or sources in mind. If the doctor cannot do the interview until tomorrow or late today, they would rather go to a different source than wait around for a callback that comes too late.

One "don't" in getting information prior to an interview: it is not a good idea to ask the "slant" of a reporter. The word sounds as if you are assuming that the reporter has a bias. Good reporters do not go into a phone interview having already decided what they want to hear or what they are going to write. The interview is part of a fact-gathering process. For a feature, the situation is slightly different. A reporter writing a feature story will generally have some idea of the "focus." So it is not unreasonable to try to establish what the feature will cover. And the reporter needs to say more than that he or she is doing a story on "breast cancer treatment," for example. If the reporter cannot be more specific, there is a good chance that he or she is either inexperienced at covering medicine or is hiding the real focus of the story.

This final point about imprecise explanations of a story's focus raises the importance of learning something about the reporter in advance. For national and even local reporters, an Internet search should provide some information about what they cover and their experience. It is also a good idea to prepare for an interview with a reporter. A doctor will want to generally identify the main points he or she hopes will be included in a story. If a public relations person is available, it may be worthwhile to go over some of the likely questions that will be asked by the reporter.

Once a doctor has an idea about deadlines, size of the news outlet, the story focus, and who the reporter is, he or she is ready to speak with a reporter. As soon as the interview starts, everything is for the record, unless the doctor specifies that something is off the record. If a reporter does not ask, the doctor should establish correct spelling of name, title, and institution. While academic titles are important to doctors they may be less so to many reporters, particularly broadcast reporters. It may be worth saying "professor of medicine," but do not be surprised if a reporter does not use it. Generally reporters would like hospital titles. It is also a good idea, if the doctor has a public relations person involved, to make sure the institution is identified in a way that will make the institution executives happy. Some doctors have academic and hospital appointments. If the public relations person comes from the medical school and not the hospital, it may be preferable to provide the medical school title. However, again a reporter would much prefer "director of surgical oncology" at the hospital than some professor title at the medical school.

Once a phone or face-to-face (no camera or audio) interview begins, there are a number of guidelines. Dan Haney, who was with the Associated Press for 30 years, including many years as medical editor, offered "A Reporters Advice to Medical Researchers" in *Clinical Cancer Research*.[39] Haney's first suggestion is critical. Use jargon-free English. Haney cites the example of "spreading" versus "metastatic." Other examples would include "lesion," "in situ," and "recurrence-free survival." Even "modality" and "therapy" are not plain English to most people.

Haney also cautions researchers against inflating the significance of what they have done. Haney said the reason not to do that is because of the tendency of the media, particularly with cancer, to "offer hope whether it is justified or not." Haney says "reporters instinctively push scientists to make the strongest possible statements about their work, because that makes the most compelling story. Scientists need not play along."[38]

Among some of Haney's other tips:

- Give reporters plenty of background and context. Tell them how this discovery fits into the larger problem of controlling disease.

- Be generous with details.
- Offer other names for interviews.
- Be reachable. Reporters often have questions that come to mind when writing.
- Disclose conflict of interest.

The circumstances are different when doing a broadcast interview. If it is a taped interview, a reporter is seeking sound bites for a story, and in many cases the story is not yet written when the interview is done. For feature stories there may be cases where a reporter has written a rough draft to be filled with sound bites.

For broadcast interviews it is also important that the doctor keep answers free of jargon, but broadcast reporters are looking for other qualities when choosing a doctor to interview. In my over 30 years of involvement with broadcast medical news, what makes a good interview subject has changed very little. The medical unit at ABC News regularly makes recommendations to ABC News programs about the on-camera ability of experts. We are constantly evaluating on-air ability of doctors all over the country, and actually have on-air ratings in our database for those we have seen. We look for people who can explain things simply, are good talkers, and have credibility and energy.

A note about each of those qualities. Broadcast reporters want doctors who can simply explain the significance of a study, or who can explain a procedure in simple terms. It is not only a matter of being jargon-free; the doctor needs to have ability to communicate in way that is easy to understand. Good talkers are people you would be interested to hear lecturing or would enjoy speaking with at a cocktail party. It is difficult to define, but most people understand what it means. "Credibility" is also a vague term when used for television. But we want the audience to feel they are getting information from someone who knows his or her subject. And finally, there is energy. Lack of energy is something that will rule out experts for an interview at the network level, particularly for live broadcasts. Energy can be "cool" or "hot." Someone may speak quietly but still communicate energy. Broadcast reporters cannot have interview subjects pausing or saying "um" every few words. They prefer fast talkers who can pack more facts into a short time. But we have put on the air plenty of doctors who do not speak quickly, but are articulate and who appear very credible.

But what if the story is not a feature or routine news story, but a story that could create a lot of negative publicity? How should a doctor or hospital deal with such a story? Gary Koops is managing director and head of the US Media Group for Burson-Marsteller, an international public relations and marketing firm. He has handled a number of crises, including the Virginia Tech shooting, the Duke transplant case, and the allegations of Medicare fraud involving the Hospital Corporation of America (HCA) Hospitals. Koops says the most important thing when faced with an explosive story is to be "open to answer all the questions even if you don't have all the facts."[39] Koops says the mistakes often made by businesses or institutions facing negative publicity are that they believe that less information is better. He says, "The more information you can share the better." Koops says that even in the case of a story that is already written, as was the case with NSABP controversy, "you want to add as much content as you can."

When asked how he would have handled the NSABP story, Koops said that you first want to identify who are the most important audiences. He says you want to know which audiences need the information right away. Once the 10 or 15 most important people who can reach the key people involved with the issue have been identified, Koops says you contact them by letter, phone, or by getting on a plane. "The sooner people can feel and touch your perspective, the sooner they can make decisions in the appropriate context." Next, Koops says you get the story out to the key people in the press, whether they are broadcast, print, or Internet journalists. He says some clients have even set up Web sites to get their message out.

Koops encourages transparency and cautions against viewing the press as out to get you, which he says is a "short sighted analysis." He says "The media reports the facts and points of view as they have them at that point in time. I don't buy that the media is responsible." He says you do not want to "put up sandbags and shut off the phone." He says the "media is either talking about you or with you. You want them talking with you." As to concerns about having to face difficult questions, Koops says "all the tough questions are legitimate questions." It is important, he says, to be willing to answer the tough questions.

His final advice is from another era, but still true today. It is not a good idea to try to fight the press. Koops says, "Never argue with a man who buys paper by the barrel and ink by the ton."

SUMMARY

Two of the most common complaints of doctors today about the press are

- Why does the press exaggerate research findings?
- Why does the press interview and quote the same doctors and ignore the research of doctors who could add a lot to the public understanding of breast cancer?

As this chapter has demonstrated, in many cases the press does have responsibility for hyped stories, overstated research, and rushes to judgement. But doctors also can do a great deal to help public understanding of breast cancer by their willingness to communicate with the press. By being accessible, talking to reporters, and making sure every effort is made to provide context, doctors can play an important role in improving the way breast cancer is reported. Reporters do want to get it right. Doctors with a simple willingness to take the time to help reporters can play an enormous role in making sure the public is well served.

Thanks to Nancy Quade, in ABC News Research, who made invaluable contributions to this chapter.

REFERENCES

1. Stadtmauer EA, O'Neill A, Goldstein LJ, et al. Conventional-dose chemotherapy compared with high-dose chemotherapy plus autologous hematopoietic stem-cell transplantation for metastatic breast cancer. *N Engl J Med*. 2000;342:1069-1076.
2. Fisher B, Anderson S, Redmond CK, et al. Reanalysis and results after 12 years of follow-up in a randomized clinical trial comparing total mastectomy with lumpectomy with or without irradiation in the treatment of breast cancer. *N Engl J Med*. 1995;333:1456-1461.

3. Gammon MD, Wolff MS, Neugut AI, et al. Environmental toxins and breast cancer on Long Island. II. Organochlorine compound levels in blood. *Cancer Epidemiol Biomarkers Prev.* 2002;11:686-697.

4. Perlmutter E. Mrs. Ford asks drive for cancer diagnosis. *New York Times.* December 2, 1976:52.

5. Lichtenfeld L. Interview. October 28, 2008.

6. Rodgers J. Interview. November 3, 2008.

7. Hogan M. *The Politics of Breast Cancer.* Washington, DC: Georgetown University Press; 2001:47.

8. Wickerham L. Interview. November 26, 2008.

9. Chapman S, McLeod K, Wakefield M, Holding S. Impact of new of celebrity illness on breast cancer screening: Kylie Minogues breast cancer diagnosis. *Medicine and the Media.* 2005;183:247-250.

10. Lane S, Poleknak A, Burg MA. The impact of the media coverage of Nancy Reagan's experience on breast cancer screening. *Am J Public Health.* 1989;79:1551-1552.

11. Schneider S, Leonard E. A matter of choice coping with breast cancer and the controversy over unorthodox treatment plans: Suzanne Somers faces the future with serene self assurance. *People.* April 30, 2001:55.

12. Cassileth B, Breu G. Let the patients beware: cancer expert Barrie Cassileth warns that alternative treatments may pose serious dangers. *People.* April 30, 2001:55.

13. Adlersburg J. E-mail. November 25, 2008.

14. Ochs R. Personal health/alternative cancer therapies: patients are leading the way. *Newsday.* June 19, 2001:C4.

15. Cohen E. *Saturday.* CNN television. May 12, 2001.

16. Kwiakowski J. Alternative path: Suzanne Somers decision to fight her breast cancer with treatments like extract of mistletoe. *Buffalo News.* May 6, 2001:E1.

17. Peck P. E-mail. November 25, 2008.

18. Savard M. E-mail. November 24, 2008.

19. Fletcher L. *Nightline.* ABC television. September 23, 2008.

20. Johnson T. *20/20.* ABC television. February 9, 1990.

21. Rettig RA, Jacobson PD, Farquhar CM, Aubrey WM. *False Hope.* New York, NY: Oxford University Press; 2007:23-24, 31, 140, 268-269.

22. Stanley D. Woman stuck in debate over cancer treatment. *Austin American-Statesman.* October 3, 1993:A1.

23. Hiltzik M. Drawing the line: an HMO dilemma. *Los Angeles Times.* January 17, 1996:1.

24. Norton L. Interview. November 26, 2008.

25. Wickerham L. Interview. November 26, 2008.

26. Love S. Interview. November 26, 2008.

27. Rodgers J. Interview. November 3, 2008.

28. Sledge G. E-mail. November 26, 2008.

29. Crewdson J. Fraud in breast cancer: doctor lied on data for decades. *Chicago Tribune.* March 13, 1994:1.

30. Mason A. *CBS Evening News.* CBS television. March 13, 1994.

31. Burnes K. *World News Tonight Sunday.* ABC television. March 13, 1994.

32. *CBS This Morning.* CBS television. March 14, 1994.

33. Adams N. *All Things Considered.* National Public Radio. March 14, 1994.

34. *The MacNeil/Lehrer NewsHour.* Public Broadcasting System. March 30, 1994.

35. Angell M, Kassirer J. Setting the record straight in the breast cancer trials. *N Engl J Med.* 1994;330:1448-1450.

36. Carpenter M. Anatomy of a scandal: science, technology and medicine. *Pittsburgh Post-Gazette.* December 26-30, 1994:1.

37. Fagin D. Tattered hopes. *Newsday.* July 28, 2002.

38. Haney DQ. A reporter's advice to medical researchers. *Clin Cancer Res.* 2005;11:6755-6756.

39. Koops G. Interview. December 3, 2008.

SECTION 1

ETIOLOGY, ASSESSING RISK, INITIAL EVALUATION, AND MANAGEMENT

Thomas B. Julian
David Euhus
Irene L. Wapnir

CHAPTER 1

Breast Carcinogenesis

Paul J. van Diest
Horst Buerger
Arno Kuijper
Elsken van der Wall

Breast cancer is an important health care problem since it is the most frequently occurring cancer (1 out of about 10 women) and among the major causes of death in women in the Western world. Despite many studies, breast carcinogenesis is still not well understood. Although many breast cancer risk factors have been identified, they do not easily translate into molecular changes that help to understand why normal breast cells derail to form early lesions that then accumulate further genetic events that make them eventually progress to cancer. Discussing these risk factors is therefore beyond the scope of this chapter. We will also stay away from providing endless lists of possibly relevant individual genetic aberrations. Rather, we will try to integrate the fairly fragmentary knowledge of genetic aberrations and changes in gene expression into progression models based on long-standing morphologic progression models. This is quite challenging, since breast cancer is a very heterogeneous disease, far beyond the so-called ductal and lobular lesions that are best known. Nevertheless, these morphologic progression models have proven to provide a proper framework to depict and understand how different early lesions may progress to cancer, and help to place relevant genetic changes into the different progression routes to cancer. Further, they have been proven to be clinically relevant, in the sense that relative risk of these lesions to progress to cancer is known from long-term follow-up studies. This has become the base for clinical management of such lesions when found in a breast biopsy, for example, after a mammographic abnormality on breast screening.

The epithelial progression routes comprise those for ductal lesions, columnar cell lesions, lobular lesions, papillary lesions, apocrine lesions, mucinous lesions, medullary lesions, metaplastic lesions, secretory lesions, and adenomyoepithelial lesions. However, in this chapter we will focus on conceptual issues that are shared by the progression routes for these different lesions, and then shortly try to place different precursors within progression routes for epithelial breast cancer. In addition, carcinogenesis in hereditary cancer syndromes will be discussed separately.

The fibroepithelial route comprises progression from fibroadenoma and related lesions to malignant phyllodes tumors. Before going into some of these individual progression routes in detail, we will provide a general framework for breast carcinogenesis, integrating morphologic, immunohistochemical, and genetic findings.

BREAST CARCINOGENESIS

The pathogenesis of invasive breast cancer has been under debate for decades, and many progression models have been proposed, incorporating the epidemiologic and genetic findings at the respective times. However, some of these models and concepts were not able to generate a global understanding for many aspects of this threatening disease.

In the general sense, (sporadic) breast carcinogenesis is not essentially different from carcinogenesis of other epithelial malignancies. Tumor suppressor gene inactivation through promoter methylation is likely among the earliest events in breast carcinogenesis.[1,2] Besides, loss of heterozygosity may occur already early in breast carcinogenesis as a means of inactivating crucial genes.[3,4]

These events will, for example, affect DNA repair, which provides a background for accumulation of more genetic events. The resulting disruption of cell cycle control mechanisms and/or apoptosis-signaling pathways leads to disturbance of the balance between proliferation and apoptosis,[5] in turn leading to growth of early lesions, which are usually polyclonal. Activating mutations in and amplifications of (proto)oncogenes, as well as chromosomal imbalances, and inactivating mutations in tumor suppressor genes (such as p53), usually kick in later, eventually leading to selective outgrowth of clones with the highest proliferation/apoptosis imbalance. Increased proliferation will lead to cells that are too far from the nearest blood vessels to sustain oxygen and nutrient supply levels, leading to hypoxia. This sets off a cellular survival program to cope with the hypoxic stress, inducing growth-factor–mediated angiogenesis and switch to anaerobic metabolism. In the stage of DCIS, angiogenesis is induced, often presenting as a network of vessels around the malignant ducts.[6] However, lymphangiogenesis does not seem to play a role.[6]

In the latest pre-invasive stages, invasion-related genes become activated, allowing cells to break down the basement membrane and extracellular matrix to invade the surrounding stroma (see Chapter 2 for an extensive overview). This provides access to lymph and blood vessels (which occurs independently), allowing cells to enter the lymphatics to pass on to lymph nodes to form locoregional metastases, as well as the bloodstream to form distant metastases (see Chapter 3 for an extensive overview). For the latter, circulating tumor cells must home to the distant site, adhere to the endothelium, invade in the local tissue, and again create the optimal microenvironment to escape dormancy and grow out to clinically manifest metastases. This may need additional genetic hits.[7] During this complex multistep process, aberrant cells must all the time escape from the immune response, in which down-regulation of Human Leukocyte Antigen (HLA) molecules plays an essential role. The concept of epithelial–mesenchymal transition (EMT), a currently very hot topic in molecular in vitro studies thought to play a main role in invasion and metastasis formation, is difficult to translate to human breast tumors, as loss of epithelial differentiation is very rare in human tumors including those from the breast.

Genes Involved

Many genes play a role in the above process, and it would be impossible to mention them all while keeping an overview. Instead, let us just mention those perhaps most important. The estrogen and progesterone receptors are highly expressed in almost all preinvasive breast lesions, stimulating proliferation. Interestingly, expression of these steroid receptors is somewhat lower in invasive cancers. Many cell-cycle control proteins are involved. Cyclin D1 may be amplified or induced in an ER-dependent manner,[8] and cyclin E is also often overexpressed.[9] Cyclin-dependent kinases like CDK4 can be overexpressed,[10] and CDK inhibitors like p27 and p21 may get deregulated.[11] Often p53 is mutated,[12] and c-myc may be amplified.[13] Several DNA repair genes may be affected by sporadic inactivating mutations like BRCA1, BRCA2, ATM, and CHEK2. Many growth factor receptors like HER2 and epidermal growth factor receptor (EGFR) are often overexpressed,[14] the former due to gene amplification, and many growth factors are overexpressed in stroma or epithelium to provide paracrine or autocrine loops.[15,16] HIF-1α mediates the hypoxia response[17] to increase cellular survival and strengthen malignant transformation.[18] The E-cadherin gene is often inactivated (especially in lobular lesions, discussed below), leading to decreased cell–cell contact, facilitating invasion and metastatic spread. hTERT must be activated to ensure proper telomere length for sustained cell division.[19] TWIST[20] and Notch1[21] seem to play a role in metastases formation. As to Wnt signaling, it appears that DNA hypermethylation leads to aberrant regulation of the Wnt pathway in breast cancer rather than mutations in, for example, APC.[22]

MiRNAs are now recognized as a highly abundant class of regulatory RNA molecules. Iorio and associates identified 29 miRNAs to be deregulated in breast cancer by microarray analysis.[23] MiRNA clusters that seem to be involved in breast carcinigenesis comprise miR-21, miR-29b-2, miR-125b, miR-145, miR-10b, miR-155, miR-17-5p, and miR-27b.[23,24]

Translocations in breast cancer occur probably rarely, but one leading to the ETV6-NTRK3 fusion gene, which encodes a chimeric tyrosine kinase, is very characteristic for the secretory type of breast cancer.[25,26]

Microarray studies have also shed light on breast carcinogenesis. Sørlie and associates analyzed 78 breast cancers by microarray analysis, and based on gene expression profiles, cancers could be classified into a basal epithelial-like group, a HER2-overexpressing group, and a group of luminal cancers that seemed to split up into at least 2 subgroups (Fig. 1-1).[27] This classification appeared to have prognostic value. This paves the way for a molecular classification of breast cancer, which is, however, paralleled by expression of common immunohistochemical markers: basal cancers (CK5 and/or CK14 positive and ER/PR/HER2 negative), a group of cancers dictated by HER2 amplification/overexpression, and a group of cancers characterized by expression of ER while HER2 negative. This latter subgroup may be heterogeneous.

Oncogenic Viruses

There is no established role for viruses in breast carcinogenesis. Some studies have suggested a role for oncogenic viruses such as human papilloma viruses (HPV) and Epstein–Barr virus (EBV), but results have been inconsistent. Some studies claim to have found EBV sequences in breast cancers by PCR, but this approach lacks specificity, since infected lymphocytes within the tumor easily lead to PCR products. Using an immunohistochemical approach, some studies have described presence of EBNA1, but the used antibody later appeared to cross-react with MAGE4.[28] Several studies have reported presence of the oncogenic HPV types 16, 18, and 33 in invasive breast cancer, including a rare case of lymphoepithelioma-like breast cancer, a type previously thought to be associated with EBV infection.[29] An association with cervical HPV induced lesions has been suggested.[30] Although one study reported that HPV 16 E6/E7 proteins converted noninvasive human breast cancer cell lines to invasive cells,[31] the etiologic role of oncogenic HPV infections remains to be proven.

Stepwise or Random Genetic Progression?

Although some of these genetic events occur more often early, or late, in carcinogenesis, breast carcinogenesis cannot be viewed as a stepwise fixed genetic progression model, as has been suggested for colorectal carcinogenesis. Rather, breast

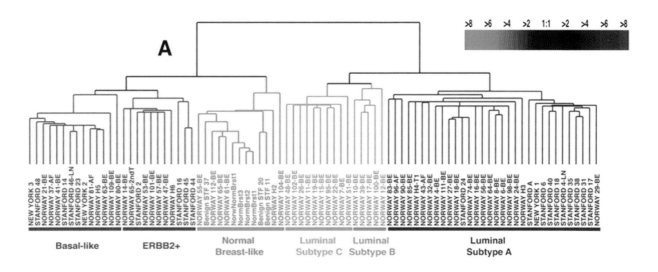

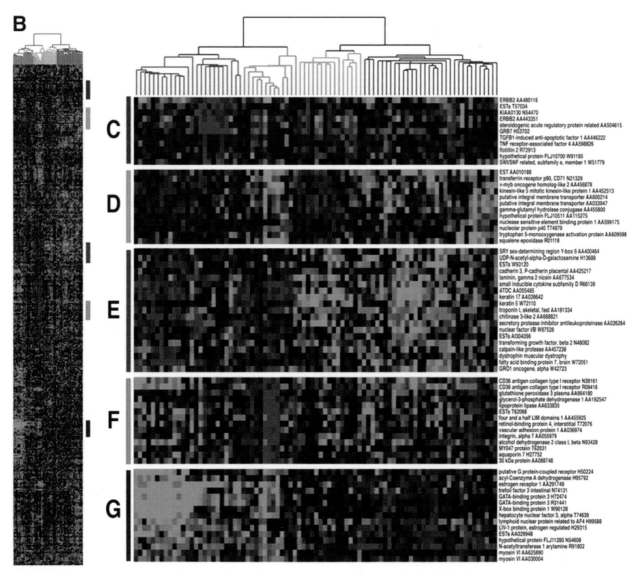

FIGURE 1-1 Gene expression patterns of 78 carcinomas, 3 benign tumors, and 4 normal tissues, analyzed by hierarchical clustering using the 476 cDNA intrinsic clone set.[27] The cluster dendrogram showed 3 main subtypes of cancer: luminal, basal-like, and HER2+. Reproduced with permission from reference 27.

cancer is to be viewed as the result of accumulation of various major and minor genetic events in a fairly random order, which we like to refer to as the "bingo principle" analogous to winning the "prize" (in this case cancer) in this popular game.

Nevertheless, these global mechanisms need adjustment to the very specific background of the normal human breast. This general concept has been challenged and needs modification according to latest genetic, morphologic, and immunohistochemical findings.

THE NORMAL BREAST

Most (pre)invasive lesions of the breast are thought to derive from the transition zone between the ducts and the functional unit of the breast, the lobule, which is composed of acini that are lined by an outer myoepithelial layer and an inner luminal or glandular layer. However, more recent studies give evidence that the inner, glandular layer contains a putative stem or progenitor cell compartment, which gives rise to the above-mentioned cells. These cells have been recently described and characterized more in detail. It is noteworthy that many characteristics of these cells are shared in mouse and human cells. A hallmark of these cells is the expression of high molecular weight cytokeratins (Ck 5/14), EGFR, and the lack of estrogen receptor expression. In contrast, more differentiated glandular cells are defined by the expression of low molecular weight cytokeratins (Ck8/18) and positivity for the estrogen receptor, whereas myoepithelial cells maintain the expression of Ck5/14 in addition to the expression of smooth-muscle actin (SMA) and p63. At present, the relationship between these cells and breast cancer–specific stem cells is unclear. Regardless of that, all these cells and presumed intermediate cells within the extremes of differentiation are targets for carcinogenic hits and potential precursor cells for the variety of morphologically different breast cancer subtypes. However, these cells can serve as a tool to explain the presence of monoclonal patches within a breast lobule or parts of the ductal tree. In addition, the description of nonrecurrent genetic changes within the morphologically normal breast tissue, requiring a large subset of affected cells, favors the idea of long-living cells as targets of the initial hit starting the genetic cascade towards an overt malignancy.

The finding of genetic changes within morphologically normal breast tissue is nowadays not only associated with an increased local recurrence risk but had also an tremendous influence on the validity of progression models of breast cancer and especially the relationship toward proposed precursor lesions. The finding of identical genetic alterations within two different precursors can therefore not automatically be interpreted as proof of a direct relationship, but might rather be regarded as a suggestion that both lesions have derived independently from a common precursor.

EVIDENCE FOR MULTIPLE GENETIC PATHWAYS IN BREAST CARCINOGENESIS

It has been a long-noted interesting phenomenon that pre-invasive lesions tend to progress while maintaining their morphologic differentiation status, usually referred to as "progression within

grade."[32] This means that well-differentiated (grade I) pre-invasive lesions tend to progress to well-differentiated invasive lesions, and that poorly differentiated (grade III) pre-invasive breast lesions usually progress to poorly differentiated invasive lesions. Even distant metastases are usually of the same grade as the primary tumor. Naturally, intermediate lesions (grade II) occur, but to discuss them would complicate the depicted concepts considerably, so for the sake of clarity we will further focus on the extreme ends of differentiation.

With the establishment of new global, genetic screening techniques such as comparative genomic hybridization (CGH), a pattern of genetic alterations, characteristic of distinct grades and morphology, has emerged. The loss of chromosomal 16q-losses occurred as the hallmark of well-differentiated intraductal as well as invasive breast cancer cases. However, this finding, as will be discussed later, was not new. The oldest descriptions of 16q losses were based on classical cytogenetic approaches using G-banding of metaphase chromosomes. It became obvious that the loss of 16q was often due to an unbalanced chromosomal translocation t(1;16)[33] and was associated with a decreased rate of lymph node metastasis, an increased expression of the estrogen and progesterone receptors[34-37], a low tumor proliferation rate and an improved overall survival[35,38-40]. In a few cases, t(1;16) was the sole cytogenetic abnormality,[41] underlining the importance of 16q losses. Since the breakpoint of the recurrent t(1;16) was located in the centromeric heterochromatin of chromosome 16, no specific genetic gene fusion transcript resulted from this chromosomal alteration, and speculation about gene dosage effects regulating the expression of respective candidate genes started. However, the consequences of this hypothesis have not been pursued, perhaps due to lack of suitable technical approaches to answer the question.

In parallel to the extensive characterization of breast cancer by conventional cytogenetics, the definition of the 16q-specific tumor suppressor gene was based on LOH analysis with a multitude of microsatellite markers covering the whole 16q arm. It was finally shown that probably 3 different shortest regions of overlap for the loss of 16q sequences in breast cancer exist. It is noteworthy that the different studies revealed partially different, and partially overlapping, results.[42] Of even higher importance was the finding that 16q losses seemed to occur as rather early events in breast carcinogenesis, shown by the detection of 16q losses in ductal (DCIS) and lobular carcinoma in situ (LCIS)[43,44] as well as in atypical hyperplasias.[4,45]

However, a part of these results might have been biased due to two circumstances. On the one hand, classical cytogenetic results could only be generated for a limited number of cases, due to technical difficulties in culturing breast cancer cells. On the other hand, the application of LOH analysis generally only allows a limited statement about the general chromosome 16q status, as discussed more extensively later in the chapter. With the introduction of technical approaches enabling a global overview of unbalanced chromosomal alterations in paraffin-embedded invasive carcinomas and their precursors, these restrictions could be overcome in a single step.

First studies on genetic changes in DCIS demonstrated that, besides gains of 1q, 16q-losses are the most recurrent changes in DCIS, already detectable at a precursor level of invasive breast cancer. However, the distribution of 16q losses in the wide morphologic spectrum of DICS showed that this distinct chromosomal alteration could predominantly be detected in well and intermediately differentiated DCIS, whereas in poorly differentiated DCIS the incidence of this change was rather low.[46-48]

In further studies it could be shown that this grade-dependent distribution of 16q losses was maintained in invasive carcinomas. Especially tubular, tubulo-lobular, and ductal invasive grade 1 breast cancers were characterized by 16q losses, whereas ductal invasive grade 3 carcinomas showed this alteration in a significant lower frequency.[49-51] More detailed studies in ductal invasive grade 3 carcinomas could further show that this chromosomal alteration is also rather uncommon in HER-2 amplified and/or overexpressing carcinomas[52] and in the recently rediscovered basal, triple-negative breast carcinomas.[53,54] Data gathered in extensive studies involving more than 100 breast cancer cases further showed that 16q was associated with prognostically favorable features, such as a low proliferation rate in invasive and in situ breast cancer, and the expression of ER and PR. However, the explanation of 16q losses in grade 3 breast cancers allows two conclusions. On one hand, it might be that this subgroup has evolved through grades 1 and 2 ER-positive carcinomas; on the other hand, some studies can lead to the conclusion that 16q losses in these tumors are a reflection of cytogenetic instability in different subclones within a tumor.[32] More recent studies of Korsching and associates support the first hypothesis.[55]

Interestingly, the underlying mechanisms of 16q losses in grades 1 and 3 ductal invasive breast cancer cases seem to differ significantly. Several studies with polymorphic markers could detect no difference in frequency of 16q LOH between invasive tumors of different histologic grades. However, by combining 16q LOH fluorescence in situ hybridization with chromosome 16–specific probes and CGH, it could be demonstrated that losses of chromosome 16q occur preferentially in well-differentiated (grade I) carcinomas, whereas in poorly differentiated grade III tumors, LOH was accompanied by mitotic recombination. These results clarified the discrepancies between CGH and LOH for 16q in breast cancer.[56]

The exceptional role of 16q in lobular differentiated breast cancer and its ultimate precursor, LCIS, was well known for years. With the routine use of global screening techniques such as different CGH methods, the genetic homology between LCIS and invasive breast cancer became even more prominent. About 60% to 70% of LCIS and lobular invasive breast cancer is characterized by a loss of 16q. Interestingly, as described also for early intraductal breast lesions such as well-differentiated DCIS and ADH, the loss of 16q has been described as the sole abnormality in synchronous, bilateral LCIS without associated invasive breast cancer.[57]

Integrating all these data into a unifying model of breast carcinogenesis, it becomes evident that the very simplified model derived from the understanding of colorectal carcinogenesis is of little help for breast cancer. Rather, the distribution of 16q loss in preinvasive or invasive breast lesions clearly points towards the existence of different pathways, associated with different malignancy grades. One could therefore propose low-grade and high-grade pathways in ductal breast carcinogenesis. The latter is characterized by a multitude of different genetic alterations and protein expression patterns (p53, HER2, CK5) in invasive breast cancer and its associated DCIS. In contrast, hallmarks of the low-grade pathway are the loss of 16q, the expression of ER, and a likewise lower degree of genetic instability.

These observations are therefore not only of tumor biological interest but also significantly influence our understanding of the classification of early breast lesions and invasive breast cancer. The most recent classification of breast cancer precursor lesions was proposed by the WHO in 2003. In analogy to a multitude of other "intraepithelial neoplasia" classification systems, such as in the cervix or squamous epithelium, these systems suggest a linear progression of grade 1 to grade 3 and finally to invasive carcinoma. However, as discussed above, this simple concept, transferred from other tumor entities, does not seem to hold true for breast cancer. Since the distribution of 16q losses changes significantly throughout grade, it is unlike that well-differentiated DCIS progresses towards poorly differentiated DCIS in a high frequency. The morphologic association of well-differentiated DCIS with tubular, tubulo-lobular, and ductal invasive grade 1 carcinomas, in contrast to the poorly differentiated DCIS/ductal invasive grade 3 carcinoma pathway, also points against this hypothesis. In consequence, our current understanding of breast cancer has to incorporate the presence of multiple genetic pathways in the progression of in situ and invasive breast cancer, as reviewed by reference.[58]

The Role of Stem Cells

The role of stem cells in the breast carcinogenetic process is not entirely clear. Breast stem cells are pluripotent, and are characterized by expression of basal cytokeratins 5, 14, and 17, EGFR, and P-cadherin, while lacking expression of HER2, ER, and CK18. They have a variable location within ducts and acini. They may differentiate into luminal cells (expressing cytokeratin 8/18) or into myoepithelial cells (retaining CK5 and CK14 expression, and acquiring expression of contractile proteins such as smooth-muscle actin and calponin). These expression patterns of stem cells and glandular cells parallel those of different types of invasive breast cancers (Fig. 1-2). In this sense, (adeno)myoepithelial carcinomas, metaplastic carcinomas, BRCA1-associated carcinomas, medullary carcinomas, and basal carcinomas have expression patterns like stem cells, being further characterized by a high frequency of EGFR amplifications, p53 mutations, and BRCA1 dysfunction (by mutation or promoter methylation) and a low frequency of 16q loss. Tubular, lobular, and non–high-grade invasive ductal carcinomas share their immunophenotype with glandular cells, usually further showing 16q loss while lacking p53 mutations, EGFR amplifications, and BRCA1 dysfunction. Basoluminal and ductal invasive grade 3 cancers fall in between, typically with HER2 amplification.

This gives rise to proposing carcinogenetic relationships between these normal breast cells and different histologic subgroups of invasive breast cancer. Two theories are possible (Fig. 1-3). In the "Linear cell of origin theory", vastly overlapping

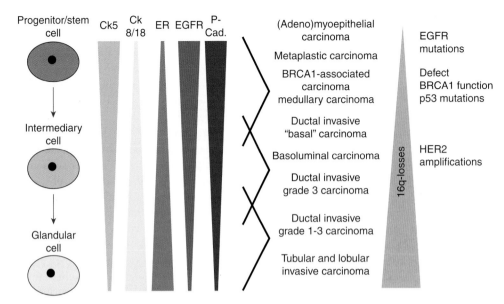

FIGURE 1-2 Associations of immunohistochemical expression patterns in physiological cellular subgroups within the normal breast and distinct subgroups of invasive breast cancer. *(Reprinted with permission from Korsching E, Jeffrey SS, Meinerz W, et al. Basal carcinoma of the breast revisited: an old entity with new interpretations.* J Clin Pathol. *2008;61:553-560.)*

expression profiles between physiological progenitor cells and invasive breast cancer supports the conclusion that the respective carcinoma subgroups originate in their respective physiological counterparts: stem cells, intermediate cells, or luminal cells. Whereas 16q-losses are rare events in breast cancer types with expression of CK5/14, the incidence increases with lower tumor grade. In contrast, EGFR amplifications, p53-mutations and defects/losses of BRCA1 are almost exclusively seen in high grade carcinomas that show CK5/14 expression. HER2-amplifications are rare in CK5/14 positive carcinomas. The "stem cell hypothesis" proposes that stem cells are the major target in the pathogenesis of different breast cancer subtypes. A multitude of genetic alterations can take place in these cells, starting distinct cellular expression programs, including the change of cytokeratin expression pattern characterizing distinct subgroups of invasive breast cancer. As often with different hypotheses, there may be truth in both of them.

CARCINOGENESIS IN GERM-LINE MUTATION CARRIERS

Not much is known about genotype and phenotype, carcinogenetic events, and precursor lesions in rare hereditary cancer syndromes such as Li-Fraumeni and Cowden syndromes. The main driving events in these syndromes are obviously the germline mutations in p53 and PTEN, respectively.

Although results between studies are not consistent, CHEK2 germ-line–associated cancers do not seem to show a clearly distinct genotype or phenotype.[59-62] Most data have been obtained for BRCA1 germ-line mutation carriers. As already partly discussed earlier, breast cancers in BRCA1 germ-line

mutated patients are often of ductal high-grade, medullary, and metaplastic types; are rather well demarcated; show solid growth, high proliferation, and apoptosis; and have prominent lymphoplasmic infiltrate in and around the tumor.[63-71] Tubular, mucinous, and lobular cancers are rare, and when they occur it is not infrequently at a higher age, which may in fact point to a sporadic carcinogenetic route in these patients. High-grade morphology and heavy inflammation are also found in DCIS lesions of these patients,[63] although DCIS itself is fairly rare. Inflammation in the form of T-cell lobulitis has even been found in the morphologically normal breast in BRCA1/2 mutation carriers.[72] The immunophenotype of BRCA1-related cancers is typically ER/PR/HER2 negative, CK5 and/or CK14 positive, and p63, EGFR, HIF-1α, P-cadherin, and p63 positive.[54-67,73] The immunophenotype of DCIS lesions in BRCA1 carriers has not been studied. Prophylactic mastectomies in BRCA1/2 germ-line mutation carriers show a higher incidence of columnar cell change, usual ductal hyperplasia, ALH, ADH, LCIS, and DCIS compared to sporadic controls.[74-76] Whether these premalignant lesions are truly part of a progression route to invasive cancer remains unclear, but for many this may be unlikely and they may rather be the result of a "sporadic" carcinogenetic process. Genetically, gene expression by microarray revealed MSH2, PDCD5, annexin 8, CX3CL1, and TRIM29 to be overexpressed in BRCA1-related cancers.[77,78] On the chromosomal level, copy number changes occurring more frequently in BRCA1-related breast cancers are gains of 8q and 3q and loss of 4p, 4q, and 5q.[79]

Altogether, this indicates that carcinogenesis in BRCA1 germ-line mutation carriers very often occurs within the "basal" progression route. Although a subclass of "basal" DCIS is a likely precursor, the earliest precursors remain to be identified.

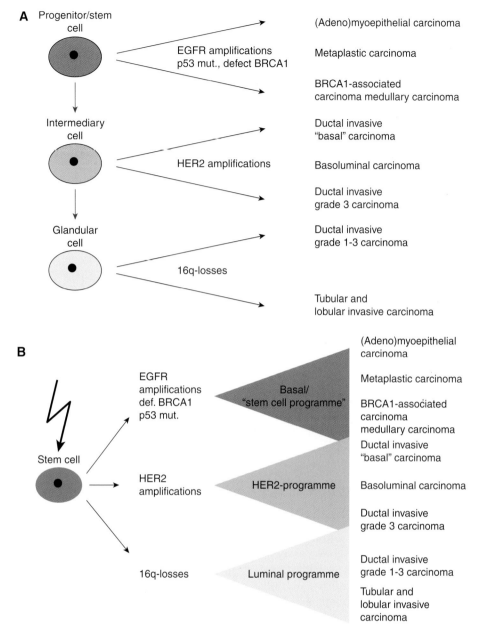

FIGURE 1-3 Different putative histogenetic models of the relationship between different subgroups of invasive breast cancer and breast stem cells. **A.** The "linear cell of origin theory" proposes that the respective carcinoma subgroups originate in their respective physiologic counterparts of the normal breast: stem cells, intermediate cells, or luminal cells. **B.** The "stem cell hypothesis" proposes that stem cells are the major target in carcinogenesis and progress after a multitude of genetic alterations that start distinct cellular expression programs to distinct subgroups of invasive breast cancer. *(Reprinted with permission from Korsching E, Jeffrey SS, Meinerz W, et al. Basal carcinoma of the breast revisited: an old entity with new interpretations. J Clin Pathol. 2008;61:553-560.)*

Whether a "basal" subclass of ductal hyperplasias exists (Fig. 1-4) is yet unclear.

The morphology and immunophenotype of BRCA2 germ-line mutation–related breast cancers is somewhat in between BRCA1-related and sporadic cancers, and is essentially unspecific.[64-66,68-70,80-82] Nevertheless, by microarray 176 genes significantly differed in their expression levels between BRCA1- and BRCA2-associated cancers.[77] Among the most interesting ones may be cyclin D1, which is expressed in BRCA2-related cancers but not in BRCA1-associated cancers. Compared to sporadic cancers, cytoplasmic RAD51 and CHEK2 expression seem to be higher in BRCA2-related cancers.[83] On the chromosomal level, gains of 8q, 17q, and 20q, and loss of 8p, 13q, and 11q, are specific for BRCA2-related breast cancer.[79]

Altogether, this indicates that in contrast to progression in BRCA1 germ-line mutation carriers, carcinogenesis and precursor lesions in BRCA2 carriers remain to a large extent to be elucidated.

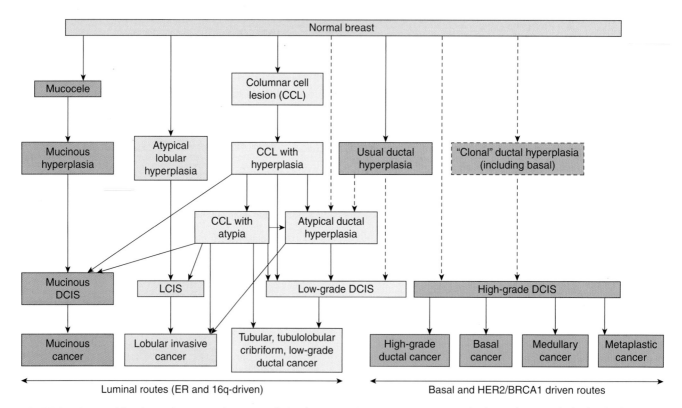

FIGURE 1-4 Proposal for the main progression routes during breast carcinogenesis. Controversial relationships are dashed. Whether a basal subclass of usual ductal hyperplasia exists is yet unknown but this would fit quite nicely. Intermediate-grade lesions are omitted for sake of clarify but naturally do occur within the gray zone of low-grade and high-grade lesions.

PRECURSOR LESIONS AND PROGRESSION ROUTES

As will be clear from earlier discussion, breast carcinogenesis is a complex molecular process, and it is not at all easy to try to depict plausible progression routes and to give established precursor lesions a proper place in these. Nevertheless, we will make an attempt (Fig. 1-4). The proposed relationships here are partially based on molecular similarities, partly on morphologic similarities, and partly on observations of close topographical associations, not further discussed here in detail. The main separation here is in the luminal and nonluminal progression routes.

The mucinous progression (luminal) route seems to occur largely from mucocele-like lesions, through stages of mucinous hyperplasia and mucinous DCIS to mucinous invasive cancer, but more advanced lesions may also derive from a subclass of mucinous columnar cell lesions that certainly exists.

One fairly clear route is from normal breast to atypical lobular hyperplasia, through LCIS to invasive lobular cancer. In this "luminal" route, early loss of 16q and loss of E-cadherin expression are key events. ER/PR expression is usually high, while HER2/EGFR amplifications are very rare. Columnar cell lesions (CCLs) may likely also progress to lobular invasive cancers through stages of hyperplasia and atypia, as may some forms of low-grade DCIS.

For the group of low-grade ductal-type cancers (tubular, tubulobular, cribriform, and low-grade ductal carcinomas),

progression from precursor lesions is far more complicated, but also in this luminal route, loss of 16q is a key event while ER/PR expression is usually high and HER2/EGFR amplifications and p53 mutations are rare. Some of these cancers may derive from LCIS, but more often columnar cell lesions (CCL) will be precursor lesions, progressing through stages of hyperplasia and perhaps atypia; while atypical ductal hyperplasia (ADH) deriving in a background of a CCL may also be an intermediate step to invasiveness, likely often thorough a stage of low-grade DCIS. The role of usual ductal hyperplasia (UDH) here is more controversial.[84] Many of these lesions are probably polyclonal dead ends, but some may turn clonal and progress to low-grade DCIS (perhaps occasionally through ADH).

Within the nonluminal routes, ER is usually low and 16q loss is rare, while expression of basal cytokeratins is frequent and HER2/EGFR amplifications, BRCA1 loss (through germline mutations and/or promoter methylation), and p53 mutations are driving forces. The earliest lesions within the nonluminal routes are controversial. A subgroup of clonal and/or basal ductal hyperplasias may exist and progress to more advanced lesions. High-grade DCIS, including a subclass with expression of basal keratins, is the most advanced pre-invasive lesion here that may progress to infiltrative basal carcinoma, medullary cancer, or metaplastic cancer.

There may be some crossover from the luminal to the nonluminal routes—for example, through intermediately differentiated lesions that certainly exist. For instance, HER2 amplification arising in a luminal precursor lesion may lead to a more basal phenotype (by some called "basoluminal"). Also, some expression of basal keratins may occasionally be found in ER-expressing cancers.

Routes not depicted and discussed here are those for papillary lesions, apocrine lesions, and secretory lesions. For papillary cancers, intracystic papillary is a precursor, and the role of papillomas as earliest precursor remains to be elucidated. Apocrine cancers will likely arise from apocrine metaplastic lesions that progress through apocrine DCIS. For secretory cancer, the precursor is yet unknown. Altogether, few data are available on events within these routes.

PROGRESSION OF FIBROEPITHELIAL LESIONS

Fibroepithelial breast lesions are composed of both a stromal and an epithelial proliferative component, arising from the epithelium and stroma of the terminal duct lobular unit. The benign end of the spectrum of fibroepithelial breast lesions comprises fibroadenoma, sclerosing lobular hyperplasia, fibroadenomatoid hyperplasia, and hamartoma; while the malignant end holds the malignant form of phyllodes tumors. The most frequent and well-known benign fibroepithelial breast lesion is fibroadenoma, so we will focus on this type of lesion.

Fibroadenoma is a well-demarcated benign fibroepithelial tumor with a relative balance between stromal and epithelial components. It contains elongated ducts surrounded by proliferative stroma that is more cellular and often myxoid than the normal breast stroma. Fibroadenomas arise within sclerosing lobular hyperplasia, which is present in the surrounding breast tissue of about 50% of fibroadenomas.[85] Fibroadenoma may also arise from the continuous expansion of only one lobule.[86] Both epithelium and stroma of fibroadenomas are polyclonal.[87] However, both the stromal and epithelial components of fibroadenoma may show progression. Fibroadenomas may develop the usual ductal hyperplasia (which is usually polyclonal)[88,89]; CIS (either ductal [DCIS] or lobular [LCIS]), which is monoclonal[87,90]; and even invasive carcinoma.[91-93] Likewise, the stromal component may expand to form benign phyllodes tumor,[87] a fibroepithelial breast lesion characterized by conspicuous stromal overgrowth. This stromal expansion may be polyclonal, but is usually clonal, underlining the potential of such lesions to recur and progress. Indeed, clonal phylloid areas within fibroadenomas have been found, and we have described a composite fibroadenoma/phyllodes tumor within the same capsule,[94] illustrating the close relationship between fibroadenoma and phyllodes tumors.[86,87,95] Lastly, there may also be expansion of both epithelial and stromal compartments of fibroadenomas to form phyllodes tumors with clonal epithelial and stromal compartments.[87] The malignant form of phyllodes tumor has a clonal stroma compartment with the morphologic features of (high-grade) sarcoma.

A graphical representation of the conceptual relations between fibroadenomas and phyllodes tumors is given in Figure 1-5.

Clinical Relevance

Several epidemiologic studies have shown that the relative risk of developing invasive breast cancer is increased in women with a history of fibroadenoma, varying from 1.6 to 2.6.[96-100] Features that further increase this risk to 3 are presence of cysts, sclerosing adenosis, calcifications, or apocrine metaplasia within the fibroadenoma, proliferative changes in the surrounding breast tissue, and a family history of breast carcinoma (relative risk of 3.7).[98,99,101] Interestingly, atypical (ductal or lobular) hyperplasia within fibroadenomas does not seem to indicate a further increased relative risk.[102] Phyllodes tumors often recur when not excised with a margin, and malignant phyllodes tumors may metastasize.

Cell Biology

The most remarkable cell biological phenomena in the progression from fibroadenoma to phyllodes tumor are increase in hypoxia, angiogenesis, proliferation, and apoptosis.[94,103,104] On the protein level, especially increased expression of collagen IV,[105] tenascin,[106] CD117,[107,108] smooth-muscle actin,[107] c-myc expression,[108] nuclear beta-catenin,[109,110] growth factors like PDGF,[111] FGF, and VEGF,[112] EGFR expression,[113,114] and stromal HIF-1alpha expression[104] seem to parallel progression to malignant phyllodes tumor.

Genetic Changes

Conventional cytogenetic studies using short-term culture and G-banding have uncovered complex and varying karyotypic changes in benign and malignant phyllodes tumors.[115-119]

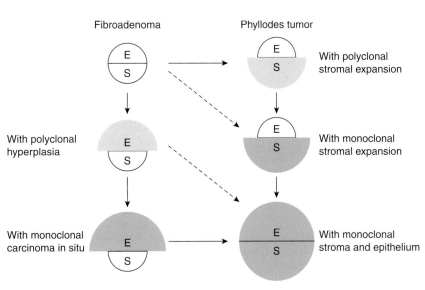

FIGURE 1-5 Concept for the progression of fibroadenoma to phyllodes tumor by (selective) progression of epithelial and stromal components of these biphasic tumors.

Karyotyping of phyllodes tumors did not result in the identification of tumor-specific alterations, however.

Copy number gains and losses as detected by comparative genomic hybridization are rare in fibroadenomas, while these changes are common in phyllodes tumors.[120-125] Several recurrent copy number changes have emerged when studying phyllodes tumors by CGH. Gain at 1q is the most prominent alteration, found in approximately 35% of tumors. In most studies, gain at 1q is not related to tumor grade, although Lu and colleagues found 1q gain to be predictive of clinical behavior,[122] but others could not confirm this.[124] Other recurrent abberations reported by most authors include losses at 10p, 13q, and 16q. However, considerable differences exist between the studies, and no specific chromosomal aberrations accompanying the progression steps of phyllodes tumors have been identified. These differences most likely reflect selection bias due to the low incidence of phyllodes tumors and intratumoral heterogeneity. Genetic instability in general, however, seems to be a characteristic of phyllodes tumors. Fibroadenomas lack genomic instability, demonstrating that this is not a general feature of fibroepithelial tumors. The amount of genomic instability—that is, the number of chromosomal alterations per case—seems to be related to tumor grade. The largest study demonstrated a significant difference in the number of genetic alterations in benign tumors on the one hand and in borderline and malignant tumors on the other hand.[121] Lae and associates also observed the segregation of benign and borderline/malignant tumors when regarding total copy number change.[123] The accumulation of copy number alterations with higher grade may suggest that genomic instability drives progression of phyllodes tumors. Indeed, when analyzing primary and corresponding recurrences, the recurrent tumors had acquired new chromosomal alterations in approximately 70% of cases.[121] Moreover, since benign phyllodes tumors are not devoid of chromosomal aberrations, genetic instability may be an early event in phyllodes tumor genesis.

Mutations of p53 are only found in phyllodes tumors and not in fibroadenomas,[126,127] usually accompanied by accumulation of nuclear p53 protein.[103] Accumulation of p53 is found more frequently at higher tumor grade and is predictive of recurrence. Also mutations in CD117 have been found in malignant phyllodes tumors.[107]

In a preliminary work we compared transcriptome-wide gene expression patterns of phyllodes tumors and fibroadenomas, resulting in further insight in the molecular mechanisms underlying development and progression of fibroepithelial tumors.[128] In phyllodes tumors, down-regulation was found of genes involved in transcription (EGR1, ELF5, LZTS1), cell adhesion (JAM2, PCDH11X, CX3CL1), apoptosis (TNFSF8, PHLDA1), and Wnt signalling (FRZB, SFRP1). Overexpression was found of factors involved in transcription (RUNX1, PTN, LHX2, PKNOX2, HOXC13), cellular integrity (SGCD, palladin), and extracellular matrix degradation (MMP11). The gene with the strongest upregulation in PT was CTAG1. CTAG1 is normally expressed only in testis but is overexpressed in a wide variety of malignancies. Although the function of this gene is currently unknown, it may aid the differentiation between fibroadenoma and benign phyllodes tumor.

FUTURE DIRECTIONS

Although progress has been made in unraveling breast carcinogenesis, many questions remain. First, few data are yet available on rare progression routes like those for papillary lesions, apocrine lesions, and secretory lesions. Second, more information is still needed on events in the luminal, basal, and HER2-driven progression routes and clinical behavior of precursor lesions, allowing a more refined classification of intermediately differentiated lesions and lesions with a mixed genotype and phenotype. Fourth, the earliest precursors within the nonluminal progression routes remain to be elucidated. Lastly, the role of usual ductal hyperplasia needs to be further explored, in search of clonal or perhaps basal subclasses that may be true precursors instead of polyclonal dead ends. All of this requires many more studies.

SUMMARY

Despite many molecular studies, breast carcinogenesis is still not well understood. Nevertheless, progress has been made in development of plausible concepts for progression of precursor lesions and the genetic events driving progression. Further, more and more data are available on morphology and immunophenotype of the different precursor lesions, allowing the pathologist to recognize them. Epidemiologic studies have yielded information on progression risk of several lesions, so that a treatment plan can be designed when precursor lesions are found in a breast biopsy.

REFERENCES

1. Evron E, Dooley WC, Umbricht CB, Rosenthal D, et al. Detection of breast cancer cells in ductal lavage fluid by methylation-specific PCR. *Lancet.* 2001;28:1335-1336.
2. Suijkerbuijk KP, van der Wall E, Vooijs M, van Diest PJ. Molecular analysis of nipple fluid for breast cancer screening. *Pathobiology.* 2008;75:149-152.
3. Visscher DW, Wallis TL, Crissman JD. Evaluation of chromosome aneuploidy in tissue sections of preinvasive breast carcinomas using interphase cytogenetics. *Cancer* 1996;77:315-320.
4. Lakhani SR, Collins N, Stratton MR, Sloane JP. Atypical ductal hyperplasia of the breast: clonal proliferation with loss of heterozygosity on chromosomes 16q and 17p. *J Clin Pathol.* 1995;48:611-615.
5. Mommers EC, van Diest PJ, Leonhart AM, Meijer CJ, Baak JP. Balance of cell proliferation and apoptosis in breast carcinogenesis. *Breast Cancer Res Treat.* 1999;58:163-169.
6. Vleugel MM, Bos R, Van der Groep P, et al. Lack of lymphangiogenesis during breast carcinogenesis. *J Clin Pathol.* 2004;57:746-751.
7. Podsypanina P, Du Y-CN, Jechlinger M, et al. Seeding and propagation of untransformed mouse mammary cells in the lung. *Science.* 2008;321:1841-1844.
8. van Diest PJ, Michalides RJ, Jannink L, et al. Cyclin D1 expression in invasive breast cancer. Correlations and prognostic value. *Am J Pathol.* 1997;150:705-711.
9. Voduc D, Nielsen TO, Cheang MC, Foulkes WD. The combination of high cyclin E and Skp2 expression in breast cancer is associated with a poor prognosis and the basal phenotype. *Hum Pathol.* 2008;39:1431-1437.
10. An HX, Beckmann MW, Reifenberger G, Bender HG, Niederacher D. Gene amplification and overexpression of CDK4 in sporadic breast carcinomas is associated with high tumor cell proliferation. *Am J Pathol.* 1999;154:113-118.
11. Mommers EC, Leonhart AM, Falix F, et al. Similarity in expression of cell cycle proteins between in situ and invasive ductal breast lesions of same differentiation grade. *J Pathol.* 2001;194:327-333.

12. O'Malley FP, Vnencak-Jones CL, Dupont WD, et al. p53 mutations are confined to the comedo type ductal carcinoma in situ of the breast. Immunohistochemical and sequencing data. *Lab Invest.* 1994;71:67-72.

13. Aulmann S, Bentz M, Sinn HP. C-myc oncogene amplification in ductal carcinoma in situ of the breast. *Breast Cancer Res Treat.* 2002;74:25-31.

14. Meijnen P, Peterse JL, Antonini N, Rutgers EJ, van de Vijver MJ. Immunohistochemical categorisation of ductal carcinoma in situ of the breast. *Br J Cancer.* 2008;98:137-142.

15. De Jong JS, Van Diest PJ, van der Valk P, Baak JPA. Expression of growth factors, their receptors and growth inhibiting factors in invasive breast cancer. I. An inventory in search of autocrine and paracrine loops. *J Pathol.* 1998;184:44-52.

16. De Jong JS, Van Diest PJ, van der Valk P, Baak JPA. Expression of growth factors, their receptors and growth inhibiting factors in invasive breast cancer II. Correlations with proliferation and angiogenesis. *J Pathol.* 1998;184:53-57.

17. Bos R, Zhong H, Hanrahan CF, et al. Levels of hypoxia-inducible factor-1 during breast carcinogenesis. *J Natl Cancer Inst.* 2001;93:309-314.

18. Koshiji M, To KK, Hammer S, et al. HIF-1alpha induces genetic instability by transcriptionally downregulating MutSalpha expression. *Mol Cell.* 2005;17:793-803.

19. Baykal A, Rosen D, Zhou C, Liu J, Sahin AA. Telomerase in breast cancer: a critical evaluation. *Adv Anat Pathol.* 2004;11:262-268.

20. Mironchik Y, Winnard PT Jr, Vesuna F, et al. Twist overexpression induces in vivo angiogenesis and correlates with chromosomal instability in breast cancer. *Cancer Res.* 2005;65:10801-10809.

21. Reedijk M, Pinnaduwage D, Dickson BC, et al. JAG1 expression is associated with a basal phenotype and recurrence in lymph node-negative breast cancer. *Breast Cancer Res Treat.* 2008;111:439-448.

22. Klarmann GJ, Decker A, Farrar WL. Epigenetic gene silencing in the Wnt pathway in breast cancer. *Epigenetics.* 2008;3:59-63.

23. Iorio MV, Ferracin M, Liu CG, et al. MicroRNA gene expression deregulation in human breast cancer. *Cancer Res.* 2005;65:7065-7070.

24. Mattie MD, Benz CC, Bowers J, et al. Optimized high-throughput microRNA expression profiling provides novel biomarker assessment of clinical prostate and breast cancer biopsies. *Mol Cancer.* 2006;5:24.

25. Diallo R, Tognon C, Knezevich SR, Sorensen P, Poremba C. Secretory carcinoma of the breast: a genetically defined carcinoma entity. *Verh Dtsch Ges Pathol.* 2003;87:193-203.

26. Tognon C, Knezevich SR, Huntsman D, et al. Expression of the ETV6-NTRK3 gene fusion as a primary event in human secretory breast carcinoma. *Cancer Cell.* 2002;2:367-376.

27. Sørlie T, Perou CM, Tibshirani R, et al. Gene expression patterns of breast carcinomas distinguish tumor subclasses with clinical implications. *Proc Natl Acad Sci USA.* 2001;98:10869-10874.

28. Hennard C, Pfuhl T, Buettner M, et al. The antibody 2B4 directed against the Epstein-Barr virus (EBV)-encoded nuclear antigen 1 (EBNA1) detects MAGE-4: implications for studies on the EBV association of human cancers. *J Pathol.* 2006;209:430-435.

29. Kulka J, Kovalszky I, Svastics E, Berta M, Füle T. Lymphoepithelioma-like carcinoma of the breast: not Epstein-Barr virus-, but human papilloma virus-positive. *Hum Pathol.* 2008;39:298-301.

30. Liang W, Tian H. Hypothetic association between human papillomavirus infection and breast carcinoma. *Med Hypotheses.* 2008;70:305-307.

31. Akil N, Yasmeen A, Kassab A, et al. High-risk human papillomavirus infections in breast cancer in Syrian women and their association with Id-1 expression: a tissue microarray study. *Br J Cancer.* 2008;99:404-407.

32. Buerger H, Simon R, Schäfer KL, et al. Genetic relation of lobular carcinoma in situ, ductal carcinoma in situ, and associated invasive carcinoma of the breast. *Mol Pathol.* 2000;53:118-121.

33. Pandis N, Jin Y, Gorunova L, et al. Chromosome analysis of 97 primary breast carcinomas: dentification of eight karyotypic subgroups. *Genes Chromosomes Cancer.* 1995;12:173-185.

34. Buerger H, Mommers EC, Littmann R, et al. Ductal invasive G2 and G3 carcinomas of the breast are the end stages of at least two different lines of genetic evolution. *J Pathol.* 2001;194:165-170.

35. Adeyinka A, Baldetorp B, Mertens F, et al. Comparative cytogenetic and DNA flow cytometric analysis of 242 primary breast carcinomas. *Cancer Genet Cytogenet.* 2003;147:62-67.

36. Tsuda H, Takarabe T, Susumu N, et al. Detection of numerical and structural alterations and fusion of chromosomes 16 and 1 in low-grade papillary breast carcinoma by fluorescence in situ hybridization. *Am J Pathol.* 1997;151:1027-1034.

37. Pandis N, Bardi G, Jin Y, et al. Unbalanced t(1;16) as the sole karyotypic abnormality in a breast carcinoma and its lymph node metastasis letter. *Cancer Genet Cytogenet.* 1994;75:158-159.

38. Tsuda H, Takarabe T, Fukutomi T, Hirohashi S. der(16)t(1;16)/der(1;16) in breast cancer detected by fluorescence in situ hybridizytion is an indicator of better patient prognosis. *Genes Chromosomes Cancer.* 1999;24:72-77.

39. Hislop RG, Pratt N, Stocks SC, et al. Karyotypic aberrations of chromosomes 16 and 17 are related to survival in patients with breast cancer. *Br J Surg.* 2002;89:1581-1586.

40. Adeyinka A, Mertens F, Idvall I, et al. Different patterns of chromosomal imbalances in metastasising and non-metastasising primary breast carcinomas. *Int J Cancer.* 1999;84:370-375.

41. Pandis N, Heim S, Bardi G, et al. Whole-arm t(1;16) and i(1q) as sole anomalies identify gain of 1q as a primary chromosomal abnormality in breast cancer see comments. *Genes Chromosomes Cancer.* 1992;5:235-238.

42. Cleton-Jansen AM, Callen DF, Seshadri R, et al. Loss of heterozygosity mapping at chromosome arm 16q in 712 breast tumors reveals factors that influence delineation of candidate regions. *Cancer Res.* 2001;61:1171-1177.

43. Lakhani SR, Collins N, Sloane J, Stratton MR. Loss of heterozygosity in lobular carcinoma in situ of the breast. *J Clin Pathol: Mol Pathol.* 1995;48:74-78.

44. Stratton MR, Collins N, Lakhani SR, Sloane JP. Loss of heterozygosity in ductal carcinoma in situ of the breast. *J Pathol.* 1995;175:195-201.

45. Gong G, DeVries S, Chew KL, et al. Genetic changes in paired atypical and usual ductal hyperplasia of the breast by comparative genomic hybridization. *Clin Cancer Res.* 2001;7:2410-2414.

46. Buerger H, Otterbach F, Simon R, et al. Comparative genomic hybridization of ductal carcinoma in situ of the breast- evidence of multiple genetic pathways. *J Pathol.* 1999;187:396-402.

47. Vos CB, ter HN, Rosenberg C, Peterse JL, et al. Genetic alterations on chromosome 16 and 17 are important features of ductal carcinoma in situ of the breast and are associated with histologic type. *Br J Cancer.* 2000;81:1410-1418.

48. Waldman F, DeVries S, Chew K, et al. Chromosomal alterations in ductal carcinomas in situ and their in situ recurrences. *J Natl Cancer Inst.* 2000;92:323-330.

49. Buerger H, Otterbach F, Simon R, et al. Different genetic pathways in the evolution of invasive breast cancer are associated with distinct morphological subtypes. *J Pathol.* 1999;189:521-526.

50. Waldman FM, Hwang ES, Etzell J, et al. Genomic alterations in tubular breast carcinomas. *Hum Pathol.* 2001;32:222-226.

51. Roylance R, Gorman P, Harris W, et al. Comparative genomic hybridization of breast tumours stratified by histological grade reveals new insights into the biological progression of breast cancer. *Cancer Res.* 1999;59:1433-1436.

52. Isola J, Chu L, DeVries S, et al. Genetic alterations in ERBB2-amplified breast carcinomas. *Clin Cancer Res.* 1999;5:4140-4145.

53. Korsching E, Packeisen J, Agelopoulos K, et al. Cytogenetic alterations and cytokeratin expression patterns in breast cancer: integrating a new model of breast differentiation into cytogenetic pathways of breast carcinogenesis. *Lab Invest.* 2002;82:1525-1533.

54. Korsching E, Packeisen J, Liedtke C, et al. The origin of vimentin expression in invasive breast cancer: epithelial-mesenchymal transition, myoepithelial histogenesis or histogenesis from progenitor cells with bilinear differentiation potential? *J Pathol.* 2005;206:451-457.

55. Korsching E, Packeisen J, Helms MW, et al. Deciphering a subgroup of breast carcinomas with putative progression of grade during carcinogenesis revealed by comparative genomic hybridisation (CGH) and immunohistochemistry. *Br J Cancer.* 2004;90:1422-1428.

56. Cleton-Jansen AM, Buerger H, Haar NN, et al. Different mechanisms of chromosome 16 loss of heterozygosity in well- versus poorly differentiated ductal breast cancer. *Genes Chromosomes Cancer.* 2004;41:109-116.

57. Lu YJ, Osin P, Lakhani SR, et al. Comparative genomic hybridization analysis of lobular carcinoma in situ and atypical lobular hyperplasia and potential roles for gains and losses of genetic material in breast neoplasia. *Cancer Res.* 1998;58:4721-4727.

58. Simpson PT, Reis-Filho JS, Gale T, Lakhani SR. Molecular evolution of breast cancer. *J Pathol.* 2005;205:248-254.

59. Kilpivaara O, Bartkova J, Eerola H, et al. Correlation of CHEK2 protein expression and c.1100delC mutation status with tumor characteristics among unselected breast cancer patients. *Int J Cancer.* 2005;113:575-580.

60. De Bock GH, Schutte M, Krol-Warmerdam EM, et al. Tumour characteristics and prognosis of breast cancer patients carrying the germline CHEK2*1100delC variant. *J Med Genet.* 2004;41:731-735.

61. Huzarski T, Cybulski C, Domagala W, et al. Pathology of breast cancer in women with constitutional CHEK2 mutations. *Breast Cancer Res Treat.* 2005;90:187-189.

62. Oldenburg RA, Kroeze-Jansema K, Meijers-Heijboer H, et al. Characterization of familial non-BRCA1/2 breast tumors by loss of heterozygosity and immunophenotyping. *Clin Cancer Res.* 2006;12:1693-1700.

63. Lakhani SR, Easton DF, Stratton MR, Consortium tBCL. Pathology of familial breast cancer: differences between breast cancers in carriers of BRCA1 or BRCA *Lancet.* 1997;349:1505-1510.

64. Quenneville LA, Phillips KA, Ozcelik H, et al. HER-2/neu status and tumor morphology of invasive breast carcinomas in Ashkenazi women with known BRCA1 mutation status in the Ontario Familial Breast Cancer Registry. *Cancer.* 2002;95:2068-2075.

65. Lakhani SR, Gusterson BA, Jacquemier J, et al. The pathology of familial breast cancer: histological features of cancers in families not attributable to mutations in BRCA1 or BRCA2. *Clin Cancer Res.* 2000;6:782-789.

66. Lakhani SR, Jacquemier J, Sloane JP, et al. Multifactorial analysis of differences between sporadic breast cancers and cancers involving BRCA1 and BRCA2 mutations. *J Natl Cancer Inst.* 1998;90:1138-1145.

67. Lakhani SR, Van De Vijver MJ, Jacquemier J, et al. The pathology of familial breast cancer: predictive value of immunohistochemical markers estrogen receptor, progesterone receptor, HER-2, and p53 in patients with mutations in BRCA1 and BRCA2. *J Clin Oncol.* 2002;20:2310-2318.

68. Armes JE, Egan AJ, Southey MC, et al. The histologic phenotypes of breast carcinoma occurring before age 40 years in women with and without BRCA1 or BRCA2 germline mutations: a population-based study. *Cancer.* 1998;83:2335-2345.

69. Palacios J, Honrado E, Osorio A, et al. Immunohistochemical characteristics de?ned by tissue microarray of hereditary breast cancer not attributable to BRCA1 or BRCA2 mutations: differences from breast carcinomas arising in BRCA1 and BRCA2 mutation carriers. *Clin Cancer Res.* 2003;9:3606-3614.

70. Eerola H, Heikkila P, Tamminen A, et al. Histopathological features of breast tumours in BRCA1, BRCA2 and mutation-negative breast cancer families. *Breast Cancer Res.* 2005;7:R93-R100.

71. Foulkes WD, Stefansson IM, Chappuis PO, et al. Germline BRCA1 mutations and a basal epithelial phenotype in breast cancer. *J Natl Cancer Inst.* 2003;95:1482-1485.

72. Hermsen BBJ, Von Mensdorff-Pouilly S, Fabry HFJ, et al. Lobulitis is a frequent finding in prophylactically removed breast tissue from women at hereditary high risk of breast cancer. *J Pathol.* 2005;206:220-223.

73. van der Groep P, Bouter A, van der Zanden R, et al. Distinction between hereditary and sporadic breast cancer on the basis of clinicopathological data. *J Clin Pathol.* 2006;59:611-617.

74. Hoogerbrugge N, Bult P, de Widt-Levert LM, et al. High prevalence of premalignant lesions in prophylactically removed breasts from women at hereditary risk for breast cancer. *J Clin Oncol.* 2003;21:41-45.

75. Kauff ND, Brogi E, Scheuer L, et al. Epithelial lesions in prophylactic mastectomy specimens from women with BRCA mutations. *Cancer.* 2003;97:1601-1608.

76. Hermsen BB, van Diest PJ, Berkhof J, et al. Low prevalence of (pre)malignant lesions in the breast and high prevalence in the ovary and Fallopian tube in women at hereditary high risk of breast and ovarian cancer. *Int J Cancer.* 2006;119:1412-1418.

77. Hedenfalk I, Duggan D, Chen Y, et al. Gene-expression profiles in hereditary breast cancer. *N Engl J Med.* 2001;344:539-548.

78. van't Veer LJ, Dai H, van de Vijver MJ, et al. Gene expression profiling predicts clinical outcome of breast cancer. *Nature.* 2002;415:530-536.

79. van Beers EH, van Welsem T, Wessels LF, et al. Comparative genomic hybridization profiles in human BRCA1 and BRCA2 breast tumors high light differential sets of genomic aberrations. *Cancer Res.* 2005;65:822-827.

80. Marcus JN, Watson P, Page DL, et al. Hereditary breast cancer: pathobiology, prognosis, and BRCA1 and BRCA2 gene linkage. *Cancer.* 1996;77:697-709.

81. Marcus JN, Watson P, Page DL, et al. BRCA2 hereditary breast cancer pathophenotype. *Breast Cancer Res Treat.* 1997;44:275-277.

82. Agnarsson BA, Jonasson JG, Bjornsdottir IB, et al. *Breast Cancer Res Treat.* 1998;47:121-127.

83. Honrado E, Osorio A, Palacios J, Benitez J. Pathology and gene expression of hereditary breast tumors associated with BRCA1, BRCA2 and CHEK2 gene mutations. *Oncogene.* 2006;25:5837-5845.

84. Abdel-Fatah TM, Powe DG, Hodi Z, et al. Morphologic and molecular evolutionary pathways of low nuclear grade invasive breast cancers and their putative precursor lesions: further evidence to support the concept of low nuclear grade breast neoplasia family. *Am J Surg Pathol.* 2008;32:513-523.

85. Kovi J, Chu H B, Leffall Jr L. Sclerosing lobular hyperplasia manifesting as a palpable mass of the breast in young black women. *Hum Pathol.* 1984;15:336-340.

86. Kasami M, Vnencak Jones CL, Manning S, et al. Monoclonality in fibroadenomas with complex histology and phyllodal features. *Breast Cancer Res Treat.* 1998;50:185-191.

87. Kuijper A, Buerger H, Simon R, et al. Analysis of progression of fibroepithelial tumors of the breast by PCR based clonality assay. *J Pathol.* 2002;197:575-581.

88. Kuijper A, Mommers EC, van der Wall E, van Diest PJ. Histopathology of fibroadenoma of the breast. *Am J Clin Pathol.* 2001;115:736-742.

89. Magda JL, Minger BA, Rimm DL. Polymerase chain reaction based detection of clonality as a non morphologic diagnostic tool for fine needle aspiration of the breast. *Cancer (Cancer Cytopathol).* 1998;84:262-267.

90. Noguchi S, Aihara T, Koyama H, et al. Clonal analysis of benign and malignant human breast tumors by means of polymerase chain reaction. *Cancer Lett.* 1995;90:57-63.

91. Persaud V, Talerman A, Jordan R. Pure adenoma of the breast. *Arch Pathol.* 1968;86:481-483.

92. Azzopardi JG. Sarcoma of the breast. In: Bennington JL, ed. *Problems in Breast Pathology.* Philadelphia, PA: Saunders; 1979:346-355.

93. Rosen PP. *Rosen's Breast Pathology.* Philadelphia, PA: Lippincott-Raven; 1997:163-200.

94. Van Diest PJ, Kuijper A, Schulz-Wendtland R, Boecker W, Van der Wall E. Fibroepithelial tumors. In: Boecker W, ed. *Preneoplasia of the Breast. A New Conceptual Approach to Proliferative Breast Disease.* Munich: Elsevier; 2006:280-315.

95. Noguchi S, Motomura K, Inaji H, Imaoka S, Koyama H. Clonal analysis of fibroadenoma and phyllodes tumor of the breast. *Cancer Res.* 1993;53:4071-4074.

96. Levi F, Randimbison L, Te VC, LaVecchia C. Incidence of breast cancer in women with fibroadenoma. *Int J Cancer.* 1994;57:681-683.

97. Carter CL, Corle DK, Micozzi MS, Schatzkin A, Taylor PR. A prospective study of the development of breast cancer in 16,692 women with benign breast disease. *Am J Epidemiol.* 1988;128:467-477.

98. McDivitt RW, Stephens JA, Lee NC, et al. Histologic types of benign breast disease and the risk of breast cancer. *Cancer.* 1992;69:1408-1414.

99. Dupont WD, Page DL, Parl FF, et al. Long-term risk of breast cancer in women with fibroadenoma. *N Engl J Med.* 1994;331:10-15.

100. Krieger N, Hiatt RA. Risk of breast cancer after benign breast diseases, variation by histologic type, degree of atypia, age at biopsy, and length of follow up. *Am J Epidemiol.* 1992;136:619-631.

101. Hutchinson WB, Thomas DB, Hamlin WB, et al. Risk of breast cancer in women with benign breast disease. *J Natl Cancer Inst.* 1980;65:13-20.

102. Carter BA, Page DL, Schuyler P, et al. No elevation in long term breast carcinoma risk for women with fibroadenomas that contain atypical hyperplasia. *Cancer.* 2001;92:30-36.

103. Kuijper A, de Vos RAI, Lagendijk JH, van der Wall E, van Diest PJ. Progressive deregulation of the cell cycle with higher tumour grade in the stroma of breast phyllodes tumours. *Am J Clin Pathol.* 2005;123:690-698.

104. Kuijper A, van der Groep P, van der Wall E, van Diest PJ. Role and prognostic relevance of HIF-1α and its downstream targets in fibroepithelial tumours of the breast. *Breast Cancer Res.* 2005;7:R808-R818.

105. Kim WH, Kim CW, Noh DY, Kim YI. Differential pattern of perivascular type IV collagen deposits in phyllodes tumors of the breast. *J Korean Med Sci.* 1992;7:360-363.

106. McCune B, Kopp J. Tenascin distribution in phyllodes tumor is distinctly different than in fibroadenoma of the breast. *Lab Invest.* 1994;70:18A.

107. Chen CM, Chen CJ, Chang CL, Hsieh HF, Harn HJ. CD34, CD117, and actin expression in phyllodes tumor of the breast. *J Surg Res.* 2000;94:84-91.

108. Sawyer EJ, Poulsom R, Hunt FT, et al. Malignant phyllodes tumours show stromal overexpression of c-myc and c-kit. *J Pathol.* 2003;200:59-64.

109. Sawyer EJ, Hanby AM, Poulsom R, et al. β-catenin abnormalities and associated insulin-like growth factor overexpression are important in phyllodes tumours and fibroadenomas of the breast. *J Pathol.* 2003;200:627-632.

110. Sawyer EJ, Hanby AM, Rowan AJ, et al. The Wnt-pathway, epithelial-stromal interactions, and malignant progression in phyllodes tumours. *J Pathol.* 2002;196:437-444.

111. Feakins RM, Wells CA, Young KA, Sheaff MT. Platelet derived growth factor expression in phyllodes tumors and fibroadenomas of the breast. *Hum Pathol.* 2000;31:1214-1222.

112. Hasebe T, Imoto S, Sasaki S, Tsubono Y, Mukai K. Proliferative activity and tumor angiogenesis is closely correlated to stromal cellularity of fibroadenoma: proposal fibroadenoma, cellular variant. *Pathol Int.* 1999;49:435-443.

113. Kersting C, Kuijper A, Schmidt H, et al. Amplifications of the epidermal growth factor receptor gene (EGFR) are common in phyllodes tumours of the breast and are associated with tumour progression. *Lab Invest.* 2006;86:54-61.

114. Agelopoulos K, Kersting C, Korshing E, et al. *EGFR* amplification specific gene expression in phyllodes tumours of the breast. *Cell Oncol.* 2007;29:443-451.

115. Dietrich CU, Pandis N, Bardi G, et al. Karyotypic changes in phyllodes tumors of the breast. *Cancer Genet Cytogenet.* 1994;76:200-206.

116. Birdsall SH, MacLennan KA, Gusterson BA. t(6;12)(q23;q13) and t(10;16)(q22;p11) in a phyllodes tumor of breast. *Cancer Genet Cytogenet.* 1992;60:74-77.

117. Ladesich J, Damjanov I, Persons D, et al. Complex karyotype in a low grade phyllodes tumor of the breast. *Cancer Genet Cytogenet.* 2002;132: 149-151.

118. Leuschner E, Meyer Bolte K, et al. Fibroadenoma of the breast showing a translocation (6;14), a ring chromosome and two markers involving parts of chromosome 11. *Cancer Genet Cytogenet.* 1994;76:145-147.

119. Woolley PV, Gollin SM, Riskalla W, et al. Cytogenetics, immunostaining for fibroblast growth factors, p53 sequencing, and clinical features of two cases of cystosarcoma phyllodes. *Mol Diagn.* 2000;5:179-190.

120. Kuijper A, Snijders AM, Berns EM, et al. Genomic profiling by array comparative genomic hybridization reveals novel DNA copy number changes in breast phyllodes tumours. *Cell Oncol* 2009;31:31-39.

121. Jones AM, MitterR, Springall R, et al. A comprehensive gentic profile of phyllodes tumours of the breast detects important mutations, intra-tumoral genetic hetreogeneity and new genetic changes on recurrence. *J Pathol.* 2008;214:533-544.

122. Lu YJ, Birdsall S, Osin P, Gusterson B, Shipley S. Phyllodes tumours of the breast analyzed by comparative genomic hybridization and association of increased 1q copy number with stromal overgrowth and recurrence. *Genes Chromosomes Cancer.* 1995;20:275-281.

123. Lae M, Vincent-Salomon A, Zavignoni A, et al. Phyllodes tumors of the breast segregate in two groups according to genetic criteria. *Mod Pathol.* 2007;20:435-444.

124. Jee KJ, Gong G, Hyun Ahn S, Mi Park J, Knuutila S. Gain in 1q is a common abnormality in phyllodes tumours of the breast. *Anal Cell Pathol.* 2003;25:89-93.

125. Ried T, Just KE, Holtgreve-Grez H, et al. Comparative genomic hybridization of formalin-fixed, paraffin-embedded breast tumours reveals different patterns of chromosomal gains and losses in fibroadenomas and diploid and aneuploid carcinomas, *Cancer Res.* 1995;55:5415-5423.

126. Gatalica Z, Finkelstein S, Lucio E, et al. p53 protein expression and gene mutation in phyllodes tumors of the breast. *Pathol Res Pract* 2001;197:183-187.

127. Kuenen Boumeester V, Henzen Logmans SC, Timmermans MM, et al. Altered expression of p53 and its regulated proteins in phyllodes tumours of the breast. *J Pathol.* 1999;189:169-175.

128. Kuijper A, Korsching E, Kersting C, Van der Wall E, Buerger H, Van Diest PJ. Gene expression signatures of breast phyllodes tumor and fibroadenoma. Submitted for publication.

CHAPTER 2

Invasion

Christopher B. Umbricht

The anatomic structures in which breast cancer invasion occurs arise as paired mammary glands developing from epithelial thickenings on the ventral surface of the 5-week fetus. A mesenchymal condensation occurs around burgeoning epithelial stalks around the 15th week. A physiologic "invasion" of this mesenchyme by cords of epithelial cells creates columns, which later give rise to the lobular organization of the mammary gland. With the onset of cyclical hormonal secretion at puberty, the hormonally responsive periductal stroma differentiates, and the epithelial columns develop into elongated lactiferous ducts terminating into terminal ducts that give rise to lobuloalveolar structures responsible for breast milk production. The adult breast consists of about 15 to 25 lobes, each associated with a major lactiferous duct terminating in the nipple. The glandular and ductal structures are embedded in specialized, hormone-responsive stromal tissue, which consists of adipose tissue admixed with collagenous and vascular elements, the relative abundance of which is largely responsible for the physical and radiographic appearance of the breast (Fig. 2-1).

There are two distinct cell types forming the epithelium of the lactiferous ducts. The majority are columnar cells lining the surface, which are interspersed with basal cells. Basal cells are thought to give rise to both columnar cells and myoepithelial cells, which separate the epithelial layer from the basal lamina in larger ducts, becoming sparser and discontinuous in the smallest branches and the lobular glands. Throughout the duct system, including terminal ductules and acini, the epithelial and myoepithelial layers are invested by a basal lamina and surrounded by delimiting fibroblasts, separating them from stromal elements of the breast.

Invasion is the second, and arguably the most consequential, of three pivotal milestones in the evolution of breast cancer. Invasion is preceded by the molecular events initiating carcinogenesis, and it may be followed by metastasis, the seeding of cancer cells to foci with no contiguous connection to the primary tumor. Before invasion occurs, the malignant cells, which

may be morphologically and biochemically very similar to invasive and metastatic cells, represent a contained, potential threat, which may be completely averted by therapeutic intervention. Significantly, as long as the *Rubicon* of epithelial organs, the basement membrane, has not been breached, *alea non jacta est*, as Caesar may have put it, and there can be certainty of cure if the local disease can be completely dealt with. This avoids the ambiguity of probabilistic risk assessments that are the usual mainstay of surgical oncology practice.

This is reflected in the histopathologic terms describing the stages of breast cancer progression, with nonproliferative and proliferative benign breast lesions, *atypical hyperplasia*, and finally *carcinoma in situ*, all reserved for cases lacking evidence of any penetration of the basement membranes surrounding these lesions. A breach is acknowledged with the term *invasive breast cancer*. Since the latter is necessary for access to lymphatic and blood vessels, before which *metastatic breast cancer* cannot occur, invasive disease is assumed as soon as a metastasis is detected, even if the actual focus has not been identified.

Unsurprisingly, much attention has been given to improve the correct classification of lesions where the determination of invasiveness is difficult, which has given rise to the term *microinvasive carcinoma,* for cases with an invasive focus of less than 0.1 cm. This category should be distinguished from *minimally invasive carcinoma,* which refers to unambiguously invasive cancers less than 1.0 cm in diameter.

Biologically, penetrating the basement membrane puts the cancer cells into contact with an entirely new microenvironment. Carcinoma in situ is devoid of vasculature, and cell interactions are limited to cells of epithelial origin. Burgeoning cells in the center of a duct or lobule may die off when distance to the basement membrane exceeds the diffusion limits for nutrient and gas exchange.

Once the basement membrane has been penetrated, cancer cells gain access to the periglandular stroma, with its entirely

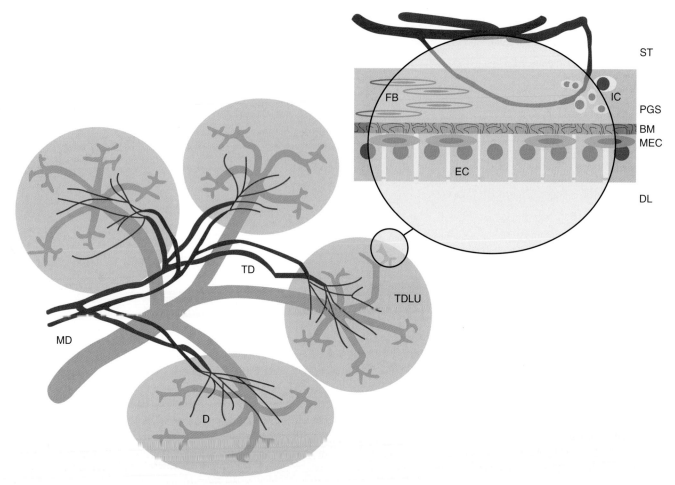

FIGURE 2-1 Diagram of breast lobular architecture. This is a stylized depiction of one of the 15 to 25 lobes, or segments, of the human breast. The duct architecture is drawn in orange, illustrating the tree like branching of the ducts into the periphery of the gland. The stromal tissue (ST) is indicated as blank space, and contains the supporting vasculature, of which only the blood vessels are drawn. The gray areas surrounding the terminal duct/lobular units (TDLU) represent the specialized, more dense stromal tissues surrounding the ductal system.

The insert shows a magnified view of a ductule (D) and its lumen (DL), with a layer of epithelial cells (EC), which are connected by intercellular tight junctions. Interspersed between the epithelium and the delimiting basement membrane (BM) are myoepithelial cells (MEC). The periglandular stroma (PGS), containing specialized myofibroblasts (FB), also known as delimiting fibroblasts, commonly harbors inflammatory cell (IC) infiltrates.

new set of cell types and molecules. This paves the way to fundamental intracellular changes induced by intense interactions with the stromal cells, growth factors, and the immune system. Vitally, the ability to induce angiogenesis, with its promise of virtually limitless nutrients and oxygen, enables potentially permanent proliferation. The organizing principle of an epithelium, the vertical stratification controlled by cells directly attached to the basement membrane, is lost.

CELL BIOLOGY OF INVASION

Epithelial to Stromal Transition

As epithelial tumors progress through progressive stages of carcinogenesis, from benign proliferative states to in situ and invasive cancer, they undergo profound architectural, cell biological, and molecular changes that have been summarized as an epithelial to mesenchymal transition (EMT).[1-3] Originally described in the context of normal embryologic development,[4] where cells from the ectodermal germ layer can detach and migrate over considerable distances to participate in the formation of various organs, EMT is now understood as a consequence of a complex set of molecular changes that allow the cancer cells to escape the structural constraints of the epithelial architecture, such as the specialized circumferential cell-to-cell adhesion complexes. These include the loss of several epithelial characteristics, such as apicobasal polarity, a term describing the marked differences in cell surface specializations at the top and bottom of an epithelial cell. Changes in cell shape from cuboidal to more spindle-shaped are associated with a reorganization of the actin cytoskeleton; and a decrease in epithelial-specific gene expression, including E-cadherin[5,6] and claudins,[7] is matched by an increase in mesenchymal gene expression, such as vimentin[8] and numerous proteases.

Fundamentally, the essential features of EMT are the disruption of intercellular, epithelial-to-epithelial contacts, and the enhancement of cell motility, which, coupled with the production of extracellular matrix-degrading enzymes, allows the escape from the confines of the breast duct and invasion into the surrounding stroma.

It should be understood, however, that the concept of EMT remains, at this point, largely an attractive but unproven concept that is still vigorously debated.[9,10] Much of the controversy revolves around the proposition that EMT necessarily implies a complete transition from an epithelial cell to a mesenchymal cell such as a fibroblast, something that has not been demonstrated in clinical tissues. A complete loss of epithelial characteristics is not observable in pathologic specimens of invasive or even metastatic breast cancer, and the appearance of abnormal, mesenchymal gene expression patterns and markers in cancer cells is not sufficient to reclassify the cells to a different lineage, since such events are a common byproduct of the genetic and epigenetic disarray in cancer cells. Indeed, most of the data supporting the existence of EMT are derived from embryologic and in vitro cancer cell-line model systems, which certainly do not perfectly mimic the in vivo situation. Nevertheless, EMT as intellectual construct to help understand and investigate these processes has been very productive, and there is little reason to abandon the model if one does not assume a complete conversion of one cell type to another.[11] Interestingly, recent evidence from a transgenic mouse model using cell-fate mapping strategies does support the possibility of true EMT, although this only occurred in association with c-MYC amplification, and a concurrent microsatellite marker analysis of human tumors suggests this to be a rare occurrence.[12]

Phenotype of EMT

At the level of the cancer cell, EMT is characterized by loss of intercellular junctions and cytoskeletal rearrangements favoring motility. Cell–cell interactions typical of stationary epithelial cells are replaced by cell–matrix interactions favoring migration and invasion, which is further enabled by reciprocal interactions with peritumoral stroma leading to an increased production of matrix-degrading proteases. The ensuing degradation and remodeling of the extracellular matrix (ECM), beginning with the basement membrane, is coupled with proliferative stimuli promoting tumor growth, recreating strands of cohesive multicellular columns. The regaining of a cohesive epithelial appearance has been termed mesenchymal–epithelial transition (MET), and is also an important feature in the establishment of metastatic disease.[3,11] It should be noted that this dynamic process leads to significant localized differences in cell function, morphology, and organization. Often, a characteristic invasive front at the advancing edge of the tumor strands can be discerned from more central parts of the tumor, at least in tumors showing more solid morphologies. This is less apparent in diffuse types of breast cancer such a lobular carcinomas, where most of the tumor mass consists of discohesive strands and scattered cells less reminiscent of epithelial cells.

Regulation of EMT

E-cadherin expression is emerging as one of the pivotal caretakers of the epithelial phenotype.[1] While E-cadherin expression is detectable in most differentiated breast cancers, there is an inverse relation with cancer grade and prognosis.[13,14] E-cadherin is a transmembrane glycoprotein that mediates homophilic interactions between its extracellular immunoglobulin domains on neighboring cells, and connects indirectly to intracellular actin filaments via cytoplasmic catenins, forming a multiprotein complex with alpha- beta-, and p120 catenins (Fig. 2-2). Clusters of E-cadherin aggregate with each other, and other specialized proteins such as claudins, into junctional complexes to establish adherens junctions and desmosomes.[1] In this way, E-cadherin is critical in establishing physical links between cells, and interconnecting them with their cytoskeleton and the basement membranes, establishing cell polarity and maintaining structural integrity and cellular signaling.

The key event promoting EMT is the down-regulation of E-cadherin, leading to a reversal of the effects listed above. In addition, decreasing levels of E-cadherin release beta-catenins from their complexed state at the cell membrane, freeing them to participate in the Wnt signaling pathway,[15] which cross talks with the hedgehog signaling cascade, including EGF/FGF, TGF-beta, and Snail.[2,3,16] The down-regulation of E-cadherin occurs during cancer progression through reversible and irreversible mechanisms, although mutations appear limited to lobular breast cancer[17] and other diffuse neoplasms such as diffuse gastric cancer,[2] where inactivating mutations are found in up to 50% of cases. More commonly, E-cadherin expression is down-regulated by promoter methylation-induced silencing, which may be dynamically reversible, as needed in the changing environment of cancer progression.[5] Loss of E-cadherin can be accompanied by an increase in N-cadherin expression, known as *cadherin switch*. N-cadherin is typically expressed in mesenchymal cells, and enhances tumor motility through its interaction with the FGF receptor.[17]

While the control of epigenetic regulation, such as promoter hypermethylation, is incompletely understood, there is an inverse relation between transcriptional activity and the likelihood of epigenetic silencing. Direct transcriptional repression by transcription factors is a likely starting point, and several signaling pathways have been implicated, including members of the basic helix-loop-helix family such as E47 and Twist; and zinc finger transcription factors such as the Snail superfamily[18] and ZEB1 and SIP1.[2] One regulatory model suggests involvement of a different set of factors for the initiation of EMT, lead by Snail and SIP1, whereas Slug and E47 would maintain the EMT phenotype.[19] Twist appears to have a critical role in enabling entry into the vasculature and favoring metastasis.[20]

Snail has been placed at the center of a hub of several signaling pathways leading to EMT, and may play a central role in breast cancer recurrence.[18] Snail is directly induced by both receptor tyrosine kinase and TGF-beta signaling, involving the PI3kinase, MAPkinase, and Smad pathways.[21] In addition to E-cadherin repression, Snail decreases desmoplakin, Muc-1, and cytokeratin-18 expression, while enhancing fibronectin and vimentin expression, all changes associated with EMT. Twist has been shown to induce Snail expression in some models,[22] although in human tissues the evidence remains correlative at this time.[23-25] Finally, Snail may play a central role in peritumoral stromal tissue as well, since serial analysis of gene

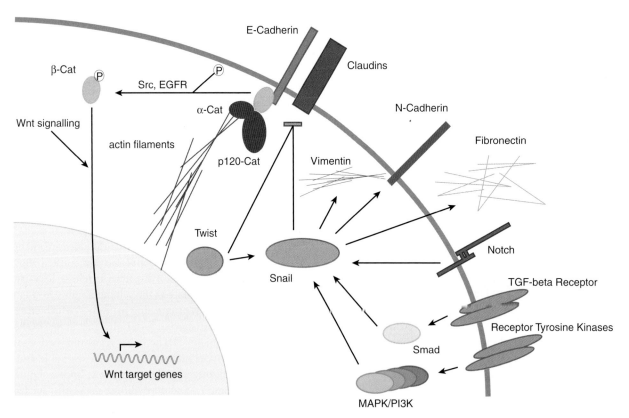

FIGURE 2-2 Simplified scheme of key regulators of epithelial-to-mesenchymal transition. The down-regulation of E-cadherin releases beta-catenins from their complexed state at the cell membrane, freeing them to participate in the Wnt signaling pathway, which cross-talks with several signaling cascades, including EGF/FGF, TGF-beta, and the hedgehog pathway. Snail has been placed at the center of a hub of several signaling pathways leading to EMT[18]. Snail is induced by numerous factors, including receptor tyrosine kinases, Notch signaling, and TGF-beta signaling, involving the PI3kinase, MAPkinase, and Smad pathways. Like Twist, another helix-loop-helix protein, it acts as direct inhibitor of E-cadherin transcription.

expression (SAGE) showed it was one of the most abundantly expressed genes in tumor endothelial cells.[26]

Two additional transcription factors induced by TGF-beta signaling have recently been described. Goosecoid (GSC), a transcription factor that plays a central role in the Spemann neuroectodermal organizer,[27] down-regulates E-cadherin and promotes metastasis in breast cells.[28] Similar effects are observed with FOXC2, with induction of mesenchymal markers such as vimentin, fibronectin, and smooth muscle actin.[29] Another homeodomain protein, HOXB7, which shows overexpression in breast cancer that increases with tumor progression to metastatic disease, has also been shown to induce EMT in breast cancer cell lines.[30,31] Overexpression of HOXB7 induces several angiogenic and growth factors seen in EMT, such as FGF, VEGF, and MMP9. Table 2-1 lists some transcription factors modulating EMT in breast epithelial cells.

Breaching the Basement Membrane

There are 3 general mechanisms responsible for the breach of the basement membrane separating the epithelial compartment from the surrounding stroma:

1. The increasing mechanical pressure arising from unrelenting proliferation

2. The increased motility of tumor cells undergoing EMT
3. The release of proteolytic enzymes breaking down the barrier

The extracellular matrix (ECM) is a product of stromal cells, and supports the adhesion and migration of cells through cell surface adhesion receptors, and provides support for the vasculature. The basement membrane is a specialized version of the ECM, separating both epithelia as well as blood vessels from the surrounding stroma. This provides a barrier to invasion by epithelial cells, and its penetration and destruction are prerequisites for invasive tumor growth. The basement membrane is 20 to 200 nm thick, consisting of self-organizing networks of laminins and type IV collagen. A variety of additional glycoproteins and proteoglycans, including CD44, are present.

In order to break through this barrier, invading cancer cells secrete a wide variety of ECM-degrading proteases. The largest group consists of the matrix metalloproteinases (MMPs), of which 28 have been described so far. They each have their own specific degradation target proteins, such as various collagen subtypes, gelatins, fibronectin, elastin, laminin, and the critical basement membrane collagens. They have a role in regulating the tumor microenvironment, given that many of the breakdown products they generate have effects of their own in attracting epithelial and stromal cell migration.

TABLE 2-1 Transcription Factors Modulating EMT in Breast Epithelial Cells

	Transcription Factor	DNA-Binding Domain	Reference
E47	Transcription factor 3	Helix loop helix	65
FOXC2	Mesenchyme forkhead 1	Forkhead domain	29
GSC	Goosecoid	Homeobox	28
HOXB7	Homeobox B7	Homeobox	31
SIP1	Smad interacting protein 1	Zinc finger motif	66
SNAI1	Snail	Zinc finger motif	67
SNAI2	Slug	Zinc finger motif	68
Twist1	Twist homolog 1	Helix loop helix	25

Unlike oncogenes, MMPs are not up-regulated by amplifications or activating mutations but by transcriptional activation by factors such as Snail, SIP1, interferons, and growth factors. Conversely, expression of MMPs can be inhibited by differentiation factors and tumor suppressors, such as retinoids, corticosteroids, or TGF-beta.[32] The expression and activation of MMPs is increased in most cancer types, including breast cancer.

A second major group of cancer invasion–associated proteases are the fibrinolytic proteinases, such as plasmin, plasminogen activators, and thrombin. These are produced remotely, such as in the liver or vasculature, and are deposited in tumors because of the hyperpermeability caused by changes in the ECM and basement membranes of tumor-associated blood vessels. They cleave fibrin and plasminogen, as well as laminin and type IV collagen. Other proteases include cathepsins, kallikreins, and elastase.

All of these proteases have counterbalancing antagonists, such as the class of tissue inhibitors of metalloproteases (TIMPs), and the serpin superfamily, which includes maspin and alpha-1 antitrypsin.[33] In analogy to the balance between oncogenes and tumor suppressor genes in the control of the cell cycle, the effect of genes mediating invasiveness and metastatic spread is balanced by these inhibitory gene products, many of which promote cell anchorage and inhibit migration. It appears that the expression of these adhesion molecules, which include cadherins, is functionally dominant over the expression of receptors promoting invasion, and they are predominantly functionally silenced, rather than mutated, in invasive cancer.[33]

The Extracellular Matrix and Tumor Stroma

As invading tumor cells penetrate the basement membrane to gain access to the periductal stroma and the ECM, they enter a fundamentally new microenvironment. They are now directly exposed to stromal influence, and can engage not only in interactions with the extracellular matrix but also extensive reciprocal cross talk with adjacent fibroblasts, immune cells, and cells lining blood and lymphatic vessels.

Fibroblasts are primarily responsible for the synthesis and remodeling of the ECM, as well as for many soluble paracrine growth factors responsible for cell proliferation and neoplastic programming of tissues.[34] Fibroblasts in peritumoral stroma are unique, and undergo dynamic changes during tumor progression.[35] They are commonly referred to as cancer-associated fibroblasts (CAFs) or myofibroblasts, exhibit a relatively high proliferative index, express smooth muscle actin, and are often surrounded by dense accumulations of fibrillar collagens in a pattern referred to as desmoplasia.[36] CAFs isolated from malignant tissue exhibit an altered phenotype characterized by enhanced production of collagens and epithelial growth factors.[36]

A link between inflammation, chronic regeneration and repair, and cancer has long been recognized.[36] Various inflammatory cells, particularly mononuclear cells, are frequently prominent components of the stroma surrounding both preinvasive and invasive cancer. These cells contribute functionally to carcinogenesis due to the release of soluble mediators promoting proliferation, remodeling, and angiogenesis.[36]

The vasculature is embedded in the stroma and maintains tissue homeostasis, and is highly responsive to the growth processes and the accompanying mediators during cancer development. Tumor angiogenesis is regulated by local changes in angiogenic molecules, inflammatory mediators, and local hypoxia.

The peritumoral stroma undergoes significant changes during the neoplastic process, both reactive and tumorigenic,[37] and early studies documented the acquired expression of numerous proteins typically associated with wound healing and inflammation, such as actin, vimentin, smooth muscle myosin, calponin, tenascin, and desmin.[36] These proteins all favor cell proliferation, inflammation, angiogenesis, and migration, and by interacting with invading tumor cells, favor tumor development.

Macrophage infiltration is a key process in wound healing, and is frequently seen in tumors, where they are referred to as tumor-associated macrophages (TAMs). They have been observed in precursor lesions of breast cancer,[38] and may aid in the invasion of cancer cells into the surrounding stroma, depending on the local levels of chemokines and the number of macrophages recruited to the area. At low levels of macrophage recruitment, angiogenesis and tumor growth are enhanced, while more robust infiltration can lead to tumor regression.[39]

In addition to these effects on tumor cell proliferation or survival, TAMs also affect tumor growth by directing tumor angiogenesis, producing vascular endothelial growth factor (VEGF)[40] as well as an array of extracellular proteases such as MMPs.[41]

TUMOR ANGIOGENESIS

Blood vessels are required to supply tissues with nutrients and oxygen, and together with lymphatic vessels, to remove waste products in order to maintain cellular homeostasis. Epithelial organs use stromal tissue as a conduit for this vascular network, while keeping epithelial cells architecturally separated from direct contact with vessels through a specialized form of the ECM, the basement membrane or basal lamina, which forms where epithelial or endothelial cells interact with the ECM. This means that maintaining epithelial homeostasis is dependent on diffusion of nutrients and gases, which can only occur over short distances, about 180 μm from the nearest arterialized blood vessel. One consequence of this architecture is that when epithelia proliferate abnormally, and start to exceed normal numbers of cell layers, diffusion fails to maintain a viable environment. The result is often a zone of central necrosis in lobules containing extensive carcinoma in situ lesions, which is known as *comedonecrosis*. Unless a cancer can break out of the confines of the surrounding basement membrane, its growth potential will remain limited to lesions several cell layers deep.

In the normal state, angiogenesis is typically limited to wound healing or the events surrounding the menstrual cycle in the uterus, is tightly regulated, and respects anatomic boundaries. Tumor angiogenesis,[42,43] on the other hand, which is induced by the chronic homeostatic stress and hypoxia of the overgrowing epithelium, is largely independent of anatomy, but is instead driven by hypoxic gradients and tissue damage.

Induction of Neovascularization

Tumor angiogenesis is a process controlled by genetic programs that are part of the stress and wound response. As in a wound, platelets release chemotactic factors such as TGF beta and PDGF, which activate CAFs to produce MMPs and growth factors, and stimulate the infiltration by TAMs. TAMs release additional chemokines and VEGF, leading to remodeling of the ECM, including neovascularization and epithelial proliferation as a form of "healing."

Since the signal for neoangiogenesis is primarily initiated by local hypoxia, local conditions will have a significant impact on both the initial foci of neovascularization, and consequently on the direction of tumor growth and expansion, since the tumor chords will proliferate preferentially around blood vessels, constrained as they are by nutrient and gas diffusion limits.

The hypoxia inducible factor-1 (HIF-1) is one of the master regulators of cellular response to hypoxia.[44-46] It is a composed of two subunits, HIF-1alpha and HIF-1beta, forming a heterodimeric transcription factor. HIF-1alpha is only stable under hypoxic conditions, and is otherwise rapidly metabolized. When stabilized by hypoxia, it translocates to the nucleus and together with reactive oxygen species (ROS), which paradoxically rise under hypoxic conditions, HIF-1alpha activates transcription of its downstream targets. These include important factors such as VEGF, EGF, and the PI3kinase pathway, and well as several μRNAs. The μRNAs (miRNAs) are endogenous, 18- to 25-nucleotide long RNA species that regulate gene expression at the posttranscriptional level. They hybridize to regions of their target messenger RNAs (mRNAs) based on sequence complementarity and induce either mRNA cleavage or suppression of its translation.[44]

Most of the hypoxia-induced signal transduction pathways support tumor proliferation and can activate genetic programs

promoting an aggressive phenotype, which is reflected in increased metastatic risk and poor survival associated with tumors showing evidence of hypoxic conditions.[46]

In responding to neovascularization stimuli, endothelial cells need to degrade their own basement membranes, develop proliferative sprouts from preexisting vessels, and invade the ECM in the direction of the hypoxic stimulus. As the new sprouts develop a lumen, capillary tubes develop with formation of tight junctions and the deposition of a new basement membrane. Notably, neovessels formed under these conditions are notoriously leaky, and offer less resistance to cell invasion than non-neoplastic vessels.

Secreted Factors

Secreted molecules regulating the formation of blood vessels include growth factors, cytokines, and guidance molecules.[32]

The VEGF/VEGF receptor system is involved early in neoangiogenesis, and acts as a selective mitogen on endothelial cells. The VEGF family consists of VEGF-A, -B, -C, and -D, and the placental growth factor PLGF, each transcribed from different genes; alternate splicing creates a large number of variant forms. In addition to direct angiogenic and lymphangiogenic effects on endothelial cells, VEGF receptor–expressing myeloid and endothelial precursors are recruited from the bone marrow.[47] Many tumor types express abundant levels of VEGF, and are often the main source of this growth factor.

There are 3 known angiopoietins (ANG-1, ANG-2, and ANG-4) that regulate endothelial cell survival. The combined action of angiopoietin and VEGF recruits pericytes and smooth muscle cells through endothelial production of PDGF, and favors loosening of the support cell interactions, which allows endothelial cells to multiply.

Fibroblast growth factors constitute a family of 20 related growth factors with varying specificities. FGF-1 and FGF-2 have angiogenic activity, and promote endothelial proliferation and migration. They also promote the release of basement membrane degrading proteases.

Platelet-derived endothelial cell growth factor (PD-ECGF) is involved in thymidine metabolism, and may have antiapoptotic effects in situations of cellular stress. PD-ECGF also induces angiogenesis and chemotaxis of endothelial cells, and is often produced at high levels in breast cancer.

Osteopontin (OPN) is a chemotactic cytokine secreted by vascular smooth muscle cells during angiogenesis. A splice variant of CD44 is an OPN receptor that induces endothelial proliferation, migration, and angiogenesis. A recent study showed that OPN was expressed in 65% of invasive breast cancers, and was negatively correlated with estrogen and progesterone receptor status, and positively correlated with her2-neu status.[48] It is also associated with poor outcome in breast cancer.[49]

Guidance molecules include a class of genes called ephrins (EFN), which are involved in providing guidance to blood vessel growth by controlling the migration and proliferation of endothelial cells. Various members of this family are specific for different types of blood and lymphatic vessels, but their role in breast cancer has not yet been proven.

Matrix-Degrading Proteases

The degradation and remodeling of the ECM surrounding budding neovasculature is necessary for tumor angiogenesis. Type I collagen is a major ECM constituent, and its cleavage is the rate-limiting step in neoangiogenesis.[50] The ECM is degraded primarily by MMPs, many of which are expressed in angiogenic tissue. In many solid tumors, MMPs are produced primarily by the peritumoral stroma and CAFs, rather than by the cancer cells. These expression patterns are regulated by tumor–stroma interactions that involve CD147, also known as EMMPRIN. CD147 mediates MMP secretion and activation,[51] as well as the release of hyaluronidase secretion to favor anchorage-independent growth,[52] which can confer resistance to anoikis.[53] Anoikis is a form of apoptosis induced by loss or alteration of cell–cell or cell–matrix anchorage.

Inhibition of Neovascularization

As discussed for the control of protease activity, the net neoangiogenic activity surrounding an invading cancer is the result of a balance of influences inducing or inhibiting angiogenesis. A number of inhibitors are stored in the ECM or as precursors in the bloodstream, and need to be released and proteolytically activated. Angiogenesis inhibitors can interact with adhesion proteins, suggesting that such complex formation might play an important role in their function. Several modes of action have been described, including binding to endothelial surface receptors, decreasing endothelial cell mobility, binding and blocking FGF and other angiogenic factors, and neutralizing heparin.[32]

Interestingly, tumors appear to produce both stimulators and inhibitors of neovascularization, with the balance of the two dictating the degree of angiogenesis both locally as well as at distant sites, if the tumor has metastasized. In such cases, the removal of a primary tumor may lead to accelerated growth of metastatic colonies. There is also overlap in the effects of inhibitors of metastasis such as the serpin family of protease inhibitors and TIMPs, which also have antiangiogenic activity.

Secreted Angiogenesis Inhibitors

Angiostatin was the first molecule isolated as specific neoangiogenesis inhibitor.[54] It is a 38kD internal fragment of plasminogen, which can be obtained proteolytically from deposited plasminogen by tumor-derived proteases. After forming complexes with fibrin and integrins in the endothelial membranes, angiostatin inhibits endothelial proliferation and can induce dormancy in metastatic deposits.[55]

Endostatin is a product of the cleavage of type XVIII collagen[56] by cathepsin-L, elastin, or matrilysin. It is a highly active endothelial cell-specific inhibitor of proliferation and migration, and forms complexes with MMPs. It also prevents VEGF binding to its receptor, without binding to VEGF itself, and reduces levels of antiapoptotic BCL proteins in endothelial cells.[57]

Thrombospondin-1 (TSP1) has antiangiogenic properties as well, inhibiting endothelial proliferation, adhesion, and migration through its binding to the CD36 receptor. TSP1 is inversely correlated with tumor grade and survival in several solid tumors, but in breast cancer it correlates with stromal response and is of little independent prognostic value.[58]

Antiangiogenic Signaling

The tumor suppressor gene PTEN regulates hypoxia-induced signal transduction. It can suppress the activity of hypoxia-inducible genes such as COX-1, PGK1, and PFK, which have been implicated in neoangiogenesis.[32] PTEN expression blocks the stabilization of HIF-1alpha by hypoxia, preventing its nuclear localization and transactivation of its downstream angiogenic genes.[59,60]

Targeting Angiogenesis

The advances in understanding tumor-associated angiogenesis over the last decade have led to a high level of interest in using this process as therapeutic target, leading to the introduction of new classes of drugs, such as small molecule blockers of VEGF, into clinical trials and clinical practice. Discussing these new approaches is beyond the scope of this chapter, but there can be no doubt that the field will progress rapidly.

PATHOLOGY OF INVASION

Microinvasive Cancer

As has been alluded to in the introduction, the diagnostic decision if invasive breast cancer is present or not is at the crux of surgical breast pathology. Since this decision rests upon the proper interpretation of the integrity of the ductal and lobular architecture at its periphery, the presence or absence of the delimiting architectural features defining benign and in situ lesions—the basement membrane and the basal myoepithelial layer—are crucial in making this determination in the presence of *microinvasive disease,* that is, in cases with an invasive focus of less than 0.1 cm.

The difficulties in identifying microinvasive disease stem from the interpretation of small areas of an indistinct basement membrane surrounding distorted ducts, which can make it difficult to exclude direct contact of cancer cells with the surrounding stroma, particularly in areas of tangential sectioning of the tissue. High-grade ductal carcinoma in situ can be distorted by periductal sclerosis and inflammation to such an extent that it will mimic irregular nests of invasive ductal carcinomas. At the opposite end of the dilemma, rounded nests of cells resembling carcinoma in situ are often found in invasive solid papillary and cribriform carcinomas,[61,62] which can cause problems if only small amounts of tissue are available for review.

In such cases, the diagnostic dilemma can often be resolved with immunohistochemical methods to detect the basal membrane.[62] Solely relying on the detection of basement membrane components such as collagen IV or laminin was soon found to be insufficient, however, since invasive breast cancer cells are capable of ectopic synthesis of basement membrane elements. The myoepithelial cell layer, however, is almost never seen adjacent to nests of invasive cancer cells, while it remains present in benign and in situ lesions. On the other hand, the detection of myoepithelial cells can be difficult using routine histologic stains, since they are often quite attenuated in the setting of in situ carcinoma.

TABLE 2-2 Immunohistochemical Markers Used to Identify Stromal Invasion [61-63,69-70]

Marker	Location	Myoepithelium	Myofibroblast	Vessels	Epithelia
SMA	Cytoplasm	+++++	+++	+++	+
Calponin	Cytoplasm	+++++	++	+++	—
SM-MHC	Cytoplasm	++++	+	+++	—
CD10	Cytoplasm	+++	++	—	+
p63	Nucleus	++++	—	—	+

Table 2-2 summarizes the features of the immunohistochemical (IH) markers most commonly used to identify stromal invasion.

Immunohistochemical staining for smooth muscle actin (SMA) is strongly positive for breast myoepithelial cells, but also stains myofibroblasts present in the reactive stroma surrounding benign and malignant breast lesions, regardless of invasiveness of the epithelium.

Calponin is a contractility protein expressed in smooth muscle cells. IH staining for calponin also strongly stains myoepithelial cells, but is less reactive for myofibroblasts.

Smooth muscle myosin heavy chain (SM-MHC) is a myosin component. IH staining shows a sensitivity for myoepithelial cells similar to that of the above two markers, but with considerably less cross-reactivity with myofibroblasts, making it an excellent choice for myoepithelial cell detection.

CD10, the common ALL antigen, is a slightly less sensitive marker for myoepithelial cells, but shows no cross-reactivity with blood vessels.[69] p63 is a p53 homologue and nuclear antigen expressed in the basal epithelia of many organs. In the breast, it is a highly specific marker for myoepithelial cells. As expected for a nuclear marker, positive staining cells produce a dotted line pattern around benign glands and in situ carcinomas, making their detection more difficult in cases of carcinoma in situ with highly attenuated numbers of myoepithelial cells. On the other hand, it does not cross-react with blood vessels. While p63 may label occasional epithelial cells in hyperplasias and carcinomas, this staining is usually weak and more focal than in myoepithelial cells,[63] and the cancer cells are rarely confused with myoepithelial cells.

A review of the contribution of immunohistochemistry in the diagnosis of invasive breast cancer concluded that the combination of SM-MHC and p63 outperformed all other markers currently available for this indication.[62]

Invasive Breast Cancer

Surgical pathologists have traditionally classified most invasive breast cancer as either ductal or lobular type. This classification is broadly based on overall cellular cohesiveness, and the presence of both morphologies in the same tumor is often identified with the catch-all term of mammary carcinoma. The most common group of breast cancers is invasive duct carcinoma (IDC). These are sometimes referred to as IDC not otherwise specified (NOS), to indicate the prognostically relevant distinction between IDCs and more specific forms of breast cancer, such as tubular, medullary, colloid, metaplastic, or adenoid

cystic variants. The relatively favorable outlook of some of the specific histologic subtypes only applies if these tumors are homogenous or largely so, while more heterogeneous tumors have less favorable outlook and should be identified as IDC, NOS. The most differentiated form of ductal carcinoma is tubular carcinoma, where over 90% of the epithelia have ductal appearance as well as lumens. It has the most favorable outlook of the IDCs, followed by the other monomorphic IDC subtypes.

IDCs are often unifocal lesions, compared to invasive lobular carcinomas (ILC), which are often multifocal. While the metastatic patterns are somewhat different between IDC and ILC, the overall mortality and disease-free survival rates appear similar.[64] Nevertheless, an accurate classification of IDC versus ILC remains desirable, since it is likely that improved prognostic and predictive stratification will be developed, and accurate assessments of pathologic features are likely to remain relevant, even in the era of genome-wide analyses.

ILC is morphologically characterized by an invasive pattern of single cells infiltrating dense fibrotic stroma. The different pattern of invasive growth can be explained by the loss of expression of E-cadherin by inactivating mutations in 50% of cases, with the effect on intercellular cohesion one would expect from the above discussion, and which are also evident at the in situ stages (Figs. 2-3 and 2-4).

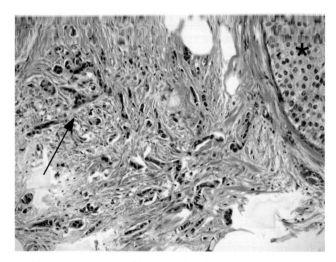

FIGURE 2-3 H&E stain of invasive ductal carcinoma (IDC) and ductal carcinoma in situ (DCIS). The *arrow* points to cohesive strands of IDC cell invading the peritumoral stroma. The *asterisk* indicates the DCIS. *(Figure courtesy of P. van Diest, Utrecht.)*

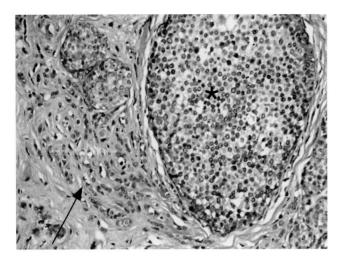

FIGURE 2-4 H&E stain of invasive lobular carcinoma (ILC) and lobular carcinoma in situ (LCIS). The *arrow* points to discohesive strands and individual ILC cells invading the peritumoral stroma. The asterisk indicates the LCIS, with its markedly decreased intercellular cohesion. *(Figure courtesy of P. van Diest, Utrecht.)*

A long-standing IH approach to differentiate IDC from ILC has involved the demonstration of strong membranous E-cadherin staining used to define IDCs. ILC shows either a complete loss of staining or abnormal localization of the stain. These differences in E-cadherin staining may reflect a permanent loss of the protein in ILC, while only transient down-regulation may be required for invasion in IDC. In about 15% of cases, the E-cadherin staining result is equivocal,[62] in which case the p120 catenin stain can be used. IDCs show a membranous pattern of staining, while in ILCs with dysfunctional E-cadherin, the p120 catenin shows strong cytoplasmic staining.[62]

FUTURE DIRECTIONS

In addition to a more refined understanding of the complex events leading to EMT-enabled invasion to metastatic progression, the study of neoangiogenesis and its inhibition by novel small molecules shows great promise for therapeutic interventions with a high level of target specificity and minimized toxicity.

SUMMARY

Invasion is the second, and arguably the most consequential, of three pivotal milestones in the evolution of breast cancer. It is preceded by the molecular events initiating carcinogenesis, and it may be followed by metastatic spread of tumor cells throughout the body. Before invasion occurs, which requires the breaching of the delimiting basement membrane, the malignant cells represent a contained, potential threat, which may be completely averted by therapeutic intervention.

Biologically, penetrating the basement membrane puts the cancer cells into contact with an entirely new microenvironment, and they gain access to the stroma, with its new set of cell types, paving the path to fundamental intracellular changes induced by intense interactions with the immune system, and

the ability to induce angiogenesis, with its promise of virtually limitless nutrients and oxygen.

In order to achieve these goals, cancer cells undergo profound architectural, cell biological, and molecular changes that have been summarized as an epithelial to mesenchymal transition (EMT). E-cadherin expression is emerging as one of the pivotal caretakers of the epithelial phenotype, and its down-regulation or genetic inactivation may be the deciding factor in allowing EMT to progress. The down-regulation may be permanent in some breast cancers, such as ILC, while only transient in others, such as IDC.

Snail has been placed at the center of a hub of several signaling pathways leading to EMT, and may play a central role in breast cancer recurrence. Once the cancer cells have entered the peritumoral stroma and ECM, a complex sequence of interactions with the new microenvironment leads to extensive remodeling of the adjacent tissues, and neoangiogenesis enables continued tumor growth as well as access to the circulation, eventually paving the way to establish metastatic disease.

REFERENCES

1. Thiery JP. Epithelial-mesenchymal transitions in tumour progression. *Nat Rev Cancer.* 2002;2:442-454.
2. Guarino M, Rubino B, Ballabio G. The role of epithelial-mesenchymal transition in cancer pathology. *Pathology.* 2007;39:305-318.
3. Hugo H, Ackland ML, Blick T, et al. Epithelial—mesenchymal and mesenchymal—epithelial transitions in carcinoma progression. *J Cell Physiol.* 2007;213:374-383.
4. Greenburg G, Hay ED. Epithelia suspended in collagen gels can lose polarity and express characteristics of migrating mesenchymal cells. *J Cell Biol.* 1982;95:333-339.
5. Graff JR, Gabrielson E, Fujii H, Baylin SB, Herman JG. Methylation patterns of the E-cadherin 5' CpG island are unstable and reflect the dynamic, heterogeneous loss of E-cadherin expression during metastatic progression. *J Biol Chem.* 2000;275:2727-2732.
6. Berx G, Van Roy F. The E-cadherin/catenin complex: an important gatekeeper in breast cancer tumorigenesis and malignant progression. *Breast Cancer Res.* 2001;3:289-293.
7. Kominsky SL, Argani P, Korz D, et al. Loss of the tight junction protein claudin-7 correlates with histological grade in both ductal carcinoma in situ and invasive ductal carcinoma of the breast. *Oncogene.* 2003;22: 2021-2033.
8. Kokkinos MI, Wafai R, Wong MK, Newgreen DF, Thompson EW, Waltham M. Vimentin and epithelial-mesenchymal transition in human breast cancer—observations in vitro and in vivo. *Cells Tissues Organs.* 2007;185:191-203.
9. Tarin D, Thompson EW, Newgreen DF. The fallacy of epithelial mesenchymal transition in neoplasia. *Cancer Res.* 2005;65:5996-6000; discussion 6000-5991.
10. Thompson EW, Newgreen DF, Tarin D. Carcinoma invasion and metastasis: a role for epithelial-mesenchymal transition? *Cancer Res.* 2005;65: 5991-5995; discussion 5995.
11. Berx G, Raspe E, Christofori G, Thiery JP, Sleeman JP. Pre-EMTing metastasis? Recapitulation of morphogenetic processes in cancer. *Clin Exp Metastasis.* 2007;24:587-597.
12. Trimboli AJ, Fukino K, de Bruin A, et al. Direct evidence for epithelial-mesenchymal transitions in breast cancer. *Cancer Res.* 2008;68:937-945.
13. Paredes J, Correia AL, Ribeiro AS, Albergaria A, Milanezi F, Schmitt FC. P-cadherin expression in breast cancer: a review. *Breast Cancer Res.* 2007; 9:214.
14. Gould Rothberg BE, Bracken MB. E-cadherin immunohistochemical expression as a prognostic factor in infiltrating ductal carcinoma of the breast: a systematic review and meta-analysis. *Breast Cancer Res Treat.* 2006; 100:139-148.
15. Nelson WJ, Nusse R. Convergence of Wnt, beta-catenin, and cadherin pathways. *Science.* 2004;303:1483-1487.
16. Katoh Y, Katoh M. Hedgehog signaling, epithelial-to-mesenchymal transition and miRNA (review). *Int J Mol Med.* 2008;22:271-275.

17. Cowin P, Rowlands TM, Hatsell SJ. Cadherins and catenins in breast cancer. *Curr Opin Cell Biol.* 2005;17:499-508.

18. Davidson NE, Sukumar S. Of Snail, mice, and women. *Cancer Cell.* 2005;8:173-174.

19. Peinado H, Portillo F, Cano A. Transcriptional regulation of cadherins during development and carcinogenesis. *Int J Dev Biol.* 2004;48:365-375.

20. Yang J, Mani SA, Donaher JL, et al. Twist, a master regulator of morphogenesis, plays an essential role in tumor metastasis. *Cell.* 2004;117:927-939.

21. Peinado H, Quintanilla M, Cano A. Transforming growth factor beta-1 induces snail transcription factor in epithelial cell lines: mechanisms for epithelial mesenchymal transitions. *J Biol Chem.* 2003;278:21113-21123.

22. Castanon I, Baylies MK. A Twist in fate: evolutionary comparison of Twist structure and function. *Gene.* 2002;287:11-22.

23. Lo HW, Hsu SC, Xia W, et al. Epidermal growth factor receptor cooperates with signal transducer and activator of transcription 3 to induce epithelial-mesenchymal transition in cancer cells via up-regulation of TWIST gene expression. *Cancer Res.* 2007;67:9066-9076.

24. Martin TA, Goyal A, Watkins G, Jiang WG. Expression of the transcription factors snail, slug, and twist and their clinical significance in human breast cancer. *Ann Surg Oncol.* 2005;12:488-496.

25. Cheng GZ, Chan J, Wang Q, Zhang W, Sun CD, Wang LH. Twist transcriptionally up-regulates AKT2 in breast cancer cells leading to increased migration, invasion, and resistance to paclitaxel. *Cancer Res.* 2007;67:1979-1987.

26. Parker BS, Argani P, Cook BP, et al. Alterations in vascular gene expression in invasive breast carcinoma. *Cancer Res.* 2004;64:7857-7866.

27. Spemann H, Mangold H. Über Induktion von Embryonalagen durch Implantation Artfremder Organisatoren. *Roux' Arch. Entw. Mech.* 1924;100: 599-638.

28. Hartwell KA, Muir B, Reinhardt F, Carpenter AE, Sgroi DC, Weinberg RA. The Spemann organizer gene, Goosecoid, promotes tumor metastasis. *Proc Natl Acad Sci USA.* 2006;103:18969-18974.

29. Mani SA, Yang J, Brooks M, et al. Mesenchyme Forkhead 1 (FOXC2) plays a key role in metastasis and is associated with aggressive basal-like breast cancers. *Proc Natl Acad Sci USA.* 2007;104:10069-10074.

30. Care A, Felicetti F, Meccia E, et al. HOXB7: a key factor for tumor-associated angiogenic switch. *Cancer Res.* 2001;61:6532-6539.

31. Wu X, Chen H, Parker B, et al. HOXB7, a homeodomain protein, is overexpressed in breast cancer and confers epithelial-mesenchymal transition. *Cancer Res.* 2006;66:9527-9534.

32. Weber GF. *Molecular Mechanisms of Cancer.* Dordrecht, Netherlands. Springer; 2007.

33. Weber GF. Invasion. In: Weber GF, ed. *Molecular Mechanisms of Cancer.* Dordrecht, Netherlands: Springer; 2007:215-282.

34. Allinen M, Beroukhim R, Cai L, et al. Molecular characterization of the tumor microenvironment in breast cancer. *Cancer Cell.* 2004;6:17-32.

35. Bhowmick NA, Moses HL. Tumor-stroma interactions. *Curr Opin Genet Dev.* 2005;15:97-101.

36. Tlsty TD, Coussens LM. Tumor stroma and regulation of cancer development. *Annu Rev Pathol.* 2006;1:119-150.

37. Ronnov-Jessen L, Petersen OW, Bissell MJ. Cellular changes involved in conversion of normal to malignant breast: importance of the stromal reaction. *Physiol Rev.* 1996;76:69-125.

38. Lin EY, Gouon-Evans V, Nguyen AV, Pollard JW. The macrophage growth factor CSF-1 in mammary gland development and tumor progression. *J Mammary Gland Biol Neoplasia.* 2002;7:147-162.

39. Nesbit M, Schaider H, Miller TH, Herlyn M. Low-level monocyte chemoattractant protein-1 stimulation of monocytes leads to tumor formation in nontumorigenic melanoma cells. *J Immunol.* 2001;166:6483-6490.

40. Barbera-Guillem E, Nyhus JK, Wolford CC, Friece CR, Sampsel JW. Vascular endothelial growth factor secretion by tumor-infiltrating macrophages essentially supports tumor angiogenesis, and IgG immune complexes potentiate the process. *Cancer Res.* 2002;62:7042-7049.

41. Coussens LM, Tinkle CL, Hanahan D, Werb Z. MMP-9 supplied by bone marrow-derived cells contributes to skin carcinogenesis. *Cell.* 2000;103: 481-490.

42. Folkman J. Anti-angiogenesis: new concept for therapy of solid tumors. *Ann Surg.* 1972;175:409-416.

43. Folkman J, Merler E, Abernathy C, Williams G. Isolation of a tumor factor responsible for angiogenesis. *J Exp Med.* 1971;133:275-288.

44. Galanis A, Pappa A, Giannakakis A, Lanitis E, Dangaj D, Sandaltzopoulos R. Reactive oxygen species and HIF-1 signalling in cancer. *Cancer Lett.* 2008;266:12-20.

45. Kimbro KS, Simons JW. Hypoxia-inducible factor-1 in human breast and prostate cancer. *Endocr Relat Cancer.* 2006;13:739-749.

46. Lundgren K, Holm C, Landberg G. Hypoxia and breast cancer: prognostic and therapeutic implications. *Cell Mol Life Sci.* 2007;64:3233-3247.

47. Lyden D, Hattori K, Dias S, et al. Impaired recruitment of bone-marrow-derived endothelial and hematopoietic precursor cells blocks tumor angiogenesis and growth. *Nat Med.* 2001;7:1194-1201.

48. Ribeiro-Silva A, Oliveira da Costa JP. Osteopontin expression according to molecular profile of invasive breast cancer: a clinicopathological and immunohistochemical study. *Int J Biol Markers.* 2008;23:154-160.

49. Patani N, Jiang W, Mokbel K. Osteopontin C mRNA expression is associated with a poor clinical outcome in human breast cancer. *Int J Cancer.* 2008;122:2646.

50. Seandel M, Noack-Kunnmann K, Zhu D, Aimes RT, Quigley JP. Growth factor-induced angiogenesis in vivo requires specific cleavage of fibrillar type I collagen. *Blood.* 2001;97:2323-2332.

51. Li QQ, Wang WJ, Xu JD, et al. Up-regulation of CD147 and matrix metalloproteinase-2, -9 induced by P-glycoprotein substrates in multidrug resistant breast cancer cells. *Cancer Sci.* 2007;98:1767-1774.

52. Tang Y, Nakada MT, Kesavan P, et al. Extracellular matrix metalloproteinase inducer stimulates tumor angiogenesis by elevating vascular endothelial cell growth factor and matrix metalloproteinases. *Cancer Res.* 2005;65: 3193-3199.

53. Yang JM, O'Neill P, Jin W, et al. Extracellular matrix metalloproteinase inducer (CD147) confers resistance of breast cancer cells to Anoikis through inhibition of Bim. *J Biol Chem.* 2006;281:9719-9727.

54. O'Reilly MS, Holmgren L, Shing Y, et al. Angiostatin: a novel angiogenesis inhibitor that mediates the suppression of metastases by a Lewis lung carcinoma. *Cell.* 1994;79:315-328.

55. Burke PA, DeNardo SJ. Antiangiogenic agents and their promising potential in combined therapy. *Crit Rev Oncol Hematol.* 2001;39:155-171.

56. O'Reilly MS, Boehm T, Shing Y, et al. Endostatin: an endogenous inhibitor of angiogenesis and tumor growth. *Cell.* 1997;88:277-285.

57. Dhanabal M, Ramchandran R, Waterman MJ, et al. Endostatin induces endothelial cell apoptosis. *J Biol Chem.* 1999;274:11721-11726.

58. de Fraipont F, Nicholson AC, Feige JJ, Van Meir EG. Thrombospondins and tumor angiogenesis. *Trends Mol Med.* 2001;7:401-407.

59. Laughner E, Taghavi P, Chiles K, Mahon PC, Semenza GL. HER2 (neu) signaling increases the rate of hypoxia-inducible factor 1alpha (HIF-1alpha) synthesis: novel mechanism for HIF-1-mediated vascular endothelial growth factor expression. *Mol Cell Biol.* 2001;21:3995-4004.

60. Phillips RJ, Mestas J, Gharaee-Kermani M, et al. Epidermal growth factor and hypoxia-induced expression of CXC chemokine receptor 4 on non-small cell lung cancer cells is regulated by the phosphatidylinositol 3-kinase/PTEN/AKT/mammalian target of rapamycin signaling pathway and activation of hypoxia inducible factor-1alpha. *J Biol Chem.* 2005;280: 22473-22481.

61. Lerwill MF. Current practical applications of diagnostic immunohistochemistry in breast pathology. *Am J Surg Pathol.* 2004;28:1076-1091.

62. Bhargava R, Dabbs DJ. Use of immunohistochemistry in diagnosis of breast epithelial lesions. *Adv Anat Pathol.* 2007;14:93-107.

63. Werling RW, Hwang H, Yaziji H, Gown AM. Immunohistochemical distinction of invasive from noninvasive breast lesions: a comparative study of p63 versus calponin and smooth muscle myosin heavy chain. *Am J Surg Pathol.* 2003;27:82-90.

64. Mersin H, Yildirim E, Gulben K, Berberoglu U. Is invasive lobular carcinoma different from invasive ductal carcinoma? *Eur J Surg Oncol.* 2003;29:390-395.

65. Perez-Moreno MA, Locascio A, Rodrigo I, et al. A new role for E12/E47 in the repression of E-cadherin expression and epithelial-mesenchymal transitions. *J Biol Chem.* 2001;276:27424-27431.

66. Comijn J, Berx G, Vermassen P, et al. The two-handed E box binding zinc finger protein SIP1 downregulates E-cadherin and induces invasion. *Mol Cell.* 2001;7:1267-1278.

67. Shen H, Qin H, Guo J. Concordant correlation of LIV-1 and E-cadherin expression in human breast cancer cell MCF-7. *Mol Biol Rep.* 2008;36: 653-659.

68. Laffin B, Wellberg E, Kwak HI, et al. Loss of singleminded-2s in the mouse mammary gland induces an epithelial-mesenchymal transition associated with up-regulation of slug and matrix metalloprotease 2. *Mol Cell Biol.* 2008;28:1936-1946.

69. Kalof AN, Tam D, Beatty B, Cooper K. Immunostaining patterns of myoepithelial cells in breast lesions: a comparison of CD10 and smooth muscle myosin heavy chain. *J Clin Pathol.* 2004;57:625-629.

70. Moriya T, Kasajima A, Ishida K, et al. New trends of immunohistochemistry for making differential diagnosis of breast lesions. *Med Mol Morphol.* 2006;39:8-13.

CHAPTER 3

Metastasis

Alison L. Allan

Breast cancer remains a leading cause of morbidity and mortality in women,[1] mainly due to the propensity of primary breast tumors to metastasize to regional and distant sites and the failure of effective clinical management of metastatic disease.[2,3] Primary therapy for breast cancer usually involves surgical resection of the tumor (lumpectomy or mastectomy), alone or in combination with local radiotherapy. As discussed in later chapters, factors such as tumor size, grade, lymph node involvement, and hormonal status provide valuable information for prognosis. If the patient is felt to have a reasonably high probability of harboring micrometastases, then adjuvant systemic drug therapy (cytotoxic or hormonal) is usually recommended.[4] This adjuvant approach has several problems, including both unnecessary treatment of patients who may have been truly cured by their primary treatment alone, as well as the fact that many patients may relapse despite treatment (adjuvant therapy typically only reduces the risk of recurrence by 25-30%).[5] A better understanding of the biology of metastasis can improve clinical management and provide the potential for developing novel prognostic and/or therapeutic strategies to combat metastatic breast cancer. This chapter will review what is currently known about the metastatic process, including the timing and steps involved the metastatic cascade, the organ-specific nature of breast cancer metastasis, the contribution of specific molecular factors to metastatic disease, and the issue of tumor dormancy.

THE METASTATIC PROCESS

Timing of Metastasis—An Early or Late Event in Breast Cancer?

The prevailing paradigm of cancer development suggests that tumor cells sequentially accumulate multiple genetic mutations that allow them to evolve from a nonmalignant epithelial cell to a highly aggressive cancer cell, a process called multistep carcinogenesis.[6,7]

Until recently, it was believed that metastasis was therefore a late event in disease progression, such that additive genetic mutations allowed cancer cells to acquire the capacity to escape from the primary tumor and disseminate to distant organs as a final step in carcinogenesis. Certainly, the clinical reality that patients with large primary breast cancers are more likely to die from metastasis than patients with small tumors[8] was believed to reflect the late onset of metastatic spread. However, experimental and clinical observations have challenged this idea, and suggested that metastatic dissemination may in fact be an early event in the overall evolution of breast cancer.[9] For example, the observation that metastases can develop in patients with small primary tumors, before the diagnosis of the primary tumor, or even in the absence of a detectable primary tumor (so-called cancers of unknown origin)[10,11] indicates that a successful metastatic cell does not necessarily need to undergo a lengthy evolution within the primary site in order to be deadly. Furthermore, recent studies have indicated that the presence of individual tumor cells in the blood or bone marrow of breast cancer patients is an important early indicator of the potential for metastatic disease and poor prognosis.[12] Finally, global gene expression analyses of primary breast cancers have identified specific molecular signatures that predict the development of distant metastases,[13,14] suggesting that the ability to metastasize can be acquired early in breast cancer development.

Steps in the Metastatic Cascade

Over the past decade or so, significant inroads have been made towards elucidating the physical steps involved in metastasis. It is now widely accepted that, similar to multistep carcinogenesis, the metastatic process is comprised of a complex series of sequential events. In order for clinically relevant metastases to form, cancer cells must successfully complete each of these steps (Fig. 3-1).[2,3]

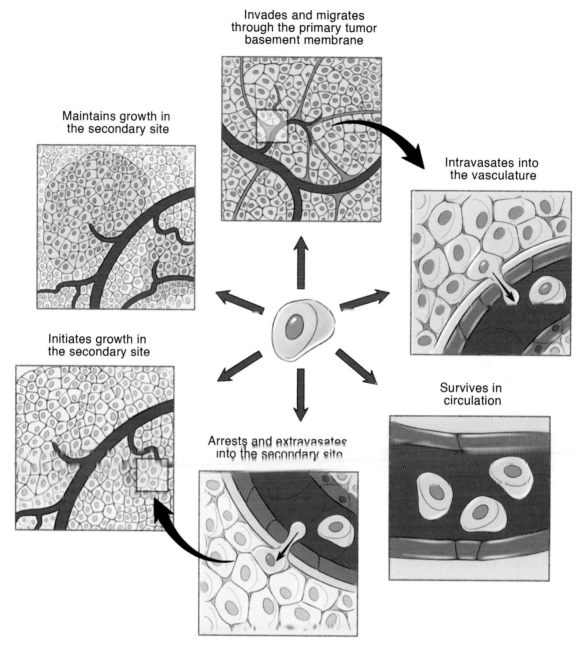

FIGURE 3-1 Metastasis is a complex, multistep process. The metastatic process is comprised of a complex series of sequential events. In order for clinically relevant metastases to form, cancer cells must successfully complete each of these steps. **(1)** Escape from the primary tumor. **(2)** Dissemination from the primary tumor via the blood or lymphatic system. **(3)** Survival within the circulation. **(4)** Extravasation into a secondary site. **(5)** Initiation of growth into micrometastases. **(6)** Maintenance of growth as a vascularized macrometastases. Based on the complexity of the metastatic process, it seems unlikely that all cancer cells would be able to successfully complete all the steps necessary to form macrometastases. Indeed, it is known that metastasis is a highly inefficient process, and that not all the steps of the metastatic process are equally inefficient. The principal rate-limiting steps are initiation of growth into micrometastases (step **5**) and maintenance of growth into macrometastases (step **6**).

Once a primary breast tumor grows beyond a certain size (~1-2 mm^3), there is a requirement for the growth of new blood vessels (angiogenesis) in order to supply the tumor with factors needed for metabolism and continued proliferation.[15] Vascularization of the primary tumor enhances the opportunity for tumor cells to enter the bloodstream, a process called intravasation. This requires cell–cell interactions between tumor cells and endothelial cells, which in turn leads to tumor cell adhesion, migration, and invasion through the extracellular matrix into the vasculature.[2,16] Since these newly formed blood vessels often lack an intact endothelial cell wall, they can provide a relatively accessible escape route for tumor cells to enter the circulation.[17] In addition, cells may also disseminate from the primary tumor through the lymphatic system. However, because there is no direct flow from the lymphatic system to other organs, cancer cells that escape via this route (a common occurrence in breast cancer) must still enter the venous system in order to be distributed to remote parts of the body.[2,3,18]

Cells that disseminate from the primary tumor and survive the challenges of host anti-tumor immune responses and hemodynamic shear stresses in the circulation are then carried to the capillary beds of secondary organs. Tumor cells are usually arrested by size restriction in the first capillary bed that they encounter, although some may pass through the first capillary bed and travel on to other secondary sites depending on regional blood pressure and deformability of the cells.[2,19] Arrested tumor cells can escape from the circulation (extravasate) by invading and migrating back through the endothelial cell wall, through the extracellular matrix, and into the secondary organ. Once in the new site, cells must initiate and maintain growth to form micrometastases, and (as with the primary tumor) these micrometastases require angiogenesis for nutrition and growth in order to grow into macroscopic tumors that are sufficiently large enough to cause physiologic effects on the patient.[15]

Metastasis Is Very Inefficient

The successful metastatic cell must therefore negotiate a number of different steps, including dissemination from the primary tumor via the blood or lymphatic system, survival within the circulation, extravasation into a secondary site, initiation of growth into micrometastases, and maintenance of growth as a vascularized macrometastases. Considering the onerous nature of this process, it is not surprising that several lines of experimental and clinical evidence indicate that metastasis is inherently inefficient[20] Experimental studies have shown that early steps in hematogenous metastasis (ie, survival in the bloodstream, extravasation) are remarkably efficient, with greater that 80% of cells successfully completing the metastatic process to this point. However, only a small subset of these cells (~ 2%,

depending on the experimental model) can initiate growth as micrometastases, and an even smaller subset (~ 0.02%, depending on the experimental model) are able to persist and grow into macroscopic tumors.[21] It is thus the later steps in metastasis involving growth at the secondary site that have been shown, at least in experimental models, to be highly inefficient. Indeed, these findings are supported by clinical observations that, despite the fact that patients diagnosed with cancer may have hundreds to thousands of single disseminated cancer cells that can be detected in the bloodstream and/or sites remote from the primary tumor, only a very small percentage progress to form overt macrometastases.[20,22]

ORGAN-SPECIFIC METASTASIS

Regulation of growth at the secondary site also differs depending on which organ the tumor cells metastasize to, and many cancers show an organ-specific pattern of metastasis. It is well established that breast cancer favors metastasis to regional lymph nodes, lung, liver, bone, and brain (Fig. 3-2).[2,3] From a pathohistologic point of view, breast tumor morphology from one metastatic site to the next can be very similar, and is often used as evidence of probable common origin when of the same morphology and grade as the primary breast tumor. It is believed that there are several factors that influence the organ-specific nature of breast cancer metastasis, and these are discussed next.

Circulatory Patterns and Mechanical Arrest

The movement of tumor cells within and between secondary organs is not random; rather, it depends to a large extent on the

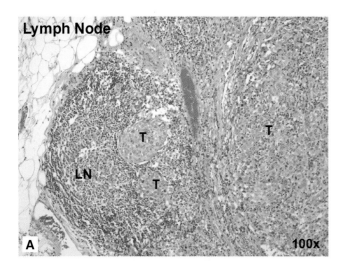
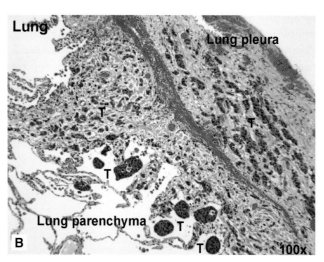

FIGURE 3-2 Breast cancer has "favorite" sites of metastasis. It is well established that breast cancer favors metastasis to specific organs including lymph node, lung, liver, bone, and brain. In breast cancer patients, pathohistologic analysis of hematoxylin and eosin (H&E) stained tissues from regional or distant organ sites can reveal the presence of metastatic tumor cells and provide a basis for prognosis and treatment decisions. **A.** Breast cancer metastasis to regional lymph node. In this patient, the metastatic breast tumor (*T*) has almost entirely occupied the node, with only a small amount of normal lymph node architecture (*LN*) still in evidence. **B.** Breast cancer metastasis to lung. In this patient, numerous nests of breast tumor cells (*T*) are evident in the lung parenchyma and invading into the pleura. It is believed that there are several factors that influence the organ-specific nature of breast cancer metastasis, including circulatory patterns, mechanical arrest, tumor cell homing, and the host tissue microenvironment. *(Images courtesy of Dr. Alan B. Tuck, London Health Sciences Centre Pathology Department, London, Ontario.)*

location of the primary tumor relative to the body's natural pattern of blood flow. For example, tumor cells that enter the circulation from most parts of the body (breast, liver, bone) are carried by the systemic venous system directly to the heart and then circulated to all organs of the body via the systemic arterial system. In contrast, cells entering the bloodstream from splanchnic organs such as the colon are circulated first through the liver via the hepatic portal vein, and then into the venous system.[16,22] In the 1920s, James Ewing proposed that blood flow patterns alone were sufficient to account for both the physical delivery of tumor cells to secondary organs and for patterns of organ-specific metastasis.[23] However, several theories have challenged this idea by proposing that there are additional, molecular-level mechanisms that explain why and how cancer cells can arrest and grow in "favorite" metastatic sites.

Metastatic Homing to Target Organs

The homing theory proposes that different organs produce chemoattractant factors, which can direct specific types of tumor cells to "home" to and arrest in a particular organ.[24] The most well-characterized of these molecules is the chemokine stromal-derived factor 1 (SDF-1) and its receptor CXCR4. In normal physiologic states, the SDF-1/CXCR4 axis is used for directed migration of several cell types, including stem cells, immune cells, and neurons.[25] SDF-1 is an ideal candidate for aiding in metastasis because of its ability to induce motility, homing responses, adhesion, and secretion of proteases and angiogenic factors in cells that express the CXCR4 receptor. Interestingly, it has been observed that CXCR4 is highly expressed in malignant breast cancer but not normal breast tissue, and that its ligand SDF-1 is expressed in organs to which breast cancer cells often metastasize (lymph node, lung, and bone).[26] In addition to chemokines, it has also been observed that endothelial cells forming the capillary beds in various organs can express a unique complement of cell surface molecules that serve as specific "homing addresses" or "vascular zip codes" for facilitating organ-specific metastasis. These molecules may offer specialized docking sites for breast cancer cells that express certain adhesion molecules on their surface, such as the integrin $\alpha v \beta 3$.[27]

Epithelial-to-Mesenchymal Transition

Another theory that has gained favor in recent years is the idea that epithelial–mesenchymal transition (EMT) can contribute to the metastatic process. First identified in embryonic development, EMT involves conversion of epithelial cells to a mesenchymal phenotype via loss of polarity, cell–cell contacts, and dramatic cytoskeletal remodeling.[28] Cells undergoing EMT also acquire expression of mesenchymal proteins and develop an enhanced ability to migrate, thus assisting in cell distribution throughout the embryo and organ development. In metastasis, it is believed that epithelial tumor cells may be able to somehow activate this primitive developmental program, thus converting differentiated epithelial cancer cells into de-differentiated cells that possess more mesenchymal characteristics. The EMT phenotype in cancer has been associated with increased resistance to apoptosis, increased motility and invasiveness,

and enhanced metastatic ability.[29] These phenotypic transitions are reversible, and it is hypothesized that once tumor cells have reached their destination, they may transform back into an epithelial phenotype (mesenchymal-to-epithelial transition; MET) in order to facilitate optimal tumor growth in the secondary site.

The Metastatic Microenvironment: "Seed and Soil"

Finally, the most central of metastasis theories is the "seed and soil" hypothesis, first proposed in 1889 by Stephen Paget.[30] Paget predicted that a cancer cell (the "seed") can survive and proliferate only in secondary sites (the "soil") that produce growth factors appropriate to that type of cell, and this theory has largely withstood the test of time.[31] In a meta-analysis of published autopsy study data, Weiss showed that, in many cases, metastases detected at autopsy were in proportion to the blood flow from the primary tumor site to the secondary organ.[22] However, in some cases, more metastases (notably breast cancer metastasis to bone) or fewer metastases were detected than would be expected by blood flow alone, indicating that the "soil" or microenvironment in the secondary organ is likely very important. In addition to mediating growth of tumor cells, it has been suggested that microenvironmental factors in the secondary site can also have significant influence on supporting tumor dormancy through suppression of immune mechanisms, angiogenesis, and alteration of growth-related signaling pathways[32] (discussed further below). Thus, the role of the microenvironment in the metastatic process is significant, particularly for the initiation/maintenance of metastatic growth and perhaps for the persistence of tumor dormancy within a secondary site.

It is unlikely that all of these theories are mutually exclusive; rather, the increasing number of molecular players that are thought to be involved in the metastatic cascade (Table 3-1) instead suggests that these various factors cooperate with mechanical influences such as blood flow in order to contribute to the ability of breast cancer cells to establish themselves as metastases in various target organs.

MOLECULAR FACTORS THAT CONTRIBUTE TO METASTASIS

Treatment for metastatic breast cancer has traditionally consisted of hormonal therapies and broad-spectrum chemotherapeutics. An improved understanding of cancer biology and the development of new technologies has led to a new generation of targeted agents directed against molecular factors involved in breast cancer progression and metastasis. A number of metastatic cell behaviors (angiogenesis, adhesion, migration, invasion, and growth) also play an important role in tightly regulated normal biological processes such as reproduction, embryogenesis, and wound healing. The fundamental difference between normal cells and cancer cells is thought to lie in their ability to be regulated at the biochemical level: in cancer cells, the molecules that start, maintain, or stop these cellular processes are often expressed at inappropriate levels or at an

TABLE 3-1 Molecular Factors That Contribute to Metastasis

Type of Molecule	Example(s)	Function in Metastasis	Targeted Therapies
Oncogenic proteins	Ras	Survival and growth at the metastatic site	Farnesyltransferase inhibitors (FTIs): Tipifarnib[a] Lonafarnib[a]
Growth factors/ receptors	EGF/EGFR	Angiogenesis, motility, survival, growth	Trastuzumab[b] Lapatinib[a]
	VEGF/VEGFR		Bevacizumab[b] Sunitinib[a] Sorafenib[a]
Integrins	αvβ3	Motility, invasion, growth	Vitaxin[a] Etaracizumab[a]
Chemokines/cytokines	CXCR4	Adhesion, motility, invasion, growth, survival, angiogenesis	AMD3100[a,c]
	OPN		??
Proteases	MMPs	Adhesion, motility, invasion, survival, organ-specific metastasis, growth	MMP inhibitors[c]
Metastasis suppressors	NM23	Initiation and maintenance of growth at the metastatic site	MPA[c]

References can be found in the appropriate sections in the text. This table shows only a representative selection of the many metastasis-associated molecules discovered to date.
[a]Investigational drug in phase I/II/III clinical trials for breast and/or other cancers.
[b]Approved drug.
[c]Preclinical investigation only.

inappropriate time and place.[7] A growing number of molecular factors have been identified as being dysregulated during metastasis.[33,34] Furthermore, the metastatic process requires the coordinated interplay of a variety of cell types, including tumor cells, endothelial cells, stromal cells, and immune cells. These critical cell–cell and cell–matrix communications are regulated by pro-metastatic and anti-metastatic molecular signals that facilitate the successful completion of the various steps of metastasis (Table 3-1). A selection of these factors and their potential as therapeutic targets are discussed below.

Metastasis-Promoting Factors

Metastasis-promoting factors can contribute to the acquisition of a metastatic cellular phenotype through increased expression and/or activation, usually as result of abnormal regulation. These include a variety of different protein types, such as oncogenic proteins, growth and angiogenic factors, integrin receptors, chemoattractant molecules, and enzymes that degrade the extracellular matrix.

Oncogenic Proteins

Oncogenes code for proteins that are important for the regulation of cellular growth control and responsiveness to extracellular signals. When these control mechanisms are constitutively up-regulated in the absence of external growth signals, the uncontrolled proliferation that is typical of cancer cells can occur.[7] Members of the Ras oncogene family provide an example of how

activated oncogenes can lead to phenotypic changes that promote metastasis.[35] Ras oncogenes encode a family of membrane-bound proteins that act as cellular transducers, relaying signals from the cell surface to the cytoplasm, which in turn activate signaling cascades that regulate the expression of a number of different genes. In addition to activating the Ras/Raf/ERK-MAPK (extracellular signal-regulated kinase/mitogen-activated protein kinase) pathway, Ras is also involved in activation other signaling pathways, such as the phosphatidylinositol 3-kinase (PI3K) pathway. Oncogenes such as Ras thus have the potential to contribute to all steps in the metastatic process via activation of angiogenic factors, adhesion molecules, proteases, growth-related genes, and/or survival factors.

Breast cancers have been reported to have a very low (< 2%) incidence of Ras mutation; however, dysregulation of Ras and its associated signaling pathways is believed to be common.[36] The rate-limiting step in Ras activation is farnesylation by farnesyl protein transferase. A class of drugs called protein farnesyltransferase inhibitors (FTIs; tipifarnib and lonafarnib) are potent inhibitors of farnesyl transferase and have shown efficacy in preclinical models of breast cancer. Clinically, phase I/II trials in breast cancer patients have also shown encouraging results with FTIs, particularly as combination therapy with taxane-based chemotherapies and endocrine therapy.[36,37] Although the particular step(s) of metastasis that are influenced by oncogenes remain to be fully elucidated, studies have demonstrated that Ras activation is important for regulating the ability of tumor cells to initiate and maintain growth of micrometastases once they have arrived at the secondary site.[35] It has been observed that the balance between proliferation and apoptosis can be tipped in favor of growth in micrometastases with activated Ras, and in favor of death in Ras-negative micrometastases, suggesting that disruption of the proliferation- to- apoptosis equilibrium to favor progressive growth is one mechanism by which oncogenic signaling can influence metastatic potential.

Growth Factors/Receptors

A number of growth/angiogenic factors and their cognate receptors have been identified as important contributors to breast cancer metastasis. The best characterized of these include members of the epidermal growth factor receptor (EGFR) family (most notably ErbB-2/HER-2), and vascular endothelial growth factors (VEGF) and their receptors (VEGFR).

The EGFR family is comprised of four closely related tyrosine kinase growth factor receptors: EGFR (ErbB-1), HER-2 (ErbB-2), HER-3 (ErbB-3), and HER-4 (ErbB-4). These receptors bind growth factor ligands such as epidermal growth factor (EGF) and transforming growth factor α (TGF α). After ligand binding, the receptor is activated by phosphorylation, which in turn initiates a cascade of downstream intracellular events via the Ras/Raf/MAPK signaling pathway. The EGFR family functionally contributes to a variety of processes that are crucial to metastasis, including cytoskeletal reorganization, adhesion, motility, invasion, angiogenesis, survival, and growth.[38]

In breast cancer, HER-2 has been found to be an important prognostic and predictive factor both in the adjuvant and metastatic settings. HER-2 is amplified/overexpressed in 20% to 25% of breast cancers, and is associated with aggressive disease and poor prognosis.[39] The HER-2 targeting monoclonal antibody trastuzumab (Herceptin) is approved for the first-line treatment of HER2-positive metastatic breast cancer in combination with chemotherapy, and provides a clear advantage in improving clinical outcome.[40,41] Trastuzumab is also approved for use as a single agent in patients who have received at least one prior chemotherapy regimen, and has shown promise in phase III investigation for use in the adjuvant and neoadjuvant settings.[42] Overall, trastuzumab and other emerging HER-2 agents such as lapatinib (which also targets EGFR) provide an exciting opportunity to provide tailored therapy and change the standard of care for this patient subset.

Another example of important growth factor/receptor pathways in breast cancer is the VEGF/VEGFR family. Through paracrine and autocrine interactions with endothelial cells, tumor cells, and immune cells, VEGF and VEGFR have been shown to play a variety of roles in the tumor microenvironment, including stimulation of angiogenesis, protection from host anti-tumor immune responses, and promotion of tumor and endothelial cell survival/growth. VEGF gene expression can be regulated by a number of stimuli, including oncogenes, tumor suppressors, other growth factors (eg, HER-2), and tumor hypoxia.[15,43] The expression of VEGF has been shown to be up-regulated in a number of different human tumor types, and has been correlated with poor prognosis in breast cancer. Studies have also indicated that there is a correlation between high VEGF levels and lack of response to radiation or chemotherapy.[44,45] The monoclonal antibody therapy bevacizumab

directly targets VEGF and has recently been approved for first-line treatment of metastatic breast cancer in combination with chemotherapy. In addition, other antiangiogenic small-molecule inhibitors targeting VEGFR are being investigated in phase II/III breast cancer trials, including sunitinib, sorafenib, and several others.[43] Because of their central role in angiogenesis, VEGF and VEGFR are therefore promising therapeutic targets in breast cancer.

Integrin Receptors

Integrins are family of dimeric transmembrane receptors comprised of α and β subunits. At least 25 different heterodimers can be formed by noncovalent associations between subunits, and integrin-ligand associations often occur through a specific RGD (arginine-glycine-aspartic acid) domain present on integrin-binding proteins. Each heterodimer can bind a wide variety of ligands, including extracellular matrix (ECM) proteins (eg, laminin, vitronectin) and the metastasis-promoting protein osteopontin (OPN). Integrins can also coordinate with growth factor pathways (eg, VEGF/VEGFR, EGF/EGFR) to activate a number of signaling cascades such as the focal adhesion kinase (FAK)-Src cascade, the PI3K cascade, and the Ras/Raf/ERK cascade. Therefore, although originally identified as important cell-surface adhesion receptors that mechanically link the cytoskeleton to the ECM or to other cells during cellular migration and invasion, integrins have more recently been recognized as key signaling receptors capable of influencing migration, growth, survival, and angiogenesis.[46] The involvement of integrins in so many aspects of cancer progression underlines the importance of these signaling receptors in regulating the metastatic process.

Integrins have been shown to have prognostic value for a number of human cancers.[46] In particular, it is believed that there is significant involvement of integrins that contain αv, α6, and/or β1 subunits. For example, increased expression of the αvβ3 integrin has been associated with metastatic breast cancer,[47] and expression of α6β1 or α6β4 integrins has been shown to increase experimental invasion and metastasis of breast cancer cells in association with various signaling pathways.[48,49] In addition, activated vascular endothelial cells express a number of integrins (most notably αvβ3) that have been found to be important for regulating angiogenesis and organ-specific metastasis.[46] Genetic polymorphisms in genes encoding integrin β4 and integrin β3 have been observed to have prognostic value in breast cancer, including an association with increased tumor grade, stage, and/or a higher risk of regional and distant metastasis.[50,51] Recently, radiolabeled RGD peptides have shown promise for clinical imaging of metastatic disease in breast cancer patients, since these peptides display increased uptake by tumors with high integrin expression.[52] Finally, monoclonal antibodies targeting the αvβ3 integrin (eg, vitaxin, etaracizumab) are currently under phase I/II clinical investigation,[53,54] and these hold promise as future targeted agents for treatment of breast cancer metastasis.

Chemokines/Cytokines

As discussed earlier, the chemokine SDF-1 and its receptor CXCR4 have been shown to play an important role in breast cancer metastasis. Experimental studies have demonstrated that breast cancer cells treated with a CXCR4 inhibitor show significantly reduced metastatic ability.[55] The CXCR4 inhibitor AMD3100 has been tested in phase I/II clinical trials for hematologic malignancies,[56] although its possible use in clinical management of breast cancer has not yet been explored.

Another well-characterized chemoattractant protein is the secreted cytokine osteopontin (OPN). Clinical studies have demonstrated that OPN is overexpressed in many human cancers, and has been associated with breast cancer progression. In particular, there is a strong correlation between elevated OPN levels in patients with breast cancer and increased tumor aggressiveness, increased tumor burden, and poor prognosis/survival.[57,58] OPN can be produced in the tumor microenvironment by both tumor cells and other surrounding cells, such as fibroblasts, inflammatory cells, or endothelial cells. The OPN protein can interact with a diverse range of factors, including integrins, growth factor/receptor pathways (VEGF/VEGFR, EGF/EGFR), and secreted proteases. These complex signaling interactions can result in changes in gene expression that ultimately lead to increased metastatic behavior.[59] Taken together with the clinical observations, these experimental studies indicate that OPN is not merely associated with breast cancer, but that it actually plays a multifaceted functional role in disease progression.

Proteases

In metastasis, the process of tissue invasion requires breakdown of the extracellular matrix, and this is facilitated by a class of proteins called proteases. One such example is the matrix metalloproteinase (MMP) family, which are produced as proenzymes that require extracellular activation through proteolytic cleavage of an amino terminal domain. Under normal physiologic conditions, the net activity of MMPs is tightly regulated by maintaining an equilibrium between levels of activated MMPs and levels of their endogenous inhibitors, known as tissue inhibitors of metalloproteinases (TIMPs). However, during cancer progression, this balance is often altered in favor of enhanced cellular invasiveness via increased production of MMPs by a number of cell types, including fibroblasts, infiltrating immune cells, endothelial cells, and tumor cells. Based on the inherent degradative activity of MMPs, it was originally believed that the major contribution of these enzymes to the metastatic process only occurred during the steps of intravasation and extravasation. However, a number of studies have suggested that their role in cancer progression is more complex than first hypothesized, including having both pro- and anti-tumor effects.[60] Although the detailed mechanisms by which MMPs can regulate the tumor growth environment remain to be elucidated, it has been proposed that they may facilitate the release of sequestered growth factors in the extracellular matrix surrounding the growing tumor. Therefore, MMPs may provide important functional contributions to breast cancer metastasis through roles in angiogenesis, intravasation, extravasation, and growth of distant metastases.

The overexpression of MMPs has been positively correlated with increasing tumor stage in many types of human cancer, and this is reflected by both an increase in the relative expression levels of individual MMPs as well as an increase in the number of different MMP family members that are expressed.[61] Unfortunately, phase III clinical trials for broad-spectrum MMP inhibitors (MMPIs) showed disappointing results, potentially due to the inadvertent inhibition of MMP activity for other physiologic processes that counterbalanced the benefits of MMP inhibition targeting the metastatic process.[60,62] However, the continued development of third-generation, highly specific MMPIs is under active preclinical investigation as a novel therapeutic strategy for breast and other cancers.

In summary, although only a small selection of the known metastasis-promoting molecules has been presented here, the studies discussed in this section representatively illustrate the important concept that the development of metastasis requires the coordinated expression and function of many different genes. Conversely, it can be theoretically predicted that only one gene might be required to block metastasis, since the failure to complete any particular step in the metastatic process could result in the loss of a cell's metastatic potential. An emerging field of study involving metastasis suppressor genes is aimed at testing this theory.

Metastasis Suppressor Genes

Metastasis suppressor genes can be broadly defined as genes that suppress the ability of metastases to form, without affecting the growth of the primary tumor.[34] These genes have been identified by their reduced or absent expression in metastatic tumor cells relative to tumorigenic but nonmetastatic cells. Similar to the paradigm of tumor suppressors such as p53 and Rb,[63] it is thought that the loss of metastasis suppressor gene function can lead to an escape from normal cellular control and the development of metastasis. Accordingly, the restoration of metastasis suppressor gene function should lead to suppression or interruption of the metastatic cascade.

Within the last two decades, at least 23 such metastasis suppressor genes have been identified. Although the molecular mechanisms by which these genes can suppress metastasis are not yet fully understood, growing evidence suggests that their main functional effect may be to inhibit the ability of tumor cells to initiate and maintain growth of metastases at the secondary site via mediation of important signal transduction pathways. Several metastasis suppressor genes have been reported to have low expression in different human tumor types, and in many cases this reduced expression can be correlated with advanced tumor stage and/or poor patient prognosis.[34] From a therapeutic perspective, metastasis suppressor genes hold promise as "drugable" targets for therapeutic intervention. Upregulation of these molecules via gene therapy approaches has been suggested as a possible strategy, although technical issues with gene delivery make this impractical at the present time. However, medroxyprogesterone acetate (MPA), a progestin that has been tested as treatment for advanced breast cancer, has been shown to elevate expression of the Nm23 metastasis suppressor gene and reduce metastasis in preclinical models of breast cancer.[64] Thus, there is potential for development of metastasis suppressor-specific drugs that may be valuable as targeted agents in the future.

Can Molecular Signatures Predict Breast Cancer Metastasis?

Dysregulation of the balance between the expression of genes that promote metastasis and the expression of genes that suppress metastasis can therefore influence a cell's ability to successfully complete all the steps in the metastatic cascade. The ongoing development of high-throughput molecular analysis tools such as DNA microarray technology may provide a more accurate picture of the relationship between genes, metastasis, and the development of tailored therapy regimes based on the individual molecular characteristics of a patient's tumor.

Several large-cohort clinical studies have illustrated the value of microarray-mediated gene profiling as a tool for predicting patient survival in different types of cancer including breast cancer. A 70-gene "signature" of primary breast tumors has been shown to more accurately predict the likelihood of metastasis development and patient outcome than current clinical and histologic criteria such as age, lymph node status, histologic tumor grade, and ER status.[13] Another 21-gene signature assay called Oncotype Dx has been shown to provide a "recurrence score" that has been validated for quantifying the likelihood of distant recurrence in tamoxifen-treated patients with node-negative, ER+ breast cancer.[65] Finally, a study by Ramaswamy and associates analyzed the gene expression profile of metastases from multiple solid tumor types (breast, uterine, ovarian, colon, prostate, and lung) relative to the gene expression profile of primary tumors from the same tumor spectrum. A 17-gene molecular signature comprised of 8 up-regulated and 9 down-regulated genes was present in some primary tumors, and these tumors were most likely to be associated with metastasis development and poor clinical outcome.[14] Not surprisingly, these molecular signatures include changes in the expression patterns of several genes that encode the functional classes of proteins already discussed. The undeniable power of microarrays as tools for high-throughput gene expression analysis is reflected by the contributions that they continue to make toward the elucidation of molecular aspects of metastasis. Moreover, the chance that these valuable tools could be used in the clinical setting for the benefit of patients is an exciting prospect, and this is discussed in further detail below.

METASTASIS AND TUMOR DORMANCY

Metastatic spread after the removal of a primary tumor can ultimately be difficult to identify, creating uncertainty in patients with regards to possible cancer recurrence. This is a particular problem in breast cancer, exemplified by the fact that recurrence can take place after decades of apparent disease-free survival.[66] This observation, referred to as clinical tumor dormancy, is also supported by studies involving individuals undergoing autopsy for other, non-cancer-related) causes of death such as accidents or trauma.[67,68] These studies, summarized by Black and Welsh,[68] report that carcinoma in situ can be found in the breasts of 39% of women age 40 to 50 years, even though only 1% of women are ever diagnosed with breast cancer during life in the same age range. The mechanisms underlying tumor dormancy in breast cancer remain poorly understood, and this presents significant challenges to both experimental investigation and clinical management of breast cancer. This final section will review what is currently known about metastasis and tumor dormancy, and consider the growing evidence that cancer stem cells may play a role in this process.

Dormancy Contributes to Metastatic Inefficiency

As discussed earlier, metastatic inefficiency can occur at two critical steps of the metastatic process: initiation of growth from single cells to micrometastases, and persistence of growth into macrometastases. Once individual tumor cells arrive in the secondary site, they may experience one of three fates: they may die, they may proliferate to form micrometastases, or they may remain viable but dormant (Fig. 3-3). These dormant solitary cells are defined by the absence of either growth or apoptosis, and this quiescent state likely conveys protection from many conventional cytotoxic drugs that only target actively cycling cells.[2] It is currently unknown whether these solitary dormant cells represent a specialized subpopulation of cells that are programmed to stay dormant, an unspecialized population of cells that are not well suited to grow in the new microenvironment, or a combination of both.[32]

If these solitary cells do begin to proliferate and go on to form micrometastases, they may again experience one of 3 fates at this next stage: they may die, they may continue to grow into vascularized macrometastases, or they may persist as "dormant" micrometastases, where dormancy at this stage is defined as a balance between proliferation and apoptosis within the cell population such that there is no net increase in the size of micrometastases (Fig 3-3).[2,69] This type of dormancy is associated with an inability to recruit new blood vessels to support further tumor growth, potentially via the protective effect of microenvironmental factors that prevent the "angiogenic switch."[67] Both these dormant micrometastases and solitary dormant cells are believed to contribute to clinical dormancy and cancer recurrence.

Clinical Evidence for Dormancy

One of the biggest challenges in studying tumor dormancy in breast cancer patients is that until recently, this phenomenon has been defined clinically as the "disease-free" period between treatment of the initial cancer and recurrence, and therefore could only be applied to patients who underwent a recurrence. Thus, the identification of patients harboring dormant cancer was close to impossible, and as a result the prevalence of clinical dormancy is likely underestimated.[66] In fact, the persistence of disease at a low or undetectable level (so-called minimal residual disease) may be a common feature of breast cancer. This is supported by the autopsy findings discussed earlier,[67,68] as well as the accumulating evidence that breast cancer patients with apparently localized disease (ie, no indication of metastatic spread by current clinical parameters) have individual tumor cells in their bone marrow and/or blood.[12]

Studies have shown that detection of isolated tumor cells in the bone marrow is an independent prognostic factor, and

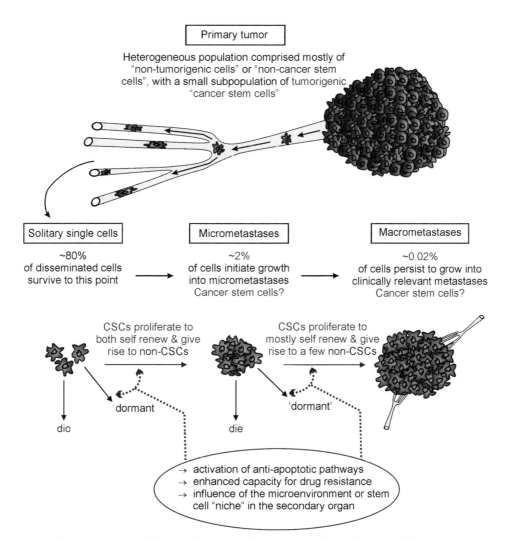

FIGURE 3-3 Cancer stem cells, metastasis, and tumor dormancy in breast cancer. The inefficiency of the metastatic process, the inherently heterogeneous nature of solid tumors, and the influence of the tumor microenvironment dictate that only a small subset of cells (shown in red) can successfully navigate the metastatic cascade and eventually reinitiate tumor growth to form life-threatening metastases. The cancer stem cell theory also predicts that only a limited number of cells within a heterogeneous tumor are capable of initiating tumorigenic growth, and that this phenotypically distinct subset of cells are cancer stem cells (CSCs). Several classical properties of normal stem cells are strikingly reminiscent of the observed experimental and clinical behavior of metastatic breast cancer cells, including a high capacity for self-renewal, activation of antiapoptotic pathways, increased drug resistance, and the requirement for a supportive "niche" or microenvironment to grow. Furthermore, experimental models of tumor dormancy have demonstrated that these influences can also play significant roles in maintaining tumor dormancy or triggering proliferation and disease progression. By applying the cancer stem cell theory to breast cancer metastasis and tumor dormancy, it can be hypothesized that the subset of cells within a primary breast tumor that are capable of initiating and maintaining metastatic growth in secondary sites (shown in red) may in fact be cancer stem cells. Understanding the role that cancer stem cells play in determining tumor dormancy and metastatic potential could have significant implications for the way we currently study and treat breast cancer. *(Reprinted from Allan AL, Vantyghem SA, Tuck AB, Chambers AF. Tumor dormancy and cancer stem cells: implications for the biology and treatment of breast cancer metastasis. Breast Dis. 2006;26:87-98.)*

approximately 30% of breast cancer patients may have micrometastatic disease in their bone marrow at initial presentation. However, only 30% to 50% of these patients will go on to develop clinically evident metastases within 5 years.[70-74] From a biological perspective, these observations suggest that the progression of dormant tumor cells to macrometastases depends on one or more factors, including the specific characteristics of individual disseminated tumor cells, the characteristics of individual patients (anti-tumor immune response), and/or the influence of

the metastatic microenvironment. Therefore, the simple presence of these cells in the bone marrow does not adequately reflect the phenotypic programming and biological heterogeneity of these cells, and is consequently unable to predict their individual potential to remain dormant or progress to clinically relevant metastases. This heterogeneity has led to the hypothesis that only a small percentage of cells in a tumor cell population are capable of reinitiating growth to form metastases in distant sites, and that these cells may in fact be so-called cancer stem cells.[32,75]

Cancer Stem Cells, Metastasis, and Tumor Dormancy

Recently, there has been increasing support for the cancer stem cell hypothesis and speculation about the role of such cells in tumor dormancy.[32,76-78] This hypothesis predicts that cancer arises from a subpopulation of tumor-initiating cells or cancer stem cells (CSC), where a CSC is defined as a cancer cell that has the ability to both self-renew to give rise to another malignant CSC, as well as undergo differentiation to give rise to the phenotypically diverse (and nonmalignant) cell population that makes up the rest of the tumor.[79] There are currently two conflicting views that attempt to explain tumor formation.[77] The classical stochastic model suggests that every cell within a tumor is a potential tumor initiator, but that entry into the cell cycle is governed by a low probability of stochastic mutations. According to this model, it would be impossible to tell which cell initiated the tumor, since each cell should have an equal ability to be malignant. In contrast, the hierarchy theory (upon which the CSC hypothesis is based) proposes that only a small subset of cells in a tumor are capable of initiating tumor growth, but that these cells all do so at a high frequency. According to this theory, it should be possible to identify the cells responsible for tumor initiation and progression (either in the primary or secondary site) because not all cells have the same phenotypic and functional characteristics.[77,78]

In breast cancer patients, prospective CSCs have been isolated from primary tumors and pleural effusions based on a CD44+CD24− phenotype.[80] Subsequent experimental studies have shown that CD44+CD24− breast cancer cells demonstrate increased expression of stem cell markers and an enhanced capacity for invasion and self-renewal.[80-83] Furthermore, clinical studies indicate that CD44+CD24− tumor-initiating cells express an invasive gene signature[84] and may be associated with aggressive basal-like (triple-negative) disease[85] and distant metastases.[86]

Metastatic inefficiency and tumor dormancy have been attributed to inability to grow in certain microenvironments; however, with the emergence of the CSC hypothesis, it is possible to add a new dimension to this concept. Since CSCs have an enhanced ability to initiate and sustain tumorigenic growth, then it is probable that the CSCs within the primary tumor also represent the successful metastatic cells (Fig. 3-3). Normal stem cells, CSCs, and metastatic cells demonstrate strikingly similar characteristics, including the requirement for a particular niche or microenvironment in which to survive and grow; enhanced resistance to apoptosis; and cell dormancy as a mechanism of survival and self-protection.[75,77,87,88] In particular, the CSC hypothesis and the idea that the most primitive CSCs may undergo periods of quiescence has major therapeutic implications for treatment of both primary and metastatic disease. Current chemotherapeutics may not be targeting the right cells; instead they may be targeting and reducing bulky disease while leaving a reservoir of the tumor cells responsible for metastatic progression untouched. It has been speculated that the proportion of CSCs within a tumor may correlate with disease stage, and may also increase with therapy as a reflection of treatment resistance.[76] Further elucidation of the role that CSCs play in determining tumor dormancy and metastatic potential will

therefore be extremely important for the way we currently study, diagnosis, and treat breast cancer.

FUTURE DIRECTIONS

Despite the fact that the majority of breast cancer deaths occur due to the physiologic effects of metastasis rather than from the consequences of the primary tumor, much remains to be learned about this deadly process. A major area of research that is needed to address this problem involves gaining a greater understanding of the metastatic process as a whole, such that current therapies can be better utilized to target metastatic disease, and new, more effective therapies can be developed that will better treat or prevent breast cancer metastasis. The section "Molecular Factors That Contribute to Metastasis" in this chapter describes some of the exciting progress being made in elucidating the molecular pathways that contribute to metastasis, and the growing number of novel targeted therapies that are showing promise in the laboratory and in clinical trials (Table 3-1). In addition, the ability to identify specific molecular characteristics of a patient's tumor will improve clinical decision-making and pave the way for tailored, individualized therapy. Two ongoing clinical trials aim to address the challenge of integrating molecular diagnostic testing into clinical practice.

MINDACT and TAILORx Trials

The purpose of the MINDACT trial is to validate the clinical use of the 70-gene profile initially identified by van't Veer and associates using the MammaPrint gene expression chip.[13,89] This is a large, multicenter, prospective randomized controlled trial that started accrual in February 2007 with a goal of recruiting 6000 node-negative breast cancer patients. Patient risk of relapse will be assessed based on both traditional clinical parameters and by the MammaPrint gene signature. If both approaches identify a patient's risk of relapse as high, then adjuvant chemotherapy will be proposed. If both approaches identify risk of relapse as low, then adjuvant chemotherapy will be withheld. If the two methods give discordant results, patients will be randomized to follow the standard clinicopathologic method or the MammaPrint results. The important subgroup of patients will be those classified as high clinical risk but low MammaPrint risk and randomly assigned to follow the MammaPrint results. It is anticipated that these women will be spared unnecessary therapy, without having any negative impact in their survival.

The TAILORx trial (ECOG PACCT-1) utilizes the 21-gene signature Oncotype Dx assay.[65] This multicenter, partially randomized trial opened in May 2006, and aims to enroll 10,000 women with recently diagnosed, node-negative, HER2-negative, estrogen-receptor and/or progesterone-receptor positive breast cancer.[90] Oncotype Dx utilizes a recurrence score (RS) system. In TAILORx, patients with RS less than 11 (low risk) will receive hormonal therapy only, patients with RS more than 25 (high risk) will receive both chemotherapy and hormonal therapy, and patients with RS from 11 to 25 (intermediate risk) will be randomized to receive either hormonal therapy alone or combination chemotherapy and hormonal therapy. Similar to the MINDACT trial, it is expected that Oncotype Dx will be

TABLE 3-2 Necessary Future Studies to Advance the Field

Description of Research Required	Future Directions
Development of molecular therapies to target breast cancer metastasis	• Continue with ongoing clinical trials (Table 3-1) • Continue with preclinical investigation and development of new agents
Development of tailored, individualized therapy approaches for breast cancer	• MINDACT trial • TAILORx trial
Development of reliable surrogate marker approaches for tracking breast cancer progression and response to therapy	• SWOG S0500 CTC trial
Improved understanding of tumor dormancy and how to exploit this for clinical management of breast cancer	• Development of better experimental model systems for studying breast cancer dormancy • Clinical drug development of agents designed to up-regulate/activate metastasis-suppressor genes
Improved understanding of the role of cancer stem cells in breast cancer metastasis and response to therapy	• Identification of reliable cancer stem cell markers and design of experimental studies investigating the role of these cells in metastasis • Clinical drug development of agents designed to target the "stem cell-like" characteristics of these cells

able to identify patients who can be spared unnecessary treatment if chemotherapy is not likely to be of substantial benefit over hormonal therapy alone. By integrating molecular diagnostic testing into the clinical decision-making process in these two trials, clinicians will be better able to stratify risk in the adjuvant setting and make more informed decisions regarding appropriate treatment options.

Circulating Tumor Cells—SWOG S0500 Trial

A second important and much needed area of metastasis research is the development of reliable surrogate marker approaches that will allow close monitoring of both disease progression and response to therapy. The SWOG S0500 trial is designed to test the strategy of changing therapy versus maintaining therapy for metastatic breast cancer patients who have elevated circulating tumor cell (CTC) levels at first follow-up.[91] Opened in October 2006, this is a multicenter, partially randomized trial that aims to enroll 500 patients with confirmed stage IV (metastatic) disease undergoing first-line chemotherapy. Patients with less than 5 CTCs at baseline (low risk) will receive standard chemotherapy without change. Patients with 5 or more CTCs at baseline will undergo a second blood draw after completion of the first course of chemotherapy. Of these patients, women with less than 5 CTCs after completing one course of chemotherapy will continue to receive the same chemotherapy regimen with no change. Patients with 5 or more CTCs after completion of one course of chemotherapy will be randomized to either continue with the same chemotherapy or switch to a different regimen. This trial will hopefully provide information regarding whether it is more effective to change treatment regimens at the time of CTC increase or wait until disease progression, thus reflecting the efficacy (or lack of efficacy) of chemotherapy in individual patients and facilitating better treatment decisions.

Looking Forward

Elucidation of the mechanisms controlling metastasis and the development of therapeutic strategies to target this deadly process remain some of the most important and provocative challenges in breast oncology. As our understanding of the cellular and molecular mechanisms of metastasis continues to evolve, this knowledge will be translated into the clinic for improved surrogate marker approaches, rational and effective drug design, individualized therapy approaches, and the ultimate goal of successful treatment of metastatic breast cancer.

SUMMARY

Breast cancer metastasis is a complex, multistep process that includes dissemination from the primary tumor, survival within the blood or lymphatic system, extravasation into a secondary organ, initiation of growth into micrometastases, and maintenance of growth into macrometastases. The metastatic process is highly inefficient, with the main rate-limiting steps being initiation and maintenance of growth at the secondary site (Fig. 3-1).

Breast cancer displays an organ-specific pattern of metastasis, favoring dissemination and growth in lymph nodes, lung, liver, brain, and bone (Fig. 3-2). Combined with blood flow patterns and homing mechanisms, it is believed that this organ-specific metastasis is dictated by the fact that a cancer cell (the "seed") can survive and proliferate only in secondary sites (the "soil") that produce growth factors appropriate to breast cancer cells.

A number of classes of pro- and anti-metastatic molecular factors have been identified as being involved in breast cancer metastasis, including oncogenic proteins, growth factor/receptors, integrins, chemoattractant molecules, and proteases. Several novel therapies targeting these factors are currently under investigation for treating metastasis (Table 3-1).

Tumor dormancy is a particular problem in breast cancer patients, and may create uncertainty with regards to disease recurrence as well as reduce the effectiveness of standard cytotoxic therapy designed to target actively cycling cells. The growing evidence supporting the cancer stem cell hypothesis suggests that breast cancer cells with "stem cell–like" characteristics may play a key role in metastasis and tumor dormancy (Fig. 3-3).

Several studies are still necessary to advance the field of metastasis, and these are summarized in Table 3-2.

ACKNOWLEDGMENTS

The author thanks members of her laboratory and her collaborators for their research work and helpful discussions. The author's work on breast cancer metastasis is supported by funding from the Canadian Breast Cancer Research Alliance, the Canada Foundation for Innovation, the Ontario Institute for Cancer Research, and the Imperial Oil Foundation. Review articles have been cited whenever possible, and readers are referred to these for citations of primary papers. Apologies to authors whose work could not be cited directly because of space restrictions.

REFERENCES

1. Jemal A, Siegel R, Ward E, et al. Cancer statistics, 2008. *CA Cancer J Clin.* 2008;58:71-96.
2. Chambers AF, Groom AC, MacDonald IC. Dissemination and growth of cancer cells in metastatic sites. *Nat Rev Cancer.* 2002;2:563-572.
3. Pantel K, Brakenhoff RH. Dissecting the metastatic cascade. *Nat Rev Cancer.* 2004;4:448-456.
4. Early Breast Cancer Trialists' Collaborative Group. Effects of chemotherapy and hormonal therapy for early breast cancer on recurrence and 15-year survival: an overview of the randomised trials. *Lancet.* 2005;365: 1687-1717.
5. Early Breast Cancer Trialists' Collaborative Group. Polychemotherapy for early breast cancer: an overview of the randomised trials. *Lancet.* 1998;352:930-942.
6. Fearon ER, Vogelstein B. A genetic model for colorectal tumorigenesis. *Cell.* 1990;61:759-767.
7. Hanahan D, Weinberg RA. The hallmarks of cancer. *Cell.* 2000;100:57-70.
8. Yamashiro H, Toi M. Update of evidence in chemotherapy for breast cancer. *Int J Clin Oncol.* 2008;13:3-7.
9. Klein CA. Gene expression signatures, cancer cell evolution and metastatic progression. *Cell Cycle.* 2004;3:29-31.
10. Engel J, Eckel R, Kerr J, et al. The process of metastasisation for breast cancer. *Eur J Cancer.* 2003;39:1794-1806.
11. van de Wouw AJ, Janssen-Heijnen ML, Coebergh JW, Hillen HF. Epidemiology of unknown primary tumours; incidence and population-based survival of 1285 patients in Southeast Netherlands, 1984-1992. *Eur J Cancer.* 2002;38:409-413.
12. Riethdorf S, Pantel K. Disseminated tumor cells in bone marrow and circulating tumor cells in blood of breast cancer patients: current state of detection and characterization. *Pathobiology.* 2008;75:140-148.
13. van't Veer LJ, Dai H, van de Vijver MJ, et al. Gene expression profiling predicts clinical outcome of breast cancer. *Nature.* 2002;415:530-536.
14. Ramaswamy S, Ross KN, Lander ES, Golub TR. A molecular signature of metastasis in primary solid tumors. *Nat Genet.* 2003;33:49-54.
15. Folkman J. Fundamental concepts of the angiogenic process. *Curr Mol Med.* 2003;3:643-651.
16. MacDonald IC, Groom AC, Chambers AF. Cancer spread and micrometastasis development: quantitative approaches for in vivo models. *Bioessays.* 2002;24:885-893.
17. Butler TP, Gullino PM. Quantitation of cell shedding into efferent blood of mammary adenocarcinoma. *Cancer Res.* 1975;35:512-516.
18. Swartz MA, Skobe M. Lymphatic function, lymphangiogenesis, and cancer metastasis. *Microsc Res Tech.* 2001;55:92-99.
19. Al-Mehdi AB, Tozawa K, Fisher AB, et al. Intravascular origin of metastasis from the proliferation of endothelium-attached tumor cells: a new model for metastasis. *Nat Med.* 2000;6: 100-102.
20. Weiss L. Metastatic inefficiency. *Adv Cancer Res.* 1990;54:159-211.
21. Chambers AF, Naumov GN, Varghese HJ, et al. Critical steps in hematogenous metastasis: an overview. *Surg Oncol Clin N Am.* 2001;10:243-255, vii.
22. Weiss L. Comments on hematogenous metastatic patterns in humans as revealed by autopsy. *Clin Exp Metastasis.* 1992;10:191-199.
23. Ewing J. *Neoplastic Diseases. A Treatise on Tumors.* London: Saunders; 1928:77-89.
24. Moore MA. The role of chemoattraction in cancer metastases. *Bioessays.* 2001;23:674-676.
25. Kucia M, Reca R, Miekus K, et al. Trafficking of normal stem cells and metastasis of cancer stem cells involve similar mechanisms: pivotal role of the SDF-1-CXCR4 axis. *Stem Cells.* 2005;23:879-894.
26. Muller A, Homey B, Soto H, et al. Involvement of chemokine receptors in breast cancer metastasis. *Nature.* 2001;410:50-56.
27. Ruoslahti E. Vascular zip codes in angiogenesis and metastasis. *Biochem Soc Trans.* 2004;32:397-402.
28. Thiery JP. Epithelial-mesenchymal transitions in tumour progression. *Nat Rev Cancer.* 2002;2:442-454.
29. Kang Y, Massague J. Epithelial-mesenchymal transitions: twist in development and metastasis. *Cell.* 2004;118:277-279.
30. Paget S. The distribution of secondary growths in cancer of the breast. *The Lancet.* 1889;1:99-101.
31. Fidler IJ. Seed and soil revisited: contribution of the organ microenvironment to cancer metastasis. *Surg Oncol Clin N Am.* 2001;10:257-269, vii–viiii.
32. Allan AL, Vantyghem SA, Tuck AB, Chambers AF. Tumor dormancy and cancer stem cells: implications for the biology and treatment of breast cancer metastasis. *Breast Dis.* 2006;26:87-98.
33. Price JT, Bonovich MT, Kohn EC. The biochemistry of cancer dissemination. *Crit Rev Biochem Mol Biol.* 1997;32:175-253.
34. Stafford LJ, Vaidya KS, Welch DR. Metastasis suppressors genes in cancer. *Int J Biochem Cell Biol.* 2008;40:874-891.
35. Varghese HJ, Davidson MT, MacDonald IC, et al. Activated ras regulates the proliferation/apoptosis balance and early survival of developing micrometastases. *Cancer Res.* 2002;62:887-891.
36. Head J, Johnston SR. New targets for therapy in breast cancer: farnesyl-transferase inhibitors. *Breast Cancer Res.* 2004;6:262-268.
37. Gligorov J, Azria D, Namer M, Khayat D, Spano JP. Novel therapeutic strategies combining antihormonal and biological targeted therapies in breast cancer: focus on clinical trials and perspectives. *Crit Rev Oncol Hematol.* 2007;64:115-128.
38. Chan SK, Hill ME, Gullick WJ. The role of the epidermal growth factor receptor in breast cancer. *J Mammary Gland Biol Neoplasia.* 2006;11:3-11.
39. Slamon DJ, Clark GM, Wong SG, et al. Human breast cancer: correlation of relapse and survival with amplification of the HER-2/neu oncogene. *Science.* 1987;235:177-182.
40. Slamon DJ, Leyland-Jones B, Shak S, et al. Use of chemotherapy plus a monoclonal antibody against HER2 for metastatic breast cancer that overexpresses HER2. *N Engl J Med.* 2001;344:783-792.
41. Romond EH, Perez EA, Bryant J, et al. Trastuzumab plus adjuvant chemotherapy for operable HER2-positive breast cancer. *N Engl J Med.* 2005;353:1673-1684.
42. Perez EA, Baweja M. HER2-positive breast cancer: current treatment strategies. *Cancer Invest.* 2008;26:545-552.
43. Marty M, Pivot X. The potential of anti-vascular endothelial growth factor therapy in metastatic breast cancer: clinical experience with anti-angiogenic agents, focusing on bevacizumab. *Eur J Cancer.* 2008;44:912-920.
44. Foekens JA, Peters HA, Grebenchtchikov N, et al. High tumor levels of vascular endothelial growth factor predict poor response to systemic therapy in advanced breast cancer. *Cancer Res.* 2001;61:5407-5414.
45. Gupta VK, Jaskowiak NT, Beckett MA, et al. Vascular endothelial growth factor enhances endothelial cell survival and tumor radioresistance. *Cancer J.* 2002;8:47-54.
46. Guo W, Giancotti FG. Integrin signalling during tumour progression. *Nat Rev Mol Cell Biol.* 2004;5:816-826.
47. Felding-Habermann B, O'Toole TE, Smith JW, et al. Integrin activation controls metastasis in human breast cancer. *Proc Natl Acad Sci USA.* 2001;98:1853-1858.
48. Shaw LM, Chao C, Wewer UM, Mercurio AM. Function of the integrin alpha 6 beta 1 in metastatic breast carcinoma cells assessed by expression of a dominant-negative receptor. *Cancer Res.* 1996;56:959-963.
49. Trusolino L, Bertotti A, Comoglio PM. A signaling adapter function for alpha6beta4 integrin in the control of HGF-dependent invasive growth. *Cell.* 2001;107:643-654.
50. Brendle A, Lei H, Brandt A, et al. Polymorphisms in predicted microRNA-binding sites in integrin genes and breast cancer: ITGB4 as prognostic marker. *Carcinogenesis.* 2008;29:1394-1399.

51. Langsenlehner U, Renner W, Yazdani-Biuki B, et al. Integrin alpha-2 and beta-3 gene polymorphisms and breast cancer risk. *Breast Cancer Res Treat.* 2006;97:67-72.

52. Kenny LM, Coombes RC, Oulie I, et al. Phase I trial of the positron-emitting Arg-Gly-Asp (RGD) peptide radioligand 18F-AH111585 in breast cancer patients. *J Nucl Med.* 2008;49:879-886.

53. Delbaldo C, Raymond E, Vera K, et al. Phase I and pharmacokinetic study of etaracizumab (Abegrin), a humanized monoclonal antibody against alphavbeta3 integrin receptor, in patients with advanced solid tumors. *Invest New Drugs.* 2008;26:35-43.

54. McNeel DG, Eickhoff J, Lee FT, et al. Phase I trial of a monoclonal antibody specific for alphavbeta3 integrin (MEDI-522) in patients with advanced malignancies, including an assessment of effect on tumor perfusion. *Clin Cancer Res.* 2005;11:7851-7860.

55. Liang Z, Wu T, Lou H, et al. Inhibition of breast cancer metastasis by selective synthetic polypeptide against CXCR4. *Cancer Res.* 2004;64:4302-4308.

56. Cashen AF, Nervi B, DiPersio J. AMD3100: CXCR4 antagonist and rapid stem cell-mobilizing agent. *Future Oncol.* 2007;3:19-27.

57. Bramwell VH, Doig GS, Tuck AB, et al. Serial plasma osteopontin levels have prognostic value in metastatic breast cancer. *Clin Cancer Res.* 2006;12:3337-3343.

58. Singhal H, Bautista DS, Tonkin KS, et al. Elevated plasma osteopontin in metastatic breast cancer associated with increased tumor burden and decreased survival. *Clin Cancer Res.* 1997;3:605-611.

59. Tuck AB, Chambers AF, Allan AL. Osteopontin overexpression in breast cancer: knowledge gained and possible implications for clinical management. *J Cell Biochem.* 2007;102:859-868.

60. Martin MD, Matrisian LM. The other side of MMPs: protective roles in tumor progression. *Cancer Metastasis Rev.* 2007;26:717-724.

61. Stetler-Stevenson WG, Hewitt R, Corcoran M. Matrix metalloproteinases and tumor invasion: from correlation and causality to the clinic. *Semin Cancer Biol.* 1996;7:147-154.

62. Overall CM, Kleifeld O. Towards third generation matrix metalloproteinase inhibitors for cancer therapy. *Br J Cancer.* 2006;94:941-946.

63. Picksley SM, Lane DP. p53 and Rb: their cellular roles. *Curr Opin Cell Biol.* 1994;6:853-858.

64. Palmieri D, Horak CE, Lee JH, Halverson DO, Steeg PS. Translational approaches using metastasis suppressor genes. *J Bioenerg Biomembr.* 2006;38:151-161.

65. Paik S, Shak S, Tang G, et al. A multigene assay to predict recurrence of tamoxifen-treated, node-negative breast cancer. *N Engl J Med.* 2004;351:2817-2826.

66. Uhr JW, Scheuermann RH, Street NE, Vitetta ES. Cancer dormancy: opportunities for new therapeutic approaches. *Nat Med.* 1997;3:505-509.

67. Folkman J, Kalluri R. Cancer without disease. *Nature.* 2004;427:787.

68. Black WC, Welch HG. Advances in diagnostic imaging and overestimations of disease prevalence and the benefits of therapy. *N Engl J Med.* 1993;328:1237-1243.

69. Holmgren L, O'Reilly MS, Folkman J. Dormancy of micrometastases: balanced proliferation and apoptosis in the presence of angiogenesis suppression. *Nat Med.* 1995;1:149-153.

70. Wiedswang G, Borgen E, Karesen R, et al. Detection of isolated tumor cells in bone marrow is an independent prognostic factor in breast cancer. *J Clin Oncol.* 2003;21:3469-3478.

71. Diel IJ, Kaufmann M, Costa SD, et al. Micrometastatic breast cancer cells in bone marrow at primary surgery: prognostic value in comparison with nodal status. *J Natl Cancer Inst.* 1996;88:1652-1658.

72. Gebauer G, Fehm T, Merkle E, et al. Epithelial cells in bone marrow of breast cancer patients at time of primary surgery: clinical outcome during long-term follow-up. *J Clin Oncol.* 2001;19:3669-3674.

73. Gerber B, Krause A, Muller H, et al. Simultaneous immunohistochemical detection of tumor cells in lymph nodes and bone marrow aspirates in breast cancer and its correlation with other prognostic factors. *J Clin Oncol.* 2001;19:960-971.

74. Braun S, Vogl FD, Naume B, et al. A pooled analysis of bone marrow micrometastasis in breast cancer. *N Engl J Med.* 2005;353:793-802.

75. Croker AK, Allan AL. Cancer stem cells: implications for the progression and treatment of metastatic disease. *J Cell Mol Med.* 2008;12:374-390.

76. Charafe-Jauffret E, Monville F, Ginestier C, et al. Cancer stem cells in breast: current opinion and future challenges. *Pathobiology.* 2008;75:75-84.

77. Reya T, Morrison SJ, Clarke MF, Weissman IL. Stem cells, cancer, and cancer stem cells. *Nature.* 2001;414:105-111.

78. Kakarala M, Wicha MS. Implications of the cancer stem-cell hypothesis for breast cancer prevention and therapy. *J Clin Oncol.* 2008;26:2813-2820.

79. Clarke MF, Fuller M. Stem cells and cancer: two faces of eve. *Cell.* 2006;124:1111-1115.

80. Al-Hajj M, Wicha MS, Benito-Hernandez A, Morrison SJ, Clarke MF. Prospective identification of tumorigenic breast cancer cells. *Proc Natl Acad Sci USA.* 2003;100:3983-3988.

81. Fillmore CM, Kuperwasser C. Human breast cancer cell lines contain stem-like cells that self-renew, give rise to phenotypically diverse progeny and survive chemotherapy. *Breast Cancer Res.* 2008;10:R25.

82. Ponti D, Costa A, Zaffaroni N, et al. Isolation and in vitro propagation of tumorigenic breast cancer cells with stem/progenitor cell properties. *Cancer Res.* 2005;65:5506-5511.

83. Sheridan C, Kishimoto H, Fuchs RK, et al. CD44+/CD24- breast cancer cells exhibit enhanced invasive properties: an early step necessary for metastasis. *Breast Cancer Res.* 2006;8:R59.

84. Liu R, Wang X, Chen GY, et al. The prognostic role of a gene signature from tumorigenic breast-cancer cells. *N Engl J Med.* 2007;356:217-226.

85. Honeth G, Bendahl PO, Ringner M, et al. The CD44+/CD24− phenotype is enriched in basal-like breast tumors. *Breast Cancer Res.* 2008;10:R53.

86. Abraham BK, Fritz P, McClellan M, et al. Prevalence of CD44+/CD24−/low cells in breast cancer may not be associated with clinical outcome but may favor distant metastasis. *Clin Cancer Res.* 2005;11:1154-1159.

87. Hendrix MJ, Seftor EA, Seftor RE, et al. Reprogramming metastatic tumour cells with embryonic microenvironments. *Nat Rev Cancer.* 2007;7:246-255.

88. Kaplan RN, Riba RD, Zacharoulis S, et al. VEGFR1-positive haematopoietic bone marrow progenitors initiate the pre-metastatic niche. *Nature.* 2005;438:820-827.

89. Cardoso F, Van't Veer L, Rutgers E, et al. Clinical application of the 70-gene profile: the MINDACT trial. *J Clin Oncol.* 2008;26:729-735.

90. Sparano JA, Paik S. Development of the 21-gene assay and its application in clinical practice and clinical trials. *J Clin Oncol.* 2008;26:721-728.

91. Southwestern Oncology Group. Available at: http://www.swog.org/. Accessed September 23, 2008.

CHAPTER 4

Epidemiology of Breast Cancer

Dezheng Huo
James Dignam

Breast cancer is the most common cancer among women both in the United States and in the world. It is the second leading cause of cancer death among women in the United States. Among U.S. women in 2009, approximately 192,370 new cases of invasive breast cancer and 62,280 carcinoma in situ will occur and 40,170 will die from breast cancer.[1] In terms of its global burden, there are about 1.05 million new cases and 373,000 deaths each year worldwide.[2]

DESCRIPTIVE EPIDEMIOLOGY

Incidence and Mortality

There is a 4- to 5-fold variation in breast cancer incidence rates worldwide, with the highest in North America (99.4/100,000) and the lowest in Asia (22.1/100,000) and Africa (23.4/100,000).[3] However, mortality rates are relatively less variable, with Africa (16.2/100,000) being similar to North America (19.2/100,000). These international variations are partly due to differences in environmental and lifestyle factors, screening practices, and treatment strategies.

In the past 50 years, breast cancer incidence has increased worldwide, including in the United States, where the highest rate is found.[4] Data from the Surveillance, Epidemiology, and End Results (SEER) program show that incidence increased in the 1980s and 1990s in the United States but decreased after 2002 mainly in white women[4] (Fig. 4-1). During the same period, 5-year survival also increased, reaching 90% at year 1997 for women 50 years or older and 87% for women under 50 at diagnosis (Fig. 4-2).[4] The continued improvement in prognosis may be attributable to both screening, which increases the diagnosis of small, localized breast tumors, and treatment effectiveness.

Age at Onset

Breast cancer incidence rates increase with age, as shown by the log scale plot of age-specific cancer incidence rates in 5-year age groups (Fig. 4-3). For estrogen receptor (ER)-positive cancer, the incidence rates increase rapidly until approximately age 50 (proportional to the seventh power of the age), and then rise slowly (proportional to the first power of the age). However, the incidence rate of ER-negative cancer increases rapidly before age 50 (proportional to the fifth power of the age) and then remains constant. As a result, ER-positive tumors are more likely to occur in postmenopausal women.

Race, Ethnicity, and Socioeconomic Status

There are racial and ethnic differences in breast cancer incidence and mortality in the United States (Fig. 4-1). In the past 30 years, incidence rates were higher in white women than in African American women. However, African American women had higher mortality rates than white women, and this racial disparity has been widening in recent years. The incidence and mortality rates in Asian, Hispanics, and Native American women are lower than those of non-Hispanic white and African American women.

African Americans are more likely to have regional and distant disease, contributing to the survival disparity (Fig. 4-4A). However, African Americans also have lower 5-year survival rates than whites within stage strata (Fig. 4-4B). In addition to later stage at diagnosis, socioeconomic factors such as limited access to quality health care and comorbidities contribute substantially to outcome disparities.[5,6] However, some degree of difference in outcomes persists between blacks and whites after accounting for these factors, suggesting that cancer biological differences might also be relevant.[7,8] Breast cancers in African Americans are more likely to be early-onset, higher-grade, and ER-negative compared with those in whites.[5,6]

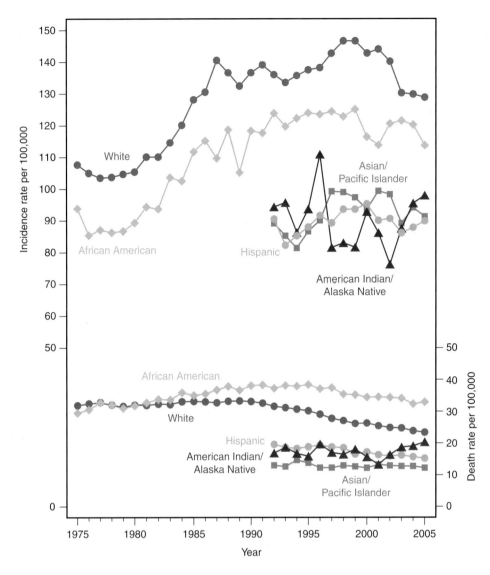

FIGURE 4-1 Trends in female breast cancer incidence and death rates by race and ethnicity, United States. Rates are age-adjusted to the 2000 U.S. standard population. *(Data from Ries L, Melbert D, Krapcho M, et al. SEER Cancer Statistics Review, 1975-2005. Bethesda: National Cancer Institute; 2008.)*

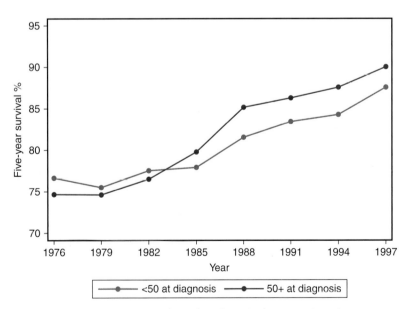

FIGURE 4-2 Breast cancer survival trends in the United States. Values shown are 5-year relative survival (survival adjusted for life expectancy—an approximation to breast cancer-specific survival). *(Data from Ries L, Melbert D, Krapcho M, et al. SEER Cancer Statistics Review, 1975-2005. Bethesda: National Cancer Institute; 2008.)*

■ Risk Factors

Reproductive Factors

Age at Menarche. Early age at menarche is a well-established risk factor for breast cancer in both premenopausal and postmenopausal women, with a reduction in risk of 5% to 10% for each year delay in age at menarche.[9] Inaccurate recall of menarcheal age, especially in older women, may underestimate the strength of this association. Several mechanisms may explain the protective effects of late menarche. Early menarche may be associated with more rapid onset of regular, ovulatory menstrual cycles and hence longer duration of lifetime exposure to endogenous hormones.[10] Estrogen levels are higher several years after menarche and remain so throughout the reproductive years in women with early menarche.[11,12]

Parity. Parous women have lower risk of breast cancer compared with nulliparous women, but

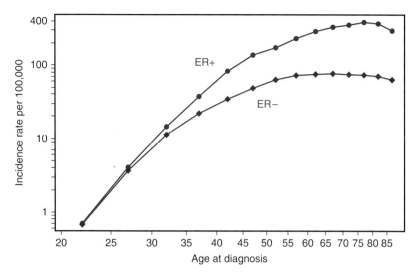

FIGURE 4-3 Breast cancer incidence rate by age and estrogen receptor status, United States, 2000-2005.[4] *(Data from Ries L, Melbert D, Krapcho M, et al.* SEER Cancer Statistics Review, 1975-2005. *Bethesda: National Cancer Institute; 2008.)*

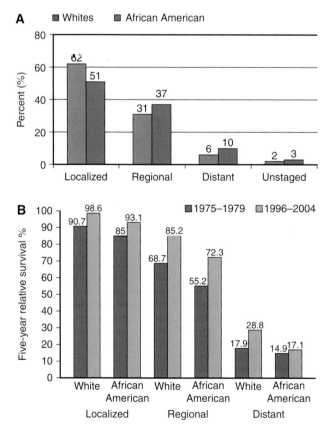

FIGURE 4-4 A. Distribution of breast cancer stage at diagnosis in African-American and white women, United States, 2000-2005. B. Five-year relative survival for African-American and white women by breast cancer stage, United States, 1975-1979 and 1996-2004.[4] *(Data from Ries L, Melbert D, Krapcho M, et al.* SEER Cancer Statistics Review, 1975-2005. *Bethesda: National Cancer Institute; 2008.)*

the relationship between pregnancy and breast cancer is complex.[10] Risk initially increases after the first pregnancy, then decreases after 10 years, and this protective effect is durable.[13] In the long run, the protective effect outweighs the transient adverse effect. The short-term increased risk is thought to be due to significant elevated hormonal levels and rapid proliferation of breast epithelial cells, whereas the mechanisms for the long-term protection involves epithelial cell differentiation, which takes place largely after the first full-term pregnancy.[14] Differentiated cells may be less sensitive to carcinogens due to longer cell cycles, allowing more time for DNA repair in the G1 phase.[14] Additional births further reduce breast cancer risk though the effect is moderate. According to the collaborative reanalysis of 47 studies, each birth reduces the relative risk of breast cancer by 7%.[15]

Age at First Full-Term Pregnancy. Women with first full-term pregnancy after 35 years of age had 40% to 60% higher risk than those who had a first child before 20 years of age.[10,16,17] However, more recent studies showed the effect was weaker,[18] or did not exist for African Americans and indigenous Africans.[18,19] For women who have later pregnancy, the transient postpregnancy risk increase mentioned earlier is more likely to manifest in epidemiologic studies, as age at delivery is closer to age at cancer diagnosis for these women. In addition, age at first birth is a less important factor among women with multiple children.[19,20]

Abortion. Whether spontaneous and induced abortion are breast cancer risk factors is controversial.[10] A meta-analysis documented an overall relative risk of 1.3 for induced abortion and no increased risk for spontaneous abortion, although there was a significant heterogeneity across studies.[21] However, two large cohort studies in Denmark and the United States demonstrated that neither spontaneous nor induced abortion was associated with breast cancer (relative risk ≈ 1.0).[22,23] A recent pooled analysis also concluded that abortions do not affect women's risk of developing breast cancer.[24] Furthermore, recent studies conducted in China, where the prevalence of induced abortion is high, found no link between induced abortion and breast cancer risk.[25,26] Taken together, available evidences does not support induced abortion increasing breast cancer risk.

Breastfeeding. Growing epidemiologic evidence supports risk reduction with prolonged breastfeeding, although studies reported varied magnitude of this protective effect.[10,15,27] In the pooled analysis of data from 47 epidemiologic studies, the relative risk of breast cancer decreased by 4.3% for every 12 months of breastfeeding.[15] There is apparently a dose–response relationship, with increasing total duration of breastfeeding decreasing the risk.[10,15,27] Inconsistent findings with respect to the comparison of ever versus never breastfeeding may be due to international variation in duration. In modern Western countries, where few women breastfed for more than 1 year, the protective effect was moderate, for example, a 22% risk reduction in premenopausal women was documented.[28] In contrast, a risk reduction of more than 50% was observed for women with at least 5 years breastfeeding in populations of China,[29] Mexico,[30] and Nigeria.[19] Several mechanisms have been postulated to explain the protective effect of breastfeeding.[10, 27] Breastfeeding delays the reestablishment of ovulation, thereby reducing lifetime endogenous hormones exposure. Breastfeeding may result in further terminal differentiation of the breast epithelium, thus making it less susceptible to carcinogenic stimuli.

Age at Menopause.

As shown in Figure 4-3, the slope of increase in breast cancer incidence slows around menopause. It is well established that late age at menopause is associated with higher risk of breast cancer. For each year delay in age of menopause, the risk for breast cancer increases by 3%.[10,31] Artificial menopause through bilateral oophorectomy also decreases breast cancer risk, while simple hysterectomy does not.[10] In women with BRCA1 or BRCA2 mutations, bilateral oophorectomy reduces the risk of breast cancer by more than 50%.[32]

Exogenous Hormones

Hormonal Contraceptives.

Many epidemiologic studies have evaluated the relationship between risk of breast cancer and oral contraceptives that contain estrogen and progestin. Generally, a positive but rather weak association has been seen. In a pooled analysis of 54 studies, current use of oral contraceptives was associated with 24% greater risk compared with never-users.[33] This elevated risk disappeared after discontinuing: the relative risks were 1.16, 1.07, and 1.01, respectively, for women 1 to 4 years, 5 to 9 years, and 10 or more years after stopping use.[33] Duration of use has no independent effect. As women usually use oral contraceptives in their second and third decade of life when the absolute risk of breast cancer is low, and the excess risk decreases after cessation of use, there are likely few breast cancer cases due to oral contraceptive use. A recent large case-control study also confirmed that former oral contraceptive use did not increase the risk later in life, when the breast cancer incidence of is higher.[34]

Postmenopausal Hormones.

Health benefits and risk of postmenopausal hormones have been evaluated by numerous studies. In a pooled analysis of 51 epidemiologic studies, the current or recent use of postmenopausal hormones was associated with increased risk of breast cancer, with a dose–response relationship based on duration of use.[35] The risk increased by 2.3% for each year of use and the relative risk was 1.35 for women who had used hormones for 5 or more years. This effect disappeared 5 years after discontinuing, regardless of duration of use. The effect of postmenopausal hormones was stronger in lean women than in obese women, a finding confirmed by later studies.[36,37] Mounting evidence suggests that estrogen plus progestin increases breast cancer risk more than estrogen alone.[31,35,37,38] Estrogen alone is associated with a relative risk of 1.3, while for estrogen plus progestin, relative risk ranges from 1.5 to 2.0 among several cohort studies.[31,35,38] In the Women's Health Initiative randomized trial, estrogen-only therapy did not increase risk, while estrogen plus progestin increased the risk by 26%.[39,40]

Anthropometric Factors

Height.

Attained height has been found to be positively associated with breast cancer in a large number of case-control and cohort studies.[41-44] Numerous hypotheses related to nutritional influence on development have been proposed, including energy intake and growth during childhood (a hypothesis supported by variations in risk based on periods of nutritional deprivation as that which occurred in World War II), the interaction of nutrition with hormones during puberty, and the relationship of insulin-like growth factor with both height and breast cancer risk.

Weight and Body Mass Index.

Excess body weight has been implicated as a risk factor, and has most often been examined via anthropometric measures such as body mass index (BMI—weight corrected for some function of total size). BMI has been convincingly correlated with breast cancer risk in numerous studies, although the relationship is often complex and involves additional modifying factors.[36,44 51] In the Nurse's Health Study involving more than 90,000 women, both high BMI and weight gain increased postmenopausal breast cancer risk.[36] A pooled analysis of 7 cohort studies estimated excess breast cancer risk of 26% for postmenopausal obese versus lean women.[44] Numerous other studies have found 1.25- to 2-fold or greater excess risk among postmenopausal obese women.[45-50] Interestingly, obesity is associated with decreased breast cancer risk in premenopausal women in most studies.[44,46,48,51]

The predominant hypothesized mechanism in postmenopausal women implicates increased endogenous estrogen resulting from conversion of androgens by the aromatase enzyme in adipose fat.[52] The association between increased circulating estrogen and breast cancer risk supports this concept,[53,54] as does the apparent protective effect of obesity on breast cancer risk in premenopausal women, in whom high BMI is associated with *decreased* serum estradiol.[55,56]

Lifestyle and Dietary Factors

Alcohol.

Alcohol intake influences breast cancer risk, with a recent large meta-analysis of studies estimating relative risk increases of 32% for consumption of 35 to 44 g/day and 46% for 45 g/day or more, compared to women with no alcohol consumption.[57]

Tobacco.

Tobacco use via smoking has not been consistently demonstrated to alter breast cancer risk, in part because this risk factor must be carefully evaluated in relation to other factors with which it may be correlated. In the above-referenced meta-analysis, the researchers identified a strong confounding influence of alcohol use on the effect of smoking, that when accounted for, resulted in no association remaining between smoking and breast cancer.[57]

Physical Activity.

Evidence from observational studies supports a modest protective effect of physical activity on breast cancer risk, with risk reductions in the range of 10% to 50%.[58] Physical activity is nearly inextricably linked with a variety of nutritional, physiologic, and social factors, and may be difficult to characterize retrospectively throughout life, leading to limited reliable inference for this observation. As a modifiable risk factor with multiple potential benefits in addition to cancer, there is great interest in prospective interventional studies. Such studies are ongoing in both breast cancer patients and women at potential risk, but results have not been reported thus far.

Soy and Phytoestrogens. Soy consumption has been suspected of providing a protective effect, based on global observations of differences in incidence that correlate with dietary patterns, coupled with the hypothesis regarding competition of phytoestrogens (known generally as isoflavones) with endogenous estrogen for binding to estrogen receptors, as well as other possible anticarcinogenic effects of these compounds.[59] Observational studies support an association between soy intake and breast cancer risk, but it is dependent on a threshold level of consumption. Specifically, results of a meta-analysis showed that in Asian countries where soy consumption is high, women with over 20 mg/day of isoflavones had a 29% lower relative risk of breast cancer compared to those who consumed 5 or fewer mg/day.[59] In the same investigation, in a synthesis of studies conducted in low soy consumption regions, where daily isoflavone intake ranged from 0.15 to 0.8 mg/day, no association could be found.

Other Dietary Factors. Dietary fat intake has long been implicated as a risk factor for breast cancer, in part as a result of the apparent strong correlation between breast cancer incidence and fat content in diet worldwide.[60] As for most putative risk factors, observational studies of fat intake and breast cancer risk show mixed results. Meta-analyses have found relative risk increases ranging from 5% to nearly 50% among individuals with the highest fat intake.[61] Different approaches and difficulties with accurate recording of fat intake, particularly in retrospective studies, likely account for some of the inconsistency in findings. For fruit, vegetable, and whole grain intake, observational study results have been similarly varied.[62]

Despite this uncertainty, diet content is one modifiable risk factor that has been evaluated in a prospective randomized study.[63] In the Dietary Modification Trial of the Women's Health Initiative, women randomized to a low-fat, higher fruit and vegetable intake diet had a 9% lower risk of breast cancer over an 8-year period (risk ratio = 0.91, 95% confidence interval 0.83-1.01).[63] Among women compliant with their assigned regimen, the effect was somewhat larger.

Environmental Factors

Ionizing Radiation. Exposure to moderate or high levels of ionizing radiation from various sources including medical treatment procedures and nuclear explosion increases the risk of breast cancer.[64] The effect of radiation on breast cancer depends on age at exposure: the risk is higher in women exposed before age 20 years and is small for exposure after age 40 years.[65] Before age 40, there is a positive correlation between radiation dose and breast cancer risk.[64-66] These radiation-induced breast cancers typically do not occur until age 30 to 35 years, but the elevated risk persists through the woman's lifetime.[64,66] The magnitude of effect can be large: an 8-fold increased risk was documented in women with Hodgkin disease who received radiotherapy dose of more than 40 Gy.[67] It is unclear whether

a low level of ionizing radiation (< 10 mGy), such as chest x-ray or mammography, increases breast cancer risk, but the cumulative dose is likely important.[68]

Other Environmental Factors. The impact of organochlorines including polychlorinated biphenyls (PCBs) and dichlorodiphenyltrichloroethane (DDT) on breast cancer have been studied extensively. A pooled analysis of 5 studies found that PCBs and DDE levels in blood were similar between breast cancer cases and healthy controls.[69] Studies that measured organochlorines using job history or residence location yielded inconsistent results.[70] Other environmental pollutants have received less attention in epidemiologic studies.

Genetic Factors

Family History. Family history is a well-established risk factor for breast cancer. Women whose mother or sisters had breast cancer are at about 2-fold increased risk compared with general population.[71] Multiple affected family members, early onset of disease, bilateral breast cancer, and affected male relatives further increase the risk. Familial risk could be attributable to shared environmental or genetic factors, or both. A twin study showed that inheritable genetic factors account for 27% of all breast cancer.[72] A conventional genetic model of breast cancer is that disease risks are affected by mutations of several high-penetrance genes and common variants of many low-penetrance genes.[71]

High-Penetrance Genes. In the 1990s, 2 major breast cancer suppressor genes, BRCA1 and BRCA2, were discovered using genetic linkage mapping and positional cloning.[71] The BRCA1 gene is located on chromosome 17q21 and the BRCA2 gene is located on chromosome 13q12-13. A deleterious mutation in the 2 genes confers an over 10-fold relative risk. A recent meta-analysis of 10 studies estimated that the cumulative risk of breast cancer by age 70 was 57% and 49% for BRCA1 and BRCA2 mutation carriers, respectively.[73] The prevalence of BRCA1 and BRCA2 mutation is generally low and varies across populations from different geographic regions and ethnicities (0.4%-7.0% for BRCA1 and 1%-3% for BRCA2).[74]

Germline mutations in P53 are linked to Li–Fraumeni syndrome, a condition characterized by increased risk of leukemias and cancers of the lung, brain, and breast.[71,75] Mutations in PTEN causes Cowden syndrome.[71,75] Both genes follow an autosomal dominant inheritance pattern and mutations are very rare. Linkage analyses using large numbers of families without BRCA1 or BRCA2 mutation failed to find additional genes, suggesting that other high-penetrance susceptibility genes, if these exist, may account for only a small fraction of the familial aggregation of breast cancer.[76]

Low-Penetrance Genes. As BRCA1 and BRCA2 are involved in the pathways of genomic integrity, DNA repair, and cell-cycle checkpoint controls, direct interrogation of these pathways have identified 6 candidates for breast cancer risk: CHEK2, ATM, BRIP1, PALB2, NBS1, and RAD50.[75] Mutations in these genes were associated with 2- to 4-fold increased risk of breast cancer.[71,75] However, mutation frequencies are very low in the general population: 1.1% have CHEK2*1100delC polymorphism,

~ 0.4% are heterozygous carriers of ATM mutations, and less than 0.1% are heterozygous carriers of BRIP1 or PALB2 mutations.[71]

Using a candidate gene approach, many studies have examined the association between breast cancer and common polymorphisms (>5%) of genes in the pathways of hormone synthesis and metabolism, carcinogen metabolism, and DNA repair. Most of the initial findings have not been replicated as the relative risks are presumably small. For example, the Breast Cancer Association Consortium has confirmed only two polymorphism in CASP8 and TGFB1, with allelic odds ratios of 0.88 and 1.08, respectively.[77]

Recently, genome-wide single-nucleotide polymorphism (SNP) association studies have found several breast cancer susceptibility loci, including FGFR2, TOX3, MAP3K1, LSP1, and 8q24.[78-80] These susceptibility loci confer only a modest risk, with allelic odds ratio of approximately 1.3 and 1.2 for FGFR2 and TOX3, although the population-attributable risk might be high.[78-80] Furthermore, both genes were found to have stronger association with ER+ than with ER– breast tumors.[81] As most of the significant SNPs fall into introns or intergenic regions, further studies are warranted to identify causative alleles.

Benign Breast Disease

History of benign breast disease is associated with breast cancer diagnosis.[82] Benign breast lesions are classified into three categories: nonproliferative breast disease (eg., fibroadenoma, cysts), proliferative breast disease without atypia (eg, adenosis, intraductal papilloma), and atypical hyperplasia.[83] Nonproliferative breast disease, the most common lesion, is associated with small increased risk or no effect (relative risk 0.9-1.6).[83-85] Women with proliferative breast disease without atypia had about 1.5- to 1.9-fold increased risk, whereas atypical hyperplasia produced about a 3- to 5-fold higher risk of breast cancer.[83-85] In the high-risk atypical hyperplasia group, atypical lobular hyperplasia conferred an even higher risk than ductal hyperplasia.[86] Of note, the subsequent breast cancer is slightly more likely to occur in ipsilateral (60%) than in the contralateral (40%) breast,[86] and the ratio of ipsilateral to contralateral breast cancer was highest in the first 5 years after benign breast disease diagnosis,[84] suggesting that benign breast disease may be both a cancer precursor and a biomarker for long-term risk.

Mammographic Density

The mammographic image is determined by the relative amounts of fat, connective tissue, and epithelial tissue.[87] Connective and epithelial tissue has a high radiologic density, whereas fat appears translucent; thus mammographic density has been consistently observed to be inversely associated with both age and obesity.[47,87-89] Women with the most extensive mammographic density (as a percentage of total area imaged) have a 2- to 6-fold greater risk, compared to those with low to absent density.[88-90] Consistent with its risk association, mammographic density has been reported to increase with hormone replacement[91,92] and to decrease with tamoxifen.[93,94] In a recent study aimed towards developing a prospective risk prediction

model using the Breast Cancer Surveillance Consortium (BCSC) cohort, breast density was found to be a strong contributor to risk, with 2- to 4-fold relative risks for extremely dense versus nondense breasts according to BI-RADS scoring.[95] Breast density also figured prominently in a subsequent extension of the original Gail Risk Model.[96] Among participants in a randomized trial for DCIS, highly dense breasts (according the area of the breast occupied with dense tissue) were associated with risk of subsequent invasive cancer.[97] However, in another study using a subset of the BCSC cohort, BI-RADS density was not significantly associated with invasive cancer after DCIS.[98]

FUTURE DIRECTIONS IN RESEARCH TO ADDRESS CURRENT QUESTIONS

Reason for Recent Change in Incidence of Breast Cancer

The recent precipitous decline in breast cancer incidence has been attributed to large numbers of women discontinuing or avoiding initiation of hormone replacement therapy,[99] motivated by findings of the Women's Health Initiative trial.[39] However, analyses of trends in national rates cannot account for other factors such as changes in use of mammography screening, which will produce apparent rate declines in some time intervals. In studies where screening use is known, it does appear that the decline persists.[100,101] Nonetheless, numerous factors will continue to influence breast cancer incidence, including adoption of new screening technology, which may contribute to the increasing incidence of DCIS. Thus, continued careful analysis of breast cancer incidence trends is needed.

Significance of Molecular Subtypes for Understanding Etiology, Prevention, and Treatment

Recent molecular analysis of breast cancer has exposed distinct classes of tumors, or subtypes, that have significance with respect to prognosis and the likely success of different treatment options.[102] These subtypes also show a differential distribution by race/ethnicity,[103,104] and thus may explain a portion of the disparity in breast cancer outcomes between; for example, African-American women and those of predominantly western European origin (ie, whites). Risk factors may differ for different subtypes,[105] but more work is needed to both fully characterize how these subtypes may differ by intrinsic and modifiable risk factors.

SUMMARY

Although much has been learned about the etiology of breast cancer, many of the established and putative risk factors are not modifiable and so are not easily translated into primary prevention. Promoting physical activity, weight reduction, breastfeeding, limited postmenopausal hormone use, and reduced alcohol intake are several important practical measures for breast cancer prevention in the general population. Physical activity, especially in early life, is an appropriate focus for reducing breast cancer risk given its role in the prevention of cardiovascular diseases and diabetes. Similarly, at least 6 months of breastfeeding should be encouraged because of its well-established protective effect against breast cancer and beneficial health effects on infant and mothers. Reducing alcohol intake and limiting postmenopausal hormone use may be a good practice in general, but the tradeoff of benefit and risk will depend on the individual woman.

Tamoxifen and other selective estrogen receptor modulators are effective primary prevention strategies for high-risk populations. Mammography is an effective method of secondary prevention of breast cancer for women older than 50, but its benefit is less clear in women younger than 50. Evaluation of an individual woman's absolute risk of breast cancer using all available risk factors described herein, is important to counseling women and identifying those potentially suitable for chemoprevention and more intensive screening.

REFERENCES

1. Jemal A, Siegel R, Ward E, et al. Cancer statistics, 2009. *CA Cancer J Clin.* 2009;59:225-249.
2. Parkin DM, Whelan SL, Ferlay J, Storm H. *Cancer Incidence in Five Continents.* Vols 1 to 8. Lyon: IARC CancerBase no. 7; 2005.
3. Kamangar F, Dores GM, Anderson WF. Patterns of cancer incidence, mortality, and prevalence across five continents: defining priorities to reduce cancer disparities in different geographic regions of the world. *J Clin Oncol.* 2006;24:2137-2150.
4. Ries L, Melbert D, Krapcho M, et al. *SEER Cancer Statistics Review, 1975-2005.* Bethesda: National Cancer Institute; 2008.
5. Eley JW, Hill HA, Chen VW, et al. Racial differences in survival from breast cancer. Results of the National Cancer Institute Black/White Cancer Survival Study. *JAMA.* 1994;272:947-954.
6. Smith-Bindman R, Miglioretti DL, Lurie N, et al. Does utilization of screening mammography explain racial and ethnic differences in breast cancer? *Ann Intern Med.* 2006;144:541-553.
7. Newman LA, Griffith KA, Jatoi I, et al. Meta-analysis of survival in African American and white American patients with breast cancer: ethnicity compared with socioeconomic status. *J Clin Oncol.* 2006;24:1342-1349.
8. Chlebowski RT, Chen Z, Anderson GL, et al. Ethnicity and breast cancer: factors influencing differences in incidence and outcome. *J Natl Cancer Inst.* 2005;97:439-448.
9. Hsieh CC, Trichopoulos D, Katsouyanni K, Yuasa S. Age at menarche, age at menopause, height and obesity as risk factors for breast cancer: associations and interactions in an international case-control study. *Int J Cancer.* 1990;46:796-800.
10. Kelsey JL, Gammon MD, John EM. Reproductive factors and breast cancer. *Epidemiol Rev.* 1993;15:36-47.
11. MacMahon B, Trichopoulos D, Brown J, et al. Age at menarche, urine estrogens and breast cancer risk. *Int J Cancer.* 1982;30:427-431.
12. Apter D, Reinila M, Vihko R. Some endocrine characteristics of early menarche, a risk factor for breast cancer, are preserved into adulthood. *Int J Cancer.* 1989;44:783-787.
13. Lambe M, Hsieh C, Trichopoulos D, et al. Transient increase in the risk of breast cancer after giving birth. *N Engl J Med.* 1994;331:5-9.
14. Russo J, Moral R, Balogh GA, Mailo D, Russo IH. The protective role of pregnancy in breast cancer. *Breast Cancer Res.* 2005;7:131-142.
15. Collaborative Group on Hormonal Factors in Breast Cancer. Breast cancer and breastfeeding: collaborative reanalysis of individual data from 47 epidemiological studies in 30 countries, including 50302 women with breast cancer and 96973 women without the disease. *Lancet.* 2002; 360:187-195.
16. Ewertz M, Duffy SW, Adami HO, et al. Age at first birth, parity and risk of breast cancer: a meta-analysis of 8 studies from the Nordic countries. *Int J Cancer.* 1990;46:597-603.
17. Layde PM, Webster LA, Baughman AL, et al. The independent associations of parity, age at first full term pregnancy, and duration of breastfeeding with the risk of breast cancer. Cancer and Steroid Hormone Study Group. *J Clin Epidemiol.* 1989;42:963-973.
18. Ursin G, Bernstein L, Wang Y, et al. Reproductive factors and risk of breast carcinoma in a study of white and African-American women. *Cancer.* 2004;101:353-362.
19. Huo D, Adebamowo CA, Ogundiran TO, et al. Parity and breastfeeding are protective against breast cancer in Nigerian women. *Br J Cancer.* 2008;98:992-996.
20. Albrektsen G, Heuch I, Hansen S, Kvale G. Breast cancer risk by age at birth, time since birth and time intervals between births: exploring interaction effects. *Br J Cancer.* 2005;92:167-175.
21. Brind J, Chinchilli VM, Severs WB, Summy-Long J. Induced abortion as an independent risk factor for breast cancer: a comprehensive review and meta-analysis. *J Epidemiol Community Health.* 1996;50:481-496.
22. Melbye M, Wohlfahrt J, Olsen JH, et al. Induced abortion and the risk of breast cancer. *N Engl J Med.* 1997;336:81-85.
23. Michels KB, Xue F, Colditz GA, Willett WC. Induced and spontaneous abortion and incidence of breast cancer among young women: a prospective cohort study. *Arch Intern Med.* 2007;167:814-820.
24. Collaborative Group on Hormonal Factors in Breast Cancer. Breast cancer and abortion: collaborative reanalysis of data from 53 epidemiological studies, including 83,000 women with breast cancer from 16 countries. *Lancet.* 2004;363:1007-1016.
25. Ye Z, Gao DL, Qin Q, Ray RM, Thomas DB. Breast cancer in relation to induced abortions in a cohort of Chinese women. *Br J Cancer.* 2002;87:977-981.
26. Sanderson M, Shu XO, Jin F, et al. Abortion history and breast cancer risk: results from the Shanghai Breast Cancer Study. *Int J Cancer.* 2001;92:899-905.
27. Lipworth L, Bailey LR, Trichopoulos D. History of breast-feeding in relation to breast cancer risk: a review of the epidemiologic literature. *J Natl Cancer Inst.* 2000;92:302-312.
28. Newcomb PA, Storer BE, Longnecker MP, et al. Lactation and a reduced risk of premenopausal breast cancer. *N Engl J Med.* 1994;330:81-87.
29. Yuan JM, Yu MC, Ross RK, Gao YT, Henderson BE. Risk factors for breast cancer in Chinese women in Shanghai. *Cancer Res.* 1988;48:1949-1953.
30. Romieu I, Hernandez-Avila M, Lazcano E, Lopez L, Romero-Jaime R. Breast cancer and lactation history in Mexican women. *Am J Epidemiol.* 1996;143:543-552.
31. Colditz GA, Rosner B. Cumulative risk of breast cancer to age 70 years according to risk factor status: data from the Nurses' Health Study. *Am J Epidemiol.* 2000;152:950-964.
32. Rebbeck TR, Lynch HT, Neuhausen SL, et al. Prophylactic oophorectomy in carriers of BRCA1 or BRCA2 mutations. *N Engl J Med.* 2002;346:1616-1622.
33. Collaborative Group on Hormonal Factors in Breast Cancer. Breast cancer and hormonal contraceptives: collaborative reanalysis of individual data on 53,297 women with breast cancer and 100,239 women without breast cancer from 54 epidemiological studies. *Lancet.* 1996;34/:1713-1727.
34. Marchbanks PA, McDonald JA, Wilson HG, et al. Oral contraceptives and the risk of breast cancer. *N Engl J Med.* 2002;346:2025-2032.
35. Collaborative Group on Hormonal Factors in Breast Cancer. Breast cancer and hormone replacement therapy: collaborative reanalysis of data from 51 epidemiological studies of 52,705 women with breast cancer and 108,411 women without breast cancer. *Lancet.* 1997;350:1047-1059.
36. Huang Z, Hankinson SE, Colditz GA, et al. Dual effects of weight and weight gain on breast cancer risk. *JAMA.* 1997;278:1407-1411.
37. Schairer C, Lubin J, Troisi R, et al. Menopausal estrogen and estrogen-progestin replacement therapy and breast cancer risk. *JAMA.* 2000; 283:485-491.
38. Million Women Study Collaborators. Breast cancer and hormone-replacement therapy in the Million Women Study. *Lancet.* 2003;362:419-427.
39. Rossouw JE, Anderson GL, Prentice RL, et al. Risks and benefits of estrogen plus progestin in healthy postmenopausal women: principal results from the Women's Health Initiative randomized controlled trial. *JAMA.* 2002;288:321-333.
40. Anderson GL, Limacher M, Assaf AR, et al. Effects of conjugated equine estrogen in postmenopausal women with hysterectomy: the Women's Health Initiative randomized controlled trial. *JAMA.* 2004;291:1701-1712.
41. Trentham-Dietz A, Newcomb PA, Storer BE, et al. Body size and risk of breast cancer. *Am J Epidemiol.* 1997;145:1011-1019.
42. van den Brandt PA, Dirx MJ, Ronckers CM, van den Hoogen P, Goldbohm RA. Height, weight, weight change, and postmenopausal

breast cancer risk: The Netherlands Cohort Study. *Cancer Causes Control.* 1997;8:39-47.

43. Tretli S. Height and weight in relation to breast cancer morbidity and mortality. A prospective study of 570,000 women in Norway. *Int J Cancer.* 1989;44:23-30.

44. van den Brandt PA, Spiegelman D, Yaun SS, et al. Pooled analysis of prospective cohort studies on height, weight, and breast cancer risk. *Am J Epidemiol.* 2000;152:514-527.

45. Hunter DJ, Willett WC. Diet, body size, and breast cancer. *Epidemiol Rev.* 1993;15:110-132.

46. Ursin G, Longnecker MP, Haile RW, Greenland S. A meta-analysis of body mass index and risk of premenopausal breast cancer. *Epidemiology.* 1995;6:137-141.

47. Lam PB, Vacek PM, Geller BM, Muss HB. The association of increased weight, body mass index, and tissue density with the risk of breast carcinoma in Vermont. *Cancer.* 2000;89:369-375.

48. Huang WY, Newman B, Millikan RC, et al. Hormone-related factors and risk of breast cancer in relation to estrogen receptor and progesterone receptor status. *Am J Epidemiol.* 2000;151:703-714.

49. Pathak DR, Whittemore AS. Combined effects of body size, parity, and menstrual events on breast cancer incidence in seven countries. *Am J Epidemiol.* 1992;135:153-168.

50. Chu SY, Lee NC, Wingo PA, et al. The relationship between body mass and breast cancer among women enrolled in the Cancer and Steroid Hormone Study. *J Clin Epidemiol.* 1991;44:1197-1206.

51. Willett WC, Browne ML, Bain C, et al. Relative weight and risk of breast cancer among premenopausal women. *Am J Epidemiol.* 1985;122:731-740.

52. Siiteri PK. Adipose tissue as a source of hormones. *Am J Clin Nutr.* 1987;45(suppl):277-282.

53. Toniolo PG, Levitz M, Zeleniuch-Jacquotte A, et al. A prospective study of endogenous estrogens and breast cancer in postmenopausal women. *J Natl Cancer Inst.* 1995;87:190-197.

54. Hankinson SE, Willett WC, Manson JE, et al. Alcohol, height, and adiposity in relation to estrogen and prolactin levels in postmenopausal women. *J Natl Cancer Inst.* 1995;87:1297-1302.

55. Potischman N, Swanson CA, Siiteri P, Hoover RN. Reversal of relation between body mass and endogenous estrogen concentrations with menopausal status. *J Natl Cancer Inst.* 1996;88:756-758.

56. Thomas HV, Key TJ, Allen DS, et al. Re: reversal of relation between body mass and endogenous estrogen concentrations with menopausal status. *J Natl Cancer Inst.* 1997;89:396-398.

57. Collaborative Group on Hormonal Factors in Breast Cancer. Alcohol, tobacco and breast cancer—collaborative reanalysis of individual data from 53 epidemiological studies, including 58,515 women with breast cancer and 95,067 women without the disease. *Br J Cancer.* 2002;87:1234-1245.

58. Friedenreich CM. Physical activity and cancer prevention: from observational to intervention research. *Cancer Epidemiol Biomarkers Prev.* 2001;10:287-301.

59. Wu AH, Yu MC, Tseng CC, Pike MC. Epidemiology of soy exposures and breast cancer risk. *Br J Cancer.* 2008;98:9-14.

60. Carroll KK. Dietary factors in hormone-dependent cancers. *Curr Concepts Nutr.* 1977;6:25-40.

61. Howe GR, Hirohata T, Hislop TG, et al. Dietary factors and risk of breast cancer: combined analysis of 12 case-control studies. *J Natl Cancer Inst.* 1990;82:561-569.

62. Smith-Warner SA, Spiegelman D, Yaun SS, et al. Intake of fruits and vegetables and risk of breast cancer: a pooled analysis of cohort studies. *JAMA.* 2001;285:769-776.

63. Prentice RL, Caan B, Chlebowski RT, et al. Low-fat dietary pattern and risk of invasive breast cancer: the Women's Health Initiative Randomized Controlled Dietary Modification Trial. *JAMA.* 2006;295:629-642.

64. John EM, Kelsey JL. Radiation and other environmental exposures and breast cancer. *Epidemiol Rev.* 1993;15:157-162.

65. Land CE, Tokunaga M, Koyama K, et al. Incidence of female breast cancer among atomic bomb survivors, Hiroshima and Nagasaki, 1950-1990. *Radiat Res.* 2003;160:707-717.

66. Preston DL, Mattsson A, Holmberg E, et al. Radiation effects on breast cancer risk: a pooled analysis of eight cohorts. *Radiat Res.* 2002;158:220-235.

67. Travis LB, Hill DA, Dores GM, et al. Breast cancer following radiotherapy and chemotherapy among young women with Hodgkin disease. *JAMA.* 2003;290:465-475.

68. John EM, Phipps AI, Knight JA, et al. Medical radiation exposure and breast cancer risk: findings from the Breast Cancer Family Registry. *Int J Cancer.* 2007;121:386-394.

69. Laden F, Collman G, Iwamoto K, et al. 1,1-Dichloro-2,2-bis (p-chlorophenyl)ethylene and polychlorinated biphenyls and breast cancer: combined analysis of five U.S. studies. *J Natl Cancer Inst.* 2001;93:768-776.

70. Brody JG, Moysich KB, Humblet O, et al. Environmental pollutants and breast cancer: epidemiologic studies. *Cancer.* 2007;109(suppl):2667-2711.

71. Stratton MR, Rahman N. The emerging landscape of breast cancer susceptibility. *Nat Genet.* 2008;40:17-22.

72. Lichtenstein P, Holm NV, Verkasalo PK, et al. Environmental and heritable factors in the causation of cancer—analyses of cohorts of twins from Sweden, Denmark, and Finland. *N Engl J Med.* 2000;343:78-85.

73. Chen S, Parmigiani G. Meta-analysis of BRCA1 and BRCA2 penetrance. *J Clin Oncol.* 2007;25:1329-1333.

74. Fackenthal JD, Olopade OI. Breast cancer risk associated with BRCA1 and BRCA2 in diverse populations. *Nat Rev Cancer.* 2007;7:937-948.

75. Walsh T, King MC. Ten genes for inherited breast cancer. *Cancer Cell.* 2007;11:103-105.

76. Smith P, McGuffog L, Easton DF, et al. A genome wide linkage search for breast cancer susceptibility genes. *Genes Chromosomes Cancer.* 2006;45: 646-655.

77. Cox A, Dunning AM, Garcia-Closas M, et al. A common coding variant in CASP8 is associated with breast cancer risk. *Nat Genet.* 2007;39:352-358.

78. Easton DF, Pooley KA, Dunning AM, et al. Genome-wide association study identifies novel breast cancer susceptibility loci. *Nature.* 2007;447: 1087-1093.

79. Stacey SN, Manolescu A, Sulem P, et al. Common variants on chromosomes 2q35 and 16q12 confer susceptibility to estrogen receptor positive breast cancer. *Nat Genet.* 2007;39:865-869.

80. Hunter DJ, Kraft P, Jacobs KB, et al. A genome-wide association study identifies alleles in FGFR2 associated with risk of sporadic postmenopausal breast cancer. *Nat Genet.* 2007;39:870-874.

81. Garcia-Closas M, Hall P, Nevanlinna H, et al. Heterogeneity of breast cancer associations with five susceptibility loci by clinical and pathological characteristics. *PLoS Genet.* 2008;4:e1000054.

82. Fitzgibbons PL, Henson DE, Hutter RV. Benign breast changes and the risk for subsequent breast cancer: an update of the 1985 consensus statement. Cancer Committee of the College of American Pathologists. *Arch Pathol Lab Med.* 1998;122:1053-1055.

83. Dupont WD, Page DL. Risk factors for breast cancer in women with proliferative breast disease. *N Engl J Med.* 1985;312:146-151.

84. Hartmann LC, Sellers TA, Frost MH, et al. Benign breast disease and the risk of breast cancer. *N Engl J Med.* 2005;353:229-237.

85. Bodian CA. Benign breast diseases, carcinoma in situ, and breast cancer risk. *Epidemiol Rev.* 1993;15:177-187.

86. Collins LC, Baer HJ, Tamimi RM, et al. Magnitude and laterality of breast cancer risk according to histologic type of atypical hyperplasia: results from the Nurses' Health Study. *Cancer.* 2007;109:180-187.

87. Saftlas AF, Szklo M. Mammographic parenchymal patterns and breast cancer risk. *Epidemiol Rev.* 1987;9:146-174.

88. Oza AM, Boyd NF. Mammographic parenchymal patterns: a marker of breast cancer risk. *Epidemiol Rev.* 1993;15:196-208.

89. Boyd NF, Lockwood GA, Byng JW, Tritchler DL, Yaffe MJ. Mammographic densities and breast cancer risk. *Cancer Epidemiol Biomarkers Prev.* 1998;7:1133-1144.

90. Saftlas AF, Hoover RN, Brinton LA, et al. Mammographic densities and risk of breast cancer. *Cancer.* 1991;67:2833-2838.

91. Stomper PC, Van Voorhis BJ, Ravnikar VA, Meyer JE. Mammographic changes associated with postmenopausal hormone replacement therapy: a longitudinal study. *Radiology.* 1990;174:487-490.

92. Persson I, Thurfjell E, Holmberg L. Effect of estrogen and estrogen-progestin replacement regimens on mammographic breast parenchymal density. *J Clin Oncol.* 1997;15:3201-3207.

93. Chow CK, Venzon D, Jones EC, et al. Effect of tamoxifen on mammographic density. *Cancer Epidemiol Biomarkers Prev.* 2000;9:917-921.

94. Brisson J, Brisson B, Cote G, et al. Tamoxifen and mammographic breast densities. *Cancer Epidemiol Biomarkers Prev.* 2000;9:911-915.

95. Barlow WE, White E, Ballard-Barbash R, et al. Prospective breast cancer risk prediction model for women undergoing screening mammography. *J Natl Cancer Inst.* 2006;98:1204-1214.

96. Chen J, Pee D, Ayyagari R, et al. Projecting absolute invasive breast cancer risk in white women with a model that includes mammographic density. *J Natl Cancer Inst.* 2006;98:1215-1226.

97. Habel LA, Dignam JJ, Land SR, et al. Mammographic density and breast cancer after ductal carcinoma in situ. *J Natl Cancer Inst.* 2004;96:1467-1472.

98. Hwang ES, Miglioretti DL, Ballard-Barbash R, Weaver DL, Kerlikowske K. Association between breast density and subsequent breast cancer following treatment for ductal carcinoma in situ. *Cancer Epidemiol Biomarkers Prev.* 2007;16:2587-2593.

99. Ravdin PM, Cronin KA, Howlader N, et al. The decrease in breast-cancer incidence in 2003 in the United States. *N Engl J Med.* 2007;356:1670-1674.

100. Kerlikowske K, Miglioretti DL, Buist DS, Walker R, Carney PA. Declines in invasive breast cancer and use of postmenopausal hormone therapy in a screening mammography population. *J Natl Cancer Inst.* 2007;99:1335-1339.

101. Glass AG, Lacey JV, Jr., Carreon JD, Hoover RN. Breast cancer incidence, 1980-2006: combined roles of menopausal hormone therapy, screening mammography, and estrogen receptor status. *J Natl Cancer Inst.* 2007;99:1152-1161.

102. Perou CM, Sorlie T, Eisen MB, et al. Molecular portraits of human breast tumours. *Nature.* 2000;406:747-752.

103. Carey LA, Perou CM, Livasy CA, et al. Race, breast cancer subtypes, and survival in the Carolina Breast Cancer Study. *JAMA.* 2006;295:2492-2502.

104. Lund MJ, Trivers KF, Porter PL, et al. Race and triple negative threats to breast cancer survival: a population-based study in Atlanta, GA. *Breast Cancer Res Treat.* 2008. Epub.

105. Millikan RC, Newman B, Tse CK, et al. Epidemiology of basal-like breast cancer. *Breast Cancer Res Treat.* 2008;109:123-139.

CHAPTER 5

Breast Cancer Screening

Haydee Ojeda-Fournier
Christopher E. Comstock

Breast cancer is the most common malignancy affecting American women excluding skin cancers. It is the second leading cause of cancer-related deaths, having been surpassed by mortality from lung cancer. The American Cancer Society estimated that there would be 182,460 new cases of breast cancer and 40,480 breast cancer-related deaths in 2008.[1] Breast cancer mortality in the United States has declined substantially over the past 30 years, from 31.4 deaths per 100,000 women per year in 1975 to 25.9 deaths per 100,000 women per year in 2001.[2] The reduction in breast cancer mortality has been attributed to advances in treatment options and the combination of increasing utilization of screening mammography and improved mammographic quality.[3,4] Mammography remains the only study proven to detect early breast cancer and decrease breast cancer–related deaths.

An additional important goal of screening mammography is to identify cancers when they are small, and subsequently at an earlier stage. In a study conducted by Barth and associates,[5] the tumor size of patients who had breast cancer detected by mammography was 1.5 cm, which was statistically significantly smaller than the cohort group whose breast cancer was detected by physical exam and in which tumor size was on average 2.9 cm. The screening-detected cancer patients were also more likely to be node negative and less likely to receive chemotherapy. Similar results have been reported in populations with high mammographic screening rates, such as in Rhode Island.[6] Ductal carcinoma in situ (DSIS), which is believed to progress to invasive carcinoma in certain patients, is clinically occult and only identified by mammography.

MAMMOGRAPHIC SCREENING TRIALS

The benefits from screening mammography for women age 40 to 70 years have been proven in 8 randomized controlled trials (RCTs) during the past 40 years.[7-14] These trials were conducted in Europe (Edinburgh, Malmö, Gothenburg, Stockholm, Swedish Two County), Canada (includes 2 trials: age 40-49 and age 50-59), and the United States (Health Insurance Plan Project). Table 5-1 summarizes the results of these trials. All but one of the RCTs report statistically significant results as measured by mortality reduction as end-point. Reported reductions in breast cancer mortality range from −2% to 32%. In addition, long-term follow-up of 3 trials (HIP, Gothenburg, and Malmö) each found statistically significant reductions in breast cancer mortality.[15-17] The only RCT to actually show mortality in the screening group is the Canadian study for women aged 40 to 49 years. This study has been highly criticized for the poor image quality and for including patients with clinically evident advanced breast cancer.[18] The benefits of mammographic screening are in general accepted as valid. Controversy remains for screening women younger than the age of 40 years; in this group there are few data from RCTs. Therefore, decisions concerning screening practice in this age group must be based on less rigorous evidence and on a more individual basis.

The Cochrane Collaboration and Other Attacks on Screening Mammography

Mammographic screening has suffered repeated attacks, some of which have made headlines in the lay media; for example the 2001 front-page coverage by *The New York Times* of the Cochrane Collaboration report.[19] The most flagrant assault on screening mammography in a reputable journal was reported in *The Lancet* by 2 members of the Cochrane Collaboration, Gotzsche and Olsen.[20,21] In their reanalysis and meta-analysis of the largest RCT, they claimed that mammography caused increased mortality. It did not take long for a number of different experts to identify the biased and faulty analysis that the

TABLE 5-1 Summary of Mammographic Screening Randomized Controlled Trials

Trial	Age (yr)	Screening Interval (mo)	Mortality Reduction (%)
Swedish Two County[13]	40–74	24–33	32
Edinburgh[7]	45–64	24	29
Malmö[8]	45–69	18–24	23
Stockholm[9]	40–64	24–28	20
Gothenburg[10]	40–59	18	23
HIP[14]	40–64	12	23
Canadian[11]	40–49	12	–3
Canadian[12]	50–59	12	–2

TABLE 5-2 Summary of American Cancer Society Breast Cancer Screening Guidelines

Annual mammogram starting at age 40
Breast clinical exam age 20-39 every 3 years, annual clinical exam beginning at age 40
Optional breast self-exam beginning at age 20
Women to be informed of the benefits and harms of mammographic screening
High-risk women: additional annual breast MRI as adjunctive to mammography

Cochrane Collaboration employed.[18,22,23] Gotzsche and Olson excluded all the trials that showed benefit because per their analysis those studies were of poor quality. Their conclusions were based on the Canadian study results, which most experts have found to otherwise be flawed. In a more recent analysis of the Swedish Two-County Trial 20-year follow-up data, Tabar and associates reported a 44% reduction in breast cancer mortality in women aged 40 to 69 years.[24] Although skepticism will reemerge regarding the benefit of screening mammography, it is doubtful that additional RCTs could be performed; it would be unethical to randomize patients to no mammographic screening when multiple large trials and clinical experience have already shown the benefits of mammographic screening.

SCREENING MAMMOGRAPHY

Recommendations

For average-risk women, the majority of professional organizations in the United States recommend screening mammography beginning at the age of 40 and to continue annually. The American Cancer Society[25] in addition recommends that women in their 20s and 30s undergo clinical breast examination once every 3 years. Although there is no evidence to recommend routine breast self-examination (SBE), the American Cancer Society recommends that women be informed about the benefits and limitations of breast self-examination to begin at age 20. If a woman chooses to do SBE, then any changes noted are to be reported to her health care provider. Table 5-2 summarizes the current American Cancer Society guidelines.

Test Interval

The time between screens is an important factor in decreasing breast cancer mortality. If too long a time were placed between screening intervals, early detection would be compromised. As noted in Table 5-1, screening intervals in all major RCTs differ, and ranged from 12 to 33 months. Most of the major American professional organizations (including the American Medical

Association, American College of Radiology, and American Cancer Society) recommend screening intervals of 12 months.

Findings at Mammography

The principal mammographic imaging findings of breast cancer include clustered microcalcifications, masses, architectural distortions, and asymmetries (Fig. 5-1). Comparison to prior mammograms is essential, as some cancers may only be detected by perceiving them as a subtle change from prior studies. In addition, the availability of prior mammograms for comparison can reduce the number of unnecessary call-backs for stable benign findings.[26] After a finding is detected in a screening mammogram, the patient is called back for diagnostic evaluation. Additional imaging evaluation is performed to determine if the lesion is real, and if real, to plan for biopsy. Imaging modalities available for diagnostic evaluation include special view mammography, ultrasound, and in selected cases, contrast-enhanced breast MRI.

Age Groups

Younger Women

The benefits of screening of younger women, defined as age 40 to 49, has been controversial because of the relatively small numbers of women in this age range who have enrolled in the individual trials. In 1997, a meta-analysis of women aged 40 to 49 years in all 5 Swedish trials found a statistically significant 29% reduction in breast cancer deaths.[27] When taking into account all 8 randomized controlled clinical trials, and with an average follow-up of 12.7 years, this same meta-analysis documented an 18% reduction in breast cancer deaths. Given that younger women have a longer life expectancy and the fact that cancers tend to grow more rapidly in younger women, earlier detection of these cancers may theoretically be advantageous. However, this must be balanced by the limitations of screening mammography in younger women, which include a lower frequency of breast cancer, reduced sensitivity of mammography, slightly increased radiation risk, and higher recall rates. Screening of younger women will be of most benefit in women at high risk, especially those known to carry the BRCA1 or BRCA2 gene mutation. Observational studies of high-risk

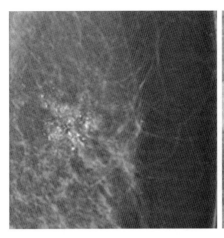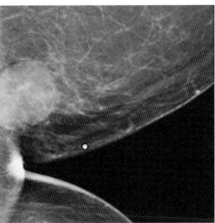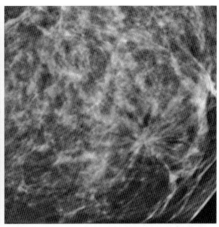

FIGURE 5-1 From left to right: spot compression magnification view of clustered pleomorphic calcifications, cleavage view of a round mass, spot compression view of architectural distortion. All of these abnormalities are biopsy-proven invasive ductal carcinomas that were identified at the time of screening mammogram.

women aged 30 to 39 years show a cancer detection rate similar to that for women aged 40 to 49 years.[28,29]

Older Women

When to stop screening evaluation is a controversial topic. There is no specific recommendation regarding at what age to stop screening mammography. In general it is agreed that when comorbidities outweigh the benefits of screening, then cessation of screening should take place. It is also agreed that age is a strong risk factor for breast cancer; the older the women, the greater the risk of breast cancer. Only 2 of the 8 RCTs (Malmö and Swedish Two-County Trials) included patients over the age of 65. There is, therefore, insufficient evidence to recommend for or against screening older women. However, since the cumulative risk of radiation is less, breast parenchymal density diminishes, and the risk of developing breast cancer increases, women should continue routine annual screening as long as there are no compromising comorbid health conditions.

Surveillance of High-Risk Women

In April 2007, the American Cancer Society published new guidelines for screening high-risk women.[30] Risk is greatest for women with genetics mutations including BRCA1 and BRCA2, p53, Cowden disease, and those women who underwent radiation therapy for lymphoma at an early age. Methods for estimating risk based on medical and family history include the Gail, Claus, and BRCAPRO mathematical models. Women who have a 20% to 25% lifetime risk for breast cancer based on family history calculated by any of these models are considered high risk. Women with a personal history of breast cancer or a prior diagnosis of atypical ductal or lobular hyperplasia also have increased risk of malignancy. Table 5-3 summarizes the factors placing women at increased risk for breast cancer. For the women with increased risk of breast cancer, in addition to annual mammography, contrast-enhanced breast MRI is recommended. One strategy that can be considered is to stagger

TABLE 5-3 Risk Factors that Place Women at Increased Risk of Breast Cancer

BRCA1 or BRCA2 mutation, or untested first-degree relative of known carrier

Chest radiation from age 10-30 for Hodgkin lymphoma

Lifetime risk of 20-25% as determined by statistical risk assessment models such as BRCAPRO or Gail

Other genetic mutations including p53 and Cowden disease

the mammogram and breast MRI so that the woman can have surveillance at a shorter interval time.

In general, screening of women under 40 years of age is restricted to high-risk subgroups (women with a 20% lifetime breast cancer risk at or before the age of 30 years, or breast cancer risk at a given age equivalent to that of the average woman at the age of 40 years).

PROTOCOLS

Standard Technique and Mammographic Quality Standards

The standard screening mammogram consists of 2 views of each breast. The mediolateral oblique (MLO) projection is usually obtained at a 45-degree angle along the border of the pectoralis major muscle (Fig. 5-2). The cranio-caudal (CC) projection is obtained with the nipple on profile and breast tissue compressed with the image receptor parallel to the floor (Fig. 5-2). The breast tissue is positioned by highly skilled technologists to maximize the breast tissue visualized and with proper compression to decrease radiation exposure.

The Mammographic Quality Standards Act of 1992 (MQSA) requires that facilities be accredited by the Food and Drug Administration (FDA) to provide high-quality screening and

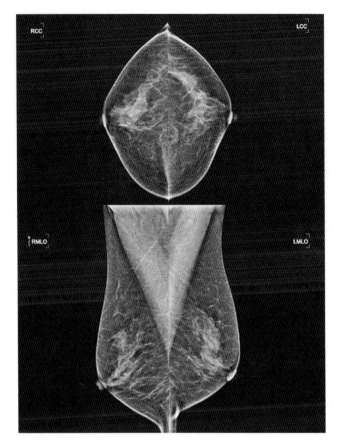

FIGURE 5-2 Routine annual screening mammogram in a patient with scattered fibroglandular densities and no mammographic abnormalities. Images in the first row are the craniocaudal projections, while images in the second row are the mediolateral oblique projections.

diagnostic mammographic services. In addition to image quality, MQSA also defines qualification standards for interpreting physicians, technologists, physicists and facility inspectors. As part of MQSA, a Breast Imaging Reporting and Data System (BIRADS) final assessment category is assigned to each interpreted study (Table 5-4). BIRADS was developed by the American College

of Radiology to standardize mammographic reporting, reduce confusion in interpretation, and facilitate monitoring of outcomes.[31] It is composed of a lexicon of descriptive terms and definitions for each of the breast imaging modalities. It also provides a standardized reporting language and provides a structure for managing the medical audit and outcomes.

Women with Implants

The presence of breast implants presents a challenge to the radiologist interpreting the mammographic screening evaluation. In addition to the standard mammographic views, women with breast implants undergo additional views in each breast in order to obtain better compression and to visualize a greater amount of breast tissue. The implant-displaced views are obtained by displacing the implant posteriorly toward the chest wall and "pinching" the breast tissue anteriorly within the image receptor area. This technique was first described by Eklund and has become standard for the mammographic evaluation of the augmented breast.[32]

Women with Transverse Rectus Abdominis Musculocutaneous (TRAM) Flap

There are few data in the mammographic screening of reconstructed breast mounds after mastectomy. Breast reconstruction is regarded as acceptable practice after mastectomy with low risk of cancer recurrence at the site of reconstruction.[33] It is accepted that there will be a small amount of residual breast tissue left after mastectomy; this raises concern that a reconstructed mound could conceal a recurrence. In a very small series by Helvie and associates,[34] mammographic evaluation detected breast cancer recurrence prior to clinical examination in 1.9% of the study population. Note that 1.9% is close to the acceptable 2% of BIRADS category 3 in which follow-up is recommended. Overall, very few cancers are expected to be identified by routine screening of the TRAM flap; nevertheless, at our institution we recommend mammographic screening of TRAM flaps.

Limitations of Mammography

Although there have been significant improvements in mammographic technique over the past 50 years, fundamental limitations

TABLE 5-4 BIRADS Final Assessment Category:

Assessment Category	Assessment	Definition
0	Incomplete	Need additional imaging evaluation or prior mammograms for comparison
1	Negative	No masses, architectural distortion, or suspicious calcifications
2	Benign	Interpreter chooses to describe a benign finding
3	Probably benign	Finding has less than 2% risk of malignancy; sequential short-term follow-up (every 6 months for 2 or more years) is recommended
4	Suspicious	Risk of malignancy is greater than category 3; biopsy is recommended
5	Highly suggestive of Malignancy	Greater than 95% probability of malignancy
6	Known cancer	Biopsy proven malignancy

remain. These include the low inherent contrast differences between tissue structures in the breast and the fact that mammographic detection of breast cancer (sensitivity) relies on the ability to visualize cancer through the background of overlying normal tissue. Mammographic specificity relies on the ability to distinguish benign from malignant breast lesions based on their margins and morphologic features.[35,36] However, malignant and benign lesions may have similar appearances, thereby reducing specificity. Data from the Breast Cancer Surveillance Consortium demonstrated that on average, screening mammography programs had a call-back rate of approximately 6.4% to 13.3% and a PPV of 3.4% to 6.2%.[37] The mean cancer detection rate was 4.7 per 1000, and the mean size of invasive cancers was 13 mm.

DIGITAL SCREENING TRIAL

Digital Mammography and DIMIST Trial

Screen-film mammography (SFM) has been the standard method used for breast cancer screening since the end of xeromammography more than 20 years ago. Advances in screen-film technology and film-processing techniques have contributed to major improvements in the quality of mammographic images. In addition to high contrast, the strength of SFM lies in its extremely high spatial resolution, often greater than 10 line pairs per millimeter (lp/mm). This allows the detection of exceedingly small clusters of microcalcifications, one of the earliest signs of breast cancer. The limitations of SFM include the detection of subtle soft-tissue lesions, especially in the presence of dense glandular tissues, and the fact that the film serves simultaneously as the image receptor, display medium, and long-term storage medium. Recent technological advances have led to the development of full field digital mammography (FFDM). One of the initial concerns of FFDM is its inherent lower spatial resolution of 5 to 10 lp/mm. However, several studies have demonstrated that despite the limited spatial resolution, the visibility of calcifications on FFDM is not significantly different from that on SFM.[38-40] The higher contrast resolution of FFDM may account for its comparable detection rates. In a recent multicenter trial of 49,528 women, Pisano and associates[40] reported that the overall diagnostic accuracy of FFDM was comparable to SFM as a means of screening for breast cancer. The study also found that digital mammography was more accurate in women under the age of 50 years, women with radiographically dense breasts, and premenopausal or perimenopausal women (Table 5-5).

Digital mammography has the potential to overcome the inherent limitations of SFM. By directly converting the detected x-ray photons to numerical values, the process of x-ray photon detection is decoupled from the image display. The digital images can be processed by a computer, displayed in multiple formats, and fed directly to computer-aided detection (CAD) software programs. In addition, there are logistical and financial advantages of FFDM, including faster patient throughput, no film or processing costs, and the ability to transmit images and to perform telemammography.

TABLE 5-5 Implications of the DIMIST Trial

Recommend Digital Mammography in:
Women younger than 50 years
Mammographically dense breasts
Premenopausal or perimenapausal women

ADVERSE CONSEQUENCES OF SCREENING

The most recent American Cancer Society guidelines for breast cancer screening recommend that women "should have the opportunity to become informed about the benefits, limitations, and potential harms associated with screening."[25] The adverse consequence of screening includes overdiagnosis, false-positive results, radiation exposure, and physical and emotional distress from the screening experience. The pain and discomfort from compression applied during screening is temporary and will vary among women from negligible to significant. A strategy to consider for premenapausal women to decrease discomfort would be to time screening evaluation for weeks 2 and 3 of the menstrual cycle; this is the time when hormonal effects and breast swelling are lowest. Radiation causes cancer, as we have learned from the atomic bombing of Hiroshima/Nagasaki and the nuclear reactor disaster in Chernobyl. At this time there is only theoretical speculation of the risk of radiation to the breast, which is considered higher for younger women.[41] Good compression and good technique aids in lowering radiation dose. The main issue with overdiagnosis and treatment of breast cancer involves DCIS. At this time there is no way to predict which DCIS will progress to invasive cancer and which will remain in situ. Finally, false-positives results are a significant issue since they lead to additional imaging evaluation, and in some cases to potentially costly biopsies. In a 2005 study by Poplack and associates,[42] only 3% of screening evaluations were referred to biopsy, but 20% of the monetary expenditure was consumed by those biopsies. Although there are limitations and risk, it is worth reiterating that screening mammography saves lives.

OTHER MODALITIES

Whole-Breast Ultrasound

Due to the inherent limitations of mammography in patients with dense parenchymal patterns, much attention has been given to ultrasound (US) as an adjuvant to screening mammography. Early studies of breast US were disappointing due to its poor detection of small cancers and excessively high false-positive rates.[43-45] With the advent of higher-megahertz (MHz) transducers, whole-breast US as a screening tool has been revisited. Small, single-institution studies have demonstrated a prevalence detection rate of 3 to 4 mammographically occult cancers per 1000 women screened.[46-51] However, a positive predictive value of less than 20% has been reported, lower than accepted for mammography.[52] Most studies have focused mainly on women with mammographically higher-density breasts.

Screening US appears to be more sensitive in detecting early invasive cancer whereas mammography is more sensitive in the detection of calcifications associated with ductal carcinoma in situ. Of the invasive cancers, US been shown to find a higher percentage of invasive lobular carcinomas than that usually found on mammography. Because of the difference in cancer types detected, whole-breast US is intended as a supplement to mammographic screening rather than a replacement.

Despite these promising early results, the use of screening US in general has not been recommend by professional organizations due to concerns regarding the scientific validity of these initial small, single-institution studies, low positive predictive value (PPV), and the lack of randomized controlled trials. In addition, most of the initial studies on whole-breast US have evaluated prevalence (initial) detection rather than incidence (subsequent) detection rates. The benefit from subsequent yearly screening US is likely to be less than the results reported for initial screening US.

The American College of Radiology Imaging Network (ACRIN) recently published the initial data on the first randomized multicenter trial evaluating whole-breast bilateral screening US in high-risk asymptomatic women with dense breasts.[53] Radiologists trained in mammographic and US interpretation, using standardized interpretive criteria, performed all of the examinations. In this study, the diagnostic yield of mammography alone was 7.6 cancer cases per 1000 women screened. This number increased to 11.8 per 1000 when US and mammogram were both used. The yield of malignancy identified by US alone was 4.2 per 1000. The positive predictive value of mammogram alone was 22.6%. However, for US alone, the positive predictive value decreased to 8.9%. Even the combination of US and mammogram decreased the positive predictive value to 11.2%. The finding is not surprising, and reiterates previously reported data. In addition to the increased false-positive rates, it is worth noting that physicians performed the scan, taking away time that can be utilized in other tasks.

Although US is less sensitive than MRI, due to its lower cost and availability, it is likely that whole-breast US will play an increasing role as a supplemental screening modality in women with dense breasts. Current postprocessing algorithms, including spatial compounding and harmonic imaging, as well as newer techniques such as elastography, may help to improve the specificity of breast US and decrease the number of false-positives and unnecessary biopsies. In addition, automated whole-breast US systems, currently being developed by several manufacturers, may help to standardize and streamline whole-breast US.

Contrast-Enhanced Breast MRI Screening

Dynamic contrast enhanced MRI of the breast has been shown to be extremely sensitive in the detection of invasive breast cancer and is not limited by the density of the breast tissue like mammography is. It is also not limited by patient positioning or lack of visualization of the posterior breast. However, because the reported sensitivity of MRI for DCIS ranges between 45% and 100%, MRI is currently not recommended as a replacement for mammography.[54] A more recent single-institution study suggests that MRI may have a higher sensitivity as compared to

TABLE 5-6 Minimum Standard for the Performance of Contrast-Enhanced Breast MRI

Field strength	Minimum 1.5 T
Resolution	3-mm slice thickness
Contrast	Gadolinium 0.1 mmol/kg
Scan time	Dynamic contrast enhancement
Coil	Dedicated breast

mammography for DCIS than previously thought, particularly for high-grade DCIS.[55]

Indications

The use of MRI in the general population has been limited by its moderate specificity. Therefore, its use has been focused on studying patients in whom the yield from MRI is likely to be higher. Multiple studies have shown that MRI is a useful tool as an adjuvant to screening mammography in women at high risk for breast cancer.[56-58] The American Cancer Society (ACS) recommends annual screening MRI for women with a 20% to 25% lifetime risk of breast cancer.[30] This includes women with the BRCA1 or BRCA2 breast cancer genes, as well as women with multiple family members with breast or ovarian cancer, and women who have undergone mediastinal irradiation for Hodgkin disease. Women whose benefit from screening MRI was considered questionable by the ACS, due to insufficient data, included women with a personal history of breast cancer, prior biopsy yielding atypia, or women with extremely dense breasts on mammography. The decision to perform screening MRI in these women should be made on a case-by-case basis.

Protocols

There is no standardized recommended protocol for performing breast MRI. Protocols will vary depending on the equipment being used and clinician's preference. For example, while some clinicians favor evaluating images in the axial planes, others will interpret in the sagittal plane. There is, however, a minimum standard for the performance of breast MRI (Table 5-6). A dedicated breast coil, minimum of 1.5 Tesla strength magnets, and dynamic contrast administration is absolutely required for the performance of breast MRI. A power injector is highly recommended to standardize contrast administration from study to study. Additionally, any breast MRI screening program should include the capability to perform MRI-guided breast biopsy, since there will be lesions identified by MRI that are not visible by other imaging modalities and not detected by physical examination.

COMPUTER-AIDED DIAGNOSIS IN MAMMOGRAPHIC SCREENING

CAD programs have been developed to assist radiologists in the interpretation of screening mammograms, and to improve cancer detection rates. These programs rely on neural networks to analyze the images and flag potentially suspicious findings that may have been overlooked. Several studies have shown improved cancer detection by radiologists using CAD versus radiologists alone, without significantly increasing call-back rates.[40,59-61] However, other studies have shown less promising results.[62,63] A recent study by Fenton and associates[63] reported that CAD decreased the accuracy of screening mammogram interpretation. This was not due to a decrease in cancer detection, but rather an increase in false-positives. In more recent study, involving 231,221 mammograms, Gromet reported increased sensitivity using CAD with only a small increase in recall rate.[64] To be effective, CAD programs should not significantly increase call-back rates and should not prolong interpretation times for screening mammograms. It is important to remember that CAD programs are tools that must be used in an appropriate manner. They should not be used to override a suspicious finding detected by a radiologist. In general, these systems tend to be more helpful for low-volume or inexperienced readers.

FUTURE DIRECTIONS

Tomosynthesis

Digital tomosynthesis, currently available for research purposes only, is a method of creating three-dimensional images of the breast using x-rays. Unlike current FFDM, in which two x-ray images of the breast are obtained from different projections, tomosynthesis is perform by taking a series of low-dose exposures (usually 9 to 15) at different angles across the breast from one projection. From these images and using mathematical methods of back projection reconstruction, a series of 1-mm slices is created in order to show the tissue structure in three dimensions. The ability of tomosynthesis to image the breast three-dimensionally may help to overcome some of the shortcomings of standard mammography caused by overlapping dense tissue. Initial results, presented by Rafferty at the 2007 meeting of the Radiological Society of North America, are promising and suggest that digital tomosynthesis imaging can potentially reduce call-back rates and increase sensitivity. However, there is still debate whether one or two tomographic projections of each breast will be necessary as well as concerns regarding radiation dose and sensitivity for DCIS. Clinical trials are currently underway to assess the utility of tomosynthesis as both a diagnostic tool and possibly as a replacement for current two-view screening mammography. However, because this technology involves multiple data sets per patient with many images each, developments in workstation display software, as well as additional reimbursement codes for increased radiologist's readout time, will be necessary for the technology to become viable.

Molecular Imaging: BSGI, PEM, and More

Unlike conventional medical imaging techniques that detect pathology based on morphologic changes, molecular imaging seeks to detect pathology based on increases in certain types of underlying metabolic activity. This may be advantageous given the fact that morphologic changes may take considerable time to manifest despite the presence of disease. Two types of molecular imaging technologies currently being explored for use in the breast are breast-specific gamma imaging (BSGI) and positron emission mammography (PEM). BSGI utilizes technetium 99m-sestamibi to target mitochondrial activity, which is presumable higher in cancerous lesions. PEM uses [F-18]-fluorodeoxyglucose (FDG) to target the glucose uptake activity of lesion. Previous attempts of breast imaging using technetium 99m-sestamibi and [F-18]-fluorodeoxyglucose (FDG) positron emission tomography (PET) were limited by the use of relatively low-resolution whole-body systems. However, newer high-resolution dedicated breast imaging systems have been developed. Their use as screening tests has not been established. Variability of uptake in primary breast tumors as well as moderate specificities has limited their potential. Randomized control trials are needed to evaluate their possible role as adjuvant screening tests in certain subgroups of women, as diagnostic tools as well as their ability to assist in determining extent of disease in patients with known cancer. However, their cost and possible radiation risks must be weighed against their potential benefits. Development of other targeted molecular imaging technologies, such as optical imaging agents, has been slow due to limitations in signal penetration, amplification, and potential toxicity.

NECESSARY FUTURE STUDIES

Breast imaging technology continues to develop and proliferate. Radiologists continually struggle to balance wanting to offer the most state-of-the-art technology while at the same time trying to protect what is in the best interests of their patients. Unfortunately, determinants for the adoption of new imaging technology into clinical practice, for the most part, are not standardized, and rigorous scientific evaluation of utility tends to follow much later than FDA approval. Given the cost and length of time needed to evaluate a new technology based on decrease in mortality, most studies evaluate cancer detection rates and assume a direct correlation. However, cancer detection cannot be evaluated in a vacuum and must incorporate factors such as cost, false-positives, radiation risk and effects and on clinical outcomes. In general, preference should be given to technology with the highest number of lives saved per dollar or the highest quality-adjusted life years (QALY) per dollar cost ratio.

Imaging techniques on the horizon—such as digital tomosynthesis, whole-breast US, molecular breast imaging, computer aided diagnosis (CADx) for mammography, US and MRI, US elastography, dedicated breast CT, and a host of new MRI techniques—will require validation through prospective randomized clinical trials. Because of mammography's proven morality reduction, high resolution, and low cost, the majority of new technologies aim to supplement rather than replace screening mammography. However, given the well-known limitations of mammography in terms of sensitivity and specificity, low cost, noninvasive adjuvant technologies that reduce false-positives or improve detection will be the most beneficial.

Automated Whole-Breast Ultrasound

With the likely advent of whole-breast screening US in selected patients, several potential issues have been raised regarding manpower, readout, and standardization. The initial results from the ACRIN 6666 trial reported an average bilateral whole-breast scanning time of approximately 19 minutes. Given the current shortages of breast imaging radiologists nationally and low reimbursement, real-time freehand whole-breast scanning may not be practical for many practices. In addition, the significant increase in the number of US images that will have to be reviewed per case, as well as issues on how to efficiently compare these to prior scans, present a challenge. Although there is currently no FDA-approved system for screening, automated whole-breast US units are currently being developed by several manufacturers. Automated techniques may help to standardize and streamline whole-breast screening US. In addition to standard reflective sonography, methods utilizing sound attenuation, transmission, and speed as well as tomographic techniques are being explored. Technical challenges remain and multicenter clinical trials will be needed to evaluate these technologies in the future.

SUMMARY

In summary, mammography is the only study to date shown to decrease breast-cancer related mortality in multiple large RCTs. Current screening guidelines recommend annual mammographic screening beginning at age 40 and continuing until the time when comorbidities do not allow for the patient to continue. Breast MRI is recommended as adjunctive study to screening for those women with a 20% to 25% lifetime risk of breast cancer and for women with known genetic mutation. New horizons in screening for breast cancer are plentiful and promising. Data from automated whole-breast US, PEM, and BSGI trials are expected in the near future with the hopes to further decrease breast cancer-related mortalities.

REFRERENCES

1. American Cancer Society. *Cancer Facts & Figures 2008*. Atlanta: American Cancer Society; 2008.
2. Ries, LAG, Eisner MP, Kosary CL, et al. *SEER Cancer Statistics Review, 1975-2001*. Bethesda, MD: Philadelphia, PA: National Cancer Institute; 2004.
3. Elkin EB, Hudis C, Begg CB, Schrag D. The effect of changes in tumor size on breast carcinoma survival in the U.S.: 1975-1999. *Cancer*. 2005;104:1149-1157.
4. Berry DA, Cronin KA, Plevritis SK, et al. Cancer Intervention and Surveillance Modeling Network (CISNET) Collaborators. *N Engl J Med*. 2005;353: 1784-1792.
5. Barth RJ Jr, Gibson GR, Carney PA, et al. Detection of breast cancer on screening mammography allows patients to be treated with less-toxic therapy. *Am J Roentgenol*. 2005;184:324-329.
6. Coburn NG, Chung MA, Fulton J, Cady B. Decreased breast cancer tumor size, stage, and mortality in Rhode Island: an example of a well-screened population. *Cancer Control*. 2004;11:222-230.
7. Alexander FE, Anderson TJ, Brown HK, et al. 14 years of follow-up from the Edinburgh randomised trial of breast-cancer screening. *Lancet*. 1999;353:1903-1908.
8. Andersson I, Aspegren K, Janzon L, et al. Mammographic screening and mortality from breast cancer: the Malmo Mammographic Screening Trial. *BMJ*. 1988; 297:943-948.
9. Frisell J, Lidbrink E, Hellström L, Rutqvist LE. Follow-up after 11 years: update of mortality results in the Stockholm mammographic screening trial. *Breast Cancer Res Treat*. 1997;45:263-270.
10. Bjurstam N, Björneld L, Duffy SW, et al. The Gothenburg breast screening trial: first results on mortality, incidence, and mode of detection for women ages 39-49 years at randomization. *Cancer*. 1997;80:2091-2099.
11. Miller AB, Baines CJ, To T, Wall C. Canadian National Breast Screening Study: 1. Breast cancer detection and death rates among women aged 40 to 49 years. Department of Preventive Medicine and Biostatistics, University of Toronto, Ont. *CMAJ*. 1992;147:1459-1476.
12. Miller AB, Baines CJ, To T, Wall C. Canadian National Breast Screening Study: 2. Breast cancer detection and death rates among women aged 50 to 59 years. *CMAJ*. 1992 Nov 15;147(10):1477-88. Erratum in: Can Med Assoc J 1993 Mar 1;148(5):718.
13. Tabar L, Fagerberg G, Duffy S, Day NE. The Swedish two county trial of mammographic screening for breast cancer: recent results and calculations of benefit. *J Epidemiol Comm Health*. 1989;43:107-114.
14. Shapiro S, Venet W, Strax P, Venet L. *Periodic Screening for Breast Cancer: The Health Insurance Plan Project and its Sequelae, 1963-1986*. Baltimore, MD Johns Hopkins University Press; 1988.
15. Chu KC, Smart CR, Tarone RE. Analysis of breast cancer mortality and stage distribution by age for the Health Insurance Plan Clinical Trial. *J Natl Cancer Inst*. 1988;80:1125-1132.
16. Bjurstam N, Björneld L, Warwick J, The Gothenburg Breast Screening Trial. *Cancer*. 2003;97:2387-2396.
17. Andersson I., Janzon L Reduced breast cancer mortality in women under 50: updated results from the Malmo Mammographic Screening Program. *J Natl Cancer Inst Monogr*. 1997;22:63-68.
18. Kopans DB. The most recent breast cancer screening controversy about whether mammographic screening benefits women at any age: nonsense and nonscience. *AJR Am J Roentgenol*. 2003 Jan;180(1):21-6. No abstract available.
19. Kolata G. Study sets off debate over mammograms' value. Bethesda, MD. *New York Times*. December 9, 2001: p A1.
20. Gotzsche PC, Olsen O. Is screening for breast cancer with mammography justifiable? *Lancet*. 2000;355:129-134.
21. Olsen O, Gotzsche PC. Cochrane review on screening for breast cancer with mammography. *Lancet*. 2001;358:1340-1342.
22. Jackson VP. Screening mammography: controversies and headlines. *Radiology*. 2002 Nov;225(2):323-6. No abstract available.
23. Freedman DA, Petitti DB, Robins JM. On the efficacy of screening for breast cancer. *Int J Epidemiol*. Berkeley, CA. 2004;33:43-55.
24. Tabar L, Yen MF, Vitak B, et al. Mammography service screening and mortality in breast cancer patients: 20-year follow-up before and after introduction of screening. *Lancet*. Falun, Sweden. 2003;361:1405-1410.
25. Smith RA, Saslow D, Sawyer KA, et al. American Cancer Society guidelines for breast cancer screening: update 2003. *CA Cancer J Clin*. Atlanta, GA. 2003;53:141-169.
26. Frankel SD, Sickles EA, Curpen BN, et al. Initial versus subsequent screening mammography: comparison of findings and their prognostic significance. *Am J Roentgenol*. San Francisco. 1995;164:1107-1109.
27. Hendrick RE, Smith RA, Rutledge JH 3rd, Smart CR. Benefit of screening mammography in women aged 40-49: a new meta-analysis of randomized controlled trials. *J Natl Cancer Inst Monogr*. 1997;22:87-92.
28. Curpen BN, Sickles EA, Sollitto RA, et al. The comparative value of mammographic screening for women 40-49 years old versus women 50-64 years old. *Am J Roentgenol*. 1995 May;164(5):1099-1103.
29. Liberman L, Dershaw DD, Deutch BM, Thaler HT, Lippin BS. Screening mammography: value in women 35-39 years old. *Am J Roentgenol*. 1993 July;161(3):53-56.
30. Saslow D, Boetes C, Burke W, American Cancer Society guidelines for breast screening with MRI as an adjunct to mammography. *CA Cancer J Clin*. 2007 Mar-Apr;57(2):75-89. Erratum in: CA *Cancer J Clin*. 2007 May-Jun; 57(3):185.
31. Bassett LW, Baum JK, Kuhl CK. American College of Radiology Breast Imaging and Reporting Data System. *Breast Imaging Atlas*. 4th ed. Reston, VA: American College of Radiology; 2003.
32. Eklund GW, Busby RC, Miller SH, Job JS. Improved imaging of the augmented breast. *Am J Roentgenol*. Portland. 1988; 151:469-473.
33. Kroll SS, Schusterman MA, Tadjalli HE, Singletary SE, Ames FC. Risk of recurrence after treatment of early breast cancer with skin-sparing mastectomy. *Ann Surg Oncol*. 1997 Apr-May;4(3):193-197.
34. Helvie MA, Bailey JE, Roubidoux MA, et al. Mammographic screening of TRAM flap breast reconstructions for detection of nonpalpable recurrent cancer. *Radiology*. 2002;224:211-216.
35. Sickles EA. Mammographic features of malignancy found during screening. *Recent Results Cancer Res*. 1990;119:88-93.
36. Sickles EA. Breast masses: mammographic evaluation. *Radiology*. 1989 Nov;173(2):297-303. Review.
37. Rosenberg RD, Yankaskas BC, Abraham LA, Performance benchmarks for screening mammography. *Radiology*. 2006 Oct;241(1):55-66.
38. Fischer U, Baum F, Obenauer S, et al. Comparative study in patients with microcalcifications: full-field digital mammography vs screen-film mammography. *Eur Radiol*. 2002;12:2679-2683.

39. Lewin JM, Hendrick RE, D'Orsi CJ, et al. Comparison of full-field digital mammography with screen-film mammography for cancer detection: results of 4,945 paired examinations. *Radiology.* 2001;218:873-880.

40. Pisano ED, Gatsonis C, Hendrick E, et al. Diagnostic performance of digital versus film mammography for breast-cancer screening. *N Engl J Med.* 2005;353:1773-1783.

41. Feig SA, Hendrick RE. Radiation risk from screening mammography of women aged 40-49 years. *J Natl Cancer Inst Monogr.* 1997;22:119-124.

42. Poplack SP, Carney PA, Weiss JE, et al. Screening mammography: costs and use of screening-related services. *Radiology.* 2005;234:79-85.

43. Egan RL, Egan KL. Automated water-path full-breast sonography: correlation with histology of 176 solid lesions. *Am J Roentgenol.* 1984;143:499-507.

44. Kopans DB, Meyer JE, Lindfors KK. Whole-breast US imaging: four-year follow-up. *Radiology.* 1985;157:505-507.

45. Sickles EA, Filly RA, Callen PW. Breast cancer detection with sonography and mammography: comparison using state-of-the-art equipment. *Am J Roentgenol.* 1983;140:843-845.

46. Gordon PB, Goldenberg SL. Malignant breast masses detected only by ultrasound. A retrospective review. *Cancer.* 1995;76:626-630.

47. Kolb TM, Lichy J, Newhouse JH. Occult cancer in women with dense breasts: detection with screening US—diagnostic yield and tumor characteristics. *Radiology.* 1998;207:191-199.

48. Crystal P, Strano SD, Shcharynski S, Koretz MJ. Using sonography to screen women with mammographically dense breasts. *AJR Am J Roentgenol.* 2003;181:177-182.

49. Buchberger W, DeKoekkoek-Doll P, Springer P, Obrist P, Dünser M. Incidental findings on sonography of the breast: clinical significance and diagnostic workup. *Am J Roentgenol.* 1999;173:921-927.

50. Kaplan SS. Clinical utility of bilateral whole-breast US in the evaluation of women with dense breast tissue. *Radiology.* 2001;221:641-649.

51. Leconte I, Feger C, Galant C, et al. Mammography and subsequent whole-breast sonography of nonpalpable breast cancers: the importance of radiologic breast density. *Am J Roentgenol.* 2003; 180:1675-1679.

52. Bassett LW, Hendrick RE, Bassford TL, et al. Quality Determinants of Mammography Guideline Panel. *Quality Determinants of Mammography.* AHCPR pub. no. 95-0632. Rockville, MD: U.S. Department of Health and Human Services, Public Health Service; 1994.

53. Berg WA, Blume JD, Cormack JB, et al. Combined screening with ultrasound and mammography vs mammography alone in women at elevated risk of breast cancer. *JAMA.* 2008;299:2151-2163.

54. Bazzocchi M, Zuiani C, Panizza P, et al. Contrast-enhanced breast MRI in patients with suspicious microcalcifications on mammography: results of a multicenter trial. *Am J Roentgenol.* 2006;186:1723-1732.

55. Kuhl CK, Schrading S, Bieling HB, et al. MRI for diagnosis of pure ductal carcinoma in situ: a prospective observational study. *Lancet.* 2007 Aug 11;370 (9586):485-92.

56. Kriege M, Brekelmans CT, Boetes C, et al. Efficacy of MRI and mammography for breast-cancer screening in women with a familial or genetic predisposition. *N Engl J Med.* 2004;351:427-437.

57. Lehman CD, Blume JD, Weatherall P, et al. Screening women at high risk for breast cancer with mammography and magnetic resonance imaging. *Cancer.* 2005;103: 1898-1905.

58. Kuhl CK, Schrading S, Leutner CC, et al. Mammography, breast ultrasound, and magnetic resonance imaging for surveillance of women at high familial risk for breast cancer. *J Clin Oncol.* 2005;23:8469-8476.

59. Freer TW, Ulissey MJ. Screening mammography with computer-aided detection: prospective study of 12,860 patients in a community breast center. *Radiology.* 2001;220:781-786.

60. Birdwell RL, Bandodkar P, Ikeda DM. Computer-aided detection with screening mammography in a university hospital setting. *Radiology.* 2005; 236:451-457.

61. Morton MJ, Whaley DH, Brandt KR, Amrami KK. Screening mammograms: interpretation with computer-aided detection—prospective evaluation. *Radiology.* 2006;239:375-383.

62. Gur D, Sumkin JH, Rockette HE, et al. Changes in breast cancer detection and mammography recall rates after the introduction of a computer-aided detection system. *J Natl Cancer Inst.* 2004;96:185-190.

63. Fenton JJ, Taplin SH, Carney PA, et al. Influence of computer-aided detection on performance of screening mammography. *N Engl J Med.* 2007;356:1399-1409.

64. Gromet M. Comparison of computer-aided detection to double reading of screening mammograms: review of 231,221 mammograms. *Am J Roentgenol.* 2008;190:854-859.

CHAPTER 6

Components of a Breast Care Program

E. Shelley Hwang
Laura J. Esserman

The last few decades have seen unprecedented advances in the screening, diagnosis, and treatment of patients with breast cancer. This prodigious growth in knowledge and information has necessitated a shift toward increased specialization within each discipline, such that those with a specific interest in breast cancer have been able to focus their efforts toward achieving a high level of expertise in their specialty. Without question, the end result of this specialization has been a greater refinement of cancer care and dramatically improved outcomes for patients with breast cancer; the 5-year survival rate for a woman diagnosed with breast cancer between 1975 and 1979 was 74.9%, compared with 87.7% for a woman diagnosed between 1995 and 2000.[1]

The growing recognition of the importance of multidisciplinary care has also mandated the creation of health care delivery systems that foster and support collaboration among specialists. The comprehensive breast center has been a model for coordinated multidisciplinary care, and this concept is even more timely now than when the Van Nuys Breast Center opened its doors almost 30 years ago. The goals of a breast center, whether real or virtual, remain excellence in the delivery of breast health care within a multidisciplinary environment, although substantial variations among centers exist around additional goals such as education, outreach, and research. Here, we will discuss the advantages favoring the treatment of breast cancer within such an infrastructure, consider the metrics by which performance and quality can be assessed, and review the individual components vital to ensuring the success of such a center, for both patient outcome and community impact.

RATIONALE FOR A COMPREHENSIVE BREAST CENTER

The increased number of treatment options coupled with the growing complexity of multidisciplinary cancer care has resulted in a growing awareness of the importance of coordinated cancer care. In addition, concurrent with these changes in medical treatment, enormous changes in the fabric of American society coalesced to create a demand for greater patient involvement in all aspects of health care decision-making and patients were empowered to seek treatment in the most comprehensive care environments. Breast cancer treatment has been at the forefront of this challenge, since the effectiveness of multidisciplinary care for breast cancer had been empirically shown for several decades in randomized clinical trials of radiation therapy for women undergoing lumpectomy as well as for systemic treatment in women with surgically resected locoregional disease. By combining access to screening, diagnosis, and multimodal therapy within one setting, comprehensive breast centers were an attractive model of care, and indeed, the emergence of coordinated breast programs has facilitated the achievement of 2 primary goals: (1) delivery of patient-centered care and (2) delivery of improved quality care for patients with breast disease.

Patient-Centered Care

Until the middle of the 20th century, the mainstay of treatment for breast cancer was the radical mastectomy described by Sir William Halsted in the 1890s.[2] However, in the 1960s and 1970s, powerful forces of social and political reform were set in motion by several seminal events that brought breast cancer and breast cancer treatment into the spotlight of public awareness. These were the exciting early years of the women's movement, where, for the first time, women's issues took center stage. Beginning in the 1960s, mammography became more widespread and this new technology was hailed for its ability to diagnose cancers that were so small that they had previously been undetectable. Then, in 1974, First Lady Betty Ford as well as Happy Rockefeller, the wife of Vice President Nelson Rockefeller, announced to the nation that they had both been diagnosed with breast cancer. Not only was such personal disclosure unprecedented in the history of presidential politics, but the public acknowledgement of breast cancer and its treatment, and the resulting increase in public awareness, mobilized the country to a heightened level of health advocacy never before encountered. Together, these powerful forces brought about a reexamination of the treatment for breast cancer. Largely as a result of public advocacy, the surgical option of lumpectomy for breast cancer was considered. Numerous prospective randomized trials subsequently confirmed that there was no significant survival advantage to mastectomy over lumpectomy and radiation.

Now more than ever, it is critical to provide a coordinated, patient-centered framework to guide patients through the complex decisions to be made when grappling with a breast cancer diagnosis. In the prior model of care, patients would be required to seek consultations from numerous providers at multiple separate medical sites. In the ideal model of a comprehensive breast center, the multidisciplinary resources and expertise required to treat the patient are all brought to bear within the same infrastructure, making for a more unified, streamlined, and coordinated experience for the diagnosis, treatment, and follow-up of patients with breast disease.

One of the first attempts to create such an environment for patients with breast cancer was exemplified by the Van Nuys Breast Care Center envisioned by a breast surgeon, Mel Silverstein (Fig. 6-1). The Van Nuys Center was a free-standing multidisciplinary outpatient clinic that incorporated breast imaging, breast surgeons, and oncologists under one roof, all sharing a deep philosophical commitment to improving the fragmented nature of breast cancer care and to creating a warm and respectful environment to support their patients. In the 19 years the center was open, over 3100 patients were treated for breast cancer, with outstanding results.[3] Although it eventually shut its doors due to declining reimbursement rates, it remains an innovative demonstration of what could be achieved in creating a patient-centered experience for breast cancer care.

■ Quality

An equally important consideration favoring treatment in multidisciplinary centers is the ongoing drive to improve the quality of breast cancer care delivery. Increasingly, the current environment puts a premium on quality benchmarks for health care. Furthermore, both patients and payors are searching for effective ways in which health care reimbursement could be tied to quality metrics. Thus, it has become essential to invest resources into the development of an efficient and cost-effective infrastructure, develop rational quality metrics, and create a system in which quality can be measured and the effects of interventions assessed. Studies of volume–outcome relationships have been reported, with large case volume often serving as a surrogate for the presence of an organized breast cancer program. When choice of surgery is evaluated as an end point, it has been clearly shown that increased rates of breast-conserving procedures are seen in larger-volume hospitals or those associated with a cancer center.[4-6] Furthermore, when adjusted for case mix, both overall survival and breast cancer–free survival were improved in large centers,

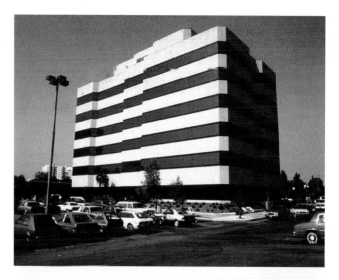

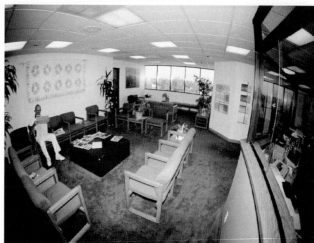

FIGURE 6-1 Van Nuys Breast Care Center, one of the first multidisciplinary breast centers in the country, opened in 1979. For almost 2 decades under the guidance of its medical director Dr. Mel Silverstein, the center was a leader in providing innovative, evidence-based, patient-centered care for women diagnosed with breast cancer and their families. **A.** The Van Nuys Breast Center Building. The center occupied the top floor and half of the floor below. **B.** Patient waiting area. Great attention to detail was taken to create a warm, patient-centered environment. *(Photos courtesy of Mel Silverstein.)*

compared to small facilities.[7,8] Such studies clearly demonstrate both a higher rate of adoption of new findings (eg, use of lumpectomy) as well as an improved outcome are associated with breast cancer treatment at large-volume centers.

REQUIREMENTS FOR A BREAST CENTER

Unlike the NCI requirements for Comprehensive Cancer Center designation, there are currently no nationally established accreditation requirements for a comprehensive breast care center. However, there has been a substantial international effort to

TABLE 6-1 ASCO/NCCN Breast Cancer Treatment Quality Measures

Numerator	Denominator	Estimated Yearly Denominator in the United States	Estimated Risk of Recurrence in the Measure: Specified Measurement Interval
Patient received tamoxifen or AI within 1 year of diagnosis	Stage I-III > 1 cm ER or PR positive > 18 years	153,302	3% node negative 9% node positive
Patient started breast radiation therapy following lumpectomy within 1 year of diagnosis	Stage I-III Age 18-70 years	134,000	1% with XRT 6% no XRT
Patient received adjuvant chemotherapy within 120 days of diagnosis	Stage II-III ER and PR negative Age 18-70 years	38,000	3%

From Desch CE, McNiff KK, Schneider EC, et al. American Society of Clinical Oncology/National Comprehensive Cancer Network Quality Measures. *J Clin Oncol.* 2008;26:3631-3637.

move toward defining standards for what constitutes a "Specialist Breast Unit." These criteria have been defined by the European Organization for the Research and Treatment of Cancer–Breast Cancer Cooperative Group (EORTC–BCCG) and the European Society of Mastology (EUSOMA) in a position paper published in 2000.[9] This paper outlined general recommendations for the essential components of a Breast Unit, including core clinical staff requirements, affiliation with a population breast screening program, and presence of outreach clinics for adjoining areas with low population density. In addition, the suggestion was made to have a case volume requirement of greater than 150 new cancer cases treated annually to ensure a sufficient caseload to maintain clinical expertise. The paper also stipulated that the unit establish written protocols for the management of each stage of breast cancer, a requirement that some in the United States have found unnecessarily rigid given the exigencies of continuous advances in treatment options and individual patient preference.[10] Nevertheless, this position paper serves as a useful template on which to design the infrastructure of multidisciplinary breast centers, and suggests guidelines upon which future accreditation of such centers can be based.

QUALITY ASSESSMENT

We are witnessing a sea change within the health care industry, where the provision of and reimbursement for care as well as the benchmarks for determining the quality of care are undergoing continuous change and ever closer scrutiny. Increasingly, quality measures will be linked to payment, and thus the selection of the best metrics for assessing the quality care are critically important and must require input from all stakeholders, including patients and health care providers. Numerous organizations have presented broad guidelines of how quality should be determined, with some outlining specific criteria by which to assess breast cancer treatment. In an effort to standardize quality measures as well as to make progress toward data collection of meaningful metrics, experts representing the American Society of Clinical Oncology (ASCO) and the National Comprehensive Cancer Network (NCCN) convened and were successful in defining quality measures for two common cancer sites: breast and colorectal.

The panel achieved consensus on three breast cancer measures (Table 6-1).[11] These standards were selected from a much larger group of measures derived from the NCCN cancer treatment guidelines as well as from the NICCQ project comparing cancer treatment practices,[12] and these 3 were selected on the basis of 2 criteria: (1) potential to impact breast cancer outcome and (2) feasibility of accurate end-point collection. These metrics have been adopted by numerous other organizations including the Cancer Program Standards of the American College of Surgeons, Commission on Cancer (ACoS), National Initiative on Cancer Care Quality (NICCQ), and the American Society for Therapeutic Radiology and Oncology (ASTRO). This represents an important first step in establishing universal quality metrics for breast cancer treatment, and these guidelines have already been implemented for ACoS Cancer Center commendation as well as individual provider performance measures. Clearly, more metrics will follow, and leadership will be required to standardize quality measures and data collection across different organizations and practice settings. Provider participation in the selection of these measures is critical to ensuring that the quality metrics remain timely, meaningful, and relevant to current breast cancer treatment. Multidisciplinary breast centers will no doubt play an important role as they will be best positioned to disseminate adherence to quality measures and to collect high-quality outcome data, since many measures will doubtless span disciplines.

THE COMPREHENSIVE BREAST CENTER TEAM

The multidisciplinary nature of breast care and cancer treatment invites collaboration and a team approach to providing care. The ideal of this team approach aspires to a goal where the whole is greater than the sum of the parts, but the quality and

TABLE 6-2 Clinical Staffing and Resource Requirements for a Comprehensive Breast Center

Administrative/Institutional Commitment	Clinical Team (Personnel)	Physical Infrastructure
Medical director	Physicians	Breast imaging facilities
Business manager	Breast imagers	Infusion center
Marketing director	Genetic counselors	Operating suites
Office for billing and collections	Oncologic surgeons/reconstructive surgeons	Radiation oncology facilities
IT support and integration	Medical oncologists	
	Cytologists/surgical pathologists	Outpatient clinic space
	Radiation oncologists	Conference facilities
	Psychologists/psychiatrists	Physician and staff office space
	Clinical nurses	Resource center
	Breast imaging technicians	Volunteer office
	Radiation oncology technicians	
	Physical therapists	
	Medical assistants	
	Scheduling staff	

expertise of each of the individual team components are of critical importance (Table 6-2).

Specialized Breast Imaging

Of the many advances made in the diagnosis and treatment of breast cancer, one of the most impactful has been the mammographic detection of early nonpalpable breast cancer. Population-based screening programs have estimated an overall mortality benefit of over 20% in favor of women undergoing screening mammography.[13,14] Thus, a critically important mission of a comprehensive breast program is to provide state-of-the-art breast imaging capabilities for screening, diagnosis, and evaluation of breast lesions. Historically, free-standing breast screening centers have been successful, but increasingly, such breast imaging programs have been incorporated into a more comprehensive multidisciplinary setting.

Screen-film mammography, the long-time mainstay of breast imaging, is being rapidly supplanted by digital mammography units. Although overall performance of digital mammography has been comparable to full field screening mammography, digital mammography can be more accurate in certain subgroups of the screened population, such as in women with dense breast tissue and in premenopausal women.[15,16] In addition, digital mammography may be more sensitive in the detection and characterization of microcalcifications.[17] However, the greatest impetus for the adoption of digital mammography has been the growing need for less cumbersome radiographic data storage and retrieval. Furthermore, image transmission has been enormously facilitated by digital mammography, such that radiologic expertise can be accessed even from the most geographically remote sites. Ultrasound technology has also improved, and must be part of the expertise provided by a dedicated breast imager. Its use has been particularly effective in the workup of benign lesions as well as for delineating the extent of mammographically occult cancers. The sensitivity of radiographic screening has improved with

the introduction of breast MRI, although arguably this gain has been achieved at the cost of reduced specificity.[18-20] However, selective use of MRI for screening high-risk women,[18,19,21] for work-up of a known cancer,[22-24] or for evaluating the breast for an axillary metastasis with unknown primary[25-27] have all been shown to be of value, and the use of breast MRI is expected to increase substantially in the coming decade.

Cancer Risk Assessment and Genetic Counseling

A team approach to the patient at risk of breast cancer must include clinicians trained in both assessing the degree of breast cancer risk as well as advising patients in how best to manage this risk. With the ability to test for cancer susceptibility genes, patients at greatest risk for hereditary breast cancers can be identified early and counseled regarding the risk-reducing strategies that best fit the patient's needs and preferences. Although BRCA1 and BRCA2 are the most commonly encountered hereditary breast cancer susceptibility genes, genetic counselors specifically trained to assess familial breast cancer risk can detect more uncommon predispositions such as Cowden syndrome (PTEN mutation), Li–Fraumeni syndrome (P53 mutation), CDH1 mutations, and CHEK2 mutations. Such testing can have beneficial implications not only for the proband tested but for family members as well. Since breast cancer syndromes are associated with increased risk of other malignancies, the genetic counseling team must include clinical expertise from other specialists including gynecologic oncologists, gastroenterologists, and dermatologists. Infrastructure to support and track these patients is vital to the most rapid adoption of screening strategies, prevention interventions, and clinical trials for these high-risk individuals.

Surgeons

As briefly mentioned above, studies have shown both more rapid dissemination of treatment advances as well as improved overall and disease-free survival among patients treated by specialist breast surgeons.[4,5,7,8,28] Over the last decade, such outcomes have engendered the recognition of breast oncologic surgery as a distinct specialty within surgical oncology. Concurrent with this development has been the establishment of an accredited program of breast surgery sponsored by the Society of Surgical Oncology (SSO). Thirty-three SSO-approved breast surgery programs now exist in the United States and participate in a fellowship match. Moreover, many surgeons currently in practice and trained before the era of breast fellowships have focused their scope to predominantly breast surgery-based activities. Professional organizations such as the SSO, the American Society of Breast Surgeons (ASBS), and the American Society of Breast Disease (ASBD) have been instrumental in fostering this specialization and have been successful in disseminating new techniques such as sentinel lymph node biopsy as well as research findings into the community.

Access to reconstructive surgeons is critical to the psychological and emotional well-being of many patients who undergo procedures that may substantially alter their physical appearance. While many women choose to decline breast reconstruction after mastectomy and are content with their decision, other women who choose mastectomy and reconstruction have been shown to experience the same long-term quality of life as those undergoing lumpectomy, a much less invasive procedure.[29] Significant advances in breast reconstruction including autologous free flap reconstructive techniques as well as nipple-sparing mastectomy procedures can result in excellent cosmesis (Fig. 6-2).[30,31] Collaboration between the oncologic and reconstructive surgeons in breast programs have allowed for better coordination of care, allowing fewer barriers to immediate breast reconstruction.

Medical Oncologists

If a breast cancer patient were asked to identify "their doctor," it would most likely be the medical oncologist. Although no single modality of treatment is dispensable, systemic treatment is clearly acknowledged to have the greatest potential impact on survival. The number of options in the breast cancer treatment armamentarium is tremendous and growing yearly. In addition, molecular prognostic and predictive tools are also proliferating, outstripping our ability to carefully consider how best to incorporate them into quality patient care.

Thus, ongoing education is particularly crucial to the specialist medical oncologist who must remain current on the most recent systemic regimens as well as on strategies to combat drug resistance. The best oncologists are able to synthesize this information, and empathetically discuss the potential risks and benefits of each option with the individual patient and her family. This can be an intellectually stimulating and emotionally rewarding pursuit, and the expertise of such a focused practice is of critical benefit to improving patient outcome.

Pathologists

An integral member of the treatment team, the breast pathologist is the arbiter of the diagnosis and thus has a profound

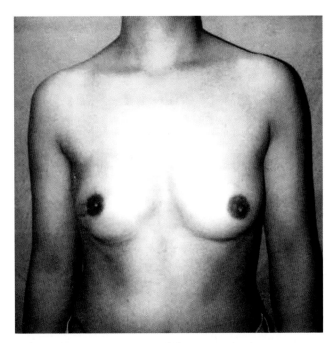

FIGURE 6-2 Cosmetic outcome following nipple-sparing mastectomy, immediate tissue expander, and implant exchange. Mastectomy was performed through a radial incision at the 9-o'clock position of the right breast. The entire skin envelope and nipple-areolar complex were preserved.

impact on driving treatment decisions. Several fundamental advances in the field have converged to make the role of the specialized breast pathologist of particular importance. In the 1980s, the widespread adoption of partial mastectomies made the accurate assessment of margin status critical to the successful outcome of these less invasive procedures and helped allow lumpectomies to gain traction. This was paralleled by national implementation of mammographic screening, which resulted in the identification of a growing number of subtle histopathologic lesions. Many of these proliferative or preinvasive lesions defy consistent diagnosis even among specialized breast pathologists.[32] The growing recognition of the heterogeneity of breast cancer, and recently the stratification of treatment based on pathologic considerations, makes the detailed pathologic assessment of breast cancers of even greater importance. In addition, the development of molecular markers that can refine diagnosis or lend prognostic information has made the accurate assessment of immunohistochemical data and genetic information firmly within the purview of the pathologist.

The breast pathologist in a multidisciplinary team has many roles. The initial diagnosis of cancer is obviously of prime importance, and in patients scheduled to undergo neoadjuvant treatment, a small core biopsy must serve to meet the needs of diagnosis, grading, and biomarker assessment. The provision of consistent radiologic/pathologic correlation is also crucial, and facilitated in an interdisciplinary environment. Pathologist participation in tumor board activities is mandatory, and provides an important basis from which clinical decisions can be made. One study showed that tumor board pathologic review resulted in a change in recommendations for surgery in 6% of cases, and in chemotherapy in 3% of cases.[33] The ability to provide a comprehensive second opinion service is also important; another study of 340 patients seeking a second opinion pathology review found that in 80% of cases, some change in pathologic diagnosis resulted.[34] Almost 8% of cases had a change in surgical recommendation as a result of the second opinion pathology review. The demand for the specialized expertise of a breast pathologist will only continue to grow, as the number, sophistication, and utility of molecular tools increase.

Radiation Oncologists

The number of options currently available for the delivery of adjuvant breast radiation is extensive, and requires that a radiation oncologist with a particular focus in breast cancer treatment be actively engaged in treatment planning. The introduction of partial breast irradiation[35-37] and brachytherapy[38] techniques, as well as accelerated hypofractionated whole-breast radiation[39] options, require that the radiation oncologist on the team be familiar with many different radiation options and be able advise the patient regarding the relative risks and benefits of each.

In addition, since surgery, systemic therapy, and radiation decisions are intertwined, early collaboration and treatment plan coordination among members of the team can have a significant impact on treatment sequencing, long-term outcome, and treatment-related morbidity. Early evaluation by the radiation oncologist can mitigate the need to alter treatment plans and is facilitated by the multidisciplinary breast center infrastructure.

Specialized Oncology Nurses

For each of the physician teams, nurses specializing in the care of cancer patients are crucial. Many nurses who work with multidisciplinary centers have considerable advanced training in perioperative care, symptom management, and patient education. They are integral team members who greatly facilitate interdisciplinary collaboration. They are often the front line for treatment and support and deserve enormous recognition for the vital work that they do. A comprehensive center can allow focus and specialization, support ongoing nursing education, and provide resources to facilitate these essential members of the treatment team.

Psychosocial, Spiritual, and Palliative Support

The diagnosis and subsequent treatment of breast cancer is one of the most difficult challenges a woman can face in her lifetime. For many patients, it is their first encounter with their own mortality. Intense fears for one's health and quality of life naturally surface. These feelings can be particularly painful for younger patients, whose distress for the projected impact of the disease on their young children can be overwhelming. On the other hand, for those who wish to have children, the decisions surrounding the possibility of treatment-related infertility are often painful to contemplate. For those families who share a known hereditary predisposition for breast cancer, feelings of anger, guilt, and blame can be common.

The breast care specialist is in a unique position to provide empathy and compassion during this vulnerable time. However, when a patient's reaction to a new diagnosis manifests in clinical depression, the team psychologist is an indispensable member of the team. It is the responsibility of the clinical staff to identify emotional distress early, and to make a referral to a psychologist as quickly as possible. Not surprisingly, there appears to be an association between psychosocial health and breast cancer survival or recurrence,[40-42] although the individual factors that lead to this improved outcome have not yet been identified. Apart from individual psychological intervention, the use of support groups, patient volunteers, and social workers can also be invaluable.

For many, spiritual faith offers a way to find hope and meaning within the context of a new cancer diagnosis. One study of 142 women diagnosed with breast cancer found an association between spiritual well-being, quality of life, and psychological adjustment.[43] At the other end of the spectrum, spirituality gives comfort and can help a patient more peacefully address end-of-life issues. In preparing for this transition, the palliative care team is indispensable in attending to physical, emotional, spiritual, and even financial needs. Early referral is essential to ensuring that a patient and her family obtain the maximal benefit from this tremendously important opportunity.

With the support of family, friends, and health care professionals, it is possible that a patient not only can endure the treatment for breast cancer but can find that her life has been enriched by the experience. Clearly it is one of our most important charges as breast cancer care providers to do our utmost to increase the chances of attaining this goal.

Survivorship Team

In recent years, excellent outcome of women treated for breast cancer has created the challenge of survivorship. This issue has achieved a national prominence that will only continue to grow as patients survive their disease only to grapple with the long-term effects of treatment-related morbidity. Important components to consider in a survivorship team are an oncologist, an internist, a pain specialist, a physical therapist, and a gynecologist. Each of these members can contribute meaningfully to the long-term follow-up of patients after the completion of acute care. We are early in the process of understanding how to best organize a comprehensive and effective follow-up program and at present have few guidelines on which to base such an initiative. Nevertheless, the effective evaluation of treatment-related symptoms and cancer survivorship issues will be an important challenge to face as we move forward into an increasingly resource-constrained environment.

Interdisciplinary Tumor Board

As treatment of breast cancer has become more complex and multidisciplinary, the number of patients who seek second opinions at comprehensive breast centers has increased. Evaluation for a second opinion consultation at a multidisciplinary center has been shown to result in a change in recommendation for many such patients.[44] The tumor board structure has evolved from a need to have an organized forum in which to discuss complex cases and design a coordinated multimodality care plan for individual patients. The American College of Surgeons as well as the NCI require that a Comprehensive Cancer Center designation must have weekly tumor boards where each discipline is represented, and all pertinent aspects of a case are reviewed. Such detailed multidisciplinary evaluation can bring about a significant change in patient treatment recommendations; in one study by Newman and colleagues, tumor board review resulted in a change in surgical management in 52% (77/149) of patients presented over a 1-year interval.[33] In this study, 29% had additional lesions seen on radiologic review, and 9% had a change in recommendations based on pathology review. Clearly, this speaks to the importance of incorporating tumor boards into patient treatment planning. Further, the tumor board is an ideal opportunity to learn from colleagues with specific expertise in their fields and to disseminate new findings among the group. Thus, the regular meeting of a tumor board with adequate representation from all disciplines will continue to be a quality metric on which multidisciplinary breast centers are evaluated. Advances in technology to facilitate worldwide data transfer will allow second opinion consultations from remote sites. In addition, it is expected that "virtual" tumor boards will be increasingly utilized.

PATIENT EDUCATION AND OUTREACH

A disproportionate breast cancer mortality burden continues to be borne by those living in disadvantaged or lower-income communities, as well as by African Americans compared to Causcasians.[45,46] Numerous factors likely contribute to this risk, including limited access to health care, differing tumor types among racial groups,[47] and differing adherence to recommended care due to differences in health literacy.[48,49]

Outreach programs are important vehicles that can mitigate the impact of factors such as access and education in the underserved population, and comprehensive breast centers with treatment expertise must lead such efforts. One initiative that has generally enjoyed success is the deployment of outreach satellite breast screening centers to increase the rate of mammographic screening among lower-income communities. This has sometimes been accomplished through the use of a mobile mammography unit. Another effective approach has been to emphasize health education among underserved communities, thereby increasing the rate of cancer screening.[50-52] An example of one such highly successful program is the New York Sate Department of Health's Healthy Women Partnership, which has collaborated with over 2300 community organizations including churches, schools, and youth clubs to promote the importance of cancer screening and health maintenance.[51] The impact of such programs can be profound: the program supported by AVON and the Georgia Cancer Center for Excellence at Grady, Emory University of Medicine, illustrates how successful implementation can affect community health.[52] In 2001, prior to the initiation of outreach activities, 16.7% of

newly diagnosed patients presented with stage IV disease; by 2004, this proportion had dropped to 9.4%. Such results indicate that patient education and outreach activities can be powerful agents of behavioral change.

Key factors contributing to the success of such initiatives are obviously tied to planning and resources. However, perhaps the most important determinant of successful implementation of outreach activities is an emphasis on community involvement through close partnerships with community-based organizations and local leaders. This extends the concept of a multidisciplinary team to include community organizers and educators to together affect significant and sustainable health reform.

RESEARCH

All meaningful advances in the treatment of breast cancer have been brought about by patient participation in clinical research. However, historically only about 3% of all breast cancer patients participate in clinical trials,[53] with only 11% participating even in an academic breast center.[54] Barriers to clinical trial accrual particularly impact enrollment in patients of lower socioeconomic status and ethnic and racial minorities; as a consequence these groups remain underrepresented in the medical literature.[55]

The infrastructure of a multidisciplinary breast care center can facilitate clinical research. There is a clear advantage with respect to case volume that is not attainable in individual private practice offices. Moreover, particularly in academic settings, the breast center is often in close proximity to research laboratories that can foster translational research. Patients who seek treatment at breast centers tend to be younger and better educated, factors shown to be associated with clinical trial participation. Nevertheless, clinical trials are difficult to conduct well even under the most ideal circumstances. The following considerations can significantly increase the ease with which patients participate in clinical trials.

Centralized Clinical Trial Support

The regulatory requirements involved in the conduct of clinical trials can be overwhelming. Programs that provide centralized clinical trial support to address Investigational Review Board (IRB) and contracting issues can vastly reduce the time required to open and complete a trial. While principle investigator (PI) oversight is necessary, the daily regulatory needs of the trial can be met by professional staff trained to respond to such needs as well as to assist in writing protocols and filing regulatory documents with local and federal agencies. Public and private vendors have created various software packages to facilitate this process and to ensure that deadlines are met and data collected in a timely manner, and will likely be increasingly incorporated into clinical trial implementation.

Integration of Clinical Trial Activities into Existing Patient Care Flow

The priority should always be patient care, and the trials least disruptive to clinic flow are likely to be the most successful.

Patient education and consent are best undertaken away from the main flow of patient traffic, ideally by a dedicated clinical trial nurse who is able to explain the rationale for the study, how it differs from usual care, and the potential risks and benefits of study participation. Physicians must always be available to answer patient questions and to support patients through the entire clinical trials process. Clear communication and respect are key components of successful recruitment and patient satisfaction.

Cancer Registries

The establishment of institutional, regional, and national cancer registries has been an important foundation on which the findings of many cancer outcome studies are based. Comprehensive breast centers must be linked to cancer registries, and must set aside resources to support the ongoing efforts of the institutional cancer registry. Although many registries are still struggling to collect reliable data for systemic therapies, data on staging, locoregional therapy, and recurrence are very robust. Registries can be a valuable repository of data for clinical research or can inform quality improvement initiatives. Many local registries upload data to regional and/or national registries such as SEER. Completeness of registry data is a quality measure by which comprehensive cancer centers are evaluated.

STRATEGIC PLANNING AND FINANCING

There is growing patient demand for breast centers and specialists who can provide the most up-to-date care. The complexities of breast cancer itself, and the many options available to treat it, require an investment of time and energy to convey this information accurately and empathetically to patients. However, in a relative value unit (RVU)-based system, the time required of providers to transmit that knowledge is undervalued. Breast cancer patients use many ancillary services, including radiology, pathology, radiation oncology, and infusion. This makes breast centers of considerable value to hospitals that associate themselves with these specialized programs. Even psychosocial services, which are an essential component of any cancer center, are now largely supported by insurance.

The finances of a center must be evaluated from the perspective of the total potential downstream revenue, including radiology, breast surgery, breast reconstruction, genetic counseling, medical and radiation oncology, as well as all of the ancillary services. The global package of breast centers is sustainable, but it requires the ability to combine revenue streams and build the infrastructure to truly invest in and support the entire enterprise of comprehensive patient care.

Going forward into the future, it is important to consider alternate financing systems. Insurance companies are increasingly imposing cost-sharing measures with patients in the form of co-pays; as the costs of ancillary tests and new treatments skyrocket, the cost to our patients will as well. Fortunately, the new diagnostic tests emerging on the market will provide us the opportunity to consider novel treatment strategies to normally treat our patients, while supporting fewer interventions for those with good-prognosis tumors, and avoiding chemotherapy in those who will most likely have an excellent prognosis with endocrine therapy alone.[56]

At present, the financial incentives currently in place may inadvertently bias toward more treatment and more testing. One example of an alternate reimbursement model to consider is that of a global capitation fee for breast cancer services. In this way, providers would look for ways that patients could safely avoid treatments, and there would be real funds to support the time expended by all providers to discuss these options. Rather than accepting low professional fees to support high RVU-based interventions, providers would have the incentive to provide shared decision-making, discuss the pros and cons of interventions with their patients, and work as teams to develop protocols to study and improve services. The key to success in such a system is transparency among providers, administrators, and patients. Outcomes will need to be collected and shared. A heavy emphasis would need to be placed on both ongoing provider education as well as patient education, and there will be a critical role for shared decision-making programs (see "Decision-Support Services" later in the chapter). Other reimbursement models exist; these alternatives will require careful review by all relevant stakeholders and such decisions will no doubt have considerable impact on whether breast centers will be able to continue to provide the comprehensive services required by our patients.

COMPREHENSIVE BREAST CENTERS: FUTURE DIRECTIONS

Although great advances have been made in breast cancer treatment as well as the infrastructure to support the administration and dissemination of these advances, there is still important progress to be made. We will discuss three key areas likely to play important roles in the breast care centers of the future.

Decision-Support Services

Since the early studies showed that lumpectomy and mastectomy were equally effective in reducing breast cancer mortality,[22,57] women have had to make decisions regarding breast cancer treatment choices. Although not all women wish to take a more active role in treatment planning, unlimited access to prodigious amounts of unfiltered medical information has created a dilemma for those seeking to be an informed partner in health care decision-making. This is particularly problematic for patients with breast cancer; at the time of this writing, a Google search using the search term "breast cancer" results in over 50,600,000 results. Further, a 1-hour consultation with a breast cancer specialist can be equally overwhelming. Additional consultations with other specialists can compound the confusion.

In this challenging environment, any assistance in making treatment decisions can be welcome. While often this function is served by a friend or family member, formal decision-support services within a cancer center can operationalize this function by having specially trained "consultation planners" on hand to meet with patients before the consultation to help articulate their information needs as well as to record and summarize the consultation for later patient review. The Consultation Planning,

Recording, and Summarizing Program (CPRS) was first piloted at the UCSF Breast Care Center in 1998. We have recently reported our initial experience with CPRS on 278 patients who agreed to participate in this study between March 2005 and December 2006.[58] In this group, we found that consultation planning resulted in an increased Decision Self-Efficacy score (3.24 to 3.53, $p < 0.001$) and reduced Decisional Conflict score (2.78 to 2.03, $p < 0.001$). Overall, the clinicians supported continuing this service for their patients, as they recognized that it provided added value to the consultation and helped to focus the discussion to specific patient concerns. We have made some modifications to streamline implementation into clinic flow and to create a more succinct summary of the consultation to the patients. We believe that such a service could be of extreme benefit to both patients and providers as more information becomes available daily and clinicians become ever more challenged in transmitting this information empathetically to patients in a time-constrained setting. Reimbursement for such services has not been explored, but these programs have the potential to add widespread utility in the multidisciplinary setting.

Although not specifically included in the decision-support model, patient navigators could play an increasing role in guiding patients not only through the decision-making process, but through the multiple provider visits and testing that are part of the challenge to any newly diagnosed patient.

Information Technology/Informatics

In order to sustain continued improvements in breast cancer care, both research and quality improvement are essential. Both efforts are heavily reliant on treatment and outcome data. Interestingly, the goals of quality assurance, performance assessment, clinical research, patient safety, and billing all require collection of similar data elements. However, the burden of developing these shared data collection systems is significant and will require shared effort both at a given center as well as across centers. The National Cancer Institute, through the Cancer BioInformatics Grid (caBIG)[59] and BIG Health,[60] is committed to developing and supporting a range of tools to support clinical trial management, tissue banking, and data analysis, and is working to develop tools for clinical data capture at the point of care. Several vendors, both small and large, are beginning to develop solutions that will not require an enormous investment in monolithic systems, and will enable all breast centers to participate in data collection to monitor their own processes.

A good example of data systems that support care are the organizational structures that developed following passage of the Mammography Quality Standards Act (MQSA). This bill mandated the notification of patients and their providers when an abnormality on a mammogram was detected. The legislation was intended to ensure notification when mammographic abnormalities were found. A beneficial unintended consequence of this act was the development of coordinated systems. Now, every mammography unit has such a system that automates the sending of letters to patients. The significant recent advances in information technology will make it possible for us to develop and use very different types of technology to support our clinical and research processes. Major Internet vendors,

such as Microsoft and Google, are providing the ability for patients to store their information, and smaller vendors are developing tools to enable patients and physicians to create shared records and communicate information among multiple providers and patients.

The future systems will involve patients providing information about themselves and their experience of care through Internet-based tools. Ideally, we will see the proliferation of open-source (or software/code that is freely available to anyone to use without a fee) solutions where data is captured and stored in a structured manner to enable data sharing. Our center has been piloting the use of Web-based surveys, in collaboration with Dartmouth Hitchcock Medical Center, to enable a summary report for providers at the time the patient arrives, and to begin to coordinate services based on patient-stated needs, making sure that genetic counselors are alerted to those patients with significant family history, and the psychosocial support teams can meet and provide assistance to those with significant psychological distress. The refinement of such tools will in future dramatically improve clinical efficiency, allow for performance assessment, and streamline clinical research efforts.

Complementary and Alternative Medicine Treatment

The growing interest in complementary and alternative medicine (CAM) in the United States has been particularly marked in patients diagnosed with cancer. CAM is defined by the NIH as incorporating four separate domains: mind-body medicine (patient support groups, cognitive-behavioral therapy, meditation, prayer); biologically based practices (herbs, dietary supplements, vitamins); manipulative/body-based practices (osteopathic manipulation, massage); and energy medicine (qi gong, electromagnetic field therapies). In addition, a separate domain that includes whole systems of practice has been defined (homeopathic medicine, naturopathic medicine, traditional Chinese medicine).[61]

Among cancer patients, the greatest use of CAM has been sought by patients with breast cancer,[62] with overall CAM use among breast cancer patients ranging from 48% to 83% across ethnic groups, predominantly in the use of dietary supplements and herbs.[63] An example of the integration of CAM into breast cancer treatment is the Osher Center for Integrative Medicine at UCSF which is housed directly adjacent to the UCSF Comprehensive Cancer Center. Practitioners in the Cancer Center work together with those at the Osher Center to provide collaborative care, incorporating CAM into the schedule of allopathic treatment regimens to reduce the effects of cancer treatment, maintain holistic health, and restore wellness. Given the highly prevalent interest in CAM among our patients, it is incumbent upon those planning future multidisciplinary breast programs to consider ways to meet this need.

SUMMARY

There are now over 500 breast centers in the United States. Whether physician-owned or academic, real or virtual, these centers continue to make important contributions to improving the delivery of health care to patients with breast disease.

Breast cancer treatment has served as a model of multidisciplinary care for the cancer community at large, and will continue to break new ground in medical discovery, patient support and advocacy, education, bioinformatics, and organizational reform of health care systems. The comprehensive breast center model allows for rapid implementation of new treatment advances and technology directly to the patients who need them, and thus these centers will become increasingly important as the complexity of treatment continues to grow. In the future, there are great opportunities for such centers to be leaders in providing "better," rather than "more," care and to disseminate these practices into the community. This is an exciting time to be part of the immense changes occurring in health care and in breast cancer treatment. Within this environment, the charge of the comprehensive breast care centers will be to advocate strongly for our patients, who deserve the best that science, human capital, and health care systems can bring to bear to overcome their disease.

REFERENCES

1. Jemal A, Clegg LX, Ward E, et al. Annual report to the nation on the status of cancer, 1975-2001, with a special feature regarding survival. *Cancer.* 2004;101:3-27.
2. Halsted WS. I. The results of operations for the cure of cancer of the breast performed at the Johns Hopkins Hospital from June, 1889, to January, 1894. *Ann Surg.* 1894;20:497-555.
3. Silverstein MJ. The Van Nuys Breast Center: the first free-standing multidisciplinary breast center. *Surg Oncol Clin N Am.* 2000;9:159-175.
4. Lee-Feldstein A, Anton-Culver H, Feldstein PJ. Treatment differences and other prognostic factors related to breast cancer survival. Delivery systems and medical outcomes. *JAMA.* 1994;271:1163-1168.
5. Iscoe NA, Goel V, Wu K, et al. Variation in breast cancer surgery in Ontario. *CMAJ.* 1994;150:345-352.
6. Samet JM, Hunt WC, Farrow DC. Determinants of receiving breast-conserving surgery. The Surveillance, Epidemiology, and End Results Program, 1983-1986. *Cancer.* 1994;73:2344-2351.
7. Bailie K, Dobie I, Kirk S, et al. Survival after breast cancer treatment: the impact of provider volume. *J Eval Clin Pract.* 2007;13:749-757.
8. Sainsbury R, Haward B, Rider L, et al. Influence of clinician workload and patterns of treatment on survival from breast cancer. *Lancet.* 1995;345:1265-1270.
9. Blamey RW, Cataliotti L. The requirements of a specialist Breast Unit. *Eur J Cancer.* 2000;36:2288-2293.
10. Silverstein MJ. Sate-of-the-art breast units-a possibility or a fantasy? A comment from the US. *Eur J Cancer.* 2000;36:2283-2285.
11. Desch CE, McNiff KK, Schneider EC, et al. American Society of Clinical Oncology/National Comprehensive Cancer Network Quality Measures. *J Clin Oncol.* 2008;26:3631-3637.
12. Malin JL, Schneider EC, Epstein AM, et al. Results of the National Initiative for Cancer Care Quality: how can we improve the quality of cancer care in the United States? *J Clin Oncol.* 2006;24:626-634.
13. Nystrom L, Andersson I, Bjurstam N, et al. Long-term effects of mammography screening: updated overview of the Swedish randomised trials. *Lancet.* 2002;359:909-919.
14. Bjurstam N, Bjorneld L, Warwick J, et al. The Gothenburg Breast Screening Trial. *Cancer.* 2003;97:2387-2396.
15. Pisano ED, Gatsonis C, Hendrick E, et al. Diagnostic performance of digital versus film mammography for breast-cancer screening. *N Engl J Med.* 2005;353:1773-1783.
16. Skaane P, Hofvind S, Skjennald A. Randomized trial of screen-film versus full-field digital mammography with soft-copy reading in population-based screening program: follow-up and final results of Oslo II study. *Radiology.* 2007;244:708-717.
17. Fischer U, Baum F, Obenauer S, et al. Comparative study in patients with microcalcifications: full-field digital mammography vs screen-film mammography. *Eur Radiol.* 2002;12:2679-2683.
18. Warner E, Plewes DB, Hill KA, et al. Surveillance of BRCA1 and BRCA2 mutation carriers with magnetic resonance imaging, ultrasound, mammography, and clinical breast examination. *JAMA.* 2004;292:1317-1325.

19. Lehman CD, Isaacs C, Schnall MD, et al. Cancer yield of mammography, MR, and US in high-risk women: prospective multi-institution breast cancer screening study. *Radiology.* 2007;244:381-388.
20. DeMartini W, Lehman C, Partridge S. Breast MRI for cancer detection and characterization: a review of evidence-based clinical applications. *Acad Radiol.* 2008;15:408-416.
21. Kuhl CK, Schrading S, Leutner CC, et al. Mammography, breast ultrasound, and magnetic resonance imaging for surveillance of women at high familial risk for breast cancer. *J Clin Oncol.* 2005;23:8469-8476.
22. Fisher B, Anderson S, Bryant J, et al. Twenty-year follow-up of a randomized trial comparing total mastectomy, lumpectomy, and lumpectomy plus irradiation for the treatment of invasive breast cancer. *N Engl J Med.* 2002;347:1233-1241.
23. Bedrosian I, Mick R, Orel SG, et al. Changes in the surgical management of patients with breast carcinoma based on preoperative magnetic resonance imaging. *Cancer.* 2003;98:468-473.
24. Schnall MD, Blume J, Bluemke DA, et al. MRI detection of distinct incidental cancer in women with primary breast cancer studied in IBMC 6883. *J Surg Oncol.* 2005;92:32-38.
25. Orel SG, Weinstein SP, Schnall MD, et al. Breast MR imaging in patients with axillary node metastases and unknown primary malignancy. *Radiology.* 1999;212:543-549.
26. Stomper PC, Waddell BE, Edge SB, et al. Breast MRI in the evaluation of patients with occult primary breast carcinoma. *Breast J.* 1999;5:230-234.
27. Henry-Tillman RS, Harms SE, Westbrook KC, et al. Role of breast magnetic resonance imaging in determining breast as a source of unknown metastatic lymphadenopathy. *Am J Surg.* 1999;178:496-500.
28. Basnett I, Gill M, Tobias JS. Variations in breast cancer management between a teaching and a non-teaching district. *Eur J Cancer.* 1992;28A:1945-1950.
29. Rowland JH, Desmond KA, Meyerowitz BE, et al. Role of breast reconstructive surgery in physical and emotional outcomes among breast cancer survivors. *J Natl Cancer Inst.* 2000;92:1422-1429.
30. Wijayanayagam A, Kumar AS, Foster RD, et al. Optimizing the total skin-sparing mastectomy. *Arch Surg.* 2008;143:38-45; discussion 45.
31. Crowe JP, Jr., Kim JA, Yetman R, et al. Nipple-sparing mastectomy: technique and results of 54 procedures. *Arch Surg.* 2004;139:148-150.
32. Schnitt SJ, Connolly JL, Tavassoli FA, et al. Interobserver reproducibility in the diagnosis of ductal proliferative breast lesions using standardized criteria. *Am J Surg Pathol.* 1992;16:1133-1143.
33. Newman EA, Guest AB, Helvie MA, et al. Changes in surgical management resulting from case review at a breast cancer multidisciplinary tumor board. *Cancer.* 2006;107:2346-2351.
34. Staradub VL, Messenger KA, Hao N, et al. Changes in breast cancer therapy because of pathology second opinions. *Ann Surg Oncol.* 2002;9:982-987.
35. Benitez PR, Keisch ME, Vicini F, et al. Five-year results: the initial clinical trial of MammoSite balloon brachytherapy for partial breast irradiation in early-stage breast cancer. *Am J Surg.* 2007;194:456-462.
36. Veronesi U, Orecchia R, Luini A, et al. A preliminary report of intraoperative radiotherapy (IORT) in limited-stage breast cancers that are conservatively treated. *Eur J Cancer.* 2001;37:2178-2183.
37. Kraus-Tiefenbacher U, Scheda A, Steil V, et al. Intraoperative radiotherapy (IORT) for breast cancer using the Intrabeam system. *Tumori.* 2005;91:339-345.
38. Arthur DW, Winter K, Kuske RR, et al. A phase II trial of brachytherapy alone after lumpectomy for select breast cancer: tumor control and survival outcomes of RTOG 95-17. *Int J Radiat Oncol Biol Phys.* 2008;72:467-473.
39. Whelan TJ, Kim DH, Sussman J. Clinical experience using hypofractionated radiation schedules in breast cancer. *Semin Radiat Oncol.* 2008;18:257-264.
40. Soler-Vila H, Kasl SV, Jones BA. Prognostic significance of psychosocial factors in African-American and white breast cancer patients: a population-based study. *Cancer.* 2003;98:1299-1308.
41. Osborne RH, Sali A, Aaronson NK, et al. Immune function and adjustment style: do they predict survival in breast cancer? *Psychooncology.* 2004;13:199-210.
42. Goodwin PJ, Ennis M, Bordeleau LJ, et al. Health-related quality of life and psychosocial status in breast cancer prognosis: analysis of multiple variables. *J Clin Oncol.* 2004;22:4184-4192.
43. Cotton SP, Levine EG, Fitzpatrick CM, et al. Exploring the relationships among spiritual well-being, quality of life, and psychological adjustment in women with breast cancer. *Psychooncology.* 1999;8:429-438.
44. Chang JH, Vines E, Bertsch H, et al. The impact of a multidisciplinary breast cancer center on recommendations for patient management: the University of Pennsylvania experience. *Cancer.* 2001;91:1231-1237.
45. Eley JW, Hill HA, Chen VW, et al. Racial differences in survival from breast cancer. Results of the National Cancer Institute Black/White Cancer Survival Study. *JAMA.* 1994;272:947-954.

46. Joslyn SA, West MM. Racial differences in breast carcinoma survival. *Cancer.* 2000;88:114-123.
47. Carey LA, Perou CM, Livasy CA, et al. Race, breast cancer subtypes, and survival in the Carolina Breast Cancer Study. *JAMA.* 2006;295:2492-2502.
48. Lund MJ, Brawley OP, Ward KC, et al. Parity and disparity in first course treatment of invasive breast cancer. *Breast Cancer Res Treat.* 2008;109: 545-557.
49. Chu KC, Lamar CA, Freeman HP. Racial disparities in breast carcinoma survival rates: seperating factors that affect diagnosis from factors that affect treatment. *Cancer.* 2003;97:2853-2860.
50. Jandorf L, Fatone A, Borker PV, et al. Creating alliances to improve cancer prevention and detection among urban medically underserved minority groups. The East Harlem Partnership for Cancer Awareness. *Cancer.* 2006;107:2043-2051.
51. Rapkin BD, Massie MJ, Jansky EJ, et al. Developing a partnership model for cancer screening with community-based organizations: the ACCESS breast cancer education and outreach project. *Am J Community Psychol.* 2006;38:153-164.
52. Gabram SG, Lund MJ, Gardner J, et al. Effects of an outreach and internal navigation program on breast cancer diagnosis in an urban cancer center with a large African-American population. *Cancer.* 2008;113:602-607.
53. Johansen MA, Mayer DK, Hoover HC Jr. Obstacles to implementing cancer clinical trials. *Semin Oncol Nurs.* 1991;7:260-267.
54. Simon MS, Brown DR, Du W, et al. Accrual to breast cancer clinical trials at a university-affiliated hospital in metropolitan Detroit. *Am J Clin Oncol.* 1999;22:42-46.
55. Swanson GM, Ward AJ. Recruiting minorities into clinical trials: toward a participant-friendly system. *J Natl Cancer Inst.* 1995;87:1747-1759.
56. Paik S, Shak S, Tang G, et al. A multigene assay to predict recurrence of tamoxifen-treated, node-negative breast cancer. *N Engl J Med.* 2004;351:2817-2826.
57. Veronesi U, Cascinelli N, Mariani L, et al. Twenty-year follow-up of a randomized study comparing breast-conserving surgery with radical mastectomy for early breast cancer. *N Engl J Med.* 2002;347:1227-1232.
58. Belkora JK, Loth MK, Chen DF, et al. Monitoring the implementation of Consultation Planning, Recording, and Summarizing in a breast care center. *Patient Educ Couns.* 2008; Dec. 73(3):536-543.
59. *About caBIG, Cancer Biomedical Informatics Grid.* National Cancer Institute. https://cabig.nci.gov/overview/.
60. BIG Health Consortium. http://www.bighealthconsortium.org/.
61. http://nccam.nih.gov/health/whatiscam/.
62. Morris KT, Johnson N, Homer L, et al. A comparison of complementary therapy use between breast cancer patients and patients with other primary tumor sites. *Am J Surg.* 2000;179:407-411.
63. DiGianni LM, Garber JE, Winer EP. Complementary and alternative medicine use among women with breast cancer. *J Clin Oncol.* 2002;20:34S-38S

CHAPTER 7

Establishing a Cancer Genetics Service

Deborah J. MacDonald

Given the accumulating evidence documenting the efficacy of genetic screening and risk-reduction interventions, genetic cancer risk assessment (GCRA) has become a medical standard-of-care option for persons with a personal and/or family history of cancer suggestive of increased cancer risk.[1-5] GCRA utilizes rapidly evolving genetic technologies along with established empiric risk models to estimate cancer risk and provide age- and risk-level appropriate cancer prevention and risk-reduction strategies for individuals and their family members. The ultimate value of GCRA is the opportunity for initiation of early detection or risk-reducing strategies that would be most effective in minimizing cancer incidence, morbidity, and mortality, by identifying persons at increased cancer risk prior to the onset of an initial or subsequent cancer.

The GCRA process includes assessing personal and family medical history and family structure[6] to determine individual cancer risks and the probability of an inherited genetic trait accounting for cancer in an individual and/or the individual's family and counseling about the appropriateness, benefits, limitations, risks, and process of genetic testing and subsequent health care implications. If genetic testing is undertaken and a deleterious mutation identified, single-site mutation testing in other at-risk family members adds relatively little cost while maximizing benefits to families by distinguishing relatives at high risk from those at modest or average risk. Relatives who did not inherit the familial mutation can then be spared the personal and economic cost of unnecessary interventions.[7]

The greatest experience and application of GCRA to date is in the evaluation of hereditary breast cancer. Quantification of risk from informative genetic testing enables women to choose among risk-reducing interventions such as chemoprevention, mastectomy, and/or bilateral salpingo-oophorectomy, enhanced and earlier surveillance, and healthier lifestyle choices.[8-20] For patients who undergo genetic testing but do not have a detectable cancer-associated mutation, who decline testing, or are unable to proceed with genetic testing due to financial or other reasons, a variety of empiric risk models may be used to quantify risk and provide individualized recommendations for cancer screening and risk-reduction. Similarly, the discovery of other single genes involved in early onset-colon cancer or other heritable cancer-associated syndromes (eg, multiple endocrine neoplasia) enables prevention, risk-reduction, or earlier diagnosis of cancer through identification of high-risk individuals. As such, GCRA has an important role in guiding patient decision-making.[4,17,18] Recognizing the value of GCRA, genetic counseling and testing was added as a supportive service to the 2004 American College of Surgeons (ACS) Commission on Cancer, Cancer Program Standards.[21] Consequently, community-based cancer centers are integrating GCRA into oncology care. State-of-the-art quality care, including access to innovative research, may be achieved by partnering with a comprehensive cancer center with a robust GCRA program.[22] This chapter describes essential components of a cancer genetics service and various models of service delivery utilized by community centers affiliated with a cancer genetics center of excellence.

PRACTICAL CONSIDERATIONS

Compliance with the ACS Cancer Program Standards and increasing consumer demand has fueled community cancer centers' interest in offering GCRA services. Prior to implementation, the purpose, goals, scope of service, and plans for operating, integrating, marketing, and evaluating the cancer genetics service must be defined. While the ultimate purpose of a cancer

The author thanks Jeffrey N. Weitzel, MD and Sharon Sand, CCRP for critical review of the chapter.

TABLE 7-1 Goals of a Cancer Genetics Service

- Identify individuals at high risk for cancer
- Provide genetic counseling for cancer risk
- Develop individualized risk management plans
- Promote appropriate screening for patients and their families
- Protect patient privacy and confidentiality
- Provide cancer genetics education to clinicians/ community
- Establish research collaborations

genetics service is to minimize cancer incidence, morbidity, and mortality, the more immediate purpose would be defined by the practice setting, considering community needs and available resources. Goals requisite for a state-of-the-art clinical cancer genetics service that respects the personal and family implications of GCRA while advancing scientific knowledge are depicted in Table 7-1 and discussed throughout this chapter. The steps in establishing a cancer genetics service are outlined in Table 7-2.

NEEDS ASSESSMENT

An essential initial step in establishing a viable GCRA program is to determine needs of the target population and potential barriers to implementation and success.[23] A culturally sensitive and linguistically appropriate anonymous survey distributed to

TABLE 7-2 Steps in Establishing a Cancer Genetics Service

- Assess community/target population needs
- Identify/educate/engage key administrative/clinician supporters
- Define purpose/goals/scope of service
- Determine clinical/support staff required
- Purchase pedigree drawing program
- Set up computer database
- Develop medical and family history data forms
- Create cancer genetics chart
- Ensure confidentiality/privacy of patients/records
- Establish consultation fees, billing procedures
- Arrange phlebotomy services
- Develop/distribute referral guidelines
- Secure consultation space/furnishings
- Determine fixed vs flexible clinic days/hours
- Establish protocol for uninsured and urgent patient consult requests
- Gain clinical cancer genetics competence
- Contract for advice from cancer genetics experts
- Develop marketing/implementation/impact/evaluation plan

patients attending oncology and general medicine clinics is a cost-effective and efficient means of obtaining information about interest in participating in cancer genetics services and uncovering potential service barriers, including psychosocial barriers related beliefs, knowledge, and risk perception.[19] For instance, a belief that cancer cannot be prevented, or lack of knowledge about genetics as a factor in cancer causation, may lessen interest in and deter uptake of genetic counseling and appropriate risk-management interventions. Educational sessions, fliers, and fact sheets could help address these barriers as well as inform the community and clinic/institution staff about the benefits of a cancer genetics service.

INSTITUTIONAL SUPPORT: ADMINISTRATORS AND CLINICIANS

Engaging institutional support for a cancer genetics service is crucial to service development and implementation. The addition of this service enhances the institution's reputation, differentiates it from its competition, and may also attract philanthropic support.[24] Further, apprising breast center administrators about expected revenue, including potential downstream revenue from cancer screening, chemoprevention, and surgical risk-reduction interventions, may help to justify under-reimbursed costs.[22,24]

Similar to other medical fee-for-service health care, most cancer genetics patients will be referred by their health care provider. Garnering clinician support from these gatekeepers and medical directors who approve requests for genetic consultations/testing will greatly influence the acceptability of a cancer genetics service. Means to do so include providing continuing medical education (CME) lectures related to the need for this service and how the service will benefit patients, families, and the breast center, and meeting with key clinicians to gain their input and enthusiasm and act as "champions" for the cancer genetics service.

SCOPE OF CANCER GENETICS SERVICES

The scope of services provided are primarily dependent upon institutional support, staff expertise and availability, practice setting, availability for consulting with genetic experts, funding, and community needs/interest. Currently, the majority of patients referred for GCRA are adult women with a personal and/or family history of premenopausal breast cancer. Given this, many community genetics programs are limited to breast cancer while more comprehensive risk assessment programs at most NCI-designated Comprehensive Cancer Centers encompass many adult- and childhood-onset cancer genetics syndromes (eg, Lynch syndrome, also known as hereditary nonpolyposis colon cancer [HNPCC] or multiple endocrine neoplasia [MEN]).[25]

MULTIDISCIPLINARY CANCER GENETICS SERVICE STAFF

Accurate risk assessment requires thorough knowledge of cancer etiology, natural history, treatment, age-specific penetrance, genotype-phenotype correlations, genetic heterogeneity, modifiers of penetrance and expression, and the availability, accuracy, and predictive value of clinical and research-based genetic tests. For example, not knowing that a reported "female" cancer at age 31 is unlikely to be an epithelial ovarian cancer could lead to inaccurate risk assessment and inappropriate interventions. Similarly, lack of awareness of breast cancer–associated germline mutations other than the BRCA genes (eg, the PTEN gene), might result in false reassurance from uninformative (negative) BRCA testing. Thus, a multidisciplinary team of genetic counselors, oncology nurses, and physicians with specialized training in clinical cancer genetics is indispensable to accurate risk assessment and appropriate risk management recommendations.[5]

Support personnel for a high-quality GCRA program would also include psychologists/social workers, research staff to coordinate related studies, and a clinic coordinator to schedule patient appointments using a standard intake form to ensure referrals are appropriate, notify referring clinicians of appointments, mail standard genetics medical and family history forms, establish and maintain patient records, and facilitate collection of pathology and/or medical reports prior to patient appointments. Considerations in staff roles/responsibilities are listed in Table 7-3.

Typical time for GCRA includes approximately 2 hours to conduct the initial appointment and 1 hour for follow-up visits, with additional time for pre- and postappointment information and medical record-gathering; completing clinical, research, and test request forms; obtaining, preparing, and sending out blood or tumor specimens for genetic tests; facilitating insurance authorization for testing and/or consultation visits; preparing clinical notes; and expert case review for consensus regarding risk assessment and management strategies.

TABLE 7-3 Physician, Counselor, Clerical Staff Roles/ Responsibilities

Define Who Will:
- Provide medical directorship
- Educate administrators, institutional leadership
- Initially communicate with new patients
- Schedule patient appointments
- Prepare patient charts
- Coordinate data collection, mailing, billing
- Request pathology reports/medical records
- See patient at initial/follow-up/test results visits
- Perform genetics focused physical examination
- Obtain informed consent for genetic tests/research
- Oversee phlebotomy process, preparation/mailing of samples
- Develop/maintain database and pedigree updates
- Generate initial/follow-up consultation note
- Sign-off on consultation notes
- Bill for services

PHYSICAL SPACE

Persons seeking cancer risk consultations often have a significant psychological burden (fear, anxiety, etc.) associated with cancer experience in their family. Consequently, a waiting area and consultation room that has limited exposure to patients in the midst of cancer treatment may minimize stress associated with GCRA. As patients often bring family members to the consultation, the room should be large enough to accommodate several family members and the genetics staff. An exam room is also needed for a genetics-focused exam (eg, performing a breast exam and teaching breast self-exam; measuring head circumference; thyroid palpation; and evaluation of other physical features characteristic of specific heritable cancer syndromes).

OPERATING EXPENSES

Given the intellectual capital and time required to provide quality GCRA, labor (professional and support staff) is the single largest institutional cost for a clinical cancer genetics service. Other costs are those related to computer programs for data entry/management and pedigree drawing, marketing, continuing education, phlebotomy, indigent patient consultations/genetic testing/risk management, research efforts, projected growth, and, if partnering with a center of excellence, consultative fees (see the "Exemplar" section later in the chapter).

BILLING FOR CANCER GENETICS SERVICES: CONSULTATION AND GENETIC TESTS

As in other fee-for-service medical care, fees for GCRA based on a physician-centered model for service delivery use E&M code billing (eg, CPT 9924x series codes, modified by extended time codes as appropriate). Non–physician counselor time is generally not separately billable as there are compliance challenges to billing "incident to" a physician visit, and lack of genetic counselor licensing in most states limits counselors' ability to bill directly.

Today, most major health insurance indemnity and managed care plans, and Medicare, have established criteria for genetic counseling/testing and for costs of risk-appropriate interventions. Many laboratory tests for hereditary cancer susceptibility are available from only a few vendors; most have reimbursement assistance programs wherein the patient deals directly with the testing vendor. Nonetheless, counselors are often burdened with time-consuming tasks required to facilitate test ordering, insurance coverage, and billing.

PROMOTING PROGRAM AWARENESS AND APPROPRIATE REFERRALS

Providing periodic cancer genetics CME presentations and tumor board or other case discussions of referred patients enables clinicians to learn first-hand of the value of cancer genetics services. Similar presentations for the lay community will also generate awareness and interest in the new service. A brochure/flyer and one-page referral guideline outlining indicators of genetic cancer risk and staff qualifications will further facilitate awareness and appropriate referrals.[22,23]

EXEMPLAR: THE CITY OF HOPE CANCER SCREENING & PREVENTION PROGRAM NETWORK (CSPPN)

The City of Hope (COH), an NCI-designated Comprehensive Cancer Center in Southern California, established the Division of Clinical Cancer Genetics and the Cancer Screening & Prevention Program (CSPP) in late 1996 as components of a multidisciplinary clinical and research program to assess individuals and families at increased cancer risk.[22] The initial clinical CSPP program, established to provide comprehensive GCRA services, was jointly developed by an MD with expertise in both medical oncology and clinical genetics, and an APN with genetic expertise. Subsequent personnel include a clinic coordinator, a laboratory research associate to conduct studies under the principal investigator's supervision and manage biospecimens from an IRB-approved Hereditary Cancer Registry protocol; a certified clinic research associate to organize the registry's relational database and pedigree drawing program[27] and assist in conducting clinical protocols; and dedicated administrative support staff, another oncologist, 3 board-certified genetic counselors, a project coordinator, 3 assistants, and an education assistant, all partly funded by research and education grants. Cancer center resources include a community health education specialist, research psychologists, and doctoral nurse scientists with expertise in education, quality of life, and survivorship research. Extramural consultants in public health and law help to support cancer genetics research in ethical, legal, and social issues. Grant support also enabled an underserved, primarily Hispanic, community outreach GCRA program. Educational outreach via CME-accredited cancer genetics presentations at regional medical centers increased the number and appropriateness of referrals.[28] A weekly multidisciplinary Clinical Cancer Genetics Working Group with experts in medical and surgical oncology, clinical genetics, genetic counseling, and clinical research allows for consensus on pedigree analysis, mutation probability, testing strategies, test results interpretation, medical management advice, and identification of candidates for research studies.

In 1998, the Cancer Screening & Prevention Program Network (CSPPN) was developed to facilitate delivery of state-of-the-art GCRA services in dispersed communities where expertise and infrastructure were needed. Community partners participate in the Working Group in-person or by Web-conferencing. To enable common pedigree structure and data collection, the Enterprise (multiclient server) version of Progeny (Progeny Software LLC, South Bend, IN) pedigree-drawing software was obtained and customized to the CSPPN clinical and research needs. Standardized scannable forms for patient medical and family history data collection enable efficient data entry. Growth of the CSPPN and innovation in technical support were catalyzed by education research grants and a technology transfer grant. An extended informatics technology-enabled network strategy was designed, enabling community-based breast centers to contract with COH for program development, specialized training, ongoing

support, and continued education for community clinicians. To date, the CSPPN has provided comprehensive GCRA services to more than 5000 individuals and their families, with nearly half of these stemming from satellite clinics.

DEVELOPING COMPETENCY IN GENETIC CANCER RISK ASSESSMENT

Conducting cancer genetics consultative services requires a higher level of practical knowledge and cancer risk assessment skills than recognizing and referring patients for GCRA.[1,29-31] Therefore, COH developed a multifaceted Cancer Genetics Education Program (CGEP) supported in part by a cancer education grant (R25 CA75131) from the NCI. The CGEP provides CME-qualified cancer genetics education for clinicians in the form of all-day seminars, 1- and 2-year career development traineeships, and an annual 8-week Web-based, 1-week on-site Intensive Course in Cancer Risk Counseling and Community Research to foster practitioner-level competence in cancer genetics for community-based clinicians.[32] Cancer genetics short courses are also available periodically through professional organizations or institutions, such as ASCO, the National Society of Genetic Counselors, the International Society of Nurses in Genetics, and the Oncology Nursing Society.

COMMUNITY BREAST CENTER–CENTER OF EXCELLENCE CONTRACTING RELATIONSHIPS AND COMPONENTS

Partnering with a GCRA center of excellence in a NCI-designated Comprehensive Cancer Center offers community breast centers access to ongoing cancer genetics education, comprehensive GCRA, education and health services research, and clinical prevention trials.[22,33] Prior to implementation, a contract of the relationship between COH and the community center describing responsibilities of each party was approved by each institution. For a monthly subscription fee to COH under a medical director agreement with the collaborating community center, COH provides expert oversight and technical support for the genetics service, as well as training and ongoing practice development (Table 7-4). Satellite cases are discussed in person or by Web-conferencing at the weekly Working Group for consensus on case evaluation and risk management, including differential diagnosis, genetic test result interpretation, empiric risk clarification, risk-management options, and in some cases identification of candidates for local or national clinical trials. Community clinicians are thus assured of providing quality care that delivers the same level of assessment to patients seen at COH and enables community centers to remain current with the progressively more sophisticated GCRA clinical science. In return, community outreach helps COH meet its NCI obligations for maintaining "comprehensive" status.

Contracted activities generally include (1) site survey and needs assessment regarding personnel (cancer risk counselor, clerical and administrative FTEs, and identification of dedicated clinician[s]), support services (eg, phlebotomy), and clinic family counseling room specifications; (2) provision of common

TABLE 7-4 Community Center/Center of Excellence Contracted Relationship Components

Assistance with Establishment of Clinical Services:

- Obtaining administrative support
- Clinic site survey and needs assessment
- Clinic family counseling room specifications
- Personnel, phlebotomy service, research collaborations
- Common data collection forms to enhance clinical/research efforts
- Professional education to augment staff skills/facilitate appropriate referrals
- Lay education to foster community awareness/interest
- IRB submission for community center participation in hereditary cancer research
- Monthly subscription fee paid to Center of Excellence under medical director agreement

data forms for medical and family history assessment to facilitate health services, clinical, and behavioral outcomes research; (3) provision of collateral materials (informational brochure, other clinical and research data collection forms, patient-oriented educational materials and printed genetic counseling aids [charts, graphs, diagrams, etc.]); (4) orientation to COH cancer genetics protocols, pedigree software, and database setup advice and assistance; (5) training for the collaborating center's cancer risk counselor(s) to augment GCRA skills; (6) lay and professional education to increase awareness in the community and promote appropriate referrals; (7) clinical research associate support for IRB submission for participation in the COH Hereditary Cancer Research Registry; and (8) a monthly subscription fee paid to the COH under a medical director agreement.

MODELS FOR CANCER GENETICS SERVICE DELIVERY IN THE COMMUNITY

In addition to GCRA via the standard 1 to 2 visits with an integrated multidisciplinary cancer genetics team at an academic cancer center, alternative modes of GCRA delivery may enable cost-effective community medical center participation. For community breast centers considering the addition of a genetics program, the use of outside expert consultants from a regional NCI-designated Comprehensive Cancer Center may be a cost-effective way to secure the required critical mass of intellectual capital to run a quality program. The length of start-up time for full program implementation is decreased through use of existing data collection forms, databases, and educational and promotional efforts. The weekly Working Group conferences promote integration rather than isolation of local GCRA teams, and provide incremental quality improvement. A variety of models, described later, operate within the CSPPN, ranging from dual providers (MD plus counselor) on site to videoconference supported telemedicine. The choice of models is dependent in part on the availability of qualified staff and the local institutional economic environment.

The first community–COH cancer center collaboration was established in 1998. At that time, there was no GCRA service within a 2-hour radius of the collaborating site. In this model, an APN cancer risk counselor conducts on-site risk assessment and initiates genetic testing/research enrollment as appropriate. The clinic operates 2 consecutive days each month, with three 2-hour appointments scheduled each day by the local clinic coordinator. The initial visit and phlebotomy are conducted at no charge as a cancer center-supported community service. Patients are seen at COH by the MD/counselor team for the required subsequent follow-up appointment for genetic test results disclosure, summary consultation, and care recommendations.

A second program operates similarly to that just described, except that the return/summary visit is conducted on-site at the community breast cancer, a 45-minute drive from COH. On clinic days, the team also attends breast tumor case conferences, providing ad hoc input on potential hereditary cases.

A third co-branded program operates in another state. In this model, an APN board-certified in genetic counseling sees patients with several of the medical center physicians. The COH program director reviews, edits, and signs the consultation notes, which are co-signed by the APN and the local physician who provided the billable services.

An additional affiliated program was initially established by an APN who attended the COH Intensive Course in Cancer Risk Assessment. To support the expanding program, a board-certified GC was hired following completion of a 1-year cancer genetics traineeship through the COH Career Development Program. A medical oncologist and a colorectal surgeon provide program support, a surgical oncologist recently completed the Intensive Course to assume a greater role in the program, and another full-time genetic counselor was brought on board to meet increasing referral requests.

TECHNOLOGY ENABLED QUALITY ASSURANCE: UNDERSERVED COMMUNITY OUTREACH

A grant-funded project targeting underserved patients allowed COH to establish a cancer genetics program at two regional health care delivery systems serving a predominantly Hispanic underserved community. The grant also provides funds for commercial genetic testing. The program is staffed in part by COH bilingual and biliterate cancer risk counselors with additional training in culturally sensitive approaches to GCRA and supported by a videoconferencing link for physician telemedicine sessions for the results disclosure visit; an on-site patient coordinator facilitates the process.[23] To ensure that referred patients receive appropriate risk management, the collaborating institutions committed to providing these patients with cancer screening and risk-reducing services, including preventive surgeries.

OPPORTUNITIES FOR RESEARCH COLLABORATION THROUGH THE CSPPN

Each affiliated center has the opportunity to participate in the City of Hope IRB-approved hereditary cancer registry enabling multiple intra- and extramural collaborations on topics as diverse as health services research; genetic epidemiology; ethical, legal and social implications; translational chemoprevention clinical trials; and behavioral science.[27,34-38]

The CSPPN team has gained considerable experience in conducting qualitative and quantitative clinical outcome studies and in cancer communications and education pertinent to GCRA.[7,18,28,35,37-42] Data from the registry enable participation in the multi-institutional consortia that are necessary to assemble enough hereditary cases for epidemiologic studies, such as a recent study demonstrating significant hormone receptor concordance in BRCA carriers with bilateral breast cancer.[40] Other collaborative studies examined the influence of oral contraceptive use on penetrance of both breast and ovarian cancers, and the effect of pregnancy on cancer risk in BRCA gene mutation carriers.[43,44]

FUTURE STUDIES

Establishing cancer genetics services in the community provides important opportunities for cancer control and behavioral and health outcomes research that might otherwise be missed, including new early detection, chemoprevention, and other risk-reduction clinical trials. Future research is needed to identify the benefits and cost-effectiveness of providing cancer genetics services in community cancer centers.

SUMMARY

Establishing a cancer genetics service in the community enables local provision of this medical standard-of-care option for individuals with a personal and/or family history of cancer suggestive of increased cancer risk. Service benefits include increased adherence to screening recommendations, reduced cancer incidence, increased detection of early-stage cancers, as well as community recognition.[8,17-20,45] Essential for the success of a cancer genetics service are determining community needs and interest, and engaging support from key genetics, oncology, and administrative professionals in the planning process. Partnering with a center of excellence facilitates delivery of state-of-the-art clinical cancer genetics services and serves as an important resource for health services delivery research.

REFERENCES

1. American Society of Clinical Oncology. American Society of Clinical Oncology policy statement update: Genetic testing for cancer susceptibility. *J Clin Oncol.* 2003;21:2397-2406.
2. Daly MB, Axilbund JE, Bryant E, et al. Genetic/familial high-risk assessment: breast and ovarian. *J Natl Compr Canc Netw.* 2006;4:156-176.
3. Weitzel JN. Evidence for advice: reduction in risk of breast or ovarian cancer after salpingo-oophorectomy in carriers of BRCA1 or BRCA2 mutations. *Breast Dis.* 2004;14:354-356.
4. Weitzel JN. Genetic cancer risk assessment: putting it all together. *Cancer.* 1999;86(suppl):2483-2492.
5. Calzone KA, Stopfer J, Blackwood A, Weber B. Establishing a cancer risk evaluation program. *Cancer Practice.* 1997;5:228-233.
6. Weitzel JN, Lagos VI, Cullinane CA, et al. Limited family structure and BRCA gene mutation status in single cases of breast cancer. *JAMA.* 2007;297:2587-2595.
7. Weitzel JN, McCahill LE. The power of genetics to target surgical prevention. *N Engl J Med.* 2001;344:1942-1944.
8. Scheuer L, Kauff N, Robson M, et al. Outcome of preventive surgery and screening for breast and ovarian cancer in BRCA mutation carriers. *J Clin Oncol.* 2002;20:1260-1268.
9. Robson M, Offit K. Clinical practice. Management of an inherited predisposition to breast cancer. *N Engl J Med.* 2007;357:154-162.
10. Robson M, Svahn T, McCormick B, et al. Appropriateness of breast-conserving treatment of breast carcinoma in women with germline mutations in BRCA1 or BRCA2: a clinic-based series. *Cancer.* 2005;103:44-51.
11. Narod SA, Offit K. Prevention and management of hereditary breast cancer. *J Clin Oncol.* 2005;23:1656-1663.
12. Hartmann LC, Degnim A, Schaid DJ. Prophylactic mastectomy for BRCA1/2 carriers: progress and more questions. *J Clin Oncol.* 2004;22:981-983.
13. Meeuwissen PA, Seynaeve C, Brekelmans CT, et al. Outcome of surveillance and prophylactic salpingo-oophorectomy in asymptomatic women at high risk for ovarian cancer. *Gynecol Oncol.* 2005;97:476-482.
14. Daly MB, Axilbund JE, Bryant E, et al. NCCN Practice Guidelines in Oncology: Genetic/familial high risk assessment: breast and ovarian. v.1.2007:http://www.nccn.org/professionals/physician_gls/PDF/genetics_screening.pdf. Accessed March 22, 2007.
15. Kauff ND, Domchek SM, Friebel TM, et al. Risk-reducing salpingo-oophorectomy for the prevention of BRCA1- and BRCA2-associated breast and gynecologic cancer: a multicenter, prospective study. *J Clin Oncol.* 2008;26:1331-1337.
16. Kuhl CK, Schrading S, Leutner CC, et al. Mammography, breast ultrasound, and magnetic resonance imaging for surveillance of women at high familial risk for breast cancer. *J Clin Oncol.* 2005;23:8469-8476.
17. Botkin JR, Smith KR, Croyle RT, et al. Genetic testing for a BRCA1 mutation: Prophylactic surgery and screening behavior in women 2 years post testing. *Am J Med Genet.* 2003;118A:201-209.
18. Weitzel JN, McCaffrey SM, Nedelcu R, et al. Effect of genetic cancer risk assessment on surgical decisions at breast cancer diagnosis. *Archives of Surgery.* 2003;138:1323-1328; discussion 1329.
19. Ricker CN, Hiyama S, Fuentes S, et al. Beliefs and interest in cancer risk in an underserved Latino cohort. *Prev Med.* 2007;44:241-245.
20. Schwartz MD, Lerman C, Brogan B, et al. Impact of BRCA1/BRCA2 counseling and testing on newly diagnosed breast cancer patients. *J Clin Oncol.* 2004;22:1823-1829.
21. Commission on Cancer: *Cancer Program Standards.* Standard 6.1, p.67. Chicago: American College of Surgeons 2004 Revised Edition.
22. MacDonald DJ, Sand S, Kass FC, et al. The power of partnership: extending comprehensive cancer center expertise in clinical cancer genetics to breast care in community centers. *Semin Breast Dis.* 2006;9:39-47.
23. Ricker C, Lagos V, Feldman N, et al. If we build it . . . will they come? Establishing a cancer genetics services clinic for an underserved predominantly Latina cohort. *J Genet Couns.* 2006;15:505-514.
24. Ho C. How to develop and implement a cancer genetics risk assessment program: clinical and economic considerations. *Oncology Issues.* 2004;19:22-26.
25. Epplein M, Koon KP, Ramsey SD, Potter JD. Genetic services for familial cancer patients: a follow-up survey of National Cancer Institute Cancer Centers. *J Clin Oncol.* 2005;23:4713-4718.
26. Hampel H, Sweet KM, Westman JA, Offit K, Eng C. Referral for cancer genetics consultation: a review and compilation of risk assessment criteria. *J Med Genet.* 2004;41:81-91.
27. Sand SR, DeRam DS, MacDonald DJ, Blazer KR, Weitzel JN. Linkage of a pedigree drawing program and database to a program for determining BRCA mutation carrier probability. *Familial Cancer.* 2005;4:313-316.
28. Blazer KR, Grant M, Sand SR, et al. Effects of a cancer genetics education programme on clinicians knowledge and practice. *J Med Genet.* 2004;41:518-522.
29. International Society of Nurses in Genetics. *Genetics/Genomics Nursing: Scope & Standards of Practice.* Sliver Spring, MD: American Nurses Association; 2007.
30. Oncology Nursing Society. The Role of the Oncology Nurse in Cancer Genetics Counseling 2004. www.ons.org. Accessed October 1, 2004.
31. Oncology Nursing Society. Cancer Predisposition Genetic Testing and Risk Assessment Counseling 2004. www.ons.org. Accessed October 1, 2004.
32. Blazer KR, Grant M, Sand SR, et al. Development of a cancer genetics education program for clinicians. *J Cancer Educ.* 2002;17:69-73.
33. Sand S, Nedelcu R, Grady I, et al. Using video conferencing to extend genetic cancer risk assessment expertise to community-based medical centers. Paper presented at the American Society of Human Genetics 51st annual meeting, San Diego, CA, 2001.
34. Jasperson KW, Lowstuter K, Weitzel JN. Assessing the predictive accuracy of hMLH1 and hMSH2 mutation probability models. *J Genet Couns.* 2006;15:339-347.
35. MacDonald DJ, Sarna L, Uman GC, Grant M, Weitzel JN. Health beliefs of women with and without breast cancer seeking genetic cancer risk assessment. *Cancer Nurs.* 2005;28:372-379.

36. MacDonald DJ, Sarna L, Uman GC, Grant M, Weitzel JN. Cancer screening and risk reducing behaviors of women seeking genetic cancer risk assessment for breast and ovarian cancers. *Oncol Nurs Forum.* 2006;33: E27–E35.

37. Palomares MR, Paz IB, Weitzel JN. Genetic cancer risk assessment in the newly diagnosed breast cancer patient is useful and possible in practice. *J Clin Oncol.* 2005;23:3165-3166.

38. Weitzel JN, Lagos V, Blazer KR, et al. Prevalence of *BRCA* mutations and founder effect in high-risk Hispanic families. *Cancer Epidemiol Biomarkers Prev.* 2005;14:1666-1671.

39. Blazer KR, MacDonald DJ, Ricker C, et al. Outcomes from intensive training in genetic cancer risk counseling for clinicians. *Genet Med.* 2005;7:40-47.

40. Weitzel JN, Robson M, Pasini B, et al. A comparison of bilateral breast cancers in *BRCA* carriers. *Cancer Epidemiol Biomarkers Prev.* 2005;14:1534-1538.

41. MacDonald DJ, Choi J, Ferrell B, et al. Concerns of women presenting to a comprehensive cancer center for genetic cancer risk assessment. *J Med Genet.* 2002;39:526-530.

42. Weitzel JN, Ding S, Larson GP, et al. The *HRAS1* minisatellite locus and risk of ovarian cancer. *Cancer Res.* 2000;60:259-261.

43. Narod SA, Dube MP, Klijn J, et al. Oral contraceptives and the risk of breast cancer in *BRCA1* and *BRCA2* carriers. *J Natl Cancer Inst.* 2002;94:1773-1779.

44. Cullinane CA, Lubinski J, Neuhausen SL, et al. The effect of pregnancy as a risk factor for breast cancer in *BRCA1/BRCA2* mutation carriers. *Int J Cancer.* 2005;117:988-991.

45. Kauff ND, Barakat RR. Risk-reducing salpingo-oophorectomy in patients with germline mutations in BRCA1 or BRCA2. *J Clin Oncol.* 2007;25:2921-2927.

CHAPTER 8

Genetic Predisposition Syndromes

Linda Robinson

In 1860, Dr. Broca, a French surgeon, reported on the pedigree of his wife's family because of her early-onset breast cancer and the striking family history of breast cancer.[1] At around the same time, in 1865, Dr. Gregory Mendel was looking at the genetics of garden peas; his work would lay the foundation for the field of genetics. In the last 150 years, the identification and recognition of the molecular genetics component of disease has advanced, and the area of breast cancer has been no exception. Molecular genetic testing is redefining familial cancer and will continue to do so for many years. This chapter will review the clinical features, causative genes, and medical management options for hereditary breast cancer syndromes.

It has been estimated that 23% of all breast cancer patients have a family history of the disease, indicating that one or more first-degree relatives have been diagnosed with breast cancer in the family (Fig. 8-1).[2] In the general population, only 2% of all women have a family history suggestive of the inheritance of an autosomal dominant, inherited high-penetrance gene for breast cancer.[2] When you look specifically at breast cancer patients, only 5% to 10% of all breast cancer cases demonstrate a clear pattern of dominant inheritance.[4] There are several highly penetrant, dominantly inherited genes associated with breast cancer predisposition syndromes, including the BRCA1, BRCA2, TP53, and PTEN genes (Fig. 8-2). Although these cancer predisposition syndromes are rare, the clinician needs to be aware of these hereditary cancer syndromes that predispose to the carcinoma of the breast, and to recognize the diversity of these unique syndromes. However, most cases of familial breast cancer are not attributed to these single-gene disorders. It is believed that may are due to unidentified, low-penetrant genetic mutations and/or variants in the genome, in combination with environmental factors. The identification of these low-penetrant alleles is the next frontier for cancer genetics.

IDENTIFICATION OF CANCER PREDISPOSITION SYNDROMES

The American Society of Clinical Oncology recommends that genetic testing be offered when three criteria are met: (1) the individual has a personal or family history suggestive of a cancer genetic susceptibility condition, (2) the test can be adequately interpreted, and (3) the results will aid in the diagnosis or influence the medical or surgical management of the patient or family members.[5] These recommendations begin with the identification of these high-risk patients. A comprehensive review of family history is key to identifying patients at increased risk for hereditary cancer. In obtaining a 3-generation family history, it is important not only to elicit the family history of breast cancer, but to also ask about other cancers, including ovarian, thyroid, sarcomas, adrenocortical carcinoma, endometrial, pancreatic, brain tumors, and dermatologic manifestations. It is critical to obtain a family history on both the maternal and paternal side of the family. Also, one must take into consideration reduced penetrance, limited family medical information, and small family size. Besides recording the types of cancer in the family, the National Comprehensive Cancer Network (NCCN) guidelines recommend that the clinician determine not only the types of cancer in the family, but the age of diagnosis, documentation of the diagnosis from medical records (particularly pathology reports of primary cancers), a history of chemoprevention and/or risk-reducing surgery, carcinogen exposure, reproductive history, hormone use, and previous breast biopsies.[6] The family and patient's medical history, in conjunction with computerized risk assessment models, can quantify the patient's risk for a genetic predisposition to breast cancer.[7-9]

Several organizations have proposed criteria for when a patient should be referred for genetic counseling and testing

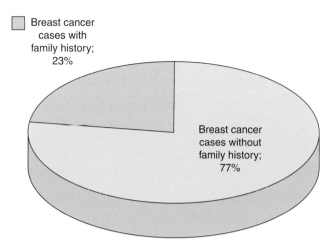

FIGURE 8-1 Percentage of breast cancer patients with a family history of breast cancer.

regarding hereditary breast and ovarian cancer. Although the criteria may vary slightly, they all recognize similar features: early-onset breast cancer (premenopausal or age 50 or less), ovarian cancer (with a family history of breast or ovarian cancer), individuals with two or more primary breast cancers, breast and ovarian cancer in the same individual, male breast cancer, and Ashkenazi Jewish ancestry. In 2006, the National Comprehensive Cancer Network published practice guidelines for *Genetic/ Familial High-Risk Assessment: Breast and Ovarian Cancer.*[6]

GENETIC COUNSELING

Cancer genetic counseling involves education regarding the characteristics of hereditary cancer, the patient's personal risk of developing cancer, and the risk that the patient carries a mutation in a cancer predisposition gene. The key components to the genetic counseling process have been outlined by the National Society of Genetic Counselors (NSGC).[10,11] Genetic counselors discuss the benefits, limitations, and risks of genetic testing, as well as options for cancer prevention and management. Genetic counseling should also include a discussion of testing sensitivity and specificity, inconclusive genetic results, and variants of uncertain clinical significance. The goal of the

process is to communicate the complex issues involved in genetic testing in a language that the patient understands and in order for the patient to make informed decisions about genetic testing and his or her health care. Attention to the psychosocial issues is critical to this process in order to initiate health care behavior changes. Genetic counseling is best offered in the context of a multidisciplinary team, which would include experts in genetic counseling, surgery, oncology, social work, nursing oncology, and psychology.

ETHNICITY AND HEREDITARY BREAST CANCER

Genetic founder mutations are defined by a genetic mutation occurring in one of the founders of a distinct population that results in a high incidence of that particular genetic mutation in a given ethnic group. The most common founder mutations in hereditary breast cancer are 185delAG, 5382insC in BRCA1, and 6174delT in the BRCA2 gene, found in the Ashkenazi Jewish population.[12] These three single mutations account for 10% of breast cancer in the Ashkenazi Jewish population; however, a Jewish woman diagnosed with breast cancer at the age of 40 has a 21% to 30% risk of a BRCA gene mutation.[13] It is important to note that 10% of Ashkenazi Jewish woman will have a BRCA mutation that is not one of the founder mutations, so in some circumstances full sequencing of the BRCA genes is recommended.[14] Due to these founder genetic mutations, the prevalence of a BRCA mutation in the Ashkenazi Jewish population is 1 in 40.[15] This can be compared to the prevalence of BRCA gene mutations in the general population of 1 in 300 to 1 in 800.[16] Additional founder mutations have been detected in the Icelandic population and other ethnic groups.[17] Due to this phenomenon, the clinician should always assess the patient's ethnicity on both the paternal and maternal side when obtaining a family history.

GENETIC TESTING FOR HEREDITARY BREAST CANCER

Genetic testing should be considered based on the medical history, as well as if the result will affect the clinical management of the patient. It is also important to test a person diagnosed with cancer first. Typically, this result will accurately predict risk for not only your patient but the family as well. If an unaffected family member were to be tested first, then a negative result is uninformative. It would be unknown if there is still a mutation in the family and the patient in question did not inherit it. Since not all the genes have been identified for hereditary breast cancer, a negative result in a high-risk family should be viewed as inconclusive or indeterminate until genetic testing sensitivity increases and can conclusively prove that the patient did not inherit a mutation.

In addition, genetic testing is often complicated by results that reveal a variant of uncertain clinical significance (VUS). This is

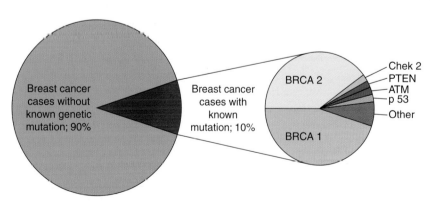

FIGURE 8-2 Percentage of breast cancer cases with a genetic mutation.

a common finding occurring in 10% to 13% of Caucasian individuals who have full BRCA gene sequencing, and it occurs at higher rates in minority populations.[18,19] These results reveal a subtle DNA sequence change where it is unknown if it is related to a change in protein function. A VUS is commonly a missense mutation or intronic mutation not known to be involved in mRNA processing. For these results, it is important to determine the number of times the particular variant has been detected, if it has been reported with another deleterious BRCA gene mutation, and if it is tracking with the cancer in the family or if additional in vitro studies have been done. Genetic variants that do not track with cancer and are seen with a proven deleterious mutation are less likely to be of clinical significance to the patient.

TABLE 8-1 BRCA1 Mutations and Associated Cancer Risks

Type of Cancer	Reported Risk by Age 70
Breast—initial	57-65%
Breast—second	3% per year
Ovarian	40%
Prostate	None to 2- to 3-fold increase
Male breast cancer	1%
Colon	Slight increase
Pancreatic cancer	1-4%

HEREDITARY BREAST AND OVARIAN CANCER SYNDROME

Hereditary breast and ovarian cancer syndrome (HBOC) is related to mutations in the BRCA1 and BRCA2 genes as well as other undefined genes. Eighty-five percent of HBOC is related to mutations in the BRCA1 and BRCA2 genes.[12] These 2 genes have a different clinical presentation, so they will be addressed separately here. However, they are both tumor suppressor genes involved in DNA repair. Over 1000 mutations have been detected to date in both of the BRCA genes. The majority of mutations detected are frameshift, nonsense, or large genomic deletions or duplications that result in premature truncation of the BRCA protein. Since 2006 genetic testing for large genomic rearrangements in the BRCA genes has revealed mutations in an additional 5% of high-risk patients.[20]

Estimates of cancer risks conferred by mutations in these genes vary according to their ascertainment. The estimated lifetime risk for breast cancer conferred by these genes has been reported to be between 35% and 87%, and the lifetime risk for ovarian cancer ranges from 16% to 60%.[14,21-23] The most frequently quoted risk for breast cancer associated with the BRCA genes comes from two studies in 1995 and 1998 by Easton and Ford. These papers give a risk for breast cancer associated with the BRCA1 gene as high as 87% and the risk with the BRCA2 gene as high as 84%.[23] It is important to note that these early studies were based on 237 families from the Breast Cancer Linkage Consortium. In order to participate in these initial studies, the research criteria were 4 cases of breast cancer, ovarian cancer at any age, and breast cancer cases at less than 60 years of age—thus these were highly penetrant families. However, a recent meta-analysis of various population-based studies of 18,432 families has estimated the cumulative risk of breast cancer by 70 years to be between 57% and 65% for BRCA1 and 45% and 49% for BRCA2, and the estimated risk for ovarian cancer in these studies was 40% for BRCA1 and 18% for BRCA2.[24]

PATIENT WITH A BRCA1 MUTATION—CLINICAL PRESENTATION AND TUMOR PROFILE

The BRCA1 gene is located on chromosome 17q11. It is a large gene with 22 coding exons and 2 noncoding exons. It encodes for 1863 amino acid polypeptide. Most BRCA1 mutation carriers have a "triple negative or basal phenotype" breast tumor profile (estrogen receptor, progesterone receptor, and HER-2/Neu overexpression all negative) with breast cancer that occurs in the third and fourth decade.[25] Thirteen percent of breast cancers with a BRCA1 mutation are medullary carcinoma compared to 2% of the general population.[26] The breast tumors from BRCA1 mutation carriers tend to be of a higher grade with faster doubling growth rate, especially in younger patients.[27] Because of the aggressive nature of these tumors, there is a reduced survival rate for BRCA1 patients. One study revealed that 57% of BRCA1 mutation carriers are diagnosed with breast cancer under the age of 50, compared to 28% of BRCA2 carriers.[23] This gene is associated with the highest rate of ovarian cancer (40%).[24] Patients with a BRCA1 mutation are reported to develop ovarian cancer at an average age of 38.6. The ovarian cancer that is associated with BRCA1 gene mutations is primarily high grade, advanced stage, and of epithelial origin. Patients with a BRCA1 mutation are reported to be at an increased risk for second breast cancer, ovarian cancer, prostate and pancreatic cancer (Table 8-1).[28-31] The risk for a second breast cancer in BRCA1 and BRCA2 mutation carriers is approximately 3% per year or 30% at 10 years.[22,28] The risk for prostate cancer in BRCA1 mutation patients is increased only if the proband was less than 65 years of age when determined to have the mutation.[29]

PATIENT WITH A BRCA2 MUTATION—CLINICAL PRESENTATION AND TUMOR PROFILE

The BRCA2 gene is located on chromosome 13q12-q13. This large gene codes for a protein of 3,418 amnio acids that are involved in DNA repair. Patients with a BRCA2 gene mutation tend to have an estrogen-positive breast cancer, later-onset disease, and increased risk for male breast cancer and other cancers as compared to patients with a BRCA1 gene mutation. Unlike the BRCA1 breast tumors, BRCA2-associated cancers have a less distinct pathologic phenotype. They are higher-grade tumors compared to sporadic breast cancer, and the estrogen and progesterone receptor status in BRCA2 cancers is similar to that in sporadic cases of breast cancer. Most tumors are invasive ductal carcinomas. The average age at the time of breast cancer diagnosis is estimated to be 43.6 years.[32] The lifetime risk for

TABLE 8-2 BRCA2 Mutations and Associated Cancer Risks

Type of Cancer	Reported Risk by Age 70
Breast—initial	45-49%
Breast—second	3% per year
Ovarian	18%
Prostate	7.5-39%
Male breast cancer	6%
Other	Low
Pancreatic	2-7%

ovarian cancer is 18%.[24] It is important to note that women with a BRCA2 gene mutation tend to develop ovarian cancer at an older age (after 50) as compared to women with a BRCA1 mutation.[33] There have been several other cancers associated with the BRCA2 gene, including pancreatic, colon, prostate, and melanoma (Table 8-2).[30,31,34-36]

MANAGEMENT CONSIDERATIONS FOR BRCA MUTATION CARRIERS

Currently the management guidelines are the same for carriers of BRCA1 and BRCA2 gene mutations. However, it is important to recognize the average age of onset of the cancers presenting in the family as well as the penetrance of the gene when developing an individualized approach to your patient. There are consensus statements for management of patients with HBOC. These published screening guidelines are based on expert opinion, but screening methods and interventions in this disorder are still unproven.[3,6] The clinical management is primarily directed toward the prevention and early detection of breast and ovarian cancer. Monthly breast self-examinations and clinical breast examinations every 6 months beginning at the age of 25 are recommended. In regards to early detection, annual mammograms should begin at the age of 25, or individualized based on the earliest breast cancer diagnosis in the family. Annual breast magnetic resonance imaging (MRI) starting at the age of 25 is also recommended.[6]

Several studies have examined the effectiveness of breast MRI in the surveillance and management of BRCA1 and BRCA2 genetic mutation carriers. In 2007, the American Cancer Society published its guidelines for breast screening with MRI only as an adjunct to mammography.[37] Annual screening with MRI is recommended to women with BRCA gene mutations as well as to high-risk women with a 20% to 25% lifetime risk for breast cancer as defined by the Gail and Claus model. These guidelines also acknowledge other cancer predisposition syndromes, such as Cowden syndrome, and high-risk families in which a genetic mutation has not yet been identified. Although the interval breast cancer rates in the breast MRI studies have been estimated to be below 10%,[37] it has been suggested to alternate MRI and mammogram every 6 months as a pattern for surveillance in these high-risk individuals because the BRCA-associated tumors are more aggressive. Patients undergoing breast MRI should be counseled regarding

the limitations and risks of this technology. They should be aware of the return rates for additional imaging and biopsy. These high-risk patients can be more anxious given their personal and family history.

Patients with a BRCA gene mutation, or patients with HBOC in which a mutation has not yet been detected, should be informed of the option of a risk-reducing mastectomy on a case-by-case basis and counseled regarding the degree of protection, reconstruction options, and risks. Decisions regarding BRCA patient management and prophylactic surgery are complex. Discussions regarding the long-term benefits, complications of surgery, degree of protection, reconstruction options, and long-term psychological impact need to be discussed with the patient. One of the reasons to offer genetic testing to breast cancer patients with a family history is to determine if they are at increased risk for a second primary cancer. The risk for developing a second primary breast cancer within 10 years has been estimated to be 30% or 3% per year.[38] The PROSE study group examined the cancer risks in BRCA mutation carriers who underwent bilateral prophylactic mastectomy.[38] The results of this study found a 90% reduction in breast cancer in women with intact ovaries and a 95% reduction in breast cancer in the BRCA carriers who had a prophylactic oophorectomy. In those patients who had a bilateral prophylactic mastectomy, 2% developed breast cancer, with the mean follow-up of 6.4 years, versus 48.7% in patients who elected not to have the prophylactic surgery.

All BRCA mutation carriers are at increased risk for ovarian cancer. It is important to convey to patients that there is no current proven methodology for surveillance and prevention of ovarian cancer. However, in women less than 35 years of age who are still considering childbirth, the management recommendations based on expert opinion are to have biannual pelvic examination beginning at the age of 35, or 5 to 10 years prior to the earliest age of first diagnosis of ovarian cancer in the family, as well as biannual CA-125 blood tests beginning at the age of 35 and annual transvaginal ultrasound with color Doppler.[6]

In women with BRCA gene mutations, the recommendation is for a bilateral salpingo-oophorectomy between the ages of 35 and 40, or when childbearing is complete. Several studies demonstrated a reduction in ovarian cancer risk up to 96% when this surgery is completed.[33,39] In addition, removing the ovaries also reduces the risk of developing breast cancer when performed in premenopausal BRCA mutation carriers. The benefit of this surgery is age-related, with the strongest benefit occurring in younger women.

Men with a BRCA gene mutation should also be aware of their increased risk for cancer based on the mutation status. For men with a BRCA gene mutation, the recommendation from NCCN guidelines is for regular monthly self-breast examinations, semiannual clinical breast examinations, and consideration of a baseline mammogram and annual mammogram if they have gynecomastia or arenchymal/glandular breast density on baseline study.[6] This is more relevant in patients with a BRCA2 gene mutation since the risk for breast cancer is greater than with a BRCA1 gene mutation (6% vs 1.2%).[31,35]

Chemoprevention via tamoxifen has been studied in BRCA mutation carriers. Several studies have shown approximately 50% reduction in breast cancer risk.[40] Although the initial data applied was found only in BRCA2 mutation carriers, it is now believed that tamoxifen may be effective in both BRCA1 and BRCA2 patients.[41] Chemoprevention is also important in lowering the risk for ovarian cancer with the use of long-term oral contraceptives. Narod and associates found a significant reduction in the rate of ovarian cancer (60%) in BRCA mutation carriers who used oral contraception for 6 years.[42] However, there may be a modest increase in risk of breast cancer in BRCA1 mutation carriers who have long-term oral contraception use.

COWDEN SYNDROME OR THE PTEN HAMARTOMA SYNDROME

The PTEN (phosphatase tensin homolog on chromosome ten) gene is a tumor suppressor gene found on chromosome 10q23. This tumor suppressor gene is involved in numerous pathways involving the cell cycle arrest. The PTEN gene is related to multiple specific syndromes including Cowden syndrome, Bannayan–Riley–Ruvalcaba syndrome, Proteus syndrome, and Proteus-like syndrome. Cowden syndrome is characterized by multiple hemartomas in various organs, specific skin findings, and increased risk for breast cancer (25%-50%), thyroid cancer (mainly follicular—10%), uterine (5%-10%), and renal cell cancer.[43-46] Adult Lhermitte–Duclos disease, facial trichilemmomas, acral keratoses, and oral papillomatous papules are pathognomonic features of this syndrome. The clinical diagnosis can be made based on the operational criteria defined by the International Cowden Consortium in 1995 and then adopted by the National Comprehensive Cancer Network (Table 8-3). It has been shown that up to 80% of patients who meet these criteria will have an identifiable PTEN gene mutation.[47] Besides having an increased risk for breast cancer, women with Cowden syndrome have a 67% to 76% risk for benign breast disease.[47,48] The benign breast findings include fibroadenomas, fibrocystic breast disease, apocrine metaplasia, microcysts, and hamartoma-like lesions.[48] The benign disease is usually bilateral. Males with Cowden syndrome are also at increased risk for breast cancer. Because of the increase risk for breast cancer in patients with Cowden syndrome, they should begin earlier cancer surveillance. The NCCN has published guidelines for the medical management of this condition.[6]

Men and women with Cowden syndrome are also at increased risk for malignant and nonmalignant conditions of the thyroid. The risk for thyroid cancer is estimated to be 10%.[47] The thyroid cancer is typically follicular and rarely papillary but never medullary. Structural problems with the thyroid gland are often present, including multinodular goiters and adenomas. There is also an increased risk for endometrial cancer with Cowden syndrome. This risk has been estimated to be between 5% and 10%.[44] Uterine fibroids have also been reported in this condition.

LI–FRAUMENI SYNDROME

Li–Fraumeni syndrome is rare, accounting for only 1% of hereditary breast cancer.[49] Li–Fraumeni syndrome (LFS) is due to germline mutations in the TP53 tumor suppressor gene, which codes for the P53 protein. This gene is located on chromosome 17p13.1 and is called the "guardian of the genome," since mutations in this gene in somatic cells are frequently associated with cancer development. This syndrome is characterized by early-onset breast cancer, bone and soft-tissue sarcomas, brain tumors, acute leukemia, lymphoma, and adrenal cortical carcinoma. The breast cancer in this syndrome can occur in the 20s. This syndrome is usually detected because of the increased incidence of pediatric cancers in a family (Table 8-4). The risk for cancer has been estimated to be 56% by the age of 45 and greater than 90% by the age of 60.[50] Most breast cancer in Li–Fraumeni syndrome occurs under the age of 40. Individuals with this syndrome often develop multiple primary cancers. Patients who meet the Li–Fraumeni criteria will have a mutation in the TP53 gene 50% to 70% of the time.[51,52] Germline mutations in the CHEK2 gene have also been reported in Li–Fraumeni families. Management for patients with this syndrome is complex given the array of tumors associated with the condition. The patient needs to be informed of the limitations of screening for the many cancers associated with this syndrome before undertaking genetic testing. The use of routine mammogram in

---

TABLE 8-3 Operational Diagnosis of Cowden Syndrome

1. Mucocutaneous lesions **alone** if there are 6 or more facial papules, of which 3 or more must be trichilemmoma or cutaneous facial papules; and oral mucosal papillomatosis or oral mucosal papillomatosis and acral keratoses or palmoplantar keratoses, 6 or more.
2. Two or more of the following major criteria: breast cancer, thyroid cancer (especially follicular), macrocephaly (head circumference 97% or ≥57 cm for women and ≥59 cm for men) **OR**
3. One major criteria (see above) and ≥ 3 minor criteria: structural thyroid lesions (adenoma, multinodular goiter), mental retardation (IQ < 75), GI hamartomous polyps, fibrocystic breast disease, lipomas, fibromas, genitourinary tumors (especially renal cell carcinoma), GU structural manifestation, uterine fibroids **OR**
4. Four or more minor criteria.

From Daly MB, Axilbund JE, Bryant E, et al. Genetic/familial high-risk assessment: breast and ovarian. *J Natl Compr Canc Netw.* 2006;4:156-176; and Eng C. Will the real Cowden syndrome please stand up: revised diagnostic criteria. *J Med Genet.* 2000;37:828-830.

TABLE 8-4 Criteria for Li–Fraumeni Syndrome

Proband with a sarcoma diagnosed ≤45 AND
First-degree relative with any cancer under the age of 45 AND
Another first- or second-degree relative with cancer ≤45 or a sarcoma at any age

women with Li–Fraumeni syndrome is controversial because of the possibility of radiation sensitivity associated with TP53 gene mutation.[53]

OTHER CANCER GENETIC SYNDROMES ASSOCIATED WITH INCREASED RISK FOR BREAST CANCER

There are other rare syndromes that have been related to hereditary breast cancer. Peutz–Jeghers syndrome is related to mutations in the STK11 (LKB1) gene encoding for a serine/threonine kinase. This disorder is characterized by perioral pigmentation and hamartomatous polyposis. Women with this syndrome have a 30% to 50% risk of developing develop breast cancer.[54] In hereditary diffuse gastric cancer syndrome, patients with a mutation in the CDH1 gene are also at increased risk for lobular breast cancer. The risk for breast cancer with this gene is estimated to be 39%.[55] For patients with breast cancer and melanoma there is an increased incidence of mutations in the CDKN2/p16 gene.[56] In addition, there are several low-penetrant genes that may increase the risk of breast cancer. These genes may also modify the penetrance of the major breast cancer genes.

FUTURE DIRECTIONS

Understanding the pathophysiology of the inherited breast cancer syndromes is leading to exciting new therapies for patients with these genetic mutations. Trials are now underway using Poly (ADP-ribose) polymerase (PARP) inhibitors to treat breast tumors in patients with a BRCA gene mutation.[57] PARP is an enzyme involved in base excision repair. If this enzyme is inhibited, the cell will have an increase in DNA lesions that are normally repaired by the BRCA1 and BRCA2 proteins. In patients with a mutation in the BRCA gene, the breast cell would be sensitive to treatment by a PARP inhibitor, thus resulting in the death of the tumor cells related to cell cycle arrest and chromosome instability. It has also been postulated that cells with a BRCA gene mutation are also more sensitive to chemotherapeutic agents that crosslink DNA, such as platinum-based drugs.[58] Future studies on specific chemotherapy regimens on BRCA mutation carriers are needed to promote individualized medicine.

SUMMARY

Genetic testing has given us the ability to identify select high-risk patients with a hereditary predisposition to breast cancer. This gives us the opportunity to educate our patients and their family members about the increased risk for breast cancer and to be proactive in their medical management. These major cancer genes have led to the identification of thousands of women at increased risk for breast cancer. However, it is important to understand that in the majority of patients with a family history of breast cancer, a genetic mutation still cannot be identified. Further research is still needed to identify other molecular or biochemical markers that are related to familial breast cancer.

REFERENCES

1. Broca PP. *Traite des tumeurs*. Paris: Asselin; 1866.
2. Lynch HT, Lynch JF. Breast cancer genetics in an oncology clinic: 328 consecutive patients. *Cancer Genet Cytogenet*. 1986;22:369-371.
3. Genetic risk assessment and BRCA mutation testing for breast and ovarian cancer susceptibility: recommendation statement. *Ann Intern Med*. 2005;143:355-361.
4. Margolin S, Johansson H, Rutqvist LE, Lindblom A, Fornander T. Family history, and impact on clinical presentation and prognosis, in a population-based breast cancer cohort from the Stockholm County. *Fam Cancer*. 2006;5:309-321.
5. American Society of Clinical Oncology policy statement update: genetic testing for cancer susceptibility. *J Clin Oncol*. 2003;21:2397-2406.
6. Daly MB, Axilbund JE, Bryant E, et al. Genetic/familial high-risk assessment: breast and ovarian. *J Natl Compr Canc Netw*. 2006;4:156-176.
7. Parmigiani G, Berry D, Aguilar O. Determining carrier probabilities for breast cancer-susceptibility genes BRCA1 and BRCA2. *Am J Hum Genet*. 1998;62:145-158.
8. Couch FJ, DeShano ML, Blackwood MA, et al. BRCA1 mutations in women attending clinics that evaluate the risk of breast cancer. *N Engl J Med*. 1997;336:1409-1415.
9. Shattuck-Eidens D, Oliphant A, McClure M, et al. BRCA1 sequence analysis in women at high risk for susceptibility mutations. Risk factor analysis and implications for genetic testing. *JAMA*. 1997;278:1242-1250.
10. Berliner JL, Fay AM. Risk assessment and genetic counseling for hereditary breast and ovarian cancer: recommendations of the National Society of Genetic Counselors. *J Genet Couns*. 2007;16:241-260.
11. Trepanier A, Ahrens M, McKinnon W, et al. Genetic cancer risk assessment and counseling: recommendations of the national society of genetic counselors. *J Genet Couns*. 2004;13:83-114.
12. Struewing JP, Hartge P, Wacholder S, et al. The risk of cancer associated with specific mutations of BRCA1 and BRCA2 among Ashkenazi Jews. *N Engl J Med*. 1997;336:1401-1408.
13. Rubinstein WS. Hereditary breast cancer in Jews. *Fam Cancer*. 2004;3:249-257.
14. King MC, Marks JH, Mandell JB. Breast and ovarian cancer risks due to inherited mutations in BRCA1 and BRCA2. *Science*. 2003;302:643-646.
15. Roa BB, Boyd AA, Volcik K, Richards CS. Ashkenazi Jewish population frequencies for common mutations in BRCA1 and BRCA2. *Nat Genet*. 1996;14:185-187.
16. Pal T, Permuth-Wey J, Betts JA, et al. BRCA1 and BRCA2 mutations account for a large proportion of ovarian carcinoma cases. *Cancer*. 2005;104:2807-2816.
17. Thorlacius S, Olafsdottir G, Tryggvadottir L, et al. A single BRCA2 mutation in male and female breast cancer families from Iceland with varied cancer phenotypes. *Nat Genet*. 1996;13:117-119.
18. Frank TS, Deffenbaugh AM, Reid JE, et al. Clinical characteristics of individuals with germline mutations in BRCA1 and BRCA2: analysis of 10,000 individuals. *J Clin Oncol*. 2002;20:1480-1490.
19. van Dijk S, van Asperen CJ, Jacobi CE, et al. Variants of uncertain clinical significance as a result of BRCA1/2 testing: impact of an ambiguous breast cancer risk message. *Genet Test*. 2004;8:235-239.
20. Walsh T, Casadei S, Coats KH, et al. Spectrum of mutations in BRCA1, BRCA2, CHEK2, and TP53 in families at high risk of breast cancer. *JAMA*. 2006;295:1379-1388.
21. Antoniou A, Pharoah PD, Narod S, et al. Average risks of breast and ovarian cancer associated with BRCA1 or BRCA2 mutations detected in case Series unselected for family history: a combined analysis of 22 studies. *Am J Hum Genet*. 2003;72:1117-1130.
22. Ford D, Easton DF, Bishop DT, Narod SA, Goldgar DE. Risks of cancer in BRCA1-mutation carriers. Breast Cancer Linkage Consortium. *Lancet*. 1994;343:692-695.
23. Ford D, Easton DF, Stratton M, et al. Genetic heterogeneity and penetrance analysis of the BRCA1 and BRCA2 genes in breast cancer families. The Breast Cancer Linkage Consortium. *Am J Hum Genet*. 1998;62:676-689.
24. Chen S, Parmigiani G. Meta-analysis of BRCA1 and BRCA2 penetrance. *J Clin Oncol*. 2007;25:1329 1333.
25. Lakhani SR, Van De Vijver MJ, Jacquemier J, et al. The pathology of familial breast cancer: predictive value of immunohistochemical markers estrogen receptor, progesterone receptor, HER-2, and p53 in patients with mutations in BRCA1 and BRCA2. *J Clin Oncol*. 2002;20:2310-2318.
26. Pathology of familial breast cancer: differences between breast cancers in carriers of BRCA1 or BRCA2 mutations and sporadic cases. Breast Cancer Linkage Consortium. *Lancet*. 1997;349:1505-1510.

27. Tilanus-Linthorst MM, Obdeijn IM, Hop WC, et al. BRCA1 mutation and young age predict fast breast cancer growth in the Dutch, United Kingdom, and Canadian magnetic resonance imaging screening trials. *Clin Cancer Res.* 2007;13:7357-7362.

28. Metcalfe K, Lynch HT, Ghadirian P, et al. Contralateral breast cancer in BRCA1 and BRCA2 mutation carriers. *J Clin Oncol.* 2004;22:2328-2335.

29. Thompson D, Easton DF. Cancer incidence in BRCA1 mutation carriers. *J Natl Cancer Inst.* 2002;94:1358-1365.

30. Burke W, Daly M, Garber J, et al. Recommendations for follow-up care of individuals with an inherited predisposition to cancer. II. BRCA1 and BRCA2. Cancer Genetics Studies Consortium. *JAMA.* 1997;277:997-1003.

31. Liede A, Karlan BY, Narod SA. Cancer risks for male carriers of germline mutations in BRCA1 or BRCA2: a review of the literature. *J Clin Oncol.* 2004;22:735-742.

32. Weitzel JN, Robson M, Pasini B, et al. A comparison of bilateral breast cancers in BRCA carriers. *Cancer Epidemiol Biomarkers Prev.* 2005;14:1534-1538.

33. Rebbeck TR, Lynch HT, Neuhausen SL, et al. Prophylactic oophorectomy in carriers of BRCA1 or BRCA2 mutations. *N Engl J Med.* 2002;346:1616-1622.

34. van Asperen CJ, Brohet RM, Meijers-Heijboer EJ, et al. Cancer risks in BRCA2 families: estimates for sites other than breast and ovary. *J Med Genet.* 2005;42:711-719.

35. Thompson D, Easton D. Variation in cancer risks, by mutation position, in BRCA2 mutation carriers. *Am J Hum Genet.* 2001;68:410-419.

36. Ozcelik H, Schmocker B, Di Nicola N, et al. Germline BRCA2 6174delT mutations in Ashkenazi Jewish pancreatic cancer patients. *Nat Genet.* 1997;16:17-18.

37. Saslow D, Boetes C, Burke W, et al. American Cancer Society guidelines for breast screening with MRI as an adjunct to mammography. *CA Cancer J Clin.* 2007;57:75-89.

38. Rebbeck TR, Friebel T, Lynch HT, et al. Bilateral prophylactic mastectomy reduces breast cancer risk in BRCA1 and BRCA2 mutation carriers: the PROSE Study Group. *J Clin Oncol.* 2004;22:1055-1062.

39. Kauff ND, Satagopan JM, Robson MF, et al. Risk-reducing salpingo-oophorectomy in women with a BRCA1 or BRCA2 mutation. *N Engl J Med.* 2002;346:1609-1615.

40. Narod SA, Brunet JS, Ghadirian P, et al. Tamoxifen and risk of contralateral breast cancer in BRCA1 and BRCA2 mutation carriers: a case-control study. Hereditary Breast Cancer Clinical Study Group. *Lancet.* 2000;356:1876-1881.

41. Gronwald J. THBCCS: tamoxifen and contralateral breat cancer in BRCA1 and BRCA2 carriers: an update. *Int J Cancer.* 2005;118:2281-2284.

42. Narod SA, Risch H, Moslehi R, et al. Oral contraceptives and the risk of hereditary ovarian cancer. Hereditary Ovarian Cancer Clinical Study Group. *N Engl J Med.* 1998;339:424-428.

43. Starink TM, van der Veen JP, Arwert F, et al. The Cowden syndrome: a clinical and genetic study in 21 patients. *Clin Genet.* 1986;29:222-233.

44. Pilarski R, Eng C. Will the real Cowden syndrome please stand up (again)? Expanding mutational and clinical spectra of the PTEN hamartoma tumour syndrome. *J Med Genet.* 2004;41:323-326.

45. Eng C. PTEN: one gene, many syndromes. *Hum Mutat.* 2003;22:183-198.

46. Eng C. Will the real Cowden syndrome please stand up: revised diagnostic criteria. *J Med Genet.* 2000;37:828-830.

47. Liaw D, Marsh DJ, Li J, et al. Germline mutations of the PTEN gene in Cowden disease, an inherited breast and thyroid cancer syndrome. *Nat Genet.* 1997;16:64-67.

48. Schrager CA, Schneider D, Gruener AC, Tsou HC, Peacocke M. Clinical and pathological features of breast disease in Cowden's syndrome: an underrecognized syndrome with an increased risk of breast cancer. *Hum Pathol.* 1998;29:47-53.

49. Sidransky D, Tokino T, Helzlsouer K, et al. Inherited p53 gene mutations in breast cancer. *Cancer Res.* 1992;52:2984-2986.

50. Nichols KE, Malkin D, Garber JE, Fraumeni JF Jr., Li FP. Germ-line p53 mutations predispose to a wide spectrum of early-onset cancers. *Cancer Epidemiol Biomarkers Prev.* 2001;10:83-87.

51. Eeles RA. Germline mutations in the TP53 gene. *Cancer Surv.* 1995;25:101-124.

52. Chompret A, Abel A, Stoppa-Lyonnet D, et al. Sensitivity and predictive value of criteria for p53 germline mutation screening. *J Med Genet.* 2001;38:43-47.

53. Nutting C, Camplejohn RS, Gilchrist R, et al. A patient with 17 primary tumours and a germ line mutation in TP53: tumour induction by adjuvant therapy? *Clin Oncol (R Coll Radiol).* 2000;12:300-304.

54. Hemminki A. The molecular basis and clinical aspects of Peutz-Jeghers syndrome. *Cell Mol Life Sci.* 1999;55:735-750.

55. Pharoah PD, Guilford P, Caldas C. Incidence of gastric cancer and breast cancer in CDH1 (E-cadherin) mutation carriers from hereditary diffuse gastric cancer families. *Gastroenterology.* 2001;121:1348-1353.

56. Monnerat C, Chompret A, Kannengiesser C, et al. BRCA1, BRCA2, TP53, and CDKN2A germline mutations in patients with breast cancer and cutaneous melanoma. *Fam Cancer.* 2007;6:453-461.

57. Evers B, Drost R, Schut E, et al. Selective inhibition of BRCA2-deficient mammary tumor cell growth by AZD2281 and cisplatin. *Clin Cancer Res.* 2008;14:3916-3925.

58. Foulkes WD. BRCA1 and BRCA2: chemosensitivity, treatment outcomes and prognosis. *Fam Cancer.* 2006;5:135-142.

CHAPTER 9

Quantitative Risk Prediction

David Euhus

THE VALUE OF QUANTITATIVE RISK ASSESSMENT

There are already several approaches available to increase the chances of diagnosing breast cancer at an early, curable stage, or of reducing the chances of getting breast cancer at all. Some examples include enhanced surveillance with periodic breast MRI, chemoprevention, or even prophylactic surgery. These interventions cannot be applied widely and indiscriminately because each exacts a cost of its own—be it financial, physiological, psychological, or social. The risks and benefits of these interventions must be considered on a case-by-case basis and this requires some sense of the balance between the risks of the proposed intervention and the risks of the disease it is trying to address.

It is well known that breast cancer can run in families, and it is not uncommon for a woman whose mother has died of breast cancer to suffer a great deal of anxiety about her own "impending" breast cancer, and even to undertake extraordinary measures, including prophylactic mastectomy, to prevent it. Individuals with a family history of breast cancer frequently overestimate their own chances of developing the disease and often experience a sense of relief when presented with quantitative information suggesting that their actual risk is quite a bit lower than they would have imagined.[1,2] Conversely, a healthy woman whose recent breast biopsy has diagnosed high-risk preneoplasia, such as atypical hyperplasia, may be spurred to effective action when presented with a quantitative estimation of her breast cancer risk over time.

Quantitative breast cancer risk assessment is also an integral component of prevention research. It can be used as a surrogate for breast cancer incidence in studies evaluating biomarkers of breast cancer risk,[3-5] and is always considered in the inclusion criteria for trials that include breast cancer incidence as an end point.[6] The value of quantitative risk assessment in the later

case cannot be overstated as these calculations permit accurate estimation of the number of end-point events that will occur. This is critical for designing the most efficient study possible.

Finally, third-party payors have begun to consider quantitative risk assessment data in their determinations of medical necessity. This is best illustrated by fairly wide adoption of recently published American Cancer Society guidelines that support screening breast MRI for women with a lifetime risk of breast cancer 20% or more.[7] The best approach for incorporating quantitative risk assessment into medical decision-making can and should be debated, but at this juncture it is reasonable to ask how one goes about estimating breast cancer risk, and whether such estimations are accurate.

RELATIVE AND ABSOLUTE RISK

A variety of metrics are available to quantify risk and each is valuable when used in the appropriate context. Relative risk is often used to identify new risk factors from case-control data and is sometimes used in calculations of absolute risk. Simply stated, relative risk expresses the strength of association between exposure to a risk factor and the presence of breast cancer. For example, the relative risk for breast cancer conferred by atypical hyperplasia is about 4.5.[8] This means that women with atypical hyperplasia develop breast cancer about 4.5 times more frequently than similar women without atypical hyperplasia. For a disease like breast cancer, which is fairly common, a high relative risk usually translates into a high absolute risk, but the concept of relative risk is foreign to most patients. Relative risk is invaluable for clinical scientists but not particularly useful in the risk-assessment clinic.

Absolute risk is the percent chance that some event will happen over some specified time. It can be observed directly and prospectively by following a cohort of individuals over time, or

TABLE 9-1 Breast Cancer Risk by Age

Current Age (yr)	+ 10 yr (%)	Eventually (%)
0	0	12.03
10	0	12.17
20	0.05	12.20
30	0.43	12.21
40	1.44	11.92
50	2.44	10.84
60	3.41	8.99
70	3.74	6.44
80	3.03	3.72

Adapted from Table IV-14, 1995-2005 SEER Data.[9]

can be estimated from disease rates measured during a single time period in a defined population. An example of the later approach is the age-specific breast cancer risk figures supplied by the NCI-sponsored Surveillance Epidemiology and End-Points (SEER) project.[9] Table IV-14 of the 1995 to 2005 SEER data shows breast cancer risk by age according to current and historical age-specific breast cancer incidence rates (Table 9-1). A quick look at this table shows that the risk of ever developing breast cancer decreases as a woman ages, but that the near-term risk (10 year risk in this case) increases as a woman ages. This is important to consider as we decide how best to apply quantitative risk calculations in medical decision-making. For example, the lifetime breast cancer risk for a 20-year old woman is 12.2%, but her near-term (10-year) risk is only 0.05%. Should intervention decisions be made based on her lifetime or near-term risk? Historically, it is near-term (5-year) risk that has been used to select women for participation in chemoprevention trials, and the threshold used to classify a woman as high risk has traditionally been 1.67%. This is simply the 5-year risk for a 60-year-old Caucasian woman calculated from the 1984 to 1988 SEER data. This threshold may be useful for ensuring that there are sufficient end-point events in a chemoprevention trial, but it is meaningless in the breast cancer risk-assessment clinic. This SEER table also tells us that, for a female born today, the risk of ever developing breast cancer in her lifetime is 12%, or 1 in 8. This is a useful metric for tracking breast cancer incidence trends over time, but is only the starting point for quantitative breast cancer risk assessment, which attempts to adjust this value based on the unique combination of risk factors operative in a specific individual.

Absolute risk can also be calculated from relative risk if certain additional information is available. In order to convert relative risk to absolute risk one must know how frequently each category of risk occurs in the population of interest and the rates of death from other causes. To be useful in the clinic this information must be known for women who are as much like the patient we are seeing as is possible (eg, same age, same race). In addition, many risk factors are not totally independent— that is, the presence of some risk factors will modulate the effects of other risk factors. A model that calculates absolute

risk from several different relative risks must consider these interactions. The Gail model is a particularly good example in this regard. This model starts with 5 separate relative risks, but accounts for the way that age and number of biopsies can interact, and for the way that age at first live birth and family history interact.[10] These 5 relative risks are combined into 3 relative risks, and then SEER incidence data, a factor to account for the prevalence of the risk factors by race, and U.S. mortality data are combined to translate these relative risks into absolute risks.[6]

TYPES OF RISK MODELS AND EXAMPLES

Cancer risk models use personal and family history information to calculate the probability that an individual carries a deleterious mutation in a cancer predisposition gene or to estimate the probability that the individual will develop cancer over time. Most quantitative risk assessment models are empiric models— that is, models that use various weighting schemes to mathematically represent an observational dataset. The Ontario Family History Assessment Tool (FHAT) is one example of a simple empiric model developed to identify women who should be referred to a genetic counselor.[11] This model was developed by having 16 clinical geneticists review 26 hypothetical pedigrees. It assigns points to a family history based on the types of cancer present, the ages at onset, and the relationship of cancer patients to the proband.

Logistic regression is commonly used to develop mathematical equations that accurately describe a set of observations that have been made in a group of individuals. A very simple example is the Finnish BRCA gene mutation prediction model, which was developed using data from 148 BRCA gene mutation-tested families with a strong history of breast and/or ovarian cancer.[12] This model uses the earliest age at breast cancer diagnosis and the number of ovarian cancers in the family to calculate the probability that the family carries a deleterious mutation in BRCA1 or BRCA2. This is the most austere logistic regression model, but also one of the most intelligent as these two variables form the core of nearly every other BRCA gene mutation prediction model. The Gail model is, perhaps, the best known and most widely used logistic regression model for calculating breast cancer risk.[10] This model was developed from a case-control study that included nearly 6000 women who had participated in the Breast Cancer Detection Demonstration Project. Dozens of risk factors were evaluated to identify the smallest number of factors providing the best risk prediction. Risk factors included in the final model were age, age at menarche, age at first live birth, number of biopsies, any history of atypical hyperplasia, and number of first-degree female relatives with breast cancer. The initial model was applicable to Caucasian women only and included both invasive and in situ cancer as end points. In preparing for the P1 Tamoxifen Breast Cancer Prevention Trial (BCPT), investigators with the National Surgical Adjuvant Breast and Bowel Project (NSABP) modified the original Gail model to include African American women and to limit the probability calculation to invasive breast cancer only.[6]

This is the model in common use today and is known as the modified Gail model or Gail2 model. Gail and colleagues have since described a revised model that excludes age at menarche but adds body weight and mammographic density.[13] Barlow and colleagues used data from 1,007,600 women enrolled in the Breast Cancer Screening Consortium to develop separate logistic regression models for premenopausal and postmenopausal women.[14] The model for premenopausal women includes age, prior breast surgery, family history of breast cancer in first-degree relatives, and mammographic density. The model for postmenopausal women includes these same factors with the addition of ethnicity, race, body mass index, age at first live birth, hormone therapy use, history of oophorectomy, and history of a "false-positive" mammogram in the prior year. Interaction between risk factors was not considered in this model.

The Claus model is another popular empiric model that grew out of efforts to find the best way to mathematically describe breast cancer family history patterns among the more than 9000 women participating in the Cancer and Steroid Hormone Study.[15] Several approaches were tried, but the model that provided the best fit to the data was one that postulated the existence of a rare autosomal dominant susceptibility gene in the population. This predated the discovery of BRCA1 by several years. The variables considered by this model are the ages at breast cancer diagnosis and the relationship of affected relatives to the proband. The model calculates the probability of developing breast cancer over time.

Mendelian models represent another major class of quantitative risk assessment models. Unlike the empiric models, which are directly derived from specific observational data, Mendelian models are based on the general rules of Mendelian inheritance. Observational data contribute to the construction of these models, but only for the purposes of estimating the allelic frequency and penetrance of the genes of interest. BRCAPRO is a Mendelian model that uses Bayes theorem to calculate the probability that an individual carries a mutation in a major autosomal dominant breast cancer susceptibility gene based on the family history of breast and ovarian cancer.[16,17] The probability that the individual will develop breast or ovarian cancer over time is then derived from this mutation probability based on age-specific incidence curves for mutation carriers and noncarriers. This model requires entry of a complete family history including all affected and unaffected relatives. Calculations are based on the ages at cancer diagnosis, the relationship of affected and unaffected relatives to the proband, results for any genetic testing that has been done, history of oophorectomy, and the characteristics (receptor status) of any primary breast cancers. Other Mendelian models, such as the Jonker model[18] and BOADICEA,[19] calculate the probability of a mutation in a major autosomal dominant breast cancer susceptibility gene, but do not provide an estimation of breast cancer risk over time.

The Tyrer–Cuzick model is an attempted synthesis of empiric and Mendelian approaches to risk modeling.[20] It first uses family history information to calculate the probability that an individual carries a mutation in an autosomal dominant breast cancer susceptibility gene and then calculates the risk of breast cancer based on this. This risk estimate is then adjusted based on age at menarche, parity, age at first live birth, age at menopause, history of atypical hyperplasia or lobular carcinoma in situ (LCIS), height, and body mass index.

STRENGTHS AND WEAKNESSES OF THE MODELS

The Gail model is the most thoroughly validated and widely used model for clinical risk assessment and breast cancer prevention research. However, its neglect of risk factors like ovarian cancer, male breast cancer, bilateral breast cancer, cancer in second-degree relatives, and LCIS means that it may not be the most appropriate model for every situation. Nevertheless, one study that included 213 women attending a breast cancer risk-assessment clinic reported that though 74% of the women had one or more risk factors likely to confound the Gail model, other models calculated a higher risk for only 13%.[21] For individuals with family histories of breast cancer in multiple generations, male breast cancer, bilateral breast cancer, or ovarian cancer, a model like BRCAPRO is more likely to provide an accurate risk assessment than the Gail model. Unfortunately, the breast cancer risk estimates provided by family history models, like BRCAPRO and Claus, have not been validated. When these models disagree it is unclear which, if either, is correct. The Tyrer–Cuzick model, which considers more risk factors than any of the other models, may provide a more widely applicable general risk assessment.[20] However, nonfamily history risk factors were not selected or combined in the same rigorous and systematic way that risk factors were added to the Gail model, and the Tyrer–Cuzick model has not been rigorously validated in the same way that the Gail model has.

▌ Model Validation: Calibration and Discrimination

The Gail model predicted that 159 of 5969 women without LCIS who were enrolled in the placebo arm of the Tamoxifen Breast Cancer Prevention trial and followed for an average of 4 years would be diagnosed with breast cancer. In fact, 155 of these women were diagnosed with breast cancer (expected/observed ratio = 1.03).[22] Similarly, the Gail model predicted that 1273 breast cancers would be diagnosed within 5 years among the 82,109 women participating in the Nurses Health Study.[23] The actual number of breast cancers diagnosed was 1354 (expected/observed ratio = 0.94). The Gail model is very well calibrated; that is, it accurately predicts breast cancer incidence for large groups of women. This makes the model invaluable for designing prevention trials that include breast cancer as an end point. Some have argued, however, that the clinical usefulness of a model is determined by its capacity to distinguish between women who will develop breast cancer and women who will not develop breast cancer. This is known as discrimination, and is quantified by the concordance statistic (C-statistic). The C-statistic tells us what proportion of women developing breast cancer will have a model probability greater than women not developing breast cancer. A value of 0.5 indicates that the model is no better than the flip of a coin for separating a group of women into

TABLE 9-2 Discrimination of the Breast Cancer Risk Prediction Models

Model and Dataset	Breast Cancers	C-Statistic
Gail, Nurses Health Study[23]	1354	0.58
Gail, San Francisco Mammography Registry (SFMR)[35]	955	0.67
Gail + MGM Density, SFMR[35]	955	0.68
Gail, Nipple Aspirate Fluid (NAF) cohort[36]	400	0.62
Gail + NAF cytology, NAF cohort[36]	400	0.64
Gail, National Cancer Institute of Naples (NCIN)[37]	558	0.55
Gail + Second-degree relatives, NCIN[37]	558	0.57
Darlow, Premenopausal, Breast Cancer Surveillance Consortium (BCSC)[14]	~432	0.63
Barlow, Postmenopausal, BCSC[14]	2325	0.62
Tyrer–Cuzick, University Hospital South Manchester[38]	64	0.76

There are many validation studies comparing the accuracy of models designed to predict BRCA1 or BRCA2 gene mutation. One recent study that compared seven models in 3342 BRCA gene mutation-tested individuals is illustrative of most other studies.[25] In general, the Mendelian models out perform the empiric models, but C-statistics for most models approach 0.8. In the aforementioned study, BRCAPRO was superior to the other 6 models (C statistic = 0.82), but not by a great deal (Fig. 9-1). Another study that presented 148 pedigrees to 8 genetic counselors found that the discrimination afforded by BRCAPRO was similar to that of the genetic counselors (0.71 vs 0.62-0.72), and that when BRCAPRO information was provided with the pedigree, discrimination improved for all but 2 of the counselors.[26] As with the breast cancer risk prediction models, efforts are underway to improve the discrimination of mutation prediction models by supplying additional information. For instance, the inclusion of grade, estrogen receptor status, and progesterone receptor status for the proband's primary breast cancer increased the discrimination of BRCAPRO from 0.84 to 0.92.[27] The current version of BRCAPRO can accept marker information for any primary breast cancers diagnosed in the family.

those who will develop breast cancer and those who will not. The C-statistic calculated for the Gail model, and a variety of related logistic regression models, ranges from 0.55 to 0.68 (Table 9-2). This rather poor discrimination challenges the utility of epidemiologic models for clinical breast cancer risk assessment and has spurred efforts to improve discrimination by adding additional risk factors to the models. Table 9-2 suggests that discrimination does not improve with the addition of more risk factors. In addition, one study found that the Gail model C-statistic was 0.6 for prediction of estrogen receptor-positive breast cancer, but only 0.5 for estrogen receptor-negative breast cancer (ie, no better than chance).[24]

Without question, the best quantitative risk assessment would accurately classify every woman as destined for breast cancer or not (C-statistic = 1.0). Our inability to improve discrimination much beyond the 0.6 mark is likely due to genetic and environmental factors yet to be identified that modify a woman's breast tissue response to established risk factors, and to the systematic approach Gail and colleagues used to include or exclude risk factors from the original model. Nevertheless, accurate estimation of breast cancer incidence (calibration) supplies the need for quantitative information useful for weighing options and making decisions about interventions.

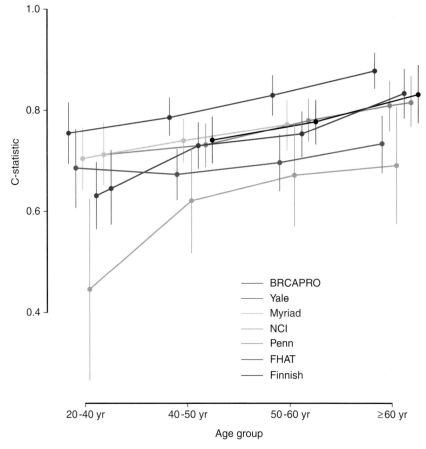

FIGURE 9-1 C-statistics calculated for various BRCA gene mutation prediction models across a range of proband ages. *(From Parmigiani G, Chen S, Iversen ESJ, et al. Validity of models for predicting BRCA1 and BRCA2 mutations. Ann Intern Med. 2007;147:441-450.)*

IMPLEMENTING QUANTITATIVE RISK ASSESSMENT IN THE CLINIC

One of the greatest barriers to implementing quantitative risk assessment in the clinic is the time it takes to input the data required by the models. BRCAPRO is the worst offender in this regard, as it requires information for all relatives whether they were affected with cancer or not. Some clinics that serve technologically savvy populations have shifted the burden of data entry to the patient. This is done using forms that patients can access on the Internet from home prior to their visit, or by handing the patient a tablet computer when they first check in. Model calculations are completed in the background, and the health care provider has immediate access to a pedigree diagram, gene mutation probabilities, and age-specific cancer risk estimates. Some clinics prefer to compartmentalize cancer risk assessment and counseling activities into dedicated risk-assessment clinics. In this case, specifically trained clinic staff can take the time to input comprehensive risk-factor information

into the computer and complete the initial counseling. Several software programs are available to facilitate this. CancerGene is one such program that provides an interface for collecting cancer family history and other risk-factor information (Fig. 9-2). It draws a pedigree, calculates probabilities of mutations in cancer susceptibility genes (BRCAPRO and other models), displays age-specific cancer risk information calculated by Gail, Claus, and BRCAPRO models, and archives the information to a database (http://www4.utsouthwestern.edu/breasthealth/cagene). Hughes RiskApps is a more comprehensive program for managing a risk assessment clinic that uses the CancerGene risk-calculation engine in the background (http://hughesriskapps.com/download.htm). The Tyrer–Cuzick model is found in the IBIS Risk Evaluator, which can be obtained at http://www.ems-trials.org/riskevaluator/ (Fig. 9-3).

For more austere settings it should be recognized that a very good initial risk screening can be accomplished using the Gail risk factors and family history information limited to the ages when each relative was diagnosed with breast cancer, any history

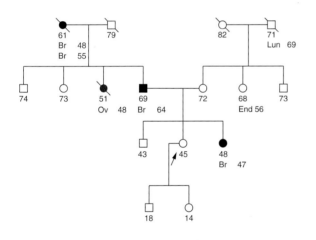

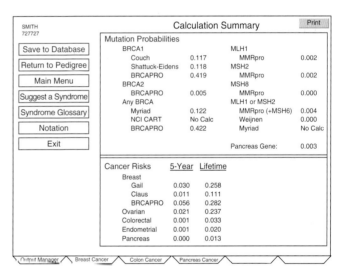

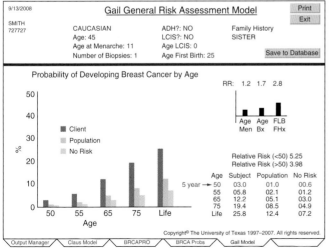

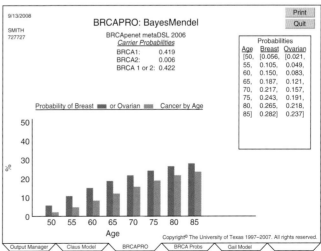

FIGURE 9-2 Sample screen shots from the CancerGene risk assessment program. *(http://www4.utsouthwestern.edu/breasthealth/cagene.)*

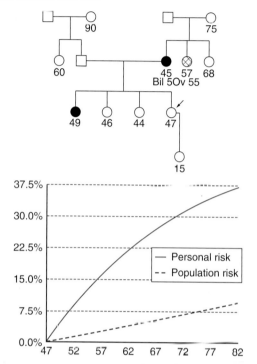

Woman's age is 47 years.
Age at menarche was 11 years.
Age at first birth was 32 years.
Person is premenopausal.
Height is 1.65 m.
Weight is 70.3 kg.
Woman has never used HRT.

Risk after 10 years is 15.85%.
10 year population risk is 2.389%.
Lifetime risk is 35.85%.
Lifetime population risk is 8.826%.
Probability of a BRCA1 gene is 17.11%.
Probability of a BRCA2 gene is 7.075%.

FIGURE 9-3 Screen shot from the IBIS Breast Cancer Risk Evaluator (Tyrer–Cuzick model). *(http://www.ems-trials.org/riskevaluator/.)*

of ovarian cancer, and any history of male breast cancer. Gail risk calculations can be performed quickly on line or using a Personal Data Assistant (http://www.cancer.gov/bcrisktool/), and BRCA gene mutation probability can be estimated from the Myriad prevalence tables (http://www.myriadtests.com/provider/brca-mutation-prevalence.htm).

Using models to quantify breast cancer risk is only the first step in risk assessment and management. This information must be communicated to the patient in an understandable way and in a way that facilitates decision-making. One way to explain absolute risk values is to say, "If I followed 100 women exactly like you for 10 years, 5 would develop breast cancer and 95 would not." There is no established threshold for classifying someone as "high risk." It could be argued that, given the current high incidence rate of breast cancer in the United States, all women are high risk. But most women do not choose to take tamoxifen or to have prophylactic surgery to reduce their risk. Patients and providers are interested in seeing how the absolute risk compares to the risk of other women, so it is often useful to also show the risk for an age- and race-matched woman from the general population. New approaches for risk communication are being developed and validated (Fig. 9-4). The emphasis is on durably influencing risk perception and facilitating medical decision-making. One promising approach is to communicate breast cancer risk in relation to competing risks an individual may face.[28] Breast cancer risk information should never be presented in isolation, but should be combined with discussion of available options for managing risk.

THE FUTURE OF QUANTITATIVE RISK ASSESSMENT

Most available risk assessment models were developed and validated in Caucasian populations, and there is reason to believe

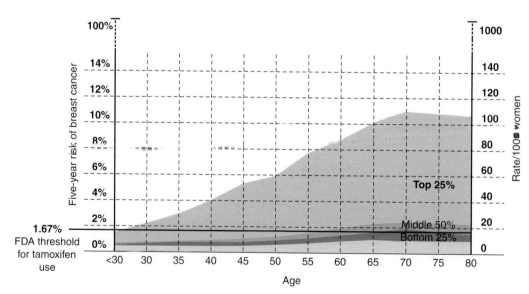

FIGURE 9-4 Gail model risk distribution of women participating in the Nurses Health Study. *(From Ozanne EM, Klemp JR, Esserman LJ. Breast cancer risk assessment and prevention: a framework for shared decision-making consultations. Breast J. 2006;12:103-113.)*

that they do not perform nearly as well for individuals who are not Caucasian. African American women, in particular, are more likely to develop high-grade triple-negative breast cancers than Caucasian women and the Gail model risk factors may not adequately account for this. Future models will make use of race-specific risk factors and breast cancer incidence data to provide a more individualized calculation. Gail and colleagues have recently moved in this direction with description of the CARE model, which attempts to adapt the usual Gail risk factors to improve prediction for African American women.[29] Future models will not stop with the generation of an absolute breast cancer risk estimate, but will include information about the competing risks an individual faces, and the risks and benefits of interventions an individual may consider to reduce breast cancer risk (Table 9-3).

Investigators will continue to address the problem of poor discrimination. It is unlikely that this problem will be solved by simply including more epidemiologic risk factors. There is justifiable interest in systematically evaluating blood and tissue biomarkers for inclusion in logistic regression models.[30] Biomarkers, like atypia identified on palpation-directed fine-needle aspiration biopsy,[31] or even molecular markers in benign breast tissue (eg, tumor suppressor gene methylation,[5] estrogen receptor expression,[32] or proliferation index[33]) may also be of value. The combination of Gail risk calculations and bone mineral density, a surrogate for cumulative estrogen exposure, was recently found to predict breast cancer risk better than the Gail model alone.[34] Biological makers of risk are particularly intriguing as they may permit individualized prevention prescriptions and may provide a ready approach for monitoring treatment effects. Identification and validation of suitable biological markers will require access to epidemiologic data and biological samples from large cohorts with sufficient follow-up.

TABLE 9-3 Future Studies Required to Advance the Field

Issue	Study Type and Objectives
Validation	Measure calibration and discrimination of the Tyrer–Cuzick model in a large population.
Race Differences	Conduct a large case-control study to identify risk factors unique to African American and other race groups.
Breast Cancer heterogeneity	Conduct a large case-control study directed at identifying risk factors for hormone receptor negative breast cancer.
Discrimination	Use case-control data to identify biological markers of risk that could be incorporated into risk prediction models.
Risk communication	Compare various approaches for communicating risk information using durability of adjusted perceived risk as an end point.

SUMMARY

Quantitative breast cancer risk assessment is invaluable for determining sample sizes for prevention trials and is already being accepted by third-party payors as evidence for the medical necessity of expensive tests like screening MRI. When combined with other risk/benefit data, breast cancer risk calculations can inform decisions about chemoprevention and prophylactic surgery and can beneficially impact a patient's perception of risk level. The Tyrer–Cuzick model is the only model in common use that addresses family history and nonfamily history variables in a comprehensive way, but definitive validation data for this model is not yet available. Implementation of risk models in the clinic can be simple or complex depending on the context and mission of the clinic. The addition of carefully selected biological markers may improve the accuracy and discrimination of quantitative risk assessment models in the future.

REFERENCES

1. Haas JS, Kaplan CP, Des Jarlais G, et al. Perceived risk of breast cancer among women at average and increased risk. *J Women's Health*. 2005;14: 845-851.

2. Mikkelsen EM, Sunde L, Johansen C, Johnsen SP. Risk perception among women receiving genetic counseling: a population-based follow-up study. *Cancer Detect Prev*. 2007;31:457-464.

3. Lewis CM, Cler LR, Bu DW, et al. Promoter hypermethylation in benign breast epithelium in relation to predicted breast cancer risk. *Clin Cancer Res*. 2005;11:166-172.

4. Euhus DM, Bu D-W, Ashfaq R, et al. Atypia and DNA methylation in nipple duct lavage in relation to predicted breast cancer risk. *Cancer Epidemiol Biomarkers Prev*. 2007;16:1812-1821.

5. Euhus DM, Bu D, Milchgrub S, et al. DNA bethylation in benign breast epithelium in relation to age and breast cancer risk. *Cancer Epidemiol Biomarkers Prev*. 2008;17:1051-1059.

6. Fisher B, Constantino JP, Wickerham DL, et al. Tamoxifen for prevention of breast cancer: report of the National Surgical Adjuvant Breast and Bowel Project P-1 Study. *J Natl Cancer Inst*. 1998;90:1371-1388.

7. Saslow D, Boetes C, Burke W, et al. American Cancer Society guidelines for breast screening with MRI as an adjunct to mammography. *CA Cancer J Clin*. 2007;57:79-89.

8. Dupont WD, Parl FF, Hartman WH, et al. Breast cancer risk associated with proliferative breast disease and atypical hyperplasia. *Cancer*. 1993;71:1258-1265.

9. Horner MJ, Ries LAG, Krapcho M, et al. (eds). SEER Cancer Statistics Review, 1975-2006, National Cancer Institute. Bethesda, MD, http://seer. cancer.gov/csr/1975_2006/, based on November 2008 SEER data submission, posted to the SEER web site, 2009.

10. Gail MH, Brinton LA, Byar DP, et al. Projecting individualized probabilities of developing breast cancer for white females who are being examined annually. *J Natl Cancer Inst*. 1989;81:1879-1886.

11. Gilpin CA, Carson N, Hunter AW. A preliminary validation of a family assessment form to select women at risk for breast or ovarian cancer for referral to a genetics center. *Clinic Genet*. 2000;58:299-308.

12. Vahteristo P, Eerola H, Tamminen A, et al. A probability model for predicting BRCA1and BRCA2 mutations in breast and breast-ovarian cancer families. *Br J Cancer*. 2001;84:704-708.

13. Chen J, Pee D, Ayyagari R, et al. Projecting absolute invasive breast cancer risk in white women with a model that includes mammographic density. *J Natl Cancer Inst*. 2006;98:1215-1226.

14. Barlow WE, White E, Ballard-Barbash R, et al. Prospective breast cancer risk prediction model for women undergoing screening. *J Natl Cancer Inst*. 2006;98:1204-1214.

15. Claus EB, Risch N, Thompson WD. Autosomal dominant inheritance of early-onset breast cancer. *Cancer*. Vol. 73; 1994;643-651.

16. Berry DA, Parmigiani G, Sanchez S, Sanchez J, Probability of carrying a mutation of breast-ovarian cancer gene BRCA1 based on family history. *J Natl Cancer Inst*. 1997;89:227-238.

17. Parmigiani G, Berry DA, Aquilar O. Determining carrier probabilities for breast cancer susceptibility genes BRCA1 and BRCA2. *Am J Hum Genet.* 1998;62:145-158.

18. Jonker MA, Jacobi CE, Hoogendoorn WE, et al. Modeling familial clustered breast cancer using published data. *Cancer Epidemiol Biomarkers Prev.* 2003;12:1479-1485.

19. Antoniou AC, Pharoah PD, McMullan G, et al. A comprehensive model for familial breast cancer incorporating BRCA1, BRCA2 and other genes. *Br J Cancer.* 2002;86:76-83.

20. Tyrer J, Duffy SW, Cuzick J. A breast cancer prediction model incorporating familial and personal risk factors. *Stat Med.* 2004;23:1111-1130. Erratum appears in *Stat Med.* 2005;24:156.

21. Euhus DM, Leitch AM, Huth JF, Peters G. Limitations of the Gail model in the specializd breast cancer risk assessment clinic. *Breast J.* 2002;8:23-27.

22. Costantino JP, Gail MH, Pee D, et al. Validation studies for models projecting the risk of invasive and total breast cancer incidence. *J Natl Cancer Inst.* 1999;91:1541-1548.

23. Rockhill B, Spiegelman D, Byrne C, et al. Validation of the Gail et al. model of breast cancer risk prediction and implications for chemoprevention. *J Natl Cancer Inst.* 2001;93:358-366.

24. Chlebowski RT, Anderson GL, Lane DS, et al. Predicting risk of breast cancer in postmenopausal women by hormone receptor status. *J Natl Cancer Inst.* 2007;99:1695-1705.

25. Parmigiani G, Chen S, Iversen ESJ, et al. Validity of models for predicting BRCA1 and BRCA2 mutations. *Ann Intern Med.* 2007;147:441-450. Summary for patients in *Ann Intern Med.* 2007;147:I38;PMID: 17909292.

26. Euhus DM, Smith KC, Robinson L, et al. Pretest prediction of BRCA1 or BRCA2 mutation by risk counselors and the computer model BRCAPRO. *J Natl Cancer Inst.* 2002;94:844-851.

27. James PA, Doherty R, Harris M, et al. Optimal selection of individuals for BRCA mutation testing: a comparison of available methods. *J Clin Oncol.* 2006;24:707-715.

28. Ozanne EM, Klemp JR, Esserman LJ. Breast cancer risk assessment and prevention: a framework for shared decision-making consultations. *Breast J.* 2006;12:103-113.

29. Gail MH, Costantino JP, Pee D, et al. Projecting individualized absolute invasive breast cancer risk in African American women. *J Natl Cancer Inst.* 2007; 99:1782-1792.

30. Santen RJ, Boyd NF, Chlebowski RT, et al. Critical assessment of new risk factors for breast cancer: considerations for development of an improved risk prediction model. *Endocr Relat Cancer.* 2007;14:169-187.

31. Fabian CJ, Kimler BF, Zalles CM, et al. Short-term breast cancer prediction by random periareolar fine-needle aspiration cytology and the Gail risk model. *J Natl Cancer Inst.* 2000;92:1217-1227.

32. Khan SA, Rogers MA, Obando JA, Tamsen A. Estrogen receptor expression of benign breast epithelium and its association with breast cancer. *Cancer Res.* 1994;54:993-997.

33. Khan QJ, Kimler BF, Clark J, et al. Ki-67 Expression in benign breast ductal cells obtained by random periareolar fine needle aspiration. *Cancer Epidemiol Biomarkers Prev.* 2005;14:786-789.

34. Chen Z, Arendell L, Aickin M, et al. Hip bone density predicts breast cancer risk independently of Gail score: results from the Women's Health Initiative. *Cancer.* 2008;113:907-915.

35. Tice JA, Cummings SR, Ziv E, Kerlikowske K. Mammographic breast density and the Gail model for breast cancer risk prediction in a screening population. *Breast Cancer Res Treat.* 2005;94:115-122.

36. Tice JA, Miike R, Adduci K, et al. Nipple aspirate fluid cytology and the Gail model for breast cancer risk assessment in a screening population. *Cancer Epidemiol Biomarkers Prev.* 2005;14:324-328.

37. Crispo A, D'Aiuto G, De Marco M, et al. Gail model risk factors: impact of adding an extended family history for breast cancer. *Breast J.* 2008;14:221-227.

38. Amir E, Evans DG, Shenton A, et al. Evaluation of breast cancer risk assessment packages in the family history evaluation and screening programme. *J Med Genet.* 2003;40:807-814.

CHAPTER 10

Chemoprevention in the Clinical Setting

Atilla Soran
Victor G. Vogel

DEFINITION OF CHEMOPREVENTION AND IDENTIFYING WOMEN AT RISK

Breast cancer is a complex disease, resulting from the interaction of nonmodifiable factors such as an individual's genome, age at menarche, menopause, and family history; along with modifiable risk factors such as environmental, hormonal, and lifestyle factors The goal of preventing breast cancer is to identify high-risk individuals who would benefit most from preventive therapies such as chemoprevention and risk-reducing surgeries. Chemoprevention can be defined as the use of natural or synthetic chemical agents to reverse, suppress, or prevent carcinogenic progression to invasive cancer.[1-5]

POPULATION BENEFITS OF CHEMOPREVENTION

In the United States, women who live to the age of 90 have a 1 in 8 chance of being diagnosed with breast cancer.[6] In 2009, breast cancer will be the most frequently diagnosed nonskin malignancy in US women, with an estimated 192,370 cases and 40,170 deaths.[7] Female breast cancer incidence rates decreased by 3.5% per year from 2001 to 2004. This decrease may reflect reduced use of hormone replacement therapy (HRT) and preventive strategies.

THE GAIL MODEL AND THE BREAST CANCER RISK ASSESSMENT TOOL

The Gail model[8] estimates the probability that a woman who engages in annual mammographic screening will develop invasive or in situ ductal or lobular cancer over a particular age interval. The risk factors were adjusted simultaneously for the presence of the other risk factors, and only 6 factors were shown to be significant predictors of the lifetime risk of breast cancer:

1. Current age
2. Age at menarche
3. Number of breast biopsies (pathologic diagnosis of atypical hyperplasia)
4. Age at first live birth (or nulliparity)
5. Family history of breast cancer in first-degree relatives
6. Race

The model may be accessed at www.cancer.gov/bcrisktool. The average American woman's Gail score is 0.3%, which represents her estimated risk for developing invasive breast cancer over the next 5 years; the lifetime risk for the average American woman is 10.1%. A previous diagnosis of atypical lobular or ductal hyperplasia nearly doubles the estimated risk.

The Breast Cancer Risk Assessment (BCRA) tool was updated from the results of the 2007 Women's Contraceptive and Reproductive Experiences (CARE) study in addition to the NCI's SEER program for more accurate risk assessment for African American women.[9]

HIGH-RISK CLINIC AND CLINICAL RISK COUNSELING

The clinician's role in identifying candidates for chemoprophylaxis should include a detailed assessment of familial breast cancer, the opportunity for genetic testing when appropriate, comprehensive quantitative risk assessment, and a specific management prescription.[10] Clinicians should also address the risks and benefits of screening, prophylactic surgery when indicated, and risk reduction using approved chemopreventive agents. In addition to genetic susceptibility, hormonally linked adult reproductive and anthropometric risk factors have been well established in the etiology of pre- and postmenopausal breast cancers.[11,12] The major steps in risk assessment of breast cancer include assessment of genetic susceptibility via genetic counseling, and quantitative risk assessment via the Gail model/BCRA tool. Women at lower risk of breast cancer qualify for routine surveillance, whereas high-risk women may qualify for chemoprevention in addition to routine and /or MRI surveillance.

CHEMOPREVENTION

Epidemiologic studies indicate that estrogen-mediated events are integral in the development of breast cancer[13-15] and support the hypothesis that intact ovarian function is required to develop breast cancer. Oophorectomy or radiation-induced ovarian ablation can reduce the incidence of breast cancer by up to 75%.[16] These observations suggest that estrogen antagonists may be instrumental in the primary prevention of breast cancer.

Chemoprevention may be recommended for certain women who are at increased risk of breast cancer based on the information cited in this chapter. Approximately 9 million women were eligible for tamoxifen chemoprevention based on criteria from the Breast Cancer Prevention Trial (BCPT).[17] Of these 9 million, approximately 2.4 million might have derived a benefit from taking tamoxifen. An estimated 58,000 cases of invasive breast cancer would develop over the ensuing 5 years with that population, and based on the 49% risk reduction associated with tamoxifen in the BCPT, if all 2.4 million women had taken tamoxifen, 24,492 cases of breast cancer might have been prevented.

TAMOXIFEN

Hormones, especially estrogens, have been linked to breast cancer,[18,19] with their role being attributed to their ability to stimulate cell proliferation. This cellular proliferation leads to the accumulation of random genetic errors that result in neoplastic transformation.[15] According to this concept, chemoprevention of breast cancer is targeted to reduce the rate of cell proliferation through administration of hormonal modulators. Tamoxifen is a triphenylethylene compound, a potential fertility agent. Demethylation to the active metabolite, N-desmethyl tamoxifen, is the principal metabolic pathway in humans. Maximum serum concentration of N-desmethyl tamoxifen is observed within 12 to 24 hours after dosing; its serum half-life is approximately 12 days,[20-23] Several mechanisms have been proposed regarding tamoxifen's ability to prevent or suppress breast carcinogenesis.[24-34]

RALOXIFENE

Raloxifene hydrochloride, like tamoxifen, is a selective estrogen receptor modulator (SERM) that has antiestrogenic effects on breast and endometrial tissue and estrogenic effects on bone, lipid metabolism, and blood clotting.[35] It is a benzothiophene with characteristics similar to but distinct from the triphenylethylene SERMs such as tamoxifen. It inhibits the growth of ER-dependent, dimethylbenzathracene-induced mammary tumors and reduces the occurrence of N-nitrosomethyl urea-induced mammary tumors in rats.

For both raloxifene and tamoxifen, minor differences in SERM–ligand interaction with specific amino acids produce different intrinsic estrogen actions. The tamoxifen-ER complex is more estrogen-like in vitro, reflecting more estrogen-like action in uterus. In contrast, the raloxifene-ER complex is much less estrogen-like and has fewer estrogen-like properties in uterus.

CHEMOPREVENTION RISK REDUCTION TRIALS

Four prospective studies evaluating tamoxifen for reducing the risk of invasive breast cancer have been published: the National Surgical Adjuvant Breast and Bowel Project (NSABP) Breast Cancer Prevention Trial (BCPT, P-1),[36,37] the Royal Marsden Hospital Tamoxifen Chemoprevention Trial,[38-40] the Italian Tamoxifen Prevention Study,[41-43] and the International Breast Intervention Study I (IBIS-I).[44,45] See Tables 10-1 and 10-2.

Breast Cancer Prevention Trial (BCPT, P-1)

The National Cancer Institute in collaboration with NSABP launched the BCPT P-1,[36] a randomized, placebo-controlled, double-blind clinical trial in 1992. The primary aim of the trial was to evaluate the effectiveness of 20 mg/day of tamoxifen (versus placebo) taken orally for 5 years for the prevention of invasive breast cancer in high-risk women. Secondary aims of the trial assessed osteoporotic fractures and cardiovascular disease in women on tamoxifen compared to the control group.

Eligible participants were 60 years or older, or 35 to 59 years of age with a 5-year predicted risk of breast cancer of at least 1.66% as indicated by the Gail model, or had a history of lobular carcinoma in situ (LCIS). The trial was terminated after a median follow-up time was 54.6 months when an interim analysis showed that statistical significance was achieved in a number of study end points. This decrease was only evident in estrogen receptor-positive breast cancers, with no significant change seen in estrogen receptor-negative tumors. The median follow-up time at the end point was 48 months, at which time a 49% ($p < 0.00001$) decreased risk of invasive breast cancer in the total study population was documented, with the greatest benefit seen in women of ages 60 and older. Overall, a total of 264 invasive cases were documented; 175 cases occurred in the placebo group, compared with 89 cases in the tamoxifen group (risk ratio, 0.51; 95% confidence interval [CI], 0.39–0.66; $p < 0.00001$). There was a 50% reduction in the rate of noninvasive breast cancer in women taking tamoxifen. The relative risks (RR) for invasive breast cancer reduction were 0.56 for women less than 50 years of age; 0.49 for women 50 to 59 years of age; and 0.45 for women 60 years of age and older.

After 7 years of follow-up in BCPT,[46] the cumulative rate of invasive breast cancer was reduced 43% in the tamoxifen group and the cumulative rate of noninvasive breast cancer was reduced 37%. The BCPT revealed that substantial net benefit accrues for women with a diagnosis of either LCIS or atypical hyperplasia who take tamoxifen. Among women with a history

TABLE 10-1 Summary of 4 Randomized Chemoprevention Trials of Tamoxifen (20 mg/day vs Placebo) for Women at Increased Risk for Breast Cancer

	Breast Cancer Prevention Trial (BCPT) (n = 13,388)	Royal Marsden Hospital Chemoprevention Trial (n = 2494)	Italian Tamoxifen Prevention Study (n = 5408)	International Breast Intervention Study I (IBIS I) (n = 7152)
Subjects	High breast cancer risk (age ≥ 60 years or a combination of risk factors using the Gail model); 39% < 50 years; ≥ 1.66% 5-year risk	Family history of breast cancer < 50 years old or 2 or more affected first-degree relatives	Women with hysterectomy (48% bilateral oophorectomy); Median age: 51 years	Women aged 35 to 70 years who were at increased risk for breast cancer; > 2-fold relative risk
Proportion who took estrogen	< 10%	26%	41%	50%
Median follow-up (y)	7	13	11	8
Invasive breast cancers	Placebo: 250 Tamoxifen: 145	Placebo: 82 Tamoxifen: 104	Placebo: 74 Tamoxifen: 62	Placebo: 168 Tamoxifen: 124
Breast cancer rates per 1000 woman years and RR of cancer (95% CI)	Invasive Placebo: 6.3 Tamoxifen: 3.6 RR: 0.57 (0.46–0.70) Noninvasive Placebo: 2.7 Tamoxifen: 1.4 RR: 0.63 (0.45–0.89)	All cases Placebo: 5.0 Tamoxifen: 4.7 RR: 0.78 (0.58–1.04)	All cases Placebo: 2.4 Tamoxifen: 2.1 RR: 0.84 (0.60–1.17) High-risk group: Placebo: 24 Tamoxifen: 6 RR: 0.2 (0.10–0.59)	Invasive Placebo: 5.8 Tamoxifen: 4.3 RR: 0.74 (0.58–0.94) DCIS Placebo: 0.94 Tamoxifen: 0.6 RR: 0.63 (0.32–1.2)
Number and RR of ER-positive breast cancer	Placebo: 182 Tamoxifen: 70 RR: 0.38 (0.28–0.50)	Posttreatment period Placebo: 47 Tamoxifen: 23 HR: 0.48 (0.29–0.79)	Placebo: 10 Tamoxifen: 8	Placebo: 132 Tamoxifen: 87 RR: 0.66 (0.50–0.87)
Risk reduction	Invasive: 43% DCIS, LCIS: 37% With prior LCIS: 46% With prior atypical hyperplasia: 75%	Overall: no reduction Posttreatment period: Invasive: 37% ER(+): 52%	Overall: no reduction; In the high-risk subset[a]: 82%	Overall: 27% DCIS: 37%

[a]The high-risk subset included women taller than 160 cm, with at least one functioning ovary, menarche at age 13 years, and no pregnancy before age 24 years.

of LCIS, the reduction in risk was 46% (RR, 0.54; 95% CI, 0.27–1.02). Among women with a history of atypical hyperplasia, the reduction in risk was 75%; tamoxifen continued to reduce the occurrence of ER-positive tumors by 62%, but no difference was seen in the occurrence of ER-negative tumors.

Secondary outcomes in the BCPT included osteoporotic fractures and cardiovascular events. Tamoxifen is known to have estrogen agonist–like effects on both mineral density and serum cholesterol levels in postmenopausal women.[47,48] Women in the tamoxifen group had a 32% reduction in hip, spine, and distal radius fractures. Most fractures (89%) occurred in women aged 50 years or older and tamoxifen reduced fractures in this group by 29%.

Adverse outcomes related to tamoxifen were significantly higher in women over the age of 50 when compared to their younger counterparts. Women on tamoxifen were found to

TABLE 10-2 Summary of Selected Adverse Eevents in 4 Randomized Chemoprevention Trials of Tamoxifen (20 mg/day vs Placebo) for Women at Increased Risk for Breast Cancer

	Breast Cancer Prevention Trial (BCPT) (n = 13,388)	Royal Marsden Hospital Chemoprevention Trial (n = 2494)	Italian Tamoxifen Prevention Study (n = 5408)	International Breast Intervention Study I (IBIS-I) (n = 7152)
Endometrial cancer	Invasive Placebo: 17 Tamoxifen: 53 RR: 3.28 (1.87–6.03)	Placebo: 5 Tamoxifen: 13 *p* = 0.06		Placebo: 11 Tamoxifen: 17 RR: 1.55 (0.68–3.65)
Stroke	Placebo: 50 Tamoxifen: 71 RR: 1.42 (0.97–2.08)	Placebo: 16 Tamoxifen: 10	*Cerebrovascular events:* Placebo: 7 Tamoxifen: 12 RR: 1.78 (0.70–4.52)	Placebo: 12 Tamoxifen: 15 RR: 1.25 (0.55–2.93)
Transient ischemic attack	Placebo: 34 Tamoxifen: 31 RR: 0.91 (0.54–1.52)	Placebo: 10 Tamoxifen: 5		Placebo: 22 Tamoxifen: 17 RR: 0.77 (0.39–1.52)
Pulmonary embolism	Placebo:13 Tamoxifen: 28 RR: 2.15 (1.08–4.51)	*Thromboembolic events:* Placebo: 9 Tamoxifen: 13	*Thromboembolic events:* Placebo: 28 Tamoxifen: 44 RR: 1.63 (1.02–2.62)	*Thromboembolic events:* Placebo: 68 Tamoxifen: 117 RR: 1.72 (1.27–2.36)
DVT	Placebo: 34 Tamoxifen: 49 RR: 1.44 (0.91–2.30)			
Cardiac	Placebo: 109 Tamoxifen: 113 RR: 1.03 (0.79–1.36)	MI and cerebrovascular Placebo: 26 Tamoxifen: 21	Placebo: 21 Tamoxifen: 35 RR: 1.73 (1.01 2.98)	Placebo: 123 Tamoxifen: 122 RR: 0.99 (0.77–1.29)
Cataracts	Placebo: 27.75 per 1000 women Tamoxifen: 22.85 per 1000 women RR:1.21 (1.10–1.34)	Placebo: 3 Tamoxifen: 12		Placebo: 54 Tamoxifen: 67 RR: 1.24 (0.87–1.77)
Osteoporotic fracture	Placebo: 116 Tamoxifen: 80 RR: 0.68 (0.51–0.92)	Placebo: 33 Tamoxifen: 28		Placebo: 235 Tamoxifen: 240 RR: 1.02 (0.86–1.21)
Hot flashes	Placebo: 65% Tamoxifen: 77.6% RR: 1.19	Placebo: 441 Tamoxifen: 671 *p* = 0.001	Placebo: 446 Tamoxifen: 635 RR: 1.78 (1.57–2.0)	*Gynecologic/Vasomotor* Placebo: 2922 Tamoxifen: 3151 RR: 108 (1.06–1.10)
Urinary disturbances		Placebo: 26 Tamoxifen: 30	Placebo: 140 Tamoxifen: 202 RR: 1.52 (1.23–1.89)	
Vaginal dryness		*Vaginal problems* Placebo: 17 Tamoxifen: 38	Placebo: 269 Tamoxifen: 295 RR: 1.14 (0.97–1.34)	
Vaginal discharge	Placebo: 34.1% Tamoxifen: 54.7% RR: 1.60	Placebo: 184 Tamoxifen: 362 *p* = 0.001	Placebo: 173 Tamoxifen: 505 RR: 3.44 (2.9–4.09)	
Breast cancer deaths	Placebo: 11 Tamoxifen: 12	Placebo: 12 Tamoxifen: 9	Placebo: 2 Tamoxifen: 2	Placebo: 13 Tamoxifen: 11
All deaths	Placebo: 114 Tamoxifen: 126 RR: 1.10 (0.85–3.08)	Placebo: 54 Tamoxifen: 54 HR: 0.99 (0.68–1.44)	Placebo: 38 Tamoxifen: 36 RR: 0.95 (0.60–1.49)	Placebo: 55 Tamoxifen: 65

have twice the incidence of pulmonary embolism compared to those on placebo. While incidences of deep vein thrombosis, stoke, and transient ischemic attack were not statistically significant, there was a higher incidence in women on tamoxifen, and thus the concern lies for development of these events in women on tamoxifen.

Women in the tamoxifen arm of the trial were found to have a 3.3 times greater risk of developing invasive endometrial carcinoma than women in the placebo arm. Of the 70 cases of endometrial cancer (17 in the placebo group and 53 in the tamoxifen froup) 67 cases were International Federation of Gynecology and Obstetrics (FIGO) stages 0 or 1 and thus had excellent clinical prognoses with treatment.

An increase of 21% in the development of cataracts was seen in women who were free of cataracts at initiation of the trial. The number of cataract surgeries was also increased by 39% in women taking tamoxifen. Vasomotor symptoms, mainly hot flashes, were reported by 46% of women on tamoxifen and only 29% of women in the placebo arm; whereas an increase in vaginal discharge was reported in 29% of women taking tamoxifen and 13% of women taking placebo. Tamoxifen was not associated with an increased risk of developing depressive symptoms comparing the tamoxifen and placebo groups in the BCPT.[49,50]

Royal Marsden Hospital (RMH) Tamoxifen Chemoprevention Trial

RMH Tamoxifen Chemoprevention Trial was a randomized, placebo-controlled clinical trial initiated in 1986 and the aim of this trial was to assess whether tamoxifen (20 mg/day for up to 8 years) would prevent breast cancer in healthy women at increased risk of breast cancer based on family history.[38-40] Eligible women were ages 30 years to 70 years with least one first-degree relative younger than 50 years with breast cancer, one first-degree relative with bilateral breast cancer, or one affected first-degree relative of any age and another affected first- or second-degree relative. Women were allowed to use HRT during the trial. In initial reports, a total of 70 invasive and noninvasive breast cancers occurred among the women in this trial, and the frequency of breast cancer was the same for women receiving tamoxifen or placebo.[38,51] After a median follow-up 13 years, the trial reported a statistically significant decrease in ER-positive tumors.[52]

Italian Tamoxifen Prevention Trial

The Italian Tamoxifen Prevention Trial was a randomized, placebo-controlled, double-blind clinical trial, initiated to evaluate the effectiveness of tamoxifen in preventing breast cancer.[41] The primary aim of this trial was to evaluate the effectiveness of 20 mg/day of tamoxifen orally for 5 years in preventing the occurrence of breast cancer versus placebo in healthy women, with the primary end points being reduction in the incidence of, and mortality from, breast cancer. Because of the potential side effect of endometrial cancer, the study was restricted to women between the ages of 35 and 70 and who had undergone a hysterectomy. More than 5400 women were randomized into either the tamoxifen 20 mg/day or the placebo group. The trial was ended prematurely because of a 26.3% dropout rate for women already randomized.

In a subgroup analysis,[41] women are at increased risk for ER-positive breast cancer. This group included women taller than 160 cm (the median height of the group), with at least one functioning ovary, who had menarche when they were no older than 13 years, and who had no full-term pregnancy before 24 years of age. This group of 702 women (13% of the trial population) was classified as high risk. Tamoxifen reduced the incidence of breast cancer in the high-risk group, but it had no effect in the low-risk group.

After 11 years of follow-up, in the group defined as "high risk" with at least one functioning ovary, there was a 77% reduction in the incidence of breast cancer.[42] This trial demonstrated that appropriate selection of women at high-risk for developing hormone receptor-positive breast cancer led to benefit from tamoxifen intervention. The update after 11 years of follow-up also confirmed the finding that tamoxifen in addition to estrogen replacement therapy is protective against breast cancer development, although this approach is not used in North America.

International Breast Cancer Intervention Study I (IBIS-I)

The IBIS-I trial was a randomized, placebo-controlled study, with design and outcomes similar to that of BCPT, initiated in 1992 to evaluate whether tamoxifen reduced the risk of invasive breast cancer in women at increased risk.[44] The primary aim of the trial was to evaluate the effectiveness of 20 mg/day of tamoxifen (versus placebo) orally for 5 years in preventing the occurrence of both invasive and in situ breast cancer in women deemed at high risk. Selection criteria for the trial's high-risk patients required that women aged 45 to 70 have at least a 2-fold RR, women aged 40 to 44 needed at least a 4-fold RR, and women aged 35 to 39 years of age had at least a 10-fold RR of developing breast cancer.[53] Risk factors involved in determining the RR of breast cancer development included family history, history of LCIS, history of atypical hyperplasia, benign breast biopsies, and nulliparity, and the primary end point was the incidence of breast cancer including ductal carcinoma in situ (DCIS).

During 9 years of recruitment, more than 7000 women were enrolled in the trial, approximately 60% had 2 or more first-degree relatives with breast cancer, and 60% of the study cohort had a 10-year risk of developing breast cancer of between 5% and 10%. One-third of women had hysterectomies previously. HRT use was permitted during the trial, and approximately 40% of women used HRT at some point during this trial. The primary end point was the incidence of breast cancer including DCIS.

After a median follow up of 50 months, 170 cases of breast cancers, including DCIS, had been diagnosed, with 32% fewer cases among the women taking tamoxifen. This risk reduction result was virtually identical to that found in the BCPT among women who did not have atypical hyperplasia. As with the BCPT, that risk reduction was only seen with estrogen receptor-positive tumors and not with estrogen receptor-negative tumors. Of women in the trial who concomitantly used HRT with tamoxifen, there was no benefit form tamoxifen. While there was no reduction in the incidence of breast cancer in women concomitantly using HRT and tamoxifen, a risk reduction was seen among women who had a history of prior HRT use and were assigned to tamoxifen in the trial: these women experienced a 57% risk reduction in their risk for breast cancer.

Additional analysis with a median follow-up of 96 months after randomization in IBIS-I revealed a continuing 27% reduction in the risk of breast cancer among the women taking tamoxifen.[45] The risk-reducing effect of tamoxifen was fairly constant for the entire follow-up period, and no lessening of benefit was observed for up to 10 years after randomization. Among women who never used HRT or who used it only before the trial, there was a statistically significant 51% reduction in ER-positive breast cancers in the tamoxifen group compared with the placebo group. For women who used HRT during any point of the trial, no clear benefit of tamoxifen was seen in reducing the risk of breast cancer. Results were similar regardless of the HRT preparations used (ie, either estrogen only or combined estrogen and progestin). HRT use was not associated with the development of ER-negative breast cancers, either during the active treatment period or during subsequent follow-up. The risk reduction observed may be smaller that that seen in the NSABP BCPT, both because patients enrolled onto IBIS-I were allowed to take HRT during the trial and because few women in IBIS-I had atypical hyperplasia where a large reduction in incidence of invasive breast cancer was seen in BCPT.

The overall risk of clotting events was increased in tamoxifen users, with a 2-fold increase in risk of venous thromboembolism. As with the BCPT, this risk was seen predominately in women over the age of 50 years and in those women with a recent history of surgery. The excess of thromboembolic events was found only in the active treatment phase. Though the risk was not significant, there was an increase in risk of endometrial cancer in women taking tamoxifen, especially among women aged 50 years or older. As observed in the BCPT, the majority cases of endometrial cancer diagnosed were FIGO stages 0 or 1.

Summary of the Tamoxifen Chemoprevention Trials

Data from all 4 trials combined concluded that tamoxifen decreased breast cancer incidence by 38% ($p < 0.0001$).[54] The risk reduction for development of estrogen receptor-positive breast cancers was 48% (RR, 0.52; 95% CI, 36-58; $p < 0.0001$). No significant risk reduction was seen in the incidence of estrogen receptor-negative breast cancers. Venous thromboembolic events were found to be nearly doubled in women using tamoxifen in all trials, with reduction in this risk seen with concomitant use of low-dose aspirin. Rates of endometrial cancer were also found to be increased in all trials in women using tamoxifen, with a reduction in this risk seen by excluding women at increased risk of endometrial cancer, and higher risks in women of the age of 50 years. Overall, there was no effect on mortality from all causes; however, these trials were not powered or designed to analyze all-cause mortality events.

INDICATIONS AND CONTRAINDICATIONS OF USING TAMOXIFEN

Women taking oral contraceptives, estrogen, progesterone, or androgens should discontinue these prior to initiation of tamoxifen therapy (Table 10-3). Women should be advised against becoming pregnant while on tamoxifen, as the drug has

---

TABLE 10-3 Indications and Contraindications of Using Selective Estrogen Receptor Modulators for Reducing the Incidence of Invasive Breast Cancer

Indications
Women with a history of one of the following:
    Lobular carcinoma in situ
    Ductal carcinoma in situ
    Atypical ductal or lobular hyperplasia
    Premenopausal women with mutations in either the BRCA1 or BRCA2 genes
    Premenopausal women at least 35 years of age with 5-year probability of breast cancer = 1.66%
    Women aged 60 years with Gail model 5-year probability of breast cancer = 5%

Absolute Contraindications
History of deep venous thrombosis, pulmonary embolus, concurrent warfarin therapy use, history of cataracts or cataract surgery, current use of hormone replacement therapy, or pregnancy

Relative Contraindications
History of transient ischemic attack or stroke, poorly controlled diabetes, hypertension, atrial fibrillation, immobility, mitral valve disease, or ischemic heart disease

Cautions
Women taking oral contraceptives, estrogen, progesterone, or androgens should discontinue these prior to initiation of tamoxifen therapy. Women should be advised against becoming pregnant while on tamoxifen as the drug has a class D pregnancy recommendation and in rats has been associated with birth defects

a class D pregnancy recommendation and in rats has been associated with birth defects. Postmenopausal women are at increased risk of adverse events; thus alternate therapy such as raloxifene should be considered.

The optimal duration of risk-reducing therapy is unknown, but adjuvant therapy studies with tamoxifen indicate that therapy of less than 5 years duration is not as effective as at least 5 years of therapy in reducing the incidence of second contralateral invasive breast cancer. Whether using tamoxifen for longer than 5 years is more effective in preventing the recurrence of breast cancer than using it for only 5 years is the subject of ongoing clinical trials; however, no trials are currently being conducted or planned to examine the ideal duration of therapy in the risk-reduction setting. The optimal age at which to start therapy is unknown.

CLINICAL MONITORING OF WOMEN TAKING TAMOXIFEN

Endometrial hyperplasia and cancer were more frequent among women taking tamoxifen than among women taking placebo in the BCPT, but there was no evidence of elevated risk from tamoxifen use in women younger than 50 (RR, 1.21; 95% CI, 0.41-3.60). The utility of endometrial cancer screening with either endometrial biopsy or transvaginal ultrasound in asymptomatic tamoxifen-treated women is limited and is not recommended outside the setting of a clinical trial. Rather, women receiving tamoxifen should have annual cervical cytology and pelvic examinations. Any abnormal bleeding should be evaluated with appropriate diagnostic testing, and women should be counseled about the risk of benign and malignant conditions associated with tamoxifen.

Routine screening with hematologic or chemical blood tests is not indicated because no hematologic or hepatic toxicities attributable to tamoxifen were demonstrated in the BCPT or in clinical trials using tamoxifen as adjuvant therapy. Because of the modest increase in risk of cataracts and cataract surgery among women using tamoxifen compared with women taking placebo, women taking tamoxifen should be questioned about symptoms of cataracts during follow-up and should discuss with their health care provider the value of periodic eye examinations.

ASSESSING RISKS AND BENEFITS OF TAMOXIFEN FOR CHEMOPREVENTION

Despite its favorable potential for breast cancer risk reduction, chemoprevention with tamoxifen is not yet routine management among physicians (Fig. 10-1). This is likely due to the perception by patients and physicians that side effects associated with tamoxifen are potentially serious and may include pulmonary embolism, deep vein thrombosis, stroke, uterine malignancy, or cataracts.

Recommendations from the NCI workshop began with calculating the 5-year risk of breast cancer in women based on the Gail model.[55] Women with a calculated risk of 1.66% or greater should be considered as high-risk individuals and potential candidates for SERM therapy. The U.S. Food and Drug Administration approved the use of tamoxifen to reduce the incidence of breast cancer in women greater than age 35 whose 5-year risk of breast cancer is 1.66% or greater as determined by the Gail model. The risks and benefits of using tamoxifen depend upon age and race, as well as on a woman's specific risk factors for breast cancer. In particular, the absolute risks of endometrial cancer, stroke, pulmonary embolism, and deep venous thrombosis associated with tamoxifen use increase with age, as does the protective effect of tamoxifen on fractures. Once women are classified for their risk of breast cancer, high-risk women should be assessed further to determine their individual specific risk-benefit profile. A woman's risk can change over time and it is important to revisit risk assessment at multiple stages during a woman's life. By using a series of risk–benefit models, tamoxifen has positive net benefit in women under the age of 50 with elevated risk of both invasive and in situ breast cancer. Women over the age of 70 have adverse events associated with tamoxifen use regardless of race or ethnicity.[56] A "high-risk" woman's risk-benefit profile, narrowed by age and race, may be helpful in determining which patients would benefit most from tamoxifen chemoprevention.

CHEMOPREVENTION WITH RALOXIFENE

The benefits of raloxifene on osteoporosis and fractures were assessed in a number of clinical trials during the last decade and after the publication of the results of the BCPT. These osteoporosis trials reported data related to the incidence of invasive breast cancer among women taking raloxifene compared to those taking the placebo (Table 10-4). The Multiple Outcomes of Raloxifene Evaluation (MORE) trial was a multicenter, randomized, double-blind trial initiated in 1994 to evaluate whether postmenopausal women with osteoporosis using raloxifene 60 or 120 mg orally daily for a period of 3 years experienced a reduced risk of fracture.[57,58]

A secondary end point of this trial was incidence of invasive breast cancer in women using raloxifene versus placebo.

Raloxifene reduced the risk of invasive breast cancer by 76% in postmenopausal women with osteoporosis; largely accounted for by a 90% reduction in estrogen receptor-positive breast cancer. There was no risk reduction seen with estrogen receptor-negative breast cancer. Overall, raloxifene decreased the risk of vertebral fractures in postmenopausal osteoporotic women. Raloxifene was also found to decrease serum levels of low-density lipoprotein cholesterol. Unlike tamoxifen, raloxifene was not found to increase the risk of endometrial cancer. Similar to tamoxifen, raloxifene was found to increase the risk of thromboembolic events almost 3-fold. Raloxifene also increased the incidence of vasomotor symptoms including hot flashes, leg cramps, and peripheral edema.

The Continuing Outcomes Relevant to Evista (CORE) trial was an extension to examine the effect of 4 additional years of raloxifene therapy on the reduction of the incidence of breast cancer in participants of the MORE trial.[59] Women in the raloxifene arm had a 59% reduction in occurrence when compared to placebo. The largest benefit (66% reduction in risk) was seen in estrogen receptor-positive tumors in women taking

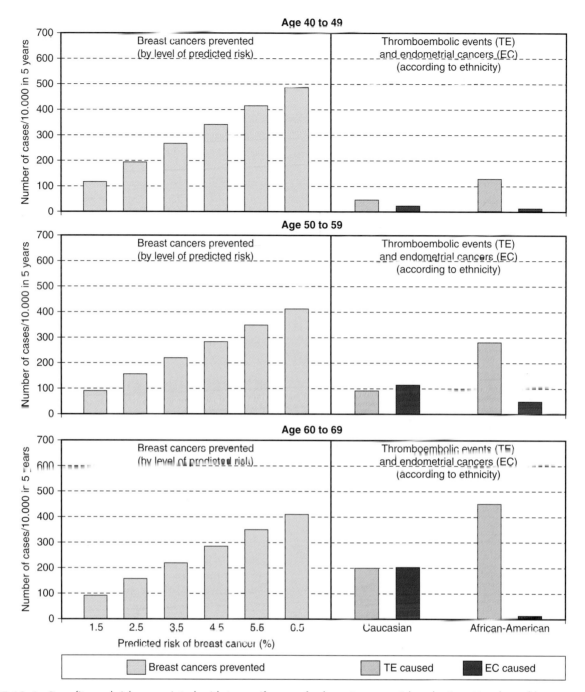

FIGURE 10-1 Benefits and risks associated with tamoxifen use for breast cancer risk reduction. Number of breast cancers prevented by tamoxifen in cases per 10,000 women over 5 years by 10-year age group and by level of predicted risk (*left*). Number of thromboembolic events and endometrial cancers caused by tamoxifen in cases per 10,000 women over 5 years, by ethnicity (*right*). (*From: Fisher B, Costantino JP, Wickerham DL, et al. J Natl Cancer Inst. 2005;97:1652-1662.*)

raloxifene compared to the placebo. As with tamoxifen chemoprevention trials, there was no reduction in the risk of developing estrogen receptor-negative breast cancer. Raloxifene at either 60 or 120 mg/day was also associated with statistically significant increases with the incidence of influenza-like symptoms, hot flashes, leg cramps, and endometrial cavity fluid.

After a period of 8 years among the 7705 participants in the MORE and CORE trials, the overall risk reduction was 66%.

Consistent with findings in the MORE trial, reductions were only seen with estrogen receptor-positive tumors (76% reduction) and no reduction in risk was seen in estrogen receptor-negative tumors. Over the 8-year period of the MORE and CORE, regardless of invasiveness, the overall incidence of breast cancer was reduced in the raloxifene arm by 58% compared with placebo.

Cardiovascular outcomes were also measured in participants of the MORE and CORE trial. Throughout the duration of the

TABLE 10-4 Prospective, Randomized, Placebo-Controlled Clinical Studies of Raloxifene with Invasive Breast Cancer as an End Point

Study	MORE[57,58] (n = 7705)	CORE[59] (n = 5213)	RUTH[60] (n = 10,101)	STAR[61] (n = 19,747)
Mean age/ study population	66.5/with at least one osteoporotic fracture	66.2/continuation of the MORE study	67.5/with a history of CHD or risk factors for CHD	58.5/postmenopausal women: increased risk of breast cancer
Primary outcome	Fractures	Fractures	CHD events and invasive breast cancer	Invasive breast cancer
Secondary outcomes	Breast cancer	Breast cancer	Death	Fracture, CHD events
Major toxicities reported	Thromboembolic events, uterine malignancy	Thromboembolic events, uterine malignancy	Thromboembolic events, uterine malignancy	Thromboembolic events, uterine malignancy, other cancers, total deaths
Formal quality-of-life study	No	No	No	Yes
Event rate in the raloxifene group (per 1000 woman-years)	0.9	1.4	1.5	4.4
No. of breast cancers in the comparison group	27	58	533	163
Event rate in the comparison group (per 1000 woman-years)	3.6	4.2	2.7	4.3
Risk reduction (hazard rate or risk ratio) and 95% confidence interval	0.24 (0.13–0.44)	0.34 (0.22–0.50)	0.56 (0.38–0.83)	Not applicable (no) placebo group

Adapted from Vogel VG. Raloxifene: a second-generation selective estrogen receptor modulator for reducing the risk of invasive breast cancer in postmenopausal women. *Women's Health.* 2007;3:139-153.

8-year analyses, there was no overall increased incidence in serious adverse cardiovascular events in the raloxifene compared to the placebo arm. There were also no statistically significant differences in either coronary or cerebrovascular events when comparing the 2 groups. Thus raloxifene offers neither an increased risk nor a benefit in regard to cardiovascular events in postmenopausal women at low risk of having an event. A subgroup analysis of women in the MORE trial also revealed that raloxifene has no effect on lipids and lipoproteins.

Both the results of the individual trial and the combined data from the MORE and CORE trial revealed an increase in the incidence of thromboembolic events in participants taking raloxifene over an 8-year period (2.2 vs 1.3 events/1000 woman-years in the raloxifene versus the placebo group, respectively). Incidence of pulmonary embolism was 0.62% in the raloxifene group with one death compare 0.16% assigned to placebo with no deaths.

The RUTH (Raloxifene Use for the Heart) trial was assembled after the observation that raloxifene was found to decrease serum levels of lipoprotein cholesterol, homocysteine, and fibrinogen in correlation with observational studies showing that treatment with estrogen decreased risk of coronary heart disease (CHD) in postmenopausal women; to assess the clinical effects of raloxifene on the reduction of coronary events in postmenopausal women.[69]

During enrollment, more than 10,000 postmenopausal women (mean age 67.5 years) with a history of CHD or with documented multiple risk factors for CHD, were randomized to either receive raloxifene 60 mg/day or placebo and were followed for a median of 5.7 years. The primary outcomes of the trial were coronary events and occurrence of invasive breast cancer. A secondary outcome in the trial was incidence of vertebral fractures.

Raloxifene reduced the risk of breast cancer in these older, postmenopausal women who were at lower risk of breast cancer by 44%; as with previous trials, this reduction was seen with estrogen receptor-positive tumors, with no effect on estrogen receptor-negative tumors. Other outcomes in the RUTH trial include risk of fracture and cardiovascular events. The risk of vertebral fracture was significantly decreased in women taking raloxifene by 35%. Despite previous documented reduction in lipoproteins, homocysteine, and fibrinogen, no decrease was found in the risk of cardiovascular events in women on raloxifene compared to placebo in the RUTH trial. Thus in the outcomes measured, there was no significant difference in the incidences of coronary event in women taking raloxifene. These findings were true for both women with a previous history of CHD and for those with multiple documented risk factors for the development of CHD.

In the raloxifene group, adverse events reported with higher frequency included arthritis, cholelithiasis, dyspepsia, hot flushes, intermittent claudication, muscle spasms, and peripheral edema. Importantly, there was no difference in the incidence of endometrial cancer between the two groups, unlike studies of similar design that employed tamoxifen as the SERM. Like tamoxifen, raloxifene increased the risk of venous thromboembolic disease 3-fold.

STUDY OF TAMOXIFEN AND RALOXIFENE (STAR) TRIAL

NSABP launched the STAR trial in 1999. Eligible women were at least 35 years old and postmenopausal, and they must have had either LCIS or a 5-year risk of invasive breast cancer of at least 1.67% as determined by the Gail model. Subjects were randomly assigned to receive either tamoxifen 20 mg/day or raloxifene 60 mg/day for 5 years in a double-blind, double-dummy design. No women in the trial received placebo alone.[61]

The primary aim of the trial was to evaluate the statistical equivalence of 20 mg/day of tamoxifen orally for over 5 years versus 60 mg/day of raloxifene in decreasing the incidence of breast cancer. Secondary aims were to assess the incidence of noninvasive breast cancer, endometrial cancer, skeletal fractures, and venous thromboembolic events in women on chemoprevention therapy. Women were evaluated as increased risk of breast cancer by using criteria from the Gail model with a mean risk in those randomized of 4%.

After a median follow-up of 3.2 years among 19,767 women (mean age 58.5 years), 331 cases of invasive breast cancer had been reported. When subpopulations in the study groups were compared based on categories of age, history of LCIS, history of atypical hyperplasia, 5-year predicted risk of breast cancer, and the number of family members with a history of breast cancer, there was no difference in the incidence of invasive breast cancer between the treatment groups. There was also no difference in tumor size, nodal status, or estrogen receptor level between compatible subgroups in the 2 treatment groups. In the tamoxifen arm of the trial, there were fewer incidences of both LCIS and DCIS over a 6-year follow-up.

The incidence of endometrial cancer, cardiovascular events, venous thromboembolic events, osteoporotic fractures, and cataracts were also analyzed in the trial. There were more cases of uterine cancer in the tamoxifen group compared to the raloxifene group. There was no significant difference in the number of cerebrovascular events between the 2 arms (53 vs 51 strokes in the tamoxifen vs raloxifene groups). The number of thromboembolic events was 30% lower in the raloxifene group, including both pulmonary embolism and deep vein thrombosis. The incidence of pulmonary embolism was 54 versus 35 women (RR, 0.64; 95% CI, 0.41-1.00); and osteoporotic fractures were comparable in the 2 groups. Women on raloxifene also experienced fewer incidences of cataracts (RR, 0.79; 95% CI, 0.68-0.92) and surgery for cataracts (RR, 0.82; 95% CI, 0.68-0.99) at 6-year follow-up.

Adverse effects experienced by patients in the STAR trial were reported by participants using a 36-item symptom check list.[62] Questionnaires were given to participants before treatment, followed by every 6 months for 5 years and then again at 6 years. Both physical and mental components were evaluated in a quality-of-life analysis, with scores worsening modestly during prolonged treatment duration, but with no significant difference seen between the 2 treatment groups. Sexual dysfunction was slightly more prominent in the raloxifene arm.

In summary, raloxifene is as effective as tamoxifen in reducing the incidence of invasive breast cancer in younger, postmenopausal women at increased risk with a reduced incidence of both endometrial cancers and thromboembolic events.

EFFECT OF CHEMOPREVENTION IN CARRIERS OF PREDISPOSING GENETIC MUTATIONS

Although BRCA1 mutation carriers are more likely to develop estrogen receptor-negative tumors,[63,64] prophylactic oophorectomy reduces the risk of breast cancer by approximately 30% in women who carry mutations in either the BRCA1 or BRCA2 genes.[65]

Tamoxifen protects against contralateral breast cancer for carriers of BRCA1 mutations.[66,67] The greater benefit of tamoxifen in carriers of BRCA1 mutations as compared with carriers of BRCA2 mutations is paradoxical given the greater prevalence of estrogen receptor-positive breast cancer reported among carriers of BRCA2 mutations. Women who used tamoxifen for 2 to 4 years had a 75% lowered risk of contralateral breast cancer. The effectiveness of tamoxifen in preventing second contralateral breast cancers is related to the high concordance of the estrogen receptor status of the first and second cancers.[68] Other data suggest a 50% reduction in the risk of contralateral, second primary breast tumors among BRCA1 mutation carriers who take tamoxifen after a first breast cancer and a 58% reduction of second cancers among BRCA2 mutation carriers.[69] These results imply that, among mutation carriers who develop breast cancer, secondary breast cancers can be prevented using tamoxifen; similar risk reductions are thus likely to be seen for primary breast cancers. However, it remains unclear whether tamoxifen has the greatest efficacy among BRCA1 or BRCA2 carriers.

The only prospective evaluation of the effect of tamoxifen among carriers of predisposing mutations was carried out in the BCPT.[70] To evaluate the effect of tamoxifen on the incidence of breast cancer among women with inherited BRCA1 or BRCA2 mutations, genomic analysis of BRCA1 and BRCA2 was performed for 288 women who developed breast cancer after entry into the trial. Of the 288 breast cancer cases, 19 (6.6%) inherited disease-predisposing BRCA1 or BRCA2 mutations. Tamoxifen reduced breast cancer incidences among healthy BRCA2 carriers by 62%, similar to the reduction in incidence of ER-positive breast cancer among all women in the trial. In contrast, tamoxifen use did not reduce breast cancer incidence among healthy women with inherited BRCA1 mutations. These results must be interpreted with caution, however, given the small number of women with mutations or either BRCA1 or BRCA2 who were identified in the trial. Larger prospective studies of women with predisposing mutations will be required to provide conclusive evidence of either protection or lack of effect by tamoxifen in women with these mutations.

FUTURE STRATEGIES: AROMATASE INHIBITORS

Although raloxifene is an acceptable alternative for many postmenopausal women, raloxifene and tamoxifen are not the ideal drugs to reduce the incidence of primary invasive breast cancer because their safety and efficacy do not reach the desired optimal agent level. Several agents are being evaluated as possibly being more suitable alternatives to tamoxifen for reducing the risk of breast cancer in high-risk women.

In postmenopausal women, the main source of estrogen is derived from the peripheral conversion of androstenedione, produced by the adrenal glands, to estrone and estradiol in breast, muscle, and fat tissue. This conversion requires the aromatase enzyme.[71,72] The selective aromatase inhibitors (AIs) markedly suppress the concentration of estrogen in plasma via inhibition or inactivation of aromatase. The use of AIs is restricted to postmenopausal women, however, because in premenopausal women, high levels of androstenedione compete with AIs at the enzyme complex such that estrogen synthesis is not completely blocked. Moreover, the initial decrease in estrogen levels causes a reflex increase in gonadotrophin levels, provoking ovarian hyperstimulation, thereby increasing aromatase in the ovary and consequently overcoming the initial blockade. Unlike tamoxifen, AIs lack partial estrogen agonist activity, and are therefore not associated with an increased risk for the development of endometrial cancer.

AIs are yet to be approved by the FDA for the chemoprevention of breast cancer, but data from the adjuvant setting have provided the rationale for study of their potential use as chemopreventive agents. Ongoing randomized, placebo-controlled trials investigating the use of third-generation aromatase inhibitors in the chemoprevention of breast cancer in postmenopausal women include the NCIC Clinical Trials Group MAP3 (ExCel) Trial (Exemestane in Preventing Cancer in Postmenopausal Women at Increased Risk of Developing Breast Cancer), and the IBIS-II trial.[71] The North American MAP3 study randomizes patients to exemestane or placebo in patients who refuse treatment with a SERM, and the international IBIS-II trial compares anastrozole for 5 years versus placebo for chemoprevention in patients at increased risk. The P4 trial to compare and contrast raloxifen with the AI letrozole is being conducted by the NSABP, and this data will not be available until 2014. Until the trials are completed, it is not appropriate to use AIs to reduce the risk of breast cancer in postmenopausal women.

SUMMARY

There is no optimal age to begin chemoprevention to reduce breast cancer risk, but chemoprevention with a SERM may be particularly beneficial to women with atypical hyperplasia, a 5-year Gail model risk of more than 5%, LCIS, or 2 or more first-degree relatives with breast cancer. Tamoxifen (20 mg/day) should be offered for breast cancer risk reduction to premenopausal women more than 35 years of age with Gail model risks of breast cancer more than 1.67% in 5 years or LCIS for the reduction of breast cancer risk. Premenopausal women at increased risk derive the greatest net benefit because of the absence of increased risks for either thromboembolic events or uterine cancer in this group. Because the risk of clotting increases with age, careful consideration must be given to risks versus benefits in older postmenopausal women who are considering tamoxifen for risk reduction. The optimum duration of tamoxifen therapy for reducing the risk of breast cancer is unknown. One study's data suggest that the benefit from tamoxifen chemoprevention extends beyond treatment into the posttreatment period.

Polymorphisms in tamoxifen-metabolizing genes affect the plasma concentration of tamoxifen metabolites, but their effect on clinical outcome is being evaluated. In tamoxifen-treated patients with breast cancer, women with the CYP2D6 *4/*4 genotype tend to have a higher risk of disease relapse and a lower incidence of hot flashes, which is consistent with the observation that CYP2D6 is responsible for the metabolic activation of tamoxifen to endoxifen.[73] Whether all women who are candidates for tamoxifen for reducing their risk of breast cancer should be screened for the CYP2D6 *4/*4 genotype has not yet been determined.

Methods to prevent thromboembolism among women receiving SERMs for breast cancer risk reduction may include early ambulation following surgery, discontinuation of tamoxifen in the perioperative setting, and the concurrent use of low-dose aspirin.

Absolute contraindications to tamoxifen use for risk reduction include a history of deep venous thrombosis, pulmonary embolus, concurrent warfarin therapy use, history of cataracts or cataract surgery, current use of HRT, and pregnancy. Women currently taking estrogen, progesterone, androgens, or birth control pills should discontinue these for 30 to 90 days before initiating tamoxifen therapy.

Among women ages 39 to 74 years and at increased risk of breast cancer, fewer than 5% elect to start taking tamoxifen based on some published resports.[74] More than one-third decline immediately, and more than 60% are undecided initially but ultimately decline. Educational sessions do not appear to influence patients decisions. Fear of side effects, including endometrial cancer, thromboembolic events, and menopausal symptoms, are the most commonly cited reason for declining tamoxifen. Therefore, most patients at increased risk for breast cancer may perceive that the risks of taking tamoxifen outweigh the benefits and decline to take it. It is not yet clear whether this is also the case for decisions about raloxifene for breast cancer risk reduction.

Raloxifene 60 mg orally daily for 5 years offers an acceptable alternative to tamoxifen for the reduction of breast cancer risk in high-risk postmenopausal women and is associated with lower associated risks of both benign and malignant uterine events as well as significantly less thromboembolic toxicity.

REFERENCES

1. Wattenberg LW. Chemoprevention of cancer. *Cancer Res.* 1985;45:1-8.
2. Lippman SM, Benner SE, Hong WK. Cancer chemoprevention. *J Clin Oncol.* 1994;12:851-873.
3. O'Shaughnessy JA. Chemoprevention of breast cancer. *JAMA.* 1996;275:1349-1353.
4. Sporn MB, Suh N. Chemoprevention of cancer. *Carcinogenesis.* 2000;21:525-530.
5. Sporn MB, Suh N. Chemoprevention: an essential approach to controlling cancer. *Nat Rev Cancer.* 2002;2:537-543.
6. Feuer EJ, Wun LM, Boring CC, et al. The lifetime risk of developing breast cancer. *J Natl Cancer Inst.* 1993;85:892-897.
7. American Cancer Society. *Cancer Facts and Figures 2009.* Atlanta: American Cancer Society; 2009. http://www.cancer.org/downloads/STT/2009CAFFfinalsecured.pdf.
8. Gail MH, Brinton LA, Byar DP, et al. Projecting individualized probabilities of developing breast cancer for white females who are being examined annually. *J Natl Cancer Inst.* 1989;81:1879-1886.
9. www.cancer.gov/bcrisktool.
10. Vogel VG. Chemoprevention: reducing breast cancer risk. In: Vogel VG, ed. *Management of Patients at High Risk for Breast Cancer.* Malden, MA: Blackwell Science; 2001.
11. Bernstein L. Epidemiology of endocrine-related risk factors for breast cancer. *J Mammary Gland Biol Neoplasia.* 2002;7:3-15.
12. Kelsey JL, Gammon MD, John EM. Reproductive factors and breast cancer. *Epidemiol Rev.* 1993;15:36-47.
13. Kelsey JL, Berkowitz GS. Breast cancer epidemiology. *Cancer Res.* 1988;48:5615.
14. Kelsey JL. A review of the epidemiology of human breast cancer. *Epidemiol Rev.* 1979;1:74-109.
15. Petrakis NL, Ernster VL, King MC. Breast. In: Schottenfeld D, Fraumeni JF Jr., eds. *Cancer Epidemiology and Prevention.* Philadelphia, PA: Saunders; 1982.
16. Henderson BE, Ross RK, Pike MC, Casagrande JT. Endogenous hormones as a major factor in human cancer. *Cancer Res.* 1982;42:3232-3239.
17. Freedman AN, Graubard BI, Rao SR, et al. Estimates of the number of U.S. women who could benefit from tamoxifen for breast cancer chemoprevention. *J Natl Cancer Inst.* 2003;95:526-532.
18. Russo J, Russo IH. Toward a physiological approach to breast cancer prevention. *Cancer Epidemiol Biomarkers Prev.* 1994;3:354-364.
19. Henderson BE, Ross RK, Pike MC. Hormonal chemoprevention of cancer in women. *Science.* 1993;259:633-638.
20. Jordan VC. Effect of tamoxifen (ICI 46,474) on initiation and growth of DMBA-induced rat mammary carcinomata. *Eur J Cancer.* 1976;12:419-424.
21. Jordan VC. Antiestrogenic and antitumor properties of tamoxifen in laboratory animals. *Cancer Treat Rep.* 1976;60:1409-1419.
22. Jordan VC, Murphy CS. Endocrine pharmacology of antiestrogens as antitumor agents. *Endocr Rev.* 1990;11:578-610.
23. Jordan VC. Chemosuppression of breast cancer with long-term tamoxifen therapy. *Prev Med.* 1991;20:3-14.
24. Motomura K, Inaji H, Imaoka S, Koyama H. Down regulation of transforming growth factor-β by tamoxifen in human breast cancer. *Cancer.* 1993;72:131-136.
25. Butta A, MacLennan K, Flanders KC, et al. Induction of transforming growth factor β in human breast cancer in vivo following tamoxifen treatment. *Cancer Res.* 1992;52:4261-4264.
26. Grainger DJ, Metcaffe JC. Tamoxifen: teaching an old drug new tricks? *Nat Med.* 1996;2:381-385.
27. Dickens TA, Colletta AA. The pharmacological manipulation of members of the transforming growth factor beta family in the chemoprevention of breast cancer. *Bioessays.* 1993;15:71-74.
28. Murphy LC, Sutherland RL. Antitumor activity of clomiphene analogs in vitro: relationship to affinity for the estrogen receptor and another high affinity antiestrogen-binding site. *J Clin Endocrinol Metab.* 1983;57: 373-379.
29. Jordan VC, Fritz NF, Tormey DC. Long-term adjuvant therapy with tamoxifen: effects on sex hormone binding globulin and antithrombin III. *Cancer Res.* 1987;47:4517-4519.
30. Berry J, Green BJ, Matheson DS. Modulation of natural killer cell activity by tamoxifen in stage I postmenopausal breast cancer. *Eur J Cancer Clin Oncol.* 1987;23:517-520.
31. Pollak MN, Huynh HT, Lefebre SP. Tamoxifen reduces serum insulin-like growth factor I (IGF-I). *Breast Cancer Res Treat.* 1992;22:91.
32. Friedl A, Jordan VC, Pollack M. Suppression of serum insulin-like growth factor-1 levels in breast cancer patients during adjuvant tamoxifen therapy. *Eur J Cancer.* 1993;29A:1368.
33. Lien EA, Anker G, Ueland PM. Influence of tamoxifen, aminoglutethimide and goserelin on human plasma IGF-I levels in breast cancer patients. *J Steroid Biochem Molec Biol.* 1992;41:533-541.
34. Loning PE, Hall K, Aakvaag A, Lien EA. Influence of tamoxifen on plasma levels of insulin-like growth factor α and insulin-like growth factor binding protein I in breast cancer patients. *Cancer Res.* 1992;52:4719.
35. Vogel VG. Raloxifene: a second-generation selective estrogen receptor modulator for reducing the risk of invasive breast cancer in postmenopausal women. *Women's Health.* 2007;3:139-153.
36. Fisher B, Costantino JP, Wickerham DL, et al. Tamoxifen for prevention of breast cancer: report of the National Surgical Adjuvant Breast and Bowel Project P-1 Study. *J Natl Cancer Inst.* 1998;90:1371-1388.
37. Fisher B, Costantino JP, Wickerham DL, et al. Tamoxifen for the prevention of breast cancer: current status of the National Surgical Adjuvant Breast and Bowel Project P-1 Study. *J Natl Cancer Inst.* 2005;97:1652-1662.
38. Powles T, Eeles R, Ashley S, et al. Interim analysis of the incidence of breast cancer in the Royal Marsden Hospital tamoxifen randomized chemoprevention trial. *Lancet.* 1998;352:98-101.
39. Powles TJ. The Royal Marsden Hospital (RMH) trial: key points and remaining questions. *Ann NY Acad Sci.* 2001;949:109.
40. Powles. TJ. Twenty-year follow-up of the Royal Marsden randomized, double-blinded tamoxifen breast cancer prevention trial. *J Natl Cancer Inst.* 2007;99:283-290.
41. Veronesi U, Ing PM, Sacchini V, Rotmensz N, Boyle P., and the Italian Tamoxifen Study Group. Tamoxifen for breast cancer among hysterectomised women. *Lancet.* 2002;359:1122-1124.
42. Veronesi U, Mariani L, Decensi A, et al. Fifteen-year results of a randomized phase III trial of fenretinide to prevent second breast cancer. *Ann Oncol.* 2006;17:1065-1071.
43. Veronesi U, Maisonneuve P, Rotmensz N, et al. Tamoxifen for the prevention of breast cancer: late results of the Italian randomized tamoxifen prevention trial among women with hysterectomy. *J Natl Cancer Inst.* 2007;99:727-737.
44. IBIS Investigators. First results from the International Breast Cancer Intervention Study (IBIS-I): a randomised prevention trial. *Lancet.* 2002;360:817-824.
45. Cuzick J, Forbes JF, Sestak I, et al. Long-term results of tamoxifen prophylaxis for breast cancer: 96-month follow-up of the randomized IBIS-I trial. *J Natl Cancer Inst.* 2007;99:272-282.
46. Fisher B, Costantino JP, Wickerham DL, et al. Tamoxifen for the prevention of breast cancer: current status of the National Surgical Adjuvant Breast and Bowel Project P-1 Study. *J Natl Cancer Inst.* 2005;97:1652-1662.
47. Love RR, Mazess RB, Barden HS, et al. Effects of tamoxifen on bone mineral density in postmenopausal women with breast cancer. *N Engl J Med.* 1992;326:852-856.
48. Love RR, et al. Effects of tamoxifen on cardiovascular risk factors in postmenopausal women. *Ann Intern Med.* 1991;115:860.
49. Day R, Ganz PA, Costantino JP, et al. Health-related quality of life and tamoxifen in breast cancer prevention: a report from the National Surgical Adjuvant Breast and Bowel Project P-1 Study. *J Clin Oncol.* 1999;17:2659-2669.
50. Powles T, Eeles R, Ashley S, et al. Interim analysis of the incidence of breast cancer in the Royal Marsden Hospital tamoxifen randomized chemoprevention trial. *Lancet.* 1998;352:98-101
51. Day R, Ganz PA, Costantino JP. Tamoxifen and depression: more evidence from the National Surgical Adjuvant Breast and Bowel Project's Breast

Cancer Prevention (P-1) randomized study. *J Natl Cancer Inst.* 2001;93:1615-1623.

52. Cuzick J, Powles T, Veronesi U, et al. Overview of the main outcomes in breast-cancer prevention trials. *Lancet.* 2003;361:296-300.

53. Powles, TJ. Twenty-year follow-up of the Royal Marsden randomized, double-blinded tamoxifen breast cancer prevention trial. *J Natl Cancer Inst.* 2007;99:283-290

54. Gail MH, Costantino JP, Bryant J, et al. Weighing the risks and benefits of tamoxifen treatment for preventing breast cancer. *J Natl Cancer Inst.* 1999;91:29.

55. Tyrer J, Duffy SW, Cuzick J. A breast cancer prediction model incorporating familial and personal risk factors. *Stat Med.* 2004;23:1111-1130.

56. McCaskill-Stevens W, Wilson J, Bryant J, et al. Contralateral breast cancer and thromboembolic events in African American women treated with tamoxifen. *J Natl Cancer Inst.* 2004;96:1762-1769.

57. Cummings SR, Eckert S, Krueger KA, et al. The effect of raloxifene on risk of breast cancer in postmenopausal women: results from the MORE randomized trial. *JAMA.* 1999;281:2189-2197.

58. Cauley JA, Norton L, Lippman ME, et al. Continued breast cancer risk reduction in postmenopausal women treated with raloxifene: 4-year results from the MORE trial. *Breast Cancer Res Treat.* 2001;65:125-134.

59. Martino S, Cauley JA, Barrett-Connor E, et al. Continuing outcomes relevant to Evista: breast cancer incidence in postmenopausal osteoporotic women in a randomized trial of raloxifene. *J Natl Cancer Inst.* 2004;96:1751-1761.

60. Barrett-Connor E, Mosca L, Collins P, et al. Raloxifene Use for the Heart (RUTH) Trial Investigators. Effects of raloxifene on cardiovascular events and breast cancer in postmenopausal women. *N Engl J Med.* 2006;355:125-137.

61. Vogel VG, Costantino JP, Wickerham DL, et al. Effects of tamoxifen vs. raloxifene on the risk of developing invasive breast cancer and other disease outcomes: The NSABP Study of Tamoxifen and Raloxifene (STAR) P-2 Trial. *JAMA.* 2006;295:2727-2741.

62. Land SR, Wickerham DL, Costantino JP, et al. Patient-reported symptoms and quality of life during treatment with tamoxifen or raloxifene for breast cancer prevention: the NSABP Study of Tamoxifen and Raloxifene (STAR) P-2 Trial. *JAMA.* 2006;295:2742-2751.

63. Berry DA, Iversen ES Jr, Gudbjartsson DF, et al. BRCAPRO validation, sensitivity of genetic testing of BRCA1/BRCA2, and prevalence of other breast cancer susceptibility genes. *J Clin Oncol.* Vol. 20; 2002;2701-2712.

64. Karp SE, Tonin PN, Bégin LR, et al. Influence of BRCA1 mutations on nuclear grade and estrogen receptor status of breast carcinoma in Ashkenazi Jewish women. *Cancer.* 1997;80:435-441.

65. Loman N, Johannsson O, Bendahl P, Steroid receptors in hereditary breast carcinomas associated with BRCA1 or BRCA2 mutations or unknown susceptibility genes. *Cancer.* 1998;83:310-319.

66. Rebbeck TR, Levin AM, Eisen A, et al. Reduction in breast cancer risk after bilateral prophylactic oophorectomy in BRCA1 mutation carriers. *J Natl Cancer Inst.* 1999;91:1475-1479.

67. Narod SA, Brunet J-S, Ghadirian P, et al. Tamoxifen and risk of contralateral breast cancer in BRCA1 and BRCA2 mutation carriers: a case-control study—Hereditary Breast Cancer Clinical Study Group. *Lancet.* 2000;356:1876-1881.

68. Narod SA. Modifiers of risk of hereditary breast cancer. *Oncogene.* 2006;25:5832-5836.

69. Weitzel JN, Robson M, Pasini B, et al. A comparison of bilateral breast cancers in BRCA carriers. *Cancer Epidemiol Biomarkers Prev.* 2005;14:1534-1538.

70. Gronwald J, Tung N, Foulkes WD, et al. Hereditary Breast Cancer Clinical Study Group. Tamoxifen and contralateral breast cancer in BRCA1 and BRCA2 carriers: an update. *Int J Cancer.* 2006;118:2281-2284.

71. Geller BA, Vogel VG. Chemoprevention of breast cancer in postmenopausal women. *Breast Dis.* 2005-2006;24:79-92.

72. Zanardi S, Serrano D, Argusti A, et al. Clinical trials with retinoids for breast cancer chemoprevention. *Endocr Relat Cancer.* 2006;13:51-68.

73. Goetz MP, Rae JM, Suman VJ, et al. Pharmacogenetics of tamoxifen biotransformation is associated with clinical outcomes of efficacy and hot flashes. *J Clin Oncol.* 2005;23:9312-9318.

74. Port ER, Montgomery LL, Heerdt AS, Borgen PI. Patient reluctance toward tamoxifen use for breast cancer primary prevention. *Ann Surg Oncol.* 2001;8:580-585.

CHAPTER 11

Prophylactic Mastectomy

Judy C. Boughey
Amy C. Degnim

Patients at increased risk of breast cancer have a range of treatment options available to decrease their risk of breast cancer development. The absolute risk reduction by any of these strategies is dependent on the individual woman's actual risk of breast cancer development. Statistical models for risk stratification, as well as the availability of genetic testing, enable women and their physicians to evaluate the risk of breast cancer. A number of risk-reducing treatment options exist for these women, and they vary in efficacy. Options include frequent surveillance with clinical examination and imaging, chemoprevention, prophylactic salpingo-oophorectomy (PSO), and prophylactic mastectomy (PM). The individuals most likely to benefit from bilateral PM are those with the highest risk—BRCA carriers and those with a strong family history of breast cancer. Women with a personal history of breast cancer are also at higher risk for a second primary breast cancer in the contralateral breast and may choose to pursue contralateral prophylactic mastectomy (CPM) to decrease this risk as well as for cosmetic and psychological reasons. As a preventive measure PM remains controversial. There are no randomized controlled trials (and likely will not be in the future) to substantiate the potential benefit or harm associated with PM. Since PM is an irreversible procedure, providers and patients must understand its consequences, benefits, limitations, and available alternatives. This chapter discusses which patients may consider prophylactic surgery and summarizes data on the efficacy of PM for the prevention of breast cancer and its effect on survival.

CANCER RISK ASSESSMENT AND PATIENT SELECTION

No Prior History of Breast Cancer

The absolute risk reduction afforded by PM is greatest in the women at highest risk of breast cancer development. The average lifetime risk of breast cancer for women in the United States is 12.7% with a lifespan of 85 years. This risk is greatest after the sixth decade of life.[1] Most women, however, tend to overestimate their risk of breast cancer.[2] It is important that women have realistic risk estimates in order to help them make informed decisions regarding risk reduction. For women without a personal or family history of breast cancer, the Gail model is the most commonly used tool to predict risk of breast cancer in women, and is viewed 20,000 to 30,000 times per month.[3] The Gail model is accurate for predicting breast cancer incidence in populations of women; however, its major limitation in terms of clinical use is its poor accuracy when used for risk prediction in individuals.[4] Also, the Gail model does not apply to women with a history of lobular carcinoma in situ (LCIS) or ductal carcinoma in situ (DCIS) and has been shown to underpredict risk for women with atypical hyperplasia.[5]

Factors associated with a generalized increased risk of breast cancer above the population average include LCIS, atypical hyperplasia, and increased breast density. Atypical ductal or lobular hyperplasia found at breast biopsy (preferably confirmed by a breast pathologist) is associated with a 4-fold increased relative risk compared to the general population,[6] with increasing foci of atypia correlating with greater risk.[7] Increasing mammographic breast density is associated with increasing risk of breast cancer[8] as well as identification of interval cancers.[9] Thus the occasional woman with combined features of very dense breast tissue, high-risk histology, and multiple prior biopsies may request PM due to concerns about inadequate detection with the use of standard imaging modalities.

Family History of Breast Cancer

Individuals with deleterious mutations of BRCA1 or BRCA2 genes are a special subset of women with highly elevated risks

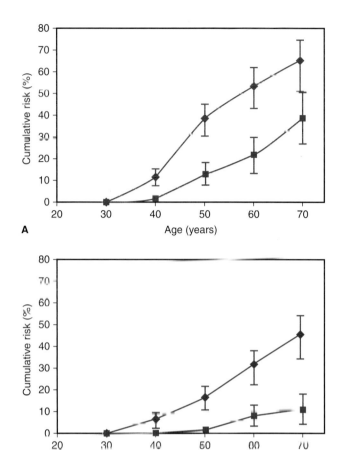

FIGURE 11-1 Cumulative risk of breast (◆) and ovarian (■) cancer in **(A)** BRCA1 mutation carriers and **(B)** BRCA2 mutation carriers. (*From Antoniou A, Pharoah PD, Narod S, et al. Average risk of breast and ovarian cancer associated with BRCA1 or BRCA2 mutations detected in case series unselected for family history: a combined analysis of 22 studies. Am J Hum Genet. 2003;72:1117-1130, with permission.*)

of breast cancer development. The average cumulative risk of breast cancer in BRCA1 and BRCA2 mutation carriers by age 70 years is 65% and 45%, respectively (Fig. 11-1).[10] These individuals are also at a higher risk of ovarian cancer, with lifetime risks of 40% and 20%, respectively, for BRCA1 and BRCA2 carriers. Some women with a strong family history may choose not to undergo BRCA testing. Additionally, some women with a strong family history may test negative for deleterious mutations, or a variant of unknown significance may be found. Claus tables can be used to provide estimates of breast cancer risk for individuals with a strong family history.[11] A negative test for a BRCA mutation is only reassuring in the presence of a positive test within the family; otherwise the possibility of an unidentified mutation remains and the risk is still dependent on the family history.

Personal History of Breast Cancer

A personal history of breast cancer is a long-established risk factor for development of a new primary breast cancer,[12] logical since the remainder of that breast and the contralateral breast have been exposed to the same genetic, environmental, and hormonal factors that led to the first breast cancer. Women with stage I and II breast cancer have a contralateral breast cancer risk of approximately 1% per year, with a cumulative risk of 17% at 20 years after first breast cancer diagnosis.[13,14] The risk of a second breast cancer is much higher in women with a strong family history of breast cancer—up to 35% by 16 years after the initial diagnosis of breast cancer.[15] The presence of a BRCA1 and BRCA2 mutation elevates the risk of contralateral breast cancer even higher, to 12% to 31% at 5 years after the primary cancer diagnosis.[16-18] In a longer-term study of BRCA carriers who underwent breast conservation, the risk of contralateral breast cancer was 39% at 15 years.[19]

Other Factors Predicting for Contralateral Breast Cancer Development

In addition to family history,[13,20] other factors associated with an increased risk of contralateral breast cancer include multicentric primary breast cancer,[21] history of radiation therapy for the first breast cancer,[22] lobular neoplasia,[23,24] and additional ipsilateral high-risk pathology.[25] Patients newly diagnosed with breast cancer who present with these features are at higher risk for developing cancer in the contralateral breast, and CPM is more justifiable in these patients. The relationship of age at diagnosis and risk of contralateral breast cancer is unclear, with two studies demonstrating increased risk in young women[23,26] and one study demonstrating the opposite.[25]

EFFICACY OF PROPHYLACTIC MASTECTOMY

The women who elect bilateral prophylactic mastectomy (BPM) and those who choose to undergo contralateral prophylactic mastectomy (CPM) are different in their characteristics, history of breast cancer, and goals for risk-reduction surgery. These scenarios will be discussed separately.

Bilateral Prophylactic Mastectomy

Impact of BPM on Breast Cancer Incidence

BRCA Mutation Carriers. Several studies confirm that BPM reduces the incidence of breast cancer in BRCA carriers. Meijers-Heijboer and associates[27] conducted a prospective study of 139 BRCA1 or BRCA2 mutation carriers. No breast cancers developed in the 76 women who underwent BPM compared to 8 breast cancers in the 63 women who pursued close surveillance with a mean follow-up of 3.0 years (*p* = 0.003). However, the risk-reduction effect of BPM could not be isolated from the effect of PSO, which also reduces breast cancer risk (see "Risk-Reduction Alternatives to PM" later in the chapter), since premenopausal PSO was more common in the BPM group (58%) compared to the surveillance group (38%).

Similarly, Hartmann and associates at the Mayo Clinic reported on 26 women with BRCA mutations who underwent BPM. At a median follow-up of 13.4 years no breast cancers developed.[28] The relative risk reduction attributed to BPM was estimated as 85% to 100% using various statistical models. In the more recent PROSE study of Rebbeck and colleagues, 105 BRCA carriers who underwent BPM were followed prospectively and compared to 378 matched BRCA controls without BPM.[29] Breast cancer developed in 2 women who underwent BPM (1.9%) compared to 184 breast cancers (48.7%) in the group who did not undergo BPM, with mean follow-up of 6.4 years. In this study, cases and controls were matched based on PSO. The relative risk reduction for breast cancer was 95% in women with PSO and 90% in those with intact ovaries. Taken together, these studies confirm a 90% to 95% relative risk reduction in breast cancer after BPM in BRCA carriers.

Non-BRCA Mutation Carriers. Some women without a known BRCA mutation, but who have other risk factors, consider BPM. For these women there are several studies providing evidence on the efficacy of BPM for high-risk women regardless of BRCA status. Hartmann and coworkers reported on a cohort of 639 high-risk women (based on a positive family history of breast cancer) who underwent bilateral subcutaneous mastectomy from 1960 to 1993 (90% with preservation of the nipple–areolar complex, 10% with removal of the nipple–areolar complex).[30] This cohort was divided into high- and moderate-risk groups based on the strength of family history. A control group of the patients' female siblings who did not undergo BPM was also followed.[30] Breast cancer incidence was reduced 90% to 94% in the high-risk group and 90% in the moderate-risk group at a median follow-up of 14 years. Breast cancer incidence was not significantly different between those women with preservation of the nipple–areolar complex and those where it was removed.

Geiger and associates evaluated the efficacy of BPM in community practices.[31] In this retrospective population-based study, BPM was found to reduce the risk of breast cancer by 95%. However, the absolute risk of breast cancer in the whole population was low, with 0.4% incidence in the BPM group compared to 4% in the control group. Borgen and colleagues also reported effective risk reduction from BPM, with less than 1% incidence of breast cancer at 14.8 years mean follow-up in 370 women who underwent BPM.[32]

Caveats. Although BPM does provide a dramatic decrease in breast cancer incidence, it is important that physicians and patients realize that breast cancers can still develop despite risk-reduction surgery. There are multiple case reports of breast cancer after BPM, with intervals from risk-reduction surgery to the diagnosis of breast cancer ranging from 3 to 42 years.[33-38] When counseling women regarding PM, the persistent long-term possibility of developing breast cancer should be discussed.

Impact of BPM on Survival

There are no data confirming an overall survival benefit in patients undergoing BPM for cancer prevention compared to similar-risk individuals who do not. While the studies on BPM in BRCA carriers clearly show reductions in breast cancer occurrence, there is no prospective clinical evidence yet that confirms a statistically significant overall survival advantage

attributable to this procedure. Among women with a family history but unknown BRCA status, the study of Hartmann and colleagues demonstrated reductions in disease-specific mortality after BPM, with an 81% to 94% reduction in mortality from breast cancer for the high-risk group and 100% reduction in breast cancer mortality for the moderate-risk group.[30]

It would be expected that successful prevention of breast cancer would translate into a survival benefit, especially for patients at a high lifetime risk of breast cancer. However, with improvements in detection and treatment of breast cancer it becomes questionable whether breast cancer prevention actually translates into improved survival. Schrag and colleagues used theoretical modeling to estimate survival gains from risk-reduction surgery for BRCA mutation carriers.[39] They calculated that on average a 30-year-old BRCA1 or BRCA2 mutation carrier would gain 2.9 to 5.3 years of life expectancy from PM and from 0.3 to 1.7 years from PSO. Another similar analysis also reported survival gains of 3.5 years for PM and 4.9 years with both BPM and PSO.[40] In both studies, gains in life expectancy declined with age and were minimal for women over 60 years of age (Fig. 11-2). The preponderance of evidence from the prospective clinical cohorts and theoretical modeling described suggest that in BRCA carriers, BPM reduces the incidence of breast cancer and in younger women likely improves longevity.

Surgical Morbidity of BPM

Surgical complication rates after BPM range from 30% to 64% and complications are more common after immediate reconstruction.[41-43] The most common complications are pain (35%), infection (17%), and seroma formation (17%).[43] Unanticipated reoperations after BPM with immediate reconstruction are common. In one report,[44] second operations were required in

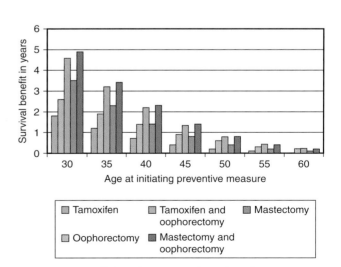

FIGURE 11-2 Effects of timing on benefits of preventive measures upon survival. *(From Grann VR, Jacobson JS, Thomason D, et al. Effect of prevention strategies on survival and quality-adjusted survival of women with BRCA1/2 mutations: an updated decision analysis. J Clin Oncol. 2002;20:2520-2529, with permission.)*

49% of patients for the following reasons: implant-related issues (46%), implant removal (37%), aesthetic concerns (32%), and immediate postoperative complications (22%).

Quality of Life after BPM

Psychosocial outcomes such as satisfaction with the decision, cosmesis, psychological well-being, and issues concerning body image and sexuality have been evaluated in patients choosing BPM. In one study, approximately 5% of women report they were dissatisfied with their decision to undergo BPM,[32] and this was more common among women reporting physician's advice as the primary reason for BPM.[32,45] Another survey study of 106 women after BPM and 62 high-risk women without BPM showed that 84% of patients choosing BPM were satisfied with their decision, and the quality of life was not different between the 2 groups.[46] Dissatisfaction with cosmetic outcomes has been reported in 16% to 40% of patients, mostly pertaining to dissatisfaction with reconstruction,[32,45,47,48] but in one study was also related to a perceived lack of information on expected outcomes.[48] Cancer-related anxiety, body image concerns, and sexuality are all associated with satisfaction or regret regarding the surgery itself.[32,45,49] On the other hand, women who forego reconstruction following BPM have high levels of satisfaction.[45] Overall, the quality of life among women undergoing BPM appears slightly better than the general population based on Quality of Life Index (QLI) scores.[50] These unexpected results likely reflect the characteristics of women who choose to undergo this preventive surgery rather than an effect of the surgical procedure. Another study affirms that survey studies of satisfaction after PM need to include open-ended questions, because closed-ended question surveys may overestimate satisfaction.[51]

■ Contralateral Prophylactic Mastectomy

Impact of CPM on Breast Cancer Incidence

Women presenting with an index breast cancer in one breast are at an increased risk of contralateral breast cancer. Similar to BPM, studies have shown a decrease in the incidence of breast cancer after CPM, both in BRCA carriers and non-BRCA carriers.

BRCA Mutations Carriers. Van Sprundel and associates reported on 148 BRCA1/2 carriers treated for unilateral invasive breast cancer stages I to IIIA.[52] Seventy-nine women underwent CPM and 69 women underwent surveillance. One contralateral breast cancer occurred in the CPM group compared to 6 in the surveillance group (*p* < 0.001). This 91% risk reduction in contralateral breast cancer was independent of PSO.

Non-BRCA Mutation Carriers. Several additional studies have evaluated breast cancer incidence after CPM in high-risk women without known BRCA mutations. McDonnell and coworkers reported a 94% to 96% risk reduction from CPM in 745 women with a first breast cancer and family history of breast or ovarian cancer after a median follow-up of 10 years compared to expected.[53] In a case-control study, CPM decreased the rate of contralateral breast cancer over 15 years follow-up,

with a rate of 4.5% in the 64 women who chose CPM compared to 27% in the 182 controls (*p* < 0.005).[54] Additionally, a retrospective cohort study of 1072 women who underwent CPM compared with 317 controls demonstrated a hazard ratio of 0.03 for contralateral breast cancer in women who underwent CPM.[55] Similar to the data in BPM, the results described here strongly support a dramatic risk reduction in contralateral breast cancer after CPM.

Impact of CPM on Survival

Although a clearly documented reduction in breast cancer occurrences is seen after CPM, data showing an overall survival advantage for CPM remain elusive, as in the setting of BPM. For patients with a primary breast cancer, the risk of death is generally higher from the primary than from a second cancer.[13,14] This is due to close surveillance resulting in a second cancer usually being detected at an early stage. However, a recent report found that 30% of contralateral breast cancers are node positive when detected despite close follow-up.[54] In the study by van Sprundel and associates of BRCA1 and BRCA2 carriers, CPM had no significant effect on overall survival by multivariate analysis adjusting for oophorectomy.[52] Another outcome study of an expanded group of the BRCA1 patients with breast cancer also did not demonstrate a survival benefit for CPM.[56]

Since the risk of contralateral breast cancer is very high in BRCA patients, it would be expected that the survival advantage of CPM should be the greatest in these patients. It is therefore somewhat surprising that the 2 studies not limited to BRCA carriers have shown survival advantages for CPM when data from BRCA carriers have not shown a survival benefit.[54,55] CPM resulted in a statistically significant improvement in disease-free survival in the case-control study of Peralta and associates.[54] Overall survival favored the CPM group, but was not statistically significant.[54] Disease-specific survival stratified by stage showed that survival was improved for early-stage (0-II) patients but did not quite meet statistical significance (*p* = 0.06). Herrinton and associates also reported statistically significant improvements in disease-specific survival and overall survival in women who underwent CPM compared to those who did not.[55]

Similarly, the data for survival benefit for patients with invasive lobular cancers undergoing CPM are mixed. In a retrospectively studied cohort from the Mayo Clinic of 419 women with invasive lobular cancer, patients with unilateral ILC who underwent CPM had a better prognosis than those with unilateral mastectomy at a mean follow-up of 6 years,[57] but this association may just reflect selection bias of patients with better prognosis for a contralateral risk-reducing procedure. In a study by Babiera and colleagues, no overall survival advantage was seen at 5 years follow-up for patients with invasive lobular cancer who underwent CPM.[58]

Discerning whether the reported survival benefits are due to CPM is complex, due to the adjuvant treatments and other prognostic factors that would be expected to impact survival. Additionally, since these studies are all retrospective, they are subject to selection bias.[59] Only 1 study by Peralta and associates controlled for prognostic factors.[54] They found CPM to be associated with improved disease-specific survival in lower-stage patients. Since prognosis is primarily determined by stage of the index tumor,[18,23] patients with better prognosis and a high risk of a second cancer are likely to benefit the most from CPM. Similar to BPM, decreasing the incidence of contralateral cancer by CPM does not necessarily translate into a survival advantage. A patient's prognosis based on the index tumor should be assessed and included in risk-benefit analysis when considering CPM.

Surgical Morbidity and Quality of Life after CPM

Surgical morbidity of CPM has not been specifically addressed in studies. When complications occur related to the CPM, such as infection and impaired wound healing, they have the potential to delay adjuvant therapy (in particular chemotherapy) for the index tumor, and this is a potential disadvantage to CPM at the time of therapeutic mastectomy. The level of satisfaction reported with the decision and cosmetic outcome post CPM have been high, ranging from 83% to 94%.[60-62] Lower satisfaction with CPM was associated with decreased satisfaction with appearance, complications with reconstruction, and increased level of stress in life.[62] A survey questionnaire reporting on quality of life found a high level of contentment with quality of life in 76% of patients. Less contentment with quality of life in this study was not associated with CPM but rather was related to physical and mental health in general and concerns regarding physical appearance.[61]

One cosmetic advantage of CPM is improved symmetry with bilateral reconstruction compared to unilateral mastectomy. Additionally, once a patient undergoes transabdominal myocutaneous (TRAM) flap for unilateral reconstruction, reconstruction options for the contralateral side at a later date are limited to other sources of autologous tissue transfer and implant-based reconstruction.

TRENDS IN PROPHYLACTIC MASTECTOMY USE

Recent data indicate that PM is being performed more frequently in recent years. An investigation of the SEER database showed that among patients undergoing mastectomy for breast cancer, the CPM rate increased significantly from 4.2% in 1998 to 11.0% in 2003.[63] A worldwide study of BRCA carriers reported that among women diagnosed with breast cancer, 27% underwent CPM. This was most common among women who chose mastectomy to treat the index cancer, and significant variation in CPM frequency was seen based upon country of residence.[64] In a survey of 2677 BRCA carriers around the world, 57% underwent bilateral prophylactic oophorectomy (BPO) and 18% had BPM, and there was wide variation in rates of preventive surgery based upon country of residence.[65]

RISK-REDUCTION ALTERNATIVES TO PM

Many high-risk women do not wish to pursue PM; only a portion of BRCA mutation carriers express interest in mastectomy for risk reduction.[66] Knowledge of all risk-reduction options is important for patients to make an informed decision, both for those considering PM and those who are not. Chemoprevention and prophylactic oophorectomy are the 2 other main breast cancer risk-reduction treatments. The NSABP P-1 study evaluated

tamoxifen for the prevention of breast cancer. In a subset analysis of NSABP P-1,[67] 288 patients who developed breast cancer were tested for BRCA mutations and 19 BRCA mutation carriers were identified. In this very small sample, it appeared that tamoxifen reduced breast cancer risk in BRCA2 carriers by 62% but not in BRCA1 carriers. This finding might be expected, since most BRCA1 tumors are estrogen–receptor negative and tamoxifen is known to decrease the incidence of estrogen–receptor positive breast cancer.[68,69]

Narod and associates reported an approximate 50% reduction in contralateral breast cancer rates associated with tamoxifen use in BRCA1/BRCA2 carriers treated prior to routine hormone receptor testing.[70] Oophorectomy also reduced contralateral breast cancer risk in this study by approximately 60%. In an update on an expanded cohort, contralateral breast cancer was reduced by more than 50% in both BRCA1 and BRCA2 carriers with tamoxifen use.[71] This finding of a significant risk reduction in the BRCA1 patients, who generally have predominantly estrogen–receptor negative tumors, is important, as physicians' recommendations about tamoxifen use in mutation carriers is highly dependent on estrogen receptor (ER) status.[72] These data suggest that tamoxifen may be effective in preventing both ER-positive and ER-negative second primary cancers in BRCA carriers.

Bilateral oophorectomy is another surgical procedure for risk reduction that significantly reduces breast cancer risk. For BRCA mutation carriers it has a dual benefit in decreasing the risk of breast cancer as well as ovarian cancer. In a prospective cohort of 170 BRCA mutation carriers, patients who underwent PSO had a lower incidence of breast cancer (4.3%) at 2 years follow-up, compared to 12.9% in women followed with close surveillance.[73] In another study with a larger sample and follow-up of 8.8 years, Rebbeck and associates reported on breast cancer rates in 99 women who had undergone PSO compared to 142 matched controls without PSO.[74] Breast cancer incidence for BRCA patients was significantly lower for women treated with PSO (21%) versus surveillance (42%). In an expanded report from the same group, an approximate 50% risk reduction for breast cancer was seen in both BRCA1 and BRCA2 subgroups, with the greatest benefit when PSO was performed before age 40.[75] Outcome modeling for BRCA carriers evaluating tamoxifen, oophorectomy, and mastectomy show that tamoxifen with oophorectomy yields almost the same survival gain as mastectomy with oophorectomy (Fig. 11-2).[40] Overall, the reductions in breast cancer risk from chemoprevention or PSO alone are not quite as high as those resulting from PM; however, they provide significant risk reductions without the body image changes of BPM and may be preferred by some women.

SURGICAL TECHNIQUE AND USE OF SENTINEL LYMPH NODE BIOPSY

Historically, total mastectomy has been considered the preferred standard surgical procedure for prophylaxis, due to the removal of the nipple–areolar complex (NAC) and its associated ductal tissue at risk for cancer development. Although subcutaneous mastectomy has been performed for surgical risk reduction, it has been criticized because of increased likelihood of retained breast tissue under the skin flaps and within the

NAC. More recent publications on skin-sparing mastectomy (SSM) in breast cancer patients report its oncologic safety and superior aesthetic results (see Chapter 66).[76,77] It is logical to extrapolate the data from these studies to the scenario of surgical prophylaxis. In addition to SSM, NAC-sparing mastectomy (NSM) techniques are also described and currently offered in highly selected patients (see Chapter on 67).[78] The current techniques of SSM and NSM are different from the historical subcutaneous mastectomy. As SSM and NSM are currently performed, the skin flaps are thinner than the subcutaneous mastectomy of the past, therefore leaving less residual breast tissue. Furthermore, in NSM, the core of ductal tissue within the nipple is excised and evaluated as a separate specimen, making it a reasonably safe option for patients undergoing PM.[79]

The possibility of finding an occult breast cancer during PM is approximately 5%,[18,23,80-82] and the risk of invasive cancer is even lower at 2% to 3%. Since the complications associated with sentinel lymph node (SLN) biopsy are 7% to 8%, the routine use of SLN biopsy in this setting is not recommended. A decision analysis model looking at the complications associated with SLN biopsy and the incidence of invasive breast cancer in PM found that routine SLN biopsy is not warranted given the large number of procedures required to benefit one patient and the potential complications associated with performing SLN in all patients.[83] However, patients older than 60 years of age, and those with invasive lobular cancer or LCIS, are at higher risk for invasive cancer at the time of PM and should be considered for SLN biopsy.[84] With increasing use of MRI the finding of an occult malignancy at the time of PM is likely to decrease further, although a study evaluating this question revealed that MRI is not cost-effective or beneficial in directing use of SLN surgery at time of PM.[85]

FUTURE DIRECTIONS

A novel nonsurgical approach to reducing breast cancer risk is linked to the protective effect of full-term pregnancy at younger ages.[86] Russo and colleagues have shown that treatment of young virgin rats with human chorionic gonadotrophin (hCG), like full-term pregnancy, induces permanent differentiation of the terminal ductal-lobular units (TDLUs), reduces proliferative activity of the mammary epithelium, induces the synthesis of inhibin (a protein with tumor-suppressor activity), and increases the expression of genes associated with programmed cell death.[87] They also observed that these genes remained activated even after the cessation of hCG administration, suggesting long-lasting genome imprinting by hCG-induced changes.[87] In theory, hCG treatment of high-risk women at young ages may reduce the long-term risk of breast cancer. Ongoing research into the biology of premalignant change will also hold promise for other novel risk-reduction strategies.

SUMMARY

Prophylactic mastectomy reduces the incidence of breast cancer, with a 90% to 95% risk reduction. However, data on survival are not proven convincingly. Undoubtedly some individuals will benefit from preventing the development of breast cancer, but the challenge remains to accurately identify them. Ironically, PM is a preventive procedure that involves more radical surgery than the surgical therapy for the majority of women with breast cancer who are eligible for breast conservation. The Society of Surgical Oncology has proposed guidelines for considering PM, but there are no absolute indications for this procedure.[88] Ideally the patient should initiate the discussion regarding PM, as this correlates with long-term satisfaction.[89] PM should only be undertaken after careful consideration and after a discussion of realistic breast cancer risk estimates in absolute terms as well as consideration of the patient's life expectancy from other causes. For women with a diagnosis of breast cancer, prognosis of the primary tumor and risk factors for contralateral breast cancer should be considerations in the risk/benefit discussion. Consultation with genetic and/or psychiatric counselors may be beneficial to assist in the decision-making process. Especially in women without a known breast cancer, the expected outcomes of surgery should be discussed in detail. For all patients considering PM, the alternative of close surveillance, as well as the risk reduction associated with chemoprevention and prophylactic oophorectomy, should be discussed, as well as any ongoing prevention trials.

REFERENCES

1. Feuer EJ, Wun LM, Boring CC, et al. The lifetime risk of developing breast cancer. *J Natl Cancer Inst.* 1993;85(11):892-897.
2. Alexander NE, Ross J, Sumner W, et al. The effect of an educational intervention on the perceived risk of breast cancer. *J Gen Intern Med.* 1996;11(2):92-97.
3. Elmore JG, Fletcher SW. The risk of cancer risk prediction: "What is my risk of getting breast cancer?" *J Natl Cancer Inst.* 2006;98:1673-1675.
4. Rockhill B, Spiegelman D, Byrne C, et al. Validation of the Gail et al. model of breast cancer risk prediction and implications for chemoprevention. *J Natl Cancer Inst.* 2001; 93(5):358-366.
5. Pankratz VS, Hartmann LC, Degnim AC, et al. Assessment of the accuracy of the Gail model in women with atypical hyperplasia. *J Clin Oncol.* 2008;26:5374-5379.
6. Hartmann LC, Sellers TA, Frost MH, et al. Benign breast disease and the risk of breast cancer. *N Engl J Med.* 2005;353:229-237.
7. Degnim AC, Visscher DW, Berman HK, et al. Stratification of breast cancer risk in women with atypia: a Mayo cohort study. *J Clin Oncol.* 2007;25(19):2671-2677.
8. Kerlikowske K, Shepherd J, Creasman J, et al. Are breast density and bone mineral density independent risk factors for breast cancer? *J Natl Cancer Inst.* 2005;97(5):368-374.
9. Mandelson MT, Oestreicher N, Porter PL, et al. Breast density as a predictor of mammographic detection: comparison of interval- and screen-detected cancers. *J Natl Cancer Inst.* 2000;92(13):1081-1087.
10. Atoniou A, Pharoah PD, Narod S, et al. Average risk of breast and ovarian cancer associated with BRCA1 and BRCA2 mutations detected in case series unselected for family history: a combined analysis of 22 studies. *Am J Hum Genet.* 2003;72(5):1117-1130.
11. Claus EB, Risch N, Thompson WD. Autosomal dominant inheritance of early-onset breast cancer: implications for risk prediction. *Cancer.* 1994;73(3):643-651.
12. Foote FW, Stewart FW. Comparative studies of cancerous versus noncancerous breast, I and II. *Ann Surg.* 1945;131:197-222.
13. Rosen PP, Groshen S, Kinne DW, Hellman S. Contralateral breast carcinoma: an assessment of risk and prognosis in stage I (T1N0M0) and stage II (T1N1M0) patients with 20-year follow-up. *Surgery.* 1989;196(5):904-910.
14. Rosen PP, Groshen S, Kinne DW. Prognosis in T2N0M0 stage I breast carcinoma: a 20-year follow-up study. *J Clin Oncol.* 1991;9(9):1650-1661.
15. Harris RE, Lynch HT, Guirgis HA. Familial breast cancer: risk to the contralateral breast. *J Natl Cancer Inst.* 1978;60(5):955-960.

16. Verhoog LC, Brekelmans CT, Seynaeve C, et al. Survival and tumour characteristics of breast cancer patients with germline mutations of BRCA1. *Lancet*. 1998;351(9099):316-321.

17. Verhoog LC, Brekelmans CT, Seynaeve C, et al. Survival in hereditary breast cancer associated with germline mutations of BRCA2. *J Clin Oncol*. 1999;17(11):3396-3402.

18. Robson M, Gilewski T, Haas B, et al. BRCA-associated breast cancer in young women. *J Clin Oncol*. 1998;16(5):1642-1649.

19. Pierce LJ, Levin AM, Rebbeck TR, et al. Ten-year multi-institutional results of breast conserving surgery and radiotherapy in BRCA1/2-associated stage I/II breast cancer. *J Clin Oncol*. 2006;24:2437-2443.

20. Anderson DE, Badzioch MD. Bilaterality in familial breast cancer patients. *Cancer*. 1985;56:2092-2098.

21. Lesser ML, Rosen PP, Kinne DW. Multicentricity and bilaterality in invasive breast carcinoma. *Surgery*. 1982;91(2):234-240.

22. Storm HH, Jensen OM. Risk of contralateral breast cancer in Denmark, 1943-80. *Br J Cancer*. 1986;54(3):483-492.

23. Healey EA, Cook EF, Oray EJ, et al. Contralateral breast cancer: clinical characteristics and impact on prognosis. *J Clin Oncol*. 1993;11(8):1545-1552.

24. Broet P, de la Rochefordiere A, Scholl SM, et al. Contralateral breast cancer: annual incidence and risk parameters. *J Clin Oncol*. 1995;13(7):1578-1583.

25. Goldflam K, Hunt KK, Gershenwald JE, et al. Contralateral prophylactic mastectomy. Predictors of significant histologic findings. *Cancer*. 2004; 101(9):1977-1986.

26. Robinson E, Rennert G, Rennert HS, Neugut AI. Survival of first and second primary breast cancer. *Cancer*. 1993;71(1):172-176.

27. Meijers-Heijboer H, van Geel B, van Putten WL, et al. Breast cancer after prophylactic bilateral mastectomy in women with a BRCA1 or BRCA 2 mutation. *N Engl J Med*. 2001;345(3):159-164.

28. Hartmann LC, Sellers TA, Schaid DJ, et al. Efficacy of bilateral prophylactic mastectomy in BRCA1 and BRCA2 gene mutation carriers. *J Natl Cancer Inst*. 2001;93(21):1633-1637.

29. Rebbeck TR, Friebel T, Lynch HT, et al. Bilateral prophylactic mastectomy reduces breast cancer risk in BRCA1 and BRCA2 mutation carriers: the PROSE study group. *J Clin Oncol*. 2004;22(6):1055-1062.

30. Hartmann LC, Schaid DJ, Woods JE, et al. Efficacy of bilateral prophylactic mastectomy in women with a family history of breast cancer. *N Engl J Med*. 1999;340(2):77-84.

31. Geiger AM, Yu O, Herrinton LJ, Barlow WE, et al. A population-based study of bilateral prophylactic mastectomy efficacy in women at elevated risk for breast cancer in community practices. *Arch Intern Med*. 2005;165(5):516-520.

32. Borgen PI, Hill AD, Tran KN, et al. Patient regrets after bilateral prophylactic mastectomy. *Ann Surg Oncol*. 1998;5(7):603-606.

33. Eldar S, Meguid MM, Beatty JD. Cancer of the breast after prophylactic subcutaneous mastectomy. *Am J Surg*. 1984;148:692-693.

34. Goodnight JE, Quagliana JM, Morton DL. Failure of subcutaneous mastectomy to prevent the development of breast cancer. *J Surg Oncol*. 1984;26:198-201.

35. Holleb A, Montgomery R, Farrow JH. The hazard of incomplete simple mastectomy. *Surg Gynecol Obstet*. 1965;121:819.

36. Jameson MB, Roberts E, Nixon J, et al. Metastatic breast cancer 42 years after bilateral subcutaneous mastectomies. *Clin Oncol (R Coll Radiol)*. 1997;9:119-121.

37. Willemsen HW, Kaas R, Peterse JH, Rutgers EJ. Breast carcinoma in residual breast tissue after prophylactic bilateral subcutaneous mastectomy. *Eur J Surg Oncol*. 1998;24:331-338.

38. Ziegler LD, Kroll SS. Primary breast cancer after prophylactic mastectomy. *Am J Clin Oncol*. 1991;14:451-454.

39. Schrag D, Kuntz KM, Garber JE, Weeks JC. Decision analysis—effects of prophylactic mastectomy and oophorectomy on life expectancy among women with BRCA1 or BRCA2 mutations. *N Engl J Med*. 1997;336(20):1465-1471.

40. Grann VR, Jacobson JS, Thomason D, et al. Effect of prevention strategies on survival and quality-adjusted survival of women with BRCA1/2 mutations: an updated decision analysis. *J Clin Oncol*. 2002;20(10):2520-2529.

41. Gabriel S, Woods J, O'Fallono M, et al. Complications leading to surgery after breast implantation. *N Engl J Med*. 1997;336(10):677-682.

42. Contant CM, Menke-Pluijmers MB, Seynaeve C, et al. Clinical experience of prophylactic mastectomy followed by immediate breast reconstruction in women at hereditary risk of breast cancer (HB(O)C) or a proven BRCA1 and BRCA2 germ-line mutation. *Eur J Surg Oncol*. 2002;28(6):627-632.

43. Barton MB, West CN, Liu I-LA, et al. Complications following bilateral prophylactic mastectomy. *J Natl Cancer Inst Monogr*. 2005;35:61-6.

44. Zion SM, Slezak JM, Sellers TA, et al. Reoperations after prophylactic mastectomy with or without implant reconstruction. *Cancer*. 2003;98(10):2152-2160.

45. Frost MH, Schaid DJ, Slezak JM, et al. Long-term satisfaction and psychological and social function following bilateral prophylactic mastectomy. *JAMA*. 2000;284:319-324.

46. Geiger AM, Nekhlyudov L, Herrington LJ, et al. Quality of life after bilateral prophylactic mastectomy. *Ann Surg Oncol*. 2007;14(2):686-694.

47. Stefanek ME, Helzlsouer KJ, Wilcox PM, Houn F. Predictors of satisfaction with bilateral prophylactic mastectomy. *Prev Med*. 1995;24(4):412-419.

48. Bresser PJC, Seynaeve C, Van Gool AR, et al. Satisfaction with prophylactic mastectomy and breast reconstruction in genetically predisposed women. *Plast Reconstr Surg*. 2006;117(6):1675-1682.

49. Metcalfe KA. Prophylactic bilateral mastectomy for breast cancer prevention. *J Women's Health*. 2004;13(7):822-829.

50. Metcalfe KA, Esplen MJ, Goel V, Narod SA. Predictors of quality of life in women with a bilateral prophylactic mastectomy. *Breast J*. 2005;11(1):65-69.

51. Altschuler A, Nekhlyudov L, Roinick SJ, et al. Positive, negative and disparate-women's differing long-term psychosocial experience of bilateral contralateral prophylactic mastectomy. *Breast J*. 2008;14(1):25-32.

52. Van Sprundel TC, Schmidt MK, Rookous MA, et al. Risk reduction of contralateral breast cancer and survival after contralateral mastectomy in BRCA1 and BRCA2 mutation carriers. *Br J Cancer*. 2005; 93(2):287-292.

53. McDonnell SK, Schaid DJ, Myers JL, et al. Efficacy of contralateral prophylactic mastectomy in women with a personal and family history of breast cancer. *J Clin Oncol*. 2001;19(19):3938-3943.

54. Peralta EA, Ellenhorn JDI, Wagman LD, et al. Contralateral prophylactic mastectomy improves the outcome of selected patients undergoing mastectomy for breast cancer. *Am J Surg*. 2000;180(6):439-445.

55. Herrinton LJ, Barlow WE, Yu O, et al. Efficacy of prophylactic mastectomy in women with unilateral breast cancer: a cancer research network project. *J Clin Oncol*. 2005;23(19):4275-4286.

56. Brekelmans CT, Seynaeve C, Menke-Pluymers M, et al. Survival and prognostic factors in BRCA1-associated breast cancer. *Ann Oncol*. 2006;17(3):391-400.

57. Lee KSU, Grant CS, Donohue JH, et al. Arguments against routine contralateral mastectomy or undirected biopsy for invasive lobular breast cancer. *Surgery*. 1995;118(4):640-648.

58. Babiera GV, Lowry AM, Davidson BS, et al. The role of contralateral prophylactic mastectomy in invasive lobular carcinoma. *Breast J*. 1997; 3(1):2-6.

59. Lostumbo L, Carbine N, Wallace J, Ezzo J. Prophylactic mastectomy in the prevention of breast cancer. *Cochrane Database of Systematic Reviews*. 2004; Issue 4, Art. No.:CD002748. DOI: 10.1002/14651858.CD002748.pub2.

60. Montgomery LL, Tran KN, Heelan MC, et al. Issues of regret in women with contralateral prophylactic mastectomies. *Ann Surg Oncol*. 1999;6:546-552.

61. Geiger AM, West CN, Nekhlyudov L, et al. Contentment with quality of life among breast cancer survivors with and without contralateral prophylactic mastectomy. *J Clin Oncol*. 2006;24(9):1350-1356.

62. Frost MH, Slezak JM, Tran NV, et al. Satisfaction after contralateral prophylactic mastectomy: the significance of mastectomy type, reconstructive complications, and body appearance. *J Clin Oncol*. 2005;23(31): 7849-7856.

63. Tuttle TM, Habermann EB, Grund EH, et al. Increasing use of contralateral prophylactic mastectomy for breast cancer patients: a trend toward more aggressive surgical treatment. *J Clin Oncol*. 2007;25(33):5203-5209.

64. Metcalfe KA, Lubinski J, Ghadirian P, et al. Predictors of contralateral prophylactic mastectomy in women with a BRCA1 or BRCA2 mutation: the Hereditary Breast Cancer Clinical Study Group. *J Clin Oncol*. 2008;26(7):1093-1097.

65. Metcalfe KA, Birenbaum-Carmeli D, Lubinski J, et al. International variation in rates of uptake of preventive options in BRCA1 and BRCA2 mutation carriers. *Int J Cancer*. 2008;122(9):2017-2022.

66. Lynch HT, Lemon SJ, Durham ST, et al. A descriptive study of BRCA1 testing and reactions to disclosure of test results. *Cancer*. 1997;79:2219-2228.

67. King M-C, Wieand S, Hale K, et al. Tamoxifen and breast cancer incidence among women with inherited mutations in BRCA1 and BRCA2: National Surgical Adjuvant Breast and Bowel Project (NSABP-P1) Breast Cancer Prevention Trial. *JAMA*. 2001;286:2251-2256.

68. Loman N, Johansson O, Bendahl P-O, et al. Steroid receptors in hereditary breast carcinomas associated with BRCA1 or BRCA2 mutations or unknown susceptibility genes. *Cancer*. 1998;83:310-319.

69. Eisinger F, Jacquemier J, Nogues C, et al. Steroid receptors in hereditary breast carcinomas associated with BRCA1 or BRCA2 mutations or unknown susceptibility genes. *Cancer*. 1999;85:2291-2295.

70. Narod SA, Brunet J, Ghadirian P, et al. Tamoxifen and risk of contralateral breast cancer in BRCA1 and BRCA2 mutation carriers: a case-control study. *Lancet*. 2000;356:1876-1881.

71. Gronwald J, Tung N, Foulkes WD, et al. Tamoxifen and contralateral breast cancer in BRCA1 and BRCA2 carriers: an update. *Int J Cancer*. 2006;118(9):2281-2284.

72. Peshkin BN, Isaacs C, Finch C, et al. Tamoxifen as chemoprevention in BRCA1 and BRCA2 mutation carriers with breast cancer: a pilot survey of physicians. *J Clin Oncol*. 2003;21:4322-4328.

73. Kauff ND, Satagopan JM, Robson ME, et al. Risk-reducing salpingo-oophorectomy in women with a BRCA1 or BRCA2 mutation. *N Engl J Med.* 2002;346:1609-1615.

74. Rebbeck TR, Lynch HT, Neuhausen SL, et al. Prophylactic oophorectomy in carriers of BRCA1 and BRCA2 mutations. *N Engl J Med.* 2002;346: 1616-1622.

75. Eisen A, Lubinski J, Klijn J, et al. Breast cancer risk following bilateral oophorectomy in BRCA1 and BRCA2 mutation carriers: an international case-control study. *J Clin Oncol.* 2005;23(30):7491-7496.

76. Newman LA, Kuerer HM, Hunt KK, et al. Presentation, treatment, and outcome of local recurrence after skin-sparing mastectomy and immediate breast reconstruction. *Ann Surg Oncol.* 1998;5(7):620-626.

77. Simmons RM, Fish SK, Gayle L, et al. Local and distant recurrence rates in skin-sparing mastectomies compared with non-skin-sparing mastectomies. *Ann Surg Oncol.* 1999;6(7):676-681.

78. Crowe JP Jr, Kim JA, Yetman R, et al. Nipple-sparing mastectomy: technique and results of 54 procedures. *Arch Surg.* 2004;139(2):148-150.

79. Garcia-Etienne CA, Borgen PI. Update on the indications for nipple-sparing mastectomy. *J Support Oncol.* 2006;4(5):225-230.

80. Bernstein JL, Thomson WD, Risch N, et al. Risk factors predicting the incidence of second primary breast cancer among women diagnosed with a first primary breast cancer. *Am J Epidemiol.* 1992;136(8):925-936.

81. Fisher ER, Fisher B, Sass R, Wickerham L. Pathologic findings from the National Surgical Adjuvant Breast Project (Protocol No. 4). XI. Bilateral breast cancer. *Cancer.* 1984;54(12):3002-3011.

82. Singletary SE, Taylor SH, Guinee VF, Whitworth PW Jr. Occurrence and prognosis of contralateral carcinoma of the breast. *J Am Coll Surg.* 1994;178(4):390-396.

83. Boughey JC, Cormier JN, Xing Y, et al. Decision analysis to assess the efficacy of routine sentinel lymphadenectomy in patients undergoing prophylactic mastectomy. *Cancer.* 2007;110(11):2542-25540.

84. Boughey JC, Khakpour N, Meric-Bernstam F, et al. Selective use of sentinel lymph node surgery during prophylactic mastectomy. *Cancer.* 2006;107(7):1440-1447.

85. Black D, Specht M, Lee JM, et al. Detecting occult malignancy in prophylactic mastectomy: preoperative MRI versus sentinel lymph node biopsy. *Ann Surg Oncol.* 2007;14(9):2477-2484.

86. MacMahon B, Cole P, Lin TM, et al. Age at first birth and breast cancer risk. *Bull Natl Health Org.* 1970;43:209-221.

87. Russo IH, Russo J. Hormonal approach to breast cancer prevention. *J Cell Biochem Suppl.* 2000;34:1-6.

88. Society of Surgical Oncology. Position statement on prophylactic mastectomy. http://www.surgonc.org/default.aspx?id=179. Accessed September 14, 2008.

89. Nekhlyudov L, Bower M, Herrinton LJ, et al. Women's decision-making roles regarding contralateral prophylactic mastectomy. *J Natl Cancer Inst Monogr.* 2005;35:55-60.

CHAPTER 12

History, Physical Examination, and Staging

Christine Laronga
Sharon Tollin
Kiran Turaga

Breast cancer is being detected at earlier stages due to improvements in imaging and increased public awareness of the breast health guidelines. The American Cancer Society recommends monthly self-breast exams, an annual clinical breast exam (CBE), and annual screening mammography for women over 40.[1] With increased compliance, primary care physicians are being overwhelmed with self-reported breast lumps or changes in the CBE or mammogram. Prompted in part by fear of litigation of missed breast cancer coupled with patient demand for expertise in breast diseases, referrals to breast specialists or diagnostic breast clinics (DBCs) are increasing. In fact, a whole new generation of breast surgeons is cropping up to meet this demand.

Despite specialization, the foundation of any new patient evaluation begins with a comprehensive history and physical examination. The information gained will then guide the ordering of appropriate imaging studies. This chapter's goal is to outline the necessary information for an appropriate evaluation of common breast problems.

DIAGNOSTIC BREAST CLINIC

Evaluation of common breast problems at our institution occurs in diagnostic breast clinic that has on-site imaging including a dedicated breast MRI. Our 3 advanced registered nurse practitioners (ARNPs) see over 1500 patients per year under the supervision of 4 breast surgeons. The ARNP performs a complete history and physical examination, has any outside films reviewed by our on-site breast radiologist, obtains any additional imaging needed, and designs a plan with the breast surgeon. Image-guided core biopsies are performed a few days later to allow for insurance approval, cessation of blood-thinning agents, and to accommodate the patient's schedule. Rarely excisional biopsies are used as the primary diagnostic procedure. Biopsy results are given by the ARNP and patients with benign results are followed for 2 years with CBE and diagnostic imaging. Excisional biopsies are performed if the core biopsy revealed atypia.

HISTORY AND PHYSICAL EXAMINATION— GENERAL

The first step in the evaluation of a new patient involves obtaining a thorough history and physical examination in a patient and supportive manner, as many women will present with significant anxiety. The patient must be considered the expert on her own body, and her concerns must be given every consideration. She must feel empowered to perform breast self-exams and feel comfortable seeking evaluation for changes. Fortunately for most, the outcome will be benign, but the initial approach is similar for all patients.

History

The essential elements of the history should include the chief complaint (symptoms) such as skin changes, nipple inversion/retraction, nipple discharge, redness, breast pain, and palpable changes. Detailed analysis of symptoms should include onset, duration, precipitating/alleviating factors, recent trauma or infection, changes in medications, changes in weight, changes in medical conditions. Additionally, previous breast history should be recorded including details of prior breast biopsies, breast augmentation/reduction, breast problems, compliance with screening guidelines, and imaging history. Exploring the past medical history can elicit relevant risk factors or comorbidities. In addition, certain conditions such as diabetes mellitus or congestive heart failure can affect the breast. Allergies are important to note. Medications can affect the breast as well, most commonly by causing nipple discharge. Coumadin and aspirin can contribute to a bloody discharge. Reproductive history includes age at menarche, menstrual and pregnancy history, breastfeeding, and use of hormones (contraception, infertility treatment, and hormone replacement). This information is important in evaluating the breast on clinical exam or imaging and assessing risk of breast cancer. The date of the last menstrual period must be taken into consideration on CBE and any diagnostic breast imaging obtained, especially breast MRI. Family history of cancer is important for individual risk assessment and potential need for genetic counseling. Social history is not unique to evaluation of breast patients, but is helpful in determining patient support and resources. Additionally, smoking is associated with poor wound healing and increases risks of infection such as a recurrent retroareolar abscess. The history of alcohol intake is important, especially when assessing males for gynecomastia. Prior breast imaging with reports should be reviewed in conjunction with current imaging. Outside films should be reviewed at the facility for concordance. Similarly, any outside pathology slides should be reviewed at the institution's pathology department to confirm diagnosis, especially when atypia are found on a core needle biopsy.

History-taking should be conducted with the woman fully clothed and preferably not on the examination table, making her more comfortable and less vulnerable. Then when it is time for the physical examination, have the gown (cape) open to the front. Consider having a chaperone for this part even if you are the same sex as the patient.

Physical Examination

Assessment begins from the first moment, whether it's observing the patient walking to the exam room or an interaction while taking vital signs. Is she cradling one of her breasts? Observe the overall demeanor of the patient, and eye contact. Is there anyone accompanying the patient for the consultation?

Although the most important part of the examination is the CBE, a thorough, relevant physical exam is ideal. Start with the patient in the sitting position and palpate the cervical region for lymphadenopathy and thyromegaly (thyroid conditions are common with breast diseases). Also include an assessment of any supraclavicular or infraclavicular lymphadenopathy. Examine the heart and lungs, and assess for peripheral edema, pulses, spinal tenderness, and costovertebral angle tenderness. While the patient is still sitting, the CBE includes elements of inspection and palpation of the breast and axillae. Stand in front of the patient, open her gown without removing it, and have her press her hands into her hips. Then have her move her arms slowly out to her side and continue moving her arms until they are above her head. Look for size, shape, symmetry (most women have slight differences), and changes in the contour of the breast (retraction, puckering, dimpling, bulging, and changes in the nipple). Inspection includes the entire breast and nipple looking for edema, erythema, rashes, and ulceration.

For palpation, begin with a superficial exam, allowing the woman to trust your touch. Watch her facial response as you do the examination. This is also an ideal opportunity to assess the comfort level of self-exams and to provide teaching in the technique. Palpation is performed by placing one hand underneath her breast for support. With your other hand palpate the entire breast mound. Relax the breast and then exam in the axilla by cradling her arm in yours and supporting the elbow. Palpate the axillary contents from the latissimus muscle, behind the pectoralis muscle, to the ribcage. Moving her arm will allow entry to the apex of the axilla. Palpation begins with the pulp of the fingers and insinuation inside the axilla with the arm initially raised, and then lower, allowing for better appreciation of the subclavicular and central group of nodes on deep palpation. Palpation along the chest wall and the subscapularis should also be routinely performed. Any palpable lymph node is evaluated for size, mobility, consistency, and for evidence of matted lymph nodes. The skin overlying the axilla and the ipsilateral arm should also be examined for presence of any sinus tracts, previous surgeries or signs of infection. Lymph nodes may be palpably enlarged from folliculitis, an arm infection, or even acrylic nails, but they should be soft and mobile. Document any palpable nodes for future reference. Suspicious lymph nodes need further assessment with imaging. Repeat your exam on the other side.

Have the patient recline for the abdominal exam and a repeat of the CBE. A variety of techniques for CBE exist, such as the radial search pattern, the concentric circular pattern, and the MammaCare method.[2-4] This latter method utilizes the vertical strip pattern and adaptations continue to be recommended today.[5] In this pattern, the pads of the 3 middle fingers are used with light, medium, and deeper levels of pressure applied at each area of tissue palpated. The key is consistency in the individual technique and that the entire breast is reliably and reproducibly examined. The area to be examined includes the tissue from the clavicle to the inframammary ridge and from mid-sternum to mid-axillary line. The superficial tissue as well as the deeper layers of breast tissue should be examined in a thorough pattern. Subtle changes may be noted, including areas of thickening, in addition to palpable masses. Nodularity of the breast tissue is usually more prominent in the upper outer quadrants and shortly before the menstrual flow. Avoid squeezing the nipple unless there is a history of spontaneous nipple discharge.

CBE is a skill that improves with experience. Standardized training with simulated breast models has been evaluated, and increased comfort levels in medical students were seen with training.[6-8] Residents' ability to detect breast masses improved utilizing a standardized vertical strip, 3-pressure method. This effort incorporated a self-study program and a trained patient surrogate in addition to the use of a silicone model.[7] The use of deep pressure and the time spent performing the exam both correlated significantly with finding a breast mass. Core components of this technique included "consistent search pattern, deep palpation, circling downward, and adequate overlap of coverage." Documentation also improved with the training initiative. In a randomized controlled trial of CBE training, Campbell and associates found duration of the exam to be an independent predictor of sensitivity.[8] The bottom line is that a thorough CBE takes time.

Documentation of the CBE should include any pertinent positive and negative findings. Any palpable areas of concern noted on CBE or by the patient should be indicated by position (clock face and centimeters from the nipple), size, shape, depth, attachment to overlying skin or chest wall, associated skin changes, and mobility. This provides pertinent information for further evaluation by diagnostic imaging, possible biopsy, and appropriate follow-up.

SIGNS AND SYMPTOMS

Most diagnoses mentioned here are discussed in detail elsewhere in this book.

Mastalgia (Breast Pain) Without Skin Changes

Pain is typically considered a "warning sign." This can vary in different cultural contexts, but most individuals in the United States consider pain to equate with a physical problem. In fact, it is the most common breast-related complaint seen in primary care clinics and affects some 70% of women.[9] An underlying fear of breast cancer is what prompts these patients to seek health care. Although the vast majority of breast cancers do not hurt, the woman may relate an anecdotal story of a friend who had breast pain for years before her cancer was detected. Thus, a significant amount of time will be spent listening, reassuring, and seeking to prove that it is not breast cancer. About 85% of women with mild to moderate mastalgia are successfully managed with just reassurance.[10]

Generalized or Focal Breast Pain Without Imaging Abnormality

Breast pain without imaging abnormality is the hardest subset of breast pain to treat, as the causative agent usually cannot be identified. In a minority of women, the pain is a result of a change in hormonal status, as with perimenopause, stopping or starting birth control pills, or hormone replacement therapy. Treatment is supportive. If the pain arises from initiating birth control pills or hormone replacement therapy and does not abate in a few months, consider switching the brand.

Cyclical Breast Pain

Next, deduce whether the pain is cyclical or noncyclical. Cyclical breast pain peaks just before the menstrual flow begins and mostly involves the upper outer quadrants of the breasts. First and foremost, treatment is reassurance and then supportive—sleep with a sports bra, intermittent anti-inflammatory medicine, and a trial of limiting caffeine intake. If persistent and significantly impacting her quality of life, one can consider medical therapy. Fortunately cyclical breast pain is more responsive to medical intervention than noncyclical mastalgia.[11]

Noncyclical Breast Pain

Supplement a general history and physical examination with an assessment of when it began, duration, aggravating and alleviating factors, whether it is unilateral or bilateral, point location or generalized through the breast, description of the character of the pain (sharp, burning, throbbing, itching, dull ache), and any new medications or health problems. This type of mastalgia is not associated with the menstrual cycle, can involve any part of the breast especially the inner breasts, and can be unilateral or bilateral. A CBE should identify areas of abnormality in terms of point tenderness, mass, or skin/nipple retraction; then a mammogram and a focused ultrasound should be performed. Treatment should be directed at any underlying factor if one is identified.

If no culprit is found, assess the impact of caffeine withdrawal and wear a sports bra while sleeping for 1 month. The belief is that the sports bra stabilizes the breast, minimizing inflammation.[12] She can repeat the cycle of wearing the sports bra as needed.

Mastalgia Management

One can also offer a trial of vitamin E 400 U/day for 1 month (Fig. 12-1). Vitamin E, a lipid-soluble antioxidant, acts as a defense against oxidative stress and has been used to treat breast pain for over 40 years. Despite this fact, only limited clinical trials using vitamin E are available, showing little or no benefit over placebo or other agents such as danazol.[12,13] In our experience, it either works or it does not. If the vitamin E does not work, try evening of primrose oil (EPO) 3 g daily for 4 months. EPO is a rich source of essential fatty acids that lessens inflammation via the prostaglandin pathway. Both vitamin E and EPO take weeks before showing any effect. Studies using EPO have shown a benefit in breast pain reduction upwards of 58% in cyclical breast pain, 38% in noncyclical mastalgia.[11] Yet a recent meta-analysis failed to show any benefit from EPO.[14] Despite conflicting results, EPO has the most tolerable side-effect profile and should be tried before prescription medications are attempted.

EPO failures commit to a daily diary recording each and every episode of pain with descriptors. She is to return for a CBE, review of the log, and repeat imaging in 2 months (6 months from presentation). Most women do not return for several reasons: (1) the pain is better; (2) realization that the pain is not as "constant" as they thought; (3) they were not compliant with keeping the log. If, however, she returns, take the time to review the log looking for a pattern or causative events that may be treatable. If no cause can be elicited and repeat CBE with imaging remains negative, embark on a trial of medical management aimed at quieting the breast via hormonal manipulation. Tamoxifen 10 mg daily, danazole 200 mg a day, or bromocriptine 1.25 mg at night can be offered. A common breast cancer treatment, tamoxifen blocks estrogen receptors and has the fewest side effects compared to danazole or bromocriptine. The success rate is upward of 80% to 90% by 6 months with a 30% relapse rate.[15] Due to a risk of endometrial cancer with use over 6 months' duration, the recommendation is to stop therapy at 6 months. Danazole, an anti-gonadotropin, acts on the pituitary–ovarian axis, and bromocriptine is an inhibitor of prolactin secretion. Both danazole (used for endometriosis) and bromocriptine (used for amenorrhea and nipple discharge) are more effective than tamoxifen but at the cost of being much less tolerable. Many women thus opt out of trialing these medications, but those that do often find that side effects are worse than the breast pain itself and self-discontinue. If they stay on the medication, 77% with cyclical breast pain will have significant benefit versus 19% in the placebo control arms.[10] The noncyclical mastalgias do not fare quite as well, with a 44%

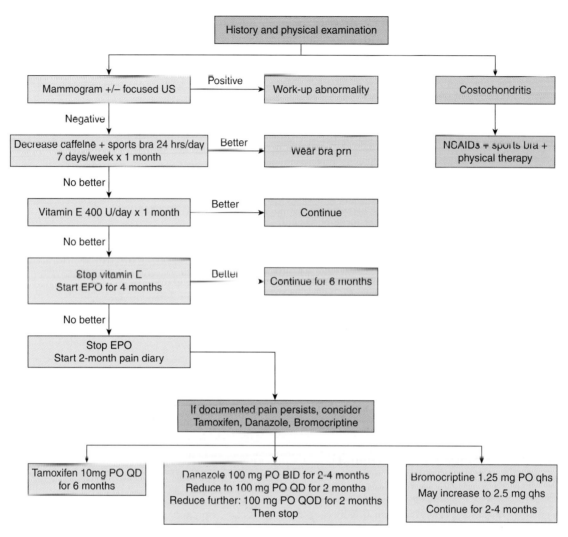

FIGURE 12-1 Mastalgia treatment algorithm.

response to drug therapy versus 9% in the placebo group.[10] If the woman fails therapy with one agent, try another drug, as about one-third of women will respond to second-line therapy. At the Cardiff Mastalgia Clinic, the women with cyclical breast pain who had an excellent or substantial response to medical management had an 80% chance of long-term reduction of significant breast pain 6 months after stopping the medication, but the women with noncyclical mastalgia had only a 40% chance of long-term benefit.[10]

Focal pain without imaging abnormality should be followed for a minimum of 1 year with CBE and imaging to confirm the localized pain was not from a very early breast cancer. Other agents such as neurontin have been used with limited success for the treatment of pain caused by herpes zoster and postmastectomy pain syndromes, but there are no controlled trials in the literature using neurontin for benign breast pain.

Costochondritis

Costochondritis (Tietze syndrome) is inflammation of the costochondral joint spaces and is common in all ages of women, especially middle-aged women. Inflammation can be trauma or

sports-related and leads to irritation of the intercostal nerves. The medial intercostal nerves that traverse these joint spaces supply sensation to the medial and central portion of the breast. Gently pushing on the joint spaces will elicit the breast pain; no abnormalities will be identified within the breast. Confirmation is obtained by lifting the breast off the chest wall while the woman is supine and palpating the breast sideways to avoid applying pressure on the joint spaces. No pain within the breast will be invoked by this maneuver. A similar phenomenon can occur laterally where the ribs curve anterior and the lateral intercostal nerves travel to get to the lateral breast. Trauma to the ribs in this area, spasm or irritation of the latissimus muscle, and herpes zoster all can lead to aggravation of these nerves and thus pain on the lateral to central aspects of the breast. On physical examination, pain can be elicited by pressing on the ribs in the anterior axillary line or latissimus muscle.

Costochondritis is predominantly a unilateral process (92% of the time) and involves either medial or lateral nerves but not both.[16] Treatment is supportive. Steroids with local injection of anesthetics are also effective therapies.[16] Duration is weeks to months long (mean time = 17 months) before symptoms resolve.

Focal Breast Pain with Imaging Abnormality

The most common cause of point tenderness with a corresponding imaging abnormality is a simple cyst. Other causes of focal mastalgia with imaging abnormalities but without skin changes include gynecomastia, fibroadenoma, diabetic mastopathy, lactating adenomas, galactoceles, and certain cancers (phyllodes tumor, adenoid cystic carcinoma, and lymphoma).

▌ Breast Pain with Skin Changes

Mastalgia with skin changes, for the most part, will have an underlying etiology. Skin changes can be a color change, skin edema or thickening, exaggeration of hair follicles, rash, or dimpling/retraction of the skin. The skin of the breast is similar to skin elsewhere and the disease process may be of skin origin, such as intradermal inclusion/sebaceous cysts, hydradenitis (usually affecting the skin on the lower half of large pendulous breast), eczema, psoriasis, contact dermatitis, and yeast infections of the inframammary fold (usually affects larger-breasted women). Chronic yeast infections result in a hyperpigmented outline of the pendulous breast on the abdominal skin.

Inflamed Breast Cyst

A simple cyst can become inflamed or infected causing pain. If that cyst is pushing on the overlying breast skin, the skin can appear red/pink. If the area is confirmed to be a cyst on ultrasound, aspiration should be performed.

Mondor Disease (Superficial Thrombophlebitis)

Mondor disease or superficial thrombophlebitis of the breast is an uncommon entity with an incidence less than 1%.[17] Common causes include trauma, tight clothing, infections, and surgical procedures of the breast, and rarely include cancer. One-third of the time no inciting event or cause can be found. The history is one of a sudden development of localized pain in the breast followed by a visible and palpable tender cordlike groove under the native breast skin. The overlying skin may be red from inflammation. These veins are usually branches of the lateral thoracic vein or thoracoepigatric vessels.[18] Interestingly, the presentation is more common in middle-aged women. On physical examination the "cord" is easily palpable as a long tubular structure. Mammogram will be normal or show a tubular density. Ultrasound will show a hyperechoic cordlike lesion with possibly an intraluminal thrombus. Fortunately, the process is self-limiting and resolves in 2 to 8 weeks. Warm compresses, anti-inflammatory medications, and loose-fitting clothes are usually all that is necessary. Rarely surgical intervention is warranted to remove the affected area or rule out cancer.

Hyperemia Versus Erythema and/or Dependent Edema (Lymphedema)

A woman presents with a pink or red heavy breast. Important to elicit in the history is duration of symptoms, insidious or abrupt onset, change or growth of the area of color over time, trauma, bug bites, nipple discharge, pain, systemic symptoms, and history of breast, axillary, or shoulder surgery. Physical exam should try to differentiate erythema (inflammation/infection) from hyperemia. With the woman supine, lift her breast off the chest wall and hold for several minutes. Observe if the pink hue fades as the breast drains (hyperemia). In inflammation (cellulitis), the redness persists and the breast is usually painful whereas hyperemia is not sensitive to touch. Anytime a woman presents with redness or a pink hue to the breast, the surgeon must eliminate inflammatory breast cancer from the differential. Most times it can be made by clinical presentation and appearance of the breast, but sometimes imaging and a punch biopsy of the affected skin are necessary.

Hyperemia can be accompanied by varying degrees of skin edema (exaggeration of the hair follicles, pitting, and thickness of the skin). The hyperemia and edema are caused by blockage of drainage (venous or lymphatic) from the breast and are usually found centrally and in the lower breast skin in pendulous breasts. Causes are seromas from breast biopsies or lumpectomies, curvilinear incisions in the upper outer quadrant of the breast, axillary surgery (sentinel lymph node biopsy, axillary node dissection), breast radiation, trauma, resolving infection, superficial vasculitis, and sometimes in young women hormonal variation. The history and physical findings will guide what diagnostic imaging to order. The mammogram is useful for identifying masses within the breast, demonstrating skin thickening and edema within the breast parenchyma, or no abnormality. The ultrasound can demonstrate a seroma/hematoma, an abscess, cancer recurrence, axillary adenopathy, or recurrence. If venous congestion is suspected (history of central venous access devices, congestive heart failure, or trauma to the shoulder/clavicular area), then ultrasound, venography, or echocardiogram may be warranted.[19] Treatment of the underlying diagnosis will alleviate the hyperemia in most cases. For women without a treatable cause, the process is usually self-limited, but breast massage by a lymphedema specialist may be beneficial. Breast compression garments are helpful but are not well tolerated by the woman.

Erythema is not dependent on the position of the breast for drainage. It can be focal from an underlying abscess or diffuse from cellulitis or mastitis. The history should attempt to decipher if the origin was within the breast spreading to the skin or vice versa. Bug bites, spider bites, cat scratches, poison ivy, and so forth should be treated as appropriate for the specific type of skin infection. Mastitis, on the other hand, originates in the breast, is most commonly pregnancy/lactationally related, and treated by the patient's obstetrician. The woman is referred if she fails to improve, if an abscess develops, or to rule out cancer as the underlying cause. An abscess less than 3 cm in greatest diameter is treated with ultrasound-guided aspiration with irrigation of the cavity.[20-21] Oral antibiotics are also given and the success rate is ~90% with a single aspiration. For those failing this treatment or having a larger abscess, the surgical treatment is incision and drainage. Mastitis in a nonlactating woman is less common and is called periductal mastitis.[22] Periductal mastitis is more common in younger women and in smokers (more than 10 cigarettes/day). Smoking increases risk of abscess and fistula formation (78% in smokers).[23,24] These women present with a red, hot, uncomfortable breast and may have systemic complaints such as fever. The cause of the infection is usually unknown but can be related to oral or hand contact to the nipple–areolar complex. Many organisms have been identified including *Staphylococcus* and rare organisms such as *Mycobacterium* species. Imaging should be aimed at identifying an abscess and allaying fears of an underlying cancer. If there is an abscess, treatment consists of ultrasound-guided aspiration. The fluid is sent for culture and sensitivity to allow for antibiotic selection. Operative management is warranted for fistulas and if conservative measures fail.

Recurrent retroareolar abcesses are associated with squamous metaplasia of the lactiferous ducts (SMOLD). SMOLD is commonly identified in smokers and leads to peri-areolar fistulous tracts despite antibiotics, incision, and drainage. The treatment includes treating the active infection and smoking cessation. The fistulous tract, the abscess, and the affected nipple duct need to be removed.[25]

BREAST MASS

Patients may also present with a chief complaint of a palpable area (lump) noted on self-exam, CBE, or by a partner/significant other. This palpable area may not be a new finding. A variety of reasons may postpone evaluation: financial hardship or access to health care, denial of breast changes, fear, anxiety, or blaming it on a past traumatic injury. Some women wait until a menstrual cycle prior to making an appointment. An abnormal mammogram or breast sonogram will prompt self-examination or recollection of previous palpable concerns. Males of all ages tend to delay seeking evaluation. Regardless, all palpable concerns merit a thorough evaluation. The majority of changes evaluated will ultimately reveal benign disease, but the patient's perception of the experience lays the groundwork for the future. A woman's breast cancer risk increases with age and she must feel comfortable seeking evaluation should another problem arise in the future.

History and Physical Exam

In conjunction with the history and physical exam, ascertain characteristics and duration of the lump. If premenopausal, ask about changes in reference to her menstrual cycle. Palpable changes can present as subtle thickening, focused nodularity, discrete mass, or as multiple palpable changes. Women of all ages may present with diffuse fibronodular changes, making the assessment challenging. Normal glandular tissue can be mistaken for a mass, but skilled CBE can help differentiate this. A common finding on ultrasound of palpable abnormalities is a prominent fat lobule.

Triple Test

Triple assessment refers to the combination of CBE, breast imaging, and biopsy. In women younger than 30 years of age, a focused breast ultrasound should be the initial diagnostic imaging study. In women aged 30 and older, both a diagnostic mammogram and focused ultrasound are recommended. The requisition for diagnostic imaging should specify the exact location of any palpable masses. Ultrasound can determine a cystic versus solid mass and may identify abnormalities not evident on mammogram.

Diagnostic mammography in symptomatic women has a higher sensitivity and lower specificity than screening mammography.[26] Negative imaging prompts a short-term follow-up with CBE and imaging in 3 to 4 months. If clinically suspicious, biopsy should not be delayed if the imaging was negative.

Solid breast masses require histocytologic diagnosis. Percutaneous core biopsy or fine-needle aspiration (FNA) offer less invasive alternatives to surgery and can further help distinguish solid from cystic lesions. Ariga and associates evaluated FNA in women with palpable breast masses in a study of 1158 FNA procedures subsequently confirmed on histopathology.[27] Sensitivity and specificity were 98%, positive predictive value 99%, and the false-negative rate 9%. In women upto 40 years, a malignancy was diagnosed in 51%, and 74% in those older than 40. Correlation of lesions seen on both mammogram and sonogram is important to avoid missing a lesion. Concordance between imaging and pathology is another critical component of the assessment. Prompt communication of the results to the patient will allay anxiety.

Cystic Lesions

Breast cysts are often seen in pre- and perimenopausal women (aged 35-50), but can be seen in women of all ages. Women often find cysts on self-exam and relate a history of a rapidly enlarging palpable change. Cysts can be single or multiple, unilateral or bilateral, tender, firm, mobile, and can vary in size from a few mm to very large. They are well circumscribed and anechoic on ultrasound. Oil cysts can be idiopathic or result from trauma or previous surgery and are confirmed on mammogram.[28] Complex cysts have both anechoic and echogenic (solid) findings on ultrasound and can be due to fibrocystic change and resolving cysts. Ultrasound-guided aspiration and/or core biopsy is recommended if a solid component or intracystic mass is seen on imaging. Hematomas and seromas are tender, palpable fluid collections seen after surgery or trauma. Fat necrosis, a very firm mass, can appear as a complex cyst on ultrasound and is common after surgical procedures here there is local destruction of fat cells. On mammogram the indeterminate calcifications, spiculated areas of increased opacity, and focal masses mimic a malignancy. A tissue diagnosis will confirm the diagnosis.[29]

Common Solid Lesions

Fibroadenomas are benign tumors of the breast that are composed of stromal and epithelial (glandular) cells and are most commonly seen in younger women, typically during their 20s and 30s, but can occur in older women. It is the most common breast lesion in adolescence and typically is a firm, rubbery, mobile mass that is well circumscribed, but can be lobulated and irregular. Multiple fibroadenomas (defined as 3 to 5 lesions in one breast) occur in 10% to 15% of patients with the diagnosis. Giant fibroadenomas by definition are greater than 5 cm or 500 g.[30]

A retrospective study of 605 women under the age of 40 with palpable breast masses detected on self-exam (n = 484) and on CBE (n = 121) found a dominant mass detected on CBE by a surgeon in 36% and 29% of the women, respectively.[31] Fibroadenoma proved to be the most common diagnosis in this group at 57%; cysts accounted for 10%. In addition, carcinoma was diagnosed in 18% of the young women in this study, including biopsies indicated for abnormal mammographic findings unrelated to any palpable mass. Vargas found fibroadenoma to be the most common diagnosis (72%) in over 500 young women and cysts accounted for 4%, fibrocystic changes 3%, and malignancy 1%.[32] Interestingly, 53% of abnormalities detected on self-exam were true masses compared to 18% detected by primary care providers.

Phyllodes tumors (formerly termed *cystosarcoma phyllodes*) are similar to fibroadenomas but much less common. They occur later in life, typically after the fourth decade, but can be seen in adolescence. In addition to a palpable, rubbery, mobile mass, these patients may present with benign lymphadenopathy. A classic presentation is a lump that suddenly popped up after a trauma. On CBE and imaging they may be impossible to differentiate from a fibroadenoma and therefore require diagnostic biopsy. A review of 443 phyllodes cases (median age of 40 years) found 64% were benign, 18% borderline, and 18% malignant.[33]

Papillomas, friable tumors with a central fibrovascular core, can be associated with palpable masses and are sometimes intracystic lesions. Solitary papillomas are often associated with nipple discharge. Multiple peripheral papillomas may appear as lobulated masses or clusters of punctuate calcifications on mammogram. Intracystic, intraductal, and solid masses can be seen on ultrasound.[28]

Adenomyoepithelioma is thought to be a variant of intraductal papilloma and presents as a well-circumscribed mass. Focal changes revealing carcinoma may not be seen on core biopsy specimens and excisional biopsy is recommended.[34]

Diabetic mastopathy is an uncommon benign condition typically seen in premenopausal women with a long history of type I diabetes mellitus. Rare cases have also been seen in women with type II diabetes and in elderly women.[35] Very firm, nontender, large, mobile masses are found on CBE in one or both breasts. The pathophysiology is unclear, but believed to be a localized autoimmune reaction resulting in inflammation and fibrosis.[36]

Pseudoangiomatous stromal hyperplasia (PASH) is a myofibroblastic lesion that can also present as a firm, mobile, palpable breast mass, typically in women of childbearing age. It has been documented in men and can resemble a fibroadenoma on CBE and imaging.[34] Typically PASH is a benign proliferation of breast stroma. A review of 26 cases found one invasive ductal carcinoma present with the PASH tumor, and one case of malignant transformation has been reported.[37,38]

Other benign etiologies include lipomas, angiolipomas, extracapsular silicone, silicone granuloma, scar tissue, and epidermal inclusion cysts (EICs). EICs of the breast tend to grow toward the deep subcutaneous tissue, unlike the protrusions typically seen in other tissue. The etiology may be due to obstructed hair follicles, trauma, or by squamous metaplasia of normal columnar cells within an ectatic duct in association with fibrocystic change.[39] Malignant transformation of EIC is possible.

Granular cell tumor typically presents as a firm, painless mass and may be fixed to the muscle or skin. Usually benign, about 8% of granular cell tumors occur in the breast. Malignant transformation has been documented and wide local excision is recommended, due to local recurrence.[40,41]

Adenosis tumors and apocrine adenomas represent pathology typically seen microscopically in the breast tissue but can present as palpable breast masses. Adenosis is a common benign, proliferative lesion arising in the terminal duct lobular unit. Adenosis tumors or nodular adenosis, typically affecting women of premenopausal age, can be suspicious on imaging. FNA is helpful. However, an additional biopsy is typically needed.[42] Apocrine adenoma is a rare epithelial tumor similar to apocrine metaplasia and occurs in women under 30 years old. Malignant variants of apocrine change include invasive apocrine carcinoma, apocrine DCIS, and apocrine adenoma adjacent to invasive ductal carcinoma.[43,44]

Other less commonly seen breast lesions are cholesterol granuloma, sparganosis, and schwannoma.[45] Schwannoma, a benign tumor of nerve sheath origin, rarely presents as a palpable breast mass.[46]

Pregnancy-Associated Lesions

Pregnancy-associated breast disease includes galactoceles. A galactocele contains milky fluid and develops during pregnancy, lactation, or even after lactation. It is the most common breast mass seen during lactation and may be due to mammary duct obstruction.[47] Due to the increased density of the breast parenchyma, mammography is less useful. An ultrasound is a more helpful in showing a galactocele as a solid mass or a simple/complex cyst.[28]

A lactating adenoma is another benign palpable breast lesion with a variable appearance on sonography. On ultrasound review of 15 biopsy-proven lactating adenomas, all were found to have an ovoid shape but varied with respect to echogenicity, posterior acoustic enhancement, and shadowing.[48] Breast abscess is common during lactation and inflammation may be absent. Ultrasound can help differentiate an abscess from carcinoma. Granulomatous mastitis is a less common finding in pregnancy.[49]

Lesions in Men and Women

Breast lesions documented as palpable masses in both males and females include hemangiomas, tuberculosis, myofibroblastoma, and desmoids tumors. Hemangiomas can be found either in the glandular breast parenchyma or in the subcutaneous fat superficial to the anterior pectoral fascia. On mammography and sonography, a well-circumscribed or microlobulated mass with an oval or lobular shape is typically noted. Image-guided biopsy is sufficient for diagnosis.[50] Mammary tuberculosis, both primary and secondary, is a chronic granulamatous disease caused by *Mycobacterium tuberculosis*. Although rare, it accounts for approximately 3% of all surgically treated breast disease in developing countries and typically presents as a tender, palpable breast mass.[51] Myofibroblastoma is a benign neoplastic proliferation of myofibroblasts.[34] Desmoid tumors of the breast, or deep fibromatoses, are rare benign tumors of infiltrative connective tissue. These tumors can be locally aggressive and tend to recur. Mammographic imaging can be negative, and sonography reveals a solid, hypoechoic mass. In a review of 32 patients, MRI findings were suspicious on most of the 8 individuals imaged and 29% developed tumor recurrence. FNA is not typically diagnostic and core biopsy is required.[40,52]

Benign Breast Disease in Males

Normal male breast tissue includes ductal elements, surrounding stroma, and adipose and subcutaneous tissue. Lobular units, necessary for lactation in women, are absent from the male breast.[53] Gynecomastia is a common, benign enlargement of the male breast due to proliferation of the glandular tissue. The etiology is commonly an increase in the ratio of estrogenic to androgenic activity. It can be an incidental finding, and is present in 30% to 50% of healthy men. There are 3 peaks in the incidence of gynecomastia: the neonatal period, puberty, and later in life.[54] The highest prevalence is in men 50 to 80 years old, "senescent gynecomastia." Approximately 25% of the cases are idiopathic, 25% persist due to puberty (physiologic), and 20% are related to drugs (Table 12-1). Other pathologic conditions associated with gynecomastia include neoplasms (testicular tumors account for 3%), primary or secondary gonadal failure, enzymatic defects of testosterone production, androgen insensitivity syndromes, true hermaphroditism, Klinefelter syndrome, liver disease, starvation, renal disease, and hypo- or hyperthyroidism.[55]

Clinical presentation consists of a tender, palpable mass of tissue at least 0.5 cm in diameter. This is usually a rubbery disk

TABLE 12-1 Drugs Associated with Gynecomastia

ACE inhibitors
Alcohol
Amiodarone
Anabolic steroids
Bicalutamide
Calcium-channel blockers (diltiazem, verapamil, nifedipine)
CNS agents (amphetamines, diazepam, methyldopa, phenytoin, reserpine, tricyclic antidepressants)
Cimetidine
Cytotoxic agents (alkylating agents; vincristine, nitrosureas, methotrexate)
Digitalis
Estrogens
Finasteride
Flutamide
Furosemide
Heroin
Hormones (androgens, estrogens, hCG)
Isoniazid
Ketoconazole; metronidazole
Marijuana
Metoclopramide
Omeprazole
Penicillamine
Phenothiazines
Protease inhibitors
Spironolactone
Theophylline
Thiazides

TABLE 12-2 Labs for Evaluation of Gynecomastia

Serum creatinine
Liver enzymes
TSH, (free T4/T3)
Testosterone, LH, FSH, estradiol, prolactin
Human chorionic gonadotrophin (may be elevated in lung, testicular, or gastric tumors)
Serum dehydroepiandrosterone sulphate/urinary 17-ketosteroids (if a feminizing adrenal tumor is part of differential diagnosis)

FSH, follicle-stimulating hormone; LH, luteinizing hormone; TSH, thyroid-stimulating hormone.

of subareolar tissue, but it can also be more diffuse, unilateral or bilateral. Nipple discharge or changes in the skin and nipple are not seen with gynecomastia. Breast pain is typically what prompts an evaluation. In adolescence, pubertal gynecomastia typically appears around the age of 13 to 14 and then regresses in 6 months or less. It can persist into the young man's 20s. The fatty breasts seen in obese males are termed "pseudogynecomastia," and are due to excess adipose tissue.[55] Clinical evaluation for gynecomastia includes a thorough review of prescription and over the counter medications, drug and alcohol history, testicular exam, and blood tests (Table 12-2). Increased hCG level or increased estradiol with a normal/decreased LH level would be an indication for referral and additional imaging evaluation, including testicular ultrasound.[55]

Sonography is indicated for palpable masses in the male breast or axilla. Prominent glandular tissue is seen on ultrasound in gynecomastia.[56] Patterson and associates reviewed imaging studies of 164 men presenting with breast symptoms; the median age for these men was 64 and the most common presentation was a mass or thickening (56%).[57] All carcinomas presented as palpable changes. Gynecomastia was the most common finding on mammography. Negative predictive value for mammography and sonography was 100%. Importantly, in this review no carcinoma was found in men with either negative mammography or findings of gynecomastia on mammogram. Focused ultrasound should be performed if the mammogram is negative. FNA or core biopsy is not required in cases of pubertal gynecomastia. However, as with women, clinically suspicious masses should be biopsied even if imaging is negative.

NIPPLE DISCHARGE

History

Nipple discharge is a frightening breast symptom that leads to prompt presentation to a physician. Questions pertaining to spontaneous versus induced discharge are paramount. Induced discharge results from pressure applied to the base of the nipple and the lactiferous sinuses. This can be the result of manual manipulation for a self-breast exam or can happen as a result of rolling over while sleeping. In the later common scenario, the woman states that she noted staining on her nightshirt in the morning when she arose. Spontaneous discharge occurs without any contact or stimulation to the nipple–areolar complex. Other discriminating factors to be addressed include the following:

1. Whether the discharge is unilateral or bilateral
2. Whether the discharge arises from a single duct or multiple ducts
3. Color of the secretion (clear, white, yellow, green, blue, red, brackish)
4. Viscosity of the fluid
5. Frequency and duration of the discharge
6. Change in character of the discharge
7. Signs of mastitis
8. Prior history of nipple discharge
9. Medical history, including a medication list

Physical Examination

A physical examination should include an attempt to reproduce the discharge. With the woman in the sitting position, stroke (massage) the breast from the periphery in each quadrant toward the nipple. GENTLY, but firmly, apply pressure to the retroareolar area (base of nipple) to elicit the discharge. If the discharge is seen, note the aforementioned discriminating factors. This is best recorded using a sheet with a grid diagram of the nipple labeling the orifice location (Fig. 12-2). If no discharge is obtained, then lay her supine for the repeat examination. Again,

stroke (massage) the breast toward the nipple and attempt to elicit the discharge. If this fails, ask her to attempt to express the fluid. When expressed, the discharge, regardless of color, should be tested for blood. Fortunately less than 10% of women with a bloody discharge will harbor a malignancy; the incidence rises with increasing age.[58]

Cytology

The role of cytology of the expressed fluid is controversial. First and foremost be selective and only send bloody discharge. Second, the technique is important. Express the discharge, touch the correct side of a glass slide to the surface of the droplet without touching the skin or any other droplets (if more than 1 duct expresses fluid), and then touch this glass slide with another (correct side only) creating a smear. Lastly, prepare properly labeled "air-dried" and "fixed" slides using the preferred fixative of your pathology department. Nipple aspirate cytology is an assessment both of the adequacy of the specimen (minimum number of ductal epithelial cells per high-powered field) and an evaluation of the individual ductal cells.

Cytology of nipple aspirate has a low sensitivity for cancer (34%-46%).[59] Regardless of the results, further workup is still needed and includes an imaging evaluation of any abnormality identified on CBE, a recent diagnostic mammogram, and an ultrasound of the retroareolar area looking for a mass or dilated ducts. Masses or calcifications identified on mammogram or ultrasound will need an image-guided biopsy.

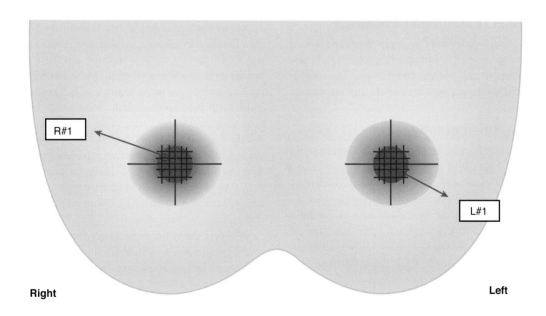

Right   **Left**

Location	Color	Spontaneous	Heme
Right #1	Yellow	No	Negative
Left #1	Brackish	Yes	Positive

FIGURE 12-2 Grid for documenting nipple discharge.

Induced (Expressed or Nonspontaneous) Discharge

Benign nipple fluid can be expressed for the majority of women and requires only reassurance. Induced nipple discharge arising from multiple ducts is considered physiologic, may have varying colors, and does not need any further treatment if the CBE and imaging were negative. If the mammogram or ultrasound demonstrate multiple dilated ducts (duct ectasia) with or without debris, no biopsy is needed, but she should be followed on a short-term basis for change. Duct ectasia typically occurs in perimenopausal and postmenopausal women and may be related to changing hormonal levels. Controversy exists around whether duct ectasia is associated with breast pain or periductal mastititis.[58,60] Regardless it is a benign condition that requires no surgical intervention.

Galactorrhea and Pregnancy-Related Discharge

Bilateral multiple ducts producing a skim-milk discharge is called galactorrhea. After eliminating pregnancy as the cause, perform a careful drug history. Many medications such as psychotropics, antihypertensives, gastrointestinal drugs, anesthetics, amphetamines, marijuana, and estrogens can elevate serum prolactin levels.[61] A prolactin level above 1000 mU/L in the absence of any drug cause should prompt a workup for pituitary adenoma.[58] Other causes of increased prolactin include bronchogenic carcinomas, hypothyroidism, head trauma, encephalitis, and hypothalamic tumors. Pregnant or lactating women can also have a nipple discharge due to the hypervascularity of the developing breast tissue; this discharge may even be bloody but requires no further therapy.

Spontaneous (Pathologic) Discharge

A spontaneous, persistent bloody or clear discharge arising from a single duct without signs of mastitis requires an invasive diagnostic procedure to rule out the small chance the etiology is cancerous. Other secretions do not need any intervention.

Ductogram/Ductography

A preoperative ductogram can be obtained demonstrating the ductal anatomy and hopefully a filling defect suggestive of a papilloma (the most common cause of a bloody discharge). Similar to cytology, a negative or benign ductogram does not preclude surgical excision of the offending duct. A potential pitfall of a ductogram is that the contrast agent used for the imaging study can solidify on drying and act as a plug, preventing future discharge. Reproduction of the nipple discharge later at surgery will be imperative if the correct duct is to be excised. A useful tip is to have the woman apply clear nail polish to her nipple every few days. This will prevent any interim leakage of fluid, increasing the chances the duct will be identified at surgery. This is also a helpful technique if the nipple discharge is self-reported but not reproducible by you. If the CBE and imaging are otherwise negative, she should follow up in 1 month for a reexamination. Just remember to remove the nail polish when trying to elicit the discharge.

Duct Excision, Ductoscopy, Ductal Lavage

At surgery, lacrimal probes or intraoperative intraductal injection of methylene blue can be used to guide removal of the correct duct. Our preferred method includes a preoperative ductogram on the day of surgery that is a 50:50 mixture of contrast material and methylene blue dye. The radiograph will identify the direction the offending duct is traveling, the branch pattern of the duct, and the distance from the orifice to any filling defect. This helps in planning the surgical incision, intraoperative identification of the duct, and the required length of duct to be excised. Alternatively, ductoscopy, a relatively new procedure, can be utilized; it has the potential to be both diagnostic and therapeutic. Ductal lavage is mostly used as a risk-assessment tool in women at high risk for the future development for breast cancer.

Failed Duct Localization

The purpose of a duct excision is to prove the etiology is *not* cancer, albeit a small chance. There is an equally small chance on the day of surgery that the offending duct cannot be identified. In this scenario, we do not advocate performing a central duct excision. Instead, a breast MRI can be obtained to look at the nipple and retroareolar space. If no abnormality is noted, then serially follow the woman at 3-month intervals with repeat imaging, such as ultrasounds, and CBE, noting if any further episodes of spontaneous bloody discharge occur. This pattern should continue for 1 year.

NIPPLE CHANGE

Nipple Inversion

Nipple inversion and nipple retraction are often used interchangeably, but they are not one and the same. Nipple inversion is when the tip of the nipple folds inwardly on itself, and is usually a benign process (3% association with cancer).[62] Some women develop with one or both nipples inverted, posing a problem later in life with breastfeeding. Acquired nipple inversion most commonly is a result of duct ectasia or periductal mastitis. Infrequently it is the result of cancer or tuberculosis.[58] The history and physical exam should document how long it has been present, associations with any other clinical breast findings including a good look at the entire nipple by everting, and an inquiry into previous breast surgery involving the nipple. Incisions on the nipple heal relatively well and may be hard to see.

Whether this is the presenting symptom or not, the imaging investigation should include a mammogram and a retroareolar ultrasound looking for cancer. Benign findings need no further investigation or treatment. Suspicious findings warrant a biopsy.

Nipple Retraction

Nipple retraction can be subtle and only involve a portion of the nipple. The result is a tilting or slanting of the nipple projection to the contralateral side. When the whole nipple is involved, the base of the nipple is retracted into the breast parenchyma and the surrounding areola sidewalls may spill over, giving an inversion appearance. Nipple retraction is usually quite frightening to the woman, and she will quickly present to your office for fear of cancer. Her fears are justified in that the etiology of retraction is cancer until proven otherwise. It is important to identify any previous breast surgery, especially a prior duct excision. After a complete history and physical exam, perform a mammogram and retroareolar ultrasound. An ultrasound is needed because CBE and mammography are not as sensitive at looking at the nipple or retroareolar space as are ultrasound and MRI.[62,63] Suspicious lesions identified must be biopsied. If no abnormality is found on imaging, then get a breast MRI. Again biopsy any abnormality found. If still negative but your clinical suspicion is high, then proceed with an open incisional biopsy.

Skin Change (Crusting, Excoriation)

When evaluating skin changes of the nipple it is important to separate the nipple from the areolar disk. The areolar disk is a skin appendage and is subject to all the conditions that can affect the skin elsewhere—contact dermatitis, eczema, psoriasis, yeast infections, inflammation, or abcess of the Montgomery glands. Discern where the rash began. In the conditions mentioned, the rash begins on the areolar disk and then extends onto the nipple. Treat the underlying etiology.

Skin changes limited to or beginning on the nipple are more concerning. The history and physical exam should provide details about a history of nipple discharge, long-standing nipple inversion, pain, associated breast masses, or recent signs of infection. Women with a history of induced nipple discharge, especially if they have nipple inversion, can get a crusty yellow film over the nipple tip. Other women can have scaly dry heaped-up skin or dried purulent discharge from mastitis on the nipple surface.

The most concerning abnormality is Paget disease of the breast. Paget disease is composed of cancerous ductal cells overflowing the nipple ducts onto the exterior surface of the nipple skin akin to a volcano spewing lava. The woman presents with a recent history of a crusty excoriated nipple tip that progresses down the nipple with time. The nipple can be subtly changed or look quite angry. The rest of the CBE is usually negative. Imaging should include a mammogram looking for calcifications and a retroareolar ultrasound looking for a mass. These abnormalities will need biopsy. As for the nipple, a scraping of the nipple (look for yeast via KOH staining) may help, but usually a biopsy of the nipple will be needed to prove Paget disease. Paget disease of the nipple is also discussed in Chapter 19.

Nipple Mass

Small frond-like protrusions from the nipple tip can represent nipple duct adenomas or papillomas and are benign. They can bleed, which is what prompts medical attention. Local excision may be necessary. Leiomyoma of the nipple proper is a rare, benign neoplasm that usually present as persistant pain and tenderness of the nipple.[64] The CBE may reveal a mass within the nipple, but more commonly the nipple feels thicker than normal. Imaging will consist of an ultrasound but the ultrasound

needs to be performed tangentially on the long axis of the nipple to assure adequate visualization. Surgical management may be required for palliation of pain.

UNILATERAL BREAST ENLARGEMENT (ASYMMETRY)

Breast asymmetry is a heterogenous group of conditions often presenting to a breast or plastic surgeon. The first historical reference to breast asymmetry was by the Ancient Greeks, when Pythagoras proposed the golden ratio (1:0.68) for asymmetry for esthetic appeal between different body parts including the breasts.[65] Patients presenting with such complaints should be treated with compassion, and reassurance plays an important role in their management. Relevant features on the history including risk factors for breast cancer should be ascertained. The physical examination should evaluate for the presence of a mass, which can often masquerade as an asymmetry, and must include a comprehensive evaluation of the spine, shoulder girdle, and chest wall. Documentation of breast asymmetry can be performed using photographic images and measurements of the breast and chest wall including ptosis. The bra cup size is a measure that most patients know and is a rough guide of asymmetry. Newer imaging modalities including lasers to scan the surface, and volumetric assessment using mammograms and 3-dimentional (3D) imaging technology, promise to make the measurement of asymmetry more objective.[66] The different components of asymmetry needing evaluation include breast mound volume, position of the inframammary fold, presence of base–diameter constriction, and symmetry and position of the nipple–areola complex. Management of asymmetries varies depending on the etiology of the breast asymmetry, but a morphologic working classification might enable better management.[67]

Bilateral asymmetric hypertrophy and unilateral hypertrophy are the most common conditions reported in the literature causing breast asymmetry.[68] After documenting asymmetry, management can range from reassurance to esthetic surgery such as reduction mammaplasty. The use of bromocriptine has been suggested for unilateral hypertrophy including juvenile mammary hypertrophy and pregnancy-related hypertrophy.[69] However, when hypertrophy is associated with hypoplasia or amastia on the contralateral side, the management is more complicated and includes a reduction mammaplasty with contralateral breast augmentation. Rare conditions such as Poland syndrome (absence of sternal head of pectoralis and other muscles, lack of subcutaneous fat and axillary hair, brachysynphalangism) can present with breast asymmetry that often requires myocutaneous flap reconstruction. Tuberous breast deformity, one of the important causes for breast asymmetry, features a constricted breast base, a constricted skin envelope, a reduction in the volume of breast parenchyma, an abnormal elevation of the inframammary fold, and herniation of the breast parenchyma into the areola. Treatment for this cause of asymmetry requires detailed planning with a plastic surgeon and potentially multiple operations. Finally, the major morphologic group of breast asymmetries includes unilateral breast ptosis, which may be idiopathic or associated with a mass such as a giant fibroadenoma or phyllodes tumor; the treatment includes elimination of the cause, a mastopexy, and an augmentation mammaplasty to achieve symmetry. Causes of asymmetry arising from scoliosis and chest wall deformities have been described and are best addressed by a neurosurgeon or orthopedic surgeon.[70]

Breast asymmetry has also been suggested in association with breast cancer development in healthy women.[71] While this association is weak, it should prompt clinicians to perform a comprehensive history and physical examination, including risk assessment, before offering any surgical procedure for asymmetry correction.

AXILLARY ADENOPATHY

The axilla is a pyramidal compartment between the chest wall and the upper extremity containing the majority of the breast lymphatic drainage. These lymph node groups are identified in 6 groups at 3 anatomic levels that are difficult to discern on physical examination. The 6 groups include the lateral group (posterior and lateral to the axillary vein), the anterior group (positioned along the lower border of the pectoralis muscle), the posterior group (against the subscapularis), the central group (in the fat of the axilla), the subclavicular or upper pectoral group, and the interpectoral group (Rotter nodes). Examination of the axilla, as mentioned earlier, is an integral part of the CBE. The clinical accuracy of the physical examination to detect a pathologic lymph node is fairly low (15%-60%), with a specificity of 68% reported in some series.[72,73]

A palpable lymph node always requires further evaluation in the setting of breast abnormalities, although a detailed history should note systemic conditions that cause lymphadenopathy such as lymphoma, human immunodeficiency virus (HIV), infectious mononucleosis, and tuberculosis.

Diagnosis of the Palpable Axillary Lymph Node

Fine-Needle Aspiration

Fine needle aspiration (FNA) cytology of an axillary lymph node is the simplest and best diagnostic test for a palpable lymph node, but should only be performed after an imaging study (ultrasound) has documented the lymph node characteristics. Cytology is reasonably accurate in the diagnosis of metastatic breast cancer and can differentiate lymphoma, melanoma, other skin cancers, and accessory breast tissue. The presence of necrotic material on an FNA may indicate a necrotizing infection. Although uncommon, this should be sent off for acid-fast bacilli staining. The sensitivity of ultrasound-guided FNA for lymph nodes ranges from 36% to 86.4%, the specificity ranges from 95.7% to 100%, the positive predictive value ranges from 92% to 100%, and the negative predictive value ranges from 67% to 70%.[74-75]

Core Needle Biopsy

Core needle biopsy for an axillary lymph node is equivalent to FNA in diagnostic capability but the risks of bleeding or injury to adjacent structures is greater. Core biopsies are used for low-lying axillary nodes and when a lymphoma diagnosis could not be made on flow cytometry of the FNA.

Ultrasound

The sonographic evaluation of the axilla is variable, like the CBE, and the sensitivity of the axillary lymph node status ranges from 35% to 82%; specificity ranges from 73% to 97.9%.[75,76] Suspicious features of a lymph node include cortical thickening, circular shape, size larger than 10 mm, absence of fatty hilum, and a hypoechoic internal echo. The overall accuracy of ultrasound varies, thus mandating histologic confirmation to rule out cancer.

Magnetic Resonance Imaging

The current role of MRI in the evaluation of the axilla is uncertain due to low sensitivity and specificity and should be used for research purposes only. Studies have relied on the use of size and morphologic characteristics to determine the potential for axillary metastasis.[77] Use of ultra-small iron superoxide contrast agents for the MRI may increase both sensitivity and specificity for metastatic disease.[78]

Evaluation of Axillary Adenopathy with an Unknown Primary

Axillary presentation of an unknown primary breast cancer is an uncommon condition (0.3%-1.0% of patients with breast cancer).[79] Originally described by Halsted in 1907 in his series of 3 cases, the evaluation of such a patient begins with a careful history and physical examination.[80] Diagnosis with FNA or core needle biopsy confirms the diagnosis of metastatic cancer with a breast primary based on special staining. To identify the primary, a diagnostic mammogram is performed but has low yield (7%-29%).[81] Ultrasound has no role in diagnosis. MRI is currently the recommended imaging modality to evaluate the breast with metastatic carcinoma in the axilla by the National Comprehensive Cancer Network.[82] An identification rate of 70% to 86% of tumors has been reported, allowing a clinician to offer breast-conserving therapy in 37% to 41% of the women.[83] PET scanning remains investigational for diagnosing the primary, although occult breast cancer detected by PET scan has been reported.[84]

ACCESSORY BREAST TISSUE

Accessory mammary tissue occurs due to failure of regression of breast tissue along the milk line in 2% to 6% of the population and may be associated with an autosomal dominant genetic defect linked to familial syndromes including the multiple neoplasia syndromes.[85,86] It is termed *supernumerary breasts* if found along the milk line (axilla to the groin) or as aberrant breast tissue if in a different position. If associated with a nipple, the person has polymastia with polythelia. This ectopic breast tissue undergoes hormonal changes like normal breasts, and can present as a mass during pregnancy/lactation, the most commons locations being the axilla and vulva (55%-65%).[87,88] This tissue can be mistaken for hidradenitis or develop benign (lipomas, fibroadenomas, and phyllodes tumors) or malignant tumors.[89] The propensity for malignant transformation may be due to retained secretions in the duct.[90] Diagnosis of accessory breast tissue is made by core biopsy or excisional biopsy performed for a presenting mass.

The management of accessory breast tissue is variable, especially if asymptomatic. Given the lack of effective screening of this accessory tissue, we recommend excision in high-risk patients. If not, routine CBE should include these nonpectoral breast tissues. Suspicious lesions must be biopsied. Treatment of invasive cancer in the accessory breast tissue is with surgery and lymph node assessment; some series report an 11% incidence of axillary metastasis.[91] Staging and the use of adjuvant radiation and hormone therapy are controversial.[92]

ABNORMAL IMAGING WITHOUT SIGNS OR SYMPTOMS

Patients often present with abnormal findings on annual imaging but with a normal CBE or self-exam. A detailed history and physical examination, review of the abnormal imaging, and risk assessment should be performed. Concordance between the imaging and the physical examination or between different imaging modalities is important and the radiologist is an essential part of the clinical team. The BIRADS (Breast Imaging Reporting and Dated System) is the communication tool used by radiologists to standardize reporting in mammography that has now been expanded to both ultrasound and MRI.[93]

MAMMOGRAPHY

Abnormalities on mammography currently account for the largest proportion of patients presenting to a breast practitioner given the large-scale application of this effective screening tool. On presentation with an abnormal report, one must interpret the lexicon and act accordingly after verifying concordance. The BIRADS 4 category often remains the equivocal category, where prediction of malignancy is still poorly defined. Currently when faced with a BIRADS 4 or higher abnormality that is nonpalpable, one must proceed with an image-guided biopsy (stereotactic core, ultrasound core, or wire-localized excisional biopsy). Pathologic results dictate the further course of care. BIRADS 3 lesions should be biopsied in high-risk women, such as genetic carriers, or if the woman is extremely anxious about knowing definitive results.

ULTRASONOGRAPHY

BIRADS classification for ultrasound has recently been advocated but does not have as much supportive data as for mammography.[94] An abnormality on mammography should be confirmed with the anatomic position on sonogram, and any abnormality must be seen on 2 orthogonal slices irrespective of compression. The BIRADS classification has prognostic value, with the BIRADS 2 having a 2% risk of malignancy; BIRADS 5 has a 95% risk.[95] BIRADS 3 and 4 have variable risk of malignancy

described in the literature, but the concordance of 2 different imaging modalities can strengthen conclusions drawn.[96]

MRI

The use of MRI in breast imaging is fairly recent and is not recommended for screening. The use of dedicated breast coils is mandatory. Again, the BIRADS lexicon will be assigned to each exam and any BIRADS 4 or 5 abnormalities need biopsy. If the abnormality is not seen on the mammogram to correspond with the MRI, a focused ultrasound should be attempted, hoping to identify the MRI abnormality. If the abnormality is only seen on MRI, then an MRI-guided biopsy will be needed.

CLINICAL TRIALS

Breast problems are very common and fortunately most are benign. As such, investigation is needed into the pathophysiology behind benign breast disease, especially mastalgia, to guide prevention and targeted therapies. Imaging modalities need to be refined (such as elastography for ultrasound) to allow better discrimination within the BIRADS 4 lexicon and better selection of who needs a diagnostic biopsy. Perhaps serum tests looking at protein profiles or immuno-antibodies will complement the BIRADS lexicon and thus further reduce the need for biopsy.

SUMMARY

New patient evaluation involves obtaining a thorough history and physical examination of the whole person, not just the breast, in a patient, supportive manner. At the end of the day, most women will have benign findings but this encounter is very important for her future. Since her risk of breast cancer increases with age, you want her to seek attention promptly for changes on self-exam or CBE and you want her to be compliant with screening guidelines.

Abnormal imaging generates fear in most women. The use of standardized reporting scales, such as BIRADS, is encouraged in general practice and hopefully will be evidence-based even for the newer imaging modalities. Concordance between CBE and imaging and between radiologists' interpretations is vital. Any discordance should prompt a detailed review. BIRAD 4 or 5 imaging studies, or suspicious clinical findings despite negative imaging, require biopsy. Concordance between imaging and pathology is equally imperative.

REFERENCES

1. Smith RA, Saslow D, Andrews Sawyer K, et al. American Cancer Society Guidelines for Breast Cancer Screening: Update 2003. *CA Cancer J Clin.* 2003;53:141-169.
2. McDonald S, Saslow D, Alciati MH. Performance and reporting of clinical breast examination: a review of the literature. *CA Cancer J Clin.* 2004;54:345-361.
3. Pennypacker HS, Naylor L, Sander AA, Goldstein MK. Why can't we do better breast examinations? *Nurse Pract Forum.* 1999;10:122-128.
4. Pennypacker HS, Pilgrim CA. Achieving competence in clinical breast examination. *Nurse Pract Forum.* 1993;4:85-90.

5. Saslow D, Hannan J, Osuch J, et al. Clinical breast examination: practical recommendations for optimizing performance and reporting. *CA Cancer J Clin.* 2004;54:327-344.

6. Pugh CM, Salud LH. Fear of missing a lesion: Use of simulated breast models to decrease student anxiety when learning clinical breast examinations. *Am J Surg.* 2007;193:766-770.

7. Steiner E, Austin DF, Prouser, NC. Detection and description of small breast masses by residents trained using a standardized clinical breast exam curriculum. *J Gen Int Med.* 2008;23:129-134.

8. Campbell HS, Fletcher SW, Pilgrim CA, et al. Improving physicians' and nurses' clinical breast examination: a randomized controlled trial. *Am J Prev Med.* 1991;7:1-8.

9. Padden DL. Mastalgia: Evaluation and Management. *Nurse Pract Forum.* 2000;11:213-218.

10. Pye JK, Mansel RE, Hughes LE. Clinical experience of drug treatments for mastalgia. *Lancet.* 1985;2:373-377.

11. Gateley CA, Miers M, Mansel RE, Hughes LE. Drug treatments for mastalgia: 17 years experience in the Cardiff mastalgia clinic. *J R Soc Med.* 1992;85:12-15.

12. Rosolowich V, Saettler E, Szuck B, et al. Mastalgia. *J Obstet Gynaecol Can.* 2006;28:49-71.

13. Ernster VL, Goodson WH III, Hunt TX, et al. Vitamin E and benign breast "disease": a double-blind, randomized clinical trial. *Surgery.* 1985;97:490-494.

14. Srivastava A, Mansel RE, Arvind N, et al. Evidence-based management of mastalgia: a meta-analysis of randomized trials. *Breast.* 2007;16:503-512.

15. Steinbrunn BS, Zera RT, Rodriquez JL. Mastalgia. Tailoring treatment to type of breast pain. *Postgrad Med.* 1997;102:183-198.

16. Maddox PR, Harrison BJ, Mansel RE, Hughes LE. Non-cyclical mastalgia: an improved classification and treatment. *Br J Surg.* 1989;76:901-904.

17. Hou MF, Huang CJ, Huang YS, et al. Mondor's disease in the breast. *Kaoshiung J Med Sci.* 1999;15:632-639.

18. Hou MF, Hwang CH, Chan HM, et al. Mondor's disease of the breast—3 case reports. *Gaoxiong Yi Xue Ke Xue Za Zhi.* 1992;8:231-235.

19. Blum C, Baker M. Venous congestion of the breast mimicking inflammatory breast cancer: case report and review of the literature. *Breast J.* 2008;14:97-101.

20. Onseler B, Ozcan UA, Rasa K, Cizmell OM. Treatment of breast abscesses with ultrasound-guided aspiration and irrigation in the emergency setting. *Emerg Radiol.* 2008;15:105-108.

21. Ulitzsch D, Nyman MK, Carlson RA. Breast abscesses in lactating women: ultrasound-guided treatment. *Radiology.* 2004;232:904-909.

22. Dixon JM. Periductal mastitis / duct ectasia. *World J Surg.* 1999;13:715-720.

23. Furlong AJ, al-Nakib L, Knox WF, et al. Periductal inflammation and cigarette smoke. *J Am Coll Surg.* 1994;179:417-420.

24. Ammarri FF, Yaghan RJ, Omari AC. Periductal mastitis. Clinical characteristics and outcome. *Saudi Med J.* 2002;23:819-922.

25. Lannin DR. Twenty-two year experience with recurring subareolar abscess and lactiferous duct fistula treated by a single surgeon. *Am J Surg.* 2004;188:401-410.

26. Barlow WE, Lehman CD, Zheng Y, et al. Performance of diagnostic mammography for women with signs of symptoms of breast cancer. *J Natl Cancer Inst.* 2002;94:1151-1159.

27. Ariga R, Bloom K, Reddy VB, et al. Fine-needle aspiration of clinically suspicious palpable breast masses with histopathologic correlation. *Am J Surg.* 2002;184:410-413.

28. Cardenosa G. Cysts, cystic lesions, and papillary lesions. *Ultrasound Clin.* 2007;1:617-629.

29. Hogge JP, Robinson RE, Magnant CM, Zuurbier RA. The mammographic spectrum of fat necrosis of the breast. *Radiographics.* 1995;15:1347-1356.

30. Park CA, David LR, Argenta LC. Breast asymmetry: presentation of a giant fibroadenoma. *Breast J.* 2006;12:451-461.

31. Morrow M, Wong S, Vena L. The evaluation of breast masses in women younger than forty years of age. *Surgery.* 1998;124:634-640.

32. Vargas HI, Vargas PM, Eldrageely K, et al. Outcomes of surgical and sonographic assessment of breast masses in women younger than 30. *Am Surg.* 2005;71:716-719.

33. Belkac Y, Bousquet G, Marsiglia H, et al. Phyllodes tumor of the breast. *Int J Radiat Oncol Biol Phys.* 2008;7:492-500.

34. Hoda SA, Rosen PP. Observations on the pathologic diagnosis of selected unusual lesions in needle core biopsies of breast. *Breast J.* 2004;10:522-527.

35. Honda M, Mori Y, Nishi T, et al. Diabetic mastopathy of bilateral breasts in an elderly Japanese woman with type 2 diabetes: a case report and a review of the literature in Japan. *Int Med.* 2007;46:1573-1576.

36. Thorncroft K, Forsyth L, Desmond S, Audisio RA. The diagnosis and management of diabetic mastopathy. *Breast J.* 2007;13:607-613.

37. Ferreira M, Albarracin CT, Resetkova E. Pseudoangiomatous stromal hyperplasia tumor: a clinical, radiologic and pathologic study of 26 cases. *Modern Pathol.* 2008;21:201-207.

38. Nash H, Elieff MP, Kronz JD, Argani P. Pseudoangiomatous stromal hyperplasia (PASH) of the breast with foci of morphologic malignancy: a case of PASH with malignant transformation? *Int J Surg Pathol.* Published online July 8, 2008. http://ijsp.sagepub.com. Accessed August 27, 2008.

39. Taira N, Aogi K, Ohsumi S, et al. Epidermal inclusion cyst of the breast. *Breast Cancer.* 2007;14:434-437.

40. Pojchamarnwiputh S, Muttarak M, Na-ChiangMai W, Chaiwun B. Benign breast lesions mimicking carcinoma at mammography. *Singapore Med J.* 2007;48:958-967.

41. Aouni NE, Laurent I, Terrier P, et al. Granular cell tumor of the breast. *Diagn Cytopathol.* 2007;35:725-727.

42. Aouni NE, Balleyguier C, Mansouri D, et al. Adenosis tumor of the breast: cytological and radiological features of a case confirmed by histology. *Diagn Cytopathol.* 2008;36:496-498.

43. Wells CA, El-Ayat GA. Non-operative breast pathology: apocrine lesions. *J Clin Pathol.* 2007;60:1313-1320.

44. Bezic J, Forempoher G, Poljicanin A, Gunjaca G. Apocrine adenoma of the breast coexistent with invasive carcinoma. *Pathol Res Pract.* 2007;203:809-812.

45. Moon HG, Jung EJ, Park ST. Breast sparganosis presenting as a breast mass with vague migrating pain. *J Am Coll Surg.* 2008;207:292.

46. Uchida N, Yokoo H, Kuwano H. Schwannoma of the breast: report of a case. *Surg Today.* 2005;35:238-242.

47. Son, EJ, Oh KK, Kim EK. Pregnancy-associated breast disease: radiologic features and diagnostic dilemmas. *Yonsei Med J.* 2006;47:34-42.

48. Rosenfield Darling ML, Smith DN, Rhei E, et al. Lactating adenoma: sonographic features. *Breast J.* 2000;6:252-256.

49. Goldberg J, Baute L, Storey L, Park P. Granulomatous mastitis in pregnancy. *Obstet Gynecol.* 2000;96:813-815.

50. Mesurolle B, Sygal V, Lalonde L, et al. Sonographic and mammographic appearances of breast hemangioma. *Am J Roentgenol.* 2008;191.W17-W22.

51. Luh SP, Chang KJ, Cheng JH, et al. Surgical treatment for primary mammary tuberculosis-report of three octogenarian cases and review of literature. *Breast J.* 2008;14:311-312.

52. Neuman HB, Brogi E, Ebrahim A, et al. Desmoid tumors (fibromatoses) of the breast: a 25-year experience. *Ann Surg Oncol.* 2007;15:274-280.

53. Hines SL, Tan W, Larson JM, et al. Evaluation of breast masses in older men. *Geriatrics.* 2008;63:19-24.

54. Niewoehner CB, Schorer AE. Gynaecomastia and breast cancer in men. *BMJ.* 2008;336:709-713.

55. Braunstein GD. Gynecomastia. *N Engl J Med.* 2007;357:1229-1237.

56. Yang W, Dempsey PJ. Diagnostic breast ultrasound: Current status and future directions. *Radiol Clin North Am.* 2007;45:845-861.

57. Patterson SK, Helvie MA, Aziz K, Nees AV. Outcome of men presenting with clinical breast problems: the role of mammography and ultrasound. *Breast J.* 2006;12:418-423.

58. Dixon JM, Bundred NJ. Management of disorders of the ductal system and infections. In: Harris JR, Lippman ME, Morrow M, Osborne CK, eds. *Diseases of the Breast.* 2nd ed. Philadelphia, PS: Lippincott Williams & Wilkins, 2000:47-55.

59. Ambrogetti D, Berni D, Catarzi S, Ciatto S. The role of ductal galactography in the differential diagnosis of breast carcinoma. *Radiol Med (Torino).* 1996;91:198-201.

60. Peters F, Diemer P, Mecks O, Behnken L. Severity of mastalgia in relation to milk duct dilatation. *Obstet Gynecol.* 2003;101:54-60.

61. Lang JE, Kuerer HM. Breast ductal secretions: clinical features, potential uses, and possible applications. *Cancer Control.* 2007;14:350-359.

62. Kalbhen CL, Kezdi-Rogus PC, Dowling MP, Flisak ME. Mammography in the evaluation of nipple inversion. *Am J Roentgenol.* 1998;17:117-121.

63. Da Costa D, Taddese A, Cure ML, et al. Common and unusual diseases of the nipple-areolar complex. *Radiographics.* 2007 Oct(suppl):S65–S77.

64. Ku J, Campbell C, Bennett I. Leiomyoma of the nipple. *Breast J.* 2006;12:377-380.

65. Amoric M. The golden number: applications to cranio-facial evaluation. *Funct Orthod.* 1995;12:18-25.

66. Losken A, Fishman I, Denson DD, et al. An objective evaluation of breast symmetry and shape differences using 3-dimensional images. *Ann Plast Surg.* 2005;55:571-575.

67. Araco A, Gravante G, Araco F, et al. Breast asymmetries: a brief review and our experience. *Aesthetic Plast Surg.* 2006;30:309-319.

68. Rohrich RJ, Hartley W, Brown S. Incidence of breast and chest wall asymmetry in breast augmentation: a retrospective analysis of 100 patients. *Plast Reconstr Surg.* 2006;118:7S,13S; discussion 14S, 15S–17S.

69. Arscott GD, Craig HR, Gabay L. Failure of bromocriptine therapy to control juvenile mammary hypertrophy. *Br J Plast Surg.* 2001;54: 720-723.
70. Iliopoulos P, Korovessis P, Koureas G, et al. Asymmetric evolution of anterior chest wall blood supply in female adolescents with progressive right-convex thoracic idiopathic scoliosis. *Eur Spine J.* 2007;16:1343-1347.
71. Scutt D, Lancaster GA, Manning JT. Breast asymmetry and predisposition to breast cancer. *Breast Cancer Res.* 2006;8:R14.
72. de Freitas R Jr., Costa MV, Schneider SV, et al. Accuracy of ultrasound and clinical examination in the diagnosis of axillary lymph node metastases in breast cancer. *Eur J Surg Oncol.* 1991;17:240-244.
73. van Rijk MC, Deurloo EE, Nieweg OE, et al. Ultrasonography and fine-needle aspiration cytology can spare breast cancer patients unnecessary sentinel lymph node biopsy. *Ann Surg Oncol.* 2006;13:31-35.
74. Krishnamurthy S, Sneige N, Bedi DG, et al. Role of ultrasound-guided fine-needle aspiration of indeterminate and suspicious axillary lymph nodes in the initial staging of breast carcinoma. *Cancer.* 2002;95:982-988.
75. Ciatto S, Brancato B, Risso G, et al. Accuracy of fine needle aspiration cytology (FNAC) of axillary lymph nodes as a triage test in breast cancer staging. *Breast Cancer Res Treat.* 2007;103:85-91.
76. Davis JT, Brill YM, Simmons S, et al. Ultrasound-guided fine-needle aspiration of clinically negative lymph nodes versus sentinel node mapping in patients at high risk for axillary metastasis. *Ann Surg Oncol.* 2006;13: 1545-1552.
77. Mameri CS, Kemp C, Goldman SM, et al. Impact of breast MRI on surgical treatment, axillary approach, and systemic therapy for breast cancer. *Breast J.* 2008;14:236-244.
78. Harada T, Tanigawa N, Matsuki M, et al. Evaluation of lymph node metastases of breast cancer using ultrasmall superparamagnetic iron oxide-enhanced magnetic resonance imaging. *Eur J Radiol.* 2007;63:401-407.
79. Fitts WT, Steiner GC, Enterline HT. Prognosis of occult carcinoma of the breast. *Am J Surg.* 1963;106:460-463.
80. Halsted WS. The results of radical operations for the cure of carcinoma of the breast. *Ann Surg.* 1907;46:1-19.
81. Baron PL, Moore MP, Kinne DW, et al. Occult breast cancer presenting with axillary metastases. Updated management. *Arch Surg.* 1990;125:210-214.
82. National Comprehensive Cancer Network. NCCN Clinical Practice Guidelines in Oncology Breast Cancer (Version 2.2008) © 2009 National Comprehensive Cancer network, Inc, Available at: NCCN.org. Accessed [8/21/2008].
83. Olson JA Jr., Morris EA, Van Zee KJ, et al. Magnetic resonance imaging facilitates breast conservation for occult breast cancer. *Ann Surg Oncol.* 2000; 7: 411-415.
84. Takabatake D, Taira N, Aogi K, et al. Two cases of occult breast cancer in which PET-CT was helpful in identifying primary tumors. *Breast Cancer.* 2008;15:181-184.
85. Osborne MP. Breast anatomy and development. In: Harris JR, Lippman ME, Morrow M, Osborne CK, eds. *Diseases of the Breast.* 2nd ed. Philadelphia, PA: Lippincott Williams & Wilkins; 2000:1-3.
86. Cohen PR, Kurzrock R. Miscellaneous genodermatoses: Beckwith-Wiedemann syndrome, Birt-Hogg-Dube syndrome, familial atypical multiple mole melanoma syndrome, hereditary tylosis, incontinentia pigmenti, and supernumerary nipples. *Dermatol Clin.* 1995;13:211-229.
87. Caceres M, Shih J, Eckert M, Gardner R. Metaplastic carcinoma in an ectopic breast. *South Med J.* 2002;95:462-466.
88. Shin SJ, Sheikh FS, Allenby PA, Rosen PP. Invasive secretory (juvenile) carcinoma arising in ectopic breast tissue of the axilla. *Arch Pathol Lab Med.* 2001;125:1372-1374.
89. Tresserra F, Grases PJ, Izquierdo M, et al. Fibroadenoma phyllodes arising in vulvar supernumerary breast tissue: report of two cases. *Int J Gynecol Pathol.* 1998;17:171-173.
90. Bland KI, Romrell LJ. *The Breast: Comprehensive Management of Benign and Malignant Diseases.* Philadelphia, PA: Saunders; 1991:69-86.
91. Rao KV, Tikku I, Kapur BM, Chopra P. Invasive primary mucinous carcinoma of the skin. *Int Surg.* 1978;63:168-170.
92. Evans DM, Guyton DP. Carcinoma of the axillary breast. *J Surg Oncol.* 1995;59:190-195.
93. Liberman L, Menell JH. Breast imaging reporting and data system (BI-RADS). *Radiol Clin North Am.* 2002;40:409-430.
94. Mendelson EB, Berg WA, Merritt CR. Toward a standardized breast ultrasound lexicon, BI-RADS: ultrasound. *Semin Roentgenol.* 2001;36:217-225.
95. Dennis MA, Parker SH, Klaus AJ, et al. Breast biopsy avoidance: the value of normal mammograms and normal sonograms in the setting of a palpable lump. *Radiology.* 2001;219:186-191.
96. Levy L, Suissa M, Chiche JF, et al. BIRADS ultrasonography. *Eur J Radiol.* 2007;61:202-211.

CHAPTER 13

Initial AJCC Staging

C. Denise Ching
Stephen B. Edge
Savitri Krishnamurthy
S. Eva Singletary

Staging is the classification used to define the risk of cancer recurrence and mortality. Cancer staging is useful for assessing prognosis and defining care for individuals and for defining the changes in cancer incidence and outcome for populations. A number of classifications systems for defining the extent or "stage" of cancer are used worldwide, each with its own historical basis and purpose. Three systems are used widely in the United States: the Extent of Disease (EOD) system used by the National Cancer Institute Surveillance, Epidemiology, and End Results Program (SEER); the Summary Stage system used primarily by state cancer registries; and the Tumor, Node, Metastases (TNM) system. The EOD and Summary Stage systems are used by population registries primarily for the purpose of population cancer surveillance. These systems generally do not change over time, allowing evaluation of temporal changes in cancer incidence and presentation.

The TNM staging system is based on the major morphologic attributes of a tumor that determine its behavior: size of the primary tumor (T), presence and extent of regional lymph node involvement (N), and presence of distant metastases (M). It includes 4 classifications: clinical, pathologic, recurrence, and autopsy. Clinical classification (cTNM) is based on evidence that is gathered before initial treatment of the primary tumor, and is used to make local/regional treatment recommendations. It includes physical examination, imaging studies (including mammography and ultrasound), and pathologic examination of the breast or other tissues as appropriate (usually needle biopsies) to establish the diagnosis of breast cancer. Pathologic classification (pTNM) includes the results of clinical staging, as

modified by evidence obtained from surgery and from detailed pathologic examination of the primary tumor, lymph nodes, and distant metastases (if present). It is used to assess prognosis and to make recommendations for adjuvant treatment. Classification of a recurrent tumor (rTNM) includes all information available at the time when further treatment is needed for a tumor that has recurred after a disease-free interval. Autopsy classification (aTNM) is used for cancers discovered after the death of a patient, when the cancer was not detected prior to death.

TNM staging is the most clinically relevant staging system and is used primarily to support clinical decision-making and for evaluation of the effectiveness of treatment. Therefore, TNM undergoes periodic revision to maintain its clinical relevance. This allows incorporation of advances in the understanding of factors affecting cancer prognosis. The TNM system is maintained and revised by the American Joint Committee on Cancer (AJCC) and the Union Interanationale de Cancer Controle (UICC). These groups empanel disease-site expert teams that recommend changes to TNM and publish TNM revisions every 6 to 8 years. The sixth edition was effective for patients diagnosed after January 1, 2003. The next revision (the seventh edition) will be published in October 2009, to be effective for cancers diagnosed on or after January 1, 2010 and is described at the end of the chapter.

Earlier in 2000, a Breast Task Force consisting of 19 internationally known experts in breast cancer management was convened to recommend revisions for the breast cancer chapter of the sixth edition of the *AJCC Cancer Staging Manual*.[1] While the general standards for defining the tumor, nodes, and metastases were largely unchanged, major changes were made in the definition of lymph nodes with minimal involvement and for the classification of nodal metastases defined by the then-new technique of sentinel lymph node biopsy (SLNB).

Undoubtedly the most controversial change in this area is the assignment of a strict size criterion to distinguish isolated tumor cells (ITCs) from micrometastases. There are conflicting data about the clinical importance of these very small entities. With increasing numbers of patients being diagnosed with very small primary tumors and minimal lymph node involvement, answering this question is more important than ever. The majority of these patients, up to 75%,[2,3] may have no need for systemic therapy, but finding the cutoff point between this group and the 25% who will prove to have more aggressive disease has been problematic.

To facilitate the collection of clinical outcome data that would be comparable across studies, the sixth edition of the AJCC defined strict quantitative criteria to separate ITCs, micrometastases, and macrometastases. Has this strategy been successful over the ensuing 5 years? To some extent it has, but problems have surfaced.

In this chapter, we will provide a brief overview of the major changes in breast cancer classification in the sixth edition of the AJCC Cancer Staging Manual, followed by a review of recent papers examining clinical outcomes as a function of size of lymph node metastases. We will assess some of the problems

that have arisen in implementing these changes, and consider what the future might hold for breast cancer staging.

REVIEW OF MAJOR CHANGES FOR BREAST CANCER STAGING IN THE SIXTH EDITION OF THE *AJCC CANCER STAGING MANUAL*

The revised staging system for breast cancer adopted for the sixth edition, has been discussed in great detail elsewhere.[4-8] The definitions relating to tumor size are unchanged from the fifth edition. Definitions related to distant metastases are largely unchanged, except that the M1 classification no longer includes metastases to ipsilateral supraclavicular lymph nodes (reclassified as N3). Overall stage groupings are also largely unchanged, except that breast disease classified as T1-4/N3/M0 has been moved from stage IIIB to a new stage IIIC.

Changes related to method of detection, size, number, and location of regional lymph node metastases are summarized in Table 13-1. The changes related to the number and location of lymph node metastases were made to reflect published data and widespread clinical consensus. On the other hand, changes related to method of detection and size of metastasis are an innovative component in the sixth edition, in that they are directed toward the future collection of data about the clinical importance of these characteristics.

TABLE 13-1 Major Changes in Breast Cancer Staging Related to Detection, Size, Number, and Location of Lymph Node Metastases in the Sixth Edition of the *AJCC Cancer Staging Manual*

Changes Related to Method of Detection[a]
Identifiers have been added to indicate the method of detection of lymph node metastases:
   Sentinel lymph node dissection—(sn)
   Molecular techniques—(mol+) or (mol−)

Changes Related to Size of Regional Lymph Node Metastases
Micrometastases are distinguished from isolated tumor cells on the basis of size:
   Micrometastases are defined as tumor deposits larger than 0.2 mm but not larger than 2.0 mm and classified as pN1mi
   Isolated tumor cells are defined as tumor deposits not larger than 0.2 mm and classified as pN0

Changes Related to Number of Axillary Lymph Node Metastases
Major classifications of lymph node status are defined by the number of affected axillary lymph nodes:
   Metastases in 1 to 3 axillary lymph nodes are classified as pN1
   Metastases in 4 to 9 axillary lymph nodes are classified as pN2
   Metastases in 10 or more axillary lymph nodes are classified as pN3

Changes Related to Location of Regional Lymph Node Metastases
Metastases to the infraclavicular lymph nodes are classified as N3
Metastases to the internal mammary nodes are classified as pN1, N2/pN2, or N3/pN3, based on the size of the lesion and the presence or absence of concurrent axillary lymph node metastases
Metastases to the supraclavicular lymph nodes are classified as N3

---

[a]The identifiers (i+) and (i−) were used in the original published version of the sixth edition to indicate lesions that were identified by immunohistochemical staining (IHC) alone. To be consistent with the updated UICC classification, the identifier (i) is now used to indicate "isolated tumor cells," regardless of method of detection.[5]

Size of Axillary Lymph Node Metastases and Outcome

In the fifth edition of the *AJCC Cancer Staging Manual*,[9] micrometastases were defined as metastatic lesions no larger than 2.0 mm and recognized as clinically relevant. While many have hypothesized that there would be a lower size limit below which lesions would no longer be clinically important, there were insufficient data to test this hypothesis. To answer this need, the sixth edition defined a new size class called "isolated tumor cells" (ITCs) that were no larger than 0.2 mm and classified as pN0(i+). Micrometastases were redefined as lesions larger than 0.2 mm but no larger than 2.0 mm and classified as pN1mi. Importantly, this size classification is the only defining characteristic used in the AJCC classification. Method of staining (immunohistochemical [IHC] or hematoxylin & eosin [H&E]) and location of the metastases were not included in the definitions for micrometastases or ITCs. (In practice, virtually all ITCs are detected by IHC, but they may be verified by H&E staining. While it is technically possible that an ITC might be detected initially by H&E, it is unlikely.) Because of this strict, quantitative definition, it was hoped that subsequent studies examining the effects of small metastases on outcome could be more easily compared.

Nine studies published from 1993 to 2008 reported outcomes associated with micrometastases and/or ITCs in any axillary lymph node (Table 13-2).[10-18] In most studies published after 2003, the size criteria specified in the sixth edition were used, while precise definitions of ITCs and micrometastases varied in earlier studies. Although most of these studies are still not strictly comparable, they support the decision to classify ITCs as pN0, with 6 of 8 studies that looked at ITCs reporting no clinical importance. The results were mixed for micrometastases: of the 7 studies that looked at micrometastases, 4 reported a significant clinical impact and 3 reported no impact. Across all 9 studies, outcomes associated with ITCs and micrometastases were not consistently related to tumor size, follow-up time, or whether patients received systemic therapy.

Since the publication of the sixth edition, SLNB has become the treatment standard for a large percentage of breast cancer patients, especially those with minimal disease. Overall, patients with no metastases detected in the sentinel node are unlikely to have metastases in other nodes, while approximately 50% of patients with sentinel node metastases will prove to have additional lesions in the non-sentinel nodes. However, it appears that the probability for non-sentinel node metastases is in part a function of the size of the sentinel node lesion. Thus, very small lesions are less likely to predict for additional metastases, and should be associated with better outcomes. This is reflected in 6 studies published since 2004 that have reported no significant effect on local recurrence, relapse-free survival, distant metastasis-free survival, or overall survival in association with ITCs in the sentinel node (Table 13-3).[19-24] Note that several of these studies define ITCs as those lesions that are positive for IHC and negative for H&E, rather than measuring the lesions.

Although these data indicate that ITCs are probably not associated with poor outcomes, it is somewhat disappointing that the recent literature continues to be highly variable, especially with respect to the clinical relevance of micrometastases. Even though the size distinctions used to define ITCs and micrometastases in the sixth edition were highly specific, there have been problems in standardizing implementation.

Problems in Assessing Axillary Lymph Nodes

Sentinel Lymph Nodes: Problems with a New Technology

When the sixth edition of the *AJCC Cancer Staging Manual* was being formulated, SLNB for breast cancer patients was still in its final validation stages, and methods had not been (and still are not) standardized. With respect to SLNB, the sixth edition specified only that if this technique was used, then a descriptor (sn) was to be added to the pathologic classification. What has become clear in the last 5 years is that there is wide variation in how SLNB is implemented among different institutions.

In the pre-SLNB era, most patients, except those whose disease was very limited, received full axillary lymph node dissections, usually removing 10 or more nodes per patient. The standard was to bivalve the retrieved nodes, examining 1 or 2 H&E-stained sections per node. With SLNB, only those nodes believed to provide the primary lymphatic drainage from the identified tumor are harvested, typically only 1 or a few nodes per patient. However, these nodes are examined in much greater detail, using multiple sections per node and employing immunohistochemical staining instead of, or in addition to, H&E staining. Not surprisingly, the number of very small lesions detected has gone up dramatically, as approximately one-third of patients who are negative on H&E evaluation will be positive on serial sectioning and IHC staining.[25]

Unfortunately, the exact methodology for pathologic examination of the sentinel nodes differs from institution to institution, and sometimes from pathologist to pathologist. There are differences in the number of sections that are examined and the thickness of the sections. Some practitioners continue to use only H&E, others use IHC only in cases that are H&E negative or for certain types of cancers (eg, lobular cancer), and still others use IHC on all patients.

Practitioners also differ in whether a completion axillary lymph node dissection (ALND) should be recommended in patients with a finding limited to ITCs or micrometastases in the sentinel node. As many as 10% of patients with ITCs may have additional metastases in non-sentinel nodes,[26] and elaborate nomograms, based on characteristics of the metastatic lesion and of the primary tumor, are being constructed to better predict the possibility of additional non-sentinel metastasis.[27] Some feel that expanding the radiation field to include the axilla will provide sufficient control. In addition, results of a limited number of studies suggest that non-sentinel node metastases are unlikely in patients with sentinel node ITCs and very small primary tumors (T1a,b).[28-33]

Pending the availability of long-term outcome data from large ongoing clinical trials (ACOSOG Z0010, ACOSOG Z0011, ALMANAC, EORTC AMAROS, and IBCSG 23-01), patients and their physicians should discuss the risk of

TABLE 13-2 Outcomes Associated with Micrometastases and Isolated Tumor Cells in any Axillary Lymph Node[a]

Study	No. Patients	Median Follow-up (mo)	% Patients Receiving Adjuvant Chemotherapy	% Patients with Tumor Size > 2 cm	Size of Nodal Deposit	Outcome
Nasser et al, 1993[10]	159	132	0%	N A	≤ 0.2 mm	Survival rate comparable to those without occult metastasis
					> 0.2 mm	Recurrence, DFS, OS significantly worse than those without occult metastasis
Colpaert et al, 2001[11]	104	92	0%	50%	ITCs vs larger deposits, all < 2 mm	No significant correlation between either type of occult metastasis and prognostically important features of the primary tumor (eg, size and grade)
Cummings et al, 2002[12]	208	120	2%	38%	No mets ≤ 0.5 mm > 0.5 mm	80% DFS; 80% OS 75% DFS, RR = 1.17; 78% OS 48% DFS, RR = 7.98; 60% OS
Millis et al, 2002[13]	477	227	<1%	50%	IHC only (0.01-0.03 mm) vs H&E (0.01-2.9 mm) vs missed (1.8-10 mm)[b]	Overall survival and relapse-free survival not related to the presence of occult metastases, regardless of size
Umekita et al, 2002[14]	148	84	61%	58%	No mets < 0.1 mm	93% DFS; 96% OS 71% DFS; 76% OS
Susnick et al, 2004[15]	48	180	10%	0%	≤ 0.2 mm > 0.2 mm and ≤ 2.0 mm	OR for distant metastasis = 2.1 (p = 0.31) OR for distant metastasis = 9.5 (p = 0.04)
Kahn et al, 2006[16]	214	96	5%	45%	≤ 0.2 mm or node negative vs > 0.2 mm and ≤ 2mm	No significant difference between groups in OS or DFS
Chen et al, 2007[17]	209,720[c]	120	N A	22% 43%[d]	No mets < 2.0 mm > 2.0 mm	76% OS 71% OS 65% OS
Tan et al, 2008[18]	368	211	0%	33%	No mets ≤ 0.2 mm > 0.2 mm and ≤ 2 mm	DFS 81% DFS 64% DFS 41%

DFS, disease-free survival; H&E, hematoxylin and eosin; IC, invasive carcinoma; IHC, immunohistochemistry; ITC, isolated tumor cells; met, metastasis; OR, odds ratio; OS, overall survival; RR, relative risk.
[a]As defined in the sixth edition of the *AJCC Cancer Staging Manual,* micrometastasis are defined as axillary metastases larger than 0.2 mm but no larger than 2.0 mm. Isolated tumor cells are defined as axillary metastases no larger than 0.2 mm.
[b]"Missed" occult metastases are those that were missed during the original axillary assessment, but were visible on the original H&E preparation when reexamined.
[c]Analysis of SEER database.
[d]Range for N0, N1mi, N1.

TABLE 13-3 Outcomes Associated with Micrometastases and Isolated Tumor Cells in the Sentinel Lymph Node (SLN)

Study	No. Patients	Median Follow-up (mo)	Size of Nodal Deposit	Outcome
Imoto et al, 2004[19]	164	53	SLN negative vs SLN IHC+/H&E–, ≤ 2.0 mm	No significant difference between SLN negative and SLN IHC+ in 6-year RFS
Chagpar et al, 2005[20]	84	40	SLN negative vs SLN IHC+/H&E–, median size of met = 0.5 mm	No significant difference between SLN negative and SLN IHC+ in 5-year OS or DMFS
Fan et al, 2005[21]	390	31	SLN negative	LR 3.3%
			SLN H&E positive, ≤ 2.0 mm	LR 2.2%
			SLN H&E positive, > 2.0 mm	LR 8.7%
Langer et al, 2005[22]	224	42	SLN negative or lesions ≤ 0.2 mm, IHC and/or H&E	LR 0.8%
			> 0.2 mm and ≤2.0 mm, IHC and/or H&E	LR 0%
			> 2.0 mm, IHC and/or H&E	LR 1.4%
Hansen et al, 2007[23]	624	73	SLN negative vs SLN IHC+/H&E– vs SLN H&E positive, ≤ 2.0 mm	No significant difference among 3 groups for 8-year OS or DFS
Herbert et al, 2006[24]	16	30	ITC	No recurrence during follow-up period

DFS, disease-free survival; DMFS, distant metastasis-free survival; H&E, hematoxylin and eosin; IHC, immunohistochemical staining; ITC, isolated tumor cells; LR, local recurrence; OS, met, metastasis; overall survival; RFS, recurrence-free survival.

non-sentinel node metastasis as a function of sentinel node status. For the patient with a small primary tumor (T1a,b) in conjunction with ITCs in a single sentinel node, the omission of axillary surgery may be suggested, with XRT used as a substitute for completion ALND, raising the tangential port to include the lower axilla. For patients with larger primary tumors with or without more extensive lesions in the sentinel node, lymph node status has little or no impact on the choice of systemic treatment options, which are primarily based on characteristics of the primary tumor (eg, size, grade, hormone, and HER2 status). However, with larger tumors, the risk of additional nodal metastases may be higher, leading most practitioners to advise full axillary dissection for women with a positive sentinel node.

Problems in Identifying ITCs and Micrometastases

The strict size criteria laid out in the sixth edition to distinguish ITCs from micrometastases were intended to assist in generating comparable data about the clinical importance of microscopic

lesions. In practice, this strategy has achieved only moderate success. There are a variety of reasons for this, broadly divided into 2 overlapping categories: (1) failure to use the recommendations of the sixth edition; and (2) confusion about how to implement the recommendations, especially in areas in which the sixth edition did not provide enough information.

Failure to Use the Recommendations of the Sixth Edition

Before the publication of the sixth edition, the classification of micrometastasis usually included all lesions smaller than 2.0 mm. When the differentiation of extremely small lesions was desired (1 or a few cells), lesions were sometimes defined by the method of detection, with IHC+/H&E–staining used as a working definition for ITCs. Unfortunately, many publications after 2002 have continued to use these designations, perhaps because of encountering difficulties in attempting to measure lesions as recommended in the sixth edition (see the next section.)

In 2004, Cserni and colleagues published the results of a survey of the European Working Group for Breast Screening

Pathology (EWGBSP) regarding current practice in the pathologic evaluation of sentinel nodes in breast cancer.[34] They reported that, for 223/240 respondents who used the term "ITC," there were 10 different definitions, only 43% of which conformed with the official classification. Some of those institutions that used the size classification also stressed the isolated or single nature of the tumor cells, some stressed localization in the sinuses, some gave a maximum number of cells that could be classified as ITCs (with that number varying from 2 to 20), some reported a definition similar to that for micrometastases, and some stressed detection by IHC. No definition was given by 22 laboratories. For 222/240 responders who reported using the term "micrometastasis," 17 different definitions were used, only 81% of which conformed to the official classification. Seventy-six laboratories used only the 2-mm upper limit (in accord with the fifth edition), 37 used heterogeneous definitions not in accord with the official classification, and 20 had no definition.

Confusion About How to Implement the Recommendations

An underlying problem contributing to this confusion is that ITCs, as defined by the sixth edition, are really a very diverse group, ranging from a single cell to clusters of cells to a large number of single cells homogeneously dispersed. Since 2002, feedback from clinicians around the world has highlighted areas that were not well addressed in the sixth edition. Several studies have now demonstrated that additional clarification in these areas can significantly improve the reproducibility of classifying these metastatic deposits.

What to do with Clusters.
The upper size limit for ITCs is 0.2 mm in diameter; a cluster of this size may contain up to 100 cells. What if there are multiple clusters? Should they be added together to estimate overall tumor burden? The standard for primary tumors as defined in the TNM classification is to use the largest tumor to designate the T classification. Most conservatively, tumors are defined as arising independently only if they occur in different quadrants. No such standards have been developed for lymph node metastases. In practice, a pathologist might look at deeper cuts of the node to see if they show a contiguous process. If they do not, opinions differ on how far apart the clusters should be in order to be classified as separate lesions.

What to do with Multiple, Evenly-Spaced, Single-Cell ITCs.
This phenomenon is sometimes seen in patients with invasive lobular carcinoma. Pathologists have frequently observed that the total volume of these individual cells, if summed together, can exceed the size of a micrometastasis. Based on this, some prefer to classify this pattern of metastasis as pN1, based on the total number of tumor cells.[35]

What to do with Metastases that are Found in Different Locations (eg, Parenchyma, Sinuses, and Vascular Spaces).
The AJCC staging system for breast cancer does not use microanatomic location as a factor in classification. Thus, ITCs, classified solely on the basis of size, can be found in the nodal parenchyma, nodal sinuses, capsular or subcapsular spaces, or extranodal lymphatic vessels. However, according to the qualitative criteria originally defined by Hermanek and associates,[36] a micrometastasis occurs when there has been arrest and implantation in the organ involved. By this definition, metastases located in the nodal parenchyma should be classified as micrometastases even if they are less than 0.2 mm in size. This is based on the assumption that the lymphatic spread of breast cancer cells has an orderly progression from the sentinel node to the non-sentinel nodes. In this model, tumor cells arrive in the subcapsular sinuses of the sentinel node via an afferent lymph vessel, followed by outgrowth into the cortical parenchyma and extension to the nodal parenchyma. Tumor cells may then follow the medullary sinuses to the efferent lymph vessels, moving to the non-sentinel lymph nodes.[37] Support for this qualitative distinction comes from a 2008 report from van Deurzen and colleagues,[38] who found that microanatomic location and penetrative depth of sentinel node metastases were significant predictors for non-sentinel node involvement ($p < 0.001$).

In terms of generating comparable data across different institutions, this means that institutions that follow the strict AJCC criteria will tend to understage some patients with ITCs compared with institutions that use the additional qualitative criterion based on microanatomic location.

What to do with borderline cases.
In studies that have looked at reproducibility of lymph node classification, a consistent trouble spot is metastases that have a borderline size near the 0.2-mm threshold.[39] The general AJCC recommendation for such situations is to select the lower-stage category, but this recommendation is not always followed. Since it is critical for comparative purposes that staging be uniformly applied, practitioners should use the internationally accepted staging standards for reporting stage. In addition, for these borderline cases, it is useful to separately classify and record the more detailed characteristics of minimal node involvement for reporting and publication. Such data will aid the future refinement of our understanding of the prognostic significance of minimal node involvement and help to direct revision of future staging standards.

APPROACHES TO REFINING THE IDENTIFICATION OF ITCs AND MICROMETASTASES

Several studies have more specifically defined ITCs and micrometastases in an attempt to improve the reproducibility of classification (Table 13-4).[39,40] Cserni and colleagues[40] used digital images of 50 cases with low-volume lymph node involvement. The images were distributed twice (before and after more specific definitions of ITCs and micrometastases were disseminated) to 24 members of the EWGBSP. For the first evaluation round, only 2 cases were classified unanimously, and the overall reproducibility was only fair ($\kappa = 0.39$). After discussion and dissemination of the refined criteria, the digital images (in a randomly rearranged order) were redistributed for evaluation. The reproducibility improved and fell into the moderate range ($\kappa = 0.49$).

Turner and coworkers[39] distributed digital images of sentinel node biopsies from 56 patients with low-volume nodal metastases

TABLE 13-4 Refinement Criteria for Classification of Isolated Tumor Cells (ITCs) and Micrometastases

Criteria Used in Cserni et al, 2005[40]	Criteria Used in Turner et al, 2008[39]
If single cells or clusters are separated by only a distance of a few cells (2 to 5), count them as one focus	Single cells or clusters of cells separated by a single benign cell or a spatial gap are measured as separate clusters, except when fibroblastic reaction to the tumor cells has caused the separation
If there are multiple foci, only the largest should be measured	ITCs are small clusters, no larger than 0.2 mm. Cells that are contiguous are measured by the largest group of contiguous cells. Mitotic activity is not considered. A single cell can be an ITC, but only when strongly CK-positive, or when otherwise identified as a carcinoma cell
If the cells or clusters are discontinuous and dispersed homogeneously across a defined area, measure the size of the defined area	Single cells in the dispersed lobular pattern are ITCs
If the cells or clusters are discontinuous and dispersed unevenly, consider as one focus if the distance between them is smaller than the smaller cluster. Otherwise, measure the size of the largest cluster	Micrometastases are clusters or confluent foci larger than 0.20 mm but no larger than 2.0 mm
Tumor cells clearly in the nodal parenchyma should be classified as micrometastases, even if they are < 0.2 mm in size. If tumor cells are in vessels or sinuses, classify according to AJCC size criteria	Microanatomic location is not considered in classification
For borderline cases, choose the lower classification	For borderline cases, choose the lower classification

to 6 experienced breast pathologists. Evaluation results were compared among the 6 pathologists and between each pathologist and a reference pathologist. The first evaluation revealed a 76.2% average agreement between the MDs and the reference pathologist ($\kappa = 0.58$), and a 71.5% agreement among the 6 MDs ($\kappa = 0.49$). After exposure to a training program containing the refined criteria (Table 13-5), the agreement between the MDs and the reference pathologist had increased to 97.3% ($\kappa = 0.95$), and the agreement among the 6 MDs had increased to 95.7% ($\kappa = 0.92$).

Although both sets of criteria led to significantly increased agreement among pathologists, there were substantial differences in the way that they defined independent cells/clusters, in how they handled the disperse pattern of ITCs seen in invasive lobular carcinoma, and in whether they considered microanatomic location in the classification. These issues need to be resolved. Any resulting set of criteria will of course be somewhat arbitrary; it might not ultimately result in the best estimate of prognosis, but diagnostic reproducibility is a critical first step in addressing that question.

SIGNIFICANT CHANGES AND CLARIFICATIONS IN THE 2010 SEVENTH AJCC CANCER STAGING MANUAL

On January 1st, 2010, the new seventh edition of the AJCC breast cancer staging took effect.[52] A summary of the new

TMN classification for Breast Cancer is shown in Table 13-5 and the corresponding anatomic stage/prognostic groups in Table 13-6. For full details about Collaborative staging, the reader is referred to the AJCC Web site (www.cancerstaging.orq). A summary of major selected changes and clarifications grouped by TNM and neoadjuvant therapy use are noted below:

Tumor (T)

- Paget's disease of the breast associated with an underlying cancer should be classified according to the underlying cancer (Tis, T1, etc). Paget's disease not associated with an underlying invasive or in situ carcinoma (DCIS or LCIS) is classified as Tis (Paget's).
- As noninvasive cancer size may influence treatment decisions, it is recommended that size of DCIS and LCIS be estimated although this feature will currently not change the T classification.
- Both "ductal intraepithelial neoplasia" (DIN) and "lobular intraepithelial neoplasia" (LIN) were recognized as uncommon and still not widely accepted terminology for DCIS/ADH and LCIS/ALH; respectively.
- Recommendation was made that all invasive cancer should utilize the Nottingham combined histologic grading system.

TABLE 13-5 AJCC Seventh Edition TMN Classification for Breast Cancer. Reproduced with permission[52]

Primary Tumor (T)

TX	Primary tumor cannot be assessed
T0	No evidence of primary tumor
Tis	Carcinoma in situ
Tis (DCIS)	Ductal carcinoma in situ
Tis (LCIS)	Lobular carcinoma in situ
Tis (Paget's)	Paget's disease of the nipple NOT associated with invasive carcinoma and/or carcinoma in situ (DCIS and/or LCIS) in the underlying breast parenchyma. Carcinomas in the breast parenchyma associated with Paget's disease are categorized based on the size and characteristics of the parenchymal disease, although the presence of Paget's disease should still be noted
T1	Tumor ≤20 mm in greatest dimension
T1mi	Tumor ≤1 mm in greatest dimension
T1a	Tumor >1 mm but ≤5 mm in greatest dimension
T1b	Tumor >5 mm but ≤10 mm in greatest dimension
T1c	Tumor >10 mm but ≤20 mm in greatest dimension
T2	Tumor >20 mm but ≤50 mm in greatest dimension
T3	Tumor >50 mm in greatest dimension
T4	Tumor of any size with direct extension to the chest wall and/or to the skin (ulceration or skin nodules). *Note*: Invasion of the dermis alone does not qualify as T4
T4a	Extension to the chest wall, not including only pectoralis muscle adherence/invasion
T4b	Ulceration and/or ipsilateral satellite nodules and/or edema (including peau d'orange) of the skin, which do not meet the criteria for inflammatory carcinoma
T4c	Both T4a and T4b
T4d	Inflammatory carcinoma

Regional Lymph Nodes (N)
*Clinical**

NX	Regional lymph nodes cannot be assessed (e.g., previously removed)
N0	No regional lymph node metastases
N1	Metastases to movable ipsilateral level I, II axillary lymph node(s)
N2	Metastases in ipsilateral level I, II axillary lymph nodes that are clinically fixed or matted; or in clinically detected* ipsilateral internal mammary nodes in the *absence* of clinically evident axillary lymph node metastases
N2a	Metastases in ipsilateral level I, II axillary lymph nodes fixed to one another (matted) or to other structures
N2b	Metastases only in clinically detected* ipsilateral internal mammary nodes and in the *absence* of clinically evident axillary lymph node metastases
N3	Metastases in ipsilateral infraclavicular (level III axillary) lymph node(s) with or without level I, II axillary lymph node involvement; or in clinically detected* ipsilateral internal mammary lymph node(s) with clinically evident level I, II axillary lymph node metastases; or metastases in ipsilateral supraclavicular lymph node(s) with or without axillary or internal mammary lymph node involvement
N3a	Metastases in ipsilateral infraclavicular lymph node(s)
N3b	Metastases in ipsilateral internal mammary lymph node(s) and axillary lymph node(s)
N3c	Metastases in ipsilateral supraclavicular lymph node(s)

*Pathologic (pN)***

pNX	Regional lymph nodes cannot be assessed (e.g., previously removed, or not removed for pathologic study)
pN0	No regional lymph node metastasis identified histologically
pN0(i−)	No regional lymph node metastases histologically, negative IHC
pN0(i+)	Malignant cells in regional lymph node(s) no greater than 0.2 mm (detected by H&E or IHC including ITC)
pN0(mol−)	No regional lymph node metastases histologically, negative molecular findings (RT-PCR)
pN0(mol+)	Positive molecular findings (RT-PCR),*** but no regional lymph node metastases detected by histology or IHC

(Continued)

TABLE 13-5 AJCC Seventh Edition TMN Classification for Breast Cancer. Reproduced with permission[52] (*Continued*)

Regional Lymph Nodes (N) (Cont.)

pN1	Micrometastases; or metastases in 1–3 axillary lymph nodes; and/or in internal mammary nodes with metastases detected by sentinel lymph node biopsy but not clinically detected****
pN1mi	Micrometastases (greater than 0.2 mm and/or more than 200 cells, but none greater than 2.0 mm)
pN1a	Metastases in 1–3 axillary lymph nodes, at least one metastasis greater than 2.0 mm
pN1b	Metastases in internal mammary nodes with micrometastases or macrometastases detected by sentinel lymph node biopsy but not clinically detected****
pN1c	Metastases in 1–3 axillary lymph nodes and in internal mammary lymph nodes with micrometastases or macrometastases detected by sentinel lymph node biopsy but not clinically detected
pN2	Metastases in 4–9 axillary lymph nodes; or in clinically detected***** internal mammary lymph nodes in the *absence* of axillary lymph node metastases
pN2a	Metastases in 4–9 axillary lymph nodes (at least one tumor deposit greater than 2.0 mm)
pN2b	Metastases in clinically detected***** internal mammary lymph nodes in the *absence* of axillary lymph node metastases
pN3	Metastases in ten or more axillary lymph nodes; or in infraclavicular (level III axillary) lymph nodes; or in clinically detected***** ipsilateral internal mammary lymph nodes in the *presence* of one or more positive level I, II axillary lymph nodes; or in more than three axillary lymph nodes and in internal mammary lymph nodes with micrometastases or macrometastases detected by sentinel lymph node biopsy but not clinically detected****; or in ipsilateral supraclavicular lymph nodes
pN3a	Metastases in ten or more axillary lymph nodes (at least one tumor deposit greater than 2.0 mm); or metastases to the infraclavicular (level III axillary lymph) nodes
pN3b	Metastases in clinically detected***** ipsilateral internal mammary lymph nodes in the *presence* of one or more positive axillary lymph nodes; or in more than three axillary lymph nodes and in internal mammary lymph nodes with micrometastases or macrometastases detected by sentinel lymph node biopsy but not clinically detected****
pN3c	Metastases in ipsilateral supraclavicular lymph nodes

Distant Metastases (M)

M0	No clinical or radiographic evidence of distant metastases
cM0(i+)	No clinical or radiographic evidence of distant metastases, but deposits of molecularly or microscopically detected tumor cells in circulating blood, bone marrow, or other nonregional nodal tissue that are no larger than 0.2 mm in a patient without symptoms or signs of metastases
M1	Distant detectable metastases as determined by classic clinical and radiographic means and/or histologically proven larger than 0.2 mm

Clinically detected is defined as detected by imaging studies (excluding lymphoscintigraphy) or by clinical examination and having characteristics highly suspicious for malignancy or a presumed pathologic macrometastasis based on fine needle aspiration biopsy with cytologic examination.

**Classification is based on axillary lymph node dissection with or without sentinel lymph node biopsy. Classification based solely on sentinel lymph node biopsy without subsequent axillary lymph node dissection is designated (sn) for "sentinel node," for example, pN0(sn).

***RT-PCR: reverse transcriptase/polymerase chain reaction.

**** "Not clinically detected" is defined as not detected by imaging studies (excluding lymphoscintigraphy) or not detected by clinical examination.

***** "Clinically detected" is defined as detected by imaging studies (excluding lymphoscintigraphy) or by clinical examination and having characteristics highly suspicious for malignancy or a presumed pathologic macrometastasis based on fine needle aspiration biopsy with cytologic examination.

TABLE 13-6 AJCC Seventh Edition Anatomic Stage/Prognostic Group. Reproduced with permission[52]

Stage 0	Tis	N0	M0
Stage IA	T1*	N0	M0
Stage IB	T0	N1mi	M0
	T1*	N1mi	M0
Stage IIA	T0	N1**	M0
	T1*	N1**	M0
	T2	N0	M0
Stage IIB	T2	N1	M0
	T3	N0	M0
Stage IIIA	T0	N2	M0
	T1*	N2	M0
	T2	N2	M0
	T3	N1	M0
	T3	N2	M0
Stage IIIB	T4	N0	M0
	T4	N1	M0
	T4	N2	M0
Stage IIIC	Any T	N3	M0
Stage IV	Any T	Any N	M1

*T1 includes T1 mi.

**T0 and T1 tumors with nodal micrometastases only are excluded from Stage IIA and are classified Stage IB.

· M0 includes M0(i+)

· The designation pM0 is not valid; any M0 should be clinical

· If a patient presents with M1 prior to neoadjuvant systemic therapy, the stage is considered Stage IV and remains Stage IV regardless of response to neoadjuvant therapy.

· Stage designation may be changed if postsurgical imaging studies reveal the presence of distant metastases, provided that the studies are carried out within 4 months of diagnosis in the absence of disease progression and provided that the patient has not received neoadjuvant therapy.

· Postneoadjuvant therapy is designated with "yc" or "yp" prefix. Of note, no stage group is assigned if there is a complete pathologic response (CR) to neoadjuvant therapy, for example, ypT0ypN0cM0.

Nodes (N)

- More stringent classification of isolated tumor cell clusters and single cells were made. Small clusters of cells not greater than 0.2 mm or nonconfluent or nearly confluent clusters of cells not exceeding 200 cells in a single histologic lymph node section are classified as isolated tumor cells.

- Stage I breast tumors have been subdivided into two groups: Stage IA and Stage IB. Stage IB includes T1 tumors with micrometastases in lymph nodes (N1 mi).

Metastases (M)

A new category of M0(i+) has been added to include either disseminated tumor cells detectable in bone marrow or circulating tumor cells or found incidentally in other tissues if not exceeding 0.2 mm (example prophylactic removal of ovaries).

Post-neoadjuvant Therapy Designations (yc or ypTNM)

- The yTNM (or posttherapy) stage documents the extent of disease for patients whose first course of therapy includes systemic therapy prior to surgical resection. Clinical stage after therapy (yC) or pathologic stage after therapy (yP) is recorded. Care must be taken to record the clinical stage prior to therapy for surveillance analysis as erroneous reports could occur (example: a patient who presents with clinical stage III breast cancer could have only residual DCIS following neoadjuvant therapy and recording of the final y stage as the original stage could lead to grossly misleading surveillance data).[52]

- Pretreatment clinical T (cT) is based on clinical and imaging findings in the setting of neoadjuvant therapy.

- Post-neoadjuvant therapy T is based on clinical or imaging (ycT) or pathologic findings (ypT).

- A subscript is added to the clinical N for both node negative and node positive patients to indicate whether the N was derived from clinical exam, fine needle aspiration, core needle biopsy, or sentinel lymph node biopsy.

- The post-treatment ypT is defined as the largest contiguous focus of invasive cancer on histopathology and a subscript to indicate the presence of multiple foci.

- Post-treatment nodal metastases are classified as ypN0(i+) if no greater than 0.2 mm. Patients with this scenario are not considered to have had a pathologic complete response (pCR)

- A description of the degree of response to neoadjuvant therapy (complete, partial, and no response) as well as the ypTNM post-treatment designation should be collected in patients receiving neoadjuvant therapy.

THE FUTURE OF BREAST CANCER STAGING

The TNM system for breast cancer staging represents our current best approach for estimating breast cancer prognosis, but it is clearly not perfect. As detailed above, for example, there are problems in the implementation of the classification system for ITCs and micrometastases. Even if the system were perfectly implemented across all laboratories, however, there are reasons why these classifications might not be well correlated with prognosis. For single cells identified by IHC, in particular, it is possible that not all such cells identified as nodal metastases have the same degree of malignant behavior. Al-Hajj and colleagues[41] suggest that most cells in a tumor permanently lack the capacity to proliferate to any significant degree; only a very small and phenotypically distinct subgroup of cells has this ability. They propose that this subpopulation of cells may derive from breast stem cells, retaining the ability for self-renewal and differentiation that is typical of normal stem cells.

It may also be that very small ITCs, single cells or clusters of only a few cells, are especially vulnerable to immune surveillance. An intriguing study by Yokoyama and colleagues[42] investigated the early development of lymph node metastasis from ITCs to micrometastases, using a gastric cancer cell line tagged with the green fluorescent protein (GFP) gene from the jellyfish, *Aequorea victoria*. This gene yields a bright, stable, green fluorescence in living cells. They found that, with the primary tumor in place, all of the ITCs present at 1 week grew continuously to develop into micrometastases by 3 weeks. However, if the primary tumor was resected 1 to 2 weeks after tumor cell inoculation, the incidence of nodal metastases at 4 weeks was significantly decreased. Additional experiments indicated that ITCs spontaneously regressed after resection of the primary tumor, apparently from attack by natural killer (NK) cells. They hypothesize that, in this mouse model, NK cells are able to destroy ITCs, unless there is a continuous recruitment of cancer cells and nutrient supply from the primary tumor through lymphatic channels.

Even if the question of the relative prognostic importance of ITCs and micrometastases can be resolved, the current staging system for breast cancer is complex and cumbersome to use, and fails to incorporate many other patient-related, tumor-related, and treatment-related factors that may influence patient prognosis.[43] Additional elements are being considered for incorporation into breast cancer staging for the upcoming seventh edition of the AJCC manual, but the inclusion of more parameters will make the staging system even more difficult to implement in day-to-day practice.

The advent of gene microarray technology and continued advances in genetic and proteomic analysis have opened up an entirely new avenue for determining breast cancer prognosis, one that may make staging based solely on clinical and histologic criteria obsolete. Researchers are now using molecular approaches to create personalized genetic or proteomic fingerprints based on the identification of genes that are actively expressed in tumor cells. For example, Van 't Veer and colleagues used RNA-based microarrays to identify a 70-gene expression profile that was strongly associated with time to distant metastasis in patients with node-negative primary breast cancer.[44,45] Recently the 70-gene profile, now being marketed as Mammaprint (Agendia, Amsterdam), was also shown to be prognostic in patients with 1 to 3 positive lymph nodes, identifying a large group of low-risk patients who might be able to avoid chemotherapy.[46] Soonmyung Paik from the NSABP's pathology division developed Oncotype DX (Genomic Health, Redwood City, CA), a 21-gene recurrence score (RS) based on monitoring mRNA expression levels in 16 cancer-related genes and 5 reference genes. In this system, RNA is extracted from paraffin-embedded tumor sections and quantified using RT-PCR. In the original validation assay, the RS was shown to be useful in determining prognosis in newly diagnosed breast cancer patients with stage I/II, ER-positive, node-negative disease who would normally receive tamoxifen as adjuvant therapy.[47] In subsequent studies, patients identified as high risk by the RS were shown to preferentially benefit from chemotherapy,[48] and the RS was shown to be useful for determining prognosis in patients with node-positive disease ($\leq$ 3 positive nodes).[49]

For both assays (Mammaprint and Oncotype DX), it is still not clear whether intermediate-risk patients can benefit from adjuvant chemotherapy. Two ongoing prospective studies should provide an answer to this question: the Microarray in Node Negative Disease May Avoid Chemotherapy Trial (MINDACT), being conducted primarily in Europe,[50] and the Trial Assigning Individualized Options for Treatment (TAILORx), being conducted primarily in the United States.[51] For both trials, patients classified as low risk will receive endocrine therapy alone, while patients classified as high risk will receive adjuvant chemotherapy in addition to endocrine therapy. Those classified as intermediate risk will be randomized to receive chemotherapy or no chemotherapy.

Such approaches to fingerprinting are rapidly being refined and brought to market. These techniques hold the promise of providing a fast and relatively inexpensive way of determining prognosis at the level of the individual cancer patient. It may be expected that these or other technologies will be incorporated into TNM staging to complement, or in some cases perhaps supplant the role of anatomic extent of disease in defining prognosis.

SUMMARY

The major changes in the sixth edition of the AJCC cancer staging system for breast cancer are related to the importance of the method of detection, size, number, and location of regional lymph node metastases. The most controversial change, and the one that has been most difficult to implement uniformly, is the assignment of a strict size criterion to distinguish ITCs from micrometastases. Available data support the decision to classify ITCs as pN0, but results are mixed for the classification of micrometastases as pN1. The major changes in the new seventh edition of the AJCC cancer staging system for breast cancer are related to the more stringent classification of isolated tumor cells not exceeding 200 cells, a new category of M0(i+) designating disseminated tumor cells detected in the blood or bone marrow, the newly described stage IA and IB designations, and the yTNM (or posttherapy) stage documentation as it relates to the prevalent use of neoadjuvant therapy for breast cancer. Molecular approaches to providing individual genetic or proteomic fingerprints that correlate with prognosis will eventually be incorporated into routine practice to supplement or perhaps supplant purely anatomic-based staging.

REFERENCES

1. Greene FL, Page DL, Fleming ID, et al., eds. *AJCC Cancer Staging Manual.* 6th ed. New York, NY: Springer; 2002.
2. Early Breast Cancer Trialists' Collaborative Group. Polychemotherapy for early breast cancer: an overview of the randomized trials. *Lancet.* 1998; 352:930-942.
3. Early Breast Cancer Trialists' Collaborative Group. Tamoxifen for early breast cancer: an overview of the randomized trials. *Lancet.* 1998;351:1451-1467.
4. Singletary SE, Connolly JL. Breast cancer staging: working with the sixth edition of the AJCC Cancer Staging Manual. *CA Cancer J Clin.* 2006;56:37-47.
5. Singletary SE, Greene FL, Sobin LH. Classification of isolated tumor cells: clarification of the 6th edition of the American Joint Committee on Cancer Staging Manual. *Cancer.* 2003;98:2740-2741.

6. Singletary SE, Greene FL. Revision of breast cancer staging: the 6th edition of the TNM Classification. *Semin Surg Oncol.* 2003;1:53-59.

7. Singletary SE, Allred C, Ashley P, et al. Staging system for breast cancer: revisions for the 6th edition of the AJCC Cancer Staging Manual. *Surg Clin North Am.* 2003;83:803-819.

8. Singletary SE, Allred C, Ashley P, et al. Revision of the American Joint Committee on Cancer staging system for breast cancer. *J Clin Oncol.* 2002;20:3628-3636.

9. Fleming ID, Cooper JS, Henson DE, et al., eds. *AJCC Cancer Staging Manual.* 5th ed, Philadelphia, PA: Lippincott Raven, 1997.

10. Nasser IA, Lee AK, Bosari S, et al. Occult axillary lymph node metastases in "node-negative" breast carcinoma. *Hum Pathol.* 1993;24:950-957.

11. Colpaert C, Vermeulen P, Jeuris W, et al. Early distant relapse in "node-negative" breast cancer patients is not predicted by occult axillary lymph node metastases, but by the features of the primary tumour. *J Pathol.* 2001;193:442-449.

12. Cummings MC, Walsh MD, Hohn BG, et al. Occult axillary lymph node metastases in breast cancer do matter. *Am J Surg Pathol.* 2002;26:1286-1295.

13. Millis RR, Springall R, Lee AHS, et al. Occult axillary lymph node metastases are of no prognostic significance in breast cancer. *Br J Cancer.* 2002;86:396-401.

14. Umekita Y, Ohi Y, Sagara Y, Yoshida H. Clinical significance of occult micrometastases in axillary lymph nodes in "node-negative" breast cancer patients. *Am J Cancer Res.* 2002;93:695-698.

15. Susnik B, Frkovic-Grazio S, Bracko M. Occult micrometastases in axillary lymph nodes predict subsequent distant metastases in stage I breast cancer: a case-control study with 15-year follow-up. *Ann Surg Oncol.* 2004;11:568-572.

16. Kahn HJ, Hanna WM, Chapman JQ, et al. Biological significance of occult micrometastases in histologically negative axillary lymph nodes in breast cancer patients using the recent American Joint Committee on Cancer Breast Cancer Staging System. *Breast J.* 2006;12:294-301.

17. Chen SL, Hoehne FM, Giuliano AE. The prognostic significance of micrometastases in breast cancer: a SEER population-based analysis. *Ann Surg Oncol.* 2007;13:3378-3384.

18. Tan LK, Giri D, Hummer AJ, et al. Occult axillary node metastases in breast cancer are prognostically significant: results in 368 node-negative patients with 20-year follow-up. *J Clin Oncol.* 2006;26:1803-1809.

19. Imoto S, Ochiai A, Okumura C, et al. Impact of isolated tumor cells in sentinel lymph nodes detected by immunohistochemical staining. *Eur J Surg Oncol.* 2006;32:1175-1179.

20. Chagpar A, Middleton LP, Sahin AA, et al. Clinical outcome of patients with lymph node-negative breast carcinoma who have sentinel lymph node micrometastases detected by immunohistochemistry. *Cancer.* 2005;103:1581-1586.

21. Fan YG, Tan YY, Wu CT, et al. The effect of sentinel node tumor burden on non-sentinel node status and recurrence rates in breast cancer. *Ann Surg Oncol.* 2005;12:705-711.

22. Langer I, Marti WR, Guller U, et al. Axillary recurrence rate in breast cancer patients with negative sentinel lymph node (SLN) or SLN micrometastases: prospective analysis of 150 patients after SLN biopsy. *Ann Surg.* 2005;241:152-158.

23. Hansen NM, Grube BJ, Ye C, et al. The impact of micrometastases in the sentinel nodes of patients with invasive breast cancer. Proceedings of the 30th Annual San Antonio Breast Cancer Symposium, 2007. Abstract 52.

24. Herbert GS, Sohn BY, Brown TA. The impact of nodal isolated tumor cells on survival of breast cancer patients. *Am J Surg.* 2007;193:571-574.

25. Cote R, Peterson H, Chaiwun B, et al. Role of immunohistochemical detection of lymph-node metastases in management of breast cancer. *Lancet.* 1999;354:896-900.

26. Singletary SE. Nanometastases in the sentinel node. *Clin Oncol News.* January 2008;1-8.

27. Van Zee KJ, Manasseh DM, Bevilacqua JL, et al. A nomogram for predicting the likelihood of additional nodal metastases in breast cancer patients with a positive sentinel node biopsy. *Ann Surg Oncol.* 2003;10:1140-1151.

28. Chu KU, Turner RR, Hansen NM, et al. Sentinel node metastasis in patients with breast carcinoma accurately predicts immunohistochemically detectable nonsentinel node metastasis. *Ann Surg Oncol.* 1999;6:756-761.

29. Reynolds C, Mick R, Donohue JH, et al. Sentinel lymph node biopsy with metastasis: can axillary dissection be avoided in some patients with breast cancer? *J Clin Oncol.* 1999;17:1720-1726.

30. Jakub JW, Diaz NM, Ebert MD, et al. Completion axillary lymph node dissection minimizes the likelihood of false negatives for patients with invasive breast carcinoma and cytokeratin positive only sentinel lymph nodes. *Am J Surg.* 2002;184:302-306.

31. Gray RJ, Pockaj BA, Conley CR. Sentinel lymph node metastases detected by immunohistochemistry only do not mandate complete axillary lymph node dissection in breast cancer. *Ann Surg Oncol.* 2004;11:1056-1060.

32. Mignotte H, Treilleux I, Faure C, et al. Axillary lymph-node dissection for positive sentinel nodes in breast cancer patients. *Eur J Surg Oncol.* 2002;28:623-626.

33. Houvenaeghel G, Nos C, Mignotte H, et al. Micrometastases in sentinel lymph node in a multicentric study: predictive factors of nonsentinel lymph node involvement—Groupe des Chirurgiens de la Federation des Centres de Lutte Contre le Cancer. *J Clin Oncol.* 2006;24:1814-1822.

34. Cserni G, Amendoeira I, Apostolikas N, et al. Discrepancies in current practice of pathological evaluation of sentinel lymph nodes in breast cancer. Results of a questionnaire based survey by the European Working Group for Breast Screening Pathology. *J Clin Pathol.* 2004;57:695-701.

35. Connolly JL. Changes and problematic areas in interpretation of the *AJCC Cancer Staging Manual,* 6th edition, for breast cancer. *Arch Pathol Lab Med.* 2006;130:287-291.

36. Hermanek P, Hutter RVP, Sobin LH, Wittekind C. Classification of isolated tumor cells and micrometastasis. *Cancer.* 1999;86:2668-2683.

37. Borgstein PJ, Meijer S, Pijpers RG, et al. Functional lymphatic anatomy for sentinel node biopsy in breast cancer: echoes from the past and the periareolar blue method. *Ann Surg.* 2000;232:81-89.

38. Van Deurzen CHM, Seldenrijk CA, Koelemij R, et al. The microanatomic location of metastatic breast cancer in sentinel lymph nodes predicts non-sentinel lymph node involvement. *Ann Surg Oncol.* 2008;15:1309-1315.

39. Turner RR, Weaver DL, Cserni G, et al. Nodal stage classification for breast carcinoma: improving interobserver reproducibility through standardized histologic criteria and image-based training. *J Clin Oncol.* 2008;26:258-263.

40. Cserni G, Bianchi S, Boecker W, et al. Improving the reproducibility of diagnosing micrometastases and isolated tumor cells. *Cancer.* 2005;103:358-367.

41. Al-Hajj M, Wich MS, Benito-Hernandez A, et al. Prospective identification of tumorigenic breast cancer cells. *PNAS.* 2003;100:3983-3988.

42. Yokoyama H, Nakanishi H, Kodera Y, et al. Biological significance of isolated tumor cells and micrometastasis in lymph nodes evaluated using a green fluorescent protein-tagged human gastric cancer cell line. *Clin Cancer Res.* 2006;12:361-368.

43. Hermanek P, Sobin LH, Fleming ID. What do we need beyond TNM? *Cancer.* 1996;77:815-817.

44. Van't Veer LJ, Dai H, van de Vijver MJ, et al. Gene expression profiling predicts clinical outcome of breast cancer. *Nature.* 2002;415:530-536.

45. Van de Vijver MJ, He UD, Van't Veer LJ, et al. A gene-expression signature as a predictor of survival in breast cancer. *N Engl J Med.* 2002;347:1999-2009.

46. Mook S, Schmidt MK, Viale G, et al. Breast cancer patients with 1-3 positive lymph nodes and a low risk 70-gene profile have an excellent survival. Proceedings of the 30th Annual San Antonio Breast Cancer Symposium, 2007. Abstract 50.

47. Paik S, Shak S, Tang G, et al. A multigene assay to predict recurrence of tamoxifen-treated, node-negative breast cancer. *N Engl J Med.* 2004;351:2817-2826.

48. Mamounas E, Tang G, Bryant J, et al. Association between the 21-gene recurrence score assay (RS) and risk of locoregional failure in node-negative, ER-positive breast cancer: results from NASBP B-14 and NASBP B-20. Proceedings of the 28th Annual San Antonio Breast Cancer Symposium, December 8-11, 2005. Abstract 29.

49. Goldstein LJ, Gray R, Childs BH, et al. Prognostic utility of 21-gene assay in hormone receptor positive operable breast cancer and 0-3 positive axillary nodes treated with adjuvant chemohormonal therapy: an analysis of Intergroup trial E2197. Proceedings of the 41st Annual Meeting of the American Society of Clinical Oncology, May 13-17, 2005, Orlando, FL. Abstract 526.

50. Mook S, Van't Veer LJ, Rutgers EJ, et al. Individualization of therapy using Mammaprint: from development to the MINDACT. *Cancer Genomics Proteomics.* 2007;4:147-155.

51. Paik S. Development and clinical utility of a 21-gene recurrence score prognostic assay in patients with early breast cancer treated with tamoxifen. *Oncologist.* 2007;12:631-635.

52. Edge SB, Byrd DR, Compton CC, et al. *AJCC Cancer Staging Manual.* 7th ed. New York, NY: Springer;2009

CHAPTER 14

Communicating a Breast Cancer Diagnosis

Walter Baile
Laura Dominici

The delivery of a diagnosis of breast cancer to a patient elicits a strong emotional response from the patient, and similarly, evokes an emotional response from the surgeon as well. The ability to deliver bad news in a way that helps improve communication and strengthen the patient–doctor relationship is a skill not often taught, although it is frequently required. Most studies have examined oncologists, and one found that 60% broke bad news to patients from 5 to 20 times per month. Fourteen percent delivered bad news more than 20 times a month. Less than 10% of those surveyed had any formal training in breaking bad news, and only 32% had any shadowing experience in watching others deliver diagnoses.[1] An American Society of Clinical Oncology survey revealed that most participants cited "traumatic experience" as the most common source of learning communication on difficult topics.[2]

Women with breast cancer, in particular, have high levels of unmet needs for health information, difficulties accessing information, and dissatisfaction with information gleaned from health care providers.[3-6] Thus, the importance of good communication in this group cannot be stressed enough. This chapter seeks to present a brief overview of delivering a breast cancer diagnosis, including the importance of the topic, barriers to communication, and strategies for the delivery of the diagnosis.

DEFINITION OF "BAD NEWS"

The delivery of a diagnosis of breast cancer falls into the category of "bad news." This is basically defined as "any information which adversely and seriously affects an individual's view of her future."[7] This is very dependent on the patient's subjective feelings and the gap between the patient's expectations of the future and the medical reality. Thus, it is key to have an appreciation for the patient's expectations and her understanding of the medical situation while delivering the diagnosis.

The delivery of the diagnosis of breast cancer involves complex communication, including a verbal component as well as the recognition and response to emotion, the involvement of the patient in the decision-making process, provision of support, and the preservation of hope.[1] Effective delivery of the diagnosis can affect a patient's compliance with treatment, better understanding of disease process, lessen stress, and improve patient satisfaction.[8] The way in which bad news is broken "influences the patient's subsequent psychosocial adjustment."[9] It has also been noted that disclosure of bad news is not universally harmful to patients but that failure of good communication may be.[10]

HISTORICAL PERSPECTIVE ON DELIVERING "BAD NEWS"

There is a level of autonomy and disclosure in medical decision-making now that was not present previously, as patients desire information about their illness. One survey revealed that 96% of participants wanted to be given their diagnosis of cancer and 85% wanted a realistic prognosis.[11] This is particularly true for breast cancer patients as well. A study by Lobb and colleagues found that 83% of women wanted as much information about their disease as possible,[3] and a similar study noted that 88% wanted increased information on the likely future of their illness.[12]

It has not, however, always been the case that the disclosure of cancer diagnoses has been this frank. In the 1950s a combination of ethical guidelines and lack of therapy combined to allow the principle of beneficence to dominate in Western society. Physicians often did not disclose a diagnosis of cancer for fear that it would cause significant psychiatric distress. As therapies improved during the 1970s, physicians became more forthcoming with cancer diagnoses.[13] This was also influenced by legislation,[14] and currently physicians practice full disclosure of cancer diagnosis. One area, however, that continues to evolve is the discussion of prognosis. This is an area of particular importance to breast cancer patients, where the study by Lobb and associates found that 91% of breast cancer patients surveyed desired more information regarding prognosis.[3] Prognosis is the focal point for the majority of patients encouraged to ask questions by their physicians.[15] Today's patients really desire as much information as possible about their diagnosis of breast cancer, and the physician plays the key role "as the main point of contact."[6]

THE PATIENT–PHYSICIAN RELATIONSHIP

The relationship between patient and physician has been studied since the time of Hippocrates, who noted in his Precepts (VI) that "some patients, though conscious that their condition is perilous, recover their health simply through their contentment with the goodness of the physician." Traditionally the patient–physician relationship took a doctor-centered approach where the visit agenda, discussions, and outcomes were under the control of the physician. Visits felt to be biomedical and physician-centered were rated least satisfying by both patients and physicians.[16] A more modern approach is that of patient-centered medicine, which recognizes the importance of the biopsychosocial factors that play into a patient's illness. The use of a 3-function model facilitates further explanation of the patient-centered approach where the following must be in place: awareness of the patient's understanding of his or her disease and role as patient, a therapeutic and cooperative relationship between physician and patient, and education of the patient regarding the disease as well as a recognition of any areas of conflict between patient and physician and awareness of the psychosocial consequences of illness.[17] The emphasis on patient-centered medicine is supported by studies that link higher patient satisfaction to patient-preferred communication features.[18]

Multiple studies have been performed that elicit how patients want their physicians to behave when disclosing a diagnosis and what aspects of patient–physician interactions are most important to them. Only 14% of patients in one survey felt that the disclosure of diagnosis was the most important part of the discussion with their physician.[19] Wright and associates did a study looking at breast cancer patients' preferences for communication with their physicians. The communication skills were found to be less important to them than their physicians' attributes. Patients placed greatest emphasis on having a doctor with expertise in breast cancer, a physician able to form individual relationships with them, and feeling that their physician respected them as "part of the team."[20] Thus, it is a means of communication that conveys these values to patients that is important for the physician to focus on when delivering the diagnosis of breast cancer.

IMPORTANCE OF COMMUNICATION

The delivery of a cancer diagnosis makes a substantial impact on patients and their treatment. It carries importance in treatment decisions and level of satisfaction with care, and can play a role in treatment outcome. Communication with a patient in an honest and effective manner also serves to reduce legal risk[21,22] and improve the patient–physician relationship.[18]

Good communication improves patient satisfaction with care, especially if the physician recognizes that patients vary in terms of the depth of information desired and the style in which their diagnosis is presented.[6,18,23] Delivery of diagnosis is meant to be performed in a way that provides patients with information about what is happening, restores to them a sense of control, and reassures them. Some degree of relief comes just with having the uncertainty relieved, and the physician plays an important role in the psychosocial adjustment of patients with a new diagnosis of cancer through this exchange of information.[23]

Receiving complete information is important to patients,[24] and it is important in allowing the patients to make informed decisions regarding their treatment. When patients have a better understanding of their diagnosis, they can better assess the variety of treatments available to them as well as their risks and benefits. This is particularly important in patients with breast cancer, given the choices of breast conservation versus mastectomy. There are also decisions to be made regarding the various reconstruction options and their timing. Disclosures including discussions about reconstruction prior to surgery may minimize the distress associated with mastectomy[25] and enable the patients to feel positively about the potential for a healthy future. It has been noted by Schain that recovery as well as feelings of being in control can come from being an active participant in one's treatment decisions.[26]

Women with breast cancer who were offered choices of treatment developed less stress than women whose physicians who determined treatment.[27] An open discussion involving options and a team approach impacts women positively even if their treatment options are limited by extent of disease or if the patient follows the clinician's recommendations.[20] Some patients, however, do not want to be active participants in their treatment decisions, and good communication depends on physicians being able to identify and adapt to such situations.[28-30] Regardless, patient outcomes can be influenced by the way in which the diagnosis is discussed with the patients. A positive correlation was found between physician interpersonal skills and low levels of anxiety and distress in patients who had undergone surgery for breast cancer.[31]

Honest and open disclosure of diagnosis carries ethical and legal implications as well. A physician is obligated to fully disclose a patient's diagnosis to comply with the standards of informed consent, patient autonomy, and case law. This, however, does not mean that blunt, insensitive passage of information should replace paternalism.[1] In this climate of increasing litigiousness, it is important to note the effects of poor communication on a physician's potential to face a lawsuit. The Harvard Medical Practice Study was performed in New York State and found that 8 times as many patients incur an injury due to negligence as file a malpractice claim.[32] Studies indicate that these suits are generally filed by families or patients who were dissatisfied with how adverse events were handled by the physician, in terms of communication.[33] Upon review of depositions in which plaintiffs discussed their reasons for filing suits, the following 4 general trends were noted: feeling deserted, felt devalued, information was delivered poorly, and the physician did not understand their perspective.[34] Thus, it can be recommended that "treating patients with respect and communicating in an honest, open, empathetic manner can reduce legal risk."[33]

BARRIERS TO COMMUNICATION

Despite the best intentions of providers to communicate in an effective manner, barriers to open communication do exist. Further exploration of these barriers raises awareness of their existence. Even if these cannot be fully overcome, an appreciation of them allows physicians to be more careful and accommodating in their delivery of a breast cancer diagnosis.

Retention of Information

It is natural for a patient given a new diagnosis of breast cancer to feel overwhelmed. A patient's ability to retain knowledge suffers in stressful situations. For example, in a study of dying patients aware of their condition, only 13% reported that their doctor had informed them of this.[35] An awareness of the patterns of patients' abilities to retain information is helpful in planning the diagnosis disclosure. Patients usually have better retention of facts provided at the beginning of an appointment. Topics that patients feel are most relevant (which may be different than what the physician feels is most relevant) are best remembered. More statements made by a physician equates to a smaller mean percentage of information retained by the patient. Patients also tend to have "flashbulb memories" of emotionally charged things they have learned, and these memories do not fade over time.[36]

Various strategies have been attempted to increase patient retention of information. Consultation planners have been used to better prepare patients for meeting with a physician in terms of preparing questions and organizing ideas.[37] This may be more helpful for patients who are meeting with a physician after their initial diagnosis has been received, although just preparing before an appointment may aid in improved retention. Community-based interventions to prepare patients for meetings with physicians as well as "coaches" to help patients prepare have also been tried with varying success.[38] Prompt sheets providing a list of questions specific to breast cancer have been tested to enhance communication, but no significant intervention effect was found. Also, there was no significant improvement in the patient's level of understanding of her illness.[39]

Attempts to give the patient a permanent transcript of her visit to the physician were also made. Several studies have tried giving both written summaries of consultation as well as audiotapes. Patients did exhibit higher satisfaction with their physician after receiving these, but there was no significant difference in terms of information recall. Even after receiving these items, patients only recalled an average of 50% of the points identified by their physician.[40,41] Still, these methods may be helpful for improving future conversations regarding treatment planning if used during the delivery of diagnosis.

Physician Factors

The physician may also feel anxiety when disclosing a new cancer diagnosis to the patient. Some of this relates to the fact that fewer than 10% of physicians receive formal training in delivery of bad news, so the anticipatory stress can be great.[1] The diagnosis of breast cancer is often emotionally charged for the patient and can be for the physician as well. The physician may respond to this emotion by giving premature reassurance or omitting important information from the disclosure.[42] Anxiety may also be related to worries about the length of discussion and what effect it will have on the physician's busy clinic. It is true that a survey found that 51% of a group of breast cancer patients replied that their physician needed to spend more time speaking with them.[6] However, it is also true that visits with less effective communication between the physician and patient were longer.[43]

Research indicates that physicians lack skill at determining the type and depth of information that patients desire during consultations.[28] Physicians do overestimate their ability to provide patients with complete information. In a study looking at surgeons responding to emotional clues during conversations, 62% missed opportunities to improve communication.[43] Another study looked at patient-initiated actions and whether they generated doctor-responsive actions. In 70% of cases, the cues were missed by the surgical oncologists.[44]

Physicians also struggle with the dilemma of having to give a patient a new diagnosis of breast cancer, but at the same time, preserve hope. Some patients felt that receiving incomplete information would harm trust and make them less hopeful, while some felt that receiving all possible information was too "blunt."[36] This reinforces the important concept that patients are quite variable in the depth and type of information they desire, and this must be taken into account. Patients noted that hopefulness was preserved by physicians who project an attitude of hope and confidence. They also gave importance to feeling like they were participating as part of a team with their surgeon and other providers.[45]

Cultural Barriers

Physicians may also struggle with delivering a diagnosis of breast cancer due to cultural factors. Across the world, patients are not necessarily told of their cancer diagnosis. Some cultures feel that such a diagnosis is both psychologically and physically detrimental to patients.[46] This causes difficulty in patient care as well as an ethical dilemma in terms of patient autonomy and informed consent. An extensive cross-cultural study looked at 90 members of the International Psycho-Oncology Society and found that oncologists from certain African countries, France, Hungary, Italy, Japan, Panama, Portugal, and Spain had less than 40% disclosure.[46] Korean Americans and Mexican Americans also favor nondisclosure.[47]

Some cultures are far less apt to disclose a diagnosis of cancer to the elder members of the family, as they feel it is their job to protect the elder.[46] To a lesser degree, this is seen in Western countries as families try to shield their elderly relatives from the emotional distress associated with a breast cancer diagnosis. A survey conducted in Taiwan revealed that families believe that truth-telling in diagnosis is not necessary in aged patients.[48]

When a diagnosis of cancer is given to a patient, it must be done in a very culturally sensitive way. Even using the word "cancer" can be received as rude, exhibiting a lack of respect, and potentially causal. Thus a careful discussion that indirectly addresses these topics is important. It may be helpful to use words such as "tumor" or "growth" in certain circumstances.[46] Again, this highlights the need for the physician to be cognizant of the patient's preferences when delivering a cancer diagnosis.

Underserved Populations

In addition to cultural differences, awareness of socioeconomic, racial, and age differences among patients is necessary. Differences in communication and treatment choices have been noted in certain groups, so it is important to keep in mind the strong impact of the patient–physician relationship. Low-income, medically underserved women with breast cancer tend to possess less medical knowledge about breast cancer, which may translate into a less favorable interaction with their physician when receiving a diagnosis.[49] It is thought that this may be counteracted by improving low-income women's knowledge in other ways, such as the Comprehensive Health Enhancement Support System (CHESS), an Internet-based health system trialed in Wisconsin and Detroit. It was shown that not only did these women spend more time on the system, but that they had significantly better scores for social support, negative emotions, participation in their care, and information competence.[50]

It has also been found that physicians tend to have more favorable interactions with patients of their race, sex, or age. One study found that racial differences occurred in nearly every communication category that was examined, and this may be significant in terms of treatment planning.[51] Race-concordant consultations tended to be longer and were correlated with more patient satisfaction.[52] Similarly, patients with higher levels of education and younger age were also found to correlate with higher levels of satisfaction after physician interaction.[51] These groups of patients were more interactive in discussions of their breast cancer with their physicians. Elderly patients were also found to be less likely to ask questions and less involved in decision-making.[52] A strong awareness of these differences can help physicians to structure their discussions with patients in a way that maximizes their receipt of knowledge and encourages their participation in treatment planning.

DEPTH OF COMMUNICATION

As has been alluded to, patients are very individual in their desires and needs for information. This is due to age, socioeconomics, culture, and personal preference. The patient-centered approach seeks to account for these differences. It is noted that although most patients desire detailed prognoses from their physicians, they also want them to be hopeful about their outcomes.[36] The knowledge that a patient will not feel abandoned by her physician is important. It is also key to note that patients may be able to feel hopeful about outcomes other than surgical cure, in that they also seek the ability to be pain free, to have anxiety relieved, and to spend time with loved ones.

It is very difficult for the physician to have a discussion of diagnosis with a patient who has advanced disease and is unlikely to be a candidate for surgical resection. Although it is rare for surgeons to be the primary doctor for these patients, a surgeon is often the first breast specialty physician to see a patient with aggressive disease. The dilemma of how much to tell and when is still an area of much discussion. It is noted that "information carefully shared is a gift to the patient and the family who want it and minimizes the risk that patients will distrust the cancer care team."[53] In these cases, it should be considered to link patients in with a palliative care team early on as well as with other services, as this can be an important resource for patient and family throughout the disease process.[53]

STRATEGIES FOR COMMUNICATION

The delivery of a diagnosis of breast cancer can be prepared for, which may improve the interaction and allow patients to participate in treatment decisions. The 4 general goals of the disclosure process are as follows: collect information from the patient to ascertain the patient's state of preparedness for news and desire for news, provide information compatible with her state of readiness, provide emotional support, and cooperatively create a treatment plan. These goals are broken down into the 6 steps of SPIKES.[1]

The first step is to **S**et up the interview. This deals with the physician's plan for discussing the diagnosis, the physical setting, and the inclusion of any family/friends who the patient desires to have involved. Be prepared for giving bad news by anticipating patient questions and the fact that they might become emotionally upset. If it will be very unexpected bad news consider having someone with you such as a member of the nursing staff. Invest in the beginning of the interview by focus on establishing rapport by introducing yourself and greeting family members. Being at eye level with the patient and making a personal connection with her is important. Pay attention to your nonverbal behavior, such as avoiding multitasking while talking. Minimize the likelihood you will be interrupted by pages or other distractions.

The next step is to assess the patient's **P**erception by getting a better idea of what the patient understands about her medical condition and why she is in the physician's office. This will allow the surgeon to begin explanation at the patient's level of understanding and to correct any misinformation or unrealistic expectations. When the patient speaks, avoid the temptation to interrupt until she is finished. Obtain the patient's **I**nvitation to give the diagnosis. This can be simply understood as "goal-setting" for the interview: "Now I'd like to discuss your test results and go over what treatment I think would be best." Following this, it is essential to give **K**nowledge to the patient at her level, in a compassionate way, checking the level of understanding throughout. In this process remember to give information in small chunks, checking periodically for comprehension. The more anxious the patient, the slower you might have to go with this process. Check with the patient by asking "are you with me" or using a similar phrase. The next step is to address the patient's **E**motions with empathic responses, letting the patient have time to speak or collect her thoughts while the physician provides support. This is usually the most stressful task for the patient, but emotions are quite normal and common after hearing bad news and an empathic response to emotions will be experienced by the patient as quite supportive. The last step involves **S**trategy and **S**ummary. This involves a team approach to decision-making and, potentially, discussion of prognosis. An important part of the strategy piece is setting realistic goals for treatment so as to avoid patient misunderstanding about the goals of care.[54] Even when the prognosis is poor, one can always "hope for the best while preparing for the worst."[55] This means that patients are greatly reassured by knowing that they will receive the best treatment available for their particular disease. Avoid explicitly negative comments such as "there is little hope for a cure" and focus on what can be done. Ask specifically what concerns the patient has. Remember that patients may recall little information once they hear the diagnosis, so this might have to be repeated. Sending patients a follow-up letter summarizing the discussion can be extraordinarily helpful. Finally, involve the family in the discussion as the patient desires, since they can be an important source of support. Using this framework will provide a means in which to approach the diagnosis delivery in an organized fashion that provides the most information and support to the patient.[1]

For information on teaching and learning communication skills, the following links may be useful:

http://depts.washington.edu/oncotalk/
www.mdanderson.org/icare

IMPROVING COMMUNICATION: FUTURE DIRECTIONS

Communication is a skill and core competency in oncology. Communication skills are best taught during the fellowship years when trainees' communication skills are challenged by clinical situations they encounter.[56]

Curricula for oncology should include basic communication skills and a knowledge of how to break bad news across the cancer trajectory including transitioning a patient to palliative care, and how to use supportive services for the patient such as psychosocial services and palliative care. Competency in this area can relieve much of the stress around giving bad news and potentially reduce burnout.[57]

Training can be accomplished in brief workshops of several days duration with reinforcement throughout the fellowship. This commitment is minimal on the part of the surgical trainee compared to time spent learning other skills but requires also faculty committed to promoting communication skills as a core competency and learning how to reinforce fellows' skills throughout their training period.

SUMMARY

The delivery of a diagnosis of breast cancer is anxiety-producing for the patient and family, as well as for the physician. Key points include recognizing the variability in patient discussion style and desired depth of information, recognizing and overcoming barriers to communication, and planning ahead for difficult discussions with patients. Also, it is important to realize the importance of the patient–physician relationship in terms of providing support and information while working together on a treatment plan. The delivery of bad news is not something that physicians are routinely taught, nor is it something that comes easily; but good methods are available to teach physicians communications skills.

REFERENCES

1. Baile WF, Buckman R, Lenzi R, et al. SPIKES—a six-step protocol for delivering bad news: application to the patient with cancer. *Oncologist.* 2000;5:302-311.
2. Foley KM, Gelband H. *Improving Palliative Care for Cancer: Summary and Recommendations.* Washington, DC: National Academy Press; 2001.
3. Lobb EA, Butow PN, Mesier B, et al. Tailoring communication in consultations with women from high risk breast cancer families. *Br J Cancer.* 2002;87:502-508.
4. Arora NK, Johnson P, Gustafason DH, et al. Barriers to information access, perceived health competence, and psychological health outcomes: test of a mediation model in a breast cancer sample. *Patient Educ Couns.* 2002;47:37-46.
5. Brake H, Sassmann H, Noeres D, et al. Ways to obtain a breast cancer diagnosis, consistency of information, patient satisfaction, and the presence of relatives. *Support Care Cancer.* 2007;15:841-847.
6. Oskay-Ozcelik G, Lehmacher W, Konsgen D, et al. Breast cancer patients' expectations in respect of the physician-patient relationship and treatment management results of a survey of 617 patients. *Ann Oncol.* 2007;18: 479-484.
7. Buckman R. *Breaking Bad News: A Guide for Health Care Professions.* Baltimore, MD: Johns Hopkins University Press; 1992:15.
8. Parker PA, Baile WF, de Moor C, et al. Breaking bad news about cancer: patients' preferences for communication. *J Clin Oncol.* 2001;19:2049-2056.
9. Ptacek JT, Ellison NM. Health care providers' perspectives on breaking bad news to patients. *Crit Care Nurs Q.* 2000;23:51-59.
10. Gigris A, Sanson-Fisher RW. Breaking bad news: consensus guidelines for medical practitioners. *J Clin Oncol.* 1995;13:2449-2456.
11. Morris B, Abram C. Making healthcare decisions. *The Ethical and Legal Implications of Informed Consent in the Practitioner-Patient Relationship.* Washington, DC: United States Superintendent of Documents, 1982:119.
12. Degner LF, Kristjanson LJ, Bowman D, et al. Information needs and decisional preferences in women with breast cancer. *JAMA.* 1997;277: 1485-1492.
13. Novack DH, Plumer R, Smith RL, et al. Changes in physicians' attitudes toward telling the cancer patient. *JAMA.* 1979;241:897-900.
14. Arber A, Gallagher A. Breaking bad news revisited: the push for negotiated disclosure and challenging practice applications. *Int J Palliative Nursing.* 2003; 10:166-172.
15. Butow PN, Dowsett S, Hagerty R, Tattersall MH. Communicating prognosis to patients with metastatic disease: what do they really want to know? *Support Care Cancer.* 2002;10:161-168.
16. Heritage J, Maynard DW. Problems and prospects in the study of physician-patient interaction: 30 years of research. *Annu Rev Sociol.* 2006;32:351-374.
17. Cohen-Cole SA, Bird J. *The Medical Interview: The Three Function Approach.* St. Louis, MO: Mosby Year Book; 1991:28-41.
18. Schofield PE, Butow PN, Thompson JF, et al. Psychological responses of patients receiving a diagnosis of cancer. *Ann Oncol.* 2003; 14: 48-56.
19. Butow PN, Kazemi JN, Beeney LJ, et al. When the diagnosis is cancer: patient communication experiences and preferences. *Cancer.* 1996;77:2630-2637.
20. Wright EB, Holcombe C, Salmon P. Doctors' communication of trust, care, and respect in breast cancer: qualitative study. *Br Med J.* 2004;328:864-868.
21. Smith ML, Forster HP. Morally managing medical mistakes. *Camb Q Healthc Ethics.* 1997;8:336-340.
22. Levinson W, Roter DL, Mullooly JP, et al. Physician-patient communication: the relationship with malpractice claims among primary care physicians and surgeons. *JAMA.* 1997;277:553-559.
23. Roberts CS, Cox, CE, Reintgen DS, et al. Influence of physician communication on newly diagnosed breast patients' psychologic adjustment and decision-making. *Cancer.* 1994;74:336-341.

24. Jenkins V, Fallowfield L, Saul J. Information needs of patients with cancer: results from a large study in UK cancer centers. *Br J Cancer.* 2001;84:48-51.

25. Reaby LL. Reasons why women who have mastectomy decide to have or not to have breast reconstruction. *Plast Reconstr Surg.* 1998;101:1810-1818.

26. Schain WS. Physician-patient communication about breast cancer: a challenge for the 1990s. *Surg Clin North Am.* 1990;70:917-936.

27. Fallowfield LJ, Hall A, Maguire GP, Baum M. Psychological outcomes of different treatment policies in women with early breast cancer outside a clinical trial. *BMJ.* 1990;301:575-580.

28. Bruera E, Willey JS, Palmer JL, Rosales M. Treatment decisions for breast carcinoma: patient preferences and physician perceptions. *Cancer.* 2002;94:2076-2080.

29. Degner LF, Krisjanson LJ, Bowman D, et al. Information needs and decisional preferences in women with breast cancer. *JAMA.* 1997;277:1485-1492.

30. Harris KA. The informational needs of patients with cancer and their families. *Cancer Pract.* 1998;6:39-46.

31. Mumford E, Schlesinger HF, Glass GV. The effects of psychological intervention on recovery from surgery and heart attacks: an analysis of the literature. *Am J Public Health.* 1982;72:141-151.

32. Harvard Medical Practice Study. *Patients, Doctors, and Lawyers: Medical Injury, Malpractice Litigation, and Patient Compensation in New York: Report of the Harvard Medical Practice Study to the State of New York.* Cambridge, MA: Harvard University Press; 1990.

33. Forster HP, Schwartz J, DeRenzo E. Reducing legal risk by practicing patient-centered medicine. *Arch Intern Med.* 2002;162:1217-1219.

34. Beckman HB, Markakis KM, Suchman AL, Frankel RM. The doctor-patient relationship and malpractice: lessons from plaintiff depositions. *Arch Intern Med.* 1994;154:1365-1370.

35. Todd CJ, Still AW. Communication between general practitioners and patients dying at home. *Soc Sci Med.* 1984;18:667-672.

36. Parker, PA, Aaron J, Baile WF. Breast cancer: unique communication challenges and strategies to address them. *Breast J.* 2009;15(1):69-75.

37. Sepucha K, Belkora J, Mutchnick S, Esserman L. Consultation planning to help patients prepare for medical consultations: effect on communication and satisfaction for patients and physicians. *J Clin Oncol.* 2002;20:2695-2700.

38. Parker PA, Davison BJ, Tishelman C, et al. What do we know about facilitating patient communication in the cancer care setting? *Psycho Oncol.* 2005;14:848-858.

39. Davison BJ, Degner LF. Feasibility of using a computer-assisted intervention to enhance the way women with breast cancer communicate with their physicians. *Cancer Nurs.* 2002;25:417-424.

40. Damian D, Tattersall MH. Letters to patients: improving communication in cancer care. *Lancet.* 1991;338:923-925.

41. Tattersall MH, Butow PN, Griffin AM, Dunn SM. The take-home message: patients prefer consultation audiotapes to summary letters. *J Clin Oncol.* 1994;12: 1305-1311.

42. Maguire P. Improving communication with cancer patients. *Eur J Cancer.* 1999;35:2058-2065.

43. Levinson W, Gorawara-Bhat R, Lamb J. A study of patient clues and physician responses in primary care and surgical settings. *JAMA.* 2000;284:1021-1027.

44. Easter DW, Beach W. Competent patient care is dependent upon attending to empathic opportunities presented during interview sessions. *Curr Surg.* 2004;61:313-318.

45. Sardell AN, Trierweiler SJ. Disclosing the cancer diagnosis: procedures that influence patient hopefulness. *Cancer.* 1993;72:3355-3365.

46. Mitchell J. Cross-cultural issues in the disclosure of cancer. *Cancer Pract.* 2001;6:153-160.

47. Gordon GH. Care not cure: dialogues at the transition. *Patient Educ Couns.* 2003;50:95-98.

48. Hu W, Chiu T, Chuang R, Chen C. Solving family-related barriers to truthfulness in cases of terminal cancer in Taiwan. A professional perspective. *Cancer Nurs.* 2002;25:486-492.

49. Chen JY, Diamant AL, Thind A, Maly RC. Determinants of breast cancer knowledge among newly diagnosed, low-income, medically underserved women with breast cancer. *Cancer.* 2008;112:1153-1161.

50. Gustafson DH, McTavish FM, Stengle W, et al. Use and impact of eHealth system by low-income women with breast cancer. *J Health Comm.* 2005;10:195-218.

51. Siminoff LA, Graham GC, Gordon NH. Cancer communication patterns and the influence of patient characteristics: disparities in information-giving and affective behaviors. *Patient Educ Couns.* 2006;62:355-360.

52. Fentiman IS. Communication with older breast cancer patients. *Breast J.* 2007;13: 406-409.

53. Harrington SE, Smith TJ. The role of chemotherapy at the end of life: when is enough, enough? *JAMA.* 2008;299:2667-2678.

54. Von Roenn JH, von Gunten CF. Setting goals to maintain hope. *J Clin Oncol.* 2003;21:570-574.

55. Back AL, Arnold RM, Quill TE. Hope for the best, and prepare for the worst. *Ann Intern Med.* 2003;138:439-443.

56. Kidd J, Patel V, Peile E, Carter Y. Clinical and communication skills. *BMJ.* 2005; 330:374-375.

57. Sharma A, Sharp DM, Walker LG, Monson JR. Stress and burnout among colorectal surgeons and colorectal nurse specialists working in the National Health Service. *Colorectal Dis.* 2008;10:397-406.

SECTION 2

PATHOLOGY OF THE BREAST AND CLINICAL MANAGEMENT

Savitri Krishnamurthy
Rache M. Simmons

CHAPTER 15

Breast Specimen Tissue Processing

Edi Brogi
Violetta Barbashina

The purpose of this chapter is to provide general guidelines on specimen evaluation and highlight some clinically relevant issues, which may help to increase the efficiency and overall quality of pathologic assessment.

As outlined in the protocol for the examination of breast specimens released by the College of American Pathologists,[1] it is important that, together with the specimen, the pathologist receives specific information identifying the patient and the anatomic site from which the specimen was obtained, including its laterality and specific location in the breast (quadrant designation, subareolar location, etc), the date and type of procedure that was performed, and the name of the treating physician to whom the final report should be addressed.

In the course of gross examination, the prosector needs to state if the specimen was received in a fresh state or in fixative and specify the latter. Usually, a breast specimen consists of only 1 piece, but if more than 1 piece is present, the number should be stated, and the size of each piece measured in 3 dimensions. A specimen consisting of 3 or more pieces should not be inked. The gross description of the specimen needs to include any orientation markings identified on the specimen (see also "Margin Evaluation" later in the chapter). If a tumor is present, its size needs to be measured and reported. It is best to give the 3 dimensions of a tumor, but no definite consensus exists on this and the CAP recommends specifying the largest diameter.[1] Description of the tumor also includes comments on its outline (eg, circumscribed, ill defined), characteristics of the cut surface (eg, bulging, retracted, papillary), consistency (eg, firm, soft, rubbery, friable, mucoid), and color (eg, white, tan, brown-red). The relation of the tumor to the surgical margin should also be clearly specified. Gross examination of a fresh specimen allows better appreciation for subtle differences in the characteristics of the tissue, and enhances both visual and tactile inspection. It also minimizes exposure to formalin fumes, although it does not protect from blood-borne pathogens.

Recently published ASCO/CAP guidelines have recommended optimal fixation times and choice of fixative for breast tissue samples, greatly contributing to protocol standardization.[2] Poor or uneven tissue fixation negatively affects tissue preservation and immunohistochemical assessment. Proteolytic tissue degradation due to delayed fixation can result in weak or absent immunoreactivity and nonspecific binding of the antibody. Shorter than optimal formalin fixation (or attempts to fix large tissue pieces without proper sectioning) can result in a mixed fixation pattern where cross-linking occurs only at the periphery of the tissue and the center is either coagulatively fixed by alcohol or remains unfixed.[3] Mixed fixation is a common cause of different staining intensities at the periphery and in the center of the same section, and can lead to difficulties in histologic diagnosis and misinterpretation of ER, PR, and HER2 results. Very long fixation should also be avoided as it may cause excessive cross-linkage and damage some epitopes.[3]

▌ Fixation of Core Biopsies

According to the current ASCO/CAP guidelines, breast core biopsies should be fixed for a minimum of 1 hour[2]; however, some published data indicate that 1-hour fixation may be insufficient for accurate receptor analysis. In a study by Goldstein and associates, very short fixation times led to unreliable results in assessment of ER expression by immunohistochemistry.[4] Most discrepancies occurred when core biopsy tissues were fixed for less than 3 hours, while excellent results were achieved after fixation of 6 hours or longer. Given the importance of receptor status in breast carcinoma, it seems prudent to fix core biopsies for at least 3 hours (preferably 6) before processing. It is also recommended to repeat ER/PR and HER2 tests on the surgical specimen if the core biopsy yielded negative or equivocal results.[5,6]

Fixation of Breast Excisions and Mastectomy Specimens

According to the current ASCO/CAP recommendations,[2] tissue sections should be fixed in 10% buffered formalin for a period of 6 to 48 hours. It is best to examine and sample the surgical specimens in the fresh state, and immediately place the tissue sections in cassettes so that they can fix more uniformly. Alternatively, the tissue can be cut into 3- to 4-mm slices and placed in a container filled with large amount of fresh formalin, with large pieces of gauze or few crumpled sheets of paper towel inserted between the slices to maximize exposure to formalin. The upper limit of fixation time is less well defined, and further studies should help to determine if it can be safely extended beyond 48 hours.

CORE BIOPSY

Percutaneous needle core biopsy is now the primary modality for diagnostic evaluation of breast lesions. Nonpalpable, radiographically suspicious areas in the breast can be targeted under stereotactic, ultrasonographic, or magnetic resonance imaging (MRI) guidance. The diagnostic accuracy of the procedure increases with increasing caliber of the needle and number of tissue cores.

Standard 14-gauge needles provide good sensitivity. The false-negative rate of ultrasound-guided 14-gauge needle biopsy was 1.6% in a recent study of 1352 cases.[1] Larger tissue samples can be obtained with 11- or 8-gauge needles coupled with vacuum-assisted devices.

Most investigators agree that a minimum of 5 cores should be collected from suspicious breast lesions to ensure accurate sampling and diagnosis.[7] In a study by Liberman and colleagues, five 14-gauge tissue cores were sufficient for diagnosis in 99% of mass lesions and 6 cores were informative in 92% of mammographic lesions with calcifications.[8] The extent of sampling is dictated by the clinicoradiologic findings, and fewer than 5 cores may be sufficient in some cases.

Core Biopsy for Mammographic Calcifications

Once collected, the core biopsy tissue is examined by a radiologist who documents the presence of the target calcifications. Pathologic evaluation is best accomplished if the cores are divided into those with and those without radiographic calcifications. Segregation of the cores allows for separate embedding and step sectioning of the appropriate block(s) if the initial levels fail to demonstrate calcifications. The pathologist should attempt to correlate histology with radiologic findings, bearing in mind that calcifications smaller than 100 μm may not be relevant as these cannot be detected radiographically,[9] unless they are clustered together. Calcifications associated with malignant lesions tend to be relatively large, ranging in size from 100 to 300 μm.[9] The pathology report needs to specify where the calcifications are located (in situ or invasive carcinoma, benign breast lesions, stroma, blood vessel wall). It is also important to review the accompanying specimen x-ray to determine if the amount of calcifications on x-ray is similar to what

is seen on the slides, and this correlation is particularly important in cases with benign histologic findings. In order to avoid false-negative results, the pathologist needs to thoroughly search for calcifications whenever necessary. The tissue blocks are usually x-rayed en face to identify calcifications still embedded in the tissue, and multiple-level sections are obtained from the index block(s). There is no advantage in leaving tissue unsampled in the block if no calcifications are identified histologically, and levels through the block(s) should be ordered as necessary. Alternatively, blocks can be x-rayed on edge, allowing to identify the calcifications and to determine their depth in the tissue; in some cases this information is useful to assess whether it is opportune to melt the block and re-embed the tissue after it has been flipped, so that the calcifications are closer to the cutting surface and the tissue is not wasted. Calcifications are rarely affected by biopsy procedure and tissue processing, but occasionally they may be displaced, shattered, or lost ("knocked off") when the paraffin block is trimmed in preparation for sectioning.[10,11] This seems to occur more commonly in cases with larger calcium deposits and/or calcium oxalate crystals. Calcium oxalate crystals are often found in apocrine cysts or adjacent stroma, where they can be associated with a giant cell reaction. These crystals are translucent and can be missed on light microscopic examination, but they are birefringent under polarized light. Calcium crystals are water-soluble, and small calcifications have been reported to disappear within 3 days if the tissue is kept in a container with aqueous solution such as 10% formalin.[12]

Core Biopsy of Mass Lesion and/or Architectural Distortion

Communication between the pathologist and the radiologist is essential and information about the radiographic appearance of the lesion and its differential diagnosis will help the pathologist to better assess adequacy of the specimen. Whenever the findings in the core biopsy are felt to be discordant or nondiagnostic, the pathologist should alert the radiologist and communicate in the final report the limitations of the specimen.

Measurement of the size of invasive carcinoma on core biopsy material may not be accurate. In many cases, the actual tumor is larger than the core fragments and its size is best measured in the excision specimen. In contrast, information about the tumor size should be provided if the invasive focus is small, such as microinvasive carcinoma, as subsequent excision may not contain additional evidence of stromal invasion.

Atypical Findings in Core Biopsy Requiring Surgical Excision

Core biopsy should be viewed as a screening method aimed to identify lesions requiring surgical intervention. For that reason, a low threshold for excision is recommended for any abnormal or suspicious finding. The goal is not to remove the atypical foci, but to rule out the presence of frank malignancy in the adjacent tissue. Surgical excision should be performed for any type of epithelial or nonepithelial atypia, including atypical ductal hyperplasia (ADH), atypical columnar cell lesions (flat epithelial atypia, FEA), and histologically suspicious stromal and vascular proliferations. No consensus exists at present on the need for excision after diagnosis of lobular neoplasia (ALH/LCIS) in a core biopsy.[13,14] Several studies have documented the association between columnar cell atypia (FEA) and lobular neoplasia on core biopsy and finding of carcinoma on subsequent surgical excision.[15-19]

Accurate diagnosis and careful wording of the report are equally important. The pathologist should be aware that even in the absence of cytologic atypia, the use of the word "papillary" in the final diagnosis of the breast core biopsy will be followed by excision of the lesion. It is reasonable to remove and evaluate in its entirety any sizable, radiologically detected papillary lesion to rule out atypia or overt malignancy; however, minute incidental papillomas or foci of florid papillary usual ductal hyperplasia should not be overinterpreted. Therefore, it is best to avoid confusing terminology, such as "papillary hyperplasia." The diagnosis of "radial scar" or "complex sclerosing lesion" is also usually followed by surgical excision, and so is the diagnosis of "fibroepithelial lesion." The latter term should be reserved for fibroepithelial proliferations characterized by increased cellularity, mitotic activity, and/or cytologic atypia, suspicious for phyllodes tumor.

BREAST EXCISION

Margin Evaluation

Surgical margin status is an important predictor of local recurrence and affects survival of early-stage breast cancer, but no consensus exists on what constitutes an optimal margin. Its definition ranges widely, from "no tumor on ink" to "at least 1.0 cm clearance." It is intuitive that a wider margin will contribute to better outcome, but even "wide negative margins" cannot guarantee complete tumor removal due to architectural complexity of the mammary ductal system, multifocality of some tumors, and limitations of margin assessment methods.

In a study of 60 mastectomy specimens, Faverly and associates explored the 3-dimensional structure of the mammary ducts and the patterns of distribution of ductal carcinoma in situ (DCIS). Each mastectomy specimen was sectioned at 5-mm intervals and x-rayed, and the slices containing radiographically or grossly suspicious areas were carefully mapped and examined by conventional microscopy and stereomicroscopy to determine the extent of intraductal carcinoma and connections between different foci. The study demonstrated that 70% of low-grade lesions were multifocal, whereas 90% of high-grade DCIS showed continuous duct involvement.[20] These findings suggest that negative margins may be easier to achieve and more reliable in cases of high-grade DCIS as compared to low-grade carcinoma. In the same study, the gaps between the foci of carcinoma ranged from 0.1 to 4 cm, but most foci (82%) were less than 0.5 cm apart; hence, a 0.5-cm margin would have been adequate for 82% of patients.[20] Studies aimed to improve the conservative management of breast carcinoma have consistently demonstrated the benefit of radiation therapy in achieving local control, and a margin smaller than 5 mm is considered adequate in this setting.[21] A recent study evaluated over 1000 patients with DCIS treated with lumpectomy

and radiation and showed that the recurrence rate at 10 years was 8% in patients with a 2-mm margin.[22]

Several methods of margin evaluation have been proposed. They are outlined next, with discussion of advantages and disadvantages of each method.

Radial (Perpendicular) Margin Evaluation

The most common method of margin assessment is the perpendicular (or radial) margin technique, which allows for precise measurement of the distance separating the tumor from the closest inked margin (Fig. 15-1). With this method, the specimen is received oriented with side specification (right vs left breast). Usually, the surgeon designates the superior margin with a short suture (or a single metal clip), and the lateral margin with a long suture (or 2 metal clips). The 6 margins are differentially inked by the prosector. Ink should be applied lightly, with gentle dabbing, so not to artificially disrupt the tissue. Excess ink should be gently removed by pressing a gauze sponge on the specimen, to reduce the problem of running ink. Brief application of acetone on the inked surface seems to enhance staining and reduce the problem of running ink.

It is best to follow an established coloring scheme for margin designation, but color-coding should be always specified in the gross description for reference. Any color scheme is acceptable, as long as it specifically identifies each of the 6 margins. Medial and lateral margins can be inked with the same color and submitted in separate tissue blocks with margin designation. The inked specimen is then sequentially cut into 2- to 3-mm slices perpendicular to its long axis, so that the perimeter of each tissue slice contains 4 margins identified by ink of different colors. The extent of margin sampling is determined by its proximity to the index lesion. Margins within 0.5 cm of the index lesion are best evaluated in their entirety, and more distant margins can be representatively sampled. Sections should be taken preferably from fibrous, not fatty areas. With this method, the pathologist can report the exact microscopic distance from the tumor to each individual margin and distinguish between a truly positive margin ("tumor on ink"), a close margin (1-2 mm), and a margin 2 mm or greater, allowing the surgeon a greater level of judgment in determining the need of reexcision.[23] The disadvantages of this method include imprecise margin orientation and seepage of ink. Breast tissue is soft and may be artifactually disrupted when the specimen is compressed to obtain a specimen radiograph, or in the course of gross examination. Seepage of ink inside the specimen and different color inks running into each other occur frequently, leading to possible overinterpretation and false-positive margins.

Shaved (En Face) Margins Obtained from the Specimen

With en face margins obtained from the specimen (Fig. 15-2), the oriented specimen can be inked entirely in 1 color, as long as the prosector is able to maintain specimen orientation, but use of different color inks for different margins is more reliable. The margins are shaved off parallel to the outer surface of the specimen (in a manner similar to peeling an orange) at a depth

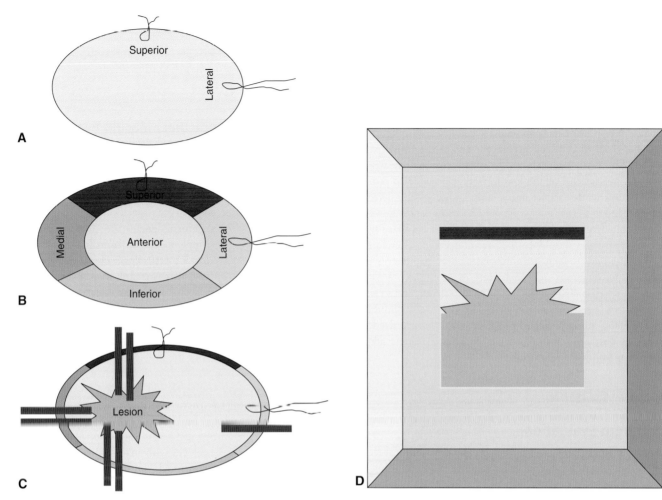

FIGURE 15-1   Perpendicular (radial) margin evaluation method. The specimen is received oriented **(A)** and the 6 margins are differentially inked **(B).** The tissue is then sequentially cut into 2- to 3-mm slices perpendicular to the long axis of the specimen, so that the perimeter of each slice contains 4 margins identified by different color inks **(C).** The margin sections are taken perpendicular to the inked surface **(C).** The extent of individual margin sampling is dictated by its proximity to the lesion. The tissue is embedded in such a manner that the distance from the lesion to the inked margin can be measured **(D).**

of 2 to 3 mm. Shaving of the margins is greatly facilitated by a short course (1-2 hours) of formalin fixation, as the outer tissue acquires firmer consistency. The shaved margins closest to the index lesion are submitted entirely, and the rest is submitted representatively. In some cases, the entire shaved surface of the specimen can be submitted for evaluation. The sections are embedded en face with the inked surface facing down, so that the histologic examination starts from the inner aspect of the shaved tissue. With this method, a margin is reported as positive when tumor is present in a section designated as shaved margin. This means that malignant cells are present within a 2- to 3-mm radius of the surgical margin, but the exact distance of the tumor to the margin cannot be assessed. If no tumor is identified, the margin is reported as negative. Microscopic examination for this method is straightforward and ink-related problems do not occur. The major disadvantage of this technique is that the pathologist cannot provide detailed information on the margin clearance, which limits the surgeon's ability to discriminate among patients with truly positive ("tumor at ink") or close margins, leading to a higher rate of reexcision.[23]

How does a shaved margin compare with a conventional radial margin? To answer this question, Guidi and associates evaluated 22 surgical specimens using both methods. The specimens were inked, and the margins were first shaved and examined microscopically. Then, the tissue was extracted from the block, cut perpendicular to the inked surface and reembedded to assess radial inked margins. The study demonstrated that a negative shaved margin was highly predictive of a negative inked margin (98% concordance), but the positive predictive value was much lower because only 61% of the positive shaved margins were called positive (tumor on ink) by the radial margin method.[24]

Cavity Shave Method

Evaluation of separate cavity shaves obtained by the surgeon likely provides the best solution to margin assessment, as it combines the advantages of the 2 methods described above and it is ideally suited for treatment of malignant tumors, when the goal is to excise the lesion with a rim of benign tissue.

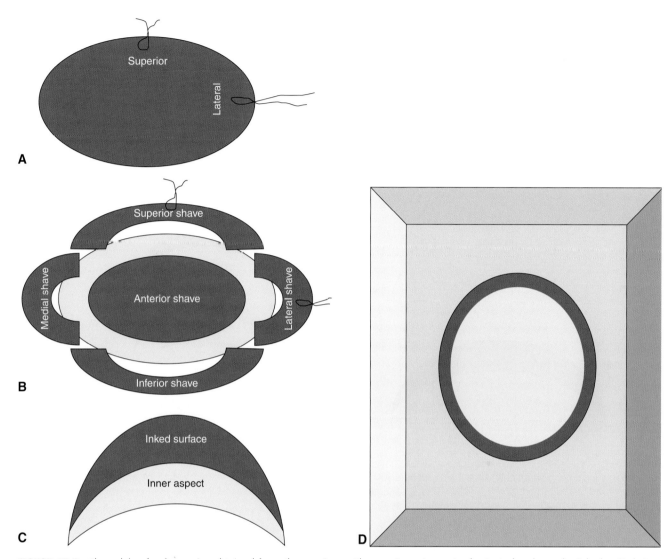

FIGURE 15-2 Shaved (en face) margins obtained from the specimen. The specimen is received oriented and may be inked entirely in one color as long as orientation is maintained **(A).** Then, the 6 margins are completely shaved off the specimen at a depth of 2 to 3 mm, parallel to the surface **(B).** Each margin is embedded en face with the inked surface facing down, so that the section for histologic examination is cut from the inner aspect of the shave **(C and D).**

With this method (Fig. 15-3), the surgeon resects the lesion and then takes separate shave margins from the surgical cavity. A separate anterior margin may or may not be submitted. The specimen containing the main tumor (central core) is received unoriented and does not necessarily need to be inked. The tumor in the central core is entirely sampled, including any prior biopsy site, if present; one or two representative sections of any grossly uninvolved breast tissue present are also submitted. Each shave specimen represents a margin, and is received oriented with a suture (or metal clip) designating the final margin surface; occasionally, 1 specimen can consist of 2 adjacent margins. Each margin is inked on the side designated with a suture, perpendicularly sectioned, and submitted either entirely or representatively in 10 blocks. This technique allows precise margin designation and accurate measurement of the margin width. These specimens are easily handled by the prosector and limited manipulation of the tissue and use of the

same color ink contribute to reduce some of the problematic artifacts described for the other methods. A significant increase in the number of blocks and slides is the main disadvantage of this technique. A group of investigators recently reported that this method significantly reduces the rate of reexcision for close margin.[25]

The cavity shave method is usually adopted by the surgeon only in patients with documented diagnosis of malignancy (by core biopsy or fine needle aspiration). Either the perpendicular margin or the shaved margin technique can be used in other cases.

Sampling of Excision Specimens

Small specimens (up to 3-4 cm) are usually submitted entirely, while larger breast excisions are selectively sampled. The extent of sampling is dictated by clinical, radiologic, and gross findings.

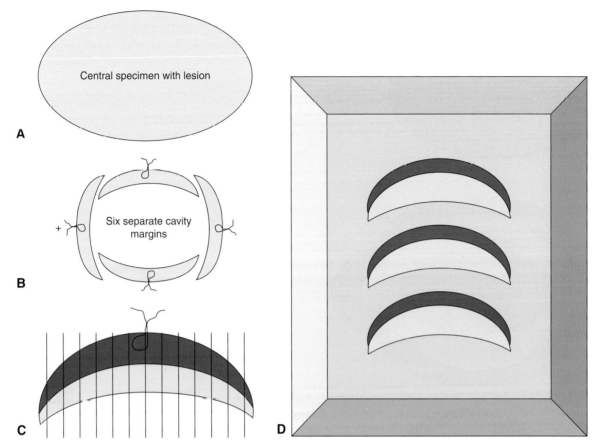

FIGURE 15-3 Cavity shave method. The surgeon first removes the lesion and then takes separate margins from the remaining cavity. Each margin should be appropriately labeled and oriented with a suture indicating the actual margin surface **(A and B).** The surface with a suture is inked, and the margins are serially sectioned and entirely submitted **(C).** Several sections can fit in one block. The tissue is embedded in such a manner that the margin width can be reported **(D).**

Palpable Lesions

If the surgeon suspects malignancy, he or she will orient the specimen to allow assessment of margin status. The lesion corresponding to a palpable abnormality should be carefully examined and, in many cases, will need to be entirely submitted. Several sections (2 or 3) representative of unremarkable breast parenchyma away from the lesions also need to be submitted.

Nonpalpable Lesions

When excision is performed for a nonpalpable abnormality, the lesion is radiographically located with the aid of one or more needle wires. The specimen is intraoperatively x-rayed to document retrieval of the index lesion and guide the surgeon as to the need for additional tissue resection. The specimen radiograph is usually sent to pathology along with the specimen to facilitate histologic sampling. If an alphanumeric specboard was used to hold the specimen during x-ray, the tissue should be kept on it during transport to maintain specimen orientation, facilitate correlation with the accompanying specimen radiograph, and guide sampling.

The excision specimen is usually received oriented for margin assessment. The prosector measures and inks the specimen (see methods above), notes the presence and number of wires, and sequentially sections the specimen (usually perpendicular

to the specimen main axis) to visualize the index lesion and/or core biopsy site. The area of interest is usually adjacent to the thick portion of the needle wire. If the lesion was previously sampled by core biopsy, a metal clip may be present, and its identification (or lack thereof) needs to be recorded. The suspicious area is widely blocked out and entirely submitted. If any gross abnormality is identified, the gross description should include its size and proximity to margin (specimen surface). Two to 3 representative sections from the grossly uninvolved parenchyma should be also submitted.

If the breast excision specimen contains calcifications, they need to be mapped and entirely submitted, noting the designation of the blocks. The remaining fibrous tissue can be representatively sampled in 2 or 3 blocks.

If no abnormality is found grossly, the entire tissue or 10 sections of its fibrous parenchyma are submitted. Schnitt and Wang studied optimal sampling of grossly benign breast lesions, and found that initial evaluation of 10 blocks of fibrous parenchyma was a cost-effective method, suitable to detect 97% of cases of microscopic atypia or carcinoma in situ.[26] The remaining tissue can be examined histologically only if carcinoma or atypical hyperplasia are found among the initial 10 blocks.

The pathologist should consider submitting all tissue if the excision is performed for a core biopsy diagnosis of atypical ductal hyperplasia (ADH) or DCIS to evaluate the morphologic spectrum of the ductal proliferation, rule out stromal invasion, and assess surgical margins status. In cases of DCIS, its extent can be calculated if the specimen is serially sectioned at 2- to 3-mm intervals and entirely submitted in sequential order.

Submission of all tissue is routinely done for breast excisions performed for

MRI-detected lesions. Selective sampling is not possible for these specimens, as no lesion is appreciated grossly.

Calcifications not amenable to core biopsy. The suspicious calcifications may be very focal and could be missed on limited sampling. These specimens are received with an accompanying specimen x-ray, and need to be sampled accordingly. If feasible, these specimens should be submitted in their entirety.

Any sizable, clinically or radiologically detected intraductal papilloma. These lesions should be examined in their entirety to exclude focal atypia or carcinoma. A papilloma usually arises in a large duct of the breast, often in a central/subareolar location. A breast excision performed for a papillary lesion is usually slightly cone-shaped and is received oriented with a stitch (metal clip) designating the apex of the specimen, which is usually the area closest to the nipple, and one designating the superior or lateral aspect of the specimen, as indicated by the surgeon. After the specimen is inked to reflect its orientation, it is best to section it from the nipple toward the deep aspect, rather than from lateral to medial. Transverse sectioning allows serial evaluation of the central ducts and maximizes the chances of identifying the papillary lesion, and of confirming its excision. In cross-section, a papilloma (or any other large papillary tumor involving a central duct) will appear as a collection of delicate fronds protruding into a cystic lumen, which consists of a dilated duct.

Discordant core biopsy and imaging findings. Atypia or malignant cells identified on fine-needle aspiration (FNA) without obvious mass on gross examination.

DOCUMENTATION OF TUMOR SIZE

Any lesion suspicious for malignancy should be carefully sampled to include at least one "full-face" section, which permits microscopic confirmation of the tumor size. Tumors measuring 2 cm or less are best submitted entirely. If the tumor is larger than 2 cm, the "full-face" section can be split and submitted in sequential, appropriately designated blocks. Gross assessment of the size may not be accurate if the tumor is poorly circumscribed and/or surrounded by fibrosis. The size, however, has important treatment implications. Accurate measurements are particularly important in very small (<1.0 cm) and very large (>5.0 cm) invasive carcinomas. The pathologist should be aware that patients with tumors smaller than 1.0 cm may be spared adjuvant chemotherapy, while those with large invasive carcinomas (>5.0 cm) are considered to have locally advanced disease requiring postsurgical chest wall radiation. Microscopic confirmation of the tumor size and correlation with imaging findings should help to ensure appropriate patient management.

REEXCISION SPECIMENS

A breast reexcision is intended to remove any residual disease from the area of interest and obtain clear margins. Reexcision usually yields 1 specimen containing the prior excision site, and it is submitted oriented using the same markings as for an excision specimen. Some surgeons submit 2 or more separate specimens (lower hemisphere, upper hemisphere), and designate the surface representing the final margin with a suture/metal clip. The prosector records the dimensions of the specimen and of the biopsy cavity, the location of the latter within the specimen, and its distance from the closest margin(s). The reexcision margin is inked and sampled according to one of the protocols described above.

The specimen is sequentially sectioned and examined. Any grossly evident abnormality is described, giving its exact location within the specimen, distance to the closest margin(s), size, color, and consistency. Sampling should focus on firmer areas. If the biopsy cavity is small (less than 3 cm), its entire wall can be submitted; larger biopsy cavities are sampled representatively (ie, every other section is submitted). More generous sampling is recommended if the prior excision contained only DCIS to rule out possible stromal invasion. Generous sampling of the margin(s) closest to the biopsy cavity is also recommended.

TYPES OF MASTECTOMY

Mastectomy (mastoid = breast and ectomy = removal) is intended to remove the breast parenchyma in its entirety, but other structures are often removed with the breast, resulting in different procedures.

Simple or total mastectomy. The entire breast is removed, but lymph nodes and surrounding muscle are left intact.

Modified radical mastectomy. This is the most common type of mastectomy performed for the treatment of breast carcinoma. The entire breast is removed together with level I and II axillary lymph nodes. The muscles of the chest wall are left intact.

Radical mastectomy. This procedure removes the entire breast, axillary lymph nodes, muscle under the breast, and some of the surrounding soft tissue. This procedure was introduced over a century ago by William Halstead for the treatment of breast carcinoma, but today it is rarely performed and only in cases of chest wall involvement.

Skin-sparing mastectomy. This procedure is less disfiguring than other types of mastectomy. The entire breast is removed through a small incision, either a "keyhole" incision around the nipple, or an incision in the inframammary fold or in the lateral breast. Nipple and areola are left in place for a more natural cosmetic result and maintained nipple sensation. To ensure that no carcinoma is left in the nipple, the ducts immediately below it are submitted for intraoperative evaluation. If DCIS and/or invasive carcinoma is present in the frozen section, a simple mastectomy is performed instead.

Recent studies have reported the use of nipple-sparing mastectomy for treatment of breast carcinoma in selected patients,[27,28] with a low rate of local recurrence.[27]

GROSS EXAMINATION OF MASTECTOMY SPECIMENS

The mastectomy is received oriented with a stitch designating either the axillary tail of the breast or the attached axillary soft tissue. With the exception of nipple-sparing procedures, a skin ellipse containing the nipple–areolar complex is situated anteriorly on the mastectomy specimen. Presence, dimensions, and appearance of skin, nipple, and areola are recorded; weighing the specimen is optional. Similarly, if any skin lesion is present, it is measured, described, and sampled. Nipple and areola are carefully evaluated for redness, scaling, and oozing, which raise the possibility of nipple/areolar involvement by adenocarcinoma (Paget disease). Histologic confirmation is necessary to render this diagnosis. Any scar present on the skin or around the areola should be described, measured, and representatively sampled.

With exception of the product of radical mastectomy, the deep aspect of the specimen is smooth and covered by a thin fascia; rarely, scattered small fragments of skeletal muscle may be present. The deep aspect of a mastectomy specimen is routinely inked to assess tumor involvement; black ink is used in most cases. At many centers, ink is also applied on the anterior surface of the specimen not covered by skin, but there is no consensus on this practice and the CAP guidelines on specimen handling do not recommend It.[1] Because carcinoma at the anterior/superficial aspect of the mastectomy specimen could potentially initiate a (sub)cutaneous chest wall recurrence, evaluation of the anterior aspect of the breast may help to prevent this scenario, but no data are available on this issue. If the anterior surface of the mastectomy specimen is inked, it is best to apply ink of a color different from that used for the deep margin (eg, blue ink).

Some prosectors also designate the axillary tail/axillary soft tissue with ink of a different color (eg, yellow ink), so that specimen orientation can easily be assessed, if additional sampling is needed at a later time.

The mastectomy specimen is sectioned into 3- to 5-mm thick longitudinal sections, which are usually kept connected anteriorly through the skin ellipse, creating a sort of "open book" for examination. Gross evaluation is best done on a fresh specimen, but if the specimen is fixed overnight before examination, it should be submerged in formalin in a large container, with crumpled sheets of paper interposed between the "pages" of the open book, to ensure proper fixation of the tissue. The exact location of all identified lesions is recorded, specifying for each the involved quadrant, o'clock designation, and distance to the nipple and/or to the closest deep margin. Description of any abnormal area includes size (3 dimensions), shape (stellate, round, irregular, etc), contour (sharply defined, ill-defined, etc), color, and consistency. Sections for microscopic evaluation are submitted from

Nipple and skin. The nipple is bi- or trisected and submitted entirely in one cassette; a section of the nipple base is also submitted.

Any grossly evident tumor/lesion, with extensive sampling.

Prior biopsy site(s). Identification of prior core biopsy sites in a mastectomy specimen with multicentric disease benefits from review of prior radiology, to determine the exact sites

of the diagnostic procedures and guide sampling. Metal clip(s) left at the time of prior biopsy need to be identified in the specimen and their location recorded.

Deep margin (including skeletal muscle, whenever present) in relation to closest tumor and/or biopsy site.

(Two) representative sections of grossly unremarkable parenchyma from each quadrant.

The anterior margin is sampled if any lesion/biopsy site is at or close to it.

In cases of complete or near complete response after neoadjuvant chemotherapy, the breast can appear unremarkable, and gross identification of residual tumor is very difficult if not impossible. In these cases, the prosector needs to review prior radiology reports and submit sections from areas of documented involvement. Extensive sampling is recommended, as residual disease can be scattered. Identification of the prior core biopsy site(s) is also extremely important.

Risk-Reducing Mastectomy

Some women at high risk of breast carcinoma (due to personal and/or family history) may elect to undergo risk-reducing mastectomy, which usually consists of a simple mastectomy, even though, more recently, nipple-sparing mastectomy has also become an option.

Nipple and skin, if present, are sampled as for any mastectomy specimen. Because of the lack of clinical or radiographic abnormalities, the product of risk reducing mastectomy needs to be more thoroughly sampled, and 4 or 5 representative sections from each quadrant should be submitted, in addition to sections from the nipple, areola, and from any grossly evident abnormality. In a patient with synchronous contralateral breast carcinoma, 2 sections per quadrant may be sufficient.

Reduction Mammoplasty Specimens

Reduction mammoplasty is intended to remove excess breast tissue. It is sometimes medically indicated, or done for cosmetic reasons, or an adjunct procedure to achieve breast symmetry in patients undergoing surgery for a malignant diagnosis in the contralateral breast. Usually access to the breast parenchyma is achieved through a T-shaped incision in the lower breast, between lower outer and lower inner quadrants. Tissue is removed through this incision from the central, medial, and lateral aspect of the gland. Some surgeons submit the tissue obtained from the 3 areas separately (central, medial, and lateral), and others combine it in one container. Strips of redundant skin are also removed. The tissue is received fragmented in multiple pieces, some with overlying skin, and cannot be inked. The specimen is weighed and measured in aggregate. The skin pieces are also measured as an aggregate, giving a size range, from smallest to largest. Representative sections of the fibrous tissue are submitted for histologic evaluation, but no specific guidelines exist regarding the extent of optimal sampling for these specimens. Some pathologists may follow the "10 blocks" rule,[26] and others may submit only 3 to 4 blocks, each containing 2 sections. If any abnormality is found histologically, additional material is submitted, but it is not possible to assess margin status.

Axillary Dissection

In the era of sentinel lymph node biopsy, axillary dissection has become a relatively uncommon procedure, and it is often performed in patients with previously proven sentinel lymph node involvement or clinically/radiologically advanced locoregional disease.

Most surgeons designate the levels of an axillary dissection with metal tags (or stitches), and this should be recorded in the gross description, with the lymph nodes from each level kept separate.

Careful gross examination of the axillary soft tissue is necessary to identify all lymph nodes present. This is best achieved by squeezing the axillary soft tissue between the tips of thumb and index/middle fingers. Lymph node(s) are recognized because they are firmer and oppose greater resistance to pressure than the surrounding fibroadipose tissue. Some fixatives containing methanol may increase the firmness of lymph nodes and also make them appear whiter than the adjacent adipose tissue, but in our experience they do not provide a substantial advantage over careful examination of the fresh specimen. The number of lymph nodes present in an axillary dissection can vary slightly. Locoregional staging of breast carcinoma requires evaluation of at least 10 axillary lymph nodes, and levels I and II combined usually contain 12 to15 nodes or more. If a level III dissection is also performed the total number of axillary lymph nodes approaches 20 or more.

The prosector needs to give an approximate count of the lymph nodes identified, and their size range, from smallest to largest. All identified lymph nodes are entirely submitted for histologic examination. Lymph nodes larger than 0.5 cm are usually longitudinally bisected. Bigger (>1.0 cm) lymph nodes are trisected or sectioned in multiple slices. The prosector needs to indicate if a lymph node is submitted as more than one section, to prevent overcounting. More than one lymph node can be submitted in a tissue block, as long as each node is designated with ink of a different color, thus enabling accurate node count.

In the postneoadjuvant setting, the lymph node yield is often reduced.[29-31]

SUMMARY

A good and thorough gross evaluation of breast surgical specimens and subsequent optimal processing of the sampled tissue is mandatory for providing the best pathologic assessment of the specimens. Knowledge of the imaging findings in a given case is important for accurate identification of the lesions in the specimen. Proper orientation of the specimen, appropriate inking, slicing as thin as possible and radiographic evaluation of specimens with suspicious calcifications are all key factors that can be instrumental in accurately identifying the lesions and/or suspicious calcifications and also for correctly evaluating the status of margins in the specimen. In the case of sentinel lymph nodes, it is mandatory to slice the lymph nodes as thin as possible so that

the majority, if not all the metastatic tumor deposits in the lymph node can be detected on histopathologic examination. A careful and thorough dissection of the adipose tissue in the case of axillary content specimens can result in the detection of all possible lymph nodes for subsequent scrutiny on pathologic examination and establishment of axillary lymph node status in patients with breast cancer. In addition to careful gross evaluation, optimal tissue fixation, processing, and staining are equally critical factors in generating high-quality tissue sections for final histopathologic evaluation and detecting prognostic and predictive markers. In essence, a coordinated team effort by pathologists, pathology assistants, and technologists involved in gross evaluation, processing, and staining of breast tissue specimens can result in high-quality pathologic assessment of breast tissue specimens, thereby aiding in appropriate management of patients with breast diseases.

REFERENCES

1. Fitzgibbons PL, Connolly JL, Page DL. Updated protocol for the examination of specimens from patients with carcinomas of the breast. Cancer Committee. *Arch Pathol Lab Med.* 2000;124:1026-1033.
2. Wolff AC, Hammond ME, Schwartz JN, et al. American Society of Clinical Oncology/College of American Pathologists guideline recommendations for human epidermal growth factor receptor 2 testing in breast cancer. *J Clin Oncol.* 2007;25:118-145.
3. Werner M, Chott A, Fabiano A, Battifora H. Effect of formalin tissue fixation and processing on immunohistochemistry. *Am J Surg Pathol.* 2000;24:1016-1019.
4. Goldstein NS, Ferkowicz M, Odish E, Mani A, Hastah F. Minimum formalin fixation time for consistent estrogen receptor immunohistochemical staining of invasive breast carcinoma. *Am J Clin Pathol.* 2003;120:86-92.
5. Hodi Z, Chakrabarti J, Lee AH, et al. The reliability of assessment of oestrogen receptor expression on needle core biopsy specimens of invasive carcinomas of the breast. *J Clin Pathol.* 2007;60:299-302.
6. Lee AH, Hodi Z, Ellis IO. False-negative assessment of oestrogen receptor on needle core biopsy of invasive carcinoma of the breast. *J Clin Pathol.* 2008;61:239-240.
7. Schueller G, Jaromi S, Ponhold L, et al. US-guided 14-gauge core-needle breast biopsy: results of a validation study in 1352 cases. *Radiology.* 2008;248: 406-413.
8. Liberman L, Dershaw DD, Rosen PP, et al. Stereotaxic 14-gauge breast biopsy: how many core biopsy specimens are needed? *Radiology.* 1994;192:793-795.
9. Dahlstrom JE, Sutton S, Jain S. Histologic-radiologic correlation of mammographically detected microcalcification in stereotactic core biopsies. *Am J Surg Pathol.* 1998;22:256-259.
10. Stein MA, Karlan MS. Calcifications in breast biopsy specimens: discrepancies in radiologic-pathologic identification. *Radiology.* 1991;179:111-114.
11. Winston JS, Geradts J, Liu DF, Stomper PC. Microtome shaving radiography: demonstration of loss of mammographic microcalcifications during histologic sectioning. *Breast J.* 2004;10:200-203.
12. Moritz JD, Luftner-Nagel S, Westerhof JP, et al. Microcalcifications in breast core biopsy specimens: disappearance at radiography after storage in formaldehyde. *Radiology.* 1996;200:361-363.
13. Cohen MA. Cancer upgrades at excisional biopsy after diagnosis of atypical lobular hyperplasia or lobular carcinoma in situ at core-needle biopsy: some reasons why. *Radiology.* 2004;231:617-621.
14. Nagi CS, O'Donnell JE, Tismenetsky M, et al. Lobular neoplasia on core needle biopsy does not require excision. *Cancer.* 2008;112:2152-2158.
15. Abdel-Fatah TM, Powe DG, Hodi Z, et al. High frequency of coexistence of columnar cell lesions, lobular neoplasia, and low grade ductal carcinoma in situ with invasive tubular carcinoma and invasive lobular carcinoma. *Am J Surg Pathol.* 2007;31:417-426.
16. Brem RF, Lechner MC, Jackman RJ, et al. Lobular neoplasia at percutaneous breast biopsy: variables associated with carcinoma at surgical excision. *AJR Am J Roentgenol.* 2008;190:637-641.
17. Cangiarella J, Guth A, Axelrod D, et al. Is surgical excision necessary for the management of atypical lobular hyperplasia and lobular carcinoma in

situ diagnosed on core needle biopsy? A report of 38 cases and review of the literature. *Arch Pathol Lab Med.* 2008;132:979-983.

18. Menon S, Porter GJ, Evans AJ, et al. The significance of lobular neoplasia on needle core biopsy of the breast. *Virchows Arch.* 2008;452:473-479.

19. Pandey S, Kornstein MJ, Shank W, de Paredes ES. Columnar cell lesions of the breast: mammographic findings with histopathologic correlation. *Radiographics.* 2007;27(suppl):S79–S89.

20. Faverly DR, Burgers L, Bult P, Holland R. Three dimensional imaging of mammary ductal carcinoma in situ: clinical implications. *Semin Diagn Pathol.* 1994;11:193-198.

21. Kell MR, Morrow M. An adequate margin of excision in ductal carcinoma in situ. *BMJ.* 2005;331:789-790.

22. Solin LJ, Fourquet A, Vicini FA, et al. Long-term outcome after breast conservation treatment with radiation for mammographically detected ductal carcinoma in situ of the breast. *Cancer.* 2005;103:1137-1146.

23. Wright MJ, Park J, Fey JV, et al. Perpendicular inked versus tangential shaved margins in breast-conserving surgery: does the method matter? *J Am Coll Surg.* 2007;204:541-549.

24. Guidi AJ, Connolly JL, Harris JR, Schnitt SJ. The relationship between shaved margin and inked margin status in breast excision specimens. *Cancer.* 1997;79:1568-1573.

25. Cao D, Lin C, Woo SH, Vang R, Tsangaris TN, Argani P. Separate cavity margin sampling at the time of initial breast lumpectomy significantly reduces the need for reexcisions. *Am J Surg Pathol.* 2005;29:1625-1632.

26. Schnitt SJ, Wang HH. Histologic sampling of grossly benign breast biopsies. How much is enough? *Am J Surg Pathol.* 1989;13:505-512.

27. Sacchini V, Pinotti JA, Barros AC, et al. Nipple-sparing mastectomy for breast cancer and risk reduction: oncologic or technical problem? *J Am Coll Surg.* 2006;203:704-714.

28. Voltura AM, Tsangaris TN, Rosson GD, et al. Nipple-sparing mastectomy: critical assessment of 51 procedures and implications for selection criteria. *Ann Surg Oncol.* Dec 2008;15(12):3396-3401. Epub 2008 Oct 16.

29. Baslaim MM, Al Malik OA, Al-Sobhi SS, et al. Decreased axillary lymph node retrieval in patients after neoadjuvant chemotherapy. *Am J Surg.* 2002;184:299-301.

30. Belanger J, Soucy G, Sideris L, et al. Neoadjuvant chemotherapy in invasive breast cancer results in a lower axillary lymph node count. *J Am Coll Surg.* 2008;206:704-708.

31. Neuman H, Carey LA, Ollila DW, et al. Axillary lymph node count is lower after neoadjuvant chemotherapy. *Am J Surg.* 2006;191:827-829.

CHAPTER 16

Benign Conditions of the Breast

Michael P. Osborne
Susan K. Boolbol
Juhi Asad

Benign breast conditions encompass nonmalignant disorders of the breast. The pathogenesis of these conditions is poorly understood, and little research is being done because most efforts are appropriately being directed toward breast cancer. However, there are large numbers of women with benign breast conditions, and the treatment of mastalgia/mastodynia is currently difficult; therefore more research is required in this area. This chapter summarizes benign breast conditions and outlines their diagnosis and management.

FIBROCYSTIC DISEASE

Fibrocystic disease has been used as a generic term to describe symptoms and fails to encompass the extent of the histologic changes.[1] The aberration of normal development and involution (ANDI)[1] was published in 1987 to help define patients' problems in terms of pathogenesis, histology, and clinical implications.[2]

The concept of the ANDI is based on the fact that benign breast disease arises from normal physiology (Table 16-1). The horizontal headings show the spectrum of benign conditions—normal to mild abnormality ("disorder") to severe abnormality ("disease"). The vertical headings define the pathogenesis of the conditions.[3]

Development Period

At the onset of puberty, estrogen is a major influence in the development of the breast by stimulating ductal growth. During the menstrual cycle, the cyclical secretion of progesterone facilitates the lobuloalveolar growth marking the developmental period. Typically, these changes are noted through the menarchal period (15-25 years old). During this period, nipple inversion, juvenile hypertrophy, and fibroadenomas are seen.[1]

Nipple Inversion

Nipple inversion can occur during the development of terminal ducts. This results in the lack of protrusion of the ducts and areola. Nipple inversion predisposes to terminal duct obstruction, which may lead to subareolar abscesses.

Juvenile Hypertrophy

Juvenile hypertrophy is a rare condition. The spectrum can range from a small breast to massive gigantomastia in peripubertal females. The etiology of juvenile hypertrophy is unknown; however, there is a hormonal basis to the condition. Baker and associates described that tamoxifen may be a useful adjunct when combined with reduction mammoplasty for the treatment of gigantomastia.[4]

Cyclical Change

The breast enlarges during the premenstrual phase and involutes before and during menstruation. The hormonal interactions during the menstrual cycle cause the epithelial and stromal activity and regression to occur regularly.

MASTALGIA/(MASTODYNIA)/NODULARITY

Breast pain is a common complaint and in most cases it is self-limiting. There is no histologic difference in patients with or without mastalgia. Breast fullness, tenderness, and nodularity are most frequent during the late luteal phase of the menstrual cycle. Treatment in most cases is reassurance. For severe pain, endocrine and nonendocrine agents have been studied, from danazol, bromocriptine, and tamoxifen to evening primrose oil and vitamin E; all have gotten variable responses.

TABLE 16-1 ANDI Classification

Reproductive Period	Normal →	Disorder →	Disease →
Development	Ductal development	Nipple inversion	Mammary duct fistula
	Lobular development	Single duct	Giant fibroadenoma
	Stromal development	Obstruction	
		Fibroadenoma	
		Juvenile hypertrophy	
Cyclical change	Hormonal activity	Mastalgia	
	Epithelial activity	Nodularity	
		Focal	
		Diffuse	
		Benign papilloma	
Pregnancy and lactation	Epithelial hyperplasia	Blood-stained nipple discharge	
	Lactation	Galactocele and inappropriate lactation	
Involution	Lobular involution	Cysts and sclerosing adenosis	
	Ductal involution	Nipple retraction	Periductal mastitis with suppuration
	Fibrosis	Duct ectasia	
	Dilatation	Simple hyperplasia micropapillomatosis	Lobular hyperplasia with atypia
	Involutional epithelial hyperplasia		Ductal hyperplasia with atypia

ANDI, aberration of normal development and involution
From Hughes LE, Mansel RE, Webster DJT. Aberrations of normal development and involution (ANDI): a new perspective on pathogenesis and nomenclature of benign breast disorders. *Lancet.* 1987;2:1316-1319.

MONDOR DISEASE

Mondor disease is a rare cause of breast pain. The clinical features are localized pain with a tender, palpable subcutaneous cord or linear skin dimpling. The cause is a superficial thrombophlebitis of the lateral thoracic vein or a tributary. It has been associated with recent surgery, trauma, and inflammatory process or carcinoma. The condition resolves spontaneously but the use of nonsteroidal anti-inflammatory drugs may help to alleviate the symptoms.

INVOLUTION

Involutional changes are usually seen by 35 years of age; thus cyclical change and involution occur simultaneously. The exact mechanism of involution is not well understood; however, orderly lobular regression depends on the coordinated involution of the epithelium and specialized connective tissue.[1] Variations of the state can result in sclerosing adenosis, microcyst formation, duct ectasia, and epithelial hyperplasia.

CYSTS

Cysts are fluid-filled, round structures that vary in size from microscopic to palpable masses (Fig. 16-1). They are most common in perimenopausal women. The cysts are derived from the terminal duct lobular unit. It has been described that if the stroma disappears too early, epithelial acini remain and may form microcysts, which then can lead to larger cysts.[1]

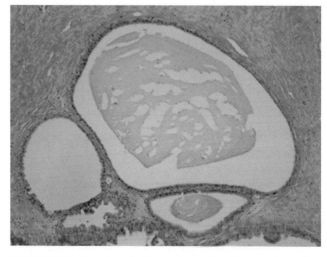

FIGURE 16-1 Breast cysts. The cysts are lined by apocrine cells, which contain abundant granular cytoplasm. Note also the presence of proteinaceous secretion in the lumen of some of the cysts. *(Courtesy of Dr Savitri Krishnamurthy, MD Anderson Cancer Center, Houston, Texas.)*

Cysts often come and go in relation to the menstrual cycle and can be exacerbated by hormonal changes. On physical exam, cysts may feel firm or rubbery and are well differentiated from normal breast tissue. Cysts that present suddenly tend to be tender. It is best to confirm the presence of a cyst by the use of ultrasound to ensure there is no underlying mass present.

Simple cysts can be observed. However, if they are symptomatic, an aspiration should be performed. A follow-up examination is recommended after an aspiration is performed to ensure resolution of the cyst. Surgical excision of a cyst is required if there is bloody aspirate, the palpable abnormality does not completely resolve with aspiration or the same cyst recurs several times within a short period of time.

FIBROEPITHELIAL LESIONS

Fibroadenoma

Fibroadenoma is a benign tumor that arises from the epithelium and stroma of the terminal duct-lobular unit (Fig. 16-2A). It is

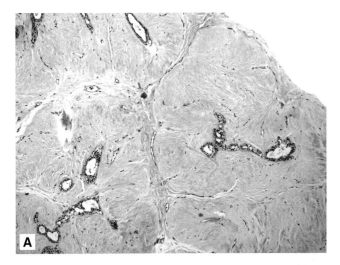

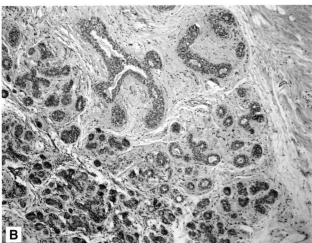

FIGURE 16-2 Classical fibroadenoma **(A)** and complex fibroadenoma **(B). A.** This benign tumor is well-circumscribed, and comprises 2 elements (as the name implies): stromal and glandular. Typically, both elements of a fibroadenoma proliferate. The tumor shown here is from an older patient. In this case, the senescent fibrous component has become somewhat sclerotic. **B.** A fibroadenoma with sclerosing adenosis, cysts larger than 3 mm, epithelium-associated calcifications, and papillary apocrine hyperplasia is termed *complex fibroadenoma*. The cumulative risk for invasive carcinoma has been stated to be approximately 3 times that of women in general population compared with a relative risk of about 1.9 times in women with noncomplex fibroadenoma. *(Courtesy of Syed A. Hoda, MD, New York Presbyterian Hospital, Cornell, New York.)*

the most common breast mass clinically and pathologically in adolescent and young women. The age distribution ranges from early teens to more than 70 years of age; however, less than 5% of women diagnosed with a fibroadenoma are postmenopausal.

The most common presentation is a painless well-circumscribed mobile mass found by the patient. Some fibroadenomas are nonpalpable and are found by imaging alone. About 10% to 20% of fibroadenomas are multiple and bilateral.

Most fibroadenomas found on ultrasound have features of a benign tumor. Some classical findings on ultrasound are an elliptical or gently lobulated shape, "wider than tall," isoechoic or mildly hypoechoic, presence of a capsule, and mobile during palpation.[5]

Most fibroadenomas are less than 3 cm in size. Tumors that are greater than 4 cm are frequently seen in patients 20 years of age and younger. A fibroadenoma greater than 6 cm in size is referred to as a *giant fibroadenoma* (Fig. 16-3). Fibroadenomas consists of epithelial and fibrous components. There are several variants of fibroadenomas, which will be discussed in the next sections.

Juvenile Fibroadenoma

Juvenile fibroadenomas account for approximately 4% of all fibroadenomas.[6] These patients tend to be younger than the average age of patients with fibroadenomas. Juvenile fibroadenomas are grossly indistinguishable from a fibroadenoma. Microscopically, they are characterized by stromal cellularity and epithelial hyperplasia (Fig. 16-4).[7]

Giant Fibroadenoma

Histologically, giant fibroadenomas are the same as conventional fibroadenomas, but it is the size of the tumor that classifies them

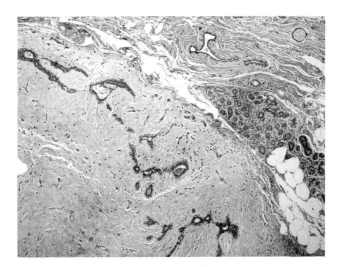

FIGURE 16-3 Giant fibroadenoma. A fibroadenoma that attains a "substantial" dimension would qualify for the designation of giant fibroadenoma. These giant fibroadenomas are rare and typically occur in adolescent girls. The stromal component can become extremely prominent and have a myxoid appearance (as seen here); however, the mitotic activity in the stromal cells is typically minimal. *(Courtesy of Syed A. Hoda, MD, New York Presbyterian Hospital, Cornell, New York.)*

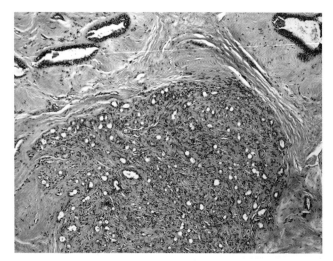

FIGURE 16-4 Juvenile fibroadenoma. The typical juvenile fibroadenoma is rapidly growing and occurs in teenage girls. This type of tumor shows increased stromal cellularity with neither overt fibrosis or myxomatous change. Mitotic activity in the stromal cells is minimal, and there is no stromal overgrowth. The epithelial component may become prominent (as shown here). *(Courtesy of Syed A. Hoda, MD, New York Presbyterian Hospital, Cornell, New York).*

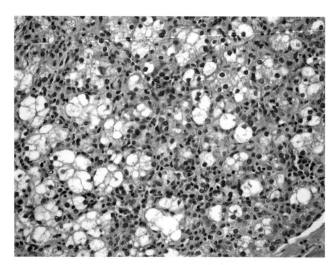

FIGURE 16-5 Lactational fibroadenoma. A circumscribed fibroepithelial nodule occurring in pregnant or postpartum women with lactational (secretory) change in the epithelial component is termed *lactational adenoma* (or *lactating adenoma*). It is debatable whether these lesions should be considered true (benign) neoplasms or a localized form of lobular hyperplasia in a gestational breast. *(Courtesy of Syed A. Hoda, MD, New York Presbyterian Hospital, Cornell, New York.)*

(Fig. 16-3). The importance of a giant fibroadenoma is the need to distinguish it from a phyllodes tumor. As compared to a phyllodes tumor, giant fibroadenomas tend to be less cellular. However, it may at times be difficult to distinguish the two.

Complex Fibroadenoma

Complex fibroadenoma is defined as a fibroadenoma with sclerosing adenosis, papillary apocrine hyperplasia, cysts, or epithelial calcifications (Fig. 16-2B). Dupont and colleagues found patients with complex fibroadenoma have a higher relative risk (3.1) for developing breast carcinoma than those who had noncomplex fibroadenomas.[8]

Lactating Adenoma

Lactating adenomas are the most prevalent breast masses in the young pregnant female.[9] During pregnancy, placental, luteal, and pituitary hormones induce ductal proliferation, which is associated with a rapid increase in the quantity and dimensions of the breast alveoli.[10] They are well-circumscribed masses measuring 2 to 4 cm in diameter with a firm rubbery texture. Infarction can occur in approximately 5% of the cases. This is due to the relative vascular insufficiency caused by the high requirement of the breast during lactation and pregnancy.[11] Histologically, lactating adenomas appear as a lobulated mass of enlarged acini surrounded by a basement membrane and edematous stroma (Fig. 16-5).[10]

Tubular Adenoma

Tubular adenoma is a variant of pericanalicular fibroadenoma with an exceptionally prominent or florid adenosis-like epithelial proliferation. The clinical presentation is similar to a fibroadenoma. These lesions are not associated with pregnancy or oral contraceptives. Microscopically, tubular adenomas are separated from the adjacent breast tissue by a pseudocapsule, and are composed of a proliferation of uniform, small tubular structures with a scant amount of intervening stroma.

Fibroadenomas can be reliably diagnosed by either fine-needle aspiration or core needle biopsy. Conservative management with short-term follow-up rather than surgical excision can be offered provided there are no associated atypia. Studies of minimally invasive techniques, such as ultrasound-guided vacuum-assisted removal and cryoablation, have been effective for fibroadenomas that were less than 2 cm in size.[12,13] These offer women who feel uncomfortable with watchful waiting an alternative to conservative management. However, if the tumor continues to grow, then surgical excision of the mass is recommended.

PHYLLODES TUMOR

In 1838, Jonathan Muller described a tumor as having a grossly fleshy appearance and emphasizing the leaflike pattern and named it *cystosarcoma phyllodes*.[14] *Phyllodes tumor* is now the preferred term, used to avoid the incorrect perception of a diagnosis of sarcoma. Phyllodes tumors account for less than 1% of all breast tumors.[15] Phyllodes tumors are fibroepithelial tumors capable of a wide range of biological behavior. Unlike a fibroadenoma, a phyllodes tumor has the potential of being malignant and can recur with distant metastases.

The age range reported for phyllodes tumor is from 10 to 80 years,[7] with the median age of about 45 years. On clinical presentation, about 80% of patients can present with a firm to hard discrete palpable mass similar to a fibroadenoma. If a patient presents with a mass greater than 4 cm or a history of a rapidly growing mass, then a diagnosis of a phyllodes tumor must be considered.

Mammographic findings of a phyllodes tumor tend to reveal a rounded, or lobulated, sharply defined high-density mass. The sonographic appearance of a phyllodes tumor is solid nodule with well-circumscribed margins. They rarely give rise to any acoustic shadowing. Horizontal striations, reflecting the presence of clefts, are characteristic of benign phyllodes tumor.[16]

The average size of a phyllodes tumor is between 4 and 5 cm, ranging from 1 to 20 cm.[7] Sometimes phyllodes tumors may become extremely large even if histologically classified as "benign," as illustrated in the patient shown in Figure 16-6. On gross examination they are well-circumscribed but not encapsulated tumors. Microscopically, phyllodes tumors contain both stroma and epithelium similar to fibroadenomas. Characteristically, the tumor is described to have a leaflike architecture. Phyllodes tumors are subclassified into 3 groups: benign, borderline, and malignant. Each is defined by 4 histologic features: stromal cellular atypia, mitotic activity, stromal overgrowth, and tumor margins.

Benign phyllodes tumor is characterized as having few mitoses in a high-power field (HPF) (< 2 per 10 HPF; Fig. 16-6). No more than mild atypia are seen, stromal overgrowth is lacking, and there is a well-circumscribed tumor. *Borderline phyllodes tumor* is described as having a greater degree of atypia, a mitotic rate between 2 and 5 per 10 HPF, no presence of stromal overgrowth, and with margins that can be infiltrative. Malignant phyllodes tumor is characterized by exhibiting marked atypia, more than 10 mitoses per HPF, infiltrative margins, and most importantly, the presence of stromal overgrowth.

The clinical management of a phyllodes tumor if possible is a preoperative core needle biopsy diagnosis, and most importantly,

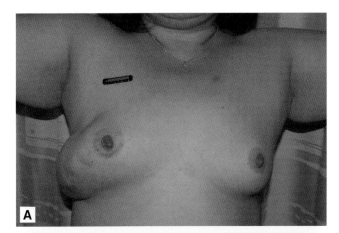
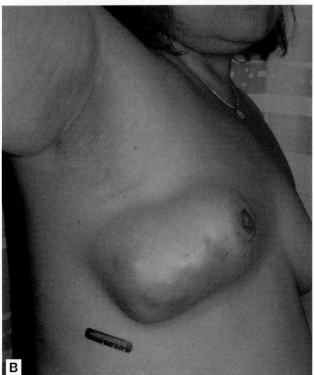
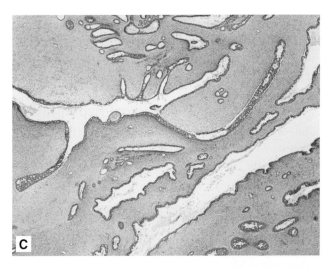
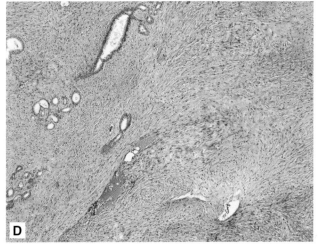

FIGURE 16-6 Benign phyllodes tumor. The patient developed a large growth in her right breast over approximately 1 year (**A** and **B**). **C.** This fibroepithelial neoplasm is composed of epithelial and stromal components. Epithelial areas have the classic leaflike configuration and intracanalicular growth pattern, consistent with phyllodes tumors. **D.** Increased stroma with increased cellularity is illustrated with occasional enlarged cells but no atypia or increase in mitosis. *(Courtesy of Constance Albaracin, MD and Henry Kuerer, MD, PhD, MD Anderson Cancer Center, Houston, Texas.)*

complete surgical excision with negative margins. There is a relatively high incidence of local recurrence, varying from 8% to 46%, especially if there are positive surgical margins.[17] Mangi and associates reported that the frequency of local recurrence correlated with the status of the surgical margin, and the incidence of local recurrence was very low in cases with 1 cm or wider margin.[18]

HAMARTOMA

Hamartoma is a benign breast lesion composed of ducts, lobules, fibrous stroma, and adipose tissue arranged in a disorganized manner. They account for 4.8% of benign breast tumors.[19] Hamartomas occur in any age group but especially between 30 and 50 year of age. Hamartomas present as a well-defined mass found on physical exam and/or mammogram. Most hamartomas found on mammogram are well-circumscribed and ovoid masses that are heterogeneous, containing breast tissue and fat. Histologically, they are predominantly comprised of fibrous tissue (Fig. 16-7). Ductal hyperplasia is usually absent but can be mild to moderate in approximately 25% of the cases.[19] If there is radiographic and pathologic correlation without evidence of atypia or carcinoma, hamartomas can be managed with observation alone.

BENIGN STROMAL LESIONS

Pseudoangiomatous Stromal Hyperplasia

Pseudoangiomatous stromal hyperplasia (PASH) was first described by Vuitch and associates[20] in 1986. PASH of the breast is a hyperplastic lesion of stromal myofibroblasts that mimics a vascular proliferation in response to hormonal stimuli.[21] The age of diagnosis ranges from the teens to mid-50s, with a median age in the mid-30s. It generally occurs in premenopausal women, but has been reported in postmenopausal women who are on hormone replacement therapy. The significance of this lesion is that it must be distinguished from angiosarcoma.

PASH often presents as a discrete painless, mobile mass, clinically indistinguishable from a fibroadenoma. Occasionally, it can cause diffuse enlargement of the breast with peau d'orange of the skin, suggesting inflammatory breast carcinoma. Peau d'orange and skin necrosis have been reported in patients who are pregnant with rapidly growing lesions.

Radiologically, PASH appears as a mass, with no associated calcifications, spiculated lesions, and/or architectural distortion. The most common mammographic abnormality is a circumscribed mass; and less common, a focal asymmetric density. Sonographic findings, as one would expect for a benign process, are a well-circumscribed hypoechoic or isoechoic oval mass with enhancement.[22] These imaging findings have the features of a benign process; pathologic diagnosis must be concordant with the imaging findings.

PASH, grossly, can range in size from 1 to approximately 7 cm. The lesion tends to be firm and rubbery with a smooth external surface. Microscopically, PASH consists of anastomosing, angulated, and slit-like spaces lined by slender spindle cells within a background of dense collagenous tissue. The spindle cells lining the spaces show no mitotic activity and occasionally contain red blood cells. The myofibroblasts of the lining tend to be positive for vimentin, CD34, and actin. Occasionally, they may show immunoreactivity for progesterone receptors.

The recommended treatment for PASH is local excision. Most patients remain well after local excision but ipsilateral

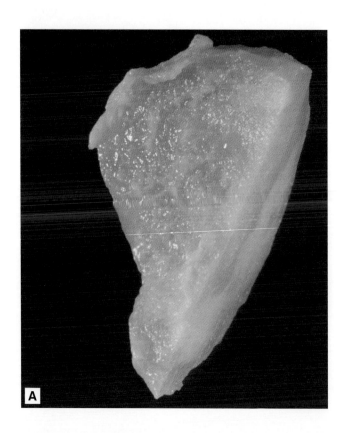

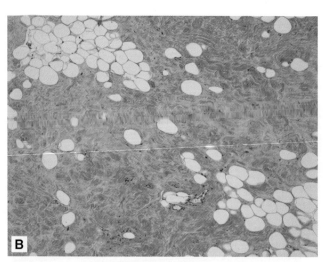

FIGURE 16-7 Breast hamartoma. **A.** Note the well-circumscribed mass with fatty appearance. **B.** Microscopically the tumor shows fibrous stroma with scattered ductal elements and adipose tissue without any lobular units. *(Courtesy of Dr Ayse Sahin, MD Anderson Cancer Center, Houston, Texas.)*

recurrence has been documented. The rates of recurrence range from 15% to 22%.[20,23] The reason for recurrence could be attributed to incomplete excision, the presence of multiple lesions that were not all excised, or de novo growth of PASH.[21] Tamoxifen use has been documented and has shown an impressive response where a patient demonstrated marked response each time tamoxifen was commenced, but PASH recurred each time she stopped the therapy.[24] Although tamoxifen appears to be effective, the long-term side effects would preclude its long-term use.

Fibromatosis

Fibromatosis of the breast is analogous to fibromatosis in other sites (eg, desmoid tumors of the abdominal wall) and is characterized as an infiltrating, well-differentiated proliferation of spindle cells. It is seen over a wide age range (13-80 years) and is much more common in women. Fibromatosis of the breast typically presents as a unilateral, painless, firm to hard palpable mass. Its clinical appearance may be suggestive of carcinoma. It may be seen in patients with a history of familial adenomatous polyposis (FAP). It is possible that trauma may have a role in the pathogenesis of some fibromatosis cases.[25]

Mammograhpic findings of fibromatosis may not reveal any abnormalities, although a spiculated lesion that can mimic carcinoma may be identified. Calcifications are rarely formed, but may be present with a benign proliferative lesion such as sclerosing adenosis.

Gross pathologic examination reveals an irregular firm area of white, tan, or gray fibrous tissue. Tumor size can vary from 1 to 10 cm. Microscopically, the tumor is composed of spindle cells surrounded by collagen with minimal pleomorphism and few to no mitoses (Fig. 16-8). The degree of cellularity may be variable, with some tumors containing very collagenous areas. The margin is infiltrative and the tumor may invade around normal structures. Lymphocytes are often seen at the edge.[25]

Preoperative diagnosis of fibromatosis is valuable. The differential diagnosis of a core biopsy includes scarring, fat necrosis, spindle-cell carcinoma, and nodular fasciitis. The proper treatment for fibromatosis is wide local excision.[26] The assessment of margins is very important because if an incomplete excision is performed there is a high risk of recurrence. Recurrence usually occurs with the first 3 years. Rarely recurrences may lead to the uncontrollable spread of fibromatosis to the chest wall. There is no role for postoperative adjuvant chemotherapy or radiation therapy in the primary treatment or to control recurrences.

Myofibroblastoma

Mammary myofibroblastoma was initially described in 1987.[27] It is a benign stromal tumor originating from mesenchymal cells. It was initially thought to be more common in men; it has now been shown to have no gender predilection. Myofibroblastoma usually presents as a single slow-growing painless mass. The average size of the lesion ranges from 1 to 4 cm, although giant myofibroblastoma have been reported.[28] There has been one documented case report of myofibromatosis seen after breast conservation surgery and radiation therapy for intraductal carcinoma.[29]

The radiologic appearance of myofibroblastoma is that of a homogenous, lobulated, well-circumscribed tumor that lacks microcalcifications. Sonographically, the findings are not specific. The lesion forms a solid nodule but does not demonstrate a capsule.[5]

Histologically, myofibroblastoma is generally well-circumscribed and composed of spindle cells arranged in short, intersecting fascicles and thick bands of eosinophilic collagen. Necrosis is absent and mitoses are rare. Myofibroblastoma of the breast characteristically expresses receptors to androgen, estrogen, and progesterone,[30] suggesting a possible role for sex hormones in the pathogenesis of the tumor.[31]

Myofibroblastoma is managed by surgical excision with clear margins. Recurrence has not been documented.

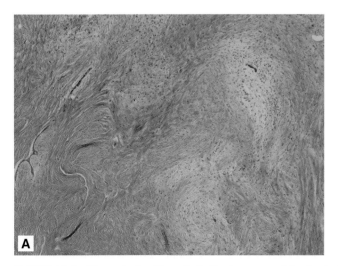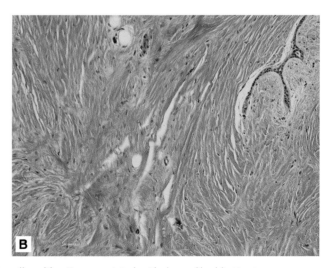

FIGURE 16-8 Fibromatosis of breast. **A.** The tumor consists of spindle-cell proliferation associated with dense fibroblastic stroma. **B.** Higher magnification demonstrates that tumor cells are uniform and lack cytologic atypia. Note that tumor cells are proliferating around breast ducts (*right upper corner*). (*Courtesy of Dr Ayse Sahin, MD Anderson Cancer Center, Houston, Texas.*)

Hemangioma

Hemangiomas are benign vascular lesions. They may occur in males or females with a wide age range of 18 months to 82 years. Hemangiomas can present as a palpable mass, imaging-detected abnormalities, or as an incidental finding. The lesions can measure from 0.3 to 2.5 cm in size.

Hemangiomas detected on mammography have been described as well-defined masses with lobulations, and sometimes with fine, punctuated or phlebolith-type calcifications.[32] Sonographically, a hemangioma is seen as a homogeneous, hypoechoic, nonattenuating lesion.[33]

Most hemangiomas have well-defined borders, but microscopically the vascular channels may blend with the surrounding breast parenchyma. Microscopically, hemangiomas can be separated into 2 common types, cavernous and capillary. Cavernous hemangiomas consist of a mesh of dilated thin-walled vessels congested with red blood cells. Capillary hemangiomas consist of a collection of small vessels that is subdivided by fibrous bands and may be arranged around a central feeding vessel.[34]

Complete surgical excision is warranted to rule out low-grade angiosarcoma. There has been no evidence of recurrence once complete excision has been performed.

SCLEROSING LESIONS

Sclerosing Adenosis

Sclerosing adenosis is a benign proliferative lesion. It is often a microscopic incidental finding in breast specimens. Sclerosing adenosis may be diagnosed at any age. However, because these lesions are sclerotic, they often contain calcifications, which may present mammographically as microcalcifications and/or architectural distortion. Occasionally, sclerosing adenosis may present as a mass lesion on palpation or by imaging.

Sclerosing adenosis arises in association with the terminal duct lobular unit composed of distorted epithelial elements surrounded by myoepithelial cells in a fibrotic stroma. This "lobulocentric" pattern, which is best appreciated at low microscopic power, is key to the correct diagnosis of sclerosing adenosis and its variants. The epithelium in this lesion may undergo apocrine metaplasia.[35] This may be confused with infiltrating carcinoma if the low-power lobulocentric pattern is not appreciated. Sclerosing adenosis may also be involved with atypical ductal hyperplasia (ADH), ductal carcinoma in situ (DCIS), atypical lobular hyperplasia (ALH), or lobular carcinoma in situ (LCIS).[51] Perineural "pseudoinvasion" may be present in approximately 2% of sclerosing adenosis and should not be misinterpreted as invasive carcinoma.[36] Immunohistochemistry may be helpful to demonstrate the presence of myoepithelial markers (eg, p63 or smooth muscle myosin-heavy chain) in difficult cases (Fig. 16-9).

Sclerosing adenosis is not a precursor of breast carcinoma. The diagnosis of sclerosing adenosis is usually a straightforward on core biopsy specimen. Therefore, patients with a diagnosis on core needle biopsy can be managed safely by observation provided that the imaging studies correlate with pathologic findings and another lesion is not present such as atypia of in situ carcinoma, in which case wide excision is indicated.

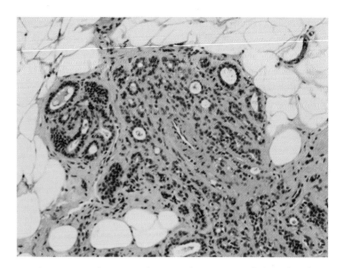

FIGURE 16-9 Sclerosing adenosis. The acini are distorted and compressed by fibrotic stroma. The lobulocentric nature of the lesion together with the presence of both epithelial and myoepithelial cells in the lesion are useful features for distinguishing sclerosing adenosis from invasive carcinoma. *(Courtesy of Dr Savitri Krishnamurthy, MD Anderson Cancer Center, Houston Texas.)*

Radial Scar

In 1928, Semb[37] referred to radial sclerosing lesions as *rosettes* or *proliferation centers* that might give rise to carcinoma. Radial sclerosing lesions have been described by a variety of names introduced in the 1970s, including sclerosing papillary proliferation, nonencapsulated sclerosing lesion, and indurative mastopathy. Hamperl[38] introduced the term *strahlige Narben* in 1975, and in 1980 Linell and associates translated the term to *radial scar*.[39] The term "complex sclerosing lesion" is sometimes used for similar lesions larger than 1 cm in size or for those lesions with several fibroelastic areas in close contiguity.[35]

Most radial scars are often microscopic in size and are incidentally found on breast biopsies. The frequency of radial scars in mastectomy specimens from patients with carcinoma has ranged between 4% and 26%. In benign breast biopsies the incidence ranges from 1.7% to 28%.[40] The presence of radial scars in both benign and malignant tissue suggests that there may be an associated increase risk of subsequent breast cancer.[41] Mammographically, radial scars tend to be spiculated lesions often with a radiolucent area. It is often difficult to distinguish from invasive carcinoma on imaging alone (Fig. 16-10).

On gross examination, if large enough to be detected mammographically, the appearance is similar to that of a small invasive carcinoma. Occasionally, dilated cysts may be seen at the periphery of larger lesions. Microscopically, radial scars are characterized by a central zone of fibroelastosis from which ducts and lobules radiate, exhibiting various benign alterations such as microcysts, apocrine metaplasia, and proliferative changes, such as florid hyperplasia and papillomas (Fig. 16-10). The "radiating" ducts and lobules expand or enlarge from the central fibroelastotic area in a "centrifugal" manner. Within the central area of fibroelastotic stroma, smaller entrapped ducts are present, and are lined by 1 or more layers of epithelium with an

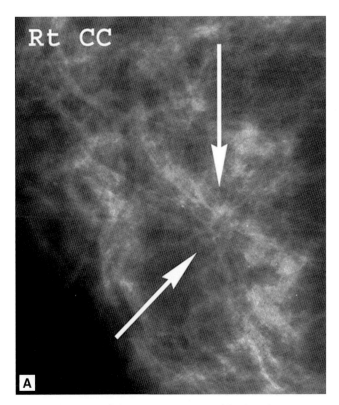

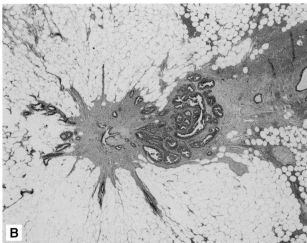

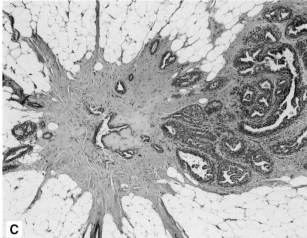

FIGURE 16-10   Radial scar. **A.** Mammographic view demonstrating a 1.5-cm area of architectural distortion (*arrows*) with radiating spicules and a central lucency. **B.** A ductal structure is seen radiating from a central fibrotic region. **C.** Higher magnification of the lesion shows that glands in the left side of the figure have flat epithelial lining and glands at right side of the figure have epithelial hyperplasia without atypia. (*Courtesy of Drs Peter Dempsey and Ayse Sahin, MD Anderson Cancer Center, Houston, Texas.*)

outer myoepithelial cell layer. Radial scars may be involved by atypical hyperplasia (ductal or lobular); LCIS, DCIS, or invasive carcinoma may rarely be present. Atypical hyperplasia and carcinoma tend to be more common in larger lesions and in radial scars in women older than 50 years of age.[35]

The literature regarding the risk of developing subsequent in situ or invasive breast carcinoma following a biopsy diagnosis of radial scar has been mixed. Berg and associates recently reported on 439 patients with radial scar found on excisional breast biopsy from the Mayo Benign Breast Disease cohort of 9262 patients. They demonstrated that there was no statistically significant difference between women with proliferative disease without atypia (PDWA) and with a radial scar (RR, 1.8; 95% CI, 1.36-2.53) and women with PDWA and no radial scar (RR, 1.57; 95% CI, 1.37-1.79). Therefore, they concluded that radial scar imparts no increased breast cancer risk.[42] Similarly, Sanders and associates examined 880 breast biopsies with radial scars, which represented 9.2% of the overall Nashville Breast Cohort of 9556 patients.[43] They found an overall relative risk of subsequent invasive breast cancer of 1.82 (95% CI, 1.2-2.7) at 10 years. They concluded that the mildly elevated risk was largely attributed to the category of coexistence of proliferative disease.[43] In contrast, Jacobs and colleagues reported that the presence of a radial scar was associated with almost a doubling

of the risk of breast cancer.[41] They showed the relative risk of breast cancer in women with PDWA with a radial scar to be 2.7 (95% CI, 1.5-5.0).[41] However, given that in situ and invasive breast carcinoma appear to be more common in larger than small radial scars,[44] the possibility that at least some radial scars represent direct cancer precursors must also be considered.

The distinction between radial scar and invasive breast carcinoma may be difficult to determine on core biopsy alone due to the limited sample size. Even if carcinoma is not found in a core biopsy specimen that shows features of a radial scar, an excisional biopsy may still be advisable to exclude the possibility of concomitant carcinoma.

NIPPLE DISCHARGE

Approximately 3% to 8% of referrals to breast clinics are due to complaints of nipple discharge.[45] Most nipple discharge is associated with a benign cause.[46] Nipple discharge usually occurs in women and rarely men of all ages. The characteristics of nipple discharge need to be defined to try to understand the underlying cause. Discharge that is unilateral, spontaneous, persistent and/or troublesome, clear, serous, blood stained or containing blood on testing tends to represent a pathologic process.

TABLE 16-2 Nonsurgical Causes of Nipple Discharge

Physiologic
    Peripartum period
    Manual stimulation
Pathologic
    Pituitary adenoma
    Primary hypothyroidism
    Ectopic production of prolactin
    Hypothalamic disorders
Pharmacologic
    Psychoactive drugs
    Antihypertensive medications
    Gastrointestinal medications
    Opiates
    Oral contraceptives or estrogen replacement therapy
Idiopathic

From Lang JE, Kuerer HM. Breast ductal secretions: clinical features, potential uses, and possible applications. *Cancer Control.* 2007;14:350-359.

However, nipple discharge that is expressed and bilateral is more consistent with a physiologic process.

The etiology of benign nipple discharge can be considered in 2 main groups: nonsurgically treated nipple discharge and surgically treated. Nonsurgically treated nipple discharge generally is placed into 4 different groups: (1) physiologic, (2) pathologic endocrine (3) pharmacologic, and (4) idiopathic causes (Table 16-2). In more than half of cases in the idiopathic category, patients present with galactorrhea.[47]

Discharge is often described as serous, milky, green, brown, bloody, cloudy, or purulent. Bloody nipple discharge may be associated with an intraductal papilloma, other papillary lesions, or carcinoma. In the majority of patients with nipple discharge it is associated with fibrocystic change, duct ectasia, drugs, hormonal effects, and other nonproliferative breast lesions.

The fluid that is physiologic can range in color from white to yellow, to green, to brown, to blue-black. About two-thirds of nonlactating women have a small amount of fluid secreted from the nipple on manual expression. The secretion usually is seen in multiple ducts. Nonspontaneous, bilateral, nonbloody secretion that is physiologic requires no treatment.[48]

Duct ectasia and benign papillomas are the commonest causes of nipple discharge in young women. Carcinoma is more common in older women. Age is an important predictor of malignancy in a patients presenting with nipple discharge as the only symptom. In one series, 3% of patients younger than 40, 10% of patients aged between 40 and 60, and 32% of patients older that 60 years had an associated malignancy when presenting with just nipple discharge alone.[49] However, an increased risk of carcinoma has been reported in women with nipple discharge associated with a palpable mass or mammographic abnormality.[47]

The evaluation of nipple discharge begins with a history, physical exam, and breast imaging. Mammogram and ultrasound are used to help identify any masses or abnormalities that may be responsible for the discharge. In a recent study, it has been shown that magnetic resonance imaging (MRI) may be useful in detecting lesions that mammography or ultrasound is unable to detect.[50] However, the use of MRI is investigational.

The standard surgical treatment of nipple discharge, once it has been determined not to be associated with a breast lesion detected by imaging, is a major duct excision. However, there are times that the causative lesion may potentially be missed on a major duct excision; studies have shown that there are other means to help identify these lesions.

Diagnostic ductography can be used for spontaneous unilateral single-duct nipple discharge. It can show the course of abnormal ducts as well as localize an intraductal lesion.[51] This allows for more selective duct excision as opposed to a major duct excision. However, there tend to be difficulties with the procedure, and its predictive role in the nonoperative setting is limited.[52]

Mammary ductoscopy is being studied in several institutions. Endoscopy is used to directly visual the ductal system of the breast through the duct orifice. The endoscope is 0.9 mm in diameter. At Beth Israel Medical Center in New York, their experience allowed for accurate visualization, analysis, and excision of intraductal abnormalities.[53] Mammary ductoscopy can be an effective tool for surgeons to allow for a limited duct excision especially for women who are of child bearing age who wish to preserve the ability to breast-feed. The experience of breast endoscopy is limited to certain academic centers and still needs more investigating before there is a definite role for the procedure.

Intraoperative intraductal injection of methylene blue dye has been described in the literature to aid visualization of discharging duct.[54] Upon performing a major duct excision, Sharma and associates describe cannulating the discharging duct and injecting it with 1 to 3 mL of methylene blue dye. The stained duct and its branches are then traced to the nipple orfice, allowing for a clean dissection of the surrounding ducts. They demonstrate the added benefit of methylene blue, which allows the surgeon to resect the involved ductal system while preserving nipple function for possible subsequent breastfeeding.[54]

PAPILLARY LESIONS

Papillary lesions of the breast cover a wide spectrum in morphology, clinical presentation, and imaging findings. Morphologically, papillary lesions can be subdivided into intraductal papillomas, papillomas with atypia, noninvasive papillary carcinoma, and papillary carcinoma.[55] Benign intraductal papillomas will be discussed.

Intraductal papillomas typically arise from central/subareolar ducts. Approximately 50% are single lesions and up to 30% present with bloody nipple discharge.[56] Multiple peripheral papillary lesions as compared to solitary papillomas are often smaller, clinically occult, and discovered as an incidental finding on imaging[57] and are more likely to be associated with breast carcinoma.[58] Papillary lesions are seen more frequently in women 30 to 50 years of age.

Papillary lesions may present radiographically as an architectural distortion, abnormal density, or mass with or without microcalcifications or microcalcifications alone. Sonographically, a papilloma may present as a well-defined hypoechoic mass that may be associated with a dilated duct.

Papillomas can range in size from less than 3 to 5 mm up to several centimeters. On gross examination, intraductal papillomas are tan-pink and tend to be friable and associated with a dilated duct or cyst. Microscopically, these lesions are composed of multiple branching papillae that are lined by epithelium (Fig. 16-11). The epithelium lining is subject to similar proliferative changes that can occur throughout the breast (papillomatosis).

The clinical management of these lesions has been controversial. With the increased use of core needle biopsy, the management of benign intraductal papillary lesions has been questioned. Prior studies have shown that core needle biopsies can accurate diagnose benign papillomas[59,60] and may not require a surgical excision. However, recent studies have shown that there is a significant upgrade of benign papillomas found on core needle biopsy after surgical excision.[55,58,61] Rizzo and associates showed an upgrade of benign lesions to DCIS in 10.5% and atypical ductal hyperplasia in 14.5%[55] of their cases. Therefore, surgical excision is recommended for all benign papillary lesions.

DUCT ECTASIA

Mammary duct ectasia is a dilation of the subareolar duct in peri- and postmenopausal women. The cause for the dilation is controversial. The dilation of the ducts may be a primary event or the result of prior periductal inflammation.[48] Duct ectasia can cause acute inflammation known as periductal mastitis (in younger women), which can be self-limiting or can lead to abscesses or mammary fistula formation.

Mild forms of duct ectasia are usually asymptomatic. Patients may complain of a cheesy, viscous, toothpaste-like nipple discharge and may have nipple retraction. Some patients can have green discharge from multiple ducts, which is considered to be physiologic. On mammogram and ultrasound, dilated ducts can be observed.

On gross pathologic examination, the subareolar ducts are dilated and contain a soft creamy or brown material. Microscopically, the epithelial lining of the ducts is thin and often contain inflammatory cells (Fig. 16-12).

Asymptomatic duct ectasia requires no treatment. Antibiotics may be needed when there are signs of infection. Duct excision is recommended when nipple discharge is persistent and troublesome and a periareolar abscess requires drainage.

BREAST INFECTIONS

Breast infections can be divided into 2 groups, lactational and nonlactational. Secondary infections such as hidradenitis sup-

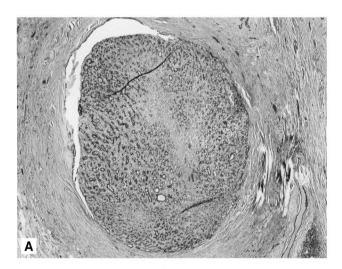

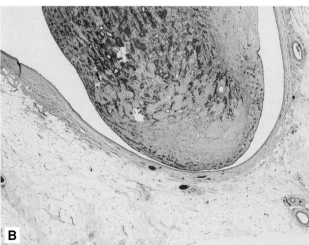

FIGURE 16-11 Intraductal papilloma. **A.** Intraductal proliferation of glands with papillary aarchitecture associated with marked stromal fibrosis. **B.** Higher magnification of the lesion shows that there is marked stromal fibrosis and the lesion can be classified as sclerosing papilloma. *(Courtesy of Dr Ayse Sahin, MD Anderson Cancer Center, Houston, Texas.)*

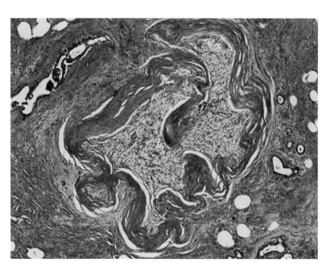

FIGURE 16-12 Duct ectasia. A markedly ectatic duct filled with foamy histocytes with focal mild chronic inflammation around the duct. *(Courtesy of Dr Savitri Krishnamurthy, MD Anderson Cancer Center, Houston, Texas.)*

puriva or sebaceous cysts can lead to breast infections. The most common organism to cause breast infections is *Staphylococcus aureus*. It has recently been noted that there has been an increase in community associated methicillin-resistant *S aureus* (MRSA) infections seen in emergency departments.[62]

Lactional Infection

Lactational infection is most commonly seen in the first 6 weeks of breast-feeding or weaning. It remains unclear whether the staphylococci are derived from the skin of the patient of from the mouth of the breast-feeding infant. The main cause of the infection is most likely from blockage of the lactiferous ducts with thickened secretions and milk, resulting in retention of milk in the peripheral lobules of the breast. The stagnant milk causes the breast to engorge and becomes a leading source of infection.

Patients often present with a swollen, tender, and erthyematous breast. A fluctuant mass may be noted at the time of presentation, indicating an abscess. Pyrexia and leukocytosis can also be associated with this presentation. If there are no signs of an abscess formation, antibiotics usually control the infection and prevent an abscess formation. Breast ultrasound may be helpful in diagnosing abscesses that cannot be appreciated on physical exam and if the patient is not improving with the antibiotics. An abscess can be managed by percutaneous needle aspiration and antibiotics with incision and drainage if it does not resolve promptly, or by incision and drainage alone.

Nonlactational Infection

Periductal Infection

Periductal infections most commonly affect younger women and are associated with smoking.[63] The pathophysiology of infection tends to be associated with duct ectasia. Secretions can stagnate within the dilated ducts, allowing for the overgrowth of bacteria to occur. This can occur distantly, causing peripheral mastitis; or near the areola, leading to periareolar infections and abscesses.

Periareolar infections can present as a mass, periareolar abscess, or a mammary duct fistula due to recurrent infections. Purulent nipple discharge has been noted as well. Treatment in these infections is similar to that for a breast infection/abscess—antibiotics and drainage of the abscess if present. If a mammary duct fistula is present, surgical treatment by excising the opening of the fistula with excision of the involved ducts is the preferred treatment.[64]

FUTURE DIRECTIONS

It is known that benign breast disease is a risk factor for breast cancer.[65,66] Various studies demonstrate variability among the actual degree of risk. Hartmann and associates followed a cohort of 9087 women with benign breast disease for a median of 15 years. They found the relative risk associated with atypia was 4.24, as compared with a relative risk of 1.88 for proliferative changes without atypia and of 1.27 for nonproliferative lesions.[65] Dupont and associates found that a family history of breast cancer had little effect on the risk in women with nonproliferative lesions. Their study also revealed that although cysts alone did not substantially elevate the risk, women with both cysts and a family history of breast cancer had a risk 2.7 times higher than that for women without either of these risk factors.[67]

It is commonly believed that the finding of simple cysts does not increase the risk of breast cancer. If this is so, why then does a woman's risk of breast cancer increase more if she has both cysts and a family history of breast cancer compared to a woman with a family history of breast cancer? This is a very interesting research protocol that potentially affects an enormous number of women.

There are many potential areas of research for benign breast disease. The authors suspect that we will continue to see research regarding the association of benign breast disease and the risk of breast cancer. There are ongoing trials now regarding the treatment of fibroadenomas. From the above-mentioned articles, it has been shown that benign breast findings without atypia may increase the risk of breast cancer. Given this fact, it is interesting that there remains a paucity of literature regarding whether removing fibroadenomas then affects the breast cancer risk.

One can surmise that the potential for research in benign breast disease is endless. It may be helpful if we continue to investigate the link between benign breast disease and breast cancer. Perhaps this will help in discovering one of the many causes of breast cancer.

SUMMARY

Most of the routine problems that are encountered in women with breast disease will not be related to breast cancer, and many findings will first present as a result of screening mammography. A thorough understanding of the presenting physical findings, imaging results, radiologic-histologic correlates, and management is essential for the practicing breast surgical oncologists to prevent under- and over-treatment of patients. The evaluation of all breast conditions begins with a history, physical exam, appropriate breast imaging, and histologic examination in almost all cases. It is also known that some benign breast disease is a risk factor for breast cancer, and studies have demonstrated variability among the actual degree of risk being related to whether the lesions are proliferative or not.

REFERENCES

1. Hughes LE, Mansel RE, Webster DJT. Aberrations of normal development and involution (ANDI): a new perspective on pathogenesis and nomenclature of benign breast disorders. *Lancet.* 1987;2:1316-1319.
2. Hughes LE. Classification of benign breast disorders: the ANDI classification based on physiological processes within the normal breast. *Br Med Bull.* 1991;47:251-257.
3. Beenken SW, Bland KI. Evaluation and treatment of benign breast disorders. In: Bland KI, Copeland EM. eds. *The Breast: Comprehensive Management of Benign and Malignant Disorders.* 3rd ed. St. Louis, MO: Saunders;223-235.

4. Baker SB, Burkey BA, Thorton P, LaRossa D. Juvenile gigantomastia: presentation of four cases and review of the literature. *Ann Plast Surg.* 2001;46:517-525.

5. Stavros TA. Benign solid nodules: specific pathologic diagnosis. In: Stavros TA, ed. *Breast Ultrasound.* Philadelphia, PA: Lippincott Williams & Wilkins; 2004:528-596.

6. Fekete P, Petrek J, Majmudar B, et al. Fibroadenomas with stromal cellularity: a clinicopathologic study of 21 patients. *Arch Pathol Lab Med.* 1987;111:427-432.

7. Rosen PP. Fibroepithelial neoplasms. In: Rosen PP, ed. *Rosen's Breast Pathology.* 2nd ed. Philadelphia, PA: Lippincott Williams & Wilkins; 2001:163-200.

8. Dupont WD, Page DL, Parl FF, et al. Long-term risk of breast cancer in women with fibroadenoma. *N Engl J Med.* 1994;331:10-15.

9. Collins JC, Liao S, Wile AG. Surgical management of breast masses in pregnant women. *J Reprod Med.* 1995;40:785-788.

10. Baker TP, Lenert JT, Parker J, et al. Lactating adenoma: a diagnosis of exclusion. *Breast J.* 2002;7:354-357.

11. Rickert RR, Rajan S. Localized breast infarcts associated with pregnancy. *Arch Pathol.* 1974;97:159-161.

12. Grady I, Gorsuch H, Wilburn-Bailey S. Long-term outcome of benign fibroadenomas treated by ultrasound-guided percutaneous excision. *Breast J.* 2008;14:275-278.

13. Nurko J, Mabry CD, Whitworth P, et al. Interim results from the Fibro-Adenoma Cryoablation Treatment Registry. *Am J Surg.* 2005;190:647-651.

14. Muller J. *Uber den feineran Bau and die Forman der krankhaften Geschwilste.* Berlin: G Reimer; 1838.

15. Reinfuss M, Mitus J, Duda K, et al. The treatment and prognosis of patients with phyllodes tumor of the breast: an analysis of 170 cases. *Cancer.* 1996;77:910-916.

16. Stavros TA. Atypical, high-risk, premalignant, and locally aggressive lesions. In: Stavros TA, ed. *Breast Ultrasound.* Philadelphia, PA: Lippincott Williams & Wilkins; 2004:689-711.

17. Taira N, Takabatake D, Aogi K, et al. Phyllodes tumor of the breast: stromal overgrowth and histological classification are useful prognosis-predictive factors for local recurrence in patients with a positive surgical margin. *Jpn J Clin Oncol.* 2007;37:730-736.

18. Mangi AA, Smith BL, Gadd MA, et al. Surgical management of phyllodes tumors. *Arch Surg.* 1999;134:487-492. Discussion 492-493.

19. Wahner-Roedler DL, Sebo TJ, Gisvold JJ. Hamartomas of the breast: clinical, radiologic, and pathologic manifestations. *Breast J.* 2001;7:101-105.

20. Vuitch MF, Rosen PP, Erlandson RA. Pseudoangiomatous hyperplasia of mammary stroma. *Hum Pathol.* 1986;17:185-191.

21. Sng KK, Tan SM, Mancer JF, Tay KH. The contrasting presentation and management of pseudoangiomatous stromal hyperplasia of the breast. *Singapore Med J.* 2008;49:e82-e85.

22. Hargaden GC, Yeh ED, Georgian-Smith D, et al. Analysis of the mammographic and sonographic features of pseudoangiomatous stromal hyperplasia. *Am J Roentgenol.* 2008;191:359-363.

23. Powell CM, Cranor ML, Rosen PP. Pseudoangiomatous stromal hyperplasia (PASH). A mammary stromal tumor with myofibroblastic differentiation. *Am J Surg Pathol.* 1995;19:270-277.

24. Pruthi S, Reynolds C, Johnson RE, Gisvold JJ. Tamoxifen in the management of pseudoangiomatous stromal hyperplasia. *Breast J.* 2001;7:434-439.

25. Lee AHS. Recent developments in the histological diagnosis of spindle cell carcinoma, fibromatosis and phyllodes tumor of the breast. *Histopathology.* 2008;52:45-57.

26. Schwartz GS, Drotman M, Rosenblatt R, et al. Fibromatosis of the breast: case report and current concepts in management of an uncommon lesion. *Breast J.* 2006;12:66-71.

27. Wargotz ES, Weiss SW, Norris HJ. Myofibroblastoma of the breast. Sixteen cases of a distinctive benign mesenchymal tumor. *Am J Surg Pathol.* 1987;11:493-502.

28. Shah SN. Giant myofibroblastoma of breast: a case report. *Indian J Pathol Microbiol.* 2007;50:583-585.

29. Yagmur Y, Prasad MJ, Osborne MP. Myofibroblastoma in the irradiated breast. *Breast J.* 1999;5:136-140.

30. Hamele-Bena D, Cranor ML, Sciotto C, et al. Uncommon presentation of mammary myofibroblastoma. *Mod Pathol.* 1996;9:786-90.

31. Meguerditchian AN, Malik DA, Hicks DG, Kulkarni S. Solitary fibrous tumor of the breast and mammary myofibroblastoma: the same lesion? *Breast J.* 2008;14:287-292.

32. Adwani A, Bees N, Arnaout A, Lanaspre E. Hemangioma of the breast: clinical, mammographic, and ultrasound features. *Breast J.* 2006;12:271.

33. Mesurolle B, Sygal V, Lalonde L, et al. Sonographic and mammographic appearance of breast hemangioma. *AJR.* 2008;191:W17-W22.

34. Rosen PP. Benign mesenchymal neoplasms. In: Rosen PP, ed. *Rosen's Breast Pathology.* 2nd ed. Philadelphia, PA: Lippincott Williams & Wilkins: 2001; 749-811.

35. Schnitt SJ, Connolly JL. Pathology of benign breast disorders. In: Harris JR, Lippman ME, Morrow M, Osborne CK, eds. *Diseases of the Breast.* 3rd ed. Philadelphia, PA: Lippincott Williams & Wilkins; 2004:77-99.

36. Gobbi H, Jensen RA, Simpson JF, et al. Atypical ductal hyperplasia and ductal carcinoma in situ of the breast associated with perineural invasion. *Hum Pathol.* 2001;32:785-790.

37. Semb C. Pathologico-anatomical and clinical investigations of fibroadenomatosis cystica mammae and its relation to other pathological conditions in the mamma, especially cancer. *Acta Chir Scand.* 1928;64(suppl): 1-484.

38. Hamperl H. Strahlige Narben und obliterierende Mastopathie: Beitrage zur pathologischen Histologie der Mamma: XI. *Virchows Arch A Pathol Anat Histol.* 1975;369:55-68.

39. Linell F, Ljungberg O, Anderson I. Breast carcinoma: aspects of early stages, progression and related problems. *Acta Pathol Microbiol Scand Suppl.* 1980;272:1-233.

40. Rosen PP. Papilloma and related benign tumors. In: Rosen PP, ed. *Rosen's Breast Pathology.* 2nd ed. Philadelphia, PA: Lippincott Williams & Wilkins; 2001:77-119.

41. Jacobs TW, Byrne C, Colditz G, et al. Radial scars in benign breast-biopsy specimens and the risk of breast cancer. *N Engl J Med.* 1999;340: 430-436.

42. Berg JC, Visscher DW, Vierkant RA, et al. Breast cancer risk in women with radial scars in benign breast biopsies. *Breast Cancer Res Treat.* 2008; 108:167-174.

43. Sanders ME, Simpson JF, Schuyler PA, et al. Interdependence of radial scar and proliferative disease with respect to invasive breast carcinoma risk in patients with benign breast biopsies. *Cancer.* 2006;106:1453-1461.

44. Sloane JP, Mayers MM. Carcinoma and atypical hyperplasia in radial scars and complex sclerosing lesions: importance of lesion size and patient age. *Histopathology.* 1993;23:225-231.

45. Arnold GJ, Neiheisel MB. A comprehensive approach to evaluating nipple discharge. *Nurse Pract.* 1997;22:96-102.

46. Mortellaro VE, Marshall J, Harms SE, et al. Breast MR for the evaluation of occult nipple discharge. *Am Surg.* 2008;74:739-742.

47. Lang JE, Kuerer HM. Breast ductal secretions: clinical features, potential uses, and possible applications. *Cancer Control.* 2007;14:350-359.

48. Dixon JM, Bundred NJ. Management of disorders of the ductal system and infections. In: Harris JR, Lippman ME, Morrow M, Osborne CK, eds. *Diseases of the Breast.* 3rd ed. Philadelphia, PA: Lippincott Williams & Wilkins; 2004:47-56.

49. Selzer MH, Perloff LJ, Kelley RI, Fitts WT Jr. The significance of age in patients with nipple discharge. *Surg Gynecol Obstet.* 1970;131:519-522.

50. Ballesio L, Maggi C, Savelli S, et al. Role of breast magnetic resonance imaging (MRI) in patients with unilateral nipple discharge: preliminary study. *Radio Med (Torino).* 2008;113:249-264.

51. Cardenosa G, Doudna C, Eklund GW. Ductography of the breast: technique and Findings. *AJR.* 1994;162:1081-1087.

52. Morrogh M, Morris EA, Liberman L, et al. The predictive value of ductography and magnetic resonance imaging in the management of nipple discharge. *Ann Surg Oncol.* 2007;14:3369-3377.

53. Kapenhas-Valdes E, Feldman SM, Cohen JM, Boolbol SK. Mammary ductoscopy for evaluation of nipple discharge. *Ann Surg Oncol* 2008; 15:2720-2727.

54. Sharma N, Huston TL, Simmons RM. Intraoperative intraductal injection of methylene blue dye to assist in major duct excision. *Am J Surg.* 2006;191:553-554.

55. Rizzo M, Lund MJ, Oprea G, et al. Surgical follow-up and clinical presentation of 142 breast papillary lesions diagnosed by ultrasound-guided core-needle biopsy. *Ann Surg Oncol.* 2008;15:1040-1047.

56. Cabioglu N, Hunt KK, Singletary SE, et al. Surgical decision making and factors determining a diagnosis of breast carcinoma in women presenting with nipple discharge. *J Am Coll Surg.* 2003;196:354-364.

57. Lewis JT, Hartmann LC, Vierkant RA, et al. An analysis of breast cancer risk in women with single, multiple, and atypical papilloma. *Am J Surg Pathol.* 2006;30:665-672.

58. Harjit K, Willsher PC, Bennett M, et al. Multiple papillomas of the breast: is current management adequate? *Breast.* 2006;15:777-781.

59. Carder PJ, Garvican J, Haigh I, Liston JC. Needle core biopsy can reliably distinguish between benign and malignant papillary lesions of the breast. *Histopathology.* 2005;46:320-327.

60. Kil WH, Cho EY, Kim JH, et al. Is surgical excision necessary in benign papillary lesions initially diagnosed at core biopsy? *Breast.* 2008;17:258-262.

61. Valdes EK, Tartter PI, Genelus-Dominique E, et al. Significance of papillary lesions at percutaneous breast biopsy. *Ann Surg Oncol.* 2006;13:480-482.

62. Pallin DJ, Egan DJ, Pelletier AJ, et al. Increased US emergency department visits for skin and soft tissue infections, and changes in antibiotic choices, during the emergence of community-associated methicillin-resistant Staphylococcus aureus. *Ann Emerg Med.* 2008;51:291-298.

63. Schafer P, Furrer C, Mermillod B. An association of cigarette smoking with recurrent subareolar breast abscess. *Int J Epidermiol.* 1988;17:810-813.

64. Dixon JM, Thompson AM. Effective surgical treatment for mammillary fistula. *Br J Surg.* 1991;78:1185.

65. Hartmann LC, Sellers TA, Frost MH, et al. Benign breast disease and the risk of breast cancer. *N Engl J Med.* 2005;353:229-237.

66. Bertelsen L, Mellemkjaer L, Balser E, et al. Benign breast disease among first degree relatives of young breast cancer patients. *Am J Epidemiol.* 2008;168:261-267.

67. Dupont WD, Page DL. Risk factors for breast cancer in women with proliferative breast disease. *N Engl J Med.* 1985;312:146-151.

CHAPTER 17

High-Risk Lesions: ALH/LCIS/ADH

Chanel E. Smart
Colin M. Furnival
Sunil R. Lakhani

PRECURSOR AND PREINVASIVE LESIONS OF THE BREAST

The multistep model for breast carcinogenesis suggests that invasive carcinomas arise from preinvasive "hyperplastic" and neoplastic proliferations. These early proliferative lesions have taken on greater significance as a result of the mammographic screening and detection programs. Pathologists are encountering these proliferative lesions with increasing frequency, and this has highlighted deficiencies in classification systems as well as a lack of data on natural history, making clinical management a challenge.

Invasive carcinomas are divided into ductal carcinoma no-special-type (IDC-NST) and the "special types," of which lobular carcinoma (ILC) is the major component. While there has been little debate or controversy about the precursor nature of ductal carcinoma in situ (DCIS), there is considerable argument regarding the role of lobular carcinoma in situ (LCIS) in progression to invasive disease. The picture is further complicated by the identification of lesions that are qualitatively the same but less developed (atypical lobular hyperplasia, ALH) and those showing intermediate features between hyperplasia and in situ carcinoma (atypical ductal hyperplasia, ADH).

The evidence for progression and the risks associated with these lesions is derived from morphology, clinical follow-up, and molecular relationships. The path from normal to invasive carcinoma is certainly not a linear one, and there is evidence that breast cancer and the evolutionary pathways are heterogeneous.[1] The overall paucity of data to stratify individual patients into meaningful risk categories and the often long time-frame to progression has created challenges in surgical management of these preinvasive lesions. This is further confounded by the diagnostic difficulties from small tissue samples in core biopsies used as part of the workup in screening programs,

In this chapter, we discuss the pathology, biology, and management of lobular neoplasia and atypical ductal hyperplasia.

ATYPICAL LOBULAR HYPERPLASIA AND LOBULAR CARCINOMA IN SITU

Historical Perspective

Foote and Stewart gave the first clear clinical-pathologic description of LCIS in 1941[2] describing the morphologic similarities between these in situ lesions and ILC. This, together with the frequent concurrent diagnosis of LCIS and ILC, suggested a progressive relationship prompting management, ultimately removal of LCIS by mastectomy. This management strategy was subsequently supported by independent clinical follow-up that demonstrated a cumulative (and bilateral) risk of carcinoma in LCIS patients.[3] Over the next 30 years, the combination of bilateral risk, the long time-frame to progression, and the identification of IDC in association with LCIS raised questions about the precursor nature of LCIS. The lesion was considered only a "risk indicator," and hence management recommendations became varied, ranging from mastectomy to surveillance only.[4-10]

ALH was introduced more recently to describe lesions that are less well-developed but morphologically similar to LCIS. In 1978 the term "lobular neoplasia" (LN) was introduced to encompass both ALH and LCIS[4]; however, the term has not gained universal acceptance.

Epidemiology

Lack of specific clinical abnormalities has made estimation of the true incidence of LN very difficult. LN is neither palpable nor usually associated with mammographic abnormalities,[11-13] nor has it any guiding macroscopic features for the pathologist sampling the specimen. As a result, diagnosis is often an incidental microscopic finding in breast biopsies taken for other reasons. Hence the prevalence of ALH and LCIS is likely to be underestimated in the general population. The incidence of LCIS in otherwise benign breast biopsy is reported as between 0.5% and 3.8%.[4-6,14-18] Compared to both DCIS and ILC, LCIS is more frequently diagnosed in younger, premenopausal women, usually between 40 and 50 years of age.[5,6,11,15,19]

Natural History

LCIS is characteristically multifocal and bilateral, with approximately 50% demonstrating multiple foci in the ipsilateral breast and 30% in the contralateral breast.[4,5,18,20-23] The multifocality of these lesions suggests an underlying genetic predisposition. There are data to link rare cases with germ-line mutations in the E-cadherin gene, but this accounts for a very small number of cases.[24] Compared to the general population, ALH has a 4- to 5-fold and LCIS an 8- to 12-fold greater lifetime risk, respectively, of developing invasive carcinoma.[16,19,25] This translates to approximately 1% per year. Furthermore, the risk of developing a contralateral invasive cancer is greater in patients with LCIS compared to DCIS.[26-29]

However, despite the bilateral risk associated with lobular neoplasias, the risk is still skewed toward the ipsilateral breast.[16,17,30] The reported time between LCIS diagnosis and the development of invasive carcinoma ranges from 15 to 30 years.[5,18] Seventy percent of invasive carcinomas reported subsequent to LCIS diagnosis are of the lobular type[5]; conversely, LCIS has been identified in up to 91% of ILC cases.[31] Wheeler and associates found that although the risk of ILC is 18-fold higher in association with LCIS, IDC is also found in association with LCIS at a 3 to 4 times higher rate than the general population.[6] IDC, found subsequent to LCIS diagnosis, is thought to be due to the coexistence of DCIS, at least in a proportion of cases.[32,33]

Histologic Features

Figure 17-1A and B show examples of ALH and classic LCIS. While overall lobular architecture is maintained in LCIS, the acini are full and distended with a monomorphic population of small loosely cohesive cells. The cells are round, polygonal, or cuboidal and have a high nuclear-to-cytoplasmic ratio. The cells contain intracytoplasmic lumina or magenta bodies. The uniform nuclei contain fine and evenly dispersed chromatin. Mitoses, calcification, or necrosis are rarely observed. The differentiation between ALH and LCIS is rather arbitrary and quantitative rather than qualitative. In ALH the acini are not completely distended and residual lumina may be present. The cells comprising these "classic" ALH and LCIS lesions are also known as type A cells, which contrast with type B cells, which have larger vesicular nuclei.[34]

Pleomorphic lobular carcinoma in situ (PLCIS) is a recently recognized variant in which there is greater nuclear polymorphism (Fig. 17-1C), prominent nucleoli, more abundant and eosinophilic cytoplasm, and apocrine differentiation.[1,35-37]

Unlike classic LCIS, necrosis and calcification can be found in PLCIS (which can be detected by mammography as suspicious for DCIS) and is associated with the cytologically similar pleomorphic invasive lobular carcinoma (PILC).

Differential Diagnosis

One of the most difficult but important differential diagnoses for classic LCIS is the low-grade, solid form of DCIS (Fig. 17-1E). PLCIS is mistaken radiologically and histopathologically for high-grade DCIS, which has different management implications for the patient. Distinguishing LCIS from low-grade solid DCIS is particularly challenging, especially when the DCIS involves the acini (cancerization of the lobules).[32,38,39] Secondary lumen formation, cellular cohesion, and greater nuclear size and pleomorphism all point to a DCIS diagnosis. Immunohistochemistry for E-cadherin can be valuable in distinguishing the lesions (Fig. 17-1D).Concurrent involvement of the lobules with LCIS and DCIS does occur, and in such instances both are recorded and the patient managed for DCIS. Cases in which LCIS arises within another type of breast lesion, such as sclerosing adenosis or radial scar, can be mistaken for invasive carcinoma. The utilization of ancillary techniques such an immunohistochemistry can be invaluable here to detect and demonstrate the integrity of the myoepithelial layer or basement membrane.

Molecular Pathology

Due to the difficulty in classification and assigning risks based on morphology, there has been a hope that molecular subtyping would provide a better means of managing patients with these early preinvasive lesions. To date, there are no molecular data that help to identify lesions that will recur or progress and hence need more aggressive therapy.

Molecular Phenotype

Over 90% of LCIS cases are immunopositive for the estrogen receptor (ER) and progesterone receptor (PgR) and do not exhibit other classic biomarkers of aggressiveness such as HER2 overexpression, p53, and/or high Ki67 index.[40-45] This immunophenotype is very similar to both ILC and low-grade DCIS/IDC, but contrasting with high-grade DCIS/IDC. Despite the higher grade, PLCIS is also usually ER and PgR positive, but more frequently shows aggressive features such as HER2 overexpression, p53 positivity, and a higher Ki67 proliferative index. A higher frequency of gross cystic disease fluid protein-15 (GCDFP-15) has also been observed in pleomorphic variants, consistent with the observation of apocrine differentiation.

One of the most distinguishing molecular features of LN is the lack of E-cadherin expression in the vast majority of cases compared to ductal lesions,[7,36,38,46-56] hence its use in clinical practice to classify these proliferations. Loss of this cell–cell adhesion protein is thought to account for the characteristic discohesive morphology of lobular neoplastic cells. E-cadherin down regulation in LN has been found to occur by a variety of

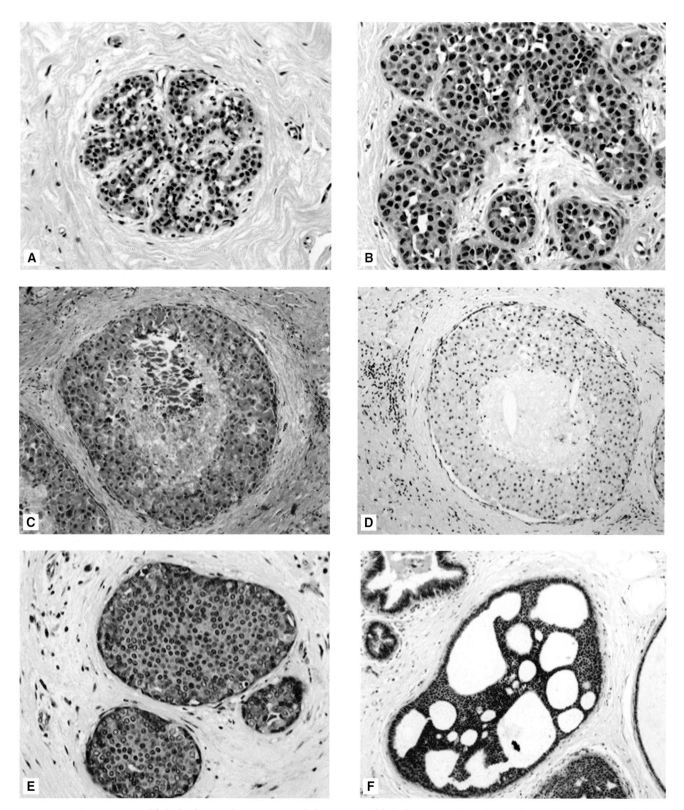

FIGURE 17-1 A. Atypical lobular hyperplasia—minimal distension of lobular unit with cells similar to those seen in lobular carcinoma in situ. **B.** Lobular carcinoma in situ—small monomorphic cells distending the terminal duct lobular unit, with no necrosis or mitoses. **C.** Pleomorphic variant of lobular carcinoma in situ—the cells are bigger with more pleomorphism, there is central comedo-type necrosis with calcification, and hence the lesion is mistaken radiologically and pathologically for high-grade ductal carcinoma in situ. E-cadherin is negative and illustrated in **(D) E.** The lesion depicted is difficult to classify; it is a solid low-grade proliferation that could be a low-grade DCIS of solid type or could also be LCIS. E-cadherin staining is useful in such cases to help classify the lesion. **F.** Atypical ductal hyperplasia. The lesion resembles low-grade DCIS but there is a retension of normal epithelium in part of the duct.

mechanisms, including the frequent loss of chromosome 16q or the more specific loss of heterozygosity of the E-cadherin locus, which is usually accompanied by truncating mutations or promoter methylation of the other allele. Reports of the same E-cadherin mutation in both LCIS and adjacent ILC has been the most direct and important evidence for the precursor role of LCIS.[49] Interestingly, although E-cadherin down regulation is observed in ALH, one paper suggests that mutations in the gene are rare, suggesting that the mutations occur after initial loss of expression.[48] Further work is required to fully understand the mechanism of LN E-cadherin loss, which may indeed be driving the tumourigenesis.

Array Comparative Genomic Hybridization (aCGH) studies that examine global genetic change further confirm that loss of 16q is a consistent and early event in the development of lobular neoplasms. The other most frequent chromosomal changes observed in LCIS include losses of 8p, 16p, 17p, 17q, and 22q, and gain of 1q and 6q. There are no significant differences in genetic alterations between ALH and LCIS, which strongly demonstrates their close relationship.[57] Interestingly there is significant overlap with changes occurring in low-grade DCIS, which suggests a close evolutionary development of lobular and low-grade ductal pathways.[56,58]

Comparison with ILC demonstrates strong concordance of genetic changes, further supporting the hypothesis of a common clonality of these lesions and suggesting that LCIS is a direct precursor to ILC.[59,60] PLCIS is also genetically similar to LCIS, demonstrating a close relationship, but also exhibits additional changes such as amplification of oncogenic loci such as MYC (0q24) and HER2 (17q12), which again suggests it is a more aggressive lesion.[36,58,61] Although of significant benefit in demonstrating the progressive relationship between these lesions, these studies have yet to provide us with new prognostic markers that assist in clinical decision-making regarding the likelihood of progression of preinvasive lesions to invasive carcinoma.

ATYPICAL DUCTAL HYPERPLASIA

Atypical ductal hyperplasia (ADH) is a very specific lesion that has cytomorphologic features both intermediate and overlapping with hyperplasia of usual type and low-grade DCIS.[62] Size criteria have also been introduced.[16,63] An example of ADH is shown in Figure 17-1F.

Epidemiology and Natural History

ADH is reported in 4% of all symptomatic benign biopsies[64] and imparts an increased risk of invasive breast cancer of 4- to 5-fold.[65,66] The reported increase in risk to 11-fold in patients with a family history of breast cancer[67] has recently been challenged by a new Mayo Clinic study[68] suggesting that the phenotype is influenced by both inherited risk and lifetime exposures. In a study by Page and associates, 12% of cases developed invasive carcinoma at an average of 16 years postdiagnosis.[16] Including DCIS as a cancer event, the Mayo Clinic recently found as many as 20% of ADH patients progressed to cancer within approximately 13 years, and this within the ipsilateral breast[68] as had already been shown for untreated DCIS.[69]

Histologic Features

ADH (Fig. 17-1F) bears high morphologic similarity to low-grade DCIS (Fig. 17-1E). It is composed of regularly arranged monotonous round, cuboidal, or polygonal cells, enclosed by a basement membrane. Mitoses are rare and nuclei are evenly distributed. Several different growth patterns have been observed, including cribriform and micropapillary patterns. Small necrotic foci may also be seen within ADH lesions. The proliferation involves part of the duct space and the secondary lumina are punched out as well as irregular. While most bridges are solid, occasional streaming of cells is also seen. Hence the features are intermediate between hyperplasia and DCIS. A size cut-off of 2 or 3 mm has also been introduced in the definition.

Intraobserver concordance for ADH diagnosis is notoriously poor,[70,71] although the work of Page, Dupont, and colleagues has done much to improve agreement amongst observers. Their methods emphasise the importance of using 3 different sets of criteria: histologic pattern, cytologic features, and anatomic extent of lesion,[16,62,72] which involves observation at both high- and low-power magnification for the features listed above.

Molecular Pathology

Expression of specific molecular markers in precursor and preinvasive lesions has been studied by multiple groups (reviewed in Zagouri et al[73]). As with LN and low-grade DCIS, ADH is uniformly positive for ER and PgR. HER2 is generally not overexpressed in the lesions.[74] HER2 amplification has been detected in a small proportion of ADH,[75] although there are conflicting reports as to whether it imparts greater risk of developing invasive carcinoma.[42,76] The well-differentiated features of ADH are further confirmed on a molecular level by low Ki-67 expression (a proliferative marker), bcl-2 positivity (a proapoptotic marker negatively correlating with aggressiveness[77]), and p53 negativity.[78] Despite these findings, no molecular markers have been found to have independent prognostic significance for ADH, indicating that more research is needed in this area.

As for lobular neoplasia, the advent of microarray technology has provided further evidence for the model of progression through ADH to DCIS and IDC. Gene expression profiling of these lesions (including multiple matched samples from the same patient) and comparison with normal breast tissue demonstrate that most alterations that distinguish invasive carcinoma from normal tissue are present in ADH.[79] This supports the notion of a clonal relationship between the distinct pathologic stages and is further supported by subsequent principal component analysis of the data.[80,81] The same study found that gene expression patterns correlated highly with grade, that is, there was more difference between samples of different grades (high or low) than between samples of different stages of progression. Notably, all ADH samples demonstrated a grade I molecular profile and clustered with low-grade DCIS and IDC.[79]

Molecular genetic analysis is consistent with the morphologic similarities between ADH and low-grade DCIS (reviewed in

Reis-Filho and Lakhani[82]). Although there are reports of ADH with no genetic change by CGH analysis,[83] others have shown recurrent loss of 16q and 17p,[84] which corroborates LOH studies of matched pairs of ADH and DCIS.[85,86] One study demonstrated that 45% of ADH lesions shared at least 1 LOH with adjacent IDC.[87] While this is very strong evidence for ADH as a precursor to DCIS in breast cancer progression, it has not, as yet, resulted in new methods for identifying those ADH lesions that will progress to invasive cancer and those that will not.

Clinical Implications and Management

From a clinical perspective, ALH, LCIS, and ADH are not life-threatening conditions. Indeed, the majority of women in whom these conditions are detected will suffer no adverse consequences throughout their lifespan. Unfortunately, a small proportion of women with each of these conditions will develop a breast cancer that may be attributable to the prior development of ALH, LCIS, or ADH.[5,20] The detection of 1 (or more) of these conditions in a breast biopsy therefore indicates an increased risk of DCIS or invasive cancer, and the clinical management must reflect the probability of a cancer developing in the ipsilateral or contralateral breast. It must be recognized that a biopsy that reveals one of these conditions implies a present risk of breast cancer as well as a risk of later breast cancer diagnosis: it is not uncommon for a breast cancer to coexist with any one of these less aggressive conditions. For example, DCIS may be present elsewhere in the breast when a biopsy reveals ADH, and ILC may exist concurrently with biopsy-detected LCIS.

The detection of ALH, LCIS, or ADH in a breast biopsy is therefore a clear indication for meticulous assessment of both breasts, using all available modalities, and (in the case of a negative result), ongoing surveillance of the breasts at a relatively short interval.

Clinical Examination and Breast Imaging

The role of clinical examination in the ongoing surveillance of women with these high-risk lesions is limited. With rare exceptions, DCIS and invasive cancers are detected on breast imaging many months before they can be clinically identified. Clinical detection of DCIS or invasive cancer is an indication of failure of either the imaging technology or the scheduling of imaging assessment.

The need for breast imaging at regular intervals cannot be overstated. There is international consensus that mammographic screening of women without high-risk lesions should be conducted at 2-year intervals, from the age of 50 onward.[88,89] In women aged 40 to 49 and for women with a strong family history of breast cancer, an annual screening interval is preferable. Annual imaging should also be the benchmark for a woman of any age with a high-risk lesion.

Options for Breast Imaging

Mammography alone is an unreliable imaging technique for the detection of small breast cancers.[90] Although it serves an invaluable role in early detection for many women, even state-of-the-art digital mammography is defeated by dense breast tissue, by very small lesions, and by DCIS that has not produced ductal calcification.

While the combination of mammography and ultrasound used in this way will detect at least 90% of existing cancers, there is little doubt that breast magnetic resonance imaging (MRI) can make a substantial contribution to the diagnosis of early lesions in these cases. Data from studies that have compared MRI with conventional imaging (mammography and breast ultrasound) are difficult to assess because *quality* is a significant variable in mammography and particularly in breast ultrasound. Setting aside this obstacle, there is no doubt that MRI can occasionally detect small cancers in breasts where meticulous mammography and ultrasound fails to show a lesion.[91] However, there is as yet no direct evidence to show that detection with MRI provides added benefit for women in terms of survival. The results of ongoing randomized clinical trials are currently awaited.[92]

This presents the clinician with a dilemma: should all women with high-risk lesions have an annual breast MRI, or does the cost of MRI exclude this modality as a routine procedure? Ultimately, this is a decision for the individual clinician (and for the woman who may have to pay for the MRI), but in examples of dense or fibrocystic breast tissue where conventional assessment with mammography and ultrasound is less than optimal, MRI should be considered as a routine investigation.

Unfortunately this is not a foolproof schedule. All specialists in this field have seen individual cancers present between annual examinations. The majority of these are rapidly growing, high-grade cancers with a poor prognosis.

Six-monthly assessment may be preferred in some circumstances (and by some women), but routine mammography is not an option at such short intervals. Annual review therefore appears to be a pragmatic solution for a difficult issue where there are no absolute benchmarks.

BIOPSY DIAGNOSIS OF ALH, LCIS, AND ADH

Notwithstanding the need for regular imaging in women with *detected* ALH, LCIS, or ADH, it must be recognized that none of these conditions has any specific appearances on mammography, ultrasound, or MRI. The initial detection of these lesions is invariably serendipitous, either because of a clinical feature that is irrelevant (eg, a fibroadenoma in tissue that is found to contain LCIS), or because a mammographic feature such as indeterminate calcification (again, often irrelevant) demands a histologic diagnosis.

Fine-needle aspiration cytology (FNAC) seldom has a role in the initial diagnosis of these lesions: occasionally cytological atypia in a perplexing ultrasound lesion will indicate the need for a tissue diagnosis but core biopsy is now the preferred first option for non-mass lesions. Standard core biopsies (14-18 gauge) are probably the most prevalent method for initial diagnosis of these high-risk lesions, although some will be identified (again probably by chance) in large-core (11-gauge), vacuum-assisted biopsies in cases where an ultrasound feature was the reason for the biopsy. Surgical biopsy, as noted, will occasionally reveal one of these conditions.

A relatively uncommon method of detection is in the routine histology of tissue excised in a breast reduction. Such lesions are managed in the same way as other lesions detected by surgical biopsy.

Surgical Management

Most of the issues for management of these high-risk lesions can be illustrated by considering three scenarios. In the first, a high-risk lesion has been detected on core biopsy; in the second, surgical excision of a benign mass (eg, fibroadenoma) reveals a high-risk lesion that appears to have been completely excised. In the third scenario, surgical excision of a high-risk lesion shows involvement of the excision margins (Fig. 17-2).

In the first case, core biopsy detection of ADH is an absolute indication for surgical excision. Since the diagnosis of ADH includes the size of the lesion as a defining criteria (less than 2 or 3 mm, depending on the criteria used), a core that shows a focus of ADH might well be a small sample of an area of DCIS. In a review of 300 vacuum-assisted biopsies that contained ADH, Foregeard and associates found DCIS in 25% of surgical excisions.[93] The mandatory surgical biopsy of core-detected ADH is therefore necessary to determine whether the lesion is indeed a small focus of ADH or part of DCIS. This procedure will either excise the lesion completely or at least give an indication of its nature and extent. When DCIS is detected in the surgical specimen, this must be treated on its merits.

Ideally, radiologic-pathologic criteria should determine the risk of DCIS or IDC when core biopsies show ADH. As yet, mostly retrospective studies have investigated the possibility of determining which patients can be spared surgery and which definitely require further excision and follow-up. Doren and colleagues proposed a method for describing atypia in ADH that correlates with the presence of cancer upon surgical excision.[94] Others have investigated whether mammographic findings can help discriminate between ADH and DCIS on core needle biopsy, and suggest that particular radiologic characteristics are associated with a lower risk of malignancy.[95] Further validation of these techniques is currently awaited.

In the previously cited study, Foregeard and associates[93] found that the size of the ADH lesion and multiple foci of ADH in the cores were related to the risk of DCIS. In 72 women with radiographic lesions larger than 20 mm in size and with more than 2 foci of ADH in the core biopsies, DCIS was present in 30% of surgical biopsies and an additional 2 cases (3%) showed IDC. By comparison, where the cores showed 2 or less than 2 foci of ADH, only 9% of surgical biopsies contained DCIS.

In the case of core-detected ALH or LCIS, the rationale for surgical excision is less clear. If the imaging features (mass, distortion, or calcification) are considered to be suspicious (BI-RADS category 4 or 5), there is a clear need for surgical excision. When the core biopsy reveals ALH or LCIS and this is considered to be compatible with the imaging features (eg, indeterminate calcification—BI-RADS category 3), surgical excision is an option (Fig. 17-2).

As in the case of ADH, the need for a surgical biopsy is based on risk—in this case, on the probability that the ALH or LCIS coexists with an invasive cancer. In a review of this risk,

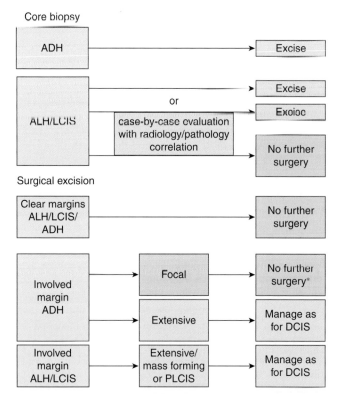

FIGURE 17-2 Diagram summarizing surgical management of ALH/LCIS and ADH. All ADH lesions on core biopsies will result in further excision, since size is a criterion for designating a lesion as ADH versus DCIS. Since size cannot be assessed on core biopsy, DCIS cannot be excluded, hence the further excision. The situation for ALH/LCIS is different since these lesions are usually incidental to the radiologic abnormality that prompted the biopsy. While many institutions excise all cases of ALH/LCIS on core biopsy, some prefer to evaluate on a case-by-case basis. Irrespective of this, most patients will go on to excision due to a radiologic-pathologic discordance. The management of involved margins in an excision specimen is also variable.
* There is no absolute consensus as to what further procedures should be carried out for focal ADH at margin in an excisional specimen. On first principle, there should be further excision; however, where the main radiologic abnormality is excised and the patient may receive radiotherapy for the primary diagnosis (eg, DCIS), many surgeons will not carry out a further excision. In contrast, when the proliferation is extensive or mass-forming, further surgery is indicated.

Elsheikh and Silverman concluded that, when a core biopsy showed LCIS, there was a 20% chance of finding a cancer in the surgical excision.[96] Although this conclusion was based on a total of 22 independent studies, 17 of these studies were comprised of fewer than 10 cases each. Furthermore, almost all were retrospective studies and the data are biased by exclusion of those cases in which surgical biopsy was not undertaken.

Although most studies support the current practice of mandatory surgical excision upon diagnosis of ALH or LCIS on core biopsy,[97] it has been suggested that excision of lobular neoplasia after biopsy diagnosis is unnecessary if careful radiographic-pathologic correlation is performed and strict histologic criteria are followed.[98]

We feel that the conclusions that can be drawn from these data are insufficient to recommend obligatory surgical biopsy for cases of core-detected ALH or LCIS. Some surgeons will be persuaded that, even in the absence of reliable evidence, the perceived risk of malignancy is sufficient to justify surgical excision of core-detected ALH or LCIS. In some institutions the decision is made on an individual, case-by-case basis: this appears to be the most rational approach, until more reliable prospective data establish the probability of finding DCIS or invasive cancer in this situation.

Where the surgical biopsy reveals ALH or LCIS, the margins of excision are paramount in determining further treatment. If the margins are clear, that is, the lesion appears to have been completely excised, no further treatment is required. The risk of subsequent cancer development must be explained clearly to the woman and regular surveillance, as detailed earlier in the chapter, is the rational option. However, there are exceptions to this rule.

Some women with a strong family history of breast cancer, but no demonstrable genetic mutation, see the detection of a high-risk lesion as a turning-point in their surveillance. In such cases, prophylactic mastectomy(ies) may be discussed, the advantages and disadvantages must be explored, and the final decision must be made by the woman herself.

Similar considerations apply in the case of a woman who has had a contralateral cancer. Specifically, if this was an invasive lobular cancer and LCIS is now detected in the untreated breast, this woman might want to consider a mastectomy as the most effective method of prevention.

Where surgical excision reveals a high-risk lesion with an involved surgical margin or margins, reexcision should be considered. The goal, of course, is complete excision, but it must be recognized that all of these lesions, particularly LCIS, can be very extensive, sometimes occupying an entire quadrant or more of the breast. If a generous diagnostic excision suggests this—usually because several margins are involved—it may be clear that a substantially wider excision would have an adverse cosmetic outcome. In such cases, provided no foci of DCIS or invasive cancer are detected, observation and surveillance as detailed may be the preferred option. Again, the patient will be fully informed of the risk of subsequent cancer and involved in this decision.

The other option, preferred by some women, is a mastectomy with or without breast reconstruction. Where the size and shape of the breast permit, our preference in this situation is for a subcutaneous ("skin-sparing") mastectomy with nipple preservation. In this procedure, an excision providing adequate access is important and the lactiferous sinuses must be cored out of the nipple. There is a small risk of nipple necrosis following this procedure.

Another scenario where margins are involved is when there is evidence of multifocal ADH, ALH, or LCIS. The only conclusion that can be drawn from this biopsy result is that other foci are likely to exist elsewhere in the same quadrant or in other quadrants of the breast. In this case, all of the preceding options (surveillance, wider excision, or mastectomy), should be considered.

In the event that a reexcision confirms substantial residual disease, particularly if the new margins are involved, it is likely that local surgical treatment will not eradicate the condition. It should be emphasized that there is no evidence to show that radiotherapy or hormone treatment is beneficial in this situation. The options are either surveillance or mastectomy.

The limited data on probability of subsequent breast cancer after excision of any of these high-risk lesions provide no evidence on the influence of clear or close margins on the risk of subsequent cancer. A study by Greene and associates found that of 155 patients with ADH on excisional biopsy, the one patient found to develop invasive carcinoma on follow-up had clear surgical margins, while no patients with positive or unknown margin status developed malignancy during the course of the study.[99] There is no information to indicate that a wide clearance (>10 mm) reduces this risk, compared with a close margin of, for example, 1 to 2 mm. Nevertheless, it is considered good surgical practice to obtain a clear margin of 10 mm or more. In cases where lesser margins are obtained, reexcision should be considered.

In resolving these difficult decisions, the surgeon may be influenced by subtypes of these lesions. One example is pleomorphic LCIS. We have recently encountered 2 cases in which a surgical biopsy for core-detected LCIS revealed PLCIS: in each case, further investigation revealed pleomorphic invasive lobular carcinoma, ultimately shown to be multicentric. In one of these cases, the premastectomy MRI demonstrated the multicentricity. We are now inclined to treat pleomorphic LCIS aggressively with an intensive search for foci of invasion, prior to surgery.

FUTURE STUDIES

There are several issues relating to high-risk lesions that require further research. These include prospective, rather than retrospective, studies that examine the association between high-risk lesions and invasive carcinoma. Most particularly, biomarkers that help stratify those lesions with higher risk of progressing to invasive carcinoma are needed to assist in clinical management. Other molecular analyses that give insight into the natural history and progression of precursor lesions to invasive carcinoma would also be invaluable.

SUMMARY

ALH, LCIS, and ADH are clonal, nonobligate precursor lesions with an increased risk of invasive carcinoma. Together with the direct epidemiologic evidence, the mounting molecular data strongly suggest a relationship between ALH, LCIS, and ILC as well as ADH, DCIS, and IDC. The evolution to invasive carcinoma may not, however, be linear and may involve multiple pathways. Clinical management of patients with ALH, LCIS, or ADH is made difficult by an inability to predict which lesions will progress to invasive stages. Most cases will never develop invasive carcinoma, but we are currently unable to differentiate the small subset that will. This poses a clinical dilemma, and future studies addressing biomarkers for predicting behavior are warranted.

The clinical management of ADH, ALH, and LCIS is challenging, often with issues and options that can be resolved only in the individual case. The involvement of the patient in these discussions is a benchmark of good clinical practice. Finally, the effective management of these high-risk lesions depends on detailed and reliable pathology reporting and a close rapport between the surgeon and the pathologist.

REFERENCES

1. Simpson PT, Gale T, Fulford LG, et al. The diagnosis and management of pre-invasive breast disease: pathology of atypical lobular hyperplasia and lobular carcinoma in situ. *Breast Cancer Res.* 2003;5:258-262.
2. Foote FW, Stewart FW. Lobular carcinoma in situ: a rare form of mammary cancer. *Am J Pathol.* 1941;17:491-496.
3. McDivitt RW, Hutter RV, Foote FW Jr., Stewart FW. In situ lobular carcinoma. A prospective follow-up study indicating cumulative patient risks. *JAMA.* 1967;201:82-86.
4. Haagensen CD, Lane N, Lattes R, Bodian C. Lobular neoplasia (so-called lobular carcinoma in situ) of the breast. *Cancer.* 1978;42:737-769.
5. Page DL, Kidd TE Jr., Dupont WD, et al. Lobular neoplasia of the breast: higher risk for subsequent invasive cancer predicted by more extensive disease. *Hum Pathol.* Dec 1991;22(12):1232-1239.
6. Wheeler JE, Enterline HT, Roseman JM, et al. Lobular carcinoma in situ of the breast. Long-term followup. *Cancer.* 1974;34:554-563.
7. Goldstein NS, Bassi D, Watts JC, et al. E-cadherin reactivity of 95 noninvasive ductal and lobular lesions of the breast. Implications for the interpretation of problematic lesions. *Am J Clin Pathol.* 2001;115:534-542.
8. Haagensen CD. Lobular carcinoma of the breast. A precancerous lesion? *Clin Obstet Gynecol.* 1962;5:1093-1101.
9. Grooff PN, Pamies RJ, Hunyadi S. Lobular carcinoma in situ: what clinicians need to know. *Hosp Pract (Off Ed).* 1993;28:122.
10. Frykberg ER, Bland KI. In situ breast carcinoma. *Adv Surg.* 1993;26:29-72.
11. Beute BJ, Kalisher L, Hutter RV. Lobular carcinoma in situ of the breast: clinical, pathologic, and mammographic features. *AJR Am J Roentgenol.* 1991;157:257-265.
12. Georgian-Smith D, Lawton TJ. Calcifications of lobular carcinoma in situ of the breast: radiologic-pathologic correlation. *AJR Am J Roentgenol.* 2001;176:1255-1259.
13. Sonnenfeld MR, Frenna TH, Weidner N, Meyer JE. Lobular carcinoma in situ: mammographic-pathologic correlation of results of needle-directed biopsy. *Radiology.* 1991;181:363-367.
14. Li CI, Anderson BO, Daling JR, Moe RE. Changing incidence of lobular carcinoma in situ of the breast. *Breast Cancer Res Treat.* 2002;75:259-268.
15. Andersen JA. Lobular carcinoma in situ of the breast. An approach to rational treatment. *Cancer.* 1977;39:2597-2602.
16. Page DL, Dupont WD, Rogers LW, Rados MS. Atypical hyperplastic lesions of the female breast. A long-term follow-up study. *Cancer.* 1985;55:2698-2708.
17. Page DL, Schuyler PA, Dupont WD, et al. Atypical lobular hyperplasia as a unilateral predictor of breast cancer risk: a retrospective cohort study. *Lancet.* 2003;361:125-129.
18. Rosen PP, Kosloff C, Lieberman PH, et al. Lobular carcinoma in situ of the breast. Detailed analysis of 99 patients with average follow-up of 24 years. *Am J Surg Pathol.* 1978;2:225-251.
19. Frykberg ER. Lobular carcinoma in situ of the breast. *Breast J.* 1999;5:296-303.
20. Bodian CA, Perzin KH, Lattes R. Lobular neoplasia. Long term risk of breast cancer and relation to other factors. *Cancer.* 1996;78:1024-1034.
21. Rosen PP, Braun DW Jr., Lyngholm B, et al. Lobular carcinoma in situ of the breast: preliminary results of treatment by ipsilateral mastectomy and contralateral breast biopsy. *Cancer.* 1981;47:813-819.
22. Rosen PP, Senie RT, Farr GH, et al. Epidemiology of breast carcinoma: age, menstrual status, and exogenous hormone usage in patients with lobular carcinoma in situ. *Surgery.* 1979;85:219-224.
23. Urban JA. Bilaterality of cancer of the breast. Biopsy of the opposite breast. *Cancer.* 1967;20:1867-1870.
24. Masciari S, Larsson N, Senz J, et al. Germline E-cadherin mutations in familial lobular breast cancer. *J Med Genet.* 2007;44:726-731.
25. McLaren BK, Schuyler PA, Sanders ME, et al. Excellent survival, cancer type, and Nottingham grade after atypical lobular hyperplasia on initial breast biopsy. *Cancer.* 2006;107:1227-1233.
26. Claus EB, Stowe M, Carter D, Holford T. The risk of a contralateral breast cancer among women diagnosed with ductal and lobular breast carcinoma in situ: data from the Connecticut Tumor Registry. *Breast.* 2003;12:451-456.
27. Habel LA, Moe RE, Daling JR, et al. Risk of contralateral breast cancer among women with carcinoma in situ of the breast. *Ann Surg.* 1997;225:69-75.
28. Webber BL, Heise H, Neifeld JP, Costa J. Risk of subsequent contralateral breast carcinoma in a population of patients with in-situ breast carcinoma. *Cancer.* 1981;47:2928-2932.
29. Haagensen CD, Lane N, Bodian C. Coexisting lobular neoplasia and carcinoma of the breast. *Cancer.* 1983;51:1468-1482.
30. Marshall LM, Hunter DJ, Connolly JL, et al. Risk of breast cancer associated with atypical hyperplasia of lobular and ductal types. *Cancer Epidemiol Biomarkers Prev.* 1997;6:297-301.
31. Abdel-Fatah TM, Powe DG, Hodi Z, et al. High frequency of coexistence of columnar cell lesions, lobular neoplasia, and low grade ductal carcinoma in situ with invasive tubular carcinoma and invasive lobular carcinoma. *Am J Surg Pathol.* 2007;31:417-426.
32. Maluf H, Koerner F. Lobular carcinoma in situ and infiltrating ductal carcinoma: frequent presence of DCIS as a precursor lesion. *Int J Surg Pathol.* 2001;9:127-131.
33. Rosen PP. Coexistent lobular carcinoma in situ and intraductal carcinoma in a single lobular-duct unit. *Am J Surg Pathol.* 1980;4:241-246.
34. Schnitt SJ, Morrow M. Lobular carcinoma in situ: current concepts and controversies. *Semin Diagn Pathol.* 1999;16:209-223.
35. Fadare O. Pleomorphic lobular carcinoma in situ of the breast composed almost entirely of signet ring cells. *Pathol Int.* 2006;56:683-687.
36. Sneige N, Wang J, Baker BA, et al. Clinical, histopathologic, and biologic features of pleomorphic lobular (ductal-lobular) carcinoma in situ of the breast: a report of 24 cases. *Mod Pathol.* 2002;15:1044-1050.
37. Eusebi V, Magalhaes F, Azzopardi JG. Pleomorphic lobular carcinoma of the breast: an aggressive tumor showing apocrine differentiation. *Hum Pathol.* 1992;23:655-662.
38. Jacobs TW, Pliss N, Kouria G, Schnitt SJ. Carcinomas in situ of the breast with indeterminate features: role of E-cadherin staining in categorization. *Am J Surg Pathol.* 2001;25:229-236.
39. Maluf HM. Differential diagnosis of solid carcinoma in situ. *Semin Diagn Pathol.* 2004;21:25-31.
40. Baqai T, Shousha S. Oestrogen receptor negativity as a marker for high-grade ductal carcinoma in situ of the breast. *Histopathology.* 2003;42:440-447.
41. Middleton LP, Perkins GH, Tucker SL, et al. Expression of ERalpha and ERbeta in lobular carcinoma in situ. *Histopathology.* 2007;50:875-880.
42. Mohsin SK, O'Connell P, Allred DC, Libby AL. Biomarker profile and genetic abnormalities in lobular carcinoma in situ. *Breast Cancer Res Treat.* 2005;90:249-256.
43. Porter PL, Garcia R, Moe R, et al. C-erbB-2 oncogene protein in in situ and invasive lobular breast neoplasia. *Cancer.* 1991;68:331-334.
44. Ramachandra S, Machin L, Ashley S, et al. Immunohistochemical distribution of c-erbB-2 in in situ breast carcinoma—a detailed morphological analysis. *J Pathol.* 1990;161:7-14.
45. Rudas M, Neumayer R, Gnant MF, et al. p53 protein expression, cell proliferation and steroid hormone receptors in ductal and lobular in situ carcinomas of the breast. *Eur J Cancer.* 1997;33:39-44.
46. De Leeuw WJ, Berx G, Vos CB, et al. Simultaneous loss of E-cadherin and catenins in invasive lobular breast cancer and lobular carcinoma in situ. *J Pathol.* 1997;183:404-411.
47. Sarrio D, Perez-Mies B, Hardisson D, et al. Cytoplasmic localization of p120ctn and E-cadherin loss characterize lobular breast carcinoma from preinvasive to metastatic lesions. *Oncogene.* 2004;23:3272-3283.
48. Mastracci TI, Tjan S, Bane AL, et al. E-cadherin alterations in atypical lobular hyperplasia and lobular carcinoma in situ of the breast. *Mod Pathol.* 2005;18:741-751.
49. Vos CB, Cleton-Jansen AM, Berx G, et al. E-cadherin inactivation in lobular carcinoma in situ of the breast: an early event in tumorigenesis. *Br J Cancer.* 1997;76:1131-1133.
50. Bratthauer GL, Moinfar F, Stamatakos MD, et al. Combined E-cadherin and high molecular weight cytokeratin immunoprofile differentiates lobular, ductal, and hybrid mammary intraepithelial neoplasias. *Hum Pathol.* 2002;33:620-627.
51. Dabbs DJ, Kaplai M, Chivukula M, et al. The spectrum of morphomolecular abnormalities of the e-cadherin/catenin complex in pleomorphic lobular carcinoma of the breast. *Appl Immunohistochem Mol Morphol.* 2007;15:260-266.
52. Droufakou S, Deshmane V, Roylance R, et al. Multiple ways of silencing E-cadherin gene expression in lobular carcinoma of the breast. *Int J Cancer.* 2001;92:404-408.

53. Gamallo C, Palacios J, Suarez A, et al. Correlation of E-cadherin expression with differentiation grade and histological type in breast carcinoma. *Am J Pathol.* 1993;142:987-993.

54. Palacios J, Sarrio D, Garcia-Macias MC, et al. Frequent E-cadherin gene inactivation by loss of heterozygosity in pleomorphic lobular carcinoma of the breast. *Mod Pathol.* 2003;16:674-678.

55. Rasbridge SA, Gillett CE, Sampson SA, et al. Epithelial (E-) and placental (P-) cadherin cell adhesion molecule expression in breast carcinoma. *J Pathol.* 1993;169:245-250.

56. Simpson PT, Reis-Filho JS, Lambros MB, et al. Molecular profiling pleomorphic lobular carcinomas of the breast: evidence for a common molecular genetic pathway with classic lobular carcinomas. *J Pathol.* 2008;215:231-244.

57. Lu YJ, Osin P, Lakhani SR, et al. Comparative genomic hybridization analysis of lobular carcinoma in situ and atypical lobular hyperplasia and potential roles for gains and losses of genetic material in breast neoplasia. *Cancer Res.* 1998;58:4721-4727.

58. Reis-Filho JS, Simpson PT, Gale T, Lakhani SR. The molecular genetics of breast cancer: the contribution of comparative genomic hybridization. *Pathol Res Pract.* 2005;201:713-725.

59. Nyante SJ, Devries S, Chen YY, Hwang ES. Array-based comparative genomic hybridization of ductal carcinoma in situ and synchronous invasive lobular cancer. *Hum Pathol.* 2004;35:759-763.

60. Shelley Hwang E, Nyante SJ, Yi Chen Y, et al. Clonality of lobular carcinoma in situ and synchronous invasive lobular carcinoma. *Cancer.* 2004;100:2562-2572.

61. Middleton LP, Palacios DM, Bryant BR, et al. Pleomorphic lobular carcinoma: morphology, immunohistochemistry, and molecular analysis. *Am J Surg Pathol.* 2000;24:1650-1656.

62. Page DL, Rogers LW. Combined histologic and cytologic criteria for the diagnosis of mammary atypical ductal hyperplasia. *Hum Pathol.* 1992;23:1095-1097.

63. Tavassoli FA, Norris HJ. A comparison of the results of long-term follow-up for atypical intraductal hyperplasia and intraductal hyperplasia of the breast. *Cancer.* 1990;65:518-529.

64. Pinder SE, Ellis IO. The diagnosis and management of pre-invasive breast disease: ductal carcinoma in situ (DCIS) and atypical ductal hyperplasia (ADH)—current definitions and classification. *Breast Cancer Res.* 2003;5:254-257.

65. Dupont WD, Parl FF, Hartmann WH, et al. Breast cancer risk associated with proliferative breast disease and atypical hyperplasia. *Cancer.* 1993;71:1258-1265.

66. Page DL, Dupont WD. Premalignant conditions and markers of elevated risk in the breast and their management. *Surg Clin North Am.* 1990;70:831-851.

67. Dupont WD, Page DL. Risk factors for breast cancer in women with proliferative breast disease. *N Engl J Med.* 1985;312:146-151.

68. Degnim AC, Visscher DW, Berman HK, et al. Stratification of breast cancer risk in women with atypia: a Mayo cohort study. *J Clin Oncol.* 2007;25:2671-2677.

69. Collins LC, Tamimi RM, Baer HJ, et al. Outcome of patients with ductal carcinoma in situ untreated after diagnostic biopsy: results from the Nurses' Health Study. *Cancer.* 2005;103:1778-1784.

70. Sloane JP, Ellman R, Anderson TJ, et al. Consistency of histopathological reporting of breast lesions detected by screening: findings of the U.K. National External Quality Assessment (EQA) Scheme. U.K. National Coordinating Group for Breast Screening Pathology. *Eur J Cancer.* 1994;30A:1414-1419.

71. Rosai J. Borderline epithelial lesions of the breast. *Am J Surg Pathol.* 1991;15:209-221.

72. Page DL, Vander Zwaag R, Rogers LW, et al. Relation between component parts of fibrocystic disease complex and breast cancer. *J Natl Cancer Inst.* 1978;61:1055-1063.

73. Zagouri F, Sergentanis TN, Zografos GC. Precursors and preinvasive lesions of the breast: the role of molecular prognostic markers in the diagnostic and therapeutic dilemma. *World J Surg Oncol.* 2007;5:57.

74. Gusterson BA, Machin LG, Gullick WJ, et al. c-erbB-2 expression in benign and malignant breast disease. *Br J Cancer.* 1988;58:453-457.

75. Xu R, Perle MA, Inghirami G, et al. Amplification of Her-2/neu gene in Her-2/neu-overexpressing and -nonexpressing breast carcinomas and their synchronous benign, premalignant, and metastatic lesions detected by FISH in archival material. *Mod Pathol.* 2002;15:116-124.

76. Rohan TE, Hartwick W, Miller AB, Kandel RA. Immunohistochemical detection of c-erbB-2 and p53 in benign breast disease and breast cancer risk. *J Natl Cancer Inst.* 1998;90:1262-1269.

77. Mustonen M, Raunio H, Paakko P, Soini Y. The extent of apoptosis is inversely associated with bcl-2 expression in premalignant and malignant breast lesions. *Histopathology.* 1997;31:347-354.

78. Viacava P, Naccarato AG, Bevilacqua G. Different proliferative patterns characterize different preinvasive breast lesions. *J Pathol.* 1999;188:245-251.

79. Ma XJ, Salunga R, Tuggle JT, et al. Gene expression profiles of human breast cancer progression. *Proc Natl Acad Sci USA.* 2003;100:5974-5979.

80. Alexe G, Dalgin GS, Ganesan S, et al. Analysis of breast cancer progression using principal component analysis and clustering. *J Biosci.* 2007;32:1027-1039.

81. Dalgin GS, Alexe G, Scanfeld D, et al. Portraits of breast cancer progression. *BMC Bioinformatics.* 2007;8:291.

82. Reis-Filho JS, Lakhani SR. The diagnosis and management of pre-invasive breast disease: genetic alterations in pre-invasive lesions. *Breast Cancer Res.* 2003;5:313-319.

83. Gong G, DeVries S, Chew KL, et al. Genetic changes in paired atypical and usual ductal hyperplasia of the breast by comparative genomic hybridization. *Clin Cancer Res.* 2001;7:2410-2414.

84. Aubele MM, Cummings MC, Mattis AE, et al. Accumulation of chromosomal imbalances from intraductal proliferative lesions to adjacent in situ and invasive ductal breast cancer. *Diagn Mol Pathol.* 2000;9:14-19.

85. Lakhani SR, Collins N, Stratton MR, Sloane JP. Atypical ductal hyperplasia of the breast: clonal proliferation with loss of heterozygosity on chromosomes 16q and 17p. *J Clin Pathol.* 1995;48:611-615.

86. Amari M, Suzuki A, Moriya T, et al. LOH analyses of premalignant and malignant lesions of human breast: frequent LOH in 8p, 16q, and 17q in atypical ductal hyperplasia. *Oncol Rep.* 1999;6:1277-1280.

87. O'Connell P, Pekkel V, Fuqua SA, et al. Analysis of loss of heterozygosity in 399 premalignant breast lesions at 15 genetic loci. *J Natl Cancer Inst.* 1998;90:697-703.

88. Andersson I. Comment on "The frequency of breast cancer screening: results from the UKCCCR Randomised Trial." *Eur J Cancer.* 2002;38:1427-1428; discussion 1465.

89. White E, Miglioretti DL, Yankaskas BC, et al. Biennial versus annual mammography and the risk of late-stage breast cancer. *J Natl Cancer Inst.* 2004;96:1832-1839.

90. Simpson WL Jr., Hermann G, Rausch DR, et al. Ultrasound detection of nonpalpable mammographically occult malignancy. *Can Assoc Radiol J.* 2008;59:70-76.

91. Houssami N, Ciatto S, Macaskill P, et al. Accuracy and surgical impact of magnetic resonance imaging in breast cancer staging: systematic review and meta-analysis in detection of multifocal and multicentric cancer. *J Clin Oncol.* 2008;26:3248-3258.

92. Houssami N, Wilson R. Should women at high risk of breast cancer have screening magnetic resonance imaging (MRI)? *Breast.* 2007;16:2-4.

93. Forgeard C, Benchaib M, Guerin N, et al. Is surgical biopsy mandatory in case of atypical ductal hyperplasia on 11-gauge core needle biopsy? A retrospective study of 300 patients. *Am J Surg.* 2008;196:339-345.

94. Doren E, Hulvat M, Norton J, et al. Predicting cancer on excision of atypical ductal hyperplasia. *Am J Surg.* 2008;195:358-361; discussion 361-362.

95. Hoang JK, Hill P, Cawson JN. Can mammographic findings help discriminate between atypical ductal hyperplasia and ductal carcinoma in situ after needle core biopsy? *Breast.* 2008;17:282-288.

96. Elsheikh TM, Silverman JF. Follow-up surgical excision is indicated when breast core needle biopsies show atypical lobular hyperplasia or lobular carcinoma in situ: a correlative study of 33 patients with review of the literature. *Am J Surg Pathol.* 2005;29:534-543.

97. Margenthaler JA, Duke D, Monsees BS, et al. Correlation between core biopsy and excisional biopsy in breast high-risk lesions. *Am J Surg.* 2006;192:534-537.

98. Nagi CS, O'Donnell JE, Tismenetsky M, et al. Lobular neoplasia on core needle biopsy does not require excision. *Cancer.* 2008;112:2152-2158.

99. Greene T, Tartter PI, Smith SR, Estabrook A. The significance of surgical margins for patients with atypical ductal hyperplasia. *Am J Surg.* 2006;192:499-501.

CHAPTER 18

Ductal Carcinoma In Situ

Melvin J. Silverstein
Michael D. Lagios

Ductal carcinoma in situ (DCIS) of the breast is a heterogeneous group of lesions with diverse malignant potential and a range of treatment options. It is the most rapidly growing subgroup among breast cancers, with more than 68,000 new cases diagnosed in the United States during 2008 (27% of all new cases of breast cancer).[1] More than 90% are nonpalpable and discovered mammographically.

It is now well appreciated that DCIS is a stage in a neoplastic continuum in which most of the molecular changes that characterize invasive breast cancer are already present.[2] Only quantitative changes in the expression of genes that have already been altered separate DCIS from invasive growth. Genes that may play a role in invasion control a number of functions, including angiogenesis, adhesion, cell motility, the composition of extracellular-matrix, and more. To date, genes that are uniquely associated with invasion have not been identified. DCIS is clearly the precursor lesion for most invasive ductal carcinomas, but not all DCIS lesions have sufficient time or the genetic ability to progress to invasive disease.[3-5]

Therapy for DCIS ranges from simple excision to various forms of wider excision (segmental resection, quadrant resection, oncoplastic resection, etc.), all of which may or may not be followed by radiation therapy. When breast preservation is not feasible, total mastectomy, with or without immediate reconstruction, is generally performed.

Since DCIS is a heterogeneous group of lesions rather than a single entity,[6,7] and because patients have a wide range of personal needs that must be considered during treatment selection, it is clear that no single approach will be appropriate for all forms of the disease or for all patients. At the current time, treatment decisions are based upon a variety of measurable parameters (tumor extent, margin width, nuclear grade, the presence or absence of comedonecrosis, age, etc), as well as physician experience and bias, and upon randomized trial data, which suggest that all conservatively treated patients should be managed with postexcisional radiation therapy.

THE CHANGING NATURE OF DUCTAL CARCINOMA IN SITU

There have been dramatic changes in the frequency, clinical importance, and treatment of DCIS in the past 30 years. Before mammography was common, DCIS was rare, representing less than 1% of all breast cancer.[8] Today, DCIS is common, representing 27% of all newly diagnosed cases and as many as 30% to 50% of cases of breast cancer diagnosed by mammography.[1,9-13]

Previously, most patients with DCIS presented with clinical symptoms, such as breast mass, bloody nipple discharge, or Paget disease.[14,15] Today, most lesions are nonpalpable and generally detected by mammography alone.

Until approximately 20 years ago, the treatment for most patients with DCIS was mastectomy. Today, almost 75% of newly diagnosed patients with DCIS are treated with breast preservation.[16] In the past, when mastectomy was common, reconstruction was uncommon; if it was performed, it was generally done as a delayed procedure. Today, reconstruction for patients with DCIS treated by mastectomy is common; when it is performed, it is generally done immediately, at the time of mastectomy. In the past, when a mastectomy was performed, large amounts of skin were discarded. Today, it is considered perfectly safe to perform a skin-sparing mastectomy for DCIS and in some instances, nipple–areola-sparing mastectomy. In the past, there was little confusion. All breast cancers including DCIS were considered essentially the same and mastectomy was the only treatment. Today, we recognize that all breast cancers are different and there is a range of acceptable treatments for every lesion. For those who chose breast conservation, there continues to be a debate as to whether radiation therapy is necessary in every case. These changes were brought about by a number of factors. Most important were increased mammographic utilization and the acceptance of breast-conservation therapy for invasive breast cancer.

The widespread use of mammography changed the way DCIS was detected. In addition, it changed the nature of the disease detected by allowing us to enter the neoplastic continuum at an earlier time. It is interesting to note the impact that mammography had on the number of DCIS cases diagnosed and the way they were diagnosed at the Breast Center in Van Nuys, California.[17]

From 1979 to 1981, the Van Nuys Group treated a total of only 15 patients with DCIS, 5 per year. Only 2 lesions (13%) were nonpalpable and detected by mammography. In other words, 13 patients (87%) presented with clinically apparent disease. Two state-of-the-art mammography units and a full-time experienced radiologist were added in 1982, and the number of new DCIS cases increased to more than 30 per year, most of them nonpalpable. When a third machine was added in 1987, the number of new cases increased to 40 new cases per year. In 1994, the Van Nuys Group added a fourth mammography machine and a prone stereotactic biopsy unit. Analysis of the entire series of 1363 patients through April 2008 shows that 1201 lesions (88%) were nonpalpable (subclinical). If we look at only those diagnosed during the last 5 years at the USC/Norris Cancer Center, 95% were nonpalpable.

The second factor that changed how we think about DCIS was the acceptance of breast conservation therapy (lumpectomy, axillary node dissection, and radiation therapy) for patients with invasive breast cancer. Until 1981, the treatment for most patients with any form of breast cancer was generally mastectomy. Since that time, numerous prospective randomized trials have shown an equivalent rate of survival for selected patients with invasive breast cancer treated with breast conservation therapy.[18-23] Based on these results, it made little sense to continue treating less aggressive DCIS with mastectomy while treating more aggressive invasive breast cancer with breast preservation.

Current data suggest that many patients with DCIS can be successfully treated with breast preservation, with or without radiation therapy. This chapter will show how easily available data can be used to help in the complex treatment selection process.

PATHOLOGY

Classification

In 1979, Azzopardi and associates aptly noted that the various architectural classifications of DCIS had no apparent significance for clinical outcome.[24] However, at that time, all DCIS was treated by total mastectomy, and therefore there was no opportunity to evaluate the impact of architectural classification on local recurrence. Grading of DCIS can be thought of as classification independent of architectural pattern. Grading was introduced for DCIS in 1989 to determine whether it had significant impact on local recurrence in conservatively treated patients. It was based on the nuclear grading component of the Scarf–Bloom–Richardson system.[25] Necrosis was included in

the grading but was not used initially to distinguish subsets. Lagios and associates were able to show significant differences in local recurrence rates with 3 grades based on the nuclear grade and presence of necrosis largely because 2 other significant prognostic variables were controlled in their study population. Tumor size (extent) was required to be 25 mm or less, and margins had to be adequate: minimally 1 mm but most were larger. Solin and colleagues, in a dichotomous classification (high grade = nuclear grade 3 with necrosis versus everything else), similarly showed significant differences at 5 years.[26]

The division by architecture alone, comedo versus noncomedo, is an oversimplification and does not work if the purpose of the division is to sort the patients into those with a high risk of local recurrence versus those with a low risk. It is not uncommon for high nuclear grade noncomedo lesions to express markers similar to those of high-grade comedo lesions and to have a risk of local recurrence similar to comedo lesions. Adding to the confusion is the fact that mixtures of various architectural subtypes within a single biopsy specimen are common. In my personal series, more than 70% of all lesions had significant amounts of 2 or more architectural subtypes, making division into a predominant architectural subtype problematic.

Numerous subsequent classifications, based on nuclear grade and necrosis, have shown a similar association of grade and local recurrence rate in conservatively treated patents. Holland and associates used surrogate nomenclature for high, intermediate, and low grades but accomplished the same thing.[27] The Van Nuys classification, which is based on nuclear grade and necrosis, has been shown to be the most reproducible in actual practice.[28,29] In the Van Nuys classification, necrosis is used in absolute terms: any zonal necrosis no matter how limited classifies the patient as exhibiting necrosis—as opposed to the NSABP-B17 randomized trial, in which a third of the ducts must exhibit necrosis to qualify as high grade. This leads to the anomalous situation that a DCIS with nuclear grade 3 but only 20% of ducts exhibiting zonal necrosis would be classified in the low-risk comparison group. DCIS with nuclear grade 1 or 2 is classified on the basis of zonal necrosis into that without necrosis (class 1 = low grade) and that with necrosis (class 2 = intermediate grade).[30] The biggest impact of grade is seen in circumstances where the other variables are controlled.[13,25] In corollary fashion in circumstances where the prognostic variables cannot be defined (B17, B24, EORTC 10853, and Swed DCIS trials), grade has a more limited impact.

In 1995, the Van Nuys Group introduced a new pathologic DCIS classification[31] based on the presence or absence of high nuclear grade and comedo-type necrosis (the Van Nuys Classification). The Van Nuys Group chose high nuclear grade as the most important factor in their classification because there was general agreement that patients with high nuclear grade lesions were more likely to recur at a higher rate and in a shorter time period after breast conservation than patients with low nuclear grade lesions.[25,26,32-35] Comedo-type necrosis was chosen because its presence also suggests a poorer prognosis[36,37] and it is easy to recognize.[38]

The pathologist, using standardized criteria, as noted in the next paragraph first determines whether the lesion is high nuclear grade (nuclear grade 3) or non–high nuclear grade (nuclear grades

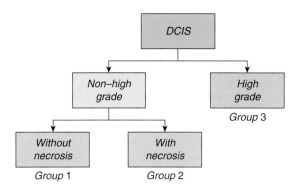

FIGURE 18-1 Van Nuys DCIS classification. DCIS patients are separated in high nuclear grade and non–high nuclear grade. Non–high nuclear grade cases are then separated by the presence or absence of necrosis. Lesions in group 3 (high nuclear grade) may or may not show necrosis.

1 or 2). Then, the presence or absence of necrosis is assessed in the non–high-grade lesions. This results in 3 groups (Fig. 18-1).

Nuclear grade is scored by previously described methods.[31] Essentially, low-grade nuclei (grade 1) are defined as nuclei 1 to 1.5 red blood cells in diameter with diffuse chromatin and unapparent nucleoli. Intermediate nuclei (grade 2) are defined as nuclei 1.5 to 2 red blood cells in diameter with coarse chromatin and infrequent nucleoli. High-grade nuclei (grade 3) are defined as nuclei with a diameter greater than 2 red blood cells, with vesicular chromatin, and one or more nucleoli.

In the Van Nuys classification, no requirement is made for a minimum or specific amount of high nuclear grade DCIS, nor is any requirement made for a minimum amount of comedo-type necrosis. Occasional desquamated or individually necrotic cells are ignored and are not scored as comedo-type necrosis.

The most difficult part of most classifications is nuclear grading, particularly the intermediate-grade lesions. The subtleties of the intermediate grade lesion are not important to the Van Nuys classification; only nuclear grade 3 need be recognized. The cells must be large and pleomorphic, lack architectural differentiation and polarity, have prominent nucleoli and coarse clumped chromatin, and generally show mitoses.[31,36]

The Van Nuys classification is useful because it divides DCIS into 3 different biologic groups with different risks of local recurrence after breast conservation therapy (Fig. 18-2). This pathologic classification, when combined with tumor size, age, and margin status, is an integral part of the USC/Van Nuys Prognostic Index (USC/VNPI), a system that will be discussed in detail.

Progression to Invasive Breast Cancer

Which DCIS lesions will become invasive and when will that happen? These are the most important questions in the DCIS field today. Currently, there is intense study of molecular and genetic factors associated with the progression of normal breast epithelium through hyperplastic and atypical hyperplastic changes to DCIS and then to invasive breast cancer. Most of the genetic and epigenetic changes present in invasive breast cancer are already present in DCIS. To date, no genes uniquely associated with invasive cancer have been identified.[2,16] As DCIS progresses to invasive breast cancer, quantitative changes in the expression of genes related to angiogenesis, adhesion, cell motility, and the composition of the extracellular matrix may occur.[2,16] Using gene-array technology, researchers are attempting to identify high-risk patterns that will require quicker and more aggressive treatment.

The retrospective studies of Page and associates[39,40] and Rosen and associates[41] provide some evidence of the natural history of untreated DCIS. In these studies, patients with non-comedo DCIS were initially misdiagnosed as having benign lesions and therefore went untreated. Subsequently, approximately 25% to 35% of these patients developed invasive breast cancer, generally within 10 years.[39,40] Had the lesions been high-grade comedo DCIS, the invasive breast cancer rate likely would have been higher than 35% and the time to invasive recurrence shorter. With few exceptions, in both of these studies, the invasive breast carcinoma was of the ductal type and located at the site of the original DCIS. These findings suggest that not all DCIS lesions progress to invasive breast cancer or become clinically significant within the patient's lifetime.[42,43]

Page and associates recently updated their series.[39,40,44] Of 28 women with low-grade DCIS misdiagnosed as benign and treated with biopsy between 1950 and 1968, 11 patients have

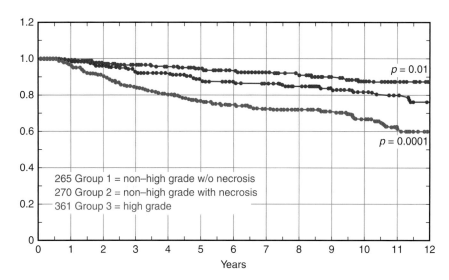

FIGURE 18-2 Probability of local recurrence-free survival for 896 breast conservation patients using Van Nuys DCIS pathologic classification.

recurred locally with invasive breast cancer (39%). Eight patients developed recurrence within the first 12 years (28%). The remaining 3 were diagnosed over 23 to 42 years. Five patients developed metastatic breast cancer (18%) and died from the disease within 7 years of developing invasive breast cancer. These recurrences and mortality rates, at first glance, seem alarmingly high. However, they are only slightly worse than what can be expected with long-term follow-up of patients with lobular carcinoma in situ, a disease that most clinicians are willing to treat with careful clinical follow-up.[45] In addition, these patients were treated with biopsy only. No attempt was made to excise these lesions with a clear surgical margin. The natural history of low-grade DCIS can extend over 40 years and is markedly different from that of high-grade DCIS.

Microinvasion

The incidence of microinvasion is difficult to quantitate because until recently there was no formal and universally accepted definition of exactly what constitutes microinvasion. The 1997 edition of *The Manual for Cancer Staging* (fifth edition) carried the first official definition of what is now classified as pT1mic, and reads as follows:

> Microinvasion is the extension of cancer cells beyond the basement membrane into adjacent tissues with no focus more than 0.1 cm in greatest dimension. When there are multiple foci of microinvasion the size of only the largest focus is used to classify the microinvasion (do not use the sum of all individual foci). The presence of multiple foci of microinvasion should be noted, as it is with multiple larger invasive carcinomas.

The reported incidence of occult invasion (invasive disease at mastectomy in patients with a biopsy diagnosis of DCIS) varies greatly, ranging from as little as 2% to as much as 21%.[46] This problem was addressed in the investigations of Lagios and associates.[25,34]

Lagios and colleagues performed a meticulous serial subgross examination correlated with specimen radiography. Occult invasion was found in 13 of 111 mastectomy specimens from patients who had initially undergone excisional biopsy of DCIS. All occult invasive cancers were associated with DCIS greater than 45 mm in extent; the incidence of occult invasion approached 50% for DCIS greater than 55 mm. In the study of Gump and associates,[47] foci of occult invasion were found in 11% of patients with palpable DCIS but in no patients with clinically occult DCIS. These results suggest a correlation between the size of the DCIS lesion and the incidence of occult invasion. The studies of de Mascarel and coworkers have also shown an association of greater disease extent and microinvasion.[48] Clearly, as the size of the DCIS lesion increases, microinvasion and occult invasion become more likely.

If even the smallest amount of invasion is found, the lesion should not be classified as DCIS. It is a T1mic (if the largest invasive component is 1 mm or less) with an extensive intraductal component (EIC). If the invasive component is 1.1 to 5 mm, it is a T1a lesion with EIC. If there is only a single focus of invasion, these patients do quite well. When there are many tiny foci of invasion, these patients have a poorer prognosis than expected.[10]

In the de Mascarel and associates study, microinvasion defined as single cells alone had no adverse impact on outcome; only those comprising small cohesive nests of cells did.[48] The latter had a small but significantly worse outcome as compared to either DCIS or microinvasion defined as single cells (91% vs 98%).

Multicentricity and Multifocality of Ductal Carcinoma In Situ

Multicentricity is generally defined as DCIS in a quadrant other than the quadrant in which the original DCIS (index quadrant) was diagnosed. There must be normal breast tissue separating the 2 foci. However, definitions of multicentricity vary among investigators. Hence the reported incidence of multicentricity also varies. Rates from 0% to 78%,[7,34,41,49-51] averaging about 30%, have been reported. Twenty years ago, the 30% average rate of multicentricity was used by surgeons as the rationale for mastectomy in patients with DCIS.

Holland and colleagues[52] evaluated 82 mastectomy specimens by taking a whole-organ section every 5 mm. Each section was radiographed. Paraffin blocks were made from every radiographically suspicious focus. In addition, an average of 25 blocks was taken from the quadrant containing the index cancer; random samples were taken from all other quadrants, the central subareolar area, and the nipple. The microscopic extension of each lesion was verified on the radiographs. This technique permitted a 3-dimensional reconstruction of each lesion. This study demonstrated that most DCIS lesions involved more than 1 quadrant by continuous extension (23%), but most importantly, were unicentric (98.8%). Only 1 of 82 mastectomy specimens (1.2%) had "true" multicentric distribution with a separate lesion in a different quadrant. This study suggests that complete excision of a DCIS lesion is possible due to unicentricity but may be extremely difficult due to larger than expected size. In a recent update, Holland reported whole-organ studies in 119 patients, 118 of whom had unicentric disease.[53] This information, when combined with the fact that most local recurrences are at or near the original DCIS, suggests that the problem of multicentricity per se is not important in the DCIS treatment decision-making process.

Multifocality is defined as separate foci of DCIS within the same ductal system. The studies of Holland and associates[52,53] and Noguchi and coworkers[54] suggest that a great deal of multifocality may be artifactual, resulting from looking at a 3-dimensional arborizing entity in 2 dimensions on a glass slide. It would be analogous to saying that the branches of a tree were not connected if the branches were cut at one plane, placed separately on a slide, and viewed in cross-section.[39] Multifocality may be due to small gaps of DCIS or skip areas within ducts, as described by Faverly and colleagues.[35]

DETECTION AND DIAGNOSIS

The importance of quality mammography cannot be overemphasized. Currently, most patients with DCIS (more than 90%) present with nonpalpable lesions. A few percent are detected as random findings during a biopsy for a breast thickening or some other benign fibrocystic change; most lesions,

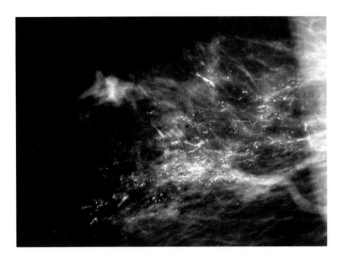

FIGURE 18-3 Mediolateral mammography in a 43-year-old woman shows irregular branching calcifications. Histopathology showed high-grade comedo DCIS, Van Nuys group 3.

however, are detected by mammography. The most common mammographic findings are microcalcifications, frequently clustered, and generally without an associated soft-tissue abnormality. More than 80% of DCIS patients exhibit microcalcifications on preoperative mammography. The patterns of these microcalcifications may be focal, diffuse, or ductal, with variable size and shape. Patients with comedo DCIS tend to have "casting calcifications." These are linear, branching, and bizarre and are almost pathognomonic for comedo DCIS (Fig. 18-3)[55]; however, nearly half of high-grade DCIS with comedo necrosis exhibits no microcalcifications

Thirty-two percent of noncomedo lesions in our personal series did not have mammographic calcifications, making them more difficult to find and the patients more difficult to follow, if treated conservatively. When noncomedo lesions are calcified, they tend to have fine psammomatous or indeterminate microcalcifications. Tabar has described these as granular powdery or crushed stone-like microcalcifications (Fig. 18-4).

A major problem confronting surgeons relates to the fact that calcifications do not always map out the entire DCIS lesion, particularly those of the noncomedo type. Even though all the calcifications are removed, in some cases, noncalcified DCIS may be left behind. Conversely, in some patients, the majority of the calcifications are benign and the calcifications "map out" a lesion bigger than the true DCIS lesion. In other words, the DCIS lesion may be smaller, larger, or the same size as the calcifications that lead to its identification. Calcifications more accurately approximate the size of high-grade comedo lesions than low-grade noncomedo lesions.[52]

Before mammography was common or of good quality, most DCIS was usually clinically apparent, diagnosed by palpation or inspection; it was gross disease. Gump and associates[47] divided DCIS by method of diagnosis into gross and microscopic disease. Similarly, Schwartz and coworkers[56] divided DCIS into 2 groups, clinical and subclinical. Both research groups thought patients presenting with a palpable mass, nipple discharge, or Paget disease of the nipple required more aggressive treatment. Schwartz and associates believed that palpable DCIS should be treated as though it were an invasive lesion. They suggested that the pathologist simply has not found the area of invasion. Although it makes perfect sense to believe that the change from nonpalpable to palpable disease is a poor prognostic sign, our group has not been able to demonstrate this for DCIS. In our series, when equivalent patients (by size and nuclear grade) with palpable and nonpalpable DCIS were compared, they did not differ in the rate of local recurrence or mortality. Lagios and coworkers had shown that patients with extensive disease (larger than 50 mm) generally present with palpable masses, nipple discharge, and so forth, and have a high frequency of microinvasion.[25,34] Complete tissue processing is required to exclude invasion, and historically this has not been a standard practice.

If a patient's mammogram shows an abnormality, most likely it will be microcalcifications, but it could be a nonpalpable mass or a subtle architectural distortion. At this point, additional radiologic workup needs to be performed. This may include compression mammography, magnification views, or ultrasonography. Magnetic resonance imaging (MRI) has become increasingly popular to map out the size and shape of biopsy-proven DCIS lesions or invasive breast cancers. I obtain a preoperative MRI on every patient with a diagnosis of breast cancer.

Biopsy and Tissue Handling

If radiologic workup shows an occult lesion that requires biopsy, there are multiple approaches: fine-needle aspiration biopsy (FNAB), core biopsy (with various types and sizes of needles), and directed surgical biopsy using guidewires or radioactive guidance. FNA is generally of little help for DCIS. With FNA, it is possible to obtain cancer cells, but because there is insufficient tissue, there is no architecture. So although the cytopathologist can say that malignant cells are present, the cytopathologist generally cannot say whether the lesion is invasive. Moreover, for DCIS of lower grades it may be impossible to distinguish ADH and low-grade invasion by cytology.

Stereotactic core biopsy became available in the early 1990s, and it is now widely used. Dedicated digital tables make this a

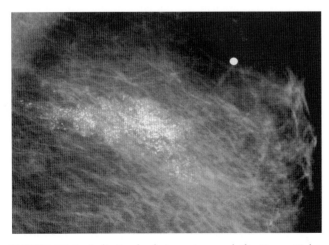

FIGURE 18-4 Left. Crushed stone-type calcifications. Right inset. Fine, granular, powdery calcifications.

precise tool in experienced hands. Currently large-gauge (11 gauge or larger) vacuum-assisted needles are the tools of choice for diagnosing DCIS. Ultrasound-guided biopsy also became very popular in the 1990s but is of less value for DCIS, since most DCIS lesions do not present with a mass that can be visualized by ultrasound. All suspicious microcalcifications, however, should be evaluated by ultrasound, since an invasive mass will be found in 5% to 15%.[9]

Open surgical biopsy should only be used if the lesion cannot be biopsied using minimally invasive techniques. This should be a rare event with current image-guided biopsy techniques.[9] Needle-localized segmental resection should be a critical part of the treatment, not the diagnosis.

Whenever needle localization excision is performed, whether for diagnosis or treatment, intraoperative specimen radiography and correlation with the preoperative mammogram should be performed. Margins should be inked or dyed and specimens should be serially sectioned at 3- to 4-mm intervals. The tissue sections should be arranged and processed in sequence. Pathologic reporting should include determination of nuclear grade, an assessment of the presence or absence of necrosis, the measured size or extent of the lesion, and the margin status with measurement of the closest margin.[57]

Tumor size should be determined by direct measurement or ocular micrometry from stained slides for smaller lesions. For larger lesions, a combination of direct measurement and calculation, based on the distribution of the lesion in a sequential series of slides, should be used. The proximity of DCIS to an inked margin should be determined by direct measurement by ocular micrometry. The closest single distance between any involved duct containing DCIS and an inked margin should be reported.

If the lesion is large and the diagnosis unproven, either stereotactic or ultrasound-guided vacuum-assisted biopsy should be the first step. If the patient is motivated for breast conservation, a multiple-wire–directed oncoplastic excision can be planned. This will give the patient her best chance at 2 opposing goals: clear margins and good cosmesis. The best chance at completely removing a large lesion is with a large initial excision. The best chance at good cosmesis is with a small initial excision. It is the surgeon's job to optimize these opposing goals. A large quadrant resection should never be performed as a diagnostic procedure. Such resections may result in significant deformity and are unwarranted without a preoperative tissue diagnosis.

Removal of nonpalpable lesions requires an integrated team of surgeon, radiologist, and pathologist. The radiologist who places the wires and interprets the specimen radiograph must be experienced, as must the surgeon who removes the lesion, and the pathologist who processes the tissue.

TREATMENT

For most patients with DCIS, there will be no single correct treatment. There will generally be a choice. The choices, although seemingly simple, are not. As the choices increase and become more complicated, frustration increases for both the patient and her physician.[58,59]

Counseling the Patient with Biopsy-Proven Ductal Carcinoma In Situ

It is never easy to tell a patient that she has breast cancer. But is DCIS really cancer? From a biologic point of view, DCIS is unequivocally cancer. But when we think of cancer, we generally think of a disease that, if untreated, runs an inexorable course toward death. That is certainly not the case with DCIS.[40] We must emphasize to the patient that she has a preinvasive cancerous lesion, which at this time is not a threat to her life. In our series of 1396 patients with DCIS, the raw mortality rate was 0.5%. Numerous other DCIS series[60-65] confirm an extremely low mortality rate.

Patients often ask why there is any mortality rate at all, if DCIS is truly a noninvasive lesion. If DCIS recurs as an invasive lesion and the patient goes on to die from metastatic breast cancer, the source of the metastases is clear. But what about the patient who undergoes mastectomy and sometime later develops metastatic disease, or a patient who is treated with breast preservation who never develops a local invasive recurrence but still dies of metastatic breast cancer? These latter patients probably had an invasive focus with established metastases at the time of their original treatment but the invasive focus was missed during routine histopathologic evaluation. The ability to detect a small invasive lesion in a large resection is dependent on the thoroughness of the pathologic examination. It is an unfortunate truth that thorough examination of large resections and mastectomies is very uncommon in current practices as it was in the randomized trials.

One of the most frequent concerns expressed by patients once a diagnosis of cancer has been made is the fear that the cancer has spread. We are able to assure patients with DCIS that if no invasion was seen microscopically, the likelihood of systemic spread is essentially zero.

The patient needs to be educated that the term "breast cancer" encompasses a multitude of lesions of varying degrees of aggressiveness and lethal potential. The patient with DCIS needs to be reassured that she has a minimal lesion and that she is likely going to need some additional treatment, which may include surgery, radiation therapy, an antiestrogen, or some combination. She needs reassurance that she will not need chemotherapy, that her hair will not fall out, and that it is highly unlikely that she will die from this lesion. She will, of course, need careful clinical follow-up.

End Points for Patients with DCIS

When evaluating the results of treatment for patients with breast cancer, a variety of end points must be considered. Important end points include local recurrence (both invasive and DCIS), regional recurrence (such as the axilla), distant recurrence, breast cancer–specific survival, overall survival, and quality of life. The importance of each end point varies depending on whether the patient has DCIS or invasive breast cancer

When treating invasive cancer, the most important end points are distant recurrence and breast cancer–specific survival; in other words, living with or dying from breast cancer. For invasive breast cancer, a variety of different systemic treatments have been shown to significantly improve survival. These include a wide range of chemotherapeutic regimens and endocrine treatments. Variations in local treatment were incorrectly thought not to affect survival.[23,66] They do, however, affect local recurrence. Recently literature has suggested that for every 4 local invasive recurrences prevented, 1 breast cancer death is prevented.[67]

DCIS is similar to invasive breast cancer in that variations in local treatment affect local recurrence, but no study to date has shown a significant difference in distant disease-free or breast cancer–specific survival, regardless of any treatment (systemic or local), and no study is likely to show a difference since there are so few breast cancer deaths in patients with pure DCIS. The most important outcome measure, breast cancer–specific survival, is essentially the same no matter what local or systemic treatment is given. Consequently, local recurrence has become the most commonly used end point when evaluating treatment for patients with DCIS.

A meta-analysis of 4 randomized DCIS trials comparing excision plus radiation therapy versus excision alone was published in 2007. It contained 3665 patients. Radiation therapy increased local control by a statistically significant 60%, but overall survival was slightly worse in the radiotherapy group, with a relative risk of 1.08.[64] These data are dissimilar to those of the Early Breast Cancer Trialists' Collaborative Group and deserve further analysis.[67] Half of the recurrences in the meta-analysis were DCIS and could not possibly affect survival. Of the remaining invasive recurrences, 80% to 90% were cured by early detection and treatment. This should result in a slight trend toward a lower survival for the excision alone group but exactly the opposite was seen, a nonsignificant trend toward a better survival. The authors of the meta-analysis feel that with longer follow-up, the higher local recurrence rate for excision alone will likely result in a lower overall survival at some point in time. But for the time being, that has not happened, and a detrimental effect secondary to radiation therapy must be considered a possibility.

Local recurrences are clearly important to prevent in patients treated with DCIS. They are demoralizing. They often lead to mastectomy, and theoretically, if they are invasive, they upstage the patient and are a threat to life. But protecting DCIS patients from local recurrence must be balanced against the potential detrimental effects of the treatments given.

Following breast-conserving treatment for DCIS, 40% to 50% of all local recurrences are invasive. About 10% to 20% of DCIS patients who develop local invasive recurrences develop distant metastases and die from breast cancer.[68,69] In the long term, this could translate into a mortality rate of about 0% to 0.5% for patients treated with mastectomy, 1% to 2% for conservatively treated patients who receive radiation therapy (if there is no mortality associated with radiation therapy), and 2% to 3% for patients treated with excision alone. In order to save their breasts, many patients are willing to accept this theoretical, and presently statistically unproven potential risk associated with breast conservation therapy.

Treatment Options

Mastectomy

Mastectomy is by far the most effective treatment available for DCIS if the goal is simply to prevent local recurrence. Most mastectomy series reveal local recurrence rates of approximately 1% with mortality rates close to zero.[70] In our series, we have had only 1 breast cancer death among 467 patients treated with mastectomy (0.2%).

But mastectomy is an aggressive form of treatment for patients with DCIS. It clearly provides a local recurrence benefit but only an indemonstrable and theoretical survival benefit. It is, therefore, often difficult to justify mastectomy, particularly for otherwise healthy women with screen-detected DCIS, during an era of increasing utilization of breast conservation for invasive breast carcinoma. Mastectomy is indicated in cases of true multicentricity (multi-quadrant disease) and when a unicentric DCIS lesion is too extensive to excise with clear margins and an acceptable cosmetic result.

Genetic positivity to 1 or more of the breast cancer–associated genes (BRCA1, BRCA2) is not an absolute contraindication to breast preservation, but many patients who are genetically positive and who develop DCIS seriously consider bilateral mastectomy.

Breast Conservation

The most recently available Surveillance Epidemiology and End Results (SEER) data reveal that 74% of patients with DCIS are treated with breast conservation. While breast conservation is now widely accepted as the treatment of choice for DCIS, not all patients are good candidates. Certainly, there are patients with DCIS whose local recurrence rate with breast preservation is so high (based on factors that will be discussed later in this chapter) that mastectomy is clearly a more appropriate treatment. However, the majority of women with DCIS diagnosed currently are candidates for breast conservation. Clinical trials have shown that local excision and radiation therapy in patients with negative margins can provide excellent rates of local control.[60,63-65,71-74] However, even radiation therapy may be overly aggressive, since many cases of DCIS may not recur or progress to invasive carcinoma when treated by excision alone.[25,40,75-78]

Rationale for Excision Alone

There are 5 lines of reasoning that suggest that excision alone may be an acceptable treatment for selected patients with DCIS:

1. *Anatomic.* Evaluation of mastectomy specimens using the serial subgross tissue-processing technique reveals that most DCIS is limited in extent, unassociated with invasion, and unicentric (involves a single breast segment and is radial in its distribution).[27,34,35,52,53,79,80] This means that in many cases, it is possible to excise the entire lesion with a segment or quadrant resection. Since DCIS, by definition, is not invasive and has not metastasized, it can be thought of in Halstedian terms. Complete excision should cure the patient without any additional therapy.

2. *Biological.* Some DCIS is simply not aggressive—for example, small well-excised low-grade lesions bordering on atypical ductal hyperplasia. Lesions like this carry a low potential for development into an invasive lesion, about 1%

per year at most.[39,40,44,75,81,82] This is only slightly more than lobular carcinoma in situ (LCIS), a lesion that is routinely treated with careful clinical follow-up.

3. *Prospective randomized data.* As will be pointed out throughout this chapter, these trials show no difference in breast cancer–specific survival, regardless of treatment after excision.[60,63,64,74] If this is true, why not strive for the least aggressive treatment?

4. *Radiotherapy may do harm.* Numerous studies have shown that radiation therapy for breast cancer may increase mortality from both lung cancer and cardiovascular disease.[83-87] More current radiotherapy techniques, which make use of CT planning, make every attempt to spare the heart and lungs from radiation exposure, but long-term data are not available. If there is no proof that breast irradiation for patients with DCIS improves survival and there is proof that radiation therapy may cause harm, it makes perfect sense to spare patients from this potentially dangerous treatment whenever possible.

5. *In the 2008 NCCN (National Comprehensive Cancer Network) Guidelines, excision without radiation therapy (excision alone) has been added as an acceptable treatment for selected patients with low risk of recurrence.*[88]

DISTANT DISEASE AND DEATH

When a patient with DCIS, previously treated by any modality, develops a local invasive recurrence, followed by distant disease and death due to breast cancer, this stepwise Halstedian progression makes sense. The patient has been upstaged by her local invasive recurrence. The invasive recurrence becomes the source of the metastatic disease and death is now a possibility.

In contrast, when a previously treated patient with DCIS develops distant disease and there has been no invasive local recurrence, a completely different sequence of events must be postulated. This sequence implies that invasive disease was present within the original lesion but was never identified pathologically and was already metastatic at the time of the original diagnosis. The best way to avoid missing an invasive cancer is with complete sequential tissue processing at the time the original lesion is treated. Although even the most extensive evaluation may miss a tiny focus of invasion, the majority of such "metastatic first events" have occurred in the randomized trials whose limited examination predisposed to missing small invasive foci at the time of treatment.

If, during histopathologic evaluation, even the tiniest invasive component is found, this patient can no longer be classified as having DCIS. She has invasive breast cancer, and she needs to be treated as such. She will need sentinel node biopsy, radiation therapy if treated conservatively, and appropriate medical oncologic consultation and follow-up.

THE PROSPECTIVE RANDOMIZED TRIALS

All of the prospective randomized trials have shown a significant reduction in local recurrence for patients treated with radiation therapy, compared with excision alone, but no trial has reported a survival benefit, regardless of treatment.[60,63,64,71-74,89,90]

Only 1 trial has compared mastectomy with breast conservation for patients with DCIS, and the data were only incidentally accrued. The National Surgical Adjuvant Breast Project (NSABP) performed protocol B-06, a prospective randomized trial for patients with invasive breast cancer.[49,91] There were 3 treatment arms: total mastectomy, excision of the tumor plus radiation therapy, and excision alone. Axillary nodes were removed regardless of the treatment assignment.

During central slide review, a subgroup of 78 patients was confirmed to have pure DCIS without any evidence of invasion.[49] After 83 months of follow-up, the percent of patients with local recurrences were as follows: 0% for mastectomy, 7% for excision plus radiation therapy, and 43% for excision alone.[92] In spite of these large differences in the rate of local recurrence for each different treatment, there was no difference among the 3 treatment groups in breast cancer-specific survival.

Contrary to the lack of trials comparing mastectomy with breast conservation, a number of prospective randomized trials comparing excision plus radiation therapy with excision alone for patients with DCIS are ongoing.[93] Four have been published: the NSABP (protocol B-17)[71]; the European Organization for Research and Treatment of Cancer (EORTC) protocol 10853[74]; the United Kingdom, Australia, New Zealand DCIS Trial (UK Trial)[63]; and the Swedish Trial.[65]

The results of NSABP B-17 were updated in 1995,[90] 1998,[73] 1999,[72] and 2001.[60] In this study, more than 800 patients with DCIS excised with clear surgical margins were randomized into 2 groups: excision alone versus excision plus radiation therapy. The main end point of the study was local recurrence, invasive or noninvasive (DCIS). The definition of a clear margin was nontransection of the DCIS. In other words, only a single fat cell or a collagen fiber needed to be present between DCIS and the inked margin to establish a clear margin. Many margins, of course, were likely much wider.

After 12 years of follow-up, there was a statistically significant, 50% decrease in local recurrence of both DCIS and invasive breast cancer in patients treated with radiation therapy. The overall local recurrence rate for patients treated by excision alone was 32% at 12 years. For patients treated with excision plus breast irradiation, it was 16%, a relative benefit of 50%.[60] There was no difference in distant disease-free or overall survival in either arm. These updated data led the NSABP to confirm their 1993 position and to continue to recommend postoperative radiation therapy for all patients with DCIS who chose to save their breasts. This recommendation was clearly based primarily on the decreased local recurrence rate for those treated with radiation therapy and secondarily on the potential survival advantage it might confer.

The early results of B-17, in favor of radiation therapy for patients with DCIS, led the NSABP to perform protocol B-24.[72] In this trial, more than 1800 patients with DCIS were treated with excision and radiation therapy, and then randomized to receive either tamoxifen or placebo. After 7 years of follow-up, 11% of patients treated with placebo had recurred locally, whereas, only 8% of those treated with tamoxifen had recurred.[60] The difference, while small, was statistically significant for invasive local recurrence but not for noninvasive (DCIS) recurrence. Data presented at the 2002 San Antonio Breast Cancer Symposium suggested that the ipsilateral benefit was seen only in estrogen receptor–positive patients and may well affect unsampled invasive disease.[94] Again, there was no difference in distant disease-free or overall survival in either arm of the B-24 Trial.

The EORTC results were published in 2000.[74,89] This study was essentially identical to B-17 in design and margin definition. More than 1000 patients were included. The data were updated in 2006.[95] After 10 years of follow-up, 15% of patients treated with excision plus radiation therapy had recurred locally compared with 26% of patients treated with excision alone, results similar to those obtained by the NSABP at the same point in their trial. As in the B-17 Trial, there was no difference in distant disease-free or overall survival in either arm of the EORTC Trial. In the initial report, there was a statistically significant increase in contralateral breast cancer in patients who were randomized to receive radiation therapy. This was not maintained when the data were updated.

The United Kingdom, Australia, New Zealand DCIS Trial (UK Trial) was published in 2003.[63] This trial, which involved more than 1600 patients, performed a 2-by-2 study in which patients could be randomized into 2 separate trials within a trial. The patients and their doctors chose whether to be randomized in 1 or both studies. After excision with clear margins (same nontransection definition as the NSABP), patients were randomized to receive radiotherapy (yes or no) and/or to tamoxifen versus placebo. This yielded 4 subgroups: excision alone, excision plus radiation therapy, excision plus tamoxifen, and finally, excision plus radiation therapy plus tamoxifen. Those who received radiation therapy obtained a statistically significant decrease in ipsilateral breast tumor recurrence similar in magnitude to the ones shown by the NSABP and EORTC. Contrary to the findings of the NSABP, there was no significant benefit from tamoxifen. As with the NSABP and the EORTC, there was no benefit in terms of survival in any arm of the UK DCIS study.

The Swedish DCIS Trial randomized 1046 patients into 2 groups: excision alone versus excision plus radiation therapy. Microscopically clear margins were not mandatory. Twenty-two percent of patients had microscopically unknown or involved margins; there was no common pathologic protocol and no size or grade determination. Radiation therapy resulted in a 67% reduction in local recurrence rate with a median follow-up of 5.2 years. There were no differences in distant metastases or deaths.[65]

Overall, these trials support the same conclusions. They all show that radiation therapy decreases local recurrence by a relative 50%, and they all show no survival benefit, regardless of treatment. The only difference is that the NSABP B-24 trial shows a significant decrease in local recurrence attributable to tamoxifen while the UK trial does not.

With all the trials, as the amount of treatment increases, the rate of local recurrence decreases; but no matter how much treatment is increased, there is no improvement in survival. In fact, there could be a slight decrease in survival if there is a negative effect from radiation therapy.[64]

Limitations of the Prospective Randomized Trials

The prospective randomized trials of irradiation for DCIS initiated in 1985, 1986, and 1987 have generated data that, however limited, are still used to mandate radiation therapy for all conservatively treated patients with duct carcinoma in situ. Yet these trials employed surgical and pathologic practices that would fall below the current standard of care for image-guided excisions. Imagine a current practice in which there was no intraoperative radiologic correlation, or specimen x-ray, no specimen orientation or identification of margins, and in which tissue sampling was often done "blindly," that is, without radiographic guidance. For those image-guided excisions confirmed as DCIS, imagine no pathologic tumor size, assessment of margins limited to "transection/nontransection" in the tissue sampled, and add in tissue sampling inadequate to exclude invasion, and the quality of the databases in B17, B24, EORTC-10853 , UK/ANZ and SweDCIS comes into sharp focus! Such data were not collected prospectively or at all in some trials, and cannot be inserted retrospectively. As a result, it is impossible to relate the outcome results of the trials to a contemporary setting in which the grade, size, and margin status are determined in an oriented specimen with careful mammographic pathologic correlation with the degree of pathologic examination adequate to exclude invasive disease.

Although the randomized trials have shown a substantial benefit for irradiation, they are entirely incapable of establishing a risk for a specific subset of given size, grade, or margin status. Moreover, there is no survival advantage for irradiation in any of the published trials, nor in subsequent nonrandomized studies. The preferential benefit of irradiation in preventing invasive recurrences as announced by NSABP-B17 was not replicated in a subsequent study, NSABP-B24, or in any other of the trials of radiation therapy. This "benefit" probably reflects the inability to exclude invasive foci admixed with the DCIS in resections, which were only sampled or incompletely removed. This is consistent with the extraordinary rate of metastatic first events in B17 at 12 years (2%), equal to the same rate for invasive breast cancers of T1b size and N0 stage.

The relative reduction in local recurrence seems to be the same in all 4 trials—about 50% for any given subgroup at any point in time. What does this relative reduction mean? If the absolute local recurrence rate is 30% at 10 years for a given subgroup of patients treated with excision alone, radiation therapy will reduce this rate by approximately 50%, leaving a group of patients with a 15% local recurrence rate at 10 years. Radiation therapy seems indicated for a subgroup with such a high local recurrence rate. But consider a more favorable subgroup, a group of patients with a 6% to 8% absolute recurrence rate at 10 years. These patients receive only a 3% to 4% absolute benefit. We must irradiate 100 women to benefit 3 or 4 individual women. Here, we must ask whether the benefits are worth the risks and costs involved, and we should make every attempt possible to identify low-risk subgroups.

Radiation therapy is expensive, time consuming, and is accompanied by significant side effects in a small percentage of patients (cardiac, pulmonary, etc).[93] Radiation fibrosis continues to occur but it is less common with current techniques than it was during the 1980s. Radiation fibrosis changes the texture of the breast and skin, makes mammographic follow-up more difficult, and may result in delayed diagnosis if there is a local recurrence. The use of radiation therapy for DCIS precludes its use if an invasive recurrence develops at a later date. The use of radiation therapy with its accompanying skin and vascular changes make skin-sparing mastectomy, if needed in the future, more difficult to perform.

Most importantly, if we give radiation therapy for DCIS, we must assume all of these risks and costs without any proven distant disease-free or breast cancer–specific survival benefits. The only proven benefit will be a decrease in local recurrence. It is important, therefore, to carefully examine the need for radiation therapy in all conservatively treated patients with DCIS. The NSABP has agreed that all patients with DCIS may not need postexcisional radiation therapy.[60] The problem is how to accurately identify those patients. If we can identify subgroups of patients with DCIS in which the probability of local recurrence after excision alone is low, they may be the patients where the costs, risks, and side effects of radiotherapy outweigh the benefits.

In spite of the randomized data, which suggest that all conservatively treated patients benefit from radiation therapy, American doctors and patients have embraced the concept of excision alone. 2003 Surveillance Epidemiology and End Results (SEER) data reveal that 74% of patients with DCIS were treated with breast conservation. Almost half of these conservatively treated patients were treated with excision alone. When all patients with DCIS are considered, 26% received mastectomy, 39% excision plus radiation therapy, and 35% were treated with excision alone. It is clear that both American doctors and American patients are not blindly following the results and the recommendations of the prospective trials. Based on data and treatment trends, in 2008, the NCCN (National Comprehensive Cancer Network) added excision alone as an alternative treatment for patients with favorable DCIS.[88] Current practice standards in pathology and radiology that require specimen radiography and intraoperative correlation, inking of margins, and thorough sequential examination—practices that were not part of the randomized trials—have played a permissive role in the selective avoidance of irradiation.

PREDICTING LOCAL RECURRENCE IN CONSERVATIVELY TREATED PATIENTS WITH DCIS

There is now sufficient, readily available information that can aid clinicians in differentiating patients who significantly benefit from radiation therapy after excision from those who do not. These same data can point out patients who are better served by mastectomy because recurrence rates with breast conservation are unacceptably high even with the addition of radiation therapy. Our research[31,96-99] and the research of others[25,26,34,36,37,76,77,82,90,100] has shown that various combinations of nuclear grade, the presence of comedo-type necrosis, tumor size, margin width, and age are all important factors that can be used to predict the probability of local recurrence in conservatively treated patients with DCIS.

The Original Van Nuys Prognostic Index (VNPI) and its Updated Version, the USC/VNPI

In 1995, the Van Nuys DCIS pathologic classification, based on nuclear grade and the presence or absence of comedonecrosis, was developed (Fig. 18-1).[31] Nuclear grade and comedo-type necrosis reflect the biology of the lesion, but neither alone nor together are they adequate as the guidelines in the treatment decision-making process. Tumor size and margin width reflect the extent of disease, the adequacy of surgical treatment, and the likelihood of residual disease, and are of paramount importance.

The challenge was to devise a system using these variables (all independently important by multivariate analysis) that would be clinically valid, therapeutically useful, and user-friendly. The original Van Nuys Prognostic Index (VNPI)[101,102] was devised in 1996 by combining tumor size, margin width, and pathologic classification (determined by nuclear grade and the presence or absence of comedo-type necrosis). All of these factors had been collected prospectively in a large series of DCIS patients who were selectively treated (nonrandomized).[103]

A score, ranging from 1 for lesions with the best prognosis to 3 for lesions with the worst prognosis, was given for each of the 3 prognostic predictors. The objective with all 3 predictors was to create 3 statistically different subgroups for each, using local recurrence as the marker of treatment failure. Cut-off points (eg, what size or margin width constitutes low, intermediate, or high risk of local recurrence) were determined statistically, using the log rank test with an optimum p-value approach.

Size Score

A score of 1 was given for a small tumors 15 mm or less, 2 was given for intermediate-sized tumors 16 to 40 mm, and 3 was given for large tumors 41 mm or more in extent. The determination of size required complete and sequential tissue processing along with mammographic/pathologic correlation Size was determined over a series of sections rather than on a single section and is the most difficult parameter to reproduce. If a 3-cm specimen is cut into 10 blocks, each block is estimated to be 3 mm thick. If a lesion measuring 5 mm in maximum diameter on a single slide appears in an out of 7 sequential blocks, it is estimated to be 21 mm (3 mm × 7) in maximum size, not 5 mm. The maximum diameter on a single slide was the way size was measured for most of the patients in the prospective randomized trials, but few patients had DCIS that appeared in a single slide.

Margin Score

A score of 1 was given for widely clear tumor-free margins of 10 mm or more. This was often achieved by reexcision with the finding of no residual DCIS or only focal residual DCIS in the wall of the biopsy cavity. A score of 2 was given for intermediate margins of 1 to 9 mm, and a score of 3 for margins less than 1 mm (involved or close margins).

Pathologic Classification Score

A score of 3 was given for tumors classified as group 3 (high-grade lesions), 2 for tumors classified as group 2 (non–high-grade lesions with comedo-type necrosis), and a score of 1 for tumors classified as group 1 (non–high-grade lesion without comedo-type necrosis). The classification is diagrammed in Figure 18-1.[31,104]

The final formula for the original Van Nuys Prognostic Index (VNPI) became

VNPI = pathologic classification score + margin score + size score

The University of Southern California/Van Nuys Prognostic Index (USC/VNPI)

By early 2001, a multivariate analysis at the University of Southern California revealed that age was also an independent prognostic factor in our database and that it should be added to the VNPI with a weight equal to that of the other factors.[98,99,105]

An analysis of our local recurrence data by age revealed that the most appropriate break points for our data were between ages 39 and 40 and between ages 60 and 61 (Fig. 18-5). Based on this, a score of 3 was given to all patients 39 years old or younger, a score of 2 was given to patients aged 40 to 60, and a score of 1 was given to patients 61 or older. The new scoring system for the USC/VNPI is shown in Table 18-1. The final formula for the USC/Van Nuys Prognostic Index became:

USC/VNPI = pathologic classification score + margin score + size score + age score

Scores range from 4 to 12. The patients least likely to recur after conservative therapy had a score of 4 (small, low-grade, well-excised lesions in older women). The patients most likely to recur had a score of 12 (large, poorly excised, high-grade lesions in younger women). The probability of recurrence increased as the USC/VNPI score increased.

Updated Results Using the USC/VNPI

Through April 2008, our group treated 1363 patients with pure DCIS. A total of 467 patients were treated with mastectomy

TABLE 18-1 The USC/Van Nuys Prognostic Index Scoring System[a]

Score	1	2	3
Size (mm)	≤15	6-40	≥41
Margins (mm)	≥10	1-9	<1
Pathologic classification	Non–high grade without necrosis	Non–high grade with necrosis	High grade with or without necrosis
Age (years)	≥61	40-60	≤39

[a]1 to 3 points are awarded for each of 4 different predictors of local breast recurrence (size, margins, pathologic classification, and age). Scores for each of the predictors are totaled to yield a VNPI score ranging from a low of 4 to a high of 12.

and are not included in any analysis that uses local recurrence as the end point. Some 896 patients were treated with breast conservation: 562 by excision alone and 334 by excision plus radiation therapy. The average follow-up for all patients was 87 months: 85 months for mastectomy, 111 months for excision plus radiation therapy, and 76 months for excision alone.

There were 161 local failures, 71 of which (44%) were invasive. The probability of local failure was reduced, overall, by 60% if radiation therapy was given, a result almost identical with the prospective randomized trials. The local, recurrence-free survival in shown by treatment in Figure 18-6. As expected, at any point in time, mastectomy had the lowest probability of local recurrence, and excision alone had the highest.

Seven patients (2.5%) treated with radiation therapy developed local recurrences and distant metastases, 6 of whom have died from breast cancer. One patient (0.2%) treated with excision alone developed local invasive recurrence and metastatic disease and died from breast cancer. Two mastectomy patients

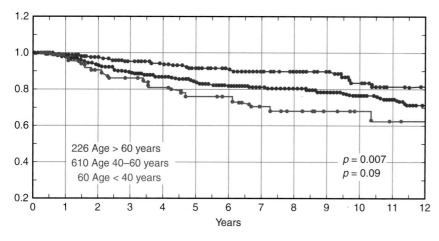

FIGURE 18-5 Probability of local recurrence-free survival by age group for 896 breast-conservation patients.

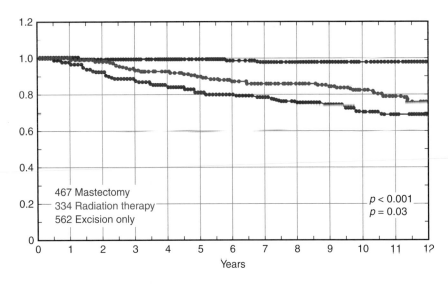

FIGURE 18-6   Probability of local recurrence-free survival by treatment for 1363 patients with DCIS.

developed distant disease after developing local invasive recurrences. One has died from breast cancer. There is no statistical difference in breast cancer–specific survival (Fig. 18-7) or overall survival (Fig. 18-8) when patients treated with excision alone, excision plus irradiation, or mastectomy are compared. There were no patients who presented as a metastatic first event, that is, a distant recurrence without a preceding loco-regional event.

Seventy one additional patients have died from other causes without evidence of recurrent breast cancer. The 12-year actuarial overall survival, including deaths from all causes, is 90%. It is virtually the same for all three treatment groups and for all three USC/VNPI groups.

The local recurrence-free survival for all 896 breast-conservation patients is shown by tumor size in Figure 18-9, by margin width in Figure 18-10, by pathologic classification in Figure 18-2, and by age in Figure 18-5.

Figure 18-11 groups patients with low (USC/VNPI = 4, 5, or 6), intermediate (USC/VNPI = 7, 8, or 9), or high (USC/VNPI = 10, 11, or 12) risks of local recurrence together. Each of these 3 groups is statistically different from one another.

Patients with USC/VNPI scores of 4, 5, or 6 do not show a local recurrence-free survival benefit from breast irradiation (Fig. 18-12) (p – NS). This has been independently confirmed by Gilleard and associates[106] Patients with an intermediate rate of local recurrence, USC/VNPI 7, 8, or 9, are benefited by irradiation (Fig. 18-13). There is a statistically significant decrease in the probability of local recurrence, averaging 15% throughout the curves, for irradiated patients with intermediate USC/VNPI scores compared to those treated by excision alone (p = 0.004). Figure 18-14 divides patients with a USC/VNPI of 10, 11, or 12 into those treated by excision plus irradiation and those treated by excision alone. Although, the difference between the 2 groups is highly significant (p = 0.0005), conservatively treated DCIS patients with a USC/VNPI of 10, 11, or 12 recur at an extremely high rate even with radiation therapy and at this time are best managed by total mastectomy.

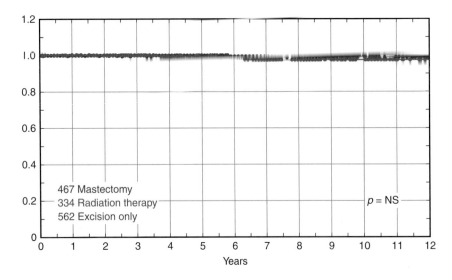

FIGURE 18-7   Probability of breast cancer–specific survival by treatment for 1363 patients with DCIS.

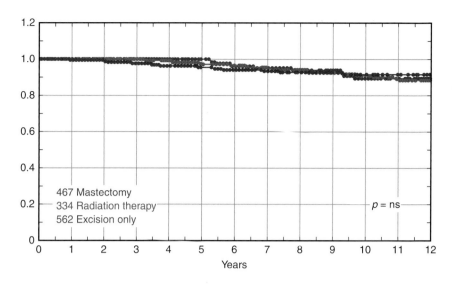

FIGURE 18-8 Probability of overall survival by treatment for 1363 patients with DCIS.

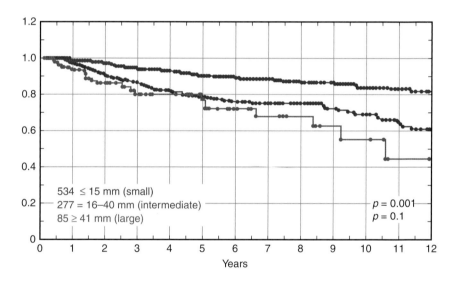

FIGURE 18-9 Probability of local recurrence-free survival by tumor size for 896 breast-conservation patients.

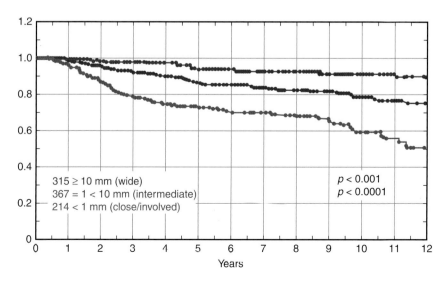

FIGURE 18-10 Probability of local recurrence-free survival by margin width for 896 breast-conservation patients.

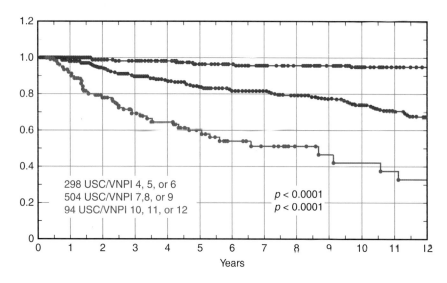

FIGURE 18-11 Probability of local recurrence-free survival for 896 breast-conservation patients grouped by USC/Van Nuys Prognostic Index score (4, 5, or 6; vs 7, 8, or 9; vs 10, 11, or 12).

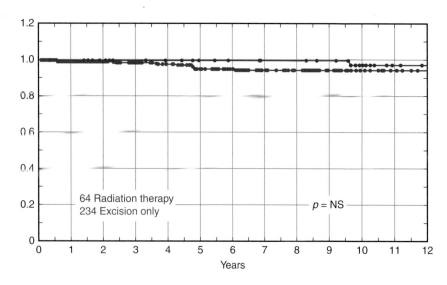

FIGURE 18-12 Probability of local recurrence-free survival by treatment for 282 breast-conservation patients with USC/Van Nuys Prognostic Index scores of 4, 5, or 6.

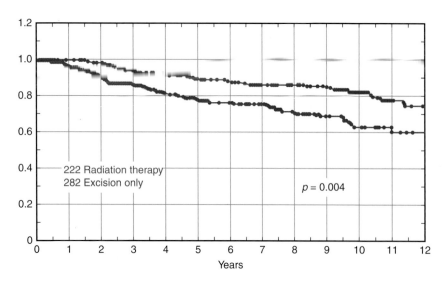

FIGURE 18-13 Probability of local recurrence-free survival by treatment for 507 breast-conservation patients with USC/Van Nuys Prognostic Index scores of 7, 8, or 9.

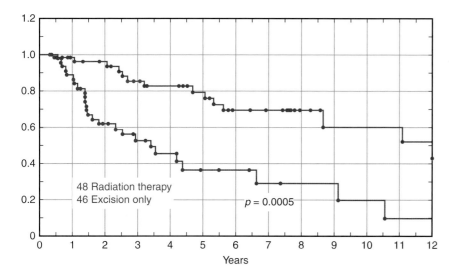

FIGURE 18-14 Probability of local recurrence-free survival by treatment for 106 breast-conservation patients with Modified USC/Van Nuys Prognostic Index scores of 10, 11, or 12.

CURRENT TREATMENT TRENDS

In the current era of evidence-based medicine, it is reasonable to interpret the prospective randomized data as support for the tenet that all conservatively treated patients with DCIS should receive postexcisional radiation therapy. However, in spite of these data, the number of patients with DCIS being treated with excision alone continues to increase. The 2003 SEER data revealed that approximately one-third of all patients with DCIS in the United States are now being treated with excision alone.[16]

As an aid to the complex treatment decision-making process, the USC/VNPI can be used as a starting point to suggest reasonable treatment options supported by local recurrence data. The USC/VNPI divides patients with DCIS into 3 groups with differing probabilities of local recurrence after breast-conserving surgery. Although there is an apparent treatment choice for each group (Table 18-2), excision alone for patients who score 4 to 6, excision plus radiation therapy for patients who score 7 to 9, and mastectomy for those who score 10 to 12, the USC/VNPI is offered only as a guideline, a starting place for discussions with patients.[106] We emphasize that the USC/VNPI requires thorough sequential tissue processing and evaluation. Application of the VNPI will not be successful if the requisite pathology has not been performed.

■ Use of Margin Width as the Sole Predictor of Local Recurrence

Determining size has always been the most difficult part of the USC/VNPI. Our method establishes size by utilizing a sequential sectioning technique. The size of the DCIS represents the extent of DCIS in a series of sequential sections (the product of the number of slides times the average thickness of the block), rather than on a single slide (unless the measurement on a single slide is larger), and correlates this with the mammographic findings. For example, if a DCIS appears in and out of 7 consecutive sections and the blocks are on average 3 mm thick, the diameter of this lesion would be recorded as a 21-mm DCIS (7 blocks × 3 mm average block width) in our database. In many other databases, it would be recorded as a 6-mm DCIS, the largest diameter on a single section.

By way of example, when the NSABP reviewed their pathologic material for the B-17 study, 75% to 90% of their cases were measured at 10 mm or less in extent.[60,107] The NSABP reported tumor size as the largest diameter on a single slide. While this is clearly the simplest and most reproducible way to measure DCIS, it is often an underestimation. Compare the NSABP sizes with our cases, where only 45% (365/806) of our conservatively treated patients had DCIS lesions measuring 10 mm or less. It is unlikely that the NSABP had twice as many smaller cases than a single group devoted to diagnosing and treating DCIS. Rather, the explanation probably lies in the way tissue was processed and the method used to estimate tumor size. In all likelihood, both groups treated tumors of similar size.

Due to the difficulty of estimating size, in 1997 we began evaluating the possibility of using margin width as the sole predictor of local recurrence, as a surrogate for the USC/VNPI.[90] The rationale was based on a multivariate analysis where patients with margin widths less than 1 mm had a 9-fold increase in the probability local recurrence compared with patients who had 10 mm or more margin widths. Narrow margin width was the single most powerful predictor of local failure.

In the current data set presented here, 315 patients had margin widths of 10 mm or more, 16 of whom (5%) have developed a local recurrence (1 in the radiotherapy group and 15 within the excision-only group). The local recurrence benefit for radiation therapy is significant ($p = 0.03$). In spite of this, the actuarial local recurrence rate at 12 years, for those treated with excision alone, was only 14%, virtually identical to that reported by the NSABP at 12 years for all patients treated with excision plus radiation therapy.[60]

TABLE 18-2 Treatment Guidelines, USAC/Van Nuys Prognostic Index

USC/VNPI Score	Recommended Treatment
4-6	Excision only
7-9	Excision + radiation
10-12	Mastectomy

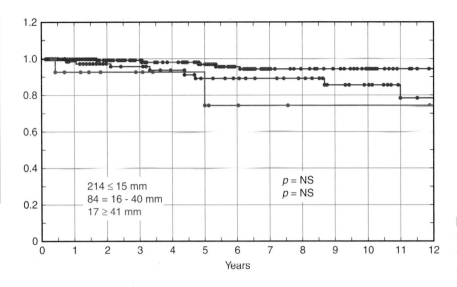

FIGURE 18-15 Probability of local recurrence-free survival by tumor size for 315 breast-conservation patients with margins widths 10 mm or more.

There were 298 patients with USC/VNPI scores of 4, 5, or 6, of whom 9 (3%) have developed a local recurrence (1 in the radiotherapy group and 8 within the excision-only group) (Fig. 18-12). The USC/VNPI is a better predictor of local recurrence than margin width alone (half as many recurrences), and it should be, since it is based on 5 predictive factors, including margin width. Nevertheless, there are so few recurrences among patients with widely clear margins that for all practical purposes, margin width can be used by itself as a suboptimal surrogate for the USC/VNPI.

When widely clear margins are obtained (larger than 10 mm), the presence of comedonecrosis nuclear grade (grade 3) and young age do not significantly increase the local recurrence rate. Figure 18-15 shows that if widely clear margins are obtained, large size does not increase the local recurrence rate, although there are too few lesions greater than 40 mm with 10 mm or more margins (n = 17) to draw firm conclusions. A final word of caution: margin width as a surrogate for the USC/VNPI will only be valid if all the resected tissue has been processed, not sampled.

Treatment of Axilla for Patients with DCIS

In 1986, our group suggested that axillary lymph node dissection be abandoned for DCIS.[108] In 1987, the NSABP made axillary node dissection for patients with DCIS optional, at the discretion of the surgeon. Since that time, we have published a series of papers that continue to show that axillary node dissection is not indicated for patients with DCIS.[96,109] To date, our group has performed a total of 634 node evaluations, 2 of which (0.3%) contained positive nodes by H&E staining. Both those patients were treated with adjuvant chemotherapy. Both were alive and well without local or distant recurrence at 8 and 10 years after their initial surgery (both had mastectomies and invasive cancer was likely missed during the serial sectioning of their specimens).

Frykberg and associates, in their review of the management of DCIS, compiled the data of 9 studies with a total of 754 patients. The incidence of axillary lymph node metastasis for patients with DCIS was 1.7%.[110]

Sentinel Node Biopsy for DCIS

Through April 2008, we have performed 234 sentinel node biopsies for patients with DCIS. All were negative by H&E; 11 (5%) were positive by IHC. In every case there were only a few positive cells (range, 4-93). In no case were any patients upstaged to stage II nor were any treated with chemotherapy. All are alive and well without distant recurrence with follow-up ranging from 0.7 to 10.4 years (average, 4.4 years).

Not all IHC-positive cells are cancer cells. Some may merely be cytokeratin positive debris. Their morphology must be closely evaluated.

Our policy for sentinel node biopsy in patients with DCIS is as follows. We perform it for all patients with DCIS who are undergoing a mastectomy. We perform it if the DCIS is an upper outer quadrant lesion and the sentinel node can be easily removed through the same incision. We also remove a sentinel node if the DCIS is palpable or greater than 4 cm on mammography and/or MRI.

THE FUTURE

Our knowledge of DCIS genetics and molecular biology is increasing at a remarkably rapid rate. Future studies are likely to identify markers that will allow us to differentiate DCIS with an aggressive potential from DCIS that is merely a microscopic finding. Once we can differentiate DCIS that will soon develop the potential to invade and metastasize from DCIS that will not, the treatment selection process will become much simpler.

SUMMARY

DCIS is now relatively common, and its frequency is increasing. Most of this is due to better and more frequent mammography by a greater proportion of the female population.

Not all microscopic DCIS will progress to clinical cancer, but if a patient has DCIS and is not treated, she is more likely to develop an ipsilateral invasive breast cancer than is a woman without DCIS.

The high-grade subtype of DCIS is more aggressive and malignant in its histologic appearance and is more likely to be associated with subsequent invasive cancer than the intermediate and low-grade subtypes. High-grade DCIS is more likely to have a high S-phase, overexpress Her-2/neu, and show increased thymidine labeling as compared with lower-grade DCIS, and is also more likely to recur locally following breast conservation. Separation of DCIS into 2 groups, comedo versus non-comedo, by histologic architecture is an oversimplification and does not reflect the biological potential of the lesion as well as separation by nuclear grade and comedo-type necrosis.

Most nonpalpable DCIS today will be detected by mammographic calcifications. It is not uncommon for DCIS to be larger than evident by mammography and to involve more than a quadrant of the breast, and to be unicentric in its distribution.

Preoperative evaluation should include film-screen mammography with compression magnification and ultrasonography. MRI is becoming increasingly more popular and we use it on every patient diagnosed with any form of breast cancer. The surgeon and the radiologist should plan the excision procedure carefully. The first attempt at excision is the best chance to get a complete excision with a good cosmetic result.

Reexcisions often yield poor cosmetic results and the overall plan should be to avoid them whenever possible. In light of this, the initial breast biopsy should be an image-guided biopsy.

After the establishment of the diagnosis, the patient should be counseled. If she is motivated for breast conservation, the surgeon and radiologist should plan the procedure carefully, using multiple wires to map out the extent of the lesion

When considering the entire population of patients with DCIS without subset analyses, the prospective randomized trials have shown that postexcisional radiation therapy can reduce the relative risk of local recurrence by about 50% for conservatively treated patients. But in some low-risk DCIS patients, the costs may outweigh the potential benefits. In spite of a relative 50% reduction in the probability of local recurrence, the absolute reduction may only be a few percent. While local recurrence is extremely important, breast cancer–specific survival is the most important end point for all patients with breast cancer, including patients with DCIS, and no DCIS trial has ever shown a survival benefit for radiation therapy when compared with excision alone. Moreover, radiation therapy is not without financial and physical cost. Because of this, in recent years, an increasing number of selected patients with DCIS have been treated with excision alone.

The University of Southern California/Van Nuys Prognostic Index (USC/VNPI) uses 5 independent predictors to predict the probability of local recurrence after conservative treatment for DCIS; these include tumor size, margin width, nuclear grade, age, and the presence or absence of comedonecrosis. In combination, they can be used as an aid to identify subgroups of patients with extremely low probabilities of local recurrence after excision alone, for example, patients who score 4, 5, or 6 using the USC/VNPI. If size cannot be accurately determined, margin width by itself can be used as a surrogate for the USC/VNPI, although it is not quite as good.

Oncoplastic surgery combines sound surgical oncologic principles with plastic surgical techniques. Coordination of the two surgical disciplines may help to avoid poor cosmetic results after wide excision and may increase the number of women who can be treated with breast-conserving surgery by allowing larger breast excisions with more acceptable cosmetic results. Oncoplastic surgery requires cooperation and coordination of surgical oncology, radiology, and pathology. Oncoplastic resection is a therapeutic procedure, not a breast biopsy, and is performed on patients with a proven diagnosis of breast cancer. New oncoplastic techniques that allow for more extensive excisions can be used to achieve both acceptable cosmesis and widely clear margins, alleviating the need for radiation therapy in many cases of DCIS.

The decision to use excision alone as treatment for DCIS should only be made if complete and sequential tissue processing has been used and the patient has been fully informed and has participated in the treatment decision-making process.

REFERENCES

1. Jemal A, Siegel R, Ward E, et al. Cancer statistics, 2008. *CA Cancer J Clin.* 2008;58:71-96.
2. Burstein HJ, Polyak K, Wong JS, et al. Ductal carcinoma in situ of the breast. *N Engl J Med.* 2004;350:1430-1441.
3. Seth A, Kitching R, Landberg G, et al. Gene expression profiling of ductal carcinomas in situ and invasive breast tumors. *Anticancer Res.* 2003;23:2043-2051.
4. Porter D, Lahti-Domenici J, Keshaviah A, et al. Molecular markers in ductal carcinoma in situ of the breast. *Mol Cancer Res.* 2003;1:362-375.
5. Ma XS, Alunga R, Tuggle J, et al. Gene expression profiles of human breast cancer progression. *Proc Natl Acad Sci USA.* 2003;100:5974-5979.
6. Page D, Anderson T. *Diagnostic Histopathology of the Breast.* New York, NY: Churchill Livingstone; 1987.
7. Patchefsky A, Schwartz G, Finkelstein S, et al. Heterogeneity of intraductal carcinoma of the breast. *Cancer.* 1989;63:731-741.
8. Nemoto T, Vana J, Bedwani R, et al. Management and survival of female breast cancer: results of a national survey by the American College of Surgeons. *Cancer.* 1980;45:2917-2924.
9. Silverstein M, Lagios M, Recht A, et al. Image-detected breast cancer: state of the art diagnosis and treatment. *J Am Coll Surg.* 2005;201:586-597.
10. Tabar L, Smith RA, Vitak B, et al. Mammographic screening: a key factor in the control of breast cancer. *Cancer J.* 2003;9:15-27.
11. Duffy SW, Tabar L, Smith RA. Screening for breast cancer with mammography. *Lancet.* 2001;358:2166; author reply 7-8.
12. Silverstein MJ, Cohlan B, Gierson E, et al. Duct carcinoma in situ: 227 cases without microinvasion. *Eur J Cancer.* 1992;28:630-634.
13. Lagios MD. Duct carcinoma in situ: pathology and treatment. *Surg Clin North Am.* 1990;70:853-871.
14. Ashikari R, Hadju S, Robbins G. Intraductal carcinoma of the breast. *Cancer.* 1971;28:1182-1187.
15. Silverstein MJ. Ductal carcinoma in situ of the breast. *Annu Rev Med.* 2000;51:17-32.
16. Baxter N, Virnig B, Durham S, Tuttle T. Trends in the treatment of ductal carcinoma in situ of the breast. *J Natl Cancer Inst.* 2004;96:443-448.
17. Silverstein MJ. The Van Nuys Breast Center—the first free-standing multidisciplinary breast center. *Surg Oncol Clin N Am.* 2000;9:159-175.
18. Veronesi U, Saccozzi R, Del Vecchio M, et al. Comparing radical mastectomy with quadrantectomy, axillary dissection and radiotherapy in patients with small cancers of the breast. *N Engl J Med.* 1981;305:6-10.
19. Van Dongen J, Bartelink H, Fentiman I, et al. Randomized clinical trial to assess the value of breast-conserving therapy in stage I and II breast cancer, EORTC 10801 trial. *Monogr Natl Cancer Inst.* 1992;11:15-18.
20. Veronesi U, Banfi A, Salvadori B, et al. Breast conservation is the treatment of choice in small breast cancer: long-term results of a randomized trial. *Eur J Cancer.* 1990;26:668-670.
21. Fisher B, Redmond C, Poisson R, et al. Eight-year results of a randomized clinical trial comparing total mastectomy and lumpectomy with or without radiation therapy in the treatment of breast cancer. *N Engl J Med.* 1989;320:822-828.

22. Veronesi U, Cascinelli N, Mariani L, et al. Twenty-year follow-up of a randomized study comparing breast-conserving surgery with radical mastectomy for early breast cancer. *N Engl J Med.* 2002;347:1227-1232.

23. Fisher B, Anderson S, Bryant J, et al. Twenty-year follow-up of a randomized trial comparing total mastectomy, lumpectomy, and lumpectomy plus irradiation for the treatment of invasive breast cancer. *N Engl J Med.* 2002;347:1233-1241.

24. Azzopardi J, Ahmed A, Millis R. *Problems in Breast Pathology.* London, UK: Saunders; 1979.

25. Lagios M, Margolin F, Westdahl P, Rose N. Mammographically detected duct carcinoma in situ. Frequency of local recurrence following tylectomy and prognostic effect of nuclear grade on local recurrence. *Cancer.* 1989;63:619-624.

26. Solin L, Yeh I, Kurtz J, et al. Ductal carcinoma in situ (intraductal carcinoma) of the breast treated with breast-conserving surgery and definitive irradiation. Correlation of pathologic parameters with outcome of treatment. *Cancer.* 1993;71:2532-2542.

27. Holland R, Peterse J, Millis R, et al. Ductal carcinoma in situ: a proposal for a new classification. *Semin Diagn Pathol.* 1994;11:167-180.

28. Bethwaite P, Smithe N, Delahunt B, et al. Reproducibility of new classification schemes for the pathology of ductal carcinoma in situ of the breast. *J Clin Pathol.* 1998;51:450-454.

29. Douglas-Jones A, Gupta S, Attanoos R, et al. A critical appraisal of six modern classifications of ductal carcinoma in situ of the breast: correlation with grade of associated invasive disease. *Histopathology.* 1996;29:397-409.

30. Consensus Conference Committee. Consensus conference on the classification of ductal carcinoma in situ. *Cancer.* 1997;80:1798-1802.

31. Silverstein MJ, Poller D, Waisman J, et al. Prognostic classification of breast ductal carcinoma-in-situ. *Lancet.* 1995;345:1154-1157.

32. Jensen J, Handel N, Silverstein M, et al. Glandular replacement therapy (GRT) for intraductal breast carcinoma (DCIS). *Proc Am Soc Clin Oncol.* 1995;14:138.

33. Jensen J, Handel N, Silverstein M. Glandular replacement therapy: an argument for a combined surgical approach in the treatment of noninvasive breast cancer. *Breast J.* 1996;2:121-123.

34. Lagios M, Westdahl P, Margolin F, Rose M. Duct carcinoma in situ: relationship of extent of noninvasive disease to the frequency of occult invasion, multicentricity, lymph node metastases, and short-term treatment failures. *Cancer.* 1982;50:1309-1314.

35. Faverly D, Burgers L, Bult P, Holland R. Three-dimensional imaging of mammary ductal carcinoma in situ: clinical implications. *Semin Diagn Pathol.* 1994;11:193-198.

36. Poller D, Silverstein M, Galea M, et al. Ductal carcinoma in situ of the breast: a proposal for a new simplified histological classification association between cellular proliferation and c-erbB-2 protein expression. *Mod Pathol.* 1994;7:257-262.

37. Bellamy C, McDonald C, Salter D, et al. Noninvasive ductal carcinoma of the breast: the relevance of histologic categorization. *Hum Pathol.* 1993;24:16-23.

38. Sloane J, Ellman R, Anderson T, et al. Consistency of histopathological reporting of breast lesions detected by breast screening: findings of the UK national external quality assessment (EQA) scheme. *Eur J Cancer.* 1994;10:1414-1419.

39. Page D, Rogers L, Schuyler P, et al. The natural history of ductal carcinoma in situ of the breast. In: Silverstein MJ, Recht A, Lagios M, eds. *Ductal Carcinoma In Situ of the Breast.* 2nd ed. Philadelphia, PA: Lippincott Williams & Wilkins; 2002:17-21.

40. Sanders M, Schuyler P, Dupont W, Page D. The natural history of low-grade ductal carcinoma in situ of the breast in women treated by biopsy only revealed over 30 years of long term follow-up. *Cancer.* 2005;103:2481-2484.

41. Rosen P, Senie R, Schottenfeld D, Ashikari R. Noninvasive breast carcinoma: frequency of unsuspected invasion and implications for treatment. *Ann Surg.* 1979;1989:377-382.

42. Nielson M, Thomsen J, Primdahl S, et al. Breast cancer and atypia among young and middle-aged women: a study of 110 medicolegal autopsies. *Br J Cancer.* 1987;56:814-819.

43. Alpers C, Wellings S. The prevalence of carcinoma in situ in normal and cancer-associated breast. *Hum Pathol.* 1985;16:796-807.

44. Page D, Dupont W, Roger L, Landenberger M. Intraductal carcinoma of the breast: Follow-up after biopsy only. *Cancer.* 1982;49:751-758.

45. Chuba P, Hamre M, Yap J, et al. Bilateral risk for subsequent breast cancer after lobular carcinoma in situ: analysis of surveillance, epidemiology and end results data. *J Clin Oncol.* 2005;23:5534-5541.

46. Schuh M, Nemoto T, Penetrante R, et al. Intraductal carcinoma: analysis of presentation, pathologic findings, and outcome of disease. *Arch Surg.* 1986;121:1303-1307.

47. Gump F, Jicha D, Ozzello L. Ductal carcinoma in situ (DCIS): a revised concept. *Surgery.* 1987;102:190-195.

48. de Mascarel I, MacGrogan G, Mathoulin-Pelissier S, et al. Breast ductal carcinoma in situ with microinvasion. A definition supported by long-term study 1248 serially sectioned ductal carcinomas. *Cancer.* 2002;94:2134-2142.

49. Fisher E, Sass R, Fisher B, et al. Pathologic findings from the National surgical Adjuvant Breast Project (Protocol 6). I. Intraductal carcinoma (DCIS). *Cancer.* 1986;57:197-208.

50. Simpson T, Thirlby R, Dail D. Surgical treatment of ductal carcinoma in situ of the breast: 10 to 20 year follow-up. *Arch Surg.* 1992;127:468-472.

51. Lagios M. Multicentricity of breast carcinoma demonstrated by routine correlated serial subgross and radiographic examination. *Cancer.* 1977;40:1726-1734.

52. Holland R, Hendriks J, Verbeek A, et al. Extent, distribution, and mammographic/histological correlations of breast ductal carcinoma in situ. *Lancet.* 1990;335:519-522.

53. Holland R, Faverly D. Whole organ studies. In: Silverstein MJ, Recht A, Lagios M, eds. *Ductal Carcinoma In Situ of the Breast.* Philadelphia, PA: Lippincott Williams & Wilkins; 2002.

54. Noguchi S, Aihara T, Koyama H, et al. Discrimination between multicentric and multifocal carcinomas of breast through clonal analysis. *Cancer.* 1994;74:872-877.

55. Tabar L, Dean P. Basic principles of mammographic diagnosis. *Diagn Imag Clin Med.* 1985;54:146-157.

56. Schwartz G, Finkel G, Carcia J, Patchefsky A. Subclinical ductal carcinoma in situ of the breast: treatment by local excision and surveillance alone. *Cancer.* 1992;70:2468-2474.

57. Lagios M. Pathology procedures for evaluation of the specimen with potential or documented ductal carcinoma in situ. *Semin Breast Dis.* 2000;3:42-49.

58. Silverstein MJ. Intraductal breast carcinoma: two thoughts of progress. *Am J Clin Oncol.* 1991;14:534-537.

59. Silverstein MJ. Noninvasive breast cancer: the dilemma of the 1990s. *Obstet Gynecol Clin N Am.* 1994;21:639-658.

60. Fisher B, Land S, Mamounas E, et al. Prevention of invasive breast cancer in women with ductal carcinoma in situ: an update of the National Surgical Adjuvant Breast and Bowel Project experience. *Semin Oncol.* 2001;28:400-418.

61. Fentiman I, Fagg N, Millis R, Haywood J. In situ ductal carcinoma of the breast: implications of disease pattern and treatment. *Eur J Surg Oncol.* 1986;12:261-266.

62. Solin L, Kurtz J, Fourquet A, et al. Fifteen year results of breast conserving surgery and definitive breast irradiation for treatment of ductal carcinoma in situ of the breast. *J Clin Oncol.* 1996;14:754-763.

63. UK Coordinating Committee on Cancer Research (UKCCCR). Ductal Carcinoma in Situ (DCIS) Working Party. Radiotherapy and tamoxifen in women with completely excised ductal carcinoma in situ of the breast in the UK, Australia, and New Zealand: randomised controlled trial. *Lancet.* 2003;362:95-102.

64. Viani GA, Stefano EJ, Afonso SL, et al. Breast-conserving surgery with or without radiotherapy in women with ductal carcinoma in situ: a meta-analysis of randomized trials. *Radiation Oncol.* 2007;2:28-39.

65. Emdin SO, Granstrand B, Ringberg A, et al. SweDCIS: radiotherapy after sector resection for ductal carcinoma in situ of the breast. Results of a randomised trial in a population offered mammographic screening. *Acta Oncol.* 2006;45:536-543.

66. Fisher B, Jeong J, Anderson S, et al. Twenty-five year follow-up of a randomized trial comparing radical mastectomy, total mastectomy, and total mastectomy followed by irradiation. *N Engl J Med.* 2002;347:567-575.

67. Group EBCTC. Effects of radiotherapy and differences in the extent of surgery for early breast cancer on local recurrence and on 15-year survival. *Lancet.* 2005;366:2087-2106.

68. Silverstein MJ, Lagios M, Martino S, et al. Outcome after local recurrence in patients with ductal carcinoma in situ of the breast. *J Clin Oncol.* 1998;16:1367-1373.

69. Romero L, Klein L, Ye W, et al. Outcome after invasive recurrence in patients with ductal carcinoma in situ of the breast. *Am J Surg.* 2004;188:371-376.

70. Swain S. Ductal carcinoma in situ—incidence, presentation and guidelines to treatment. *Oncology.* 1989;3:25-42.

71. Fisher B, Costantino J, Redmond C, et al. Lumpectomy compared with lumpectomy and radiation therapy for the treatment of intraductal breast cancer. *N Engl J Med.* 1993;328:1581-1586.

72. Fisher B, Dignam J, Wolmark N, et al. Tamoxifen in treatment of intraductal breast cancer: National Surgical Adjuvant Breast and Bowel Project B-24 randomized controlled trial. *Lancet.* 1999;353:1993-2000.

73. Fisher B, Dignam J, Wolmark N, et al. Lumpectomy and radiation therapy for the treatment of intraductal breast cancer: findings from National Surgical Adjuvant Breast and Bowel Project B-17. *J Clin Oncol.* 1998;16:441-452.

74. Julien J, Bijker N, Fentiman I, et al. Radiotherapy in breast conserving treatment for ductal carcinoma in situ: first results of EORTC randomized phase III trial 10853. *Lancet.* 2000;355:528-533.

75. Page D, Dupont W, Rogers L, et al. Continued local recurrence of carcinoma 15-25 years after a diagnosis of low grade ductal carcinoma in situ of the breast treated only by biopsy. *Cancer.* 1995;76:1197-2000.

76. Zafrani B, Leroyer A, Fourquet A, et al. Mammographically detected ductal in situ carcinoma of the breast analyzed with a new classification. A study of 127 cases: correlation with estrogen and progesterone receptors, p53 and c-erbB-2 proteins, and proliferative activity. *Semin Diagn Pathol.* 1994;11:208-214.

77. Schwartz G. The role of excision and surveillance alone in subclinical DCIS of the breast. *Oncology.* 1994;8:21-26.

78. Schwartz G. Treatment of subclinical ductal carcinoma in situ of the breast by local excision and surveillance: an updated personal experience. In: Silverstein MJ, Recht A, Lagios M, eds. *Ductal Carcinoma In Situ of the Breast.* 2nd ed. Philadelphia, PA: Lippincott Williams & Wilkins; 2002:308-321.

79. Holland R, Faverly D. *Whole Organ Studies.* Baltimore, MD: Williams & Wilkins; 1997.

80. Holland R, Hendriks J. Microcalcifications associated with ductal carcinoma in situ: mammographic-pathologic correlation. *Semin Diag Pathol.* 1994;11:181-192.

81. Page D, Dupont W, Roger L, Rados M. Atypical hyperplastic lesions of the female breast. A log-term follow-up study. *Cancer.* 1985;55:2698-2708.

82. Lagios M. Controversies in diagnosis, biology, and treatment. *Breast J.* 1995;1:68-78.

83. Group EBCTC. Favorable and unfavorable effects on long-term survival of radiotherapy for early breast cancer: an overview of the randomized trials. *Lancet.* 2006;2000:1757-1570.

84. Giordano S, Kuo Y, Freeman J, et al. Risk of cardiac death after adjuvant radiotherapy for breast cancer. *J Natl Cancer Inst.* 2005;97:419-424.

85. Darby S, McGale P, Taylor C, Peto R. Long-term mortality from heart disease and lung cancer after radiotherapy for early breast cancer: prospective cohort study of about 300,000 women un U.S. SEER cancer registries. *Lancet Oncol.* 2005;6:557-565.

86. Zablotska L, Neugut A. Lung carcinoma after radiation therapy in women treated with lumpectomy or mastectomy for primary breast carcinoma. *Cancer.* 2003;97:1404-1411.

87. Darby S, McGale P, Peto R, et al. Mortality from cardiovascular disease more than 10 years after radiotherapy for breast cancer: nationwide cohort study of 90,000 Swedish women. *BMJ.* 2003;326:256-257.

88. NCCN Clincal Practice Guidelines in Oncology: Breast Cancer. 2008. www.nccn.org. Accessed 2008.

89. Bijker N, Peterse J, Duchateau L, et al. Risk factors for recurrence and metastasis after breast-conserving therapy for ductal carcinoma in situ: analysis of European Organization for Research and Treatment of Cancer Trial 10853. *J Clin Oncol.* 2001;19:2263-2271.

90. Fisher E, Constantino J, Fisher B, et al. Pathologic findings from the National Surgical Adjuvant Breast Project (NSABP) Protocol B-17. *Cancer.* 1995;75:1310-1319.

91. Fisher B, Bauer M, Margolese R, et al. Five-year results of a randomized clinical trial comparing total mastectomy and lumpectomy with or without radiation therapy in the treatment of breast cancer. *N Engl J Med.* 1985;312:665-673.

92. Fisher E, Lemming R, Andersen S, et al. Conservative management of intraductal carcinoma (DCIS) of the breast. *J Surg Oncol.* 1991;47:139-147.

93. Recht A. Randomized trial overview. In: Silverstein MJ, Recht A, Lagios M, eds. *Ductal Carcinoma In Situ of the Breast.* 2nd ed. Philadelphia, PA: Lippincott Williams & Wilkins; 2002:414-419.

94. Allred D, Bryant J, Land S, et al. Estrogen receptor expression as a predictive marker of effectiveness of tamoxifen in the treatment of DCIS: findings from NSABP Protocol B-24. *Breast Cancer Res Treat.* 2003;76:36.

95. Bijker N, Meijnen P, Peterse J, et al. Breast conserving treatment with or without radiotherapy in ductal carcinoma in situ: ten-year results of European Organization for Research and Treatment of Cancer Randomized Phase III Trial 10853—a study by the EORTC Breast Cancer Cooperative Group and EORTC Radiotherapy Group. *J Clin Oncol.* 2006;24:1-8.

96. Silverstein MJ, Barth A, Poller D, et al. Ten-year results comparing mastectomy to excision and radiation therapy for ductal carcinoma in situ of the breast. *Eur J Cancer.* 1995;31A:1425-1427.

97. Silverstein MJ, Lagios M, Groshen S, et al. The influence of margin width on local control in patients with ductal carcinoma in situ (DCIS) of the breast. *New Engl J Med.* 1999;340:1455-1461.

98. Silverstein MJ, Buchanan C. Ductal carcinoma in situ: USC/Van Nuys Prognostic Index and the impact of margin status. *Breast.* 2003;12:457-471.

99. Silverstein MJ. The University of Southern California/Van Nuys Prognostic Index for ductal carcinoma in situ of the breast. *Am J Surg.* 2003; 186:337-343.

100. Ottesen G, Graversen H, Blichert-Toft M, et al. Ductal carcinoma in situ of the female breast. Short-term results of a prospective nationwide study. *Am J Surg Pathol.* 1992;16:1183-1196.

101. Silverstein MJ, Lagios M, Craig P, et al. The Van Nuys Prognostic Index for ductal carcinoma in situ. *Breast J.* 1996;2:38-40.

102. Silverstein MJ, Poller D, Craig P, et al. A prognostic index for ductal carcinoma in situ of the breast. *Cancer.* 1996;77:2267-2274.

103. Silverstein MJ, Lagios M, Recht A, eds. *Ductal Carcinoma In Situ of the Breast.* 2nd ed. Philadelphia, PA: Lippincott Williams & Wilkins; 2002.

104. Poller D, Silverstein MJ. The Van Nuys ductal carcinoma in situ: an update. In: Silverstein MJ, Recht A, Lagios M, eds. *Ductal Carcinoma In Situ of the Breast.* 2nd ed. Philadelphia, PA: Lippincott Williams & Wilkins; 2002:222-233.

105. Silverstein MJ. The University of Southern California/Van Nuys Prognostic Index. In: Silverstein MJ, Recht A, Lagios M, eds. *Ductal Carcinoma In Situ of the Breast.* 2nd ed. Philadelphia, PA: Lippincott Williams & Wilkins; 2002:459-473.

106. Gilleard O, Goodman A, Cooper M, et al. The significance of the Van Nuys Prognostic Index in the management of ductal carcinoma in situ. *World J Surg Oncol.* 2008;6:61-66.

107. Fisher E, Dignam J, Tan-Chie E, et al. Pathologic findings from the National Adjuvant Breast Project (NSABP) eight-year update of Protocol B-17: intraductal carcinoma. *Cancer.* 1999;86:429-438.

108. Silverstein MJ, Rosser R, Gierson E, et al. Axillary Lymph node dissection for intraductal carcinoma—is it indicated? *Cancer.* 1987;59:1819-1824.

109. Silverstein MJ. An argument against routine use of radiotherapy for ductal carcinoma in situ. *Oncology.* 2003;17:1511-1546.

110. Frykberg E, Masood S, Copeland E, Bland K. Duct carcinoma in situ of the breast. *Surg Gynecol Obstet.* 1993;177:425-440.

CHAPTER 19

Paget Disease of the Breast

Nimmi Arora
Rache M. Simmons

An English surgeon by the name of Sir James Paget reported on a condition of eczematous change of the nipple–areola complex associated with underlying breast malignancy in 1874.[1] It is now recognized that Paget disease denotes an entity of intraepithelial adenocarcinoma within the epidermis of the nipple–areola complex that is associated with underlying in situ or invasive mammary carcinoma in 92% to 100% of cases.[2-4] Paget cells, large cells with pale cytoplasm and prominent nucleoli, identified within nipple epidermis on histology confirm diagnosis. Ninety percent of these will overexpress Her-2/neu.

EPIDEMIOLOGY

Paget disease represents only 0.5% to 5% of all breast cancer, with average age of onset in the 50s to 60s. The majority of patients are postmenopausal women; however, a few cases have been documented in men, with a ratio of 1:50-200 men to women.[5,6]

CLINICAL PRESENTATION

Paget disease usually presents as a scaling, erythematous, eczematous lesion of the nipple that can be mistaken as a benign condition leading to delayed diagnosis (Fig.19-1). Usually the disease is unilateral, beginning at the nipple, and may spread to the areola; however, there are instances where only the areola may be affected. Late stages may be associated with ulceration, crusting, serous or bloody nipple discharge, and nipple retraction or flattening (Fig. 19-2). Patients may complain of pain, burning, and/or itching. Physical exam may reveal an underlying breast mass in 30% to 50% of cases. Rarely, Paget disease will be identified on a mastectomy specimen without clinical signs of disease (no skin lesion).

PATHOGENESIS

The pathogenesis of Paget disease has been long debated, with 2 main competing theories: the epidermotrophic theory and the transformation theory. The epidermotrophic theory, currently the more favored theory, states that neoplastic ductal epithelial cells migrate through the ductal system of the breast into the epidermis of the nipple. Evidence for this lies in the observation that both the underlying mammary carcinoma and the intraepithelial nipple lesion will have similar staining of markers such as CEA, c-erb-B2, and Her-2/neu,[6,7] suggesting that the nipple lesion arose from the breast malignancy. In addition, there is some research pointing to the ability of the Her2/neu receptor acting as an agent that induces chemotaxis of tumor cells, allowing for migration of malignant cells to the nipple, thus giving a mechanistic explanation supporting the epidermotrophic theory.[8,9]

On the other hand, the transformation theory suggests that epidermal keritinocytes within the nipple transform into malignant Paget cells, implying that Paget disease is actually an in situ carcinoma. Evidence for this lies in the fact that not all intraepithelial malignant lesions are associated with underlying mammary carcinoma. In addition, some breast cancers are located peripheral to the nipple lesion, suggesting 2 concurrent but separate processes. Electron microscopy studies of cell junctions have been able to identify tight junctions between adjacent Paget cells, suggesting that they may not have migrated from underlying breast tissue.[10] Additional evidence for the transformation theory lies in the detection of a "pre-Paget" cell—half keritinocyte, half Paget, also known as a Toker cell.[11]

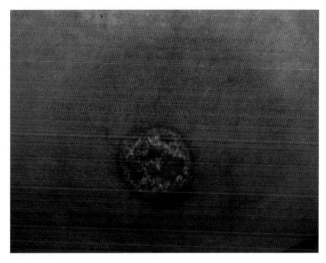

FIGURE 19-1 Clinical presentation of early Paget disease. Note eczematous change of nipple–areola complex. *(Courtesy of Kelly Hunt, MD, Department of Surgical Oncology, MD Anderson Cancer Center.)*

This cell could represent an intermediate or precursor to Paget, in line with the transformation theory.

Both the epidermotrophic theory and the transformation theory have credible evidence, and it remains to future research to delineate the actual pathogenesis.

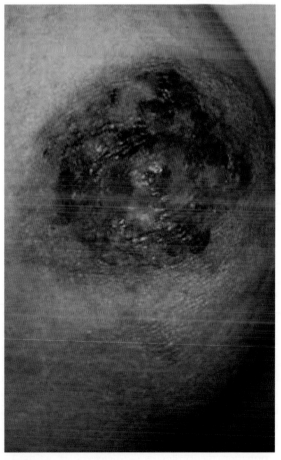

FIGURE 19-2 More advanced stage of Paget disease. *(Courtesy of Kelly Hunt, MD, Department of Surgical Oncology, MD Anderson Cancer Center.)*

DIFFERENTIAL DIAGNOSIS

The differential diagnosis for Paget disease includes a variety of other benign and malignant conditions, including atopic or contact dermatitis, erosive adenomatosis (nipple adenoma), psoriasis, hyperkeratosis of the nipple–areola, eczema, Bowen disease, basal cell carcinoma, superficial spreading malignant melanoma, and pemphigus vulgaris. Immunohistochemistry stains can differentiate these various pathologies (CEA, c-erb-B2, Her-2/neu).

DIAGNOSIS

The diagnosis of Paget disease is made with a full-thickness wedge biopsy of the nipple–areola complex. On histology, Paget cells can be identified within the epidermis of the nipple (Fig. 19-3). In lower epidermal layers, Paget cells can form gland-like structures. Immunohistochemical stains for CEA, keratin 7, androgen receptor, c-erb-B2, and other oncoproteins and cell cycle–related antigens may be positive and can aid in diagnosis.

IMAGING

Any patient with suspected Paget disease should undergo mammography to identify breast lesions. Fifty percent of patients with Paget disease will have a mammographic abnormality, and in some cases tumors can be multifocal or distant from the nipple.[12,13] The most common findings include microcalcifications, architectural distortion, and mass. Ultrasonography can also be useful in identifying lesions, especially when mammography is negative. Other imaging modalities that have been useful in detecting lesions associated with pagetoid change of the nipple include magnetic resonance imaging (MRI), positron emission tomography (PET), and even ^{99m}Tc-MIBI in some cases.

PROGNOSIS

The prognosis of Paget disease is based on that of the underlying mammary carcinoma. In general, due to delay in diagnosis, prognosis is often worse for men and worse for patients with a palpable breast mass, as this usually indicates invasive disease (90% of patients) and often axillary metastasis (50%-65% of patients).[5,6]

TREATMENT

The historical management of patients with Paget disease was a modified radical mastectomy with lymph node dissection. This allowed for complete excision of the disease process as well as any associated underlying malignancy and local lymph node spread. The following is a brief overview of other alternatives for the management of Paget disease of the breast.

Breast Conservation

In an attempt to preserve breast parenchyma for improved cosmetic results, a number of studies have reviewed the oncologic results after limited resection in Paget disease. In general, surgical

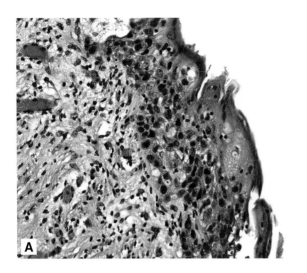

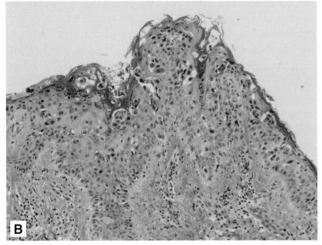

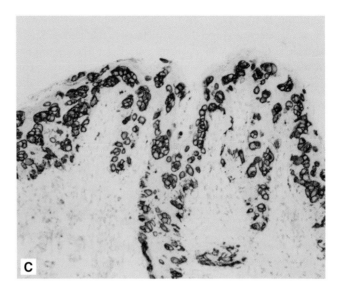

FIGURE 19-3 Histologic appearance of Paget disease. **A.** High-power view showing the surface of the nipple with neoplastic epithelial cells, which are histologically similar to the high-grade intraductal carcinoma cells present in the underlying lactiferous ducts. **B.** Tissue section of nipple shows presence of neoplastic epithelial cells distributed singly and in clusters (*arrows*). **C.** Some of the tumor cells contain brownish pigment derived from ingestion of melanin pigment from adjacent melanocytes. The tumor cells demonstrate strong and diffuse membranous staining for Her-2/neu, a commonly noted feature in Paget disease. *(Courtesy of Dr Syed A. Hoda, Department of Pathology, New York Presbyterian Hospital—Cornell [**A**] and Dr Savitri Krishnamurthy, Department of Pathology, MD Anderson Cancer Center [**B** and **C**].)*

resection of the nipple–areola complex is usually a minimal requirement to remove all diseased tissue (Fig. 19-4). When local excision alone is performed in patients with Paget disease and documented ductal carcinoma in situ (DCIS), recurrence rates can be as high as 30% to 50% at 10 years.[14,15] Local recurrence rates can be reduced when ensuring complete excision of any suspicious associated microcalcifications, obtaining negative histologic margins, and with the use of adjuvant radiation.

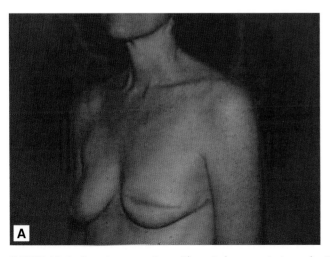

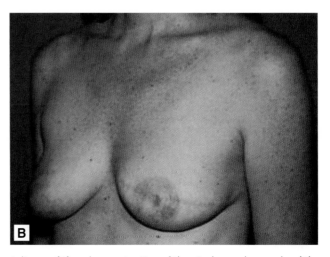

FIGURE 19-4 Breast conservation with central segmentectomy for Paget disease **(A)** and reconstruction of the nipple–areola complex **(B)**. *(Courtesy of Kelly Hunt, MD, Department of Surgical Oncology, MD Anderson Cancer Center.)*

In the 1980s, studies on the use of radiotherapy alone for the management of Paget disease surfaced in the literature, with variable results.[16-19] When patients with Paget disease confined to the nipple are treated with radiotherapy alone, local recurrence rates can be as low as 16% to18%.[17,19] On the other hand, when palpable disease was present, distant metastasis and death can occur after treatment with radiation alone secondary to missed concurrent untreated invasive carcinoma.[18,19]

In an attempt to improve patient outcome, whole breast irradiation was added to local excision, and in select cases, the rate of recurrence at 10 years decreased to 16% to 19%.[18,20,21] The key in these studies, however, was selecting the group of patients to fit this treatment regimen. In the majority of cases, patients were required to have no palpable mass and no mammographic abnormality prior to treatment. In one prospective European trial of 61 patients who mostly fit into the above criteria and were managed with wide local excision followed by whole-breast irradiation, the estimated 5-year local recurrence was 5.2%.[22] Table 19-1 lists features associated with Paget disease that are more likely to be amenable to breast-conserving therapy.

There are few instances, however, when breast conservation may not be an appropriate strategy for the management of Paget disease. Local excision of the nipple–areola complex and immediate underlying breast tissue for treatment of patients with Paget disease of the breast presumes 2 things: (1) physical exam and mammography are reliable tests for identification of malignancy and (2) any malignancy present will be in this excised tissue. In one retrospective review of women with Paget disease, physical exam findings and mammography were correlated with final pathologic diagnosis.[23] Of 40 women without a palpable mass and a negative mammogram, 5% had an invasive malignancy and 68% had DCIS. While women with a mass and a positive mammogram in this study had overall worse survival than women without these findings, this study shows that physical exam and mammography may be unreliable in detecting all cancer in Paget disease.

Another study reviewed pathologic findings of patients undergoing excision for Paget disease and found that while 61% of malignancies were indeed centrally located as predicted, 29% of patients with no associated palpable mass had a peripherally located tumor, greater than 2 cm from the areolar margin.[24] This suggests that wide local excision for patients may not always be an adequate resection. In yet another study of 70 women who underwent mastectomy for Paget disease, only

25% of malignancies were confined to the retroareolar space, and mammography was found to underestimate extent of disease in 43% of patients.[3]

One way of avoiding this conundrum, however, would be to obtain frozen sections intraoperatively to insure negative surgical margins in the event that a breast-conserving strategy is chosen. Future studies in the applicability of MRI in the detection of Paget-associated breast malignancy may prove useful in preoperative workup for these patients to better plan the surgical procedure of choice, as some isolated case reports have already been able to demonstrate its usefulness in this area.[25,26]

Management of the Axilla

While breast conservation is still a debated topic for Paget disease, management of the axilla seems to be less controversial in the literature at this time. With the widespread use of sentinel lymph node biopsy (SLNB), there is less need for initial axillary lymph node dissections (ALNDs) in patients with Paget disease. As with other malignancies of the breast, patients with Paget disease and without palpable or suspicious axillary lymph nodes and without a history of prior axillary surgery to preclude use of sentinel node detection, SLNB has replaced the need for ALND. Several studies have shown that the use of SLNB in the axillary management of Paget disease patients is adequate and comparable to ALND in terms of diagnosis, recurrence, and survival.[27,28]

On the other hand, entirely neglecting the axilla in a patient with suspected Paget disease would be inappropriate. Theoretically, SLNB is usually reserved for patients with suspected invasive cancer, and Paget disease is occasionally not even associated with any underlying malignancy (6.8% in one recent study), let alone invasive disease.[20] Numerous studies, however, have demonstrated the association of axillary nodal involvement with Paget disease both with and without an associated palpable breast mass. In patients with a palpable mass associated with Paget disease, as many as 45% to 57% will have axillary nodal involvement; and in patients without a palpable mass or mammographic abnormality, 11% will have axillary nodal involvement.[23,28] Thus, some would recommend performing a SLNB for every patient with Paget disease of the breast.

Adjuvant Systemic Therapy

Use of adjuvant systemic therapy in Paget disease depends solely on the pathology of the underlying malignancy. In the absence of underlying malignancy, adjuvant therapy is not indicated. Tamoxifen, however, may be applicable in some of these cases for the prevention of cancer, but future trials will be needed in this area.

NECESSARY FUTURE STUDIES TO ADVANCE THE FIELD

There is still controversy in the pathogenesis of Paget disease, with credible lines of evidence in support of both the epidermotrophic theory and transformation theory. Further research in

TABLE 19-1 Patients Likely to Be Candidates for Breast-Conserving Therapy in Paget Disease

Absence of palpable mass
Absence of mammographic density
Absence of multicentric disease, if lesion is present
Absence of extensive or multicentric in situ carcinoma
Tumor appropriate distance from nipple–areola complex to allow complete excision with negative histologic margins

this area will better elucidate the mechanism of disease progression and may allow for physicians to further tailor treatment regimens. In addition, current use of mammography with physical exam can often underestimate the diffuse underlying malignant component associated with Paget disease, and further imaging modalities such as MRI may be needed to better identify these lesions. The use of tamoxifen in the management of Paget disease alone (in the absence of underlying malignancy) needs to be further investigated, as do other adjuvant therapies in this unique disease entity.

SUMMARY

Paget disease is an uncommon entity accounting for fewer than 5% of all diseases of the breast. Delay in diagnosis is common due to the fact that it resembles other benign entities such as eczema and dermatitis. Nonetheless, Paget disease should be managed as any other breast malignancy, since carcinoma is associated with this process in over 90% of cases. All patients with suspected Paget disease should undergo physical exam and mammography to detect underlying tumors. While the standard of treatment has been modified radical mastectomy and ALND, there are select cases in which a breast-conserving approach coupled with radiation therapy may be applied. Adjuvant systemic therapy needs to be tailored to the underlying malignancy, and prognosis is entirely based on the stage of this malignancy.

REFERENCES

1. Paget J. On the disease of the mammary areola preceding cancer of the mammary gland. *St Bartholomew Hosp Rep*. 1874;10:87-89
2. Caliskan M, Gatti G, Sosnovskikh I, et al. Paget's disease of the breast: the experience of the European institute of oncology and review of the literature. *Breast Cancer Res Treat*. 2008.
3. Kothari AS, Beechey-Newman N, Hamed H, et al. Paget disease of the nipple: a multifocal manifestation of higher-risk disease. *Cancer*. 2002;95:1-7.
4. Yim JH, Wick MR, Philpott GW, et al. Underlying pathology in mammary Paget's disease. *Ann Surg Oncol*. 1997;4:287-292.
5. Ascenso AC, Marques MS, Capitao-Mor M. Paget's disease of the nipple. Clinical and pathological review of 109 female patients. *Dermatologica*. 1985;170:170-179.
6. Chaudary MA, Millis RR, Lane EB, Miller NA. Paget's disease of the nipple: a ten year review including clinical, pathological, and immunohistochemical findings. *Breast Cancer Res Treat*. 1986;8:139-146.
7. Cohen C, Guarner J, DeRose PB. Mammary Paget's disease and associated carcinoma. An immunohistochemical study. *Arch Pathol Lab Med*. 1993;117:291-294.
8. de Potter CR, Eeckhout I, Schelfhout AM, et al. Keratinocyte induced chemotaxis in the pathogenesis of Paget's disease of the breast. *Histopathology*. 1994;24:349-356.
9. Schelfhout VR, Coene ED, Delaey B, et al. Pathogenesis of Paget's disease: epidermal heregulin-alpha, motility factor, and the HER receptor family. *J Natl Cancer Inst*. 2000;92:622-628.
10. Sagebiel RW. Ultrastructural observations on epidermal cells in Paget's disease of the breast. *Am J Pathol*. 1969;57:49-64.
11. Toker C. Further observations on Paget's disease of the nipple. *J Natl Cancer Inst*. 1967;38:79-92.
12. Ikeda DM, Helvie MA, Frank TS, et al. Paget disease of the nipple: radiologic-pathologic correlation. *Radiology*. 1993;189.89-94.
13. Sawyer RH, Asbury DL. Mammographic appearances in Paget's disease of the breast. *Clin Radiol*. 1994;49:185-188.
14. Dixon AR, Galea MH, Ellis IO, et al. Paget's disease of the nipple. *Br J Surg*. 1991;78:722-723.
15. Lagios MD, Margolin FR, Westdahl PR, Rose MR. Mammographically detected duct carcinoma in situ. Frequency of local recurrence following tylectomy and prognostic effect of nuclear grade on local recurrence. *Cancer*. 1989;63:618-624.
16. Bulens P, Vanuytsel L, Rijnders A, van der Schueren E. Breast conserving treatment of Paget's disease. *Radiother Oncol*. 1990;17:305-309.
17. Fourquet A, Campana F, Vielh P, et al. Paget's disease of the nipple without detectable breast tumor: conservative management with radiation therapy. *Int J Radiat Oncol Biol Phys*. 1987;13:1463-1465.
18. Pierce LJ, Haffty BG, Solin LJ, et al. The conservative management of Paget's disease of the breast with radiotherapy. *Cancer*. 1997;80:1065-1072.
19. Stockdale AD, Brierley JD, White WF, et al. Radiotherapy for Paget's disease of the nipple: a conservative alternative. *Lancet*. 1989;2:664-666.
20. Kawase K, Dimaio DJ, Tucker SL, et al. Paget's disease of the breast: there is a role for breast-conserving therapy. *Ann Surg Oncol*. 2005;12:391-397.
21. Marshall JK, Griffith KA, Haffty BG, et al. Conservative management of Paget disease of the breast with radiotherapy: 10- and 15-year results. *Cancer*. 2003;97:2142-2149.
22. Bijker N, Rutgers EJ, Duchateau L, et al. Breast-conserving therapy for Paget disease of the nipple: a prospective European Organization for Research and Treatment of Cancer study of 61 patients. *Cancer*. 2001;91:472-477.
23. Zakaria S, Pantvaidya G, Ghosh K, Degnim AC. Paget's disease of the breast: accuracy of preoperative assessment. *Breast Cancer Res Treat*. 2007;102:137-142.
24. Kollmorgen DR, Varanasi JS, Edge SB, Carson WE III. Paget's disease of the breast: a 33-year experience. *J Am Coll Surg*. 1998;187:171-177.
25. Amano G, Yajima M, Moroboshi Y, et al. MRI accurately depicts underlying DCIS in a patient with Paget's disease of the breast without palpable mass and mammography findings. *Jpn J Clin Oncol*. 2005;35:149-153.
26. Echevarria JJ, Lopez-Ruiz JA, Martin D, et al. Usefulness of MRI in detecting occult breast cancer associated with Paget's disease of the nipple-areolar complex. *Br J Radiol*. 2004;77:1036-1039.
27. Laronga C, Hasson D, Hoover S, et al. Paget's disease in the era of sentinel lymph node biopsy. *Am J Surg*. 2006;192:481-483.
28. Sukumvanich P, Bentrem DJ, Cody HS III, et al. The role of sentinel lymph node biopsy in Paget's disease of the breast. *Ann Surg Oncol*. 2007;14:1020-1023.

CHAPTER 20

Invasive Breast Carcinoma

David R. McCready,
Naomi A. Miller
Bruce J. Youngson

The term *invasive breast carcinoma* refers to a heterogeneous group of epithelial malignancies that originate in breast tissue and are characterized by their ability to invade adjacent normal tissue, and metastasize to body sites distant to the breast. The vast majority of these tumors are adenocarcinomas, and they are thought to arise from mammary epithelial cells in the terminal ductulo lobular unit (TDLU) of the breast.

The traditional histologic classification of invasive breast carcinoma provides prognostic and predictive information about the biological behavior of a particular tumor that supplements the other major prognostic indicators such as lymph node status, histologic tumor grade, tumor size, and lymphovascular invasion. In the future, it is likely that new technologies that allow for the rapid genetic and expression profiling of specific tumors will provide information that will aid and refine the existing traditional morphologic classification of tumors. The World Health Organization (WHO) classification of breast tumors is probably the most widely used morphologic classification schema today, and will be used throughout this chapter.[1]

GRADING OF INVASIVE CARCINOMA

The grade of invasive carcinoma is a reflection of the degree of differentiation of the carcinoma. It is generally recognized that histologic grading provides prognostically important information and should be routinely performed for all types of invasive carcinomas of the breast.

The most widely used grading system for invasive breast carcinoma was developed in Nottingham, United Kingdom[2] and is commonly referred to as the Nottingham Combined Histologic Grade.[3] This grading system is a modification of the Bloom and Richardson grading system. There are 3 components of the histologic grade for invasive breast carcinoma:

1. Degree of tubule (gland) formation
2. Degree of nuclear pleomorphism (atypia)
3. Mitotic count

Each component is given a numerical score of 1 to 3, with a score of 1 reflecting prominent gland formation, little nuclear atypia, and little mitotic activity, and 3 reflecting little or no gland formation, prominent nuclear atypia, and prominent mitotic activity. To obtain the overall grade, the score in each category is added to give a total out of 9 (Figs. 20-1 to 20-3):

Total 3 to 5: grade I
Total 6 or 7: grade II
Total 8 or 9: grade III

Grading is performed after evaluation of all sections of carcinoma, and incorporates assessment of tubule formation throughout the carcinoma, degree of nuclear atypia from the most atypical areas, and mitotic activity from mitotic count of 10 high-power-fields from the most mitotically active area. Any combination of scores from these 3 features may exist. The high-power pictures in Figures 20-1 to 20-3 are representative of the invasive carcinomas; it should be remembered that accurate grading cannot be assigned from a single high-power view such as these.

The authors of this updated grading schema provide detailed criteria for assessment of the components of the grade, such as size of microscope field for counting of mitoses. Strict adherence to these criteria is necessary to attempt to reduce subjectivity and optimize reproducibility.[3] Critics of grading stress its subjectivity,

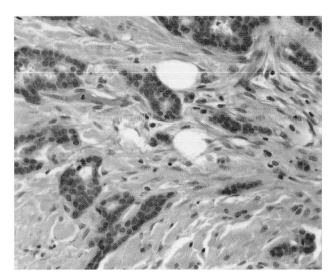

FIGURE 20-1 Invasive duct carcinoma, Nottingham histologic grade I/III (H&E stain, 400×). This invasive carcinoma demonstrates some tubule formation (2/3), mild nuclear atypia (1/3), and no mitotic activity (1/3). The cumulative score is 4/9.

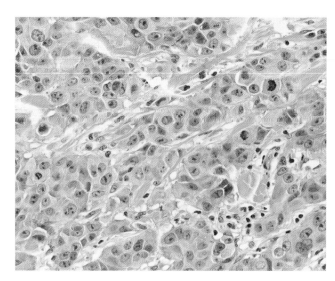

FIGURE 20-3 Invasive duct carcinoma, Nottingham histologic grade III/III (H&E stain, 400×). This invasive carcinoma demonstrates no tubule formation (3/3), marked nuclear atypia (3/3), and frequent mitoses (3/3). The cumulative score is 9/9.

and many studies on reproducibility exist with wide-ranging results; however, pathology studies have shown that concordance in grading ranging up to 80% to >90% can be attained by strict adherence to uniform criteria.[3,4] All references to grade within this chapter employ this grading scheme.

The proportion of carcinomas in the three grades (I, II, and III) is not equal, and the ratio of grade I:II:III is reported as 2:3:5.[5]

Certain factors are known to influence grading; these include tissue fixation, tumor heterogeneity, and size of sample.

Tissue Fixation

Optimal tissue handling with prompt fixation is essential for preservation of histologic detail and to optimize grading. A decline in the number of recognizable mitotic figures in tissue has been correlated with delays in fixation, with a 30% reduction in mitotic figures with 2-hour delay in fixation and a 50% reduction with 6-hour delay in fixation.[6] A reduction in mitotic count as a result of delayed fixation may result in underestimation of the grade of the invasive carcinoma. As formalin penetrates only a short distance into tissue (3.8 mm in 24 hours[5]), proper slicing of breast specimens to allow formalin penetration is essential. Submerging an intact specimen in formalin will not allow penetration of formalin into the tissue and will result in tissue changes secondary to delayed fixation.

Tumor Heterogeneity and Size of Sample

There may be variation in the appearance of a tumor in different areas, particularly in the amount of mitotic activity. Assessment of grade on a small tissue sample such as a core biopsy may therefore be different from that assessed on the excised specimen.

LYMPHOVASCULAR TUMOR EMBOLI IN INVASIVE BREAST CARCINOMA

Peritumoral lymphovascular tumor emboli are identified in approximately 15% of invasive breast carcinomas after tissue examination by H&E staining (Fig. 20-4). While most patients with lymphovascular tumor emboli will also have axillary lymph node metastases, approximately 5% to 10% of patients

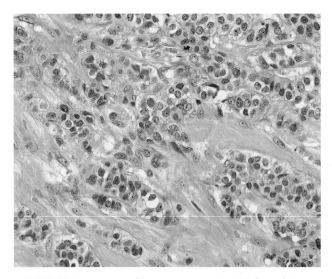

FIGURE 20-2 Invasive duct carcinoma, Nottingham histologic grade II/III (H&E stain, 400×). This invasive carcinoma demonstrates no tubule formation (3/3), moderate nuclear atypia (2/3), and occasional mitoses (1/3). The cumulative score is 6/9.

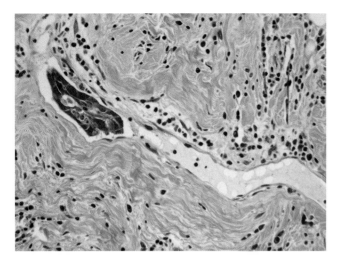

FIGURE 20-4 Tumor embolus in a lymphatic channel (H&E stain, 200×). An extratumoral endothelially lined vascular channel containing a carcinomatous tumor embolus and lymphatic fluid.

who are axillary lymph node-negative by H&E have peritumoral lymphovascular tumor emboli. Multiple studies have shown that peritumoral lymphovascular tumor emboli are prognostically unfavorable.[7-9] Care must be taken by the pathologist not to confuse spaces created by fixation retraction artifact around nests of tumor cells, with tumor in lymphovascular channels. Immunohistochemical stains for specific endothelial cell markers such as factor VIII, D2-40, or YLYVE-1 may assist in confirming the presence of lymphovascular channels, but we do not use these stains routinely, preferring to rely on routine H&E staining and strict morphologic criteria (ie, extratumoral location and convincing endothelial cell morphology) for this diagnosis.

Use of Immunohistochemistry in the Diagnosis of Invasive Breast Carcinoma

Some routine immunohistochemical stains can be of great practical utility in the interpretation of breast carcinoma in identifying the presence of invasive/microinvasive carcinoma and assisting in the determination of the type of invasive carcinoma.[10]

Identifying the Presence of Invasive/ Microinvasive Carcinoma

There are situations in which the surgical pathologist has difficulty either making a diagnosis of invasive carcinoma or ruling it out, when using routine hematoxylin and eosin staining alone. Reasons for this include a complex morphology in which a benign process or in situ carcinoma may be mistaken for invasive carcinoma (for example, radial scar versus tubular carcinoma, or in situ carcinoma within sclerosing adenosis versus invasive carcinoma), or the presence of fibrosis and inflammation obscuring histologic detail. Particular difficulty may be experienced with certain pathologic entities such as papillary lesions, and with

small biopsies such as cores in which the architectural context of the lesion is absent.

Immunohistochemical stains that are helpful in this context are markers of myoepithelium and epithelial cells. Myoepithelial cells are virtually always absent from around nests of invasive carcinoma, and present around benign and in situ lesions. Thus the absence of myoepithelium is very helpful in confirming suspected invasive carcinoma, and in contrast, its presence supports a lesion being either benign or in situ carcinoma. Commonly used myoepithelial markers include smooth muscle myosin heavy chain, calponin, smooth muscle actin, and P63. Epithelial markers such as LMWK and CK7 stain both benign and malignant epithelium and are very useful in demonstrating small numbers of invasive carcinoma cells obscured by inflammation, or in identifying small bland cells as being carcinoma, for example, with invasive lobular carcinoma.

Determining the Type of Invasive Carcinoma

E-Cadherin to Confirm Invasive Lobular Carcinoma. E-cadherin is an epithelial specific cell–cell adhesion molecule[11] encoded by a gene on chromosome 16q22.[11] E-cadherin can be demonstrated in tissue by staining with anti–E-cadherin antibodies, and in the normal breast there is strong staining of the cell membranes of ducts and lobules.[11] Ductal and lobular types of invasive carcinoma show different expression with anti–E-cadherin antibodies, with most invasive duct carcinomas showing strong membrane staining and most lobular carcinomas showing complete loss of membrane staining.[11]

Types of Keratins. Cytokeratins are intermediate filaments present in all epithelial and some nonepithelial cells. The type of cytokeratin may differ in carcinomas from different sites of origin, and in different morphologic patterns from the same tumor site. There is increasing interest in luminal- and basal-type cytokeratins in breast carcinoma. The following are luminal-type cytokeratins: CK7, CK8, CK18, and CK19. The following are basal-type cytokeratins: CK5/6, CK14, and CK17.[12]

Gene Expression in the Classification of Breast Carcinoma

Gene expression studies have revealed that breast carcinoma can be classified based on patterns of gene expression, and that this classification has clinical relevance.

Analysis of cDNA microarrays of samples of breast carcinoma by hierarchical clustering of patterns of gene expression has shown that breast carcinoma can be classified into groups based on profiles of gene expression.[13-15] Two main subsets have been identified, an estrogen receptor (ER)-positive group characterized by higher expression of a panel of genes typically expressed by breast luminal cells (luminal cancer) and an ER-negative group that encompasses 3 subgroups: one group overexpressing ERBB2 (HER-2), one expressing genes characteristic of breast basal/myoepithelial cells (basal or basal-like cancer), and one with gene expression profile similar to normal breast tissue (normal breast-like).[13-16] The ER-positive group is further subdivided into 2 or 3 subgroups—Luminal A, B, C in some classifications[14,15]; however, others have not defined 3 groups.[16] This classification system has been found to have prognostic significance. Most studies show the best prognosis is in the luminal A group and the worst prognosis in the HER-2 and basal groups. The biologic significance of the normal breast-like group is not yet clear.[16]

Breast carcinomas do not all fit neatly into this classification: up to 50% of HER-2–positive tumors are hormone receptor–positive and up to 17% of hormone receptor–positive tumors are HER-2–positive.[16]

Basal, Basal-Like Breast Carcinoma

Use of the terminology "basal" and "basal-like" is not consistent; sometimes these terms are used interchangeably in the literature,[17] while at other times the term "basal" is used to describe carcinoma identified by gene expression analysis studies, and "basal-like" or "with basal phenotype" to describe carcinomas with a particular immunostaining profile.

Expression of genes usually found in normal basal/myoepithelial cells of the breast remains the gold standard for identification of the basal type of breast carcinoma.[17] As defined by gene microarray analysis, this accounts for up to 15% of breast cancer, often occurs in younger patients, is more frequent in African American women, and frequently shows lack of expression of hormone receptors and HER-2.[17]

These carcinomas usually express high-molecular-weight "basal" cytokeratins CK5/6, CK14, and CK17. Demonstration of staining with basal cytokeratins may be used as a surrogate for gene expression analysis to identify this type of carcinoma. There is no consensus as to what stain or stains should be used; however, the commonly used immunostains are cytokeratin 14 either alone or in combination with CK 5/6, ER, HER-2.[16-18] Basal-like carcinoma is positive with cytokeratins 5/6 and 14 and usually negative with ER and HER-2.

Basal-like breast cancers are characterized by these morphologic features: high histologic grade with high mitotic index, pushing margin, central necrosis, metaplastic elements (squamous or spindle), and lymphocytic infiltrate.[17,18] Several of these morphologic features are present in metaplastic and medullary types of invasive carcinoma, and it has been shown that >90% of metaplastic breast carcinomas and most medullary carcinomas show a basal-like phenotype.[17]

Basal-like breast cancers have been shown to have a more aggressive clinical behavior than non–basal-like breast cancers in some studies; however, other studies do not show a poorer outcome relative to either ER-negative non–basal-like cancer or grade-matched non–basal-like cancers.[17] Some studies show basal-like breast cancers have a different pattern of metastatic spread, spreading to axillary nodes and bone less frequently, and showing hematogenous spread to brain and lung more frequently than the non-basal type.[17,18]

Breast carcinoma occurring in the BRCA1 germline mutation carrier, especially diagnosed before age 50, often has morphologic and immunostaining features similar to those described in basal-like breast cancer and is triple negative (ER, [progesterone receptor] PR, HER-2 negative).[17]

Triple-Negative Breast Carcinoma

Triple-negative breast carcinomas account for 10% to 17% of breast carcinomas, occur more frequently in younger patients (< 50), are more prevalent in African American women, and often present as interval cancers[17] in breast-screening programs. These carcinomas are mainly high-grade invasive duct carcinoma of no special type, metaplastic carcinoma, and medullary carcinomas.[17]

There is overlap between triple-negative and basal breast cancers. The groups are not the same[17] as expression of at least one of ER, PR, and HER-2 is reported in 15% to 54% of basal-like breast cancers identified by microarray-based expression analysis. Furthermore, the triple-negative subgroup is not homogeneous; it includes the subset of breast cancer with "normal" gene expression pattern, which has a better prognosis than the basal-cell type.[17]

INVASIVE BREAST CARCINOMA—USUAL OR COMMON TYPES

Invasive Ductal Carcinoma of No Special Type/Not Otherwise Specified Type

Clinical Features

Invasive breast carcinoma of the "no special type" (NST) or "not otherwise specified" (NOS) variety makes up the largest single category of invasive breast carcinomas, accounting for between 47% and 75% of all invasive breast cancers, depending on the series.[19,20] These tumors may present as a clinical lump, or be clinically inapparent and detected by a variety of imaging techniques including mammography, ultrasonography, or magnetic resonance imaging. The designation of a particular invasive mammary carcinoma as NST/NOS type is one of exclusion, and does not refer to a particular type of invasive ductal carcinoma but rather to an invasive ductal carcinoma that cannot be classified histologically as a particular special type of invasive ductal carcinoma based on current morphologic classification schemes (ie. the subtypes described later in the chapter). As such, NST tumors are a heterogeneous group of carcinomas of varying histologies and grades. The WHO definition of an NST tumor requires a nonspecial-type pattern to be present in greater than 50% of the tumor after a thorough examination of representative histologic sections. If an NST pattern is present in 10% to 49% of the tumor, the carcinoma is classified as mixed NST and special type. For an invasive carcinoma to classify as a special-type tumor, at least 90% of the tumor must show the appropriate special-type histomorphology. NST tumors appear to make up a lower proportion (approximately 40%) of small, screen-detected invasive carcinomas, and there may be a slightly increased frequency of NST tumors below the age of 35 years compared with older patients, who have an increased proportion of lobular and other special-type carcinomas.[21]

Gross and Microscopic Pathologic Findings

Generally, NST carcinomas form a solid, gray-white nodular mass that may be well circumscribed or have ill-defined, infiltrative borders on cut section. The descriptive terms "scirrhous" or "stellate" carcinoma refer to a carcinoma with extensive fibro-elastosis that manifests grossly as firm yellow-white streaks on cut section.

Scirrhous carcinomas demonstrate a central solid mass that radiates irregularly into the surrounding fatty breast tissue. Tumor necrosis may be found in large, rapidly growing tumors that are outgrowing their blood supply, and this necrosis grossly presents as soft, white chalky areas. Gross cystic degeneration in NST tumors is rare.

The size of these tumors varies greatly, ranging from a few millimeters to over 10 centimeters; on average, the size of these tumors is approximately 2 cm in maximal dimension.

Microscopically, NST invasive ductal carcinoma is characterized by a growth of malignant epithelial cells organized into cohesive cords, nests, sheets, and tubules that infiltrate breast stroma in a disorganized and irregular fashion. The stroma within a particular tumor may be densely fibrotic or minimal in amount. The tumor cells of NST tumors show a varying degree of cytologic atypia, and variable amounts of inflammation may be present within/around the tumor mass. Immunostaining for myoepithelial cells (ie, with smooth-muscle myosin heavy-chain, calponin, or P63) or basement membrane (collagen IV) is often a useful adjunctive diagnostic technique to confirm the lack of a myoepithelial cell layer or basement membrane, a finding critical to the diagnosis of stromal invasion. Ductal carcinoma in situ (DCIS) is found in approximately 80% of cases either within or around the tumor mass, and is usually of intermediate or high grade.[22] Approximately 70% to 80% of NST tumors are ER positive, 60% PR positive, and 15% to 30% are HER-2/neu positive.

Prognosis and Treatment

The prognosis of a particular NST tumor is dependent on the traditional prognostic indicators such as size, tumor grade, lymphovascular invasion, and lymph node status. Overall, NST tumors show a 35% to 50% 10-year survival without adjuvant treatments. Following surgical excision with clear margins, treatment specifics (ie, postoperative radiation and chemotherapy) are determined by the traditional prognostic indicators noted earlier, as well as ER, PR, and HER-2/neu status of the tumor.

■ Invasive Lobular Carcinoma

Clinical Features

Invasive lobular carcinoma is the second most common type of invasive breast carcinoma after NST invasive duct carcinoma. The reported frequency is between 5% and 15%.[23,24] Factors that contribute to this range include the wide range of morphologic features represented by invasive lobular carcinoma and differing criteria used for diagnosis, and the impact of mammographic screening and hormonal therapy. The incidence of invasive lobular carcinoma increased over the time period 1987 to 1999 while the incidence of invasive duct carcinoma remained stable. This increase occurred at a time of increased use of combined replacement hormonal therapy and it is postulated that the increased incidence of invasive lobular carcinoma

is associated with this use.[25] An increased proportion of lobular carcinoma has been reported in populations at higher risk of breast cancer.[26]

Several morphologic patterns of invasive lobular carcinoma are recognized, with the most common type termed the classic type. Other types are termed variants of invasive lobular carcinoma and include mixed, solid, alveolar, signet ring, histiocytoid, tubulolobular, and pleomorphic carcinoma. The types are differentiated based on histologic morphology, and some subtypes appear to be associated with differences in clinical outcome.

Patients with invasive lobular carcinoma tend to be slightly older than those with nonlobular invasive carcinoma (mean age reported as 57 years[23] and 64 years[27]). On mammography, architectural distortion is more common and microcalcification less common with invasive lobular carcinoma compared to invasive duct carcinoma.[1]

Gross and Microscopic Pathologic Findings

Invasive lobular carcinoma tends to be larger at diagnosis than nonlobular invasive carcinoma,[23] with 19% of invasive lobular carcinoma larger than 5 cm in one series.[23] Increasing tumor size has been correlated with increasing grade.[27] The gross appearance may be indistinguishable from invasive duct carcinoma with formation of a stellate mass, or may be more ill defined resulting in an area of vague induration that is difficult to delineate on gross examination. In the latter situation the invasive carcinoma may be much more extensive on microscopic examination than anticipated from gross examination.

A number of morphologic features distinguish invasive lobular from invasive duct carcinoma on microscopic examination; however, it is the combination of features that allows this distinction, as individually none of these features are specific for a lobular type in routine stains.[28] Some invasive carcinomas (approximately 3-4%[28]) have features indeterminate between ductal and lobular type on routine stains. To accommodate this difficulty in classification, some pathologists have used terms such as "invasive carcinoma with both ductal and lobular features." This is in addition to, and distinct from, mixed type of invasive carcinomas with features that can be identified as ductal in type in some areas and lobular in type in other areas—estimated to be 5% of invasive carcinoma.[1] E-cadherin immunostaining is proving increasingly helpful in assigning a morphologic type since the majority of invasive lobular carcinomas do not show cytoplasmic membrane staining while invasive ductal carcinomas do.[11,27]

To qualify as an invasive lobular carcinoma, more than 90% of the carcinoma must show one of more patterns of lobular carcinoma, in keeping with the classification of other types of invasive mammary carcinoma. To qualify for a particular subtype there are not uniformly agreed-upon criteria, although an 80% threshold has been suggested (>80% of a particular pattern required for a particular subtype designation, if <80% considered mixed type).[29]

The most common subtypes of invasive lobular carcinoma are classical and mixed subtypes, representing 55% and 34% of a series of invasive lobular carcinoma, respectively.[24]

Some components of the grading scheme appear less applicable to invasive lobular carcinoma than nonlobular since the majority of invasive lobular carcinomas have a solid growth pattern and little mitotic activity.[24] It is, however, recommended that invasive lobular carcinoma is graded using the same grading scheme as nonlobular carcinoma. The majority of invasive lobular carcinomas are grade II (76%[7]) with a small proportion being grade I or III (12% each[24]). Tubulolobular carcinoma and some classic invasive lobular carcinoma are grade I, pleomorphic invasive lobular carcinoma is grade II or III, and other classic invasive lobular carcinoma and variants are grade II. Invasive lobular carcinoma has been reported to be associated with an increased risk of multicentricity and bilaterality; however, some studies, both clinical and imaging, have not shown a significant difference in the incidence of multicentricity and bilaterality between invasive lobular carcinoma and invasive duct carcinoma.[1,23] Invasive lobular carcinoma is more frequently ER positive than nonlobular carcinomas; the positivity rate ranges from 70% to 100%.[1,27] PR positivity is similar to invasive duct carcinoma, in some reports positive in 60% to 70% of cases[1]; however, in some series invasive lobular carcinoma is more frequently PR positive than invasive duct carcinoma (positive in 85-90%[27]). HER-2 protein overexpression is less likely than with invasive duct carcinoma, with some reported series of invasive lobular carcinoma entirely negative (0% of 50 cases[27]); however, HER-2 protein overexpression have been reported in 81% of 38 cases of pleomorphic variant of invasive lobular carcinoma.[30]

Classic Invasive Lobular Carcinoma.

Classic invasive lobular carcinoma is the most common type of invasive lobular carcinoma. The tumor cells are small, uniform, and monotonous and infiltrate in a dispersed, noncohesive manner (Fig. 20-5). The cells often show a linear growth pattern (referred to as "single file") and grow around structures in concentric lines of cells referred to as a "targetoid" growth pattern. The cells may

percolate into fatty tissue between fat cells without associated stromal fibrosis. This growth pattern may result in the invasive carcinoma being more extensive than grossly estimated.

Small numbers of invasive tumor cells, particularly if admixed with lymphocytes or reactive changes, may easily be overlooked. These cells are keratin positive, which can be very helpful both to identify the existence of these cells and confirm that these are epithelial in nature.

Pleomorphic Variant of Invasive Lobular Carcinoma.

The tumor cells have the pattern of infiltration of classic lobular carcinoma but are larger, more pleomorphic, and have a tendency to aggregate, with features that may overlap with invasive ductal carcinoma (Fig. 20-6).[30,31] Apocrine features may occur in invasive lobular carcinoma; this tends to be present in the pleomorphic variant,[31] and these cells will be GCDFP-15 positive. Histiocytic features are also described in this variant.[31]

There are no specific criteria for how large or atypical the tumor cells should be to qualify for this type, which will account for some variability in diagnosis. In general, the degree of mitotic activity identified is greater than with classic type. The use of E-cadherin stain allows identification of this as lobular type, which may otherwise have been interpreted as ductal type.

Tubulolobular Variant of Invasive Lobular Carcinoma.

The tubulolobular variant of invasive lobular carcinoma is a rare variant with features of both tubular and lobular carcinoma. The pattern of infiltration is reminiscent of invasive lobular carcinoma with an infiltrative growth pattern and cells arranged in single file or in a targetoid growth pattern; however, the tumor cells also form small cohesive cell groups and microtubules.[32] This has traditionally been classified as a variant of invasive lobular carcinoma; however, recently this type of invasive carcinoma has been found to show a ductal staining pattern

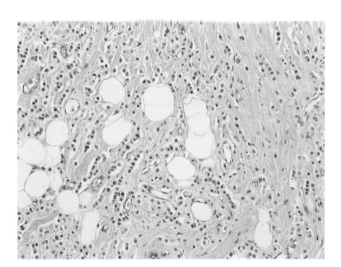

FIGURE 20-5 Invasive lobular carcinoma, classic type (H&E stain, 200×). The malignant cells are small and bland. The cells do not form cohesive cell groups; in areas the cells are in linear arrangement (single file). In one area tumor cells can be seen extending into fat.

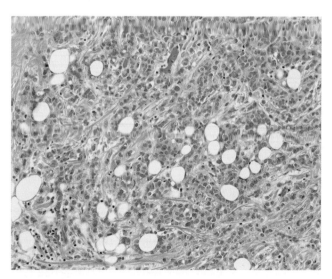

FIGURE 20-6 Invasive lobular carcinoma, pleomorphic type (H&E stain, 200×). In contrast to Figure 20-5, the tumor cells are more cohesive, forming small cell groups, and are larger with more nuclear variability and atypia.

with E-cadherin stain.[32] Further studies will clarify if this should continue to be considered a variant of invasive lobular carcinoma or should be reclassified.[1]

Signet Ring Cell Carcinoma.

The presence of some signet ring cells is frequent in forms of invasive lobular carcinoma, but extensive signet ring formation is much less frequent, representing 0.1% to 0.3% of invasive breast carcinoma.[28]

Solid and Alveolar Variants.

In the solid pattern the tumor cells are arranged in loose sheets, while in the alveolar pattern the tumor cells are in small, circumscribed aggregates of 20 or more cells and may simulate in situ lobular carcinoma.

Prognosis

The prognosis for invasive lobular carcinoma has been reported as worse, better, or the same as for invasive duct carcinoma.[23] The prognostic value associated with tumor stage and lymph node status is applicable with invasive lobular carcinoma,[23] but some have found less prognostic value with grade for invasive lobular carcinoma than with nonlobular types,[23] possibly due to difficulty applying the grading scheme. With strict adherence to the criteria for grading, others have found histologic grade to be of independent prognostic value.[24]

The pleomorphic variant of invasive lobular carcinoma is associated with more aggressive clinical behavior than the classic type.[31]

Other Comments

Lymphoma is in the differential diagnosis of a breast mass composed of an infiltrate of noncohesive tumor cells. Staining with immunostains for keratin and lack of staining with lymphoid markers will allow this distinction.

Metastatic lobular carcinoma within lymph nodes is less easily recognizable than metastatic ductal carcinoma, as the cells may resemble histiocytes and be misinterpreted as a reactive change. Identification of metastatic lobular carcinoma at frozen section may be particularly difficult. Keratin immunostains may be very helpful in confirming metastatic lobular carcinoma in lymph node.

Tubular Carcinoma

Clinical Features

Tubular carcinoma is a special type of invasive duct carcinoma, which is well differentiated and has a favorable prognosis.

Overall, tubular carcinoma accounts for < 2% of invasive breast cancer.[1] The proportion of invasive carcinomas of this type in different series is influenced both by the criteria used for histologic diagnosis and also the method of detection of the carcinoma. Tubular carcinoma is more common in cancers detected by mammographic screening than detected clinically, with the proportion of screen-detected cancers that are tubular carcinomas ranging from 9% to 19%.[33] The majority of tubular carcinomas are detected mammographically[34] as either a small spiculated mass or parenchymal deformity.[35] Patients with tubular carcinoma are similar in age to patients with well-differentiated (grade I) invasive duct carcinoma.[36,37]

Gross and Microscopic Pathologic Findings

The majority of tubular carcinomas are 1 cm or less in maximum dimension.[1,33,36] The mean dimension of tubular carcinoma has not changed over time; however, the mean dimension of invasive duct carcinomas has decreased over time,[36] and currently the size of tubular carcinomas is similar to well-differentiated (grade I) invasive duct carcinoma.[36]

There are no distinguishing characteristics on gross examination.

On microscopic examination, the invasive carcinoma is composed of glands (tubules) within stroma that is cellular and fibroblastic. The glands are open, irregular, and angulate in shape, and are lined by a single layer of epithelial cells, which may have protrusions into the lumen known as "apical snouts." The tumor cells are small and uniform, without high-grade nuclear features, and mitoses are unusual (Fig. 20-7).

All tubular carcinomas are grade I invasive carcinomas, but the reverse is not so (not all grade I invasive carcinomas are tubular). Tubular carcinoma is differentiated from grade I invasive duct carcinoma mainly by the extent of tubule formation; there has not been uniformity in the proportion of carcinoma required to form tubular structures for a diagnosis of tubular carcinoma, which has ranged from at least 75% to 100%.[1,37] The dominant current view is that at least 90% of the invasive carcinoma must form tubules to qualify for the designation of pure tubular carcinoma.[1,3,37] Invasive carcinoma that is >50% tubular and the remainder cribriform is also classified as pure tubular carcinoma.[33] Invasive carcinoma that is 50% to 90% tubular and the remainder of non-cribriform type is classified as mixed type of invasive carcinoma.[1,33] Recent attempts have been made to refine the criteria for diagnosis by further evaluating tubule formation and also nuclear atypia and mitotic activity.[36,38]

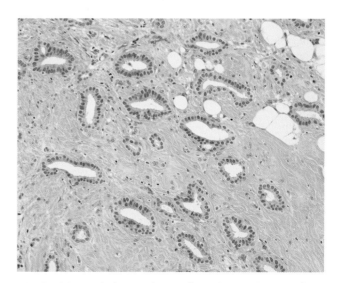

FIGURE 20-7 Tubular carcinoma (invasive carcinoma of tubular type) (H&E stain, 200×). The malignant cells are very bland in appearance and form well-defined glands. In some areas, the inner (luminal) surface of the glands have protrusions—"apical snouts." The stroma shows some increased cellularity.

Tubular carcinoma has been associated with a high risk of multicentricity (56%) and bilaterality (38%).[39] The majority of tubular carcinomas are ER and PR positive, and negative for HER-2 protein over expression.[1,39] The differential diagnosis of tubular carcinoma includes benign entities such as sclerosing adenosis and radial scar, and other forms of invasive carcinoma, particularly grade I invasive duct carcinoma of no special type, and also tubulolobular carcinoma. Differentiation from benign entities may be particularly challenging on core biopsies and is greatly assisted by the use of immunohistochemical stains for myoepithelium.

Prognosis

When uniform criteria for diagnosis are used, in comparison with well-differentiated (grade I) invasive duct carcinoma, patients with tubular carcinoma have a lower proportion of axillary node involvement at presentation (12.9% compared to 23.9%), a statistically significant lower rate of local recurrence, and a trend to lower rate of systemic relapse.[37] The more restrictive the diagnostic criteria, the better the clinical outcome associated with a diagnosis of tubular carcinoma, with 100% 10-year disease-free survival reported in one series using the most restrictive diagnostic criteria.[36]

◼ Mucinous (Colloid) Carcinoma

Mucinous carcinomas (also referred to as colloid carcinoma, gelatinous carcinoma, mucous carcinoma, or mucoid carcinoma) contain "large amounts of extracellular epithelial mucous sufficient to be visible grossly, and recognizable microscopically, surrounding and within tumor cells."[1] The tumor cells within this mucinous material must also demonstrate a low nuclear grade. As noted previously, by current WHO criteria, at least 90% of tumor must show this histomorphology to be classified as a pure mucinous carcinoma. Tumors that show mucinous differentiation in 50% to 90% of the tumor and/or high-grade nuclear cytology are classified as mixed NST/mucinous tumors, or NST tumors showing mucinous features, a diagnosis that does not connote an improved prognosis as does a pure mucinous carcinoma.

Clinical Features

Pure mucinous carcinomas are relatively uncommon, accounting for approximately 2% of invasive ductal carcinomas when strict diagnostic criteria are applied.[40] Most studies have noted a higher mean age for women with mucinous carcinoma as compared to patients with nonmucinous carcinoma. Mucinous carcinoma accounts for about 7% of carcinomas in women 75 years or older and only approximately 1% of women younger than 35 years of age.[41] The majority of mucinous carcinomas present as a breast mass with mammographically detected microcalcifications occurring in a minority (ie, approximately 40%) of the tumors.[42]

Gross and Microscopic Features

Grossly, these tumors tend to be relatively well circumscribed and lobulated, with a glistening, mucoid-appearing cut surface. Histologically, the tumor consists of small clusters, nests, and acini of cytologically low-grade malignant epithelial cells floating within lakes of mucin (Fig. 20-8). The mucous is composed of both neutral and acidic mucopolysaccharides. The tumor cells have granular eosinophilic and hyaline cytoplasm, and intracellular mucin may be identified. Argyrophilia (ie, neuroendocrine differentiation) has been identified in up to 25% of mucinous carcinoma on histochemical or immunohistochemical staining, and electron microscopy, but this finding appears to be of no prognostic significance.[43] An associated ductal carcinoma in situ component is found in 60% to 75% of cases.[44] Immunohistochemical studies have shown that almost 90% of mucinous carcinomas are positive for ER,[45] while they tend to be negative for HER-2/neu.

Prognosis and Treatment

Relative to stage-matched NST invasive ductal carcinoma, mucinous carcinoma has a relatively favorable prognosis. These tumors tend to be axillary lymph-node negative, with the reported frequency of axillary node positivity in series reported in the past 2 decades ranging from 0% to 29%.[46] The 15-year disease-free survival rates have been cited in the range of 85% for pure mucinous carcinoma, compared to 63% for invasive ductal carcinomas NST with a mucinous component.[47]

◼ Metaplastic Carcinoma

Metaplasia is the process by which one adult cell type changes into another adult cell type that is not normally present within that tissue. As invasive ductal carcinoma arises from the glandular epithelium of the breast, it usually shows the morphologic features of an adenocarcinoma. In less than 5% of invasive breast carcinomas, some or all of the malignant cells exhibit a nonepithelial or nonglandular growth pattern.[48]

The term "metaplastic carcinoma" refers to this uncommon, heterogenous group of breast carcinomas, which show a mixed, biphasic (ie, glandular and nonglandular) morphology, or a

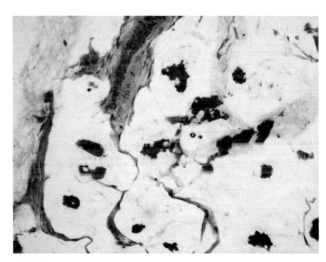

FIGURE 20-8 Mucinous (colloid) carcinoma (H&E stain, 100×). Clusters of cytologically low-grade malignant epithelial cells floating in lakes of abundant mucin.

pure nonglandular morphology with immunohistochemical staining evidence of epithelial differentiation.

Traditionally, metaplastic carcinomas have been divided into 2 groups, those with squamous differentiation and those with pseudosarcomatous differentiation; however, some tumors exhibit both types of differentiation. The metaplastic differentiation may be quite focal or extensively present within an individual tumor, and does not require the 90% or more metaplastic subtype morphology that other special-type carcinomas require for diagnosis.

Squamous differentiation is the most frequent type of metaplasia that has been observed in these lesions, but a variety of mesenchymal differentiation may also be present.

Due to their relative rarity, the diversity of the type and amount of metaplasia that may be present, and a lack of consensus as to terminology, a clinically meaningful pathologic classification system for this group of tumors has proven to be somewhat elusive. The following subclassification of metaplastic breast carcinoma is based largely on morphology and the empiric findings that the specific type of metaplasia present within a tumor influences its biological behavior.

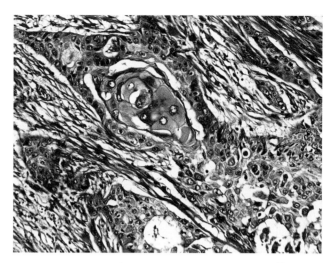

FIGURE 20-9 Metaplastic carcinoma, squamous cell type (H&E stain, 100×). Malignant ductal epithelium exhibiting focal squamous metaplasia. The squamous cells have "glassy" eosinophilic cytoplasm with intercellular bridges.

Metaplastic Carcinoma, Squamous Cell Type

Clinical Features. There are no clinical features that are specific for metaplastic squamous cell carcinoma of the breast. The age at diagnosis is similar to the age at diagnosis of breast carcinoma generally, and ranges from 31 to 83 years.[49] A diagnosis of squamous metaplastic breast carcinoma requires exclusion of cutaneous origin and metastasis from other primary sites, which may include lung, uterine cervix, and urinary bladder. Invasion into the skin and chest wall may make differentiation of secondary skin involvement by a primary breast carcinoma from a carcinoma of cutaneous origin difficult, and requires clinicopathologic correlation. While there are no pathognomonic imaging findings, calcifications may be present associated with tumor necrosis, and cystic degeneration may occur.

Gross and Microscopic Features. Squamous carcinomas tend to be somewhat larger on presentation than other types of breast carcinoma, with nearly half of the tumors being 5 cm or more in maximal dimension.[50] These tumors often show central cystic degeneration with necrosis and hemorrhage. Histologically, these lesions are not different from squamous cell carcinomas of other primary sites, most being moderately differentiated (Fig. 20-9). A spindle-cell component may be present that stains positively for either high- or low-molecular-weight keratins. There may be an associated ductal carcinoma in situ component present that helps confirm the primary nature of the tumor. Most tumors have been reported to be ER negative.[49,51]

Prognosis and Treatment. Overall, the prognosis of mammary squamous carcinoma does not appear to be different from stage-matched, NST breast carcinomas[52]; that is, the presence of squamous metaplasia does not appear to significantly influence prognosis.

Metaplastic Carcinoma, Low-Grade Adenosquamous Carcinoma Type

Clinical Features. The mean age at presentation in the largest series yet published[51] was 54 years, with a range of 33 to 88 years. All patients presented with a palpable mass. The average size of the tumors was 2.5 cm.

Gross and Microscopic Features. The tumors tended to be irregular, tan or pale-yellow mass lesions that were often poorly circumscribed with a stellate, infiltrative character. Histologically, the tumors are composed of infiltrating, compressed, often comma-shaped glandular structures with varying proportions of squamous and glandular elements that sometimes merge into a single structure. The lumina of these structures may contain eosinophilic material and keratinous debris associated with squamous differentiation. The tumor cells are bland with little cytologic atypia and infrequent mitoses. The epithelial components of this neoplasm are typically widely separated by a cellular collagenous stroma that may have an edematous appearance and have a mild lymphocytic infiltrate. An association with sclerosing/papillary lesions and adenomyoepithelioma has been noted. These tumors tend to show no ER or PR positivity. HER-2/neu positivity has been described in less than half of the cases.

Prognosis and Treatment. Low-grade adenosquamous carcinoma is considered to have a relatively good prognosis compared to NST tumors, with a low rate of lymph node and/or distant metastases noted.[53]

Metaplastic Carcinoma, Mixed Spindle Cell and Monophasic Spindle Cell Type

Clinical features. This type of metaplastic carcinoma presents as a mass lesion and occurs mainly in postmenopausal females.

Gross and Microscopic Features. These tumors tend to be fairly large, solid, and have a gritty, gray-white appearance, sometimes with foci of necrosis. In Fletcher's series of 29 cases, the tumor size ranged from 1.5 to 15 cm, with a median size of 4.0 cm.[54] The tumors may be grossly circumscribed or poorly defined and infiltrative with areas of cystic degeneration/necrosis. The nuclear grade of the spindle cells may be variable, ranging from low-grade to high-grade. The spindle cells tend to be arranged in interlacing fascicles sometimes with a storiform appearance (Figs. 20-10 and 20-11). A component of invasive ductal carcinoma of NST type, or squamous cell carcinoma may be present, and DCIS is identified in a minority of cases. Immunohistochemical staining is pivotal in establishing the epithelial nature of the spindle cells, and may require the use of a wide range of keratin stains (ie, both high- and low-molecular-weight keratins), and often coexpression of vimentin or other mesenchymal markers may be seen. The degree of keratin positivity in the spindle cells ranges from rare scattered cells to diffuse staining of the spindle cells.

Immunohistochemical evidence suggesting myoepithelial differentiation has also been noted. These tumors tend to be negative for ER, PR, and HER-2/neu.

Prognosis and Treatment. Most patients with spindle-cell metaplastic carcinoma have been treated with mastectomy, usually with axillary dissection. Several studies have noted a decreased propensity for axillary lymph node metastases for metaplastic carcinomas in which the spindle-cell component predominates over the epithelial component when compared with usual adenocarcinoma of the breast, and some authors have questioned the utility of axillary lymph node dissection in

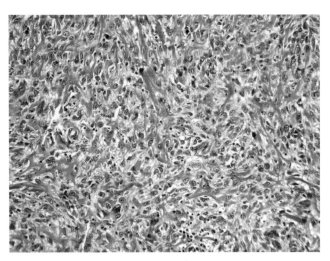

FIGURE 20-11 Metaplastic carcinoma, pure spindle-cell type (H&E stain, 100×). This breast carcinoma consists virtually entirely of malignant spindle cells, which exhibit areas of keratin positivity by immunohistochemistry.

patients without clinical lymphadenopathy.[54,55] Overall, the presence of extensive spindle cell metaplasia may have an adverse influence on prognosis. Spindle-cell metaplastic carcinomas appear to behave aggressively and have a propensity for pulmonary and other visceral metastases.[54,55] The effect of radiation and adjuvant chemotherapy on metaplastic carcinoma has not been determined,[56] but there is no evidence that they would behave differently than other breast cancers with adjuvant treatment.

Metaplastic Carcinoma, Mixed Epithelial Mesenchymal Type

Clinical Features. The patients tend to be postmenopausal and present with a palpable mass.

Gross and Microscopic Features. This group of tumors includes invasive ductal carcinomas with heterologous differentiation that may include a variety of mesenchymal elements such as chondrosarcoma, osteosarcoma, liposarcoma, rhabdosarcoma, fibrosarcoma, or angiosarcoma (Fig. 20-12). Once again, epithelial differentiation may be focal, and require confirmatory immunohistochemical staining. The presence of a DCIS component is helpful in confirming the diagnosis of metaplastic carcinoma. ER, PR, and HER-2/neu tend to be negative.

Prognosis and Treatment. It appears that heterologous metaplasia does not seem to have negative impact on prognosis, with these tumors appearing to behave like a high-grade invasive ductal carcinoma. Most patients in the literature have been treated with mastectomy and axillary dissection, but this diagnosis should not dissuade one from lumpectomy and sentinel lymph node biopsy if caught at an early stage. The effect of radiation and adjuvant chemotherapy on metaplastic carcinoma has not been determined.[56]

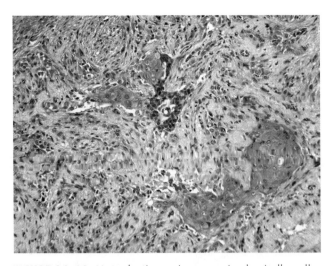

FIGURE 20-10 Metaplastic carcinoma, mixed spindle cell and squamous type (H&E stain, 100×). This tumor demonstrates malignant spindle cells (which showed keratin positivity by immunohistochemistry) with interspersed areas of squamous differentiation. A focus of ductal epithelial differentiation that is merging with a focus of squamous metaplasia is noted centrally.

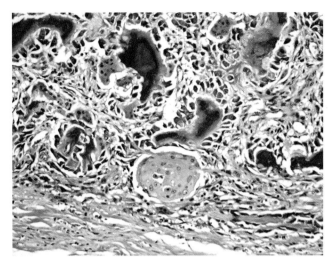

FIGURE 20-12 Metaplastic carcinoma, mixed epithelial/ mesenchymal type (H&E stain, 100×). This invasive breast carcinoma demonstrates both osteosarcomatous differentiation (a malignant spindle-cell proliferation with osteoid and bony trabeculae formation) and focal squamous metaplasia (a focus of squamous metaplasia is seen in the mid-central portion of the photograph).

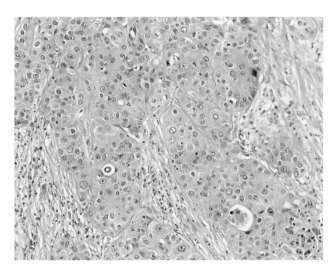

FIGURE 20-13 Apocrine carcinoma (invasive carcinoma of apocrine type) (H&E stain, 200×). The tumor cells resemble apocrine cells—that is, relative to the usual invasive duct carcinoma the tumor cells are larger, the cytoplasm is more abundant and pinker, and the nuclei are larger with more prominent nucleoli.

INVASIVE BREAST CARCINOMA—UNCOMMON TYPES

Invasive Apocrine Carcinoma

Clinical Features

Invasive apocrine carcinoma is classified as a special type of invasive carcinoma in the WHO classification,[1] although some consider this a variant of invasive duct carcinoma.[57] The reported frequency depends on the criteria used for diagnosis. In the WHO fascicle more than 90% tumor cells should have both cytologic and immunohistochemical features of apocrine cells for this classification.[1] While invasive duct carcinoma with apocrine features insufficient to meet criteria for apocrine carcinoma is reported in 12% to 57% of invasive duct carcinoma,[57] invasive carcinoma easily recognized as being apocrine type is much less common, likely representing from 0.3% to 0.4% of invasive breast carcinoma.[58] Apocrine differentiation is also observed in some invasive lobular carcinoma.

Invasive apocrine carcinoma and invasive duct carcinoma of no special type are not clinically distinguishable.[57]

Gross and Microscopic Pathologic Findings

No characteristic gross features are described.

On microscopic examination, the tumor cells of the invasive carcinoma resemble apocrine cells, with nuclear and cytoplasmic features that differ from the usual ductal carcinoma cell: the cells are larger; the cytoplasm is both more abundant and pinker (eosinophilic) and may be granular, homogenous, or vacuolated; while the nuclei are enlarged and contain prominent and often multiple nucleoli, with hyperchromatic nuclear membranes (Fig. 20-13). Gross cystic disease fluid protein (GCDFP-15) is a glycoprotein present in apocrine epithelium,[59]

and although regarded as a functional marker of apocrine cells,[60] GCDFP-15 expression does not correlate completely with apocrine morphology as it is expressed in 75% of apocrine breast carcinomas and in 23% of non-apocrine breast carcinomas.[60] Ultrastructurally (on electron microscopic examination) in limited series, apocrine features have been reported to correspond to several features: cytoplasmic vesicles or granules[59] or abundant mitochondria. The majority of invasive apocrine carcinomas are grade II/III.

Most apocrine lesions are negative for ER and PR protein expression, and positive for androgen receptor expression, but while this profile is present in benign apocrine lesions and apocrine in situ duct carcinoma, the profile is more variable in invasive apocrine carcinoma[57] in which there is a wide range in reported staining: ER positive in 3.8% to 60%, PR positive in 5.8% to 40%, and androgen receptor positive in 56% to 100% cases.[58] There is limited data on HER-2 status, with HER-2 protein overexpression being reported in 16% to 50% of cases.[58,61]

Prognosis

Lymphatic invasion and metastatic carcinoma to axillary nodes is reported as being less common in invasive apocrine carcinoma than invasive duct carcinoma, with 27% axillary lymph node positive, and 18% showing lymphovascular invasion in one series.[61] There is no significant difference in relapse-free survival or overall survival compared to invasive duct carcinoma of no special type.[61]

Other Comments

Recognizing invasive carcinoma as being of apocrine type is not currently important in patient management. Recognizing apocrine differentiation is of more importance in the correct identification of some benign lesions and forms of in situ carcinoma with apocrine differentiation. For example, apocrine metaplasia within sclerosing adenosis may contain significant cellular atypia that should not be overinterpreted as in situ carcinoma, and correspondingly in situ carcinoma of apocrine type should not be underdiagnosed as apocrine metaplasia with epithelial hyperplasia.

Invasive Micropapillary Carcinoma

Clinical Features

Invasive micropapillary carcinoma is a recently described uncommon type of invasive carcinoma. It may occur in pure form, but more commonly occurs as a component of invasive duct carcinoma of other type. A micropapillary component has been reported in from 2.6% to 12% of invasive carcinomas[62-65]; however, micropapillary carcinoma making up more than 80% of the invasive carcinoma is less common, reported in 0.7% of invasive carcinoma.[62] In one series in which race was recorded, 44/72 patients were African American and 28/72 were Caucasian.[62] The mean age of patients is no different from NST invasive duct carcinoma. No significant difference in age of patient, mean tumor size, grade, ER positivity, or axillary node status when the proportion of micropapillary carcinoma ranged from less than 20% to more than 80% has been observed.[62]

Gross and Microscopic Pathologic Findings

Micropapillary carcinoma ranges in size from 0.1 mm to 10 cm[64] with mean tumor size between 2 and 4.9 cm.[62-65] Invasion of skin has been reported in 22%,[62] but no characteristic gross features are reported.

The term "micropapillary" refers to the architectural pattern in which one or a small number of tumor-cell groups lie within clear spaces within the tissue, which has a spongy appearance. The cell groups may be solid or form tubular structures (Fig. 20-14). In one series there were 15 cases of corresponding frozen-section slides and permanent-section slides, and the clear spaces present in the permanent-section slides were not evident in any of the frozen-section slides, suggesting the spaces are artifactual.[64] There may be associated psammoma body–like microcalcification. Micropapillary carcinomas may be admixed with NST invasive duct carcinoma[62] or papillary or mucinous types.[63] Most carcinomas of this type are grade II or III, and the proportions that are grade III have ranged from 11% to 82% in series.[62-65]

This pattern of invasive carcinoma is associated with a high propensity for both lymphovascular permeation and lymph node involvement. Lymphovascular permeation is reported in 15% to 76% cases.[62-65]

Micropapillary invasive carcinomas are ER positive in 68% to 91% of cases,[62,64,65] and PR positive in 61% to 70% of cases.[63,65] HER-2 protein overexpression is reported in 54% to 59% of cases.[64,65]

Prognosis

There is a high propensity for involvement of axillary nodes, with positive nodes reported in 69% to 100% of cases.[62-65] The

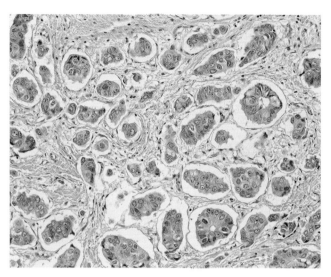

FIGURE 20-14 Micropapillary carcinoma (invasive carcinoma of micropapillary type) (H&E stain, 200×). The striking feature of this invasive carcinoma is that the tumor cells are lying in spaces within the tissue. The tumor cell groups are mainly solid, but focally form a gland. The spaces are not lined by endothelium and are therefore not lymphatics or blood vessels.

tendency to show lymphovascular involvement and nodal involvement has been found independent of the proportion of the carcinoma with micropapillary morphology,[62] and is also independent of size of primary carcinoma, occurring even in very small carcinomas with micropapillary morphology.[64] The extensive lymph node involvement is also independent of age, associated histologic type, histologic grade, and presence or absence of lymphovascular permeation.[63]

Studies suggest that micropapillary morphology is associated with an aggressive clinical course and poor outcome, regardless of whether a small component or a majority of the carcinoma has this morphology.[63] In one study, 46% of 83 patients died of disease, with mean interval to death 36 months[62]; however, the authors noted that patient survival was similar to that of infiltrating duct carcinoma of similar nodal status.[62]

In view of the association of this morphologic pattern with lymph node status and outcome, any proportion of invasive carcinoma that shows micropapillary features should be noted in a pathology report.

The main differential diagnoses are nonmicropapillary carcinoma and nonmammary carcinoma.

Nonmicropapillary Carcinoma. The presence of groups of tumor cells lying within spaces may be confused with either shrinkage of tumor cells or involvement of lymphovascular spaces by carcinoma. Shrinkage of tumor cells may occur with suboptimal tissue processing either secondary to an issue with the processing within the pathology laboratory, or due to tissue degeneration as a result of delayed fixation. Recognition of lymphovascular permeation may be assisted by the use of immunostains to identify lymphatics (eg, D2-40) and blood vessels (eg, factor VIII).

Nonmammary carcinoma. Micropapillary carcinoma arising in the breast must be differentiated from metastatic papillary carcinoma from an extramammary site, particularly papillary serous carcinoma of the ovary.

Invasive Papillary Carcinoma

Clinical Features

The entity invasive papillary carcinoma is included in the classification of special types of invasive breast carcinoma[1] and is reported as representing 1% to 2.1% of invasive breast cancers.[1,66] In a series by Fisher and associates,[66] this occurred predominantly in postmenopausal and non-Caucasian women. The term "papillary carcinoma" may be used for either invasive or in situ carcinoma, and this may cause clinical confusion. There are also forms of papillary carcinoma, namely encapsulated papillary carcinoma and solid papillary carcinoma, in which it is unclear whether the entity should be regarded as invasive or in situ carcinoma. Therefore, when the term "papillary carcinoma" is used it is essential that the reporting pathologist qualifies this term to reflect the presence or absence of unequivocal invasive carcinoma.

The term "invasive papillary carcinoma" has also been used to describe invasive carcinoma with formation of papillary structures, and even to describe invasive carcinoma arising in the context of in situ papillary carcinoma even though the invasive carcinoma in this context usually does not have a papillary architecture.

Gross and Microscopic Pathologic Findings

Invasive papillary carcinoma as defined by the presence of papillary architecture in the invasive carcinoma is uncommon. In the series by Fisher and associates of 1603 invasive mammary cancers, only 35 demonstrated this morphology.[66] The distinguishing feature is the presence of papillae, that is, the presence of finger-like structures with a fibrovascular core covered with malignant epithelium (Fig. 20 15). This is rarely a pure type of invasive carcinoma. It is usually mixed with other patterns of invasive duct carcinoma.[33] The papillary structures may be closely packed and difficult to identify or may lie in pools of mucin, in which case the differential diagnosis includes mucinous carcinoma or invasive duct carcinoma with mucinous features.[66]

The lack of uniformity in the use of the term invasive papillary carcinoma may influence the characteristics reported for this type of carcinoma. The gross appearance is reported as being mainly well circumscribed,[33,66] or indistinguishable from ductal no special type.[33] In the small numbers of reported cases it is ER positive[67] and negative for HER-2 protein overexpression.[68] The prognosis is reported as favorable.[66]

Encapsulated ("Intracystic") Papillary Carcinoma

Clinical Features

Encapsulated papillary carcinoma usually occurs as a subareolar lesion in elderly women and nipple discharge may be present.

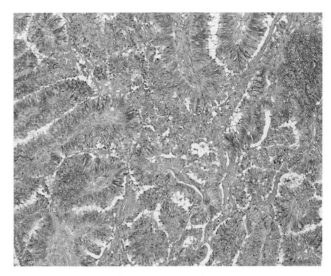

FIGURE 20-15 Papillary carcinoma (invasive carcinoma of papillary type) (H&E stain, 100×). This relatively low-power picture is from a solid area of carcinoma. The tumor cells form well-defined papillary structures—that is, finger-like structures with a core of fibrovascular tissue covered in epithelium. There is intervening fibrous tissue present.

Gross and Microscopic Pathologic Findings

On gross examination this carcinoma may form a friable mass within a cystic space,[69] or a lesion composed of hemorrhagic friable tissue lining a cystic space. The mean size is 1.3 cm[70]; however, these lesions may be substantially larger and may form a palpable mass.

On microscopic examination there is usually one and occasionally more than one nodule of papillary carcinoma surrounded by a rim of fibrous connective tissue. The carcinoma within the nodules usually has a papillary architecture composed of fibrovascular cores covered in malignant epithelium, but may in areas have a cribriform architecture.[69,70] There is no myoepithelium within the fibrovascular cores of the lesion, and recent studies show absence of myoepithelium around the periphery of the lesion.[70] The nodules of papillary carcinoma may occur alone or be associated with in situ duct carcinoma of low to intermediate grade type in the surrounding breast tissue.[69] Unequivocal invasive carcinoma, usually of ductal type, may be seen in association with encapsulated papillary carcinoma.[69] Fibrosis at the periphery of the nodules may result in entrapment of epithelium within dense fibrous tissue, which may simulate invasive carcinoma.

This entity has previously been called intracystic papillary carcinoma, and has traditionally been considered a form of in situ duct carcinoma. The finding of a lack of myoepithelium around the periphery of this lesion has recently suggested that this may in fact be a form of invasive carcinoma. In view of this, a change in name from intracystic papillary carcinoma to encapsulated papillary carcinoma was suggested,[70] and this name change is being adopted.[69]

Prognosis

When there is no unequivocal invasive carcinoma, this entity has an excellent prognosis with local treatment only. Therefore it is suggested that in the absence of definitive invasive carcinoma, the pathologist should diagnose this entity as encapsulated papillary carcinoma, and include a comment in the pathology report to indicate that although recent studies have suggested that this may represent circumscribed low-grade invasive carcinoma rather than in situ carcinoma, this should be managed in a manner similar to DCIS.[69]

Solid Papillary Carcinoma

Clinical Features

Solid papillary carcinoma is a lesion that usually occurs in older women as soft, well-circumscribed masses.[71]

Gross and Microscopic Pathologic Findings. Microscopically this consists of solid circumscribed nodules of epithelial cells with fibrovascular cores within the nodules. There are no discrete papillary structures present. The tumor cells may show spindling and neuroendocrine differentiation. These circumscribed nodules have traditionally been considered in situ duct carcinoma.[72] While some entities with this morphology have a peripheral myoepithelium,[72] there is often no peripheral myoepithelium around the nodules,[69,72] prompting consideration that at least some forms may represent invasive carcinoma rather than in situ duct carcinoma.

This entity is frequently found with overt invasive carcinoma but may occur without it.[77] When there is no overt invasive carcinoma, solid papillary carcinomas appear to have an indolent clinical course.[69,72]

Cribriform Carcinoma

Clinical Features

A special type of invasive duct carcinoma, cribriform carcinoma is well differentiated and has a favorable prognosis. Pure cribriform invasive carcinoma accounts for 0.01% to 0.6% of invasive breast carcinoma in reported series[35,73,74]; whereas invasive carcinoma with a cribriform component is more common, accounting for 6.2% to 9% of invasive carcinoma.[74] In comparison to invasive carcinoma with a cribriform component, patients with pure invasive cribriform carcinoma are younger, with a mean age of 53 years.[35,73] The mammographic appearance is that of a spiculated mass, which may contain punctate calcification, similar to that of invasive ductal carcinoma of no special type, but it may be mammographically occult.[35]

Gross and Microscopic Pathologic Findings

The average tumor size of pure invasive cribriform carcinoma is smaller than invasive carcinomas with a cribriform component in an older series in which the average size was 3.1 cm[73]; the imaging size has been reported as 20 to 35 mm.[35] There are no characteristic gross features.

On microscopic examination the tumor cells are similar to those of tubular carcinoma but are arranged in a cribriform architecture, similar to the pattern of cribriform in situ duct carcinoma.[73]

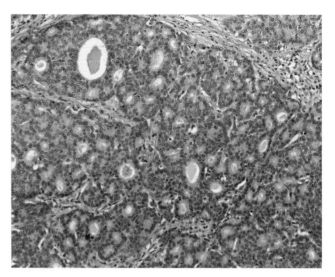

FIGURE 20-16 Invasive cribriform carcinoma (H&E stain, 200×). The malignant cells are low grade and form cribriform groups of tumor cells.

The tumor cells are small and regular, lack high-grade features, may have apical snouts, and have infrequent mitoses. The associated stroma may be fibroblastic (Fig. 20-16).[35,73,74] This pattern may be found admixed with tubule formation or invasive duct carcinoma of no special type. For a designation of pure invasive cribriform carcinoma, or the alternate term classic cribriform carcinoma, the invasive carcinoma must be at least 90% cribriform carcinoma, or at least 50% cribriform carcinoma, with the rest tubular carcinoma.[35,73,74] Invasive carcinomas with 50% to 90% cribriform architecture and the remainder invasive carcinoma of other than tubular type are considered mixed type of invasive carcinoma.[73,74] Multifocality is reported in one-fifth of cases.[73] Invasive cribriform carcinoma is ER positive in 100% cases, PR positive in 69%,[74] and negative for HER-2 protein overexpression in 100%[08] in limited series.

The main differential diagnoses are in situ duct carcinoma of cribriform type and other forms of invasive carcinoma. Invasive cribriform carcinoma can be differentiated from in situ duct carcinoma by the use of myoepithelial immunostains, which will be absent from the periphery of the nests of cribriform invasive carcinoma. Because of its favorable prognosis, this should be differentiated from other forms of invasive carcinoma such as mixed type, invasive duct carcinoma of no special type, and adenoid cystic carcinoma.

Prognosis

Metastatic carcinoma to lymph nodes is reported in pure cribriform carcinoma but usually involves only a small number of nodes (1 to 3), and this has not seemed to influence the prognosis.[74] The prognosis for pure cribriform carcinoma is excellent, better than that of invasive carcinoma of no special type, with no patients dying as a result of their invasive carcinoma in limited series.[73,74]

Medullary Carcinoma

Clinical Features

Medullary carcinoma is a rare subtype of invasive ductal carcinoma that, depending on the series cited, and the diagnostic criteria used, represents between 1% and 7% of invasive breast carcinomas.[75,76] In our experience, less than 1% of invasive ductal carcinomas would qualify for the diagnosis of medullary carcinoma if there was strict adherence to the diagnostic histologic criteria described in the next section. The mean age at diagnosis ranges from 45 to 52 years.[1] Given the well-circumscribed soft, nodular nature of medullary carcinoma, it may be confused clinically and radiologically with a fibroadenoma. The average size at presentation is usually between 2 and 3 cm. An association of medullary and medullary-like breast carcinoma morphology with BRCA1 mutations has been noted.[77]

Gross and Microscopic Features

The gross morphology of medullary carcinoma is quite distinctive. These tumors are sharply circumscribed, with a soft fleshy consistency, and although most have a uniform, tan to gray-white cut surface, small foci of necrosis may be present. They usually measure between 1 and 4 cm in diameter. There are 5 well-recognized histologic criteria for diagnosis,[1] and as the differential diagnosis is a high histologic grade NST tumor, it is critical that these criteria be strictly adhered to.

1. A syncytial architecture in more than 75% of the tumor (ie, sheets of tumor cells usually more than 4 or 5 cells thick with indistinct cell borders separated by small amounts of loose connective tissue). Small amounts of necrosis may be present.
2. Absence of glandular or tubular structures.
3. Diffuse lymphoplasmacytic tumor infiltrate, ranging from sparse to dense.
4. Round tumor cells with abundant cytoplasm, vesicular nuclei with one or more nucleoli and moderate to marked nuclear pleomorphism (nuclear grade 2 to 3), and numerous mitoses.
5. Complete histologic circumscription with pushing margins that may produce a compressed fibrous zone at the periphery of the tumor.

All medullary carcinomas are high grade (ie, grade III; Fig. 20-17). Ductal carcinoma in situ may be found at the periphery of the tumor.

The term "atypical medullary carcinoma" has been applied to those tumors in which some but not all of the 5 criteria are present, but this terminology is confusing, and we do not use that term, preferring to use a high-grade NST designation for these cases. Patients with medullary carcinoma tend to have a lower overall rate of axillary lymph node metastases than patients with NST ductal carcinomas. Medullary carcinomas tend to be ER and PR negative (ie, approximately 90% of medullary carcinomas are ER/PR negative), and HER-2/neu negative.

Prognosis and Treatment

Medullary carcinoma has been reported to have a significantly better prognosis than NST tumors, with one series reporting a

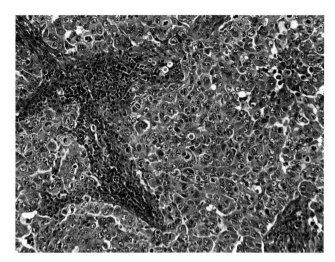

FIGURE 20-17 Medullary carcinoma (H&E stain, 100×). Despite its poorly differentiated histologic appearance (ie, pleomorphic, high-grade nuclei arranged in syncytial sheets with no tubule formation and a high mitotic rate), medullary carcinoma has a good prognosis relative to stage-matched NST tumors. Rigid adherence to strict diagnostic criteria is required for proper diagnosis.

90% 5-year survival when treated with breast-conserving surgery and radiation.[78]

Adenoid Cystic Carcinoma

Clinical Features

Adenoid cystic carcinoma of the breast is an extremely rare tumor representing approximately 0.1% of all invasive breast carcinomas.[79] It is histologically indistinguishable from the adenoid cystic carcinoma that may be seen in other body sites such as salivary glands, upper respiratory tract, and genitourinary tract.[80] However, in contrast to those occurring in other body sites, the prognosis of adenoid cystic carcinoma of the breast is excellent. In the vast majority of cases, the patients are postmenopausal, with a mean age at diagnosis between 50 and 63 years depending on the series cited.[81] Adenoid cystic carcinoma of the breast typically presents as a palpable, discrete firm mass lesion between 1 and 3 cm in size, and a predilection for the subareolar or periareolar location has been noted.[58]

Gross and Microscopic Features

Although grossly these tumors form discrete nodules that tend to be well circumscribed, microscopically, approximately 50% of adenoid cystic carcinomas invade the surrounding breast tissue beyond the confines of the grossly apparent tumor nodule.[81] In a minority of cases, there may be an associated ductal carcinoma in situ component. Histologically, adenoid cystic carcinoma of the breast is characterized by a mixture of proliferating glands (the adenoid component), and stromal basement membrane elements (the pseudoglandular or cylindromatous component), and as such may show a tubular, cribriform, or solid architecture, or mixtures thereof (Fig. 20-18). The tumor

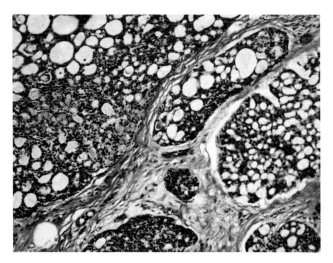

FIGURE 20-18 Adenoid cystic carcinoma (H&E stain, 100×). The infiltrating malignant cell nests of adenoid cystic carcinoma demonstrate 2 cell types, central basaloid cells and in some areas, larger, more eosinophilic cells at the periphery of the cell nests. True glandular lumina and cylindromatous areas containing pink, basement membrane material are present. This histomorphology is identical to adenoid cystic carcinomas that occur in other body sites.

demonstrates 2 basic cell types, a small, hyperchromatic basaloid cell with scanty cytoplasm that is grouped in nests or lines the pseudocysts or cribriform spaces of the cylindromatous component that contain amorphous eosinophilic basement membrane material, and a less common cell type that has round nuclei, abundant eosinophilic cytoplasm, and lines small ductule-like, but true glandular structures. The latter cells may uncommonly undergo squamous metaplasia. The basement membrane material in the pseudocysts of the cylindromatous component stains positively for Alcian Blue and negatively for PAS, while the material in the true glandular lumena is PAS positive. The basaloid cells show a generally myoepithelial phenotype, staining positively for vimentin, cytokeratin 14, collagen IV, and laminin, with focal staining for S100, smooth-muscle actin, calponin, and P63. The epithelial cells lining the true glandular spaces stain positively for cytokeratin 7 and E-cadherin. Ro and associates[80] have suggested that adenoid cystic carcinoma be stratified into 3 grades based on the proportion of solid growth within the tumor (grade I, no solid elements; grade II, less than 30% solid; grade III, more than 30% solid), with the higher grades correlating with a worse prognosis. Strict adherence to the recognized diagnostic criteria for adenoid cystic carcinoma, especially the requirement for a cylindromatous component, is vital, as some NST forms of breast carcinoma with prominent cribriform components may be misdiagnosed as adenoid cystic carcinoma.[82] Perineural invasion is found in a minority of cases, and lymphovascular tumor emboli are extremely uncommon.

Prognosis and Treatment

As noted, adenoid cystic carcinoma of the breast behaves like a low-grade malignancy and has an excellent prognosis. Even in

those very rare cases where distant metastases have occurred, these patients may live for many years—death from adenoid cystic carcinoma of the breast is extremely unusual. In contrast to NST breast carcinomas, routine sampling of axillary lymph nodes at the time of initial surgery has not been considered by some to be useful in either providing prognostic information or contributing to local disease control.[83] In a review of over 140 cases, Page and associates found only 3 cases of adenoid cystic carcinoma of the breast that involved axillary lymph nodes.[84] Adenoid cystic carcinoma of the breast is typically ER and PR negative. Prognostic data on adenoid cystic carcinoma are based mainly on surgical treatment with mastectomy, which has been curative in virtually all cases. Recurrence in the breast has been described after treatment by local excision alone, and most cases are best managed by wide excision and radiation if mastectomy is not performed.[81]

Glycogen-Rich (Clear-Cell) Carcinoma

Clinical Features

Glycogen-rich or clear-cell carcinoma is another rare subtype that comprises approximately 1% to 3% of invasive breast carcinomas.[85,86] An age range of 41 to 78 years with a median age of 57 years has been described.[87] The clinical presentation is not dissimilar from NOS tumors with most patients presenting with a palpable mass.

Gross and Microscopic Features

This tumor type does not exhibit any distinctive gross features. Microscopically, more than 90% of the tumor must show cells with predominantly clear (and occasionally finely granular) cytoplasm (Fig. 20-19) that contains PAS-positive, diastase-labile

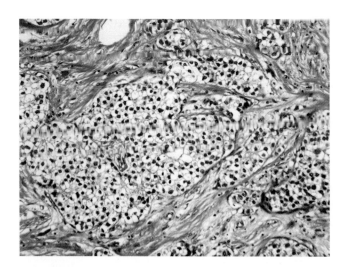

FIGURE 20-19 Glycogen-rich (clear-cell) carcinoma (H&E stain, 100×). The tumor cells demonstrate clear cytoplasm with small, hyperchromatic nuclei. A periodic acid Schiff (PAS) stain will demonstrate abundant intracellular pink speckling (intracellular glycogen) that disappears following diastase digestion (a PAS-d stain).

material (ie, glycogen). Because clear, transparent cytoplasm may result from a variety of different cytoplasmic contents (including lipid), the use of PAS/PAS-d stains to confirm the presence of glycogen is critical to the diagnosis. The tumor cells tend to be polygonal rather than round and have sharply defined borders with small, relatively uniform, hyperchromatic nuclei. The cells are usually arranged in cords, solid nests, and sheets. If an in situ ductal carcinoma component is present, it often is also of the clear-cell glycogen-rich variety. Patchy areas of necrosis are often present in large tumors. The possibility of metastasis, particularly metastatic renal-cell carcinoma, should be considered.

Prognosis and Treatment

Most studies suggest that glycogen-rich clear-cell carcinoma behaves more aggressively than tumors of the NST type.[88] Approximately 30% of patients have been reported as axillary lymph-node positive. Most reported cases (from older literature series that predated wide local excision and radiotherapy) have been treated with mastectomy and axillary lymph node dissection; however, there are no data to suggest that wide local excision followed by radiotherapy is not appropriate therapy for these patients. Approximately 50% of these tumors are ER positive, and virtually all cases have been PR negative.[88]

Lipid-Rich (Lipid-Secreting) Carcinoma

Clinical Features. Lipid-rich or lipid-secreting carcinoma is an extremely rare subtype of breast carcinoma of which only a few examples have been described. Over a 12-year period at the U.S. Armed Forces Institute of Pathology, only 4 cases were seen,[89] and it is one of the least frequently diagnosed variants of breast carcinoma. Most patients have presented with palpable nodules, with the tumor size ranging from 1.2 to 15 cm.[90]

Gross and Microscopic Features. Lipid-rich carcinomas have been described grossly as being poorly circumscribed with a firm cut surface. The diagnosis of lipid-rich carcinoma requires that approximately 90% of the tumor cells contain abundant neutral lipid in their cytoplasm, and that the cells have clear-cell morphology on H&E staining. In formalin-fixed, paraffin-embedded tissue, the cytoplasm of the cells is clear and vacuolated, as the lipid has been removed during tissue processing, and the cells have small, hyperchromatic nuclei. Confirmation of the presence of neutral lipid (which may require Oil-Red O staining on frozen tissue), and the absence of glycogen and mucin, support the diagnosis. In most cases reported, the tumors have been high grade.

Prognosis and Treatment

There have been insufficient numbers of patients with lipid-rich breast carcinoma reported with limited follow-up, and thus it is not possible to definitively comment on prognosis/treatment. The data on hormone receptor status are also very limited, but in one series, all of the tumors were ER/PR negative.[90]

Further studies with larger numbers of patients and longer follow-up will be required to establish whether lipid-rich

carcinomas in fact represent a clinically distinct subtype of breast carcinoma.

Secretory (Juvenile) Carcinoma

Clinical Features

Secretory carcinoma is another extremely uncommon subtype of breast carcinoma, representing less than 0.15% of all breast cancers.[91] Athough originally described in children (hence the term "juvenile carcinoma"), it is well recognized to occur in adults, and therefore the term "secretory carcinoma" is preferred. There is a wide reported age range of between 3 and 87 years, with a median age of 25 years. About 60% of the patients have been older than 20 years. The majority of cases have occurred in females, but several cases have been reported in prepubertal and adult males. Most cases have presented as a palpable breast mass, often in the sub- or periareolar area.

Gross and Microscopic Features

These tumors are generally firm, well-circumscribed nodules that often mimic a fibroadenoma and have the usual grayish-white to yellow-tan cut surface of a carcinoma. The median tumor size at diagnosis is approximately 2.5 to 3 cm. Most tumors show central fibrosis with a more cellular periphery, and the architecture in the cellular areas may be tubular, microcystic/follicular, papillary, solid, or show variable combinations of the preceding. The individual tumor cells lack significant atypism, having relatively uniform ovoid nuclei with small nucleoli, and a large amount of pale pink to amphophilic staining cytoplasm with H&E staining (Fig. 20-20). Intracytoplasmic lumina of variable size are frequent. Mitoses are generally scanty and necrotic areas very rare.

The prominent intracellular and extracellular secretions are PAS-d positive and also stain positively with Alcian Blue at pH 2.5. The tumor cells tend to be positive for S-100 protein, EMA, polyclonal CEA, and alpha lactalbumin, and negative for

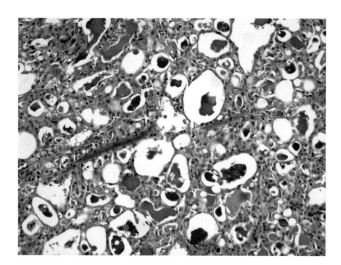

FIGURE 20-20 Secretory (juvenile) carcinoma (H&E stain, 100×). Tumor cells with vacuolated cytoplasm and adjacent microcystic spaces containing abundant pale pink secretion.

GCDFP-15. Ductal carcinoma in situ of similar morphology may be present in or around the tumor.

Prognosis and Treatment

Secretory breast carcinoma has an extremely favorable prognosis in children and adolescents. Although the risk of lymph node involvement is similar in young and older patients (ie, axillary lymph node metastases are found in approximately 15% of patients[92]), systemic metastases/deaths attributable to secretory carcinoma are unknown in childhood.[93] Secretory carcinoma in adults behaves in a slightly more aggressive manner,[94] with late recurrences and deaths having been described. Local excision, with consideration to preserving the breast bud, is the preferred treatment in children, however, technically this may not be possible, and subsequent breast development can be affected.[95] Axillary nodal dissection is indicated if clinical examination suggests nodal disease, however, as a significant number of children with nodal metastases did not have palpable axillary lymph nodes, sentinel lymph node mapping may be the best method for initial staging of the axilla. There is no evidence that post-lumpectomy radiation is of value in adults, and in children it may inhibit normal breast development. Experience with systemic chemotherapy in patients with secretory breast carcinoma has been very limited and its role in this type of breast cancer is unclear at this time. ER/PR status of secretory carcinoma has been predominantly negative, and HER-2/neu overexpression also mainly negative.

In summary, overall, secretory carcinoma is considered to have a better prognosis than NST tumors, with death from metastatic disease unusual.

Small-Cell (Oat-Cell) Carcinoma

Clinical Features

Primary small-cell carcinoma of the breast is extremely rare, with only a small number of cases reported in the literature. The largest series of 9 patients[96] reported an age range of 43 to 70 years. This diagnosis requires that the possibility of metastasis from a lung primary (or other nonmammary sites) to the breast be conclusively ruled out. The lung is the commonest primary site for small-cell carcinoma metastatic to the breast.[97]

Gross and Microscopic Features

In the series of 9 patients by Shin and associates,[96] the tumors were ill-defined firm mass lesions with a mean size of 2.6 cm. On cut surface, the tumors were tan-white to tan/pink-gray without prominent calcification, hemorrhage, or necrosis evident on gross examination. Primary small-cell carcinoma of the breast is histologically indistinguishable from small-cell carcinomas of other sites. The tumor cells are approximately twice the size of lymphocytes and demonstrate minimal cytologic or nuclear pleomorphism. The cells have scant cytoplasm and hyperchromatic oval nuclei without prominent nucleoli (Fig. 20-21). Nuclear molding with crush and streaming due to nuclear disruption may be seen. In the largest series published to date,[96] all primary small-cell carcinomas of the breast were positive for cytokeratin (AE1/AE3), and neuroendocrine

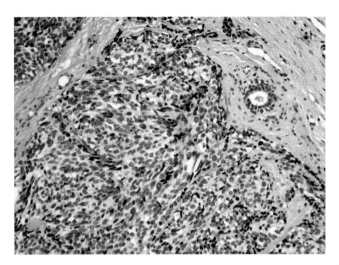

FIGURE 20-21 Small-cell carcinoma (hematoxylin/phloxin/saffron stain, 100×). The tumor cells consist of sheets and nests of small "oat-like" cells with hyperchromatic nuclei. Note the benign breast ductule to the upper right of the photograph.

markers (chromogranin, synaptophysin) were positive in 6 of the 9 cases. Dimorphic features (ie, an abrupt transition from small-cell histomorphology to one with adenocarcinomatous, lobular, or focal squamous features) may be seen in these cases. There is often an associated ductal carcinoma in situ component with a high nuclear grade present, which is helpful in confirming breast as the primary site of the carcinoma.

Prognosis and Treatment

Approximately 50% of the published cases had axillary lymph node metastases present at the time of diagnosis. The most recent results suggest that the prognosis of relatively early-stage small-cell carcinoma may be more favorable than that reported in the older literature, which is largely based on patients with higher-stage disease. Mammary small-cell carcinoma has been responsive to chemotherapy used for small-cell carcinoma of other sites such as VP-16 and cisplatin.[98] In the series by Shin and associates,[96] 5 of the 9 patients' tumors were ER and PR positive and all were HER-2/neu protein-overexpression negative.

FUTURE DIRECTIONS

The phenotypic or histologic classification of invasive breast cancer is able to tell us much about an individual's presentation, prognosis, and response to treatments. It is an amazing compilation of empiric observation and evidence. However, the next 20 years will likely herald the age of genetic subtyping, and new pharmaceuticals will be developed against specific targets within breast cancer genotypic subgroups.

Current commercially available RNA- and DNA-typing platforms can help guide the use of general chemotherapeutic regimens, and it is likely that the utility of these methodologies will increase as they become more sophisticated and hopefully less expensive. In the future the automated evaluation of tumors will be commonplace, where sections of tumor are introduced into an apparatus, the DNA/RNA extracted and measured, and an analytic report that will guide individualized treatment will be the output. Whether morphologically based classification of breast cancer will be clinically valuable in 20 years is a thought-provoking question.

Necessary Future Studies

There are few breast cancer trials that have been or will be based on specific pathologic entities. Treatment trials based on what are now the accepted predictive factors such as ER, PR, and HER-2/neu have generally been completed.

The results from the NCI TailoRx trial are awaited, as this randomized clinical trial is using the Oncotype DX RNA platform to help decide prognosis in ER-positive, node-negative breast cancer patients. Those with an intermediate prognosis are randomized to systemic chemotherapy or not. Studies that utilize the prognostic and predictive abilities of different genetic platforms will increase in the future as we learn more about the genetic make-up of cancer cells and try to use this information to choose specific and individualized chemotherapeutic and endocrine treatments.

SUMMARY

Invasive carcinoma of the breast is comprised of a group of pathologically heterogenous entities whose classification is based on specific histologic criteria. This chapter presents the salient points that help discriminate the various pathologic entities, from the most common—invasive duct carcinoma of no specific type, to the rare—secretory or juvenile carcinoma. The many distinguishing points of differentiation between these subtypes, whether in clinical presentation, prognosis, or potential for metastases, are discussed.

However, despite the heterogenous morphologic subtypes, the commonalities are more important than the diversities when deciding upon the surgical treatment. That is, the tumor size and patient variables are the primary determinants of whether a patient is a candidate for breast conservation and not the histologic variant. The prognostic factors of tumor size, grade, presence of lymphovascular invasion, and nodal status also cross most histologic boundaries. Finally, predictive factors such as the presence or absence of the estrogen receptor, progesterone receptor, and Her-2\neu overexpression are biological tumor characteristics to help guide adjuvant systemic treatments for breast cancer of all types.

REFERENCES

1. Ellis IO, Schnitt SJ, Sartre-Garau X, et al. Invasive breast carcinoma. In: Tavassoli FA, Devilee P, eds. *World Health Organization Classification of Tumours. Pathology and Genetics of Tumours of the Breast and Female Genital Organs.* Lyon: IARC Press; 2003:13-59.
2. Elston CW, Ellis IO. Pathological prognostic factors in breast cancer. 1. The value of histological grade in breast cancer: experience from a large study with long-term follow-up. *Histopathology.* 1991;19:403-410.
3. Fitzgibbons PL, Page DL, Weaver D, et al. Prognostic factors in breast cancer. College of American Pathologists Consensus Statement 1999. *Arch Pathol Lab Med.* 2000;124:966-78.
4. Robbins R, Pinder S, de Klerk N, et al. Histological grading of breast carcinomas: a study of interobserver agreement. *Hum Pathol.* 1995;26:873-879.
5. Ellis IO and Elston CW. Histologic grade. In O'Malley FP and Pinder SE, eds. *Foundations in Diagnostic Pathology; Breast Pathology.* Churchill Livingstone:2006:225-240.
6. Cross SS, Start RD, Smith JHF. Does delay in fixation affect the number of mitotic figures in processed tissue. *J Clin Pathol* 1990; 43:597-599.
7. Rosen PP. Tumor emboli in intramammary lymphatics in breast carcinoma: pathologic criteria for diagnosis and clinical significance. *Pathol Annu.* 1983;18:215-232.
8. Lauria R, Perrone F, Carlomagno C, et al. The prognostic value of lymphatic and blood vessel invasion in operable breast cancer. *Cancer.* 1995;76:1772-1778.
9. Clemente CG, Boracchi P, Andreola S, et al. Peritumoral lymphatic invasion in patients with node-negative mammary duct carcinoma. *Cancer.* 1992;69:1396-1403.
10. Lerwill MF. Current practical applications of diagnostic immunohistochemistry in breast pathology. *Am J Surg Pathol.* 2004;28:1076-1091.
11. Moll R, Mitze M, Frixen UH, Birchmeier W. Differential loss of E-cadherin expression in infiltrating ductal and lobular breast carcinomas. *Am J Pathol.* 1993;143:1731-42.
12. Yeh IT, Mies C. Application of immunohistochemistry to breast lesions. *Arch Pathol Lab Med.* 2008;132:349-358.
13. Perou CM, Sorlie T, Eisen MB, et al. Molecular portraits of human breast tumours. *Nature.* 2000;406:747-752.
14. Sorlie T, Perou CM, Tibshirani R, et al. Gene expression patterns of breast carcinomas distinguish tumor subclasses with clinical implications. *Proc Natl Acad Sci USA.* 2001;98:10869-10874..
15. Sorlie T, Tibshirani R, Parker J, et al. Repeated observation of breast tumor subtypes in independent gene expression data sets. *Proc Natl Acad Sci USA.* 2003;100: 8418-8423..
16. Rakha EA, El-Sayed ME, Reis-Filho JS, Ellis IO. Expression profiling technology: its contribution to our understanding of breast cancer. *Histopathology.* 2008;52:67-81.
17. Reis-Filho JS, Tutt ANJ. Triple negative tumours: a critical review. *Histopathology.* 2008;52:108-118.
18. Fulford LG, Easton DF, Reis- Filho JS, et al. Specific morphological features predictive for the basal phenotype in grade 3 invasive ductal carcinoma of the breast. *Histopathology.* 2006;49:22-34.
19. Sakamoto G, Sugano H, Hartmann WH. Comparative pathological study of breast carcinoma among American and Japanese women. In: McGuire WK, ed. *Breast Cancer: Advances in Research and Treatment.* Vol 4. New York, NY: Plenum; 1981:211-231.
20. Rosen PP. The pathological classification of human mammary carcinoma: past, present and future. *Ann Clin Lab Sci.* 1979;9:144-156.
21. O'Malley FP, Pinder SE, eds. In: *Breast Pathology.* A volume in the series Foundations in Diagnostic Pathology. Philadelphia, PA: Elsevier; 2006:202.
22. Azzopardi JG. *Problems in Breast Pathology.* Philadelphia, PA: Saunders; 1979:244.
23. Sastre-Garau X, Jouve M, Asselain B, et al. Infiltrating lobular carcinoma of the breast: clinicopathological analysis of 975 cases with reference to data on conservative therapy and metastatic patterns. *Cancer.* 1996; 77:113-20.
24. Rakha EA, El-Sayed ME, Menon S, et al. Histologic grading is an independent prognostic factor in invasive lobular carcinoma of the breast. *Breast Cancer Res Treat.* 2008;111:121-127.
25. Li CI, Anderson BO, Daling JR, Moe RE. Trends in incidence rates of invasive lobular and ductal breast carcinoma. *JAMA.* 2003;289:1421-1424.
26. Stalsberg H, Thomas DB, Noonan EA, WHO Collaborative Study of Neoplasia and Steroid Contraceptives. Histologic types of breast carcinoma in relation to international variation and breast cancer risk factors. *Int J Cancer.* 1989;44:399-409.
27. Bane AL, Tjan S, Parkes RK, et al. Invasive lobular carcinoma: to grade or not to grade. *Mod Pathol.* 2005;18:621-628.
28. Azzopardi JG. Classification of primary breast carcinoma. *Problems in Breast Pathology.* WB Saunders; 1979: 240-257.
29. Dixon LM, Anderson TJ, Page DL, et al. Infiltrating lobular carcinoma of the breast. *Histopathology.* 1982;6:149-161.
30. Middleton LP, Palacios DM, Bryant BR et al. Pleomorphic lobular carcinoma: Morphology, immunohistochemistry, and molecular analysis. *Am J Surg Pathol.* 2000;24:1650-1656.
31. Eusebi V, Magalhaes F, Azzopardi JG. Pleomorphic lobular carcinoma of the breast: an aggressive tumor showing apocrine differentiation. *Hum Pathol.* 1992;23:655-662.
32. Esposito NN, Chivukula M, Dabbs DJ. The ductal phenotypic expression of the E-cadherin/catenin complex in tubulolobular carcinoma of the breast: an immunohistochemical and clinicopathologic study. *Modern Pathology.* 2007. 20:130-138.

33. Pinder SE, Elston CW, Ellis IO. Invasive carcinoma–usual histological types. Elston CW and Ellis IO, eds. *Systemic Pathology: The breast*. 3rd ed. Vol 13. Churchill Livingstone. 1998:283-337.

34. Newcomer LM, Newcomb PA, Trentham-Dietz A, et al. Detection method and breast carcinoma histology. *Cancer*. 2002;95:470-477.

35. Stutz JA, Evans AJ, Pinder S, et al. The radiological appearances of invasive cribriform carcinoma of the breast. *Clin Radiol* 1994;49:693-5.

36. Goldstein NS, Kestin LL, Vicini FA. Refined morphologic criteria for tubular carcinoma to retain its favorable outcome status in contemporary breast carcinoma patients. *Am J Clin Pathol*. 2004;122:728-739.

37. Kader HA, Jackson J, Mates D, et al. Tubular carcinoma of the breast: a population-based study of nodal metastases at presentation and of patterns of relapse. *Breast J*. 2001;7:8-13.

38. Stalsberg H, Hartmann WH. The delimitation of tubular carcinoma of the breast. *Hum Pathol*. 2000;31:601-607.

39. Lagios MD, Rose MR, Margolin FR. Tubular carcinoma of the breast: association with multicentricity, bilaterality, and family history of mammary carcinoma. *Am J Clin Pathol*. 1980;73:25-30.

40. Avisar E, Khan MA, Axelrod D, Oza K. Pure mucinous carcinoma of the breast: a clinicopathologic study. *Ann Surg Oncol*. 1998;5:447-451.

41. Rosen PP, Lesser ML, Kinne DW. Breast carcinoma at the extremes of age: a comparison of patients younger than 35 years and older than 75 years. *J Surg Oncol*. 1985;28:90-96.

42. Cardenosa G, Doudna C, Eklund GW. Mucinous (colloid) breast cancer: clinical and mammographic findings in 10 patients. *AJR*. 1995;165:285-289.

43. Rasmussen BB, Rose C, Thorpe SM, et al. Argyrophilic cells in 202 human mucinous carcinomas. Relation to histopathologic and clinical factors. *Am J Clin Pathol*. 1985;84:737-740.

44. Fentiman IS, Millis RR, Smith P, et al. Mucoid breast carcinomas: histology and prognosis. *Br J Cancer*. 1997;75:1061-1065.

45. Shousha S, Coady AT, Stamp T, et al. Estrogen receptors in mucinous carcinoma of the breast: an immunohistochemical study using paraffin wax sections. *J Clin Pathol*. 1989;41:902-905.

46. Rosen PP. In: *Rosen's Breast Pathology*. 2nd ed. Philadelphia, PA: Lippincott Williams & Wilkins, 2001.479.

47. Toikkanen S, Kujari H. Pure and mixed mucinous carcinomas of the breast: a clinicopathologic analysis of 61 cases with long-term follow-up. *Hum Pathol*. 1989;20:758-764.

48. Rosen PP. In: *Rosen's Breast Pathology*. 2nd ed. Philadelphia, PA: Lippincott Williams & Wilkins; 2001;425.

49. Rostock RA, Bauer TW, Eggleston JC. Primary squamous carcinoma of the breast: a review. *Breast*. 1984:10:27-31.

50. Rosen PP. In: *Rosen's Breast Pathology*. 2nd ed. Philadelphia, PA: Lippincott Williams & Wilkins; 2001:457.

51. Drudis T, Arroyo C, Van Oveven K, et al. The pathology of low grade adenosquamous carcinoma of the breast. *Pathol Annu*. 1994;181-197.

52. Eggers JW, Chesney TMC. Squamous cell carcinoma of the breast: a clinicopathologic analysis of eight cases and review of the literature. *Hum Pathol*. 1984;15:526-531.

53. Van Hoeven KH, Drudis T, Cranor ML, et al. Low grade adenosquamous carcinoma of the breast: a clinicopathological study of 32 cases with ultrastructural analysis. *Am J Surg Pathol*. 1993;17:248

54. Carter MR, Hornick JL, Lester S, Fletcher DW. Spindle cell (sarcomatoid) carcinoma of the breast. A clinicopathologic and immunohistochemical analysis of 29 cases. *Am J Surg Pathol*. 2006;30:300-309.

55. Davis WG, Hennessy B, Bariera G, et al. Metaplastic sarcomatoid carcinoma of the breast with absent or minimal overt invasive carcinomatous component. A misnomer. *Am J Surg Pathol*. 2005;29:1456-1463.

56. Rosen PP. In: *Rosen's Breast Pathology*. 2nd ed. Philadelphia, PA: Lippincott Williams & Wilkins; 2001:452.

57. O'Malley FP, Bane A. An update on apocrine lesions of the breast. *Histopathology*. 2008;52: 3-10.

58. Azzopardi JG. Tumours analogous with tumours of the salivary and sweat glands. *Problems in breast pathology*. WB Saunders; 1979;334-345.

59. Eusebi V, Millis RR, Cattani MG, et al. Apocrine carcinoma of the breast. A morphologic and immunocytochemical study. *Am J Pathol*. 1986;123:532-541.

60. Honma N, Takubo K, Akiyama F, et al. Expression of GCDFP-15 and AR decreases in larger or node-positive apocrine carcinomas of the breast. *Histopathology*. 2005;47:195-201.

61. Tanaka K, Imoto S, Wada N, et al. Invasive apocrine carcinoma of the breast: clinicopathologic features of 57 patients. *Breast J*. 2008;14:164-168.

62. Nassar H, Wallis T, Andea A, et al. Clinicopathologic analysis of invasive micropapillary differentiation in breast carcinoma. *Mod Pathol*. 2001;14:836-841.

63. Luna-More S, Gonzalez B, Acedo C, et al. Invasive micropapillary carcinoma of the breast. A new special type of invasive mammary carcinoma. *Pathol Res Pract*. 1994;190:668-674.

64. Walsh MM, Bleiweiss IJ. Invasive micropapillary carcinoma of the breast: eighty cases of an underrecognized entity. *Hum Pathol*. 2001;32:583-589.

65. Zekioglu O, Erhan Y, Ciris M, et al. Invasive micropapillary carcinoma of the breast: high incidence of lymph node metastasis with extranodal extension and its immunohistochemical profile compared with invasive ductal carcinoma. *Histopathology*. 2004;44:18-23.

66. Fisher ER, Palekar AS, Redmond C, et al. Pathologic findings from the National Surgical Adjuvant Breast Project (Protocol no. 4): VI. Invasive papillary cancer. *AJCP*. 1980;73:313-322.

67. Reiner A, Reiner G, Spona J, et al. Histopathologic characterization of human breast cancer in correlation with estrogen receptor status: a comparison of immunocytochemical and biochemical analysis. *Cancer*. 1988;61:1149-1154.

68. Soomro S, Shousha S, Taylor P, et al. C-erbB-2 expression in different histological types of invasive breast carcinoma. *J Clin Pathol*. 1991;44;211-214.

69. Collins LC, Schnitt SJ. Papillary lesions of the breast: selected diagnostic and management issues. *Histopathology*. 2008;52:20-29.

70. Collins LC, Carlo VP, Hwang H, et al. Intracystic papillary carcinomas of the breast: a reevaluation using a panel of myoepithelial cell markers. *Am J Surg Pathol*. 2006;30:1002-1007.

71. Maluf HM, Koerner FC. Solid papillary carcinoma of the breast: a form of intraductal carcinoma with endocrine differentiation, frequently associated with mucinous carcinoma. *Am J Surg Pathol*. 1995;19:1237-1244.

72. Nicolas M M, Wu Y, Middleton LP, Gilcrease MZ. Loss of myoepithelium is variable in solid papillary carcinoma of the breast. *Histopathology*. 2007;51: 657-665.

73. Page DL, Dixon JM, Anderson TJ, et al. Invasive cribriform carcinoma of the breast. *Histopathology*. 1983;7:525-536.

74. Venable JG, Schwartz AM, Silverberg SG. Infiltrating cribriform carcinoma of the breast: a distinctive clinicopathologic entity. *Hum Pathol*. 1990;21:333-338.

75. Bloom HJ, Richardson WW, Field JR. Host resistance and survival in carcinoma of breast: a study of 104 cases of medullary carcinoma in a series of 1,411 cases of breast cancer followed for 20 years. *Br Med J*. 1970;3.181-188.

76. Rapin V, Contesso G, Mouriesse H, et al. A reevaluation of 95 cases of breast cancer with inflammatory stroma. *Cancer*. 1988;61:2503-2510.

77. Armes JE, Egan AJ, Southey MC, et al. The histologic phenotype of breast carcinoma occurring before age 40 years in women with and without BRCA1 or BRCA2 germline mutations: a population-based study. *Cancer*. 1998;83:2335-2345.

78. Fourquet A, Vilcoq JR, Zefani B, et al. Medullary breast carcinoma, the role of radiotherapy as primary treatment. *Radiother Oncol*. 1987;10:1-6.

79. Lamovec J, Us-Krasovec M, Zidar A, Kljun A. Adenoid cystic carcinoma of the breast: a histologic, cytologic, and immunohistochemical study. *Semin Diagn Pathol*. 1989;6:153-164.

80. Ro JY, Silva EG, Gallager HS. Adenoid cystic carcinoma of the breast. *Hum Pathol*. 1987;18:1276-1281.

81. Rosen PP. Adenoid cystic carcinoma of the breast: a morphologically heterogeneous neoplasm. *Path Annu*. 1989;24:237-254.

82. Sumpio BE, Jennings TA, Merino MH, Sullivan PD. Adenoid cystic carcinoma of the breast: data from the Connecticut Tumor Registry and a review of the literature. *Ann Surg*. 1987;20,22 9-301.

83. Page DL. Adenoid cystic carcinoma of breast, a special histopathologic type with excellent prognosis. *Breast Cancer Res Treat*. 2005;93:189-190.

84. Nicholson BP, Kasami M, Page DL, Johnson DH. Adenoid cystic carcinoma of the breast. In: Raghavan D, Brechner ML, Johnson D, eds. *Textbook of Uncommon Cancer*. Chichester, UK: Wiley; 1999:719-724.

85. Fisher ER, Tavares J, Bulatao IS, et al. Glycogen-rich, clear cell breast cancer: with comments concerning other clear cell variants. *Hum Pathol*. 1985;16:1085-1090.

86. Hull MT, Warfel KA. Glycogen-rich clear cell carcinomas of the breast. A clinicopathologic and ultrastructural study. *Am J Surg Pathol*. 1986;10:553-559.

87. Tavassoli FA. Glycogen-rich (clear-cell) carcinoma. In: *Pathology of the Breast*. Stamford, CT: Appleton & Lang; 1999:527-529.

88. Hayes MM, Seidman JD, Ashton MA. Glycogen-rich clear cell carcinoma of the breast. A clinicopathologic study of 21 cases. *Am J Surg Pathol*. 1995;19:904-911.

89. Tavassoli FA. Lipid-rich Carcinoma. In: *Pathology of the Breast*. Stamford, CT: Appleton & Lang; 1999:519-522.

90. Wrba F, Ellinger A, Reiner G, et al. Ultrastructural and immunohistochemical characteristics of lipid-rich carcinoma of the breast. *Arch A Pathol Anat Histopathol*. 1988;413:381-385.

91. Lamovec J, Bracko M. Secretory carcinoma of the breast: Light microscopical, immunohistochemical, and flow cytometric study. *Mod Pathol*. 1994;7:475-479.

92. Sullivan JJ, Magee HR, Donald KJ. Secretory (juvenile) carcinoma of the breast. *Pathology.* 1977;9:341-346.

93. Krausz T, Jenkins D, Grontoft O, et al. Secretory carcinoma of the breast in adults:emphasis on late recurrence and metastasis. *Histopathology.* 1989;14:25-36.

94. Tavassoli FA, Norris HJ. Secretory carcinoma of the breast. *Cancer.* 1980;45:2404-2413.

95. Rosen PP, Cranor ML. Secretory carcinoma of the breast. *Arch Pathol Lab Med.* 1991;115:141-144.

96. Shin SJ, DeLellis RA, Ying L, Rosen PP. Small cell carcinoma of the breast: a clinicopathologic and immunohistochemical study of nine patients. *Am J Surg Pathol.* 2000;24:1234-1238.

97. Kelly C, Henderson D, Corris P. Breast lumps: rare presentation of oat cell carcinoma of the lung. *J Clin Pathol.* 1988;41:171-172.

98. Sebenik M, Nair SG, Hamati HF. Primary small cell anaplastic carcinoma of the breast diagnosed by fine needle aspiration cytology: a case report. *Acta Cytol.* 1998;42:1199-1203.

CHAPTER 21

Male Breast Cancer

Mahmoud El-Tamer
Benjamin Pocock

Males infrequently develop breast cancer; hence the dearth of prospective randomized trials in male breast cancer. Our knowledge of the disease has been derived mostly from retrospectives studies. Due to the similarities of disease behavior in men and women with breast cancer, the management and treatment of male breast cancer has been guided by conclusions drawn from studies conducted in women.

PREVALENCE

Breast cancer represents less than 1% of all cancers in men[1]; the male to female ratio is 1:100.[2] Since 1973 there has been a gradual increase in the incidence of male breast cancer, the reasons for which are unclear. Nonetheless the overall incidence remains low, at about 1 case per 100,000 population per year.[3] Unlike women, where breast cancer displays a bimodal distribution, the disease in men increases exponentially with age. The median age at presentation for male breast cancer is 65 to 71, unlike with women, in whom breast cancer is seen about 5 to 10 years earlier.[4] The epidemiology of breast cancer in men is similar to that in women, such that North America and Europe see the highest incidences, while Japan has the lowest.[5] Interestingly, in sub-Saharan countries in Africa where infectious liver damage is common, such as in Zambia[6] and Uganda,[7] 7% to 14% of breast cancer cases occur in men. In the United States, tumor registries indicate that male breast cancer is most common in African American men, intermediate in non-Hispanic Caucasian men and Asian-Pacific Islanders, and lowest in Hispanic men. In 2009, the American Cancer Society estimated that 1910 men will have been diagnosed with breast cancer in the United States, with 440 deaths.[8]

RISK FACTORS

Similarly to women, hormonal factors seem to play an important role in the development of breast cancer in men. A frequently cited risk factor is Klinefelter syndrome, where an extra X chromosome is inherited in these male patients. The risk of developing breast cancer in patients with Klinefelter syndrome is increased by 58-fold, with an absolute risk of 3%.[9] Patients with this syndrome have atrophic testes with high levels of gonadotropins, low levels of testosterone, and normal to low levels of estrogen, leading to a high estrogen to testosterone ratio. Also suggestive that hormonal factors may play a role, male breast cancer is seen in hermaphrodites, men having undergone feminizing surgery, and men who have received exogenous estrogen for prostate cancer, where cases of bilateral breast cancer have been described.[10,11] As Klinefelter syndrome and male breast cancer are both rare diseases, it is very unlikely that a health care provider will encounter this situation; however, a breast lesion in a patient with Klinefelter syndrome must be considered suspiciously. It has been reported that 4% of men with breast cancer have Klinefelter syndrome.[12]

It has been suggested that male breast cancer and gynecomastia represent different ends of the same spectrum, or that gynecomastia may be a premalignant lesion. This assumption was based on the observation that men with breast cancer have the clinical and histologic diagnosis of gynecomastia in 4% to 23% and 26.5% to 88%, respectively.[13] In autopsy studies of men dying from other causes than breast cancer, gynecomastia was found in 40% to 55% cases.[14] Currently there is no conclusive evidence to support a causal relationship between male breast cancer and gynecomastia; it is possible, however, that both are the result of a hormonal imbalance.

Other risk factors cited in the literature include liver disorders (cirrhosis and bilharziasis), testicular injury, orchitis, history of head injury with resulting hyperprolactinemia, and prostate cancer.[15] Male breast cancer has been seen more frequently in boys being treated with chest irradiation for lymphoma as well as in men exposed to nuclear fallout, such as Japanese men following World War II. Additionally, it has been proposed that electromagnetic fields and the exposure of the testis to heat may be occupational hazards.[16]

As in women, a family history of breast cancer is a risk factor in men. A history of breast cancer in a mother or sister confers respectively a 2.33 or 2.23 relative risk of developing breast cancer in men.[17] This risk increases if the affected first-degree female relative developed breast cancer before the age of 45 years. Furthermore, 30% of men with breast cancer have a history of one or more affected first-degree relatives. Genetic predisposition to the development of male breast cancer has also been identified.[18] Men who carry the BRCA1, and particularly the BRCA2, gene mutations may not only transmit them to their offspring, but are also at increased risk of developing breast cancer themselves.[19] Men with the BRCA2 mutation have a 100-fold increased risk of developing breast cancer, with a lifetime risk of approximately 7% by age 80. BRCA2 is thought to represent about 15% of breast cancer in men. Men with the BRCA1 mutation are at increased risk but to a lesser degree, with a 1.2% risk by age 70.[20] Men of Ashkenazi Jewish descent have a higher prevalence of BRCA1 and BRCA2, and therefore an increased risk of developing male breast cancer.[21] Currently there are no established screening guidelines for men with higher risk of breast cancer.[22]

PRESENTATION AND WORKUP

The most common presentation of male breast cancer (75%-95%) is a palpable mass. The lump is discovered by the patient in 60% of these cases.[23,24] On physical exam the breast mass is painless, eccentric, and ill-defined. In as many as 80% of cases, the mass may be associated with nipple discharge. On the other hand, serosanguinous nipple discharge in a male patient is associated with breast cancer in 75% of cases. Due to the smaller size of the male breast, involvement of the skin and nipple–areola complex or the underlying chest wall is more frequently seen in men than in women. Skin fixation and ulceration is seen in 44% and 13% of cases, respectively.[25]

The most frequent breast complaints for which men seek medical advice are breast enlargement, a palpable mass, or breast pain.[26] History and physical exam are very helpful in differentiating benign from malignant disease. Age is important, as men younger than 40 years rarely develop breast cancer. The most common diagnosis of men, even the older patients, presenting with a palpable mass remains gynecomastia.[27] In a review of more than 800 male breast biopsies, 96% were benign, gynecomastia being the most common (91%) entity.[28] In this series, other benign findings included lipoma, fibrosis, inflammatory changes, and normal breast tissue. Medications such as cimetidine, antipsychotics, and antihypertensives, as well as recreational drugs such as anabolic steroids and marijuana, have been implicated as causes for gynecomastia.[29]

Clinically, patients with gynecomastia are often seen to have diffusely enlarged and frequently tender breasts bilaterally, rather than a carcinoma, which is usually a hard palpable mass involving one breast. Nipple discharge is not a physiologic condition in men; it is most likely associated with malignancy, and requires further workup. Masses associated with skin ulceration or fixation are highly suspicious and necessitate a biopsy. The differential diagnosis of breast enlargement may also include pseudogynecomastia, which is breast enlargement due to adiposity. While no clinical finding is pathognomic of cancer or gynecomastia, those listed in Table 21-1 may be helpful in rendering a diagnosis.

Mammography is a useful tool in the diagnosis of male breast cancer. The mammographic findings seen in breast cancer, in order of frequency, are mass, architectural distortion, or microcalcifications.[27] False-negative mammography is seen more commonly in men than in women (10%-20%).[30] Sonography is recommended as an adjunct to mammography, in order to further define a breast mass or to examine the breast in the case of a negative mammogram. Solid and complex cystic masses are suspicious findings at sonography.[16] Sonography may also be used to assess the axillary lymph nodes. Sonography and mammography are both useful in differentiating cancer from gynecomastia. Unlike women who have or are at high risk for breast cancer, the use of breast magnetic resonance imaging (MRI) in the male patient remains to be defined. The extent of systemic disease may be ascertained as clinically appropriate, by using laboratory evaluation, chest radiography, bone scan, computed tomography of the abdomen and pelvis, or positron emission tomographic/computed tomographic (PET/CT) scan.

Pathologic evaluation of a breast mass in men can be easily performed with fine-needle aspiration (FNA) or core needle biopsy (CNBx).[31] FNA is a cytologic test performed with a 10-mL syringe and a 22-gauge needle. It is important to note

TABLE 21-1 Clinical Findings Suggestive of Gynecomastia or Carcinoma

Feature	Gynecomastia	Carcinoma
Age	Young	Old
Mass	Diffuse	Localized
	Mobile	Fixed
	Rubbery/smooth	Hard
	Centered nipple–areola	Frequently eccentric
Pain	Occasionally	Uncommon
Skin fixation	Rare	Frequent
Ulceration	None	Frequent
Nipple discharge	Infrequent	Common
Nipple deformity	None	Common
Bilateral	Common	Rare
Skin	Normal	Thickened, red, or ulcerated
Axilla	Normal	Axillary adenopathy

that the reliability of an FNA depends on the experience of the institution and the cytopathologist. CNBx is a histologic test and is performed percutaneously through a 2-mm skin incision, requiring a dedicated device. We prefer a 14-gauge needle and retrieve 5 or 6 cores of tissue. We also prefer to perform CNBx to FNA, as the former renders more tissue, which allows the differentiation between invasive and in situ cancer, as well as the estrogen receptors (ER) and progesterone receptors (PR), in addition to HER-2/neu oncogene status. This subsequently allows for definitive surgery to be planned. The incidence of a false-negative result with either FNA or CNBx ranges from to 3% to 10%.[31] The rate of an equivocal, atypical, or inadequate specimen, however, depends on the experience of the person performing the needle biopsy and/or the pathologist.

While the gold standard of managing a palpable male breast mass is excisional biopsy, the similarities to women have seen the application of the triple test (clinical exam, imaging evaluation, and pathologic assessment) to men. Should all 3 tests be consistent with a benign process, and the pathologic results are concordant with the imaging features, the patient may be observed and an excisional biopsy avoided. Furthermore, if pathologic evaluation reveals a malignant process, definitive surgery can be planned.

Men in whom breast cancer is diagnosed may develop clinically significant anxiety or depression. There are no psychosocial studies in this regard, but there is evidence that men, like women diagnosed with breast cancer, may benefit from psychosocial interventions.[32] Unfortunately, there is little sex-specific information or support for the male patient.[33]

HISTOLOGY

Within the male breast there is ductal architecture, but virtually no lobular development. Lobular development may occur as a response to increased estrogen exposure. The ductal epithelium is the most common site for malignant transformation. Rare cases of lobular carcinoma have been described in the male patient. Invasive ductal carcinoma represents the most common histology (80%), while ductal carcinoma in situ (DCIS) is seen in 5% to 15% of cases.[34] When present, DCIS is usually papillary and low to intermediate grade.[35] Other types of breast cancer—such as lobular, medullary, tubular, papillary, small cell, and mucinous carcinoma, as well as Paget disease—are rarely seen. Similarly to women, tubular and papillary cancers portend a better prognosis. Lobular carcinoma in situ (LCIS) has been seen in the rare cases where it is associated with invasive lobular cancer.[36]

Unlike women, men more frequently develop malignant lesions arising from cells other than the ductal epithelium, such as sarcomas, lymphomas, overlying skin cancers, and metastatic lung, prostate, and liver cancers, all of which must be ruled out during the workup.[37]

Male breast cancer is more frequently positive for ER and PR than in women. ER positivity is seen in 85% to 90% and PR in 70% to 80% of men, and may relate to the older age at presentation of men. Similarly to women, male breast cancer ER and PR positivity increases with age.[38] A proportion of male breast cancer displays overexpression of c-erbB-2 (HER-2/neu oncogene), reflecting an increase in proliferative activity, the importance of which, however, is unclear in the male patient. The HER-2/neu oncogene is less likely to be overexpressed in men than in women with breast cancer.[39]

Male breast cancer is staged as in women, by following the TNM staging system as set by the American Joint Committee on Cancer and the Union International Contre le Cancer.

TREATMENT

Surgery

The treatment of male breast cancer, similarly to women, remains surgical. While the classic procedure was the radical mastectomy,[40] recent extrapolation of outcomes in women has seen the modified radical mastectomy become the standard.[41] These studies have failed to show any difference in disease recurrence or survival rates between patients treated with radical and modified radical mastectomies. It is important to remember that the male breast is a small organ beneath the nipple–areola complex. As such, male breast cancer tends to be adjacent to the skin, nipple–areola complex, and chest wall.

The surgical resection of choice begins with an elliptical incision that includes skin and the nipple–areola complex overlying the mass. Flaps are raised in all directions similarly to the female patient, in order to separate the breast from the skin and subcutaneous tissue. The specimen is resected en bloc with pectoralis major fascia. Enbloc resection of overlying skin, breast, and underlying pectoralis major muscle is limited to patients where the tumor is adherent to the underlying fascia or muscle. We have avoided full resection of the pectoralis major muscle and have limited our resection in cases of fascial or muscle involvement to the underlying segment with a margin of 2 to 3 cm.

Axillary lymph node dissection remains the gold standard for male breast cancer, and usually includes resecting level I and II lymph nodes in continuity with the breast specimen. Extrapolating from the experience in female patients, the sentinel lymph node biopsy (SLNB) technique has become a viable option in selected cases.[42-44] Currently, total mastectomy with SLNB has become the procedure of choice for male breast cancer, limiting axillary dissection to patients with a positive sentinel node. Postmastectomy reconstruction may be considered for interested patients, and is limited to nipple reconstruction and tattooing for the areola.

The role of breast conservation treatment (BCT) in men remains a question of debate. In some small, uncontrolled series, similar local recurrence, survival, and morbidity outcomes have been reported in men undergoing either mastectomy or lumpectomy with radiation therapy.[45,46] Other studies have not confirmed such observation.[47-49] BCT in men has been questioned, as mastectomy in men may not carry the same psychosocial implications as it does in women.[50] Furthermore, lumpectomy may not be feasible due to the smaller volume of the male breast, the frequent involvement of the nipple, and the presence of nipple discharge.

Radiation

The use of postoperative radiation therapy in men is based on data from female patients. Men may benefit from adjuvant radiation therapy, given the central location of male breast cancer with frequent involvement of the skin and chest wall, and high rate of axillary metastasis. Given these facts, some authors have recommended the routine usage of postmastectomy radiation therapy in all male breast cancers including the chest wall, axilla, and supraclavicular and internal mammary lymph nodes.[51] Currently postmastectomy radiation in men follows the same guidelines as in women and is limited to T3 and T4 lesions, for 4 or more positive axillary lymph nodes, and positive or close margins.

Hormonal Therapy

The role of hormonal therapy in male breast cancer, like many other aspects of this disease, has not been evaluated in prospective, randomized trials. Nonetheless, as most male breast cancers display ER and PR positivity, the rational for hormonal manipulation is similar to that in women.[52] Historically, orchiectomy was the standard treatment, affording an approximately 80% response rate. Adrenalectomy and hypophysectomy were commonly recommended in the past, though no longer practiced. These ablative surgical options have been replaced by the use of the ER modulator, tamoxifen. Tamoxifen (20 mg/day for 5 years) is generally well tolerated, though associated with side effects such as weight gain, hot flashes, and loss of libido.[53] Such side effects have been suggested as reasons for noncompliance in some patients. The use of tamoxifen and orchiectomy are not mutually exclusive, such that men who fail tamoxifen may nonetheless respond to orchiectomy. Other hormonal agents used as second- or third-line therapies include androgens, estrogens, progestins, anti-androgens, aminoglutethimide, and luteinizing hormone-releasing hormone (LHRH) analogs.

Adjuvant hormonal therapy has been recommended in men with locally advanced disease, positive axillary nodes, and distant metastasis.[46] In a nonrandomized trial, tamoxifen significantly improved the disease-free survival in men with stage I and II disease.[27] Currently hormonal therapy is frequently recommended for men with breast cancer. Hormonal therapy is considered the first line of therapy in metastatic disease, affording an approximately 30% response rate.[54] Tamoxifen may also have a preventive role for the contralateral breast in men undergoing ipsilateral mastectomy.

The role of aromatase inhibitors in the male breast cancer patient remains to be defined, as there are only a handful of small series or case reports.[30] In addition, 20% of circulating estrogen is produced by the testis and is independent of aromatase enzyme activity; therefore for aromatase inhibitors to be effective would require gonadal ablation.

Chemotherapy

There is a lack of prospective randomized trials and limited retrospective data examining the use of chemotherapy for male breast cancer. Extrapolating from the experience in female breast cancer, chemotherapy is usually used for stage II, III, and IV disease.[55,56] Treatment consists of multiple cycles of cyclophosphamide, methotrexate or doxorubicin, and 5-fluorouracil. In one study, for node-positive stage II patients, adjuvant chemotherapy resulted in

5-year survival rates exceeding 80%. In contrast, fewer than 50% of men with metastatic breast cancer responded to chemotherapy, with a median survival rate of 4 to 23 months. The role of taxanes and dose dense chemotherapy has not been established in male breast cancer patients. Chemotherapy, used as second- or third-line treatment, may provide palliation in metastatic male breast cancer that is refractory to hormonal therapy or rapidly progressive. Advanced age at presentation has precluded adjuvant chemotherapy in men with breast cancer.[57]

There are no studies that have assessed the effectiveness of trastuzumab in HER-2/neu–overexpressing male breast cancer. Given the evidence in support of its use in women, however, it remains an option in selected male cases.

PROGNOSIS

It was often thought that men with breast cancer had a worse prognosis than their female counterparts. Men are more likely to present with a more advanced stage than women. However, recent studies have matched men and women for stage and number of positive lymph nodes, and have shown that men and women with breast cancer have similar overall survival rates.[58,59] Due to the older age at presentation, however, male breast cancer patients often have comorbid disease, and more frequently die of causes unrelated to the breast cancer. In one series, 39.5% of deaths were unrelated to the breast cancer. At Columbia-Presbyterian Medical Center, 52 men were diagnosed with breast cancer over an 10 year period, only 25% of deaths being related to the breast cancer itself. In a further 25% of cases, the death was related to another cancer, and the remaining 50% died of other, noncancer causes.[4] When comparing prognosis in well-matched groups of men and women with breast cancer, men tend to have a better disease-specific survival.[4] Similarly to women, the most important prognostic factor is the number of positive lymph nodes. Ten-year survival rates for patients with histologically negative nodes range from 77% to 100%, compared to patients with positive nodes ranging from 37% to 61%. Estimates for the overall 5-year survival are 40% to 65%.[60] The size of the tumor is also important prognostically, though the estrogen and progesterone status does not seem to be. Distant metastasis in men is similar to women, with bone, lung, liver, and brain being the most common sites.

Male breast cancer survivors, like their female counterparts, have an increased risk of developing a metachronous breast cancer. The risk of a contralateral breast cancer is about 93-fold greater than in men with no history of breast cancer, with an absolute risk of 1.75%.[16] Screening guidelines for the contralateral breast remain to be defined, though yearly mammography and 6-monthly clinical breast exam are reasonable options.[22] Those men who undergo genetic testing and are found to be BRCA1 or BRCA2 positive may be offered a prophylactic contralateral mastectomy.

CONCLUSIONS

Male breast cancer is a rare disease, whose diagnosis and management is greatly influenced by the data gained from women. Surgery remains the primary treatment, though radiation therapy, hormonal manipulation, and chemotherapy are important adjuncts. The prognosis and outcome in men with breast cancer is similar to those seen in women. Further work in the field of male breast cancer, as well as further research in female breast cancer from which data can be extrapolated, will aid in improving the survival of men with this disease.

REFERENCES

1. Sasco AJ, Lowenfels AB, Pasker-de Jong P. Review article: epidemiology of male breast cancer. A meta-analysis of published case-control studies and discussion of selected aetiological factors. *Int J Cancer.* 1993;53:538-549.
2. Weiss JR, Moysich KB, Swede H. Epidemiology of male breast cancer. *Cancer Epidemiol Biomarkers Prev.* 2005;14:20-26.
3. Jemal A, Murray T, Ward W, et al. Cancer statistics 2005. *Cancer J Clin.* 2005;55:10.
4. El-Tamer MB, Komenaka IK, Troxel A, et al. Men with breast cancer have a better disease-specific survival than women. *Arch Surg.* 2004;139:1079-1082.
5. Stierer M, Rosen H, Weitenfelder W, et al. Male breast cancer: the Austrian experience. *World J Surg.* 1995;19:687-693.
6. Bhagwandin S. Carcinoma of the male breast in Zambia. *East Afr Med J.* 1972;49:176-179.
7. Ojara EA. Carcinoma of the male breast in Mulago Hospital, Kampala. *East Afr Med J.* 1978;55:489-491.
8. American Cancer Society. Cancer Statistics 2005 Presentation. Available at http://www.cancer.org/docroot/CRI/content/CRI_2_4_1X_What_are_the_key_statistics_for_male_breast_cancer_28.asp
9. Agrawal A, Ayantunde AA, Rampaul R, et al. Male breast cancer: a review of clinical management. *Breast Cancer Res Treat.* 2007;103:11-21.
10. McClure JA, Higgins CC. Bilateral carcinoma of the male breast after estrogen therapy. *JAMA.* 1951;146:7-9.
11. Symmers WSC. Carcinoma of breast in trans-sexual individuals after surgical and hormonal interference with the primary and secondary sex charateristics. *Br Med J.* 1968;2:83-85.
12. Swerdlow AJ, Schoemaker MJ, Higgins CD, et al. Cancer incidence and mortality in men with Klinefelter syndrome: a cohort study. *J Natl Cancer Inst.* 2005;97:1204-1210.
13. Niewoehner CB, Schorer AE. Gynaecomastia and breast cancer in men. *BMJ.* 2008;336:709-713.
14. Andersen JA, Gram JB. Male breast at autopsy. *Acta Path Microbiol Immunol Scand.* 1982;90:191-197.
15. Memon MA, Donohue JH. Male breast cancer. *Br J Surg.* 1997;84:433-435.
16. Fentiman IS, Fourquet A, Hortobagyi GN. Male breast cancer. *Lancet.* 2006;367:595-604.
17. Ewertz M, Holmberg L, Tretli S, et al. Risk factors for male breast cancer, a case-control study from Scandinavia. *Acta Oncol.* 2001;40:467-471.
18. Thomas DB. Breast cancer in men. *Epidemiol Rev.* 1993;15:220-231.
19. Couch FJ, Farid LM, DeShano ML, et al. BRCA2 germline mutations in male breast cancer cases and breast cancer families. *Nat Genet.* 1996;13:123-125.
20. Tai YC, Domchek S, Parmigiani G, et al. Breast cancer risk among male BRCA1 and BRCA2 mutation carriers. *J Nat Cancer Inst.* 2007;99:1881-1884.
21. Struewing JP, Hartge P, Wacholder S, et al. The risk of cancer associated with specific mutations of BRCA1 and BRCA2 among Ashkenazi Jews. *N Eng J Med.* 1997;336:1401-1408.
22. Estala SM. Proposed screening recommendations for male breast cancer. *Nurse Pract.* 2006;31:62-63.
23. Appelqvist P, Salmo M. Prognosis in carcinoma of the male breast. *Acta Chir Scand.* 1982;148:499-502.
24. Erlichman C, Murphy KC, Elhakim T. Male breast cancer: a 13-year review of 89 patients. *J Clin Oncol.* 1984;2:903-909.
25. Crichlow RW. Carcinoma of the male breast. *Surg Gynecol Obstet.* 1972;134:1011-1019.
26. Heller KS, Rosen PP, Schottenfeld D, et al. Male breast cancer: a clinicopathologic study of 97 cases. *Ann Surg.* 1978;188:60-65.
27. Giordano SH, Buzdar AU, Hortobagyi GN. Breast cancer in men. *Ann Intern Med.* 2002;137:678-687.
28. Gough DB, Donohue JH, Evans MM, et al. A 50-year experience of male breast cancer: is outcome changing? *Surg Oncol.* 1993;2:325-333.
29. Donegan WL, Redlich PN, Lang PJ, et al. Carcinoma of the breast in males. *Cancer.* 1998;83:498-509.
30. Giordano SH. A review of the diagnosis and management of male breast cancer. *Oncologist.* 2005;10:471-479.
31. Lilleng R, Paksoy N, Vural G, et al. Assessment of fine needle aspiration cytology and histopathology for the diagnosing of male breast masses. *Acta Cytol.* 1995;39:877-881.
32. France L, Michie S, Barrett-Lee P, et al. Male breast cancer: a qualitative study of male breast cancer. *Breast.* 2000;9:342-348.
33. Williams BG, Iredale R, Brain K, et al. Experiences of men with breast cancer: an exploratory focus group study. *Br J Cancer.* 2003;89:1834-1836.
34. Muir D, Kanthan R, Kanthan SC. Male versus female breast cancers. A population-based comparative immunohistochemical analysis. *Arch Path Lab Med.* 2003;127:36-41.
35. Hittmair AP, Lininger RA, Tavassoli FA. Ductal carcinoma in situ (DCIS) in the male breast. *Cancer.* 1998;83:2139-2149.
36. Hultborn R, Friberg S, Hultborn KA. Male breast carcinoma: a study of the total material reported to the Swedish Cancer Registry 1958-1967 with respect to clinical and histopathological parameters. *Acta Oncol.* 1987;26:241-256.
37. Ribeiro GG. Carcinoma of the male breast: a review of 200 cases. *Br J Surg.* 1977;64:381-383.
38. Bezwoda WR, Hesdorffer C, Dansey R, et al. Breast cancer in men: clinical features, hormone receptor status, and response to therapy. *Cancer.* 1987;60:1337-1340.
39. Bloom KJ, Govil H, Gattuso P, et al. Status of HER-2 in male and female breast carcinoma. *Am J Surg.* 2001;182:389-392.
40. Williams WL, Powers M, Wagman LD. Cancer of the male breast: a review. *J Natl Med Assoc.* 1996;88:439-443.
41. Borgen PI, Wong GY, Vlamis V. Current management of male breast cancer: a review of 104 cases. *Ann Surg.* 1992;215:451-457.
42. Albo D, Ames FC, Hunt KK, et al. Evaluation of lymph node status in male breast cancer patients: a role for sentinel lymph node biopsy. *Breast Cancer Res Treat.* 2003;77:9-14.
43. Cimmino VM, Degnim AC, Sabel MS, et al. Efficacy of sentinel lymph node biopsy in male breast cancer. *J Surg Oncol.* 2004;86:74-77.
44. Goyal A, Horgan K, Kissin M, et al. Sentinel lymph node biopsy in male breast cancer patients. *Eur J Surg Oncol.* 2004;30:480-483.
45. Crichlow RW, Galt SW. Male breast cancer. *Surg Clin North Am.* 1990;70:1165-1177.
46. Jaiyesimi IA, Buzdar AU, Sahin AA, et al. Carcinoma of the male breast. *Ann Intern Med.* 1992;117:771-777.
47. Goss PE, Reid C, Pintilie M, et al. Male breast carcinoma: a review of 229 patients who presented to the Princess Margaret Hospital during 40 years: 1955-1996. *Cancer.* 1999;85:629-639.
48. Lipshy KA, Denning DA, Wheeler WE. A statewide review of male breast carcinoma. *Contemp Surg.* 1996;49:71-75.
49. Yildirim E, Berberoglu U. Male breast cancer: a 22-year experience. *Eur J Surg Oncol.* 1998;24:548-552.
50. McLachlan SA, Erlichman C, Liu FF, et al. Male breast cancer: an 11 year review of 66 patients. *Breast Cancer Res Treat.* 1996;40:225-230.
51. Cutuli B, Lacroze M, Dilhuydy JM, et al. Male breast cancer: results of the treatments and prognostic factors in 397 cases. *Eur J Cancer.* 1995;31A:1960-1964.
52. Ribeiro GG. Tamoxifen in the treatment of male breast carcinoma. *Clin Radiol.* 1983;34:625-628.
53. Anelli TFM, Anelli A, Tran KN, et al. Tamoxifen administration is associated with a high rate of treatment-limiting symptoms in male breast cancer patients. *Cancer.* 1994;74:74-77.
54. Griffith H, Muggia FM. Male breast cancer: update on systemic therapy. *Rev Endocr Rel Cancer.* 1989;31:5-11.
55. Paatel HZ, Buzdar AV, Hortobayi GN. Role of adjuvant chemotherapy in male breast cancer. *Cancer.* 1989;64:1583-1585.
56. Bagley CS, Wesley MN, Young RC, et al. Adjuvant chemotherapy in males with cancer of the breast. *Am J Clin Oncol.* 1987;10:55-60.
57. Ribeiro GG, Swindell R, Harris M, et al. A review of the management of male breast carcinoma based on an analysis of 240 treated cases. *Breast.* 1996;5:141-146.
58. Robinson R, Montague ED. Treatment results in males with breast cancer. *Cancer.* 1982;49:403-406.
59. Guinee VF, Olsson H, Moller T. The prognosis of breast cancer in males: a report of 335 cases. *Cancer.* 1993;71:154-161.
60. Scott-Conner CE, Jochimsen PR, Menck HR, et al. An analysis of male and female breast cancer treatment and survival among demographically identical pairs of patients. *Surgery.* 1999;126:775-780.

CHAPTER 22

Prognostic and Predictive Factors in Breast Cancer

Celina G. Kleer
Michael S. Sabel

Early detection and improvement in adjuvant systemic therapy has resulted in a decrease in breast cancer mortality. However, each year 500,000 women still die of breast cancer worldwide. It is clear that more work is needed to identify which breast cancers have a high propensity to metastasize, and to guide clinicians in selecting the most appropriate therapies.

Prognostic factors reflect the biology of the cancer and are defined as those factors associated with outcome without consideration of treatment. Predictive factors reflect the tumor sensitivity or resistance to a particular treatment, and are defined as those factors that predict which patients are likely to respond to a specific therapy. The relative worth of predictive factors will obviously differ with varying treatments. While some factors are primarily prognostic, some tumor markers are both prognostic and predictive. The classic example is the overexpression of HER-2/neu, which is associated with a worse outcome (prognostic), but also associated with response to treatment with trastuzumab (predictive).

The relative benefit of a predictive or prognostic factor can be classified as weak, moderate, or strong. For prognostic factors, the relative strength is related to the difference in the likelihood of an adverse event (recurrence, death) between a patient with the prognostic factor and one who is negative. An example of a strong prognostic factor is lymph node status, as a node-positive patient is 2 to 3 times more likely to have an event than a lymph node-negative patient. An example of a weak prognostic factor is estrogen receptor (ER) expression, as patients with ER-positive cancers have only slightly better outcomes than ER-negative patients. Predictive factors can also be classified as weak, moderate, and strong based on the likelihood that a patient with the factor will respond to treatment compared to that of a patient without the factor. While ER expression is a weak prognostic factor, it is a strong predictive factor for hormonal therapy, as ER-positive patients may realize a

50% reduction in the risk of recurrence with hormonal therapy, while ER-negative patients obtain almost no benefit from hormonal therapy.

When discussing prognostic and predictive factors, it is crucial to separate the statistical significance of a factor from the clinical significance. As an independent factor, many measurable factors may correlate with outcome. However, when examined in the context of other prognostic or predictive factors (multifactorial analysis), they may lose statistical significance. So while there may be biological significance to the factor it may provide little help to the clinician in estimating the likelihood of death or the benefit of therapy. Moreover, even if a factor retains statistical significance on multifactorial analysis, this still does not guarantee clinical significance. If the absence or presence of the factor is relatively rare among breast cancer patients, its clinical utility is severely limited. One example is tumor grade. While grade III (poorly differentiated) patients may have worse outcomes than grade I (well-differentiated) patients, the great majority of patients are either grade III or II (moderately differentiated), greatly limiting the clinical utility of grade as a prognostic factor.

More importantly, the measurement of that factor must be technically reliable and reproducible. The more variation there is in its interpretation, the less useful it is. Again, grade is a good example, as the subjective labeling of tumors as grade I, II, or III allows for significant variation among pathologists. Recent changes to the grading system have attempted to increase the objectivity and decrease variation, but differences in interpretation can never be fully eliminated. Even for "standard" tumor markers, such as ER expression or HER-2/neu overexpression, there can be variability in the assays used for measurement. Researchers and clinicians can use different assays to measure the factor (immunohistochemistry [IHC], Western blotting, or enzyme-linked immunosorbent assay [ELISA] for protein expression; Northern blotting or reverse transcriptase-polymerase chain reaction [RT-PCR] for RNA expression; or florescence in situ hybridization [FISH] for DNA amplification) and different reagents for the assay (such as different antibodies for IHC). Even minor technical differences such as the concentration of a reagent or the method by which the specimen is procured and processed can impact the results of the test. Finally, whenever visual assays are used for the final interpretation, intra and interobserver variability will always be a concern. For example, several studies have demonstrated significant discordance for HER-2/neu overexpression between laboratories.[1,2]

It is important to realize that true estimations of prognosis are dependent upon weighing the relative impact of all known prognostic factors. One extremely useful method of determining the risk of recurrence and of death based on multiple prognostic factors is the use of computer programs. The most popular is the Web-based Adjuvant Online. The prognostic information was created based on prognosis estimates derived mainly from the Surveillance, Epidemiology, and End Results (SEER) data, which are then adjusted using a Bayesian method on the relative risks conferred and the prevalence of positive test results. After entering in patient and tumor data, a 10-year risk of recurrence and 10-year risk of death are calculated. In addition, estimates of the benefit of hormonal therapy and chemotherapy, based on the Oxford Overviews and other sources, are also presented. This information and program have been extremely useful in facilitating physician–patient communication regarding outcome and the benefits of adjuvant therapy.

This chapter will review several factors presently used to gauge prognosis and predict response to therapy. We will discuss individual factors and emphasize the practical and controversial aspects associated with them.

PROGNOSTIC FACTORS

Tumor Size

One of the first described and still most important prognostic factors in breast cancer is the size of the primary tumor. Many studies have demonstrated a linear correlation between the diameter of the primary tumor and both the presence of lymph node metastases and clinical outcome. Among node-negative patients, tumor size is the single most important prognostic factor.[3]

The reasons that tumor size is so strongly associated with outcome are multifactorial. Part of this is explained by the increased presence of metastases in the regional lymph nodes with increasing tumors size. However, tumor size is still an independent prognostic factor; small tumors associated with positive nodes have a better prognosis than large tumors with positive nodes. Larger tumor size appears to be associated with increased occult blood vascular dissemination. It must always be remembered, however, that there may be a detection bias at play. More aggressive tumors are typically found when they are large given the intervals at which we screen, while slow-growing tumors have an inherent favorable prognosis *and* are found at a small size.[4]

Practical Considerations

For the most precise prognostic information, tumor size should be obtained from the pathologic specimen. The correlation with the clinical assessment (physical examination, radiographic studies) may be inaccurate.

Although reporting of pathologic size has not yet been standardized, numerous studies have demonstrated that it is the size of the invasive component that is associated with outcome. There are some relevant practical considerations in reporting tumor size; especially the determination of microinvasion, multifocal tumors, and tumors removed in more than one specimen.

Microinvasion is defined by the current AJCC *Cancer Staging Manual* (sixth edition) as "the extension of tumor cells beyond the basement membrane into the adjacent tissues with no focus more than 0.1 cm in greatest dimension." When multiple foci of microinvasion are present, it is the size of only the largest focus that is used, not the sum of the microinvasive foci. Most studies have shown that the prognosis of ductal carcinoma in situ (DCIS) with microinvasion is similar to the prognosis of DCIS alone.[5,6]

When more than one focus of invasive carcinoma is present, the largest focus is used for staging purposes. Similarly, when invasive carcinomas are removed in more than one specimen, pathologists measure the size of the largest tumor. In difficult cases, radiologic correlation can be very helpful in determining tumor size.[7] A few studies have demonstrated that invasive carcinomas with multiple foci of invasion have higher rates of lymph node metastasis and that the number of lymph node metastasis is predicted best by the aggregate size of the invasive foci.[8,9] Even though at this time size determination is based on the size of the largest focus, emerging data may result in revisions to our current staging system in the future.

Lymph Node Status

The most powerful prognostic factor in breast cancer remains the presence of disease in the regional lymph nodes. Repeated studies show an inferior outcome when disease is identified in the lymph nodes and the more nodes involved, the worse the outcome.

Breast cancer can metastasize to both the axillary lymph nodes and the internal mammary (IM) lymph nodes (as well as the supraclavicular nodal basins, although this is less common). Metastases to either the IM or axillary nodes are associated with a poor outcome compared to lymph node-negative patients. However the presence of regional disease in both the IM and axillary lymph nodes portends a worse prognosis than disease in either basin alone.[10-14] The majority of these data come from the era of the extended radical mastectomy. At that time, it was thought that including an IM lymph node dissection with the radical mastectomy might improve outcomes. This was not the case, and support for the extended radical mastectomy has faded. However, the importance of staging the IM nodes has reemerged with the introduction of radioactive colloid for intraoperative lymphatic mapping. Depending on the method of injection, drainage to the IM nodes is often identified on lymphoscintigraphy. Whether the prognostic information and potential therapeutic benefit of excising SLN in the IM chain justifies the morbidity of the procedure is an area of ongoing debate.

Practical Considerations

The SLN biopsy was introduced in the 1990s. As pathologists were faced with fewer lymph nodes to evaluate, we began using multiple levels and/or IHC in the routine evaluation of SLN.

Before we can discuss the impact of SLN biopsy on prognosis we need to define two commonly used terms: micrometastasis and isolated tumor cells. *Micrometastases* are foci of cancer in a lymph node that are greater than 0.2 mm but with none greater than 2.0 mm. In the most recent AJCC staging system for breast cancer, these are designated as pN1mi. *Isolated tumor cells* are defined as single cells or small clusters of cells smaller than 0.2 mm. These are staged as pN0. As compared with micrometastases, which often show evidence of proliferation or stromal reaction, isolated tumor cells or small cell clusters usually do not show such evidence of malignant activity.

Although more definitive evidence is needed, available literature suggests that micrometastasis not only are associated with a risk of additional disease in the non-SLN (justifying complete axillary lymph node dissection) but also provide prognostic information.[15,16] Until recently, there have been no convincing data suggesting that patients with isolated tumor cells in SNL have a worse prognosis.[7] However, a recent study found that isolated tumor cells or micrometastasis in the SLN were associated with a reduced 5-year disease-free survival compared to node negative patients, and that disease-free survival was improved with adjuvant therapy.[16B] Additional data from prospective studies of SLN biopsy (NSABP B-32, ACOSOG Z-10) are pending.

There are practical with applying the strict size definitions of the AJCC that arise in daily pathology practice. Those issues include methods to measure very small metastasis, how to assess the diffuse single-cell pattern of metastasis of invasive lobular carcinomas, and the presence of multiple clusters of tumor cells.

To measure accurately the size of isolated tumor cells, pathologists need to employ a calibrated ocular micrometer, or estimate from field sizes.

Invasive lobular carcinomas have long been recognized to metastasize in a diffuse, sometimes single-cell pattern. In this pattern, there can be thousands of cells, but no cell cluster larger than 0.02 mm. Sometimes the identification of rare metastatic cancer cells is extremely hard on routine hematoxylin and eosin staining, and the use of cytokeratin stains is recommended. The designation of isolated tumor cells and N0 classification seems inappropriate for such cases, and several pathologists have advocated classifying these cases as N1, based on the number of tumor cells. This will likely be addressed in the upcoming seventh edition of the AJCC.

Another difficulty that pathologists face is the presence of multiple clusters of tumor cells in a lymph node. In this instance, if 2 or more clusters are separated by normal lymph node tissue, the distance between the clusters should not be included in the measurement. Sometimes a lymph node may contain over 5 clusters smaller than 0.2 cm. Is this best classified as a micrometastasis or a bonafide metastasis? Some of these issues need clarification in the very near future. We recommend that pathologists communicate with the surgeons and clinicians when these cases arise to be considered in clinical decision-making.

Histologic Grade and Type

Both histologic grade and type are routinely used to make clinical recommendations.

Practical Considerations

The most common method of determining histologic grade is the Nottingham combined histologic grade (the Elston-Ellis modification of the Scarff-Bloom-Richardson grading system). This system is based on scoring 3 factors: tubule formation, degree of pleomorphism, and mitotic count. While this modification is more objective than previous methods of determining grade, there are still issues of variability in tissue fixation and observer interpretations.

Histologic grade correlates with survival independent of lymph node status and tumor size.[17] Additionally, some studies have demonstrated that histologic grade can be prognostic among certain subsets of breast cancer patients. Among patients with tumors smaller than 1.0 cm (and primarily node negative), Stierer et al[18] found that high histologic grade was a significant predictor of recurrence and death. Winchester et al[19] found histologic grade to be a significant predictor of disease-free survival among aneuploid tumors. Grade was the most powerful prognostic factor in a multiple regression analysis of 654 reported patients by Sundquist et al.[20]

It is important to note that in addition of being a powerful prognostic factor, histologic grade may have predictive value. Adjuvant chemotherapy may produce a greater benefit in high-grade tumors than in low-grade tumors, particularly among node-negative patients.[21-23] For this reason, histologic grade is commonly used in adjuvant therapy decision-making.

Certain histologic types of invasive breast carcinoma including tubular, mucinous, cribriform, adenoid cystic, and medullary are associated with favorable outcome. Pathologists need to apply strict criteria in order to make these diagnoses. If strict diagnostic criteria are used, the 20-year disease-free survival of these favorable histologic tumor types measuring up to 3.0 cm is similar to that of invasive ductal carcinomas of 1.0 cm or smaller.[24] The College of American Pathologists (CAP) recommends using the World Health Organization classification for the determination of histologic type.[25]

Angiolymphatic Invasion

The prognostic importance of angiolymphatic invasion has been investigated with mixed results. Angiolymphatic (or vascular lymphatic) invasion is defined as invasion of lymphatic or blood vessels by a primary tumor. Several studies have demonstrated independent prognostic significance of angiolymphatic invasion.[26-28] The major drawback to using angiolymphatic invasion as a prognostic factor is the subjectivity and variation in methods of detection. While some pathologists search for vessel invasion on routine H&E, others routinely use IHC to identify the vessels, which may increase the detection rate of angiolymphatic invasion.

Practical Considerations

The distinction between angiolymphatic invasion from retraction artifact (tissue shrinkage during processing) around foci of invasive carcinoma can be difficult for the pathologist. Analysis of angiolymphatic invasion at the periphery of the tumor is thus suggested. Although the CAP recommends reporting of angiolymphatic invasion, no defining criteria are described.

The assessment of angiolymphatic invasion, is the least reproducible prognostic factor among pathologists, with many possibilities for misinterpretation. In our practice, we follow the criteria proposed by Rosen.[29] These include that (1) angiolymphatic invasion should be diagnosed outside the border of invasive carcinoma and (2) endothelial cell nuclei should be seen lining the space. The experience using endothelial cell markers has not been compelling to date, and should be used with caution.

Age and Comorbidities

A young age at diagnosis has emerged as a poor prognostic factor for breast cancer. Young women, particularly in their 30s, exhibit a poor survival compared with older women.[30,31] Much of this is related to a worse biology. Tumors among young women are more likely to be node-positive, hormone-receptor negative, and possess worse molecular features.[32,33] Adjuvant systemic treatment appears to diminish the poor prognosis associated with young age.[33] Older age and comorbidities are also associated with higher breast cancer mortality rates; however, this is likely related to less extensive treatment.

Race

Another poor prognostic sign in breast cancer is race. Although breast cancer incidence is lower in African American women, overall age adjusted mortality rates are higher as compared to Caucasian women.[34,35] A 1.5 to 2.2 fold difference in mortality was first noted in the 1970s, and has unfortunately been increasing.[36,37] Certainly socioeconomic factors account for a proportion of breast cancer outcome disparities. This ranges from suboptimal breast cancer screening, resulting in a more advanced stage of disease at diagnosis; to disparities in delivery of treatment. However, meta-analysis of multiple studies examining race and breast cancer demonstrate that even after adjusting for socioeconomic status and stage and age at diagnosis, there is still a 22% higher mortality risk among African American patients.[38] Two studies of breast cancer survival rates among African American and Caucasian women in the US Department of Defense health care system, where medical care is accessible and available at no cost, also showed that African American women still have a worse overall survival.[39,40] Therefore, socioeconomic factors do not completely explain the poor prognosis associated with ethnicity; biological factors also play a role. Tumors of African American breast cancer patients are more likely to be higher grade, hormone-receptor negative, aneuploid, and node positive, even after controlling for tumor size and age.[41] Several molecular and genetic differences have also been identified.[42] Continued research is necessary and ongoing, but until the complex interactions between genetic, socioeconomic, and cultural features associated with breast cancer and race are dissected out, ethnicity remains a poor prognostic factor.

PREDICTIVE FACTORS

Standard predictive factors include hormone receptor status for selection of endocrine therapy and HER-2/neu amplification and/or overexpression for selection of targeted therapy. Available predictive factors may spare patients from ineffective treatment and unnecessary side effects of systemic therapy. However, so far predictive factors cannot guarantee treatment response. For example, while negative ER status is associated with lack of response to endocrine manipulation, not all patients with ER-positive tumors respond to this treatment. This is a reflection of our incomplete understanding of the complexities of breast cancer genetics and biology.

Estrogen and Progesterone Receptors

While the prognostic effect of hormone receptor expression is modest, their predictive value is strong. ER expression is probably the most powerful individual predictive factor in breast cancer. Data from the National Surgical Adjuvant Breast Project (NSABP), the National Cancer Institute (NCI), and the Early Breast Cancer Trialists' Collaborative (EBCTC) Overview show that the benefits of hormonal treatment are confined to those patients whose tumors express hormone receptors.

Progesterone receptor (PR) is an estrogen-regulated gene; its expression therefore thought to indicate a functioning ER pathway.[43] There are studies suggesting that tumors positive for PR are more likely to respond to hormonal treatment.[44,45] The predictive value of PR in the absence of ER is controversial in the literature, but perhaps PR positivity identifies a group of patients responsive to hormonal therapy.

Practical Considerations

The analysis of hormonal receptors, particularly of ER, is an essential component of the evaluation of breast cancers. Therefore, the use of clinically validated, reproducible, and standardized cutoffs for determining the scoring of positive results is critical. IHC is the standard method for determining ER and PR status. IHC can be applied to core biopsy and surgical excision specimens. A wide range of arbitrary cutoffs (eg, 5% or 10% of tumor cells) have been employed by different laboratories to report ER and PR. Only one cutoff for both ER and PR IHC has been clinically validated as predicting response to endocrine therapy. In the landmark study of Harvey and coworkers[46] a 9-point semiquantitative "Allred" score (ranging from 0 to 8) was performed on a large group of patients and results were correlated with response to adjuvant endocrine therapy. The authors found strong direct association between the level of ER expression and response to hormonal therapy. More recent studies have supported this cutoff for IHC analysis of PR.[47] These studies emphasize the importance of clinical validation before a cutoff is implemented. At this time, the value of further quantification of ER and PR is uncertain. Recent data showed a dichotomized, bimodal distribution of ER expression, which has called into question the clinical utility of quantifying ER expression. These studies suggested that ER is almost always either completely positive or completely negative.[48,49]

Advances in computers have led to the development of computerized image analysis systems to more accurately provide a percentage of ER-positive cells. Although sophisticated, using a cutoff of greater than 1% to be considered ER positive, this system yielded results almost identical to traditional visual pathologist scoring.[50] In the future, other techniques might prove more efficacious than IHC in quantifying ER. Further clinically validated studies are need to define whether ER should be reported as a continuous or a dichotomized variable.

Human Epidermal Growth Factor Receptor 2 (HER-2)

The human epidermal growth factor receptor 2 gene (ERBB2, referred to as HER-2) is expressed at low levels in a variety of normal epithelia, including breast duct epithelium, but is amplified in approximately 18% to 20% of breast cancers.[51] Amplification is the predominant mechanism of gene overexpression and abnormal high levels of the 185-kDa glycoprotein are associated with worse prognosis; but most importantly, they are highly predictive of response to therapies that target HER-2. Trastuzumab (Herceptin; Genentech, South San Francisco, California), a humanized monoclonal antibody against HER-2, is effective in both the metastatic and adjuvant settings.[52] This drug can be used alone or in combination with chemotherapy.[53-55]

HER-2 status is also predictive for several systemic therapies. HER-2 positivity appears to be associated with resistance to endocrine therapy, and with resistance or sensitivity to different types of chemotherapeutic agents.[52] Taken together, all available data indicate that HER-2 is a useful predictive marker for clinical decision-making for women with breast cancer.

Practical Considerations

For the aforementioned reasons, HER-2 testing is. an essential part of the clinical evaluation of all breast cancer patients in the United States, and accurate HER-2 results are critical in identifying patients for whom this targeted therapy is appropriate. Recently, the American Society of Clinical Oncology together with the College of American Pathologists reported improved guidelines for HER-2 testing.[52] A positive HER-2 result is defined as IHC staining of 3+ of more than 30% of invasive tumor cells, a FISH result of more than 6 HER-2 gene copies per nucleus, or a FISH ratio of more than 2.2. A negative result is defined as an IHC staining of 0 or 1+, a FISH result of less than 4 HER-2 gene copies per nucleus, or a FISH ratio of less than 1.8. The recommendation also provides guidelines to deal with equivocal cases.[52]

Importantly, the new guidelines establish testing validation requirements by all laboratories performing HER-2 testing. This entails specifically documenting 95% concordance rates between cases that are IHC 3+ and FISH-amplified, and between cases that are IHC 0/1+ and non-FISH-amplified. HER-2 FISH is reported as amplified (HER-2/CEP17 ratio > 2.2), equivocal (ratio 1.8-2.2), or negative (ratio < 1.8).

Although attaining near-perfect correlation between assessment of HER-2 status by IHC and FISH is a goal, discordance between these two assays may be due to biology as well as laboratory error. For example, Pauletti and associates[56] have demonstrated that at least 3% of breast cancers show protein overexpression in the absence of concomitant gene amplification, implying that such cancers manifest high levels of protein expression through a mechanism other than gene amplification.

Several investigators have shown that polysomy of chromosome 17 can account for a small subset of breast cancers showing 3+ levels of HER-2 immunostaining but no amplification by FISH when the HER-2/chromosome 17 ratio is evaluated.[57-59]

Newer Factors

Over 100 promising breast cancer prognostic factors have been reported in the last decade. However, most have not been validated to date. Recently, the American Society of Clinical Oncology met and discussed new tumor marker tests. The article was published in the *Journal of Clinical Oncology.*[60] In addition to ER, PR, and HER-2, urokinase plasminogen activator (uPA) and plasminogen activator inhibitor (PAI-1) were recommended by the panel. These 2 markers are measured by ELISA on fresh or frozen breast cancer tissues, and may be used for prognostication in patients with newly diagnosed, node-negative breast cancer. At this time, IHC for these markers is not as accurate as desired, and has not been validated. Experimentally, uPA and PAI-1 have been shown to regulate invasion, angiogenesis, and metastasis.[61] In addition, the panel recommended the use of multiparameter gene expression analyses, which are discussed in a separate chapter of the book, including Oncotype DX.

SUMMARY

Considerable progress has been made in recent years in elucidating the molecular alterations that contribute to the development of breast cancer. However, except for the evaluation of ER, PR, and HER-2, very little of this information has had any real impact on the clinical management of breast cancer. Most of the clinically relevant information is obtained through the careful histopathologic evaluation of resected breast specimens.

Translation of laboratory results into the clinical field is necessary to improve our ability to predict outcome and apply more specific and effective treatments to women with breast cancer. Ideally, prognostic and predictive markers that can be tested in paraffin-embedded tissue sections would be desirable and easily implemented in the clinic. Several such factors are being investigated. One of those makers is the Polycomb group protein EZH2. This protein has been shown to be overexpressed in aggressive and metastatic invasive breast carcinomas by several independent groups.[62-64] EZH2 overexpression detected by IHC was an independent prognostic marker.[55] Ongoing work is focused on determining whether EZH2 overexpression in T1 breast cancers can identify which tumors have high propensity to metastasize.

It is reasonable to expect that in coming years the combined power of new high-throughput technologies and bioinformatics will result in the identification of molecular markers capable of guiding treatment interventions. The recently reported 70-gene prognosis profile, found to be superior to standard clinical and histologic evaluation, is one example of the power of these novel technologies applied to cancer prognosis and prediction.[65] The close cooperation of basic scientists, clinicians, and pathologists is required for the evaluation of novel prognostic and predictive assays to determine when and if they should be incorporated into routine clinical use.

REFERENCES

1. Perez EA, Suman VJ, Davidson NE, et al. HER2 testing by local, central and reference laboratories in teh NCCTG N9831 INtergroup Adjuvant Trial. *J Clin Oncol.* 2004,22.567a.

2. Press MF, Hung G, Godolphin W, et al. Sensitivity of HER 2/neu antibodies in archival tissue samples: potential source of error in immunohistochemical studies of oncogene expression. *Cancer Res.* 1994;54:2771-2777.

3. Carter CL, Allen C, Henson OE. Relation of tumor size, lymph node status and survival in 24,730 breast cancer cases. *Cancer.* 1989;63:181-187.

4. Spratt JS. Realities of breast cancer control, public expectations and the law. *Surg Oncol Clin North Am.* 1994;3:25-44.

5. de Mascarel I, MacGrogan G, Mathoulin-Pelissier S, et al. Breast ductal carcinoma in situ with microinvasion: a definition supported by a long-term study of 1248 serially sectioned ductal carcinomas. *Cancer.* 2002;94: 2134-2142.

6. Padmore RF, Fowble B, Hoffman J, et al. Microinvasive breast carcinoma: clinicopathologic analysis of a single institution experience. *Cancer.* 2000;88:1403-1409.

7. Connolly JL. Changes and problematic areas in interpretation of the AJCC *Cancer Staging Manual,* 6th edition, for breast cancer. *Arch Pathol Lab Med.* 2006;130:287-291.

8. Andea AA, Bouwman D, Wallis T, Visscher DW. Correlation of tumor volume and surface area with lymph node status in patients with multifocal/multicentric breast carcinoma. *Cancer.* 2004;100:20-27.

9. Coombs NJ, Boyages J. Multifocal and multicentric breast cancer: does each focus matter? *J Clin Oncol.* 2005;23:7497-7502.

10. Caceres E. An evaluation of radical mastectomy and extended radical mastectomy for cancer of the breast. *Surg Gynecol Obstet.* 1967;123:337-341.

11. Urban JA, Marjani MA. Significance of internal mammary lymph node metastases in breast cancer. *Am J Roentgenol Radium Ther Nucl Med.* 1971;111:130-136.

12. Bucalossi P, Veronesi U, Zingo L, Cantu C. Enlarged mastectomy for breast cancer: review of 1213 cases. *Am J Roentgenol Radium Ther Nucl Med.* 1971;111:119-122.

13. Veronesi U, Cascinelli N, Bufalino R, et al. Risk of internal mammary lymph node metastases and its relevance on prognosis of breast cancer patients. *Ann Surg.* 1983;198:681-684.

14. Li KYY, Shen ZZ. An analysis of 1,242 cases of extended radical mastectomy. *Breast.* 1984;10:10-19.

15. Dowlatshahi K, Fan M, Snider HC, Habib FA. Lymph node micrometastases from breast carcinoma: reviewing the dilemma. *Cancer.* 1997;80:118811-97.

16. Liberman L. Pathologic analysis of sentinel lymph nodes in breast carcinoma. *Cancer.* 2000;88:971-977.

16B. de Boer M, van Deurzen CH, van Dijck JA, et al. Micrometastases or Isolated Tumor Cells and the Outcome of Breast Cancer. *New England Journal of Medicine.* 2009;361(7):653-663.

17. Elston CW, Ellis IO. Pathological prognostic factors in breast cancer. I. The value of histological grade in breast cancer: experience from a large study with long-term follow-up. *Histopathology.* 1991;19:403-410.

18. Seidman JD, Schnaper LA, Aisner SC, et al. Long-term analysis of factors influencing the outcome in carcinoma of the breast smaller than one centimeter. *Surg Gynecol Obstet.* 1992;175:151-160.

19. Winchester DJ, Duda RV, August CZ, et al. The importance of DNA flow cytometry in node-negative breast cancer. *Arch Surg.* 1990;125: 886-889.

20. Sundquist M, Thorstenson S, Brudin L, et al. A comparsion between flow cytometric assessment of S-phase fraction and Nottingham histologic grade as prognostic instruments in breast cancer. *Breast Cancer Res Treat.* 2000;63:11-15.

21. Fisher B, Fisher ER, Redmond C, Brown A. Tumor nuclear grade, estrogen receptor and progesterone receptor: their value alone or in combination as indicators of outcome following adjuvant therapy for breast cancer. *Breast Cancer Res Treat.* 1986;7:147-60.

22. Fisher ER, Redmond C, Fisher B. Histologic grading of breast cancer. *Pathol Annu.* 1980;15:239-251.

23. Davis BW, Gelber RD, Goldhirsh A, et al. Prognostic significance of tumor grade in clinical trials of adjuvant therapy for breast cancer with axillary lymph node metastasis. *Cancer.* 1986; 8:2662-2670.

24. Rosen PP, Groshen S, Kinne DW, Norton L. Factors influencing prognosis in node-negative breast carcinoma: analysis of 767 T1N0M0/T2N0M0 patients with long-term follow-up. *J Clin Oncol.* 1993;11:2090-2100.

25. World Health Organization Classification of Tumours. *Pathology and Genetics of Tumours of the Breast and Female Genital Organs.* Lyon, France: IARC Press; 2003.

26. De Mascarel I, Bonichon F, Durand M, et al. Obvious peritumoral emboli: an elusive prognostic factor reappraised. Multivariate analysis of 1320 node-negative breast cancers. *Eur J Cancer.* 1998;34:58-65.

27. Lauria R, Perrone F, Carlomagno C, et al. The prognostic value of lymphatic and blood vessel invasion in operable breast cancer. *Cancer.* 1995;76:1772-1778.

28. Pinder SE, Ellis IO, Galea M et al. Pathological prognostic factors in breast cancer III. Vascular invasion: relationship with recurrence and survival in a large study with long-term follow-up. *Histopathology.* 1994;24:41-47.

29. Rosen PP. Tumor emboli in intramammary lymphatics in breast carcinoma: pathologic criteria for diagnosis and clinical significance. *Pathol Annu.* 1983;18:215-232.

30. Arriagada R, Le MG, Dunant A, et al. Twenty-five years of follow-up in patients with operable breast carcinoma: correlation between clinicopathologic factors and the risk of death in each 5-year period. *Cancer.* 2006;106: 743-750.

31. Fisher ER, Anderson S, Tan-Chiu E, et al. Fifteen year prognostic discriminants for invasive breast carcinoma. National Surgical Adjuvant Breast and Bowel Project protocol-06. *Cancer.* 2001;91:1679-1687.

32. Kollias J, Elston CW, Ellis IO, et al. Early onset breast cancer- histopathological and prognostic considerations. *Br J Cancer.* 1997;75:1318-1323.

33. Kroman N, Jensen MB, Wohlfahrt J, et al. Factors influencing the effect of age on prognosis in breast cancer: population based study. *BMJ.* 2000;320:474-478.

34. Brawley OW. Disaggregating the effects of race and poverty on breast cancer outcomes. *J Natl Cancer Inst.* 2002;94:471-473.

35. Ries L, Eisner M, Kosary M. *SEER Cancer Statistics Review, 1975-2000.* Bethesda, MD: National Cancer Institute; 2003.

36. Eley JW, Hill HA, Chen VW, et al. Racial differences in survival from breast cancer. Results of the National Cancer Institute Black/White Cancer Survival Study. *JAMA.* 1994;272:947-954.

37. Jatoi I, Anderson WF, Rao SR, Devesa SS. Breast cancer trends among black and white women in the United States. *J Clin Oncol.* 2005;23:7836-7841.

38. Newman LA, Mason J, Cote D, et al. African-American ethnicity, socioeconomic status and breast cancer survival: a meta-analysis of 14 studies involving over 10,000 African American and 40,000 white American patients with carcinoma of the breast. *Cancer.* 2002;94:2844-2854.

39. Wojcik BE, Spinks MK, Stein CR. Effects of screening mammography on the comparative survival rates of African American, white, and hispanic beneficiaries of a comprehensive health care system. *Breast J.* 2003;9:175-183.

40. Jatoi I, Becher H, Leake CR. Widening disparity in survival between white and African-American patients with breast carcinoma treated in the US Department of Defense Healthcare System. *Cancer* 2003;98:894-899.

41. Shavers VL, Harlan LC, Stevens JL, et al. Racial/ethnic variation in clinical presentation, treatment, and survival among breast cancer patients under age 35. *Cancer.* 2003;97:134-147.

42. Newman LA. Breast cancer in African-American women. *Oncologist.* 2005;10:1-14.

43. Horwitz KB, Koseki Y, McGuire WL. Estrogen control of progesterone receptor in human breast cancer: role of estradiol and antiestrogen. *Endocrinology.* 1978;103:1742-1751.

44. Bardou VJ, Arpino G, Elledge RM, et al. Progesterone receptor status significantly improves outcome prediction over estrogen receptor status alone for adjuvant endocrine therapy in two large breast cancer databases. *J Clin Oncol.* 2003; 21:1973-1979.

45. Ravdin PM, Green S, Dorr TM, et al. Prognostic significance of progesterone receptor levels in estrogen receptor-positive patients with metastatic breast cancer treated with tamoxifen: results of a prospective Southwest Oncology Group study. *J Clin Oncol.* 1992;10:1284-1291.

46. Harvey JM, Clark GM, Osborne CK, Allred DC. Estrogen receptor status by immunohistochemistry is superior to the ligand-binding assay for predicting response to adjuvant endocrine therapy in breast cancer. *J Clin Oncol.* 1999;17:1474-1481.

47. Mohsin SK, Weiss H, Havighurst T, et al. Progesterone receptor by immunohistochemistry and clinical outcome in breast cancer: a validation study. *Mod Pathol.* 2004;17:1545-1554.

48. Nadji M, Gomez-Fernandez C, Ganjei-Azar P, Morales AR. Immunohistochemistry of estrogen and progesterone receptors reconsidered: experience with 5,993 breast cancers. *Am J Clin Pathol.* 2005;123:21-27.

49. Collins LC, Botero ML, Schnitt SJ. Bimodal frequency distribution of estrogen receptor immunohistochemical staining results in breast cancer: an analysis of 825 cases. *Am J Clin Pathol.* 2005;123:16-20.

50. Turbin DA, Leung S, Cheang MC, et al. Automated quantitative analysis of estrogen receptor expression in breast carcinoma does not differ from expert pathologist scoring: a tissue microarray study of 3,484 cases. *Breast Cancer Res Treat.* 2008;110:417-426.

51. Slamon DJ, Clark GM, Wong SG, et al. Human breast cancer: correlation of relapse and survival with amplification of the HER-2/neu oncogene. *Science.* 1987;235:177-182.

52. Wolff AC, Hammond ME, Schwartz JN, et al. American Society of Clinical Oncology/College of American Pathologists guideline recommendations for human epidermal growth factor receptor 2 testing in breast cancer. *J Clin Oncol.* 2007;25:118-145.

53. Cobleigh MA, Vogel CL, Tripathy D, et al. Multinational study of the efficacy and safety of humanized anti-HER2 monoclonal antibody in women who have HER2-overexpressing metastatic breast cancer that has progressed after chemotherapy for metastatic disease. *J Clin Oncol.* 1999;17:2639-2648.

54. Slamon DJ, Leyland-Jones B, Shak S, et al. Use of chemotherapy plus a monoclonal antibody against HER2 for metastatic breast cancer that overexpresses HER2. *N Engl J Med.* 2001;344:783-792.

55. Vogel CL, Cobleigh MA, Tripathy D, et al. Efficacy and safety of trastuzumab as a single agent in first-line treatment of HER2-overexpressing metastatic breast cancer. *J Clin Oncol.* 2002;20:719-726.

56. Pauletti G, Godolphin W, Press MF, Slamon DJ. Detection and quantitation of HER-2/neu gene amplification in human breast cancer archival material using fluorescence in situ hybridization. *Oncogene.* 1996;13:63-72.

57. Ma Y, Lespagnard L, Durbecq V, et al. Polysomy 17 in HER-2/neu status elaboration in breast cancer: effect on daily practice. *Clin Cancer Res.* 2005;11:4393-4399.

58. Varshney D, Zhou YY, Geller SA, Alsabeh R. Determination of HER-2 status and chromosome 17 polysomy in breast carcinomas comparing HercepTest and PathVysion FISH assay. *Am J Clin Pathol.* 2004;121:70-77.

59. Lal P, Salazar PA, Ladanyi M, Chen B. Impact of polysomy 17 on HER-2/neu immunohistochemistry in breast carcinomas without HER-2/neu gene amplification. *J Mol Diagn.* 2003;5:155-159.

60. Harris L, Fritsche H, Mennel R, et al. American Society of Clinical Oncology 2007 update of recommendations for the use of tumor markers in breast cancer. *J Clin Oncol.* 2007;25:5287-5312.

61. Stephens RW, Brunner N, Janicke F, Schmitt M. The urokinase plasminogen activator system as a target for prognostic studies in breast cancer. *Breast Cancer Res Treat.* 1998;52:99-111.

62. Kleer CG, Cao Q, Varambally S, et al. EZH2 is a marker of aggressive breast cancer and promotes neoplastic transformation of breast epithelial cells. *Proc Natl Acad Sci USA.* 2003;100:11606-11611.

63. Collett K, Eide GE, Arnes J, et al. Expression of enhancer of zeste homologue 2 is significantly associated with increased tumor cell proliferation and is a marker of aggressive breast cancer. *Clin Cancer Res.* 2006;12:1168-1174.

64. Bachmann IM, Halvorsen OJ, Collett K, et al. EZH2 expression is associated with high proliferation rate and aggressive tumor subgroups in cutaneous melanoma and cancers of the endometrium, prostate, and breast. *J Clin Oncol.* 2006;24:268-273.

65. van de Vijver MJ, He YD, van't Veer LJ, et al. A gene-expression signature as a predictor of survival in breast cancer. *N Engl J Med.* 2002;347:1999-2009.

CHAPTER 23

Nonepithelial Neoplasms of the Breast

Tina W. F. Yen
Jennifer D. Lorek
Zainab Basir

The disease processes discussed in this chapter are uncommon tumors: phyllodes tumors, sarcomas, lymphomas, melanomas, and metastases to the breast. As a group, these tumors are rare and heterogeneously diverse. Given their small numbers, there have been few large patient series or trials, and no large prospective trials will likely be performed. The majority of the literature consists of single-institution, retrospective studies/case reports with small numbers, varied follow-up, and inherent biases. Furthermore, these studies are difficult to compare as the definition, management, and treatment of these tumors have changed over time. Therefore, there are no established guidelines for the treatment of these uncommon tumors; patients with these rare tumors should be managed in a multidisciplinary fashion.

PHYLLODES TUMORS

Phyllodes tumors represent a spectrum of fibroepithelial neoplasms that have biological behavior that is diverse and unpredictable. They account for less than 1% of all breast neoplasms.[1,2] These tumors have also been referred to as *cystosarcoma phyllodes*, *phylloides tumors*, and *periductal stromal tumors*. The term *cystosarcoma phyllodes* was first introduced in 1838 by Johannes Mueller; "sarcoma" for the fleshy nature of the tumor and "phyllodes" for its leaf-like architecture.[3] Mueller emphasized the benign nature of this tumor. The first report of histologically malignant features in these tumors was by Lee and Pack in 1931.[4] In 1960, Lomonaco proposed the name *tumor phyllodes* to avoid any implications of biological behavior.[5] The World Health Organization proposed *phyllodes tumor* to emphasize the putative origin of these tumors from specialized periductal stroma and to avoid the designation of sarcoma with its deceptive implication of malignancy for a majority of these tumors.[6]

These tumors can arise de novo, and less frequently from preexisting fibroadenomas or from the malignant transformation of benign phyllodes tumors.[2]

Clinical Presentation

Phyllodes tumors occur over a wide age range from adolescents to the elderly, with the majority of tumors occurring in women in their 40s to 50s.[1,2,7,8] These tumors can occur in young children and men. Women usually present with a palpable, firm-hard, discrete, mobile mass with an average size of 4 to 5 cm. Most tumors are unilateral and painless. Some women may give a history of a stable mass that grows rapidly. Larger tumors may cause stretching of the overlying skin and ulceration. All of these findings can be seen in both benign and malignant tumors. Compared with fibroadenomas, phyllodes tumors are seen more frequently in older patients and those with a history of rapid tumor growth and/or larger tumors. Palpable axillary lymphadenopathy can be identified in up to 20% of patients but is usually due to reactive changes as metastatic involvement is rare.[9-11] In some instances, tumors may be multifocal, bilateral, or occur in ectopic breast tissue. In 1% to 2% of cases, an in situ or invasive breast carcinoma occurs within a phyllodes tumor.[12] Also, patients can have a concurrent phyllodes tumor with a noninvasive or invasive breast carcinoma.[1,2]

Radiographically, there are no distinct imaging characteristics that can reliably distinguish a fibroadenoma, a benign phyllodes tumor, or a malignant phyllodes tumor.[2,13,14] On mammography, most tumors are indistinguishable from fibroadenomas. They are round, well-circumscribed densities with smooth borders. Calcifications are uncommon but can be seen in both benign and malignant phyllodes tumors. On ultrasound, these lesions are discrete, hypoechoic, solid structures that may have scattered cystic regions. On magnetic resonance imaging (MRI), tumors are oval, round, or lobulated circumscribed masses with rapid enhancement and high signal intensity on T2-weighted images.[14]

A fine-needle aspiration and/or percutaneous core needle biopsy of the lesion can be performed.[7] However, the cytologic and limited histologic features obtained from a small biopsy may sometimes by difficult to interpret due to sampling artifact and the varied nature of the tumor. For these reasons, the distinction between a fibroadenoma from a phyllodes tumor may be difficult and surgical excision is recommended, especially in older patients and those with a large tumor or history of rapid growth of the tumor. Since these lesions resemble fibroadenomas clinically and radiographically, the clinical suspicion for a phyllodes tumor is important. Furthermore, most phyllodes tumors are not diagnosed preoperatively and therefore are shelled out/enucleated at initial surgery, usually resulting in inadequate surgical margins. Therefore, all surgical specimens should be oriented and a close examination of the margins should be performed.

Pathology

Phyllodes tumors are highly variable in their gross appearance.[2] The majority are well-circumscribed, solid, grayish white, yellow, or pink fleshy masses with cystic areas. Foci of necrosis and hemorrhage may be seen in larger tumors (Fig. 23-2A). Tumors range in size from 1 to 45 cm, but on average are 4 to 5 cm in diameter. A true histologic capsule is absent. On gross examination, these tumors do not appear distinctly different from fibroadenomas.

Histologically, these biphasic fibroepithelial tumors are composed of benign epithelial elements and mixed connective tissue (stroma). These tumors arise from the periductal stroma. They have a broad range of appearances, but the hallmark is the hypercellular mesenchymal component with stromal overgrowth. This stromal overgrowth accounts for the characteristic leaflike architecture produced by large areas of stroma surrounding clefts lined by epithelial cells (Fig. 23-1). The degree

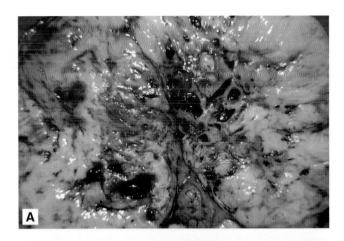

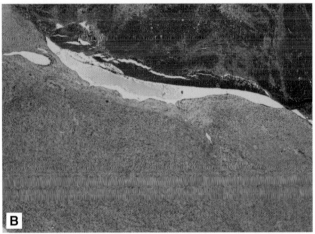

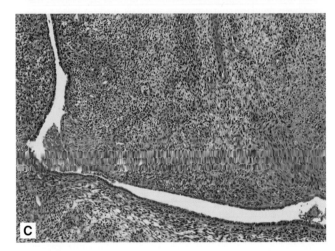

FIGURE 23-2 Malignant phyllodes tumor. **A.** The cut surface of a phyllodes tumor demonstrating a cleft appearance, resulting from the prominent intracanalicular growth pattern that is usually present. Usually firm and rubbery, phyllodes tumors may have gelatinous areas with foci of necrosis and hemorrhage as seen here. These features are suggestive of malignancy. **B.** A histologic section from the same tumor shows a dilated, blood-filled space adjacent to an area of marked stromal overgrowth. Note the absence of an epithelial component in this low-power view. **C.** Other areas of this tumor show the diagnostic biphasic architecture. This densely cellular stroma shows nuclear hyperchromasia, pleomorphism, and increased mitotic figures.

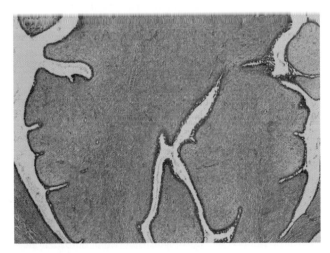

FIGURE 23-1 Phyllodes tumor. This low-power view demonstrates the prominent leaflike intracanalicular growth pattern and increased stromal cellularity, which is most obvious adjacent to the epithelial layer.

of stromal cellularity and stromal overgrowth resulting in the presence of a leaflike architecture distinguishes a phyllodes tumor from a fibroadenoma. These tumors must be differentiated from juvenile fibroadenomas, cellular fibroadenomas, metaplastic carcinomas, and primary breast sarcomas.

Phyllodes tumors are classified as benign, borderline/low-grade malignant, or malignant based on the mitotic activity, type of margin (infiltrative or pushing), stromal overgrowth, and cellular pleomorphism (Table 23-1).[12,15] Overall, more than 50% of tumors are benign and approximately 25% are malignant.[1] Although this classification system is widely used, the clinical course of a phyllodes tumor cannot be accurately predicted by its histopathologic features.[9,11,16,17] The degree of stromal overgrowth may be the most important histologic feature for predicting the metastatic behavior of a phyllodes tumor (Fig. 23-2A, B, and C).[10,16-18]

In general, benign phyllodes tumors have an approximately 5% to 20% local recurrence rate but do not metastasize.[9,11,19] Recurrences are usually benign. Borderline tumors have a greater than 25% risk of local recurrence, usually within the first 2 years; these recurrences may be malignant.[11] The risk for distant metastases is less than 5%. Malignant tumors have a 20% to 40% risk of local recurrence and distant metastases.[9,19] These recurrences usually occur earlier after the initial treatment than for borderline and benign cases. Distant metastases can occur without an antecedent local recurrence.[1,2,11] Less than 1% of patients have axillary lymph node involvement.[11,17] The clinical course, in most cases, is indolent. Overall 5-year survival rates are 75% to 88% and 10-year survival rates are 57% to 80%.[8,9,16]

Treatment

Phyllodes tumors are treated surgically by wide local excision with negative margins, preferably more than 1 cm for definitive local control.[1,2,9,11,16,18,20] Since these tumors are surrounded by a pseudocapsule of dense, compressed, normal surrounding tissue that contains microscopic projections of the lesion, achieving a 1-cm histologic margin will often require a gross 2- to 3-cm margin. Since mastectomy and wide local excision with adequate margins have similar local recurrence rates and overall survival rates, mastectomy should be reserved for large tumors or lesions with infiltrating margins and aggressive histologic features that would not allow for local excision with an adequate margin and/or acceptable cosmetic result.[1,2,8,16] Since phyllodes tumors rarely metastasize to axillary lymph nodes, there is no role for routine axillary lymph node dissection.

As most phyllodes tumors are diagnosed after excisional biopsy, the margin status of many cases may be suboptimal, and the decision to undergo a reexcision must be determined. Positive/close margin status is the most powerful independent predictor of local recurrence.[9-11,18-20] The local recurrence rates for tumors that are excised "locally" with positive margins or margins of only a few millimeters are 21%, 46%, and 65% for benign, borderline, and malignant tumors, respectively; local recurrence rates for tumors that are widely excised with 1 to 2 cm margins are 8%, 29%, and 36% for benign, borderline, and malignant tumors, respectively.[21] Some authors advocate reexcision in all patients with a less than 1-cm margin, especially those with malignant tumors, while others propose close observation, especially in those patients with benign/borderline tumors in whom reexcision may be technically difficult or cosmetically deforming.[9,20,21]

There is no clearly defined role for adjuvant radiation therapy, as most studies are anecdotal case reports and no series has shown a clear benefit for radiation therapy in the primary treatment of phyllodes tumors.[16,19,22] Adjuvant radiation therapy (50-60 Gy) has been recommended for malignant tumors and tumors greater than 5 cm; it has also been considered in patients for whom negative margins have not been attained.[7,10,16,19] Similarly, there is no proven role for adjuvant chemotherapy or hormonal therapy in reducing recurrences or deaths.[1,2,7] Given the high rate of distant metastases in patients with excessive stromal overgrowth, especially if the tumor size is greater than 5 cm, Chaney and associates recommend considering chemotherapy in this cohort.[16]

Given the risk of local recurrence, patients should be followed closely with a clinical breast examination and baseline mammography within 4 to 6 months of surgery. Clinical breast examination and imaging (mammography with or without ultrasonography) should be recommended every 6 months for 5 years, and annually thereafter.[7] For patients with malignant phyllodes tumors, biannual chest/abdominal CT scans for 2 to 5 years can be considered, although the benefits of this screening regimen are unproven.

TABLE 23-1 Histologic Classification of Phyllodes Tumors

| Criteria | HISTOLOGIC TYPE | | |
	Benign	Borderline	Malignant
Mitotic rate (per 10 hpf)	< 5	5-9	≥10
Tumor margins	Pushing	Pushing–infiltrative	Infiltrative
Stromal cellularity	Low	Moderate	High
Pleomorphism	Mild	Moderate	Severe

From Azzopardi JG. Sarcoma in the breast. In: Bennington J, ed. *Problems in Breast Pathology.* Vol. 2. Philadelphia, PA: Saunders; 1979:355-359; and Salvadori B, Cusumano F, Del Bo R, et al. Surgical treatment of phyllodes tumors of the breast. *Cancer.* 1989;63:2532-2536.

Management of Local Recurrence

Overall, local recurrence occurs in 15% to 30% of patients, usually within the first 2 to 3 years after initial diagnosis.[9,20] Time to local recurrence is shortest among those with malignant tumors.[15] Generally, most recurrences recur with the same histology as that of the initial tumor; however, cases of transformation to a more aggressive tumor have been reported.[1,16,20] Recurrences can be managed by reexcision with wide margins or total mastectomy with or without reconstruction. Salvage mastectomy for recurrent disease does not affect overall survival.[16] Adjuvant radiation therapy to the breast/chest wall after reexcision with negative margins can be considered.[23]

Management of Metastatic Disease

Overall, distant metastasis occurs in about 5% to 10% of patients; however, it occurs in up to 20% to 40% of patients with malignant tumors. Metastases occur via hematogenous spread, most commonly to lung, liver, bone, mediastinum, and brain. Metastases usually occur within the first 3 years of diagnosis; death occurs approximately 2 to 3 years after the development of metastatic disease.[1,8,9,17] The degree of stromal overgrowth may be the most important histologic feature for predicting the metastatic behavior of a phyllodes tumor.[10,16-18] Due to limited numbers and experiences, the optimal treatment (chemotherapy, hormonal therapy, palliative radiation therapy) of metastatic disease has not been determined.[9,10,17,21] Chemotherapeutic agents have included cyclophosphamide, ifosfamide, cisplatin and doxorubicin, and etoposide and cisplatin.[1,17] Responses, when they occur, are usually of short duration. Given such limited experience, the management of metastatic phyllodes tumors should follow the guidelines for treatment of advanced extremity/truncal sarcoma.[24]

Summary

Phyllodes tumors are uncommon, heterogeneously diverse tumors that are often misdiagnosed as fibroadenomas. These tumors are biphasic, composed of an epithelial and stromal component, and can be classified as benign, borderline, or malignant based on histology. Overall, these tumors have a propensity to recur locally. Distant metastases may develop in 5% to 15% of patients overall but in over 20% of patients with malignant tumors. Phyllodes tumors, including those that are malignant, have a long-term survival > 90%. Definitive treatment is wide local excision with a 1-cm or larger margin. The role of adjuvant radiation therapy and systemic therapy remains unproven and must be considered, especially in those patients with excessive stromal overgrowth, on an individual basis in a multidisciplinary fashion. Patients with local recurrences should be managed with wide excision with or without subsequent radiation therapy. Patients with metastatic disease should be managed according to treatment guidelines similar to patients with metastatic extremity soft-tissue sarcomas.

SARCOMA

Sarcomas of the breast include a heterogeneous group of malignant tumors that arise from the mammary stroma. These mesenchymal tumors account for less than 1% of all malignant breast neoplasms and less than 5% of all soft-tissue sarcomas.[25-27] The most common subtypes are angiosarcoma, liposarcoma, leiomyosarcoma, undifferentiated high-grade sarcoma (malignant fibrous histiocytoma, MFH), and fibrosarcoma. The etiology of primary breast sarcomas is largely unknown; saline prostheses have been previously implicated as a possible risk factor, but most recent data do not appear to support a relationship.[27] Previous radiation therapy to the breast/chest wall and/or a history of lymphedema to the breast or upper extremity are established risk factors for angiosarcomas (discussed later in the chapter). As with sarcomas originating in other areas of the body, these tumors rarely spread to regional lymph nodes, and distant metastases occur most commonly to the lung, bone, and liver.[25,26,28-31] Treatment is primarily surgical.

Clinical Presentation

Primary breast sarcomas are typically seen in women in their 40s to 50s (range, 16 to 81 years).[25-32] Most women present with a well-circumscribed, firm, mobile, painless, unilateral mass, which may be difficult to distinguish from a fibroadenoma. The suspicion for a primary breast sarcoma should be raised if there is a history of rapid tumor growth.[25,28,30] These tumors vary in size but typically are 5 to 6 cm in diameter.[26,27,30-32] Other features, such as nipple discharge, nipple inversion, and skin changes (excluding angiosarcomas), are rarely seen.

On mammography and ultrasonography, these lesions are typically well-circumscribed, solid, nonspiculated masses.[27,33] Breast CT/MRI and whole-body PET scans have not been extensively studied in primary breast sarcomas but could potentially be used in the evaluation of these patients.[24,33] Preoperative chest x-ray should be performed in all patients given the risk of hematogenous spread to the lungs, especially from a high-grade sarcoma.[24]

Pathology

Primary sarcomas of the breast represent a heterogeneous group of tumors. Grossly, these tumors are usually fleshy, moderately firm tumors with varying degrees of hemorrhage and necrosis. The specific histologic findings for the more common mesenchymal tumors are summarized below. In general, given the heterogeneous nature of these tumors, the importance of adequate sampling for accurate diagnosis must be emphasized. Histologic evaluation and immunohistochemical stains can help distinguish primary breast sarcomas from sarcomatous overgrowth in a phyllodes tumor, sarcomatoid carcinoma/carcinosarcoma, fibromatosis, metaplastic carcinoma, and malignant myoepithelioma.[34]

Tumors are staged by the 2002 American Joint Committee on Cancer (AJCC) TNM staging system; staging is dependent on tumor location/depth, tumor size, histologic grade, and presence of nodal or distant metastases (Table 23-2).[24,35] Tumor grade plays an important role in prognosis.

Treatment

There are currently no consensus guidelines or randomized trials that have specifically addressed primary breast sarcomas. The mainstay of treatment remains wide local excision with histologically negative margins (optimally 2-3 cm); en bloc

TABLE 23-2 2002 AJCC Staging System for Soft-Tissue Sarcoma

TNM Definitions

Primary Tumor (T)

TX	Primary tumor cannot be assessed
T0	No evidence of primary tumor
T1	Tumor 5 cm or less in greatest dimension
T1a	Superficial tumor*
T1b	Deep tumor
T2	Tumor more than 5 cm in greatest dimension
T2a	Superficial tumor*
T2b	Deep tumor

Regional Lymph Nodes (N)

NX	Regional lymph nodes cannot be assessed
N0	No regional lymph node metastasis
N1	Regional lymph node metastasis

Distant Metastases (M)

MX	Distant metastasis cannot be assessed
M0	No distant metastasis
M1	Distant metastasis

Histologic Grade

GX	Grade cannot be assessed
G1	Well differentiated
G2	Moderately differentiated
G3	Poorly differentiated
G4	Poorly differentiated or undifferentiated (four-tiered systems only)

Stage	T	N	M	Grade		
I	T1a, 1b, 2a, 2b	N0	M0	G1-2	G1	Low
II	T1a, 1b, 2a	N0	M0	G3-4	G2-3	High
III	T2b	N0	M0	G3-4	G2-3	High
IV	Any T	N1	M0	Any G	Any G	High or low
	Any T	N0	M1	Any G	Any G	High or low

AJCC, American Joint Committee on Cancer; M, metastasis; N, node; T, tumor.

*Superficial tumor is located exclusively above the superficial fascia without invasion of the fascia; deep tumor is located exclusively either beneath the superficial fascia, superficial to the fascia with invasion of or through the fascia, or both superficial yet beneath the fascia.

Used with the permission of the American Joint Committee on Cancer (AJCC), Chicago, Illinois. The original source for this material is the AJCC Cancer Staging Manual, Sixth Edition (2002) published by Springer Science and Business Media LLC, www.springerlink.com. From Soft tissue sarcoma. In: Greene FL, Page DL, Fleming ID, et al, eds. *AJCC Cancer Staging Manual,* Sixth Edition. New York, NY: Springer, 2002:195.

resection of underlying muscle may be required. If negative margins can be achieved by breast-conserving surgery, there is no additional benefit to patients who undergo a mastectomy.[25,26,28-32] Therefore, attempts at breast preservation are reasonable; however, total mastectomy may be required to achieve negative margins depending on tumor size, type, and/or location.[27] Since tumors rarely metastasize to the regional lymph nodes, there is no role for routine axillary lymph node dissection. Local recurrences are typically treated with reexcision and radiation therapy, if not previously administered.

Potential prognostic features that have been studied include tumor grade, tumor size, cellular appearance, presence of infiltrating borders, mitotic activity, stromal atypia, and margin status.

Although not universally replicated, prognostic factors that have more consistently been shown to have an adverse outcome (local recurrence and distant metastasis) include high histologic grade, larger tumor size (> 5 cm), and inadequate margins.[25-32,36]

Few data exist on the use of radiation therapy and/or chemotherapy in a neoadjuvant or adjuvant setting.[25,26,28-32,35,37] A few retrospective studies have shown that adjuvant radiation therapy provides excellent local control and improves disease-free survival but not overall survival.[26,28,38] Although there is no definitive evidence, some have proposed that adjuvant radiation therapy be considered in patients with high-grade tumors, especially those larger than 5 cm, and those with positive margins in whom repeat surgery may not be feasible.[25,29,30] As there are no adjuvant chemotherapy studies that have been completed in breast sarcoma patients, chemotherapy regimens for these patients have been based on data from other soft-tissue sarcomas.[39,40] The results from the Sarcoma Meta-Analysis Collaboration of 14 randomized trials (1568 patients) showed that doxorubicin-based chemotherapy prolongs relapse-free survival and decreases recurrence rates in adults with localized, resectable soft-tissue sarcomas of the extremity.[39] For breast sarcoma patients, those with high-grade tumors, especially those greater than 5 cm in size, should be considered for chemotherapy given their high risk for recurrent/metastatic disease.[30,32,36] The use of neoadjuvant chemotherapy for breast sarcomas has not been recommended routinely given the fact that response rates are limited and most sarcomas are amenable to surgical resection at the time of presentation.[30]

Overall, it appears that patients with primary mammary sarcoma have a similar natural history, prognostic factors, and outcome after multimodality therapy as those with extremity sarcoma; 5-year overall survival rates range from 45% to 66%.[25-28,30-32,36] The 5-year disease-free survival rates range from 28% to 52% and most failures occur within the first 1 to 3 years.[25-32,36] Local recurrences occur in up to one-third of patients, highlighting the importance of a negative surgical margin. Breast sarcomas metastasize most commonly to the lung, bone, and liver. Other sites of metastases include the brain, skin, subcutaneous tissue, spleen, and adrenal glands.[27,68] Management of metastatic disease may include surgery, chemotherapy, radiation therapy, and ablative or embolization procedures.[24] In general, most patients with advanced primary breast sarcoma should be managed by established guidelines for patients with extremity sarcoma.[24,32,36]

Patients with stage I disease should be followed every 3 to 6 months for 2 to 3 years then annually; chest x-ray can be considered every 6 to 12 months. Patients with stage II to IV disease should undergo clinical examinations and chest x-ray or CT scan every 3 to 6 months for 2 to 3 years, and then every 6 months for the next 2 years, and then annually.[24] For all patients, baseline ipsilateral mammography should be performed 6 months postoperatively in those who undergo breast-conserving surgery, and then bilateral mammography should be performed annually.

Angiosarcoma

Angiosarcomas are malignant vascular neoplasms of the breast that typically have a more aggressive clinical course with higher recurrence rates and lower overall survival than other breast sarcomas.[25,27,30-32,36,41] These tumors have also been called hemangiosarcoma, hemangioblastoma, malignant hemangioendothelioma, angioblastoma, and benign metastasizing hemangioma. Angiosarcomas arise in the breast more frequently than any other organ. They may arise de novo within the breast parenchyma (primary angiosarcoma) or as a secondary tumor associated with lymphedema (Stewart–Treves syndrome due to postmastectomy changes, congenital lymphedema, or parasitic infections) or radiation therapy to the breast, skin, or chest wall.[42,43] Women with primary angiosarcomas are typically young, in their third to fourth decade, and usually have high-grade tumors with a rapid clinical course.

Postmastectomy angiosarcomas arise in the skin and soft tissues of the arm due to chronic lymphedema after mastectomy and/or radiation therapy.[42,43] The etiology of this form of angiosarcoma is likely (1) chronic lymphatic obstruction leading to collateralization and neovascularization that eventually escape tissue control mechanisms or (2) absence of immunologic surveillance as a result of loss of afferent lymphatic circulation.[43] These tumors arise from the endothelial lining of lymphatic channels. The majority of angiosarcomas occur within 10 years following mastectomy and typically occur in the upper inner or medial arm. The initial lesion is usually a focal purple discoloration of the skin, which rapidly evolves into plaques and nodules that may ulcerate and bleed easily in the ipsilateral arm, chest wall, or residual breast. These lesions are typically high grade.[44]

Postradiation angiosarcomas arise in the skin overlying the breast and chest wall and rarely in the breast parenchyma. These tumors typically present in older women (40s-80s), on average 3 to 7 years after radiation therapy.[42-45] Reddish/blue discolored macules/nodules are identified on the skin within the radiation portals. The majority of lesions are high grade; there is no difference in outcome (disease-free survival or overall survival) when compared to radiation-naïve patients with angiosarcomas.[44]

Clinically, angiosarcomas may present insidiously, often with a painless discrete mass that grows rapidly and becomes painful.[43,46] The typical finding is a bluish-purple-red discoloration of the overlying skin, reflecting the hemorrhage and vascularity of the lesion (Fig. 23-3). Given the aggressive nature of these lesions, the clinical suspicion for an angiosarcoma must be very high. Mammography findings are unrevealing in a third of patients and ultrasound findings are nonspecific.[33,43] Breast MRI may demonstrate a mass with low signal intensity on T1-weighted images but high signal intensity on T2-weighted images.[33,43] A diagnosis of angiosarcoma by fine-needle aspiration cytology and/or limited biopsy may be difficult.[33,46]

Pathology of Angiosarcoma

Grossly, angiosarcomas vary in size (average about 5 cm) and have a spongy/friable consistency often with irregular hemorrhagic areas and poorly defined margins.[47,48] A rim of congested, thin-walled vessels surrounds the main mass; cystic or necrotic areas may be present in large, high-grade sarcomas. These tumors may involve the overlying skin but rarely extend posteriorly into the pectoralis major fascia/muscle. Histologically, these heterogeneous tumors proliferate around and into the lobular stroma and infiltrate the surrounding adipose tissues.[47-49] These tumors are composed of irregular anastomosing vascular channels/spaces in the dermis and superficial subcutaneous fat, which are lined by 1 or more layers of malignant endothelial cells.[47-49]

Angiosarcomas are graded by the appearance and behavior of the endothelial cells based on nuclear atypia, mitotic activity, and the proportion of solid aggregates of spindle cells (Table 23-3).[48,49] Low-grade (well-differentiated, grade I) lesions occur in approximately one-third of breast angiosarcomas and have a favorable prognosis. Intermediate-grade (moderately

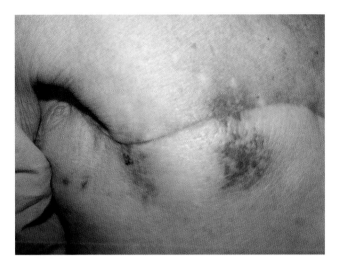

FIGURE 23-3 Angiosarcoma. A 90-year-old female with a history of stage IIA invasive ductal carcinoma in 2000, status post segmental mastectomy and negative sentinel lymph node biopsy, radiation therapy, and tamoxifen who developed an angiosarcoma in the radiation field in 2006, which was treated by mastectomy. She developed a recurrent angiosarcoma, shown here with its typical features, in 2007.

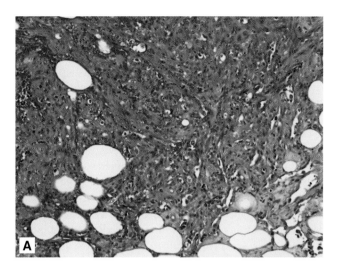

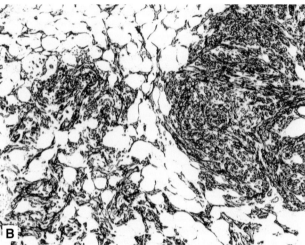

FIGURE 23-4 Angiosarcoma, high grade. **A.** This tumor shows an almost solid mass composed of plump endothelial cells. These cells are pleomorphic and hyperchromatic with increased mitotic activity. Red blood cells are present in some of the anastomosing vascular channels. **B.** An immunohistochemical stain for CD-31 highlights the plump endothelial cells.

differentiated, grade II) lesions are similar to low-grade lesions but have focal areas of more cellular proliferation and papillary configurations scattered throughout the tumor. High-grade (poorly differentiated, grade III) lesions are a mixture of interanastomosing vascular channels with solid areas of spindle cells. Areas of hemorrhage accompanied by necrosis (blood lakes) are usually present. More than 50% of the total neoplasm is composed of solid and spindle-cell components without evidence of vascular spaces (Fig. 23-4).

The proportion and distribution of the well-formed vascular spaces and papillary and solid areas vary significantly in different tumors and within a given tumor, emphasizing the importance of adequate sampling of large lesions and complete processing of smaller lesions to avoid under-diagnosis and allow accurate grading of the angiosarcoma. On immunohistochemistry, angiosarcomas are typically negative for cytokeratins and positive for CD31, CD34, and FVIII; these markers may be lost in high-grade tumors.[43,49] Angiosarcomas must be differentiated from benign hemangiomas, atypical vascular lesions, and angiolipomas, which are usually smaller lesions (less than 2 cm) with sharply demarcated, well-circumscribed margins.

Treatment of Angiosarcoma

As with other breast sarcomas, treatment remains surgical. However, unlike most other breast sarcomas, given the extensive involvement of the skin, most patients with angiosarcomas require mastectomy with possible coverage by a split-thickness skin graft or myocutaneous flap.[42,44,46] Routine axillary dissection

TABLE 23-3 Grading System for Angiosarcomas

Tumor Grade	HISTOLOGIC FINDING			
	Nuclear Atypia	Mitotic Activity	Papillary Formations	Blood Lakes
Low	Mild	Rare	Absent	Absent
Intermediate	Moderate	Infrequent	Infrequent	Absent
High	Severe	Frequent	Frequent (> 50%)	Present

is not indicated, as few patients develop axillary metastases. Although there are no definitive data, given the relatively high risk for local recurrence, adjuvant radiation therapy to the breast/chest wall should be considered. Chemotherapy has provided minimal improvement in outcome, but should be considered in high-grade lesions and patients with metastatic disease; vascular targeting agents are under investigation.[42,43,47,48]

As with other sarcomas, tumor grade predicts prognosis.[47-49] In one study, 5-year disease-free survival was 76%, 70%, and 15% for well-, moderately-, and poorly-differentiated lesions.[49] The majority of angiosarcomas are either intermediate- or high-grade lesions and are thus highly lethal neoplasms.[44] Tumors recur locally in about 75% of patients and the majority occur within 1 year of surgery; distant metastases also develop shortly after diagnosis, most commonly to the lung, liver, skin, bone, and contralateral breast.[42-44,46,47] Most patients die of disseminated disease within 2 years of diagnosis.[29,30,44,46,48,49]

As the number of patient receiving radiation therapy to the breast for treatment of breast cancer increases, it is anticipated that the number of cases of radiation-induced sarcomas, particularly angiosarcoma, of the breast will increase.[45] Given the poor prognosis of angiosarcomas, long-term follow-up for skin changes is imperative and attention to postradiation skin lesions and timely diagnostic interventions including biopsies are encouraged.

Liposarcoma

Liposarcomas of the breast are malignant lipomatous tumors containing lipoblasts and are identical to their soft-tissue counterparts in other parts of the body. These tumors can be a component of a malignant phyllodes tumor or arise directly from the mammary adipose tissue.[50,51] Mammographic findings depend on the histologic type of liposarcoma; well-differentiated liposarcomas are radiolucent while the other types are radio-opaque.[50,52] Ultrasound usually reveals a solid mass with irregular internal echoes and margins. CT scans will show extremely variable patterns of enhancement. Well-differentiated liposarcomas on MRI are largely fatty masses with nonspecific irregularly thickened linear septa that show decreased intensity on T1-weighted imaging and increased intensity on T2-weighted imaging.[50,52]

Microscopically, these tumors have a histopathology similar to liposarcomas at other sites. The World Health Organization classification identifies 3 categories: well-differentiated, myxoid, and pleomorphic.[50,52,53] The well-differentiated type has mature lipocytes without nuclear atypia and few lipoblasts. These tumors are often low-grade and have the potential to recur locally but rarely metastasize. The well-differentiated type can sometimes progress to a dedifferentiated liposarcoma. The myxoid variant, which is the most common type of liposarcoma found in the breast, displays an abundant myxoid matrix, lipoblasts of varying stages of differentiation, and a characteristic delicate, plexiform capillary stromal pattern (Fig. 23-5). These tumors are intermediate grade. A myxoid liposarcoma can progress to a round-cell liposarcoma, which is characterized by proliferating small, uniform-shaped round cells. The pleomorphic variant is a highly cellular tumor that displays a disorderly growth pattern with numerous lipoblasts and mitotic figures,

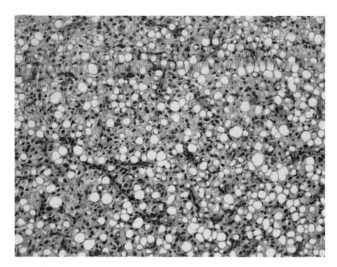

FIGURE 23-5 Myxoid liposarcoma. This tumor is characterized by a myxoid matrix and a delicate "chicken-wire" capillary network providing support for the proliferating lipoblasts.

including bizarre giant cells. Pleomorphic liposarcomas are high-grade tumors. Liposarcomas must be differentiated from changes related to silicone implants, fat necrosis, signet ring cell carcinoma, myxoma, myxoid variant of undifferentiated high-grade sarcoma (MFH), and pleomorphic lipoma.[51]

Treatment involves complete excision with a 2-cm margin; given the infiltrative nature of these tumors, many patients may require mastectomy.[50,51] The majority of recurrences occur with the pleomorphic and myxoid types, usually within the first 2 years of diagnosis. Death usually occurs in 18 months.[50-52]

Leiomyosarcoma

Leiomyosarcomas originate from the smooth muscle of blood vessels or the nipple–areolar complex.[54-56] Nearly half of these lesions are present in or near the nipple–areolar complex. Histologically, these tumors are characterized by interlacing bundles of fusiform, spindle-shaped cells with pleomorphism, cytologic atypia, hyperchromatism, and numerous mitoses.[56] Tumor cell necrosis may be present.[57] These tumors must be differentiated from a poorly differentiated carcinoma, metaplastic carcinoma, or malignant phyllodes tumor.[54,55]

Treatment is typically total mastectomy; there are a few reported cases of wide local excision.[56] Local recurrences and metastases are rare but can occur late (16-20 years).[57,58] These tumors may behave less aggressively than other breast sarcomas.[57]

Pleomorphic/Undifferentiated High-Grade Sarcoma

Pleomorphic or undifferentiated high-grade sarcomas were previously called malignant fibrous histiocytomas (MFH). These tumors typically arise de novo in the breast parenchyma; however, they can arise as a component of a phyllodes tumor or be associated with radiation therapy.[59-61] Pleomorphic high-grade sarcomas are tumors composed of varying proportions of fibroblasts, myofibroblasts, histiocyte-like cells, and undifferentiated cells, resulting in a wide range of histologic features. Most of the spindle cells are arranged randomly with numerous mitotic figures, bizarre giant cells, and inflammatory cells. These tumors must be differentiated from a fibrosarcoma, metaplastic carcinoma, fibromatosis, a phyllodes tumor with stromal overgrowth, nodular fasciitis, malignant schwannoma, and pleomorphic liposarcoma.[62]

Treatment is the same as for other breast sarcomas. Pleomorphic high-grade sarcomas behave aggressively with a high rate of local recurrence.[60,62] As with other sarcomas, high-grade lesions more frequently metastasize and have a worse prognosis.[62] Most patients die of disseminated disease, usually within 3 years of diagnosis.[32,59,62]

Other Sarcomas

Other rare sarcomas that have occurred in the breast include fibrosarcomas, osteosarcoma (osteogenic sarcoma), stromal sarcomas, rhabdomyosarcomas, hemangiopericytomas, dermatofibrosarcoma protuberans, and malignant peripheral nerve sheath tumors.[34]

Summary

Primary sarcomas of the breast are rare malignancies and should be managed by a multidisciplinary approach. Surgery with a wide local excision of 2- to 3-cm margins remains the mainstay of treatment. Routine axillary node dissection is not required. Adjuvant radiation therapy and chemotherapy should be considered in patients at high risk for recurrent disease, especially high-grade tumors that are greater than 5 cm in size. As primary breast sarcomas behave in a similar fashion to extremity sarcomas, management of advanced primary breast sarcomas should be similar to that of extremity sarcomas. As the number of patients receiving radiation therapy to the breast for treatment of breast cancer increases, it is anticipated that the incidence of radiation-induced breast sarcomas, particularly angiosarcomas, will increase.

PRIMARY BREAST LYMPHOMA

A malignant lymphoid neoplasm of the breast may be either a primary or, more commonly, a secondary tumor. There are no morphologic criteria to separate a primary from a secondary lymphoma; the distinction is made on clinical criteria after excluding a lymphoma involving other organs. The diagnostic criteria for a primary breast lymphoma, described by Wiseman and Liao in 1972, include (1) breast as the site of presentation, (2) an absence of a history of previous lymphoma or evidence of widespread disease at the time of diagnosis, (3) lymphoma is demonstrated in close association with breast tissue in the pathologic specimen, and (4) ipsilateral lymph nodes may be involved if they develop simultaneously with the primary breast tumor.[63] Therefore, all primary breast lymphomas are either stage I (breast only) or stage II (breast and axillary nodes); all other breast lymphomas not meeting these 4 criteria are considered secondary breast lymphomas.

Primary lymphomas of the breast are rare, representing about 2% of extranodal lymphomas and less than 0.5% of breast malignancies.[64] The origin of primary breast lymphoma may be from lymphatic tissue within the breast parenchyma, an intramammary lymph node, or from mucosal-associated lymphoid tissue (MALT).[64] The most common type of either primary or secondary lymphoma is diffuse large B-cell lymphoma. Both non-Hodgkin and Hodgkin lymphomas occur. Hodgkin lymphomas and T-cell lymphomas are very rare.[64]

Clinical Presentation

Non-Hodgkin lymphoma of the breast usually occurs in females in their 40s to 50s (age range, 14-90 years).[64,65] These tumors are usually unilateral but bilateral diffuse involvement with overlying skin changes or diffuse infiltration has been reported in younger women who are pregnant or lactating.[64] Most women present with a breast mass or pain. About 10% have constitutional "B" symptoms of night sweats, fever, and weight loss. Approximately 30% have axillary nodal involvement.[64,66]

Mammographically, these lesions are relatively circumscribed benign-appearing, homogeneous masses with smooth margins or are characterized by focal or diffuse thickening and densities. Typically, these lesions lack calcifications, spiculations, and skin retraction, findings that are often associated with primary breast carcinomas.[33,66,67] Diffuse infiltration and multiple ill-defined lesions are radiologic clues suggestive of the possible diagnosis of lymphoma; however, overall the mammographic findings are nonspecific.[67] Ipsilateral axillary adenopathy may be seen in up to 50%.[33,66] On ultrasound, these lesions may be well-defined and hypoechoic or present as diffuse hypoechogenicity within the breast parenchyma that infiltrates through the tissues.[33,67] Fine-needle aspiration may be performed and is diagnostic in about 65% of cases or higher, if material for flow cytometry is also obtained.[65] However, core needle biopsy or excisional biopsy is often required to provide adequate tissue for histopathologic evaluation and immunophenotyping.

Pathology

Primary breast lymphomas are usually solitary, well-circumscribed, lobulated, soft or firm tumors that are usually 3 to 4 cm in size (range, 1-20 cm).[64,65] Histologically, there is diffuse infiltration of the mammary parenchyma by a uniform population of neoplastic lymphocytes. These neoplastic cells typically form a well-circumscribed mass, but there may be variable degrees of marginal irregularity. Lymphomatous infiltration into the epithelium of ducts and lobules, especially in poorly differentiated lymphocytic lymphoma, may mimic an in situ carcinoma. Signet-ring cell lymphoma may bear a striking resemblance to signet-ring cell lobular mammary carcinoma and may require immunostains for lymphoid and epithelial markers to distinguish these entities. Distinguishing large-cell lymphoma from poorly differentiated carcinoma may also be difficult, especially if the carcinoma lacks a classic intraductal component. In addition, unusual inflammatory conditions with prominent lymphocytic infiltration or pseudolymphoma (atypical lymphocytic infiltrate) should always be considered in the differential diagnosis.

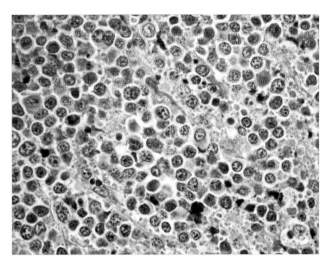

FIGURE 23-6 Diffuse large B-cell lymphoma. The infiltrate is composed of sheets of discohesive large atypical lymphocytes without an admixture of inflammatory cells or histiocytes.

The most common type of primary breast lymphoma is the diffuse large B-cell lymphoma, which typically has a diffuse infiltrative pattern showing large tumor cells, commonly centroblastic (Fig. 23-6). Other types of non-Hodgkin primary breast lymphomas include Burkitt lymphoma, extranodal marginal zone B-cell lymphoma of MALT, follicular lymphoma, and small lymphocytic lymphoma. T-cell lymphomas are rare.[64]

Treatment

The prognosis of primary breast lymphoma confined to the breast is comparable to that of other localized extranodal lymphomas. Patients with stage I disease and histologically low-grade lesions have the best prognosis[64,68,69]; bilateral breast involvement may portend a worse prognosis.[65,70] In the past, radical surgery (lumpectomy or mastectomy with axillary node dissection) followed by radiation therapy and/or chemotherapy was the treatment of choice.[64] Today, there remains no clear consensus for the management of primary breast lymphoma. However, limited surgery for tissue diagnosis and tumor classification followed by systemic therapy with or without radiation therapy for local control is now commonly recommended.[64,65,68,72-74] Excellent local control in the breast and axillary nodes can be achieved with radiation therapy after lumpectomy; mastectomy should be reserved for specific clinical situations, such as bulky, ulcerated, local disease.[72]

Progression and/or relapse, usually to other extranodal regions or the contralateral breast, occurs in approximately 50% of patients with primary breast lymphoma.[65,70,71] Some reports demonstrate a 5% to 29% incidence of central nervous system involvement. The use of central nervous system prophylaxis with intrathecal chemotherapy is debatable.[65,69,70,73,74]

The most common chemotherapeutic regimen for diffuse large B-cell lymphoma has been cyclophosphamide, adriamycin, vincristine, and prednisone (CHOP). For primary breast lymphoma, one prospective study randomized 96 primary breast lymphoma patients to chemotherapy (6 cycles of CHOP), radiation therapy (45 Gy to the breast/chest wall and axillary and supraclavicular lymphatics), or chemotherapy followed by radiation therapy.[73] Ten-year event-free survival and actuarial survival was significantly better in those patients who received both chemotherapy and radiation therapy (83% and 76%, respectively) compared with those who received only radiation therapy (50% and 50%) or only chemotherapy (57% and 50%). In one retrospective study of 204 patients with diffuse large B-cell lymphoma of the breast, 89% of patients treated with anthracycline-base chemotherapy had a complete response.[65] Rituximab, a monoclonal antibody, has been added to chemotherapeutic regimens for B-cell lymphomas with significant improvements in outcomes; however, its role in the treatment of primary breast lymphoma has yet to be described.[64,65] Five-year overall survival rates for primary breast lymphoma vary widely, up to 89% for stage I and 50% for stage II disease.[64,71,74] In the study by Ryan and associates, the median overall survival was 8 years, with 5- and 10-year overall survival rates of 63% and 47%, respectively.[65]

Summary

Primary breast lymphoma is a rare tumor that can be managed with limited surgery for tissue diagnosis and tumor classification followed by systemic therapy with or without radiation therapy for local control. Relapses usually occur to other extranodal locations and the contralateral breast; the use of prophylactic intrathecal chemotherapy is controversial. Systemic therapy typically involves CHOP; the addition of rituximab in the management of primary breast lymphoma has not yet been described. Prospective trials should be performed to determine whether the impact of rituximab and/or other targeted therapies on the patterns of relapse and outcome parallels that of diffuse large B-cell lymphoma presenting in other sites.[65]

PRIMARY MALIGNANT MELANOMA

Primary malignant melanoma of the skin or glandular tissue of the breast is extremely rare and accounts for less than 5% of malignant melanomas.[75] The majority of these lesions are cutaneous, arising in the skin and subcutaneous tissues overlying the breast, but cases of primary melanoma arising from the breast parenchyma have been reported.[76,77]

Clinical Presentation

Primary cutaneous melanomas of the breast occur more frequently in males than females with an average age in the 30s to 40s.[78,79] Risk factors for melanoma include a positive family history of melanoma, a personal history of prior melanoma or multiple clinically atypical moles or dysplastic nevi, certain inherited genetic mutations, and sun exposure.[80] All histologic types of malignant melanoma can arise in the skin of the breast. Lymph node metastases may be found in the axillary (60% of patients) and supraclavicular locations[78]; there has been only one documented case of metastases to the internal mammary nodes.[81]

Careful attention should be paid to the axillary and supraclavicular draining lymph node basins. If suspicious lymphadenopathy is present, ultrasound-guided fine-needle aspiration or excisional biopsy should be performed to rule out metastatic disease. A complete skin examination should be performed to rule out a nonmammary malignant melanoma primary lesion.

Diagnosis/Pathology

The histologic diagnosis of malignant melanoma of the breast is based on the same criteria used to assess nonmammary cutaneous lesions. Malignant melanomas are composed of round to polyhedral or spindle cells (Fig. 23-7A). Any suspicious pigmented skin lesion should be removed by a diagnostic full-thickness, excisional biopsy, ideally with 1- to 3-mm margins.[80] If a diagnostic biopsy is inadequate, rebiopsy may be appropriate. At the minimum, the Breslow thickness, presence of histologic ulceration, Clark level, mitotic rate per mm^2, and peripheral and

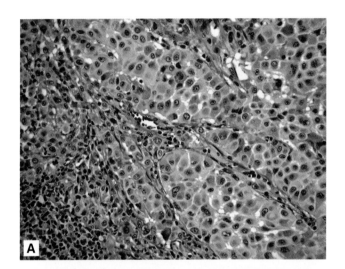

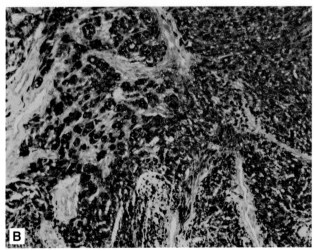

FIGURE 23-7 Malignant melanoma. **A.** Malignant melanoma demonstrating nests of tumor cells. The tumor cells display severe cytologic atypia and the characteristic eosinophilic macronucleoli. **B.** Malignant melanoma cells highlighted by an immunohistochemical stain for S-100 protein.

deep margin status should be reported in the pathology report. In addition, the presence of regression, tumor infiltrating lymphocytes, vertical growth phase, angiolymphatic invasion, neurotropism, and histologic subtype should also be consistently reported.

The diagnosis of a primary breast melanoma should be made only after exclusion of a metastatic melanoma or a mammary carcinoma with melanin phagocytosis. Immunohistochemical staining can help differentiate a melanoma from a mammary carcinoma (Fig. 23-7B). Most melanomas stain positive for S-100, HMB-45, and Melan A, and negative for cytokeratins; while mammary carcinomas stain positive for cytokeratins but negative for S-100, HMB-45, and Melan A.

The diagnosis of a nipple–areolar complex malignant melanoma can be difficult; the presence of melanin pigment is not sufficient to distinguish a malignant melanoma from Paget disease, because Paget cells may acquire melanin pigment. A diagnosis of Paget disease is supported by the presence of a noninvasive or invasive mammary carcinoma in the breast and reactivity to 1 or more of the epithelial markers.

Tumors are staged according to the 2002 AJCC TNM staging system, which is dependent on tumor thickness, presence of ulceration, regional nodal status, and the presence of in-transit or satellite metastasis and distant disease (Table 23-4).[80,82] Distant metastases usually occur to lung, liver, other visceral sites, bone, and brain.

Treatment

Surgical management of a primary breast malignant melanoma is the same as the management of a nonmammary cutaneous lesion. Since the 5-year disease-free survival is similar for patients undergoing an adequate wide local excision versus mastectomy, wide local excision, including the breast parenchyma and pectoralis major fascia, with primary closure is the treatment of choice; mastectomy is generally not required.[78-80] The recommended surgical margin depends on the tumor thickness (Table 23-5).[80] As with any malignant melanoma, appropriate axillary staging should be considered/performed for all melanomas except for cases of melanoma in situ or stage IA tumors with no adverse features (positive deep margin, extensive regression, and mitotic rate greater than zero). Clinically node-negative patients should undergo a sentinel lymph node biopsy procedure. Patients with a positive sentinel lymph node and patients with known nodal involvement should undergo a metastatic workup (chest x-ray, CT ± PET scan, MRI) as well as complete dissection of the involved regional nodal basin. There is no role for internal mammary node dissection as internal mammary metastases are rare and elective dissection does not improve loco-regional control or survival.[75,78,81]

For patients with stage IIB or higher disease, systemic adjuvant treatment with interferon-alpha or a clinical trial should be considered. Treatment of local scar recurrence, satellitosis, and/or in-transit recurrence, nodal recurrence, and distant metastatic disease is beyond the scope of this chapter and is summarized in the National Comprehensive Cancer Network practice guidelines for melanoma.[80]

TABLE 23-4 2002 AJCC Staging System for Melanoma

TNM Definitions

Primary Tumor (T)

TX	Primary tumor cannot be assessed (eg, shave biopsy or regressed melanoma)
T0	No evidence of primary tumor
Tis	Melanoma in situ
T1	Melanoma ≤ 1.0 mm in thickness with or without ulceration
T1a	Melanoma ≤ 1.0 mm in thickness and level II or III, no ulceration
T1b	Melanoma ≤ 1.0 mm in thickness and level IV or V or with ulceration
T2	Melanoma 1.01-2.0 mm in thickness with or without ulceration
T2a	Melanoma 1.01-2.0 mm in thickness, no ulceration
T2b	Melanoma 1.01-2.0 mm in thickness, with ulceration
T3	Melanoma 2.01-4.0 mm in thickness with or without ulceration
T3a	Melanoma 2.01-4.0 mm in thickness, no ulceration
T3b	Melanoma 2.01-4.0 mm in thickness, with ulceration
T4	Melanoma > 4.0 mm in thickness, with or without
T4a	Melanoma > 4.0 mm in thickness, no ulceration
T4b	Melanoma > 4.0 mm in thickness, with ulceration

Regional Lymph Nodes (N)

NX	Regional lymph nodes cannot be assessed
N0	No regional lymph node metastasis
N1	Metastasis in 1 lymph node
N1a	Clinically occult (microscopic) metastasis
N1b	Clinically apparent (macroscopic) metastasis
N2	Metastasis in 2 or 3 regional nodes or intralymphatic regional metastasis without nodal metastases
N2a	Clinically occult (microscopic) metastasis
N2b	Clinically apparent (macroscopic) metastasis
N2c	Satellite or in-transit metastasis without nodal metastasis
N3	Metastasis in four or more regional lymph nodes, or matted metastatic nodes, or in-transit metastasis or satellite(s) with metastasis in regional node(s)

Distant Metastases (M)

MX	Distant metastasis cannot be assessed
M0	No distant metastasis
M1	Distant metastasis
M1a	Metastasis to skin, subcutaneous tissue, or distant lymph nodes
M1b	Metastasis to lung
M1c	Metastasis to all other visceral sites or distant metastasis at any site associated with an elevated lactic dehydrogenase (LDH)

Clinical Stage Grouping

Stage	T	N	M
0	Tis	N0	M0
IA	T1a	N0	M0
IB	T1b, T2a	N0	M0
IIA	T2b, T3a	N0	M0
IIB	T3b, T4a	N0	M0
IIC	T4b	N0	M0
III	Any T	N1, N2, or N3	M0
IV	Any T	Any N	M1

Clinical staging includes microstaging of the primary melanoma and clinical/radiological evaluations for metastases. By convention, it should be used after complete excision of the primary melanoma with clinical assessment for regional and distant metastases.

(Continued)

TABLE 23-4 2002 AJCC Staging System for Melanoma (*Continued*)
Pathologic Stage Grouping

Stage	T	N	M
0	Tis	N0	M0
IA	T1a	N0	M0
IB	T1b, T2a	N0	M0
IIA	T2b, T3a	N0	M0
IIB	T3b, T4a	N0	M0
IIC	T4b	N0	M0
IIIA	T1-4a	N1a or N2a	M0
IIIB	T1-4b	N1a or N2a	M0
	T1-4a	N1b or N2b	M0
	T1-4a/b	N2c	M0
IIIC	T1-4b	N1b or N2b	M0
	Any T	N3	M0
IV	Any T	Any N	M1

Pathologic staging includes microstaging of the primary melanoma and pathologic information about the regional lymph nodes after partial or complete lymphadenectomy. Pathologic stage 0 or stage IA patients are the exception; they do not require pathologic evaluation of their lymph nodes.
Used with the permission of the American Joint Committee on Cancer (AJCC), Chicago, Illinois. The original source for this material is the AJCC Cancer Staging Manual, Sixth Edition (2002) published by Springer Science and Business Media LLC, www.springerlink.com. From Melanoma of the skin. In: Greene FL, Page DL, Fleming ID, et al, eds. *AJCC Cancer Staging Manual*, Sixth Edition. New York, NY: Springer, 2002:211-212.

TABLE 23-5 Recommended Surgical Margins for Wide Excision of Primary Melanoma

Tumor Thickness	Surgical Margin (cm)
In situ	0.5
≤ 1.0 mm	1.0
1.01-2 mm	1.0-2.0
2.01-4 mm	2.0
> 4 mm	2.0

Reproduced with permission from The NCCN (2.2009) Melanoma Clinical Practice Guidelines in Oncology. © National Comprehensive Cancer Network, 2009. Available at: www.nccn.org. Accessed [August 20, 2009]. To view the most recent and complete version of the guideline, go online to www.nccn.org.

For follow-up, patients should undergo lifelong skin examinations. The frequency of examination is dependent on tumor stage.[80] Routine laboratory work or imaging studies are not recommended for asymptomatic patients. As with nonmammary cutaneous lesions, the prognosis of malignant melanoma of the breast depends on the tumor stage (nodal involvement, tumor thickness).[80] In general, those with localized disease and tumors 1.0 mm or less in thickness achieve long-term survival in more than 90%. Survival rates vary from 50% to 90% for patients with melanomas more than 1.0 mm in thickness, depending on regional nodal involvement. Long-term survival

in patients with distant metastatic disease is less than 10%. In the largest series of 115 patients with primary cutaneous melanomas of the breast, approximately 60% of patients remained disease-free at 5 years. When axillary lymph nodes were not involved, the 5-year disease-free survival was nearly 90% but it dropped to about 25% when axillary metastases were present.[78]

Summary

Primary malignant melanomas of the breast are extremely rare tumors that typically involve the skin overlying the breast. The clinical presentation, workup, management, and prognosis of these lesions do not differ from primary cutaneous malignant melanomas arising elsewhere in the body. Surgical treatment includes wide local excision and appropriate axillary staging/surgery. Prognosis is dependent on tumor stage, most importantly lymph node status. For patients with stage IIB or higher disease, systemic adjuvant treatment with interferon-alpha or a clinical trial should be considered.

METASTASES TO THE BREAST

Metastatic lesions to the breast from an extramammary malignancy account for approximately 0.2% to 6.6% of all malignant mammary tumors.[83,84] Up to 40% of patients with breast metastases from an occult extramammary malignancy initially present with a breast lesion.[83-86] The time interval from the diagnosis of an extramammary primary cancer to the diagnosis of breast metastases varies widely (1 month to 15 years), but on average occur within 2 years of the previously treated cancer.[83,87]

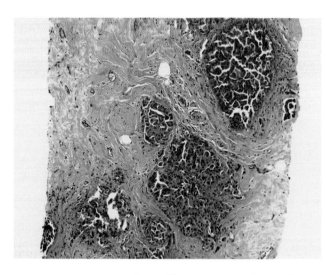

FIGURE 23-8 Metastatic papillary serous carcinoma from an ovarian primary. The glandular epithelium displays pseudostratification, nuclear hyperchromasia, and pleomorphism. Small papillae are also seen invading the fibrous tissue of the breast. Without a clinical history, this tumor could easily be confused with a primary breast tumor.

In most cases, extramammary metastases have been previously noted or are present at the time of diagnosis of the breast metastasis, signifying widespread disease. Isolated metastases limited to the breast are uncommon but do occur.[88]

Excluding metastatic lesions from hematopoietic and lymphatic malignancies and the contralateral breast, the most common cancers metastasizing to the breast are malignant melanoma and lung.[85,86] In males, the prostate is a common source; in children, the most common cancer is rhabdomyosarcoma.[89,90] Metastatic lesions to the breast can originate from any organ in the body, including the gastrointestinal tract, ovary, uterine cervix and endometrium, kidney, pancreas, thyroid, pharynx, salivary glands, and retina (Fig. 23-8).[85,86] Tumor types include melanomas, carcinomas, sarcomas, and neuroendocrine tumors.[91-93]

A metastatic breast lesion should be considered when a patient has a history of a previously treated extramammary cancer, especially melanoma, lung, or any adenocarcinoma. This history of a previous cancer should be conveyed to the pathologist. A metastatic breast tumor should also be considered with any breast lesion that has unusual clinical, radiographic, gross, or histologic features. The recognition of a breast lesion as a metastatic lesion rather than a primary breast tumor is extremely important, as the correct diagnosis of a metastatic lesion will avoid unnecessary breast surgery and direct appropriate attention to the treatment of the primary extramammary tumor.

Clinical Presentation

Metastatic tumors to the breast have been documented in both females and males usually in their fourth or fifth decades (age range, 12-90 years).[85,86] These lesions usually present as palpable, superficial, painless, firm, well-circumscribed masses, which may grow rapidly.[84,86,94] Lesions may be solitary, multiple,

bilateral, or diffuse; multiple and diffuse lesions are usually seen with more advanced disease.[81,83-85] Metastases to the ipsilateral axillary lymph nodes may be seen in 25% to 50% of patients.[83,84] In the majority of patients, extramammary metastases have been previously noted or are present at the time of diagnosis of the breast metastasis, signifying disseminated disease. Most patients succumb to their disease within 1 to 2 years.[83-86,94]

On mammography, metastatic lesions typically are round, discrete nodules with well-defined or slightly irregular margins without spiculations; microcalcifications are rarely seen with the exception of serous papillary carcinoma of the ovary/peritoneum.[33,86] Metastatic lesions are not usually distinguishable from circumscribed primary breast carcinomas or benign lesions. On ultrasonography, the lesions are typically hypoechoic masses with circumscribed, indistinct, or irregular margins.[33,86] There is usually a close correlation between the clinical and radiographic size of the lesion.

The distinction of a primary breast tumor versus a metastasis in the breast is critical. Any patient with a history of cancer and a breast abnormality should undergo tissue sampling. Most metastatic breast lesions can be diagnosed with a core biopsy, but some may require excisional biopsy to ensure accurate identification.[94] When a patient with an occult extramammary neoplasm presents with a breast metastasis, the workup for the primary lesion will be influenced by the morphologic features of the tumor.

Pathology

Metastatic lesions to the breast are usually sharply demarcated tumors. A search should be made for an intraepithelial component, as the presence of in situ disease is the only absolute proof of a primary breast carcinoma. If a tumor has unusual histology and lacks an in situ component, the possibility of a metastatic lesion should be considered and excluded. The presence of elastosis is common in primary mammary carcinomas but is rare in extramammary tumors.[94] Certain histologic patterns present especially difficult problems, as tumors of similar or identical appearance arise in the breast as well as other organs. Immunohistochemistry may play a helpful role in differentiating the etiology of certain lesions (Table 23-6).[94] However, no marker is 100% sensitive or specific, and the choice of antibodies used should be based on the history and morphology of the tumor. Histologic and immunohistochemical features of the breast lesion and the primary cancer should be compared to confirm the diagnosis of a breast metastasis.

Treatment

Emphasis should be placed on systemic treatment of the primary lesion as metastatic involvement to the breast is a manifestation of disseminated disease in virtually all cases. Surgery has a limited role in these situations. Diagnostic excisional biopsy may be necessary to ensure an accurate diagnosis. Surgery with curative intent (lumpectomy with or without radiation therapy or mastectomy) can be considered in patients with isolated breast metastases and indolent disease.[87]

TABLE 23-6 Common Histologic and Immunohistochemical Features of Various Cancers

Cancer	IHC-Positive	IHC-Negative	Histologic Features
Breast	CK7, CAM 5.2, ER, GCDFP-15, PR	CK20	
Lung (small cell)	CD56, TTF-1		Speckled chromatin with prominent nucleoli, scant cytoplasm, necrosis, and frequent mitoses
Lung (adenocarcinoma)	TTF-1		Acinar cell growth pattern or mucin-secreting columnar cells
Melanoma	HMB45, S100		Cytoplasmic pigment, intranuclear inclusions, spindle cells
Ovarian (serous papillary)	CA-125, mesothelin, WT-1	GCDFP-15	Papillary architecture
Prostate	PSA, prostatic acid phosphatase	CK7, ER, GCDFP-15, PR	
Stomach	CDX2, CK20	CK7, ER, GCDFP-15	Columnar mucin-secreting cells. Intestinal pattern may resemble an invasive ductal carcinoma of the breast, and diffuse gastric pattern may resemble an invasive lobular carcinoma of the breast
Renal cell	CD10, renal cell carcinoma marker		Abundant clear or granular cytoplasm with prominent fine vessels
Carcinoid tumors	CDX2, CK20 if GI source, TTF-1 if pulmonary source		Cannot differentiate from primary carcinoid tumor of breast

ER, estrogen receptor; GCDFP, gross cystic disease fluid protein-15; IHC, immunohistochemistry; PR, progesterone receptor; PSA, prostate-specific antigen; TTF-1, thyroid transcription factor-1; WT-1, Wilms tumor-1.
From Lee AH. The histological diagnosis of metastases to the breast from extramammary malignancies. *J Clin Pathol.* 2007;60:1333-1341.

Mastectomy may be required for local control of lesions that are symptomatic and/or bulky, ulcerated, or necrotic. The prognosis depends on the clinical characteristics of the primary lesion but most patients die within 1 to 2 years of their diagnosis of breast metastases.[83,86,94] Prolonged survival can occur with non-aggressive malignancies, such as carcinoid tumors.[86,91]

Summary

The differentiation of a metastatic breast lesion from a primary breast tumor is critical. A careful history with special attention to concurrent or previous malignancies, combined with clinical examination and appropriate imaging and pathologic evaluations, is needed to ensure the correct diagnosis and management of these patients. Surgery plays a limited role, as the majority of these patients have widely disseminated disease and a poor prognosis. Although metastatic disease to the breast remains rare, as systemic treatments and therefore overall survival for patients with metastatic malignancies improve, the number of patients with breast metastasis will increase. The appropriate surgical management for these patients will remain difficult as it is hard to predict patient longevity and whether local complications from the breast metastases will occur.

Patients with breast metastases should be managed on an individual basis using a multidisciplinary approach.

SUMMARY

For phyllodes tumors, sarcomas, and melanomas, the primary treatment remains surgery with negative margins; the role of adjuvant therapies (radiation and systemic treatment) remains unproven and must be considered on a case-by-case basis. Primary breast lymphomas and metastases to the breast are managed by limited surgery for tissue diagnosis and tumor classification followed by systemic therapy. Because of the rarity of these tumors, no established guidelines for the management of these nonepithelial breast tumors exists. The treatment of patients with these uncommon tumors should be accomplished by a multidisciplinary team approach.

REFERENCES

1. Telli ML, Horst KC, Guardino AE, et al. Phyllodes tumors of the breast: natural history, diagnosis, and treatment. *J Natl Compr Canc Netw.* 2007;5:324-330.

2. Parker SJ, Harris SA. Phyllodes tumours. *Postgrad Med J.* 2001;77:428-435.

3. Mueller J. *Ueber den feinern Bau und die Formen der krankhaften Geschwuelste.* Berlin, Germany; G. Reiner; 1838:54-57.

4. Lee BJ, Pack GT. Giant intracanalicular myxoma of the breast: the so-called cystosarcoma phyllodes mammae of Johannes Muller. *Ann Surg.* 1931;93:250-268.

5. Lomonaco F. Phyllode tumors of the breast (cystosarcoma phyllodes of J. Muller). *Tumori.* 1960;46:156-184.

6. Histological typing of breast tumors. *Tumori.* 30 1982;68:181-198.

7. August DA, Kearney T. Cystosarcoma phyllodes: mastectomy, lumpectomy, or lumpectomy plus irradiation. *Surg Oncol.* 2000;9:49-52.

8. Macdonald OK, Lee CM, Tward JD, et al. Malignant phyllodes tumor of the female breast: association of primary therapy with cause-specific survival from the Surveillance, Epidemiology, and End Results (SEER) program. *Cancer.* 2006;107:2127-2133.

9. Reinfuss M, Mitus J, Duda K, et al. The treatment and prognosis of patients with phyllodes tumor of the breast: an analysis of 170 cases. *Cancer.* 1996;77:910-916.

10. Mangi AA, Smith BL, Gadd MA, et al. Surgical management of phyllodes tumors. *Arch Surg.* 1999;134:487-492; discussion 492-483.

11. Grimes MM. Cystosarcoma phyllodes of the breast: histologic features, flow cytometric analysis, and clinical correlations. *Mod Pathol.* 1992;5:232-239.

12. Azzopardi JG. Sarcoma in the breast. In: Bennington J, ed. *Problems in Breast Pathology.* Vol. 2. Philadelphia, PA: Saunders; 1979:355-359.

13. Chao TC, Lo YF, Chen SC, Chen MF. Sonographic features of phyllodes tumors of the breast. *Ultrasound Obstet Gynecol.* 2002;20:64-71.

14. Farria DM, Gorczyca DP, Barsky SH, et al. Benign phyllodes tumor of the breast: MR imaging features. *AJR Am J Roentgenol.* 1996;167:187-189.

15. Salvadori B, Cumumano F, Del Bo R, et al. Surgical treatment of phyllodes tumors of the breast. *Cancer.* 1989;63:2532-2536.

16. Chaney AW, Pollack A, McNeese MD, et al. Primary treatment of cystosarcoma phyllodes of the breast. *Cancer.* 2000;89:1502-1511.

17. Hawkins RE, Schofield JB, Fisher C, et al. The clinical and histologic criteria that predict metastases from cystosarcoma phyllodes. *Cancer.* 1992;69:141-147.

18. Barrio AV, Clark BD, Goldberg JI, et al. Clinicopathologic features and long-term outcomes of 293 phyllodes tumors of the breast. *Ann Surg Oncol.* 2007;14:2961-2970.

19. Belkacemi Y, Bousquet G, Marsiglia H, et al. Phyllodes tumor of the breast. *Int J Radiat Oncol Biol Phys.* 2008;70:492-500.

20. Zurrida S, Bartoli C, Galimberti V, et al. Which therapy for unexpected phyllode tumour of the breast? *Eur J Cancer.* 1992;28:654-657.

21. Barth RJ Jr. Histologic features predict local recurrence after breast conserving therapy of phyllodes tumors. *Breast Cancer Res Treat.* 1999;57:291-295.

22. Pandey M, Mathew A, Kattoor J, et al. Malignant phyllodes tumor. *Breast J.* 2001;7:411-416.

23. National Comprehensive Cancer Network. Clinical Practice Guidelines in Oncology. Breast Cancer. v.2.2000. Available at: http://www.nccn.org/professionals/physician_gls/f_guidelines.asp. Fort Washington, PA. Accessed September 9, 2008.

24. National Comprehensive Cancer Network. Clinical Practice Guidelines in Oncology. Soft Tissue Sarcoma. v.2.2008. Available at: http://www.nccn.org/professionals/physician_gls/f_guidelines.asp. Fort Washington, PA. Accessed September 9, 2008.

25. Blanchard DK, Reynolds CA, Grant CS, Donohue JH. Primary nonphylloides breast sarcomas. *Am J Surg.* 2003;186:359-361.

26. McGowan TS, Cummings BJ, O'Sullivan B, et al. An analysis of 78 breast sarcoma patients without distant metastases at presentation. *Int J Radiat Oncol Biol Phys.* 2000;46:383-390.

27. Lum YW, Jacobs L. Primary breast sarcoma. *Surg Clin North Am.* 2008;88:559-570.

28. Gutman H, Pollock RE, Ross MI, et al. Sarcoma of the breast: implications for extent of therapy. The M.D. Anderson experience. *Surgery.* 1994;116:505-509.

29. Barrow BJ, Janjan NA, Gutman H, et al. Role of radiotherapy in sarcoma of the breast—a retrospective review of the M.D. Anderson experience. *Radiother Oncol.* 1999;52:173-178.

30. Zelek L, Llombart-Cussac A, Terrier P, et al. Prognostic factors in primary breast sarcomas: a series of patients with long-term follow-up. *J Clin Oncol.* 2003;21:2583-2588.

31. Confavreux C, Lurkin A, Mitton N, et al. Sarcomas and malignant phyllodes tumours of the breast—a retrospective study. *Eur J Cancer.* 2006;42:2715-2721.

32. Pollard SG, Marks PV, Temple LN, Thompson HH. Breast sarcoma. A clinicopathologic review of 25 cases. *Cancer.* 1990;66:941-944.

33. Yang WT. Sonography of unusual breast neoplasms. *Ultrasound Clin.* 2007;1:661-672.

34. Tavassoli FA. Mesenchymal lesions. In: *Pathology of the Breast.* 2nd ed. Stamford, CT: Appleton & Lange; 1999:675-729.

35. Soft tissue sarcoma. In: Greene FL, Page DL, Fleming ID, et al., eds. *AJCC Cancer Staging Manual.* 6th ed. New York, NY: Springer-Verlag; 2002:193-200.

36. Bousquet G, Confavreux C, Magne N, et al. Outcome and prognostic factors in breast sarcoma: a multicenter study from the rare cancer network. *Radiother Oncol.* 2007;85:355-361.

37. Pandey M, Mathew A, Abraham EK, Rajan B. Primary sarcoma of the breast. *J Surg Oncol.* 2004;87:121-125.

38. Johnstone PA, Pierce LJ, Merino MJ, et al. Primary soft tissue sarcomas of the breast: local-regional control with post-operative radiotherapy. *Int J Radiat Oncol Biol Phys.* 1993;27:671-675.

39. Adjuvant chemotherapy for localised resectable soft-tissue sarcoma of adults: meta-analysis of individual data. Sarcoma Meta-analysis Collaboration. *Lancet.* 1997;350:1647-1654.

40. Pisters PW, Leung DH, Woodruff J, et al. Analysis of prognostic factors in 1,041 patients with localized soft tissue sarcomas of the extremities. *J Clin Oncol.* 1996;14(5):1679-1689.

41. McGregor GI, Knowling MA, Este FA. Sarcoma and cystosarcoma phyllodes tumors of the breast—a retrospective review of 58 cases. *Am J Surg.* 1994;167:477-480.

42. Sher T, Hennessy BT, Valero V, et al. Primary angiosarcomas of the breast. *Cancer.* 2007;110:173-178.

43. Monroe AT, Feigenberg SJ, Mendenhall NP. Angiosarcoma after breast-conserving therapy. *Cancer.* 2003;97:1832-1840.

44. Vorburger SA, Xing Y, Hunt KK, et al. Angiosarcoma of the breast. *Cancer.* 2005;104:2682-2688.

45. Cha C, Antonescu CR, Quan ML, et al. Long-term results with resection of radiation induced soft tissue sarcomas. *Ann Surg.* 2004;239:903-909, discussion 909-910.

46. Chen KT, Kirkegaard DD, Bocian JJ. Angiosarcoma of the breast. *Cancer.* 1980;46:368-371.

47. Rosen PP, Kimmel M, Ernsberger D. Mammary angiosarcoma. The prognostic significance of tumor differentiation. *Cancer.* 1988;62:2145-2151.

48. Donnell RM, Rosen PP, Lieberman PH, et al. Angiosarcoma and other vascular tumors of the breast. *Am J Surg Pathol.* 1981;5:629-642.

49. Merino MJ, Carter D, Berman M. Angiosarcoma of the breast. *Am J Surg Pathol.* 1983;7:53-60.

50. Parikh BC, Ohri A, Desai MY, et al. Liposarcoma of the breast—a case report. *Eur J Gynaecol Oncol.* 2007;28:425-427.

51. Austin RM, Dupree WB. Liposarcoma of the breast: a clinicopathologic study of 20 cases. *Hum Pathol.* 1986;17:906-913.

52. Mazaki T, Tanak T, Suenaga Y, et al. Liposarcoma of the breast: a case report and review of the literature. *Int Surg.* 2002;87:164-170.

53. WHO Classification of Soft Tissue Tumours. In: Fletcher CD, Unni KK, Mertens F, eds. *World Health Organization Classification of Tumours. Pathology and Genetics of Tumours of Soft Tissue and Bone.* Lyon, France: IARC Press; 2002:9-18.

54. Gupta RK, Kenwright D, Naran S, et al. Fine needle aspiration cytodiagnosis of leiomyosarcoma of the breast. A case report. *Acta Cytol.* 2000;44:1101-1105.

55. Szekely E, Madaras L, Kulka J, et al. Leiomyosarcoma of the female breast. *Pathol Oncol Res.* 2001;7:151-153.

56. Munitiz V, Rios A, Canovas J, et al. Primitive leiomyosarcoma of the breast: case report and review of the literature. *Breast.* 2004;13:72-76.

57. Chen KT, Kuo TT, Hoffmann KD. Leiomyosarcoma of the breast: a case of long survival and late hepatic metastasis. *Cancer.* 1981;47:1883-1886.

58. Nielsen BB. Leiomyosarcoma of the breast with late dissemination. *Virchows Arch Pathol Anat.* 1984;403:241-245.

59. van Niekerk JL, Wobbes T, Holland R, van Haelst UJ. Malignant fibrous histiocytoma of the breast with axillary lymph node involvement. *J Surg Oncol.* 1987;34:32-35.

60. Iellin A, Waizbard E, Levine T, Behar A. Malignant fibrous histiocytoma of the breast. *Int Surg.* 1990;75:63-66.

61. Ajisaka H, Maeda K, Uchiyama A, Miwa A. Myxoid malignant fibrous histiocytoma of the breast: report of a case. *Surg Today.* 2002;32:887-890.

62. Jones MW, Norris HJ, Wargotz ES, Weiss SW. Fibrosarcoma-malignant fibrous histiocytoma of the breast. A clinicopathological study of 32 cases. *Am J Surg Pathol.* 1992;16:667-674.

63. Wiseman C, Liao KT. Primary lymphoma of the breast. *Cancer.* 1972;29:1705-1712.

64. Jennings WC, Baker RS, Murray SS, et al. Primary breast lymphoma: the role of mastectomy and the importance of lymph node status. *Ann Surg.* 2007;245:784-789.

65. Ryan G, Martinelli G, Kuper-Hommel M, et al. Primary diffuse large B-cell lymphoma of the breast: prognostic factors and outcomes of a study by the International Extranodal Lymphoma Study Group. *Ann Oncol.* 2008;19:233-241.

66. Paulus DD. Lymphoma of the breast. *Radiol Clin North Am.* 1990;28:833-840.

67. Liberman L, Giess CS, Dershaw DD, et al. Non-Hodgkin lymphoma of the breast: imaging characteristics and correlation with histopathologic findings. *Radiology.* 1994;192:157-160.

68. Domchek SM, Hecht JL, Fleming MD, et al. Lymphomas of the breast: primary and secondary involvement. *Cancer.* 2002;94:6-13.

69. Gholam D, Bibeau F, El Weshi A, et al. Primary breast lymphoma. *Leuk Lymphoma.* 2003;44:1173-1178.

70. Ryan GF, Roos DR, Seymour JF. Primary non-Hodgkin's lymphoma of the breast: retrospective analysis of prognosis and patterns of failure in two Australian centers. *Clin Lymphoma Myeloma.* 2006;6:337-341.

71. Decosse JJ, Berg JW, Fracchia AA, Farrow JH. Primary lymphosarcoma of the breast. A review of 14 cases. *Cancer.* 1962;15:1264-1268.

72. DeBlasio D, McCormick B, Straus D, et al. Definitive irradiation for localized non-Hodgkin's lymphoma of breast. *Int J Radiat Oncol Biol Phys.* 1989;17:843-846.

73. Aviles A, Delgado S, Nambo MJ, et al. Primary breast lymphoma: results of a controlled clinical trial. *Oncology.* 2005;69:256-260.

74. Ganjoo K, Advani R, Mariappan MR, et al. Non-Hodgkin lymphoma of the breast. *Cancer.* 2007;110:25-30.

75. Lee YT, Sparks FC, Morton DL. Primary melanoma of skin of the breast region. *Ann Surg.* 1977;185:17-22.

76. Gatch WD. A melanoma, apparently primary in a breast; its single known metastasis in the small bowel. *AMA Arch Surg.* 1956;73:266-268.

77. Stephenson SE Jr., Byrd BF Jr. Malignant melanoma of the breast. *Am J Surg.* 1959;97:232-235.

78. Papachristou DN, Kinne DW, Rosen PP, et al. Cutaneous melanoma of the breast. *Surgery.* 1979;85:322-328.

79. Roses DF, Harris MN, Stern JS, Gumport SL. Cutaneous melanoma of the breast. *Ann Surg.* 1979;189:112-115.

80. National Comprehensive Cancer Network. Clinical Practice Guidelines in Oncology. Melanoma. v.2.2008. Available at: http://www.nccn.org/professionals/physician_gls/f_guidelines.asp. Fort Washington, PA. Accessed September 10, 2008.

81. Lise M, Kinne DW, Fortner JG. Internal mammary node dissection for melanoma of the anterior chest wall. *Proc Am Soc Clin Oncol.* 1974:193.

82. Melanoma of the skin. In: Greene FL, Page DL, Fleming ID, et al., eds. *AJCC Cancer Staging Manual.* 6th ed. New York, NY: Springer-Verlag; 2002:209-220.

83. Toombs BD, Kalisher L. Metastatic disease to the breast: clinical, pathologic, and radiographic features. *AJR Am J Roentgenol.* 1977;129:673-676.

84. Hajdu SI, Urban JA. Cancers metastatic to the breast. *Cancer.* 1972;29:1691-1696.

85. Georgiannos SN, Chin J, Goode AW, Sheaff M. Secondary neoplasms of the breast: a survey of the 20th Century. *Cancer.* 2001;92:2259-2266.

86. Bartella L, Kaye J, Perry NM, et al. Metastases to the breast revisited: radiological-histopathological correlation. *Clin Radiol.* 2003;58:524-531.

87. Vaughan A, Dietz JR, Moley JF, et al. Metastatic disease to the breast: the Washington University experience. *World J Surg Oncol.* 2007;5:74.

88. Wood B, Sterrett G, Frost F, Swarbrick N. Diagnosis of extramammary malignancy metastatic to the breast by fine needle biopsy. *Pathology.* 2008;40:345-351.

89. Salyer WR, Salyer DC. Metastases of prostatic carcinoma to the breast. *J Urol.* 1973;109:671-675.

90. Rogers DA, Lobe TE, Rao BN, et al. Breast malignancy in children. *J Pediatr Surg.* 1994;29:48-51.

91. Upalakalin JN, Collins LC, Tawa N, Parangi S. Carcinoid tumors in the breast. *Am J Surg.* 2006;191:799-805.

92. Ravdel L, Robinson WA, Lewis K, Gonzalez R. Metastatic melanoma in the breast: a report of 27 cases. *J Surg Oncol.* 2006;94:101-104.

93. Recine MA, Deavers MT, Middleton LP, et al. Serous carcinoma of the ovary and peritoneum with metastases to the breast and axillary lymph nodes: a potential pitfall. *Am J Surg Pathol.* 2004;28:1646-1651.

94. Lee AH. The histological diagnosis of metastases to the breast from extramammary malignancies. *J Clin Pathol.* 2007;60:1333-1341.

CHAPTER 24

Cytology in Breast Care Management

Savitri Krishnamurthy

Cytopathology is a specialized branch of pathology related to the study of cells derived from either fine-needle aspiration biopsy (FNAB) or exfoliation including effusions, washings, brushings, or body fluids. FNAB is performed using a 23- or 25-gauge hypodermic needle attached to a 10-mL plastic syringe. FNAB can be performed blindly for palpable masses or under radiologic guidance including ultrasound (US), computed tomography (CT), or magnetic resonance imaging (MRI) for nonpalpable lesions. Specimens obtained from any of these sources can be prepared in several ways for conventional cytopathologic evaluation and ancillary studies. Smears can be made directly or from the cell pellet obtained after centrifugation of the specimen following admixture with a liquid base such as RPMI or Cytolyt solution. Monolayer preparation of the specimen can also be made using different techniques such as Thin Prep and Sure Path. Smears prepared by any of the techniques are usually fixed in alcohol for Papanicalaou staining, or air-dried for Diff-Quik staining. In addition, aspirated material from FNA or exfoliative specimens can be rinsed in RPMI or Cytolyt solution to prepare tissue blocks that are fixed in formalin, processed routinely similar to surgical tissues, embedded in paraffin, and subsequently cut at 5 μm and finally stained by the hematoxylin and eosin (H&E) method.

The popularity of core needle biopsy (CNB) has to a large extent reduced the performance of FNAB in many centers. CNB produces cores of breast tissue that are generated by introduction of automated spring-loaded devices that activate a 14- to 18-gauge cutting needle into the localized site. Unlike FNAB, CNB not only provides tissue architecture that facilitates interpretation but also adequate tissue for performing ancillary studies. In contrast to CNB, FNAB is however better tolerated, less

invasive, and allows more effective sampling of small-sized lesions. Moreover, the possibility of sampling multiple sites in a large-sized lesion is an added advantage. FNAB is also the preferred technique for investigating breast lesions close to the chest wall because of fear of causing pneumothorax with a CNB or for investigating lesions occurring in breast with any type of tissue expander because of the risk of puncturing the latter. FNAB, however, may yield very minimal material insufficient for diagnosis particularly in sclerotic lesions necessitating the performance of CNB. For primary breast masses, the inability of FNAB to distinguish in situ from invasive carcinomas is a major disadvantage, which has essentially led CNB to replace FNAB for initial investigation of index breast lesions that are deemed to be very suspicious for malignancy on clinical examination and imaging findings. It should be noted, however, that FNAB and CNB are complementary techniques and can be used alone interchangeably or in conjunction based on the requirement of individual cases for preoperative diagnosis. The golden rule for the interpretation of breast FNAB is to always correlate the cytologic findings with clinical and imaging findings, commonly referred to as the triple test. Any discrepancy between the 3 components of the triple test should lead to obtaining a CNB or surgical excision for definite diagnosis of the abnormality. The results of FNAB should be categorized into 1 of 5 categories: benign, atypical/indeterminate, suspicious, malignant, or nondiagnostic/unsatisfactory.[1] The overall sensitivity and specificity of FNAB in comparison to CNB and surgical excision is high and ranges from 85% to 100% in different reports.[2-8] The role of cytology including FNAB of primary breast masses and metastatic tumors and exfoliative specimens such as nipple aspirate fluid, ductal lavage, and effusions is discussed in the following sections.

INVESTIGATION OF BREAST MASSES

Diagnosis of Nonneoplastic Lesions

Breast Cysts

Most breast cysts are encountered in premenopausal women. They can be single or multiple, of variable size, and may mimic solid masses on imaging. FNAB of breast cysts yields foamy histiocytes, few benign ductal epithelial cells, and cells with abundant granular cytoplasm referred to as apocrine cells in a background of proteinaceous material.[9-10] Cytologic examination of breast cysts may be optional if the cyst yields clear yellow fluid and collapses following aspiration. However, cysts that yield brownish or reddish fluid, do not collapse following aspiration, or are associated with a residual mass should be aspirated again or subjected to further investigation to exclude cancer.

Fat Necrosis

FNAB is useful for confirming lesions highly suspicious for fat necrosis on imaging or for those cases of fat necrosis that may closely mimic malignant lesions clinically and on imaging.[11] It is to be noted however that fat necrosis and malignancy can coexist, and therefore proper sampling of the lesion, careful cytologic examination, recognition of the pitfalls, and strict adherence to the triple test can avoid the occurrence of a false-positive or false-negative diagnosis. Fat necrosis yields fragments of degenerated adipose tissue, foamy histiocytes including multinucleated giant cells, conglomeration of red blood cells resulting in structures resembling a bag of grapes referred to as myospherulosis, hemosiderin pigment deposition, and variable degrees of acute and chronic inflammation, granulation tissue, and fibrosis. Figure 24-1 illustrates multinucleated giant cells and myospherules on direct smears of FNAB from a case of fat necrosis of the breast. Reactive atypia may be encountered in the macrophages, myofibroblasts, and epithelial cells, which can lead to an erroneous diagnosis of malignancy.

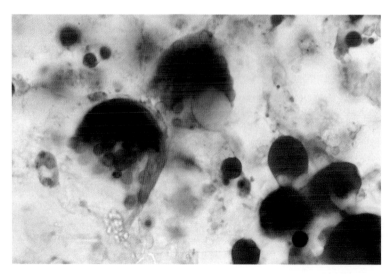

FIGURE 24-1 Direct smear of FNAB of a case of fat necrosis of the breast. Note the presence of multinucleated giant cells and conglomeration of red blood cells forming myospherules (*reddish structures and greenish structures*).

Breast Abscess

FNAB can be utilized not only for making a diagnosis but also for obtaining material for microbiologic culture studies from breast abscesses. Breast abscesses are commonly encountered in lactating women. The aspirated material is yellow, purulent, and shows abundant neutrophils, granulation tissue, and cellular debris.[12] Epithelial and mesenchymal cells may exhibit reactive atypia, which should not be mistaken for malignancy.

Subareolar abscess is a distinct type of breast abscess that occurs over a wide age range, is not related to lactation, and results from squamous metaplasia of lactiferous ducts resulting in keratin plugging and rupture of the duct.[13] The resultant squamous material in the stroma elicits acute inflammation and eventually may lead to fistula formation. FNAB shows abundant squames, acute inflammation, and the characteristic finding of multinucleated giant cells with ingested squames.

Granulomatous mastitis, caused by organisms such as mycobacterium tuberculosis, fungus, actinomyces, cat scratch disease, and foreign bodies such as sutures following surgery or silicon leakage from breast implants, can result in a breast mass that may be suspicious for malignancy on clinical examination and on imaging. FNAB shows clusters of epithelioid macrophages and multinucleated giant cells with or without associated necrosis. Silicone may be dissolved during processing resulting in empty spaces or it may be noted as homogenous refractile droplets on the smears.

Fibrocystic Changes

Women in the reproductive age group show variable degrees of epithelial proliferation, stromal fibrosis, and cystic change resulting in ill-defined thickening and/or masses that are often investigated by FNAB to exclude malignancy. FNAB in these cases yields few fragments of benign ductal epithelial cells with or without evidence of proliferation, apocrine cells, scattered individual nuclei derived from myoepithelial cells, foamy histiocytes, and stromal fragments of fibrosis. Proliferative changes involving ductal epithelial cells result in moderate- and large-sized fragments comprised of sheets of epithelial cells including both ductal and myoepithelial types. There may be mild pleomorphism of the nucleus, presence of small nucleoli, and mild nuclear enlargement. There is evidence of cellular streaming with nuclear overlap, crowding, and presence of irregular slit-like spaces within the fragments. Presence of punched-out spaces with focal cribriforming and evidence of monotony in the epithelial cells are worrisome features for presence of atypical ductal hyperplasia. Further investigation of lesions demonstrating findings of atypia on FNAB is warranted to exclude the presence of low-grade carcinoma in situ.

Diagnosis of Neoplastic Lesions

Fibroadenoma

Fibroadenoma is a benign fibroepithelial tumor, characterized by the proliferation of benign epithelial and stromal elements. These lesions are noted as a moveable well-defined mass in women in their 20s and 30s, which may be either easily palpable or nonpalpable and detected on imaging alone. Direct smears of classical cases of FNAB of fibroadenoma show clusters and sheets of benign ductal epithelial cells with associated myoepithelial cells that often form antler hornlike clusters, few fibromyxoid fragments of low cellularity, and many individual naked nuclei in the background.[14] Figure 24-2 illustrates the presence of many individually distributed naked nuclei, associated with a cluster of benign ductal cells obtained from FNAB of a case of fibroadenoma. The majority of the latter are myoepithelial in origin. Fibroadenomas are one of the most common causes of a false-positive diagnosis on FNAB of breast. High cellularity of the epithelial elements, nuclear atypia, presence of dispersed epithelial cells, and myxoid/mucoid background can all lead to misdiagnosis of fibroadenoma as a malignant lesion. Definite diagnosis of fibroadenoma should only be made on FNAB if the lesion exhibits all the three characteristic cytologic features and correlates with imaging findings of a well-defined mass with no irregularity or lobulations of the edges, absence of increased vascular flow, and no history of increased growth. Lesions not fulfilling the criteria or any discordance between cytologic imaging and clinical findings should be investigated further with either a CNB or preferably with surgical excision.

Phyllodes Tumor

Phyllodes tumors are fibroepithelial tumors that by definition are associated with a benign epithelial component and a cellular stromal component that exhibits variable degrees of atypia. At the lower end of the spectrum, the stromal fragments exhibit a mild increase in cellularity without any evidence of atypia or presence of mitotic figures and no evidence of stromal overgrowth or necrosis. Because of overlapping features between low-grade phyllodes tumors and cellular fibroadema, FNAB of these lesions is categorized as indeterminate and surgical excision is recommended for a definite diagnosis.[15,16] FNAB, however, can clearly establish the diagnosis of malignant phyllodes tumor. Stromal fragments on FNAB of malignant Phyllodes tumor clearly exhibit not only increased cellularity but also stromal atypia, pleomorphism, and mitotic figures. In addition, atypical stromal cells are also distributed in the background of the smears. There may be necrosis. The epithelial fragments in all cases of Phyllodes tumors is essentially benign with the presence of both epithelial and myoepithelial cells.

Papillary Neoplasms

Papillary neoplasms by definition exhibit a fibrovascular core with proliferation of epithelial cells around them. Papillary neoplasms can be benign or malignant. When they occur in the lactiferous ducts, they are usually associated with a bloody nipple discharge. Intraductal papillomas are benign tumors that demonstrate proliferation of benign ductal epithelial cells including myoepithelial cells around the fibrovascular cores.[17] Three-dimensional papillary clusters of the same cells, foamy and hemosiderin-laden macrophages, and a proteinaceous material in the background are usually noted. In some cases, the fragments may be bordered by tall columnar cells and similar cells may be distributed in the background. Papillary carcinomas, on the other hand, demonstrate atypical epithelial cells around the fibrovascular cores and in the background without the presence of myoepithelial cells.[17-19] While the distinction between benign and malignant papillary tumors may be possible in many cases, it is recommended to designate these lesions as papillary neoplasms and categorize them as indeterminate on cytology.

Mucinous Carcinoma

Mucinous carcinoma exhibits abundant extracellular mucin in direct smears. These tumors must be distinguished from mucocele-like lesions on FNAB, which range from benign to atypical in morphology. Unlike mucinous carcinomas, mucocele-like lesions are generally associated with reduced cellularity and

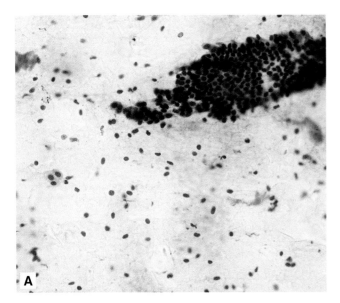

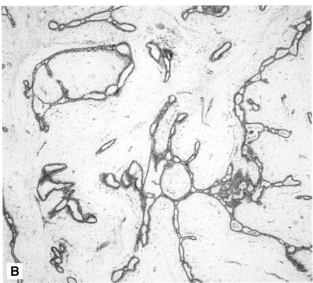

FIGURE 24-2 Illustration of a case of fibroadenoma on FNAB **(A)** and CNB **(B)**. Note the cluster of benign ductal cells with associated myoepithelial cells and presence of many naked nuclei in the background of the smear. The corresponding CNB **(B)** shows classic features of a fibroadenoma including the proliferation of benign ductal and stromal elements.

show few sheets of benign ductal epithelial cells including myoepithelial cells. On the other hand, mucinous carcinoma demonstrate increased cellularity with 3-dimensional epithelial cell clusters and individually distributed atypical epithelial cells of varying degrees of atypia.[19,20] Most importantly, the clusters do not contain myoepithelial cells. Therefore, while a distinction of mucocele-like lesions from mucinous carcinomas is possible on FNAB majority of times, lack of typical features and inability to definitely distinguish these lesions on FNAB with confidence should lead to surgical excision.

Ductal and Lobular Carcinoma

Ductal tumors are associated with increased cellularity and are comprised of 3-dimensional and loose clusters of epithelial cells with varying degrees of atypia.[21] Figure 24-3 is an illustration of a case of ductal carcinoma on FNAB. Unlike benign clusters of epithelial cells, these clusters do not demonstrate the presence of myoepithelial cells. In addition, there are several individually distributed atypical cells in the background. There may be mitotic figures in the atypical cells and necrosis in the background. Distinction of carcinoma in situ from invasive

carcinoma cannot be reliably made on FNAB because of overlapping features between in situ and invasive carcinoma, particularly those of high nuclear grade including the presence of necrosis.[22,23] The presence of atypical cell clusters of low nuclear grade and with prominent cribriforming generally raises the suspicion for low-grade DCIS. Well-differentiated invasive ductal carcinomas including tubular carcinomas exhibit small clusters of tightly cohesive ductal epithelial cells with abnormal angulated contours without the presence of myoepithelial cells in the clusters.[24] Such clusters are often admixed with clearly benign groups, a few naked nuclei in the background, and fragments of fibrosis. FNAB of such cases can be mistaken for fibroadenomas or adenosis. Careful attention to cytologic details, adhering to the triple test and performing CNB and/or surgical excision in difficult cases can avoid misdiagnosis of such cases.

Lobular carcinoma is commonly associated with single individually scattered tumor cells with minimal atypia and presence of mucin vacuoles in many if not all cases.[21] Figure 24-4 shows the features of lobular carcinoma on FNAB. In addition, small groups or linear rows of cells, referred to as "Indian filing," may also be noted. Occasionally signet-ring cells may be encountered.

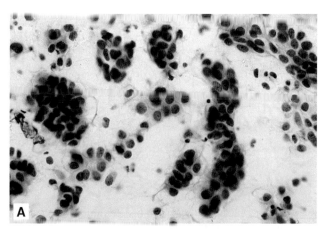

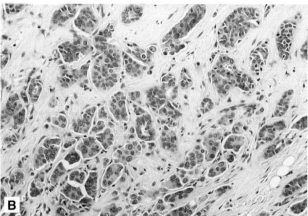

FIGURE 24-3 FNAB of breast mass **(A)** showing features of a ductal carcinoma, intermediate nuclear grade including many loosely cohesive clusters of atypical ductal epithelial cells with a relatively high nuclear to cytoplasmic ratio. Note the absence of myoepithelial cells in the clusters of tumor cells. The corresponding CNB **(B)** shows features of invasive ductal carcinoma, moderately differentiated.

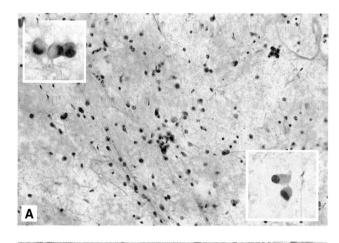

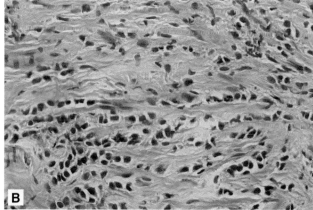

FIGURE 24-4 FNAB of a breast mass **(A)** showing features of a lobular carcinoma including many scattered relatively bland single cells, some of which contain mucin vacuoles **(A,** *inset*). The corresponding CNB **(B)** shows features of invasive lobular carcinoma, classic type.

The cellularity of these tumors is invariably low due to the occurrence of significant fibrosis in most of the tumors, which often results in a false-negative diagnosis on FNAB.[25]

In summary, except for well-differentiated invasive ductal carcinomas, the distinction of in situ from invasive ductal and lobular carcinomas cannot be made with absolute confidence due to overlapping cytomorphologic features between the two components as well as the usual occurrence of both components in a given tumor mass. Therefore, for primary index masses, CNB is generally preferred over FNAB because of the need for a definite preoperative distinction for selecting the appropriate management option.

Diagnosis of Metastatic Tumors

Metastatic tumors to breast account for up to 3% of all mammary tumors.[26] In general, involvement of the breast by hematologic malignancies, including malignant lymphoma and or leukemia, is the most common type of metastatic involvement of the breast in women. Metastasis from a primary mammary tumor in the contralateral breast is more common than metastases from other solid organ primaries. Small-cell carcinoma of the lung, signet-ring cell carcinoma of the stomach, renal cell carcinoma, and melanoma are the most common types of tumors that metastasize to the breast. In men, metastasis from prostatic adenocarcinoma is the most common cause of metastatic tumor in the breast. The accurate diagnosis of a breast tumor as metastatic and not primary is important, and is possible by FNAB majority of the times. Familiarity with the clinical history of the case, accurate cytologic interpretation, comparison of cytomorphologic features with the primary tumor and appropriate usage of ancillary immunostaining may all be helpful in avoiding the misdiagnosis of a metastatic tumor as a primary breast malignant tumor.

Just as FNAB is useful for diagnosis of metastatic tumors to breast from other sites, FNAB is also a useful technique for the diagnosis of metastasis from breast tumors to any site in the body including visceral organs, bone, and body cavity effusions.

EVALUATION OF PROGNOSTIC AND PREDICTIVE MARKERS

FNAB of breast and metastatic sites including regional or distant sites can be utilized for ascertaining prognostic and predictive markers. There are several reports in the literature that have demonstrated comparable results of the evaluation of estrogen and progesterone receptors between FNAB and corresponding breast tissue, the latter being regarded as the gold standard.[27,28] In today's era, where CNB is performed on all suspicious index lesions, the need for performing prognostic markers in primary breast cancer does not arise any very often. In addition, because of the inability to distinguish in situ from invasive carcinoma on FNAB, determination of prognostic markers on FNAB of primary breast tumors is generally not recommended. However, FNAB of regional and distant metastatic breast tumors can be reliably utilized for determining prognostic and predictive markers. Figure 24-5 shows an example of estrogen immunostaining performed on destained direct smears from a case of

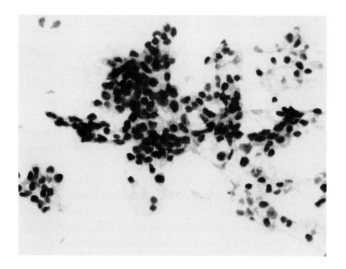

FIGURE 24-5 Immunostaining for estrogen receptor performed on a destained Papanicalaou-stained direct smear obtained from FNAB of an axillary lymph node, positive for metastatic carcinoma. Note that all of the tumor cells show strong nuclear positivity for estrogen receptor.

FNAB of axillary lymph node positive for metastatic carcinoma. Direct smears fixed in formalin, destained Pap smears, as well as thin prep slides and cell block sections can be used for estrogen and progesterone receptor staining. For the evaluation of HER-2 protein overexpression, however, only cell blocks and not smears are recommended because of lack of reliability in determining the accurate extent of complete membranous staining on the cells on smears. Air-dried smears either unstained or stained with Diff-Quik are, however, ideal specimens for determining HER-2 gene amplification status by fluorescence in situ hybridization.[29] Figure 24-6 illustrates HER-2 gene amplification as evidenced by fluorescence in situ hybridization performed on an air-dried smear of metastatic breast carcinoma in the lymph node.

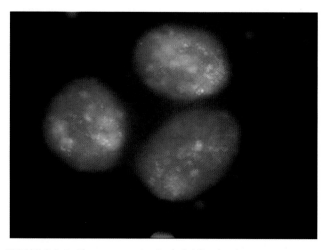

FIGURE 24-6 Fluorescence in situ hybridization for HER-2 performed on an air-dried direct smear obtained from FNAB of a case of metastatic carcinoma in the axillary lymph node. Note the increased copy numbers of HER-2 (orange signal) indicating HER-2 gene amplification.

INITIAL STAGING OF BREAST CARCINOMA

Imaging modalities such as ultrasound (US), being more sensitive than physical examination alone, are commonly used to evaluate axillary lymph nodes in the initial staging of patients with a diagnosis of breast carcinoma. Due to the overlap of sonographic features between benign/reactive and indeterminate/suspicious lymph nodes, FNAB is often performed on axillary lymph nodes so as to obtain a more definite diagnosis than US alone. FNAB of palpable and nonpalpable axillary lymph nodes is a simple, minimally invasive, and reliable technique for the initial determination of axillary lymph node status in breast carcinoma.[30,31] The results of FNAB can be useful to confirm the sonographic impression of a benign or malignant lymph node and for further categorization of sonographically indeterminate/suspicious lymph nodes. The results of FNAB of axillary lymph nodes determine management options in individual cases. In patients with early breast cancer, a negative result leads to selection of the patient for sentinel lymph node biopsy; a positive result for complete axillary dissection. In patients with locally advanced breast cancers, who are candidates for receiving neoadjuvant chemotherapy, FNAB of the lymph nodes can be used to monitor response of a malignant lymph node. False-negative results of FNAB are generally due to failure to visualize all the axillary lymph nodes on US, small size of metastasis and preoperative neoadjuvant chemotherapy. The overall sensitivity of US-guided FNAB ranges from 55% to 86% and specificity from 95% to 100%.

RISK ASSESSMENT AND CHEMOPREVENTION

Three different types of cytology specimens, including nipple aspiration fluid (NAF), ductal lavage (DL), and random periareolar fine-needle aspiration (RPFNA), can be utilized for risk stratification . The utility of these specimens in this regard is, however, largely investigational and should not be considered as the standard of care. NAF is collected following breast massage with or without the use of breast pump for providing suction. NAF production has been reported in 39% to 66% of women without regard to risk and in 50% to 95% of high-risk women. Women producing NAF and exhibiting proliferative epithelium with or without atypia have been shown to have a 2.4- to 2.8-fold risk of breast cancer compared with those who did not produce NAF after a median follow-up of 21 years.[32] NAF cytomorphology may also stratify risk, based on the Gail model. Both NAF production and NAF cytomorphology have been associated with elevated risk in prospective trials. Although easy and inexpensive, it should be noted that up to 50% of high-risk women fail to produce NAF, and up to 73% of NAF samples have insufficient cells for cytomorphologic evaluation, which limits its utility.

Ductal lavage is a relatively new technique wherein lactiferous ducts are cannulated with a microcatheter followed by infusion of saline or other physiologic solution. The effluent is subsequently collected and evaluated for epithelial morphology. The results of DL in a large multi-institutional study found adequate cellularity in 78%, in contrast to 27% in NAF; median number of epithelial cells from NAF was only 120 in comparison to 13,500 on DL.[33] Ductal lavage detected abnormal cells 3.2 times more than NAF. Women with DL atypia are presumed to be at increased risk of breast cancer based on elevated risk observed with NAF or RPFNA atypia. However, the impact of DL-detected atypia on short- and long-term risk of cancer is currently not known. The sensitivity of DL for cancer detection is low, 13% to 42%, and therefore DL should not be used for this purpose. It is to be noted that studies that directly compared DL with RPFNA report superiority of the latter with respect to number of epithelial cells as well as detection of hyperplastic and atypical cells, casting doubt regarding the future of DL for risk stratification and utilization for chemoprevention trials. However, unlike RPFNA, an advantage of DL is that ducts showing atypia or malignant cells can be further investigated by ductoscopy.

RPFNA is a commonly used technique for nonlesion-directed breast tissue sampling for risk stratification and chemoprevention trials. RPFNA attempts to detect a field change in the breast. Women who have atypia detected in RPFNA have the highest probability of containing precancerous lesions in the breast tissue and therefore a higher short-term risk of breast cancer than those in whom atypia are not detected. RPFNA is a minimally invasive technique that produces very little discomfort and yields more cells than NAF or DL.[34] Cytologic evidence of atypia confers a 5-fold increase in risk compared with the absence of atypia and allows stratification of women with elevated Gail risk. RPFNA is less expensive than DL and produces more evaluable specimens. The primary drawback of the procedure is the difficulty in exactly localizing the site of marked atypia for further investigation.

PROCUREMENT OF MATERIAL FOR MOLECULAR AND PROTEOMIC STUDIES

Cytology specimens, including FNAB and exfoliative specimens, are excellent sources of tumor cells, as they are devoid of stromal cells, which makes them suitable for any type of molecular or proteomic studies. Except for the determination of HER-2 by FISH on FNAB specimens, all the molecular and proteomic studies using cytology specimens are currently investigational and not utilized for patient care. Several molecular tests such as FISH for chromosomal aneusomy, polymerase chain reaction (PCR) for allelotyping, and methylation-specific PCR and clonality studies for the distinction of benign from malignant lesions have been reported. Both FNAB and CNB are reported to provide equivalent amounts of RNA.[35] FNAB of breast has been used successfully for transcriptional profiling in several studies with variable success.[36-39] Serial FNAB of breast has been used to study sequential changes in molecular events in the breast such as transcriptional profiling before and after neoadjuvant chemotherapy to identify candidate genes that can predict response to chemotherapy, and effectiveness of gene transfer of adenoviral p53 (Advexin) gene therapy by showing increases in p53 mRNA levels in locally advanced breast cancer.[40]

Proteomic studies such as SELDI-TOF mass spectrometry have been performed using NAF specimens to identify possible protein signatures for risk assessment and early detection of cancer.[41,42] Proteomic studies using cytology specimens of breast and metastatic tumors are in their infancy.[43] The potential of using these specimens for such studies is, however, tremendous.

SUMMARY

FNAB of breast has an important role in the management of patients with breast diseases even in the current era where CNB is increasingly popular. The success of FNAB as a diagnostic test for the investigation of palpable and nonpalpable breast lesions is heavily dependent on always correlating the cytologic findings with the results of clinical and radiologic examination, that is, following the rules of the triple test. It is preferable that the cytology and radiology suites are in close proximity, allowing immediate assessment of the FNAB specimens by the cytopathologists, and communication of the preliminary diagnosis to the radiologist in the case of nonpalpable lesions. Immediate correlation of the cytologic features with the imaging findings is thereby made possible, which can lead to the performance of CNB in the same sitting when needed. Similarly, immediate assessment of the specimen for adequacy can improve the contribution of FNAB in the investigation of palpable breast lesions.

FNAB of indeterminate and suspicious axillary lymph nodes is valuable in the initial staging of patients with breast carcinoma and in the selection of the appropriate management based on the results of cytologic evaluation. When positive for metastatic carcinoma, FNAB of axillary lymph nodes also allows the evaluation of prognostic and predictive markers on the metastatic tumor.

FNAB is also an excellent modality for obtaining a pure population of tumor cells for molecular and proteomic research studies and for studying the changes in normal and diseased sites following therapeutic manipulation.

REFERENCES

1. The uniform approach to breast fine needle aspiration biopsy. A synopsis. *Acta Cytol.* 1996;40:1120-1126.
2. Boerner S, Fornage B, Singletary E, et al. Ultrasound-guided fine needle aspiration (FNA) of nonpalpable breast lesions. *Cancer.* 1999;87:19-24.
3. Westenend PJ, Sever AR, Beekman-De Volder HJ, Liem SJ. A comparison of aspiration cytology and core needle biopsy in the evaluation of breast lesions. *Cancer.* 2001;93:146-150.
4. Ariga R, Bloom K, Reddy VB. Fine-needle aspiration of clinically suspicious palpable breast masses with histopathologic correlation. *Am J Surg.* 2002;184:410-413.
5. Liao J, Davey DD, Warren G, et al. Ultrasound-guided fine-needle aspiration biopsy remains a valid approach in the evaluation of nonpalpable breast lesions. *Diagn Cytopathol.* 2003;30:325-331.
6. Ishikawa T, Hamaguchi Y, Tanabe M, et al. False-positive and false-negative cases of fine needle aspiration cytology for palpable breast lesions. *Breast Cancer.* 2007;14:388-392.
7. Vimpeli SM, Saarenmaa I, Huhtala H, Soimakallio S. Large-core needle biopsy versus fine-needle aspiration biopsy in solid breast lesions: comparison of costs and diagnostic value. *Acta Radiol.* 2008;10:1-7.
8. Willis SL, Ramzy I. Analysis of false results in a series of 835 fine needle aspirates of breast lesions. *Acta Cytol.* 1995;39:858-864.
9. Sterns EE. The natural history of macroscopic cysts in the breast. *Surg Gynecol Obstet.* 1992;174:36-40.
10. Frable WJ. Fine-needle aspiration biopsy. *Va Med.* 1982;109:452-455.
11. Orson LW, Cigtay OS. Fat necrosis of the breast: characteristic xeromammographic appearance. *Radiology.* 1983;146:35-38.
12. Das DK, Sodhani P, Kashyap V, et al. Inflammatory lesions of the breast: diagnosis by fine needle aspiration. *Cytopathology.* 1992;3:281-289.
13. Silverman JF, Lannin DR, Unverferth M, Norris HT. Fine needle aspiration cytology of subareolar abscess of the breast. Spectrum of cytomorphologic findings and potential diagnostic pitfalls. *Acta Cytol.* 1986;30:413-419.
14. Kollur SM, El Hag IA. FNA of breast fibroadenoma: observer variability and review of cytomorphology with cytohistological correlation. *Cytopathology.* 2006;17:239-244.
15. Veneti S, Manek S. Benign phyllodes tumor vs. fibroadenoma: FNA cytological differentiation. *Cytopathology.* 2001; 2:321-328.
16. Krishnamurthy S, Ashfaq R, Shin HJ, Sneige N. Distinction of phyllodes tumor from fibroadema: a reappraisal of an old problem. *Cancer.* 200;90:342-349.
17. Jayaram G, Elsayed EM, Yaccob RB. Papillary breast lesions diagnosed on cytology. Profile of 65 cases. *Acta Cytol.* 2007;51:3-8.
18. Kumar PV, Talei AR, Malekhusseini SA, et al. Papillary carcinoma of the breast. Cytologic study of nine cases. *Acta Cytol.* 1999;43:767-770.
19. Haji BE, Das DK, Al-Ayadhy B, et al. Fine-needle aspiration cytologic features of four special types of breast cancers: mucinous, medullary, apocrine, and papillary. *Diagn Cytopathol.* 2007; 5:408-416.
20. Dawson AE, Mulford DK. Fine needle aspiration of mucinous (colloid) breast carcinoma. Nuclear grading and mammographic and cytologic findings. *Acta Cytol.* 1998;42:668-672.
21. Greeley CF, Frost AR. Cytologic features of ductal and lobular carcinoma in fine needle aspirates of the breast. *Acta Cytol.* 1997;41:333-340.
22. Shin HJ, Sneige N. Is a diagnosis of infiltrating versus in situ ductal carcinoma of the breast possible in fine-needle aspiration specimens? *Cancer.* 1998;84:186-191.
23. Cangiarella J, Waisman J, Shapiro RL, Simsir A. Cytologic features of tubular adenocarcinoma of the breast by aspiration biopsy. *Diagn Cytopathol.* 2001;25:311-315.
24. Chhieng DC, Fernandez G, Cangiarella JF. Invasive carcinoma in clinically suspicious breast masses diagnosed as adenocarcinoma by fine-needle aspiration *Cancer.* 2000;90.96-101.
25. Lerma E, Fumanal V, Carreras A, et al. Undetected invasive lobular carcinoma of the breast: review of false-negative smears. *Diagn Cytopathol.* 2000;23:303-307.
26. Georgiannos SN, Aleong JC, Goode AW, Sheaff M. Secondary neoplasms of the breast. *Cancer.* 2001;92:2259-2266.
27. Tafford S, Bohler PJ, Risberg B, Torlakovic E. Estrogen and progesterone hormone receptor status in breast carcinoma: comparison of immunocytochemistry and immunohistochemistry. *Diagn Cytopathol.* 2002;26:137-141.
28. Konofaos P, Kontzoglou K, Georgoulakis J. The role of ThinPrep cytology in the evaluation of estrogen and progesterone receptor content of breast tumors. *Surg Oncol.* 2006;15:257-266.
29. Krishnamurthy S. Applications of molecular techniques to fine needle aspiration biopsy. *Cancer.* 2007;111:106-122.
30. Krishnamurthy S, Sneige N, Bedi DG, et al. Role of ultrasound-guided fine-needle aspiration of indeterminate and suspicious axillary lymph nodes in the initial staging of breast carcinoma. *Cancer.* 2002;95:982-988.
31. Koelliker SL, Chung MA, Mainiero MB, et al. Axillary lymph nodes: US-guided fine-needle aspiration for initial staging of breast cancer—correlation with primary tumor size. *Radiology.* 2008;246:81-89.
32. Wrensch MR, Petrakis NL, Miike R, et al. Breast cancer risk in women with abnormal cytology in nipple aspirates of breast fluid. *J Natl Cancer Inst.* 2001;93:1791-1798.
33. Dooley WC, Ljung BM, Veronesi U, et al. Ductal lavage for detection of cellular atypia in women at high risk for breast cancer. *J Natl Cancer Inst.* 2001;93;1624-1632.
34. Fabian CJ, Kimler BF, Mayo MS, Khan SA. Breast tissue sampling for risk assessment and prevention. *Endocr Relat Cancer.* 2005;12:185-213.
35. Symmans WF, Pusztai L, Ayers M, et al. RNA yield from needle biopsies for cDNA microarray analysis of breast cancer prior to neoadjuvant chemotherapy. *Cancer.* 2003;97:2960-2971.
36. Assersohn L, Gangi L, Zhao Y, et al. The feasibility of using fine needle aspiration from primary breast cancers for CDNA microarray analysis. *Clin Cancer Res.* 2002;8:794-801.
37. Pusztai L, Ayers M, Stec J. Gene expression profiles obtained from fine needle aspirations of breast cancer reliably identify routine prognostic markers and reveal large scale molecular differences between estrogen-negative and estrogen-positive tumors. *Clin Cancer Res.* 2003;9:2406-2415.
38. Ayers M, Symmans WF, Stec J, et al. Gene expression profiling of fine needle aspirations of breast cancer identifies genes associated with complete pathologic response to neoadjuvant. Taxol/FAC chemotherapy. *J Clin Oncol.* 2004;22:2284-2293.

39. Sotiriou C, Powles T, Dowsett M, et al. Gene expression profiles derived from fine needle aspiration correlate with response to systemic chemotherapy in breast cancer. *Breast Cancer Res.* 2002;4:R3.

40. Cristofanilli M, Krishnamurthy S, Guerra L, et al. A nonreplicating adenoviral vector that contains the wild type p53 transgene combined with chemotherapy for primary breast cancer. *Cancer.* 2006;107:935-944.

41. Alexander H, Stegner AL, Wagner-Mann C, et al. Proteomic analysis to identify breast cancer biomarkers in nipple aspirate fluid. *Clin Cancer Res.* 2004;22:7500-7510.

42. Pawlik TM, Hawke DH, Liu Y, et al. Proteomic analysis of nipple aspirate fluid from women with early stage breast cancer using isotope coded affinity tags and tandem mass spectrometry reveals differential expression of vitamin D binding protein. *BMC Cancer.* 2006;6:68.

43. Fowler LJ, Lovell MO, Izbicka E. Fine-needle aspiration in PreservCyt: a novel and reproducible method for possible ancillary proteomic pattern expression of breast neoplasms by SELDI-TOF. *Mod Pathol.* 2004; 17:1012-1020.

CHAPTER 25

Pathology Post-Neoadjuvant Therapy

W. Fraser Symmans

DEFINITION OF PATHOLOGIC COMPLETE RESPONSE

A central tenet of neoadjuvant clinical trials is that tumor response, as a surrogate end point, should be strongly correlated with long-term patient survival.[1,2] Otherwise, the value of neoadjuvant treatment would be to convert a tumor to operability or to increase the probability of conservative surgery. However, a close association between pathologic response to treatment and subsequent survival establishes neoadjuvant treatment as a method for clinical trials including operable disease to evaluate promising treatments more purely in terms of direct tumoricidal activity and without confounding variables of natural history and subsequent treatments. Indeed, pathologic complete response (pCR) has been adopted as the primary end point for neoadjuvant trials because it has consistently been associated with long-term survival in neoadjuvant trials using different chemotherapy regimens of variable treatment duration.[3-12] If pCR is achieved using current therapies, one can anticipate more than 90% probability of disease-free survival within the first decade of follow-up.

Communication between surgeon, radiologist, and pathologist is very important for accurate definition of pathologic response of a patient's breast cancer. The macroscopic appearance of residual tumor can be deceptive in a resected breast specimen, so pCR could be falsely ascribed if the residual tumor bed was not correctly identified and sampled, such that a different area of breast tissue was submitted for histopathologic study. Effective use of the pathology requisition form (clinical history section), electronic medical record, placement of metallic indicators in the tumor bed at the beginning of treatment, and conservative surgical resection (lumpectomy) contribute to more accurate gross and microscopic pathologic assessment of response in the primary tumor bed. We find that specimen radiography with radiologic-pathologic correlation is particularly helpful to identify the tumor bed and to map its extent and margin status, particularly if metallic indicators have been placed in the tumor bed.

Although it is generally held that a definition of pCR should include patients without residual invasive carcinoma in the breast (pT0), the presence of nodal metastasis, minimal residual cellularity, and residual in situ carcinoma are not consistently defined as pCR or residual disease (RD).[12-15] When there is no residual invasive cancer in the breast, the number of involved axillary lymph nodes is inversely related to survival.[11] Conversely, patients who convert to node-negative status after treatment have improved survival, even if there is RD in the breast.[16] This supports the concept that pathologic response in the regional lymph nodes is as important as response in the primary tumor bed. Consequently, the combination of tumor size and nodal status after neoadjuvant treatment is prognostic.[17] No evidence indicates that residual in situ carcinoma alone increases risk of future distant relapse.[12,18,19] However, residual ductal carcinoma in situ (DCIS) is relevant for local control, and so resection specimens are carefully evaluated for residual DCIS and margin status just like any breast cancer specimen. Therefore, the most appropriate definition of pCR with respect to prognosis is lack of residual invasive cancer and node-negative status after neoadjuvant therapy.

IMPROVEMENTS IN PATHOLOGIC COMPLETE RESPONSE RATE TRANSLATE TO IMPROVED SURVIVAL

Patients who achieve pCR from neoadjuvant (preoperative) systemic therapy have excellent 5-year overall survival that is independent of treatment regimen or tumor phenotype.[2,7,9,11,12,20-22] However, it remains difficult to calculate improvements in overall survival for a particular study arm based on observed improvement in the pCR rate. This is

TABLE 25 1 Changes in Pathologic Complete Response in Neoadjuvant Trials Predicted Survival Difference in Adjuvant Trials

NEOADJUVANT TREATMENT					ADJUVANT TREATMENT				
Trial	Treatment Arms	N	pCR (%)	p	Treatment Trial	Arms	N	5-yr DFS	p (HR)
NSABP-B27	AC + Tam	802	13		NSABP-B27	AC + Tam	802	67.7%	
	AC/Dx4 + Tam	803	26	<0.0001		AC/Dx4 + Tam	803	71.1%	0.22 (0.90)
					NSABP-B28	AC + Tam	1529	72%	
						AC/Tx4 + Tam	1531	76%	0.006 (0.83)
					CALGB-9344	AC	1551	65%	
						AC/Tx4	1570	70%	0.002 (0.83)
MDACC	3-weekly Tx4/FAC	131	16		E1199	3-weekly Tx4/AC	1253	65%	
	weekly Tx12/FAC	127	28	0.02		weekly Tx12/AC	1231	70%	0.006 (0.79)
MDACC	Tx4/FEC	19	26		N9831 + NSABP-B31	AC/Tx4	1679	1253	
	Tx4/FEC + Herceptin	23	65	0.016		AC/Tx4 + Herceptin	1672	1231	0.0001 (0.48)
	Tx4/FEC + Herceptin	22	55						

DFS, disease free survival, HR, hazard ratio, pCR, pathologic complete remission.

because many other variables influence overall survival in addition to the achievement of pCR, including baseline prognosis, use and efficacy of endocrine therapy, and length of follow-up. These complexities are illustrated by the findings of the National Surgical Adjuvant Breast and Bowel Project (NSABP)-B27 study.[23] The addition of docetaxel (3 times weekly for four cycles) to AC chemotherapy increased the pCR rate by 13% (breast only), but this did not translate to significantly improved 5-year survival for this arm (Table 25-1). Patients in either treatment arm who achieved pCR had excellent survival, but the B27 study was only powered to detect a difference in pCR rate between the treatments and was not powered to detect a survival difference.[11] Furthermore, Table 25-1 illustrates how improvement in pCR observed in a neoadjuvant trial anticipated a survival difference in a phase III adjuvant trial for 3 recent treatment advances: addition of a taxane to anthracycline-based chemotherapy (white),[11,23,24] more frequent paclitaxel dosing schedule (gray),[25,26] and the addition of trastuzumab (Herceptin) to sequential anthracycline-taxane chemotherapy (blue).[27-29] Therefore, neoadjuvant chemotherapy trials provide a valid clinical model in which to test for further improvements in adjuvant treatment.

PATHOLOGIC RESPONSE AND HORMONE RECEPTOR STATUS

There is current debate about whether pathologic response from preoperative chemotherapy is a useful end point for hormone receptor (HR)-positive breast cancer. A potential disadvantage of relying solely on pCR is that the frequency of this outcome is comparatively low in HR-positive breast cancer, usually in the range of 3% to 9%.[30,31] Indeed, HR-positive disease constitutes the majority of breast cancers, and the extent of receptor positivity can have confounding effects on results of chemotherapy trials.[32] Nonetheless, it is clear that the incremental improvements in adjuvant chemotherapy (such as inclusion of anthracyclines, addition of taxanes, and dosing schedule of paclitaxel) do benefit patients with HR-positive breast cancer with acceptable reduction in the relative risk of disease recurrence in the range of 20% to 30%.[31,33,34] Therefore, it is reasonable to conclude that less than complete remission from chemotherapy for HR-positive breast cancer can provide a survival benefit. It is possible that some degree of tumor response to adjuvant chemotherapy effectively reduces tumor burden and improves the duration of benefit from subsequent adjuvant endocrine therapy: in essence, partial efficacy from chemotherapy, followed by partial efficacy from endocrine therapy, to achieve full adjuvant efficacy. In that context, an end point of pCR would have a favorable prognosis, but the other category of RD would also include patients with an excellent prognosis, essentially blurring the distinction between categories of pathologic response.

RESIDUAL PATHOLOGIC STAGE (AJCC Y-STAGE)

The American Joint Committee on Cancer (AJCC) staging system for breast cancer was revised to designate with a "y" prefix when stage has been obtained from the pathologic evaluation of a surgical resection specimen that was obtained after a patient received neoadjuvant therapy.[35] Of course, y-Stage 0 is identical to pCR. The main purpose of this is to distinguish between the prognosis of pathologic stage in breast cancer with and without prior systemic therapy. Two reports that evaluated AJCC y-Stage categories after neoadjuvant chemotherapy have both demonstrated a prognostic association.[17,36] The pathologic stage of RD can also be combined with pretreatment tumor clinical and pathologic characteristics to define 5 categories of clinical-pathologic score (CPS) or also combined with estrogen receptor (ER) and grade (CPS+EG) to define 7 categories of response.[37] This approach estimates the extent of down-staging after neoadjuvant treatment as well as biologic characteristics of the disease that are known to be associated with response to chemotherapy. It was developed from 932 patients at the MD Anderson Cancer Center (MDACC) who were variably treated. A potential advantage of this approach is that it enriched the proportion of patients in the good prognosis category, from 14% with pCR to 22% with CPS score 0 and 24% with CPS+EG score 0 or 1 (Fig. 25-1). However, relatively few patients were identified with high (more than 50%) risk of relapse following poor response to neoadjuvant therapy (3% with CPS score 4, and 6% with CPS+EG score 5 or 6). Those results might reflect the effects of adjuvant hormonal therapy in those with ER-positive disease and that many of the earlier patients in this cohort underwent surgery midway through their adjuvant chemotherapy regimen. The published work to date represents the development of an index, and therefore independent validation of this new method will be necessary. However, the method could become clinically useful as a nomogram to summarize information about tumor response that combines an estimate of tumor response with biologic features of the tumor.

REGIONAL LYMPH NODES

It appears that the prognostic relevance of a micrometastases in a regional lymph node after neoadjuvant chemotherapy is different from a micrometastasis when surgery is performed before chemotherapy, suggesting that any residual metastatic disease in the regional lymph nodes is important.[38] However, those data were obtained from an era before sentinel lymph node (SLN) procedures became available, with more thorough gross and microscopic evaluation of those nodes. Therefore, the implication of those results should be interpreted with caution at this time. Other data from the era before the sentinel biopsy indicate that conversion from pathologic node-positive status at diagnosis (confirmed by needle biopsy at the time) to pathologic node-negative status after neoadjuvant chemotherapy is associated with an excellent survival that is significantly better than failure to down-stage from positive- to negative-node status.[16] Those results, and the results described later, support an opinion that evaluation of nodal status after neoadjuvant treatment provides more prognostic information than nodal status before neoadjuvant treatment. It is therefore prudent to have a consistent approach to the timing of SLN biopsy for clinical trials of neoadjuvant chemotherapy that intend to use pathologic response, or survival, as an end point.

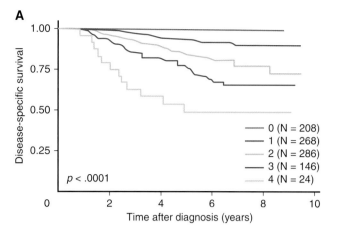

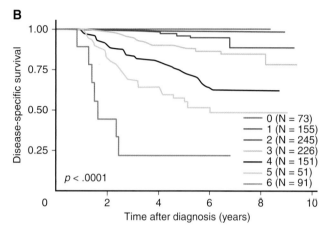

FIGURE 25-1 Disease-specific survival curves for categories of clinicopathologic score (CPS) alone **(A),** or combined with estrogen receptor status and grade as the CPS+estrogen grade (EG) score **(B).** (*Reproduced, with permission, from Jeruss JS, Mittendorf EA, Tucker SL, et al. Combined use of clinical and pathologic staging variables to define outcomes for breast cancer patients treated with neoadjuvant therapy. J Clin Oncol. 2008;26:246-252.*)

However, there is currently controversy about whether SLN sampling should be routinely performed to stage the axilla before neoadjuvant treatment or after the treatment has been completed. Is it more useful prognostic information to know the pathologic extent of nodal cancer burden before or after adjuvant chemotherapy? At MDACC we prefer posttreatment SLN evaluation because it reduces the number of surgeries and we believe it has stronger prognostic value, but there are clinical concerns about the accuracy of sampling at that time and the potential information for radiation therapy planning. The issue remains controversial and may be the subject of a prospective randomized trial.

OTHER PATHOLOGIC CHANGES

Other changes occur in the tissues after neoadjuvant chemotherapy. The number of cancer cells within a tumor mass can decrease, and that reduction in cancer cellularity can be highly variable within a tumor mass. Decreased cancer cellularity is usually associated with fibrosis and some degree of chronic inflammatory infiltrate. Indeed, the Miller and Payne classification ignores tumor size and nodal status altogether, and it estimates only the decrease in cancer cellularity by comparing the initial diagnostic core biopsy with the residual cellularity in the tumor bed after treatment.[10] The Miller and Payne classification includes 5 categories: grade 1, no reduction; grade 2, minor loss (less than 30%); grade 3, moderate loss (30%-90%); grade 4, marked loss (more than 90%); and grade 5, complete loss of cellularity. This was reported to be prognostic in 170 patients, with the largest separation in disease-free survival observed between grade 5 and the other grades.[10] It has also been demonstrated that the reduction in cellularity is often greatest when the residual tumor is small, suggesting a relationship between residual size and cellularity.[39] However, there was considerable variability in the extent of cytoreduction within any residual y-Stage category.[39] This suggests that tumor shrinkage and cytoreduction are associated but not uniformly correlated. Although microscopic RD, altered cytologic appearance, and estimated tumor volume less than 1 cm³ also indicate good response, these tend to be descriptive parameters and are also difficult to apply to tumor beds with dispersed microscopic foci of carcinoma.[3-6,9,40]

RESIDUAL CANCER BURDEN AFTER NEOADJUVANT TREATMENT

RD after neoadjuvant treatment includes a broad range of actual responses from near pCR to frank resistance. We developed a method to measure RD by combining histopathologic components of RD (cellularity, overall diameter, and number and extent of nodal involvement) into a numerical index of residual cancer burden (RCB).[36] A free Web site is available to calculate RCB from the histopathologic variables (http://www.mdanderson.org/breastcancer_RCB). A detailed description of the rationale and methods is included here. We developed the RCB index in 241 patients who received 6 months of neoadjuvant chemotherapy with T/FAC, and validated it in a separate cohort of 141 patients who received 3 months of preoperative chemotherapy with FAC followed by an additional 3 months of postoperative adjuvant chemotherapy (FAC in 129, other in 12).[36] In the T/FAC cohort, RCB was independently prognostic for distant relapse-free survival in a multivariate model that included age, pretreatment clinical stage, HR status and hormonal therapy, and pathologic response (pCR versus RD) (hazard ratio, 2.50; confidence interval, 1.70 to 3.69; $p < 0.001$) (Fig. 25-2). The bias-adjusted C-index for RCB as a prognostic factor was 0.77. The generalizability of RCB for prognosis of distant relapse was confirmed in the FAC-treated validation cohort, with a C-index of 0.70.[36]

It should be noted that minimal RD (RCB-I) in 17% of patients in the study carried the same prognosis as pCR, even in HR-negative breast cancers (Fig. 25-3A).[36] Furthermore, extensive RD (RCB-III) in 13% of patients was associated with poor prognosis (Fig. 25-3).[36] Even for ER-positive breast cancer, patients with RCB-III had a 5-year distant relapse rate of 40%, despite ongoing treatment with adjuvant hormonal treatment (Fig. 25-3B).[36] This identifies an important subset of

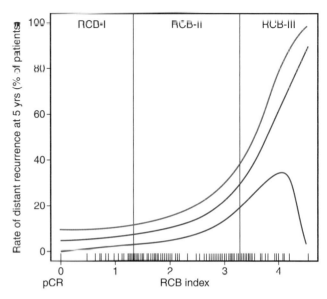

FIGURE 25-2 Residual cancer burden provides a continuous estimate of RD that can be described as pathologic complete response (pCR) when residual cancer burden (RCB) = 0; and 3 classes of increasing amounts of RD (RCB-I to RCB-III) that were defined by 2 thresholds (vertical lines) based on 5-year distant metastasis-free survival. (*Reproduced, with permission, from Symmans WF, Peintinger F, Hatzis C, et al. Measurement of residual breast cancer burden to predict survival after neoadjuvant chemotherapy.* J Clin Oncol. *2007;25:4414-4422.*)

patients with either combined insensitivity to chemotherapy and hormonal therapy, or with RD (after surgery) that is too extensive to be controlled by hormonal therapy alone, and it illustrates how identification of the subset of receptor-positive patients who might correctly be spared (denied) adjuvant chemotherapy despite consensus treatment recommendations will require very careful selection based on the tumor's predicted chemosensitivity and the predicted endocrine sensitivity.[33,41] RCB incorporates the information from pCR, represents the extent of RD, more strongly predicts distant relapse-free survival, and can define clinically relevant subsets with near-pCR (RCB-I) or resistance (RCB-III).

DETAILED PATHOLOGY METHODS FOR USING RESIDUAL CANCER BURDEN

RCB is estimated from routine pathologic sections of the primary breast tumor site and the regional lymph nodes after the completion of neoadjuvant therapy. Six variables are included in a calculation formula (Fig. 25-4) that is freely available at a dedicated Web site located at http://www.mdanderson.org/breastcancer_RCB, which can be found using Internet search engines.

Relevant information can be included within a pathology report (diagnoses or comment) without need for reporting calculated RCB index results. For example, all the necessary relevant information from a report would be as follows:

- Residual invasive carcinoma with chemotherapy effect.
- Residual carcinoma measures 2.4 × 1.8 cm and contains approximately 10% cancer cellularity.

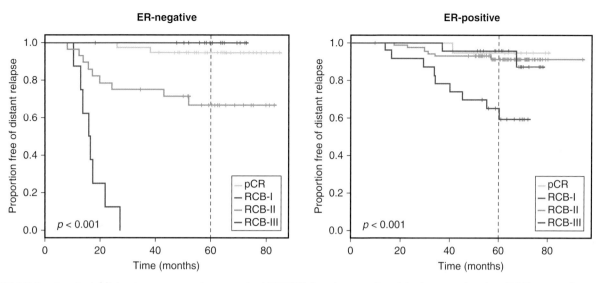

FIGURE 25-3   Survival (distant recurrence-free survival [DRFS]) for classes of residual cancer burden (RCB), according to estrogen receptor (ER) status (Kaplan-Meier plots, log-rank test). (*Reproduced, with permission, from Symmans WF, Peintinger F, Hatzis C, et al. Measurement of residual breast cancer burden to predict survival after neoadjuvant chemotherapy.* J Clin Oncol. *2007;25:4414-4422.*)

- Residual intraductal carcinoma, solid type with necrosis, comprising 5% of the residual carcinoma.
- Metastatic carcinoma involving 3 of 14 axillary lymph nodes (3/14).
- The largest metastasis measures 4 mm in greatest dimension.

One can then enter the results just listed to calculate RCB as follows: primary tumor bed area = 24 mm × 18 mm, overall cancer cellularity = 10%, percentage of cancer that is in situ

disease = 5%, number of positive lymph nodes = 3, diameter of largest metastasis = 4 mm.

Primary Tumor Bed

In general terms, pathologic evaluation of the primary tumor bed in the breast requires that the pathologist make 3 judgments about the primary tumor bed:

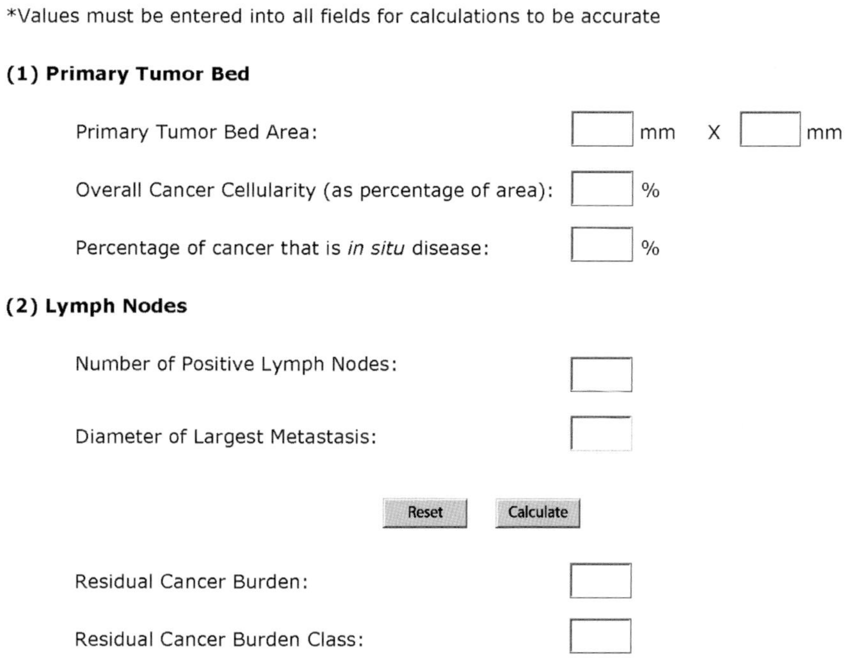

*Values must be entered into all fields for calculations to be accurate

(1) Primary Tumor Bed

Primary Tumor Bed Area: ☐ mm   X   ☐ mm

Overall Cancer Cellularity (as percentage of area):   ☐ %

Percentage of cancer that is *in situ* disease: ☐ %

(2) Lymph Nodes

Number of Positive Lymph Nodes: ☐

Diameter of Largest Metastasis: ☐

[Reset]   [Calculate]

Residual Cancer Burden: ☐

Residual Cancer Burden Class: ☐

FIGURE 25-4   Online calculation tool for residual cancer burden, provided as both an index score and a category.

1. Identify the cross-sectional dimensions of the residual tumor bed (d_1 and d_2)
2. Estimate of the proportion of that residual tumor bed area that is involved by cancer (%CA)
3. Estimate the proportion of the cancer that is an in situ component (%CIS)

Defining the Tumor Bed

In cases of multicentric disease, the RCB measurements are from the largest residual tumor bed. In cases where the extent of residual cancer under the microscope does not correlate with the gross measurement of the residual tumor bed, the tumor bed dimensions are to be revised according to the microscopic findings. Schematic diagrams are shown here to illustrate how gross residual tumor bed dimensions are first estimated from the gross findings (pink area) but may be revised after review of the slides from the gross tumor bed area according to the extent of residual cancer (blue).

Using the illustrations in Figure 25-5, the macroscopic tumor bed dimensions in examples A, C, and D also define the final dimensions of the residual tumor bed after microscopic review. However, the macroscopic tumor bed dimensions in example B overestimates the extent of residual cancer, and so the dimensions of the residual tumor bed (d_1 and d_2) would be revised after microscopic evaluation of the extent of residual cancer in the corresponding slides from the gross tumor bed. In a different example (E), microscopic residual cancer extends beyond the confines of the macroscopic tumor bed. Again, the dimensions of the residual tumor bed (d_1 and d_2) would be revised after microscopic evaluation of the recognizable extent of residual cancer beyond the macroscopic tumor bed. It should be noted that would also be necessary to measure residual tumor diameter in order to correctly assign y-T stage. The defined area of tumor bed is the area that should be evaluated for cancer cellularity. This approach accounts for differences in the concentration and distribution of residual cancer within a tumor bed. In the illustration here, the estimated %CA in example A would be high (in a small area), whereas the estimated %CA for examples C and D would be lower (in a larger area). In examples C and D, the estimated %CA would likely be similar, even though the distribution of cancer within the residual tumor bed is different in those two examples.

Estimating Cellularity Within the Tumor Bed

The proportion of cancer (%CA) and the proportion of in situ component (%CIS) in the residual tumor bed are estimated from microscopic evaluation of the slides representing the largest area of the residual tumor bed, as illustrated in Figure 25-6. The most effective way to obtain this information is to measure and submit for histology the largest cross-sectional area of residual tumor bed, and to designate in the report which slides represent the cross section of the tumor bed (Fig. 25-6, slides A1 to A5). After reviewing those slides, the pathologist can estimate the average cellularity in the tumor bed on each slide in order to estimate the overall average cellularity of the tumor bed area. A practical way to estimate the percentage cancer cellularity in a single slide is to encircle with ink dots the tumor bed within the tissue section on that slide, and then use the microscope to estimate the cellularity within the designated area of tumor bed on that slide. Within the area identified on a slide as residual tumor, percentage cancer cellularity can be estimated by averaging the proportion of residual tumor bed area containing cancer (invasive or in situ) in a series of representative fields across the tumor bed area on that slide (Fig. 25-6, slide A1, circular microscopic fields). The same can be done for in situ component (%CIS) of the identifiable cancer, using the same method of interpretation that is routine for estimation of the in situ component of any invasive breast cancer. Estimates of cellularity are to the nearest 10%, but include 0%, 1%, and 5% for areas with low cellularity. The Web site contains computer-generated diagrams of exact cellularity per area, to assist pathologists with an accurate estimation of the cellularity in a microscopic field. An average for the readings for percentage cancer cellularity per microscopic field across residual tumor in a single section can then be estimated (Fig. 25-6, lower center). The average of the average cancer cellularity estimates from each slide of the largest residual tumor bed area can then be estimated (Fig. 25-6, lower right).

In summary, the key elements to pathologic evaluation of the primary tumor bed are to simply:

1. Define the gross tumor bed as the largest cross-sectional area
2. Submit sections representing that tumor bed area as individual slides
3. Review those slides to estimate the %CA and %CIS within the residual tumor bed

Regional Lymph Nodes

Pathologic evaluation of the primary tumor bed in the breast requires that the pathologist make 2 judgments:

1. Count the number of positive lymph nodes (LN)
2. Measure the diameter of the largest nodal metastasis (d_{met})

It is standard pathologic practice to obtain an accurate lymph node count for staging. In addition, the measurement of residual cancer burden requires a measurement of the largest metastasis. If the largest metastasis is identified from a slide, one can measure the distance between 2 ink dots placed at each end of the metastatic deposit or use a micrometer. If there is a large metastasis, the diameter should be recorded as part of the macroscopic description. Sometimes there are marked treatment changes in the lymph nodes and only rare scattered tumor or histiocytoid cells are identified. In that setting, one does not need to estimate cellularity of the metastasis but must record the diameter of extent of those cells, having confirmed that the cells of concern represent metastatic carcinoma.

SPECIAL CIRCUMSTANCES AND ESTIMATION OF RESIDUAL CANCER BURDEN

Inoperable or Progressive Disease

The RCB index cannot be accurately calculated for patients whose disease remains inoperable at the completion of the neoadjuvant treatment course (eg, requiring subsequent additional treatments before surgical resection is possible) or those who experience disease progression and so do not undergo surgical

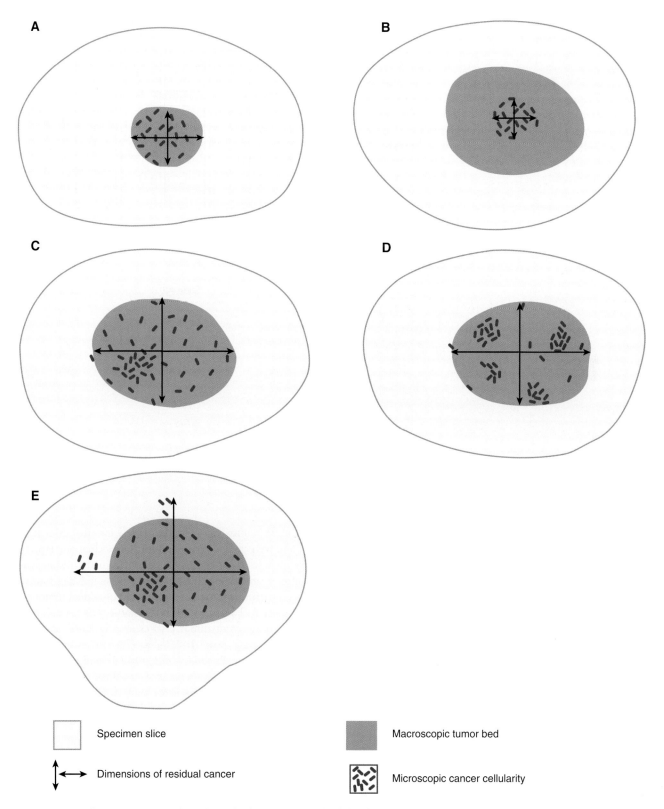

FIGURE 25-5 Illustrative examples of residual gross tumor bed (pink area) within slices of a resection specimen (white area). The measurement of the largest 2 diameters of the residual gross tumor bed (pink area) would be recorded in the macroscopic description of the pathology report. Thereafter, the corresponding slides from the pink area and adjacent tissues would be evaluated microscopically for histologic evidence of residual cancer (blue shapes), and the final tumor bed dimensions might then be revised accordingly.

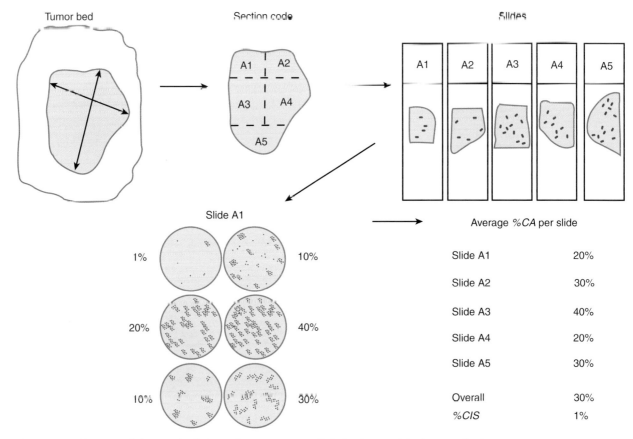

FIGURE 25-6 Diagram of the methods to estimate cancer cellularity in a residual tumor bed.

resection at the completion of the neoadjuvant treatment course. For those patients, RCB is assigned as extensive (ie, RCB-III).

Internal Mammary Lymph Node Metastasis

There were no examples of internal mammary nodal metastasis in the published study that evaluated the prognostic value of RCB. However, it is reasonable to include internal mammary nodes with the other regional (axillary) nodes in the assessment of RCB.

Pretreatment Sentinel Lymph Node Biopsy

Surgical excision of a positive SLN before the neoadjuvant treatment would invalidate the accuracy of measuring RCB after the treatment to assess response. If all SLNs were negative before treatment began, this would not affect the assessment of RCB after treatment ended.

PATHOLOGIC RESPONSE TO NEOADJUVANT HORMONAL THERAPY

A multiparameter index, named the preoperative endocrine prognostic index (PEPI) score, has been developed for assessment of RD after neoadjuvant endocrine therapy.[42] The model was developed from a cohort of 158 patients who received

neoadjuvant tamoxifen or letrozole for 4 months, prior to surgery, and were able to receive postoperative chemotherapy. The index includes pathologic information from the tumor before and after treatment and is a weighted scoring index of four variables as prognostic for relapse-free survival: residual tumor stage (1 1/2 score 0, 13/4 score 3), nodal status (N0 score 0, N ≥ 1 score 3), the percent tumor cells expressing Ki-67 after treatment (Ki67 < 2.7, score 1; 2.7 < Ki67 ≤ 19.7, score 1; 19.7 < Ki67 ≤ 53.1, score 2; Ki67 > 53.1, score 3), and the ER immunohistochemistry status after treatment (Allred score 4-8 score 0; Allred score 0-3 score 3). This index was then divided into 3 classes: group 1, total score 0; group 2, total score 1 to 3; and group 3, total score 4 or more. The PEPI score was then validated in a cohort of 203 patients who received adjuvant tamoxifen, anastrozole, or the combination for 3 months before surgery and did not receive adjuvant chemotherapy. The bias-adjusted C-index for PEPI compared to relapse-free survival was 0.72 in the developmental cohort (a result similar to the C-index for RCB after chemotherapy) and was not reported in the validation cohort.[42] This form of index combines residual tumor stage with functional indicators of endocrine response, namely reduction in cellular proliferation and retention of ER expression. Presumably this PEPI score will be independently evaluated in the American College of Surgical Oncology Group (ACOSOG) Z-1031 clinical trial of neoadjuvant hormonal therapy, when the follow-up of those patients is sufficiently mature.

PATHOLOGIC RESPONSE TO NEOADJUVANT CHEMOTHERAPY AND HER2-TARGETED THERAPY

In a pronounced example, the inclusion of trastuzumab (Herceptin) in the thrice weekly T/FAC regimen for HER2-positive breast cancer dramatically improves the rate of pCR from 26% to about 60% (Table 25-1).[27,28] However, it was also reported that HER2-positive breast cancers achieved a pCR rate of 45% from weekly T/FAC.[30] Indeed, an unplanned subset analysis of HER2-positive breast cancer patients from the E-1199 trial confirmed that weekly paclitaxel improved disease-free survival, compared to every 3-weekly paclitaxel in the AC/T regimen.[26] This suggests that HER2-positive breast cancer is generally chemosensitive, improvements in chemotherapy further improve responsiveness, and the addition of trastuzumab also improves response. We retrospectively evaluated RCB in 199 patients with HER2-positive breast cancer who had received 1 of 3 different regimens: every 3-weekly T/FAC (n = 47), weekly T/FAC (n = 63), or every 3-weekly T/FEC with concurrent trastuzumab (n = 89).[43] It should be noted that the cohort included patients from the original neoadjuvant studies reported by Buzdar et al.[27,28] Rates of pCR, and combined pCR/RCB-I, were 28% and 41% for every 3-weekly T/FAC, 44% and 57% for weekly T/FAC, and 54% and 72% for every 3-weekly T/FEC with concurrent trastuzumab. Treatment with T/FEC with concurrent trastuzumab achieved higher rates of pathologic response (pCR/RCB-I), compared with weekly T/FAC (likelihood ratio [LR] test, p = 0.03) or every 3-weekly T/FAC (LR test, p < 0.0001).[43] It was interesting to observe, from this nonrandomized retrospective cohort, that the use of weekly paclitaxel in T/FAC had the most effect on pathologic response (pCR/RCB-I) in HR-negative cancers,

whereas concurrent trastuzumab with every 3-weekly T/FEC improved the rate of pCR/RCB-I to parity with the response rate in HR-negative breast cancers (Fig. 25-7). The results are provocative to consider that HR-positive breast cancers might be rendered more chemosensitive by concurrent treatment with an appropriate molecular agent. Of course, a properly designed, prospective clinical trial would be required to prove this hypothesis. Nevertheless, the example illustrates how carefully evaluated pathologic response after neoadjuvant treatment can potentially be very informative.

FUTURE DIRECTIONS

It is likely that neoadjuvant studies will become more common in the future and that with increased experience there will be trials of additional treatments for patients who have a significant amount of RD at the completion of neoadjuvant treatment. This approach promises to offer treatment options for those whose adjuvant treatment is likely to be insufficient. These so-called post-preoperative therapy trials will likely need to have clearly defined eligibility criteria, so that the novel therapeutics to be used are tested in patients at a significant risk of relapse. In addition, such studies will need to be randomized to ensure that the extent of RD is likely to be balanced among different treatment arms.

Response measurements might be improved if better methods can be developed to measure pretreatment tumor burden more accurately. One should expect that improvements would be likely, but they are probably currently hampered by limitations to the accuracy of information about the extent of tumor when using standard breast imaging of mammography and ultrasound. Ongoing studies from the Investigations of Serial

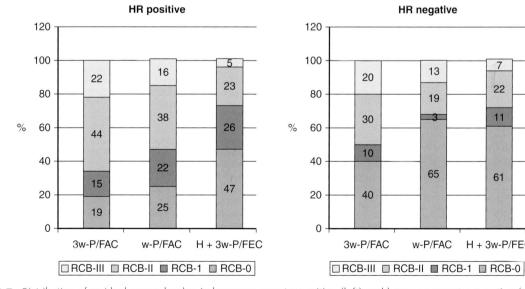

FIGURE 25-7 Distribution of residual cancer burden in hormone receptor-positive (left) and hormone receptor-negative (right) cases. (*Reproduced, with permission, from Peintinger F, Buzdar AU, Kuerer HM, et al. Hormone receptor status and pathologic response of HER2-positive breast cancer treated with neoadjuvant chemotherapy and trastuzumab. Ann Oncol. 2008;19:2020-2025.*)

studies to Predict Your Therapeutic Response with Imaging And molecular analysis (I-SPY) trial group are likely to shed light on whether changes in the primary tumor observed with magnetic resonance imaging will provide useful information to predict response and/or survival.

SUMMARY

The lack of uniform methods to report pathologic response is a contributing factor in the recent erosion of confidence in the value of neoadjuvant trials to anticipate the results of larger adjuvant trials. Although pCR (including node-negative status) has consistently imparted an excellent prognosis in published studies, meaningful reporting of RD has been an elusive goal. This problem is accentuated when evaluation of pathologic response is limited to the review of archival pathology reports. This is because asymmetry of RD and variable hypocellularity after treatment are not usually quantified in the report, and they are not captured by tumor diameter and nodal status alone. We have attempted to combine relevant pathologic characteristics of RD into a composite index of residual cancer burden (RCB). Each variable in the equation for RCB has prognostic significance, and the calculated primary and metastatic terms in the equation are equivalently and independently prognostic.

The key points for pathologic assessment of the primary tumor bed are as follows:

1. *Gross.* Identify the probable tumor bed and describe this macroscopic finding:
   a. Report the measurements of the largest gross dimensions (prefer three dimensions, but minimum is two dimensions).
   b. Submit the largest cross-sectional area for histology and specifically describe those blocks in the Section Code:
      i. Try to indicate how they are oriented by photography, radiography, photocopy, or intelligent description (eg, "sections B1 – B7 cross section of tumor bed in rows from anterosuperior to posteroinferior").
      ii. If additional sections are from surrounding tissues, then describe those as well.
      iii. Five representative sections from a big, obvious tumor bed should be sufficient.
2. *Microscopy.* Review the slides that correspond to the tumor bed (+/– surrounding tissues):
   a. Estimate the extent of spread of residual cancer relative to the gross tumor bed.
      i. If similar to the gross description, then keep the original measurements.
      ii. If obviously different, then revise the dimensions of the tumor bed based on the microscopic review of the tumor bed.
      iii. Suggestion: Dotting the perimeter of cancer in each slide can be helpful to reconstruct the tumor extent across multiple slides (see point 1-b-i).
   b. Using the microscope, make visual snapshots of cancer cellularity as you go from field to field across the defined tumor bed from one end to the opposite (eg, left to right, then top to bottom) to estimate the

   i. Average cancer cellularity (%) across the entire tumor bed. This is all cancer, whether invasive or in situ.
   ii. Average percent of the cancer within the tumor bed that is in situ.
   iii. Cellularity estimates are to the nearest 10%, with additional selections of 1% and 5% for very low cellularity. For reference there are images of computer-generated examples linked to our Web site, http://www.mdanderson.org/breastcancer_RCB.
   iv. The usual misunderstanding is only to make estimates in foci of the tumor bed that contain lots of cancer. *The estimates are supposed to represent the average across the entire residual tumor bed area.*

REFERENCES

1. Feldman LD, Hortobagyi GN, Buzdar AU, et al. Pathological assessment of response to induction chemotherapy in breast cancer. *Cancer Res.* 1986;46:2578-2581.
2. Hortobagyi GN, Ames FC, Buzdar AU, et al. Management of stage III primary breast cancer with primary chemotherapy, surgery, and radiation therapy. *Cancer.* 1988;62:2507-2516.
3. Chevallier B, Roche H, Olivier JP, et al. Inflammatory breast cancer. Pilot study of intensive induction chemotherapy (FEC-HD) results in a high histologic response rate. *Am J Clin Oncol.* 1993;16:223-238.
4. Sataloff DM, Mason BA, Prestipino AJ, et al. Pathologic response to induction chemotherapy in locally advanced carcinoma of the breast: a determinant of outcome. *J Am Coll Surg.* 1995;180:297-304.
5. Honkoop AH, Pinedo HM, De Jong JS, et al. Effects of chemotherapy on pathologic and biologic characteristics of locally advanced breast cancer. *Am J Clin Pathol.* 1997;107:211-218.
6. Honkoop AH, van Diest PJ, de Jong JS, et al. Prognostic role of clinical, pathological and biological characteristics in patients with locally advanced breast cancer. *Br J Cancer.* 1998;77:621-626.
7. Bonadonna G, Valagussa P, Brambilla C, et al. Primary chemotherapy in operable breast cancer: eight-year experience at the Milan Cancer Institute. *J Clin Oncol.* 1998;16:93-100.
8. Fisher B, Bryant J, Wolmark N, et al. Effect of preoperative chemotherapy on the outcome of women with operable breast cancer. *J Clin Oncol.* 1998;16:2672-2685.
9. Kuerer HM, Newman LA, Smith TL, et al. Clinical course of breast cancer patients with complete pathologic primary tumor and axillary lymph node response to doxorubicin-based neoadjuvant chemotherapy. *J Clin Oncol.* 1999;17:460-469.
10. Ogston KN, Miller ID, Payne S, et al. A new histological grading system to assess response of breast cancers to primary chemotherapy: prognostic significance and survival. *Breast.* 2003;12:320-327.
11. Bear HD, Anderson S, Smith RE, et al. Sequential preoperative or postoperative docetaxel added to preoperative doxorubicin plus cyclophosphamide for operable breast cancer: National Surgical Adjuvant Breast and Bowel Project Protocol B-27. *J Clin Oncol.* 2006;24:2019-2027.
12. Kaufmann M, Hortobagyi GN, Goldhirsch A, et al. Recommendations from an international expert panel on the use of neoadjuvant (primary) systemic treatment of operable breast cancer: an update. *J Clin Oncol.* 2006;24:1940-1949.
13. Kurosumi M: Significance of histopathological evaluation in primary therapy for breast cancer—recent trends in primary modality with pathological complete response (pCR) as endpoint. *Breast Cancer.* 2004;11:139-147.
14. Kuroi K, Toi M, Tsuda H, et al. Unargued issues on the pathological assessment of response in primary systemic therapy for breast cancer. *Biomed Pharmacother.* 2005;59:S387-S392.
15. von Minckwitz G, Raab G, Caputo A, et al. Doxorubicin with cyclophosphamide followed by docetaxel every 21 days compared with doxorubicin and docetaxel every 14 days as preoperative treatment in operable breast cancer: the GEPARDUO study of the German Breast Group. *J Clin Oncol.* 2005;23:2676-2685.
16. Hennessy BT, Hortobagyi GN, Rouzier R, et al. Outcome after pathologic complete eradication of cytologically proven breast cancer axillary node metastases following primary chemotherapy. *J Clin Oncol.* 2005;23:9304-9311.

17. Carey LA, Metzger R, Dees EC, et al. American Joint Committee on Cancer tumor-node-metastasis stage after neoadjuvant chemotherapy and breast cancer outcome. *J Natl Cancer Inst.* 2005;97:1137-1142.

18. Jones RL, Lakhani SR, Ring AE, et al. Pathological complete response and residual DCIS following neoadjuvant chemotherapy for breast carcinoma. *Br J Cancer.* 2006;94:358-362.

19. Mazouni C, Peintinger F, Wan-Kau S, et al. Residual ductal carcinoma in situ in patients with complete eradication of invasive breast cancer after neoadjuvant chemotherapy does not adversely affect patient outcome. *J Clin Oncol.* 2007;25:2650-2655.

20. Feldman LD, Hortobagyi GN, Buzdar AU, et al. Pathological assessment of response to induction chemotherapy in breast cancer. *Cancer Res.* 1986;46:2578-2581.

21. Fisher B, Bryant J, Wolmark N, et al. Effect of preoperative chemotherapy on the outcome of women with operable breast cancer. *J Clin Oncol.* 1998;16:2672-2685.

22. Guarneri V, Broglio K, Kau SW, et al. Prognostic value of pathologic complete response after primary chemotherapy in relation to hormone receptor status and other factors. *J Clin Oncol.* 2006;24:1037-1044.

23. Mamounas EP, Bryant J, Lembersky B, et al. Paclitaxel after doxorubicin plus cyclophosphamide as adjuvant chemotherapy for node-positive breast cancer: results from NSABP B-28. *J Clin Oncol.* 2005;23:3686-3696.

24. Henderson IC, Berry DA, Demetri GD, et al. Improved outcomes from adding sequential paclitaxel but not from escalating doxorubicin dose in an adjuvant chemotherapy regimen for patients with node-positive primary breast cancer. *J Clin Oncol.* 2003;21:976-983.

25. Green MC, Buzdar AU, Smith T, et al. Weekly paclitaxel improves pathologic complete remission in operable breast cancer when compared with paclitaxel once every 3 weeks. *J Clin Oncol.* 2005;23:5983-5992.

26. Sparano JA, Wang M, Martino S, et al. Weekly paclitaxel in the adjuvant treatment of breast cancer. *N Engl J Med.* 2008;358:1663-1671.

27. Buzdar AU, Ibrahim NK, Francis D, et al. Significantly higher pathologic complete remission rate after neoadjuvant therapy with trastuzumab, paclitaxel, and epirubicin chemotherapy: results of a randomized trial in human epidermal growth factor receptor 2-positive operable breast cancer. *J Clin Oncol.* 2005;23:3676-3685.

28. Buzdar AU, Valero V, Ibrahim NK, et al. Neoadjuvant therapy with paclitaxel followed by 5-fluorouracil, epirubicin, and cyclophosphamide chemotherapy and concurrent trastuzumab in human epidermal growth factor receptor 2-positive operable breast cancer: an update of the initial randomized study population and data of additional patients treated with the same regimen. *Clin Cancer Res.* 2007;13:228-233.

29. Romond EH, Perez EA, Bryant J, et al. Trastuzumab plus adjuvant chemotherapy for operable HER2-positive breast cancer. *N Engl J Med.* 2005;353:1673-1684.

30. Rouzier R, Perou CM, Symmans WF, et al. Breast cancer molecular subtypes respond differently to preoperative chemotherapy. *Clin Cancer Res.* 2005;11:5678-5685.

31. Mazouni C, Kau SW, Frye D, et al. Inclusion of taxanes, particularly weekly paclitaxel, in preoperative chemotherapy improves pathologic complete response rate in estrogen receptor-positive breast cancers. *Ann Oncol.* 2007;18:874-880.

32. Pusztai L, Broglio K, Andre F, et al. Effect of molecular disease subsets on disease-free survival in randomized adjuvant chemotherapy trials for estrogen-receptor positive breast cancer. *J Clin Oncol.* 2008;26:4679-4683.

33. Berry DA, Cirrincione C, Henderson IC, et al. Estrogen-receptor status and outcomes of modern chemotherapy for patients with node-positive breast cancer. *JAMA.* 2006;295:1658-1667.

34. Andre F, Broglio K, Roche H, et al. Estrogen receptor expression and efficacy of docetaxel-containing adjuvant chemotherapy in patients with node-positive breast cancer: results from a pooled analysis. *J Clin Oncol.* 2008;26:2636-2643.

35. Singletary SE, Allred C, Ashley P, et al. Revision of the American Joint Committee on Cancer staging system for breast cancer. *J Clin Oncol.* 2002; 20:3628-3636.

36. Symmans WF, Peintinger F, Hatzis C, et al. Measurement of residual breast cancer burden to predict survival after neoadjuvant chemotherapy. *J Clin Oncol.* 2007;25:4414-4422.

37. Jeruss JS, Mittendorf EA, Tucker SL, et al. Combined use of clinical and pathologic staging variables to define outcomes for breast cancer patients treated with neoadjuvant therapy. *J Clin Oncol.* 2008;26:246-252.

38. Fisher ER, Wang J, Bryant J, et al. Pathobiology of preoperative chemotherapy: findings from the National Surgical Adjuvant Breast and Bowel (NSABP) protocol B-18. *Cancer.* 2002;95:681-695.

39. Rajan R, Poniecka A, Smith TL, et al. Change in tumor cellularity of breast carcinoma after neoadjuvant chemotherapy as a variable in the pathologic assessment of response. *Cancer.* 2004;100:1365-1373.

40. Thomas E, Holmes FA, Smith TL, et al. The use of alternate, non-cross-resistant adjuvant chemotherapy on the basis of pathologic response to a neoadjuvant doxorubicin-based regimen in women with operable breast cancer: long-term results from a prospective randomized trial. *J Clin Oncol.* 2004;22:2294-2302.

41. Swain SM. A step in the right direction. *J Clin Oncol.* 2006;24:3717-3718

42. Ellis MJ, Tao Y, Luo J, et al. Outcome prediction for estrogen receptor-positive breast cancer based on postneoadjuvant endocrine therapy tumor characteristics. *J Natl Cancer Inst.* 2008;100:1380-1388.

43. Peintinger F, Buzdar AU, Kuerer HM, et al. Hormone receptor status and pathologic response of HER2-positive breast cancer treated with neoadjuvant chemotherapy and trastuzumab. *Ann Oncol.* 2008;19:2020-2025.

CHAPTER 26

Axillary and Sentinel Lymph Node Evaluation

Roderick R. Turner
Helen Mabry
Armando E. Giuliano

In the current era, many patients present with a small primary breast cancer detected by mammography or other screening procedures. In recent decades, the median size of nodal metastases has decreased, paralleling the decrease in primary tumor size. The median size of nodal metastases is now approximately 6 mm,[1] and 70% to 80% of patients have negative nodes after surgical and pathologic nodal staging. A systematic approach to the evaluation of lymph nodes is needed today to reliably identify metastatic carcinoma.

Sentinel lymph node (SLN) biopsy has led to the use of more sensitive pathologic techniques to reliably detect small metastases and reduce the risk of false-negative results. The nature of SLNs as first-draining lymph nodes, combined with the use of multilevel sections and cytokeratin immunohistochemistry, has significantly increased the number of patients with nodal micrometastases or isolated tumor cells[2] and intensified the debate over the therapeutic benefit of axillary dissection and the clinical impact of minimal metastases on patient prognosis and choices for adjuvant therapies. Clinicians, including pathologists, need to understand that minimal nodal disease, when present, should be considered in the context of the primary tumor characteristics and the patient's clinical status. A multidisciplinary breast conference discussion helps to optimize individual patient care recommendations.

SLN biopsy performed by an experienced surgeon provides prognostic and staging information equivalent to that provided by axillary dissection. Validation studies, with comprehensive pathologic analysis of both SLNs and non-SLNs, have confirmed the accuracy and safety of SLN biopsy. [2-4] The accuracy of SLN biopsy compared with complete level I and II axillary dissection is greater than 95% at major centers.[5] Axillary recurrence rates for patients with negative SLN biopsy followed by adjuvant therapies appear similar to recurrence rates for patients who have had complete axillary dissection.[6]

Nonsurgical alternative approaches to axillary staging have recently focused on ultrasound evaluation to determine whether SLN biopsy is indicated.[7,8] Patients with a large primary tumor[9,10] or suspicious axillary clinical examination may benefit from preoperative axillary ultrasound with fine-needle aspiration cytology or core biopsy of suspicious nodes (Chapter 24). Patients with a positive needle biopsy result can proceed to complete axillary dissection, whereas those with a negative or nondiagnostic result undergo SLN biopsy. Studies with fine-needle aspiration cytology have demonstrated a high level of accuracy for ultrasound-detected macrometastases, with a reduction of SLN procedures by 10% to 15% and resultant cost savings.[9] Pathologists should be careful to avoid a false-positive result, which has been reported rarely.

Primary tumor typing with phenotypic and molecular genotypic assays, under investigation today,[11] may help in the future to determine which patients benefit from SLN biopsy and complete axillary node dissection (CLND).

Optimal patient care derives from a well-functioning surgeon–pathologist team. Sentinel nodes should be submitted to pathology preferably as single nodes dissected free of adipose tissue and with a description as hot or blue. Individual institutions and physicians need to decide whether intraoperative pathologic examination is a good management approach in their practice setting, and, if so, which methods would be best with the available personnel, facilities, and instruments.

SIGNIFICANCE OF MICROMETASTASIS

The clinical significance of axillary node micrometastases and isolated tumor cells continues to be debated, because in population-based statistical comparisons, the prognostic impact of nodal micrometastases is relatively small. Recent studies using more thorough lymph node embedding and improved immunohistochemical methods have reported a significant association between micrometastases and poor survival compared with that of node-negative patients.[12,13] However, the prognostic significance of nodal micrometastases remains unclear,[14] particularly in adjuvant therapy–treated patients. Ongoing clinical trials will further help to define the clinical impact of nodal micrometastases and isolated tumor cells.

The goal for the pathologist in current practice is to minimize the risk of missing macrometastases and micrometastases in SLNs. Because the likelihood of identifying metastases is related to the number and depth of histologic sections, the use of cytokeratin-immunohistochemistry (CK-IHC) stains, and the size of metastases, it is now well accepted that SLNs should be examined more thoroughly than other lymph nodes. The detection of early metastasis helps to reduce the false-negative rate of the SLN staging procedure.[15] Nevertheless, it should be recognized that detection of all cases with only isolated tumor cells is an unrealistic goal with the available techniques and resources.

SENTINEL LYMPH NODE PROCESSING

Gross Handling

Variations in gross and microscopic sectioning methods for SLNs account, in part, for substantial differences in rates of metastasis detection reported in the literature. Longitudinal sections are recommended,[5] since afferent lymphatics generally enter the node in the midline plane of the long axis, and small metastases are most likely to be found near that entry point.[16,17] Placement of the central nodal surfaces at the bottom of the cassette will result in the highest yield of metastasis detection in the first histologic levels.[18,19] It is also important to cut thin gross sections, no thicker than 2 mm, which is accomplished with simple longitudinal bisection of most SLNs (Figs. 26-1 and 26-2). When gross sections are thick, additional deep histologic levels may be needed for sufficient sampling. Histologic

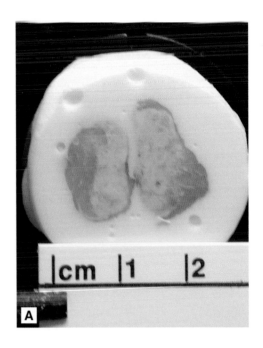

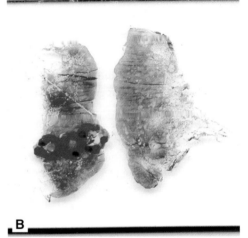

FIGURE 26-2 A. Bisected SLN with focal blue dye in preparation for frozen section. **B.** Micrometastases were found at the blue-dye-stained end, opposite half (frozen section).

examination of only half of the SLN, as occurs with rapid molecular assays, may cause a histologic false negative result.[20]

Paraffin Section Levels

There is no consensus among pathologists regarding how many hematoxylin and eosin (H&E) and CK-IHC levels should be examined. Conflicting data on this subject may be explained, at least in part, by differences in methods applied to gross sections and the number of cytokeratin levels examined, in addition to the absence of an accepted standard for metastasis detection. The studies that have supported limited (2 to 4) step sections have generally utilized longitudinal gross sections with both CK-IHC and H&E at each microscopic level. Comprehensive examination with CK-IHC has demonstrated that positive lymph nodes nearly always have multiple clusters/deposits and that limited sections are sufficient to detect some of them in

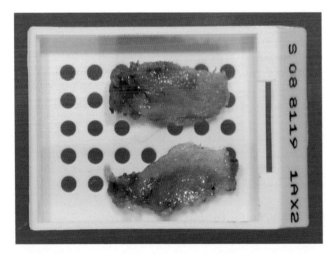

FIGURE 26-1 Longitudinal bisection of an SLN. Cut surface placed at bottom of cassette will appear at the top of the paraffin block for initial histologic sections.

TABLE 26-1 Selected References Supporting the Accuracy of Limited Step Section Examination of Sentinel Lymph Nodes With Cytokeratin Immunohistochemistry

Study	Limited Sections	Accuracy Versus Deeper Levels
Turner et al (1999)[18]	Two levels, 40 μm, each with CK-IHC	98% (41/42)
Cserni (2002)[19]	Five levels, 50-100 μm, no CK-IHC	90% (111/123)
Freneaux et al (2002)[21]	Three levels, 150 μm, with CK-IHC	97% (72/74)
Yared et al (2002)[22]	Three adjacent levels with one CK-IHC	98% (94/96)

CK-IHC = cytokeratin immunohistochemistry.

nearly all patients with metastasis (Table 26-1).[18,19,21-23] Institutions that have applied transverse gross sections or utilized predominantly H&E stains in histologic evaluation have generally concluded that more numerous levels of the paraffin block are needed to identify cases with small metastases.

Before publication of the sixth edition of the *AJCC Cancer Staging Manual*,[24] isolated tumor cells (ITCs) were commonly considered micrometastases; therefore, the early SLN studies tended to overstate the frequency of micrometastasis compared with current practice because the minimal findings on cytokeratin stains or step sections are commonly ITCs, classified as N0(i+). The goal today should be to detect all cases with nodal macrometastasis and the large majority of cases with micrometastasis as currently defined by the 0.2-mm threshold. Several histologic levels (2 to 4) with CK-IHC accomplish that goal with a high degree of accuracy. In clinical practice, the pathologist who encounters multiple ITC clusters, in a limited section protocol, may choose to examine deeper levels to exclude fusion of those clusters as a micrometastasis or macrometastasis deeper in the paraffin block.

The Protocol

Both superficial and limited deeper histologic sections are needed to reduce variations in gross sections, to ensure adequate examination of the capsular–subcapsular areas, and to control different sizes and shapes of lymph nodes. It is best for an institution to have a single protocol with a limited number of histologic and CK-IHC levels, usually 2 to 4 levels separated by a specified interval in the paraffin block, so that histotechnologists can follow the protocol systematically. The levels are typically separated by 100 or 200 μm, but may be up to 500 μm or as little as 50 μm apart. Both H&E and CK-IHC stains should be examined at each level so that any cytokeratin-positive finding can be closely scrutinized on the corresponding H&E section and any suspicious finding on H&E stain can be discounted when the adjacent cytokeratin stain is negative.

HISTOLOGIC EXAMINATION

Use of Immunohistochemistry

Standard H&E examination of lymph nodes reliably detects macrometastases but commonly fails to identify small metastases,

which are easily missed because their shapes and colors may not be obvious in the background of reactive lymphoid tissue (Fig. 26-3). CK-IHC provides a sharp contrast between metastases and lymph node cellular constituents and permits consistent

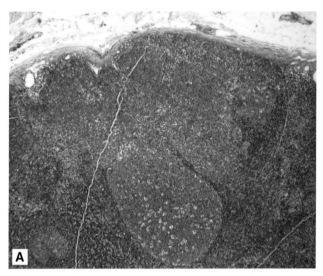

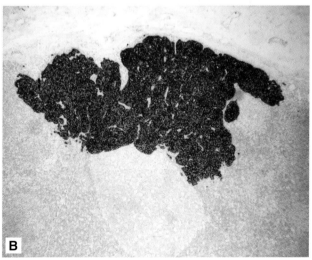

FIGURE 26-3 / Micrometastasis difficult to see on **(A)** H&E-stained section, but readily identified on **(B)** CK-IHC stain.

identification and measurement of tumor cell deposits. The value of adding IHC to the SLN work-up is to avoid missing metastases that should have been seen on H&E stains; this promotes reproducible pathology reporting and assures patients that their SLN results are accurate.

The American Joint Committee on Cancer (AJCC) staging system[24] provides a framework for consistent diagnosis of nodal metastases, with measurement thresholds up to 0.2 mm for ITCs (pN0[i+]), up to 2.0 mm for micrometastasis (pN1mi), and greater than 2.0 mm for macrometastasis (pN1a). However, histologic criteria for classification of multiple clusters or single dispersed tumor cells, as commonly seen with lobular carcinomas (Fig. 26-4), are unclear in the sixth edition of the *AJCC Cancer Staging Manual*, which has led to variable application among pathologists. The new category of ITC, plus the use of different terminology in the International Union Against Cancer system, has contributed to diagnostic variation.[25,26]

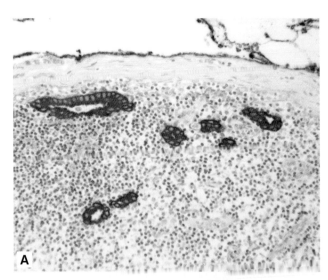

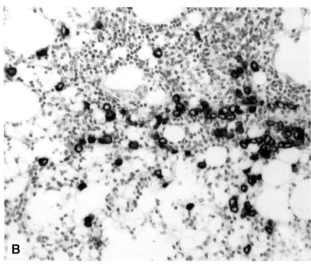

FIGURE 26-4 Isolated tumor cells in SLNs. **A.** Ductal carcinoma cells with cohesive pattern, largest cluster 0.15 mm. **B.** Lobular carcinoma cells in dispersed pattern, largest contiguous grouping 0.10 mm.

Reproducible Reporting

Reproducible reporting is readily achievable using strict, simple criteria for measurement of tumor cluster size. In the presence of multiple clusters and single cells, the greatest dimension of the largest cluster is used for classification, irrespective of the number of clusters. These criteria have demonstrated a high level of reproducibility among pathologists, without which valid statistical comparisons between institutions and pathologists would not be possible. The proposed clarification of the AJCC system[26] may have a bias toward a lower nodal stage and more ITC diagnoses, with a trend toward a higher frequency of non-SLN positivity in patients with SLN ITCs, but this may not be statistically significant.[27] A basic tenet of the AJCC system is that clinicians faced with a borderline finding should select the lower stage category. Understaging is appropriate with minimal nodal disease and causes substantially less diagnostic variation than the overstaging that occurs when tumor cells clusters are summed or spanned in adjusted measurements.

Benign Epithelial Rests

Pathologists experienced in the interpretation of CK-IHC of lymph nodes have little difficulty excluding keratinous debris or other floater artifacts that may appear on these slides. The use of a low-molecular-weight keratin antibody, instead of a broad-spectrum antibody, is preferred to prevent staining of fibroblastic reticular cells, a normal constituent in lymph nodes. One caveat with a low-molecular-weight keratin is that basal-like carcinomas may infrequently cause a false-negative IHC stain.

Benign epithelial inclusions are rare in axillary lymph nodes, less than 0.5% of axillary dissections,[28] and are readily identified in H&E examination (Fig. 26-5). Small squamous inclusion cysts, rare benign apocrine or ciliated glands, and normal lobules have been described. In the setting of SLN biopsy for breast cancer staging, it is more likely to encounter a micrometastasis mimicking a benign epithelial rest than a true benign epithelial rest (Fig. 26-6).

Needle Biopsy Displacement

Epithelial cell displacement within the breast after needle biopsy is well-described and readily identified by pathologists as clusters or single cells in the hemorrhagic core track or associated granulation tissue. This observation has led to a concern that some cells iatrogenically displaced by biopsy or massage could drain to the regional lymph nodes and cause a false-positive ITC finding.[29,30] However, because many breast cancers shed tumor cells into the lymphatic circulation, ITCs in the SLN are far more likely to reflect a true metastatic process. Clusters of needle-displaced epithelial cells are commonly seen in excised breast tissue because they are too big to drain out of the interstitial space and are retained in the healing reaction. Although this remains a debated issue,[31] a large Austrian study has concluded that preoperative biopsy does not increase the risk of SLN metastasis.[32]

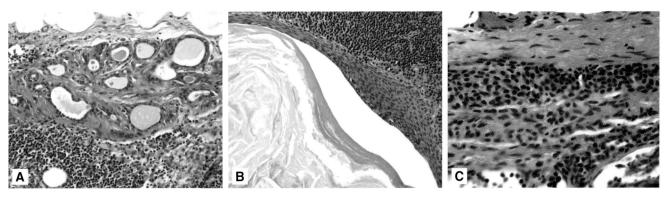

FIGURE 26-5 Benign epithelial rests in SLNs. **A.** Normal-appearing ectopic breast lobule in SLN capsule. **B.** Benign squamous inclusion with keratin. **C.** Nodal nevus cell aggregate in SLN capsule.

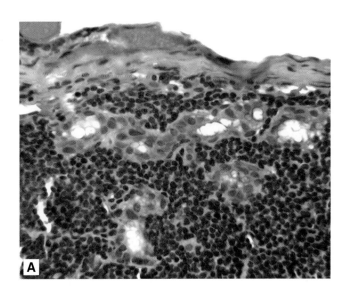

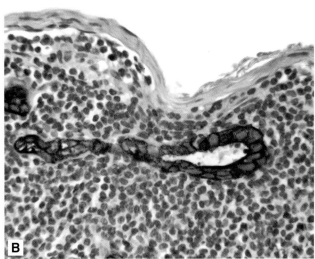

FIGURE 26-6 Micrometastasis mimics a benign apocrine epithelial rest. **A.** H&E stain. **B.** CK-IHC stain.

INTRAOPERATIVE EXAMINATION OF THE SLN

General

Rapid, intraoperative diagnosis of SLNs allows further axillary dissection at the same surgery and spares some patients surgical reoperation. Several determinants are cited by physicians and institutions to support different approaches taken in today's clinical practice before a consensus on the therapeutic benefit of axillary node dissection.

Axillary node dissection is most likely to be beneficial for patients with SLN macrometastasis, and macrometastases are reliably detected by standard intraoperative (IO) techniques for frozen section (FS) and/or touch imprint cytology (TIC). These standard techniques fail to detect most cases with micrometastasis or ITCs, potentially subjecting patients with a false-negative IO result to return to surgery. A concern with FS and newer molecular detection techniques is that some of the SLN tissue is consumed with rapid diagnostic procedures that could cause a false-negative final result, although studies with FS indicate that it can be safely utilized.[2,33] Another concern with FS is that surgical scheduling may be disrupted and anesthesia prolonged by a delay from pathology testing. Lastly, the final size of metastases may not be known at surgery, which would preclude the surgeon, patient, and family from having a fully informed discussion of the benefit and risks of axillary dissection.

Economic Analysis

Studies that have evaluated the costs of surgical care have reported economic support for IO pathologic examination with immediate dissection for SLN-positive patients.[34,35] Even a small reduction in the number of patients scheduled for reoperation may justify the relatively minor costs of pathology evaluation.

A complicating factor in determining the benefit of IO exam is that some patients with nodal metastases undetected at surgery, either because IO exam was not requested or the pathologist's IO result was falsely negative, would have a second surgery for positive lumpectomy margins.[36] This factor tends to negate the benefit of SLN IO exam, the magnitude of which would depend on the surgeon's frequency of take-back to surgery for positive breast margins.

Technical Considerations

Practice patterns vary widely on the use and techniques for intraoperative examination, which range from all cases to none (paraffin sections only). A few institutions have explored a selective use of IO exam in an effort to concentrate resources and time for patients most likely to have SLN metastases.[37,38] Strategic approaches may target younger patients (age < 60 years), larger primary tumor size (T2/3), peritumoral lymphatic vascular invasion, surgeon's suspicion at SLN biopsy, or pathologist's suspicion at gross examination. The false-negative rate of IO exam is lower for patients with a large primary tumor because of the more frequent association with SLN macrometastases. A nomogram weighs some of these risk factors.[39]

The pathologist presented with a request for IO exam has an expanding list of available techniques. Standard techniques, in addition to careful gross examination, are TIC, FS, or both. Scrape smear cytology enhances the cell yield in cytologic preparations and may be particularly useful in cases with a suspicious focus in gross sections. Comparisons of FS and TIC have found that FS offers a higher level of sensitivity, approximately 80% to 90% versus H&E paraffin sections, compared with TIC sensitivity of approximately 70% to 80%.[40-48] Both techniques commonly fail to detect micrometastasis and ITCs. Rapid CK-IHC stains may reduce IO false-negative cases, but require additional time, personnel, and costs.[49,50]

Comprehensive Analysis

Molecular techniques for rapid diagnosis are under investigation because of their high sensitivity. They consume about half of the SLN and require carefully controlled assay conditions to avoid false-positive results. Test manufacturers have set cut-off levels at the lower limit of micrometastasis, 0.2 mm, with generally favorable results. Early studies have reported that rapid molecular techniques detect approximately 10% more cases of metastasis than FS analysis, with few if any false positive results.[51-53] Although the assay sensitivity is described as comparable to multilevel paraffin sections, current commercially available tests miss approximately half of cases with micrometastases.[51-53] Moreover, they typically take 35 to 45 minutes, which may delay surgery (Table 26-2).

The European Institute of Oncology group performs FS analysis of the entire SLN in multiple step sections separated by 50 μm; sensitivity is high[54,55] and comparable to that of reverse transcriptase polymerase chain reaction results.[56] This FS method, however, leaves no residual tissue for paraffin section analysis and therefore is unlikely to be widely adopted.

COMPLETE AXILLARY NODE DISSECTION

Determining Potential Benefit

The size of metastases in the SLNs, the number of positive and negative nodes removed at sentinel lymphadenectomy, and extranodal invasion are helpful predictors of the likelihood and bulk of metastases in non-SLNs.[57,58] Primary tumor characteristics are also important, particularly tumor size and peritumoral lymphatic vascular invasion. An argument in favor of axillary dissection as a reoperation after SLN biopsy is that these data can be compiled and discussed with the patient to make a fully informed decision on the therapeutic role of CLND. The use of a nomogram may help to quantify the risk of non-SLN disease and potential benefit of further surgery.[59,60] Patient age and primary tumor characteristics, such as hormone receptor status, are also relevant factors.[61,62] The current trend is toward less CLND for patients with small SLN metastases.[63] Ongoing clinical trials will help determine which patients with SLN metastases have a low risk of axillary clinical recurrence without CLND and therefore can be safely treated with adjuvant therapies.

Pathologic Evaluation of Non-SLNs

The apical node, marked by a surgeon's stitch, should be separately inked or embedded, because it may affect fields for radiation therapy. Careful visual inspection of fat and manual palpation is widely regarded as sufficient for lymph node identification. Grossly negative axillary dissections should have all nodal tissue embedded for histologic evaluation with standard H&E-stained sections. Multiple histologic levels and/or CK-IHC are generally not performed on non-SLN in the absence of H&E suspicious findings. Because the IHC detection of small metastases is higher for lobular carcinomas than ductal carcinomas, some pathologists use CK-IHC routinely to examine non-SLNs of patients with lobular carcinomas. In general, the pathology protocol should be uniform for all cancers and systematically applied within an institution.

TABLE 26-2 Intraoperative Techniques for Detection of Sentinel Lymph Node Micrometastases and Macrometastases

Technique	Estimated Time Required	Approximate Sensitivity
Cytology	10 minutes	70-80%
Frozen section	20 minutes	80-90%
Complete frozen section	30-40 minutes	95-100%
Stat CK-IHC	30-40 minutes	90-95%
Rapid molecular assays	35-45 minutes	95-100%

CK-IHC = cytokeratin immunohistochemistry.

PROGNOSTIC AND STAGING INFORMATION

The pathologist must carefully correlate the gross sectioning methods with the microscopic findings for total and positive SLN and non-SLN counts necessary for accurate nodal staging. It should be remembered that lymph nodes with ITCs only are considered negative according to AJCC sixth edition criteria and are not factored into N1, N2, or N3 categorization. In contrast, lymph nodes with micrometastases are counted toward final nodal stage classification provided that another node contains macrometastasis, which further emphasizes the importance of reproducible distinction between ITC and micrometastasis. Size criteria for micrometastasis (currently > 0.2 to 2.0 mm) may be refined with follow-up data from ongoing clinical trials.

FUTURE DIRECTIONS

- Clinical trial data will help pathologists set protocols for detection of specific size metastases.
- Pathology organizations will establish expected standards for diagnostic evaluation.
- SLN biopsy will be used more selectively: ultrasound and directed needle biopsy for high-risk patients, no surgical staging for a few low-risk patients.
- Primary tumor phenotypic and genotypic studies will determine which patients are likely to develop clinically significant axillary disease to better determine which SLN-positive patients benefit from therapeutic axillary dissection.

SUMMARY

- A systematic approach to the diagnosis of SLNs is needed to reliably detect macrometastases and micrometastases.
- Cytokeratin immunohistochemistry is a helpful adjunct for the pathologist to consistently detect and accurately measure small metastases using a practical limited step sections protocol.
- Classification of small metastases based solely on the size of the largest cohesive cluster promotes reproducible nodal staging.
- Intraoperative examination of the SLN spares some patients a second surgery, but positive rates and efficacy are impacted by multiple patient, surgeon, and institutional variables.
- The risk of non-SLN metastases may be predicted from the patient's primary tumor characteristics and SLN findings.
- Clinical trial data will help to direct the use of therapeutic axillary dissection.

ACKNOWLEDGMENTS

The authors are supported by funding from QVC and the Fashion Footwear Association of New York Charitable Foundation (New York, NY), the Margie and Robert E. Petersen Foundation (Los Angeles, CA), Mrs. Lois Rosen (Los Angeles, CA), and the Associates for Breast and Prostate Cancer Studies (Santa Monica, CA).

REFERENCES

1. Weaver DL. Handling and evaluation of sentinel lymph nodes. In: O'Malley FP, Pinder SE. *Breast Pathology*. Philadelphia, PA: Churchill Livingstone Elsevier: 2006:249-256.
2. Giuliano AE, Dale PS, Turner RR, et al. Improved axillary staging of breast cancer with sentinel lymphadenectomy. *Ann Surg.* 1995;222:394-401.
3. Turner RR, Ollila DW, Krasne DL, Giuliano AE. Histopathologic validation of the sentinel lymph node hypothesis for breast carcinoma. *Ann Surg.* 1997; 226:271-278.
4. Weaver DL, Krag DN, Ashikaga T, Harlow SP, O'Connell M. Pathologic analysis of sentinel and nonsentinel lymph nodes in breast cancer. A multicenter study. *Cancer.* 2000;88:1099-1107.
5. Lyman GH, Giuliano AE, Somerfield MR, et al. American Society of Clinical Oncology guideline recommendations for sentinel lymph node biopsy in early-stage breast cancer. *J Clin Oncol.* 2005;23:7703-7720.
6. Langer I, Marti R, Guller U, et al. Axillary recurrence rate in breast cancer patients with negative sentinel lymph node (SLN) or SLN micrometastases. Prospective analysis of 150 patients after SLN biopsy. *Ann Surg.* 2005;241:152-158.
7. Krishnamurthy S, Sneige N, Bedi DG, et al. Role of ultrasound-guided fine-needle aspiration of indeterminate and suspicious axillary lymph nodes in the initial staging of breast carcinoma. *Cancer.* 2002;95:982-988.
8. Deurloo EE, Tanis PJ, Gilhuijs KGA, et al. Reduction in the number of sentinel lymph node procedures by preoperative ultrasonography of the axilla in breast cancer. *Eur J Cancer.* 2003;39:1068-1073.
9. Davis JT, Brill YM, Simmons S, et al. Ultrasound-guided fine-needle aspiration of clinically negative lymph nodes versus sentinel node mapping in patients at high risk for axillary metastasis. *Ann Surg Oncol.* 2006;13:1545-1552.
10. Koelliker SL, Chung MA, Mainiero MB, Steinhoff MM, Cady B. Axillary lymph nodes: US-guided fine-needle aspiration for initial staging of breast cancer: correlation with primary tumor size. *Radiol.* 2008;246:81-89.
11. Nakagawa T, Huang SK, Martinez SR, et al. Proteomic profiling of primary breast cancer predicts axillary lymph node metastasis. *Cancer Res.* 2006;66:11825-11830.
12. Tan LK, Giri D, Hummer AJ, et al. Occult axillary node metastases in breast cancer are prognostically significant: results in 368 node-negative patients with 20-year follow-up. *J Clin Oncol.* 2008;26:1803-1809.
13. Chen SL, Hoehne FM, Giuliano, AE. The prognostic significance of micrometastases in breast cancer: a SEER population-based analysis. *Ann Surg Oncol.* 2007;14:3378-3384.
14. Hansen NM, Grube B, Ye X, et al. Impact of micrometastases in the sentinel node of patients with breast cancer. *J Clin Oncol.* 2009; in press.
15. Jacub JW, Diaz NM, Ebert MD, et al. Completion axillary lymph node dissection minimizes the likelihood of false negatives for patients with invasive breast carcinoma and cytokeratin positive only sentinel lymph nodes. *Am J Surg.* 2002;184:302-306.
16. Cserni G. Mapping metastases in sentinel lymph nodes of breast cancer. *Am J Clin Pathol.* 2000;113:351-354.
17. Diaz LK, Hunt K, Ames F, et al. Histologic localization of sentinel lymph node metastases in breast cancer. *Am J Surg Pathol.* 2003;27:385-389.
18. Turner RR, Ollila DW, Stern S, Giuliano AE. Optimal histopathologic examination of the sentinel lymph node for breast carcinoma staging. *Am J Surg Pathol.* 1999;23:263-267.
19. Cserni G. Complete sectioning of axillary nodes in patients with breast cancer. Analysis of two different step sectioning and immunohistochemistry protocols in 246 patients. *J Clin Pathol.* 2002;55:926-931.
20. Daniele L, Annaratone L, Allia E, et al. Technical limits of comparison of step-sectioning, immunohistochemistry and RT-PCR on breast cancer sentinel nodes: a study on methacarn fixed tissue. *J Cell Mol Med.* 2008 Jul 30; Epub ahead of print.
21. Freneaux P, Nos C, Vincent-Salomon A, et al. Histologic detection of minimal metastatic involvement in axillary sentinel nodes: a rational basis for a sensitive methodology usable in daily practice. *Mod Pathol.* 2002;15:641-646.
22. Yared MA, Middleton LP, Smith TL, et al. Recommendations for sentinel lymph node processing in breast cancer. *Am J Surg Pathol.* 2002;26:377-382.
23. Falconieri G, Pizzolitto S, Gentile G. Comprehensive examination of sentinel lymph node in breast cancer: a solution without a problem? *Int J Surg Pathol.* 2006;14:1-8.
24. Greene FL, Page DL, Fleming ID, eds. *AJCC Cancer Staging Manual*. 6th ed. Chicago, IL: Springer: 2002:223-240.
25. Cserni G, Bianchi S, Boecker W, et al. Improving the reproducibility of diagnosing micrometastases and isolated tumor cells. *Cancer.* 2005;103:358-367.

26. Turner RR, Weaver DL, Cserni G, et al. Nodal stage classification for breast carcinoma: improving interobserver reproducibility through standardized histologic criteria and image-based training. *J Clin Oncol.* 2008;26:258-263.

27. Cserni G, Bianchi S, Vezzosi V, et al. Variations in sentinel node isolated tumor cells/micrometastasis and non-sentinel node involvement rates according to different interpretations of the TNM definitions. *Eur J Cancer.* 2008;44:2185-2191.

28. McGuckin MA, Cummings MC, Walsh MD, et al. Occult axillary metastases in breast cancer: their detection and prognostic significance. *Br J Cancer.* 1996;73:88-95.

29. Carter BA, Jensen RA, Simpson JF, Page DL. Benign transport of breast epithelium into axillary lymph nodes after biopsy. *Am J Clin Pathol.* 2000;113:259-265.

30. Diaz NM, Cox CE, Ebert M, et al. Benign mechanical transport of breast epithelial cells to sentinel lymph nodes. *Am J Surg Pathol.* 2004;28:1641-1645.

31. Turner RR, Giuliano AE. Does breast massage push tumor cells into sentinel nodes? *Am J Surg Pathol.* 2005;29:1254-1255.

32. Peters-Engl C, Konstantiniuk P, Tausch C, et al. The impact of preoperative breast biopsy on the risk of sentinel lymph node metastases: analysis of 2502 cases from the Austrian sentinel lymph node biopsy study group. *Br J Cancer.* 2004;91:1782-1786.

33. Aurora N, Martins D, Huston T, et al. Sentinel node positivity rates with and without frozen section for breast cancer. *Ann Surg Oncol.* 2007;15:256-261.

34. Ronka R, v. Smitten K, Sintonen H, et al. The impact of sentinel node biopsy and axillary staging strategy on hospital costs. *Ann Oncol.* 2004;15:88-94.

35. Jeruss JS, Hunt KK, Xing Y, et al. Is intraoperative touch imprint cytology of sentinel lymph nodes in patients with breast cancer cost effective? *Cancer.* 2006;107:2328-2336.

36. McLaughlin SA, Ochoa-Frongia LM, Patil SM, et al. Influence of frozen-section analysis of sentinel lymph node and lumpectomy margin status on reoperation rates in patients undergoing breast-conserving therapy. *J Am Coll Surg.* 2008;206:76-82.

37. Klepchick PR, Dabbs DJ, Bonaventura M, et al. Selective intraoperative consultation for the evaluation of sentinel lymph nodes in breast cancer. *Am J Surg.* 2004;188:429-432.

38. Weiser MR, Montgomery LL, Susnik B, et al. Is routine intraoperative frozen-section examination of sentinel lymph nodes in breast cancer worthwhile? *Ann Surg Oncol.* 2000;7:651-655.

39. Bevilacqua JL, Kattan MW, Fey JV, et al. Doctor, what are my chances of having a positive sentinel node? A validated nomogram for risk estimation. *J Clin Oncol.* 2007;25:3670-3679.

40. Creager AJ, Geisinger KR, Shiver SA, et al. Intraoperative evaluation of sentinel lymph nodes for metastatic breast cancer by imprint cytology. *Mod Pathol* 2002;15:1140-1147.

41. Dabbs DJ, Fung M, Johnson R. Intraoperative cytologic examination of breast sentinel lymph nodes: test utility and patient impact. *Breast J.* 2004;10:190-194.

42. Tew K, Irwig L, Matthews A, Crowe P, Macaskill P. Meta-analysis of sentinel node imprint cytology in breast cancer. *Br J Surg.* 2005;92:1068-1080.

43. Motomura K, Nagumo S, Komoike Y, Koyama H, Inaji H. Accuracy of imprint cytology for intraoperative diagnosis of sentinel node metastases in breast cancer. *Ann Surg.* 2008;247:839-842.

44. van Diest PJ, Torrenga H, Borgstein PJ, et al. Reliability of intraoperative frozen-section and imprint cytological investigation of sentinel lymph nodes in breast cancer. *Histopathology.* 1999;35:14-18.

45. Turner RR, Hansen NM, Stern SL, Giuliano AE. Intraoperative examination of the sentinel lymph node for breast carcinoma staging. *Am J Clin Pathol.* 1999;112:627-634.

46. Mori M, Tada K, Ikenaga M et al. Frozen section is superior to imprint cytology for the intra-operative assessment of sentinel lymph node metastasis in stage I breast cancer patients. *World J Surg Oncol.* 2006;4:26.

47. Langer I, Guller U, Berclaz G, et al. Accuracy of frozen section of sentinel lymph nodes: a prospective analysis of 659 breast cancer patients of the Swiss multicenter study. *Breast Cancer Res Treat.* 2009;113:129-136.

48. Krishnamurthy S. Intraoperative evaluation of axillary sentinel lymph nodes in breast cancer. *Breast Diseases: A Year Book Quarterly.* 2008;19:211-217.

49. Choi YJ, Yun HR, Yoo KE, et al. Intraoperative examination of sentinel lymph nodes by ultrarapid immunohistochemistry in breast cancer. *Jpn J Clin Oncol.* 2006;36:489-493.

50. Holm M, Paaschburg B, Balslev E, et al. Intraoperative immunohistochemistry staining of sentinel nodes in breast cancer: clinical and economical implications. *Breast.* 2008;17:372-375.

51. Blumencranz P, Whitworth PW, Deck K, et al. Sentinel node staging for breast cancer: intraoperative molecular pathology overcomes conventional histologic sampling errors. *Am J Surg.* 2007;194:426-432.

52. Tsujimoto M, Nakabayashi K, Yoshidome K, et al. One-step nucleic acid amplification for intraoperative detection of lymph node metastasis in breast cancer patients. *Clin Cancer Res.* 2007;13:4807-4816.

53. Visser M, Jiwa M, Horstman A, et al. Intra-operative rapid diagnostic method based on CK19 mRNA expression for the detection of lymph node metastasis in breast cancer. *Int J Cancer.* 2008;122:2562-2567.

54. Viale G, Bosari S, Mazzarol G, et al. Intraoperative examination of axillary sentinel lymph nodes in breast carcinoma patients. *Cancer.* 1999;85:2433-2438.

55. Viale G, Maiorano E, Mazzarol G, et al. Histologic detection and clinical implications of micrometastases in axillary sentinel lymph nodes for patients with breast carcinoma. *Cancer* 2001;92:1374-1384.

56. Viale G, Dell'Orto P, Biasi MO, et al. Comparative evaluation of an extensive histopathologic examination and a real-time reverse-transcription-polymerase chain reaction assay for mammaglobin and cytokeratin 19 on axillary sentinel lymph-nodes of breast carcinoma patients. *Ann Surg.* 2008;247:136-142.

57. Turner RR, Chu KU, Qi K, et al. Pathologic features associated with nonsentinel lymph node metastases in patients with metastatic breast carcinoma in a sentinel lymph node. *Cancer* 2000;89:574-581.

58. Degnim AC, Griffith KA, Sabel MS, et al. Clinicopathologic features of metastasis in non sentinel lymph nodes of breast carcinoma patients. *Cancer.* 2003;98:2307-2315.

59. Lambert LA, Ayers GD, Hwang RF, et al. Validation of a breast cancer nomogram for predicting nonsentinel lymph node metastases after a positive sentinel node biopsy. *Ann Surg Oncol.* 2006;13:310-320.

60. Pal A, Provenzano E, Duffy SW, Pinder SE, Purushotham AD. A model for predicting non-sentinel lymph node metastatic disease when the sentinel lymph node is positive. *Br J Surg.* 2008;95:302-309.

61. International Breast Cancer Study Group. Randomized trial comparing axillary clearance versus no axillary clearance in older patients with breast cancer: first results of International Breast Cancer Study Group Trial 10-93. *J Clin Oncol.* 2006;24:337-344.

62. Evans SB, Gass J, Wazer DE. Management of the axilla after the finding of a positive sentinel lymph node: a proposal for an evidence-based risk-adapted algorithm. *Am J Clin Oncol.* 2008;31:293-299.

63. Park J, Fey JV, Naik AM, et al. A declining rate of completion axillary dissection in sentinel lymph node-positive breast cancer patients is associated with the use of a multivariate nomogram. *Ann Surg.* 2007;245:462-468.

CHAPTER 27

Minimal Residual Cancer

Stephan Braun
Bjorn Naume
Elin Borgen

The genesis of overt metastases in breast cancer is based on the idea that tumor cells that dissociate from the primary cancer get access to circulation either directly into blood vessels or after transit in lymphatic channels. Thus detection of such cells in patients with newly diagnosed solid tumors has been an appealing strategy to provide evidence for future metastases.

In the past, several models have been constructed to explain the presence of individual tumor cells in secondary organs and their influence on the subsequent course of the disease. Currently, according to most recent transcriptome and genome analyses, tumor cells circulating in the bloodstream (CTCs) and those already disseminated to secondary organs (DTCs) are viewed as rare and much earlier indicators of tumor cell spread than generally assumed from the typical year-long course of cancerous diseases, such as breast cancer. Despite the observation that the numerous genetic alterations found so far in such cells are rarely identical or even similar, the idea that some of these cells might be progenitor cells with self-renewing properties that give rise to most of the tumor mass that is dealt with clinically is supported by the following: (1) the long interval between dissemination and clinical manifestation of metastases, (2) the frequently observed relative resistance of some cells to chemotherapy, and (3) their significant effect on disease progression, despite their low abundance in secondary organs.

Beyond the discussion of such models and opinions, the actual presence of tumor cells outside the primary tumor and in organs relevant for subsequent metastasis formation, such as bone and bone marrow, would serve 3 purposes that could be clinically useful:

1. As unambiguous evidence for an early occult spread of tumor cells
2. As a relevant risk factor for subsequent metastasis and thus a poor prognosis
3. As a marker for monitoring treatment susceptibility

Finally, and perhaps as importantly in the long run, genotyping and phenotyping of these cells should provide detailed insight into the metastatic process and permit direct exploration of targeted treatment strategies.

TECHNICAL ADVANCEMENTS

The 2 main approaches for the assessment of minimal residual cancer—both for DTCs and CTCs—are immunologic assays using monoclonal antibodies directed against histogenetic proteins and polymerase chain reaction (PCR)–based molecular assays exploiting tissue-specific transcripts. In review of the last decades, the immunologic approach emerged in the first place due to the technological availability, whereas molecular techniques seem to have taken over in the last few years.

Detection of Tumor Cell Dissemination

Tumor cells evaded or shed to the blood circulation may be detectable in peripheral venous blood and, in principle, all body organs, as shown in a few elegant experiments during the 1960s and 1970s.[1,2] When specific monoclonal antibodies became broadly available in the 1980s, the interest in the identification of spread tumor cells was renewed. The first study groups,[3-8] however, did not investigate peripheral blood, presumably due to pathophysiologic considerations, the presence of tumor cells in circulation was thought to be merely temporary. For similar theoretical reasons, the initial studies did not investigate epithelial parenchymous organs, such as lung, liver, or brain, known to be frequently colonized by epithelial cancer cells, because specific antibodies available at that time largely only discriminated between the histogenetic origin of cells, although they were raised against tumor-associated antigens. The ability to detect nonautochthonous epithelial breast cancer cells in a mesenchymal organ environment, characterized by a physiologic absence of epithelial cells, its relevance for breast cancer metastases, and the clinical convenience to explore (ie, diagnose) the organ site of interest led to numerous studies investigating the presence and significance of hematogenously disseminated tumor cells in bone marrow samples.[9-18]

Immunologic Approaches

Protocols for the direct analysis of unprocessed samples exist, but most approaches require an enrichment of DTCs and/or CTCs before application of the detection technology. Enrichment is usually based on either density-gradient centrifugation or immunomagnetic procedures[19,30] since its introduction in the early 1980s[20] and validation thereafter.[21-23]

Of particular note, we have to appreciate the varying quality of immunologic stainings, as we learned our lessons from the HER-2 and the hormone receptor stories during the past decade. Nevertheless, the first question that arises is that of the putative origin of the detected cells, as "positive" staining may have multiplex reasons. The strongest and most likely unequivocal reason to accept that DTCs are of epithelial origin stems from analysis of control samples. Among various series of either healthy candidates or patients with benign disease conditions, reports of positively stained cells usually aroused skepticism on the validity of the approach. Sorting out unspecific staining by both adherence to morphologic criteria and exclusion of immunologic artifacts (both factors we address in details below), the true false-positive rate ranges between 1% and 5% in the hands of experienced and devoted laboratory experts.[14,24-26] The currently accepted benchmark technology for the detection of DTCs and CTCs implies Ficoll-Hypaque density centrifugation, collection of mononucleated cells from the interphase layer, and subsequent preparation of cytospins by using a cytocentrifuge, most often applying 5 to 10 × 10[5] mononucleated cells per slide, followed by immunostaining for epithelial cells on cytospins. Crucial steps in this process are sampling techniques and the methods used for immunostaining, including the choice of antibodies.[27,28] The proof of concept and the demonstration of the clinical utility of this approach has been shown in a recent pooled analysis.[29] The most widely used monoclonal antibodies are A45-B/B3[31] and AE1/AE3,[32] for which clinical significance is well documented in numerous clinical trials.[17,29,33-36]

The alkaline phosphatase anti-alkaline phosphatase (APAAP) visualization system,[37] in combination with the red chromogen New Fuchsin, represents the immunostaining method most widely used. It is known that false-positive staining of hematopoietic cells (HCs) does occur.[24] Mechanisms for such unintended reactions include direct binding of alkaline phosphatase (as part of the APAAP detection system) to plasma/preplasma cells,[26] cross-reactivity of the primary anti-epithelial antibodies with HC epitopes, and interactions with Fc receptors present on leukocytes. Morphologic evaluation of immunocytochemistry-visualized cells is feasible[25,38]; however, it is noteworthy that morphologic overlap between tumor cells and false-positive

HCs exists.[24-26,39] To exclude such unspecific interference, high quality approaches usually incorporate parallel immunostaining in which, for control purposes, additional sample slides are incubated with immunoglobulin isotype-identical antibodies directed against irrelevant antigens. Figure 27-1 exemplifies the analytical algorithm according to guidelines implemented by the European International Society for Hemotherapy and Graft Engineering (ISHAGE) Working Group for Standardization of Tumor Cell Detection.[25] The clinical validation on 817 patients with breast cancer[33] confirmed that only cells classified as "tumor cell" or "probable tumor cell" (Fig. 27-1A through 27-1D), and tumor cells despite signs of degeneration (Fig. 27-1I and 27-1J) signified poor prognosis, as compared with presence of cells classified as HC (Fig. 27-1E through 27-1H).

PCR-Based Approaches

PCR methods targeting tissue-specific gene expression initiated a competitive race against immunocytochemistry for the detection of DTCs and CTCs in the beginning of the 1990s.[40-42] PCR-based assays are extremely sensitive and are able to detect a single cell in a sample of 2 × 10[7] or more white blood cells.[43] However, a few transcripts—for example, by either illegitimate low-level expression of the targeted mRNA in hematopoietic cells[44] or amplification of DNA-reassembling sequences[45] ("pseudogenes"), down-regulation of the actual gene in DTC/CTC, and possibly the presence of rare normal epithelial cells[46,47]—cause false-positive signals in noncancer controls, and only since the introduction of the quantitative real-time PCR (qPCR) methods has this problem been addressed.[48] In view of the lack of true cancer-specific molecular targets, qPCR became more or less the state-of-the-art quantitative method, allowing one to determine cut-off values of marker transcript numbers in samples of noncancer controls,[49-51] above which transcripts can be considered as tumor cell–derived. Moreover, the expression level of all known marker genes varies between tumors from different patients and even among cells of the same tumor. This cancer heterogeneity points to the use of multiple marker mRNAs.[57,58] Consequently, the discovery of sensitive mRNA markers has been approached using specific differential gene expression screening of primary tumors and normal tissue. The technical problems have been substantially reviewed and are beyond the scope of this section.[19,48,52] Nevertheless, recent data suggest prognostic significance for molecular CTC detection in breast cancer patients in various stages,[53-55] including patients with lymph node–negative disease.[56]

BIOLOGY OF HEMATOGENOUS TUMOR CELL DISSEMINATION

Biological Characteristics

In order to investigate the underlying biology of DTCs and CTCs, antibodies against tumor-associated antigens—in parallel with the (usually anticytokeratin) detection antibody—are used to profile these cells, predominantly to, among various reasons, determine what percentage of these cells are actually of neoplastic origin. Using such immunocytochemical procedures, it has

"TC"
(pathognomonic
TC features)

"TC?"
(final conclusion
depends on
negative
control findings)

Hematopoietic
cells
("false positives")

Hematopoietic
cells
("false positives")

Degenerated/
destroyed
tumor cells

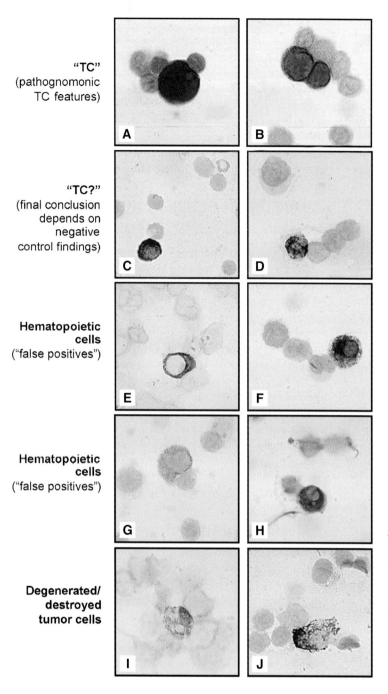

FIGURE 27-1 Categorization of immunostained cells for the detection of breast carcinoma cells in bone marrow and peripheral blood. "Tumor cell," pathognomonic features of epithelial tumor cell nature, with a clearly enlarged nucleus compared with the size of neighboring hematopoietic cells (**A**) and/or the formation of clearly immunostained tumor cell doublets/clusters (**B**), a morphology never observed in false-positive hematopoietic cells or in negative control specimens. "Probable tumor cells" represent a morphologic overlap between tumor cell and hematopoietic cell, lacking pathognomonic features of tumor cells, but morphologic signs of hematopoietic cell are also absent; typically cytoplasmic staining is strong (**C,D**), often irregularly distributed (**D**), and clearly overlaying the nucleus (**C,D**). "Hematopoietic cells" (so-called false positives): typical hematopoietic cell features include a small, hematopoietic cell-sized nucleus (**E–H**) with an even or regularly distributed cytoplasmic staining (**G,H**), which often is microvacuolar (**G**) and not overlying the nucleus (**E,G,H**); a small, pin-point vacuole is typically seen in the hematopoietic cell cytoplasm (**H**), whereas larger vacuoles may be present in actual tumor cells (**A**). "Destroyed/degenerated tumor cells" are tumor cells that show morphologic signs of degeneration and or destruction (**I,J**). *(Adapted and reproduced with permission from Borgen E, Naume B, Nesland JM, et al. Standardisation of the immunocytochemical detection of cancer cells in bone marrow and blood: I. Establishment of objective criteria for the evaluation of immunostained cells. Cytotherapy. 1999;1:377-388. and Naume B, Wiedswang G, Borgen E, et al. The prognostic value of isolated tumor cells in bone marrow in breast cancer patients: evaluation of morphological categories and the number of clinically significant cells. Clin Cancer Res. 2004;10:3091-3097.)*

been possible to identify frequent expression of urokinase-type plasminogen activator receptor (uPAR) in gastric cancer[59] and HER-2 (also known as ERBB2 or HER-2/neu) in breast cancer (Meng, 2004 #1582; Meng, 2004 #1584; Solomayer, 2006 #1627).[60] In both cases, the (over) expression was associated with poor clinical outcome, and uPAR and HER-2, as a consequence, might be important for the survival and growth of DTCs.[59,60]

Detailed examination of the genome was made possible by recent technical developments, such as the combination of immunocytochemistry and fluorescence in situ hybridization, which led to the demonstration that the bone marrow contains disseminated epithelial cells of malignant origin.[61] By developing a new procedure for whole-genome amplification and

subsequent comparative genomic hybridization of single immunostained cells, Klein and coworkers demonstrated that cytokeratin-positive cells in the bone marrow of patients with epithelial breast cancer without clinical signs of overt metastases (stage M0) are genetically heterogeneous.[62] This heterogeneity was strikingly reduced with the emergence of clinically evident metastasis (stage M1). Similar to these genomic analyses of DTCs, research groups showed the malignant nature and viability of CTCs from peripheral blood samples.[38,63-67]

The stage at which individual cells leave the primary tumor is unclear. In patients with early-stage invasive breast cancer, the cytokeratin-positive cells isolated from the bone marrow had few features in common with those found in their respective primary tumors.[68] A provocative interpretation of this surprising finding is that the DTCs separated from their primary tumor at a very early stage. This hypothesis is also supported by the finding that only a few DTCs in these patients had TP53 mutations, which are associated with the later stages of tumorigenesis.[62,69] DTCs might therefore evolve independently into overt metastases, driven by the specific selective pressures of the bone marrow environment.[70]

Genetic analyses that compared paired primary and metastatic breast tumor samples confirm the hypothesis that DTCs evolve independently from the primary tumor. The patterns of genetic alterations that are observed in overt metastases are often discordant with those of the primary tumor and differ almost completely in approximately one-third of the cases.[71] During genetic progression of the primary breast tumor, cancer cells might disseminate continuously, acquiring additional genetic alterations after migration into secondary organs such as the bone marrow.

Minimal Residual Cancer and the Concept of Targeted Therapy

The advent of targeted therapy in oncologic treatment of patients with breast cancer was praised as the major momentum of the last decade. Surprisingly enough, review of the literature and both ongoing and completed clinical trials show the discrepancy between pretension and reality. The approaches rarely ever seek to demonstrate that the target is present on residual tumor—it is without saying that assessment of protein expression of primary tumor cells does not fulfill the criteria to call a patient "target-positive" because neither residual tumor cells may be present nor residual tumor cells may express the target. The data for the latter hypothesis stem from DTC and CTC characterizing studies. The most prevalent therapeutic targets—such as estrogen receptor and HER-2—are heterogeneously expressed in DTCs and/or CTCs, and extrapolation from the corresponding primary tumor to the spread tumor cell pool usually failed to confirm concordance. Fehm and colleagues[72] showed that primary tumor cells and DTCs had a concordant estrogen receptor status in only 28% among 38 patients with DTCs in bone marrow and an estrogen receptor positive primary tumor. Similarly, Schardt et al[73] and Solomayer et al[65] recently showed in their molecular and immunologic analyses, respectively, that a concordant HER-2 status may be observed in as few as 4% of the patients. In addition to these data, Balic et al[74] analyzed similarities between the proposed stem cell phenotype and the phenotype of DTCs in breast cancer patients. The results indicated that almost all patients with DTCs have stem cell–like DTCs in the detectable pool of their DTCs and, moreover, that the majority of DTCs have a stem cell–like phenotype.[74] These findings support the previous data on both estrogen receptor negativity and HER-2 heterogeneity, which are usually found in tumor cells with stem cell or progenitor cell characteristics.

Obviously, such data are strong arguments to explain failure of obviously effective treatment strategies for which efficacy has been demonstrated in clinical trials of metastatic breast cancer patients in which—at least sometimes—the biology of the metastatic lesion is assessed, but where the response is almost always monitored according to Response Evaluation Criteria in Solid Tumors (RECIST). This principle has been left out of adjuvant treatment approaches, most likely because of the lack of (or perhaps ignorance to) an appropriate surrogate marker.

Given the clinical evidence for the prognostic importance of viable tumor cell dissemination, the emerging data on the heterogeneity, and differential phenotypic and genotypic pattern of CTCs and DTCs as compared with the parental tumor cells, the observations on biological characteristics of such cells are immediately indicative of the clinical need to rethink current treatment decision algorithms and future study designs.

TUMOR CELL DETECTION IN THE CLINICAL CONTEXT

When Steven Paget published his theory of "seed and soil" in 1889,[75] the idea of hematogenous tumor cell dissemination was born. More than a century later, with molecular tools being available, new clinical findings explained hitherto unexplainable phenomena, such as donor-derived cancer in recipient organ allografts[76] or detection of viable single tumor cells in secondary organs being both descendants of a known primary tumor[77] and potential precursors of subsequent metastasis.[29] The fulfillment of the request for factors enabling individual risk assessment seems to be on the horizon. Yet, in breast cancer, recent guidelines for adjuvant systemic therapy still foresee treatment recommendations for more than 90% of patients, even in case of a negative lymph node status.[78-80] The risk of tumor relapse in these patients is considered high enough to recommend adjuvant therapy, even though up to 70% of early-stage breast cancer patients are cured by locoregional surgery alone.

Staging Revisited

For their broad utilization, markers need to be implemented into current risk classification systems, such as the Tumor-Node-Metastasis (TNM) classification. Although the decision upon implementation appears to be pending since the 1990s, when DTCs were mentioned for the first time in the TNM Supplement,[81,82] a useful proposal for an appropriate TNM terminology has recently been made by the International Union Against Cancer.[83] The most recent TNM classification for breast cancer[84] does not qualify the presence of single cancer cells in peripheral blood or bone marrow as metastasis (stage M0), but it optionally reports the presence of such cells together with their detection method (eg, M0[i+] or [mol+]) in analogy to its use for description of the presence of micrometastasis or isolated tumor cells in lymph nodes. CTCs and DTCs were only recently cited for the first time in the American Society of Clinical Oncology's 2007 recommendations on the use of tumor markers.[85]

Prognostic Value of Tumor Cell Detection

In order to determine the actual significance of DTCs in bone marrow for the outcome and survival of breast cancer patients, the literature basis is ample. To date, most experience with bone marrow screening for DTCs exists for immunocytochemical analyses. Numerous studies reported a strong prognostic impact of the presence of DTCs,[8,11-18,86-88] whereas other investigations failed to do so.[5,6,10,89-91] One reason for the discrepant results of clinical follow-up studies is a substantial methodologic variation (eg, sensitivity and specificity of detection antibody, lower detection rate of bone marrow biopsy as compared with bone marrow aspiration, and considerable variation in the number of cells analyzed) resulting in a wide range of detection rates between study populations.

However, even if only large, well-designed, and controlled studies are now considered for a summarizing statement on the prognostic significance of DTCs, at least 3 confounding technical factors varied considerably: (1) consistent and blinded analysis of noncarcinoma control patients, (2) diversity of antibodies used for identification of epithelial cells in bone marrow, and (3) number of cells analyzed per patient sample.

In the past, 2 studies therefore attempted to solve this dilemma, performing meta-analyses of the published studies.[92,93] However, several authors suggested that the ideal way to perform a meta-analysis of survival data would be to use individual patient data.[94,95] Using individual patient data instead

would have the advantage of including information on patient characteristics, accounting for differences in immunoassays, and considering variability in treatment over time. Therefore, a large pooled analysis of individual patient data of 4703 breast cancer patients from 8 large studies[13-18,86] now provides conclusive data on the adverse prognostic influence of presence of DTCs on the clinical outcome and survival of patients with stage I, II, and III breast cancer.[29] DTCs are present in up to one-third of patients with stage I, II, and III breast cancer. As compared with women without DTCs, patients with DTCs had larger tumors, tumors with a higher histologic grade, lymph node metastases, and hormone receptor–negative tumors (for all variables, $p < 0.001$). The presence of DTC was a significant prognostic factor for poor overall and breast cancer–specific survival and disease-free and distant metastasis–free survival during the 10-year observation period (univariate mortality ratios, 2.15, 2.44, 2.13, and 2.33, respectively; for all, $p < 0.001$) (Fig. 27-2). In multivariable analysis, presence

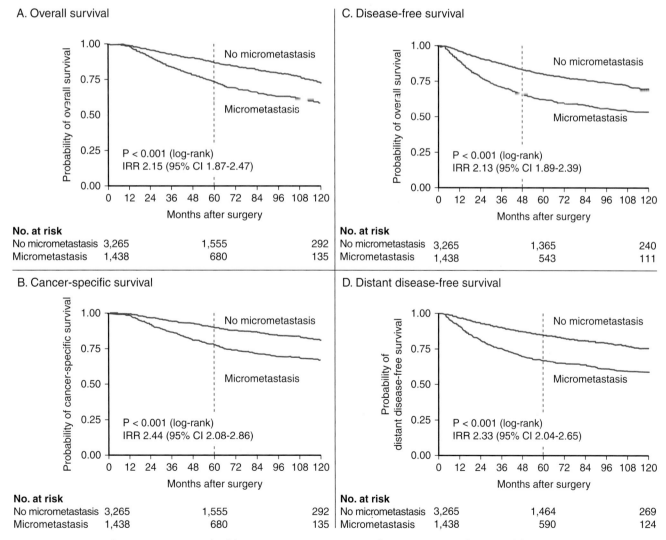

FIGURE 27-2 Kaplan-Meier estimates of long-term patient outcome by presence or absence of bone marrow micrometastasis. Panels show estimates of overall **(A)**, cancer-specific **(B)**, disease-free **(C)**, and distant disease-free survival **(D)** for the complete patient group. The vertical dotted lines in **A-D** divide the time intervals used for piecewise Cox regression modeling. CI, confidence interval; IRR, incidence rate ratio. *(Reproduced with permission from Braun S, Vogl FD, Naume B, et al. A pooled analysis of bone marrow micrometastasis in breast cancer. N Engl J Med. 2005;353:793-802.)*

TABLE 27-1 Multivariable Hazard Ratios for Overall and Cancer-Specific Survival at Different Time Intervals (Adjusted for Center)

	HR (95% CI)	p	HR (95% CI)	p
Overall survival*	Follow-up interval years 0-5 (N=3974)		Follow-up interval years 6-10[†] (N=1674)	
Bone marrow micrometastasis	1.81 (1.51-2.16)	<0.001	1.58 (1.12-2.22)	0.009
Tumor size	1.70 (1.50-1.94)[†]	<0.001	—	
Lymph node metastasis	1.63 (1.50-1.77)[†]	<0.001	1.88 (1.61-2.21)[†]	<0.001
Tumor grade	1.72 (1.44-2.06)	<0.001	—	
Hormone receptor	0.56 (0.47-0.68)	<0.001	—	
Cancer-specific survival*	Follow-up interval, years 0-5 (N=3974)		Follow-up interval, years 6-10[‡] (N=1674)	
Bone marrow micrometastasis	1.93 (1.58-2.36)	<0.001	1.63 (1.07-2.47)	0.022
Tumor size	1.67 (1.44-1.94)[†]	<0.001	—	
Lymph node metastasis	1.71 (1.55-1.89)[†]	<0.001	1.98 (1.64-2.40)[†]	<0.001
Tumor grade	1.75 (1.43-2.15)	<0.001	—	
Hormone receptor	0.50 (0.41-0.61)	<0.001	—	

*Comparison of variable categories: Bone marrow micrometastasis, negative versus positive; tumor size, T1 versus T2 versus T3/T4; lymph node metastasis, N0 versus N1 versus N2 versus N3; tumor grade: G1/G2 versus G3; hormone receptor, negative versus any receptor positive.

[†]Hazard ratio (HR) for linear trend test across categories.

[‡]A separate model was fit for the second interval; blanks indicate that no risk estimates are available for variables that dropped from the final model according to the selection process. Modified with permission from Braun S, Vogl FD, Naume B, et al. A pooled analysis of bone marrow micrometastasis in breast cancer. *N Engl J Med.* 2005;353:793-802.

of DTCs was an independent predictor of poor patient outcome (Table 27-1).

Predictive Value of Tumor Cell Detection

Beyond merely adding another prognostic factor to the plethora of such markers in breast cancer, it must be emphasized that assessment of occult hematogenous tumor cell spread inherits the potential for a tool for prediction and monitoring of efficacy of systemic therapy.[96-100] In contrast to lymph nodes, which are generally accepted as "indirect" markers of hematogenous tumor cell spread and, hence, risk of systemic spread, but which are also generally removed at primary surgery and unavailable for follow-up evaluations, bone marrow and blood can be obtained repeatedly in the postoperative course of the patient. Of all clinically utilized and/or established factors, the only prognostic factors available for follow-up risk assessment, in principle, are DTCs or CTCs. For DTCs, the clinical value of such examinations has been strongly suggested by clinical studies on a total of almost 500 patients in which the prognostic relevance of DTCs present in bone marrow several months after diagnosis or treatment when no relapse has occurred until that date has been identified.[35,99,101] The potential of a surrogate marker assay that permits immediate assessment of therapy-induced cytotoxic effects on occult metastatic cells is therefore evident, as indicated previously.[99] Because repeated bone marrow sampling might not be easily implemented into clinical study protocols for breast cancer, serial examinations of blood for CTC or tumor cell–associated nucleic acids might be

more acceptable for most patients and clinical investigators[30] than repeated bone marrow aspirations. The detection and characterization of CTCs in peripheral blood of patients with cancer has therefore received much attention in recent years and could lead to strategies for evaluation of therapeutic efficacy. This approach has been successfully realized in metastatic breast cancer[30,102] and in lungcancer,[103,104] but no data is available for those patients in which adjuvant therapy is applied in a curative intent.

For the time being, and with validated assays being available for the evaluation of bone marrow only, prospective clinical studies are now required to evaluate whether eradication of DTCs in bone marrow and CTCs in blood after systemic therapy translates into a longer disease-free period and overall survival. In translational research approaches, the question should be addressed whether number of DTCs before, during, and after randomized treatment is indicative of patient outcome or whether assessments of tumor-specific mutations in CTCs,[103] as well as disseminated or circulating methylated DNA,[105] could provide similar information that might be available from more convenient and perhaps even more reliable analytical approaches.

Monitoring of Minimal Residual Cancer

Although current treatment decisions are scheduled in review of the primary tumor material, which is usually removed during primary surgery and represents a frozen view on the tumor biology at that time, repeated bone marrow aspirations and blood sampling provide a window for continuous assessment of the presence[35,99,101,106] and biology of the residual tumor load. In a first explorative study, we showed that the presence of DTCs after taxane- and/or anthracycline-containing chemotherapy in advanced breast cancer patients was associated with poor prognosis and that response to treatment was unpredictably heterogeneous.[99]

FUTURE DIRECTIONS

Biology: Self-Seeding

In synopsis of the data on DTCs and CTCs presented here, and in knowledge of the work by Norton and Massagué,[107] the analogy between both research concepts becomes clearly visible. Features of tumor progression, such as high cell density, rapid growth rate, and large population size, which contribute to a pathologically high ratio of cell production to cell death, might also or instead result from inappropriate cell movement, already understood to underlie invasion and metastasis. The integrating concept for numerous research findings, including gene signatures for organ-specific metastasis,[108,109] is the concept of self-seeding, which postulates that partially overlapping mediators exist for both self-seeding in the primary site (which contributes to growth of the primary tumor and circulation and dissemination of tumor cells) and in the secondary site (which contributes to growth of the metastatic lesion, tumor-type–specific metastasis patterns, and sequences). Apparently, CTCs and DTCs are actors in this concept, and their biologic characteristics seem to be a suitable script for their role in a self-seeding scenario. Further research on the DTC/CTC phenotype and genotype will help to elucidate the actual role of CTCs and DTCs in metastatic progression.

Clinical Trials

The clinical utility of translational research findings on DTCs and CTCs will have to be demonstrated in classic randomized clinical trials. The time gap between statements on the readiness of DTCs and CTCs for clinical implementation[30,102,110-113] and the initiation of such trials reflects the difficulties to convince stakeholders of current oncologic treatment strategies and in the pharmaceutical industry. The data are there and the risks of novel and modified trials have to be undertaken. There is no doubt that the risks are high, which is shown by the history of trials failing to complete recruitment[100] (see also http://www.abcsg.at for further information). Currently, there are at least 4 trials underway to examine the clinical utility of DTC/CTC assessment and monitoring in patients with breast cancer. The Norwegian cooperative SATT trial (NBCG9) (see http://www.cancer.gov/clinicaltrials/NBCG9/ for further information) has completed inclusion of 1128 patients. The trial investigates presence of DTCs after 6 cycles of fluorouracil, epirubicin, and cyclophosphamide and offers an additional 6 cycles of docetaxel in case of a positive DTC status, thereby assessing the rate of DTC eradication and clinical outcome to support the use of DTCs as a surrogate for clinical outcome if the baseline risk of recurrence associated with the presence of DTCs is altered by therapeutic intervention. The SWOG S0500 randomized trial, led by the

Southwest Oncology group (see http://www.cancer.gov/clinicaltrials/SWOG-S0500/ for further information), examines whether patients with metastatic breast cancer and increased levels of CTCs after 3 weeks of first-line chemotherapy show an improved survival and progression-free survival when changing to an alternative chemotherapy regimen rather than waiting for clinically manifest progression. The GEPARQuattro trial (see http://www.germanbreastgroup.de/geparquattro/ for further information) investigates the efficacy of primary chemotherapy in locally advanced, nonmetastatic breast cancer patients and the impact of persisting CTCs after chemotherapy. The significance of persisting CTCs after postsurgical adjuvant chemotherapy is an objective of the SUCCESS trial (see http://www.success-studie.de/ for further information).

Although the latter 2 trials are classic randomized clinical trials and the objectives of CTC assessment are merely secondary study objectives, the SWOG S0500 trial, besides the prematurely terminated Austrian Breast and Colorectal Cancer Study Group (ABCSG) trial 21 (@fame), is the only ongoing trial with the primary study objective directly linked to the concept of CTC assessment and monitoring. Consequently, this is the only trial as of now that will deliver an answer on the clinical utility of CTC examination in the setting of metastatic breast cancer. Clinical trials for both DTCs and CTCs in the adjuvant setting are still to be designed and conducted before the concept of minimal residual cancer can be implemented in the armamentarium of treatment modalities against breast cancer.

SUMMARY

The currently available data unequivocally show that level 1a evidence exists for the prognostic value of DTC detection. DTCs and CTCs appear to be relevant for metastatic progression, can survive current chemotherapy, might indicate failure of therapeutic interventions, and provide a diagnostic source of the residual tumor cell load, allowing for considerations to switch to alternative treatment modalities. Prospective randomized clinical phase III trials are now needed to investigate the predictive value of CTCs and DTCs.

REFERENCES

1. Zeidman I. The fate of circulating tumors cells. I. Passage of cells through capillaries. *Cancer Res.* 1961;21:38-39.
2. Fidler IJ. Quantitative analysis of distribution and fate of tumor emboli labeled with ^{125}I-5-iodo-2 -desoxyuridine. *J Natl Cancer Inst.* 1970;145:773-782.
3. Mansi JL, Berger U, Easton D, et al. Micrometastases in bone marrow in patients with primary breast cancer: evaluation as an early predictor of bone metastases. *Br Med J.* 1987;295:1093-1096.
4. Untch M, Harbeck N, Eiermann W. Micrometastases in bone marrow in patients with breast cancer. *Br J Med.* 1988;296:290.
5. Porro G, Menard S, Tagliabue E, et al. Monoclonal antibody detection of carcinoma cells in bone marrow biopsy specimens from breast cancer patients. *Cancer.* 1988;61:2407-2411.
6. Salvadori B, Squicciarini P, Rovini D, et al. Use of monoclonal antibody MBr1 to detect micrometastases in bone marrow specimens of breast cancer patients. *Eur J Cancer.* 1990;26:865-867.
7. Kirk SJ, Cooper GG, Hoper M, et al. The prognostic significance of marrow micrometastases in women with early breast cancer. *Eur J Surg Oncol.* 1990;16:481-485.

8. Cote RJ, Rosen PP, Lesser ML, Old LJ, Osborne MP. Prediction of early relapse in patients with operable breast cancer by detection of occult bone marrow micrometastases. *J Clin Oncol*. 1991;9:1749-1756.

9. Mansi JL, Berger U, Wilson P, Shearer R, Coombes RC. Detection of tumor cells in bone marrow of patients with prostatic carcinoma by immunocytochemical techniques. *J Urology*. 1988;139:545-548.

10. Funke I, Fries S, Rolle M, et al. Comparative analyses of bone marrow micrometastases in breast and gastric cancer. *Int J Cancer*. 1996;65:755-761.

11. Diel IJ, Kaufmann M, Costa SD, et al. Micrometastatic breast cancer cells in bone marrow at primary surgery: prognostic value in comparison with nodal status. *J Natl Cancer Inst*. 1996;88:1652-1664.

12. Landys K, Persson S, Kovarik J, Hultborn R, Holmberg E. Prognostic value of bone marrow biopsy in operable breast cancer patients at the time of initial diagnosis: results of a 20-year median follow-up. *Breast Cancer Res Treat*. 1998;49:27-33.

13. Mansi JL, Gogas H, Bliss JM, et al. Outcome of primary-breast-cancer patients with micrometastases: a long-term follow-up. *Lancet*. 1999;354: 197-202.

14. Braun S, Pantel K, Müller P, et al. Cytokeratin-positive cells in the bone marrow and survival of patients with stage I, II or III breast cancer. *N Engl J Med*. 2000;342:525-533.

15. Gebauer G, Fehm T, Merkle E, et al. Epithelial cells in bone marrow of breast cancer patients at time of primary surgery: clinical outcome during long-term follow-up. *J Clin Oncol*. 2001;19:3669-3674.

16. Gerber B, Krause A, Muller H, et al. Simultaneous immunohistochemical detection of tumor cells in lymph nodes and bone marrow aspirates in breast cancer and its correlation with other prognostic factors. *J Clin Oncol*. 2001;19:960-971.

17. Wiedswang G, Borgen E, Karesen R, et al. Detection of isolated tumor cells in bone marrow is an independent prognostic factor in breast cancer. *J Clin Oncol*. 2003;21:3469-3478.

18. Pierga J-Y, Bonneton C, Vincent-Salomon A, et al. Clinical significance of immunocytochemical detection of tumor cells using digital microscopy in peripheral blood and bone marrow of breast cancer patients. *Clin Cancer Res*. 2004;10:1392-1400.

19. Pantel K, Brakenhoff RH, Brandt B. Detection, clinical relevance and specific biological properties of disseminating tumour cells. *Nat Rev Cancer*. 2008;8:329-340.

20. Sloane J, Ormerod M, Imrie S, Coombes R. The use of antisera to epithelial membrane antigen in detection micrometastases in histological sections. *Br J Cancer*. 1980;42:392-398.

21. Muller V, Stahmann N, Riethdorf S, et al. Circulating tumor cells in breast cancer: correlation to bone marrow micrometastases, heterogeneous response to systemic therapy and low proliferative activity. *Clin Cancer Res*. 2005;11:3678-3685.

22. Dearnaley D, Ormerod M, Sloane J. Micrometastases in breast cancer: long-term follow-up of the first patient cohort. *Eur J Cancer*. 1991;27:236-239.

23. Boyum A, Lovhaug D, Tresland L, Nordlie E. Separation of leucocytes: improved cell purity by fine adjustments of gradient medium density and osmolality. *Scand J Immunol*. 1991;34:697-712.

24. Borgen E, Pantel K, Schlimok G, et al. A European interlaboratory testing of three well-known procedures for immunocytochemical detection of epithelial cells in bone marrow. Results from analysis of normal bone marrow. *Cytometry B Clin Cytom*. 2006;70B:400-409.

25. Borgen E, Naume B, Nesland JM, et al. Standardisation of the immunocytochemical detection of cancer cells in bone marrow and blood: I. Establishment of objective criteria for the evaluation of immunostained cells. *Cytotherapy*. 1999;1:377-388.

26. Borgen E, Beiske K, Trachsel S, et al. Immunocytochemical detection of isolated epithelial cells in bone marrow: non-specific staining and contribution by plasma cells directly reactive to alkaline phosphatase. *J Pathol*. 1998;185:427-434.

27. Riethdorf S, Fritsche H, Muller V, et al. Detection of circulating tumor cells in peripheral blood of patients with metastatic breast cancer: a validation study of the CellSearch system. *Clin Cancer Res*. 2007;13:920-928.

28. Fehm T, Braun S, Muller V, et al. A concept for the standardized detection of disseminated tumor cells in bone marrow from patients with primary breast cancer and its clinical implementation. *Cancer*. 2006;107:885-892.

29. Braun S, Vogl FD, Naume B, et al. A pooled analysis of bone marrow micrometastasis in breast cancer. *N Engl J Med*. 2005;353:793-802.

30. Cristofanilli M, Budd GT, Ellis MJ, et al. Circulating tumor cells, disease progression and survival in metastatic breast cancer. *N Engl J Med*. 2004;351:781-791.

31. Karsten U, Widmaier R, Kunde D. Monoclonal antibodies against antigens of the human mammary carcinoma cell line MCF-7. *Arch Geschwulstforsch*. 1983;53:529-536.

32. Woodcock-Mitchell J, Fichner R, Nelson W, Sun T. Immunolocalization of keratin polypeptides in human epidermis using monoclonal antibodies. *J Cell Biol*. 1982;95:580-588.

33. Naume B, Wiedswang G, Borgen E, et al. The prognostic value of isolated tumor cells in bone marrow in breast cancer patients: evaluation of morphological categories and the number of clinically significant cells. *Clin Cancer Res*. 2004;10:3091-3097.

34. Wiedswang G, Borgen E, Kåresen R, et al. Isolated tumor cells in bone marrow three years after diagnosis in disease free breast cancer patients predict unfavourable clinical outcome. *Breast Cancer Res Treat*. 2003,82: S8. Abstract 8.

35. Wiedswang G, Borgen E, Kåresen R, et al. Isolated tumor cells in bone marrow 3 years after diagnosis in disease free breast cancer patients predict unfavorable clinical outcome. *Clin Cancer Res*. 2004;10: 5342-5348.

36. Wiedswang G, Borgen E, Schirmer C, et al. Comparison of the clinical significance of occult tumor cells in blood and bone marrow in breast cancer. *Int J Cancer*. 2006;118:2013-2019.

37. Cordell JL, Falini B, Erber WN, et al. Immunoenzymatic labeling of monoclonal antibodies using immune complexes of alkaline phosphatase and monoclonal anti-alkaline phosphatase (APAAP-complexes). *J Histochem Cytochem*. 1984;32:219-229.

38. Meng S, Tripathy D, Frenkel EP, et al. Circulating tumor cells in patients with breast cancer dormancy. *Clin Cancer Res*. 2004;10:8152-8162.

39. Borgen E, Naume B, Nesland JM, et al. Use of automated microscopy for the detection of disseminated tumor cells in bone marrow samples. *Cytometry*. 2001;46:215-221.

40. Benoy IH, Elst H, Van der Auwera I, et al. Real-time RT-PCR correlates with immunocytochemistry for the detection of disseminated epithelial cells in bone marrow aspirates of patients with breast cancer. *Br J Cancer*. 2004;91:1813-1820.

41. Slade MJ, Smith BM, Sinnett HD, Cross NCP, Coombes RC. Quantitative polymerase chain reaction for the detection of micrometastases in patients with breast cancer. *J Clin Oncol*. 1999;17:870-879.

42. Datta YH, Adams PT, Drobyski WR. Sensitive detection of occult breast cancer by the reverse-transcriptase polymerase chain reaction. *J Clin Oncol*. 1994;12:475-482.

43. Brakenhoff RH, Stroomer JGW, Brink Ct, et al. Sensitive detection of squamous cells in bone marrow and blood of head and neck cancer patients by E48 reverse transcriptase-polymerase chain reaction. *Clin Cancer Res*. 1999;5:725-732.

44. Traweek ST, Liu J, Battifora H. Keratin gene expression in non-epithelial tissues. Detection with polymerase chain reaction. *Am J Pathol*. 1993;142:1111-1118.

45. Ruud P, Fodstad Ø, Hovig E. Identification of a novel CK-19 pseudogene that may interfere with reverse-transcriptase-polymerase chain reaction assays used to detect micrometastatic tumor cells. *Int J Cancer*. 1999;80:119-125.

46. Krismann M, Todt B, Schröder J, et al. Low specificity of cytokeratin 19 reverse transcriptase-polymerase chain reaction analyses for detection of hematogenous lung cancer dissemination. *J Clin Oncol*. 1995;13:2769-2775.

47. Schoenfeld A, Luqmani Y, Smith D, et al. Detection of breast cancer micrometastases in axillary lymph nodes by using polymerase chain reaction. *Cancer Res*. 1994;54:2986-2990.

48. van Houten VMM, Tabor MP, van den Brekel MWM, et al. Molecular assays for the diagnosis of minimal residual head-and-neck cancer: methods, reliability, pitfalls, and solutions. *Clin Cancer Res*. 2000;6:3803-3816.

49. Molloy T, Bosma A, van't Veer L. Towards an optimized platform for the detection, enrichment, and semi-quantitation circulating tumor cells. *Breast Cancer Res Treat*. 2008;112:297-307.

50. Slade M, Coombes R. The clinical significance of disseminated tumor cells in breast cancer. *Nat Clin Pract Oncol*. 2007;4:30-41.

51. Ring AE, Zabaglo L, Ormerod MG, Smith IE, Dowsett M. Detection of circulating epithelial cells in the blood of patients with breast cancer: comparison of three techniques. *Br J Cancer*. 2005;92:906-912.

52. Nolan T, Hands RE, Bustin SA. Quantification of mRNA using real-time RT-PCR. *Nat Protoc*. 2006;1:1559-1582.

53. Ignatiadis M, Kallergi G, Ntoulia M, et al. Prognostic value of the molecular detection of circulating tumor cells using a multimarker reverse transcription-PCR assay for cytokeratin 19, mammaglobin A, and HER2 in early breast cancer. *Clin Cancer Res*. 2008;14:2593-2600.

54. Ignatiadis M, Georgoulias V, Mavroudis D. Circulating tumor cells in breast cancer. *Curr Opin Obstet Gynecol*. 2008;20:55-60.

55. Ignatiadis M, Xenidis N, Perraki M, et al. Different prognostic value of cytokeratin-19 mRNA positive circulating tumor cells according to estrogen receptor and HER2 status in early-stage breast cancer. *J Clin Oncol*. 2007;25:5194-5202.

56. Xenidis N, Perraki M, Kafousi M, et al. Predictive and prognostic value of peripheral blood cytokeratin-19 mRNA-positive cells detected by real-time polymerase chain reaction in node-negative breast cancer patients. *J Clin Oncol.* 2006;24:3756-3762.

57. Nagrath S, Sequist LV, Maheswaran S, et al. Isolation of rare circulating tumour cells in cancer patients by microchip technology. *Nature.* 2007;450:1235-1239.

58. Krivacic RT, Ladanyi A, Curry DN, et al. A rare-cell detector for cancer. *Proc Natl Acad Sci USA.* 2004;101:10501-10504.

59. Heiss MM, Allgayer H, Gruetzner KU, et al. Individual development and uPA-receptor expression of disseminated tumour cells in bone marrow: a reference to early systemic disease in solid cancer. *Nat Med.* 1995;1:1035-1039.

60. Braun S, Heumos I, Schlimok G, et al. ErbB2 over-expression on occult metastatic cells in bone marrow predicts poor clinical outcome of stage I-III breast cancer patients. *Cancer Res.* 2001;61:1890-1895.

61. Solakoglu O, Maierhofer C, Lahr G, et al. Heterogeneous proliferative potential of occult metastatic cells in bone marrow of patients with solid epithelial tumors. *Proc Natl Acad Sci USA.* 2002;99:2246-2251.

62. Klein CA, Blankenstein TJF, Schmidt-Kittler O, et al. Genetic heterogeneity of single disseminated tumour cells in minimal residual cancer. *Lancet.* 2002;360:683-689.

63. Schwarzenbach H, Müller V, Beeger C, et al. A critical evaluation of loss of heterozygosity detected in tumor tissues, blood serum and bone marrow plasma from patients with breast cancer. *Breast Cancer Res.* 2007;9:R66.

64. Smirnov DA, Foulk BW, Doyle GV, et al. Global gene expression profiling of circulating endothelial cells in patients with metastatic carcinomas. *Cancer Res.* 2006;66:2918-2922.

65. Solomayer EF, Becker S, Pergola-Becker G, et al. Comparison of HER2 status between primary tumor and disseminated tumor cells in primary breast cancer patients. *Breast Cancer Res Treat.* 2006;98:179-184.

66. Meng S, Tripathy D, Shete S, et al. HER-2 gene amplification can be acquired as breast cancer progresses. *Proc Natl Acad Sci USA.* 2004;101:9393-9398.

67. Fehm T, Sagalowsky A, Clifford E, et al. Cytogenetic evidence that circulating epithelial cells in patients with carcinoma are malignant. *Clin Cancer Res.* 2002;8:2073-2084.

68. Schmidt-Kittler O, Ragg T, Daskalakis A, et al. From latent disseminated cells to overt metastasis: Genetic analysis of systemic breast cancer progression. *Proc Acad Natl Sci USA.* 2003;100:7737-7742.

69. Offner S, Schmaus W, Witter K, et al. p53 mutations are not required for early dissemination of cancer cells. *Proc Natl Acad Sci USA.* 1999;96:6942-6946.

70. Gray JW. Evidence emerges for early metastasis and parallel evolution of primary and metastatic tumors. *Cancer Cell.* 2003;4:4-6.

71. Kuukasjarvi T, Karhu R, Tanner M, et al. Genetic heterogeneity and clonal evolution underlying development of asynchronous metastasis in human breast cancer. *Cancer Res.* 1997;57:1597-1604.

72. Fehm T, Krawczyck N, Solomayer E, et al. ER alpha-status of disseminated tumor cells in bone marrow of primary breast cancer patients. *Breast Cancer Res.* 2008;10:R76.

73. Schardt JA, Meyer M, Hartmann CH, et al. Genomic analysis of single cytokeratin-positive cells from bone marrow reveals early mutational events in breast cancer. *Cancer Cell.* 2005;8:227-239.

74. Balic M, Lin H, Young L, et al. Most early disseminated cancer cells detected in bone marrow of breast cancer patients have a putative breast cancer stem cell phenotype. *Clin Cancer Res.* 2006;12:5615-5621.

75. Paget S. Distribution of secondary growths in cancer of the breast. *Lancet.* 1889;1:571.

76. Loh E, Couch FJ, Hendricksen C, et al. Development of donor-derived prostate cancer in a recipient following orthotopic heart transplantation. *JAMA.* 1997;277:133-137.

77. Klein CA, Schmidt-Kittler O, Schardt JA, et al. Comparative genomic hybridization, loss of heterozygosity, and DNA sequence analysis of single cells. *Proc Natl Acad Sci USA.* 1999;96:4494-4499.

78. Goldhirsch A, Glick JH, Gelber RD, Coates AS, Senn HJ. Meeting highlights: international consensus panel on the treatment of primary breast cancer. *J Clin Oncol.* 2001;19:3817-3827.

79. Goldhirsch A, Wood WC, Gelber RD, et al. Meeting highlights: updated international expert consensus on the primary therapy of early breast cancer. *J Clin Oncol.* 2003;21:3357-3365.

80. Goldhirsch A, Glick JH, Gelber RD, et al. Meeting highlights: international expert consensus on the primary therapy of early breast cancer 2005. *Ann Oncol.* 2005;16:1569-1583.

81. Hermanek P. What's new in TNM? *Pathol Res Pract.* 1994;190:97-102.

82. Hermanek P, Henson DE, Hutter RV, Sobin LH. *TNM Supplement 1993.* Berlin, Germany: Springer: 1993.

83. Hermanek P, Hutter RV, Sobin LH, Wittekind C. Classification of isolated tumor cells and micrometastases. *Cancer.* 1999;86:2668-2673.

84. Singletary SE, Allred C, Ashley P, et al. Revision of the American Joint Committee on Cancer Staging System for Breast Cancer. *J Clin Oncol.* 2002;20:3628-3636.

85. Harris L, Fritsche H, Mennel R, et al. American Society of Clinical Oncology 2007 update of recommendations for the use of tumor markers in breast cancer. *J Clin Oncol.* 2007;25:5287-5312.

86. Wong GYC, Yu QQ, Osborne MP. Bone marrow micrometastasis is a significant predictor of long-term relapse-free survival for breast cancer by a non-proportional hazards model. *Breast Cancer Res Treat.* 2003;82(suppl 1): S99. Abstract.

87. Braun S, Cevatli BS, Assemi C, et al. Comparative analysis of micrometastasis to the bone marrow and lymph nodes of node-negative breast cancer patients receiving no adjuvant therapy. *J Clin Oncol.* 2001;19:1468-1475.

88. Harbeck N, Untch M, Pache L, Eiermann W. Tumour cell detection in the bone marrow of breast cancer patients at primary therapy: results of a 3-year median follow-up. *Br J Cancer.* 1994;69:566-571.

89. Courtemanche DJ, Worth AJ, Coupland RW, Rowell JL, MacFarlane JK. Monoclonal antibody LICR-LON-M8 does not predict the outcome of operable breast cancer. *Can J Surg.* 1991;34:21-26.

90. Singletary SE, Larry L, Trucker SL, Spitzer G. Detection of micrometastatic tumor cells in bone marrow of breast carcinoma patients. *J Surg Oncol.* 1991;47:32-36.

91. Mathieu MC, Friedman S, Bosq J, et al. Immunohistochemical staining of bone marrow biopsies for detection of occult metastasis in breast cancer. *Breast Cancer Res Treat.* 1990;15:21-26.

92. Weinschenker P, Soares HP, Otavio Clark O, Del Giglio A. Immunocytochemical detection of epithelial cells in the bone marrow of primary breast cancer patients: a meta-analysis. *Breast Cancer Res Treat.* 2004;87:215-224.

93. Funke I, Schraut W. Meta-analysis of studies on bone marrow micrometastases: an independent prognostic impact remains to be substantiated. *J Clin Oncol.* 1998;16:557-566.

94. Hunink MG, Wong JB. Meta-analysis of failure-time data with adjustment for covariates. *Med Decis Making.* 1994;14:59-70.

95. Clarke MJ, Stewart LA. Obtaining data from randomised controlled trials: how much do we need for reliable and informative meta-analyses? *BMJ.* 1994;309:1007-1010.

96. Schlimok G, Pantel K, Loibner H, Fackler-Schwalbe I, Riethmüller G. Reduction of metastatic carcinoma cells in bone marrow by intravenously administered monoclonal antibody: towards a novel surrogate test to monitor adjuvant therapies of solid tumours. *Eur J Cancer.* 1995;31A:1799-1803.

97. Pantel K, Enzmann T, Köllermann J, et al. Immunocytochemical monitoring of micrometastatic disease: reduction of prostate cancer cells in bone marrow by androgen deprivation. *Int J Cancer.* 1997;71:521-525.

98. Braun S, Hepp F, Kentenich CRM, et al. Monoclonal antibody therapy with edrecolomab in breast cancer patients: monitoring of elimination of disseminated cytokeratin-positive tumor cells in bone marrow. *Clin Cancer Res.* 1999;5:3999-4004.

99. Braun S, Kentenich CRM, Janni W, et al. Lack of effect of adjuvant chemotherapy on the elimination of single dormant tumor cells in bone marrow of high-risk breast cancer patients. *J Clin Oncol.* 2000;18:80-86.

100. Thurm H, Ebel S, Kentenich C, et al. Rare expression of epithelial cell adhesion molecule on residual micrometastatic breast cancer cells after adjuvant chemotherapy. *Clin Cancer Res.* 2003;9:2598-2604.

101. Janni W, Rack B, Schindlbeck C, et al. The persistence of isolated tumor cells in bone marrow from patients with breast carcinoma predicts an increased risk for recurrence. *Cancer.* 2005;103:884-891.

102. Cristofanilli M. The "microscopic" revolution in breast carcinoma. *Cancer.* 2005;103:877-880.

103. Maheswaran S, Sequist LV, Nagrath S, et al. Detection of mutations in EGFR in circulating lung-cancer cells. *N Engl J Med.* 2008;359:366-377.

104. Schiller JH. Noninvasive monitoring of tumors. *N Engl J Med.* 2008;359:418-420.

105. Widschwendter M, Siegmund KD, Muller HM, et al. Association of breast cancer DNA methylation profiles with hormone receptor status and response to tamoxifen. *Cancer Res.* 2004;64:3807-3813.

106. Slade MJ, Singh A, Smith BM, et al. Persistence of bone marrow micrometastases in patients receiving adjuvant therapy for breast cancer: results at 4 years. *Int J Cancer.* 2005;114(1):94-100.

107. Norton L, Massagué J. Is cancer a disease of self-seeding? *Nat Med.* 2006;12:875-878.

108. Minn AJ, Gupta GP, Siegel PM, et al. Genes that mediate breast cancer metastasis to lung. *Nature.* 2005;436:518.

109. Minn AJ, Kang Y, Serganova I, et al. Distinct organ-specific metastatic potential of individual breast cancer cells and primary tumors. *J Clin Invest.* 2005;115:44-55.

110. Braun S, Vogl F, Schneitter A, et al. Disseminated tumor cells: are they ready for clinical use? *Breast.* 2007;16:51-54

111. Braun S, Naume B. Circulating and disseminated tumor cells. *J Clin Oncol.* 2005;23:1623-1626.

112. Braun S, Marth C. Circulating tumor cells in metastatic breast cancer: toward individualized treatment? *N Engl J Med.* 2004;351:824-826.

113. Braun S, Vogl FD, Janni W, et al. Evaluation of bone marrow in breast cancer patients: prediction of clinical outcome and response to therapy. *Breast.* 2003;12:397-404.

SECTION 3

IMAGING

Pat W. Whitworth
Terri-Ann Gizienski

CHAPTER 28

Mammography

Ian Grady
Pat Hansen

PERFORMANCE OF MAMMOGRAPHY: HISTORICAL PERSPECTIVE

The first mammogram was performed in 1913 by Albert Salomon, a surgeon in Berlin, using a standard x-ray machine on an excised breast and axilla. Dr. Salomon wanted to show that the cancer spread to the axillary lymph nodes from the breast. Unfortunately, Dr. Salomon's work was cut short by political turmoil in Germany, and we do not hear of radiographs of breast specimens again until 1927 when another German surgeon, Otto Kleinschmidt, describes a technique for imaging the breast that he attributed to his mentor, the plastic surgeon Dr. Erwyn Payr.

It was not until 1930 that a radiologist, Stafford L. Warren, from Rochester University, in New York, described an in vivo technique to image the breast preoperatively. He used a relatively sophisticated stereoscopic system with a grid mechanism to cut down on noise and intensifying screens to amplify the image. Little or no compression was used in these first mammograms. Still, Dr. Warren claimed to be correct 92% of the time when using this technique to predict malignancy.

In 1931, Walter Vogel, and subsequently Paul Seabold, described methods to distinguish benign from malignant lesions with mammography. Shortly thereafter, in 1938, radiologists named Jacob Gershon-Cohen and Albert Strickland published an article describing the radiographic changes in a woman's breast throughout her menstrual cycle and life history. Dr. Gershon-Cohen tirelessly correlated mammographic images and pathologic specimens throughout his career, in an attempt to convince his colleagues of the utility of mammography. Dr. Gerson-Cohen emphasized the importance of compression and image contrast, using 2 films to collect data from both the thicker posterior breast tissue and the thinner peripheral breast.

Despite his efforts, mammography was not used with any frequency until the 1950s.

In 1949, Raul Leborgne, in Uruguay, reported seeing microcalcifications in 30% of breast cancers using mammography. This rekindled interest in mammograms. Leborgne was the father of modern mammography, emphasizing good compression and spot/magnification to better see small structures. His large cone-shaped compression devices and careful descriptions of positioning, as well as calibration for exposure times, set the stage for our current techniques.

It was Robert Egan, however, who pulled all the technology together. By using high milliampere, low-kilovolt x-rays on industrial film with grids, he was able to effectively standardize screening mammography in the early 1960s.

In May 1963, the Cancer Control Program of the US Department of Public Health held a conference on mammography at M.D. Anderson Hospital to report the results of an initial national mammography study involving 24 institutions. The results showed a 21% false-negative rate and a 79% true-positive rate for screening studies using Egan's technique.[1] This was a milestone for women's imaging in the United States. Screening mammography was off to a tentative start.

STANDARD SCREENING VIEWS AND POSITIONING

Standard screening views have evolved from the original positions of Leborgne, with the woman lying on her side, to Egan's technique, where the woman stands or sits upright for her mammogram. This saves room in mammography departments, where space is usually at a premium and departments must be

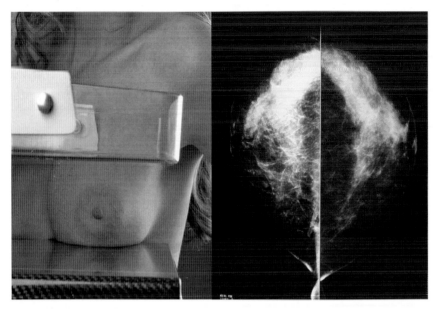

FIGURE 28-1 Patient in craniocaudad (CC) view on left, with CC mammogram on right.

border of the pectoralis major muscle. This angle varies with every patient; hence the adjustable arm of the mammography machine and the virtual 360 degree rotation of the device. The MLO view should always include some pectoralis muscle. Ideally, the pectoralis muscle should be seen to the level of the nipple (Fig. 28-4). The MLO view is the most inclusive view, especially for the upper outer quadrant of the breast, which includes the most cancers. The Swedish Two-County Trial was performed using only MLO views.[2] The MLO should be able to show about 95% of the breast tissue. Remember, the breast tissue can be found anywhere below the clavicles to the anterior stomach and from the midaxillary line to the sternum. Therefore 100% of breast tissue will not be covered, even by the best mammogram.

cost effective. The American College of Radiology (ACR) describes the standard screening mammographic views as craniocaudad (CC), mediolateral oblique (MLO), and mediolateral (ML). The patient positioning and position of the mammography machines are always the same for CC and ML views. The MLO view, however, varies based on a woman's body habitus.

The CC view is achieved with the woman facing the horizontal mammogram bucky and compression device, which should be at the level of her inframammary fold (Fig. 28-1). She must then lean into the bucky while the technologist elevates her breast into the compression space (Fig. 28-2). The compression paddle is lowered with the foot control by the technologist (Fig. 28-3). It is useful to tighten the device manually after automatic compression to achieve the most optimum pressure on the breast and to maximize visualization of small structures such as microcalcifications and small spiculated masses. An experienced technologist can palpate a woman's compressed breast and know if it has an appropriate amount of compression.

The ML view is not used in all cases. It is considered an additional view on screening cases unless the patient has augmentation or reconstructive breast implants in place. The ML view is achieved by placing the patient facing the vertical bucky and compression device. The technologist stands behind and to the outside of the patient as she is placed in the compression. The patient's arm is extended over the bucky to the body of the mammography machine. She leans into the bucky (on the outside of her breast), and the compression paddle closes in on her breast from the medial side (Fig. 28-4). It is important for the technologist to elevate the breast during positioning because this causes the breast tissue to stretch out and flatten in the most advantageous fashion.

The MLO view must be tailored to the woman's pectoralis muscle position. In the MLO view, the compression plates and bucky are angled from the vertical to be parallel to the lateral

TECHNICAL ASPECTS OF EXPOSURE AND RADIATION DOSE

The carcinogenic risk associated with low-dose mammography is small but not negligible. Accordingly, attempts have been made to lower mammographic dose over the years while continuing to improve the quality of mammographic imaging.

Initially, mammograms were performed with standard x-ray machines using a tungsten target and standard x-ray filter and film. Low-dose mammography (using 18 to 40 keV) was started by Egan, using molybdenum targets and filters and higher

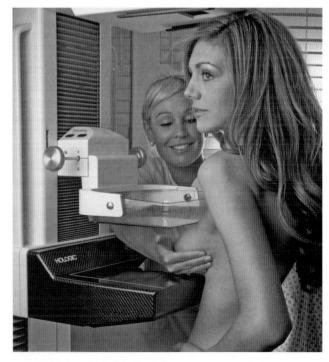

FIGURE 28-2 Placing the breast in the craniocaudad position.

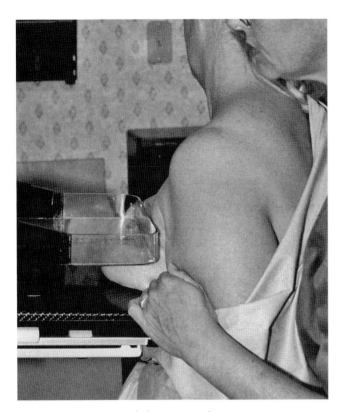

FIGURE 28-3 Craniocaudad position with compression.

resolution film. Despite reducing the x-ray dose, Egan's technique resulted in the ability to discern 10 to 15 line pairs/mm, a significant improvement over the 3 to 5 line pairs/mm seen on plain film.

In addition to instrumentation, the amount of compression of the breast and the density of the gland combine to affect the radiation dose to the individual patient. Thinner tissue is penetrated more readily by the beam, causing less scatter and less absorption of the dose. Therefore, compression is not only a necessity for accurate reading of the films but is paramount to safe mammography technique. Dense glandular tissue also can cause increased beam scatter and elevate glandular dosage. The use of rhodium anodes and targets, common in digital mammography systems, is used to increase the penetration of the beam with some necessary increase in the glandular dosage in dense breasts. Overall, however, total exposure is decreased because less callback studies are required to complete the radiographic evaluation.

Magnification views may have a higher mean glandular dose than that of standard screening views. A typical magnification view creates a mean glandular dose of approximately 4 mGy, compared with about 1.5 mGy for screening views. Magnification views are generally performed with a nongrid technique because the "air gap" or distance from the tube absorbs most of the scatter radiation. Because the air gap also attenuates the beam, higher beam energy is required.

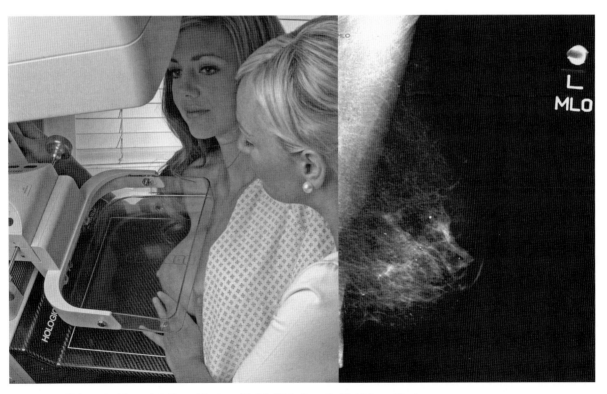

FIGURE 28-4 Mediolateral oblique (MLO) positioning. (Right) MLO view. (Left) MLO positioning.

Radiation exposure with current standard mammograms is between 1 and 2 mGy per image, or about 3 mGy per breast. In contrast, a pulmonary computed tomography angiogram yields a 20 mGy/breast exposure.[3] Additionally, standard whole-breast radiation therapy produces an exposure of approximately 50 Gy. The lifetime exposure of an average woman beginning at age 40 to 90 for yearly mammograms will be 0.2 to 0.4 Gy.

Although there is no low level of radiation exposure that does not increase the risk of breast cancer, in the average woman the benefit of detecting preclinical breast cancer far outweighs the risk of excess cancer obtained through standard screening mammography exposure.[4] It is, however prudent to minimize radiation dose during mammographic screening by using a low-exposure technique and minimizing callback studies. Minimizing exposure is an important component of the Mammographic Certification program administered by the ACR.

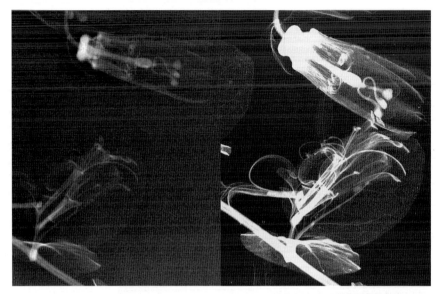

FIGURE 28-5 Improvements in imaging have made the difference in detail you see here. (Right) Digital mammogram. (Left) Analog x-ray film. Note the enhanced detail on the digital mammogram film.

ANALOG VERSUS DIGITAL MAMMOGRAPHY

Up to this point we have been discussing film-screen mammography. Standard film screen mammography (analog imaging) has greatly aided in the detection of breast cancer, and it has lowered breast cancer deaths by as much as 30% over the past 50 or 60 years. Improvements in imaging techniques continue to arise, and full-field digital mammography has recently been introduced. The first digital mammography system prototype was exhibited at the Radiological Society of North America annual meeting in Chicago in 1995 with the first commercial unit becoming available in 2000. Full field digital mammography has been credited with finding more breast cancers in younger women than analog, is more efficient, and more cost-effective than analog imaging.[5]

Like film-screen mammography, digital mammography (Fig. 28-5) uses x-rays to produce images of breast tissue. The difference is that digital images are formed on a phosphor screen rather than a film screen. The phosphor screen converts photons to light, which passes through a fiberoptic cable to a device that converts the light to a digitized signal for display on the computer monitor. This enables the viewer to manipulate the orientation, magnification, brightness, and contrast of the image as desired.

In contrast to analog imaging, which uses x-ray film to acquire, store, and display images (Fig. 28-6), digital mammography separates these functions. Digital mammography enables the reader to manipulate the images using specially optimized computer workstations and monitors, thus increasing the conspicuity of small tumors and microcalcifications. This postprocessing manipulation decreases callbacks. Digital techniques also minimize repeat imaging related to poor exposure by increasing the signal to noise ratio of an image over a broad range of keV.

As with analog imaging, appropriate positioning and compression are vital in producing a diagnostic film. From the patient's standpoint, a digital mammogram is exactly like an analog mammogram, except she will wait a shorter time to know if the images are satisfactory. This is useful in situations such as high-volume screening programs and when doing needle localizations. As opposed to a 3- to 5-minute wait between views, the mammogram is available to evaluate within about

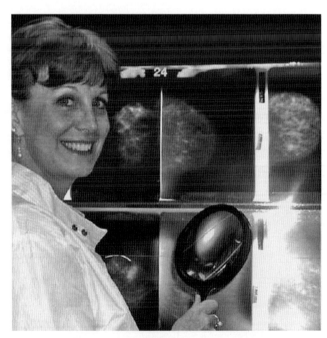

FIGURE 28-6 Analog mammography reading requires films, film processing, a film viewing station, and a magnifying glass.

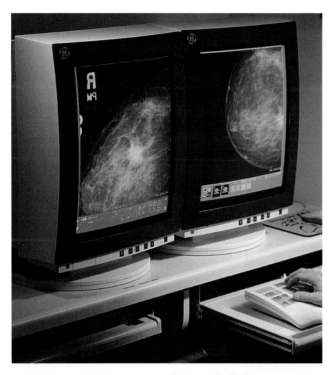

FIGURE 28-7 Digital mammography is read off of computer screens (soft copy) with the added benefits of image manipulation.

30 seconds. There is also no need for quality assurance of the film processing and developer fluid monitoring. Studies can be read at different locations from where they have been obtained, and with archiving; there is no need for hard copy (Fig. 28-7).

Results of the Digital Mammography Imaging Screening Trial (DMIST) were published on September 16, 2005, by the *New England Journal of Medicine*.[5] This large-scale, multicenter trial was designed to measure differences in diagnostic accuracy between analog and digital mammography. It showed that, for the entire population of women studied, analog and digital mammography had very similar accuracy. However, the study showed that digital mammography was superior to analog in women <50 years of age, irrespective of glandular density, in women of any age with dense breast tissue, and in women who are pre- or perimenopausal.

The disadvantage of digital mammography is that the units are 3 to 4 times more expensive than analog units, and they are more sensitive to ambient temperature than are analog units. In addition, film-screen mammography is still superior to digital imaging in detail (line pairs/mm). Also, with slightly smaller bucky sizes, in a very large breast, the digital images must be taken in a patchwork pattern, which is more difficult to read.

SPECIAL VIEWS

Some women require additional mammographic imaging beyond the usual standard views to image their breast tissue completely. Mammography technicians are trained to obtain these views in women who have special screening needs. Typically, women with large breasts, augmented breasts, or who

have undergone mastectomy require special views as a routine part of their screening. Special views are also required for the diagnostic evaluation of clinical or imaging abnormalities.

In some cases, additional imaging modalities are used to completely visualize all of the patient's breast tissue. These modalities can include ultrasound, magnetic resonance imaging (MRI), and molecular imaging. This type of imaging is referred to as secondary screening. Women with dense breasts may also benefit from secondary screening.

Special Views for the Large Breast

If a patient's breast is larger than average and cannot be completely imaged using standard mammogram films, extra views are recommended. At times, up to 4 additional images of each breast are recommended, in a patchwork fashion, to include all breast tissue.

Typically, women who require multiple views are still imaged using CC and MLO projections. If more than 1 image is required per projection to image the breast completely, these are labeled according to the quadrant of the view.

In centers that perform analog imaging, large-format mammographic films are available to image women with large breasts more completely. Unfortunately, large-format imaging is not available in digital systems.

Special Views for the Augmented Breast

For the augmented breast, implant displacement views are required to adequately visualize breast tissue anterior to the implant. These views are performed by pushing the implant back, allowing compression of the natural breast tissue. These views are obtained in the standard prescreening projections and are labeled with "ID" in addition to CC, MLO, and ML. The standard CC, MLO, and ML views must also be included to evaluate each breast completely.

Despite the use of implant displacement views, the presence of the opaque implant obscures portions of the breast tissue, particularly if the implant is subglandular. This is graphically shown in Figure 28-8. Some imaging centers perform an additional ML screening view to minimize this problem.

Special Views for the Diagnostic Evaluation of Abnormalities

As opposed to screening studies, diagnostic mammography involves the use of special views to work up either physical findings or findings from a previous screening study (Fig. 28-9).

Diagnostic mammography uses spot/compression views, magnification views, tangential views, retromammary views, and anything else needed to better image areas of concern. In addition, ancillary imaging techniques such as ultrasound, MRI, and nuclear medicine imaging are also used at times. These latter techniques are discussed in other chapters.

Spot/compression views are performed with a smaller compression paddle, in the shape of a small circle or square, depending on the manufacturer. The smaller surface area compresses more effectively and therefore brings the tissue closer to

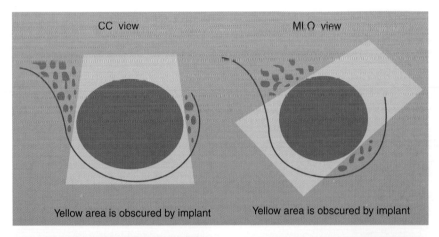

CC view   MLO view

Yellow area is obscured by implant   Yellow area is obscured by implant

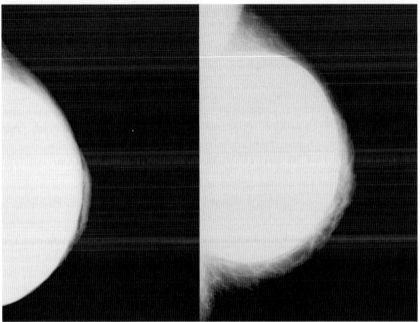

FIGURE 28-8 Implants obscure the shaded areas in both the craniocaudad (CC) and mediolateral oblique (MLO) views. Some centers perform a mediolateral view on all patients with implants to see more of the obscured tissue.

the bucky and yields a clearer image of the area of concern. This is used for areas of architectural distortion, spiculation, small masses, and ill-defined densities. Densities that efface under compression tend to be benign, whereas densities that persist under compression are more suspicious.

Magnification views are images taken with a smaller focal spot than standard images. In general mammography, the focal spot is 0.3 mm and with magnification imaging, the focal spot is 0.1 mm and uses an air gap. This enables magnifications of up to ×2.5 with associated improved contrast resolution. This technique is used primarily for microcalcifications; however, it is also useful for small masses of any sort because it elucidates the borders of these lesions.

Tangential views are images taken with the palpable area of concern or calcifications centered along the surface of the breast and the x-ray beam coming perpendicular to the surface. These views are very helpful in distinguishing skin lesions from lesions deep in the breast. In general, skin lesions are considered less likely to be breast cancers.

Retromammary views are views of the deep tissue of the breast adjacent to the chest wall, used primarily in imaging of implants (Fig. 28-10). This is useful to see the retromammary tissues, looking behind the posterior wall of implants.

MAMMOGRAPHIC INTERPRETATION

The Radiographic Workup and Auditing

Although radiologists' talents are no longer limited solely to diagnosis, diagnosis remains the core of their work. In all areas of image-based diagnosis, the key functions the radiologist must perform are perception, interpretation, and action.

Mammography remains one of the most difficult areas in radiology primarily because of difficulty with the perception and, to a lesser extent, interpretation of mammograms. This is, unfortunately, a fundamental limitation of mammography. Mammographic studies are simply difficult to read.

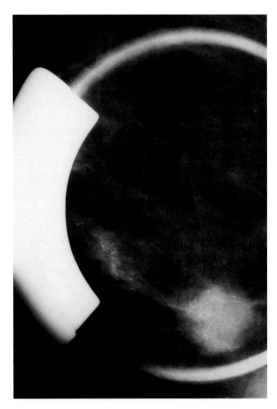

FIGURE 28-9 Spot compression view of a spiculated mass and associated malignant microcalcifications.

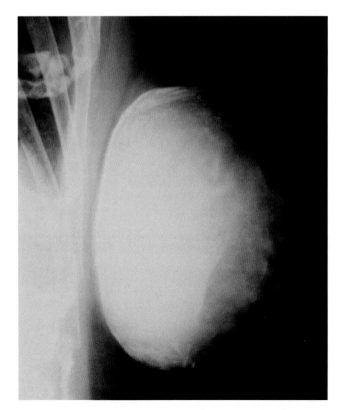

FIGURE 28-10 Retromammary view of an encapsulated, calcified implant.

Perception is the most difficult radiologic process to teach. To a certain extent, good mammographic readers are born, not made. Talent is definitely a factor in recognizing small and subtle lesions. The other primary factor is image quality. Maximizing mammographic image quality has been and remains a major focus of the ACR through their mammography certification program.

Interpretation can also be a challenge but is easier to teach. Teaching interpretation is, in our experience, a good way to teach perception. By working with the findings, students are often better able to recognize them.

More than other areas of radiology, mammographic interpretation is highly dependent on subtle pattern recognition and 3-dimensional visualization. Interpretation of mammograms is best performed in a quiet, darkened room. The only distractions or interruptions physicians should have while interpreting screening mammograms is the necessity of dealing with an emergency.

There is a positive correlation between reading volume and sensitivity in mammography as described by Moss et al.[6] In the UK National Health Service screening program, a minimum of 5000 mammograms are required per year per interpreting physician. In the United States, federal law requires interpretation of at least 480 mammograms a year. Although every physician must meet these minimum requirements in the United States, there remains tremendous variability in the quality of mammographic reading. To become proficient in mammographic interpretation, many more studies than the minimum should be interpreted. A recent peer-reviewed study indicated that breast cancer detection is improved with mammography specialists who read > 4000 mammograms per year.

Ideally, an internal audit of each radiologist should be performed. The Mammography Quality Standards Act (MQSA) requires that each facility keep an audit of the performance of each reading physician. The number of cases read, the positive predictive value (PPV), the recall rates, cancer detection rate, which may include the number of minimal cancers, the number of node-positive cancers, and the number of false-negative cases should be included in the audit. The definition of the PPV varies among authors, but one of the most useful numbers to calculate in clinical practice is the number of cancers found/ number of biopsies recommended (PPV2). This number is a guide to the aggressiveness and accuracy of the interpreting physician. This number should be >25% and < 40%. A cancer detection rate will vary for the community being screened, but a rate of between 2 and 15 per 1000 would be considered normal. A callback rate of around 5% to 10% is ideal and a false-negative rate of <0.5% in a screening population is strived for as defined by Linver et al.[7] Figure 28-11 shows an example of an audit by 6 radiologists.

THE INTERPRETATION OF SPECIFIC FINDINGS

Findings on screening mammography tend to fall into specific categories that the radiologist can analyze using a variety of special views or studies. Generally, in the United States, women who undergo screening mammography do not have their

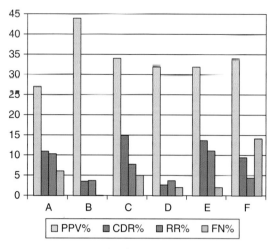

FIGURE 28-11 An example of an internal audit of a 6-physician group, with variability between members but all conforming to Mammography Quality Standards Act MQSA standards.

studies read immediately. Women who need additional views or special studies are asked to return to the imaging center for these. Studies performed on this basis are referred to as callbacks.

As discussed earlier, Callback studies are a reportable quality indicator. An increased number of callback studies have a positive effect on mammographic sensitivity but increased radiation exposure. Accordingly, the ACR has set standards for the number of callback studies performed to minimize this exposure.

Callback studies may be indicated to evaluate specific mammographic findings, including calcifications, circumscribed lesions, stellate lesions, radial scars, parenchymal asymmetry, or various indirect signs. The specific workup of these abnormalities is summarized in Table 28-1 and discussed later.

Calcifications

Because microcalcifications can be one of the earliest signs of breast cancer, detecting them remains a mainstay of mammography. One

of the most basic aspects of the interpretation of mammography is the recognition and evaluation of breast calcifications. There are some hard and fast rules to distinguish benign from malignant, however, there will always be exceptions to these rules.

In general, benign calcifications can be defined as calcifications that form in normal structures within the breast or from benign processes such as fat necrosis, cyst formation, vascular atheromas, and duct ectasia. The vast majority of these calcifications have a typical appearance and can be recognized easily as nonmalignant. Some examples of benign calcifications are shown in Figure 28-12.

Malignant calcifications are associated with calcified intraductal carcinoma. Their appearance is variable, and their shapes are pleomorphic. Because they form inside ductal structures, they have a tendency to form in a linear arrangement and to have branching elements as shown in Figure 28-13.

Circumscribed Lesions

Circumscribed lesions, meaning lesions of which the borders are well defined and smooth, are considered predominantly benign. There are cases of well-circumscribed cancers, but if properly imaged, with small focal spot magnification views, almost always cancers can be distinguished by their irregular margins. Most of these lesions are ovoid in shape or smoothly lobular, with less than 3 lobulations. The majority of these lesions in the breast are cysts, fibroadenomas, or lymph nodes. Other well-circumscribed structures that may be seen include granulomas, fat necrosis, oil collections or "oily cysts," or extracapsular silicone collections. Many of these calcify and are illustrated in Figure 28-12.

Stellate Lesions and Radial Scars

Stellate lesions are lesions with irregular, spiculated margins and are usually associated with cancer. Exceptions to this rule are radial scars and posttraumatic scars. The process of stellate lesion formation is similar with both the benign and malignant

TABLE 28-1 Diagnostic Evaluation of Screening Mammographic Findings

Finding	Special Views	Benign	Suspicious	Ancillary Studies
Calcifications	Magnification	Nonbranching	Branching pleomorphic casting	MRI
Circumscribed	Magnification	Smooth	Microlobulated	Ultrasound
Stellate	Compression	Effaces	Persists	Ultrasound MRI
Radial scar	Compression	Effaces	Persists	Ultrasound MRI
Asymmetry	Compression retromammary	Effaces	Persists	Ultrasound MRI
Indirect signs	—	—	—	Ultrasound MRI
Density	—	—	—	Ultrasound molecular MRI

MRI = magnetic resonance imaging.

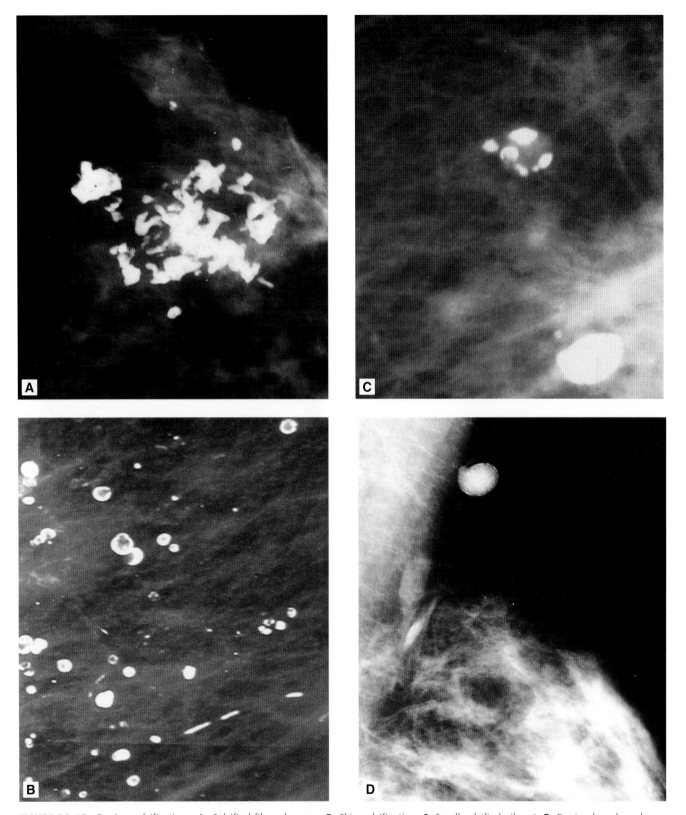

FIGURE 28-12 Benign calcifications. **A.** Calcified fibroadenoma. **B.** Skin calcification. **C.** Small calcified oil cyst. **D.** Benign lymph node calcifications. **E.** Milk of calcium cysts. **F.** Multiple calcified acinar structures. **G.** Large calcified oil cysts. **H.** Vascular calcification.

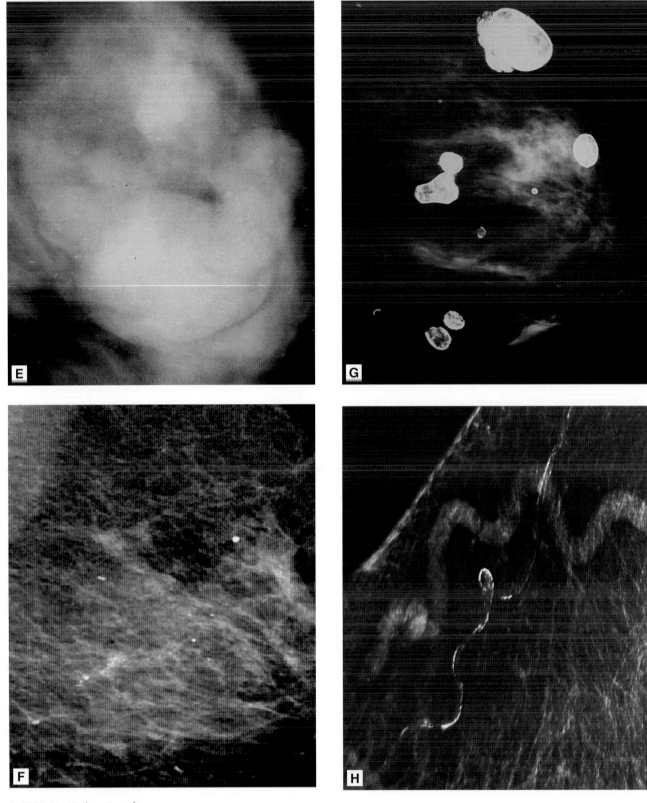

FIGURE 28-12 (Continued)

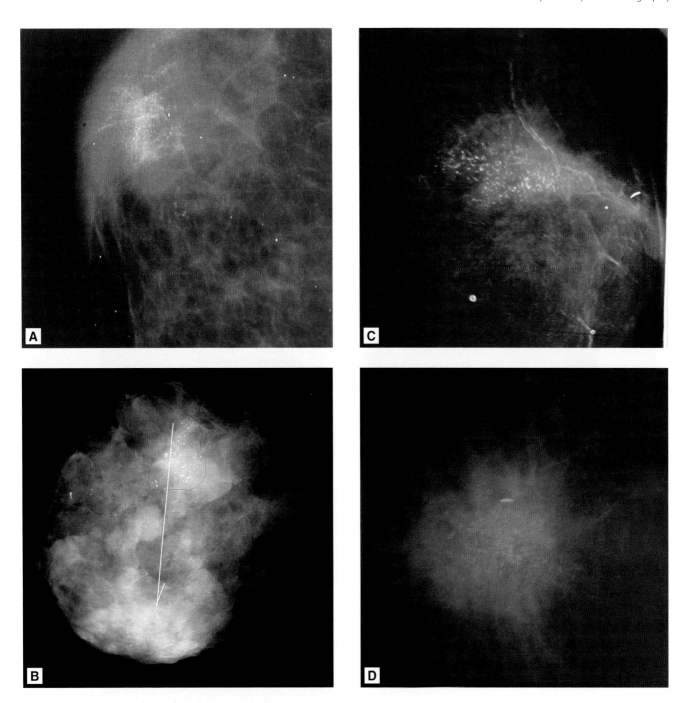

FIGURE 28-13 Multiple examples of malignant calcifications. **A.** Cribriform ductal carcinoma in situ (DCIS). **B.** Excisional biopsy with DCIS. **C.** Comedocarcinoma. **D.** Spiculated mass with DCIS.

causes, and relates to fibrosis. In the case of benign scar formation, fibrosis is part of the healing process and involves the deposition of fibrin and collagen. In the case of a radial scar, which is a complex sclerosing lesion that appears de novo from a presumed nidus of inflammation, or sclerosing adenosis, the spiculations are caused by fibrotic strands extending outward from the central lesion. In the case of carcinoma, the spiculations are formed by a desmoplastic reaction the body forms around the growing cancer cells. Figure 28-14 shows examples of spiculated lesions.

Cancers that present as stellate lesions tend to be low-grade carcinomas because the formation of the inflammatory desmoplastic response takes time. High-grade cancers, which are fast growing, tend to present as circumscribed lesions.

Parenchymal Asymmetry

Parenchymal asymmetry refers to mammographic densities that occur in one breast but not the other, or in the areas such as the retromammary space, where breast tissue is not normally

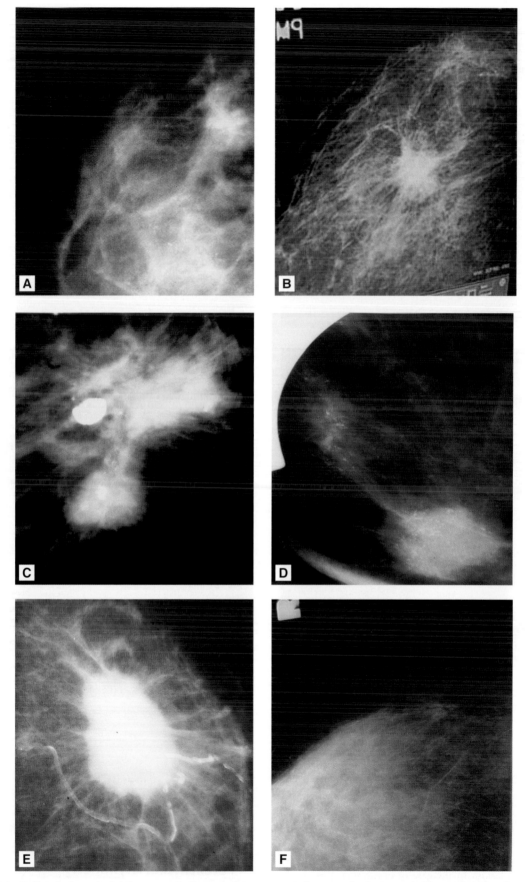

FIGURE 28-14 Stellate lesions. **A.** Subtle cancer. **B.** More obvious cancer. **C.** Fat necrosis. **D.** Cancer with associated malignant microcalcifications. **E.** Large malignancy. **F.** Radial scar.

present. Of all the mammographic findings suggestive of malignancy, parenchymal asymmetry is considered the least suspicious.

Printable asymmetry is usually worked up with additional views to ensure there is no malignancy causing this asymmetry. Some patients have a significant amount of accessory fibroglandular tissue (as discussed earlier under polymastia) and, similarly, this may need to be addressed with additional imaging to rule out occult malignancy. Figure 28-15 shows examples of normal asymmetric breast tissue.

Indirect Signs

Skin thickening, nipple retraction, subtle increasing or decreasing breast size, tenting, and sharp angulation are indirect signs

of malignancy. Other indirect mammographic findings include a sharply defined skin line, folded or asymmetrically angled nipple, or an increasingly dense breast on one side. These findings may be subtle and only well appreciated when compared with films from several years back. They may, however, be all there is to see in a developing cancer, especially in a subtle infiltrating lobular cancer. Again, these findings should be corroborated with ancillary imaging methods such as ultrasound, which may be able to detect a subtle mass causing these changes.

THE BI-RADS STAGING SYSTEM

At the conclusion of the interpretive process, the reader must summarize findings seen on the mammogram for the other health care providers who are involved in the patient's treatment. Referred to as *reporting*, this process was identified as having potential for error as far back as the congressional hearings that led to development of the MQSA of 1992.

As part of implementation of the mammography certification process, the ACR developed a standardized reporting system for mammographic findings that is in worldwide use today. Called the breast imaging, reporting, and data system (BI-RADS), the system mandates the use of a standardized descriptive vocabulary, or lexicon, to describe radiographic findings, as well as a standardized outcome measure that recommends actions to be taken on the part of the screen to patient and their health care providers.

The ACR recommends that a final BI-RADS stage should be assigned only after the entire radiographic workup is completed. In other words, the BI-RADS stage does not just apply to a mammogram, but to any and all imaging studies needed to reach a conclusion as to any abnormalities that may be present. If a study must be reported before completion of the entire workup the BI-RADS category 0 may be used to indicate an incomplete workup that requires further evaluation.

The fourth edition BI-RADS system for reporting radiographic findings is as follows[8]:

Category 0: Incomplete
Category 1: Negative
Category 2: Benign
Category 3: Probably benign
Category 4: Suspicious; biopsy should be considered
Category 5: Highly suspicious; appropriate action should be taken
Category 6: Known malignancy; appropriate action should be taken

Categories 1 and 2 are considered negative for malignancy. Category 1 refers to a normal workup, without any abnormal findings. Category 2 refers to studies that have findings that are known to be benign, such as simple cysts. The majority of mammographic screening workups fall within either category 1 or 2.

Category 3 refers to findings that are probably benign. Generally, category 3 findings have <2% probability of being malignant. Although this is somewhat subjective, most readers are fairly conservative, making category 3 findings safe to follow. As a rule, category 3 findings are reevaluated in 6 months.

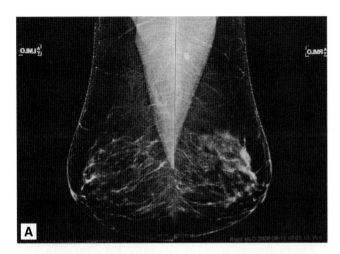

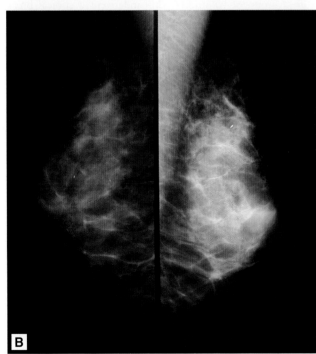

FIGURE 28-15 Examples of parenchymal asymmetry. In both cases the mammogram on the right is denser than the left one.

Category 4 findings have a higher suspicion of malignancy, which exceeds 2%, but most of these findings are also benign. Some readers divide category 4 lesions into 3 subcategories, A, B, and C. Because category 4 findings cover a broad range, with the probability of malignancy anywhere between 3% and 90%, subcategorization can provide a better estimate of the suspicious nature on the lesion. Most category 4 lesions are further evaluated through needle biopsy.

Category 5 lesions are highly suspicious, with a probability of malignancy >90%. These lesions can undergo needle biopsy or open surgical biopsy at the discretion of the treating physician.

Category 6 findings are lesions that are known to be malignant through previous tissue biopsy. This is an administrative category to facilitate reporting of imaging studies performed after a diagnosis, such as a staging MRI.

The great strength of BI-RADS staging is that it provides both the patient and her health care provider clear direction as to what action should be taken. This has greatly decreased errors related to misunderstanding of significant radiologic features that were common prior to the ACR mammographic certification program.

The BI-RADS Lexicon

In addition to the staging system, BI-RADS also specifies a lexicon of terms to be used in the description of imaging findings. This is especially important because diagnostic radiographic workups commonly employ multiple different types of imaging technologies such as ultrasound and MRI, in addition to mammography.

The lexicon is designed in a way that the same terms have the same significance when used in different imaging studies. For example, a circumscribed lesion has the same significance when described on a mammographic report as it does in an ultrasound report. Also, standardization results in more consistent reports that can be understood by any qualified reader. This facilitates correlation between imaging studies, which is important in reaching a final interpretive conclusion. Currently the BI-RADS lexicon can be applied to mammographic, sonographic, and MRI studies.

MAMMOGRAPHIC SCREENING

Population-Based Mammographic Screening and Mortality

By the early 1960s, clinical experience with breast cancer had led to the appreciation that women with early-stage breast cancer had better outcomes than women with advanced disease. Programs were initiated to promote breast self-examination as well as clinical breast examination in an effort to detect breast cancer before it became locally advanced. Initial reports of success in detecting cancer in a more localized form were initially treated with some skepticism and did not result in a significant, nationwide change in practice until these techniques were adopted and advocated by the American Cancer Society in the 1970s.[9]

Mammography, under development since the early 20th century, had been demonstrated by that time to facilitate the diagnosis of breast cancer. This led to the possibility of using mammography to detect breast cancer before it was clinically apparent. Robert Egan, working at M.D. Anderson Hospital in Houston, Texas, conducted a multicenter clinical trial of a new technique of performing mammography. His method was found to be reproducible and forms the basis of screening mammography today.[1,9]

The first prospective evaluation of mammography as a systematic screening technique began in 1963 with a trial sponsored by the Health Insurance Plan of Greater New York (HIP) and the National Cancer Institute. The HIP Trial randomized 62,000 women, 40 to 64 years of age, who were subscribers of the insurance plan to receive or not receive an invitation to 4 rounds of breast cancer screening at 18-month intervals. Each round consisted of a bilateral 2-view mammogram using Egan's technique and a clinical breast exam. Standard x-ray equipment was used to obtain the mammograms because dedicated mammography units did not become available until the mid-1970s. Age and socioeconomic criteria were used to stratify the randomization of the study with respect to matched controls. All deaths within the trial were reviewed for cause by a committee blinded to which arm the participants had been randomized.[9]

Initial results for the HIP trial were published in the *Journal of the American Medical Association* in 1971[10] with updated results in 1997.[11] The trial found an overall relative mortality risk of 0.78 (0.6 to 1.0) in women invited for screening. In women <50 years of age, the results were approximately the same, with a relative mortality risk of 0.77, but with confidence intervals of 0.5 to 1.1.

There followed 6 additional trials of mammographic screening over the next 10 years. Slightly different methodologies in patient selection, randomization, and imaging were used as shown in Table 28-2.[9]

The Canadian National Breast Screening Trial was unique in that all patients who were entered into the trial were recruited from a group of volunteers who underwent a clinical breast exam and training in breast self-examination. As a result, the screening rate was virtually 100%. The trial participants were separated into 2 separate cohorts, women ages 40 to 49 and women ages 50 to 59 to evaluate the effect of age at entry.[12,13]

Results of these trials were similar to the HIP trial. Except for the Canadian trial, which did not show a clear benefit, all of the trials found a decreased relative mortality risk in women who had been invited for screening. The effect was more conclusive in women ≥50 years of age. These results are shown in Table 28-3.[11,14-19]

Breast Density and Contrast Resolution

Contrast resolution refers to the ability on a screening study to differentiate between the background of normal tissue and the cancer we are looking for. With high-contrast resolution, findings are easy to perceive. Unfortunately, mammography has a low-contrast resolution in women with radiographically dense breast tissue (Fig. 28-16). Fundamentally this occurs because both cancers and dense breast tissue show up as white densities on mammogram. One of us (PH) sometimes refers to mammography in women with dense breasts as "Looking for a polar bear in a snowstorm. By the time you see it, it's much too late."

The use of secondary screening, that is, the use of ancillary imaging techniques in addition to mammography to screen for

TABLE 28-2 Design of the Breast Cancer Screening Trials

Trial	Year	Age, yr	Comparison	Interval	Attendance	Views	N	Follow-up
HIP	1963	40-64	M+ CBE vs usual	12	67	2	60,995	18
Malmo	1976	43-70	M vs usual	18-24	75	1 or 2	60,076	16
Two County	1977	40-74	M vs usual	24	89	1	133,065	20
Edinburgh	1978	45-64	M+ CBE vs usual	24	61	2	44,268	13
Canadian	1980	40-59	M+CBE+BSE vs CBE+BSE*	12	100*	2	50,430	13
Stockholm	1981	40-64	M vs usual	28	81	1	60,117	15
Gothenburg	1982	39-59	M vs usual	18	84	1 or 2	51,611	14

*Recruited from volunteers invited for clinical breast examination (CBE) and breast self-examination (BSE) education.
M, Mammography.
Source: Reproduced, with permission, from Smith RA, Duffy SW, Gabe R, et al. The randomized trials of breast cancer screening: what have we learned? *Radiol Clin North Am.* 2004;42(5):793-806.

TABLE 28-3 Results of the Breast Cancer Screening Trials

Trial	Year	Age 39-49 yr (Confidence Intervals)	Age 50+ yr (Confidence Intervals)	Overall
HIP[11]	1963	0.77 (0.52-1.13)	0.79 (0.58-1.08)	0.78 (062-1.00)
Malmo[14]	1976	0.70 (0.49-1.00)	0.83 (0.66-1.04)	0.78 (0.65-0.95)
Two County[15]	1977	0.93 (0.63-1.37)	0.65 (0.55-0.77)	0.68 (0.59-0.80)
Edinburgh[16]	1978	0.75 (0.48-1.18)	0.79 (0.60-1.02)	0.78 (0.62-0.97)
Canadian*[17,18]	1980	0.97 (0.74-1.27)	1.02 (0.78-1.33)	—
Stockholm[14]	1981	1.52 (0.80-2.88)	0.70 (0.46-1.07)	0.90 (0.63-1.28)
Gothenburg[19]	1982	0.65 (0.40-1.05)	0.91 (0.61-1.36)	0.79 (0.58-1.08)

* Recruited from volunteers invited for clinical breast examination (CBE) and breast self-examination (BSE) education.
Source: Reproduced, with permission, from Smith RA, Duffy SW, Gabe R, et al. The randomized trials of breast cancer screening: what have we learned? *Radiol Clin North Am.* 2004;42(5):793-806.

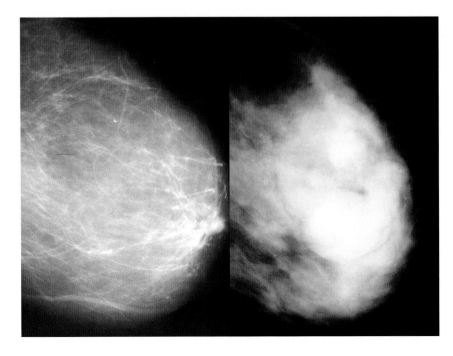

FIGURE 28-16 The image on the right is of a dense breast, the one on the left is of a fatty breast. Mammography is much less sensitive in detecting cancers in the dense breast tissue.

breast cancer, has been recommended in the evaluation of women with dense breasts. Ultrasound,[20] MRI,[21-23] and molecular imaging[24] can improve sensitivity in these patients. Secondary screening is currently a subject of intense research. Mammography is still recommended as the initial screening study to find microcalcifications in women with dense breasts. Microcalcifications cannot be optimally imaged with other techniques.

Interval Cancers

Despite the best efforts of well-trained radiologists, breast cancers are occasionally missed, which can result in a delay of diagnosis. Ideally, all breast cancers are diagnosed at a presymptomatic stage during regularly scheduled screening examinations. When a breast cancer is diagnosed between scheduled rounds of screening examinations, it is referred to as an interval cancer.

The diagnosis of an interval cancer does not mean that a screening film was necessarily misread. Some cancers, such as invasive lobular carcinomas, are simply difficult to detect at an early stage. It is, however, important to review cases of interval cancers to assess the quality of a screening program and to provide feedback to mammographic readers so that they may improve.

The European Union has established a method for review of interval cancers that has been adopted worldwide.[25] First, a bilateral diagnostic mammogram is obtained at the time of diagnosis of the interval cancer. Then, the initial screening films are examined. This is referred to as a *blind review* and is ideally performed by three or more radiologists. Next, the diagnostic films are compared to the initial screening views and a final assessment is made. This is called the *informed review*. The assessment categories are shown in Table 28-4.[25]

This 2-phase assessment guards against retrospective bias. Accordingly, the initial phase can be used for quality assurance, and the informed review can be used for educational purposes. This is especially true of cases with minimal signs. False-negative cases should not exceed 20% of interval cancers. Note that women who are late for their prescribed screening and develop a cancer are not considered to have an interval cancer.

Overdiagnosis

Overdiagnosis is a risk present in any population-based screening effort. Overdiagnosis refers to the diagnosis of disease that never becomes symptomatic or, in other words, the diagnosis of disease that does not need to be treated. Overdiagnosis must be differentiated from the lead-time effect, where presymptomatic disease is encountered during an initial round of screening. As far as breast cancer is concerned, overdiagnosis applies to low-grade ductal carcinoma in situ (DCIS) and possibly small, grade 1 invasive cancer, particularly in the elderly.

Rates of overdiagnosis in clinical screening trials must be ascertained by statistical estimation because it is not possible, a priori, to determine which cancers will or will not progress. The way that rates of overdiagnosis are evaluated is to compare rates of cancer diagnosis during screening with those that occurred when screening is not performed. Although screening will detect cancers sooner, excess cancers are suspicious for overdiagnosis. In practice, estimates of overdiagnosis are difficult to perform. Large numbers of women in well-designed trials are required to determine reliable numbers of excess cancers. Confounding factors such as lead-time bias, sojourn time, and rising incidence all contribute to excess cancers and must be estimated and adjusted for. Small adjustments can make a large difference, and there is not universal agreement in how they should be performed. As a result, estimates of overdiagnosis are somewhat subjective. Fortunately, rates of overdiagnosis in major screening studies are small, as shown by the estimates listed in Table 28-5.[26-28]

As can be seen, overdiagnosis is a very minor problem in mammographic service screening. Certainly, concerns of overdiagnosis should not dissuade anyone from participating in mammographic service screening.

Sojourn Time, Lead Time, and Screening Interval

Breast cancers, if not discovered and treated, eventually become symptomatic. The whole point of screening, of course, is to

TABLE 28-4 Evaluation of Interval Cancers

Categories	Subtypes	Screening	Diagnostic
True interval		Negative	Positive
Occult		Negative	Negative
Minimal signs		Minimal signs	Minimal signs or positive
False negative	Reading error	Positive	Positive
	Technical error	Negative*	Positive
Unclassifiable		Any	Not available

*For technical reasons (ie, inadequate image quality).
Source: Data from Perry N, Broeders M, de Wolf C, et al. *European Guidelines for Quality Assurance in Breast Cancer Screening and Diagnosis*. 4th ed. European Union, Health and Consumer Protection Directorate-General: 2006.

TABLE 28-5 Overdiagnosis Estimates from Population-Based Screening Trials

	N*	Model	DCIS	Invasive	Overall
Impact[26]	13,999	Poisson regression	—	3.2%	4.6%
Dutch NSP[27]	Not stated	Microsimulation	—	—	3%
Two-County[28]	77,080	Markov chain	1%	0	1%
Gothenburg[28]	21,650	Markov chain	2%	2%	2%

*Number screened. DCIS = ductal carcinoma-in-situ.
Source: Data compiled from Paci E, Miccinesi G, Puliti D, et al. Estimate of overdiagnosis of breast cancer due to mammography after adjustment for lead time. A service screening study in Italy. *Breast Cancer Res.* 2006;8(6):R68; de Koning HJ, Draisma G, Fracheboud J, de Bruijn A. Overdiagnosis and overtreatment of breast cancer: microsimulation modelling estimates based on observed screen and clinical data. *Breast Cancer Res.* 2006;8(1):202; Duffy SW, Agbaje O, Tabar L, et al. Overdiagnosis and overtreatment of breast cancer: estimates of overdiagnosis from two trials of mammographic screening for breast cancer. *Breast Cancer Res.* 2005;7(6):258-265.

reduce morbidity and mortality by detecting cancers while they are in a preclinical phase. When designing a program for service screening, it is helpful to know how long a cancer will stay in a preclinical phase. This time interval, the time from when a cancer is first detectable to when it becomes symptomatic, is called the *sojourn time*. It must be distinguished from *lead time*, which is the time from when a tumor is actually detected to the point at which it becomes symptomatic.

Lead time cannot exceed sojourn time, but we would like lead time to be as long as possible. To be effective in reducing breast cancer mortality, the time between screening examinations must be less than the sojourn time.

Within a screening program, lead time can be measured, but sojourn time must be estimated through statistical techniques. Although there are different methods of estimating sojourn time, they all agree to a surprising extent. Sojourn time is usually expressed as a mean (mean sojourn time, or MST) and is estimated from the ratio of true interval cancers to the incidence of new cancers detected at screening. A similar technique can be used to estimate the sensitivity of mammographic screening. The technique to estimate sojourn time is complex, but the principle is clear: A higher number of true interval cancers between screening exams indicates a shorter sojourn time.

Sojourn times have been estimated for a number of screening trials. Table 28-6 shows an example from the Swedish Two-County Trial.[29]

Note that sojourn time is shorter in women <50 years of age. This has been noted in other trials as well. A combination of smaller sojourn time combined with less mammographic sensitivity in younger women is believed by some experts to be one reason that screening in this population has a smaller mortality benefit. As a result, there have been calls to screen women <50 years of age more often than every 2 years.

As mammographic and other screening techniques continue to improve, it is hoped that, with increasing sojourn times, we will see further improvements in mortality in younger women.

TABLE 28-6 Estimates of Sojourn Time in the Two-County Trial

Age, yr	Mean Sojourn Time (yr)
40-49	1.7
50-59	3.3
60-69	3.8
70-74	2.6

Source: Data from Tabar L, Fagerberg G, Chen HH, et al. Efficacy of breast cancer screening by age. New results from the Swedish Two-County Trial. *Cancer.* 1995;75(10):2507–2517.

Double Reading and Computer-Aided Diagnosis

One of the oldest methods used to decrease the incidence of interval cancers is double reading. The idea here is simple: Two pairs of eyes are often better than one. In a radiology centers that perform double reading, mammograms undergo an initial read, and then are examined again by a different radiologist who is blinded to the results of the initial interpretation.

Double reading has been shown to improve the overall accuracy of mammographic interpretation without significant increases in callback rates. Although double reading is commonly performed in the United Kingdom, its use in the United States has been limited due to a lack of reimbursement for the service. Widespread use of double reading also requires a much larger mammographic workforce, which further limits its use. In the United States, double reading has largely been replaced by computer-aided detection (CAD) systems that have recently been shown to be just as effective.[30]

Computer-aided detection (CAD) systems process digitized mammographic images to look for suspicious areas that might be missed by a radiologist. These systems place a mark near suspected abnormalities, which are then reexamined by the radiologist. These systems have undergone continuous improvement since their inception in the early 1990s. As a result, CAD literature that is more than 2 to 3 years old is generally out of date and does not reflect the current accuracy of these systems.

That being said, several studies have shown that the use of computers to overread mammograms can increased the cancer detection rates by up to 15%. Freer found when comparing the radiologist's performance without CAD with that when CAD was used, recall rate was slightly increased (from 6.5% to 7.7%), the PPV remained about 38%, but a 19.5% increase in the number of cancers detected, and an increase in the number of early-stage breast cancers was found.[31]

The use of CAD-based systems in the United States is well reimbursed, contributing to their widespread adoption.

INTERVENTIONAL MAMMOGRAPHY

Interventional mammography refers to the use of mammographic images as a guidance mechanism for the performance of further diagnostic or therapeutic procedures. Traditionally, these procedures fall into 1 of 3 categories: needle-localization procedures, galactography, or stereotactic biopsy.

Needle-localization procedures are commonly used for the placement of J wires as an aid to surgical resection of malignant tumors. Needle localization is rarely used for diagnostic purposes these days because it has largely been replaced by stereotactic biopsy. Galactography is a diagnostic tool that allows the evaluation and localization of intraductal lesions for study or surgical excision.

Stereotactic biopsy uses mammographic guidance to localize suspicious lesions in three dimensions so that they can be biopsied using either a core-needle or a vacuum-assisted technique. Stereotactic techniques are discussed in another chapter.

Needle-Localization Procedures

Needle localizations are performed to guide the surgeon to lesions within the breast (Fig. 28-17). They can be performed with mammographic or stereotactic guidance. Needle-localization procedures can also be carried out under ultrasound guidance.

The mammographic method is the more traditional but is now being largely replaced by stereotactic localization. The radiologist should consult with the surgeon first, before performing a localization, because each surgeon has his or her preference as to how to localize the lesion. Some use "bracketing" technique, whereby the lesion is surrounded by up to four needles. Others want a "peri-areolar" approach, to minimize scarring.

For mammographic localization, a special compression plate with multiple small holes is used to facilitate placement of the J-wire while the patient is in compression. Once the mammographic lesion is localized,

a needle containing the J-wire is placed into the lesion from the skin using the shortest distance possible. The J wire is then deployed as compression is released. An orthogonal view confirms placement of the J-wire within the vicinity of the lesion. The J-wire should be imaged in 2 projections to ensure that the lesion is actually located near the desired target in 3-dimensional space.

Galactography

Galactograms are performed for spontaneous, clear, or bloody discharges. Dark or bright red blood is most commonly associated with papillomas. Clear discharge is most often associated with cancer. Milky or greenish discharges are considered benign. The former is associated with galactorrhea, and the latter with fibrocystic changes in the breast.

Galactography is performed with a modified sialogram catheter (20 to 25 g). The patient lies in the supine position on the table, and the nipple is rubbed with topical lidocaine. This not only relieves nipple tenderness but relaxes the smooth muscle of the nipple prior to the procedure. A magnifying glass or headset is used to see the nipple ducts. The catheter is filled with an x-ray-visible contrast material, and all bubbles are removed. The catheter is inserted into the discharging duct, and contrast is gently administered. An abnormal discharging duct will be somewhat patulous, and the catheter should fall into it without much pressure. In cases of true spontaneous nipple discharge, galactography is almost always positive. Small intraductal papillomas or small intraductal cancers can be seen as filling defects.

When performed for preoperative localization of intraductal filling defects, the x-ray-visible contrast is mixed with methylene blue, which can be visualized at surgery. At the time of surgery, periareolar incision can be performed with dissection carried out toward the nipple until the blue duct is localized. The duct is then followed distally until all visible methylene blue has been excised. Most intraductal defects causing nipple discharge are located within 2 cm of the nipple. Figure 28-18 shows a galactogram of an intraductal papilloma found at surgery.

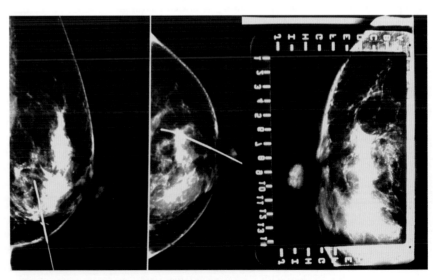

FIGURE 28-17 Needle wire localization uses a grid system and orthogonal views to pinpoint the area of concern for the surgeon.

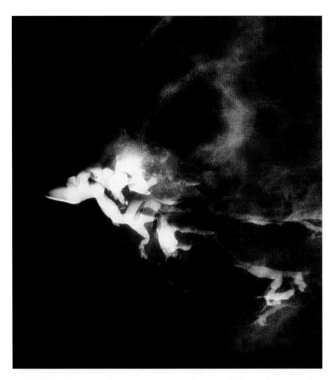

FIGURE 28-18 A galactogram. Note the tip of the galactography catheter in the duct. A large irregular filling defect representing a papilloma is seen highlighted by linear marks.

GOVERNMENT REGULATION OF MAMMOGRAPHY

▪ The Mammography Quality Standards Act

By the late 1980s, there was widespread concern among policymakers, women's health advocates, and the public that poor-quality screening mammographic examinations were leading to unnecessary biopsies and, in some cases, delays in diagnosis of breast cancer. Partly in response to public concern about the reliability of mammography, the ACR developed a voluntary mammography accreditation program in 1987.[32]

In 1991, hearings on improving the quality of mammography were conducted by the US House Committee on Energy and Commerce and the Subcommittee on Aging of the Senate Committee on Labor and Human Relations. Their reports, issued in late 1991, found that problems in the perception and interpretation of mammographic findings led to most mammographic errors. Nonstandard reporting and errors in notifying patients and their health care providers were also found to contribute to delays in diagnosis, even when mammographic findings were noted and correctly interpreted.[32]

The congressional hearings commended the ACR's accreditation program but found that, because it was voluntary, it was insufficient to guarantee adequate mammographic quality. At that time, <25% of mammography facilities were accredited through the ACR program and >50% of the centers that had applied had failed. Several witnesses testifying before the committees also expressed concern that a then recent decision providing

Medicare funding for screening mammography was leading to a proliferation of low-cost, low-quality mammogram machines that would cause further quality problems in the future.[32]

Following the hearings, work began on legislation to improve mammographic quality. These efforts culminated in the passage of the MQSA in October 1992. Enjoying broad congressional and public support, the act was unprecedented at that time in regulating the practice of medicine at the federal level, a power previously reserved to the states.[32]

The act amended the Public Health Service Act to delegate federal authority to the secretary of the Department of Health and Human Services to develop regulations pertaining to mammographic services and equipment. All mammographic centers, except Veterans Administration facilities, were required to obtain a certificate of operation from the secretary by October 1, 1994, in order to continue operation. To obtain this certificate, the act required each center to undergo accreditation by an agency approved by the secretary. The act did not specify the requirements of accreditation but directed the secretary to develop standards that mandated the use of radiological equipment specifically designed for mammography, set licensing guidelines for personnel who perform mammograms and qualification standards for interpreting physicians, and specified the establishment and maintenance of a quality assurance and quality control program at each mammographic facility. The act also provided for a National Mammography Quality Assurance Advisory Committee, composed of radiologists, other health care providers, and members of the public to advise the secretary as to the adoption of specific standards.[32,33]

In June 2003, the secretary delegated to the commissioner of the Food and Drug Administration (FDA) to implement the MQSA. The FDA recognized that with insufficient time to develop comprehensive standards by the October 1994 deadline, interim regulations would be required. These regulations were published on December 14, 1993. In the interim regulations, standards relating to mammographic equipment and technique, reader training and qualification, and facility-based quality assurance that had been part of the voluntary ACR accreditation program were adopted and made mandatory.[32,33]

On April 3, 1996, the FDA published a set of proposed rules that eventually became known as the MQSA Final Regulations.[34] After a period of public comment, they were formally issued on October 28, 1997, to become effective on April 28, 1999.[35] The MQSA regulations that are currently in effect are, to a large part, unchanged since that time.

The MQSA has been amended twice since the final regulations were implemented. The necessity of legislative reauthorization of the MQSA every 5 years was written into the original 1992 act. The Mammography Quality Standards Reauthorization Act of 1998 added requirements for mammography centers to send copies of the patient's final mammographic interpretation to referring health care providers as well as a letter, written in lay terms, to women who had undergone a mammographic study detailing the significance of their results. The reauthorization act of 2004 provided additional funds for research into mammography standards as well as making minor changes to the process by which state governments can become FDA-approved accreditation agencies. Currently, the MQSA is overdue for reauthorization.[36] There have been calls for broadening the scope of the act to include all breast imaging, as well as tighter regulation of stereotactic procedures in particular.[37] Current FDA regulation of mammography will continue in its present form until passage of the next reauthorization act.

As currently written, the MQSA Final Regulations are divided into 3 main sections. Section A deals with the application process a nongovernmental entity must follow to become an FDA-approved accreditation body. Section B details the minimum national quality standards that approved mammography centers must meet in order to become accredited. Section C establishes procedures by which a state government can become an FDA-approved accreditation body. Other sections of the act established penalties for noncompliance with FDA-mandated standards and other administrative issues.[34,35] Currently, approved accreditation agencies include the ACR and the states of Arkansas, California, Iowa, Wisconsin, Ohio, and Texas.

The Role of the American College of Radiology

The ACR has had a pivotal role in the development of the MQSA legislation and regulations since their inception in the early 1990s. The majority of the members of the National Mammography Quality Assurance Advisory Committee, which is still providing recommendations to the FDA on mammographic standards, are radiologists who are also members of the ACR. Additionally, the basis of the Interim Regulations, and subsequently the MQSA Final Regulations, were originally developed by the college as part of their voluntary accreditation program in the late 1980s.

The college is an FDA-approved accreditation agency and provides certification and inspection for mammography centers throughout the country. Currently, the majority of mammographic facilities, >8000, are accredited through the ACR. The college is active in providing support to accredited centers, including continuing medical education programs, materials on quality control, templates for patient letters, and workflow-related software to administer quality control programs and reporting requirements. Without the efforts of ACR members volunteering their time, the current system of accreditation and inspection would be impossible to administer.

In recent years, the ACR has developed additional accreditation programs in breast ultrasound, stereotactic biopsy, and MRI. Beginning in October 2007, the college developed an additional level of accreditation for imaging centers that complete the mandatory MQSA certification as well as voluntary certification in stereotactic biopsy and breast ultrasound. Centers that complete this process are designated by the college as Breast Imaging Centers of Excellence.

Of course, the major contribution of the ACR has been the development and standardization of BI-RADS. The BI-RADS system was devised to facilitate standardized reporting of mammographic findings, as well as to facilitate clear recommendations for action to the referring health care providers. BI-RADS was developed by the Breast Task Force Committee of the ACR in the late 1980s. The system was a component of the original ACR voluntary accreditation program and was based, in part, on an earlier reporting system used at Massachusetts General Hospital.

BI-RADS is designed to facilitate outcome research. The standardized lexicon supports comparison between different studies, readers, and mammographic centers. BI-RADS classifications have been shown to be reproducible among different readers. As a result, the majority of multicenter trials conducted today by the radiology community currently use BI-RADS to support their outcome data and statistical reporting.

Currently the system is used worldwide, and its use is mandated by the MQSA. The ACR continues to support development of the system with educational publications, administrative software, and continuing extensions to the system to cover new imaging modalities. Currently, BI-RADS has a standardized lexicon of not only mammographic findings, but also findings under ultrasound and MRI, all of which are integrated into a comprehensive assessment system. The overall system is organized in such a way that sonographic or MRI findings that have similar appearances to mammographic findings all have the same descriptive terms. This facilitates the correlation of different imaging modalities that are part of the overall radiologic workup.

The ACR continues to be the driving force behind quality-related regulation of breast imaging. They have, over a period of >20 years, consistently worked to improve issues related to breast image quality, reader training, and continuing education. Although it is difficult to quantitate the outcomes of their work, their contribution has unquestionably improved the quality and consistency of breast imaging throughout the world.

Requirements for MQSA Reader Qualification

The essence of the radiologic process can be summed up in 3 words: perception, interpretation, and action. From the beginning, the MQSA was intended to improve the accuracy of mammography by improving quality in all these areas. Perception was improved by first mandating high image quality with dedicated, high-resolution film techniques. Action was improved through the standardization of reporting using the BI-RADS system. Finally, it was recognized that further improvements in both perception and interpretation would have to come through setting minimum standards for the reader.[34]

Accordingly, the final regulations mandated training in mammography equaling 3 months, the amount provided in most radiology residency programs, including radiation physics specific to mammography and radiation protection. This requirement can be met by board certification in radiology, independent study continuing medical education (CME), or a formal training course in the United States or Canada. Additionally, 60 hours of CME specific to mammography are required, with 15 of these within 1 year of accreditation. As part of this training, 240 mammograms must be read under the supervision of an MQSA-qualified radiologist within a 6-month period prior to accreditation.

Once initial qualifications are met, 15 hours of continuing medical education are required every 3 years, and 960 mammograms must be read every 2 years. Before interpreting studies obtained using a new modality, such as digital mammography, an additional 8 hours of CME are required in that modality.[34]

Regulation of Interventional Mammography

In the proposed MQSA final rules published by the FDA on April 3, 1996, the definition of mammography in 21 CFR § 900.2 was amended specifically to exclude "Radiography of the breast performed during invasive interventions for localization or biopsy procedures." This sentence, which has been present in the regulations since the final rules became effective in 1999, has effectively excluded stereotactic biopsy, stereotactic needle localization, mammographic needle localization, and galactography from regulation by the FDA under the MQSA. Note that this exclusion is present only in the final regulations; it was not mentioned in the MQSA itself.[33,36]

The reason for this exemption, as stated in the preamble of the proposed final rules, was that the FDA believed that "science had not advanced to the point where effective national quality standards could be developed for these devices." However, the preamble also stated that "eventually, FDA does expect to develop standards for interventional mammography devices, and for research devices that come into standard use."[34]

Soon after the publication of the final rules, the ACR developed and began accreditation under a new voluntary stereotactic biopsy certification program. The program borrowed many of the same quality standards used in the MQSA regulations, including submission outcome data and site inspections. In 1997, the ACR extended this certification program to surgeons through a cooperative program administered by both colleges.

Response to voluntary stereotactic certification has been poor, as it was for the ACR voluntary mammography certification program in the 1980s. As of November 2007, the ACR had accredited a total of 459 stereotactic facilities, an estimated 20% of the total in operation nationwide.[36] The ACR found that 25% of facilities initially failed certification, but that only 6% failed a second attempt at certification, suggesting that the certification process itself was resulting in an improvement in quality for centers applying for certification. Many of the initial failures were related to overexposure, a problem that initially was common in the mammography certification experience but is now virtually unknown. The American College of Surgeons (ACS), through the cooperative ACS-ACR program, has accredited just 4 stereotactic units.[36] On a personal note, we are proud to say that one of them is ours.

In 2005, the Committee on Improving Mammography Quality Standards, of the Institute of Medicine in cooperation with the ACR, issued a report, "Improving Breast Imaging Quality Standards." The report looked at issues relating to reader training, the use of expanded outcome data to improve interpretation, the adequacy of the breast cancer screening workforce, and the certification of readers. The report listed 10 recommendations pertaining to technical modifications of the MQSA regulations, workforce recruitment, and further research into barriers to accurate mammographic interpretation.[37]

The fifth recommendation was to remove the regulatory exemption for stereotactic biopsy but not for other forms of interventional mammography, including mammographic and stereotactic needle-localization procedures. This recommendation was based on the improved compliance with process-related standards that was seen during the ACR mammography, ultrasound, and stereotactic certification programs. The Institute of Medicine (IOM), in the full text of their report, proposed specific regulatory language that would require MQSA reader qualification for all physicians performing stereotactic biopsies, effectively excluding all nonradiologists from performing these procedures.

Other interventional mammography procedures were not included in this recommendation because "FDA should not require accreditation specifically for non-stereotactic biopsy interventional procedures (e.g., wire needle localization), since accreditation programs do not exist for these procedures." The IOM did recommend, however, that the machines used to perform these procedures be included under MQSA regulation.[37]

In November 2007, the National Mammography Quality Assurance Advisory Committee took up the recommendation of the IOM in relation to removing the exclusion for stereotactic biopsy from regulation. A public hearing was held on November 5, with testimony given by representatives of the ACR, the ACS, the American Society of Breast Surgeons, the Society of Breast Imaging, device manufacturers, and various members of the public.[36]

Representatives from the ACR and the Society of Breast Imaging recommended removing the exemption based on the data from their certification experience, which was presented. Representatives from the ASBS, the ACS, and the industry recommended against removing the exemption. Their argument was essentially that more study was needed to determine if there was a difference in outcome between voluntarily accredited facilities and nonaccredited facilities. Also pointed out was the fact that >25% of stereotactic biopsies are performed by surgeons. Concern was expressed that removing the exemption, as proposed by the IOM, would effectively exclude surgeons from performing these procedures, leading to an increase in open surgical biopsies.[36]

In the end, the National Mammography Quality Assurance Advisory Committee was not persuaded and voted to recommend to the FDA that the stereotactic exemption be removed. Several committee members, although voicing their support for removing the exemption, stated that they hoped this would be done in such a way that surgeons would not be excluded from these procedures. The committee did not express an opinion on other interventional mammography procedures.[36]

At this time, there has been no word from the FDA as to any changes in the current MQSA regulations. We believe it is likely that the stereotactic exemption will eventually be removed. We tend to believe the National Mammography Quality Assurance Advisory Committee when they assure us that when this is done there will still be an opportunity for surgeons to perform stereotactic procedures. Time, of course, will tell.

Interventional Mammography Certification for Surgeons

Stereotactic certification for surgeons is currently available through either the cooperative ACS-ACR program or through a new program initiated in 2007 by the American Society of Breast Surgeons (ASBS). Both programs require initial and continuing experience, continuing medical education, and dedicated equipment.

The principal difference between them is that there is no defined role for radiologists in the ASBS program. The ASBS program is also somewhat more rigorous in that it requires a written and practical examination.

The ACS-ACR Cooperative Certification Program

After the ACR developed its stereotactic certification program for radiologists in the late 1990s, the ACS formed a Committee on Stereotactic Breast Biopsy Accreditation to evaluate development of a stereotactic certification program for surgeons. This occurred as a result of the concerns at the time of radiologists, fellows of the ACS, government agencies, and the public that stereotactic procedures performed improperly were resulting in delays of diagnosis.

Negotiations with the ACR brought about a cooperative ACS-ACR certification program in 1997. Similar to the voluntary ACR stereotactic certification program and the mammographic certification program, the cooperative program was designed to maximize both image quality and needle placement accuracy while ensuring that patient radiation dose was minimized through the use of proper exposure technique.

Requirements were specified for surgeon continuing education in a variety of practice settings and qualifications set for surgeon stereotactic instructors. It was recognized that most surgeons would be practicing in a collaborative hospital or clinic setting with radiologists performing supervision and interpretive services for the surgeon. In this event, experience and CME requirements for the surgeon were fairly minimal.

Surgeons in higher volume or academic practices without radiologist support are also able to obtain certification, but in this circumstance higher levels of experience and education are required. Surgeons in this setting are also responsible for maintaining procedural logs for quality assurance purposes.

As in the mammography certification program, on-site inspections and physicist reviews of exposure settings are required. Cases must be submitted for review to show accurate needle placement. The equipment used must be designed specifically for stereotactic biopsy and be approved by the program.

Lastly, requirements for mammography reading are specified for surgeons who practice independently. In this setting the surgeon must "have evaluated" 480 mammograms every 2 years. Evaluating a mammogram is defined as reviewing the images with an authenticated report prepared by an MQSA-qualified radiologist. This requirement was specified to ensure adequate interpretive skills.

Overall, we found that certification under this program was not burdensome and easy to attain. We benefited from the process because our site inspector, a very knowledgeable radiologist from the ACR, provided us with several tips that we have used to this day to minimize patient exposure while maintaining excellent image quality.

The American Society of Breast Surgeons Certification Program

Within the last year, partly in response to the regulatory initiatives just described, the ASBS established a certification program

of its own. The program is divided into a Stereotactic Breast Procedures Certification for individual surgeons and a Stereotactic Facility Accreditation. This is to accommodate different practice scenarios. In some cases, surgeons will practice in hospital- or radiologist-owned facilities, and in some cases they will own the facilities where they practice. In the case of surgeon ownership, facility certification is encouraged.

The procedures certification program requires both a written and a practical examination, which are offered twice a year. Under the program, there is no provision for cooperative certification with a radiologist as in the ACS-ACR cooperative program. Surgeon qualifications for certification include between 5 or 15 hours of CME, depending on level of prior experience, evaluating 480 mammograms every 2 years, and performing 20 procedures per year. Certification covers both stereotactic biopsies as well as other interventional procedures such as needle localization.

Facility accreditation specifies qualifications for technicians and radiation physicists. At least 1 surgeon must be accredited under the procedures certification program per facility before facility accreditation can be obtained. Surgeons not certified under the procedures certification program must be proctored by a surgeon who is certified. There is no on-site inspection requirement, but equipment used must be approved, and maintenance and medical physics documentation must be submitted. Overall, the program is very similar to the ACS-ACR cooperative program but somewhat more rigorous.

The Proposed Breast-Imaging Quality Standards Act

The last recommendation in the 2005 IOM report was to bring all breast diagnostic and interventional imaging, including ultrasound and MRI, under federal regulation and accreditation. With the exception of interventional mammography, this would require new legislation. The IOM recommended that this occur during the current reauthorization cycle of the MQSA and the new act be renamed the Breast Imaging Quality Standards Act, or BIQSA.[37]

Again, this recommendation was based on successful certification programs that demonstrate improvements in facilities that occur during, and presumably as a result of the certification process. Currently, the ACR and the American Institute of Ultrasound in Medicine offer certification programs in breast ultrasound. Both of these programs are mentioned in the IOM report and presumably would be models for potential regulations. A program in breast MRI certification is currently under development by the ACR.

At the present time, there are no written proposals for the BIQSA. The IOM recommends that, at a minimum, it include breast MRI and ultrasound under its mandate.[37] The role of the proposed act in regulating other imaging technologies such as thermography or elastography is not clear. Nor is it clear what the standards specified in the BIQSA might be. Most of the final regulations will likely be determined by the FDA after a period of public comment, if the proposed legislation passes.

Despite a variety of future regulatory changes in the performance of diagnostic or interventional imaging, we feel that the future for surgeons is bright. The available data shows that obtaining certification results in improvements in process, which probably results in improvements in accuracy. The ACS and the ASBS recognizes this by offering certification programs in both breast ultrasound and stereotactic biopsy. Certification and increased regulation are in our future. By embracing these programs we can be ready for that future.

FUTURE DIRECTIONS

Secondary Screening

As discussed earlier, population-based service screening has resulted in significant improvements in both cancer-specific and overall mortality. However, mammography is not a perfect screening technology. False-negative studies remain a problem, principally because mammograms are difficult to interpret. The root cause of false-negative mammographic studies is low-contrast resolution, particularly in women with dense breasts.[38] Digital techniques, although decreasing callbacks, have not significantly improved overall accuracy. Accordingly, current research is not aiming to improve mammographic accuracy but instead is focusing on improving contrast resolution through secondary screening.

Secondary screening is essentially a second-look imaging study using a different imaging modality in women who are most at risk for false-negative mammography. Two principal risk groups for false-negative studies have been identified: women with mammographically dense breasts and women with an increased risk of developing breast cancer.[38-40]

In practice, there is overlap between these two groups. Women at high risk, including BRCA mutation carriers, often have increased breast density, and women with increased density are known to be at higher risk of developing breast cancer.[39]

Research is now centering on the efficacy of different imaging technologies in secondary screening. The leading contenders, so far, include contrast-enhanced MRI, ultrasound (handheld and automated), and breast-specific gamma imaging. Other technologies are currently in the preliminary stages of evaluation.

Contrast-Enhanced Magnetic Resonance Imaging

Contrast-enhanced MRI is especially useful in evaluating women at increased risk of breast cancer.[41,42] The technique is also used for preoperative staging prior to definitive surgery for breast cancer diagnosed by needle biopsy.[43,44]

Breast MRI uses gadolinium, a rare earth, to image blood flow around breast ductal and lobular structures on the microcapillary level. Anatomic structures are imaged with and without contrast. Digital subtraction is then performed to identify areas of suspicion based on the washout kinetics of the contrast.

MRI can reliably spot areas of in situ or invasive cancer. Because areas of proliferative fibrocystic chance can also exhibit abnormal capillary flow, the specificity of the technique is relatively low. Accordingly, positive results must be confirmed by needle biopsy.[45,46] Sensitivity, however, is very high.[43,47]

Needle biopsies can be performed under MRI guidance using either a core-needle or vacuum-assisted technique.[48,49]

Because suspicious lesions identified under MRI can often also be identified under ultrasound, ultrasound guidance can also be used in most cases.

MRI has the principal disadvantage of being expensive when compared with other imaging techniques. Gadolinium contrast requires an intravenous (IV) start and cannot be used in patients with renal insufficiency. Some women cannot be examined because of claustrophobia.

Overall, MRI has a high sensitivity and the largest body of supporting literature of any secondary screening technique.

Ultrasound

Ultrasound has been used for the diagnostic evaluation of breast lesions since the advent of high-resolution scanning probes in the 1990s. Sonographic changes associated with malignancy are well described.[50] Although studies performed in the 1990s showed little benefit from sonographic secondary screening, the recently reported American College of Radiology Imaging Network (ACRIN) 6666 study showed a significant increase in early-operative cancer diagnoses using a handheld scanning technique. In the ACRIN study, screening was performed using very high-resolution probes and was physician performed.[20]

Within the last 2 years, automated breast ultrasound units have been developed to improve the screening process. A 3-dimensional large volume of data is obtained and reformatted in coronal tomographic slices for interpretation on a separate workstation. A typical study takes 10 minutes to complete and does not require physician attendance.

Sonographic tomography using an automatic breast ultrasound unit has the advantages of low cost and no contrast use, and imaging is performed in the supine position. In typical handheld ultrasound studies, the reader only performs the interpretation of selected images. The function of perception and image selection is performed by the scanner, typically a technologist. This may be why physician-performed ultrasound seems more accurate. Automated units provide an advantage in this respect because the technologist can perform the study but the reader examines the entire breast.

Unfortunately, there is not a large body of literature on ultrasound for secondary screening. Also, DCIS is notoriously difficult to evaluate with ultrasound. Studies are currently underway to evaluate secondary screening by sonographic tomography using automated units.

Breast-Specific Gamma Imaging

Breast-specific gamma imaging is a new technique that uses radioactive technetium 99 (^{99m}Tc)-sestamibi to image breast carcinomas.[24,51] Essentially, the technique is contrast-enhanced mammography. Sestamibi is used for cardiac studies but also is preferentially taken up by adenocarcinomas.

After sestamibi injection, a gamma camera obtains images of the breast. The camera is designed to mimic the standard mammographic projections as well as special views. The gamma images can then be directly compared to the corresponding mammographic views. Gamma-imaged "hot-spots" can then be identified on the mammogram and biopsied under stereotactic guidance. Alternatively, sestamibi hot spots can be easily localized intraoperatively for open surgical excision using a gamma probe.

The sensitivity of the technique has been reported to be high and comparable with MRI. Specificity may be better than MRI, but the amount of available data on this is limited. Brem et al have recently reported a sensitivity of 95% and a specificity of 60%. The study is relatively inexpensive when compared with MRI.[24]

The required dose of sestamibi per study is on the order of 30 mCi. Because many women have mammograms that are difficult to interpret for their entire lives, yearly studies may be required. In this setting, the cumulative tracer dose may become an issue. An IV start is required for each study, which may also limit patient acceptance.

Other Technologies

Several other imaging technologies are under development that may prove useful in the secondary screening of breast cancer. These include nuclear medicine techniques such as positron emission mammography (PEM), which uses a fluorodeoxyglucose (FDG) tracer to produce gamma scintigraphy images of the breast, and mammotomography in which thin-slice mammographic tomograms are prepared using a moving mammographic gantry.

These technologies, and probably more, are currently undergoing preliminary study.

FUTURE STUDIES TO ADVANCE MAMMOGRAPHY

Because the primary purpose of mammography is screening, we would recommend that future studies concentrate on new screening technologies to complement mammography. Although advancements are difficult to predict, the lack of significant progress in mammographic accuracy over the last 15 years argues that the technology may be reaching its limits.

We would encourage researchers to perform studies of new imaging techniques, combined with standard screening mammography to improve screening accuracy. The ACR or the US FDA could make yet another contribution to population-based service screening by standardizing criteria for the performance of these studies. Companies that wish to apply for FDA approval of their screening devices would then design their device studies to comply with these standards as a condition of FDA approval. In this way, the results of the studies of different imaging technologies would be comparable.

The IOM has also called for further studies to define improved outcome measures for mammographic imaging and reading performance.[37] We would favor pursuing studies along these lines as well. Although large improvements in accuracy would probably not result from improved outcome measures, the size of the population being screened would make small improvements significant in terms of overall mortality.

SUMMARY

Mammography and mammographic service screening have significantly decreased mortality in women, particularly in women >50 years of age. Through the efforts of researchers

throughout the world, the dedication of the ACR, and the unprecedented involvement of the federal government, mammographic screening has become one of the greatest public health advances of the 20th century and a model for other cancer-screening programs.

The HIP trial in New York in the 1960s and the 6 large screening trials that followed clearly demonstrated that large-scale population-based service screening using mammography reduced breast cancer–specific, as well as overall mortality in women who are invited to screening. This effect was more pronounced in women >50 years of age. Different mammographic findings have been well described, and their workup is now standardized. Additional studies have helped to define appropriate mammographic technique and screening intervals. Potential screening errors, including overdiagnosis, have been found to be minor and not of significant concern in pursuing decreased mortality through screening.

With the assistance of the ACR, a standardized lexicon has been developed to describe mammographic findings. In addition, the BI-RADS staging system has helped to standardize the significance of mammographic findings and decrease errors related to reporting. In cooperation with the FDA, the ACR has developed a nationwide mammography certification program, which has resulted in significant improvements in the performance and reading of mammographic studies.

Mammography has also revolutionized the treatment of breast cancer. The identification of tumors while small has facilitated the conservative treatment of cancer as well as improving survival. The advent of digital mammographic techniques, although not significantly improving accuracy beyond that achieved with film screening techniques, have decreased callback repeat views, resulted in improved ease of reading, and allowed automatic reporting.

Interventional mammography techniques such as stereotactic biopsy have resulted in a decrease in open surgical biopsy and its attended cost and a great benefit in relation to the cosmetic and psychological outcome of breast biopsy. Although currently interventional mammography is not regulated by the federal government, recommendations from the IOM and the ACR may result in such regulation. The exact form that this regulation will take for surgeons is not clear at this time.

Secondary screening promises to further extend the accuracy and usefulness of mammography for breast cancer screening. New technologies, when combined with traditional mammography, hold great promise for improving the overall accuracy of breast cancer screening within the community. This, we believe, will further decrease mortality among women with breast cancer.

Few technologies have had as great an impact in the practice of medicine as mammography. For the foreseeable future, mammography will remain our primary screening tool for women at risk for breast cancer.

REFERENCES

1. Clark RL, Copeland MM, Egan RL, et al. Reproducibility of the technic of mammography (Egan) for cancer of the breast. *Am J Surg.* 1965;109:127-133.
2. Tabar L, Akerlund E, Gad A. Five-year experience with single-view mammography randomized controlled screening in Sweden. Recent Results. *Cancer Res.* 1984;90:105-113.

3. Parker MS, Hui FK, Camacho MA, et al. Female breast radiation exposure during CT pulmonary angiography. *AJR Am J Roentgenol.* 2005;185(5):1228-1233.

4. Zheng T, Holford TR, Mayne ST, et al. Radiation exposure from diagnostic and therapeutic treatments and risk of breast cancer. *Eur J Cancer Prev.* 2002;11(3):229-235.

5. Pisano ED, Gatsonis C, Hendrick E, et al. Diagnostic performance of digital versus film mammography for breast-cancer screening. *N Engl J Med.* 2005;353(17):1773-1783.

6. Moss SM, Blanks RG, Bennett RL. Is radiologists' volume of mammography reading related to accuracy? A critical review of the literature. *Clin Radiol.* 2005;60(6):623-626.

7. Linver MN, Osuch JR, Brenner RJ, Smith RA. The mammography audit: a primer for the mammography quality standards act (MQSA). *AJR Am J Roentgenol.* 1995;165(1):19-25.

8. American College of Radiology. *American College of Radiology Breast Imaging Reporting and Data System (BI-RADS).* 4th ed. Reston, VA: American College of Radiology: 1998-2008.

9. Smith RA, Duffy SW, Gabe R, et al. The randomized trials of breast cancer screening: what have we learned? *Radiol Clin North Am.* 2004;42(5):793-806, v.

10. Shapiro S, Strax P, Venet L. Periodic breast cancer screening in reducing mortality from breast cancer. *JAMA.* 1971;215:1777-1785.

11. Shapiro S. Periodic screening for breast cancer: the HIP Randomized Controlled Trial. Health Insurance Plan. *J Natl Cancer Inst Monogr.* 1997(22):27-30.

12. Miller AB, Baines CJ, To T, Wall C. Canadian National Breast Screening Study: 2. Breast cancer detection and death rates among women aged 50 to 59 years. *CMAJ.* 1992;147(10):1477-1488.

13. Miller AB, Baines CJ, To T, Wall C. Canadian National Breast Screening Study: 1. Breast cancer detection and death rates among women aged 40 to 49 years. *CMAJ.* 1992;147(10):1459-1476.

14. Nystrom L, Andersson I, Bjurstam N, et al. Long-term effects of mammography screening: updated overview of the Swedish randomised trials. *Lancet.* 2002;359(9310):909-919.

15. Tabar L, Vitak B, Chen HH, et al. The Swedish Two-County Trial twenty years later. Updated mortality results and new insights from long-term follow-up. *Radiol Clin North Am.* 2000;38(4):625-651.

16. Alexander FE, Anderson TJ, Brown HK, et al. 14 years of follow-up from the Edinburgh randomised trial of breast-cancer screening. *Lancet.* 1999;353(9168):1903-1908.

17. Miller AB, To T, Baines CJ, Wall C. Canadian National Breast Screening Study-2: 13-year results of a randomized trial in women aged 50–59 years. *J Natl Cancer Inst.* 2000;92(18):1490-1499.

18. Miller AB, To T, Baines CJ, Wall C. The Canadian National Breast Screening Study-1: breast cancer mortality after 11 to 16 years of follow-up. A randomized screening trial of mammography in women age 40 to 49 years. *Ann Intern Med.* 2002;137(5 Part 1):305-312.

19. Bjurstam N, Bjorneld L, Warwick J, et al. The Gothenburg Breast Screening Trial. *Cancer.* 2003;97(10):2387-2396.

20. Berg WA, Blume JD, Cormack JB, et al. Combined screening with ultrasound and mammography vs mammography alone in women at elevated risk of breast cancer. *JAMA.* 2008;299(18):2151-2163.

21. Yoshikawa MI, Ohsumi S, Sugata S, et al. Comparison of breast cancer detection by diffusion-weighted magnetic resonance imaging and mammography. *Radiat Med.* 2007;25(5):218-223.

22. Rubinstein WS, Latimer JJ, Sumkin JH, et al. Prospective screening study of 0.5 Tesla dedicated magnetic resonance imaging for the detection of breast cancer in young, high-risk women. *BMC Womens Health.* 2006;6:10.

23. Bluemke DA, Gatsonis CA, Chen MH, et al. Magnetic resonance imaging of the breast prior to biopsy. *JAMA.* 2004;292(22):2735-2742.

24. Brem RF, Floerke AC, Rapelyea JA, et al. Breast-specific gamma imaging as an adjunct imaging modality for the diagnosis of breast cancer. *Radiology.* 2008;247(3):651-657.

25. Perry N, Broeders M, de Wolf C, et al. *European Guidelines for Quality Assurance in Breast Cancer Screening and Diagnosis.* 4th ed. Brussels, Belgium. European Union, Health and Consumer Protection Directorate-General; 2006.

26. Paci E, Miccinesi G, Puliti D, et al. Estimate of overdiagnosis of breast cancer due to mammography after adjustment for lead time. A service screening study in Italy. *Breast Cancer Res.* 2006;8(6):R68.

27. de Koning HJ, Draisma G, Fracheboud J, de Bruijn A. Overdiagnosis and overtreatment of breast cancer: microsimulation modelling estimates based on observed screen and clinical data. *Breast Cancer Res.* 2006;8(1):202.

28. Duffy SW, Agbaje O, Tabar L, et al. Overdiagnosis and overtreatment of breast cancer: estimates of overdiagnosis from two trials of mammographic screening for breast cancer. *Breast Cancer Res.* 2005;7(6):258-265.

29. Tabar L, Fagerberg G, Chen HH, et al. Efficacy of breast cancer screening by age. New results from the Swedish Two-County Trial. *Cancer.* 1995;75(10):2507-2517.

30. Gilbert FJ, Astley SM, Gillan MG, et al. Single reading with computer-aided detection for screening mammography. *N Engl J Med.* 2008;359(16)1675-1684.

31. Freer TW, Ulissey MJ. Screening mammography with computer-aided detection: prospective study of 12,860 patients in a community breast center. *Radiology.* 2001;220(3):781-786.

32. Wheeler CD. *The Mammography Quality Standards Act: Misread Mammograms, Malpractice, and the Politics of Regulation.* Boston, MA: Legal Electronic Document Archive, Harvard Law School: 2003.

33. HR 6182: Mammography Quality Standards Act of 1992, United States Code 42: Sec. 263b, §263b (1992).

34. United States Department of Health and Human Services Mammography Quality Standards; Proposed Rules: Federal Register. Apr 3, 1996;61(65): 14856.

35. The Mammography Quality Standards Act Final Regulations, United States Food and Drug Administration; Federal Register. Mar 1999;64(53):13590-13591.

36. Proceedings of the National Mammography Quality Assurance Advisory Committee, United States Food and Drug Administration; Rockville, MD, Nov 5, 2007.

37. Nass S, Ball J, eds. *Improving Breast Imaging Quality Standards.* Washington, DC: National Academy of Sciences: 2005.

38. Mandelson MT, Oestreicher N, Porter PL, et al. Breast density as a predictor of mammographic detection: comparison of interval- and screen-detected cancers. *J Natl Cancer Inst.* 2000;92(13):1081-1087.

39. Boyd NF, Guo H, Martin LJ, et al. Mammographic density and the risk and detection of breast cancer. *N Engl J Med.* 2007;356(3):227-236.

40. Harvey JA, Bovbjerg VE. Quantitative assessment of mammographic breast density: relationship with breast cancer risk. *Radiology.* 2004;230(1):29-41.

41. Griebsch I, Brown J, Boggis C, et al. Cost-effectiveness of screening with contrast enhanced magnetic resonance imaging vs x-ray mammography of women at a high familial risk of breast cancer. *Br J Cancer.* 2006;95(7):801-810.

42. Wright H, Listinsky J, Rim A, et al. Magnetic resonance imaging as a diagnostic tool for breast cancer in premenopausal women. *Am J Surg.* 2005;190(4):572-575.

43. Hollingsworth AB, Stough RG. Preoperative breast MRI for locoregional staging. *J Okla State Med Assoc.* 2006;99(10):505-515.

44. Fischer U, Zachariae O, Baum F, et al. The influence of preoperative MRI of the breasts on recurrence rate in patients with breast cancer. *Eur Radiol.* 2004;14(10):1725-1731.

45. Kim do Y, Moon WK, Cho N, et al. MRI of the breast for the detection and assessment of the size of ductal carcinoma in situ. *Korean J Radiol.* 2007;8(1):32-39.

46. Kneeshaw PJ, Lowry M, Manton D, et al. Differentiation of benign from malignant breast disease associated with screening detected microcalcifications using dynamic contrast enhanced magnetic resonance imaging. *Breast.* 2006;15(1):29-38.

47. Hollingsworth AB, Stough RG, O'Dell CA, Brekke CE. Breast magnetic resonance imaging for preoperative locoregional staging. *Am J Surg.* 2008;196(3):389-397.

48. Liberman L, Holland AE, Marjan D, et al. Underestimation of atypical ductal hyperplasia at MRI-guided 9-gauge vacuum-assisted breast biopsy. *AJR Am J Roentgenol.* 2007;188(3):684-690.

49. Chen X, Lehman CD, Dee KE. MRI-guided breast biopsy: clinical experience with 14-gauge stainless steel core biopsy needle. *AJR Am J Roentgenol.* 2004;182(4):1075-1080.

50. Stavros AT, Thickman D, Rapp CL, et al. Solid breast nodules: use of sonography to distinguish between benign and malignant lesions. *Radiology.* 1995;196(1):123-134.

51. Brem RF, Rapelyea JA, Zisman G, et al. Occult breast cancer: scintimammography with high-resolution breast-specific gamma camera in women at high risk for breast cancer. *Radiology.* 2005;237(1):274-280.

CHAPTER 29

Stereotactic Breast Biopsy

Rand Stack
Arthur Lerner

Minimally invasive breast biopsies are rapidly replacing open surgical biopsy. Percutaneous breast biopsy can be performed with several possible guidance technologies. Other chapters in this book describe techniques for ultrasound-guided minimally invasive biopsy of lesions detected with ultrasound, and for percutaneous biopsy of palpable breast lesions based upon palpation. Stereotactic breast biopsy is a minimally invasive technique for the sampling of nonpalpable breast lesions detected on mammography.[1,2] If the lesion is only visualized on one imaging modality, that modality should be used for guidance during the biopsy procedure. In cases where the lesion is visualized by more than 1 imaging modality, the modality utilized for guiding the biopsy device should be the modality expected to afford the least complicated biopsy. Stereotactic breast biopsy technology was introduced into the United States by Dr. Kambiz Dowlat, a surgeon at Rush University Medical College, in the late 1980s (Fig. 29-1).[3]

This technology enables the surgeon to consistently obtain sufficient tissue for the pathologist to establish a diagnosis, as well as allowing for the determination of any relevant receptors in malignant lesions.[4,5] In contrast to open surgical breast biopsy, stereotactic biopsy takes less time, needs only local anesthetic, requires only a minimal incision without the potential for significant parenchymal and skin scarring, and is more cost-effective. Following stereotactic biopsy, there is essentially no recovery period, and there is no breast deformity at the biopsy site. An additional advantage of stereotactic biopsy over traditional needle localization and open surgical biopsy is that stereotactic biopsy can be performed on a lesion seen in only one mammographic view, in contrast to traditional needle localization, which is only possible for a lesion seen in 2 orthogonal mammographic views. (It is possible to use stereotactic guidance for needle localization of a lesion seen in only 1 mammographic view.)

The term "stereotactic" comes from the same root as the terms "stereophonic" and "stereoscopic." The word "stereophonic" refers to the presentation of sound from 2 speakers to create the illusion of 3-dimensional sound, and the word "stereoscopic" refers to the presentation of 2 images simultaneously to create the illusion of a 3-dimensional image. Stereotactic breast imaging involves taking 2 digital x-ray images of the breast from different angles and using a computer to analyze the information from these 2 images to reconstruct the location of a breast lesion in 3-dimensional space. The computer then uses the data to help the physician guide a needle to the precise location of the lesion in the breast.

The principle of stereotactic imaging can best be understood by analogy to human vision and depth perception. The basis of experiencing 3-dimensional vision is depth perception. Depth perception gives humans the ability to judge the distance to objects in the visual field. To experience depth perception requires vision in both eyes. The slight difference in the position of the 2 eyes results in a slightly different image being seen by each eye. The brain is able to synthesize these 2 different views into a 3-dimensional reconstruction of the visualized scene. A simple demonstration of the difference between the images seen by the right eye and the left eye is to hold up a finger 1 ft in front of your nose and rapidly alternate between closing the left eye and the right eye. The finger appears to jump from side to side, because its location in each eye's visual field is different (parallax). Individuals who are blind in 1 eye lack 3-dimensional vision and are handicapped in judging depth or distance.

In stereotactic imaging,[6,7] 2 mammographic images of the breast are obtained 30 degrees apart (the x-ray tube is first rotated 15 degrees to the right of midline and then 15 degrees to the left of midline). The 2 images are viewed on a monitor, and the physician uses a cursor to select the target lesion on both images. The computer software performs a triangulation function using the selected points on the 2 images to determine

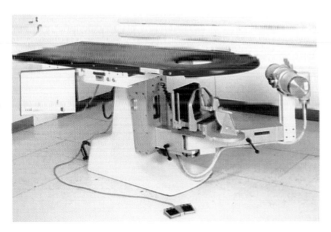

FIGURE 29-1 First stereotactic table in the United States. (*Used with permission of Dr. Kambiz Dolatshahi.*)

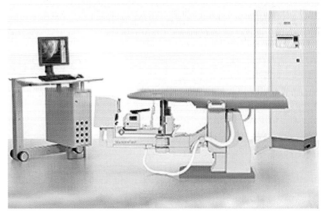

FIGURE 29-3 Prone stereotactic table originally manufactured by Fischer Imaging (Denver) as Mammotest, and now by Siemens (New York). A unidirectional table utilizing a polar coordinating system for targeting.

the horizontal x, vertical y, and depth z coordinates of the lesion in 3-dimensional space. These coordinates are transmitted to the needle holder, which is moved to the exact position that will place the tip of the biopsy probe at the lesion.

There are 2 targeting systems utilized in stereotactic biopsy equipment. Stereotactic equipment manufactured by Siemens utilizes a polar coordinate system (Fig. 29-2), and equipment

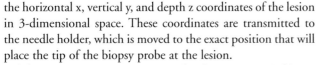

manufactured by Hologic utilizes a Cartesian coordinate system (Fig. 29-3). The polar coordinate system defines a target by distances from a fixed point and angular distances from a reference line (Fig. 29-4). The depth of the targeted lesion is determined from the back compression plate. The horizontal and vertical axes are expressed in degrees while the depth of the lesion is in mm.

The Cartesian system defines the exact position of the target lesion in 3-dimensional space in millimeters in 3 axes that intersect at right angles: z (depth), x (horizontal), and y (vertical). The depth is determined from a reference point in front of the breast on the front compression plate (Fig. 29-5). The z-coordinate indicates the depth of the target lesion between the superficial skin surface and the deep skin surface on the opposite side of the compressed breast. A z-value of 0 indicates the level of a reference point on the compression plate in front of the breast (this is the plate constructed with the opening through which the biopsy is performed). The z-value corresponding to the level of the image receptor behind the breast will, by definition, equal the thickness of the compressed breast.

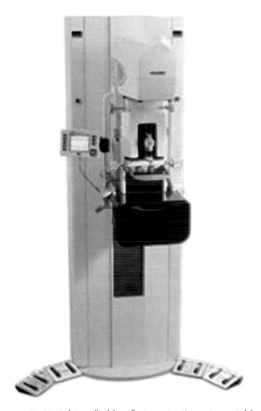

FIGURE 29-2 Upright or "add-on" stereotactic system. Added to an existing mammography unit. When stereotactic procedures are not being done, functions as a mammography system for screening or diagnostic studies. (*Used with permission from Siemens, New York.*)

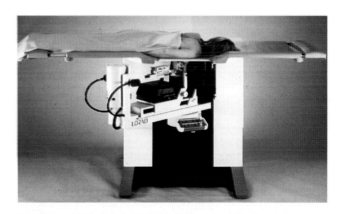

FIGURE 29-4 Prone stereotactic table (Lorad Multicare Platinum, Hologic; Bedford, Massachusetts). Utilizes a Cartesian coordinating system for targeting.

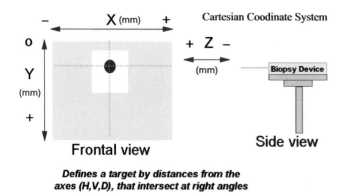

FIGURE 29-5 Depiction of the Cartesian coordinating technology. All coordinates are derived from a reference point on the front compression paddle. All coordinates are given in millimeters.

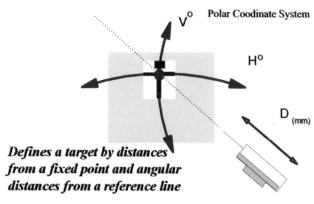

FIGURE 29-6 Depiction of the polar coordinating technology. Depth from the back of the breast to the lesion is expressed in millimeters, while the horizontal and vertical axes are given in degrees.

For example, if the breast compresses to a thickness of 35 mm, the skin surface through which the biopsy needle enters will have a z-value of 0, and the opposite skin surface, against the image receptor, will have a z-value of 35; a point with a z-value of 45 lies beyond the breast in the image receptor. One should never attempt to biopsy any lesion with a calculated z-value greater that the compression thickness of the breast for 2 reasons. First, if a lesion is real, it cannot lie outside of the breast. Second, extending the biopsy device into the image receptor will damage both the biopsy probe and the back breast support.

INDICATIONS

Indications for stereotactic breast biopsy are suspicious microcalcifications and masses (or densities) seen on mammography but not identifiable on ultrasound. At many institutions percutaneous core needle biopsy has replaced open surgical biopsy of the breast in the majority of cases. In the future, minimally invasive core needle biopsy promises to become the standard of care for the biopsy of breast lesions.[8]

CONTRAINDICATIONS

Contraindications for stereotactic biopsy include patient characteristics that make lying prone on the biopsy table for the duration of the procedure (about 45 minutes) impossible, medications that make needle biopsy dangerous, and factors related to individual breast geometry.

Contraindications related to the biopsy table are patient weight greater than the weight limit of the table (currently 300 lb); extreme kyphosis, making it impossible to position the breast deep enough through the hole in the biopsy table; and orthopnea, making it impossible for the patient to lie prone. These factors related to the biopsy table can be overcome by use of a stereotactic biopsy attachment that attaches to an upright mammography unit. These units are less popular than table-mounted

dedicated sterotactic biopsy units, but they are less expensive, and are useful in settings where there is not sufficient room available to dedicate to a stereotactic biopsy table (Fig. 29-6).

Contraindications that make an intervention dangerous include bleeding diathesis and anticoagulants such as Plavix (*clopidogrel bisulfate*) and Coumadin (*warfarin sodium*). Careful planning for the procedure may include reversing a bleeding disorder, the temporary interruption of anticoagulants, or the substitution of short-acting anticoagulants.

Contraindications to stereotactic breast biopsy that are the result of individual breast geometry can be the most difficult obstacles to overcome. If the breast compresses to less than 2.8 cm (2.2 cm for a highly experienced team), the patient is likely not a candidate for stereotactic breast biopsy with currently available equipment. When reviewing a patient's mammogram prior to scheduling a biopsy, it is often possible to determine the compressed thickness of the breast simply by reading the demographic information included on the corner of each mammogram image. It is also possible for a breast to be so thick (9 cm) that a lesion in the center of the breast is not accessible to the biopsy probe. Finally, some lesions are so close to the chest wall or to the skin that they are not accessible for stereotactic biopsy. Despite these diverse contraindications, the vast majority of breast lesions identified on mammography can be successfully sampled with stereotactic breast biopsy.

PROCEDURE

Under ideal circumstances, stereotactic breast biopsy is considered a team endeavor, with essential functions performed by the surgeon, the radiologist, the pathologist, the x-ray technologist, and the histologic technologist. The first step in preparation for a stereotactic core needle breast biopsy is selecting the approach to the breast for the needle insertion (ie, lateral, medial, cranial, or caudal). The shortest approach is usually preferable, as the biopsy probe passes through the smallest volume of breast tissue. In some cases, if the patient intends to wear bikinis or clothing with very low necklines, the physician may choose the caudal or lateral approach in preference to the shortest approach, so that the small incision needed to pass the biopsy device into the breast tissue and resulting scar will not be on an exposed area of the breast. If the surgeon plans to biopsy multiple lesions in the same breast at the same sitting, it may be preferable to choose an approach that allows optimal access to all of the lesions with minimal repositioning of the patient rather than choosing a different approach for each of the multiple lesions and repositioning the patient for each lesion. One should keep in mind that to biopsy different lesions in the same breast from both the lateral and the medial approaches requires taking the patient off the table in between biopsies to reverse the positions of the patient's head and feet.

After choosing an approach, and positioning the patient on the biopsy table, a 0-degree scout image is obtained with the stereotactic equipment to confirm the presence of the lesion within the field of view (Fig. 29-7). If the lesion does not fall within the small field of view, the compression plate must be repositioned so that the lesion is clearly identified on the image. One of the greatest challenges in performing a stereotactic biopsy can be deciding where to reposition the compression plate so that the lesion falls within the field of view. One can save time by carefully studying the screening mammogram image looking for landmarks such as a vessel or a macrocalcification that can aid the physician in identifying the lesion to be biopsied.

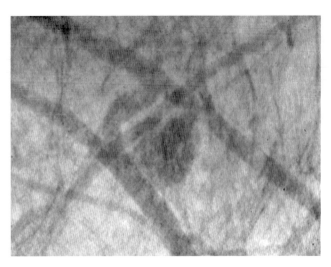

FIGURE 29-8 The relationship of vessels to the abnormality to be biopsied is evaluated on the scout image. The patient may have to be repositioned to obtain a clear path for the biopsy device to reach the lesion. Vessels may be targeted like the lesion to determine the depth to the vessels, which may be in front of or behind the abnormality.

Once the target lesion has been identified, if it is located in the periphery of the field of view, the compression plate should be repositioned so that the lesion is closer to the center of the field of view. An important fact that can be learned from the planar image is the proximity of blood vessels to the target lesion (Fig. 29-8). If the vacuum-assisted biopsy probe is positioned in proximity to a blood vessel, there is danger of injuring the vessel with the biopsy needle, resulting in hemorrhage that might require suturing or surgical exploration. Therefore, a different approach might be necessary to avoid excessive bleeding during the biopsy. Following this, a stereo pair of images is obtained. In some cases when there is not complete confidence that the correct lesion has been identified, the stereo pair itself may be helpful in confirming the identity of a finding as the correct target.

The physician identifies the lesion on both images of the stereo pair and selects the point on each image with a computer cursor (Fig. 29-9). The computer software triangulates from these 2 data points to calculate the exact position of the target lesion in 3-dimensional space. This position is expressed on the computer display as 3 coordinates (in the Cartesian coordinate system, these are labeled x, y, and z). The physician must first confirm that the coordinates of the target lie within the breast. If the z value lies beyond the breast, a different skin surface should be selected to approach the lesion; for example, if the z-value is greater than the compressed thickness of the breast when targeted from a lateral approach, consider a caudal approach.

Second, the physician must determine that there is sufficient breast tissue in front of the lesion and behind the lesion to use the available biopsy device. For instance, one brand of biopsy probe requires that the z-value must be at least 15 because sampling a lesion less than 15 mm from the external skin surface would risk sampling skin resulting in a gaping entry wound,

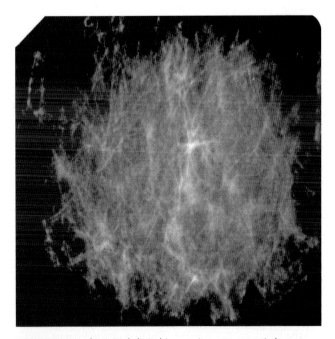

FIGURE 29-7 The initial digital image in a stereotactic breast biopsy. The scout image identifies the target. The image abnormality must be in the center one-third of the image in the vertical plane. The patient may have to be repositioned until the abnormality is identified and is located in the proper area of the image.

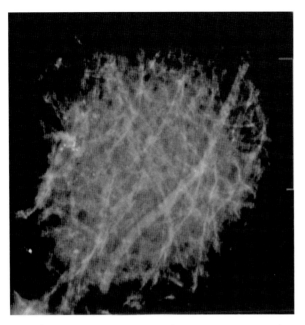 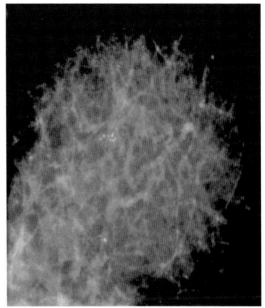

FIGURE 29-9 The stereotactic images, 30 degrees apart, are used to target the lesion.

and allowing air to freely enter the biopsy cavity, breaking the vacuum that is necessary for a vacuum-assisted biopsy device to function. The same biopsy probe requires that the z-value plus an additional 5 mm must, in combination, total less than the compression thickness. This determination is referred to as the stroke margin, which is defined as the distance from the tip of the biopsy needle to the back of the breast once the needle is in position for tissue sampling. If the stroke margin is too small, the biopsy needle will pierce the back of the breast, injuring the patient and damaging the back compression plate.

Only after the lesion has been targeted and it has been determined that the depth of the lesion in the breast is compatible with the biopsy device, does the biopsy procedure continue. Following application of an antiseptic solution to the skin, local anesthetic is injected into the skin at the intersection of the x- and y-coordinates corresponding to the location of the target. The automated needle holder of the stereotactic biopsy system can be used to introduce a spinal needle into the breast through the lesion. Anesthetic is injected through the spinal needle to the level of the target lesion. An alternative method of delivering local anesthetic to the intended biopsy site is to introduce a needle "free handed," approximating the depth of the lesion and injecting anesthetic into the vicinity of the lesion.

While a stereotactic breast biopsy can be performed utilizing several biopsy techniques including fine-needle aspiration biopsy, multiple-insertion spring-operated "biopsy gun" biopsy, single-insertion vacuum-assisted biopsy, or intact radiofrequency extraction devices, it is now recommended that fine-needle aspiration and spring-loaded biopsy needles should be replaced by the more advanced sampling devices such as a vacuum device or a radiofrequency biopsy tool, which yield larger samples.

The next step in the biopsy procedure is dependent upon which biopsy probe is utilized. For some biopsy probes, it is necessary to nick the skin with a scalpel, spread the skin, and retract the skin nick with a pair of eyelid retractors. Other biopsy probes are designed with a cutting tip on the probe, and can be advanced directly into the breast without a skin nick. The biopsy device is then advanced to the prefire position in the breast or the biopsy position if the device is fired (extended) outside the breast. A pair of prefire stereo images is obtained to confirm that the biopsy probe is in the correct position prior to sampling (Fig. 29-10). If necessary, the position of the probe can be adjusted to assure that the target lesion is optimally sampled. Strategies for correcting for suboptimal prefire position are covered thoroughly elsewhere. If the biopsy device is fired outside of the patient, the next paragraph does not apply.

After confirming that the prefire position of the biopsy probe is correct (ie, the tip is aimed at the target lesion), the probe is fired, and a postfire pair of stereo images is obtained (Fig. 29-11). The postfire images are evaluated to confirm that the biopsy probe is positioned within or alongside the lesion. If necessary, the probe position can be adjusted, and the new position confirmed with a pair of stereo images.

SAMPLING AND SPECIMEN PROCESSING

Sampling of the lesion varies depending upon the biopsy device. Vacuum-assisted core biopsy devices are usually rotated to take between 4 and 12 samples located at different positions along the probe designated according to the numbers on a clock face, such as 12:00, 3:00, 6:00, and so forth.

The handling of the biopsy sample is an important phase of the procedure. If the target lesion was a cluster of microcalcifications, the specimen is radiographed to establish whether there are calcifications in the biopsy sample (Fig. 29-12).[9] If there are no calcifications on the specimen radiograph, then additional biopsy samples are obtained. When calcifications have been identified in the specimen, the specimen radiograph is studied, and those

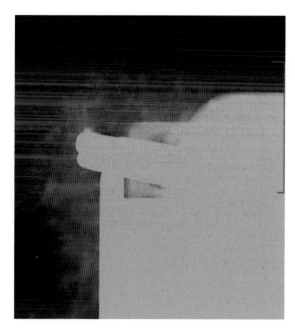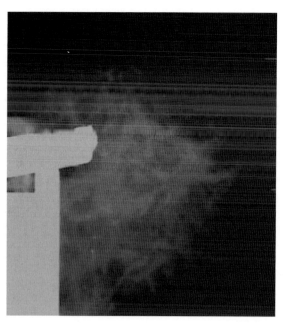

FIGURE 29-10 All vacuum-assisted biopsy devices can be "fired" in the breast or before insertion into the breast. If fired in the breast, prefire stereotactic images are always obtained to evaluate the position of the lesion relative to the needle. Repositioning of the needle may be necessary if during insertion of the needle the lesion moved or "snow-plowed" away from the needle far enough so that the lesion will not be captured unless repositioning takes place.

cores that contain calcium should be separated into one labeled container of preservative and those cores that do not contain calcium are placed into a second separate labeled container of preservative. This technique tells the pathologist which set or cores should be the most diagnostic, although all cores, with and without calcification, must be examined microscopically.

Upon confirming the presence of calcium in the biopsy sample, a radiopaque marker is placed through the biopsy probe to permanently mark the biopsy site (Fig. 29-13). This is particularly important if the target lesion represented calcifications that were completely removed by the biopsy device. In the event that the pathologic diagnosis is malignant or premalignant, then

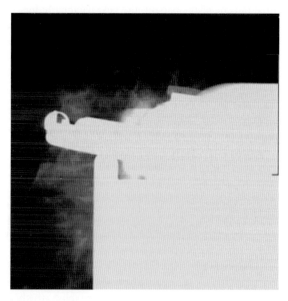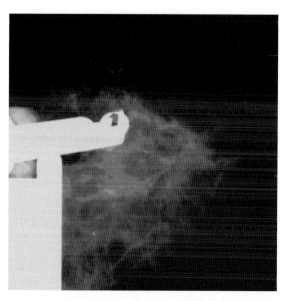

FIGURE 29-11 Postfire stereotactic images are obtained after the device is fired in the breast or if the device was fired outside the breast and inserted in the fired position. These images allow the biopsy sequence to be planned utilizing the rotational capability of all of the vacuum-assisted or rotating cutter needles. Recognizing the special relationship of the lesion to the sampling trough of the needle at any "hour" of the clock allows for sampling an area most likely to have the lesion at the star of the biopsy sequence.

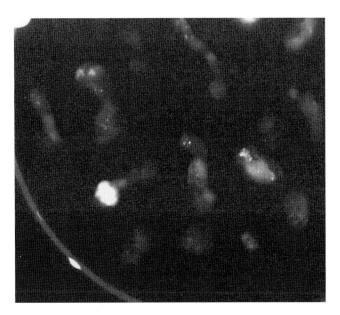

FIGURE 29-12 Example of a specimen radiograph confirming the presence of microcalcifications in the sample cores.

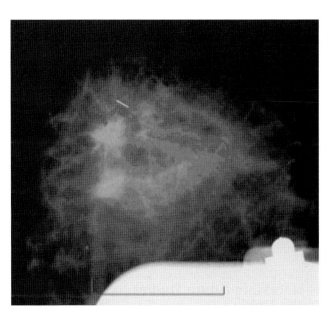

FIGURE 29-13 This post-procedure image confirms proper deployment of a marker (clip) placed at the conclusion of the stereotactic biopsy procedure. A stereo pair of images would confirm that the marker was deployed at the proper depth, as well.

the marker serves as a target for future needle localization and open surgery.

If more than 1 lesion is biopsied, or if there are preexisting biopsy markers in the breast resulting from previous biopsies, it is wise to use a different-shaped marker for each biopsy site. The shape of the marker should be noted on the pathology requisition for the specimen from each biopsy site, and the pathologist should record the shape of the marker on the pathology report as well. In this way, if one biopsy site is positive and others are negative, it is possible to localize the correct site for lumpectomy.

COMPLETION OF PROCEDURE

Before the patient is released from compression, a stereo pair of images should be obtained to confirm that the marker has been successfully deployed and is at the approximate depth of the lesion. A single postprocedure image is not adequate to confirm marker placement, because one might mistakenly believe that the marker is at the biopsy site, even if it has migrated along the track of the biopsy probe and has been left just under the skin at the entry site. Following stereotactic biopsy, the patient is taken out of the biopsy device and pressure is applied to the breast until it has been determined that there is no bleeding. Then 2 standard mammographic images are obtained of the involved breast to document the marker location and confirm that the correct lesion was biopsied. If mammography is not available at the location of the biopsy, then in a timely fashion the patient should be sent to an imaging facility for a postbiopsy 2-view mammogram of the biopsied breast. It is a good policy to have printed postprocedure instruction sheets to give to patients following the biopsy.

Prior to leaving the biopsy room, the small incision in the skin can be closed with self-adhesive strips and covered with a small gauze dressing. It is recommended that a disposable ice pack be used over the dressing for about 1 hour. In some centers the chest is wrapped for compression with an Ace bandage or a commercially available wrap to try to reduce bruising and postprocedure bleeding.

It is incumbent on the surgeon to evaluate the pathology report following each biopsy and confirm that the pathologic diagnosis is concordant with the imaging findings. Recognizing a discordant biopsy result and appreciating that a repeat biopsy is necessary is the key to preventing a false-negative biopsy—that is, missing a breast cancer.

FUTURE DIRECTIONS

Digital mammography technology has made enormous strides since the introduction of stereotactic biopsy equipment.[10] Full-field digital mammography equipment is now widely available, and it should be possible in the near future to produce a stereotactic biopsy device that images the entire breast, including the opening through which the biopsy probe is placed. This advance would greatly simplify repositioning the patient if the target lesion does not fall in the field of view of the opening in the compression plate.

Stereotactic guidance may be used in the future to treat breast cancers measuring 1 cm or less with minimally invasive in situ thermal ablation, or noninvasive focused microwave energy. Clinical trials are underway at the time of this writing to evaluate laser ablation, cryoablation, and radiofrequency ablation to treat small breast cancers. To date, laser ablation is most easily adapted to stereotactic guidance. Employing the prone table or upright stereotactic systems, a laser probe is inserted into the malignancy and an array of thermisters is situated juxtaposed to the tumor, also placed using stereotactic guidance. Once the laser is in place, it is energized, resulting in thermal destruction of the cancer. The temperature array provides constant readouts of the temperature. Tissue dies at approximately 60°C. Tissue around the tumor must also be ablated to provide an acceptable margin around the tumor to minimize local recurrences.

Cryoablation and radiofrequency ablation are being studied using ultrasound as the image-guidance technology. Noninvasive focused high-density ultrasound ablations are being studied utilizing MR guidance. In the future, it is possible that stereotactic guidance will be applied to these ablation technologies as well.

Necessary Future Studies to Advance the Field

Stereotactic breast biopsy is currently a diagnostic technique, not a treatment for breast cancer. Even if the mammographic finding is completely removed by the vacuum-assisted biopsy device, the standard of care is to perform an open surgical lumpectomy. In the future, it is possible that physicians may perform stereotactic "lumpectomy" as a replacement for open surgical lumpectomy. This would be a potential treatment for the smallest malignant breast lesions. This would be possible using intact extraction devices that have recently been developed. These devices use stereotactic guidance and have the potential to resect and extract small cancers from the breast with a measurable margin of intact normal tissue around the cancer. Clinical trials would be necessary to show the equivalence of stereotactic lumpectomy to traditional open lumpectomy. These trials would have to demonstrate consistent histologically negative margins. The recurrence rate and complication rate would have to be favorable compared to traditional open lumpectomy.

SUMMARY

Stereotactic breast biopsy has almost completely replaced open surgical biopsy at many institutions. Stereotactic biopsy has several important advantages compared to open surgical biopsy. It is a minimally invasive technique, and the procedure is much more rapid than open biopsy. If a mammographically detected lesion is visible in only one mammographic view, it can be biopsied using stereotactic guidance, whereas needle localization for surgical biopsy requires that a lesion be visible in 2 mammographic views.

The procedure for performing stereotactic breast biopsy follows a logical sequence of standardized steps. The tissue obtained is prepared into histology slides for pathologic diagnosis. A marker is placed at the biopsy site to mark the location for future lumpectomy, in the event that the biopsy sample proves to be malignant. It is critical that pathology review demonstrates histologic and radiologic concordance. Future developments in this field may include stereotactic guidance for thermal ablation of tumors and minimally invasive, nonsurgical intact extraction lumpectomy for small breast cancers.

REFERENCES

1. Bolmgren J, Jacobson B, Nordenstrom B. Stereotaxic instrument for the needle biopsy of the mamma. *Am J Roentgenol.* 1977;129:121-125.
2. Elvecrog EL, Lechner MC, Nelson MT. Nonpalpable breast lesions: correlation of stereotactic large-core needle biopsy and surgical results. *Radiology.* 1993;188:453-455.
3. Dowlatshahi K, Jokich PM, Schmidt R, et al. Cytologic diagnosis of occult breast lesions using stereotaxic needle aspiration. *Arch Surg.* 1987;122:1343-1346.
4. Gisvold J, Goellner J, Grant C, et al. Breast biopsy: a comparative study of stereotaxically guided core and excisional techniques. *Am J Roentgenol.* 1994;193:91-95.
5. Kopans D. Review of stereotaxic large-core needle biopsy and surgical biopsy results in nonpalpable breast lesions. *Radiology.* 1993;189:665-666.
6. Parker SH, Lovin JD, Jobe WE, et al. Nonpalpable breast lesions: stereotactic automated large core biopsies. *Radiology.* 1991;180:403-407.
7. Fajardo LL, Willison KM, Pizzutiello RJ. *A Comprehensive Approach to Stereotactic Breast Biopsy.* Blackwell Science, Inc. Cambridge, MA. 1996.
8. Silverstein MJ, Recht A, Lagios M, et al. Image-detected breast cancer: state of the art diagnosis and treatment, International Breast Cancer Consensus Conference. *J Am Coll Surg.* 2001;193:297-302.
9. Liberman L, Evans WP III, Dershaw DD, et al. Radiography of microcalcifications in stereotaxic mammary core biopsy specimens. *Radiology.* 1994;190:223-225.
10. Pisano ED, Gastonis C, Hendrick E, et al. Diagnostic performance of digital versus film mammography for breast-cancer screening. *N Engl J Med.* 2005;353:1773-1183.

CHAPTER 30

Anatomy and Ultrasound of the Breast and Atlas of Ultrasound Findings

Jay K. Harness

ANATOMY AND ULTRASOUND OF THE BREAST

The contemporary practice of breast surgery requires an in-depth understanding of breast anatomy and imaging. Ultrasound of the breast has emerged over the past decade as an essential component of the evaluation of patients with breast disease and as an important tool in the operating room (OR).

Surgeons are natural imagers since they are use to thinking 3-dimensionally. Once they understand how ultrasound machines create images, what the images mean, and how the images correlate with benign and malignant breast conditions, they become "sonographic clinicians." Surgeons synthesize the patient's history with their physical, mammographic, ultrasound, and magnetic resonance imaging (MRI) findings into a clearer understanding of the probable diagnosis and a future course of action. In the OR, ultrasound is an important tool to facilitate wire-localization excisional biopsies or partial mastectomies. Ultrasound can be used to localize nonpalpable benign or malignant lesions in the OR or map the location of a cancer prior to starting a mastectomy.

This chapter offers an introduction to understanding ultrasound anatomy of the breast. The chapter also includes a discussion on how to characterize the sonographic appearances of benign and malignant breast lesions as well as an atlas of common benign and malignant lesions of the breast.

BREAST ANATOMY

There are literally thousands of drawings of the breast, its blood supply, lymphatic drainage, and regional nerves that can be found in anatomy books and textbooks on breast disease. The breast is composed of 15 to 20 lobes in most women. Within each lobe are numerous lobules and small ducts that join to form larger ducts, which then progress to form a single major lobar duct. The major lobar ducts come together beneath the nipple and widen as the lactiferous sinus (Figs. 30-1 and 30-2).

In general, the central lobar ducts course away from the nipple in a radial pattern (Fig. 30-3). However, these ducts may be tortuous. Lobes vary in size and overlap each other. The central lobar ducts lie nearer the chest wall than the skin of the breast. Arising from the central lobar ducts are rows of lobules that are circumferential.[1] Most of the lobules are oriented anteriorly or anterolaterally (Fig. 30-1).

The terminal ductolobular unit (TDLU) is the functional unit of the breast (Fig. 30-1). It is composed of a lobule and its terminal duct. Most lobules arise from smaller, more peripheral branch ducts. However, they may arise from larger central ducts, but rarely from the lactiferous sinus portion of main lobar ducts.[2] Most ductal carcinomas are thought to arise within the TDLU or more centrally from an intraductal papilloma.

The breast is roughly elliptical in shape with an extension toward the axilla called the tail of Spence. The length and volume of the tail of Spence is variable, and its resection must not be missed during the performance of a mastectomy. The nipple is usually somewhat medial and inferior to the center of the breast. This asymmetry of the breast means that more lobular volume is in the upper outer quadrant with less lobular volume in the lower quadrants (Fig. 30-3). The greater number of breast cancers in the upper outer quadrant is at least partially due to the greater lobular volume in that quadrant plus the slower involution of tissue in that quadrant with aging.

The breast is a modified sweat gland that lies between 2 layers of the superficial fascia: a superficial layer beneath the dermis and a deep layer overlying the pectoralis fascia and chest wall (Fig. 30-2). There are 3 major zones within the breast: the

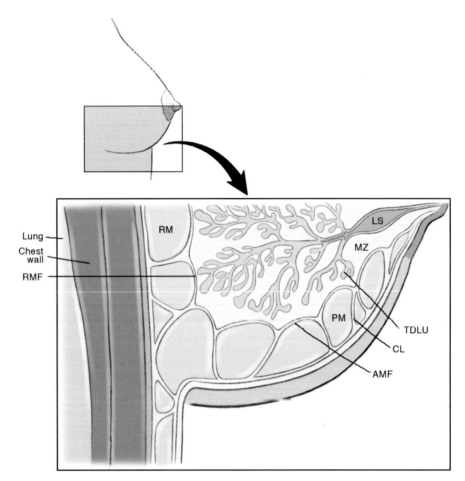

FIGURE 30-1 There are 3 zones within the breast. The premammary (PM) or subcutaneous fat zone contains Cooper ligaments (CL), and in some cases, a small number of peripheral ducts and lobules. The mammary zone (MZ) contains all of the central ducts and most of the peripheral ducts and lobules. The retromammary zone (RM) is the deepest of the 3 zones and contains only fat and ligaments. The anterior mammary fascia (AMF) and the retromammary fascia (RMF) encase the mammary zone. The lactiferous sinus (LS) is the dilated end of a main lobar duct. *(Redrawn with permission from Stavros AT. Breast Ultrasound. Philadelphia, PA: Lippincott Williams, & Wilkins; 2004.)*

premammary, mammary, and retromammary zones (Fig. 30-1).[1] Most TDLUs lie within the mammary zone, but (importantly) a few TDLUs may extend into the Cooper ligaments and thus lie in the premammary (subcutaneous fat) zone.

The areola and nipple are covered by pigmented skin. The areola also contains sweat glands that lubricate it during lactation. The epithelium of the nipple skin (squamous) transitions through the outer ducts of the nipple to the epithelium of the lactiferous sinus and ductal system as 1 to 2 cell layers stuck to a thinner "basal membrane." That basal membrane is then stuck onto myoepithelial cells, loose connective tissue, and fat.[2]

■ Variations in Breast Anatomy over Time

Ductal growth is stimulated by estrogen production. Full lobular development requires both estrogen and progesterone stimulation. Initial breast development begins with estrogen stimulation during the onset of puberty (around 11-14 years

of age). Lobular proliferation and maturation do not occur until progesterone production stabilizes in late the teens or early 20s. Under age 20, connective tissue is the major component of the breast, representing over 50% of the total breast organ volume.

Pregnancy causes significant changes in the breast. In the first trimester, there is marked estrogenic stimulation of the breasts. During the second and third trimesters, there is a proliferation in both number and size of the TDLUs with an increase in the number of ductules (acini). Ultimately, nearly all of the fibrous tissue is replaced by glandular tissue during pregnancy.

After each pregnancy and lactation period, there is a regression of the lobules. The number of ductules within each TDLU decreases and the number of lobules also decreases. The volume of epithelial cells peaks at age 30 years, when it can be 30% of the total breast volume. Thereafter, it rapidly falls off. The percentage of fat in the breast increases from around 30% of the breast volume at age 30 to 65% at 75 years.[2]

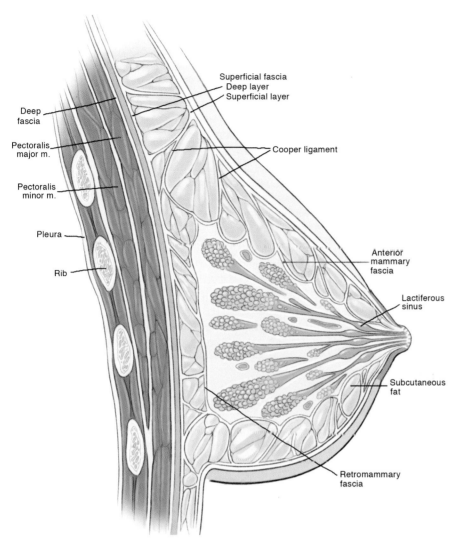

Deep fascia

Pectoralis major m.

Pectoralis minor m.

Pleura

Rib

Superficial fascia
Deep layer
Superficial layer

Cooper ligament

Anterior mammary fascia

Lactiferous sinus

Subcutaneous fat

Retromammary fascia

FIGURE 30-2 Cross-sectional anatomy of the breast showing important landmarks. *(Reproduced with permission from Harness JK, Wisher DB, eds. Ultrasound in Surgical Practice—Basic Principles and Clinical Applications. New York, NY: Wiley-Liss; 2001: 159-236.)*

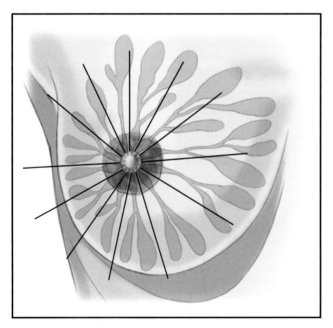

FIGURE 30-3 Ellipsoid shape of the breast with a generally radial pattern of the lobar ducts. *(Reproduced with permission from Stavros AT. Breast Ultrasound. Philadelphia, PA: Lippincott Williams, & Wilkins; 2004:56-79.)*

There is a process of involution that takes several years after menopause. Very few mature lobules remain in the breast. Hormone replacement therapy (HRT) will alter the process of involution. Combined estrogen-progesterone HRT may cause postmenopausal persistence or development of mature lobules. Estrogen-alone HRT will not result in persistence of fully developed lobules, but may slow their regression.[1] With normal involution of the breast, the volume of epithelial cells falls off after peaking at age 30 years (30%) to around 10% at 50 years and 5% at 75 years. It is replaced primarily by fat.[2]

LYMPHATIC DRAINAGE OF THE BREAST

The lymphatics of the breast drain primarily to the axilla and much less frequently to the internal mammary lymph nodes. Documented cases of drainage to the opposite axilla are quite rare. Most quadrants of the breast drain first superficially in a rich layer of lymphatics just superficial to the anterior mammary fascia, which flows to the periareolar plexus and then to the axilla. Injection of blue dye and/or a radioisotope in the subareolar region has proven to be a very accurate way to perform sentinel lymph node biopsies.

The axillary lymph nodes are classified by regions. Level I nodes are lateral and inferior to the pectoralis minor muscle. Level II nodes are deep to the pectoralis minor, while level III nodes lie medial and superior to the pectoralis minor. It is felt that lymphatic drainage can only reach the supraclavicular nodes after first passing through subclavian or deep jugular chains.

Intramammary lymph nodes are most common in the axillary segment or far lateral aspects of the breast.[1] They can also occur in the far medial aspect of the breast or any quadrant. Intramammary lymph nodes can be sentinel nodes and are occasionally found to be the only positive lymph node with invasive cancers.

Newly diagnosed patients with invasive breast cancer should have their axillae carefully examined not only by physical examination but also by ultrasound. The finding of a suspicious lymph node(s) should lead to a prompt ultrasound-guided biopsy (see Chapter 34).

BLOOD SUPPLY TO THE BREAST

The blood supply to the breast is very rich. Medially, there are perforating branches of the internal mammary arteries. Additional blood supply comes from intercostal perforators and by lateral thoracic and thoracoabdominal branches of the axillary artery. A network of small arteries also connects the skin with the glandular portion of the breast via branches running with some Cooper ligaments.

The venous drainage of the breast is more variable than the arterial inflow. Much of the venous drainage of the breast parallels the lymphatic drainage with superficial branches that are not accompanied by arteries. The deeper arteries supplying the breast are accompanied by veins. Preserving more subcutaneous fat during mastectomy helps to insure flap viability by preserving the subcutaneous plexus of veins and small arteries that supply the skin of the breast.

INDICATIONS FOR BREAST ULTRASOUND

Table 30-1 lists the generally accepted indications for breast ultrasound. In the United States, ultrasound is not yet indicated as a screening procedure for the detection of nonpalpable breast cancers. Mammography cannot distinguish between solid breast lesions and cyst. Ultrasound can differentiate these. Ultrasound identifies characteristics of a lesion that suggest whether it is benign or malignant. The evaluation and diagnosis of mammographically and/or MRI indeterminate lesions (both palpable and nonpalpable) is one of the most important uses of breast ultrasound.

SCANNING TECHNIQUES

The patient is positioned for an ultrasound examination the same way she (he) is for a physical examination: supine with the ipsilateral hand behind the head (Fig. 30-4). This position allows the

TABLE 30-1 Indications for Breast Ultrasound

Palpable breast mass
Mammographically indeterminate lesion
Second-look ultrasound for MRI indeterminate lesion
Radiographically dense breast
Axillary lymph nodes
Pregnancy and lactation
Oncologic follow-up
  After mastectomy
  After breast-conserving surgery
Postoperative follow-up
  Hematomas
  Seromas
  Prostheses
Ultrasound-guided interventions
  Cyst aspirations
  Biopsy of solid lesions
  Preoperative needle localization
  Axillary lymph node fine-needle aspiration
  Peritumoral injection for sentinel lymph node biopsy

breast to be thinned to the greatest extent possible and the tissue planes of the breast are pulled parallel with the skin.

The patient is rolled medially (obliquely) to a degree that minimizes breast thickness in the quadrant being scanned. Lesions in the lateral quadrants require the greatest degree of oblique positioning, while lesions in the medial quadrants may be best scanned with the patient in a straight supine position (Fig. 30-5).

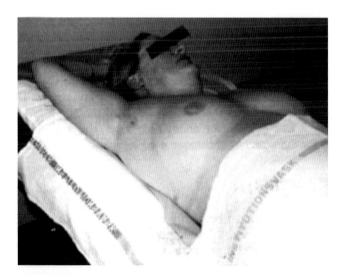

FIGURE 30-4 The standard position for breast ultrasound. *(Reproduced with permission from Harness JK, Wisher DB, eds.* Ultrasound in Surgical Practice—Basic Principles and Clinical Applications. *New York, NY: Wiley-Liss; 2001:159-236.)*

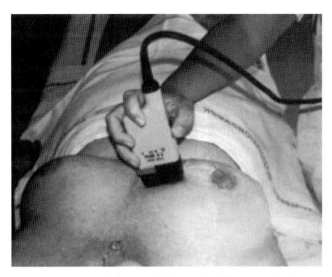

FIGURE 30-5 Radial scan of the medial breast with the patient in the supine position. *(Reproduced with permission from Harness JK, Wisher DB, eds.* Ultrasound in Surgical Practice—Basic Principles and Clinical Applications. *New York, NY: Wiley-Liss; 2001:159-236.)*

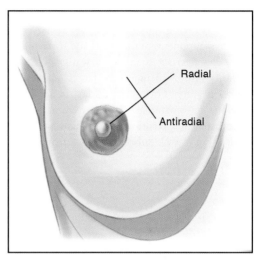

FIGURE 30-7 Transducer placement for radial and antiradial scanning. *(Reproduced with permission from Harness JK, Wisher DB, eds.* Ultrasound in Surgical Practice—Basic Principles and Clinical Applications. *New York, NY: Wiley-Liss; 2001:159-236.)*

Imaging the nipple–areolar complex and its underlying ducts requires special maneuvering of the transducer because of the dense connective tissue in this area. The nipple–areolar complex may cause strong posterior shadowing as a result of the attenuation of the ultrasound beam. To avoid the shadowing problem, place the transducer adjacent to the nipple and angle the ultrasound beam into the retroareolar region (Fig. 30-6).

Most breast ultrasound examinations performed by surgeons target a specific clinical and/or mammographic finding. Such examinations are usually limited to the general area of abnormality. Solid and cystic lesions of the breast should be scanned in 2 planes (usually the radial and antiradial) (Fig. 30-7). The location should be documented using a clock notation, identifying both the hour location and the distance from the nipple.

LEARNING A NEW LANGUAGE

When describing an ultrasound image, it is important for surgeons to use a standardized nomenclature. The following key words are essential for describing ultrasound images:

Hyperechoic: A shade of gray that is bright white or brighter than surrounding structures; for example, Cooper ligaments of the breast are hyperechoic compared to the subcutaneous fat.

Hypoechoic: A shade of gray that is dark or less bright than surrounding structures; for example, the subcutaneous fat of the breast is always hypoechoic.

Anechoic: Without internal echoes (black); for example, a simple cyst is anechoic (black) because it has no internal echoes.

Echogenic: A bright white appearance when scanning with a darker background; for example, microcalcifications in a cancer (which is usually hypoechoic) are very bright white dots.

Homogeneous: Uniform shades of gray throughout a lesion; for example, the internal echoes of a fibroadenoma are usually homogeneous.

Heterogeneous: Nonuniform shades of gray throughout a lesion; for example, the internal echoes of most cancers are heterogeneous.

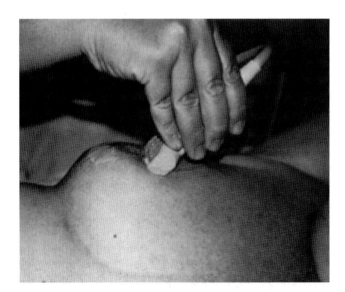

FIGURE 30-6 Transducer angled to view under the nipple–areolar complex. *(Reproduced with permission from Harness JK, Wisher DB, eds.* Ultrasound in Surgical Practice—Basic Principles and Clinical Applications. *New York, NY: Wiley-Liss; 2001:159-236.)*

NORMAL BREAST SONOGRAPHIC ANATOMY

The anatomic components of the breast and surrounding structures display characteristic sonographic features. These components include skin, subcutaneous fat, Cooper ligaments, superficial fascia, anterior mammary fascia, parenchyma, nipple areolar region, retromammary fascia, retromammary space, pectoralis muscles, ribs, pleura, and intramammary and axillary lymph nodes (Fig. 30-2). Subcutaneous, retromammary, and intramammary fat are hypoechoic compared to glandular tissue.

Skin

The skin usually measures 1 to 2 mm in thickness. It is best seen when employing a fluid standoff pad. The skin is generally thicker in the inframammary fold. The thickness of the skin may change as a result of inflammatory disease, irradiation, lymphatic obstruction, or infiltration by cancer (Fig. 30-8).

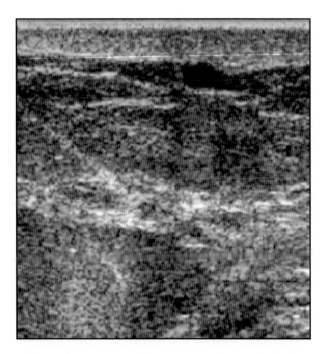

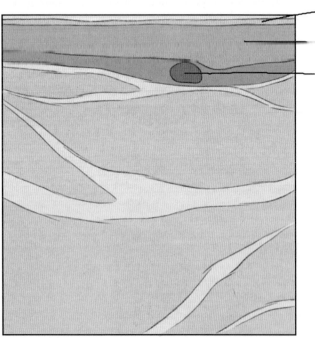

— Emergence echo of transducer

— Skin

— Vein

FIGURE 30-8   Image of a breast that is primarily fatty replaced showing the skin line. *(Reproduced with permission from Harness JK, Wisher DB, eds.* Ultrasound in Surgical Practice—Basic Principles and Clinical Applications. *New York, NY: Wiley-Liss; 2001:159-236.)*

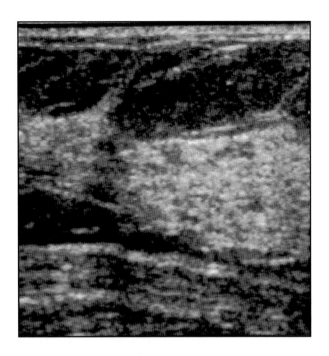

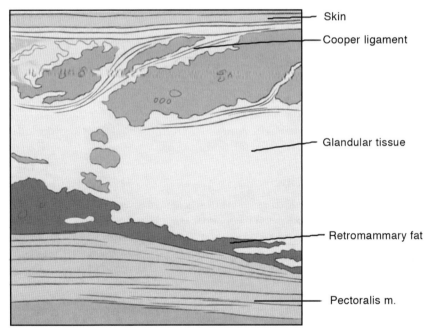

Skin

Cooper ligament

Glandular tissue

Retromammary fat

Pectoralis m.

FIGURE 30-9 Normal breast showing several important landmarks. *(Reproduced with permission from Harness JK, Wisher DB, eds.* Ultrasound in Surgical Practice—Basic Principles and Clinical Applications. *New York, NY: Wiley-Liss; 2001:159-236.)*

Superficial Layer of the Superficial Fascia

The superficial fascia of the thorax divides around the breast into superficial and deep layers. The superficial layer runs under the skin and is seen as a distinct hyperechoic line. Cooper ligaments insert into the superficial layer of the superficial fascia (Fig. 30-9).

Fat

The fat content of the breast varies with age, body weight, and parity. Younger, thinner women may have little subcutaneous or intraparenchymal fat, while postmenopausal women may have breasts that have been nearly completed replaced by fat (Fig. 30-10). Fat lobules are oval in one plane and elongated in the opposite plane.

Cooper Ligaments

Cooper ligaments are the suspensor support for the breast. They are a continuation of the anterior mammary fascia that insert into the superficial layer of the superficial fascia (Fig. 30-11).

Glandular tissue may extend up the Cooper ligaments. With real-time scanning, Cooper ligaments can cause a considerable amount of acoustic shadowing.

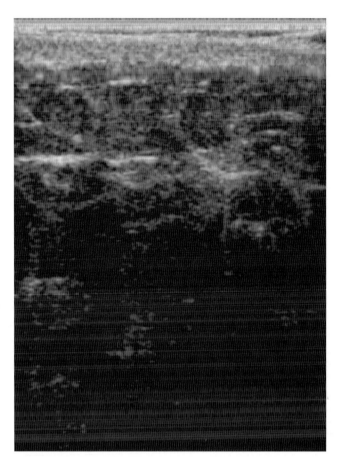

FIGURE 30-10 Fatty replaced breast showing anterior mammary fascia (horizontal hyperechoic line) separating the subcutaneous fat from the fatty replaced mammary zone. (*Reproduced with permission from Harness JK, Wisher DB, eds.* Ultrasound in Surgical Practice—Basic Principles and Clinical Applications. *New York, NY: Wiley-Liss; 2001:159-236.*)

Anterior and Retromammary Fasciae

Each mammary lobe is encased within a fascial sheath. The fascia that lies on the anterior surface of the lobe and separates it from the subcutaneous fat is called the anterior mammary fascia (Fig. 30-12).

The fascia, that lies on the posterior surface of the lobe and separates the lobe from the retromammary fat is termed the retromammary fascia. The glandular or parenchymal portion of the breast lies between these 2 fascial planes (Fig. 30-13).

Breast Parenchyma

Breast parenchyma appears homogenously echogenic compared to fat, but may have hypoechoic zones caused by fat. The glandular tissue is often interlaced with small hypoechoic mammary ducts. Four major parenchymal patterns can be identified: juvenile, premenopausal, postmenopausal, and pregnancy.[3]

The juvenile breast is markedly hyperechoic with little fat. The premenopausal breast is often partially involuted and areas of parenchyma are replaced by fat (Fig. 30-14). The subcutaneous and retromammary fat may also be increased. Postmenopausal

breasts are usually replaced by fat unless a woman has been on hormone replacement therapy. During pregnancy and lactation, a significant increase in glandular tissue occurs along with increases in intramammary ducts (Fig. 30-15).

Nipple–Areolar Region

The nipple–areolar region has dense connective tissue in the nipple and envelopes the lactiferous ducts. The dense connective tissue causes a shadow deep to the nipple if the transducer is placed directly over the nipple (Fig. 30-16). The skin of the areola is less echogenic than the rest of the breast skin. The lactiferous ducts are radially arranged around the nipple. The ducts progressively enlarge as they approach the nipple and form the lactiferous sinuses. The ducts appear as anechoic tubular or round structures that measure 1 to 8 mm in diameter (Fig. 30-17).

Retromammary Fat

Retromammary fat fills the space behind the parenchyma and retromammary fascia (Fig. 30-9). This space usually appears smaller during ultrasound examinations because the patient is supine with ultrasound, which collapses this space.

Pectoralis Muscles

These muscles can be best imaged in the direction of their fibers which is the transverse position of the transducer. The muscles have echogenic fascial planes and fibrous septa. The muscle bundles are hypoechoic (Fig. 30-18). Visualization of the pectoralis muscles ensures that the breast has been adequately penetrated at the site of examination.

Ribs

Ribs are hypoechoic to anechoic structures behind the pectoralis muscles. Longitudinal (sagittal) scans through the medial parasternal portion of the ribs show them as oval structures with homogeneous internal echoes. Ribs attenuate sound causing a deep posterior shadow (Figs 30-19 and 30-20).

Pleura

The pleura images as a bright hyperechoic line behind the ribs and often move with respiration seen with real-time scanning (Fig. 30-19).

Lymph Nodes

Lymph nodes may be seen in the breast parenchyma and the axilla. Normal lymph nodes are usually oval, have an echogenic hilus, and a hypoechoic cortex (Fig. 30-21).

DIAGNOSTIC SONOGRAPHIC DISCRIMINANTS

Benign and malignant breast lesions manifest a wide range of ultrasound appearances. No characteristic is 100% specific. Combinations of ultrasound features are better predictors of malignancy than any one feature. Figure 30-22 lists the 6 major characteristics used by most breast sonographers to suggest that

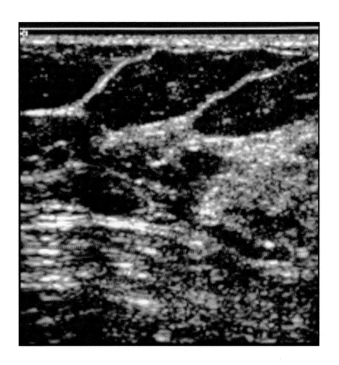

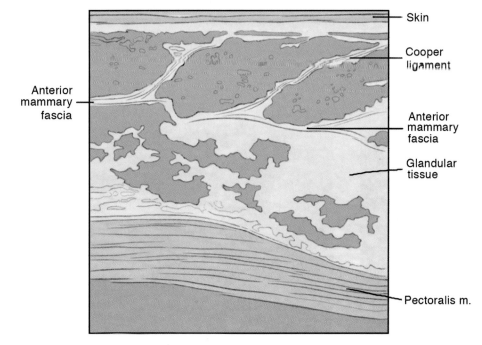

FIGURE 30-11 Cooper ligaments image as bright, hyperechoic, tentlike arcs from the anterior mammary fascia to the superficial layer of the superficial fascia. *(Reproduced with permission from Harness JK, Wisher DB, eds.* Ultrasound in Surgical Practice— Basic Principles and Clinical Applications. *New York, NY: Wiley-Liss; 2001:159-236.)*

a sonographic lesion is benign, malignant, or indeterminate.[4] For each of these characteristics, there are different findings for benign, malignant, and indeterminate features. The shape of the lesion is also an important finding that can suggest whether a lesion is benign or malignant.

The evaluation of margins represents an important step, because the process identifies the lesion's demarcation with respect to its surrounding tissue. Border sharpness results from little interaction between the native tissue and the lesion at its margins. An indistinct border suggests a host response (desmoplastic reaction) has occurred. Cysts and fibroadenomas usually display sharp borders with an abrupt transition from the lesion to the surrounding glandular tissue. Malignancies usually fade

into the surrounding tissue. A hyperechoic rim results from the desmoplastic reaction and is most often associated with malignancy. It also may be associated with breast abscesses and some forms of fibrocystic changes of the breast.

There are several acoustic phenomena that may be observed deep to a sonographic lesion. These include posterior shadowing, posterior enhancement, edge shadowing, and no change in the echoes relative to its surroundings. Posterior enhancement represents a brightening of the tissue behind a lesion and results from enhanced transmission of the ultrasound beam because there is little or no absorption or reflection of the ultrasound beam compared to the adjacent tissue. The brightness behind a cyst is a classic example of posterior enhancement.

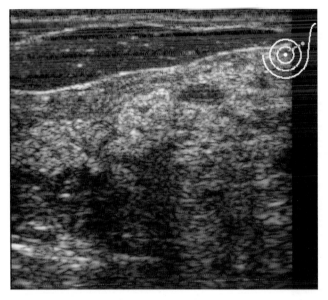

FIGURE 30-12 The bright hyperechoic anterior mammary fascia lies on the anterior surface of the mammary zone.

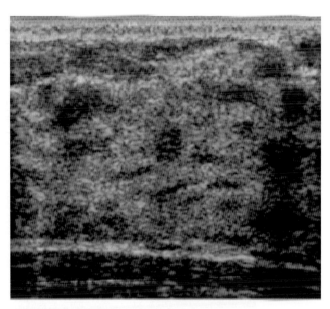

FIGURE 30-14 Breast of a 41-year-old woman who has normal skin, subcutaneous fat, and an early mixed glandular pattern. *(Reproduced with permission from Harness JK, Wisher DB, eds.* Ultrasound in Surgical Practice—Basic Principles and Clinical Applications. *New York, NY: Wiley-Liss; 2001:159-236.)*

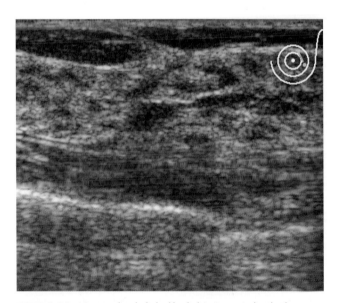

FIGURE 30-13 In the left half of this image, both the anterior mammary fascia and the retromammary fascia can be clearly seen encasing the mammary zone.

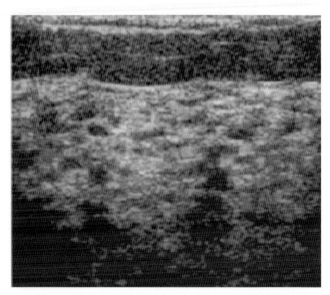

FIGURE 30-15 The normal breast during pregnancy. Note the increased density of the parenchyma and the many dilated ducts. *(Reproduced with permission from Harness JK, Wisher DB, eds.* Ultrasound in Surgical Practice—Basic Principles and Clinical Applications. *New York, NY: Wiley-Liss; 2001:159-236.)*

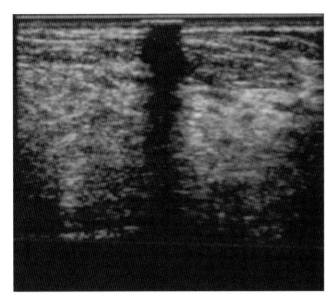

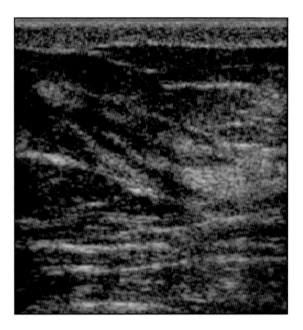

FIGURE 30-16 A posterior acoustic shadow is seen when the transducer is placed over the nipple. *(Reproduced with permission from Harness JK, Wisher DB, eds. Ultrasound in Surgical Practice—Basic Principles and Clinical Applications. New York, NY: Wiley-Liss; 2001:159-236.)*

Posterior shadowing represents a deflection of the ultrasound beam away from the lesion (ie, shadowing behind the rib) and should always be looked upon as a clue that something is going on at the origin of the shadow. A desmoplastic reaction (hyperechoic rim) around a cancer will cause dense posterior shadowing behind a cancer.

Edge shadowing represents an artifact resulting from the reflection of an ultrasound beam off a smooth edge, like the edges of a cyst or a fibroadenoma. Bilateral edge shadowing is associated usually with benign breast lesions and often unilateral shadowing is associated with malignancies.

Taller-than-wide indicates that a lesion has a greater AP dimension than a transverse or craniocaudal dimension. The tissue planes in the breast course horizontally in the position in which the patient is scanned. Lesions that are taller-than-wide are growing across tissue planes and are more likely to be malignant than are lesions growing within the planes. Wider-than-tall is usually associated with benign lesions, which tend to grow within the planes of the breast and therefore appear to be wider-than-tall. Ellipsoid is another term for the appearance of a benign lesion that is wider-than-tall. Fibroadenomas are often ellipsoid.

The internal echo pattern of lesions is important in differentiating benign from malignant. Typically benign lesions have homogeneous internal echoes, while malignancies tend to have few to no echoes or are heterogeneous. A complete absence of echoes (anechoic) is seen with simple cysts. Malignancies can have a broad spectrum of differing degrees of heterogeneity.

LIMITATIONS AND PITFALLS OF ULTRASOUND

There are certainly limitations and pitfalls associated with the use of breast ultrasound. Most importantly, the quality of the

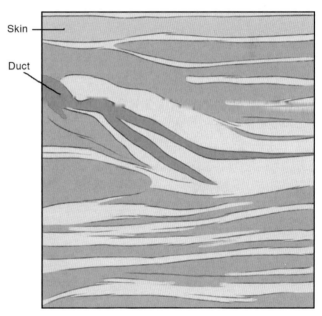

FIGURE 30-17 Radial scan near the nipple demonstrating a lactiferous sinus and normal ducts. *(Reproduced with permission from Harness JK, Wisher DB, eds. Ultrasound in Surgical Practice—Basic Principles and Clinical Applications. New York, NY: Wiley-Liss; 2001:159-236.)*

ultrasound image is everything and is related to several factors: the quality (and expense) of the machine, the quality and design of the transducer, the proper use of the equipment, and the experience and knowledge of the operator. Breast ultrasound requires high-quality equipment and high-frequency transducers, now available up to 15 MHz. In general, the more expensive the equipment the higher the quality of the image and the greater the number of features available with the equipment. The advent of digital ultrasound and the creation of smaller machines have made ultrasound more affordable without trading off much in the way of image quality.

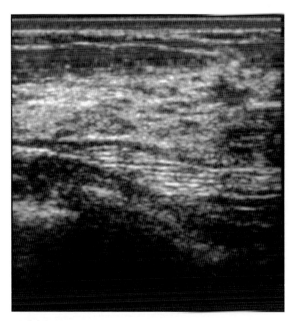 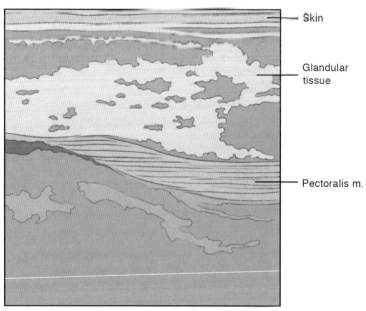

Skin

Glandular tissue

Pectoralis m.

FIGURE 30-18 Pectoralis muscle deep to dense glandular tissue. *(Reproduced with permission from Harness JK, Wisher DB, eds. Ultrasound in Surgical Practice—Basic Principles and Clinical Applications. New York, NY: Wiley-Liss; 2001:159-236.)*

Breast sonographers have to clearly understand the intricacies of their equipment and how to maximize image quality, including ensuring that there is uniformity of the gray scale throughout the image. Scanning techniques should be learned by attending courses on breast ultrasound, practicing on phantoms and live models, and working with experienced breast sonographers. Surgeons typically learn breast ultrasound quickly because of their inherently good hand–eye coordination and their ability to think in 3 dimensions.

Beginning breast sonographers must remember that even a single or atypical sonographic characteristic means that there is a less than 100% chance that a lesion is benign. Therefore, ultrasound-guided biopsy (needle or core) is indicated to prevent false-negative interpretation. In addition, it is important to avoid missing a lesion seen on a mammogram, to prevent inadvertently identifying a second lesion with ultrasound, and to avoid missing the primary lesion altogether. Careful comparison of the mammographic and ultrasound examinations is essential.

FUTURE DIRECTIONS

The "Holy Grail" of breast imaging has yet to be invented. The combination of digital mammography, digital ultrasound, and breast MRI are as close as we can come today to both high sensitivity and high specificity. The search for a single technology that can differentiate benign from malignant lesions continues.

Ultrasound elasticity imaging (USEI) is a modification of standard ultrasound to incorporate tissue compression and elasticity measurements to the scan results. Data are collected using the ultrasound device both before and after tissue compression. The manner in which various components of the tissue respond to compression results in a slightly different ultrasound echogenicity. This can be visualized in real time in a

similar way to conventional ultrasound. Malignant masses are stiffer and, therefore, deform less than benign masses. Malignant masses appear darker than benign masses on the elasticity image. In addition, benign masses have better-delineated boundaries between the mass and the surrounding tissue while malignant masses appear larger as the indefinite boundaries are enhanced visually under compression increasing the apparent size of the mass.[5] Initial reports indicate an increased specificity of USEI in distinguishing between benign from malignant lesions.[6] USEI is now being further evaluated in multi-institutional trials.

Ultrasound of the breast will remain a basic tool for years to come. Matrix array transducers (in place of linear array transducers) are emerging as the future of 3D and 4D ultrasound. Both 3D and 4D ultrasound have current important roles in fetal and cardiac scanning. Once this technology is designed for small-parts applications, there will likely be multiple uses for it in breast ultrasound. Such applications could include guiding large tissue acquisition devices for the percutaneous resection of benign and malignant breast lesions or the ablation of these lesions with either heat or cold.

SUMMARY

Breast ultrasound is an essential basic tool for the general and breast surgeon. It should be viewed as an important adjunct to the physical examination and the clinical decision-making process. It is an invaluable asset in guiding biopsies (both needle and core), placing partial breast irradiation devices, and guiding breast procedures in the OR. It is a technology that will be around for years to come and whose applications will expand in the future. It behooves surgeons to learn ultrasound and incorporate it into everyday practice. For those who want to be true students of breast ultrasound, the classic work on this subject is Tom Stavros's *Breast Ultrasound.*[1]

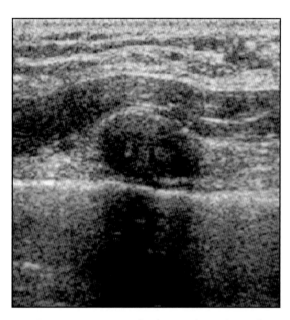 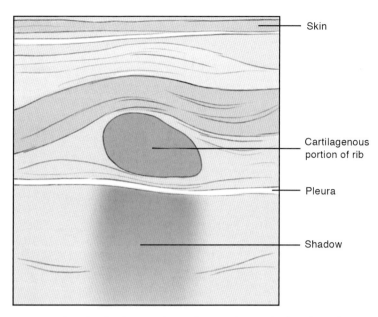

FIGURE 30-19 Longitudinal scan through cartilaginous portion of a rib. The hyperechoic pleura is beneath the rib and there is a posterior shadow from the rib. *(Reproduced with permission from Harness JK, Wisher DB, eds.* Ultrasound in Surgical Practice—Basic Principles and Clinical Applications. *New York, NY: Wiley-Liss; 2001:159-236.)*

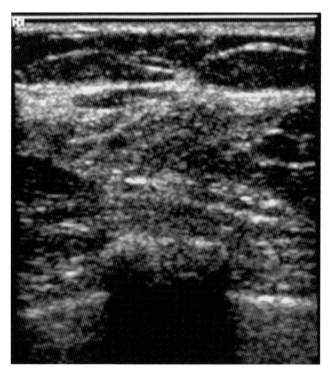 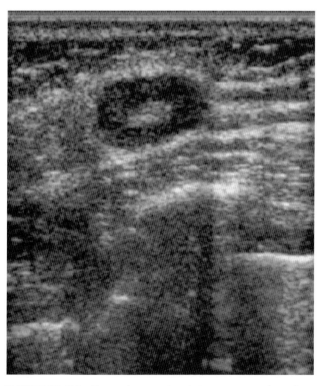

FIGURE 30-20 Longitudinal scan through the bony portion of a rib with a deep posterior shadow and no pleura seen behind the rib. *(Reproduced with permission from Harness JK, Wisher DB, eds.* Ultrasound in Surgical Practice—Basic Principles and Clinical Applications. *New York, NY: Wiley-Liss; 2001:159-236.)*

FIGURE 30-21 Normal appearing intramammary lymph node with a hypoechoic cortex and a hyperechoic fatty hilus. *(Reproduced with permission from Harness JK, Wisher DB, eds.* Ultrasound in Surgical Practice—Basic Principles and Clinical Applications. *New York, NY: Wiley-Liss; 2001:159-236.)*

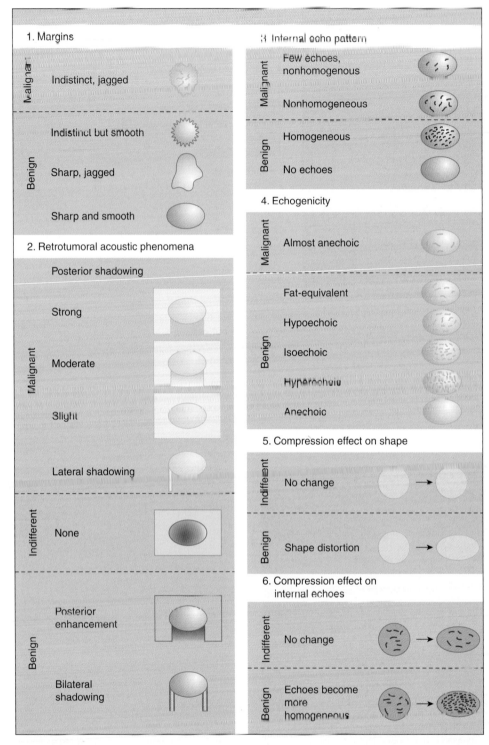

FIGURE 30-22 Analytic criteria for the interpretation of focal breast sonographic lesions.

ATLAS OF ULTRASOUND FINDINGS

Benign Conditions Examples

Abscesses

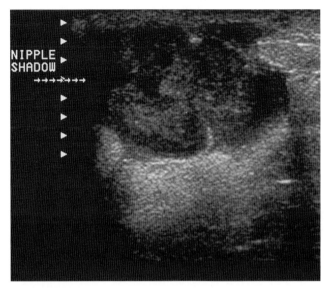

FIGURE 30-23 Example of a loculated abscess adjacent to the nipple–areolar complex. Note the posterior acoustic enhancement and the heterogeneous internal echoes of the abscess.

Cysts (Simple)

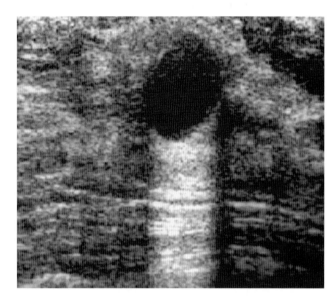

FIGURE 30-25 Classic appearance of a cyst. Note the smooth margins. It is anechoic, and has reverberation artifact in the cyst, edge shadows, and posterior enhancement. *(Reproduced with permission from Harness JK, Wisher DB, eds.* Ultrasound in Surgical Practice—Basic Principles and Clinical Applications. *New York, NY: Wiley-Liss; 2001:159-236.)*

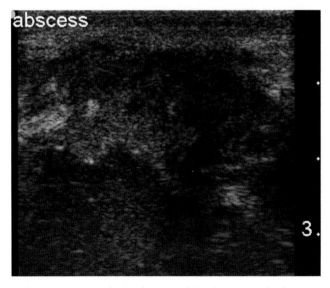

FIGURE 30-24 Diffuse abscess of the breast with skin thickening and marked heterogeneity of the internal echoes.

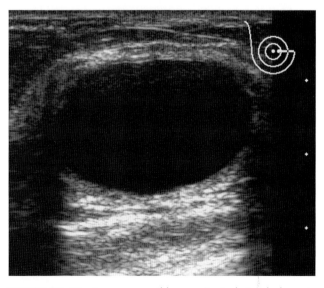

FIGURE 30-26 Large, smoothly marginated simple breast cyst with bright posterior enhancement and reverberation artifact in the anterior one-fourth of the cyst.

Cysts (Complex)

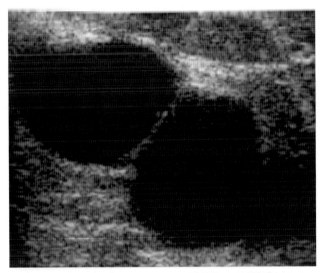

FIGURE 30-27 Complex cyst with internal septation. *(Reproduced with permission from Harness JK, Wisher DB, eds. Ultrasound in Surgical Practice—Basic Principles and Clinical Applications. New York, NY: Wiley-Liss; 2001:159-236.)*

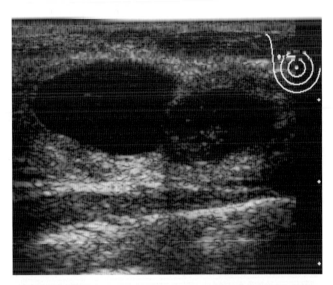

FIGURE 30-29 Septated, complex cyst with hyperechoic internal echoes.

Duct Ectasia

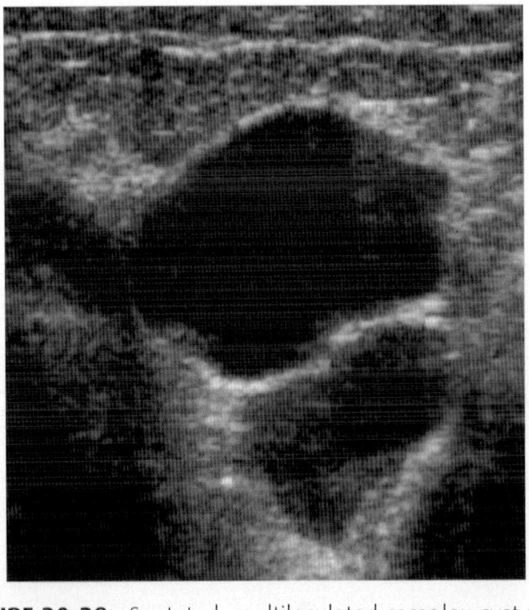

FIGURE 30-28 Septated, multiloculated complex cyst with hyperechoic internal echoes. *(Reproduced with permission from Harness JK, Wisher DB, eds. Ultrasound in Surgical Practice—Basic Principles and Clinical Applications. New York, NY: Wiley-Liss; 2001:159-236.)*

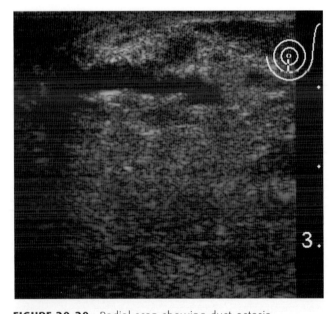

FIGURE 30-30 Radial scan showing duct ectasia.

Fibroadenomas

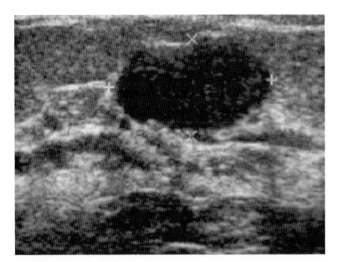

FIGURE 30-31   Smoothly marginated fibroadenoma. *(Reproduced with permission from Harness JK, Wisher DB, eds. Ultrasound in Surgical Practice—Basic Principles and Clinical Applications. New York, NY: Wiley-Liss; 2001: 159-236.)*

Gynecomastia

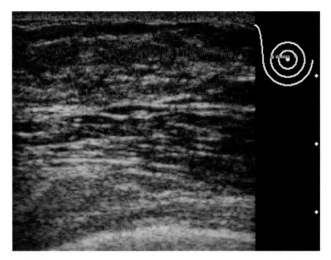

FIGURE 30-33   Male gynecomastia. Hyperechoic breast tissue mixed with fat is below the anterior mammary fascia and above the pectoralis muscle.

Intracystic Papillomas

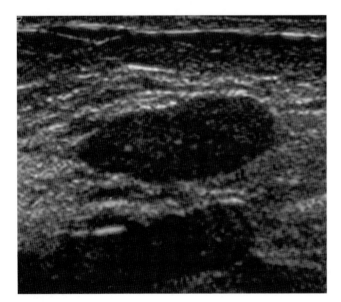

FIGURE 30-32   Wider-than-tall, smoothly marginated fibroadenoma with homogeneous internal echoes.

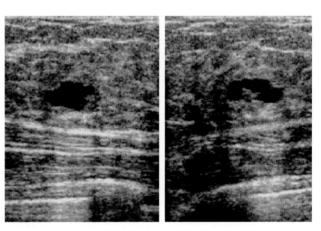

FIGURE 30-34   Two different views of a cyst with an intracystic papilloma. *(Reproduced with permission from Harness JK, Wisher DB, eds. Ultrasound in Surgical Practice—Basic Principles and Clinical Applications. New York, NY: Wiley-Liss; 2001: 159-236.)*

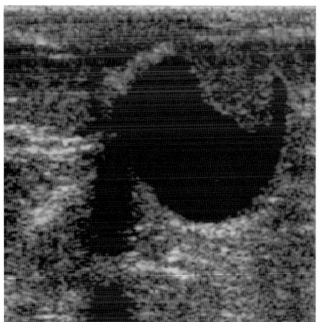

FIGURE 30-35 Intracystic papilloma in an anechoic cyst. *(Reproduced with permission from Harness JK, Wisher DB, eds. Ultrasound in Surgical Practice—Basic Principles and Clinical Applications. New York, NY: Wiley-Liss; 2001:159-236.)*

Intraductal Papilloma

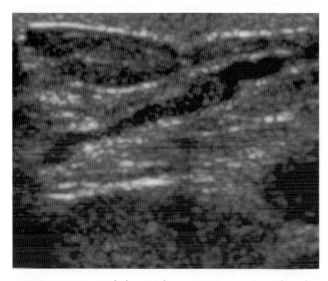

FIGURE 30-36 Radial scan demonstrating an intraductal papilloma. *(Reproduced with permission from Harness JK, Wisher DB, eds. Ultrasound in Surgical Practice—Basic Principles and Clinical Applications. New York, NY: Wiley-Liss; 2001:159-236.)*

Subcutaneous Lesion

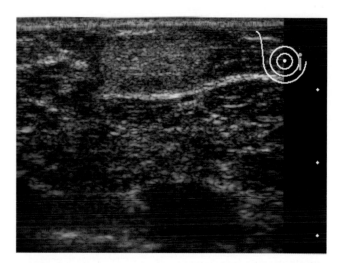

FIGURE 30-37 A hyperechoic, smoothly marginated subcutaneous lesion (anterior to the anterior mammary fascia) that likely represents a lipoma or an unusual hyperechoic sebaceous cyst.

Cancer Examples

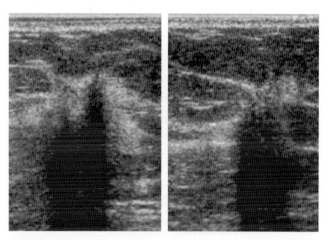

FIGURE 30-38 A hyperechoic rim and posterior shadow from a nearly anechoic, infiltrating cancer seen on 2 different views. *(Reproduced with permission from Harness JK, Wisher DB, eds. Ultrasound in Surgical Practice—Basic Principles and Clinical Applications. New York, NY: Wiley-Liss; 2001:159-236.)*

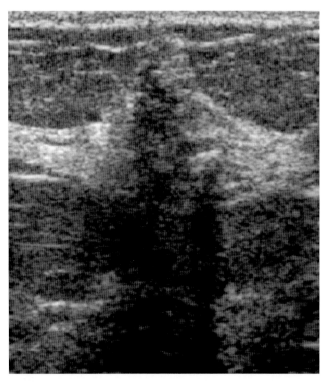

FIGURE 30-39 Taller-than-wide carcinoma that is growing into a Cooper's ligament with irregular margins, heterogeneous internal echoes, and posterior shadow. *(Reproduced with permission from Harness JK, Wisher DB, eds. Ultrasound in Surgical Practice—Basic Principles and Clinical Applications. New York, NY: Wiley-Liss; 2001:159-236.)*

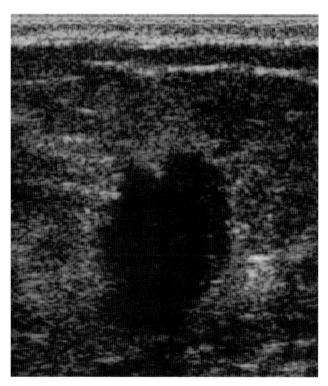

FIGURE 30-41 Carcinoma demonstrating an anechoic internal echo pattern. *(Reproduced with permission from Harness JK, Wisher DB, eds. Ultrasound in Surgical Practice—Basic Principles and Clinical Applications. New York, NY: Wiley-Liss; 2001:159-236.)*

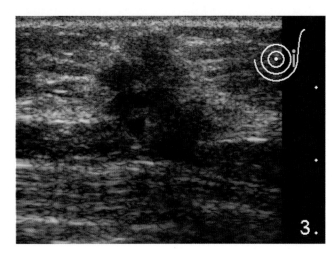

FIGURE 30-40 Taller-than-wide, irregularly marginated lesion with a hyperechoic rim and heterogeneous internal echoes. This is a classic cancer.

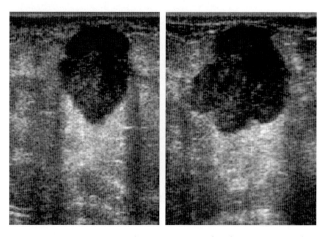

FIGURE 30-42 Heterogeneous internal echo pattern, edge shadows, and posterior enhancement from a cancer seen on 2 different views. The posterior enhancement is the result of considerable necrosis of the cancer. *(Reproduced with permission from Harness JK, Wisher DB, eds. Ultrasound in Surgical Practice—Basic Principles and Clinical Applications. New York, NY: Wiley-Liss; 2001:159-236.)*

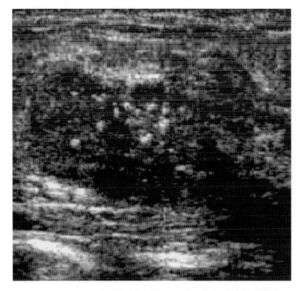

FIGURE 30-43 Multiple microcalcifications are seen in a carcinoma with an isoechoic, heterogeneous internal echo pattern. *(Reproduced with permission from Harness JK, Wisher DB, eds. Ultrasound in Surgical Practice—Basic Principles and Clinical Applications. New York, NY: Wiley-Liss; 2001:159-236.)*

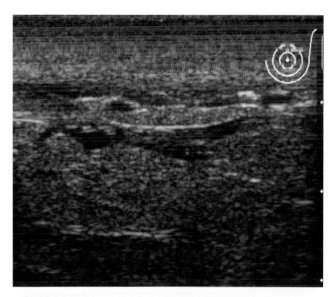

FIGURE 30-45 Inflammatory breast cancer with marked thickening of the skin and dilation (hypoechoic) of the subdermal lymphatics.

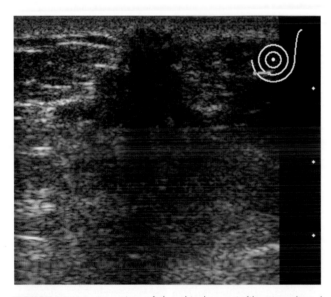

FIGURE 30-44 Invasion of the skin by an infiltrating ductal carcinoma.

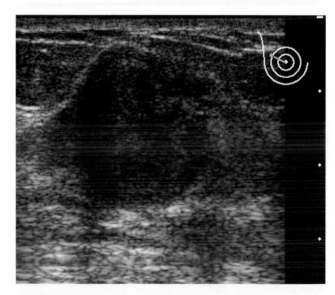

FIGURE 30-46 Somewhat smoothly marginated cancer pushing the anterior mammary fascia towards the superficial layer of the superficial fascia.

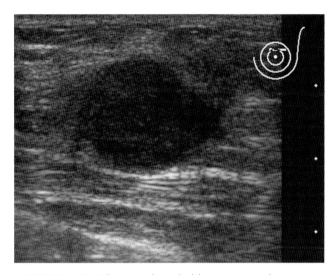

FIGURE 30-47 Ultrasound-guided lumpectomy for cancer with specimen margins evaluated in Figure 30 48.

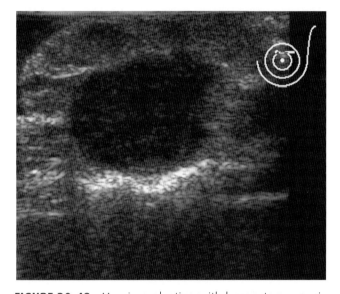

FIGURE 30-48 Margin evaluation with lumpectomy specimen from Figure 30-47 scanned in sterile water.

REFERENCES

1. Stavros AT. *Breast Ultrasound.* Philadelphia, PA: Lippincott Williams, & Wilkins; 2004:56-79.
2. Teboul M, Halliwell M. *Atlas of Ultrasound and Ductal Echography of the Breast.* Oxford, UK: Blackwell Science; 1995:49-79.
3. Harness JK, Wisher DB, eds. *Ultrasound in Surgical Practice—Basic Principles* and *Clinical Applications.* New York, NY: Wiley-Liss; 2001:159-236.
4. Leucht D, Madjar H. *Teaching Atlas of Breast Ultrasound.* New York, NY: Thieme Medical; 1996.
5. Sehgal CM, Weinstein SP, Arger PH, Conant EF. A review of breast ultrasound. *J Mammary Gland Biol Neoplasia.* 2206;11(2):113-123.
6. Thomas A, Fischer T, Frey H. Real-time elastography—an advanced method of ultrasound: first results in 108 patients with breast lesions. *Ultrasound Obstet Gynecol.* 2006;28(3):335–340.

Basic Breast Ultrasound, Certification, and Accreditation for the Surgeon

Howard Snider

Breast ultrasound has become an indispensable tool for surgeons who wish to provide state-of-the-art care to patients with diseases of the breast. Surgeons depend daily on their interpretation of the images to make diagnoses and to guide interventional procedures. To understand the ultrasound images properly, the surgeon must have a thorough understanding of the physics involved in the generation of those images.

ULTRASOUND PHYSICS

Sound is a form of mechanical energy that travels at varying speeds through different materials by causing temporary compression and rarefaction of the molecules of those materials. Consequently, unlike electromagnetic radiation, sound cannot travel through a vacuum. Sound travels in waves, and there is an inverse relationship between the wavelength (the distance from one point on the wave to the same point on the next wave) and the frequency of the waves. A human with perfect hearing might hear frequencies between 20 and 20,000 cycles per second or 20 Hz to 20 kHz. Sound with a higher frequency than audible sound is referred to as ultrasound. Diagnostic medical ultrasound is generally somewhere between 2 and 30 million cycles per second, or 2 to 30 MHz.

Piezoelectric Effect

The fundamental operating principle of all ultrasound transducers is the piezoelectric effect, discovered by Pierre Curie and his less famous brother, Jacques. There are crystals that occur in nature and others that can be created that have the ability to transform electrical energy into sound and vice versa. A linear array transducer used in breast ultrasound has a series of tiny piezoelectric crystals extending from one end of the footplate to the other, each of which can be fired individually or in groups. When a voltage is applied to the piezoelectric crystal, the crystal is deformed and the electrical energy is converted into mechanical energy in the form of sound. A damping material adjacent to the crystal acts like a finger on a tuning fork to immediately stop the sound, resulting in a very short pulse. Operating according to the pulse-echo principle, the transducer is generating ultrasound less than 1% of the time. Greater than 99% of the time it is "listening" to returning echoes, which are in turn converted back into electrical energy and recorded.

Echogenicity

When sound meets an interface between tissues with different acoustic impedances (an acoustic mismatch), part of the sound is transmitted into the second tissue, and part is reflected as an echo. The impedance of the tissue is simply the product of the density of the tissue and the rate at which sound travels in it. The greater the acoustic mismatch between adjacent tissues, the greater the echoes produced at that interface. The returning echoes are recorded on a scale in proportion to their strength or amplitude with a varying degree of brightness. Ultrasound using this scale is called B-mode scanning (the B stands for brightness). The highest strength echoes are displayed as white, the absence of echoes as black, with different shades of gray in between. Thus the other name for B-mode scanning is gray scale. The degree of echogenicity is compared with the surrounding tissues, usually the breast parenchyma, although some authors use the subcutaneous fat as the reference area.[1] Tissues that generate the same degree of echogenicity as the reference area are referred to as *isoechoic*. Those that generate more echoes are *hyperechoic*, and fewer echoes are *hypoechoic*. The absence of echoes is referred to as *anechoic*. Because sound travels through most soft tissues at a rate of around 1450 to 1550 m/s, only low-level echoes are produced at most of the interfaces where there are only slight differences in acoustic impedance. Where dense tissue is adjacent to much less dense areas, there is a greater acoustic mismatch and more echoes are generated. Air is a poor conductor of sound with a speed in the range of 330 m/s, whereas bone conducts sound at speeds in excess of 4000 m/s. When sound meets an interface between soft tissue and either bone or air, there is a large acoustic mismatch, and high-level echoes are seen.

Generation of the Image

Each crystal in the transducer fires several thousand times a second and interrogates the breast tissue underneath it as the ultrasound beam travels through the tissues. Multiple echoes return from each pulse of sound as it travels deeper and deeper. After each 100 or so crystal firings, all of the echoes from all of the tissues are combined into an image, or "frame," and displayed on the screen. With a frame rate of about 30 per second, the human eye cannot detect the individual images, and it appears that the scanning is being done in real time, like a motion picture. If the frame rate is significantly lower and the transducer is moved fairly rapidly across the patient's breast, the individual images can be perceived, and a flickering pattern appears on the screen, much like an old-time silent movie.

Time-Space Conversion

Part of the sound that strikes a smooth acoustic interface perpendicular or nearly perpendicular to the path of the ultrasound beam (at right angles to the footplate of the transducer) is reflected back to the transducer and recorded. The pixels are displayed on the screen at a depth commensurate with the amount of time that has elapsed from the firing of the crystal until the return of the echoes. The longer the interval of time, the deeper (lower) the pixel is displayed on the screen, the so-called time-space conversion.

Attenuation

As the sound goes deeper into the tissues, it gradually weakens or attenuates for 4 different reasons.[2] The most significant of these is that the tissues absorb the sound and the mechanical energy is converted into heat, albeit a negligible amount in diagnostic ultrasound.[3] The second factor is that some of the energy is reflected back to the transducer as echoes. Third, when the sound strikes an irregular surface it is scattered through the tissues without returning to the transducer, further attenuating it. The final thing that attenuates the sound is the refraction (or bending) of the sound at the side of smooth surfaces such as cysts or fibroadenomas.

Time-Gain Compensation

Overall gain refers to the amplification of the returning echoes, making the entire screen brighter. If the echoes throughout the screen were amplified to the same degree, the near field (top of image) would be very bright and the far field very dark as the sound attenuates in the deeper tissues. Built into the ultrasound

equipment is a function known as time-gain compensation (TGC). The longer the time elapsed from the time the crystal fires until the echo returns to the transducer, the greater the amplification of the echoes. There are also individual slide pods that allow the sonographer to further fine-tune the amplification at each level, adjusting the image so that relative echogenicity is the same throughout the image. When TGC is set appropriately, fat in the near field has the same echogenicity as fat in the far field.

Resolution

Axial Resolution

Resolution of the image refers to the ability of the equipment to distinguish 2 separate reflectors in the tissues and display them as 2 separate pixels on the screen. If the reflectors are side by side, parallel to the footplate of the transducer and perpendicular to the ultrasound beam, the resolution is referred to as *lateral*. If they are at different depths on the y-axis of the screen, parallel to the beam and perpendicular to the footplate, the resolution is *axial*. The higher the frequency of the ultrasound beam, the greater the resolution, both axial and lateral. A short pulse length is also an important contributor to good axial resolution. If one imagines 2 reflectors in an axial (vertical) plane with a short pulse of high frequency ultrasound passing through them from the transducer, it is easy to imagine that pulse fitting between them and distinguishing them as separate. However, if either the pulse length increases or the frequency decreases (lengthening the wave length), the pulse will overlap the reflectors and not be able to distinguish them as separate. The reflectors will be merged and displayed as one reflector on the image, decreasing axial resolution (Fig. 31A-1).

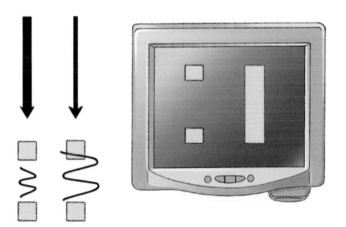

FIGURE 31A-1 If the wavelength and pulse width are short enough to fit between 2 axial reflectors, they will be distinguished and displayed as separate pixels on the image, increasing axial resolution. If the wavelength or pulse width is long enough to overlap the reflectors, they will be merged and displayed as 1, decreasing axial resolution.

Lateral Resolution and Focal Zones

The ultrasound beam can be electronically focused (narrowed) by varying the sequencing of the groups of crystals that are fired together. Most instruments have a mechanism that allows the sonographer to move the depth of the focal zones to the area of interest or to add additional focal zones. If 2 lateral reflectors are close enough together that they can both fit within the width of the unfocused beam, they will be merged and displayed as 1. However, if the focal zone is placed at the level of the reflectors, narrowing the beam such that the 2 can no longer fit within it, they will be recognized and displayed as separate, increasing lateral resolution (Fig. 31A-2).

Frame Rate

As mentioned previously, a high frame rate allows the sonographer to see an image in real time as though it were a motion picture. When there is 1 focal zone, the beam is focused at that depth each time the crystals fire, allowing the highest frame rate. If another focal zone is added, the beam is focused alternately at each of the 2 levels when the crystals are fired. The resolution is the same at both levels, but it takes twice as long to acquire the same amount of information. Thus the number of frames that can be acquired in a given period of time is cut in half. As additional focal zones are added, the frame rate continues to decrease proportionally, such that the human eye can better perceive the individual frames, yielding a flickering pattern as the transducer is passed across the breast. It is a matter of individual preference as to whether the sonographer prefers to accept the flickering pattern with numerous focal zones or move an individual focal zone to the depth of the lesion as different areas of the breast are examined.

Penetration

The reason one cannot always use a high-frequency transducer is that the penetration of the beam decreases as frequency

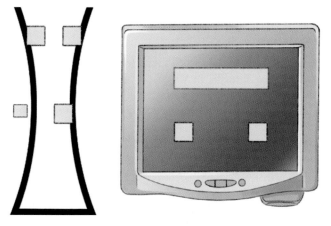

FIGURE 31A-2 If 2 lateral reflectors are close enough together that they can both fit within the width of the unfocused beam, they will be merged and displayed as 1. However, if the focal zone is placed at the level of the reflectors, narrowing the beam such that the 2 can no longer fit within it, they will be recognized and displayed as separate, increasing lateral resolution.

increases. Thus to examine structures deep in the abdomen one might have to use a 3-MHz transducer, whereas examination of most breasts can be done quite well with a 10- to 14-MHz transducer because there is less tissue to penetrate. Think of a thunderstorm. If lightning strikes nearby, there is a loud, high-pitched (high-frequency) clap of thunder. However, if the storm is 10 miles away, the high-frequency thunder has attenuated, and one hears only the low-frequency rumble that has penetrated much further. The same principle is true if one listens to a band playing down the street or a stereo from down the hall. The sound from the high-pitched flute has attenuated and is not heard. Only the low-frequency bass drum and other low-pitched instruments are audible.

Artifacts

Shadowing

When the ultrasound beam encounters a strongly attenuating structure, there will be a relative decrease in the amount of sound that continues to pass into the deeper structures. There will be fewer echoes returning from the depths of the image below the structure, and the image there will appear more hypoechoic or even anechoic. This is referred to as *posterior shadowing*. An extreme example would be the very high acoustic mismatch between soft tissue and rib. Almost all of the sound is reflected from the surface of the rib and appears on the screen as a bright hyperechoic rim at the anterior surface of the rib. The remainder of the rib and the deeper tissues below it are not well seen because there is essentially no sound there, resulting in an almost anechoic shadow (Fig. 31A-3).

Posterior Enhancement

When the ultrasound beam encounters a weakly attenuating structure, there will be a relative increase in the amount of sound (relative to the adjacent tissue) that continues to pass into the deeper structures. There will be more echoes returning to the transducer, and this will result in a brighter (more hyperechoic) area deep to the structure, sometimes referred to as "good through transmission." Cysts with clear fluid are classic examples of weakly attenuating structures because there are no acoustic mismatches when the sound passes through the fluid. Other relatively homogeneous structures can also be weakly attenuating and cause posterior enhancement, including medullary, colloid (mucinous), or high-grade carcinomas.[1] The tissues immediately below all of these structures appear hyperechoic relative to the adjacent tissue because there has been more attenuation of the sound in the adjacent tissues by the time it reaches that depth. In addition, the area immediately beneath these weakly attenuating structures appears brighter than the tissue immediately superficial to the structure, even though the amount of sound (and echoes) are essentially the same. This phenomenon is caused by the fact that the deeper tissues are amplified more due to time-gain compensation (Fig. 31A-4).

Reverberation

Reverberation echoes are often mistakenly thought of as being generated by a cyst. In fact, the cyst has nothing to do with

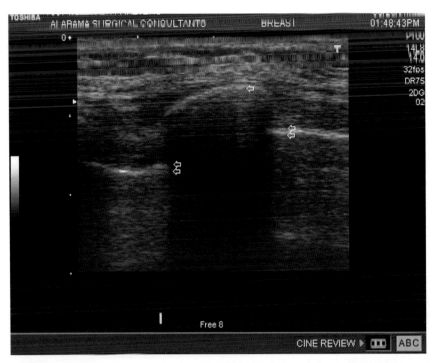

FIGURE 31A-3 The high acoustic mismatch between the soft tissue and rib results in near-total reflection of sound, seen as the hyperechoic rim at the superficial surface of the rib (single arrow). The posterior shadowing obscures the remainder of the rib and underlying structures including the pleura (double arrows).

their creation. Reverberation echoes are occurring all of the time throughout the ultrasound image. They are lost in the myriad of other echoes, and we just don't see them until an otherwise anechoic window is opened on the screen, such as a large cyst. To understand reverberation, look at the needle in

the tissue parallel to the footplate of the transducer at a depth of 0.6 cm (Fig. 31A-5). The strong acoustic mismatch creates a very hyperechoic structure on the screen at 0.6 cm, placed at that level by the amount of time that elapsed before the echoes returned to the transducer. The transducer itself, however, represents a very strong acoustic mismatch with the skin, so part of the returning beam is reflected back into the tissue of the breast. When the beam that is reflected back into the tissue strikes the needle again, the echoes return a second time to the transducer, part of which are recorded and part of which make another trip into the tissue, and so on. The part that is recorded took twice as long to return as the original echoes, so the computer displays them at twice the depth, or 1.2 cm, according to the time-space conversion principle. Look closely and you will see a somewhat weaker replica of the needle at that depth. Between and below those 2 "needles" are numerous other weaker copies of the needle, regularly spaced very close to each other. These reverberations are being caused by the fact that the anterior and posterior walls of the needle also serve as reflectors, and sound is continuously bouncing back and forth between them. With each bounce, some of the sound travels back to the transducer and arrives slightly later than the previous echo and is recorded slightly deeper on the screen. The evenly spaced reverberation echoes that are seen in the superficial aspect of a cyst are being caused by some reflectors just superficial to the cyst. If one looks closely, an area of fibrous tissue, or perhaps a thick cyst wall, can usually be identified as the cause of the echoes (Fig. 31A-4). Whereas it is true that sound bounces between the anterior and posterior walls of the cyst, those echoes are displayed deep to the cyst and are generally lost in the tissue and not seen.

Refraction

According to Snell's law, when sound (or light) crosses an interface between 2 media in which the speed of transmission is different, the change in velocity will cause the transmitted beam to travel at a different angle relative to the interface, thus causing the wave to bend. This phenomenon is called *refraction* and explains why a pole placed into a swimming pool will appear to be bent. When ultrasound passes into a relatively round structure such as a cyst or fibroadenoma, the closer the beam gets to the edge of the structure, the greater the angle of incidence. If the rounded structure has different acoustic properties from the surrounding tissues, the sound wave will be bent once as it enters the structure and again as it exits. This bending of the sound wave deflects sound away from the edge of the structure, resulting in the relative absence of sound deep to the edges of the structure. This usually causes bilateral, fairly symmetric shadows called *edge shadowing* or *edge effect*.

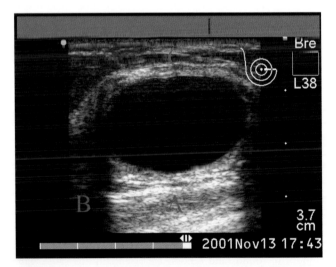

FIGURE 31A-4 Posterior enhancement is seen deep to the cyst. The area marked B is darker than A because more of the sound has been attenuated as it passed through the superficial tissues. The area marked A is brighter than the area marked C because there is more amplification of those echoes from time-gain compensation (TGC). Note the reverberation echoes in the superficial aspect of the cyst being caused by the thickened anterior cyst wall.

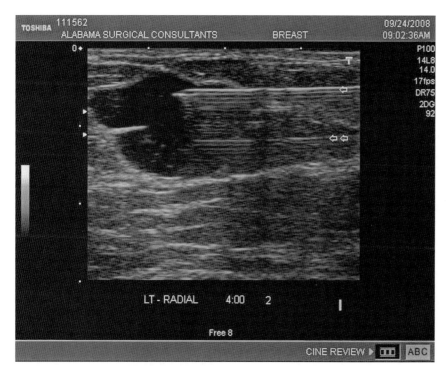

FIGURE 31A-5 The needle in this image is adjacent to the cancer at a depth of 1 cm. The first reverberation caused by reflection from the transducer can be seen at a depth of 1.2 cm. The multiple closely spaced weaker reverberations are caused by the small delay in the echoes that return to the transducer each time the sound bounces between the acoustic mismatches at the anterior and posterior walls of the needle.

INDICATIONS FOR BREAST ULTRASOUND

Improvements in ultrasound technology and image interpretation over the last decade or so have made ultrasound an invaluable tool in the evaluation and characterization of various breast problems. Indications for breast ultrasound include palpable masses, mammographic masses and densities, abnormalities detected on magnetic resonance imaging (MRI), problems with implants, nipple discharge, focal pain, and the evaluation of response of cancers to preoperative therapy. Ultrasound is also an important tool in the evaluation of the extent of disease and in excluding multicentricity and bilaterality in patients with known breast cancer.

Palpable Mass

In past decades traditional surgical teaching was that most palpable masses that could not be resolved with aspiration should be biopsied. Ultrasound has fundamentally changed that recommendation, significantly decreasing the incidence of biopsy, but it is critical for the physician to palpate the abnormality at the time of scanning to be certain the findings correlate with what is being felt. For large masses this might mean placing a finger alongside the transducer and rolling it over the mass as the transducer is painted across the lesion. Smaller masses can be trapped between the long and index fingers and

the transducer placed between them. Alternatively, an opened gem clip or small straw can be placed beneath the transducer overlying the palpable mass. The reverberation artifact from the marker allows the sonographer to be sure the palpable mass is being interrogated.

Often the palpable mass can be dismissed as completely benign without further intervention. If the mass is shown to be a simple cyst there is no need to aspirate it unless the cyst is symptomatic and aspiration might alleviate pain. Frequently what the patient and referring physician feel is a ridge of normal fibroglandular tissue that comes close to the skin (Fig. 31A-6). The patient may have been previously told that a mammogram and ultrasound show nothing, leaving her anxious about the mass that she continues to feel. It is important for the physician to show the images to the patient, reassuring her that what is seen on the ultrasound correlates with what she is feeling and is completely normal tissue.

If the palpable mass cannot be conclusively dismissed as benign, the findings help to characterize its nature. In young women, rubbery masses that have findings typical for a fibroadenoma can be safely followed if they have no findings suggestive of malignancy.[1] If there are any suspicious characteristics on ultrasound, the diagnosis can usually be obtained with an ultrasound-guided core biopsy.

Mammographic Abnormalities

Mammography and sonography are complementary examinations. Little useful information is obtained by ultrasounding a completely fatty replaced breast, but it is extremely unlikely that a significant lesion would be missed on mammography in such a breast. In contrast, ultrasound is most useful in dense breasts where the density of the breast tissue might obscure lesions on the mammogram. Abnormalities found on mammography can frequently be dismissed as benign by using ultrasound to assess them further, but the physician must be certain that what is seen sonographically is the same as the area of concern on the mammogram. It is not sufficient to find a cyst in the same quadrant and conclude that the mammographic lesion is benign. The best way to be sure the lesions are the same is to compare the lesion's appearance on a transverse ultrasound scan with the craniocaudad mammographic view.[1] The location, size, shape, and surrounding tissue density should be the same on ultrasound and mammogram before the examiner concludes that the lesions are the same. When there is still uncertainty, a marker can be placed on the skin or within the breast at the site of the sonographic lesion and a confirmatory mammogram obtained.

Ultrasound is most useful in characterizing masses and asymmetric densities in breasts with a large amount of residual

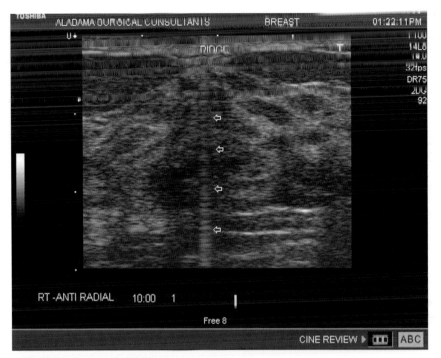

FIGURE 31A-6 Note the ridge of normal breast tissue that comes closer to the skin than the surrounding tissue. It is firmer than the adjacent fatty tissue and gives the sensation of a mass. An opened gum clip over the mass produces reverberation echoes (arrows) that overlie the ridge, leaving no doubt that the palpable mass and the sonographic ridge are the same.

fibroglandular tissue. In such breasts, significant lesions are usually seen sonographically. The findings usually suggest whether the lesion is benign, malignant, or indeterminate. Although calcifications are best seen with mammography, modern high-frequency transducers make it possible for them to often be seen as specular reflectors on ultrasound as well.

Magnetic Resonance Imaging Abnormalities

MRI has been increasingly used in recent years both in screening high-risk patients and in evaluating the extent of disease in patients with known breast cancer. When a morphologic or enhancing abnormality is detected on MRI, the next step is usually a focused (or "second look") ultrasound of the region in question. If a corresponding abnormality is seen, it is easiest to biopsy the lesion with ultrasound guidance. If a lesion is not seen, depending on the degree of suspicion of the MRI abnormality, an MRI-guided biopsy might be necessary.

Implants

Breast ultrasound can, of course, be performed in patients with implants to evaluate palpable, mammographic, or MRI abnormalities. It can also be used to evaluate the integrity of the implants as well. Although MRI is perhaps more definitive in determining implant rupture, a skilled sonographer can gain much valuable information from ultrasound evaluation of implants. A distinction between intracapsular and extracapsular rupture can usually be made.[1]

Nipple Discharge

Most nipple discharges are benign, but those that are spontaneous, copious, persistent, unilateral, from a single duct, and clear, serous, or bloody demand evaluation. Ultrasound plays an important role in the evaluation of these pathologic nipple discharges. Frequently a filling defect can be seen within a dilated duct, prompting either percutaneous or open biopsy.[4] If ultrasound by an experienced sonographer is normal, it is very unlikely that the offending lesion is malignant, and some authors recommend observation in that situation.[5]

Focal Pain

Ultrasound is not generally useful when patients have a diffuse cyclical or noncyclical breast pain. However when the pain is focal and persistent, ultrasound will sometimes reveal a cause, such as a tense or inflamed cyst, a finding that might lead to aspiration for alleviation of the patient's symptoms. Some authors believe that the sonographic findings in acute periductal mastitis are definitive enough to make a specific diagnosis of the cause of the pain.[1]

Evaluation of Response to Preoperative Therapy

Many patients now undergo systemic treatment with either chemotherapy, hormonal manipulation, or both prior to surgical resection of breast cancers. Ultrasound is an easy and relatively inexpensive way of monitoring the response to therapy, especially when the tumor has well-defined borders. Periodic measurements can be taken, reassuring the patient and medical oncologist that the therapy is effective or prompting a therapeutic change if the tumor progresses. If a periodic evaluation is done as the tumor shrinks, it is usually possible to tell sonographically where the tumor was even if the response is nearly complete and only subtle changes persist. This allows either intraoperative localization of the tumor or at least preoperative localization with ultrasound, obviating the need for an unpleasant and inconvenient wire localization using mammographic guidance.

Screening

Screening ultrasound is sometimes used in high-risk patients or to evaluate the remainder of the breast tissue in patients with known cancer. Screening is covered elsewhere in this textbook.

PATIENT POSITIONING AND TECHNIQUES OF SCANNING

Positioning

In general, the goal of positioning of the patient for a breast ultrasound examination is to have the area of the breast being examined flat against the chest wall, thinning the breast to give the shortest distance possible between the skin and underlying musculature. For lesions lateral in the breast, this usually requires that the patient be rotated slightly medially (contralateral posterior oblique position), placing a pillow or other supporting device beneath the shoulder and the ipsilateral arm beneath the head. For medial lesions, a supine position usually works best. For some superior lesions, particularly in large or pendulous breasts, it is preferable to perform the examination with the patient in a seated position.

Scanning

When the breast is scanned, the transducer can be moved at right angles to its long axis, sometimes called *painting* because of the similarity of the movement of a paint brush (Fig. 31A-7). This movement causes lesions to appear and disappear at the same location on the image as the transducer is painted across a lesion. Movement of the transducer along its long axis is sometimes called *skiing* because of the similarity in the movement of skis. This movement causes a lesion to move across the screen at a given depth from right to left or vice versa.

When one examines a palpable lesion, there is no problem finding the area of concern. However, when examining for a nonpalpable mammographic abnormality, it is best to cover a large area of breast tissue in an efficient manner in order to find the lesion of concern. One way of accomplishing this is to use a sweep of the transducer with a painting motion. For any transverse scan, by international convention the transducer should be oriented transversely with the patient's right side to the left of the screen. For a sagittal (longitudinal) scan, the long axis of the transducer is in line with the long axis of the body with the patient's head to the left of the screen. For a transverse sweep, the transducer is oriented transversely and moved from cephalad to caudad or vice versa, overlapping each sweep slightly as if mowing the lawn in order not to miss any area. For a sagittal sweep, the transducer is oriented in a sagittal plane and moved from left to right or vice versa.

Surgeons frequently prefer to scan in radial and antiradial planes because of the generally radial orientation of the ducts. For a radial scan, the long axis of the transducer is oriented like the spoke of a wheel, but there is no international convention as to whether the nipple should be to the left or right of the screen. In courses taught by the American Society of Breast Surgeons and also the American College of Surgeons, it is suggested that the nipple be to the left of the screen, but all sonographers do not adhere strictly to this routine. For an antiradial scan, the transducer is rotated 90 degrees into an orthogonal plane. The sonographer should develop a consistent way of rotating either clockwise or counterclockwise for antiradial scans. When the transducer is oriented in an antiradial plane, a painting sweep of the transducer from central to peripheral is an efficient way of covering a large area of breast tissue. If the transducer is moved from central to peripheral in a radial plane, only a small area of breast tissue is covered with each sweep. The transducer can be rotated 360 degrees around the nipple areolar complex in concentric circles, but this is somewhat awkward. Some sonographers "rock" the transducer back and

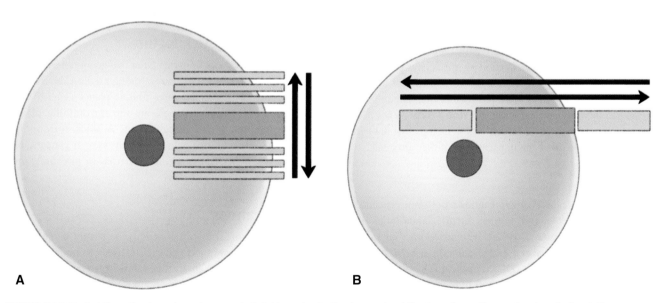

A   **B**

FIGURE 31A-7 A. When the transducer is moved at right angles to the long axis of the transducer, the motion is called *painting* because of the similarity in the movement of a paint brush. **B.** When it is moved in the direction of the long axis, it is called *skiing* because of the similarity in the movement of skis. Painting across a lesion causes it to appear and disappear at the same location on the screen. Skiing causes a lesion to move at a fixed depth across the screen.

forth in a radial plane as the transducer is moved from central to peripheral in order to cover more breast tissue. This maneuver is to be discouraged because the superficial tissue on each side of the transducer is not examined when the probe is rocked. A final way of scanning is to paint the transducer back and forth over a given zone of tissue as the transducer is moved from central to peripheral in a radial plane.

Regardless of the planes of scanning, any lesion should be viewed in 360 degrees and measured in its longest diameter, whether that is radial, antiradial, transverse, or sagittal. The lesion should then be measured at right angles to that plane before rotating the transducer into an orthogonal plane for the final horizontal measurement. The images should be captured in either radial and antiradial planes or transverse and sagittal. It is incorrect to mix terminology and capture a lesion, for example, in radial and transverse planes.

BENIGN VERSUS MALIGNANT FINDINGS

Size

Although it is often said that it is safe to follow well-circumscribed lesions less than a centimeter in size, it is really not the size that is important in determining whether a lesion is malignant. Regardless of the size of the lesion, if it has any malignant characteristics it should be biopsied. It is no longer unusual for cancers ≤5 mm to be diagnosed with ultrasound. Frequently the dimensions of lesions, whether benign or malignant, can be accurately measured sonographically. This is particularly true for most benign masses and for well circumscribed malignant lesions as well. However, it is often impossible to measure the exact size of some cancers, most notably infiltrating lobular carcinomas and duct carcinomas with lobular features.

Shape

In general, a round or oval shape is thought of as a benign finding, but it is actually quite common for some malignant lesions to have a relatively round shape. Cancers that are commonly round include mucinous (colloid), medullary, intracystic papillary, or any high-grade carcinoma. Although not a hard and fast rule, lesions that are taller than wide and smaller than about 1.5 cm are frequently malignant. Lesions larger than 1.5 cm do not necessarily continue to conform to that shape. Lesions that are wider than tall are frequently benign, particularly if they are small.

Margins

Smooth margins favor a benign diagnosis, but some cancers can actually have rather smooth borders. Gentle, larger lobulations of the margin are usually seen in benign lesions, but microlobulations are suggestive of either micronodular invasive cancer or ductal carcinoma in situ (DCIS) in the ducts or lobules. Any angular margin is suggestive enough of malignancy to demand biopsy. Low- to intermediate-grade cancers frequently have spicules that can be seen sonographically because the growth is slow enough to evoke a desmoplastic stromal reaction around the infiltrating cancer cells. The spicules will be seen as bands radiating from the lesion. They may be either hyperechoic or hypoechoic, depending on the density of the surrounding stroma. Spiculations are very suggestive of cancer but can also be seen in scar tissue, complex sclerosing lesions, and fat necrosis. More rapidly growing cancers do not generally allow time for a desmoplastic reaction, and their borders are usually smoother without spicules. Hypoechoic extensions into the duct away from the main tumor mass are highly suggestive of DCIS.

Echogenicity

Most cancers are hypoechoic or extremely hypoechoic, but it is not uncommon to have significant isoechoic, or even hyperechoic, components to the tumor mass. Rarely, if ever, are cancers purely hyperechoic. Occasionally, special types of cancers, such as medullary, can be so smooth walled and almost anechoic that they can easily be mistaken by the unwary for cysts.[1]

Artifacts

Shadowing is often thought of as an indicator of malignancy, and its presence demands biopsy of most lesions unless an unequivocally benign cause can be found such as a heavily calcified fibroadenoma. Actually only a little more than a third of cancers have shadowing, a third have normal sound transmission, and almost a third have posterior enhancement.[1] Most low-grade carcinomas, including infiltrating lobular carcinoma, usually have intense, irregular, posterior shadowing. High-grade infiltrating duct carcinomas, medullary, colloid (mucinous), and papillary carcinomas, typically cause posterior enhancement. Cancers smaller than 1.5 cm and also intermediate-grade tumors may not have enough desmoplasia or cellularity and inflammatory reaction to cause either shadowing or enhancement. They may have normal through transmission of sound. Symmetric shadowing on each side of a lesion due to refraction, the so-called edge effect, is usually associated with benign cysts or fibroadenomas, but it can also be seen with smooth-walled carcinomas.

Surrounding Architecture

Clues as to whether a lesion is benign or malignant can sometimes be gleaned by looking at the surrounding tissue. Cancers grow through and distort surrounding fibrous planes (Fig. 31A-8). Benign lesions may push or elevate the surrounding planes, but they do not grow through them. A thick surrounding hyperechoic capsule, or "halo," is often seen in cancers, but they can also be indicative of inflammatory or infectious processes as well.

Calcifications

On mammograms some calcifications are clearly benign; others, clearly malignant; and still others, indeterminate. Clusters are more worrisome than scattered and isolated calcifications. Coarse calcifications are usually benign, whereas powdery ones can be benign or malignant. Irregular, pleomorphic, so-called crushed-stone calcifications are suggestive of malignancy. Linear, branching, "casting" calcifications are highly suggestive of malignancy. Although calcifications are not as reliably seen and characterized on ultrasound as on mammography, they

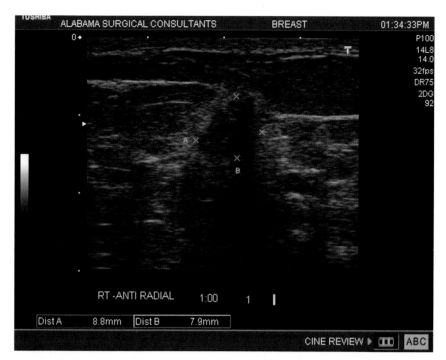

FIGURE 31A-8 The cancer can be seen growing through and disrupting the anterior mammary fascia. Note the intense, irregular shadowing deep to the cancer.

commonly appear as bright specular reflectors. Ultrasound shows malignant calcifications against the hypoechoic background of cancers better than it does benign calcifications, which are frequently in hyperechoic areas. Large, course, benign calcifications are easily seen because they cause intense posterior shadowing. Fine malignant calcifications may appear as specular reflectors against a hypoechoic background but do not cause shadowing because they are smaller than the diameter of the ultrasound beam and thus do not block the transmission of the sound.[1]

DOCUMENTATION

Surgeons frequently perform ultrasound examinations and ultrasound-guided biopsies on their own patients, and the images and report may not necessarily be going to a referring physician as is the case when a radiologist performs the procedure. Nevertheless, each ultrasound study should be permanently stored in some retrievable format, either printed or electronic. Along with a set of images there should be a written report that becomes a part of the patient's permanent medical record.[6,7]

Image Documentation

Images should generally include the facility name, date of examination, patient's first and last name, and an identification number, if applicable. All images should contain a notation of left or right breast in addition to the location of the lesion in the breast. Diagnostic images should also indicate transducer orientation. All of these notations should be made using the icon or the annotation script capability of the instrument. The distance of the lesion from the nipple should be noted either in centimeters or by zone using the instrument's script.

Handwritten notes on the images should be used only to correct errors on previously printed images.

Written Documentation

All diagnostic and interventional procedures should be accompanied by a written report describing the salient features of each study. The report may be written or dictated as a separate document or may be included in the body of the office note. Standard forms or checklists may be used so long as they are comprehensive and include all necessary information.

The report of a diagnostic ultrasound should contain a clear indication for the study, regardless of whether it is a mammographic, palpable, or some other abnormality that prompted the study. The technique of the study should be included in an optimal report including scanning location, transducer orientation, and frequency of the transducer. A description of the findings should be made using standard sonographic terminology. The findings should include the size, shape, borders, and echogenicity of the lesion along with a description of physics artifacts. The impression should be given as specifically as possible, preferably including a Breast Imaging-Reporting and Data System (BI-RADS) classification. A recommendation should be made incorporating the physical, mammographic, sonographic, and other imaging findings, if applicable.

The report of an ultrasound-guided interventional procedure should include the location of the lesion as well as the approach (lateral to medial, etc.) taken to biopsy the lesion. This is particularly important when someone other than the person who biopsied the lesion needs to determine its location. A notation should be made of the type of preparation and local anesthesia used along with a skin incision, if any. The type of device and gauge of needle should be specified along with at least an approximate number of cores taken. A notation should be made if a clip is placed, including the type of clip. If a specimen radiograph is done, the information should also be recorded in the report. After the pathology report is available, a written note should be made documenting concordance (or discordance) of imaging findings with pathology, complications (if any), and a disposition based on correlation of physical, imaging, and pathology findings.

CERTIFICATION AND ACCREDITATION

During the last decade or so, the use of ultrasound has become important to a variety of disciplines in providing optimum patient care. It can no longer be considered a procedure that belongs only in the domain of radiologists. The American Medical Association (AMA) recognized the need for appropriately trained physicians of any specialty to be able to use this

TABLE 31A-1 H-230.960 Privileging for Ultrasound Imaging

(1) AMA affirms that ultrasound imaging is within the scope of practice of appropriately trained physicians

(2) AMA policy on ultrasound acknowledges that broad and diverse use and application of ultrasound imaging technologies exist in medical practice

(3) AMA policy on ultrasound imaging affirms that privileging of the physician to perform ultrasound imaging procedures in a hospital setting should be a function of hospital medical staffs and should be specifically delineated on the Department's Delineation of Privileges form

(4) AMA policy on ultrasound imaging states that each hospital medical staff should review and approve criteria for granting ultrasound privileges based upon background and training for the use of ultrasound technology and strongly recommends that these criteria are in accordance with recommended training and education standards developed by each physician's respective specialty (Res. 802, I-99; Reaffirmed: Sub. Res. 108, A-00)

vital technology in the care of patients.[8] A resolution was passed in 1999 by the AMA House of Delegates supporting that position (Table 31A-1).[9] There remains a need to ensure that physicians in all specialties perform ultrasound properly and with appropriate training. Thus pathways for certification or accreditation have become available for surgeons who perform breast ultrasound. *Certification* refers to the competence of an individual, whereas *accreditation* refers to the competence of a facility.

There are a variety of reasons why surgeons should become certified in breast ultrasound, their practices accredited, or both. Going through a rigorous process of certification or accreditation of necessity ensures that the surgeon must pay attention to the details of generating high-quality images with proper settings for depth, focal zones, gain, and TGC. The experience helps the surgeon develop good habits in image annotation and chart documentation. These things help to ensure that the patient receives the high-quality examination she has a right to expect when she has a breast ultrasound. From a practical point of view, it is becoming more important to be certified or accredited as we move into the pay-for-performance era because more and more insurance carriers will require some type of proof of competence for reimbursement.

Certification and Accreditation Programs

American College of Radiology

To set quality standards for practices and help them continuously improve on the quality of care they give to their patients, the American College of Radiology (ACR) initiated a breast ultrasound accreditation program in 1998.[10] The program evaluates and provides peer review and constructive feedback to the facility concerning their staff's qualifications, equipment, quality control, quality assurance, image quality, and accuracy of needle placement for diagnostic procedures. It is difficult for surgeons' practices to qualify for ACR accreditation. Consequently, there are currently no surgeons' practices accredited by ACR.

American Institute of Ultrasound in Medicine

The American Institute of Ultrasound in Medicine (AIUM) is a multidisciplinary association dedicated to advancing the safe and effective use of ultrasound in medicine through professional and public education, research, development of guidelines, and accreditation. It is composed of a diverse population of members who share an interest in medical ultrasound. Physicians include radiologists, obstetricians and gynecologists, surgeons, endocrinologists, and others. In addition, engineers, scientists, technologists, and representatives of manufacturers are members.

In 1999, AIUM instituted a breast ultrasound accreditation program and began accrediting facilities.[11] Surgeons' practices are eligible for accreditation, and a limited number have been accredited. Physicians must be board certified in some specialty to be eligible for consideration. In the absence of formal residency training in ultrasound, a physician can meet the training guidelines for accreditation eligibility by documenting 100 AMA PRA Category 1 continuing medical education (CME) credits dedicated to breast ultrasound and by being involved with the performance, evaluation, and interpretation of the images of at least 300 sonograms within a 3-year period. In most circumstances the examinations must be done under the supervision of a qualified physician. Alternatively, certification in breast ultrasound by the American Society of Breast Surgeons (ASBS) is accepted as adequate proof of training for consideration for practice accreditation (see later).

For a facility or practice to be accredited by AIUM, one physician in the practice must be designated as director of ultrasound and accept responsibility for overseeing the breast ultrasound program. To maintain accreditation, all physicians in the practice who perform breast ultrasound must obtain 10 hours of AMA-PRA Category 1 CME credits every 3 years. All nonphysician sonographers who perform breast ultrasound in the practice must be certified by the American Registry of Diagnostic Medical Sonography (ARDMS) when the practice reaccredits in 3 years.

For accreditation by AIUM, information must be submitted to document proper selection and maintenance of equipment, storage, reports, and record-keeping policies. Also required are descriptions of policies and procedures for safeguarding patients, personnel, and equipment in addition to a description of the facilities' quality improvement program. Images from five diagnostic cases and five interventional cases must be submitted along with proper reports, mammography and pathology reports, and follow-up where applicable. Interventional images must show a lesion clearly, an image with the needle in proper biopsy position, and a postprocedure image.[12]

American Society of Breast Surgeons

The ASBS is an organization of more than 2800 international members that was founded in 1999 to encourage the study of breast surgery, to promote research and development of advanced surgical techniques, and to improve standards of practice for breast surgery and serve as a forum for the exchange of ideas.[13] Active membership is open to surgeons with a special interest in breast disease. Associate membership is open to nongeneral surgeons or nonsurgeon physicians with a demonstrated interest in breast surgery. Affiliate membership is open to allied health care professionals, researchers, and scientists who are engaged in the care of breast surgery patients. Candidate membership is offered to general surgery residents, surgical oncology fellows, and breast fellows currently enrolled in a residency/fellowship program.

Although the AIUM provides a very reasonable mechanism for a surgeon's practice to become accredited, the accreditation is specific for the practice and not the individual. Consequently, if the surgeon changes practice locations or arrangements, a fairly common occurrence for surgeons, the accreditation is not portable, and it is necessary for the surgeon to reapply for accreditation of the new practice. Because this format is not ideally suited to surgeons' practices, the ASBS developed a breast ultrasound certification program in 2002 that is individual specific and portable if the surgeon changes practice locations. As of September 2009, 95 surgeons have certified in breast ultrasound and 31 have recertified after 5 years of certification.

To become certified by ASBS, a surgeon must be board certified by the American Board of Surgery, the American Board of Osteopathic Surgery, or the International equivalent. Surgeons certified in obstetrics and gynecology are eligible if they complete a breast fellowship recognized by ASBS, the Society of Surgical Oncology, and the American Society of Breast Diseases. One year of experience in breast ultrasound is required prior to application, and a minimum of 80 diagnostic and 20 interventional cases per year must be performed. Documentation must be provided reflecting the use of proper equipment along with maintenance records for the equipment, and quality assurance policies must be submitted for review. Complications from procedures must be listed and described.

A minimum of 15 AMA-PRA category 1 CME credits in breast ultrasound is required for ASBS certification. Of these, a minimum of 7 credits in breast ultrasound must be obtained during the 18 months prior to submission of the application. The applicant must document successful completion of a full-day course, including a didactic portion on the principles of ultrasound as well as a hands-on portion demonstrating ultrasound-guided procedures. Recertification occurs every 5 years and requires a total of 15 hours of CME credit, 5 of which must be AMA-PRA Category 1.

A comprehensive written examination must be passed (passing score = 80) covering a wide range of breast ultrasound topics, including physics, image quality, image interpretation, pathology, patient management, scanning techniques, breast ultrasound anatomy, recognition of BI-RADS categories on ultrasound, concordance/discordance, and interventional ultrasound. The examination is given at least twice a year and must be passed within 18 months of the time of submission of the application. The application includes submission of 5 diagnostic cases and 5 interventional cases. High-quality images are required with proper documentation (Table 31A-2). The case submissions must include a correlation of the physical and

TABLE 31A-2 Proper Submission of Images
American Society of Breast Surgeons' Ultrasound Certification

1. **All Cases**—The images must be technically acceptable with respect to proper transducer selection, gain, depth, focal zone placement, and annotation. Each ultrasound image must document "Right" or "Left" side, and the location of the imaged lesion in the breast using diagram or clock notation. Centimeter distance from the nipple or zone of the lesion must be indicated on the images.

2. **Diagnostic Cases**—Examinations must include *2 orthogonal views* of the lesion in which the lesion is clearly visible and must show at least 2 orthogonal dimensions measured. Each image must document the transducer orientation in addition to the above required annotation. Documentation must include indications for study, mammographic correlation when applicable, findings, impression and recommendation. Description of the ultrasound findings must include reference to the lesion's echogenicity, shape characteristics, and physics artifacts.

3. **Interventional Procedures**—Images should show *the long axis of the needle* demonstrating the needle's location with respect to the sonographic lesion as specifically described below. Coaxial views may be submitted in addition, but must be clearly labeled.

    a. **Cyst Aspirations**—Must include at least 1 view demonstrating the needle within the cyst, as well as at least 1 view of the breast parenchyma following complete aspiration of the cyst just prior to removal of the needle.

    b. **Fine-Needle Aspiration of Solid Lesions**—Must include an image showing the needle longitudinally with the needle's tip clearly within the lesion.

    c. **Core Needle Biopsy**—Must include images along the long axis of the needle demonstrating both the pre- and post-fire position of the needle relative to the sonographic lesion.

    d. **Vacuum-Assisted / Rotational-Cutter Biopsy**—Must include at least 2 images along the long axis of the needle, 1 showing the needle in pre-biopsy position, and 1 demonstrating the post-biopsy appearance of the lesion. Please note that the appropriate "pre-biopsy" position is different for the various biopsy devices: ie single insertion vacuum-assisted devices are generally positioned deep to the lesion before beginning the biopsy, whereas rotational-cutter devices are positioned within or through the lesion

The procedure note should include specifics such as the location of the lesion, the type of prep and anesthesia, the needle type, the number of cores taken, and the approach (lateral to medial, etc).

imaging findings, mammogram and pathology reports, and documentation of proper interpretation of studies and disposition recommendations. Each of the 10 cases must score at least 85 to pass. For recertification, 3 cases with both diagnostic and interventional components are required.

In 2008, in response to the threat that the Food and Drug Administration (FDA) might bring stereotaxis under the Mammography Quality Standards Act (MQSA) and regulate it in a manner that might make it difficult for surgeons to continue performing stereotactic breast biopsies,[14] the ASBS developed a voluntary program to certify individuals and accredit facilities in stereotactic biopsy. The Institute of Medicine (IOM) had previously recommended to Congress that MQSA be changed to the Breast Imaging Quality Standards Act (BIQSA) and that breast ultrasound be regulated as well.[15] The ASBS leadership thought it would be prudent to expand the breast ultrasound certification program and develop an accreditation component for the surgeon's facility as well. The accreditation component was added and, along with the stereotactic certification and accreditation programs, was submitted to the ACS for endorsement. On June 13, 2008, the ACS Board of Regents approved all of the programs including the accreditation of physicians' practices in breast ultrasound.

Surgeons can now apply for individual certification alone or for both individual certification and practice accreditation through ASBS.[16] The accreditation program is designed to ensure that facilities receiving such accreditation have met the applicable requirements regarding the equipment, personnel (physicians, ultrasound technologists, physician assistants, nurse practitioners, and nurses), quality control and quality assurance programs, and accuracy of examinations and procedures being performed. One surgeon must be certified and accept responsibility for the ultrasound program in order for a practice to be accredited. If the responsible surgeon moves to a different practice location, he or she remains certified by the ASBS for the duration of the certification or recertification, but further application is required to maintain accreditation for the former facility or to obtain accreditation for the new practice facility. All other personnel who perform breast ultrasound in the practice must be actively working toward certification and attain it within a 3-year period for the practice to remain accredited. Appropriate certification is through ASBS for surgeons and ARDMS or the American Registry of Radiologic Technologists (ARRT) for all other nonphysician personnel who perform breast ultrasound. Quality assurance data including number of procedures, biopsy results, concordance/discordance and follow-up must be tracked and reported when applying for reaccreditation in 5 years. A Web-based tracking system is being developed by the society and should be available for use in 2009.

FUTURE DIRECTIONS

Ultrasound Technology

Improvements in transducers and software, including compounding of images, have improved ultrasound substantially in the last decade, but there is still much room for further advancement. It remains an operator-dependent examination

that evaluates only small amounts of tissue at a time, and image resolution and clarity remain suboptimal in fatty replaced breasts. Evaluation of fatty breasts is so good with mammography that there is not as much of a need to refine ultrasound for that population of patients as there is for those with dense breasts in which ultrasound has distinct advantages over mammography. Elastography, which compares the relative stiffness of lesions to that of surrounding tissue, will likely contribute to the analysis of sonographic abnormalities, but it, or any other modality, is unlikely to be specific enough in the foreseeable future to obviate the need for biopsy. However, because ultrasound-guided core biopsy is so easy and accurate, there is really not a pressing need to develop mechanisms for making a diagnosis without tissue acquisition. Far more important is the development of ways to perceive subtle lesions that are currently missed, and to do so in a cost-effective, widely available manner. Improvements in contrast imaging and the availability of less expensive contrast agents may afford better detection of subtle lesions. An even more promising avenue is the development of a system that provides rapid, cost-effective breast scanning in which a single-sweep automated acquisition technique produces reproducible 3-dimensional (3D) images for evaluation. An integrated display system allows advanced 3D reconstruction of images resulting in better visualization, especially in a coronal plane.[17] This combination offers hope for a mass screening tool for women with dense breasts in whom mammography is woefully inadequate.

Certification and Accreditation

Currently only a small percentage of radiology practices are accredited, and a small percentage of surgeons who perform breast ultrasound are certified or their practices accredited. This will almost surely change in the near future, hopefully as a result of the recognition by surgeons and radiologists of the value in voluntarily going through the process. If not, it will surely be mandated by the government to try to ensure that patients get high-quality exams or by third-party payers for the facility or physician to be reimbursed.

NECESSARY FUTURE STUDIES

Studies are needed to evaluate the emerging ultrasound technologies to determine the benefit in detecting subtle lesions that are currently being missed. What are the characteristics of lesions that are initially missed on ultrasound but are later seen when a second-look ultrasound is prompted by abnormalities on MRI? Would better contrast agents, elastography, or full-field automated screening with 3D reconstruction allow them to be seen before an MRI is done? Is there a role for ultrasound fusion with mammography or MRI as there is for computed tomography/positron computed tomography (CT/PET) fusion? Studies to answer these important questions should be given high priority.

SUMMARY

Modern breast ultrasound has become an indispensable tool for the surgeon who wishes to provide state-of-the-art care to patients with breast problems. The surgeon should have a thorough understanding of the physics of ultrasound in order to interpret the generated images properly. Breast ultrasound should be used for generally accepted indications, and the indication for the procedure clearly documented in the patient's record, along with the findings, interpretation, and recommendation. A comprehensive knowledge of findings that suggest benign or malignant disease is vital for the surgeon to properly use the device to decrease the necessity for biopsies, particularly open surgical procedures, without significantly increasing the miss rate for carcinomas. Obtaining individual certification and/or practice accreditation is important to ensure that breast ultrasound is being done well and that patients are receiving optimal examinations. It will likely become more important in the future in order to obtain reimbursement.

ACKNOWLEDGMENT

The author would like to thank a special colleague, Dr Eva Rubin, for her willingness to share her ideas and her remarkable expertise in the preparation of this chapter.

REFERENCES

1. Stavros AT. *Breast Ultrasound*. Philadelphia, PA. Lippincott Williams & Wilkins: 2004:66.
2. Fry WR. In: Harness JK, Wisher DB, eds. *Ultrasound in Surgical Practice: Basic Principles and Clinical Applications*. New York, NY: Wiley-Liss:2001:8.
3. Kremkau FW. *Diagnostic Ultrasound: Principles and Instruments*. 6th ed. Philadelphia, PA: WB Saunders: 2002:32-33.
4. Rissanen T, Reinikainen H, Apaja-Sarkkinen M. Breast sonography in localizing the cause of nipple discharge: comparison with galactography in 52 patients. *J Ultrasound Med*. 2007;26(8):1031-1039.
5. Gray RJ, Pockaj BA, Karstaedt PJ. Navigating murky waters: a modern treatment algorithm for nipple discharge. *Am J Surg*. 2007;194(6):850-855.
6. American Institute of Ultrasound in Medicine. AIUM Practice Guideline for the Performance of a Breast Ultrasound Examination. Available at: http://www.aium.org/publications/clinical/breast.pdf. Accessed August 29, 2008.
7. American Society of Breast Surgeons: Performance and practice guidelines for breast ultrasound. Available at: http://www.breastsurgeons.org/official-stmts/Performance_Practice_Guidelines_BreastUltrasound_4-29-2008.pdf. Accessed August 29, 2008.
8. Harness JK, Wisher DB. *Ultrasound in Surgical Practice: Basic Principles and Clinical Applications*. New York, NY: Wiley-Liss: 2001:515.
9. American Medical Association: House resolution 230.960. Available at: http://www.ama-assn.org/apps/pf_new/pf_online?f_n=resultLink&doc=policyfiles/HnE/H-230.960.HTM&s_t=ultrasound&catg=AMA/HnE&catg=AMA/BnGnC&catg=AMA/DIR&&nth=1&&st_p=0&nth=2&Accessed August 5, 2008.
10. American College of Radiology: Breast ultrasound accreditation program history. Available at: http://www.acr.org/accreditation/breast/b_history.aspx. Accessed August 29, 2008.
11. American Institute of Ultrasound in Medicine: History of the AIUM. Available at: http://www.aium.org/aboutAIUM/timeline/1990.asp. Accessed August 29, 2008.
12. American Institute of Ultrasound in Medicine: Application for ultrasound Practice Accreditation: Available at: http://www.aium.org/. Accessed August 30, 2008.
13. American Society of Breast Surgeons: Mission statement: Available at: http://www.breastsurgeons.org/index.html. Accessed August 29, 2008.
14. American College of Radiology: FDA Mammography Advisory Committee votes to include stereotactic breast biopsy under MQSA Regulations. Available at: http://www.acr.org/accreditation/FeaturedCategories/Articles-Announcements/FDAtoIncludeSBBinMQSARegulations.aspx. Accessed August 30, 2008.
15. Institute of Medicine: Improving breast imaging quality standards (2005). Available at: http://books.nap.edu/openbook.php?record_id=11308&page-15. Accessed August 30, 2008.
16. American Society of Breast Surgeons: breast ultrasound certification and facility accreditation program. Available at: http://www.breastsurgeons.org/certification.shtml. Accessed August 30, 2008.
17. Siemens and U-Systems Announce Worldwide Distribution Agreement for U-Systems' SomoVu Automated Breast Ultrasound System. Available at: http://findarticles.com/p/articles/mi_m0EIN/is_2007_March_23/ai_n27191706. Accessed September 13, 2008.

Screening Breast Ultrasound

Edgar D. Staren

For at least 2 decades, the role of breast ultrasound (US) has continued to evolve. Initially proposed to differentiate the cystic versus solid nature of indeterminate masses identified on mammogram, the indications have grown to include evaluation of palpable breast masses, pregnancy and lactation, postoperative follow-up for hematomas, seromas, prosthesis, and recurrence, evaluation of axillary lymph nodes, US-guided interventions: cyst aspiration, biopsy of solid lesions, needle localization, and most recently, screening, especially of the high-risk and/or dense breast.[1]

RATIONALE FOR SCREENING BREAST ULTRASOUND

There is considerable rationale to support the concept of screening US. If one considers the impact of screening mammogram, it alone is thought to have decreased breast cancer deaths by at least 15% to 20% in women ≥40 years of age with some studies reporting substantially higher benefits.[2] Unfortunately, approximately a third of screening mammograms are classified as American College of Radiology-Breast Imaging-Reporting Data System (ACR-BI-RADS) density protocol 3 to 4, defined as heterogeneously dense (51%-75% glandular) or even homogeneously dense; such results may dramatically lower the sensitivity of the mammogram.[3,4] Although recent data have suggested that digital mammography improves the sensitivity in such dense breasts, this limitation is not obviated.[5] Conversely, screening breast US actually has its visualization capability improved in dense breast tissue.[6] Moreover, screening US is well tolerated by patients, is noninvasive, exposes the patient to no radiation, and is relatively inexpensive. When performed in the clinician's office, it becomes a logical extension to a thorough physical breast examination.[7]

HISTORICAL ORIGINS OF SCREENING BREAST ULTRASOUND

The origins for screening breast US go back to the late 1970s when Bailar suggested that radiation from mammography might be carcinogenic.[8] This in turn led to efforts to replace mammography with US. As one might expect given the quite limited quality of US in general at the time, these initial studies yielded relatively poor results and particularly were associated with very high false positives.[9,10] Not to be deterred, several studies were performed in the decade subsequent to the mid-1980s that identified patients' breast cancers that were incidentally discovered by screening breast ultrasound.[11] Part of the difficulty in comparing these studies rests with the various techniques and equipment used in performing the evaluations. Nonetheless, the results were such that the concept of screening breast US as a viable entity was gaining momentum. This was further supported by 2 large studies, the first performed by Gordon and Goldenberg on 12,706 women who were identified by having a palpable mass or a mammographic abnormality.[12] In this study, use of optimal equipment and reliable technique resulted in a 0.3% detection of incidental cancers by US alone; of note, most were in women who had dense breast parenchyma. These data were substantiated in another large study by Kolb et al in which 11,220 women with negative mammograms as well as a normal clinical breast examination (3626 "dense" breasts on mammogram) underwent bilateral whole breast US.[13] There were 74 cancers detected, 11 by US only (0.3%). In women viewed as "high risk," the incidence was 6 of 1043 (0.6%).

Taking the concept of screening for incidental breast cancer a step further, 2 studies evaluated patients (by screening US) who had already been diagnosed with breast cancer.[14,15] Berg and Gilbreath performed ipsilateral US only and despite a relatively small patient cohort, found a 14% incidence (9 of 64) of cancer by US alone. Moon et al performed bilateral screening breast US and identified 36 of 237 cancers (15%) by US alone; of note, 28 of these were ipsilateral and 8 were contralateral.

REASONS FOR LACK OF ACCEPTANCE OF SCREENING BREAST ULTRASOUND

Given these results, why has there been a general lack of acceptance of screening breast US? The reasons for this are many but include the only fair spatial resolution (fine detail) associated with even the most technically advanced piece of US equipment, the inability to detect (or at least do so quantitatively) most calcium deposits (calcifications) on breast lesions, the high operator dependence associated with performing breast US examinations, and the inability to document reliably how much breast tissue has been imaged, leading to questions about thoroughness of the examination.[1] Although with repetition the total examination time does decrease, it certainly is more time consuming for the clinician than image interpretation alone. Perhaps even more limiting to the expanded use of screening breast US has been the recent increased use of magnetic resonance imaging (MRI) to evaluate the breast and particularly those at high risk and in whom the mammographic examination might be compromised (eg, dense breast parenchyma), exactly the population presumed to benefit by the performance of screening breast US in the first place.[16-19]

AMERICAN COLLEGE OF RADIOLOGY IMAGING NETWORK (ACRIN 6666) STUDY

Fortunately, in 2004, the American College of Radiology Imaging Network (ACRIN 6666) initiated a study aimed at clarifying the role of annual screening US in a 3-year multicenter trial in high-risk women with dense breasts and in whom the investigators were blinded to the mammographic results.[20,21] In this ongoing study, women with dense breast tissue in at least one quadrant were scanned; 2637 (96.8% of eligible participants) have completed at least 12 months of follow-up. Forty patients were diagnosed with cancer (41 breasts): 8 suspicious on both US and mammogram, 12 on US alone, 12 on mammogram alone, and 8 (9 breasts) on neither. The diagnostic yield for US plus mammogram versus mammogram alone was 11.8 versus 7.6 of 1000, respectively; the diagnostic accuracy was 91% versus 78%, respectively. However, long the Achilles heel of screening breast US, the combined tests yielded a false-positive rate of 10.4% as compared with 4.4% for mammogram alone. Moreover, the time required for physicians to perform the examination approached a median of 20 minutes. Taking this alone into account, not to mention the time required to compare studies, follow protocols for thoroughness, and so on, has even led some to suggest that MRI may in fact be less expensive than screening breast US, and if not less, insignificant in difference. This issue is exacerbated by Medicare reimbursement rates that do not cover the costs of performing and interpreting the examination. Perhaps some of these points will be addressed by additional and properly trained examiners as well as perhaps automated whole-breast ultrasound capabilities, but this remains

to be seen. For the time being, however, although the ACRIN study may have well supported the already documented increased detection benefit of screening breast US, it has not clarified the role of screening breast US. As in the past, numerous limitations to its routine adoption persist, and until these are better defined or addressed the quote by Kopans in the *American Journal of Roentgenology* (2003) still stands: "Breast sonographic screening is not ready for prime time."[22]

SUMMARY

There is considerable rationale to support the concept of screening US. Approximately a third of screening mammograms will be classified as ACR-BI-RADS density protocol 3 to 4, defined as heterogeneously dense (51%-75% glandular) or even homogeneously dense; such results may dramatically lower the sensitivity of the mammogram. Although recent data have suggested that digital mammography improves the sensitivity in such dense breasts, this limitation is not obviated. Conversely, screening breast US actually has its visualization capability improved in dense breast tissue. Screening US is well tolerated by patients, is noninvasive, exposes the patient to no radiation, and is relatively inexpensive. When performed in the clinician's office, it becomes a logical extension to a thorough physical breast examination.

The expanded use of screening breast US has been limited by the recent increased use of MRI to evaluate the breast and particularly those at high risk and in whom the mammographic examination might be compromised (eg, dense breast parenchyma). The current role of screening breast US is debated and remains to be clarified universally by breast surgical oncologists and radiologists.

REFERENCES

1. Staren ED, O'Neill TP. Breast ultrasound. *Surg Clinics North Am.* 1998; 78:219-235.
2. Humphrey LL, Helfand M, Chan BK, Woolf SH. Breast cancer screening: a summary of the evidence for the US Preventive Services Task Force. *Ann Intern Med.* 2002;137:347-360.
3. Stomper PC, D'Souza DJ, DiNitto PA, Arredondo MA. Analysis of parenchymal density on mammograms in 1353 women 25–79 years old. *Am J Roentgenol.* 1996;167:1261-1265.
4. D'Orsi CJ, Bassett LW, Berg WA, et al. *Breast Imaging Reporting and Data System, BI-RADS: Mammography.* 4th ed. Reston, VA: American College of Radiology: 2003.
5. Pisano ED, Gatsonis C, Hendrick E, et al. Diagnostic performance of digital versus film mammography for breast cancer screening. *N Engl J Med.* 2005;237:1075-1080.
6. Kolb TM, Lichy J, Newhouse JH. Comparison of the performance of screening mammography, physical examination, and breast US and evaluation of factors that influence them: an analysis of 27,825 patient evaluations. *Radiology.* 2002;225:165-175.
7. Velez N, Earnest D, Staren ED. Diagnostic and interventional ultrasound for breast disease. *Am J Surg.* 2000;180:284-287.
8. Bailar JC III. Mammography: a contrary view. *Ann Intern Med.* 1976;84: 77-84.
9. Sickles EA, Filly RA, Callen PW. Breast cancer detection with sonography and mammography: comparison using state-of-the-art equipment. *Am J Roentgenol.* 1983;140:843-845.
10. Kopans DB, Meyer JE, Lindfors KK. Whole-breast US imaging: four-year follow-up. *Radiology.* 1985;157:505-507.
11. Bassett LW, Kimme-Smith C, Sutherland LK, et al. Automated and hand-held breast US: effect on patient management. *Radiology* 1987;165:103-108.

12. Gordon PB, Goldenberg SL. Malignant breast masses detected only by US: a retrospective review. *Cancer*; 1995;76:626-630.

13. Kolb TM, Lichy J, Newhouse JH. Occult cancer in women with dense breasts: detection with screening US-diagnostic yield and tumor characteristics. *Radiology*. 1998;207:191-199.

14. Berg WA, Gilbreath PL. Multicentric and multifocal cancer: whole-breast US in preoperative evaluation. *Radiology*. 2000;214:59-66.

15. Moon WK, Noh DY, Im JG. Multifocal, multicentric, and contralateral breast cancers: bilateral whole-breast US in the preoperative evaluation of patients. *Radiology*. 2002;224:569-576.

16. Kuhl CK, Schrading S, Leutner CC, et al. Mammography, breast ultrasound, and magnetic resonance imaging for surveillance of women at high familial risk for breast cancer. *J Clin Oncol*. 2005;23:8469-8476.

17. Liberman L. Breast MR imaging in assessing extent of disease. *Mag Reson Imaging Clinics North Am*. 2006;14:339-349.

18. Smith RA. The evolving role of MRI in the detection and evaluation of breast cancer. *N Engl J Med*. 2007;356(13):1362-1364.

19. Lehman CD, Isaacs C, Schnall MD, et al. Cancer yield of mammography, MR, and US in high-risk women: prospective multi-institutional breast cancer screening study. *Radiology*. 2007;244:381-388.

20. Berg WA. Rationale for a trial of screening breast ultrasound: American College of Radiology Imaging Network (ACRIN) 6666. *Am J Roentgenol*. 2003;180:1225-1228.

21. Berg WA, Blume JD, Cormack JB, et al. Combined screening with ultrasound and mammography vs. mammography alone in women at elevated risk of breast cancer. *JAMA*. 2008;299:2151-2163.

22. Kopans DB. Breast sonographic screening is not ready for prime time. *Amer J Roentgenol*. 2003;181:1426-1428.

CHAPTER 32

Selection of Ultrasound Machine and Office Setup

Eric B. Whitacre

Breast ultrasound has become an essential tool for the breast surgeon. Traditionally, however, it has not been a part of the general surgical curriculum, and many practicing surgeons are still struggling with how to incorporate breast ultrasound into their practice. This chapter will outline the steps to facilitate this transition.

SELECTION OF THE ULTRASOUND MACHINE

The minimum requirements for a functional breast ultrasound machine are listed in Table 32-1. Fortunately, because of recent advances in software, solid-state circuitry, and probe technology, machines that are more sophisticated are now available, and a more suitable choice of features would include some of the additional features listed. The most important aspect of the machine itself is the probe, which ideally would be a multifrequency 8 to 14 MHz linear array probe (although a 7.5-10 MHz probe will also work well). Today, almost any unit that will accommodate this type of probe will include the other features required for high-quality scanning.

Other requirements include a large, high-quality black and white display, or color display if color Doppler is available, and the ability to record information about the scan on the recorded image, including patient name and/or unique identifier, the date, the location of the scanned image as an icon or text, as well as other information about the mechanics of the scan (depth, Time-Gain Compensation settings probe MHz, and frame rate). Ideally, the machine would allow for digital storage of images in addition to the standard printer port for creation of small black and white glossy prints.

For most surgeons, the main criterion for deciding which machine to purchase is whether the unit needs to be portable. This is important because it is essential to have access to a suitable high-quality unit in the operating room. Although many hospitals have ultrasound equipment available for use in the operating room, the unit may be cumbersome to transport from the radiology department, or if already available in the operating suite, may not have a suitable probe for breast scanning. The availability of intraoperative ultrasound is important not only for margin assessment and localization of nonpalpable lesions, but also because it provides an excellent venue to develop and to continue to improve ultrasound skills. The ability to visualize gross anatomic and pathologic findings minutes after performing a scan provides immediate feedback about interpretation of the study and can considerably shorten the learning curve for new users and improve skills of more experienced imagers.

Portability is also an important consideration for surgeons working in multiple office locations. In a small office or clinic, however, it is often easier to dedicate an exam room to ultrasound scanning than to move the scanner from room to room, because it is disruptive to patient flow and because of the other room modifications listed below. Fortunately, there is little, if any, significant difference in quality between the portable and fixed ultrasound machines available today. Figure 32-1 shows 2 state-of-the-art machines available today, which are comparable with regard to scanning features and quality and are in the same price range.[1,2]

LOCATION

The optimal location for an ultrasound machine in the breast clinic is almost always in the room where most breast patients are examined. There is a strong inclination to locate a newly acquired ultrasound machine in the "procedure room" where there already may be other equipment, such as suction or cautery. For breast ultrasound, however, this is not necessarily the best location because of the benefits of ready access to ultrasound scanning for evaluation of almost any breast problem. In

TABLE 32-1 Requirements for a Breast Ultrasound Machine

Minimum Requirements

7.5-MHz linear array probe
High-quality black and white monitor, > 10-in diagonal
Adjustable focal zone
Controls to modify scanning depth and TGC curve
Ability to document details of the scan, including patient name or identifier, date, time, location and orientation of the probe, MHz, and frames per second

Desirable Features

8–14-MHz linear array probe
High-quality color monitor, > 14-in diagonal
Color and power Doppler

Available Useful Options (price-dependent)

Compound imaging
Harmonic imaging
3-dimensional scanning

most busy surgical practices, if the ultrasound equipment is not available for immediate scanning, the opportunity to perform the ultrasound is lost. Instead, it is better to make small modifications to a standard office examination room to make it suitable for diagnostic scanning as well as for most percutaneous

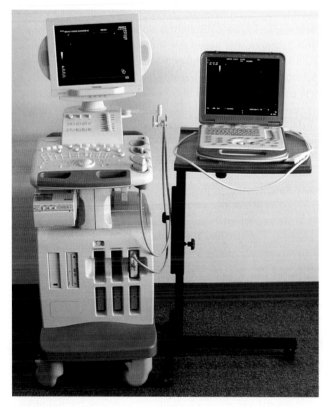

FIGURE 32-1 These 2 ultrasound machines are comparable in quality, features, and price. The laptop-style unit is completely portable; the fixed unit is more cumbersome to transport, but has more options that are upgradeable.

ultrasound-guided procedures. Figure 32-2 shows how a stationary ultrasound unit can be located in a typical 10 × 12 ft examination room and still leave space for a console to perform percutaneous procedures.

ADDITIONAL EQUIPMENT

In addition to the ultrasound unit, which should include a small printer to record selected images from the scanning process, it is essential to have an x-ray view box in the room to be able to compare outside imaging studies with the real-time ultrasound scan. Also, because an increasing number of outside studies are available on CD-ROM instead of printed film, it is important to consider equipping the room with a computer with a CD/DVD drive and high-quality monitor. The ability to compare the live scan with outside studies (as well as your own prior imaging) is critical for accurate interpretation of the imaging and its correlation with the history and physical examination.

A gel warmer is an inexpensive addition that patients will greatly appreciate. Removing the gel after the scan is also an important and often overlooked issue—the doctor can easily rinse hands at the sink, whereas a patient will require soft paper or cloth wipes to remove the gel from the breast. Gowns or capes made from soft cloth, instead of the traditional paper, are a nice addition to the examination overall and can be used later by patients to help remove gel.

If you are planning to perform ultrasound-guided procedures, then the room should have adequate storage space for supplies. For convenience and safety, you must also ensure disposal and waste bins large enough to accommodate the supplies you will use. Figure 32-3 shows that a small work light installed over the sink is useful to help an assistant work when the room lights are dimmed and can double as a room "dimmer" if the room is not equipped with a rheostat to dim the lights for better viewing of the ultrasound image.

If invasive procedures are not currently being performed in the office, but ultrasound-guided interventions are going to be added in addition to diagnostic ultrasound scanning, then all of the required Occupational Safety and Health Administration (OSHA) policies and procedures must be in place, including appropriate barrier protection items for employees (gloves, gowns, masks, etc).[3] In addition, because invasive procedures will generate "medical waste" as defined by the Environmental Protection Agency, each office will need to arrange for appropriate disposal of contaminated materials according to state and local guidelines.[4] The ombudsman of your local medical society, or the risk management department of your medical liability insurance carrier, are excellent places to begin to investigate these requirements.

DOCUMENTATION AND CHARTING

A complete breast ultrasound consists not only of the scanning process itself, but also a record of selected images from the scan and a dictated report of the scan with interpretation of the findings and recommendations for further management. This is critical for billing (as a record of the scan is required by Current Procedural Terminology [CPT] description of the diagnostic

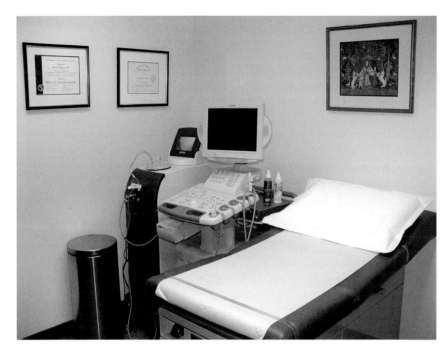

FIGURE 32-2 A standard 10 × 12 ft examination room will accommodate a fixed ultrasound machine and still have room for a console to perform vacuum-assisted biopsies or other percutaneous procedures. It is generally preferable to locate the ultrasound unit where most patients are examined and then make small modifications to accommodate the scanner and to perform percutaneous ultrasound-guided procedures. (Note the large wastebasket, which is useful if procedures are performed due to the large amount of disposable material generated.)

breast scanning code[5]), but is also expected medical practice. There are published guidelines concerning the elements of a breast ultrasound scan and the accompanying report from the American College of Radiology,[6] the American Institute of Ultrasound in Medicine,[7] and the American Society of Breast Surgeons.[8] The American Society of Breast Surgeons recommendations for the written report are reproduced in Table 32-2. An example of a paper template that can be used to record

information from a simple diagnostic scan showing discrete ultrasound lesions is shown in Figure 32-4. Although this template is useful for recording the information "on the fly," a more detailed report and interpretation is desirable in the permanent patient record.

It can be a challenge to incorporate ultrasound images into individual patient charts when working in a facility that does not have a sophisticated electronic medical record integrated with a

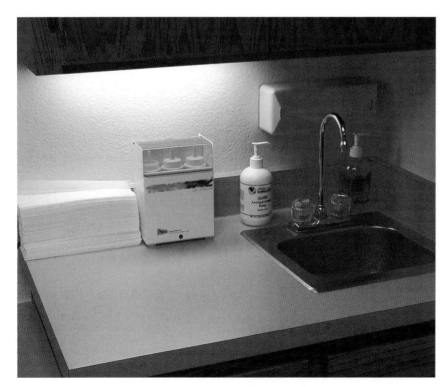

FIGURE 32-3 A small work light installed over the sink not only provides light for an assistant to help label and process biopsy specimens, but can be used as a "dimmer" to improve visualization of the ultrasound image. Patients appreciate use of a gel warmer and the availability of soft paper wipes to remove gel.

TABLE 32-2 American Society of Breast Surgeons Guidelines for Breast Ultrasound Scanning Written Reports

A. Each ultrasound study should have a permanent written record along with the accompanying set of images in retrievable image storage format. The images and report should become a part of the patient's permanent medical record.

B. Each individual image should include the facility name, date of examination, patient's first and last name, and identification number, if applicable. A notation of left or right breast and the location of the lesion should be shown on all images. Diagnostic images should also indicate transducer orientation within the breast. *All of the above notations should be made using the icon or the annotation script capability of the instrument.* The distance of the lesion from the nipple should be noted either in centimeters or by zone using the instrument's script. *Handwritten notes on the images should be used only to correct errors on previously printed images.*

C. Standard form reports may be used as long as they are comprehensive in nature.

D. Reports of diagnostic procedures should include the indication for the study (including correlation with physical and/or imaging studies), description of technique, findings (including size, shape, echogenicity, and physics artifacts), impression (with provisional diagnosis, if possible), and recommendation.

E. Reports of ultrasound-guided interventional procedures should include the location of the lesion; the approach (lateral to medial, etc); the type of prep and local anesthesia; skin incision, if any; type of device used; the number of cores taken; and the type of clip placed, if any. If specimen radiographs or sonograms are done, the information should be recorded in the report.

F. Final reports should be completed and sent to the referring clinician in a timely manner, if indicated.

G. A written note should be made documenting concordance (or discordance) of imaging findings with pathology, complications (if any), and a disposition based upon correlation of physical, imaging, and pathology findings.

H. Optional classification of breast ultrasound lesions may be used employing the American College of Radiology Breast Imaging Reporting and Data System, or BI-RADS.

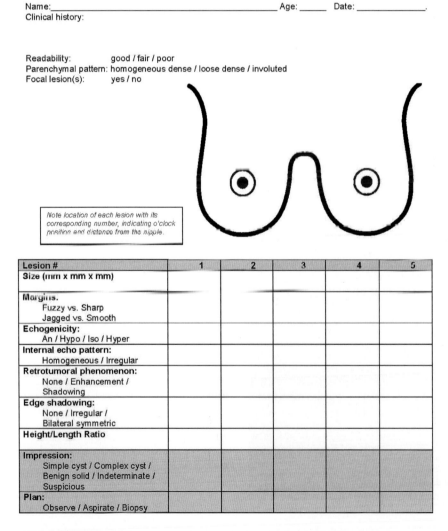

Breast Ultrasound Report

Name:_____ Age: _____ Date: _____.
Clinical history:

Readability: good / fair / poor
Parenchymal pattern: homogeneous dense / loose dense / involuted
Focal lesion(s):   yes / no

Note location of each lesion with its corresponding number, indicating o'clock position and distance from the nipple.

Lesion #	1	2	3	4	5
Size (mm x mm x mm)					
Margins: Fuzzy vs. Sharp Jagged vs. Smooth					
Echogenicity: An / Hypo / Iso / Hyper					
Internal echo pattern: Homogeneous / Irregular					
Retrotumoral phenomenon: None / Enhancement / Shadowing					
Edge shadowing: None / Irregular / Bilateral symmetric					
Height/Length Ratio					
Impression: Simple cyst / Complex cyst / Benign solid / Indeterminate / Suspicious					
Plan: Observe / Aspirate / Biopsy					

FIGURE 32-4 A simple template can be used to record real-time findings quickly. Ideally, however, this information would later be incorporated into a more detailed report to be placed in the patient record.

picture archiving and communication system (PACS). Offices with paper charts can use small plastic pockets or envelops available from most office supply companies to hold the 3 × 5 inch glossy prints; practices with independent electronic medical records can store the images digitally on the ultrasound unit at the time of the procedure and then transfer them to the patient record. Whatever the technique, it is important to be able to retrieve the images for review during subsequent patient visits and be capable of sharing the images with other outside facilities for comparison.

FINANCES AND BILLING

In the current practice environment, the cost of a new ultrasound unit appears considerable, and it is essential to become familiar with the details of coding in order to make ultrasound available in your practice. Fortunately, appropriate CPT codes and modifiers exist to cover the practice expense and professional work associated with ultrasound scanning and procedures (Tables 32-3 and 32-4). Although there is not sufficient

TABLE 32-3 CPT Codes for Breast Ultrasound Scanning and Procedures[5]

Code	Ultrasound Imaging Codes	Description
76645	Ultrasound, breast(s) (unilateral or bilateral), real time with image documentation	Diagnostic ultrasound of the breast
76880	Ultrasound, extremity, nonvascular, real time with image documentation	Diagnostic ultrasound of the axilla
76942	Ultrasonic guidance for needle placement (eg, biopsy, aspiration, injection, localization device), imaging supervision and interpretation	Code with any ultrasound-guided procedure (except 19105 and 19296)
76970	Ultrasound study follow-up (specify)	For interval follow-up targeted scan
76998	Ultrasound guidance, intraoperative	Intraoperative scanning that does not include device placement
Ultrasound-Related Procedure Codes (Code with 76942 in Addition to the Procedure Code)		
10022	Fine-needle aspiration, with image guidance	For solid lesions in the breast or axilla
19000	Puncture aspiration of cyst of breast	For cyst aspiration (code with 76942 if performed under image guidance)
+19001	Puncture aspiration of cyst of breast, each additional cyst (list separately in addition to code for primary procedure)	For each additional cyst
19102	Biopsy of breast, percutaneous, needle core, using imaging guidance	For "Tru-cut"–type needle biopsies
19103	Biopsy of breast, percutaneous, automated vacuum-assisted or rotating biopsy device, using imaging guidance	For "Mammotome"-type needle biopsies
19290	Preoperative placement of needle localization wire, breast	For placement localization wires and other similar devices
+19291	Preoperative placement of needle localization wire, breast, each additional lesion (list separately in addition to code for primary procedure)	For each additional lesion (not wire) localized
+19295	Image-guided placement, metallic localization clip, percutaneous, during breast biopsy (list separately in addition to code for primary procedure)	For placement of a radiographic marker
Ultrasound-Related Procedure Codes (Do Not Add 76942 as This is Included in the Code)		
19105	Ablation, cryosurgical, of fibroadenoma, including ultrasound guidance, each fibroadenoma	Per fibroadenoma
19296	Placement of radiotherapy afterloading expandable catheter (single or multichannel) into the breast for interstitial radioelement application following partial mastectomy, includes imaging guidance; on date separate from partial mastectomy	For delayed insertion of a "MammoSite"-type device

TABLE 32-4 Important CPT Modifiers for Breast Ultrasound Scanning and Procedures

Modifiers to Apply to Imaging Codes 76XXX		
26	Professional component	Add this to the imaging code when you do not own the equipment being used
–TC	Technical component	The facility which owns the equipment where the procedure is performed will bill this
Modifiers to Apply to Evaluation and Management (E&M) Codes 99XXX		
–25	Significant, separately identifiable evaluation and management service by the same physician on the same day of the procedure or other service	Add this to the E&M code for the visit if you perform a procedure on the same day. This does not apply to diagnostic ultrasound codes that do not require an E&M modifier.

space in this chapter to review all the intricacies of ultrasound coding, there are important principles that are different from coding for either evaluation and management or procedural CPT codes. These are listed in Table 32-5. In addition, because the details of coding can change so quickly, it is very important to update your knowledge with use of the most updated references, including the most current CPT materials.

FUTURE DIRECTIONS

Although excellent breast ultrasound can be performed using a simple linear array probe and a black and white monitor, there are constant advances in ultrasound technology, some of which will eventually require upgrading from a basic unit. Assessment of Doppler flow is not currently a standard technique for evaluation of breast lesions, but Doppler capability is required for assessment of "vocal fremitus," which has been reported to help distinguish normal breast tissue from subtle lesions.[9] Doppler capability is also very beneficial for assessment of vascular anatomy of the axilla and of selected lesions before ultrasound-guided procedures. It will become essential if intravenous contrast techniques become important in routine breast ultrasound evaluation in the future.[10]

In addition, other sophisticated scanning techniques such as compound and harmonic imaging[11] have been developed and are incorporated into many of the very high-end scanners because they

TABLE 32-5 Important Principles of Coding for Breast Ultrasound and Ultrasound-Guided Procedures

1. Imaging codes do not use procedural modifiers, only the professional/technical modifiers based on whether or not you own the equipment used.
2. You are permitted to bill for diagnostic breast ultrasound during initial and follow-up evaluations or consultations. This can be in addition to a procedure utilizing an ultrasound guidance code.

   For example, if you see a patient in consultation for a newly noted area of tenderness and vague fullness in the right breast and perform an ultrasound to diagnose a symptomatic cyst, and then aspirate the cyst under ultrasound guidance, your final coding would look like the following:

99243-25	Intermediate level consultation (with -25 modifier for cyst aspiration same visit)
76645	Diagnostic breast ultrasound
19000	Cyst aspiration (in this instance under ultrasound guidance)
76942	Ultrasound guidance for the cyst aspiration

3. Many, but not all, procedure codes, exist in code "pairs"—one code for the image-guided version and another for the same procedure without image guidance:

For example:	10021	Fine-needle aspiration without image guidance
	10022	Fine-needle aspiration with image guidance
and		
	19100	Core-needle biopsy without image guidance
	19102	Core-needle biopsy with image guidance

   Cyst aspiration is the same code regardless of image guidance, and vacuum-assisted biopsy exists only with image guidance.
4. More recently developed procedure codes (such as 19105, cryoablation of fibroadenoma, and 19296, delayed insertion of a brachytherapy catheter) have been valued to include the work of ultrasound guidance and should not be billed with the ultrasound guidance code 76942. Because this is not apparent from the CPT numerical coding sequence, it is important to pay close attention to the instructions for code use.
5. For all these reasons, always refer to the latest coding references.

help refine the diagnostic image. Integration of these software enhancements, together with the possibility of 3-dimensional whole breast ultrasound scanning[12] with use of intravenous contrast enhancement, may herald a new era for ultrasound evaluation of the breast. Computer-assisted diagnostic (CAD) software for ultrasound is under development to assist with Breast Imaging Reporting and Data System (BI-RADS) classification of lesions.[13]

SUMMARY

Breast ultrasound has become an indispensable tool in the evaluation and management of breast disease. Improvements in technology have made high-quality machines very affordable, so there is little reason not to have ultrasound readily available for the assessment of almost any breast condition. Successful integration of breast ultrasound into the surgical practice can be accomplished with only minor changes to the office environment, but does require a commitment to developing and constantly improving ultrasound imaging skills. Integration of breast ultrasound into the breast practice is essential.

REFERENCES

1. Toshiba America Medical Systems: Toshiba Nemio XG ultrasound unit. Available at: http://www.medical.toshiba.com/products/ul/product-lineup.php Accessed September 14, 2008.
2. Shenzhen Mindray Bio-Medical Electronics Co. Mindray M5 ultrasound unit. Available at: http://www.mindray.com/main/products/show.jsp?catalogID=63&id=173. Accessed September 14, 2008.
3. U.S. Department of Labor, Occupational Safety and Health Administration. Standards. Available at: http://www.osha.gov/pls/oshaweb/owastand.display_standard_group. Accessed September 14, 2008.
4. U.S. Environmental Protection Agency. Medical waste, basic information. Available at: http://www.epa.gov/osw/nonhaz/industrial/medical/index.htm. Accessed September 14, 2008.
5. American Medical Association. CPT 2008 Electronic Professional Edition (CD-ROM version). Chicago, IL: American Medical Association: 2008. CPT code 76645.
6. American College of Radiology. ACR Practice Guideline for the Performance of a Breast Ultrasound Examination. Available at: http://www.acr.org/SecondaryMainMenuCategories/quality_safety/guidelines/breast/us_breast.aspx. Accessed September 14, 2008.
7. American Institute of Ultrasound in Medicine. AIUM Standard for the Performance of Breast Ultrasound Examination, 2002. Available at: http://www.jultrasoundmed.org/cgi/content/long/28/1/105. Accessed September 14, 2008.
8. American Society of Breast Surgeons. The American Society of Breast Surgeons Performance and Practice Guidelines for Breast Ultrasound. Available at: http://www.breastsurgeons.org/statements/PDF_Statements/Perf_Guidelines_Breast_US.pdf. Accessed September 14, 2008.
9. Weinstein SP, Conant EF, Sehgal C. Technical advances in breast ultrasound imaging. *Semin Ultrasound CT MRI.* 2006;27:273-283.
10. Forsberg F, Goldberg BB, Merritt CRB, et al. Diagnosing breast lesions with contrast-enhanced 3-dimensional power doppler imaging. *J Ultrasound Med.* 2004;23:173-182.
11. Sehgal CM, Weinstein SP, Arger PH, et al. A review of breast ultrasound. *J Mammary Gland Biol Neoplasia.* 2006;11:113-123.
12. U-Systems, Inc. Automated Breast Ultrasound View with Somo.v. Available at: http://www.u-systems.com/Healthcare_Professionals/index.cfm/1. Accessed September 14, 2008.
13. Medipattern Corporation, B-CAD V1. Available at: http://www.medipattern.com/section.asp?section_id=26. Accessed September 14, 2008.

CHAPTER 33

Image-Guided Percutaneous Breast Biopsy

Pat W. Whitworth

Image-guided percutaneous biopsy is the technique of choice for the diagnosis of breast lesions. The transition from open to percutaneous techniques as the favored approach in this setting began in the mid-1990s and was complete by January 2005, at the time of the second international consensus conference on the diagnosis and management of image-detected breast cancer, organized by Silverstein.[1]

ADVANTAGES OF THE PERCUTANEOUS ROUTE

Percutaneous diagnosis is the optimal strategy for planning the management of malignant lesions. The open biopsy of the past has several disadvantages: (1) it usually requires an additional operating room procedure for breast cancer patients; (2) it yields unclear resection margins about twice as often as resection after percutaneous diagnosis; (3) it can complicate or even compromise oncoplastic surgical planning; and (4) it can eliminate options for neoadjuvant treatment.

With percutaneous diagnosis, both palpable and nonpalpable benign lesions may be left in place if the pathology results fully explain the imaged findings. For patients with benign breast biopsy results, representing approximately 80% of breast biopsies, the percutaneous route avoids the expense, distress, and morbidity of an open operation. For the informed patient who requests that a mass with benign features be removed, percutaneous excisional biopsy is ideal as well.

The vast majority of breast cancers and benign breast lesions can be diagnosed accurately with percutaneous large-core needle biopsy.[2] Since the goal is diagnosis rather than therapy, surgeons performing image-guided biopsies usually leave most of the target lesion in place; any cancers found are later removed by lumpectomy. Percutaneous management of benign lesions (sampling or excisional biopsy) has several benefits. The patient is spared significant physical and emotional trauma as well as

considerable cost. In addition, precious operating room time is reserved for the patients who need it most, enhancing the efficient use of hospital facilities and improving the care of those patients. It is important to note that the efficiency of percutaneous diagnosis can be nullified by the subsequent open surgical removal of a benign lesion already diagnosed by image-guided core biopsy. In retrospect, the surgeon, the patient, and her health insurance provider regret that the lesion was not removed with excisional biopsy (percutaneous or open) in the first place.

CONCORDANCE IS ESSENTIAL

In certain circumstances it is critically important to proceed with open excision after image-guided percutaneous biopsy yields benign findings. The most common and the most important reason that benign lesions are removed after percutaneous core biopsy is a lack of concordance between breast imaging findings and the histopathology report. To avoid excision, the surgeon must be satisfied that the findings reported by the pathologist fully explain those on mammographic, sonographic, and physical examination. This rule should be followed without exception to avoid a false-negative result, since a missed diagnosis of breast cancer is unacceptable. In many cases, the experienced breast surgeon can weigh the pathologic findings in light of imaging results on mammography and sonography and determine whether they agree. Any doubt should spur a discussion with the pathologist, the consulting radiologist, or both until a firm conclusion has been reached. Holding clinical–pathologic correlation conferences at regular intervals improves safety and the efficiency of care in any breast care program.

For example, on occasion the surgeon may be surprised to hear from the pathologist that a discrete lesion seen on ultrasound of the breast can be fully accounted for by some form of benign sclerosing adenosis. In other cases, the pathologist will doubt the ability of the histologic findings to explain the imaged abnormality. In the latter case, the lesion must either be excised or an attempt can be made at percutaneous biopsy again to obtain concordant results. Thus the surgeon must work cooperatively with the pathologist and radiologist to prevent false-negative findings in a variety of situations involving a lack of concordance.

CLINICAL CONSIDERATIONS AND DIAGNOSTIC TECHNIQUE

While available technology permits almost all lesions to be adequately sampled, and many selected lesions to be removed (by percutaneous excisional biopsy), the surgeon must select the most appropriate instrumentation and biopsy type for each case. Sampling biopsy is ideal for suspicious lesions that are large enough to be targeted with certainty. The residual imaged signature of the lesion can then be used to precisely guide the ultimate removal of a malignant process with intraoperative ultrasound or mammographic needle localization.

Although traditional 14-gauge devices can be used to achieve accurate histologic diagnosis, radiologists, surgeons, pathologists, and oncologists agree that more substantial specimens obtained with the larger, vacuum-assisted/rotational core devices offer advantages. In the first place, upgrades in diagnosis (from atypical hyperplasia to cancer or from ductal carcinoma in situ [DCIS] to invasive cancer) and discordance between imaging and histology are reduced when more tissue is obtained at image-guided core biopsy.[2,3] Furthermore, in the modern era, much depends on accurate biological characterization of the individual breast cancer, including hormone receptor status, genomic profile, and protein expression. The initial tissue sampling event can provide the best opportunity to obtain this key biological information for 2 reasons: first, tissue preservation can be optimized; and second, in selected cases neoadjuvant treatment permits alterations in tumor size and biology to guide further treatment and to help the surgeon predict outcome.

The choice of device is also important when percutaneous excisional biopsy is planned. Devices that remove a very large single-core specimen are most suitable when pathologic examination of the entire intact lesion is desirable. Devices that permit the percutaneous multi-core excision of even larger lesions are ideal when the patient wants a larger lesion removed entirely even though the diagnosis is expected to be benign.

Lesions Visible on Mammography Only

Suspicious lesions (Breast Imaging-Reporting and Data System [BI-RADS] category 4 or 5)[4] that are visible only on mammography are best approached with stereotactic biopsy (Fig. 33-1). Clustered microcalcifications comprise the vast majority of these ultrasound-invisible lesions. Mass lesions and architectural distortions seen more clearly on mammography than on ultrasound also call for stereotactic biopsy.

Modern stereotactic biopsy technique employs the use of a directional vacuum-assisted/rotational core device such as the

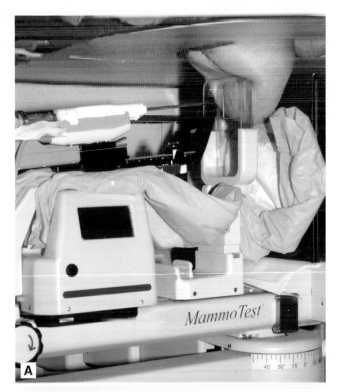

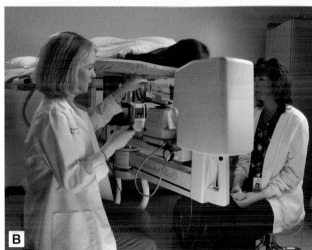

FIGURE 33-1 Modern stereotactic biopsy employs a hinged arm that allows images to be taken from −15 degrees and +15 degrees, producing a "stereo" pair of images. The platform provides a mount that will accommodate a broad variety of biopsy devices **(A)**. The prone position stabilizes the patient and is well tolerated **(B)**. *(Courtesy of SenoRx, Irvine, California [A], and Ethicon Endo-Surgery, Cincinnati, Ohio [B].)*

Mammotome Breast Biopsy System (Ethicon Endo-Surgery, Cincinnati, Ohio), the Automated Tissue Excision and Collection (ATEC) Breast Biopsy and Excision System (Suros Surgical Systems, Indianapolis, Indiana), or a large single-core device such as the Site Select Stereotactic Breast Biopsy System (Site Select Medical Technologies, Pharr, Texas; Fig. 33-2), the Intact Breast Biopsy System (Intact Medical Corporation, Natick, Massachusetts; Fig. 33-3), or the Halo Breast Biopsy

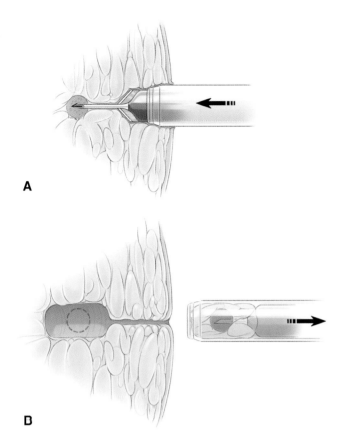

FIGURE 33-2 A flat blade at the tip of the Site Select allows the operator to advance the device to the target without removing intervening tissue. The coring cylinder is then advanced to capture the targeted lesion. *(Main photograph and drawing from which inset was adapted courtesy of Site Select Medical Technologies, Pharr, Texas.)*

Device (Rubicor Medical, Redwood City, California; Fig. 33-4). Understanding similarities and differences in available technology enables the surgeon to select the most appropriate device and application.

Confirming the Diagnosis

Concordance confirmation for stereotactic biopsy of calcifications is straightforward and rests on three key safeguards. First, specimen x-ray of the core samples must show the targeted calcifications convincingly. Next, the image of the biopsy site must demonstrate the removal of a representative portion of the target calcifications. Finally, the pathology report must note the presence of calcifications in the processed tissue; if not, recuts should be requested. Occasionally the target calcifications are composed of calcium oxalate, which can be seen only under polarized light.

Mass Lesions and Architectural Distortions

When stereotactic biopsy is used for mass lesions or architectural distortions, the surgeon must take greater care than usual to ensure that the targeted lesion is adequately represented in the core samples. Specimen x-rays are usually less helpful in such cases. Careful comparison of prebiopsy and postbiopsy mammograms, however, will confirm that a representative portion of the lesion has been sampled. Discussion with the pathologist and radiologist further establishes concordance. If doubt persists, excision is the rule.

LESIONS VISIBLE ON ULTRASOUND

When a lesion is seen clearly on ultrasound, most surgeons with the requisite skills prefer to use ultrasound guidance for sampling.

Advantages of Ultrasound Guidance

At least 2 advantages pertain to ultrasound guidance over the stereotactic approach. First, the patient is more comfortable supine than in the prone compression required for stereotactic guidance. Second, sonography is more likely than stereotactic equipment to be available in the surgeon's clinic. Using the equipment at hand minimizes expense, scheduling delays, and patient inconvenience.

IMAGE EVALUATION

Benign solid lesions tend to have characteristic features on ultrasound evaluation. Analyzing these features affords the surgeon an opportunity to determine whether the pathologic findings are in accord with the imaging features. This analysis is not intended to help determine whether to biopsy a BI-RADS 4 or 5 lesion; biopsy for such lesions is indicated by definition.

The 4 fundamental features that contribute to the reliable analysis of most lesions are the margins, internal echo pattern, shadowing, and height versus width of the mass (Table 33-1). Smooth, well-defined margins suggest that a lesion is benign, whereas irregular, vague margins suggest malignancy. A homogeneous internal echo pattern implies a benign diagnosis, while internal heterogeneity is seen in most cancers. Bilateral corner shadows are consistent with a smooth-walled benign lesion; any other shadow pattern is suspicious. Enhanced transmission of sound through the lesion (causing a brighter echo pattern beneath the lesion than in adjacent tissue) is relatively reassuring, since it results from homogeneous tissue within the mass. Finally, benign lesions tend to be wider than they are tall (width greater than anteroposterior diameter). In contrast, cancers tend to violate the natural tissue planes and to grow taller than they are wide.

By understanding and integrating these features, the surgeon can anticipate the histologic findings that adequate lesion sampling will provide. Any discordance between image analysis and pathologic findings requires excision of the mass.

TECHNICAL CONSIDERATIONS

Breast ultrasound requires the use of a transducer of 7.5 MHz or greater. Although a full description of diagnostic ultrasound techniques is beyond the scope of this chapter, 4 fundamental

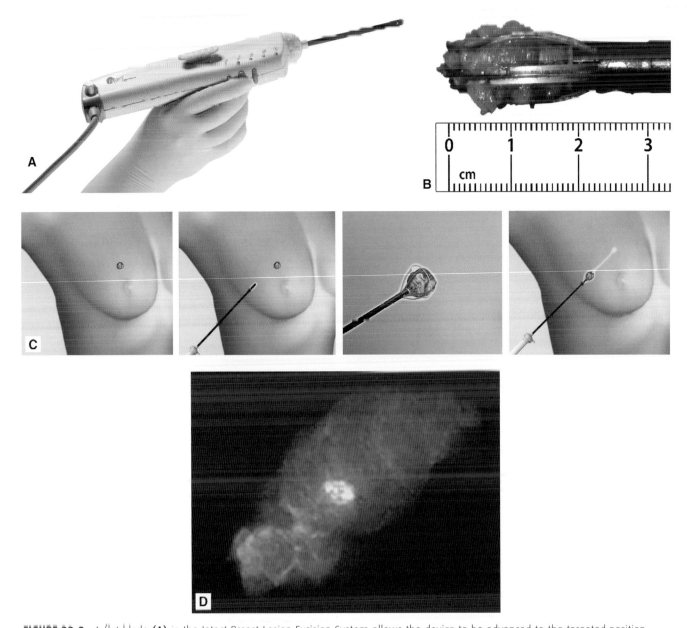

FIGURE 33-3 A flat blade **(A)** in the Intact Breast Lesion Excision System allows the device to be advanced to the targeted position, where the capture basket **(B)** is deployed, cutting through tissue with radiofrequency current **(C)**. The mammograph **(D)** reveals the target lesion within the specimen. *(Courtesy of Intact Medical Corporation, Natick, Massachusetts.)*

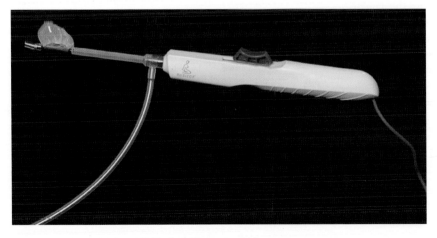

FIGURE 33-4 The Halo device is placed under the lesion. The collection pouch is deployed with radiofrequency current. The device is rotated manually to capture the lesion within the pouch. *(Courtesy of Rubicor Medical, Inc., Redwood City, California.)*

TABLE 33-1 Ultrasound Lesion Analysis—Key Features

Characteristic	Likely Diagnosis	
	Benign	Malignant
Margins	Smooth, well defined	Irregular, vague margins
Internal echo pattern	Homogeneous	Heterogeneous
Shadowing	Bilateral	Nonbilateral
Sound transmission through lesion	Enhanced	Attenuated
Proportion of width to anteroposterior diameter	Greater	Less

targeting techniques deserve mention: "skiing," "painting," transducer–device alignment, and confirmation scanning.

With the lesion in view, the surgeon, sliding the transducer footplate in line with its long axis, performs the "skiing" motion, which moves the image of the lesion from side to side on the monitor (Fig. 33-5). This motion allows the surgeon to place the lesion image in an area of the screen that will be optimal for biopsy access. The "painting" motion, in which the transducer footplate is moved perpendicular to its long axis, brings the lesion into and out of view at a given position on the monitor, permitting the lesion's widest portion to be targeted for the best sample (Fig. 33-6).

The most common error made by surgeons who are gaining skill in ultrasound device guidance is failure to align the device with the transducer (Fig. 33-7). Small alignment deviations result in failure to visualize the tip of the device and to be able to anticipate the trajectory of the advancing tip. Frequent direct visual checks of device–transducer alignment will help to prevent this dangerous situation. Further alignment is required if the full length of the device is not well seen.

Once proper alignment with the widest portion of the lesion has been achieved and the device has advanced, the surgeon confirms that the device is in its target location, inside the lesion (Fig. 33-8), or under the lesion for percutaneous excisional biopsy with a vacuum-assisted/rotational core biopsy device. First the device is seen traversing the lesion. The transducer is then "painted" a short distance to one side to permit visualization of the lesion on that side of the device, so that the device disappears but the lesion is still seen.

Next, the transducer is painted back across the device so that it first briefly reimages the device within the lesion and then shows the lesion alone on the other side of the device. Seeing the lesion on both sides of the device confirms that the device is inside the lesion and rules out the "image averaging" artifact that can occur when the device is immediately adjacent to the lesion. Finally, the surgeon can obtain further confirmation by turning the transducer perpendicular to the device and imaging a cross-section of the device within the lesion. With this orientation, the device appears as a small bright dot within the mass.

TECHNIQUES

The surgeon who has acquired the fundamental analytical and hands-on skills described above may choose from a number of technical options.

Fine-Needle Aspiration

The accurate diagnosis of benign and malignant primary breast lesions with fine-needle aspiration (FNA) has been reported.[5-7] Unfortunately, even in the hands of a surgeon with specialized experience and profound expertise, in general FNA yields

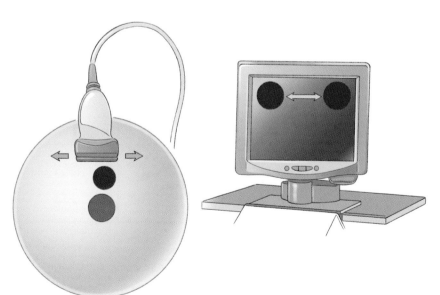

FIGURE 33-5 "Skiing" mode: The ultrasound transducer is moved in line with the long axis of the footplate. The operator may position the image of the lesion anywhere on the screen from left to right at a fixed depth.

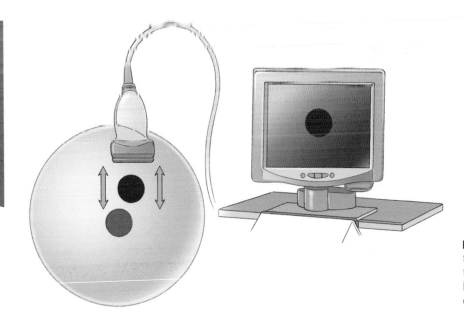

FIGURE 33-6 "Painting" mode: The operator moves the transducer perpendicular to the long axis of the footplate, bringing the lesion in and out of view at a fixed location on the screen.

higher false-negative primary breast cancer diagnosis rates compared to those obtained with core biopsy. Centers whose staff have extensive experience and documented accuracy may employ FNA with outstanding results. In contrast to its great value in ultrasound-guided axillary lymph node biopsy (see Chapter 34), however, FNA cannot be recommended for general use with primary breast lesions when the possible diagnoses include breast cancer.

Under restricted circumstances, palpation-guided FNA can provide reassurance or guidance when used as part of a modified negative triple test. This modified version of the negative triple test holds that the chance of malignancy is exceedingly low under 3 simultaneous circumstances: (1) the area of thickening is not a discrete 3-dimensional mass on clinical examination;

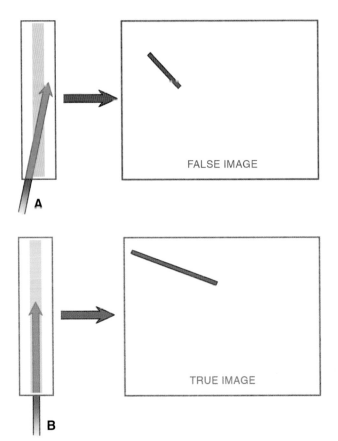

FIGURE 33-7 Misalignment of the length of the biopsy device with the long axis of the transducer, the most common error made by physicians performing ultrasound-guided biopsy, produces a misleading image **(A)**, making control of the sharp tip of the device impossible. In contrast, proper (parallel) alignment of the beam **(B)** produces a true image of the full length of the biopsy device, including the sharp tip.

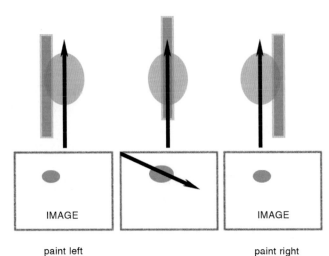

FIGURE 33-8 In a confirmation scan, the operator visualizes the lesion on both sides of the biopsy device by "painting" the transducer a short distance on either side (see Fig. 33-6).

(2) no lesion is seen on imaging studies; and (3) the FNA result is benign—that is, benign epithelial cells are found, or adipose tissue is found when lipoma was suspected.

Core Biopsy

Image-guided core biopsy represents the state of the art for the diagnosis of both benign and malignant breast lesions, whether the mass is palpable or nonpalpable.

Indications: Palpable Masses

A diagnosis of cancer obtained by palpation-guided core biopsy can be trusted; however, a benign diagnosis obtained with palpation-guided biopsy is less reliable. For this reason the American Society of Breast Surgeons published the following Position Statement on Image-Guided Percutaneous Biopsy of Palpable Breast Lesions, defining "percutaneous" as "needle core biopsy with Tru-cut [sic] style devices or vacuum-assisted or rotating cutter type devices introduced through a small cutaneous incision" (January 29, 2001)[8]:

> Image-guidance is an extremely useful adjunct in the performance of percutaneous biopsy of palpable breast lesions. Image-guidance confirms the proper placement of the biopsy device into the lesion (when core needle device is used), or immediately below the lesion (when vacuum-assisted device is used). Performing percutaneous breast biopsy procedures without the use of image-guidance may lead to false negative results since the biopsy device cannot be confirmed to be in the proper position to obtain tissue from the suspect mass. In most, if not all instances of image-guided biopsy of palpable breast lesions, ultrasound is the preferred image-guidance modality.

In many deeply placed, palpable tumors, the location of the margin of the lesion is not discernible (Fig. 33-9). In such cases, the biopsy needle inserted without ultrasound guidance may easily be misdirected into the compressed adjacent tissue.

Devices

Percutaneous biopsy devices are available in 2 forms: (1) devices that remove multiple cores through a very small incision and (2) those that remove a single large block of tissue through an incision that is slightly larger, but small compared with incisions used for open excision. Each approach has advantages and drawbacks.

14-Gauge Spring-Loaded Core Biopsy Needle

The 14-gauge spring-loaded core biopsy needle (Fig. 33-10) has been the mainstay of ultrasound-guided biopsy of solid lesions at most centers since the mid-1990s. This device remains the most commonly used type for ultrasound-guided core sampling. Devices with smaller gauges were often adequate in the initial series reported by Parker and associates.[9] However, because a few false-negative results occurred when smaller needles were used, Parker's group recommended 14-gauge core sampling.

Ultrasound-guided 14-gauge core biopsy is tried and true. It is adequate in most circumstances. Nevertheless, newer devices offer certain advantages (outlined above under "Clinical

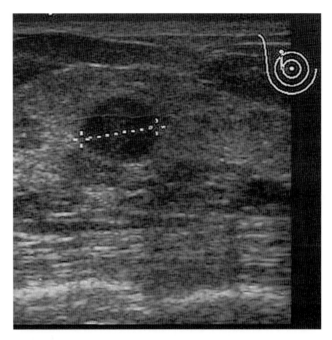

FIGURE 33-9 Compression of surrounding parenchyma by an expanding lesion produces a palpable mass larger than the lesion. In such circumstances, palpation is not a reliable guide to ensure accurate sampling. *(Reproduced with permission from Whitworth PW. Percutaneous biopsy of benign breast masses. Prob Gen Surg 2003;20:71.)*

Considerations and Diagnostic Technique") over this cornerstone technique.

Vacuum-Assisted and Rotational Core Biopsy Devices

These are available in 2 forms: those that remove multiple cores and those that remove a single larger core of tissue.

Devices That Remove Multiple Cores Per Pass. This category includes a number of vacuum-assisted/rotational core directional core biopsy devices. Those most commonly used are the Mammotome, ATEC, and EnCor. Others are discussed as well.

The advent of the Mammotome (Fig. 33-11) indisputably represented an advance in the technology for stereotactic biopsy of microcalcifications. The surgeon can overcome small targeting deviations by directing the biopsy aperture, which may be rotated 360 degrees, toward the lesion as seen on postplacement stereotactic images. Samples obtained with the standard 11-gauge Mammotome are considerably larger than those obtained via the ordinary 14-gauge needle used without vacuum assistance.

Perhaps the greatest advantage of the Mammotome is its ability to collect multiple samples with a single placement of the probe. In contrast, a one-core-per-pass needle used for stereobiopsy of microcalcifications must be placed, fired, removed, and replaced for each of 10 to 20 cores obtained. As a result, procedure time, patient discomfort, and targeting difficulty are increased.

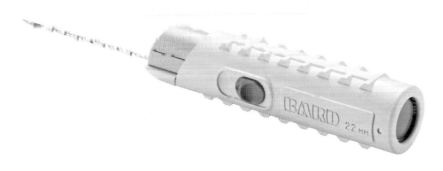

FIGURE 33-10 Many different manufacturers provide a wide variety of spring-loaded 14-gauge core biopsy devices. Among the most commonly used is the MaxCore, Bard Biopsy Systems. *(Courtesy of Bard Biopsy Systems, Tempe, Arizona.)*

Three newer vacuum-assisted/rotational core devices (Fig. 33-12) offer the same advantages as the Mammotome. The ATEC, pneumatically driven and lightweight, obtains cores faster than the Mammotome and collects them in a closed chamber. The EnCor (SenoRx, Irvine, California) offers 10- and 7-gauge versions, the latter is the largest currently available in this category. The Flash (Rubicor) offers these features in a self-contained disposable unit requiring no capital cost. All three employ a closed collection chamber.

The Mammotome, ATEC, EnCor, and Flash are capable of removing all imaged evidence of an entire lesion (percutaneous excisional biopsy), such as a benign fibroadenoma (see further discussion below). In addition, all 9 devices are available in handheld versions for ultrasound-guided procedures and in versions that are compatible with MRI-guided biopsy.

The larger core samples obtained with vacuum-assisted and rotational core devices afford more extensive pathologic and biologic analysis than the 14-gauge spring-loaded needle simply in collecting more tissue for the pathologist's review. Authors who studied the use of multiple devices in large series (14-gauge

spring-loaded needle, Mammotome, and others) have shown that use of the vacuum-assisted larger gauge devices reduces the upgrade rate from atypical ductal hyperplasia (ADH) on core biopsy to DCIS or infiltrating carcinoma (IC), or from DCIS to IC, on excision.[2,10] As discussed, another clear advantage of improved pretreatment characterization (receptor status, genomic and proteomic analysis) of breast lesions obtains in the case of locally advanced breast cancers destined for preoperative chemotherapy.

Other currently available devices designed to remove larger core samples (Fig. 33-13) include the Cassi Rotational Core Biopsy System (Sanarus Medical, Pleasanton, California), EnCor 360 (formerly the SenoCor 360; SenoRx), and Celero (Hologic, Bedford, Massachusetts) spring-loaded handheld breast biopsy devices and the Vacora Breast Biopsy System (Bard Biopsy Systems, Tempe, Arizona). These devices require less capital expense for the practicing surgeon than the Mammotome, ATEC, or EnCor while providing the diagnostic advantage of being able to capture larger tissue specimens. They require reinsertion for each core sample, however, and do not generally provide percutaneous excisional capability. Device technology can be expected to advance, serving the needs and intentions of the patient and surgeon more completely.

Devices That Remove a Single Large Block of Tissue.
Three devices now on the market were designed to remove a single large block of tissue: the Site Select Stereotactic Breast Biopsy System (Site Select; Fig. 33-2), the Intact Breast Biopsy System (Intact Medical; Fig. 33-3), and the Halo Breast Biopsy Device (Rubicor; Fig. 33-4). The main advantage of these devices is that they make it possible to excise a single larger sample of intact tissue than with the other vacuum-assisted devices described above. This capability provides maximal diagnostic certainty and may prove particularly helpful in removing such challenging lesions as radial scar and ADH.

Site Select is available in 10- to 22-mm probes; Intact, in 10- to 30-mm probes; and Halo, in 15- to 20-mm probes. The larger versions may permit the complete removal of a small intact lesion (see the next section, "Percutaneous Excisional Biopsy").

Data are limited regarding outcomes when these devices are used with the goal of complete removal of imaged evidence of the lesion. More information is available concerning lesion removal in series whose primary goal was accurate diagnosis.[11-13] Trials under way at the time of writing, in late 2008, were based on small, successful pilot studies[14,15] evaluating the Intact device for definitive removal of lesions containing atypical ductal hyperplasia and small cancers

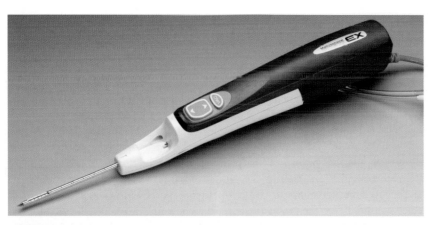

FIGURE 33-11 The Mammotome device is available in 11 gauge, best suited to focused sampling, and 8 gauge, best suited to wider tissue removal. *(Courtesy of Ethicon Endo-Surgery, Cincinnati, Ohio.)*

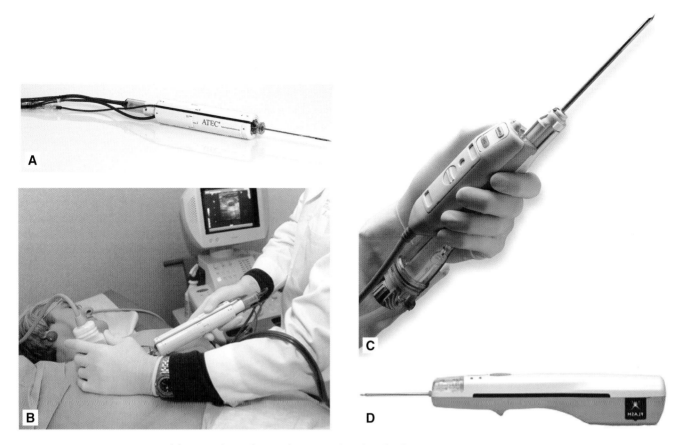

FIGURE 33-12 Vacuum-assisted/rotational core biopsy devices with a closed collection chamber and many of the advantages of the Mammotome include **(A,B)** the ATEC, **(C)** EnCor, and **(D)** Flash. All are available in handheld versions for ultrasound-guided procedures and in styles that are compatible with MRI-guided biopsy. *(Courtesy of Hologic, Bedford, Massachusetts. **[A,B]**; SenoRx, Irvine, California **[C]**; and Rubicor Medical, Redwood City, California **[D]**.)*

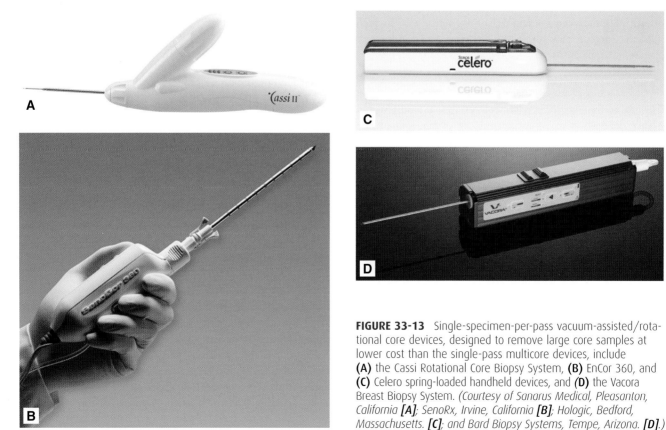

FIGURE 33-13 Single-specimen-per-pass vacuum-assisted/rotational core devices, designed to remove large core samples at lower cost than the single-pass multicore devices, include **(A)** the Cassi Rotational Core Biopsy System, **(B)** EnCor 360, and **(C)** Celero spring-loaded handheld devices, and **(D)** the Vacora Breast Biopsy System. *(Courtesy of Sanarus Medical, Pleasanton, California **[A]**; SenoRx, Irvine, California **[B]**; Hologic, Bedford, Massachusetts. **[C]**; and Bard Biopsy Systems, Tempe, Arizona. **[D]**.)*

(see "Future Directions, Desirable Studies" at the end of this chapter).

Percutaneous Excisional Biopsy

Historically, excisional biopsy (CPT code 19120)[16] has been defined as the removal of a palpable mass; in contrast, incisional biopsy consists of the removal of a portion of a palpable mass. Discrimination between excisional and incisional is based on palpation, not on histology. Since the advent of screening mammography, excisional biopsy has also referred to the removal of a nonpalpable imaged lesion, usually with needle localization (CPT code 19125),[16] based on imaged findings. Similarly, image-guided percutaneous excisional biopsy is defined as the removal of the imaged evidence of the lesion by means of a percutaneous approach. In late 2008, percutaneous excisional biopsy and percutaneous sampling biopsy still used the same CPT code, 19103; revised coding is anticipated.

Indications

Percutaneous excisional biopsy makes sense when the surgeon knows in advance that a lesion with benign features is very likely to require removal. The most clear-cut case is that of a palpable mass that is bothersome to the patient. While surgeons tend to discourage patients from pursuing the excision of benign palpable fibroadenomas, most respect the patient's wishes if she is well informed and understands the benign nature of the lesion.

Another common reason for excisional biopsy of a benign lesion is diagnostic uncertainty, such as with suspected papilloma. When papilloma is diagnosed via sampling biopsy, further excision is recommended to rule out atypia or malignancy. Considerable clinical experience and judgment may be required to anticipate the need for removal of a given lesion; in such cases, the surgeon may regain the efficiency and kindness of image-guided diagnosis via percutaneous excisional biopsy.

Devices

The ideal technology for percutaneous excisional biopsy would balance the need to maximize the amount of removable tissue while minimizing the incision required to do so. Several innovative devices were designed in an attempt to solve this problem in different ways. Many such devices are still in clinical trials; several are available now. Once data exist to aid the surgeon in proper patient selection and to establish levels of efficacy and patient acceptance, complication rates, and device reliability, percutaneous excisional biopsy will begin to replace open excisional biopsy in routine practice.

Clinical trial results addressing these important parameters have begun to be reported for individual devices. As of late 2008, however, no comparative studies had been carried out. This chapter will review the currently available technologies and the clinical results reported for each. Finally, the chapter will consider recommendations for current practice and anticipate future developments.

Tumor Types

Prior to biopsy, the surgeon employs careful, informed image analysis (usually involving ultrasound and/or mammogram) to anticipate the most likely diagnosis. As discussed above, the most important reason to analyze imaged features of the lesion with care before biopsy is to specify a list of potentially likely lesions — that is, explanations satisfying the concordance rule, which states that histologic findings must fully explain the image abnormality. With these possibilities in mind, the surgeon can select the device (multi-core versus larger single core) and technique (sampling versus excision) that best suit the situation.

Benign Tumors. Except when the surgeon wishes to remove the lesion as an intact specimen (see "Intact Benign Lesions," the next section), the Mammotome, ATEC, and EnCor combine the features ideal for allowing maximal tissue removal through the smallest possible incision. Because these devices are designed to remove multiple cores in a given procedure, the size of the resulting biopsy cavity is limited only by the mechanical properties of the patient's breast. Thus a sizable tissue sample may be obtained through a diminutive incision (about 4-6 mm in length) that requires no sutures.

The Mammotome is the current benchmark for image-guided percutaneous tissue excision. A wealth of data are available regarding clinical outcomes after use of the Mammotome in the diagnostic setting.[2,17,18] Results have also been reported for clinical trials in which the researchers evaluated outcomes of procedures performed with the goal of removing the lesion.

In the first of these trials, Fine and associates attempted excision of 50 lesions (using stereotactic guidance for 38 and ultrasound for 12) in 45 patients.[19] After twelve to sixteen 11-gauge core samples had been taken from each lesion, 45 (90%) of the lesions were judged, immediately after the procedure, to have been percutaneously excised. Of those 45 lesions, 41 (90%) showed no evidence of residual abnormality on mammogram or ultrasound scan at 6-month follow-up.

The second trial evaluating outcomes after lesion removal was a multi-institutional investigation of ultrasound-guided 11- and 8-gauge Mammotome excision of palpable masses under 15 mm and 15 to 30 mm, respectively.[20] Biopsies were performed in 127 patients with the 8-gauge probe; the 11-gauge probe was used in 89 patients. At 6-month follow-up, 98% of the lesions remained nonpalpable, including 73% with no ultrasound-visible abnormality at the biopsy site. Though some imaged abnormality would be expected in a proportion of patients after open excisional biopsy, no directly comparable data regarding imaging findings after open biopsy are available.

Complications were mild and anticipated. Most patients (98%) were satisfied with incision appearance; 92% of patients said they would recommend the procedure to others.

Intact Benign Lesions. When diagnostic uncertainty indicates removal of the lesion, as is the case with radial scars and papillomas, current practice usually requires open excisional biopsy. Now that devices such as the Site Select, Intact, and Halo are available, surgeons and their patients have another option in selected cases. In particular, when the pathologist confirms that the entire lesion has been removed intact, it makes no difference which technology was used to accomplish the excision. In such cases, these newer image-guided approaches are superior to old-fashioned wire localization because of the precise targeting and tissue conservation they provide as well as the cost saving obtained by avoiding operating room charges.

Special Benign Lesions. The management of 6 types of benign lesion—stromal fibrosis, papilloma, pseudoangiomatous stromal hyperplasia, radial scar, ADH, and atypical lobular hyperplasia—deserves special comment.

Stromal fibrosis may or may not account for a given 3-dimensional lesion seen on ultrasound examination. This is the paradigmatic example of necessity for communication between surgeon and pathologist. Sometimes this communication will occur via a high-quality pathology report that comments on possible concordance with ultrasound or mammographic findings, often as a result of clinical information provided to the pathologist. In many other cases the matter of concordance between an imaged mass and a pathology report of stromal fibrosis will be settled by a simple phone call to the pathologist. The breast surgeon should know this phone number by heart.

Papillary lesions often cause concern because of their potential for malignant transformation. In a large series reported by Rosen and associates,[21] image-guided core biopsy provided reliable, accurate diagnosis for selected papillary lesions. Excision of lesions associated with atypia, or when recommended by the pathologist, identified all malignant papillary lesions. Follow-up without open excision provided safe management when the diagnosis on core biopsy was benign. The authors recommend extensive sampling of such lesions. Use of a device that provides larger cores is advantageous for papillary lesions. Percutaneous excisional (removal of all imaged evidence) biopsy is ideal.

Although pseudoangiomatous stromal hyperplasia (PASH) can be found in microscopic form in up to 25% of breast biopsies,[22] this is a relatively unusual and benign finding in reported image-guided biopsy series.[23] Unless PASH presents as an enlarging mass, it may be safely managed with follow-up imaging.

Radial scar, originally a large, mammographically defined abnormality, is considered a high-risk lesion[24] because it must be examined intact to be safely distinguished from low-grade carcinoma. Some programs mandate open excision for all such cases, whether defined mammographically or histologically. However, if the pathologist can confidently state that a small, histologically defined lesion has been completely removed intact, whether by a vacuum-assisted device, by a rotational core device that removes an intact block of tissue, or by open excision, this concern is safely put to rest.

Because ADH cannot reliably be distinguished from low-grade DCIS on core biopsy and because of its frequent association with DCIS, it must be removed as an intact specimen. As discussed above, small foci of ADH might be safely evaluated, in selected cases by targeted reexcision with one of the devices that removes a large, intact single-core specimen. This approach is the subject of the Intact Percutaneous Excision Trial (I-PET; Intact Medical), wherein blinded pathology and radiologic review are carried out to determine whether outcome on open excision can be predicted with certainty. In a retrospective series of patients who underwent ultrasound-guided percutaneous biopsies, the upgrade rate from ADH to carcinoma was reduced to zero with percutaneous excisional biopsy.[10] If confirmatory

studies such as I-PET should define reproducible clinical and pathologic criteria for definitive diagnosis of ADH, pathologic confirmation of percutaneous removal may save the patient and her surgeon an unnecessary trip to the operating room.

Reports in the radiology and surgery literature in the early 2000s altered the management of atypical lobular hyperplasia (ALH).[25] Long considered a marker of elevated risk for the development of breast cancer,[26] lobular neoplasia has been reported in association with DCIS or carcinoma with increasing frequency.[27-29] For this reason, a finding of ALH on core biopsy should usually lead to excision of an intact specimen containing the core biopsy site (excisional biopsy). Clinical judgment may affirm concordance between a benign lesion seen on pathology and the imaged abnormality in certain cases. Perfect concordance in such a case may allow safe selection of a patient with incidental ALH for follow-up and risk counseling. However, such decisions should be individualized in light of contemporary and future reports.

FUTURE DIRECTIONS, DESIRABLE STUDIES

Currently the majority of image-guided biopsies yield benign results. A number of new imaging technologies are under active investigation to reduce the number of "false-positive" imaging studies (those that lead to benign biopsy); examples include computed tomographic laser mammography and computed breast impedance measurements. Other studies employ breast MRI with the same goal.[30] So far none have shown an ability to identify conventional BI-RADS 4 or 5 patients who do not require biopsy. Tremendous cost savings and kinder patient management will be possible if the promise of these investigations is fulfilled.

Clinical decision-making based on image-guided core biopsy will continue to evolve. Currently, most biopsies yielding "high-risk" findings such as atypical hyperplasia or lobular neoplasia lead to a costly second procedure, such as open surgical biopsy. Though the vast majority of these second procedures demonstrate benign findings, they are required because a significant minority (10%-20%) will be associated with malignant findings on open excision of the biopsy site. This current practice is based on extensive retrospective studies.

Those studies are limited because the key parameters that might support accurate patient selection for surveillance or resection cannot be controlled retrospectively. Therefore, the most pressing need is for prospective studies that control lesion characteristics, device selection, extent of biopsy, and radiologic and pathologic parameters to precisely identify which combinations warrant further tissue removal and which support surveillance alone. The I-PET study[10] is among the first of the many prospective studies needed to define clinical, procedural, radiologic, and pathologic criteria that will allow clinicians to identify more accurately which patients need a second procedure.

Advances in percutaneous biopsy set the stage for more ambitious percutaneous intervention. Percutaneous treatment of breast cancer is one of the most enthusiastically anticipated surgical advances at the beginning of the 21st century. The National Cancer Institute–funded Z1072 trial from the American College of Surgeons Oncology Group, evaluating the management of small breast cancers with percutaneous cryoablation, opened in late 2008. The Evaluation of Margin Assessment Trial (EMAT), begun in early 2009, investigates the percutaneous removal of small breast cancers using the large version of the Intact device described earlier. More such investigations with devices in the large, intact sample category are expected.

SUMMARY

Ideal management of breast lesions now usually begins with image-guided percutaneous biopsy. For sonographically visible lesions, ultrasound-guided biopsy is preferred because it costs less, can be accomplished in less time than mammographically guided biopsy, and grants more comfort to patients. For lesions that are not visible on ultrasound, mammographically guided stereotactic biopsy must be used.

Benign lesions, whether palpable or not, may be left alone if the pathologic evaluation is concordant with the imaged abnormality. If the informed patient still desires excision of a mass with benign features, percutaneous excisional biopsy is often preferable. Any question of concordance between imaged abnormality and pathology findings must be settled by a discussion with the pathologist or excisional biopsy.

Device technology can be expected to advance, serving the needs and intentions of the patient and surgeon more completely.

ACKNOWLEDGMENT

The author thanks Marcia Ringel for her editorial support.

REFERENCES

1. Silverstein MJ, Lagios MD, Recht A, et al. Image-detected breast cancer: state of the art diagnosis and treatment. *J Am Coll Surg.* 2005;201:586-597.
2. Meyer JE, Smith DN, Lester SC, et al. Large-core needle biopsy of nonpalpable breast lesions. *JAMA.* 1999;281:1638-1641.
3. Liberman L, Kaplan JB, Morris EA, et al. To excise or to sample the mammographic target: what is the goal of stereotactic 11-gauge vacuum-assisted breast biopsy? *AJR Am J Roentgenol.* 2002;179:679-683.
4. American College of Radiology. *Breast Imaging Reporting and Data System (BI-RADS).* 3rd ed. Reston, VA: American College of Radiology; 1998.
5. Ariga R, Bloom K, Reddy VB, et al. Fine-needle aspiration of clinically suspicious palpable breast masses with histopathologic correlation. *Am J Surg.* 2002;184:410-413.
6. Litherland JC. Should fine needle aspiration cytology in breast assessment be abandoned? *Clin Radiol.* 2002;57:81-84.
7. Ljung BM, Drejet A, Chiampi N, et al. Diagnostic accuracy of fine-needle aspiration biopsy is determined by physician training in sampling technique. *Cancer.* 2001;93:263-268.
8. American Society of Breast Surgeons. Position Statement on Image-Guided Percutaneous Biopsy of Palpable Breast Lesions. January 29, 2001. Available at: http://breastsurgeons.org/officialstmts/image-guided_perc _biopsy.html/. Accessed December 5, 2008.
9. Parker SH, John WE, Dennis MA, et al. US-guided automated large-core breast biopsy. *Radiology.* 1993;187:507-511.
10. Grady I, Gorsuch H, Wilburn-Bailey S. Ultrasound-guided, vacuum-assisted, percutaneous excision of breast lesions: an accurate technique in the diagnosis of atypical ductal hyperplasia. *J Am Coll Surg.* 2005;201:14-17.
11. Schwartzberg BS, Goates JJ, Kelley WE. Minimal access breast surgery. *Surg Clin North Am.* 2000;80:1383-1398.
12. Schwartzberg BS, Goates JJ, Keeler SA, Moore JA. Use of advanced breast biopsy instrumentation while performing stereotactic breast biopsies: review of 150 consecutive biopsies. *J Am Coll Surg.* 2000;191:9-15.
13. Velanovich V, Lewis FR Jr., Nathanson SD, et al. Comparison of mammographically guided breast biopsy techniques. *Ann Surg.* 1999;229:625-630; discussion 630-633.
14. Killebrew LK, Oneson RH. Comparison of the diagnostic accuracy of a vacuum-assisted percutaneous intact specimen sampling device to a vacuum-assisted core needle sampling device for breast biopsy: initial experience. *Breast J.* 2006;12:302-308.
15. Sie A, Bryan DC, Gaines V, et al. Multicenter evaluation of the breast lesion excision system, a percutaneous, vacuum-assisted, intact-specimen breast biopsy device. *Cancer.* 2006;107:945-949.
16. American Medical Association. *CPT 2008 Standard Edition.* Chicago, IL: American Medical Association; 2008.
17. Fine R, Boyd BA, Whitworth PW, et al. Percutaneous removal of benign breast masses using a vacuum-assisted hand-held device with ultrasound guidance. *Am J Surg.* 2002;184:332-336.
18. Burbank F, Parker SH, Fogarty TJ. Stereotactic breast biopsy: improved tissue harvesting with the Mammotome. *Am Surg.* 1996;62:738-744.
19. Fine RE, Israel PZ, Walker LC, et al. A prospective study of the removal rate of imaged breast lesions by an 11-gauge vacuum-assisted biopsy probe system. *Am J Surg.* 2001;182:335-340.
20. Fine RE, Whitworth PW, Kim JA, et al. Low-risk palpable breast masses removed using a vacuum-assisted hand-held device. *Am J Surg.* 2003;186:362-367.
21. Rosen EL, Bentley RC, Baker JA, Soo MS. Imaging-guided core needle biopsy of papillary lesions of the breast. *AJR Am J Roentgenol.* 2002;179:1185-1192.
22. Powell CM, Cranor ML, Rosen PP. Pseudoangiomatous stromal hyperplasia (PASH). A mammary stromal tumor with myofibroblastic differentiation. *Am J Surg Pathol.* 1995;19:270-277.
23. Schoonjans JM, Brem RF. Fourteen-gauge ultrasonographically guided large core needle biopsy of breast masses. *J Ultrasound Med.* 2001;20:967-972.
24. Philpotts LE, Hooley RJ, Lee CH. Comparison of automated versus vacuum-assisted biopsy methods for sonographically guided core biopsy of the breast. *AJR Am J Roentgenol.* 2003;180:347-351.
25. Dmytrasz K, Tartter PI, Mizrachy H, et al. The significance of atypical lobular hyperplasia at percutaneous breast biopsy. *Breast J.* 2003;9:10-12.
26. Page DL, Dupont WD, Rogers LW, Rados MS. Atypical hyperplastic lesions of the female breast. A long-term follow-up study. *Cancer.* 1985;55:2698-2708.
27. Cohen MA. Cancer upgrades at excisional biopsy after diagnosis of atypical lobular hyperplasia or lobular carcinoma in situ at core-needle biopsy: some reasons why. *Radiology.* 2004;231:617-621.
28. Brem RF, Lechner MC, Jackman RJ, et al. Lobular neoplasia at percutaneous breast biopsy: variables associated with carcinoma at surgical excision. *AJR Am J Roentgenol.* 2008;190:637-641.
29. Mahoney MC, Robinson-Smith TM, Shaughnessy EA. Lobular neoplasia at 11-gauge vacuum-assisted stereotactic biopsy: correlation with surgical excisional biopsy and mammographic follow-up. *AJR Am J Roentgenol.* 2006;187:949-954.
30. Bazzocchi M, Zuiani C, Panizza P, et al. Contrast enhanced breast MRI in patients with suspicious microcalcifications on mammography: results of a multicenter trial. *AJR Am J Roentgenol.* 2006;186:1723-1732.

CHAPTER 34

Ultrasound Evaluation of the Lymphatic Spread of Breast Cancer

Bruno D. Fornage

In patients with breast cancer, the presence of nodal metastases limits the therapeutic options and also indicates worse prognosis. When a potentially "early" curable cancer has been detected, the next most critical step is therefore to determine whether the nodal basins are involved as part of the staging process. The TNM classification system has been revised to better reflect the prognostic implications of the discovery of lymph node metastasis in the various nodal basins draining the cancer-containing breast.[1]

Ultrasound (US) is more sensitive than physical examination in the detection of axillary nodal metastases and can visualize high axillary, infraclavicular, and internal mammary lymphadenopathy that cannot be assessed with palpation and mammography.

GENERAL CONSIDERATIONS

A few points must be kept in mind when using imaging modalities in general and US in particular to detect lymph node metastases from breast cancer:

- With all recent imaging modalities, the criteria for the diagnosis of lymph node metastasis remain to be defined (and evaluated).
- There are multiple nodes in the axilla, and a one-to-one correlation between the nodes imaged in vivo and the nodes examined pathologically from the axillary node dissection surgical specimen is rarely—if ever—possible, which may lead to errors in the reporting of an imaging modality's diagnostic accuracy. A satisfactory solution would be to perform an image-guided needle biopsy of any abnormal node with placement of a metallic marker for subsequent identification during the pathologic examination of the surgical specimen from axillary node dissection.
- Imaging techniques that rely on blood perfusion cannot be used for ex vivo examination of surgical specimens from axillary node dissection.
- Currently, no imaging modality can detect micrometastases (< 2 mm in diameter), the significance of which remains controversial. Although micrometastases possibly affect long-term survival, there is debate about whether their presence should alter patient management.

A few common-sense tips are useful in the evaluation of nodal basins:

- Multiple mildly abnormal nodes in the same nodal basin are probably benign.
- If similar mildly abnormal nodes are found in the contralateral basin, then the indeterminate nodes in question are probably benign (with the exception of lymphoma or leukemia).
- If only one or a few nodes are abnormal and other adjacent nodes appear completely normal, then these nodes are suspicious for metastasis until proven otherwise, usually via US-guided fine-needle aspiration (FNA).

INSTRUMENTATION

Recent advances in US equipment used for small body parts include very-high-frequency and multiarray transducers that operate at peak frequencies of up to 17 MHz and provide exquisite spatial resolution. Such transducers allow visualization of lymph node metastases as small as a few millimeters.

Among recent image-processing techniques, real-time compound scanning, which was initially predicted to provide higher-quality images than those attainable with conventional

US, has not proved as beneficial as hoped. In fact, in our experience, the significant blurring associated with this technique has a negative effect on image quality.

Tissue harmonic imaging slightly increases spatial resolution and boosts contrast. In our experience, though, it does not provide any substantial benefit in the US evaluation of nodal metastases.

Three-dimensional US is still investigational and is not expected to provide a breakthrough in the evaluation of the nodal basins in the near future.[2] It might be helpful in facilitating the guidance of percutaneous needle biopsy.

Over the last decade, the sensitivity of power Doppler US (PDUS) systems has greatly increased, allowing not only detection of the mere presence of Doppler signals within a node but also detailed mapping of the normal versus disturbed nodal vascularity. This is expected to help differentiate between benign and malignant nodes.

Recently, elasticity imaging with US (elastography) has been reported as a promising adjunct imaging modality to conventional US.[3] When several elastography-capable scanners became available in our section 2 years ago, our expectations were that elastography might help discriminate between firm metastatic nodes and soft benign nodes. However, our hopes did not materialize and our preliminary experience of elastography of axillary nodes with current equipment has been disappointing. This issue should be reevaluated when more refined equipment is available.

EXAMINATION TECHNIQUE

Examination of the nodal basins is performed with the patient supine. The arm is elevated for examination of the axilla and brought back down for examination of the infraclavicular region, supraclavicular fossa, and low neck. Examination of the internal mammary nodes is done by scanning along the edge of the sternum. For the last 15 years at MD Anderson Cancer Center, we have included systematic examination of the ipsilateral axilla and internal mammary chains in the US breast examination of patients who have or have had breast cancer. If suspicious nodes are demonstrated, examination of the nodal basins is extended to include the supraclavicular fossa and the low neck.[4]

At the least doubt, examination of the contralateral nodal basin is performed. This usually (although not always) provides a reference for normality.

PDUS should be used in most cases to evaluate the internal vascularity of the nodes, especially when they are indeterminate on grayscale sonograms.

NORMAL ULTRASOUND ANATOMY

In normal adults, the axillary lymph nodes appear as ovoid or elongated (sometimes sausage-shaped) structures containing a large amount of fat, which is usually (but not always) echogenic (Fig. 34-1). PDUS shows harmonious vascular branching, which radiates from the hilum toward the periphery of the node.

During breast-feeding and for a few months afterward, axillary nodes become moderately swollen and hypoechoic. Such an appearance may be confusing and misinterpreted as suspicious

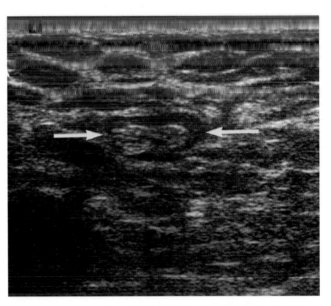

FIGURE 34-1 Sonogram shows a normal axillary node (*arrows*), which is nearly completely replaced by mildly echogenic fat.

for metastasis in a woman diagnosed with breast cancer postpartum.

A special mention must be given to intramammary nodes. They frequently appear on mammograms in the outer breast with a characteristic appearance. However, when they grow, a US examination may be required to confirm their benign nature. The demonstration of a small rounded structure with a central echogenic component and hilar vascularization on PDUS is pathognomonic of a benign intramammary node.

Normal internal mammary nodes are not usually visible on US, but tiny fat-containing oval nodes are occasionally seen in the supraclavicular fossa and, more commonly, in the low neck.

ULTRASOUND DIAGNOSIS OF LYMPH NODE METASTASES

The US diagnosis of a lymph node metastasis is based on the enlargement and/or focal deformity (bulge) at the periphery of the node and—at least as important—on the marked decrease in echogenicity exhibited by an intranodal metastatic deposit. Because the lymph circulates from the periphery to the hilum of the node, early metastatic deposits develop preferentially at the periphery.

Axillary Nodes

Minute (measuring at least 4 or 5 mm) metastatic foci can be detected at the periphery of a totally echogenic node or if they produce a focal hypoechoic bulge on the surface of the node (Fig. 34-2). Even when the central fat is hypoechoic, metastatic deposits appear darker than the hypoechoic fat. Lymph nodes that are massively involved with metastatic tumor are easily recognized on US as rounded (when small) or irregularly shaped (when large) masses with little or no residual central echogenic fat (Fig. 34-3).

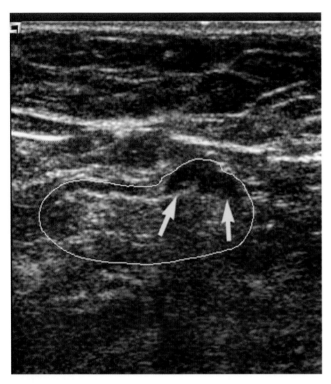

FIGURE 34-2 Sonogram of an early axillary lymph node metastasis. The metastatic deposit (*arrows*), which measures about 0.7 × 0.4 cm, creates a bulge at the surface of an otherwise normal appearing, fat-replaced node.

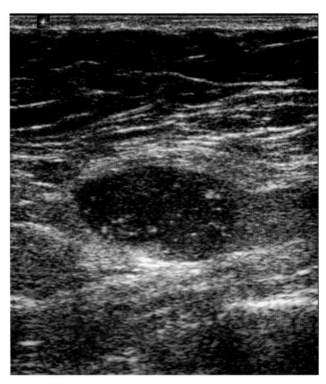

FIGURE 34-4 Metastatic axillary node with microcalcifications. Sonogram shows numerous punctate echoes within the node reflecting the presence of microcalcifications.

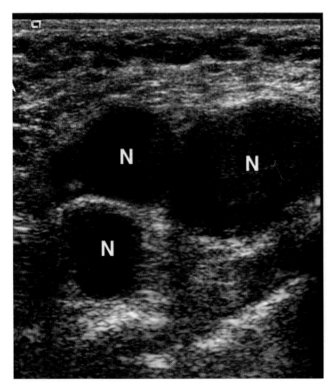

FIGURE 34-3 Massive metastatic involvement of axillary nodes. Sonogram shows complete replacement of 3 nodes (*N*) by markedly hypoechoic tumor.

If the primary tumor contains microcalcifications, identification of microcalcifications within a node is synonymous with metastatic involvement (Fig. 34-4).

On PDUS, the Doppler signals associated with metastatic nodes range from absent to numerous and disorganized. This wide range of PDUS appearances of malignant nodes considerably limits the role of PDUS in the diagnosis of nodal metastases—at least of small ones. On the other hand, the demonstration on PDUS of a dense harmonious vascular network covering the thickened cortex of a moderately enlarged node in a fashion similar to the cortical perfusion of a kidney (ie, with fine, parallel, hair-like vessels nearly reaching the capsule) correlates well with a diagnosis of BRH (Fig. 34-5).

Although US with state-of-the-art equipment can reliably detect lymph node metastases larger than 7 or 8 mm, it cannot, like other "nonfunctional" imaging modalities, demonstrate metastases that are only a few millimeters in size.

Because of the paucity of the cellular component of the metastatic deposit, nodal metastases from invasive lobular carcinomas, like the primary tumors from which they derive, can also have a deceptive US appearance and be very difficult to recognize. It is not unusual for such metastatic nodes to appear with an evenly thickened cortex and residual central fat, suggesting a benign node (Fig. 34-6). On cytology, only a few scattered cell groups are seen, and cytokeratin stain is often required for confirmation of the metastatic involvement.

Internal Mammary Nodes

The internal mammary chains constitute the second pathway for lymphatic drainage of the breast. US examination of the

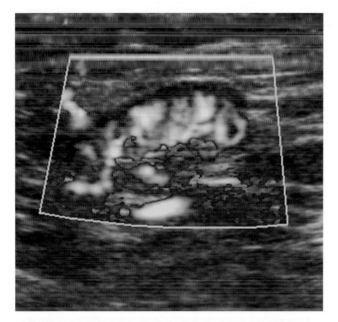

FIGURE 34-5 Benign reactive hyperplasia. Power Doppler sonogram shows a dense harmonious vascular network covering the thickened hypoechoic cortex.

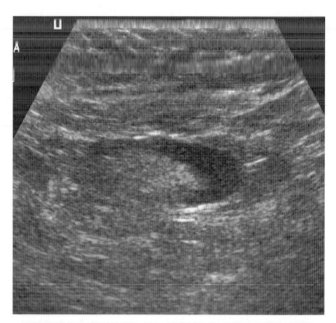

FIGURE 34-6 Metastatic axillary node from infiltrating lobular carcinoma. Sonogram shows grossly even thickening of the hypoechoic cortex. This appearance can be seen with benign reactive hyperplasia.

parasternal region is a simple, fast, and effective method of detecting internal mammary lymphadenopathy.[5] Because normal internal mammary nodes are too small to be visible on US, any hypoechoic mass seen along the internal mammary chains in a patient with breast cancer should be viewed as a potential metastasis (Fig. 34-7).

Metastatic internal mammary nodes are classified as N2 (in the *absence* of clinically evident axillary lymph node metastasis) or N3b (in the *presence* of clinically evident axillary lymph node metastasis). Detection of an internal mammary nodal metastasis (in addition to axillary metastases) therefore qualifies the disease as stage IIIC. (See Chapter 13 for cancer staging tables.)

enlarged, deformed, and completely hypoechoic (a "black node") is metastatic until proven otherwise. A hypoechoic node seen in an area where nodes are not normally seen (eg, internal mammary chains, supraclavicular fossa) is suspicious until proven otherwise.

Other Nodes

Affected infraclavicular nodes are important to detect and confirm by FNA because their adverse prognostic significance is worse than that of axillary nodes.[6]

The presence of metastatic infra (N3a) or supraclavicular nodes (N3c) qualifies the disease as stage IIIC.

Intramammary Nodes

When they are involved with metastatic disease, intramammary nodes are coded as axillary nodes. Any suspicious intramammary node in a cancer containing breast should be sampled with FNA. However, the remote possibility of metastatic axillary nodes coexisting with a benign intramammary node in the vicinity of a cancer should be kept in mind. Therefore, a benign result of the FNA biopsy of an intramammary node should prompt the verification of any additional indeterminate axillary node.

In general and in simpler terms, a node that is completely replaced by echogenic fat (a "white node") is benign. A node that is

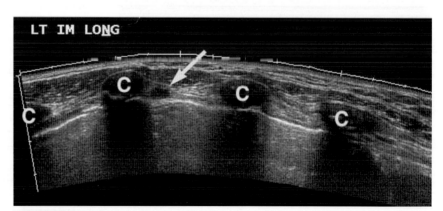

FIGURE 34-7 Internal mammary metastatic node. Longitudinal extended-field-of-view grayscale sonogram along the left internal mammary chains shows a small metastatic node (*arrow*). (C, sternocostal cartilage.)

Metastasis to any other lymph node, including the cervical or contralateral internal mammary lymph nodes, is coded as a distant metastasis (M1).

IMPACT OF THE DETECTION OF UNSUSPECTED METASTATIC NODES

The effect of the US detection of clinically occult metastases in the regional nodal basins on breast cancer staging is substantial. For example, the detection of a nonpalpable metastatic lymph node in the axilla makes the disease at least stage II. The detection of a metastasis in ipsilateral infraclavicular lymph node(s) (N3a), in ipsilateral internal mammary and axillary node(s) (N3b), or in ipsilateral supraclavicular lymph node(s) (N3c) makes the disease stage IIIC.

Also, at a time when efforts are being made to reduce unnecessary axillary lymph node dissections, the US detection of a nonpalpable metastasis in an axillary node (confirmed with US-guided FNA) makes the sentinel lymph node biopsy unnecessary in up to 25% of patients.[7-10]

ULTRASOUND-GUIDED FNA BIOPSY OF INDETERMINATE AND/OR SUSPICIOUS NODES

US-guided FNA biopsy readily permits ruling out or confirmation of metastatic involvement of enlarged lymph nodes in any of the nodal basins, including the internal mammary chains (Fig. 34-8).[11] FNA of lymph nodes is easy to perform because of their rich cellularity; as a rule, a single pass is sufficient to obtain an adequate specimen from a lymph node—benign or malignant—and there is never a need for core biopsy, unless the services of a cytopathologist are not available.

In a review of 103 cases of US-guided FNA biopsy of nonpalpable indeterminate or suspicious/metastatic-appearing

lymph nodes, the sensitivity of US combined with US-guided FNA was 86%, the specificity was 100%, the overall accuracy was 79%, the positive predictive value was 100%, and the negative predictive value was 67%.[12]

Possible causes of discrepancies (essentially false-negative results) in US-guided FNA biopsies of axillary nodes include small size of the metastasis (metastases $\leq$ 5 mm cannot be visualized); the small number of metastases; and human error, such as incomplete examination of the axilla, the operator's failure to see the abnormality or to interpret it, and improper technique in performing US-guided FNA (eg, error in targeting the lesion or inadequate aspiration, resulting in insufficient specimen). Because nodes are easy to aspirate, the rate of obtaining nondiagnostic specimens from lymph nodes should be close to 0%.

EVALUATION OF RESPONSE TO NEOADJUVANT CHEMOTHERAPY

At MD Anderson, we have used US to quantify the response of breast cancer to preoperative chemotherapy by measuring the volumes of both the primary breast tumor and the metastatic nodes before, during, and after the treatment. The formula for calculating the volume of a prolate ellipsoid (0.52 times the product of the 3 longest diameters) is used to obtain the volumes of the primary tumor and the metastatic nodes, which can then be compared with the volumes of the same lesions calculated on the previous study. This allows the breast imager to provide the clinician with a percentage decrease in volume that accurately reflects the response of the tumor to chemotherapy. Usually, the nodal metastases regress faster and resume a normal appearance sooner than the primary tumor does.

As shown in studies correlating sonographic with pathologic findings after adjuvant chemotherapy, and because of the known size limit in sonographic detection of nodal metastases,

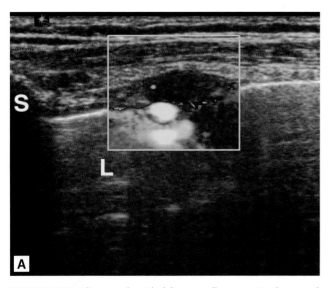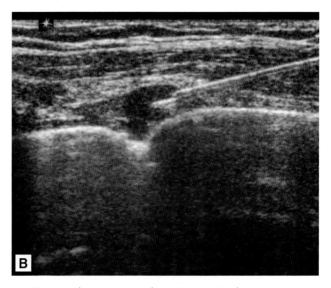

FIGURE 34-8 Ultrasound-guided fine-needle aspiration biopsy of a metastatic internal mammary node. **A.** Power Doppler transverse sonogram of the first left intercostal space shows a suspicious hypoechoic node anterior to the internal mammary artery in close proximity to the pleura. (S, left edge of the sternum; L, lung.) **B.** Sonogram obtained during the ultrasound-guided fine-needle aspiration shows the tip of the echogenic needle within the node.

the complete sonographic disappearance of metastatic nodes does not mean complete healing of the nodes. However, the residual pathologic disease in those patients without residual abnormal nodes on US after neoadjuvant chemotherapy has been shown to be of low volume, including micrometastases.[13,14]

FUTURE OF SONOGRAPHIC IMAGING OF LYMPH NODES

It has been shown that contrast-enhanced US with microbubble agents can be used to differentiate benign from malignant superficial nodes.[15] A 25% albumin solution has been used as a negative contrast agent for sentinel lymph node imaging; 5 mL of the solution was injected superficial to the breast primary tumor. Grayscale US was able to identify the sentinel node on the basis of the hypoechogenicity generated by the arrival of the albumin solution in the sentinel node.[16]

Oddly, US has received very little attention to date as a molecular imaging tool. However, the use of a lymph node–specific microbubble agent, which incorporates an antibody that targets the *L*-selectin ligand expressed in lymph node venules, has been reported.[17]

SUMMARY

Ultrasound examination of the breast in a patient with a suspicion or history of breast cancer must include the regional nodal basins, namely the axilla, infra- and supraclavicular regions, and internal mammary chains. At the present time, US with US-guided FNA remains the most practical and cost-effective technique for evaluating the lymphatic involvement of breast cancer.

REFERENCES

1. Sobin LH, Wittekind C, eds. UICC International Union Against Cancer. *TNM Classification of Malignant Tumours*. 6th ed. New York, NY: Wiley; 2002.
2. Białek EJ, Jakubowski W, Szczepanik AB, et al. 3D ultrasound examination of the superficial lymph nodes—does it provide additional information? *Ultraschall Med*. 2006;27:467-472.
3. Itoh A, Ueno E, Tohno E, et al. Breast disease: clinical application of US elastography for diagnosis. *Radiology*. 2006;239:341-350.
4. Fornage BD. Sonography of breast cancer. In: Winchester DJ, Winchester DP, Hudis CA, et al, eds. *Breast Cancer*. 2nd ed. Hamilton, Ontario: Decker; 2006:137-161.
5. Scatarige JC, Hamper UM, Sheth S, Allen HA III. Parasternal sonography of the internal mammary vessels: technique, normal anatomy, and lymphadenopathy. *Radiology*. 1989;172:453-457.
6. Newman L, Kuerer H, Fornage B, et al. Adverse prognostic significance of infraclavicular lymph nodes detected by ultrasonography in patients with locally advanced breast cancer. *Am J Surg*. 2001;181:313-318.
7. De Kanter AY, van Eijck CH, van Geel AN, et al. Multicentre study of ultrasonographically guided axillary node biopsy in patients with breast cancer. *Br J Surg*. 1999;86:1459-1462.
8. Deurloo EE, Tanis PJ, Gilhuijs KG, et al. Reduction in the number of sentinel lymph node procedures by preoperative ultrasonography of the axilla in breast cancer. *Eur J Cancer*. 2003;39:1068-1073.
9. Sahoo S, Sanders MA, Roland L, et al. A strategic approach to the evaluation of axillary lymph nodes in breast cancer patients: analysis of 168 patients at a single institution. *Am J Surg*. 2007;194:524-526.
10. Gilissen F, Oostenbroek R, Storm R, et al. Prevention of futile sentinel node procedures in breast cancer: ultrasonography of the axilla and fine-needle aspiration cytology are obligatory. *Eur J Surg Oncol*. 2008;34:497-500.
11. Fornage BD, Sneige N, Edeiken BS. Interventional breast sonography. *Eur J Radiol*. 2002;42:17-31.
12. Krishnamurthy S, Sneige N, Bedi DG, et al. Role of ultrasound-guided fine-needle aspiration of indeterminate and suspicious axillary lymph nodes in the initial staging of breast carcinoma. *Cancer* 2002;95:982-988.
13. Kuerer HM, Newman LA, Fornage BD, et al. Role of axillary lymph node dissection after tumor downstaging with induction chemotherapy for locally advanced breast cancer. *Ann Surg Oncol*. 1998;5:673-680.
14. Vlastos G, Fornage BD, Mirza NQ, et al. The correlation of axillary ultrasonography with histologic breast cancer downstaging after induction chemotherapy. *Am J Surg*. 2000;179:446-452.
15. Rubaltelli L, Khadivi Y, Tregnaghi A, et al. Evaluation of lymph node perfusion using continuous mode harmonic ultrasonography with a second generation contrast agent. *J Ultrasound Med*. 2004;23:829-836.
16. Omoto K, Hozumi Y, Omoto Y, et al. Sentinel node detection in breast cancer using contrast-enhanced sonography with 25% albumin—initial clinical experience. *J Clin Ultrasound*. 2006;34:317-326.
17. Hauff P, Reinhardt M, Briel A, et al. Molecular targeting of lymph nodes with L-selectin ligand-specific US contrast agent: a feasibility study in mice and dogs. *Radiology*. 2004;231:667-673.

CHAPTER 35

Breast Magnetic Resonance Imaging

Elizabeth Morris
Elisa Port

Breast magnetic resonance imaging (MRI) has attained a solid position in the evaluation of the breast, and many believe it is currently a necessary component of any breast imaging practice. In the past decade, many advances have contributed to the more routine use of this robust tool for cancer detection, including newer faster imaging sequences with improved image quality as well as new biopsy equipment that allows percutaneous needle biopsy of suspicious lesions. Additionally, societies have created guidelines for breast MRI, thus improving standardization in the performance, interpretation, and recommended use of this technology. Many of our current algorithms in the detection and treatment of breast cancer have been changed by the availability of breast MRI.

CLINICAL INDICATIONS

Clinical indications for breast MRI[1] include screening for breast cancer in the high-risk patient (Fig. 35-1), assessing response to chemotherapy in the patient with known breast cancer undergoing new-adjuvant chemotherapy (Fig. 35-2), assessing residual disease in a conserved breast with positive margins (Fig. 35-3), assessing possible recurrence in the treated breast when there is clinical or imaging suspicion (Fig. 35-4), screening the contralateral breast in the patient with known breast cancer (Fig. 35-5), and assessing for underlying cancer in a patient with occult primary breast cancer (Fig. 35-6). Breast MRI can also be valuable in the evaluation of inconclusive findings on conventional imaging (Fig. 35-7). The final clinical indication where MRI may be helpful but where there is less clinical evidence is assessing extent of disease in the preoperative setting (Fig. 35-8).

SENSITIVITY AND SPECIFICITY ISSUES IN BREAST MRI

Breast MRI uses an intravenous contrast agent for cancer detection and therefore relies almost exclusively on the associated neovascularity associated with carcinomas.[2,3] The administration of an intravenous contrast agent such as gadolinium-diethylenetriamine pentaacetic acid (Gd-DTPA) allows these lesions to be well visualized. Leaky capillaries and arteriovenous shunts allow contrast agents to rapidly accumulate and then rapidly leave the lesion over time, resulting in the characteristic washout time intensity curves that can be seen with some but not all malignancies (Fig. 35-9). Detection of invasive breast carcinoma is extremely reliable on MRI as the sensitivity approaches 100%.[4,5] Because the sensitivity for cancer detection is high, the negative predictive value of breast MRI is high. If no enhancement is present in the breast, and any possible technical mishap such as intravenous contrast extravasation has been excluded, there is an extremely low likelihood that invasive carcinoma (but not ductal carcinoma in situ[DCIS], as discussed in the following paragraph) is present. Specificity is lower than sensitivity, and therefore false positives can pose a problem in interpretation.

FALSE POSITIVES

False positives can be caused by high-risk lesions such as lobular carcinoma in situ (LCIS) (Fig. 35-10), atypical ductal hyperplasia (ADH) (Fig. 35-11), and atypical lobular hyperplasia (ALH), as well as benign masses such as fibroadenomas (Fig. 35-12), papillomas (Fig. 35-13), and lymph nodes (Fig. 35-14). Additionally,

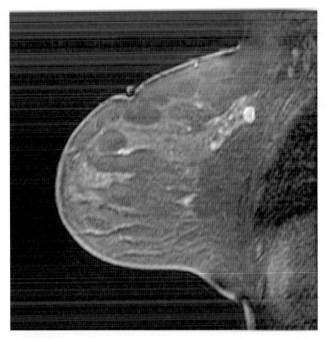

FIGURE 35-1 High-risk screening. A 37-year-old high-risk woman with suspicious rim-enhancing mass with surrounding clumped enhancement in the posterior breast that proved to represent a 4-mm invasive carcinoma with surrounding ductal carcinoma in situ.

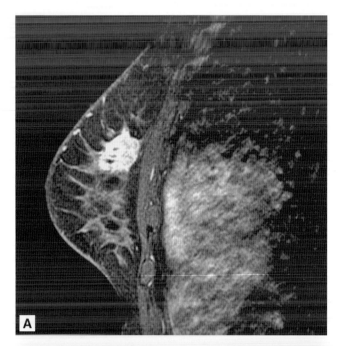

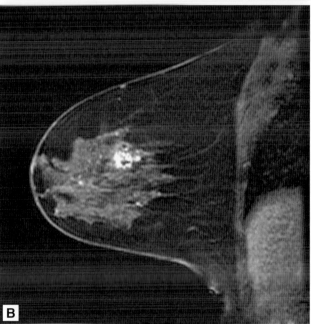

FIGURE 35-2 Response to chemotherapy. A 37-year-old woman with recent diagnosis of left breast and left axillary nodal metastases. **(A)** Pre- and **(B)** post-neoadjuvant chemotherapy.

fibrocystic changes (Fig. 35-15), sclerosing adenosis (Fig. 35-16), duct hyperplasia (Fig. 35-17), and fibrosis (Fig. 35-18) can result in a benign biopsy. With experience, many of these lesions can be diagnosed as benign; however, false positives will always be an issue on MRI as they are on mammography and sonography. Despite the reputation of high detection of cancer, false-negative examinations with MRI do exist. It should be noted that false negatives have been reported with some well-differentiated invasive ductal carcinomas as well as invasive lobular carcinoma.[6]

SPECIAL CONSIDERATIONS REGARDING DUCTAL CARCINOMA IN SITU

Not all DCIS is detected on MRI. Despite the sensitivity being very high for invasive carcinoma, the sensitivity of detection of DCIS has been reported in prior literature to be somewhat lower,[7] possibly secondary to more variable angiogenesis associated with DCIS lesions. But more recent evidence[8] suggests that the sensitivity for DCIS detection may actually be higher than previously reported now that high-resolution scanning techniques are more available and widely used and the patterns of DCIS on MRI are more recognized (Fig. 35-19). However, the sensitivity is still below that of invasive carcinomas.[9] Morphology may be more important than kinetics in the evaluation of DCIS; thus a slightly modified interpretation approach is taken when evaluating for DCIS.[10] Although more work needs to be performed in the MR assessment of in situ disease, MRI does not currently have as high a negative predictive value for DCIS as with invasive cancer. Therefore, MRI is not able to exclude DCIS with current technology and cannot be used to exclude the need for biopsy of suspicious calcifications. Nevertheless, MRI can detect mammographically occult DCIS and is able to play a valuable role possibly in the preoperative assessment of DCIS, where extent of disease may be underestimated by mammography (Fig. 35-20).

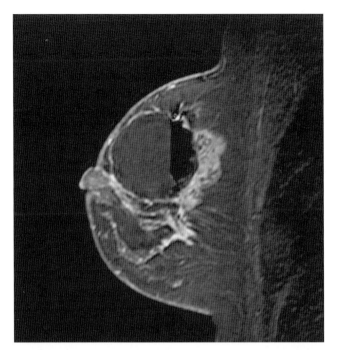

FIGURE 35-3 Residual disease assessment. Postoperative magnetic resonance imaging was performed for widely positive margins a few days following surgery. A seroma cavity is identified in the central breast with an air fluid layer (the patient is scanned prone). Along the posterior aspect of the seroma cavity toward the chest wall, there is lobular enhancement that represents residual disease. The amount of residual disease proved too much for reexcision (proved first by percutaneous biopsy), and the patient underwent mastectomy.

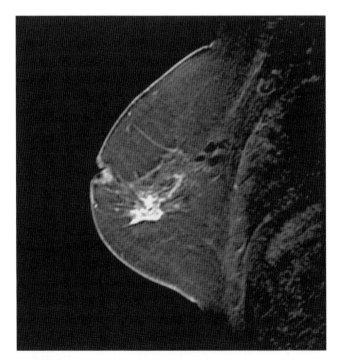

FIGURE 35-4 Recurrence following breast conservation. A 63-year-old woman with a history of ductal carcinoma in situ in the posterior breast (lumpectomy site clips are visible as black signal void) 2 years ago was treated with surgery and radiation. Screening magnetic resonance imaging demonstrates a new suspicious irregular mass in the anterior breast that proved to represent invasive mammary carcinoma with ductal and lobular features.

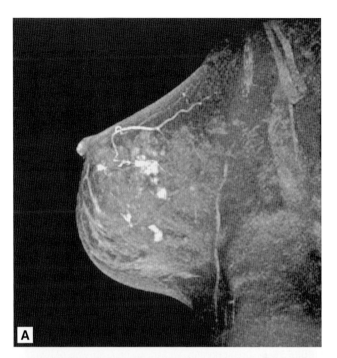

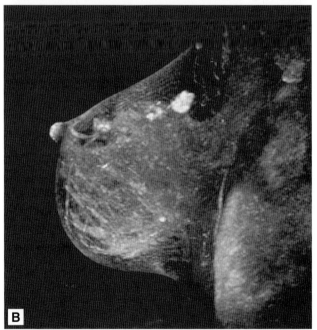

FIGURE 35-5 Screening of the contralateral breast. **A.** A 38-year-old woman with biopsy-proven moderately differentiated invasive ductal carcinoma of the right breast demonstrated on 3-dimensional magnetic resonance imaging (MRI) underwent bilateral MRI for preoperative staging. MRI demonstrated multiple additional findings in the index breast that proved to represent multicentric disease on biopsy. **B.** Contralateral MRI breast screening demonstrates an unsuspected mass with satellite lesions that proved to represent moderately differentiated ductal carcinoma of the opposite breast as well. The patient elected to undergo bilateral mastectomy.

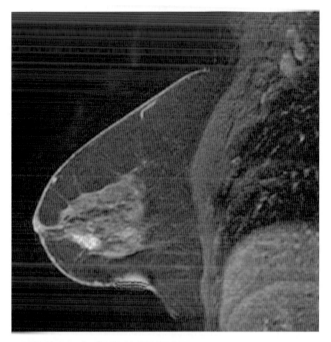

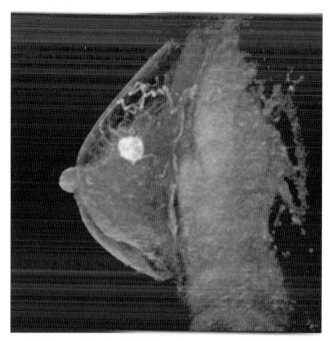

FIGURE 35-6 Occult primary breast cancer. A 60-year-old woman status postexcision of enlarged right axillary node showing metastatic adenocarcinoma from breast primary. Clinical examination, mammogram, and ultrasound of the breast were negative without suspicious findings. MRI demonstrated the underlying small primary cancer in the anterior breast.

FIGURE 35-8 Preoperative evaluation of disease extent. A 44-year-old woman with palpable moderately to poorly differentiated invasive ductal cancer identified and biopsied under ultrasound guidance. Mammogram was dense without suspicious finding. Magnetic resonance imaging performed for assessment of disease extent demonstrates a unifocal cancer without additional suspicious finding. Breast conservation confirmed a 1.5-cm cancer with associated ductal carcinoma in situ, and margins were free of tumor.

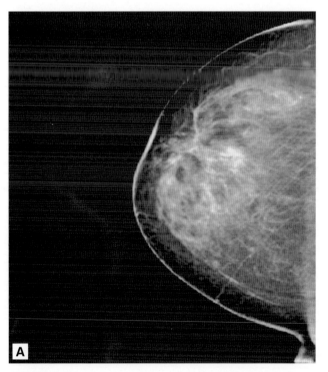

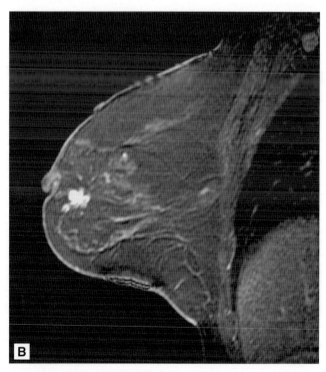

FIGURE 35-7 Inconclusive findings on mammography. A 66-year-old woman with increased distortion on mammography at a site of prior benign biopsy that yielded lobular carcinoma in situ (LCIS). Magnetic resonance imaging demonstrates suspicious mass at the prior benign biopsy site. Pathology yielded LCIS with several foci of invasive lobular carcinoma measuring 2 mm with negative sentinel nodes.

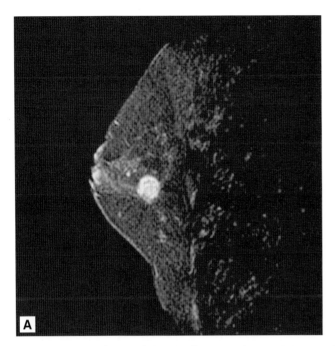
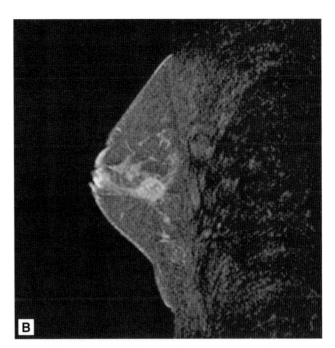

FIGURE 35-9 Washout with invasive breast carcinoma. A 41-year-old woman with invasive ductal carcinoma of the breast demonstrates **(A)** intense enhancement on the first postcontrast image followed by **(B)** rapid decrease in enhancement as demonstrated on the delayed third postcontrast image.

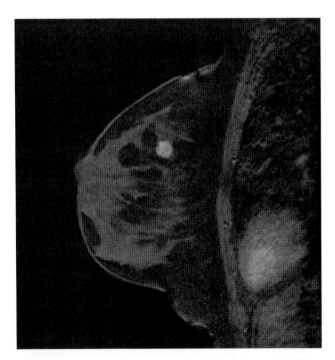
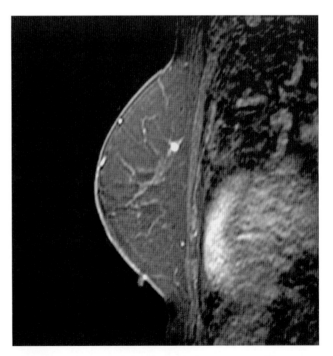

FIGURE 35-10 Lobular carcinoma in situ (LCIS). A 55-year-old woman with a prior history of benign breast biopsy for calcifications yielding LCIS undergoes screening magnetic resonance imaging examination. An enhancing mass was identified that was biopsied yielding LCIS.

FIGURE 35-11 Atypical duct hyperplasia. A 49-year-old woman with a prior history of benign biopsy yielding lobular carcinoma in situ and atypical ductal hyperplasia (ADH) undergoes screening magnetic resonance imaging (MRI) examination. An enhancing mass in the superior breast was identified that underwent MR intervention yielding ADH.

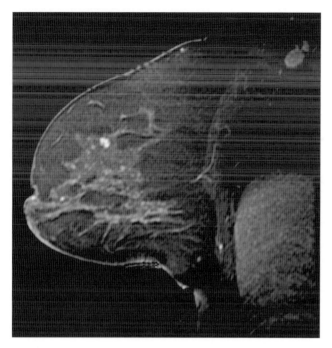

FIGURE 35-12 Fibroadenoma. A 65-year-old woman undergoing preoperative staging magnetic resonance imaging for invasive ductal carcinoma of the contralateral breast. An enhancing mass is identified that proved to be a fibroadenoma at biopsy.

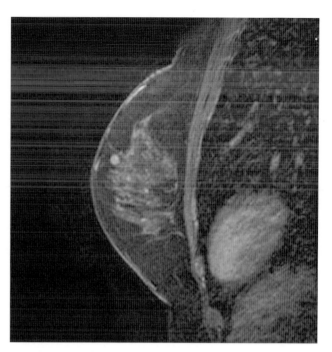

FIGURE 35-14 Lymph node. A 38-year-old woman with a prior history of benign biopsy yielding lobular carcinoma in situ, intraductal papillomas, and pseudoangiomatous stromal hyperplasia undergoes screening magnetic resonance imaging. In the supraareolar region there is an enhancing mass that represents a lymph node.

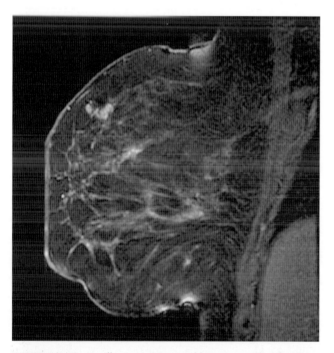

FIGURE 35-13 Papilloma. A 51-year-old woman with a family history of breast cancer undergoes screening magnetic resonance imaging. In the superior breast several small enhancing foci are identified. Biopsy yielded multiple papillomas with associated atypia.

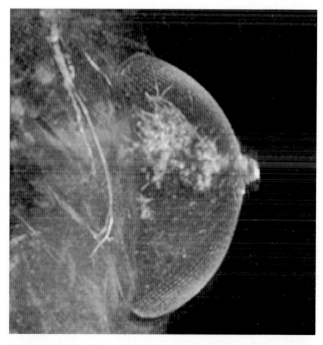

FIGURE 35-15 Fibrocystic change. A 30-year-old woman with a strong family history of breast cancer undergoes screening magnetic resonance imaging. Three-dimensional volumetric image demonstrates central enhancement compatible with marked fibrocystic change.

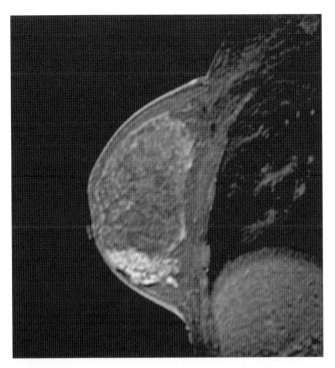

FIGURE 35-16 Sclerosing adenosis. A 33-year-old with a family history of breast cancer and personal history of ovarian cancer undergoes screening magnetic resonance imaging. Regional enhancement in the lower breast was identified that yielded florid sclerosing adenosis at biopsy.

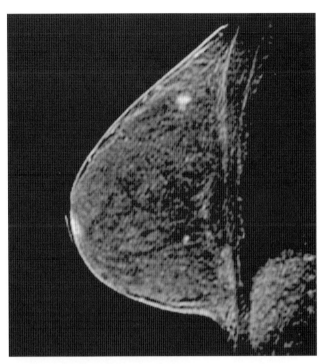

FIGURE 35-18 Fibrosis. A 41-year-old woman BRCA2 positive undergoes screening magnetic resonance imaging. Enhancing mass in the superior breast yielded fibrosis at biopsy.

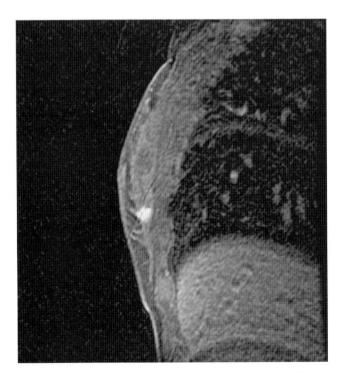

FIGURE 35-17 Duct hyperplasia. A 36-year-old woman with a family history of breast cancer undergoes screening magnetic resonance imaging. Mass in the lower breast proved to represent duct hyperplasia.

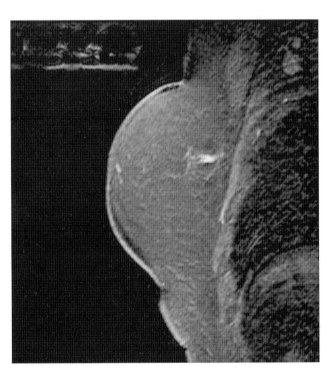

FIGURE 35-19 Appearance of ductal carcinoma in situ (DCIS) on magnetic resonance imaging. Linear enhancement is highly suspicious for DCIS, which was found at biopsy.

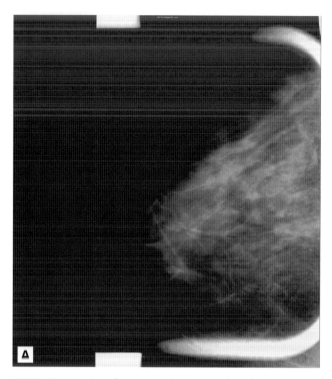
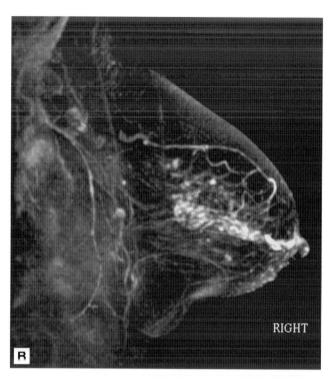

FIGURE 35-20   Ductal carcinoma in situ (DCIS) underestimated on mammography. **A.** Few calcifications are seen in the retroareolar region of the breast on mammography. **B.** Three-dimensional magnetic resonance imaging of the breast demonstrated more extensive ductal enhancement that corresponded to the full extent of DCIS.

INTERPRETING MRI IN CONJUNCTION WITH MAMMOGRAPHY AND SONOGRAPHY

Because of the potential issue of a false-negative examination, a negative MRI examination should not deter biopsy of a suspicious lesion (BI-RADS 4 or 5) on mammography or ultrasound. Mammographically suspicious findings, such as suspicious calcifications, spiculated masses, or areas of distortion, warrant appropriate biopsy, regardless of a negative MRI examination. The MRI should ideally be interpreted in conjunction with all other pertinent imaging studies such as the mammogram and the ultrasound to arrive at the best treatment option for the patient. With these limitations, breast MRI is best used as an adjunct test to conventional imaging, complementing but never replacing basic mammography and sonography.

RECENT GUIDELINES AND RECOMMENDATIONS

During the past few decades, as breast MRI has been incorporated into the clinical evaluation of the breast, it became apparent that standardization of image acquisition and terminology is extremely important. The American College of Radiology (ACR) Committee on Standards and Guidelines published a document for the indications and performance of breast MRI in 2004. Recently, the Breast Imaging Reporting and Data System (BI-RADS) lexicon[11] has added a section regarding breast MRI that has already been revised, and further revisions are in progress. These efforts have been important in establishing the standards of reporting and the standards for patient selection. The

existence of standardized guidelines in image acquisition and interpretation has helped disseminate this technology from academic centers into the community.[12,13] Furthermore, the ACR is supporting efforts to establish a voluntary accreditation process for performing breast MRI. The accreditation process will further standardize the acquisition of the MRI examination and will ensure that high-quality imaging will be performed on referred patients to the accredited centers.

In 2006, the American Cancer Society (ACS) modified for the first time the screening recommendations to include screening of high-risk women with breast MRI.[14]

HIGH-RISK SCREENING

An important recent recommendation of breast MRI is in the screening of high-risk patients who have at least a ≥20% lifetime risk of developing breast cancer. Because mammography has an overall false-negative rate of up to 15% in the general population, it is evident that all cancers are not detected by conventional means. The rate of false-negative examinations may be even higher in premenopausal women with dense breasts (reaching 50%),[15] and therefore exploration into alternative screening methods such as MRI has occurred. MRI has high-resolution capabilities, full documentation of the examination, and the potential to detect preinvasive DCIS and small invasive cancers that are usually node negative (Fig. 35-21). Studies that include patients with an overall cumulative lifetime risk of developing breast cancer of approximately 30% show that MRI is able to detect cancer in approximately 1% to 3% of patients.[16-23] There

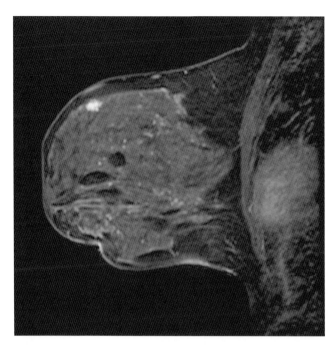

FIGURE 35-21 Screen detected cancer on magnetic resonance imaging (MRI). A 43-year-old woman with history of LCIS undergoes MRI screening. A new enhancing mass was identified in the superior breast that could not be seen on mammography or with targeted ultrasound. MR intervention demonstrated invasive ductal carcinoma. At surgery a 9-mm cancer was found with negative sentinel nodes.

are clear-cut indications for MRI screening in a small minority of patients at the highest risk of developing breast cancer. For the remaining majority, more data is needed to determine who benefits from this additional screening test.

THE AMERICAN COLLEGE OF SURGERY RECOMMENDATIONS

The use of breast MRI in the high-risk population is limited to those women with the documented BRCA1 or BRCA2 gene or those women with a family member who is a documented carrier but they themselves are untested; any woman with a greater than 20% to 25% lifetime risk (as defined by the BRCAPRO or other models dependent on family history); women with a history of mantle radiation; women with a breast cancer syndrome such as Li-Fraumeni, Cowden, and Bannayan-Riley-Ruvalcaba. There is very little published clinical information that exists for screening patients who are at increased risk based on a prior benign biopsy yielding LCIS, ADH, or ALH. The ACS did not issue a recommendation for or against screening in these clinical scenarios because there is not yet enough compelling clinical data. The decision whether or not to screen patients with these high-risk lesions should be made on an individual basis by the referring clinician.

BRCA Heterozygotes

Approximately 0.1% of the general population and 2% of the Ashkenazi Jewish population are BRCA heterozygotes, harboring

a mutation in either the BRCA1 or BRCA2 mutations. These genetic predispositions herald a lifetime risk of breast cancer of approximately 80%. This group is therefore deemed to be at the highest possible estimated risk of developing breast cancer. Because of this increased risk, and the predisposition to developing breast cancer at younger ages when breasts are denser, patients with known or suspected BRCA mutations are one group in whom screening MRI is clearly recommended based on both ACS and National Comprehensive Cancer Network (NCCN) guidelines. Although many studies evaluating MRI screening in the high-risk population involve heterogeneous groups of patients, most focus on those at high risk based on known or suspected BRCA heterozygosity. Results from the studies focusing on those with genetic predisposition demonstrate a 1% to 7% incidence of cancer detection with MRI (see Table 35-1). Furthermore, evidence indicates that in this specific population of patients at genetic predisposition, MRI is more sensitive than mammography and ultrasonography or the combination of these two tests in detecting cancer (Fig. 35-22).[20]

Previous Thoracic Radiation Therapy

Patients who undergo previous radiation treatment to the chest wall, such as mantle radiation for Hodgkin disease, are at increased risk for breast cancer. The magnitude of this risk is related to age at treatment. Those treated between 12 and 16 years of age are estimated to be at the highest risk, a 37- to 40-fold increased risk over the general population, presumably because of exposure to radiation during the critical years of pubertal breast development.[24] Screening recommendations for this group of patients include annual mammography for patients aged 25 years or more, beginning 8 to 10 years after radiation treatment or at 40 years of age (whichever comes first). Consideration of screening MRI is recommended as an adjunct to mammography, given the high risk of developing breast cancer in this group and the frequency with which it develops in the young age group.

Lobular Cancer In Situ/Atypia

For patients with LCIS or ADH/ALH, the absolute risk of developing breast cancer ranges from 15% to 30% . Most studies describing MRI screening in high-risk populations focus on patients with genetic predisposition, as mentioned earlier, or those with strong family histories and therefore suspected of harboring gene mutations. Some studies have looked at MRI screening in a more heterogeneous mix of patients at increased risk, and therefore include subgroups of patients whose increased risk for breast cancer is attributable to a previous biopsy demonstrating atypical hyperplasia or LCIS. These patients typically represent just a small subgroup of patients in few studies. Port et al described the only current series in the literature looking at MRI screening specifically in patients with LCIS and atypia.[25] This retrospective study described the results of the MRI screening experience at Memorial Sloan-Kettering Cancer Center for patients with LCIS and atypia. Of 378 patients identified, 182 (48%) underwent MRI screening. Patients with LCIS/atypia who chose or were recommended by their physicians to undergo MRI were younger and more likely

TABLE 35-1 Summary of MRI Screening Studies Performed to Date

Investigator	Year	Institute	N	Mean Age	Risk	Bx (%)	PPV (%)	No. CA MRI Only (%)	No. DCIS (%)
Kuhl	2000	U Bonn	192	39	Gene carriers	14 (7%)	9/14 (64%)	6/192 (3%)	1/6 (7%)
Tilanus-Linthorst	2000	Erasmus MC Rotterdam	109	43	High risk	9 (8%)	3/9 (33%)	3/109 (3%)	0/3 (0%)
Warner	2001	U Toronto	196	43	High risk	23 (12%)	6/23 (26%)	4/196 (2%)	0/4 (0%)
Stoutjesdijk	2001	Nijmeger	179	NS	High risk	30 (17%)	13/30 (43%)	8/170 (4%)	2/8 (25%)
Lo	2001	U Penn	157	43	High risk	28 (18%)	5/28 (18%)	5/157 (3%)	NS
Robson	2003	MSKCC	54 (129 rounds)	44	Gene carriers	15 (12%)	3/15 (20%)	3/129 (2%)	NS
Kriege	2003	Erasmus MC Rotterdam	1869 (3280 rounds)	40	High risk	NS	NS	39/3280 (1%)	5/39 (13%)
Kuhl	2003	U Bonn	359 (583 rounds)	39	Gene carriers	63 (11%)	21/63 (34%)	21/583 (4%)	NS
Morris	2003	MSKCC	367	50	High risk	64 (17%)	14/59 (24%)	14/367 (4%)	8/14 (57%)
Leach	2002	UK	1236	<50	High risk	NS	NS	15/1236 (1%)	NS
Podo	2002	Italy	105	46	Gene carriers	3 (8%)	7/8 (88%)	7/105 (7%)	3/7 (43%)
Sardanelli	2007	Italy	278	46	Gene carriers	33 (12%)	18/33 (54%)	6/278 (2%)	3/6 (50%)
Lehman	2007	Seattle	171	46	High risk	16 (22%)	6/16 (37%)	4/171 (2%)	0/6 (0%)

Bx = biopsy; CA = cancer; DCIS = ductal carcinoma in situ; MRI = magnetic resonance imaging; MSKCC = Memorial Sloan-Kettering Cancer Center; NS = not significant; PPV = positive predictive value; Risk = risk factor for entrance into the screening study.

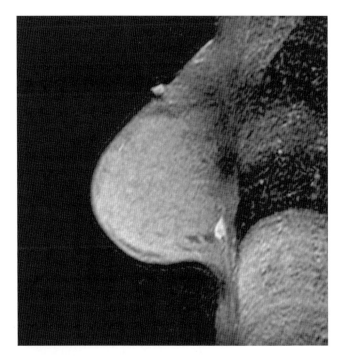

FIGURE 35-22 Screen detected cancer on magnetic resonance imaging. A 41-year-old woman BRCA2 positive undergoes MRI screening . In the posteroinferior breast, a rim enhancing mass is identified that was not detected at mammography or screening ultrasound. Biopsy yielded a 9-mm invasive ductal carcinoma with negative sentinel nodes.

to have a concomitant family history of breast cancer than those who did not have an MRI. Overall, MRI generated additional biopsies in 25% of patients who underwent MRI screening, and cancer was identified in 13% of biopsies performed based on MRI alone. MRI-identified cancers were only identified in patients with LCIS (4%), with no cancers detected in patients with atypia. This study led to the conclusion that in patients with LCIS or atypia selected to undergo MRI screening, MRI generated a larger proportion of biopsies than cancer diagnoses but may be warranted in highly selected patients with LCIS. Currently, ACS and NCCN guidelines indicate that MRI may be considered as an adjunct to screening in this patient population.

Additional High-Risk Screening Criteria

Lastly, patients who did not fit into the specific high-risk categories just described may nevertheless qualify as being at increased risk for breast cancer based on one of the models designed to assess breast cancer risk. The Gail model, for example, incorporates a variety of risk factors including family history and evaluates an individual woman's risk of developing breast cancer over the ensuing 5-year period and over her lifetime. Women with a 5-year risk of developing breast cancer more than 1.7% or a lifetime risk more than 20% are categorized as high risk based on this model, and they are therefore eligible for risk reduction strategies such as tamoxifen. Although the Gail model does incorporate significant risk factors, such as

family history in determining risk, other risk factors, such as age at menarche, age at first live birth, and patient age, are also incorporated into this model, such that a patient more than 60 years of age by itself allows a patient to meet the criteria for increased risk for breast cancer based on the definitions just described. At this time, MRI screening is not recommended for the heterogenous group of women whose risk for breast cancer is determined to be increased solely based on meeting Gail model criteria for increased risk.

Average-Risk Women

Moreover, no information exists for screening "dense, difficult to examine" breasts. There is evidence that women with dense breasts are at increased risk of developing breast cancer,[26] and therefore these recommendations may change in the future as more data accumulates. Screening by MRI in this population where the incidence of breast cancer is low would very likely result in too many false-positive biopsies to justify its use although no data exist to support this view. Furthermore, no screening studies have been performed on the average-risk population to determine if the cancer detection rate is too low and if any benefit is outweighed by the possibility of a false-positive biopsy. The recommendation not to screen average-risk women with MRI is based solely on expert opinion.

NEOADJUVANT CHEMOTHERAPY RESPONSE

Neoadjuvant chemotherapy is given preoperatively to shrink the tumor before definitive surgery is performed. It is nearly always given in cases of locally advanced breast cancer, yet in recent years it is being used to decrease tumor size in earlier stage cancer as well. The benefit of giving the chemotherapy up front is that one has the ability to determine whether the tumor is going to respond to that particular chosen chemotherapy regimen. A complete pathologic response (elimination of tumor) following neoadjuvant therapy is strongly predictive of excellent long-term survival (Fig. 35-23). Minimal response suggests a poor long-term survival regardless of postoperative therapy (Fig. 35-24).

Assessing response to neoadjuvant chemotherapy cancer can be complicated clinically and on mammography. MRI can be useful to overcome the limitations of breast density and fibrosis.[27] MRI may find a role in being able to predict at an earlier time point, perhaps after several cycles of chemotherapy, which patients are responding to neoadjuvant chemotherapy.[28] Early knowledge of suboptimal response may allow switching to alternative treatment regimens earlier rather than later. Unless the response is dramatic, it currently takes longer to predict response because one must wait to see a volume change in the tumor that is measurable. Volume change may be difficult to assess on the mammogram and physical examination because fibrosis, a response to chemotherapy, can mimic residual disease. Investigators[29,30] have demonstrated that residual tumor measurements on MRI correlate with the pathologic residual disease following neoadjuvant chemotherapy. Patterns of response are being evaluated in the hope that these findings

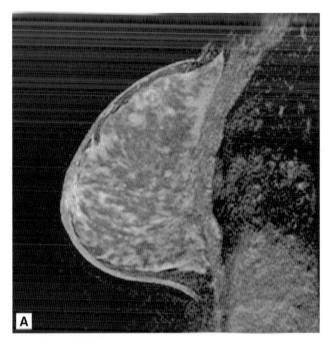
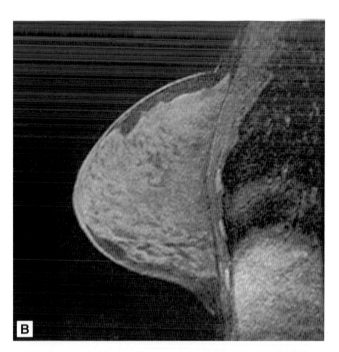

FIGURE 35-23   Complete response on magnetic resonance Imaging (MRI) to neoadjuvant chemotherapy. A 36-year-old woman with inflammatory breast carcinoma. **A.** MRI before chemotherapy demonstrates diffuse enhancement throughout the breast. **B.** After 3 cycles of chemotherapy, a repeat MRI examination demonstrates no residual enhancement. At pathology small isolate foci of invasive cancer were demonstrated in all quadrants of the breast.

may predict recurrence and survival. Patterns of response may hold more information because the mere presence or absence of enhancement may be misleading because fibrosis, a consequence of treatment, may enhance or residual tiny islands of tumor may exist after treatment that are below the detection level of MRI.

Magnetic Resonance Spectroscopy in the Evaluation of Response

Besides volumetric measurements, MRI is able to exploit functional information about the tumor. Kinetic changes occur early in the tumors before volume alterations, and another

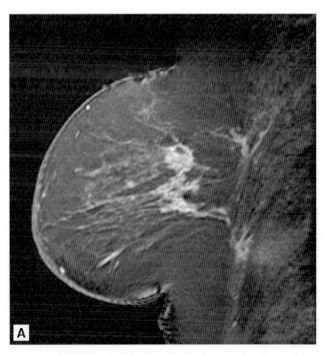
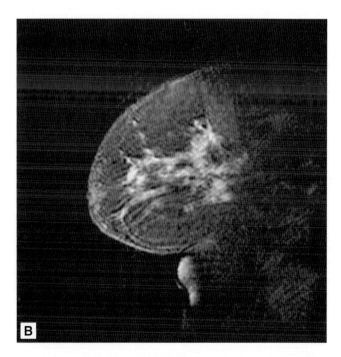

FIGURE 35-24   No response on magnetic resonance imaging to neoadjuvant chemotherapy. A 43-year-old woman with locally advanced breast carcinoma invading the chest wall **(A)** before chemotherapy and **(B)** after chemotherapy. The dominant tumor mass in the central breast has increased in size, and the breast has become retracted.

important application that MRI can provide to evaluate response is the use of magnetic resonance spectroscopy (MRS). MRS evaluates the choline content in the cancer. Several preliminary studies[31] have shown that choline can decrease prior to a change in the size or morphology of the cancer. It is proposed that choline may be able to predict very early on—perhaps in a day or two—following the first dose of chemotherapy whether or not the patient will have a response.[32] Information that is helpful to the oncologist in deciding the optimal chemotherapy regimen will hopefully give the patient the best chance for response.

ASSESSMENT OF RESIDUAL DISEASE

For patients who have not had a preoperative MRI examination and have undergone lumpectomy with positive margins, postoperative MRI can be helpful in the assessment of residual tumor load.[33] Postoperative mammography may be also indicated and is able to detect residual calcifications, although it is very limited in the evaluation of residual uncalcified DCIS or residual mass. MRI is able to detect bulky residual disease at the lumpectomy site as well as residual disease in the same quadrant (multifocal) (Fig. 35-25) or different quadrant (multicentric) (Fig. 35-26). Determination whether the patient would be best

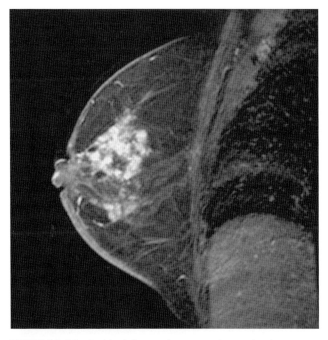

FIGURE 35-26 Residual disease in a separate quadrant. A 56-year-old woman with invasive ductal carcinoma in the upper outer quadrant status post initial attempt at conservation has marked residual enhancement throughout the breast (suspicious regional enhancement is shown in the anterior breast).

served with directed reexcision (residual disease at the lumpectomy site or multifocal disease) or whether the patient warrants mastectomy (multicentric disease) is where MRI can be helpful. Evaluation for microscopic residual disease directly at the lumpectomy site is not the role of MRI because the surgeon will perform reexcision based on pathologic margins and not based MRI results. The role of MRI is to define whether the patient should return to the operating room for a reexcision or would be better served with a mastectomy. Traditionally, patient can have several trips to the operating room prior to the decision to perform mastectomy. Therefore, MRI may save some patients from these repeated surgical procedures. If multicentric disease is identified on MRI prior to mastectomy, it is important to sample the lesion to document and verify this impression.

When to Perform MRI After Surgery

Due to conflicting literature, there is confusion about when to image following surgery for cancer to determine whether residual disease is present.[34] The most appropriate time for scanning a patient to assess for residual disease is as soon as possible after surgery. Immediately after surgery there is a postoperative seroma cavity that is low in signal. Surrounding the cavity there is usually enhancement in the granulation tissue that is formed due to the surgical procedure. The enhancement is generally thin and uniform when there is no residual disease or if there is minimal/microscopic residual disease. Bulky residual disease will be easily seen as bulky asymmetric enhancement around the cavity (Fig. 35-27). More importantly, however, is the assessment of the remainder of the breast for

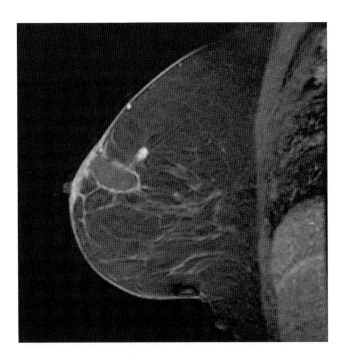

FIGURE 35-25 Residual disease in the same quadrant. A 54-year-old woman underwent surgical excision of a palpable mass yielding invasive ductal carcinoma with positive margins. Postoperative magnetic resonance imaging demonstrates a seroma cavity on the supraareolar region anteriorly. Immediately superior to the seroma there is a suspicious irregular enhancing mass that represented residual disease. The patient underwent localization of this mass, and subsequent reexcision yielded negative margins.

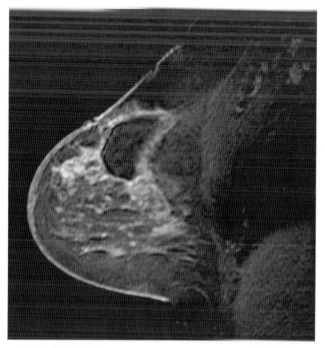

FIGURE 35-27 Bulky disease at the surgical margin. Postoperative magnetic resonance imaging for widely positive margins demonstrates bulky residual disease along the anterior aspect of the seroma cavity as well as the inferoposterior aspect. Percutaneous biopsy proved that the enhancement represented residual disease, and the patient then went to mastectomy.

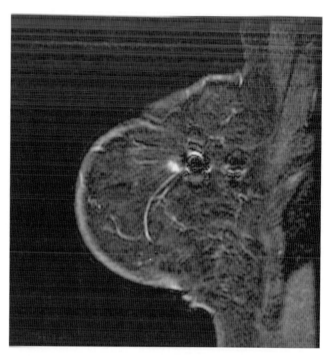

FIGURE 35-28 Recurrence. A 56-year-old woman with prior history of invasive lobular carcinoma 13 years ago treated with surgery, chemotherapy, and radiation therapy. Screening magnetic resonance imaging demonstrates a new enhancing mass anterior to the lumpectomy site. Biopsy proved to represent recurrent invasive lobular carcinoma.

additional disease that would preclude the patient from receiving conservation therapy. The longer one waits following surgery, the more chance there is for the seroma cavity to collapse and cause diagnostic difficulties. Once the seroma cavity collapses the enhancing seroma wall is all that is left, and the appearance can mimic a spiculated mass or area of distortion with suspicious morphology and enhancement. When the breast is imaged early following surgery, these diagnostic dilemmas usually do not arise.

TUMOR RECURRENCE AT THE LUMPECTOMY SITE

Tumor recurrence after breast conservation occurs at an overall rate of 1% per year. Recurrence directly at the lumpectomy site occurs earlier than elsewhere in the breast and usually peaks several years following conservation therapy. Early recurrence is generally thought to represent untreated disease that was present at the time of lumpectomy. Evaluation of the lumpectomy site by mammography may be limited due to postoperative scarring, and physical examination has been reported to have greater sensitivity than mammography in the detection of recurrence. Mammography is an important tool though and should be performed because it is able to detect 25% to 45% of recurrences. Mammography is more likely to detect recurrent tumors associated with calcifications than recurrences without calcifications because the postsurgical distortion limits evaluation for residual masses.

MRI is able to detect recurrent disease that may not be detected mammographically (Fig. 35-28).[35] When to image for

potential recurrence has been reported as problematic because the scar can enhance for years following surgery.

OCCULT PRIMARY BREAST CANCER

Patients presenting with axillary metastases suspicious for breast primary and a negative physical examination and negative mammogram should undergo breast MRI. In patients with this rare clinical presentation, MRI has been able to detect cancer in 90% to 100% of cases, if a tumor is indeed present. The tumors are generally small in size, less than 2 cm, thus they may evade detection by conventional imaging and physical examination (Fig. 35-29).[36,37]

The identification of the site of malignancy is important therapeutically. Patients traditionally undergo mastectomy because the site of malignancy is unknown. Whole-breast radiation can be given, although it is generally not recommended because survival is equal but the recurrence rate is higher, up to 23%. Thus if a site of malignancy can be identified, the patient can be spared mastectomy and offered breast conservation therapy, thereby having a significant impact on patient management. In one study, the results of the MR examination changed therapy in approximately half of the cases, usually allowing conservation in lieu of mastectomy.

PREOPERATIVE STAGING

Breast MRI can give helpful information for staging on tumor size, presence or absence of multifocal or multicentric disease, as well as whether the chest wall or pectoralis muscle is invaded

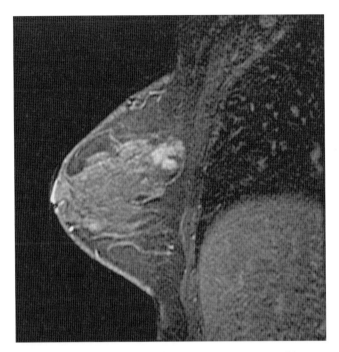

FIGURE 35-29 Occult primary breast cancer. A 28-year-old woman with palpable axillary lymph node that demonstrated adenocarcinoma suggestive of breast primary at biopsy. Mammogram and physical examination were unremarkable. Magnetic resonance imaging evaluation demonstrated the underlying occult cancer in the posterior breast superiorly.

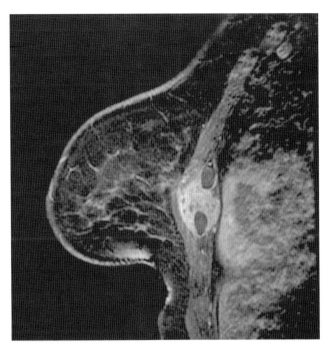

FIGURE 35-30 Chest wall invasion. A 43-year-old woman with a family history of breast cancer recently diagnosed with invasive ductal carcinoma of the breast. Preoperative magnetic resonance imaging demonstrates chest wall invasion (mass in the breast not included on sagittal slice) as demonstrated by the enhancement within the pectoralis muscle and intercostal muscles.

(Fig. 35-30). It has been well documented that MR defines the anatomic extent of disease more accurately than mammography.[38] Many studies have shown that MRI is able to detect additional foci of cancer in the breast that has been overlooked by our conventional techniques.[39-42] Several investigators have shown that MRI is able to detect additional disease (Fig. 35-31) in up to a third of patients, possibly resulting in a treatment change.[43-45] MRI can potentially provide valuable information for preoperative planning in the single-stage resection of breast cancer. By using breast MRI as a complementary test to the conventional imaging techniques, more precise information can be obtained about the extent of breast cancer. No evidence indicates that the additional cancer found by MRI is any different or less significant that the cancer found by mammography ultrasonography or physical examination.

CONTROVERSIES IN USING BREAST MRI IN CANCER STAGING

Controversy exists regarding the use of MRI to stage breast cancer.[46-48] Because breast cancer treatment has been successfully refined over the past decades, there is appropriate concern about addition of MRI to the preoperative workup of the known cancer. The general argument is that with breast conservation surgery followed by radiation therapy, recurrence rates are low: reported recurrence rates at 10 years are in some centers less than 10%. It had been thought that because MRI detects more

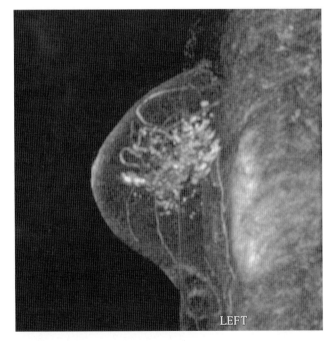

FIGURE 35-31 Additional disease in preoperative staging. A 60-year-old woman underwent stereotactic biopsy of a small cluster of calcifications yielding invasive lobular carcinoma. No suspicious additional suspicious findings were identified on mammography. Magnetic resonance imaging demonstrates abnormal enhancement throughout the breast suspicious for multicentric disease. Biopsy confirmed multicentric invasive lobular carcinoma prior to mastectomy.

cancer the recurrence rate must be positively affected in those patients undergoing breast MRI; however, there is a paucity of data to support this. In fact, a recent retrospective study[49] looking at early-stage breast cancer found that MRI had no effect on the recurrence rate.

Breast radiation therapy developed to fill a need to treat residual disease and has become a mainstay of the treatment of breast conservation of most patients whether or not residual disease exists. It has been well documented that radiation reduces local recurrence. However, until the use of MRI, it has not been possible to reliably identify those patients who harbor additional multifocal or multicentric cancer and who may be at increased risk of recurrence. From the radiology perspective, these issues raise many questions such as what lesion size can we safely ignore on MRI. If we are committed to using radiation on all patients, perhaps MRI is too sensitive in detecting cancer in general. On the one hand, for our current treatment algorithms that involve the use of radiation, MRI is likely detecting subclinical disease that radiation therapy would treat adequately. On the other hand, MRI may detect additional disease that would not be treated with adjuvant therapy. The challenge for the radiologist is identifying what is and what is not significant disease. At this time, identification of significant disease that will not be treated with radiation therapy is not possible, and all additional disease is treated surgically. Performing breast MRI to possibly prevent recurrence may have benefit to the minority of breast conservation patients, namely those who will recur (at least 10% by 10 years). Trials that involve radiologists as well as radiation oncologists and surgeons are needed to answer these perplexing questions.

It is thought that breast MRI may be helpful in decreasing positive margin rates because it outlines more precisely the minimum extent than other modalities; however, no studies or outcomes support this claim.

EXAMINING THE CONTRALATERAL BREAST IN THE STAGING MRI EXAMINATION

Probably the most compelling reason to perform breast MRI in the patient with known cancer is the assessment of the contralateral breast (Fig. 35-32). It has been well documented that MRI is able to detect occult contralateral breast cancer in approximately 4% to 6% of patients.[50-52] These cancers are sometimes the more significant lesion and may alter the staging of the patient. Furthermore, knowledge of the extent of disease in both breasts allows optimal treatment options to be discussed at the outset with the patient instead of many years later when the patient develops her contralateral primary.

WHO SHOULD UNDERGO PREOPERATIVE BREAST MRI?

All patients with a new diagnosis of breast cancer should arguably undergo bilateral MRI examination preoperatively. There are several reasons for this statement. First, the high rate of contralateral carcinoma justifies the use of routine bilateral MRI. Also for those patients with true multicentric disease, the appropriate therapy can be done upfront. A conservative recurrence rate of 10% at 10 years certainly justifies the use of a single MRI examination at the time of treatment planning to identify those patients who may benefit from mastectomy. Lastly, the index lesion is better defined on MRI so that the

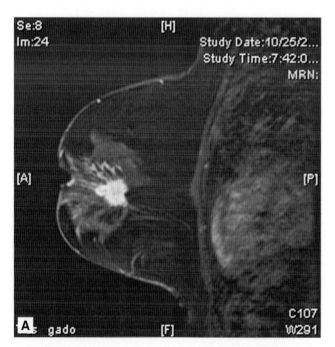
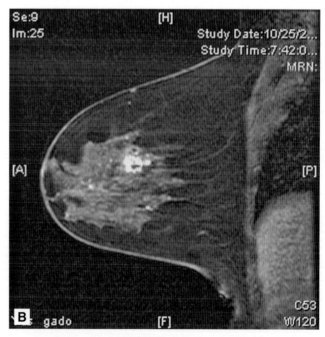

FIGURE 35-32 Occult contralateral carcinoma in preoperative staging. A 62-year-old woman with **(A)** known moderately differentiated invasive ductal carcinoma of the left breast. **(B)** Contralateral breast magnetic resonance imaging demonstrates an irregular mass that proved to represent ductal carcinoma in situ with microinvasion.

surgeon may have a better chance at obtaining negative margins at the first attempt of conservation. One study[53] showed that bracketing of the lesion by MRI may facilitate complete removal of the lesion if a large DCIS component is not present. Therefore performing preoperative MRI may increase the chance that the surgeon obtains a negative margin at the initial surgery. More data are needed to address this potential use of MRI to decrease the positive margin rate.

At the very least, perhaps the best patients for preoperative MRI are those that are known to have high rates of positive margins and recurrence: for example, young patients, all patients with dense or moderately dense breasts, and patients with difficult tumor histology such as infiltrating lobular carcinoma, DCIS, and tumors with an extensive intraductal component, where tumor size assessment is difficult on mammography or ultrasound. Additionally, an extensive intraductal component (EIC) is associated with positive margins and high recurrence rates. EIC is described when the invasive carcinoma has an associated greater than 25% component of DCIS. EIC is associated with residual carcinoma and positive margins after lumpectomy, and there is some evidence that the presence of an EIC may indicate an increased risk of local recurrence (Fig. 35-33). Interestingly, because MRI is more sensitive to DCIS detection than mammography, it may become the test of choice to evaluate patients preoperatively. Several trials are underway to assess this potential use of MRI.

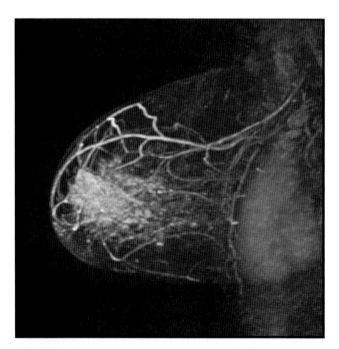

FIGURE 35-33 Magnetic resonance imaging (MRI) demonstrates extensive intraductal component. A 45-year-old woman with a new cluster of calcifications on mammography underwent stereotactic biopsy yielding invasive ductal carcinoma and ductal carcinoma in situ. Preoperative MRI was performed that demonstrated diffuse clumped enhancement in the superior breast involving more than 2 quadrants that proved to represent an extensive intraductal component. MRI demonstrated the need for further biopsy to prove multicentric disease. The patient underwent mastectomy.

POTENTIAL PITFALLS IN OVERUSE/OVERRELIANCE ON MRI

As with any examination, breast MRI interpretation depends on the experience of the reader. A real concern is when inexperienced interpreters generate large numbers of false-positive biopsies. Examination of the literature, however, demonstrates that the positive biopsy rate of MR recommended biopsies is quite high, approaching 45%.[54] However, these numbers come from centers with a lot of experience in MRI interpretation. And the reputation of MRI as generating too many false-positive biopsies is unjustified if one looks at the positive predictive values for biopsy. Indeed, even in a community practice just starting out in their biopsy practice, a positive biopsy rate indicating cancer detection was found in 25% of women recommended for biopsy on the basis of MRI.[55] The biopsy rate is similar to that generated by routine mammography and is certainly better than that generated by ultrasonography. What is interesting about the analysis of these biopsy studies is that many of the lesions recommended for biopsy under MRI guidance turned out to be high-risk lesions such as ALH, ADH, and LCIS, in 10% to 15% of reported biopsies. Often the presence of a high-risk lesion is an important data point for the patient and referring clinician.

Concern has also been raised about the possibility of inexperienced readers recommending close interval follow-up or biopsies in too many patients. Short-term follow-up recommendation of breast MRI examinations varies in the literature from 5% to 30%. It is clear that the more experience a radiologist has, the fewer follow-ups are recommended. Additionally, the more comparison MRI examinations a patient has, the lower the recommendation for short-term follow-up. As with mammography, being able to document the stability of a particular finding allows the reader to assign a benign interpretation to the examination in lieu of short-term follow-up or even biopsy. Because patients undergoing breast MRI examination are likely high risk, there may be more of a tendency by the reader to recommend biopsy over short-term follow-up. A minimal number of MRI examinations should be performed by an individual radiologist to gain experience and recognize normal enhancement versus suspicious enhancement. That number has not yet been defined, but it is evident that the more examinations a radiologist is responsible for the more comfortable he or she becomes with benign enhancement. What these data indicate is that it is important to audit your practice to document the positive biopsy rate as well as the follow-up rate.

BENIGN FINDING: HORMONE-RELATED ENHANCEMENT

Because MRI is performed with intravenous contrast, normal fibroglandular parenchyma can demonstrate contrast enhancement. Background enhancement refers to the normal enhancement of the patient's fibroglandular parenchyma. In general, background enhancement is bilateral, symmetric, and diffuse; however, sometimes it may be focal, regional, and/or asymmetric.[56] Background enhancement can occur regardless of the menstrual cycle or menopausal status of the patient. The background enhancement may not be directly related to the amount of fibroglandular parenchyma present. Patients with extremely dense breasts may demonstrate little or no background enhancement, whereas patients with mildly dense breasts may demonstrate marked background enhancement. Nevertheless, younger patients with dense breasts are more likely to demonstrate background enhancement.

Background enhancement on MRI is analogous to density on mammography insofar as it can "obscure" suspicious possibly malignant enhancing lesions by decreasing conspicuity of enhancing cancers. In general, background enhancement is more prominent in the luteal phase of the cycle if the patient is premenopausal. Therefore, for elective examinations (ie, high-risk screening), every effort should be made to schedule the patient in the second week of her cycle (days 7 to 14) to minimize the issue of background enhancement. Despite scheduling the patient at the optimal time of her cycle, enhancement may still occur. Women in whom cancer has been diagnosed and MRI is performed for staging (ie, diagnostic) should be imaged with MRI regardless of the timing of the menstrual cycle or menstrual status.

FUTURE DIRECTIONS

As MRI becomes more integrated into practice, it will become important for centers that perform this examination to perform it at the highest level of quality so that breast cancer diagnosis will be optimized. When screening patients the goal is to detect small in situ or invasive cancer with negative nodes with an acceptable positive biopsy rate—when MRI is performed with high standards this can be achieved. There will be a voluntary accreditation process that will require high-resolution imaging be done by an experienced radiologist who will be able to offer percutaneous biopsy to the patient.

The use of breast MRI in the preoperative setting needs to be optimized. There likely are groups of patients who could greatly benefit, although the data are not yet available. To whom should we offer this test? Our algorithms for breast cancer treatment need to be examined. For example, do all patients, particularly those who demonstrate a discrete unicentric mass on MRI need to undergo a complete course of whole-breast radiation if the margins are negative and the remainder of the breast has no suspicious enhancement? Perhaps we could tailor our therapies to make the treatments more individualized and more therapeutic, decreasing morbidity and ultimately cost of treatment.

In a similar fashion, does the patient with 2 separate cancers in different quadrants require mastectomy if each is removed with negative margins and good cosmesis and there is no additional suspicious enhancement on MRI in the remainder of the breast? Perhaps more women could save their breast instead of having a mastectomy. Similarly, when there is a small recurrence in a treated breast detected on MRI, does the patient require mastectomy? Perhaps these patients could undergo complete surgical removal with negative margins and be followed with serial MRI examinations, conserving their breast.

NECESSARY FUTURE STUDIES

1. Prospective randomized trial of preoperative MRI versus no MRI measuring recurrence as end point. Effect, if any, on positive margin rates could be assessed.
2. Unifocal cancer on MRI removed surgically with negative margins and no radiation therapy versus standard radiation therapy with recurrence as end point.
3. Unifocal recurrent breast cancer treated with surgical excision alone versus standard treatment of mastectomy with recurrence as end point.

SUMMARY

Breast MRI is a well-established tool in many centers. The majority of breast MRI performed today is for high-risk screening. Other well-established indications such as occult primary breast cancer, assessment of residual disease, assessment of recurrence, and problem solving are other important uses of breast MRI. Where there is controversy is in the use of MRI for all patients with a new diagnosis of breast cancer for staging. It seems paradoxical that once the patient has been diagnosed with breast cancer, the information on MRI may lead to too many additional procedures (biopsies, follow-ups, mastectomies) that may or may not affect the outcome (positive margin rates, recurrence rates, survival) of the patient.

REFERENCES

1. Kuhl CK. Current status of breast MR imaging. Part 2. Clinical applications. *Radiology.* 2007;244:672-691.
2. Hylton NM. Vascularity assessment of breast lesions with gadolinium-enhanced MR imaging. *Magn Reson Imaging Clin N Am.* 1999;7:411-420.
3. Knopp MV, Weiss E, Sinn HP, et al. Pathophysiologic basis of contrast enhancement in breast tumors. *J Magn Reson Imaging.* 1999;10:260-266.
4. Heywang SH, Wolf A, Pruss E, et al. MR imaging of the breast with Gd-DTPA: use and limitations. *Radiology.* 1989;171:95-103.
5. Kaiser WA, Zeitler E. MR imaging of the breast: fast imaging sequences with and without Gd-DTPA. *Radiology.* 1989;170:681-686.
6. Boetes C, Strijk SP, Holland R, et al. False-negative MR imaging of malignant breast tumors. *Eur Radiol.* 1997; 7:1231-1234.
7. Orel SG, Mendonca MH, Reynolds C, et al. MR imaging of ductal carcinoma in situ. *Radiology.* 1997;202:413-420.
8. Hwang ES, Kinkel K, Esserman LJ, et al. Magnetic resonance imaging in patients diagnosed with ductal carcinoma-in-situ: value in the diagnosis of residual disease, occult invasion and multicentricity. *Ann Surg Oncol.* 2003;10:381-388.
9. Menell JH, Morris EA, Dershaw DD, et al. Determination of the presence and extent of pure ductal carcinoma in situ by mammography and magnetic resonance imaging. *Breast J.* 2005;11:382-390.
10. Raza S, Vallejo M, Chikarmane SA, Birdwell RL. Pure ductal carcinoma in situ: a range of MRI features. *AJR Am J Roentgenol.* 2008;191:689-699.
11. American College of Radiology. *Breast Imaging Reporting and Data System (BI-RADS).* Reston, VA: American College of Radiology: 2003.
12. Ikeda DM, Baker DR, Daniel BL. Magnetic resonance imaging of breast cancer: clinical indications and breast MRI reporting system. *J Magn Reson Imaging.* 2000;12(6):975-983.
13. Mann RM, Kuhl CK, Kinkel K, Boetes C. Breast MRI: guidelines from the European Society of Breast Imaging. *Eur Radiol.* 2008;18:1307-1318.
14. Saslow D, Boetes C, Burke W, et al. American Cancer Society guidelines for breast screening with MRI as an adjunct to mammography. *CA Cancer J Clin.* 2007;57:75-89.
15. Kolb TM, Lichy J, Newhouse JH. Occult cancer in women with dense breasts: detection with screening US-diagnostic yield and tumor characteristics. *Radiology.* 1998;207:191-199.
16. Kuhl CK, Schmutzler RK, Leutner CC, et al. Breast MR imaging screening in 192 women proved or suspected to be carriers of a breast cancer susceptibility gene: preliminary results. *Radiology.* 2000;215:267-279.

17. Warner E, Plewes DB, Shumak RS, et al. Comparison of breast magnetic resonance imaging, mammography, and ultrasound for surveillance of women at high risk for hereditary breast cancer. *J Clin Oncol.* 2001;19:3524-3531.

18. Podo F, Sardanelli F, Canese R, et al. The Italian multi-centre project on evaluation of MRI and other imaging modalities in early detection of breast cancer in subjects at high genetic risk. *J Exp Clin Cancer Res.* 2002;21:115-124.

19. Morris EA, Liberman L, Ballon DJ, et al. MRI of occult breast carcinoma in a high-risk population. *AJR Am J Roentgenol.* 2003;181:619-626.

20. Kuhl CK, Schrading S, Leutner CC, et al. Mammography, breast ultrasound, and magnetic resonance imaging for surveillance of women at high familial risk for breast cancer. *J Clin Oncol.* 2005;23:8469-8476.

21. Kriege M, Brekelmans CT, Boetes C, et al; Magnetic Resonance Imaging Screening Study Group. Efficacy of MRI and mammography for breast-cancer screening in women with a familial or genetic predisposition. *N Engl J Med.* 2004;351:427-437.

22. Lehman CD, Blume JD, Weatherall P, et al; International Breast MRI Consortium Working Group. Screening women at high risk for breast cancer with mammography and magnetic resonance imaging. *Cancer.* 2005;203:1898-1905.

23. Leach MO, Boggis CR, Dixon AK, et al; MARIBS Study Group. Screening with magnetic resonance imaging and mammography of a UK population at high familial risk of breast cancer: a prospective multicentre cohort study (MARIBS). *Lancet.* 2005;365:1769-1778.

24. Basu SK, Schwartz C, Fisher SG, et al. Unilateral and bilateral breast cancer in women surviving pediatric Hodgkin's disease. *Int J Radiat Oncol Biol Phys.* 2008;72:34-40.

25. Port ER, Park A, Borgen PI, Morris E, Montgomery LL. Results of MRI screening for breast cancer in high-risk patients with LCIS and atypical hyperplasia. *Ann Surg Oncol.* 2007;14:1051-1057.

26. Boyd NF, Guo H, Martin LJ, et al. Mammographic density and the risk and detection of breast cancer. *N Engl J Med.* 2007;356:227-236.

27. Schott AF, Roubidoux MA, Helvie MA, et al. Clinical and radiologic assessment to predict breast cancer pathologic complete response to neoadjuvant chemotherapy. *Breast Cancer Res Treat.* 2005;92:231-238.

28. Bolan PJ, Nelson MT, Yee D, Garwood M. Imaging in breast cancer: magnetic resonance spectroscopy. *Breast Cancer Res.* 2005;7:149-152.

29. Hylton N. MR imaging for assessment of breast cancer response to neoadjuvant chemotherapy. *Magn Reson Imaging N Am.* 2006;14:383-389.

30. Partridge SC, Gibbs JE, Lu Y, et al. MRI measurements of breast tumor volume predict response to neoadjuvant chemotherapy and recurrence-free survival. *AJR Am J Roentgenol.* 2005;184:1774-1781.

31. Bartella L, Morris EA, Dershaw DD, et al. Proton MR spectroscopy with choline peak as malignancy marker improves positive predictive value for breast cancer diagnosis: Preliminary study. *Radiology.* 2006;239:686-692.

32. Meisamy S, Bolan PJ, Baker EH, et al. Neoadjuvant chemotherapy of locally advanced breast cancer: predicting response with in vivo (1) H MR spectroscopy—a pilot study at 4T. *Radiology.* 2004;233:424-431.

33. Orel SG, Reynolds C, Schnall MD, et al. Breast carcinoma: MR imaging before re-excisional biopsy. *Radiology.* 1997;205:429-436.

34. Frei K, Kinkel K, Bonel HM, et al. MR Imaging of the breast in patients with positive margins after lumpectomy: influence of the time interval between lumpectomy and MR imaging. *AJR Am J Roentgenol.* 2000; 175:1577-1584.

35. Preda L, Villa G, Rizzo S, et al. Magnetic resonance mammography in the evaluation of recurrence at the prior lumpectomy site after conservative surgery and radiotherapy. *Breast Cancer Res.* 2006;8:R53.

36. Morris EA, Schwartz LH, Dershaw DD, et al. MR imaging of the breast in patients with occult primary breast cancer. *Radiology.* 1997;205:437-440.

37. Orel SG, Weinstein SP, Schnall MD, et al. Breast imaging in patients with axillary node metastases and unknown primary malignancy. *Radiology.* 1999;212:543-549.

38. Houssami N, Ciatto S, Macaskill P, et al. Accuracy and surgical impact of magnetic resonance imaging in breast cancer staging: systematic review and meta-analysis in detection of multifocal and multicentric cancer. *J Clin Oncol.* 2008;29:3248-3258.

39. Berg WA, Gutierrez L, NessAiver MS, et al. Diagnostic accuracy of mammography, clinical examination, US, and MR imaging in preoperative assessment of breast cancer. *Radiology.* 2004;233:830-849.

40. Van Goethem M, Schelfout K, Dijckmans L, et al. MR mammography in the preoperative staging of breast cancer in patients with dense breast tissue: comparison with mammography and ultrasound. *Eur Radiol.* 2004;14:809-816.

41. Liberman L, Morris EA, Dershaw DD, Abramson AF, Tan LK. MR imaging of the ipsilateral breast in women with percutaneously proven breast cancer. *AJR Am J Roentgenol.* 2003;180:901-910.

42. Sardanelli F, Giuseppetti GM, Panizza P, et al; Italian Trial for Breast MR in Multifocal/Multicentric Cancer. Sensitivity of MRI versus mammography for detecting foci of multifocal, multicentric breast cancer in fatty and dense breasts using whole breast pathologic examination as a gold standard. *AJR Am J Roentgenol.* 2004;183:1149-1157.

43. Bedrosian I, Mick R, Orel SG, et al. Changes in the surgical management of patients with breast carcinoma based on preoperative magnetic resonance imaging. *Cancer.* 2003;98:468-473.

44. Esserman L, Hylton N, Yassa L, et al. Utility of magnetic resonance imaging in the management of breast cancer: evidence for improved preoperative staging. *J Clin Oncol.* 1999;17:110-119.

45. Bilimoria KY, Cambic A, Hansen NM, Bethke KP. Evaluating the impact of preoperative breast magnetic resonance imaging on the surgical management of newly diagnosed breast cancers. *Arch Surg.* 2007;142:441-445.

46. Morrow M. Magnetic resonance imaging in the cancer patient: Curb your enthusiasm. *J Clin Oncol.* 2008;26:352-353.

47. Schnall M. MR imaging evaluation of cancer extent: is there clinical relevance? *Magn Reson Imaging N Am.* 2006;14:379-381.

48. Kuhl CK, Kuhn W, Braun M, Schild H. Pre-operative staging of breast cancer with breast MRI: one step forward, two steps back? *Breast.* 2007;16:34-44.

49. Solin LJ, Orel SG, Hwang WT, Haris EE, Schnall MD. Relationship of breast magnetic resonance imaging to outcome after breast-conservation treatment with radiation for women with early stage invasive breast carcinoma or ductal carcinoma in situ. *J Clin Oncol.* 2008;26:386-391.

50. Lehman CD, Gatsonis C, Kuhl CK, et al; ACRIN Trial 6667 Investigators Group. MRI evaluation of the contralateral breast in women with recently diagnosed breast cancer. *N Engl J Med.* 2007;356:1295-1303.

51. Liberman L, Morris EA, Kim CM, et al. MR imaging findings in the contralateral breast of women with recently diagnosed breast cancer. *AJR Am J Roentgenol.* 2003;180:333-341.

52. Lee SG, Orel SG, Woo IJ, et al. MR imaging screening of the contralateral breast in patients with newly diagnosed breast cancer: preliminary results. *Radiology.* 2003;226:773-778.

53. Wallace AM, Daniel BL, Jeffrey SS, et al. Rates of reexcision for breast cancer after magnetic resonance imaging-guided bracket wire localization. *J Am Surg Coll.* 2005;200:527-537.

54. Liberman L, Bracero N, Morris E. Thornton C, Dershaw DD. MRI-guided 9-gauge vacuum assisted breast biopsy: initial clinical experience. *AJR Am J Roentgenol.* 2005;185:183-193.

55. Friedman P, Sanders L, Russo J, et al. Detection and localization of occult lesions using breast magnetic resonance imaging: initial experience in a community hospital. *Acad Radiol.* 2005;12:728-738.

56. Kuhl CK, Bieling HB, Gieseke J, et al. Healthy premenopausal breast parenchyma in dynamic contrast-enhanced MR imaging of the breast: normal contrast medium enhancement and cyclical phase dependency. *Radiology.* 1997;203:137-144.

CHAPTER 36

Systemic Staging and the Radiologic Work-Up of Abnormal Findings

Tanya W. Stephens
Eleni Andreopoulou

Despite important therapeutic innovations within the past several years, the odds of patients with metastatic breast cancer achieving complete response remain extremely low. Judiciously applied multiple endocrine, chemotherapeutic, or biologic therapies attempt to induce a series of remissions and ultimately adequate palliation. Patients with localized breast or chest wall recurrences, however, may be long-term survivors with appropriate therapy. At present, there is a lack of both a consensus management algorithm and an ideal treatment model of specific subsets of women. Before treatment selection for recurrent or metastatic cancer, restaging to evaluate extent of disease is indicated. In the absence of symptomatic disease, the usefulness of a routine diagnostic work-up is not evidence-based. Diagnostic tests and staging procedures are directed by the organ sites most frequently involved in metastatic breast cancer and by patient signs and symptoms. Documentation of initial metastatic sites is helpful in treatment planning and in later assessment of response to treatment. Over the past 45 years, the American Joint Committee on Cancer has regularly updated its staging standards to incorporate advances in prognostic technology.[1,2] However, until the development of prognostic indices based on molecular markers are incorporated, Tumor-Node-Metastasis (TNM) staging continues to quantify only the physical extent of the disease. Anatomic staging continues to play a major role in guiding treatment decisions. Clinical decision-making still involves a number of patient and tumor characteristics.[3-5] Pretreatment prognostic (measures of tumor burden or hormonal receptor status) and predictive factors (hormonal receptor and HER-2/neu status) are considered in order to select a therapy most likely to benefit patients.[6]

Given the biologic heterogeneity of the disease in primary and metastatic settings, the potential for continued mutation, and the variety of treatment options available, the information obtained at the initial diagnosis of breast cancer may not be as relevant to planning the treatment for recurrence in women who have recurrent metastatic breast cancer years after their initial diagnosis. Appropriate risk and biologic stratification in breast cancer will offer the unique opportunity for development of more effectively tailored targeted therapies.

HISTORY AND PHYSICAL EXAMINATION

Obtaining a comprehensive *history* is essential to provide pertinent information of primary diagnosis, treatment management, toxicity complications, and interval period to disease recurrence. Comorbidity, current medications, allergies, and menopause status is important for management planning and treatment selection. There is a great heterogeneity in the clinical presentation of metastatic breast cancer. Certain characteristics can be used to predict favorable clinical course, including long disease-free interval, hormone receptor positivity, response to prior endocrine therapy or chemotherapy, single site of metastases, and lack of liver, parenchymal lung, or central nervous system involvement. Early failure (< 6 months) on hormone therapy suggests that cytotoxic chemotherapy should be the next modality employed.

In metastatic breast cancer, maintenance of quality of life and elimination of cancer-related symptoms is the major objective. Patients with estrogen receptor–positive tumors are especially unlikely to suffer recurrence initially in the brain or liver. Routine brain and liver imaging procedures are expensive and are not indicated in the absence of symptoms, physical findings, or laboratory values suggesting involvement.

Physical examination should focus on the detection of metastases on the chest wall, skin, remaining breast, regional and distant lymph nodes, axial skeleton, lungs, liver, and central nervous system. One-third of patients with recurrent breast cancer present initially with local recurrence involving regional lymph nodes or the chest wall, with the diagnosis of recurrence made on clinical examination with subsequent biopsy confirmation. Local chest wall recurrence after mastectomy is usually the harbinger of widespread disease. In a subset of patients, it may be the only site of recurrence and surgery and/or radiation therapy may be curative. Patients with chest wall recurrences of less than 3 cm, axillary and internal mammary node recurrence (not supraclavicular, which has a poorer survival), and a greater than 2-year disease-free interval before recurrence have the best chance for prolonged survival.[7-10]

LABORATORY TESTS

Laboratory evaluation should include a complete blood count, a platelet count, serum calcium, and liver and renal function studies.

NATIONAL COMPREHENSIVE CANCER NETWORK IMAGING GUIDELINES

A complete diagnostic imaging evaluation is a major component of the staging workup of breast cancer patients. Imaging determines the extent of disease (tumor size, multifocality, multicentricity) in the breast(s), excludes or identifies additional areas of malignancy in the contralateral breast, and excludes or identifies nodal involvement and/or distant metastases.

The National Comprehensive Cancer Network (NCCN) provides guidelines for the imaging staging workup of breast cancer patients.[11] In general practice, a diagnostic bilateral mammogram is required for the workup of stages 0 to IV. By excluding axillary nodal metastases, ultrasound and ultrasound-guided biopsy of indeterminate lymph nodes will support the diagnosis of stage I disease and will evaluate the extent of regional nodal involvement in stages II to IV. Ultrasound and magnetic resonance imaging (MRI) will exclude stage IIB and IIIA disease and confirm stage IIIB disease with the exclusion or identification of skin and chest wall involvement.

Bone scans, chest x-rays, and abdominal ultrasound, computed tomography (CT), or MRI are generally recommended only in the presence of symptoms for patients with stage I, II, and IIIA breast cancer and for patients who present with stage IIIB or IIIC disease with or without the presence of symptoms. The diagnosis of stage IV disease will be supported by plain films of the chest and axial skeleton; bone scans; chest CT or MRI; abdominal ultrasound, CT, or MRI; and/or pelvis ultrasound, CT, or MRI and biopsy confirmation that suspicious findings represent distant metastases. In spite of these formal recommendations from the NCCN, many surgeons and oncologists consider and perform systemic imaging, often positron emission tomography (PET)/CT, abdominal and chest CT, for patients with node-positive, stage II or greater extent of disease. The necessity of these tests is a subject of debate, and current guidelines should be discussed within the multidisciplinary group in which the patient is treated. Additionally, many systemic therapy clinical trials may have specific criteria for staging patients before initiation of therapy.

IMAGING WORKUP OF ABNORMAL FINDINGS

Mammography

Mammography is the backbone imaging modality of breast cancer staging and is most commonly the first test that is interpreted. With consultations, the radiologist must review all prior imaging studies from outside institution(s) and determine whether the submitted images are adequate to make an appropriate diagnosis. If inadequate, the images must be repeated. The radiologist must also determine whether additional imaging studies are needed. In the case of a suspected incomplete or unsuccessful excision, residual calcifications and mass lesions will be noted on mammography. Ultrasound and MRI are helpful in the evaluation of residual mammographically occult uncalcified tumor.

In general, mammography (or any imaging study) cannot completely exclude cancer, but mammography is consistently able to detect unsuspected breast cancer, even in women whose clinically suspicious finding is proven benign.[12] All findings must be adequately imaged and thoroughly documented in the radiology report. The 9 o'clock position or location and the distance from the nipple of the suspicious finding(s) are recorded. If multiple suspicious findings are noted, then percutaneous biopsies are performed to determine multifocality or multicentricity. Any secondary signs of malignancy are recorded. With suspicious calcifications, the full extent of the calcifications is assessed, which includes measuring the volume of calcifications and the distance from the calcifications to the closest overlying skin margin and to the nipple (Fig. 36-1). A large volume of calcifications may prohibit breast conservation. Completely documented mammogram findings can then be correlated with findings seen on additional imaging studies.

Ultrasound

Ultrasound is used in the evaluation of mammographically occult uncalcified tumor, mammographically identifiable tumor, the evaluation of palpable masses, and to thoroughly evaluate the regional nodal basins. A good routine breast ultrasound study includes evaluation of the whole breast and the infraclavicular, axillary, and internal mammary nodal regions. If indeterminate or suspicious infraclavicular lymph nodes are identified, the supraclavicular nodal region should be scanned. All sonographic findings are correlated with all mammographic findings and other findings seen on additional imaging studies. Suspicious masses and the highest level lymph nodes are biopsied.

Metastatic involvement of regional nodes is an important prognostic parameter. The presence or absence of axillary metastases is the strongest prognostic indicator available for breast cancer.[13-15] Although no imaging method can detect or exclude microscopic metastases, a positive diagnosis obtained with cytologic or histologic confirmation is quite reliable and

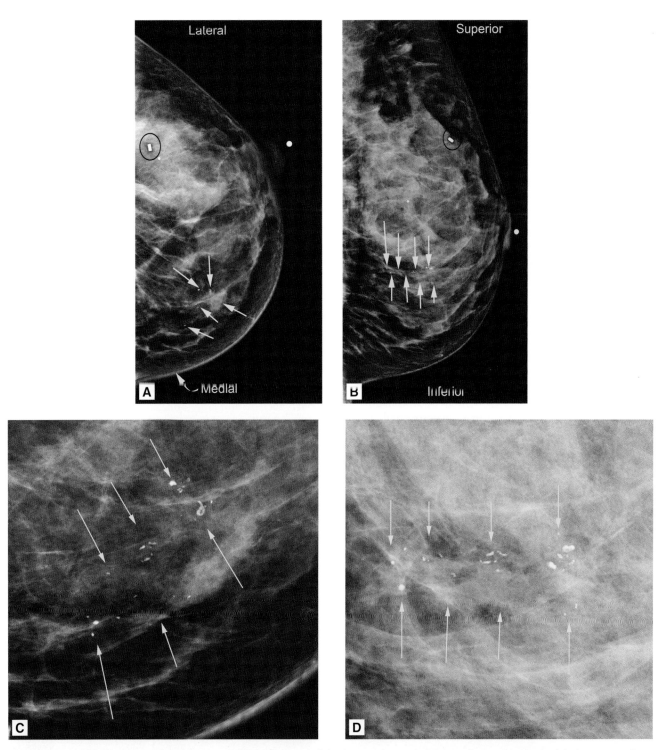

FIGURE 36-1 **(A)** Cranial-caudal (CC) view and **(B)** lateral-medial (LM) view show calcifications *(arrows)* in the 9 o'clock position of the left breast located 5 cm from the nipple. The approximate volume of calcifications is 1.8 cm (LM measurement) × 1.7 cm (anterior-posterior measurement) × 1 cm (superior-inferior measurement). The medial skin margin is closest *(curved arrow)*. The circle annotates a marker clip that denotes a prior benign biopsy. **(C)** CC magnification view and **(D)** LM magnification view characterize the calcifications *(arrows)* as heterogeneous, warranting biopsy.

can be used to influence treatment decisions. Some sonographic features that favor benignity include lymph nodes that are predominantly hyperechoic, the presence of a thin homogeneous symmetrical cortical rim around the hyperechoic hilar fat (Fig. 36-2), and symmetric cortical lobulations similar to

contralateral axillary lymph nodes.[16] Suspicious or metastatic-appearing sonographic features would include thickening or eccentric lobulation of the hypoechoic cortical rim, compression or displacement of the fatty hyperechoic hilum, and/or complete replacement of the hilar fat by hypoechoic tissue (Fig. 36-3).[16]

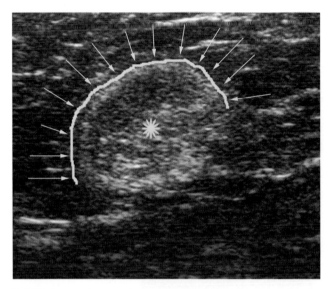

FIGURE 36-2 Ultrasound of a normal lymph node with a thin cortical rim *(arrows)* and hyperechoic *(bright)* hilar fat *(asterisk)*.

Fine needle aspiration of indeterminate, suspicious, or metastatic-appearing lymph nodes (Fig. 36-4) can provide a more definitive diagnosis than ultrasound alone. Krishnamurthy et al[4] found that the overall sensitivity of ultrasound-guided fine-needle aspiration was 86.4%, the specificity was 100%, the diagnostic accuracy was 79%, the positive predictive value was 100%, and the negative predictive value was 67%. Bedrosian et al[17] reported a sensitivity of 25% and specificity of 100%. Overall, suspicious or indeterminate lymph nodes were more likely to contain metastases at final pathology than benign-appearing lymph nodes.[17] Core biopsy of indeterminate, suspicious, or metastatic-appearing lymph nodes may also be done, particularly when dedicated cytopathology is unavailable. In the case of core biopsy of axillary lymph nodes, the imager must be careful to avoid the axillary vasculature.

Berg et al[18] found that in women with increased risk for breast cancer, adding a screening ultrasound examination to routine mammography revealed 28% more cancers than with mammography alone. However, the additional ultrasound

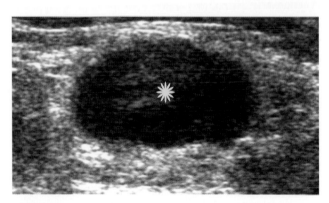

FIGURE 36-3 Ultrasound of a malignant-appearing lymph node with complete replacement of the hilar fat by hypoechoic *(dark)* tissue *(asterisk)*.

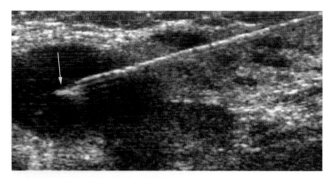

FIGURE 36-4 Ultrasound-guided fine-needle aspiration of a malignant-appearing lymph node with a 21-gauge needle *(arrow)*.

examination substantially increased the rates of false-positive findings and unnecessary biopsies.[18]

Magnetic Resonance Imaging

Although MRI is a valuable imaging tool with the ability to detect occult multifocal (Fig. 36-5) and multicentric malignancies, there is no consensus on whether the detection of additional foci within the affected breast improves patient outcomes.[18-21]

This scholarly evaluation of the use and role of MRI in breast cancer staging was initiated in part to the results of one of the first large series describing the surgical management of breast cancer patients on the basis of preoperative MRI. In this study, the rate of conversion to mastectomy exceeded the reported local recurrence rates after breast conservation.[22]

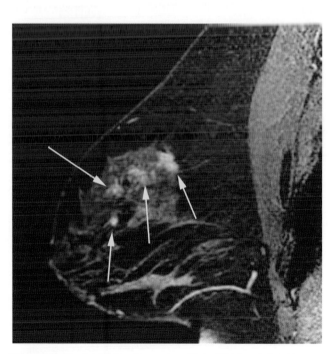

FIGURE 36-5 Contrast-enhanced sagittal MRI image shows multifocal malignancies *(arrows)*.

Although the controversy continues, it is clear that MRI often identifies more extensive disease than may be detected using conventional imaging. Also, the ability of MRI to detect contralateral malignancy may be more straightforward, as treatment for unilateral malignancy is not appropriate for patients with synchronous malignancies.

The results of the multi-institutional American College of Radiology Imaging Network (ACRIN) Trial 6667 reported a 3.1% probability of discovering occult contralateral cancer missed by clinical examination and mammography with preoperative staging with MRI.[23] The detection of these cancers was not influenced by breast density, menopausal status, or the histologic features of the primary cancer. Clearly the detection of contralateral invasive cancer or ductal carcinoma in situ can reduce the total number of treatments.

It should be noted that the negative predictive value of MRI was extremely high in the population studied in ACRIN Trial 6667. The risk of detecting an occult cancer in the contralateral breast 1 year after a negative MRI was estimated at 0.3%, and all the cancers detected at 1 year were ductal carcinoma in situ measuring 4 mm or less in diameter.[23] This information can give patients with unilateral cancer greater confidence in choosing breast conservation over bilateral mastectomies.

Benign and malignant lesions can have overlapping postcontrast MRI enhancement morphology and kinetic patterns. This overlap leads to additional biopsies and increased patient anxiety. MRI-ultrasound correlation with second-look ultrasound aids the dismissal of benign findings and allows for ultrasound-guided biopsy of indeterminate or suspicious lesions. Suspicious MRI findings without an identifiable correlate on second-look ultrasound must be biopsied using MRI guidance. Breast cancer staging with MRI should not be performed in settings without access to MRI-guided biopsies.

MRI provides an accurate characterization of the size and extent of tumor, which can reduce the rates of positive margins and the number of reexcisions after breast-conserving surgery. Complete excision eliminates recurrence secondary to residual disease. MRI can assess disease extent in patients with posterior breast masses who are suspected to have tumor invasion into the underlying musculature. Involvement of the pectoralis muscles and the serratus and intercostal muscles (chest wall) is well delineated due the anatomic detail demonstrated by MRI.[24] Extension of adjacent tumor into underlying musculature is indicated by abnormal muscle enhancement. Violation of the fat plane between tumor and muscle, without other findings, is not indicative of tumor involvement.[24] Knowledge of the size and extent of tumor and tumor invasion into the underlying musculature improves patient selection for breast conservation.

18F-Fluorodeoxyglucose Positron Emission Tomography/Computed Tomography

The information provided by mammography, ultrasound, CT, and MRI is structural, whereas the information provided by 18F-fluorodeoxyglucose (FDG)–PET is functional, reflecting the degree of metabolic activity of the malignancy.[25] Increased tumor uptake of 18F-FDG reflects elevated glucose consumption by tumor cells, evidenced by the overexpression of glucose

transporter proteins at the surface of the cells and increased levels of active hexokinase demonstrated in many tumors.[26,27] The degree of tumor 18F-FDG uptake is expressed with the use of a semiquantitative measure, the standardized uptake value (SUV).[27]

The limited anatomical information obtained from 18F-FDG PET alone can cause inconclusive interpretations or mislocalization of disease (Fig. 36-6A). The CT portion of 18F-FDG PET/CT provides anatomical mapping images for PET. Thus 18F-FDG PET/CT provides PET, CT, and high-quality fused imaging of both function and anatomy at the same location of the body (Figs. 36-6B and 36-6C).[28] This imaging modality, as a noninvasive, all-in-one technique, has been reported to be useful in whole-body staging, restaging, and monitoring of treatment response in breast cancer patients.[29-31] The primary role of 18F-FDG PET/CT has been for the evaluation of distant metastasis; however, its impact on the assessment of primary breast lesions and of the axilla for nodal metastases not been validated in larger cohorts.[31]

Given the ease of ultrasound-guided biopsies, abnormal SUVs suspicious for axillary nodal metastases may be best evaluated and biopsied using sonography. Abnormal SUVs suspicious for liver metastases may biopsied with sonography or CT. Correlation with plain films and/or MRI is imperative for SUVs suspicious for skeletal metastases, and biopsies of suspicious findings may be performed using CT or MRI.

Other routine perioperative studies include chest x-ray, bone scan, and abdominal CT. This practice in asymptomatic patients with newly diagnosed breast cancer has been challenged because these tests uncommonly yield positive results.

Chest X-Ray

NCCN guidelines regarding chest x-ray are discussed in the following section. The lungs are not as common a site as bone for breast metastases but are routinely evaluated in the staging of breast cancer. Any suspicious findings noted on chest x-ray will require further evaluation with chest CT, and metastatic disease can be confirmed with biopsy (Fig. 36-7). Additionally, the chest x-ray is used to evaluate the cardiopulmonary status of the patient for the anesthesiologist's workup.

Technetium-99m Radionuclide Bone Scans

Technetium-99m radionuclide bone scans are used in the evaluation of skeletal metastases and are indicated if localized symptoms are present or in the case of elevated alkaline phosphatase.[11] Sensitivity rates as high as 98% have been reported.[32] Bone scans can also detect benign processes such as degenerative joint disease, and false-positive rates have ranged from 10% to 22%.[33] The false-negative rate is about 10%.[24] Bone scans (Fig. 36-8A) are best interpreted in conjunction with plain film images of the skeleton (Fig. 36-8B). Equivocal findings suggestive of skeletal metastases will require additional evaluation with MRI and biopsy confirmation.

Abdominal Computed Tomography

The liver is one the most common sites of metastatic spread of epithelial cancers, second only to regional lymph nodes.[34] Contrast-enhanced abdominal CT is superior to liver ultrasound

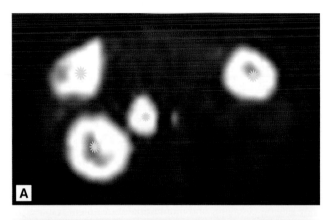

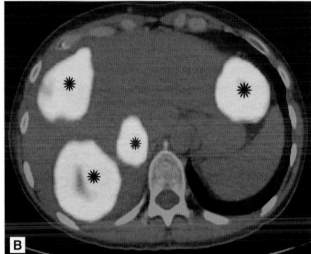

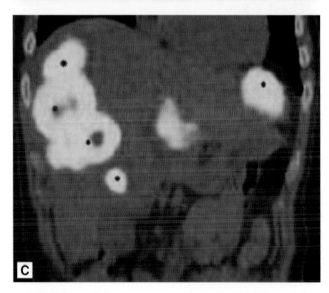

FIGURE 36-6 **(A)** PET shows metastases *(asterisks)* but provides limited anatomical information, whereas **(B)** axial PET/CT and **(C)** coronal PET/CT views provide high-quality fused imaging of both function and anatomy at the same location of the body.

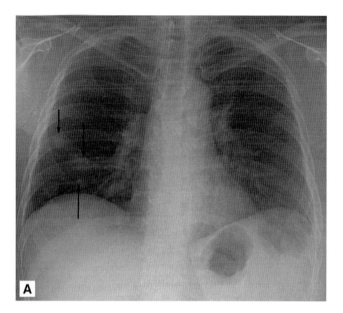

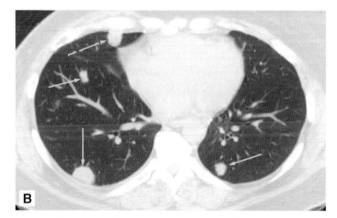

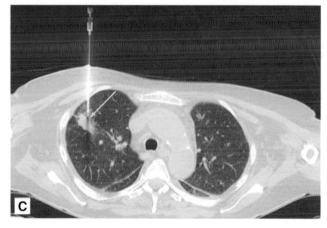

FIGURE 36-7 **A.** Chest x-ray shows pulmonary nodules *(arrows)* suggestive of metastases. **B.** Chest CT further evaluates the nodules *(arrows)*. **C.** Needle biopsy of a nodule *(arrow)* using CT guidance.

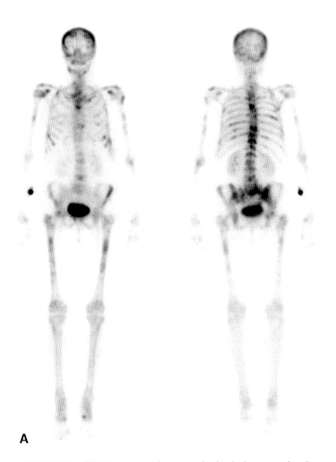
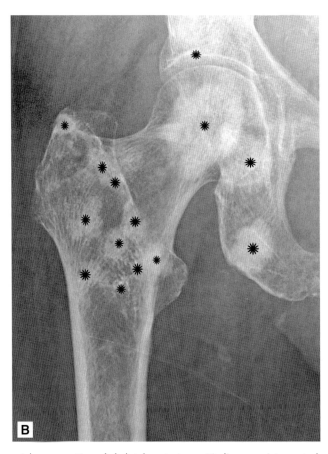

A

B

FIGURE 36-8 **(A)** Bone scan shows multiple dark areas of radiotracer uptake suggestive of skeletal metastases. Findings are interpreted in conjunction with a **(B)** plain film of the right hip, which confirms skeletal metastases *(asterisks)*.

in the evaluation of the liver for liver metastases (Fig. 36-9). The detection of liver lesions on ultrasound is limited due to similar echogenicities of liver metastases and the surrounding liver. Although the majority of liver metastases have a target appearance on CT or appear as an area of low attenuation during the portal venous phase of contrast enhancement, liver metastases may have a varied spectrum of appearances on CT.[35] Metastases are confirmed with percutaneous biopsy.

BIOPSY

Patients with previous diagnosis of breast cancer who present with findings suspicious for recurrent metastatic disease should be strongly considered for diagnostic biopsy. Although in the majority of cases the presentation of metastases is almost certain to be related to breast cancer spread, careful history taking and physical examination may suggest that other primary sites could be responsible for such findings, especially if there has been a long disease-free interval. Certain presentations that suggest metastases justify tissue diagnosis to exclude another cause of malignancy, including isolated lung lesions and isolated liver and central nervous system lesions.

Cytologic or histologic documentation of recurrent or metastatic disease should be obtained whenever possible to redetermine hormone receptor and HER-2/neu status. Estrogen

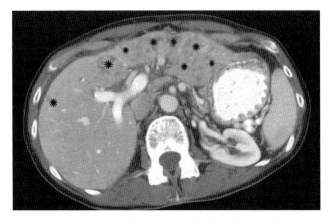

FIGURE 36-9 Abdominal CT shows multiple enhancing liver metastases *(asterisks)*.

receptor and progesterone receptor status enables appropriate identification of patients most likely to benefit from endocrine forms of therapy in the metastatic disease setting.

Given the predictive importance of hormone receptors and HER-2, it is currently recommended that they should be determined as part of diagnostic routine on every primary tumor.

HER-2 amplification, overexpression, and the presence of HER-2 extracellular domain are generally associated with poorer prognosis.[36] Although the use of HER-2 to determine prognosis is not recommended, high levels of tissue HER-2 expression or HER-2 gene amplification principally indicates for anti-HER-2–based therapy. However, changes in receptor status over the course of disease progression have been described.[37-42] Several studies have addressed the issue of concordance/discordance in expression of individual receptors between primary tumor and tumor recurrence/metastases, with discordance rates varying substantially from study to study. In a single small study by the Cancer and Leukemia Group B, 36% of hormone receptor–positive tumors were found to be receptor negative in biopsy specimens isolated at the time of recurrence.[43]

SERUM MARKERS

Serial monitoring of levels of tumor markers such as carcinoembryonic antigen (CEA), CA 15-3, and CA 27-29 may be helpful in assessing systemic treatment efficacy in the metastatic setting.[44] Prior studies suggested that levels of classic serum markers such as antibodies to epithelial MUC are related to tumor burden. However, the clinical utility of serum markers in predicting prognosis and monitoring treatment still remains controversial. CA 15-3 and CA 27-29 are well-characterized assays that allow the detection of circulating MUC-1 antigen in peripheral blood and are used as surrogate markers for breast cancer. CEA levels are less commonly elevated than are levels of the MUC-1 assays, with CEA levels minimally complementary to MUC-1 levels. These markers can be used in conjunction with diagnostic imaging, history, and physical examination. Present data are insufficient to recommend the use of these markers alone for monitoring response to treatment, but in the absence of readily measurable disease, an increasing marker may be used to indicate treatment failure.

Optimal monitoring of bone lesions during therapy should include symptoms, tumor markers (CA 27-29, CA 15-3, CEA), and radiographs or MRI of the involved areas.

BASELINE MULTIPLE-GATED ACQUISITION SCAN/ECHOCARDIOGRAM EVALUATION

The potential for doxorubicin-induced cardiotoxicity should be considered in the selection of chemotherapeutic regimens for an individual patient. Recognized risk factors for cardiac toxicity include advanced age, prior chest wall radiation therapy, prior anthracycline exposure, hypertension, diabetes, and known underlying heart disease.

FUTURE DIRECTIONS

As traditional approaches are confounded by inaccuracies and limitations, simpler, more effective means of staging are needed to allow optimal management of individual patients and to serve as surrogate measure of activity for novel therapies.

Future studies are needed to develop sonographic and MRI criteria that more accurately distinguish between benign and malignant findings. This would substantially decrease the rates of false-positive findings and unnecessary biopsies. Studies are also needed to determine which groups of patients would benefit most from preoperative staging with MRI and to determine the clinical significance of multicentricity noted on MRI.

Advances in technology have facilitated the detection of even very small numbers of circulating tumor cells in the peripheral blood of cancer patients. The demonstration of the prognostic implication of circulating tumor cells in patients with both localized and metastatic breast cancer raises the possibility that this method will modify the existing staging system by providing a true biologic staging of breast cancer.[45-48] Important questions about the biological characteristics of these cells and the reasons for the reduced capacity of systemic treatment to arrest or eradicate the cancer need to be answered to advance the field and increase cure rates.

SUMMARY

The workup of abnormal findings in breast cancer patients is directed by the organ sites most commonly involved in metastatic breast cancer and by patient signs and symptoms. Careful documentation of initial metastases directs treatment planning and will guide assessment of response to therapy. The components of the workup include history and physical examination, laboratory tests, imaging, biopsy of suspicious finding, monitoring serum markers, and obtaining a baseline multiple-gated acquisition scan/echocardiogram evaluation.

REFERENCES

1. International Union Against Cancer (UICC). *TNM Classification of Malignant Tumours.* 1st ed. Geneva, Switzerland: UICC: 1968.
2. Greene FL, Fritz AG, Winchester DP, eds. *AJCC Cancer Staging Manual.* 6th ed. New York, NY: Springer: 2002.
3. Swenerton KD, Legha SS, Smith T, et al. Prognostic factors in metastatic breast cancer treated with combination chemotherapy. *Cancer Res.* 1979;39:1552-1562.
4. Hortobagyi GN, Smith TL, Legha SS, et al. Multivariate analysis of prognostic factors in metastatic breast cancer. *J Clin Oncol.* 1983;1:776-786.
5. Kataja V, Castiglione M. Locally recurrent or metastatic breast cancer: ESMO clinical recommendations for diagnosis, treatment and follow-up. *Ann Oncol.* 2008;19(suppl 2):ii11-ii13.
6. Andreopoulou E, Hortobagyi GN. Prognostic factors in metastatic breast cancer: successes and challenges toward individualized therapy. *J Clin Oncol.* 2008;26:3660-3662.
7. Al-Husaini H, Amir E, Fitzgerald B, et al. Prevalence of overt metastases in locally advanced breast cancer. *Clin Oncol (R Coll Radiol).* 2008;20:340-344.
8. Schneider C, Fehr MK, Steiner RA, et al. Frequency and distribution pattern of distant metastases in breast cancer patients at the time of primary presentation. *Arch Gynecol Obstet.* 2003;269:9-12.
9. Bafford AC, Burstein HJ, Barkley CR, et al. Breast surgery in stage IV breast cancer: impact of staging and patient selection on overall survival. *Breast Cancer Res Treat.* 2009;115:7-12.
10. Clarke M, Collins R, Darby S, et al. Early Breast Cancer Trialists' Collaborative Group (EBCTCG). Effects of radiotherapy and of differences in the extent of surgery for early breast cancer on local recurrence and 15-year survival: an overview of the randomised trials. *Lancet.* 2005;366:2087-2106.
11. National Comprehensive Cancer Network (NCCN): Clinical Practice Guidelines in Oncology, Breast Cancer. Available at: http://www.nccn.org Fort Washington, PA. Accessed November 21, 2008.

12. Kopans DB, Meyer JE, Cohen AM, et al. Palpable breast masses: the importance of preoperative mammography. *JAMA*. 1981;246:2819-2822.

13. Adair F, Berg J, Joubert J, et al. Long-term follow-up of breast cancer patients: the 30-year report. *Cancer*. 1974;33:1145-1150.

14. Veronesi U, Galimberti V, Zurrida S, et al. Prognostic significance of number and level of axillary node metastases in breast cancer. *Breast*. 1993;2:224-228.

15. Krishnamurthy S, Sneige N, Bedi DG, et al. Role of ultrasound-guided fine-needle aspiration of indeterminate and suspicious axillary lymph nodes in the initial staging of breast carcinoma. *Cancer*. 2002;95:982-988.

16. Krishnamurthy R, Bedi DG, Krishnamurthy S, et al. Ultrasound of axillary lymph nodes: classification based on cortical morphology. *Radiology*. 2001;21(suppl P):646.

17. Bedrosian I, Bedi D, Kuerer HM, et al. Impact of clinicopathological factors on sensitivity of axillary ultrasonography in the detection of axillary nodal metastases in patients with breast cancer. *Ann Surg Oncol*. 2003;10:1025-1030.

18. Berg WA, Blume JD, Cormack JB, et al. Combined screening with ultrasound and mammography vs mammography alone in women at elevated risk of breast cancer. *JAMA*. 2008;299:2151-2163.

19. Morrow M, Freedman G. A clinical oncology perspective on the use of breast MR. *Magn Reson Imaging Clin N Am*. 2006;14:363-378.

20. Hillman BJ. Do we need randomized controlled clinical trials to evaluate the clinical impact of breast MR imaging? *Magn Reson Imaging Clin N Am*. 2006;14:403-409.

21. Houssami N, Ciatto S, Macaskill P, et al. Accuracy and surgical impact of magnetic resonance imaging in breast cancer staging: systematic review and meta-analysis in detection of multifocal and multicentric cancer. *J Clin Oncol*. 2008;26:3248-3258.

22. Bedrosian I, Mick R, Orel SG, et al. Changes in the surgical management of patients with breast carcinoma based on preoperative magnetic resonance imaging. *Cancer*. 2003;98:468-473.

23. Lehman CD, Gatsonis C, Kuhl CK, et al. MRI evaluation of the contralateral breast in women with recently diagnosed breast cancer. *N Engl J Med*. 2007;356:1295-1303.

24. Morris EA, Schwartz LH, Drotman MB, et al. Evaluation of pectoralis major muscle in patients with posterior breast tumors on breast MR images: early experience. *Radiology*. 2000;214:67-72.

25. Cermik TF, Mavi A, Basu S, et al. Impact of FDG PET on the preoperative staging of newly diagnosed breast cancer. *Eur J Nucl Med Mod Imaging*. 2008;35:475-483.

26. Bos R, van Der Hoeven JJ, van Der Wall E, et al. Biologic correlates of (18)fluorodeoxyglucose uptake in human breast cancer measured by positron emission tomography. *J Clin Oncol*. 2002;20:379-387.

27. Juweid JE, Cheson BD. Positron-emission tomography and assessment of cancer therapy. *N Engl J Med*. 2006;354:496-507.

28. Tatsumi M, Cohade C, Mourtzikos KA, et al. Initial experience with FDG-PET/CT in the evaluation of breast cancer. *Eur J Nucl Med Mol Imaging*. 2006;33:254-262.

29. Zangheri B, Messa C, Picchio M, et al. PET/CT and breast cancer. *Eur J Nucl Med Mol Imaging*. 2004;31(suppl 1):S135-S42.

30. Reddy DH, Mendelson EB. Incorporating new imaging models in breast cancer management. *Curr Treat Options Oncol*. 2005;6:135-145.

31. Heusner TA, Kuemmel S, Umutlu L, et al. Breast cancer staging in a single session: whole-body PET/CT mammography. *J Nucl Med*. 2008;49:1215-1222.

32. Meyers RE, Johnston M, Pritchard K, et al. Baseline staging tests in primary breast cancer. *CMAJ*. 2001;164:1439-1444.

33. Wikenheiser KA, Silberstein EB. Bone scintigraphy screening in stage I-II breast cancer: is it cost-effective? *Cleve Clin J Med*. 1996;63:43-47.

34. Schima W, Kulinna C, Langenberger H, et al. Liver metastases of colorectal cancer: US CT or MR? *Cancer Imaging*. 2005;5:S149-S155.

35. Roach H, Whipp E, Virjee J, et al. A pictorial review of the varied appearance of atypical liver metastasis from carcinoma of the breast. *Br J Radiol*. 2005;78:1098-1103.

36. Slamon DJ, Clark GM, Wong SG, et al. Human breast cancer: correlation of relapse and survival with amplification of the HER-2/neu oncogene. *Science*. 1987;235:177-182.

37. Li BD, Byskosh A, Molteni A, et al. Estrogen and progesterone receptor concordance between primary and recurrent breast cancer. *J Surg Oncol*. 1994;57:71-77.

38. Vincent-Salomon A, Jouve M, Genin P, et al. HER2 status in patients with breast carcinoma is not modified selectively by preoperative chemotherapy and is stable during the metastatic process. *Cancer*. 2002;94:2169-2173.

39. Simon R, Nocito A, Hübscher T, et al. Patterns of her-2/neu amplification and overexpression in primary and metastatic breast cancer. *J Natl Cancer Inst*. 2001;93:1141-1146.

40. Edgerton SM, Moore D 2nd, Merkel D, et al. erbB-2 (HER-2) and breast cancer progression. *Appl Immunohistochem Mol Morphol*. 2003;11:214-221.

41. Gancberg D, Di Leo A, Cardoso F, et al. Comparison of HER-2 status between primary breast cancer and corresponding distant metastatic sites. *Ann Oncol*. 2002;13:1036-1043.

42. Kuukasjärvi T, Kononen J, Helin H, et al. Loss of estrogen receptor in recurrent breast cancer is associated with poor response to endocrine therapy. *J Clin Oncol* 1996;14.2584-2589.

43. Perry MC, Kardinal CG, Korzun AH, et al. Chemohormonal therapy in advanced carcinoma of the breast: Cancer and Leukemia Group B protocol 8081. *J Clin Oncol*. 1987;5:1534-1545.

44. Harris L, Fritsche H, Mennel R, et al. American Society of Clinical Oncology 2007 update of recommendations for the use of tumor markers in breast cancer. *J Clin Oncol*. 2007;25:5287-5312.

45. Cristofanilli M, Budd GT, Ellis MJ, et al. Circulating tumor cells, disease progression, and survival in metastatic breast cancer. *N Engl J Med*. 2004;351:781-791.

46. Budd GT, Cristofanilli M, Ellis MJ, et al. Circulating tumor cells versus imaging—predicting overall survival in metastatic breast cancer. *Clin Cancer Res*. 2006;12:6403-6409.

47. Cristofanilli M, Broglio KR, Guarneri V, et al. Circulating tumor cells in metastatic breast cancer: biologic staging beyond tumor burden. *Clin Breast Cancer*. 2007;7:471-479.

48. Dawood S, Broglio K, Valero V, et al. Circulating tumor cells in metastatic breast cancer: from prognostic stratification to modification of the staging system? *Cancer*. 2008;113:2422-2430.

SECTION 4

LANDMARK CLINICAL TRIALS IN BREAST SURGICAL ONCOLOGY

Eleftherios P. Mamounas

CHAPTER 37

Statistical Design and Analysis of Phase III Clinical Trials

Joseph P. Costantino
Stewart Anderson
Greg Yothers

The purpose of this chapter is to describe key aspects of the design and analysis of phase III clinical trials focusing on the treatment of breast cancer. Phase III clinical trials are 1 of 5 basic hierarchical phases of human research activity designed to ascertain information regarding the biological processing, safety, and efficacy of a new treatment.[1,2] Details regarding phase III trials are provided later in the chapter. To provide a perspective from which to understand the relative importance of the type of information that is gained from a phase III clinical trial, before we begin our presentation on the design and analysis of phase III trials, we present a synopsis of all of the different phases of clinical trial research. We use the term "new treatment" as a general term to refer to the use of one or several methods for treating a disease or condition with a new surgical technique, a new medical device, or a new form of chemical, physical, or biological agent.

TYPES OF CLINICAL TRIALS

Phase 0 Trials

Phase 0 trials are a relatively newly defined type of trial involving the administration of a subtherapeutic dose of a new treatment to a single group of usually 10 to 15 human subjects. The purpose of this type of trial is to determine early in the development process if a new treatment has the pharmacokinetic and pharmacodynamic properties in humans as would be anticipated from the findings from laboratory and animal studies. Because the dosing is subtherapeutic, these trials are also referred to as microdosing trials. Due to the subtherapeutic nature of the dosing, phase 0 trials are not intended to provide relevant information on safety or efficacy. Discussions on the methodology and issues in phase 0 trials are presented by Takimoto, Murgo and associates, and others.[2-5]

Phase I Trials

Phase I trials also involve the administration of a new treatment to a single group of human subjects in the range of 20 or more, but rarely over 100. The purpose of this phase of research is to obtain some initial information regarding the therapeutic dosing of the treatment. Until the point of initiating a phase 1 trial, information has been limited to that from laboratory investigations, studies among animals, and perhaps the pharmacokinetics in humans of subtherapeutic doses. The objectives of a phase I trial can include obtaining information on the best mode of treatment delivery, determining adequate dosing levels, describing the nature of side effects from treatment and detecting some signal that the new treatment has activity on the disease or condition for which the treatment is planned to be used. Eisenhauer and coworkers, Miller, Horstmann and colleagues, and others present discussions regarding methodology and issues in phase1 trials.[6-11]

Phase II Trials

If the findings from phase I research show some promise and are within safety parameters, phase II trial research is initiated. This type of trial typically involves 100 or more participants and can, but does not always, include a control group with randomization of treatment assignment to the control treatment or new treatment. The goals of phase II studies are to learn more about the method of delivery, best dosing levels, safety, and effectiveness the new treatment. Herson and associates, Fleming and colleagues, Simon and coworkers, and several others provide more discussion regarding the design and analysis issues in phase II trials.[12-25]

Phase III Trials

A new treatment will be taken into a phase III trial only if the results from phase I and phase II research demonstrate that the new treatment is within safety parameters and has good potential to be an effective treatment. This type of trial involves many hundreds or even many thousands of human subjects, and always includes a control group with randomized treatment assignment. The control group could be one receiving the treatment that represents the current standard of care or, if there is no standard, one receiving a placebo. If possible, the treatments administered are done so in a double-blinded fashion where neither the participant nor the treating health care provider is aware of which treatment (new or control) the participant is receiving. The primary goals of a phase III trial are to definitively determine the efficacy of the new therapy and refine safety information. In some circumstances, the goal regarding efficacy is to show that the new treatment is better than the current treatment. In other circumstances, the goal is to show that the new therapy is as effective as the current treatment, but may be less costly, have fewer or less intense side effects, and/or is easier to administer. Results from phase III trials are the primary information used by the U.S. Food and Drug Administration (FDA) and other similar agencies throughout the world to approve a new treatment for general use among individuals who have a specific disease or condition. Methodologic issues involved with phase III studies are the focus of this chapter.

Phase IV Trials

Phase IV trials are conducted after a new treatment has been approved by the FDA and are often referred to as post-marketing surveillance trials. This type of trial is usually conducted by the company that developed the new treatment. The primary purpose of phase IV research is to obtain long-term information on side effects of the new treatment or learn more about rare side effects of the new treatment. Sometimes phase IV research involves the continued follow-up of the participants in a phase III trial that was used as the basis for FDA approval of the new treatment. Phase IV research can also involve the establishment of a surveillance system to collect data from the general population who begin taking the new treatment or the establishment of other activities needed to collect information to refine risk/benefit profile of the treatment or to identify subgroups for whom treatment should be limited or withheld.

DESIGNING PHASE III TRIALS

Defining the Primary Hypothesis and the Primary End Point

Defining the primary hypothesis of a trial is the first step to designing the trial. The primary hypothesis is meant to reflect the main objective of the trial. Most often the primary objective is to compare effects of 2 treatments. In this case, the primary hypothesis would be to evaluate the efficacy of a new treatment as compared to the control treatment in terms of some undesirable health outcome. However, trials can involve the comparison of more than 2 treatments, and in this circumstance the hypothesis would identify more than one comparison of a new treatment to a control treatment and/or comparisons among several of the new treatments. The undesirable health outcome that is used as the basis for comparing treatment is referred to as the primary end point. When dealing with phase III breast cancer treatment trials, possible end points include breast cancer recurrence-free interval, invasive disease-free survival, overall survival, or one of several others.[26] Once the primary end point has been selected, one must define the specific types of events that are to be included as part of the end point. For example, events under disease-free survival would include cancer recurrence at the original anatomic site of diagnosis, recurrence at a different anatomic site, diagnosis of a second primary cancer, and death without evidence of recurrence at any anatomic site or a second primary cancer. A lack of standardization of the specific types of events included as part of a particular end point has caused difficulty when comparing results across trials evaluating similar treatments. In an effort to rectify this situation, there have been recent harmonization efforts to standardize the types of events included as part of end points used in the cancer clinical trials.[26,27] The recommendations from these efforts should be used as the basis for defining the health outcomes selected for trials.

Most often, the anticipated results from testing the study hypothesis is that the new treatment would be superior to the control treatment. This type of hypothesis is referred to a superiority hypothesis. In some circumstances, one may not wish to demonstrate the superiority of a new treatment, but rather to demonstrate the new treatment is no less effective that a control treatment. This type of hypothesis is known as a non-inferiority hypothesis. It would be considered when it is anticipated that, within a given tolerance, the new and control treatments may have similar efficacy but the new treatment would be more desirable because it may have fewer or less severe side effects, may be less costly, and/or may be easier to administer.[28-31]

It is rare that there is only one objective of a phase III clinical trial. Thus, as must be accomplished for the primary hypothesis, end points for secondary objectives must also be defined. This should be accomplished using the same considerations as those for the primary objective.

Establishing the Parameters for the Trial Design

Once the primary hypothesis has been defined there are several key parameters that must be established. These parameters are key factors that taken together become the basis for determining the sample size of participants needed to perform a statistically adequate test of the primary hypothesis. There are 2 types of parameters that must be established; those that are statistical in nature and those that are operational in nature.

The statistical parameters that must be established before the trial is initiated are the α-level, the statistical power, the baseline rate of the primary end point for the control group, and the effect size. The α-level is also referred to as the type I error rate. It is the threshold *p*-value that is used for determining statistical significance in hypothesis testing. It represents the likelihood of concluding that there is a difference between the new and control treatments when there really is no difference. As one wants to minimize the probability of such an error, one usually chooses a low α-level. Traditionally, the α-level that is used for hypothesis testing is set at 0.05. In situations where there are more than 2 treatments being compared or formal testing of secondary hypotheses is planned, the α-level for any particular comparison would be reduced or the testing would be performed in an hierarchical, conditional manner to maintain the experiment-wise α-level at the 0.05 level.[32] The statistical power for the test of hypothesis is the likelihood of concluding that there is a difference between the new and control treatments when a difference of a specific magnitude really does exist. As one wants to maximize this circumstance, one chooses a high statistical power. Practically speaking, the statistical power is usually set in the range of 0.8 to 0.9. A value of less than 0.8 is not recommended. The baseline rate of the primary end point is the anticipated rate of the end point among those receiving the control treatment. This can be determined from reports in the literature for populations similar to that which is likely to be accrued to the trial. The effect size is the magnitude of the difference in rates of the primary end point that is anticipated between the new and control treatments. For example, if the hypothesis involves evaluating the rate of breast cancer recurrence and one anticipates that the rate among those receiving the new treatment will be 25% less than the rate among those receiving the control treatment, then the effect size is a 25% reduction. The effect size that is chosen must be one that is biologically meaningful and also one that can be justified as a reasonable magnitude of effect that could be achieved with the new treatment.

The key operational parameters that must be established include the anticipated participants lost to follow-up rate, nonadherence rate, and patient accrual pattern. To the extent that is possible, these can be determined from prior experiences in trials of a similar nature. The lost to follow-up rate is the proportion of those randomized who formally withdraw their consent to participate, cannot be located, or decide to discontinue returning for clinical assessments. The nonadherence rate is the proportions of those randomized who continue participation in clinical assessments, but discontinue the study treatment to which they were randomly assigned before the full planned course is completed. The determination of these 2 rates is important, as these parameters could affect the observed rate of the study outcome and therefore increase the sample size needed to be studied. The projected patient accrual pattern is the anticipated number of individuals who would be randomized over a specified unit of time. Consideration should be given to the time-dependent nature of accrual in that accrual for a clinical trial will often start out at a less than maximum level and that it may be several months before reaching a peak level and possibly staying constant or dropping thereafter.

Determination of Sample Size and Power

A fundamental part of the design of any clinical trial is the consideration of the number of individuals who are required to appropriately conduct the trial. Once the trial parameters are set, the investigators then calculate a sample size based on the power requirement. In a few cases, due to cost constraints, ethical considerations, and so forth, one can only obtain a fixed sample size for a study. In this latter case, one may wish to calculate the power of a test, given the prespecified sample size.

An important distinction that must be made in calculating sample size and power is whether or not the investigators wish to frame their results in terms of confidence intervals or in terms of hypothesis testing. Another consideration is whether or not the investigators hope to establish that one treatment is more efficacious than other treatments or, alternatively, whether or not 2 or more treatments are equivalent. In the latter case, one would hope that one of the treatments or interventions would have fewer side effects than the other.

In this section, we focus on issues related to sample size and power calculations when hypothesis testing is employed and when the question of interest is that of whether or not efficacy is different between 2 treatments or interventions. Also, we focus on issues related to time to event outcomes, although we recognize that one must also consider power for other types of end points. However, in most phase III trials, the primary interest is to determine whether one treatment as compared to another increases the time to some event (eg, death, relapse, adverse reaction). Such studies are analyzed using "survival" analysis. In most such studies, at the time of the definitive analysis, the outcome (time to event) is not observed for all of the individuals. Those observations for which no event is observed are considered to be "censored." In analyzing such data, each individual is still "at risk" up until the time he or she was observed to have an event or censoring has occurred. In survival analysis, the power and sample size are determined by the number of events observed in the study. From the timing of these events, one can estimate hazard rates. The hazard rate is related to the instantaneous failure rate in a time interval $(t, t + \Delta t)$ given that an individual is still at risk at the beginning of the interval (ie, at time t). In studies of chronic diseases, it is often the case that the hazard rate, denoted λ, is constant over time, that is the risk of failure for those who have not yet had the event of interest does not change as time goes on. In such studies, the hazard rate for a cohort can be approximated simply by taking the number of events and dividing through by the total number of person-years in the cohort, that is,

$$\hat{\lambda} = n_e \Big/ \sum t_i \, .$$

Notational Note Z_α denotes that value Z of a normal distribution having the property that Pr $(Z < z) = \alpha$. For example, Pr $(Z < Z_{1-\alpha/2}) = 1 - \alpha/2$. In the case that $\alpha = 0.05$, $Z_{1-\alpha/2} = 1.96$. Also, "Φ" represents the cumulative standard normal distribution, that is, $\Phi(z) = \mathrm{Pr}(Z \le z)$, where Z follows a standard normal distribution, that is, $Z \sim N(0,1)$. For example, $\Phi(1.645) = 0.95$, $\Phi(0) = 0.50$, $\Phi(-\infty) = 0$ and $\Phi(\infty) = 1$.

In a clinical trial where the outcome of interest is time to an event, the sample size is driven by the number of events. Hence, for example, the power associated with observing 300 events will be the same regardless if the trial has 5000 or 500 subjects. Of course, there would be a big difference in the cost of the trial depending on how many individuals are accrued. Consequently, it is important to be able to estimate the hazard or failure rate of at least the control arm of the trial. For comparing the event-free rates in 2 groups, where the hazard rates, λ_1 and λ_2 are assumed to be constant, George and Desu[33] and Piantadosi[34] showed that the total number of events in the study is given by

$$n_e = \frac{(Z_{1-\alpha/2} + Z_{1-\beta})^2}{[pq \ln\Delta]^2} \qquad (1)$$

where p and q are the proportions of patients in each treatment arm, "ln" denotes the natural logarithm, $\Delta = \lambda_2/\lambda_1$, and the α-level and power, $1 - \beta$, are prespecified. From equation [1], we can derive a formula for power as

$$1 - \beta = \Phi\left\{\frac{\sqrt{n_e}}{2}|\ln(\Delta)| - Z_{1-\alpha/2}\right\}. \qquad (2)$$

Example 1 In a breast cancer trial among women who have at least one axillary node with cancer, an experimental agent is only expected to reduce the hazard rate of mortality by 25%. Thus, $\Delta = \lambda_2/\lambda_1 = 0.75$. Often the mortality rates in such a population are approximately exponential. In order to have 80% power to detect the above-mentioned 25 reduction in hazard rates for a 2-sided test, one must observe

$$n_e = \frac{4(1.96 + 0.8416)^2}{[\ln(0.75)]^2} \approx 379.4 \to 380 .$$

Consequently, in order to ensure 80% power to detect such a difference, one would need to observe 380 deaths in the study.

In cases where there is no assumption about the event time distributions but where the hazards are assumed to be proportional, that is, $\Delta = \lambda_1(t)/\lambda_2(t)$ is a constant for all t, Freedman[35] derived an expression for the total number of deaths as

$$n_e = (Z_{1-\alpha/2} + Z_{1-\beta})^2\left[\frac{\Delta+1}{\Delta-1}\right]^2. \qquad (3)$$

This latter expression gives a slightly more conservative estimate than the expression in equation [1] for determining the number of events needed to achieve a specified power.

Example 1 (Continued) In the breast cancer clinical trial described above, one would need to observe

$$n_e = (1.96 + 0.8416)^2 \frac{1.75^2}{0.25^2} \approx 384.6 \to 385$$

so that 385 deaths would have to be observed to achieve 80% power to detect a 25% mortality reduction.

From equation [3], an expression for power can be derived as

$$1 - \beta = \Phi\left\{\sqrt{n_e}\,\frac{\Delta-1}{\Delta+1} - Z_{1-\alpha/2}\right\}. \qquad (4)$$

The above equations are written with the assumption that the alternative hypotheses are 2-sided. For a 1-sided alternative hypothesis, $Z_{1-\alpha/2}$ is replaced by $Z_{1-\alpha}$, which results in an increased power but which must be further justified based on scientific and ethical considerations.

To get a quick estimate of the total number of patients to achieve one's power goals assuming a fixed follow-up time for each patient, one can use a formula from Freedman[35]:

$$N_{p,i} = \frac{(Z_{1-\alpha/2} + Z_{1-\beta})^2}{2 - p_1 - p_2}\left[\frac{\Delta+1}{\Delta-1}\right]^2, \qquad (5)$$

where $N_{p,i}$ is the total number of patients in group i, $i = 1,2$; and p_1 = the proportion of patients in group 1 who are event free at a given time t, p_2 = the proportion of patients in group 2 who are event free at t and $\Delta = \ln(p_1)/\ln(p_2)$.

Example 2 Suppose that the projected proportion of patients alive in the control group at 5 years is 77.9% based on an average annual mortality rate of 5%. Suppose also that we wish to test a 2-sided hypothesis with $\alpha = 0.05$ and that we wish to calculate the number of patients needed per group to have 80% power to detect a difference if the hazard rate is reduced by 25%. The number of patients per group needed in this trial is approximately:

$$N_{p,1} = N_{p,2} = \frac{(1.96 + 0.8416)^2}{2 - p_1 - p_2}\left[\frac{0.75+1}{0.75-1}\right]^2$$

$$= \frac{7.849 \times 49}{2 - 0.7788 - 0.8290} \approx 981 \text{ per group,}$$

This calculation does not take into account the accrual time it would take to recruit our patient population.

Consideration of Follow-Up Time and Accrual Rates

Another practicality in designing a clinical trial is that it may take months or years to accrue patients to the trial. Suppose, for example, that a trial accrues patients over the interval $(0, T)$ where T is the time interval from the beginning of the accrual period to the end of the accrual period. Obviously, the follow-up time, τ, to achieve a specified power would be longer in this case than a (hypothetical) trial that accrued its complete population instantaneously. In addition, one would expect that, as in most clinical studies, there would be a proportion, μ, of patients who are lost to follow-up. Using these parameters and the assumption of Poisson accrual rates, Rubinstein and associates[36] showed that the study parameters must satisfy

$$\sum_{i=1}^{2} \frac{2\lambda_i^*}{N\lambda_i} \frac{1}{\lambda_i^* T - e^{-\lambda_i^*\tau}(1-e^{-\lambda_i^* T})} = \frac{(Z_{1-\alpha/2} + Z_{1-\beta})^2}{[\ln\Delta]^2} \qquad (6)$$

where N is the total accrual into the study, $\lambda_i^* = \lambda_i + \mu$, and the other parameters are defined as earlier. Numerical techniques are often needed to solve for parameters of interest in this equation. Programs such as PASS, PROC POWER (in SAS), and Survpower use such techniques in solving for these parameters.

To facilitate discussion about how large a clinical trial should be, it is useful to construct plots of power curves. To produce a power curve plot one usually graphs the power to detect a difference of interest versus a range of parameters. For example, one might be interested in relating power to the magnitude of the differences or ratios being projected, the number of events in each arm, the sample size of the overall population, or the by how long one wishes to follow a particular cohort. Examples of how power over calendar time relates to the time of accrual and loss to follow-up are given below.

Example 3 Suppose that the projected annual failure rates in the control and experimental groups of proposed study are 3% and 4%, respectively. Suppose also that we wish to test a 2-sided hypothesis with $\alpha = 0.05$ and that we wish to compare the power curves over time of one scenario in which the patient accrual takes 1 year and another scenario in which the accrual takes 2 years. A plot of these 2 curves from the time of study initiation is given in Figure 37-1.

Loss to Follow-Up

A potentially greater issue affecting power is that involving loss to follow-up. In cases where insufficient funding of resources is

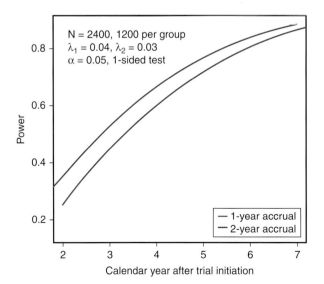

FIGURE 37-1 Plot of statistical power over time by years of accrual.

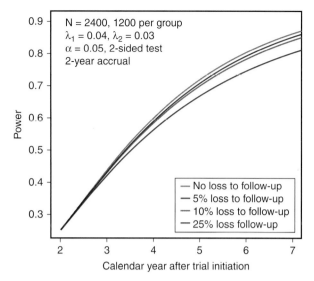

FIGURE 37-2 Plot of statistical power over time by loss to follow-up.

available for adequate follow-up, or where a large proportion of patients withdraw their consent to be followed, diminished power to detect treatment differences occurs. Moreover, biases in assessing treatment comparisons can emerge because the balance among treatment groups obtained by randomization can be compromised due to differential drop-out rates among the groups. This is a particularly acute problem if there a high proportion of early consent withdrawals.

Example 4 Consider the situation in Example 3 where the annual failure rates in the control and experimental groups of proposed study are 3% and 4%, respectively, $\alpha = 0.05$, and we wish to perform a 2-sided test and that we wish to compare the power curves over time by how much loss to follow-up. The loss to follow-up here is assumed to be uniform over time (Fig. 37-2).

Other Considerations

Other considerations such as nonuniform drop-out rates, drop-in rates, and hazard rates that are not proportional must be considered to appropriately power a trial.[36-38] These issues must be approached with great care as a priori assumptions regarding nonuniform parameter values may be sensitive to small changes in the trial design. Such considerations become even more complex if there are more than 2 groups being compared.[39] A good strategy is to use conservative but simple assumptions regarding design parameters to ensure that adequate power is achieved even if minor variations from the original values are observed after trial initiation.

A Short Note about Equivalence Trials

Equivalence trials are employed when a standard therapy is considered to be adequate for efficacy but when a new therapy is introduced that is thought to be equally efficacious but that may have fewer side effects, be less costly, be easier to administrate, or result in a higher quality of life for patients. In equivalence trials, the "null hypothesis" may be that the treatments are different whereas the "alternative hypothesis" may be that the treatments are the same.

Consequently, the roles of type I and type II errors may be reversed and power calculations may be based on one-sided tests. In addition, the values of α and β may be different in power and sample size calculations than are typically used in efficacy trials. Furthermore, a "range of equivalence" must be established based on biological principles. Once these parameters are established, sample size and power formulas can be modified accordingly.

Possible Need for Reevaluation of Protocol Design Parameters and Sample Size

Occasionally there is uncertainty in the accuracy of the protocol design parameters for a study because there may be no good historical precedent for estimating the parameters. For example, the baseline rate of the primary end point, the rate of accrual, or how either parameter may vary with time. An inaccurately specified parameter will cause a discrepancy between the power calculated for a trial and the actual power of the trial. In such cases, it is good practice to prespecify in the study protocol that the parameters of interest be estimated from the current trial at a specified time-point in the trial. The updated parameter estimates can be used to amend the required sample size for the trial as necessary to ensure the design power is maintained. In blinded trials, event rates may need to be estimated from the pooled treatment arms to avoid un-blinding. Any updating of design parameter for an active trial should generally be completed early in the monitoring phase of the trial and, if possible, prior to the initiation of any planned interim end point analyses of efficacy. The design parameters considered for reevaluation would not include those that would change the a priori defined hypothesis test such as the effect size, α level, statistical power, or 1- versus 2-sided test. It is also good practice to have the need to modify the sample size certified by the data monitoring committee for the trial.

Randomization and Stratification Factors for Randomization

Until the 1950s, the most common method for comparing different treatments or therapies was via the use of observational studies. Many authors pointed out that such studies were often associated with selection bias, over enthusiastic investigator reports, inconsistency in end point definitions, changes of treatment administration over time, and a plethora of other methodologic problems.[40-43] The use of randomization procedures to randomly allocate patients to 1 of 2 or more therapies has gained wide acceptance.[43-46] Some of the consequences of the use of randomized, prospective clinical trials are that (1) investigator bias regarding inclusion criteria is minimized, (2) definitions of outcomes and other aspects of a study are standardized, (3) the effects of calendar time on treatment administration when assessing a new treatment are minimized, (4) the type and length of follow-up of patients in each of the

treatment arms is balanced, and (5) a beginning point in each patient's course of therapy can be established.[42,43]

One problem encountered in the design and analysis of a clinical trial is how to minimize the confounding of treatment effects by other variables. Confounding, in the statistical sense, refers to the masking or biasing of an effect. Confounding can be due to not accounting for, or not properly accounting for, covariates related to the outcome of interest. For example, in a cancer clinical trial involving the treatment of patient with solid tumors, the stage of the disease should be accounted for in any assessment of treatment effect in a heterogeneous population. This is done by controlling for demographic variables (eg, race, age, sex) that may affect outcomes, clinical variables (eg, type of surgery), and variables (eg, nodal status, histologic type, hormone receptor status, and tumor size) that are used to determine the stage of the patient's disease. In a prospective randomized clinical trial, covariates that are known to be confounders can be controlled for in the design phase. In very large trials, one can do this partially by the process of simple randomization.[45] However, in trials with moderate sample sizes where simple randomizations are employed, imbalances with respect to variables other than treatment often occur.[47] If the variables are strong predictors of the outcome of interest, then such imbalances lead to biased assessments of the true treatment effect. To alleviate this problem, an attempt is made to allocate treatments equally within each stratum, thus ensuring that the overall proportion of each level of a confounding variable is somewhat balanced across treatments.

A seemingly optimal strategy for ensuring that an unbiased treatment assessment is made is to stratify by every conceivable variable that may have some association with the outcome of interest. However, such a strategy is not recommended because it leads to another competing bias due to over-stratification. One reason for this is that, due to the fact the number of strata (or "cells") defined by the combination of stratification variables increases by at least a factor of 2^r where r is the number of variables, the chances of imbalance within some of the strata (cells) increase greatly due to the small numbers of observations within each stratum. This rule is actually quite conservative, as in many trials the stratification variables have more than 2 levels as was assumed above. Thus, due to these imbalances of observations across treatment arms, a biased assessment of treatment effect can occur. Consequently, Therneau[48] recommends that studies that use stratified allocation should only attempt to balance on a few of the very important factors related to the outcome of interest. A further reason for limiting the number of stratification variables in phase III clinical trials relates to the analysis of the data. In the case of time to event outcomes, the "observations" being analyzed refer to the events reported. Two types of analyses recommended for comparison of treatments are the stratified log-rank test, which sums the treatment comparisons over all of the strata; and using a Cox proportional hazards model, which compares treatments while adjusting for the stratification variables. In either case, over-stratification should be avoided because empty "cells" can occur when there are many levels of the combined stratification variables. In addition to biasing the comparisons as described earlier, the empty cell phenomenon can also lead to a loss of power to detect treatment differences as well as leading to biased results. Finally, authors such as Meier[49] argue that stratification can sometimes put undue burdens on institutions in correctly classifying patients and this problem is intensified when too many stratification variables are introduced.

In recent years, a popular approach to the allocation of patients to treatment arms with or without stratification factors employs a "biased coin" principle first proposed by Efron.[47] This principle is based on the idea that treatment assignment realizations can have numerical imbalances even when the allocation procedure is theoretically equal between treatment arms. When such an imbalance is observed in 1 or more strata in a randomization scheme, the technique allows one to make corrections by increasing the probability of new allocations of patients to the arm of the trial that has a smaller number of individuals. This provides more assurance than simple randomization of balancing the different treatment arms with respect to each other and with respect to other variables related to the outcome of interest.

A more involved method of allocation of patients to treatment groups when one wants to also balance patient assignment among stratification variables was developed by White and Freedman.[50] They discussed both deterministic and stochastic algorithms for achieving such balance in patient allocation.

STATISTICAL ANALYSIS OF PHASE III TRIALS

The statistical analysis plan for a phase III trial should be prespecified. The plan should describe the statistical tests to be used for each hypothesis, the definition of the patient cohorts to be used for each test of hypothesis, the statistical procedures to be used for estimating the absolute outcomes in each treatment arm and the relative outcomes between treatments (effect size), optionally plans for reevaluation of protocol design parameters, and the plan for interim monitoring of end points. Prespecification of the analysis plan ensures that knowledge gained from the trial does not bias the selection of the statistical test, patient cohort, or estimation procedure.

Hypothesis Testing and Estimation of Effects

The primary efficacy end point and many secondary end points in phase III breast cancer trials are frequently time-to-event end points.[51] In this situation, the absolute measure of outcome is usually the proportion of patients event-free at a given time as estimated by the method of Kaplan and Meier.[52] The relative measure of outcome or the treatment effect is usually estimated by the hazard ratio from a Cox proportional hazards model.[53] Even when the proportional hazards assumption does not apply, this is a useful statistic for summarizing the treatment effect observed in a trial.

In addition to time-to-event end points, hypothesis testing can involve end points measured by binary or categorical outcomes. In these situations simple proportions are normally adequate for estimating the absolute outcome in each arm. These can be analyzed with chi-square tests or related tests for

ordinal data or exact inference.[54] Hypothesis tests of categorical data are often applied to safety-related end points, such as the presence or absence of an adverse event or the grade of adverse event experienced. The sample mean or median is typically used to estimate the absolute outcome in each arm for end points measured by a continuous variable. The difference in means or medians is commonly used to summarize the treatment effect. One may wish to use a t-test (when there is reason to believe the data will be normally distributed) or the nonparametric Mann–Whitney test for hypothesis testing. When other covariates besides the treatment(s) of interest are related to the end point, power may be improved by using a stratified test of hypothesis. Stratified tests are practical when continuous covariates can be categorized into a small number of levels and the total number of strata is not too large. When stratified tests are impractical due to too many strata or continuous covariates, one may use statistical modeling to test hypotheses while controlling for covariates. The Cox proportional hazards model is widely used for time-to-event end points, and logistic regression models are commonly used for binary outcomes.[53] Linear and nonlinear regression models or their nonparametric counterparts may be used for continuous end points.

Recent advances in our ability to quantify genomic and proteomic expression have resulted in the inclusion of microarray results as a secondary outcome in phase III trials. Such data are evaluated for association between specific markers and patient outcomes such as relapse-free survival or overall survival. Statistical techniques to minimize the number of false-positive findings when screening the markers for association are used to control the false discovery rate.[55,56] Once a pool of markers that have association with outcome have been identified, statistical modeling can be used to combine information from multiple covariates to produce and validate genomic/proteomic-based algorithms for predicting prognosis or response to treatment.[57,58]

Patient Cohorts for Analysis

The proper patient cohort to be used for a particular test of hypothesis depends on the type of hypothesis and the type of end point. Commonly, 2 primary cohorts are used in analysis; the full analysis cohort and the perprotocol cohort.[59] The full analysis cohort typically includes all patients who were randomized and followed, including them in their randomly assigned treatment group without regard to the treatment they actually received. Patients with major eligibility violations, particularly those violations that would make the patient not at risk for the primary end point, are sometimes excluded if they comprise a small portion of the total number of patients randomized. The perprotocol cohort typically excludes patients who do not begin (or complete some other prespecified portion of) their randomly assigned treatment, and also excludes patients with prespecified eligibility violations and patients without a measurement of the end point of interest. Because patients who fail to fully comply with their assigned treatment are included in the full analysis cohort, one might expect that the difference between treatments would be diminished in the full analysis cohort as compared to the perprotocol cohort.

In a typical trial, one would generally use the full analysis cohort to test the primary efficacy outcome. The use of the full analysis cohort is intended to reflect the intention-to-treat principal[60,61] to the extent that is possible in practice, and thereby preserve the protection against biased treatment comparisons that is provided by the use of randomized treatment assignment. The perprotocol cohort is not the primary choice for testing efficacy because the exclusion of those who do not initiate treatment or complete a full course of treatment is likely to result in a biased subset of the study population. However, in many instances, an analysis of efficacy is performed using both the full analysis cohort and the perprotocol cohort as a form of sensitivity analysis. This type of sensitivity analysis is particularly important in non-inferiority trials where treatment noncompliance may cause treatments to appear more similar than they actually are. In addition, the perprotocol cohort is often used for the evaluation of safety end points, as this cohort includes only those who actually received their assigned treatment and those who would meet the eligibility criteria for patients who are appropriate candidates to receive the treatment. While the use of this cohort is often anticonservative for preserving the α-level of the test, we accept this method in this situation because it is preferred to err on the side of over estimating safety problems as opposed to underestimating such problems.

Statistical Aspects of the Interim Monitoring Plan

Interim monitoring of a trial should be accomplished by a data monitoring committee composed of individuals who are not involved in the implementation of the trial management or implementation of the trial. These individuals are charged with the responsibility of reviewing outcome and safety data, making recommendations to the trial management team regarding continuing the trial as planned, modifying the trial to ensure the safety of the trial participants or to sustain the scientific integrity of the trial, or stopping the trial earlier than stated in the trial protocol. The interim monitoring plan is specified in the trial protocol as a guide for key decision-making with which the data monitoring committee is charged.

Recommendations to stop a trial or to divulge trial results earlier than planned can be made for 3 primary reasons. First, findings from the interim analysis may indicate that there is some serious safety issue requiring the discontinuation of the trial. Second, findings indicate that there is little or no efficacy evident for the new treatment and even if the trial is continued for the planned duration there is very little likelihood that the new treatment will show efficacy that is better than, that of the control treatment. This is referred to as stopping for futility. Lastly, the findings may indicate the magnitude of efficacy for the new treatment is much greater than anticipated and the primary test of hypothesis has already been proven beyond any reasonable doubt. The primary reason for early stopping or early divulgence of trial results is ethical in nature. Stopping early when the hypothesis is proven beyond a reasonable doubt will allow the experimental intervention to be made available to patients outside of the trial as soon as possible. In addition,

sometimes patients on the control arm of the trial can cross over to the new treatment and benefit directly from the better treatment. Stopping early for futility will allow patents on the new, less effective treatment to cross over to the effective control treatment, and will prevent subjecting the patients on the ineffective treatment to the risk of future toxicities when there is no longer an expectation of a gain. The "stopping" of a trial in this context usually means that the protocol therapy is stopped and/or that the results of the analysis of treatment comparisons are divulged. Patient follow-up may be continued, however.

Interim monitoring can be applied to any of the end points discussed in this chapter: time-to-event, categorical, or continuous. However, it is usually applied to the primary end point. The timing of interim analyses is described in terms of information time.[62] Information time varies from 0 to 1, where 1 is all the information necessary to perform the planned definitive analysis. For categorical or continuous end points, information is usually measured in terms of the number of patients. In a trial expected to accrue 100 patients for the planned definitive analysis, an interim analysis with 30 patients would occur at information time $i = 30 / 100 = 0.3$. For time-to-event end points, information time is measured in terms of events rather than patients. In a trial where the planned definitive analysis is to occur after the 200th event is observed, an interim analysis with 50 events would occur at information time $i = 50 / 200 = 0.25$. In order to use tabulated critical values, interim analyses were historically equally spaced over information time so that a trial with 2 interim analyses and a definitive analysis would conduct them at $i = 0.33, 0.66,$ and 1.0, while a trial with 4 interim analyses would time them at $i = 0.2, 0.4, 0.6, 0.8$ and 1.0. Modern computation allows us to relax the requirement for equal spacing of analyses, but equal spacing remains the most efficient use of information. Normally 2 to 5 total analyses are sufficient to provide adequate monitoring of a trial's progress. More than 5 analyses can begin to increase the total number of events/patients required depending on the chosen monitoring boundaries.

Simple monitoring boundaries for the case of analyses spaced equally in terms of information have been proposed by Pocock[63] and O'Brien and Fleming.[64] Wang and Tsiatis[65] proposed a more general family of monitoring boundaries that includes the Pocock and O'Brien and Fleming boundaries as special cases. Wieand and associates[66] proposed a simple yet effective rule for futility monitoring that has little impact on power in superiority trials. Lan and DeMets[67] proposed that a predefined α-spending function be used to allow flexibility in the timing and number of interim analyses. The Lan and DeMets approach is sometimes referred to as a "maximum information" approach since the definition of the α-spending function requires the maximum number of patients (categorical or continuous end point) or events (time-to-event) be prespecified. Jennison and Turnbull[62] give a comprehensive review of issues related to interim monitoring of clinical trials. For a standard phase III breast cancer trial testing the superiority of a new treatment using a time-to-event end point, good practice would dictate a plan for 2 to 5 analyses (perhaps more for a very long duration trial) with separate monitoring boundaries for superiority and futility.

SUMMARY

There are 5 sequential phases of clinical trial research recognized by the FDA as steps in the process to approve and monitor new treatments in the United States. The phases encompass trials designed to obtain information from the administration of subtherapeutic doses of new treatments (phase 0) to those designed primarily to enhance the safety database for a treatment once it has been approved by the FDA (phase IV). Phase III clinical trials are designed to provide the definitive test of efficacy for a new treatment for which FDA approval is being sought. A key feature that differentiates a phase III trial from other phases of trials is that phase III trials always include a control group and employ randomized treatment assignment. Also, if possible, phase III trials employ blinded treatments.

When designing a phase III clinical trial to assess the efficacy of a new treatment for breast cancer or any disease, there are several items to be considered. The first step is to specify the primary and secondary hypotheses to be tested and to define the end points that will be used to test these hypotheses. The next step is to establish the key statistical and operation parameters needed to determine the sample size. The statistical parameters include the α-level used for hypothesis testing (usually 0.05), the statistical power for the test of hypothesis (usually 0.8 or 0.9), the expected rate of the outcome of interest in the group receiving the control treatment, and the magnitude of reduction in the outcome rate in the group receiving the new treatment group compared to the outcome rate in the group receiving the control treatment (effect size). The operational parameters include the anticipated loss to follow-up rate, the nonadherence rate, and the patient accrual pattern. Once the key study parameters are established, one can then proceed with the determination of the sample size required for the trial using established algorithms to do so.

Another item of design consideration for phase III clinical trials is the nature of the method that will be used for randomized treatment assignment. Randomization enhances the scientific integrity of the trial by assigning patients to treatments in a manner that is not subject to bias and substantially increasing the likelihood that the patients within the treatment groups are comparable with regard to host factors that may be associated with prognosis or the magnitude of treatment effect. Complex methods of randomization using stratification and dynamic, biased coin allocation can be employed to maximize the likelihood of treatment group comparability and thereby the likelihood of unbiased treatment group comparisons.

The analysis plan for phase III trials should be prespecified and documented by including the description of the plan as part of the trial protocol. The analysis plan should include a description of the methods for interim monitoring, as well as the methods for hypothesis testing. Interim monitoring methods should identify the rules for triggering each interim analysis and the critical values to be used as guidelines for making a decision to stop the trial early for efficacy or futility. Hypothesis testing related to assessing the efficacy of a new treatment should be based on the intention-to-treat principle. Most often the end point being assessed is time-to-event in nature and is analyzed using Kaplan–Meier methods or Cox proportional hazard modeling. End points that are not time-to-event in nature are analyzed by a range of statistical methods as appropriate for the end point, encompassing t-test, chi-square, and one or more of many available regression procedures. Assessments to identify a pool of genomic or proteomic markers that are associated with outcome are performed using techniques to control for false discovery, and modeling methods are used to develop genomic/proteomic-based algorithms to predict prognosis or response to therapy.

REFERENCES

1. Temple R. Current definitions of phases of investigation and the role of the FDA in the conduct of clinical trials. *Am Heart J.* 2000;139:S133-S135.
2. Takimoto CH. Phase 0 clinical trials in oncology: a paradigm shift for early drug development. *Cancer Chemother Pharmacol.* Published online July 10, 2008.
3. Murgo AJ, Kummar S, Rubinstein L, et al. Designing phase 0 cancer trials. *Clin Cancer Res.* 2008;14:3675-3682.
4. Doroshow JH, Parchment RE. Oncologic phase 0 trials incorporating clinical pharmacodynamics from concept to patient. *Clin Cancer Res.* 2008;14:3658-3663.
5. Calvert AH, Plummer R. The development of phase 1 cancer trial methodologies: the use of pharmacokinetic and pharmacodynamic end points set the scene for phase 0 cancer clinical trials. *Clin Cancer Res.* 2008;14:3664-3669.
6. Eisenhauer EA, O'Dwyer PJ, Christian M, Humphery JS. Phase I clinical trial design in cancer drug development. *J Clin Oncol.* 2000;18:648-692.
7. Miller M. Phase I cancer trials: a crucible of competing priorities. *Int Anesthesiol Clin.* 2001;39:13-33.
8. Horstmann E, McCabe MS, Grochow L, et al. Risks and benefits of phase 1 oncology trials, 1991 through 2002. *N Engl J Med.* 2005;352:895-904.
9. Sekine I, Yamamoto N, Kunitoh H, et al. Relationship between objective responses in phase I trials and potential efficacy of nonspecific cytotoxic investigational new drugs. *Ann Oncol.* 2002;13:1300-1306.
10. Roberts TG Jr, Goulart BH, Squitieri L, et al. Trends in the risk and benefits to patients with cancer participating in phase 1 clinical trials. *JAMA.* 2004;292:2130-2140.
11. Kurzrock R, Benjamin RS. Risks and benefits of phase 1 oncology trials, revisited. *N Engl J Med.* 2005;352:930-932.
12. Herson J. Predictive probability early termination plans for phase II trials. *Biometrics.* 1979;35:775-783.
13. Fleming TR. One sample multiple testing procedure for phase II clinical trials. *Biometrics.* 1982;38:143-151.
14. Simon R. Optimal two-stage designs for phase II clinical trials. *Contol Clin Trials.* 1989;10:1-10.
15. Green SJ, Dahlberg S. Planned versus attained design in phase II clinical trials. *Stat Med.* 1992;11:853-862.
16. Ratain MJ, Mick R, Schilsky RL, Siegler M. Statistical and ethical issues in the design and conduct of phase I and II clinical trials of new anticancer agents. *J Natl Cancer Inst.* 1993;85:1637-1643.
17. Thall PF, Simon R. Practical Bayesian guidelines for phase IIB clinical trials. *Biometrics.* 1994;50:337-349.
18. Chen TT. Optimal three-stage designs for phase II cancer clinical trials. *Stat Med.* 1997;16:2701-2711.
19. Heitjan DF. Bayesian interim analysis of phase II cancer clinical trials. *Stat Med.* 1997;16:1791-1802.
20. Herndon JE II. A design alternative for two-stage, phase II, multicenter cancer clinical trials. *Control Clin Trials.* 1998;19:440-450.
21. Chen TT, Ng TH. Optimal flexible designs in phase II clinical trials. *Stat Med.* 1998;17:2301-2312.
22. Case LD, Morgan TM. Duration of accrual and follow-up for two-stage clinical trials. *Lifetime Data Analysis.* 2001;7:21-37.
23. Cheung YK, Thall PF. Monitoring the rates of composite events with censored data in phase II clinical trials. *Biometrics.* 2002;58:89-97.
24. Vickers AJ, Ballen V, Scher HI. Setting the bar in phase II trials: the use of historical data for determining "go/no go" decision for definitive phase III testing. *Clin Cancer Res.* 2007;13:972-976.
25. Owzar K, Jung S. Designing phase II studies in cancer with time-to-event endpoints. *Clin Trials.* 2008;5:209-221.
26. Hudis CA, Barlow WE, Costantino JP, et al. Proposal for standardized definitions for efficacy end points in adjuvant breast cancer trial: the STEEP system. *J Clin Oncol.* 2007;25:2127-2132.

27. Punt CJA, Buyse M, Kohne C, et al. Endpoints in adjuvant treatment trials: a systemic review of the literature in colon cancer and proposed definitions for future trials. *J Natl Cancer Inst.* 2007;99:998-1003.

28. Pocock SJ. The pros and cons of non-inferiority (equivalence) trials. In: Guess HA, Kleinman A, Kusek JW, EngLw, eds. *The Science of Placebo: Toward an Interdisciplinary Research Agenda.* London, UK: BMJ Books: 2000:236-248.

29. D'Agostino RB, Massaro JM, Sullivan LM. Non-inferiority trials: design concepts and issues – the encounters of academic consultants in statistics. *Stat Med.* 2003;22:169-186.

30. Lester LL, Johnson MF. Non-inferiority trials: the "at least as good as" criterion. *Stat Med.* 2003;22:187-200.

31. Rothman M, Li N, Chen G, et al. Design and analysis of non-inferiority mortality trials in oncology. *Stat Med.* 2003;22:239-264.

32. Bauer P. Multiple testing in clinical trials. *Stat Med.* 1991;10:871-890.

33. George SL, Desu MM. Planning the size and duration of a clinical trial studying the time to some critical event. *J Chron Dis.* 1974;27:15-24.

34. Piantadosi S. *Clinical Trials: A Methodologic Perspective.* New York, NY: Wiley; 1997:169-174.

35. Freedman LS. Tables of the number of patients required in clinical trials using the logrank test. *Stat Med.* 1982;1:121-129.

36. Rubinstein LV, Gail MH, Santner TJ. Planning the duration of a comparative clinical trial with loss to follow-up and a period of continued observation. *J Chron Dis.* 1981;34:469-479.

37. Lachin JM, Foulkes MA. Evaluation of sample size and power for analyses of survival with allowance for nonuniform patient entry, losses to follow-up, noncompliance, and stratification. *Biometrics.* 1986;42:507-516.

38. Lakatos E. Sample sizes based on the log-rank statistic in complex clinical trials. *Biometrics.* 1988;44:229-241.

39. Ahnn S, Anderson S. Sample size determination in complex clinical trials comparing more than two groups for survival endpoints. *Stat Med* 1998;17:2525-2534.

40. Hill AB. Medical ethics and controlled trials. *Br Med J.* 1963;1:1043-49.

41. Byar DP. Why data bases should not replace randomized clinical trials. *Biometrics.* 1980;36:337-342.

42. Byar DP. Problems with using observational databases to compare treatments. *Stat Med.* 1991;17:663-666.

43. Pocock S. *Clinical Trials: A Practical Approach.* Chichester, England: Wiley; 1983:14-27.

44. Greenberg BG. Why randomize? *Biometrics.* 1951;7:309-322.

45. Peto R, Pike M, Armitage P, et al. Design and analysis of randomized clinical trials requiring prolonged observation of each patient. I. Introduction and design. *Br J Cancer.* 1976;34:585-612.

46. Green S, Benedetti J, Crowley J. *Clinical Trials in Oncology.* 2nd ed. Boca Raton, FL: Chapman & Hall; 2003:4-5.

47. Efron B. Forcing a sequential experiment to be balanced. *Biometrika.* 1971;58: 403 417.

48. Therneau TM. How many stratification factors are "too many" to use in a randomization plan?. *Control Clin Trials.* 1993;14:98-108.

49. Meier P. Stratification in the design of a clinical trial. *Control Clin Trials.* 1981;1:355-361.

50. White SJ, Freedman LS. Allocation of patients to treatment groups in a controlled clinical study. *Br J Cancer.* 1978;37:849-857.

51. Klein JP, Moeschberger ML. *Survival Analysis: Techniques for Censored and Truncated Data.* New York, NY: Springer; 2003:191-214.

52. Kaplan E, Meier P. Nonparametric Estimation from incomplete observations. *JASA.* 1958;53:457-481.

53. Cox DR. Regression models and life tables. *J R Stat Soc B.* 1972;34: 87-220.

54. Agresti A. *Categorical Data Analysis.* New York, NY: Wiley; 1996:47-65.

55. Lee MT. *Analysis of Microarray Gene Expression Data.* Boston, MA: Kluwer; 2004:143-155.

56. Simon RM, Korn EL, McShane LM, et al. *Design and Analysis of DNA Microarray Investigations.* New York, NY: Springer; 2003:75-84.

57. Paik S, Shak S, Tang G, et al. A multigene assay to predict recurrence of tamoxifen-treated, node-negative breast cancer. *N Engl J Med.* 2004;351:2817-2826.

58. Paik S, Tang G, Shak S, et al. Gene expression and benefit of chemotherapy in women with node-negative, estrogen receptor-positive breast cancer. *J Clin Oncol.* 2006;24:3726-3734.

59. ICH E9 Expert Working Group. ICH harmonised tripartite guideline: statistical principles for clinical trials. *Stat Med.* 1999;18:1905-1942.

60. Fisher L, Dixon D, Jerson J, et al. Intention to treat in clinical trials. In: Peace K, ed. *Statistical Issues in Drug Research and Development.* New York, NY: Marcel Dekker; 1990: 331-350.

61. Gillings D, Koch G. The application of the principle of intention-to-treat to the analysis of clinical trials. *Drug Info J.* 1991;25:411-424.

62. Jennison C, Turnbull B. *Group Sequential Methods with Applications to Clinical Trial.* Boca Raton, FL: Chapman and Hall;2000:159-160.

63. Pocock SJ. Group sequential methods in the design and analysis of clinical trials. *Biometrika.* 1977;64:191-199.

64. O'Brien PC, Fleming TR. A multiple testing procedure for clinical trials. *Biometrika.* 1979;35:549-556.

65. Wang SK, Tsiatis AA. Approximately optimal one-parameter boundaries for group sequential trials. *Biometrics.* 1987;43:193-200.

66. Wieand S, Schroeder G, O'Fallon JR. Stopping when the experimental regimen does not appear to help. *Stat Med.* 1994;13:1453-1458.

67. Lan KKG, DeMets DL. Discrete sequential boundaries for clinical trials. *Biometrika.* 1983;70:659-663.

CHAPTER 38

Study Conduct

Walter M. Cronin

The purpose of this chapter is to define and describe the factors that an investigator needs to consider in conducting a multi-center, randomized clinical trial evaluating various treatments in breast surgical oncology. Many examples and experiences will be drawn from the National Surgical Adjuvant Breast and Bowel Project (NSABP), which has had a 50-year history of conducting such evaluations.

The goals of this chapter are to make the reader aware of the principles that lead to a verifiable scientific discovery via the conduct of a clinical trial and to direct the reader to other resources that further elucidate and educate. Additional goals are to increase the reader's awareness of the potential obstacles and pitfalls that can be associated with the study conduct, to provide real-world examples, and to characterize the mindset and skill sets that are valuable in the conduct of a clinical trial. Because of the complexity and the breadth of topics, no single book chapter can extensively describe all the information that is necessary for an investigator to embark on a study.

In its simplest form, a clinical trial is an experiment in humans designed to compare treatments. All the major land-mark surgical oncology trials have been "controlled clinical trials," which are defined by Meinert and Tonascia as "a clinical trial involving one or more test treatments, at least one control treatment, and concurrent enrollment, treatment and follow-up of all patients in the trial."[1] The conduct of that trial comprises a sequence of steps necessary to bring that trial to completion. It requires the recruitment of a sufficient sample size of evaluable study population, the administration of the assigned therapies, and the construction of a database of sufficiently high integrity that will be available for analysis by the study statisticians and the drawing of conclusions by the study scientists.

If the "conduct" of a clinical trial were a simple matter, it would not have evolved into the major industry that it has become today, with thousands of books, peer-reviewed articles, and other scientific publications devoted to the subject and with hundreds of contract research organizations promoting their services. When considering the factors necessary to mount a clinical trial, investigators must have access to all available information and proceed in a systematic, controlled, methodologic progression.

RELATIONSHIP BETWEEN THE PROTOCOL DOCUMENT AND STUDY CONDUCT

The clinical trial protocol document serves as the plan for how the trial is to be conducted. There should be a strong relationship between this document and the ensuing conduct of the protocol. The successful conduct of the trial will be enhanced if the individuals responsible for carrying out the trial participate in the development of the protocol document. Review by these individuals should concentrate on the logistical aspects of the protocol, including eligibility assessment, subject recruitment, treatment administration, and follow-up surveillance. Their review should ensure that the protocol is internally consistent with respect to these factors and that the protocol clearly defines the logistics of entry, treatment, and follow-up.

PARTICIPANT RECRUITMENT

Before mounting a clinical trial, a formal recruitment plan should be established. The recruitment plan will be influenced by whether the study population as defined in the protocol exists in sufficient numbers and whether the population of eligible patients can be readily ascertained by the investigators at the time when they would meet protocol eligibility criteria.

The recruitment of participants into a clinical trial should be approached as a specialized discipline. Much rests on the success of the recruitment effort, so the trial organizers need to take advantage of any available related literature, discuss the trial expectations with others who have had experience recruiting similar subjects, and consult with individuals who have the general knowledge, recognized skills, and practical experiences in patient recruitment to clinical trials.

To establish the expected recruitment pattern, trial organizers might elect to conduct a pretrial survey of investigators to determine whether they have access to potentially eligible patients and interest in the proposed trial. The survey can also serve to increase awareness of the planned trial among the investigators. Any pretrial estimates and plans for recruitment must address the "recruitment funnel,"[2] the phenomenon that more patients need to be approached about clinical trial recruitment than the number that eventually end up consenting to participate.

To the extent possible, trial leaders must attenuate any logistical and fiscal burdens placed on the investigators and participants during the recruitment process. Early during the recruitment phase, it might also be beneficial for the trial leaders to survey participants who have enrolled in the trial and their investigators in order to establish what successful mechanisms were employed and why the participants agreed to trial enrollment. If the survey results point to procedural or logistical changes that could positively impact recruitment, consideration should be given to modifying the recruitment plan.

It is essential that any recruitment plan does not coerce or influence the investigators such that their potential participants are not fully informed, committed, and willing to participate in the study. The recruitment of participants who are not fully committed to completing the treatment and/or follow-up phase of the trial may adversely affect the trial outcome.

SITE AND INVESTIGATOR SELECTION

The team responsible for conducting a clinical trial needs to be fully apprised of the qualifications and reputations of the sites and investigators that will be involved in the study. Additionally, depending on the required sample size, it might be prudent to select from among a larger group of sites and investigators those that are most qualified to participate.

This screening step may involve an application that needs to be submitted by the local investigator. The application form should establish that the local site and investigator possess the following:

- A track record in the conduct of similar trials
- A recruitment plan specifically directed at the population that is being studied
- A plan for maintaining adequate patient adherence to the treatment and follow-up schedule
- A team of qualified coinvestigators that will be involved in the conduct of the trial
- A team of support personnel (including nurses and clinical research associates) who will be trained in the study conduct

The review of applications should be a formal step in the trial initiation process and may involve a panel of investigators experienced with the conduct of clinical trials. After the selection process, the selected sites and investigators need to fulfill all established regulatory requirements and trial sponsor requirements before beginning study participation.

DATA COLLECTION AND MANAGEMENT

In the conduct of clinical trials, the need for well-established procedures for data collection and data management is self-evident; the completeness and efficiency of these processes will largely determine the adequacy and availability of study outcomes.

Planning for case report form (CRF) design should begin early in the protocol development process. The design of CRFs should involve the trial developers (both clinicians and statisticians), as well as representatives from data management, programming, and other areas involved in the day-to-day logistics of conducting the trial. To a large extent, the structure of the CRFs is strongly influenced by the selection of the database software and by the computer system used for data collection, as well as whether or not the data will be collected by remote data capture versus conventional methods (faxing or mailing of CRFs). Nonetheless, several basic principles should always be applied to the design of CRFs:

- The forms should be simple, easy to understand, and relate directly to the protocol document.
- The collection of extraneous information (ie, details that do not relate specifically to protocol eligibility, treatment, and follow-up) should not be allowed.
- A plan for adjudicating differences of opinion regarding CRF content should be established and followed consistently.

A centralized database to store information is integral to the conduct of a trial. The trial also needs to be supported with well-specified software that enables the following:

- Data management and medical review staff need to conduct prospective evaluations of quality control, data completeness, and data timeliness.
- Study organizers need periodic reports in order to perform study monitoring of recruitment, adverse events, data submission, and protocol end points. These reports will enable an assessment of whether or not the trial is proceeding as planned. Variations of these reports may be reviewed by the independent data and safety monitoring committee, if one has been established.

QUALITY ASSURANCE

In the context of clinical trial conduct, quality assurance is defined as "any procedure, method or philosophy for collecting, processing or analyzing data that is aimed at maintaining or improving the reliability or validity of the data."[1] Adoption of a broad definition reinforces that every aspect of clinical trials conduct needs to be rooted in quality assurance.

A quality assurance program should be designed to ensure compliance to the extant guidelines that govern the research, including such standards as the Code of Good Clinical Practice and, where applicable, any federal or pharmaceutical company guidelines.[3] Quality assurance programs should be the responsibility of designated staff members, although any member of the clinical trial coordinating team may be able to suggest new quality assurance procedures. To that end, quality assurance programs should be

- Broad-based to cover the wide spectrum of clinical trials conduct.
- Designed to assist program management and institutional members in their efforts to monitor and improve data quality.
- Dynamic to address the changing requirements of a clinical trial.

The cornerstone of a quality assurance program is the comparison of a centralized database with source documentation (eg, pathology reports, operative reports, history, and physical exam reports), which is summarized on the case report forms. Periodic monitoring visits and site audits are necessary to ensure that the data in the central database accurately represent the data at the participating site.

Periodic feedback to the participating investigators regarding the quality of data submitted is important for fostering a common understanding about the need for complete and accurate data. Also, the use of established criteria that define institutional data quality and the incorporation of incentives or sanctions based on performance can be effective tools for promoting data quality.

SPECIAL FEATURES IN LANDMARK BREAST CANCER SURGICAL TRIALS OF THE NSABP

There have been 3 hallmarks that have distinguished the surgical trials of the NSABP and have contributed to their ability to maintain a database with high integrity:

- Centralized collection of source documents: The NSABP clinical trial protocols have required the submission of key source documents, such as pathology and operative reports. This has enabled study staff to ensure the accuracy of the case report forms and the integrity of the central database.
- Centralized, prospective medical review: Source documents are reviewed by trained medical staff who follow defined standard operating procedures in the definition of study end points. This ensures consistency across the database. Furthermore, performing these assessments prospectively ensures that an up-to-date database is readily available for interim analysis.
- Specialized investigator training: Since NSABP Protocol B-06 (evaluating lumpectomy) and through the most recent surgical trial involving sentinel node biopsies, the NSABP has recognized the need for surgical training programs and workshops.[4,5] These serve to ensure that the investigators are indoctrinated with the required protocol procedures.

It is strongly suggested that these features be considered for implementation when a multicenter breast surgery oncology trial is being mounted.

SUGGESTIONS FOR THE PRACTICING ONCOLOGIST PARTICIPATING IN MULTICENTER CLINICAL TRIALS

The quality of the conduct of a clinical trial, and the integrity of the resultant data, is largely determined by how closely the protocol is followed by its investigators and the reliability of the reported data. To that end, it is imperative that participating investigators implement procedures and practices to enhance the quality of their participation in multicenter trials. Some of the most common problems associated with clinical trial conduct (eg, failure to follow the protocol, keep adequate and accurate records, report adverse events in a timely manner, and accounting for the disposition of study drug) can be avoided by implementing the following suggestions at the local participating sites:

- Have dedicated and trained staff in place from the beginning of participation. Begin slowly, working with a limited number of phase III trials that have clinical and scientific importance. Do trials that are supported by the federal government or pharmaceutical industry, from whom resources are available for training, recruitment, and data submission.
- Ensure that investigators and staff take advantage of training opportunities. Resources include numerous books on how to conduct clinical trials,[6,7] how to participate responsibly in research,[8,9] as well as educational programs offered through the government and private vendors.
- Maintain documented study management within the practice setting related to the clinical research activities. These include procedures for patient screening, the informed consent process, documentation of serious adverse events, the use of source documents, research chart maintenance, obtaining medical records from other physicians, and so on.
- Continue to evaluate your local clinical research program. Perform internal, independent quality assurance audits, looking for problems in charting, CRF corrections, undocumented events, and so on. Communicate to others involved in research activities about the findings and put corrective action plans in place.

In general, the local investigator needs to foster an environment of and an understanding that everyone involved in the research project locally is critical to the scientific process and needs to understand the benefits of quality participation and ramifications of failing to do so.

SUMMARY

This chapter provides basic principles that should be considered when conducting a multicenter clinical trial. Several themes should be apparent:

- Equipoise in the conduct of a clinical trial is essential. For example, devoting too much emphasis or resources to "recruitment" without an adequate counterbalance involving "patient compliance" may adversely affect data integrity and disrupt the delicate balance necessary to bring a trial to closure.
- The conduct of a clinical trial requires skilled and experienced representation from various disciplines and practices. It is imperative that the clinical research team is involved early in the protocol development process and continues to be intimately involved throughout the conduct of the study.
- The conduct of clinical trials requires the adherence to established rules and regulations, with which the investigators and their colleagues must be knowledgeable.

Clinical trials can be a daunting undertaking, but they are a necessary step in the medical discovery process. The conduct of clinical trials is an evolving field, and although new technologies and cost-effectiveness strategies may drive the direction of the field, the successful conduct of a clinical trial will always rely on compliance with the clinical trial protocol, adherence to the established guidelines, and frequent/open communication among those involved in conducting the trial.

REFERENCES

1. Meinert CL, Tonascia S. *Clinical Trials Design, Conduct, and Analysis.* New York, NY: Oxford University Press: 1986.
2. Spilker B, Cramer J. *Patient Recruitment in Clinical Trials.* New York, NY: Raven Press: 1992.
3. McFadden E. *Management of Data in Clinical Trials.* New York, NY: John Wiley & Sons: 1998.
4. Margolese R, Poisson R, Shibata H, et al. The technique of segmental mastectomy (lumpectomy) and axillary dissection: a syllabus from the National Surgical Adjuvant Breast and Bowel Project workshop. *Surgery.* 1987;102: 828-834.
5. Harlow S, Krag D, Julian T, et al. Pre-randomization surgical training for the National Surgical Adjuvant Breast and Bowel Project (NSABP) B-32 trial: a randomized phase III clinical trial to compare sentinel node resection to conventional axillary dissection in clinically node-negative breast cancer. *Ann Surg.* 2005;241:48-54.
6. Liu M, Davis K. *Lessons From a Horse Named Jim.* Durham, NC: Duke Clinical Research Institute: 2001.
7. Green S, Benedetti J, Crowley J. *Clinical Trials in Oncology.* Boundary Row, London, UK: Chapman & Hall: 1997.
8. Steneck N. *ORI Introduction to the Responsible Conduct of Research.* Revised ed. Washington DC: Health and Hyman Services Department Office of Research Integrity: 2004.
9. *On Being a Scientist: Responsible Conduct in Research.* 2nd ed. Washington DC: National Academy Press: 1995.

CHAPTER 39

Protocol Components and Production

Alice Matura
Aurora Madrigal

Protocol development is a meticulous process that requires a team of professionals who are proficient in the performance of the tasks involved. Proper implementation and coordination of the protocol is managed by the research team, which is headed by the principal investigator, who develops the protocol and oversees the overall management of the study. The research nurse or research coordinator is responsible for implementation and coordination of the study according to the protocol requirements. Another important member of the team is a program coordinator, who is knowledgeable about regulatory requirements and ensures that proper documents and updates are submitted to the institutional review board (IRB) in a timely fashion. All members must have a good understanding of the Code of Federal Regulations and International Conference on Harmonisation Guideline for Good Clinical Practice.[1]

COMPONENTS OF A PROTOCOL DOCUMENT

The National Cancer Institute and their Cancer Therapy Evaluation Program (CTEP) have developed aids for assistance with protocol development, as well as a listing of specific protocol elements that should be included in clinical protocols, which are also generally summarized below. This exceptional resource is available on the CTEP Web site (http://ctep.cancer.gov/protocolDevelopment/default.htm#protocol_development).[2]

Protocols containing complex scientific information can be organized and simplified by utilizing protocol templates, which can also expedite the review process. Using the CTEP protocol template as an example,[2] the major components of a protocol are listed below:

- Title Page—lists the title of the study, version date, contact information of the principal investigator, coinvestigators, and other study personnel.

- Treatment Schema—provides a summary of the proposed treatment plan.
- Table of Contents—includes page numbers.
- Objective(s)—description of the primary protocol objectives and secondary objectives.
- Background and Rationale—background information on the various currently accepted treatments available and investigational study agent(s), including the mechanism of action, summaries of clinical and nonclinical studies and pharmacokinetics, safety profile, the rationale for the proposed starting doses and dose-escalation scheme, and the results of other clinical studies using a brief overview. Also included is background information on the study disease and the background and rationale for evaluating the study agent in the study disease.
- Patient Eligibility Criteria—specifically states the conditions under which a patient is eligible to join the study. Includes references to diagnosis, prior therapies, age, performance status, and organ and marrow function. This section will also include criteria that make a patient ineligible for the study, such as treatment with other agents, allergies to the class of agent under study, pregnancy, brain metastasis, and HIV infection. CTEP has also developed guidelines that can be used during the protocol writing process that outline the inclusion of various populations. These guidelines are posted on the CTEP Web site (http://ctep.cancer.gov/guidelines/templates.html).[3]
- Pharmaceutical Information—The Pharmaceutical Management Branch (PMB) has posted a primer recommending how this section should be completed on the CTEP Web site (http://ctep.cancer.gov/protocolDevelopment/policies_pharm.htm).[4] The PMB pharmaceutical data sheet for the CTEP-held investigational new drug agent(s) will be provided with the concept approval letter.

- Treatment Plan—a detailed description of the treatment that enrolled patients will receive. CTEP uses the treatment plan to derive the Treatment Assignment Codes and Descriptors (TACs/TADs). CTEP has posted to the Web site a guide for the development of TACs and TADs (http://ctep.cancer.gov/protocolDevelopment/docs/TreatmentAssignment.pdf).[5]
- Procedures for Patient Entry on Study—describes how eligible patients, as indicated by the protocol, are registered in the study according to the procedure set by the sponsor or the institution or both.
- Dose Modifications for Adverse Events—describes how the principal investigator will modify the administration of the agent under study in the event that an adverse event (AE) is experienced. This modification is specified by nature and grade of the AE (see "Adverse Event Reporting" section later in the chapter).
- Criteria for Response Assessment—the CTEP Web site contains information about the use of the Response Evaluation Criteria in Solid Tumors (http://ctep.cancer.gov/protocolDevelopment/docs/recist_guideline.pdf).[6]
- Monitoring of Patients—specifically describes how patients will be monitored and at what frequency.
- Off Study Criteria—describes the conditions under which a subject will need to be taken off the study due to certain adverse events or conditions that may not be beneficial to the subject if he/she continues to participate. Also addresses how patients will be followed once off-study.
- Adverse Event Reporting—see "Adverse Event Reporting" section later in the chapter.
- Tissue Handling, Laboratory, and Correlative Science Studies—describes what materials if any are needed to be processed for analysis and how these materials are to be handled and stored.
- Statistical Considerations—this is an essential component that is used in the formulation of the most basic hypothesis and objectives for the trial, the analyses, and eventual publication of the study.
- Informed Consent—see the separate section on "Informed Consent" later in the chapter.

INSTITUTIONAL REVIEW BOARD

The IRB can be a local hospital or university-based, independent, or central IRB. Independent IRBs are generally for-profit organizations and are most often used by industry-sponsored clinical trials. The central IRB is sponsored by the National Cancer Institute and used for cooperative group studies. An IRB is an administrative body established to protect the rights and welfare of human subjects recruited to participate in research activities conducted under the auspices of the institution with which it is affiliated. The IRB has the authority to approve, require modifications in, or disapprove all research activities that fall within its jurisdiction as specified by both federal regulations and institutional policy. The involvement of human subjects in research will not be permitted until the IRB has reviewed and approved the research protocol and informed consent document. IRB members may include physicians, scientists, pharmacists, a chaplain, a social worker, a retired nurse, an attorney, and a patient. The IRB reviews new protocols, ongoing protocols, protocol amendments, and any adverse reactions experienced by protocol patients. The IRB Guidebook on the Web site of the Office for Human Research Protections (OHRP) is an excellent resource that provides OHRP's interpretation of the federal regulations regarding the function of IRBs. The guidebook discusses many aspects of how IRBs function (http://www.hhs.gov/ohrp/irb/irb_guidebook.htm).[7]

ROLE OF THE RESEARCH NURSE

The safe and effective delivery of a clinical research trial is dependent on key research personnel who conduct the day-to-day "hands-on" functions of the clinical trial. One such key research personnel in the majority of academic and private clinics is the research nurse (RN), who is responsible for conducting the daily activities of the clinical trial, ensuring patient safety, and maintaining a large body of specialized knowledge. Historically, for example, at The University of Texas MD Anderson Cancer Center, before the late 1970s the role of the RN in clinical research trials was mainly that of a data manager (collect the data, enter the data), with occasional administration of treatment. However, over the last 2 decades, the role of the RN has undergone a significant evolution to that of a broader role due to the increasing volume. The clinical RN frequently performs multiple roles all throughout the conduction of the clinical research trial that incorporate the nursing process: educator, patient advocate, direct care provider, coordinator of care, data manager, and protocol manager. The RN's role in clinical research today is critical, requiring the daily performance of a set of multiple and complex tasks while having a large body of specialized knowledge in order to promote patient safety and effectiveness of the clinical trial.

Overall, the primary focus and responsibility of the clinical RN is to conduct and manage the clinical research trial. There are 3 distinct stages of participation in a clinical trial that require the RN's involvement: (1) before study implementation, (2) study implementation, and (3) after study.

Before Study Implementation

The clinical RN's initial responsibilities in the prestudy preparation phase include a range of responsibilities, from reviewing the protocol for clarity and consistency, identifying study collaborators and sponsors, and preparing the logistics of the study, to completing all regulatory forms and documents.

A detailed outline of role responsibilities for prestudy is described in Table 39.1.

During Study Implementation

Once the study has been approved by the IRB, the clinical RN will work very autonomously to conduct daily hands-on work for the assigned study. The range of responsibilities is broad and can include recruiting and screening potential participants, obtaining the informed consent, coordinating tests and procedures, evaluating, and following patient participation in the clinical trial. A detailed outline of role of responsibilities for study implementation is described in Table 39.2. If a study

TABLE 39-1 Research Nurse Responsibilities Prior to Study Implementation

- Review the protocol for clarity and consistency
- Identify study collaborators and sponsors
- Create regulatory binder
- Schedule site initiation visits
- Coordinate protocol-related activities
  - special labs
  - specimen/s
  - treatments
- Develop preprinted protocol materials
  - teaching
  - patient calendars
  - in/out patients orders
  - prescriptions
  - special lab requests
- Develop study tools
  - eligibility criteria checklist
  - patient instruction sheet
  - patient diary
  - medication administration record
- Ensure all regulatory forms and documents are completed
  - Form 1572
  - Financial Disclosure Form
  - Investigator Agreement Form
  - Investigator Confidentiality Form
  - Supplemental Data Form
  - Signed and dated Curriculum Vitae
  - Medical License
- Write informed consent and study abstract
- Create specialized data report forms if applicable
- Process and submit all study documents (protocol, abstract, informed consent, and appendices) to the Institutional Review Board (IRB) for approval
- Identify research related costs versus standard of care costs
- Develop, design, and negotiate budget issues, in collaboration with the principal investigator and/or study drug sponsor

TABLE 39-2 Research Nurse Responsibilities During Study Implementation

- Maintain regulatory binder
- Ensure annual reviews completion
- Recruit and screen potential participants
- Review medical record and/or computer based data to ensure patient's eligibility
- Obtain informed consent
  - Review content of the informed consent with the patient and obtain signatures
- Document the informed consent process and study entry
- Order pertinent laboratory tests
- Schedule procedures
- Collect specimens (blood, fluid, and/or tissue)
- Process specimens if required
  - centrifuge blood
  - package and ship blood and/or tissue
- Monitor and/or operate research devices and/or machines during surgery
- Record data obtained from research device and/or machines during surgery or procedures
- Monitor drug responses and grade level of toxicities (adverse events/side effects)
- Administer study medications
- Provide ongoing education to the patient and family
- Enter data in specialized data base and/or case report forms
- Review and perform basic statistics on study data
- Plan, design, and provide professional and ancillary staff in-services on the study overview
- Consult specialists as required on study specifics
- Maintain close communication with research team
- Schedule audits and/or monitor visits for internal and external sources
  - order medical records
  - order diagnostic imaging films
  - ensure regulatory binder updated
  - print applicable data

sponsor is involved in the research endeavor, either financially or by providing a testable drug or a medical device, there are usually case report forms that must be completed and reviewed by a study monitor hired by the sponsoring entity. In addition to all that has been mentioned, the research nurse is also responsible for arranging and scheduling the visits with the study monitors. These visits are in frequency depending on the study data accrual and level of complexity.

INFORMED CONSENT AND REFUSAL

Clinical investigators may not involve a human being as a subject in research without obtaining informed consent of the subject or the subject's legally authorized representative. Investigators should seek consent only under circumstances that provide the prospective subject or the representative sufficient opportunity to consider whether or not to participate and that minimize the possibility of coercion or undue influence. The information that is given to the subject or the representative shall be in language understandable to the subject or the representative. No informed consent, whether oral or written, may include any exculpatory language through which the subject or the representative is made to waive or appear to waive any of the subject's legal rights, or releases or appears to release the investigator, the sponsor, the institution or its agents from liability for negligence.

Basic Elements of Informed Consent

1. A statement that the study involves research, an explanation of the purposes of the research and the expected duration of the subject's participation, a description of the procedures to be followed, and identification of any procedures that are experimental
2. A description of any reasonably foreseeable risks or discomforts to the subject
3. A description of any benefits to the subject or to others that may reasonably be expected from the research
4. A disclosure of appropriate alternative procedures or courses of treatment, if any, that might be advantageous to the subject
5. A statement describing the extent, if any, to which confidentiality of records identifying the subject will be maintained, and a disclosure of who will have access to the medical records, such as monitors, auditors, IRB, or other regulatory authorities
6. For research involving more than minimal risk, an explanation regarding whether any compensation and an explanation of whether any medical treatments are available if injury occurs and, if so, what they consist of, or where further information may be obtained
7. An explanation of whom to contact for answers to pertinent questions about the research and research subjects' rights and whom to contact in the event of a research-related injury to the subject
8. A statement that participation is voluntary, refusal to participate will involve no penalty or loss of benefits to which the subject is otherwise entitled, and the subject may discontinue participation at any time without penalty or loss of benefits to which the subject is otherwise entitled

When appropriate, additional elements of informed consent may include 1 or more of the following elements of information:

1. A statement that the particular treatment or procedure may involve risks to the subject (or to the embryo or fetus, if the subject is or may become pregnant) that are currently unforeseeable
2. The responsibilities of the subjects and any anticipated circumstances under which the subject's participation may be terminated by the investigator without regard to the subject's consent
3. Any additional costs to the subject that may result from participation in the research
4. The consequences of a subject's decision to withdraw from the research and procedures for orderly termination of participation by the subject
5. A statement that significant new findings developed during the course of the research that may relate to the subject's willingness to continue participation will be provided to the subject
6. The approximate number of subjects involved in the study and duration of time that each subject is expected to participate

ADVERSE EVENT REPORTING

An adverse event (AE) is defined as any untoward or unfavorable medical occurrence in a human subject—including any abnormal sign (eg, abnormal physical exam or laboratory finding), symptom, or disease—temporally associated with the subject's participation in the research, whether or not considered related to the subject's participation in the research. For minimal risk studies, such as behavioral science, laboratory, and epidemiologic protocols, as well as chart reviews, reasonable judgment must be used to determine what constitutes an AE.

Expected AE

Any AE with specificity or severity that is consistent with the current Investigator Brochure (IB) or consistent with the risk information described in the Informed Consent Document (ICD) or general investigational plan is considered an expected AE. All clinical protocols should include a list of the expected and anticipated events or hospitalizations relating to the study treatment.

Unexpected (Unanticipated) AE

An unexpected AE occurs if it is specifically not described in the current IB or not consistent with the risk information described in the ICD or general investigational plan.

Serious Adverse Event (SAE)

Any AE associated with the subject's participation in research that

- Results in death
- Is life-threatening (places the subject at immediate risk of death from the event as it occurred)
- Results in inpatient hospitalization or prolongation of existing hospitalization
- Results in persistent or significant disability/incapacity
- Results in a congenital anomaly/birth defect
- Based on appropriate medical judgment, may jeopardize the subject's health, and may require medical or surgical intervention to prevent one of the other outcomes listed in this definition

Study Related and Unrelated AEs

A "related" AE is an event directly or indirectly attributed to study drug, device, or procedures and/or study participation and occurs with sufficient frequency to suggest that it is not random. An "unrelated" AE occurs regardless of study participation, including events that are clearly random occurrences. If the frequency of the event suggests a possible connection to the study intervention, then it generally should be considered related.

AE Attribution

The attribution determination describes whether an AE is related to the research (medical treatment or intervention):

- Definite—it is clearly related
- Probable—it is likely related
- Possible—it may be related
- Unlikely—it is doubtfully related
- Unrelated—it is clearly *not* related

AE Severity

AE severity refers to the intensity (grading) of a specific AE. Most clinical trials use the Common Terminology Criteria for Adverse Events (CTCAE) scale. The CTCAE v3.0 scale may be viewed on the CTEP Web site (http://ctep.cancer.gov/protocol Development/electronic_applications/ctc.htm).[8]

SUMMARY

Developing a protocol and conducting the clinical trial may seem laborious and demanding, but there is always a sense of accomplishment when a study is over and published and the research findings advance our understanding of breast cancer and improve the quality of treatments for our patients. There are many resources available to assist anyone who is willing to venture in this endeavor. The availability of electronic transmission has made the wealth of information easier to obtain anytime and anywhere. The components of the protocol and elements presented in this chapter are basic and presented in very simple way. Exploring the references and Web sites listed is highly encouraged to have a more in-depth understanding of each component. The creation of a research team knowledgeable of the regulations involved will determine the success of every clinical trial. The information obtained as defined by the purpose of each protocol will always be regarded as an important contribution to the advancement of science and medicine.

ACKNOWLEDGMENT

The authors are appreciative for Ms Shunice Edwards efforts in coordinating material for this chapter.

REFERENCES

1. U.S. Food and Drug Administration: Guidances, Information Sheets, and Notices. Available at: http://www.fda.gov/oc/gcp/guidance.html. Accessed January 11, 2009.
2. Cancer Therapy Evaluation Program: Protocol Development. Available at: http://ctep.cancer.gov/protocolDevelopment/default.htm#protocol_development. Accessed January 11, 2009.
3. Cancer Therapy Evaluation Program: Protocol Development: Protocol Templates and Guidelines. Available at: http://ctep.cancer.gov/guidelines/templates.html. Accessed January 11, 2009.
4. Cancer Therapy Evaluation Program: Protocol Development: Guidelines for Preparing Pharmaceutical Sections. Available at: http://ctep.cancer.gov/protocolDevelopment/policies_pharm.htm. Accessed January 11, 2009.
5. Cancer Therapy Evaluation Program: Treatment Assignment Instructions and Guidelines. Available at: http://ctep.cancer.gov/protocolDevelopment/docs/TreatmentAssignment.pdf. Accessed January 11, 2009.
6. Cancer Therapy Evaluation Program: Protocol Development: RECIST Quick Reference. Available at: http://ctep.cancer.gov/protocolDevelopment/docs/recist_guideline.pdf. Accessed January 11, 2009.
7. U.S. Department of Health and Human Services: Office for Human Resource Protections (OHRP): IRB Guidebook. Available at: http://www.hhs.gov/ohrp/irb/irb_guidebook.htm. Accessed January 11, 2009.
8. Cancer Therapy Evaluation Program: Protocol Development: CTC v2.0 and Common Terminology Criteria for Adverse Events (CTCAE). Available at: http://ctep.cancer.gov/protocolDevelopment/electronic_applications/ctc.htm. Accessed January 11, 2009.

CHAPTER 40

Tissue Acquisition and Banking for Breast Cancer

Soonmyung Paik

The promise of personalized therapies for breast cancer can only be fulfilled through tissue-based correlative science studies. Unfortunately, access to a tissue bank has been the major barrier to the development of prognostic or predictive tests. This chapter describes issues related to tissue acquisition and banking for breast cancer in the multicenter clinical trial setting.

BARRIERS TO TISSUE ACQUISITION AND BANKING IN CLINICAL TRIALS

Although survival outcome of patients has improved greatly over the past 2 decades due to incremental benefits achieved from systemic therapies, it has become quite clear that molecular heterogeneity of breast cancer dictates treatment response and not every patient derives significant benefit from a given therapy.[1,2] Development of assays that enable assessment of baseline risk and expected degree of benefit from systemic therapy in specific clinical contexts has become a top priority in the research agenda for breast cancer.

These kinds of correlative science studies need tumor tissue with good clinical annotation. Best source of such materials is from randomized phase 3 clinical trials. Unfortunately, tissue procurement is most difficult in such a setting. Ideally every single tumor operated should be snap frozen according to a uniform standard operating procedure and archived in a proper environmental condition. However, reality is that in a typical practice setting in North America, procurement of snap frozen biopsy tissue in expectation of future correlative science studies is often difficult, if not impossible. Because patients usually are presented with the option of enrolling into a clinical trial only after cancer diagnosis is made, the window of opportunity to procure snap frozen tumor tissue often gets lost. National infrastructure to procure snap frozen tissue samples from all tumors operated and store in an ideal environment before shipping to a central bank does not exist, and liquid nitrogen or dry ice may not be readily available in a community oncology setting. For this reason, frozen tissue procurement in large phase 3 multicenter adjuvant clinical trials has not been successful.

Surprisingly, even procurement of formalin-fixed paraffin-embedded tumor blocks has been lacking in phase 3 adjuvant clinical trials until only recently, which is now mandated by many clinical trial groups. Although the utility of archived formalin-fixed paraffin-embedded tumor tissue has been limited by technological barriers, recent development of gene expression analysis methods enabled National Surgical Adjuvant Breast and Bowel Project (NASBP) investigators to use these nonideal materials from already completed trials for the development of the OncotypeDx assay (Genomic Health Inc., Redwood City, California), which is now widely used in the prognostication of outcome in patients with estrogen receptor positive, node-negative breast cancer.[1,3] Therefore there is now a clear scientific rationale to mandate tumor block collection in all clinical trials.

PROCUREMENT OF FROZEN TUMOR TISSUE

Most molecular profiling methods dictate the importance of using snap frozen tissue as the starting material. This has especially been the norm for gene expression profiling studies using microarrays. Ideally in an academic setting with active clinical investigation, dedicated personnel such as pathology assistants should be on call to procure specimens immediately after they were removed from patients. A staff pathologist should be available to grossly examine the specimens, to triage them according to study and banking requirements, and to aliquot them into various fixing and storage conditions. How much time lapse can be tolerated between the removal of tissue from the body and freezing is still the subject of debate. There are few published studies that addressed the impact of time delay on RNA integrity. For normal breast tissue, up to 3 hours was tolerable in one study.[4]

There are now methods that allow gene expression profiling of archived formalin-fixed paraffin-embedded blocks, but proteomics studies still require frozen tumor tissue.[5] How much time lapse can be tolerated for proteomics studies is not clear. It is generally believed that immediate freezing is required for studies interrogating the phosphorylation status of proteins.

PROCUREMENT IN RNAlater

In a community setting with lack of infrastructure, one alternative to snap freezing is the use of the RNAlater solution (Applied Biosystems; Ambion, Austin, Texas).[6] This is a high-salt solution that enables procurement of tumor tissue at room temperature and shipping and storage at 4°C before going into a permanent storage at −20°C. Therefore, RNAlater can be used at institutions where deep freezers or liquid nitrogen tanks are not available for long-term storage of frozen specimens. RNAlater is also useful in a multicenter trial setting when frozen tumor tissue needs to be procured at local sites and shipped to the central bank. Studies demonstrated that tumor tissue specimens procured and stored in RNAlater can be used for microarray gene expression analyses.[6,7] However, in one study using colon and tonsil tissue, RNAlater was found to impact on expression level of a gene, whereas simple transportation in ice preserved expression levels up to 16 hours.[8] Because for breast tissue up to 3 hours at room temperature is tolerated,[4] it may be a good idea not to use RNAlater purely for the purpose of preventing RNA degradation during time delay between surgical procedure and freezing.

In one of the trials conducted by the NSABP, 66 of 76 core biopsies (88%) procured and shipped using RNAlater yielded high-quality RNA adequate for microarray gene expression analyses.[9] In NSABP neoadjuvant trials, RNAlater is routinely used to procure and ship core biopsy specimens. Figure 40-1 shows the components of a custom made RNAlater shipping package. It includes two polypropylene bottles containing 5 mL of RNAlater solution, blotting papers, vinyl gloves, freezer pack, and instructions on how to handle the specimen and package it into a plastic foam and corrugated box, compliant with transportation regulations.

One disadvantage of using RNAlater is that tumor tissue becomes too hardened and, as a result, preparing cryosections from such tissue is very difficult. One solution to this problem is to wash the tissue in saline before cutting[6] or blot dry the tissue to remove excess RNAlater before embedding and cut the tissue at below −20°C.[9] After cutting a few sections for microscopic examination and assessment of tumor cellularity, the tumor-rich area can be manually dissected and homogenized immediately or stored in RNAlaterICE solution (Applied Biosystems) at −20°C before batch processing to extract RNA.

RNAlater can be also used to prevent RNA degradation during the processing of the cryosections from archived frozen tumors that were not preserved in RNAlater.[10]

Although RNAlater preserves RNA and DNA, some proteins such as S-100 protein do get affected by this high-salt solution, and therefore RNAlater is not recommended for proteomics studies.[11]

NEOADJUVANT TRIALS AS A SETTING TO PROCURE TISSUE FOR CORRELATIVE SCIENCE STUDIES

Difficulties of collecting frozen tumors from adjuvant trials and sample size considerations have resulted in a proliferation of neoadjuvant trials as a biomarker research tool in recent years.[12] Neoadjuvant trials provide a unique setting, in which surgical

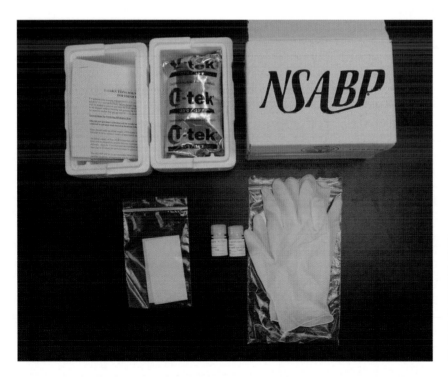

FIGURE 40-1 Components of the RNAlater tissue procurement and shipping kit used in the NSABP trials. It includes 2 polypropylene bottles containing 5 mL of RNAlater solution, blotting papers, vinyl gloves, freezer pack, and instructions on how to handle the specimen and package it into a plastic foam and corrugated box compliant with transportation regulations.

oncologists can control the acquisition of pretreatment tumor tissue samples and the molecular profile of these samples can be correlated with response to preoperative therapy. Pathologic complete response (pCR) to neoadjuvant therapy eventually correlates with clinical outcome and thus provides a convenient alternative to long-term follow-up. Because the same statistical power can be achieved with much smaller sample sizes than in the adjuvant setting, many clinical investigators favor neoadjuvant trials over adjuvant trials as a correlative science research platform. However, for high-throughput discovery approaches such as gene expression microarrays or proteomics, the typical sample sizes of neoadjuvant trials are grossly underpowered when the issue of multiple comparisons is considered. Furthermore, neoadjuvant trials do not consider the effect of additional adjuvant therapies such as tamoxifen on baseline risk because only response is measured. Therefore, the clinical utility of markers discovered in the neoadjuvant trials needs eventually to be tested in the adjuvant setting. Because the predictive algorithm for predicting pCR, developed in the neoadjuvant setting, cannot be directly applied into the adjuvant setting, where time-dependent end points are analyzed, it may make more sense to use materials from adjuvant trials even for the discovery step. The fact that the only multigene-based predictor of chemotherapy benefit in clinical use (OncotypeDx) was developed purely through use of archived tumor blocks from adjuvant trials attest to the latter point.

PROCUREMENT OF FORMALIN-FIXED PARAFFIN-EMBEDDED TUMOR TISSUE BLOCKS

For clinical trial groups in the United States, even collecting paraffin blocks in the multicenter clinical trial setting has been difficult. Pathologists are inherently reluctant to part with diagnostic blocks, and hospital administrators and lawyers, fearing legal liability, have instituted policies to prevent block submission. The procurement rate for tissue blocks in NSABP trials is approximately 85% to 90% of enrolled patients, even though the submission of blocks is mandated. However, this is a greatly improved figure compared with what used to be a rate of submission of approximately ≤50%. This has hampered the study of prognostic and predictive markers, which already suffers from lack of sufficient statistical power.

Most phase III multicenter clinical trials now mandate block submission and permanent banking of collected blocks at the central pathology banks. According to current trend, in the near future, participation in NCI funded multicenter phase III clinical trials may be conditional on the commitment of the institution to submit tumor tissue blocks. Therefore, it is recommended that investigators arrange with their local pathology departments for the preparation of at least one additional tumor block for research use at the time of the initial processing of the biopsy specimens, especially if the institution has a policy against the release of diagnostic blocks to outside pathology banks or investigators.

One method we have developed to deal with noncompliant institutions is the use of a 2-mm skin biopsy device (Miltex Inc., York, Pennsylvania). A 2-mm core sampling of the tumor area

in the paraffin block is now accepted as an alternative to block submission. From a 2-mm core we can sample three 0.6-mm cores for tissue array construction. The acceptance of this alternative has been quite remarkable within the NSABP membership institutions.

Although rare, if the institution refuses to submit even 2-mm cores, then it may be a good idea to get at least fresh-cut sections and process them immediately to isolate RNA and DNA and go through at least the first round of RNA amplification or initial cDNA synthesis because stored precut slides are not ideal material for gene expression analyses. If immediate extraction is not an option, it is probably a good idea to coat the unstained section with paraffin for long-term storage, although this has not been studied systemically. Due to the need to extract the nucleic acid immediately upon receiving the slides, this alternative creates significant burden on the tissue bank and should be only used as a last resort.

STORAGE OF PARAFFIN BLOCKS

Studies have shown a significant decrease in antigenicity during storage of unstained precut sections. Jacobs et al performed a systemic examination of the impact of storage of cut sections at room temperature or refrigerated condition on immunoreactivity for p53, estrogen receptor, Bcl-2, and factor VIII.[15] Regardless of storage conditions, there was a significant decrease in antibody staining compared with time zero. Coating of slides with paraffin did not prevent this effect. Therefore blocks rather than slides should be collected for banking at any cost.

No data are available regarding the ideal storage conditions for paraffin blocks. Ideally the blocks have to be stored airtight under nitrogen gas to prevent oxygen-induced damage. In practice, however, this is difficult to set up and maintain, and almost all banks store blocks at room temperature. The NSABP tissue bank stores all blocks in a refrigerated room to prevent temperature variations, but there is no clear scientific basis for this practice.

Cronin et al have examined the effect of long-term storage of paraffin-embedded tumor blocks on RNA.[14] Old blocks tend to have much more fragmented RNA, and absolute signal from real-time reverse transcription polymerase chain reaction was significantly lower compared with newly made blocks. However, this could be compensated by normalizing with housekeeping genes from the same samples.

PROCESSING OF BANKED TISSUE BLOCKS

For archived tumor blocks that are usually less than 3 mm thick, preservation of the tissue is of maximum priority. To achieve this, the initial processing step is of utmost importance. Figure 40-2 shows the standard operating procedure at the NSABP tissue bank. We use a microtome equipped with a histocollimator, an optical alignment device that aids histologists in aligning the angle of the surface of the block to that of the knife on the microtome (Fig. 40-3). Use of the histocollimator helps minimize the loss of tissue at the initial attempt at sectioning by aligning the angle of the block to that of the knife. Otherwise, depending on the expertise level of the histologist, loss of tissue can be significant.

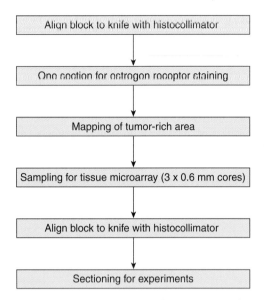

Align block to knife with histocollimator

↓

One section for estrogen receptor staining

↓

Mapping of tumor-rich area

↓

Sampling for tissue microarray (3 x 0.6 mm cores)

↓

Align block to knife with histocollimator

↓

Sectioning for experiments

FIGURE 40-2 Flowchart for tissue block processing at the NSABP. Tissue conservation is a top priority. A histocollimator is used to align the block with the knife before cutting sections. Estrogen receptor staining is used to map tumor-rich area in the block, and tissue microarray cores are sampled before cutting any more sections.

Once the block is aligned to the knife, a single section is made to stain for estrogen receptor with hematoxylin counterstaining. Estrogen receptor stained slides are then used to map the tumor-rich areas on the tissue blocks. Permanent marker is used to map four tumor rich spots on the block, and 0.6 mm cores are extracted and seeded to tissue microarray blocks. We generate 3 replica arrays containing one 0.6-mm core from each case and save one additional core in a tube for future nucleic acid extraction.

TISSUE MICROARRAY CONSTRUCTION

Although it is possible to examine multiple markers on individual cases by serial sectioning of paraffin blocks, at some point it becomes too costly and time consuming. Tissue microarray (TMA) solves this problem of throughput. Once constructed, assay cost is reduced >100-fold, so screening of multiple markers becomes a reality. Screening 100 cases for 70 markers requires staining and reading of 7000 individual slides, whereas tissue arrays containing cores from 100 cases in each array block reduces this to only 70 slides.

The idea of generating a block that contains multiple tissue types was pioneered by Dr. Battifora but was not widely used due to the tedious process involved in the generation of such blocks.[15] In 1990, Lampkin and Allred devised a novel method of creating a tissue array without the need to deparaffinize the donor samples by using a skin biopsy punch 3 to 6 mm in diameter, resulting in up to 40 samples per array.[16] Further improvement of this method has resulted in a method that used a 2-mm-diameter skin biopsy punch resulting in an array containing 60 cores. In 1998, Kononen et al improved this method further by reducing the core diameter to 0.6 mm, using a high-throughput manual device.[17] Owing to the affordability of the instrument and increased density of the array, the tissue array has become widely accepted as a high-throughput screening method for candidate molecular markers.

Although the method developed by Kononen et al can generate much higher density array, in reality it may be unnecessary to put so many cores into one array block. Design of an array with >100 cores often results in the need for creating subarrays or subsections within the array, which creates problems when navigating between the cores, especially when using fluorescence markers. However, the Kononen method may be preferable to the Allred method because the latter leaves a large hole

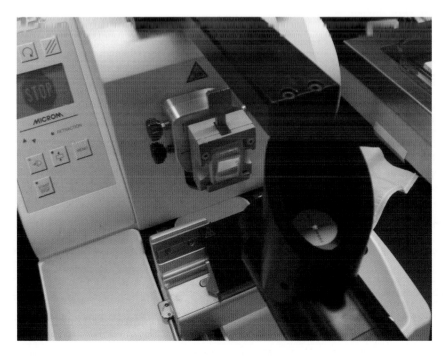

FIGURE 40-3 Histocollimator. A histocollimator is an optical device attached to a microtome that uses light reflection from a mirror overlaid on top of the tissue block to orient the surface of the block to the angle of the knife.

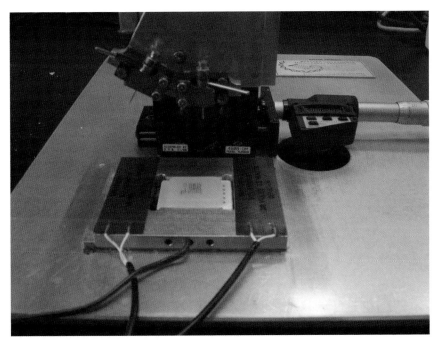

FIGURE 40-4 Manual tissue microarrayer with modification to heat the recipient block. There are 2 needles in the vertical tower. One needle is used to take out a 0.6-mm core from the recipient block to generate an empty hole. The other needle is used to take out a 0.6-mm tissue core from donor block and seed it into the empty hole in the recipient block. There are 2 controllers attached to micrometers that control movements of the vertical tower in the x- and y-axis. The recipient array block is held in a heated holder.

in the donor block. This defect may create legal or political problems with the pathology department from which the block was provided.

At the NSABP tissue bank, we routinely generate tissue arrays containing single 0.6-mm core samples from 100 cases in 3 replicas. For studies of markers that are expected to be homogeneously expressed, only 1 block is used among 3 replicas. For markers that are more heterogeneous in expression within a tumor, all 3 are used.

The original commercialized version of the method described by Kononen et al by Beecher Instrument has popularized the use of tissue array (Fig. 40-4). This simple device uses a micrometer to move the recipient block in a precise manner. It has 2 vertical arms with 0.6-mm punches. The donor punch is slightly bigger in diameter so that the tissue core squeezes into the smaller sized hole in the recipient block. The cores are seeded slightly above the recipient block surface and then later pressed, after incubation at 37°C, so that the height of the seeding can be adjusted to an even surface level.

When creating a high-density array, the center of the block tends to bulge significantly owing to the increased volume (the diameter of the donor core is slightly larger than that of the recipient hole). In their excellent review of the tissue array technique, Jensen and Hammond suggested that keeping the recipient block at approx 100°F using 2 heating strips attached to the recipient block holder will prevent this compression effect and greatly improve the quality of the array.[18] Figure 40-4 shows a manual tissue microarrayer device with heat strips attached to the recipient array block holder according to Jensen's modification.

RNA EXTRACTION

RNA extraction can be achieved with relative ease using commercial kits and can also be automated with ease using magnetic separation devices. It is a routine practice to check the quality of extracted RNA using Bioanalyzer (Agilent) when fresh, snap frozen, or RNAlater procured tissue samples are used as source materials and routine procedures are used for microarray gene expression profiling. When using RNA from formalin-fixed paraffin-embedded blocks as starting materials, Bioanalyzer profile does not provide any meaningful information because RNA is degraded.

There are many ready-made RNA extraction kits available from vendors, but homogenization reagents included in those kits do not work well with RNAlater-procured tissue because the tissue is too hard. Mechanical homogenization devices using glass beads should be used to homogenize RNAlater-procured tissue.

REVERSE PHASE PROTEIN ARRAY

Many investigators are also interested in examining expression levels of proteins—especially phosphorylated proteins—to assess drug targets in the tissue samples. Although procedures such as immunostaining can be used to assess a single target or few targets at a time on a single microscopic section, it is desirable to assess many targets at once quantitatively. Reverse phase protein array is a technique in which tissue lysates are spotted on a slide in a microarray format so that many cases are printed on a single slide in serial dilutions.[19] Antibody staining of these slides generates quantitative information for many cases at a time. This method could prove quite useful in assessing targets and pathways in trials evaluating targeted therapies.

HUMAN SUBJECT PROTECTION

Control of the flow of materials and data files is a very important issue due to the regulatory requirements for human subject

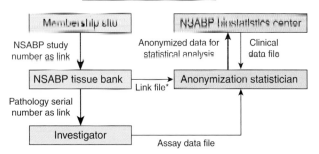

Flow of material and data files

* Also with assay data file if assay is done at tissue bank.

FIGURE 40-5 Human subject protection. A third-party anonymization office is used to comply with all regulations regarding human subject protection. Tumor blocks are collected with only the study number as an identifier. Tissue sections are provided to the investigators with a new serial number. Assay data file, link file for serial number and study number, and clinical data file are sent to the anonymization office. The assembled linked data set is purged from the study number and sent to the biostatistical center for analysis.

protection. There are 2 different models in tissue banking. The usual model is that the tissue bank does not conduct any research using the collected materials and simply provides the tissue to investigators. In this model, the bank is allowed to keep patient identifiers but is not allowed to provide patient identifiers to investigators. Investigators have to send assay data to the group biostatistician for correlation with clinical outcome data. If the informed consent of the clinical trial does not clearly cover the assay under investigation, use of a third-party anonymization office to link clinical data with assay data is required. In the NSABP model, the tissue bank also conducts research in addition to providing banked tissue to outside investigators (Fig. 40-5). Therefore the bank also functions as an investigator. In this setting, the bank is not allowed to keep any patient identifiers. Because the bank has to keep the protocol study numbers in order to be able to return tissue blocks for clinical care in some cases, a third party anonymization office is used to link experimental data with clinical data (Fig. 40-2). The assay data with a link file that connects the sample number and the study number are sent to the anonymization office. At the same time the clinical data file with the study number is sent from the biostatistics center to the anonymization office. A linked dataset file that contains the lab assay data and the clinical outcome data is created, and the study number is purged from the linked dataset file and sent to the biostatistician for analysis.

FUTURE DIRECTIONS

Ideally a national tissue banking system should be in place to freeze every tumor removed from patients. In the absence of such infrastructure, it will be difficult to construct a meaningful frozen tumor bank from phase III adjuvant trials. In the absence of such system, the neoadjuvant platform provides opportunity to procure fresh or snap frozen tumor tissue for correlative science studies. However, with the current practice of neoadjuvant studies having relatively small sample sizes, the usefulness of collected tumor specimens may be limited. Ultimately, prognostic and predictive markers are most useful when developed for a specific clinical context. Therefore there will be increasing demand for archived tumor tissue blocks from phase III adjuvant clinical trials as newer technologies are developed that allow interrogation of macromolecules contained in those blocks.

SUMMARY

Tissue acquisition and banking have become an important aspect of clinical trials for breast cancer. Although snap frozen specimens remain the gold standard, alternatives exist that provide realistic solutions in a large multicenter clinical trial setting. RNAlater solution stabilizes nucleic acids and enables specimen procurement and shipping at suboptimal conditions. Gene expression profiling can be performed with RNA extracted from formalin-fixed paraffin-embedded tumor blocks. Stored precut sections are not ideal for many assays and therefore not recommended for banking.

REFERENCES

1. Paik S, Tang G, Shak S, et al. Gene expression and benefit of chemotherapy in women with node-negative, estrogen receptor-positive breast cancer. *J Clin Oncol.* 2006;24(23):3726-3734.
2. Rouzier R, Perou CM, Symmans WF, et al. Breast cancer molecular subtypes respond differently to preoperative chemotherapy. *Clin Cancer Res.* 2005;11(16):5678-5685.
3. Paik S, Shak S, Tang G, et al. A multigene assay to predict recurrence of tamoxifen-treated, node-negative breast cancer. *N Engl J Med.* 2004;351(27):2817-2826.
4. Ohashi Y, Creek KE, Pirisi L, Kalus R, Young SR. RNA degradation in human breast tissue after surgical removal: a time-course study. *Exp Mol Pathol.* 2004;77(2):98-103.
5. Paik S. Methods for gene expression profiling in clinical trials of adjuvant breast cancer therapy. *Clin Cancer Res.* 2006;12(3 Pt 2):1019s-1023s.
6. Ellis M, Davis N, Coop A, et al. Development and validation of a method for using breast core needle biopsies for gene expression microarray analyses. *Clin Cancer Res.* 2002;8(5):1155-1166.
7. Mutter GL, Zahrieh D, Liu C, et al. Comparison of frozen and RNAlater® solid tissue storage methods for use in RNA expression microarrays. BMC Genomics 2004; 5(1):88.
8. Micke P, Ohshima M, Tahmasebpoor S, et al. Biobanking of fresh frozen tissue: RNA is stable in nonfixed surgical specimens. *Lab Invest.* 2006;86(2):202-211.
9. Hamm JT, Wilson JW, Rastogi P, et al. Gemcitabine/epirubicin/paclitaxel as neoadjuvant chemotherapy in locally advanced breast cancer: a phase II trial of the NSABP Foundation Research Group. *Clin Breast Cancer.* 2008;8(3):257-263.
10. Guo D, Catchpoole DR. Isolation of intact RNA following cryosection of archived frozen tissue. *BioTechniques.* 2003;34(1):48-50.
11. Florell SR, Coffin CM, Holden JA, et al. Preservation of RNA for functional genomic studies: a multidisciplinary tumor bank protocol. *Mod Pathol.* 2001;14(2):116-128.
12. Paik S. Incorporating genomics into the cancer clinical trial process. *Semin Oncol.* 2001;28(3):305-309.
13. Jacobs TW, Prioleau JE, Stillman IE, Schnitt SJ. Loss of tumor marker-immunostaining intensity on stored paraffin slides of breast cancer. *J Natl Cancer Inst.* 1996;88(15):1054-1059.
14. Cronin M, Pho M, Dutta D, et al. Measurement of gene expression in archival paraffin-embedded tissues: development and performance of a 92-gene reverse transcriptase-polymerase chain reaction assay. *Am J Pathol.* 2004;164(1):35-42.

15. Battifora H. The multitumor (sausage) tissue block: novel method for immunohistochemical antibody testing. *Lab Invest.* 1986;55(2):244-248.

16. Lampkin SR, Allred DC. Preparation of paraffin blocks and sections containing multiple tissue samples using a skin biopsy punch. *J Histotechnol.* 1990;13:121-123.

17. Kononen J, Bubendorf L, Kallioniemi A, et al. Tissue microarrays for high-throughput molecular profiling of tumor specimens. *Nat Med.* 1998;4(7):844-847.

18. Jensen TA, Hammond E. The tissue microarray—a technical guide for histologist. *J Histotechnol.* 2003;24:283-287.

19. Wulfkuhle JD, Aquino JA, Calvert VS, et al. Signal pathway profiling of ovarian cancer from human tissue specimens using reverse-phase protein microarrays. *Proteomics.* 2003;3(11):2085-2090.

CHAPTER 41

Funding for Clinical Trials

Edward L. Trimble
Andrea Denicoff
Jeffrey Abrams

Breast cancer investigators must contend with the critical issue of how to fund their trials, including what costs should be included in the budget for a trial. We have divided this chapter into 2 sections: first, a discussion of the various components associated with clinical trials that require funding, and, second, potential funding sources to fund the proposed trial costs.

CENTRAL COSTS

The costs of a clinical trial include both central costs, related to protocol development and management, as well as the institutional costs, related to the regulatory review and the actual conduct of the trial at participating sites. If a clinical trial is to be conducted at only one location, then all these costs will be incurred at that site. If the trial will take place in multiple locations, then the central and institutional costs will be incurred at different locations.

Protocol Design and Development

The guiding text for a trial is the protocol document and associated appendices. Drafting a functional protocol document requires input from a variety of disciplines, including all those treatment modalities used in the trial, as well as biostatistics, nursing, pharmacy, and ancillary clinical disciplines such as pathology and radiology. Wherever possible, investigators should use an appropriate template to streamline the task of developing a new protocol. Model templates are available at the National Cancer Institute's Cancer Therapy Evaluation Program (NCI CTEP) Web site, as well as through the NCI-sponsored Clinical Trials Cooperative Groups.[1] In general, a face-to-face meeting involving representatives of the appropriate disciplines is required to initiate protocol development. Follow-up work

may be conducted via e-mail, telephone, and conference calls. The trial budget should include, therefore, the costs of face-to-face meetings, as well as the time of key investigators, biostatisticians, and protocol coordinators.

DATA COLLECTION

Before the trial begins, the investigators must also develop case report forms and a system for data collection. This process requires time and potentially money. The requirement for time and money can be lessened by the use of existing case report forms and a data collection system that is already in place. For multi-institutional trials, remote data capture via a secure Web site may prove less time consuming and expensive than the traditional paper-based system in which forms are mailed or faxed to a central location. We also recommend that all case report forms use the standard Common Data Elements, which the NCI and the Clinical Trials Cooperative Groups jointly developed.[2] We also encourage the collection of clinical trial data through electronic means using consistent definitions and formats across trials. Compliance with data collection standards and electronic data reporting standards, as developed by 2 international groups, the Clinical Data Standards Interchange Consortium (CDISC) and Health Level 7 (HL7), can further increase clinical trials efficiency and speed up regulatory review.[3,4]

CDISC and HL7 are the 2 principal groups that have taken on the task of creating clinical-research reporting standards. CDISC has created models to standardize the submission of data to regulators, and HL7 produces standards for clinical and administrative data. To promote interoperability among applications using CDISC or the HL7 standard, the US Food and Drug Administration (FDA), NCI, CDSIC, and HL7 created the Biomedical Research Integrated Domain Group (BRIDG). The BRIDG model, released in 2007, has been adopted by the NCI's Cancer Biomedical Informatics Grid (CaBIG) initiative.[6]

CaBIG, an open-source, open-access, open-development, and federated platform that facilitates the collection and sharing of standardized data across participating sites, shows great potential for increasing the pace of innovative in cancer treatment. CaBIG offers participants tools that aid clinical trials management, integrate and analyze various types of data, and assure secure data-sharing connections among the NCI-designated cancer centers and 16 community health centers in the network. Of particular interest will be the forthcoming proposed rule for Electronic Submission of Data from Studies Evaluating Human Drugs and Biologics, expected in September 2008 (but still pending as of September, 2009).

Regulatory Review and Oversight

Once the protocol document has been finalized, it must be submitted for regulatory review. This review may include the local institutional review board (IRB), in some cases, a central or national IRB, and/or the FDA. In addition, at NCI-designated cancer centers, the protocol must be reviewed by a scientific review committee. Submission of these documents requires additional time and effort on the part of the principal investigator and protocol coordinator at each site. Some sites require that investigators partially defray the institutional costs of protocol and amendment submission. The protocol coordinator at each site must maintain meticulous records documenting approval by the local and/or central IRB of the protocol, amendments, and yearly reviews. For multi-institutional studies, a central coordinating office will also need to confirm regulatory approval at all participating sites. In addition, all investigators participating in a trial sponsored by the NCI or by a pharmaceutical company planning to submit trial data to the FDA must complete and file the FDA 1572 investigator registration form.[7] The NCI's CTEP maintains these forms for CTEP sponsored trials, including those conducted by the Clinical Trials Cooperative Groups. Certain trials may also require certification of expertise and/or protocol orientation. Examples might include expertise in sentinel lymph node assessment, intensity-modulated radiation therapy (IMRT), and so on. The budget may need to include costs of training and orientation programs, as well as the cost of maintaining a registry of those certified to participate in the trial.

Patient Registration

The process of patient registration also requires an investment of time and resources. Certain trials may require verification of eligibility, such as with real-time review of pathology. Budgets for such trials will need to cover the costs of such verification, as well as that of registration and randomization, if required by study design. For large Phase 2 and 3 trials, most trial networks, including the NCI-supported Cooperative Groups, have developed centralized online registration and randomization systems to enable 24-hour availability to the trial by investigators in different time zones.

Distribution of Experimental Agents

Trials evaluating novel experimental agents generally require support for a central research pharmacy, the time of research pharmacists, and, for multi-institutional studies, shipment of the experimental agent to participating sites. For trials sponsored by the NCI's CTEP in which CTEP holds the Investigational New Drug (IND) application for the investigational agent, the NCI's CTEP maintains the central pharmaceutical repository and ships drugs to participating sites. The NCI core grants to NCI-designated cancer centers may partially support the cost of a research pharmacy.

Correlative Science and Ancillary Studies

Tumor and Specimen Banking

Many trials now require or encourage collection of slides confirming histologic diagnoses, fixed and/or frozen tumor tissue, serum, whole blood, and other specimens. The budget for multi-institutional trials, therefore, may need to include the costs of preparing and shipping specimen collection kits to participating sites, sites coordinating and obtaining specimens from trial participants, shipping specimens to central tumor banks and/or core laboratories, and central tumor banking activities. The NCI's Cancer Diagnosis Program partially supports the tumor and specimen-banking activities of the Clinical Trials Cooperative Groups. CTEP and the Clinical Trials Cooperative Groups have jointly developed a guidance document that outlines various correlative science and ancillary studies with suggested payment tiers for such studies.[8]

Correlative Scientific Studies

In many trials, analysis of specimens collected from patients may be useful for the development and/or validation of diagnostic, prognostic, and predictive markers. Other potential studies may include more research into tumor biology, intermediate biomarkers, pharmacogenomics, pharmacokinetics, and other areas. The NCI's CTEP supports the cost of some core laboratories through parent grants to the Clinical Trials Cooperative Groups. The NCI has also earmarked funds, available on a competitive basis, to support the costs of correlative science components that are integral to a specific clinical treatment trial. In some cases, for trials sponsored or cosponsored by industry, the industry partner may be willing to support the cost of the correlative science or perform the laboratory analyses in house. Investigator-initiated grants may also be used to support these laboratory analyses. The NCI's Division of Cancer Treatment and Diagnosis has worked to strengthen collaboration in such correlative scientific analyses between the Specialized Programs of Research Excellence (SPOREs) and Clinical Trials Cooperative Groups. The NCI does sponsor an ongoing program announcement indicating the NCI's interest in receiving grant applications for correlative science linked to clinical trials.[9]

Health-Related Quality of Life, Health Services Research, and Other Ancillary Studies

Breast cancer investigators also collaborate with a variety of other disciplines interested in studying secondary end points on treatment trials, including aspects of health-related quality of life, health services, epidemiology, psychosocial, and/or behavioral studies. These studies may be either companion studies to or embedded studies within treatment trials, most commonly phase 3 trials, but also some large phase 2 studies. The NCI's Division of Cancer Prevention (DCP) may assign additional monetary credits for cancer control companion studies of NCI-sponsored phase 3 trials, whether incorporated within the trial or as a stand-alone companion protocol. The NCI has also earmarked funds, available competitively, to support the costs of health-related quality-of-life (HRQOL) components that are integral to a specific clinical treatment trial. Industry may also provides funding for these types of ancillary studies because treatment effects on patient quality of life is now even more important to measure and intervene, given the long-term survival of many patients. The budget for these trials may include the costs for programs to train members of the research team how to use and administer patient surveys and various measurement tools, personnel time to coordinate the additional data collection and quality control, along with the central costs of data collection, statistical analysis, and reporting of results.

Quality Assurance/Quality Control

Investigators must also budget for the cost of ensuring quality assurance/quality control in clinical trials. This may include review of operative notes, videos, and pathology reports to confirm the quality of surgery, review of planning films for radiation therapy, central pathology review, and review of original source documentation to confirm accuracy of trial data and compliance with regulatory requirements. Costs can include collection of materials for review, travel for on-site audits, as well as the time of the appropriate experts to perform these reviews. The NCI funds the Quality Assurance Review Center (QARC) to perform quality assurance for radiation therapy and the Radiological Physics Center to monitor and standardize radiation dosimetry for the Clinical Trials Cooperative Groups.[10] In addition, the NCI's CTEP also funds the Clinical Trials Cooperative Groups to conduct on-site audits of each site's participating Cooperative Group studies and also conducts audits at the NCI's Comprehensive Cancer Centers nationwide. These audits must take place at least every 3 years, with the audit to include charts for at least 10% of patients accrued to trials at that site.

INSTITUTIONAL COSTS

Institutional Review Board Activity

Institutions participating in clinical trials generally maintain an ethics committee (institutional review board). In some cases, as mentioned earlier, they charge investigators for protocol review, amendments, and yearly reviews to defray some of their costs for these activities. Filing the appropriate forms and cover materials for initial and ongoing review of the institutional level requires a major investment of time from the principal investigator and trial staff. Some institutions have decided to use commercial IRBs instead of maintaining their own local board.

Costs for this activity must be budgeted. For phase 3 cooperative group trials, the NCI has developed a Centralized Institutional Review Board (CIRB) that should alleviate, to some degree, the costs associated with these trials. The CIRB is able to perform the initial protocol review as well as all continuing reviews, amendment reviews, and reviews of adverse events, sparing local boards the need to perform a full board review on these phase 3 trials.

Staff Time

Beyond these efforts to comply with regulatory requirements, conduct of a trial at the institutional level requires a major commitment of time by the clinical investigators, research nurses, data managers, and research pharmacists. The time commitment of the clinical investigators and their team includes their efforts to educate health care providers and potential trial participants about the trial, screen patients for trial eligibility, counsel patients and their families about the trial, obtain informed consent, administer protocol therapy, collect and report required data, perform surveillance for and manage potential toxicity arising from protocol therapy, and conduct the required schedule of follow-up after completion of protocol therapy. In addition, the trial may require additional work by hospital pathologists for specimen preparation and radiologists for trial-specific review of imaging. The NCI, working with the Clinical Trials Cooperative Groups, has worked to standardize recommendations for reimbursement of these services. Emanuel et al recently surveyed 21 sites active in clinical trials and asked them to estimate the number of hours required for a mock phase 3 randomized placebo-controlled trial of a new chemotherapeutic trial. The participating sites estimated that they would need on average 200 hours per patient, of which 68% was clinical and 32% nonclinical.[11] C-Change, which is a forum of cancer leaders from government, industry and non-profit sectors, has recently issued the "Guidance Document for Implementing Effective Cancer Clinical Trials," which includes an extensive discussion of staff time requirements for clinical trials.[12] It also describes a commissioned survey of 14 cancer clinical trials sites across the United States that were asked to estimate their costs of implementing mock federal and industry-sponsored phase 2 and 3 treatment trials. The median study cost per subject based on the mock protocols for the government-sponsored randomized phase 2 study was $6266, whereas the cost of the industry-sponsored randomized phase 2 study was $8240. The median cost per subject for the government-sponsored phase 3 study was $3427, whereas the cost of the industry-sponsored phase 3 study was $4696. Industry trials were found to be more labor intensive than government trials.

Indirect Costs

Nongovernmental institutions commonly negotiate with the US General Services Administration an "indirect-cost rate" to cover the institutional overhead costs associated with research, including clinical trials. Trialists should be aware of the indirect-cost rate their individual institution charges and what institutional resources are supported by the indirect costs. When government and nongovernmental funding sources make decisions to fund grant applications, they generally commit to paying both direct and indirect costs.

POTENTIAL FUNDING SOURCES

We have organized this section into funding for clinical trials at the level of the local institution, funding from foundations and professional societies, funding from industry, and finally funding from federal sources, including the NIH, the NCI, and the Department of Defense. Investigators should understand that they may well need to assemble financial support from a variety of different sources to support their clinical trials.

Institutional Funding for Clinical Trials

Investigators seeking to start trials for women with breast cancer at their home institution should first find out what resources exist to support and manage trials. Collegial relationships with the staff of the institutional Clinical Research Office and IRB are critical. New investigators should find out whether there is institutional support for trial biostatistics, data management, research pharmacy services, core laboratories, trial education, and community outreach for trials. As noted earlier, in some cases, the indirect costs associated with grants or contracts may cover all or part of these activities. In addition, many institutions do have small grant programs that provide seed money for new investigators.

Foundation and Professional Society Funding for Clinical Trials

A number of foundations and professional societies have ongoing programs to support cancer research, including clinical trials. Some of those most likely to support breast cancers trials are shown in Tables 41-1 and 41-2. Funding mechanisms, dollars, and deadlines can change from year to year, so investigators should check for updates regularly with these organizations. The Community of Science provides a comprehensive electronic database of funding sources for scientific research.[13] Many institutions have research offices that can provide guidance on potential funding sources from all sites, including foundations.

Industry

Pharmaceutical and biotechnology companies provide a large amount of support for research, including clinical trials. The

TABLE 41-2 Partial List of Professional Societies with Grant Programs That May Be Appropriate for Support of Clinical Trials in Breast Cancer

American College of Surgeons (http://www.facs.org)
American Society for Clinical Oncology (http://www.asco.org)
American Society for Therapeutic Radiology and Oncology (http://www.astro.org)
Society of Surgical Oncology (http://www.surgonc.org)

Pharmaceutical and Manufacturers Research Association estimated that in 2007 research and investment in new drugs totaled at least $55.8 billion.[14] These include both company-sponsored trials, as well as investigator-initiated trials. Some large companies have grant programs to provide experimental agents and, in some cases, additional financial support for investigator-initiated trials. Investigators undertaking clinical trials under contract with industry should ensure that the contracts include appropriate funding at the institutional levels for the costs described in the first section of this chapter.

Federal Funding Sources

National Institutes of Health

Through the National Center for Research Resources, the NIH has 2 major programs of importance to clinical trialists. These both provide support at the institutional level for aspects of clinical trials. The General Clinical Research Centers help pay for the costs of research nurses, data managers, biostatisticians, hardware, and software, as well as underwriting patient care costs associated with clinical trials that are not part of routine patient care, including additional overnight stays, imaging studies, and laboratory studies. A list of those 78 institutions that have General Clinical Research Center grants may be found at the National Center for Research Resources Web site.[15] In general, each institution has an application process by which an investigator can apply for funds to cover the additional patient care costs associated with clinical trials. The Clinical and Translational Science Awards (CTSA) program provides institutional funding to strengthen clinical and translational research at academic health centers.[16] The funding will be used to train new investigators, design new informatics tools for clinical trials, support outreach to the public and health care

TABLE 41-1 Partial List of Foundations Which May Consider Supporting Clinical Trials in Breast Cancer

American Cancer Society (http://www.cancer.org)
Breast Cancer Research Foundation (http://www.bcrfcure.org)
Carol M. Baldwin Breast Cancer Research Foundation (http://www.findacure.org)
The Inflammatory Breast Cancer Research Foundation (http://www.ibcresearch.org)
International Breast Cancer Foundation (http://www.ibcrf.org)
National Breast Cancer Research Foundation (http://nationalbreastcancer.org)
Susan G. Komen Breast Cancer Foundation (http://www.komen.org)

providers, build interdisciplinary research teams, and build new partnerships with public and private health care organizations, including the pharmaceutical companies, the Veterans Administration hospitals, health maintenance organizations, as well as state health agencies. Currently, the CTSA consortium includes 38 academic centers in 23 states. In 2012, when the program is fully implemented, the consortium will include approximately 60 CTSAs with an annual budget of $500 million.

National Cancer Institute

NCI funding for clinical trials can be divided into support for training in clinical research, support for investigator-initiated clinical trials, and ongoing support for clinical trials network. The NCI currently supports Institutional Research Training Grants for young investigators at many sites.[17] NCI individual grants for training in clinical trials span early, transition, and mid-career. A list of the various grant mechanisms may be found at the NCI Cancer Training Web site.[18] Another useful Web site is the NIH Career Award Wizard.[19] The NCI has also earmarked money to support the training of underrepresented minorities in clinical trials through the Comprehensive Minority Biomedical Program, using both institutional and individual award programs.[20]

The NCI supports investigator-initiated clinical research through a variety of grant mechanisms. The smallest is the R03, which can be used to support correlative science linked to a clinical trial. Next comes the R21, which is used to support small developmental trials. A larger grant, which could incorporate both clinical trials and the associated translational research, would be the R01. The largest grants are the Program Project (PO1), which consists of several related projects, and the cancer-site-specific SPORE. Currently the NCI funds 11 SPOREs in breast cancer.[21] Many of these have undertaken early-phase clinical trials in breast cancer. Investigators should check the NCI Web site for relevant program announcements, indicating NCI interest (but not earmarked money) and requests for applications (RFAs), for which the NCI has set aside money.[22] Two Program Announcements that breast cancer investigators should note are the Quick Trials program announcement for small trials of novel cancer therapies and the program announcement for correlative studies from multisite clinical trials.[5,23] It is important to note that due to budgetary limitations, NIH and NCI grants have been cut back to 85% of approved funds, highlighting the need for investigators to put together funding from a variety of sources for an individual clinical trial.

The NCI also funds several ongoing consortia for clinical trials. These include sites that conduct phase 1 trials of novel agents for cancer treatment under contract, as well as a larger consortium that conducts phase 2 trials of novel agents for cancer treatment. Definitive phase 3 cancer treatment trials are largely conducted by the NCI's Clinical Trials Cooperative Groups. Table 41-3 shows those groups that conduct trials in breast cancer. The NCI has established a separate but overlapping consortium, composed of academic centers linked to community physicians to develop and conduct trials in cancer control and prevention.[24] Sites that are funded to develop such trials, termed Community Clinical Oncology Program (CCOP) Research Bases, include the Clinical Trials Cooperative Groups marked with an asterisk in Table 41-3, as well as the institutions listed in Table 41-4. Community sites that are funded to participate in cancer control, prevention, and treatment trials through the CCOP and Minority-Based CCOP program are listed at the NCI CCOP Web site.[25]

We encourage breast cancer investigators to take advantage of the ongoing support for research infrastructure from NIH and NCI described here. Trialists should explore what NIH and NCI support for clinical research exists at their current institution, as well as at institutions where they may be seeking employment. The extensive clinical trials infrastructure represented by the NCI's Clinical Trials Cooperative Groups and

---

TABLE 41-3 NCI-Sponsored Clinical Trials Cooperative Groups That Conduct Trials in Breast Cancer

American College of Radiology Imaging Network (http://www.acrin.org)
American College of Surgeons Oncology Group (http://www.acosog.org)
Cancer and Leukemia Group B* (http:// www.calgb.org)
Eastern Cooperative Oncology Group* (http://ecog.dfci.harvard.edu)
National Cancer Institute of Canada Clinical Trials Group (http://www.ctg.queensu.ca)
National Surgical Adjuvant Breast and Bowel Project* (http://nsabp.pitt.edu)
North Central Cancer Treatment Group* (http://ncctg.mayo.edu)
Radiation Therapy Oncology Group* (http://www.rtog.org)
Southwest Oncology Group* (http://www.swog.org)

*Also an NCI CCOP research base.

TABLE 41-4 Additional Community Clinical Oncology Program Research Bases

Fox-Chase Cancer Center (http://www.fccc.edu)
H. Lee Moffitt Cancer Center and Research Institute (http://www.moffitt.org)
University of Michigan Cancer Center (http://www.mcancer.org)
University of Rochester Cancer Center (http://www.urmc.rochester.edu/cancer-center/)
University of Texas MD Anderson Cancer Center (http://www.mdanderson.org)
Wake Forest University School of Medicine (http://www1.wfubmc.edu/cancer)

CCOP program is ideal for conducting breast cancer prevention, treatment, and symptom control trials.

Department of Defense

The Department of Defense sponsors research in breast cancer through the Congressionally Directed Medical Research Programs.[26] Funding mechanisms and priorities can change from year to year, so investigators should check for updates with Congressionally Directed Medical Research Program staff and the Web site.

SUMMARY

Investigators designing breast cancer trials should be aware of the costs associated with various components of a trial and include a budget appropriate for those costs. Potential funding sources include institutions, foundations, charities, industry, and government. The US NCI provides extensive support for the various components of breast cancer clinical trials. NCI support includes both grants for individual trials and the cooperative agreements that support an ongoing research infrastructure for clinical trials through the Clinical Trials Cooperative Groups and the Clinical Community Oncology Program research bases.

REFERENCES

1. Cancer Therapy Evaluation Program. National Cancer Institute. Available at: http://ctep.cancer.gov/guidelines/templates.html. Accessed September 8, 2008.
2. Cancer Therapy Evaluation Program. National Cancer Institute. Available at: http://ctep.cancer.gov/reporting/cde.html. Accessed September 8, 2008.
3. Clinical Data Standards Interchange Consortium. Available at: http://cdisc.org. Accessed September 22, 2008.
4. Health Level 7. Available at: http://www.hl7.org. Accessed September 22, 2008.
5. Biomedical Research Integrated Domain Group. National Cancer Institute. Available at: https://cabig.nci.nih.gov/inventory/infrastructure/bridg. Accessed September 22, 2008.
6. Cancer Biomedical Informatics Grid. National Cancer Institute. Available at: https://cabig.nci.nih.gov. Accessed September 22, 2008.
7. Cancer Therapy Evaluation Program. National Cancer Institute. Available at: http://ctep.cancer.gov/resources/investigator3.html. Accessed September 8, 2008.
8. Cancer Therapy Evaluation Program. National Cancer Institute. Available at: http://ctep.cancer.gov/forms/cie_ancillary_studies.pdf. Accessed September 19, 2008.
9. Division of Cancer Treatment and Diagnosis. National Cancer Institute. Available at: http://dctd.cancer.gov/ProgramPages/CTEP-FundOpp_MultiInstitutional_Trials.htm. Accessed September 19, 2008.
10. Quality Assurance Review Center. Available at: http://www.qarc.org; http://rpc.mdanderson.org/rpc/. Accessed September 8, 2008.
11. Emauel EJ, Schnipper LE, Kamin DY, et al. The costs of conducting clinical research. *J Clin Oncol.* 2003;21:4145-4150.
12. C-Change. Available at: http://www.c-changetogether.org/pubs/pubs/GuidanceDocument.pdf.
13. Community of Science. Available at: http://www.cos.com. Accessed September 8, 2008.
14. Pharmaceutical and Manufacturers Research Association. Available at: http://www.phrrma.org/about_phrma/. Accessed September 8, 2008.
15. General Clinical Research Centers. Available at: http://www.gcrconline.org. Accessed September 8, 2008.
16. Clinical and Translational Science Awards. National Cancer Institute. Available at: http://www.ctsaweb.org. Accessed September 8, 2008.
17. National Cancer Institute. Available at: http://www.cancer.gov/researchandfunding/training/T32/page3. Accessed September 8, 2008.
18. National Cancer Institute. Available at: http://www.cancer.gov/researchandfunding/training/awards. Accessed September 8, 2008.
19. National Institutes of Health. Available at: http://grants.nih.gov/training/kwizard/index.htm. Accessed September 8, 2008.
20. National Cancer Institute. Available at: http://minorityopportunities.nci.nih.gov/index.html. Accessed September 8, 2008.
21. Specialized Programs of Research Excellence. National Cancer Institute. Available at: http://spores.nci.nih.gov/current/breast/breast.html. Accessed September 8, 2008.
22. National Cancer Institute. Available at: http://www.cancer.gov/researchandfunding#fundingopportunities. Accessed September 8, 2008.
23. National Institutes of Health. Available at: http://grants.nih.gov/grants/guide/pa-files/par-04-155.html. Accessed September 8, 2008.
24. Loprinzi CL, Barton DL, Jatoi A, et al. Symptom control trials: a 20-year experience. *J Support Oncol.* 2007;5:119-125.
25. Community Clinical Oncology Program. National Cancer Institute. Available at: http://prevention.cancer.gov/program-resources/programs/ccop. Accessed September 8, 2008.
26. Congressionally Directed Medical Research Programs. US Department of Defence. Available at: http://cdmrp.army.mil/bcrp/default.htm. Accessed September 8, 2008.

CHAPTER 42

The NSABP Experience

Eleftherios P. Mamounas
D. Lawrence Wickerham
Bernard Fisher
Charles E. Geyer
Thomas B. Julian
Norman Wolmark

Over the past 50 years, the National Surgical Adjuvant Breast and Bowel Project (NSABP) has made significant contributions in reducing the extent of surgical resection and in improving the outcome of patients with early-stage breast cancer through the conduct of large, randomized clinical trials evaluating various aspects of local and systemic therapy. Some of these trials have been instrumental in establishing new standards of care in the locoregional and adjuvant systemic therapy for these patients. The rationale, design, and updated results from those pivotal trials are reviewed in this chapter. In addition, the design and rationale for newer trials put forth by the NSABP and other major cooperative groups in an attempt to refine several aspects of adjuvant therapy and introduce new promising drugs are also reviewed. Finally, current and future research directions of the NSABP in the context of other developments in the surgical and adjuvant breast cancer therapy are discussed.

PIVOTAL LOCOREGIONAL THERAPY TRIALS FOR INVASIVE CARCINOMA

Trials Evaluating Less Radical Breast Surgery in Patients with Invasive Carcinoma

The National Surgical Adjuvant Breast and Bowel Project (NSABP) has been instrumental in changing the paradigm of the surgical management of both invasive and noninvasive breast cancer that was founded on Halstedian principles of tumor growth and dissemination. Several randomized trials (B-04, B-06, B-17) have demonstrated that the extent of local therapy

is not paramount to patient's survival.[1-3] As a result of these trials as well as those conducted by other groups,[4,5] disfiguring operations developed a century ago, such as radical mastectomy, have now been replaced in the majority of cases by the more cosmetically acceptable and less function-impairing lumpectomy.

NSABP B-04

The NSABP B-04 trial was set up as 2 companion trials conducted in parallel, one for patients with clinically node-negative breast cancer and the other for those with clinically node-positive disease. Since radical mastectomy was the standard of care at that time, this operation was included as the control arm for both trials. One thousand seventy-nine patients with clinically node-negative disease were randomized to radical mastectomy (362 patients), total mastectomy plus local-regional/axillary irradiation (352 patients), or total mastectomy alone, with no targeted axillary treatment (365 patients). For patients presenting with clinically suspicious disease in the axilla, 586 patients were randomized to radical mastectomy (292 patients) or total mastectomy plus radiation (294 patients). The most recent update from the B-04 trial after 25 years of follow-up[6] continues to demonstrate no significant differences in long-term outcome between clinically node-negative patients who received radical mastectomy and those who received total mastectomy with or without nodal irradiation, or between clinically node-positive patients who received radical mastectomy and those who received total mastectomy with nodal irradiation. Among women with clinically negative nodes, the hazard ratio for death among those who were treated with total mastectomy and irradiation as compared with those who underwent radical mastectomy was 1.08 (95% CI 0.91–1.28, p = 0.38), and the hazard ratio for death among those who had total mastectomy without irradiation as compared with those who underwent radical mastectomy was 1.03 (95% CI 0.87–1.23, p = 0.72). Among women with clinically positive nodes, the hazard ratio for death among those who underwent total mastectomy and radiation as compared with those who underwent radical mastectomy was 1.06 (95% CI 0.89–1.27, p = 0.49). These findings validate earlier results showing no advantage from radical mastectomy.[1] Although differences in outcome of a few percentage points cannot be excluded with this sample size, these findings do not demonstrate a clinically significant survival advantage from removing occult positive nodes at the time of initial surgery or from the addition of locoregional radiation to total mastectomy. In patients presenting with clinically node-negative disease, pathologic evaluation of the radical mastectomy specimen revealed that 40% of cases were pathologically node positive. Because of randomization, one would assume that 40% of the patients randomized to total mastectomy with or without radiation were also node positive at presentation and had disease that was either radiated or not treated at all. However, the axillary failure rate in the TM alone arm was only 19%, indicating that microscopic, occult disease in the axilla may not always progress into clinically overt disease. Furthermore, the similar overall (OS) survival between the 3 arms suggests that an axillary node dissection for the clinically-negative axilla is largely prophylactic, and that outcome is not likely to be significantly compromised by deferring the dissection until there is clinical evidence of disease in the axilla.

Perhaps more importantly, the initial results from the B-04 trial helped pave the way for the conduct of the NSABP B-06 trial evaluating even less radical surgical procedures for the treatment of early-stage breast cancer.

NSABP B-06

The NSABP B-06 trial compared lumpectomy and axillary node dissection with or without breast irradiation with modified radical mastectomy in patients with tumors 4 cm or less in greatest diameter. Between 1976 and 1984, 2163 patients were randomized to modified radical mastectomy, lumpectomy plus axillary node dissection plus breast irradiation, or lumpectomy and axillary node dissection. Similar to prior reports,[2,7] the last update from that trial continues to demonstrate the value of lumpectomy and breast irradiation as the preferred treatment for the majority of patients with invasive operable breast cancer. After 20 years of follow-up,[8] there continue to be no significant differences in OS, disease-free survival (DFS), or distant disease-free survival between the total mastectomy group and the groups treated with lumpectomy with or without breast irradiation. The hazard ratio (HR) for death with lumpectomy alone compared to total mastectomy was 1.05 (95% CI 0.90–1.23, p = 0.51). The hazard ratio (HR) for death with lumpectomy plus breast irradiation compared to total mastectomy, was 0.97 (95% CI 0.83–1.14, p = 0.74). Among lumpectomy-treated women with tumor-free margins, the hazard ratio for

death among those who received postoperative breast irradiation compared to those who did not was 0.91 (95% CI 0.77–1.06, p = 0.23). Radiation therapy was associated with a marginally significant decrease in deaths due to breast cancer. However, this decrease was partially offset by an increase in deaths from other causes.

Despite lack of significant differences in overall survival, significant differences in local control of the disease were observed among the 3 arms of the B-06 trial. In-breast recurrence occurred in 39.2% of the patients randomized to lumpectomy alone compared to 14.3% in those randomized to lumpectomy plus breast irradiation. Chest wall recurrence was observed in 10.2% of the patients in the mastectomy group. Nearly three-quarters of the local recurrences in the lumpectomy-alone group occurred within the first 5 years after surgery, compared to the lumpectomy and breast irradiation group, in which only 40% of recurrences occurred within the first 5 years.

The NSABP B-06 trial, along with other trials including those conducted by the Milan group evaluating quadrantectomy,[4,5] were instrumental in establishing breast-conserving surgery plus breast irradiation as the preferred method for the local treatment of patients with operable breast cancer.[9] These results were further confirmed in a meta-analysis of all the randomized clinical trials.[10]

Effect of Radiotherapy and Tamoxifen in Patients with Tumors upto 1 cm

NSABP B-21

One of the commonly asked questions following disclosure of the results from the NSABP B-06 and the Milan trials was whether all patients with invasive breast cancer undergoing lumpectomy need postoperative radiotherapy. It was hypothesized that patients with small tumors (≤1 cm) could potentially be spared from radiotherapy because they have lower rates of local recurrence. It was further argued at the time (1990 NIH Consensus Development Conference) that patients with negative nodes and tumors upto 1 cm may not even need adjuvant systemic therapy because of their good prognosis. Since the NSABP B-06 trial (as well as the NSABP B-14 trial, described later in the chapter) did not include a sufficient number of patients with tumors upto 1 cm, to adequately address the radiotherapy or the tamoxifen questions respectively, the NSABP designed protocol B-21 to address these questions in a randomized prospective trial (Fig. 42-1). The primary aims of the trial were to examine whether tamoxifen was as effective as breast irradiation in preventing in-breast recurrence, and whether the addition of tamoxifen to breast irradiation was superior to breast irradiation alone in terms of local and systemic control of the disease. Women with node-negative invasive breast cancer upto 1 cm in diameter treated with lumpectomy and axillary dissection were randomized to tamoxifen alone, breast irradiation plus tamoxifen for 5 years, or breast irradiation plus placebo for 5 years. A total of 1009 patients were randomized (tamoxifen: n = 336; radiation and placebo: n = 336; radiation and tamoxifen: n = 337). Although the B-21 trial did not reach the originally required sample size of 2000 patients, recently published results[11] demonstrated that radiation and

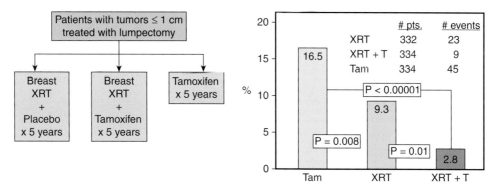

FIGURE 42-1   A. Schema of the NSABP B-21 trial evaluating the role of tamoxifen, breast radiotherapy (XRT), and a combination of the 2 in patients with invasive breast cancer ≤ 1 cm in size treated with lumpectomy. **B.** Comparison of the 8-year cumulative incidence of ipsilateral breast tumor recurrence (IBTR) rates between the 3 groups. *(Reproduced with permission from Mamounas EP. NSABP breast cancer clinical trials: recent results and future directions.* Clin Med Res. 2003;1:309-326.)

placebo resulted in a 49% lower hazard rate of in-breast recurrence compared to tamoxifen alone; radiation and tamoxifen resulted in a 63% lower rate of in-breast recurrence compared to radiation and placebo. When compared with tamoxifen alone, radiation and tamoxifen resulted in an 81% reduction in hazard rate of in-breast recurrence. Cumulative incidence of in-breast recurrence through 8 years was 16.5% with tamoxifen alone, 9.3% with breast irradiation and placebo, and 2.8% with breast irradiation and tamoxifen (Fig. 42-1). Breast irradiation reduced in-breast recurrence below the level achieved with tamoxifen alone, regardless of estrogen receptor (ER) status. Distant treatment failures were infrequent and not significantly different among the 3 groups (*p* = 0.28). When tamoxifen-treated women were compared with those who received breast irradiation and placebo, there was a significant reduction in contralateral breast cancer (hazard ratio 0.45, *p* = 0.039). Overall survival was not different between the 3 groups (93%, 94%, and 93%, respectively; *p* = 0.93). Thus, this trial demonstrated that in node-negative patients with small invasive tumors treated with lumpectomy, tamoxifen was not as effective as breast irradiation in controlling the disease in the breast. It further showed that the combination of tamoxifen and breast irradiation resulted in better local control of the disease in the breast than either modality alone.

Trial Evaluating Sentinel Node Biopsy in Patients with Invasive, Operable Breast Cancer

Despite several decades of clinical investigations on prognostic factors for recurrence in patients with operable breast cancer, the status of the axillary lymph nodes has remained the single most important independent prognostic factor. None of the newer imaging modalities (such as magnetic resonance imaging [MRI], positron emission tomographic [PET] scan, or sestamibi scan) has been shown to be as accurate as pathologic examination of the axillary nodes in predicting nodal status. Thus, surgical excision of the axillary nodes still represents the gold standard for staging the axilla.

As mentioned above, initial randomized trials evaluating less radical procedures for the surgical treatment of operable breast cancer have demonstrated that elective axillary dissection did not impact survival when compared to delayed axillary dissection (if and when the axillary lymph nodes became clinically palpable).[1,6] Thus, for several years it has been accepted that elective axillary dissection is mainly performed for staging purposes, to aid in the selection of appropriate adjuvant therapy, and for local control of the disease in the axilla. Recent randomized trials, however, have demonstrated a small but statistically significant survival advantage by adding locoregional radiation postmastectomy, in patients with positive axillary nodes who receive adjuvant chemotherapy.[12,13] As an alternative to radiotherapy, axillary dissection provides excellent local control of the disease in the axilla in patients with positive axillary nodes. Whether axillary dissection is performed merely for staging purposes or whether it is performed for a possible small therapeutic benefit in patients with positive nodes, the axillary nodes are found to be histologically negative in the majority of patients with operable breast cancer (about 75%) at the time of surgery. These patients do not derive any therapeutic benefit from the axillary dissection but could experience significant postoperative morbidity. The desire to avoid an axillary dissection in these node-negative patients without losing the prognostic information derived from knowledge of the nodal status has led to the development of lymphatic mapping and sentinel node biopsy.

During the past decade, sentinel node biopsy (SNB) has become the procedure of choice for staging the axilla in patients with operable breast cancer. The feasibility and accuracy of this technique has been demonstrated in multiple single-institution,[14-20] multicenter,[21-25] and randomized clinical trials,[26-31] as well as in a meta-analysis that included 69 studies and over 10,000 patients.[32] Although outcome results from large randomized trials comparing SNB with axillary node dissection are not available yet, results from a smaller randomized trial—including 516 patients with a median follow-up of 46 months—have shown no differences in axillary recurrence or overall survival between patients receiving SNB alone and those receiving a completion axillary dissection.[31] However, due to the small number of patients included in this trial, the confidence intervals around the estimates of outcome are wide.

NSABP B-32

The NSABP B-32 trial was developed to definitively compare SNB alone to SNB followed by an axillary dissection in clinically node-negative patients with operable breast cancer.[33] Patients were randomized to undergo SNB with mandatory concomitant axillary dissection (group 1) or SNB followed by axillary dissection only if the sentinel node revealed metastatic disease (group 2) (Fig. 42-2). Patients in the SNB-alone group who were found to have a positive sentinel node were required to also undergo full axillary dissection. In addition to its main objective, which is to compare the 2 procedures in terms of outcome, the study addresses a number of important biological and clinical questions such as the prognostic significance of immunohistochemically detected tumor cells in the SN when a routine H&E stain is negative, and quality-of-life factors related to lymphedema and arm function. Between 1999 and 2004, 5611 patients were randomized. Although the trial is not mature yet for survival analysis, technical reports on the performance of the procedure have shown an identification rate of 97% and a false-negative rate of 9.7%. The proportion of patients with metastatic sentinel nodes was 26% for both arms of the study. In nearly two-thirds of the cases, the sentinel nodes were the only sites of metastatic adenopathy.[33-35]

◼ Trial Evaluating Partial Breast Irradiation in Patients with Operable Breast Cancer

Whole-breast irradiation (delivered in 5-days-per-week fractions over a 5/6-week period) represents the standard approach for patients with early-stage breast cancer treated with lumpectomy.

However, most in-breast recurrences occur near the lumpectomy scar, and in-breast events that occur in separate quadrants are frequently new primary breast tumors that develop with longer follow-up. The incidence of these second primaries is not necessarily affected by the delivery of postlumpectomy breast irradiation. These patterns of local failure following lumpectomy have provided the rationale for exploring the use of accelerated partial-breast irradiation (APBI) techniques. Possible advantages of APBI include the feasibility of completing adjuvant breast irradiation in a shorter time interval (usually within a week) and the potential for repeating breast-sparing surgery when an in-breast event occurs outside of the irradiated lumpectomy bed. In addition, given the short duration of the regimen, breast irradiation can precede the administration of adjuvant chemotherapy in patients who require both. APBI may also increase the use of breast-conserving therapy in women who may be reluctant to have whole-breast irradiation. However, before APBI can be considered in place of whole-breast irradiation, large-scale randomized clinical trials must demonstrate comparable clinical safety and efficacy between APBI and whole-breast irradiation.

NSABP B-39

One such trial, currently conducted in North America by the NSABP and the Radiation Treatment Oncology Group (RTOG) is NSABP B-39/RTOG 0413 (Fig. 42-3).[33,36] This trial will randomize a total of 4300 women to receive either conventional whole-breast irradiation or APBI. Eligible patients must have stage 0 ductal carcinoma in situ (DCIS) or stage I or II invasive adenocarcinoma of the breast, 3 cm or less in size, with no evidence of metastatic disease. For patients with positive axillary nodes, eligibility is restricted to those with 1 to 3 positive nodes. Women must have undergone a lumpectomy with histologically free margins. Participating institutions have the option of delivering APBI via high-dose multi-catheter brachytherapy, high-dose single-catheter balloon brachytherapy, or 3-dimensional conformal external beam irradiation. The primary end point of the trial is in-breast recurrence. The study will also compare the overall survival, recurrence-free survival, and distant disease-free survival between women receiving APBI and

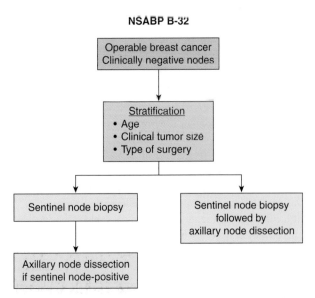

NSABP B-32

FIGURE 42-2 Schema of the NSABP B-32 trial evaluating the safety and efficacy of sentinel node biopsy in patients with operable breast cancer and clinically negative axillary nodes.

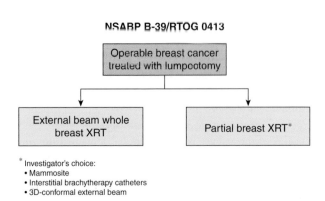

NSABP B-39/RTOG 0413

FIGURE 42-3 Schema of NSABP B-39/RTOG 0413 comparing external-beam whole-breast irradiation to accelerated partial-breast irradiation (XRT) in patients with operable breast cancer treated with lumpectomy.

those receiving whole-breast irradiation. It will also examine quality-of-life issues related to cosmesis, fatigue, treatment-related symptoms, and perceived convenience of care. The trial opened to accrual in March 2005 with a target sample size of 3000 patients. In December 2006, accrual was closed to the low-risk cohorts of patients (women over the age of 50 with node-negative and ER-positive invasive tumors and women over the age of 50 with DCIS). In addition, the total sample size was increased to 4300. As of August 2009, more than 3550 patients have been entered and randomized.

Trial Evaluating "Adjuvant" Chemotherapy in Patients Who Develop In-Breast Recurrence or Other Locoregional Recurrence

The increasing use of lumpectomy as the preferred surgical procedure for operable breast cancer has resulted in a corresponding increase in the number of in-breast recurrences despite a reduction in the rate of recurrence secondary to improvements in surgery, radiotherapy, and the expanded use of adjuvant systemic therapy. As a result, there continues to be a need to further improve our understanding of the biological and clinical significance of in-breast recurrence and, more importantly, to further explore new therapeutic strategies for this group of patients. The need for the latter has become increasingly important since several reports published during the past decade have identified in-breast recurrence as an independent predictor of distant metastases. Following in-breast recurrence, the 5-year overall survival rate is in the range of 45% to 79%. In a recent report from 5 NSABP node-positive trials, the overall annual mortality rate for the first 5 years after an in-breast recurrence was about 14%, again underscoring the poor outcome of these patients.[37]

Adequate surgical management, the addition of locoregional radiotherapy, and the widespread use of adjuvant systemic therapy, have also resulted in a substantial decrease in the rate of locoregional recurrence (chest wall recurrence after mastectomy or regional lymph node recurrence irrespective of surgical procedure). However, approximately 10% to 20% of breast cancer patients with stages I to IIIa will have a locoregional recurrence alone, or as a component of distant failure within 10 years of undergoing mastectomy. Development of locoregional recurrence as the first event has long been associated with poor prognosis, with the majority of patients developing distant disease in a relatively short period of time. For node-positive patients, the average annual mortality rate in the first 5 years following locoregional recurrence ranges from 21.8% to 29.0%.[37]

Thus, it is quite evident that patients who develop an in-breast recurrence after lumpectomy, chest wall recurrence after mastectomy, or regional nodal recurrence irrespective of surgical procedure, are at significant risk for subsequent development of distant metastases and death from breast cancer. This information provides justification for focusing our research efforts to identify ways to improve the outcome of these patients. There is scant information regarding the worth of systemic therapy at the time of local or regional recurrence,[38] and most of the available information relates to the use of hormonal

therapy.[39] To date, there have been no reported prospective randomized trials evaluating the worth of chemotherapy at the time of in-breast or other locoregional recurrence. As a result, there is widespread variability in the use of systemic chemotherapy at the time of locoregional recurrence. Data from 5 NSABP studies in node-positive patients indicate that "adjuvant" chemotherapy use at the time of in-breast recurrence varied between 18% and 40% of the cases.[37] One of the reasons for not evaluating additional "adjuvant" chemotherapy at the time of in-breast or other locoregional recurrence is that, until the development of taxanes, there were no candidate non–cross-resistant regimens with promising activity that could be tested in this setting. However, the demonstration of significant antitumor activity with taxanes in patients resistant to anthracyclines and alkylating agents, as well as the recent successful results with sequential anthracycline-taxane regimens in the adjuvant and neoadjuvant settings,[40-43] provided the opportunity to test this question in a randomized clinical trial.

NSABP B-37

One such currently ongoing trial is the IBCSG (International Breast Cancer Study Group) 27-02/NSABP B-37 trial, which randomizes patients with resected in-breast recurrence or other locoregional recurrence to "adjuvant" chemotherapy or observation, in addition to hormonal therapy for hormone-receptor-positive tumors (Fig. 42-4).[33] Eligible patients are randomized within 6 weeks of resection and treated within 4 weeks after randomization. Locoregional treatment consists of surgery and radiotherapy whenever possible. Radiotherapy is mandatory for patients who have not received prior adjuvant radiotherapy. Patients allocated to chemotherapy will preferentially receive combination chemotherapy with 2 or more drugs for at least 3 cycles. All patients with hormone-receptor-positive (ER+ and/or PgR+) recurrences will receive hormonal treatment. Trastuzumab therapy is permissible for HER-2/neu (HER-2)–positive patients, but this should be declared prior to randomization. A total of 977 patients will need to be randomized in this currently ongoing trial, and the primary end point is disease-free survival. Over 130 patients have been randomized to date.

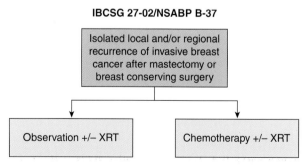

FIGURE 42-4 Schema of IBCSG 27-02/NSABP B-37 evaluating "adjuvant" chemotherapy in patients with isolated local and/or regional recurrence of invasive breast cancer after mastectomy or breast-conserving surgery.

PIVOTAL NSABP TRIALS IN PATIENTS WITH DUCTAL CARCINOMA IN SITU

As randomized trials demonstrated the value of breast-conserving surgery in patients with invasive breast cancer, the obvious question arose relative to the value of this procedure in patients with noninvasive disease. In addition, the introduction and widespread use of mammography has contributed to a dramatic increase in the incidence of small, localized, nonpalpable DCIS, an entity with excellent prognosis after local therapy alone. According to SEER data, DCIS accounts for approximately 20% of all breast cancers diagnosed in the United States, with age-adjusted incidence rates of 30 cases per 100,000 women, and approximately 47,000 cases detected each year.[44] Following the results of the B-06 and other trials described above, in the early 1980s there was a paradox in the surgical treatment of early-stage breast cancer, with invasive disease being treated progressively more with lumpectomy, whereas mastectomy remained the recommended surgical treatment for noninvasive disease. Thus, it became imperative at the time to test the value of breast conservation in patients with DCIS. The NSABP was the first group to conduct such a prospective randomized trial.

NSABP B-17

The NSABP B-17 trial compared lumpectomy alone to lumpectomy plus breast irradiation in 818 patients with localized DCIS (Fig. 42-5).[3,45-47] A mastectomy control group was not included, given the acceptance of lumpectomy based on the results of the B-06 trial, as well as the excellent prognosis of patients with localized DCIS. Recently updated results from the B-17 trial, after 12 years of follow-up,[47] continue to indicate—as previously reported[3,45]—that radiotherapy significantly decreases the rate of invasive and noninvasive ipsilateral breast tumor recurrence. The cumulative incidence of noninvasive ipsilateral breast cancer recurrence as a first event was significantly reduced with breast irradiation from 14.6% to

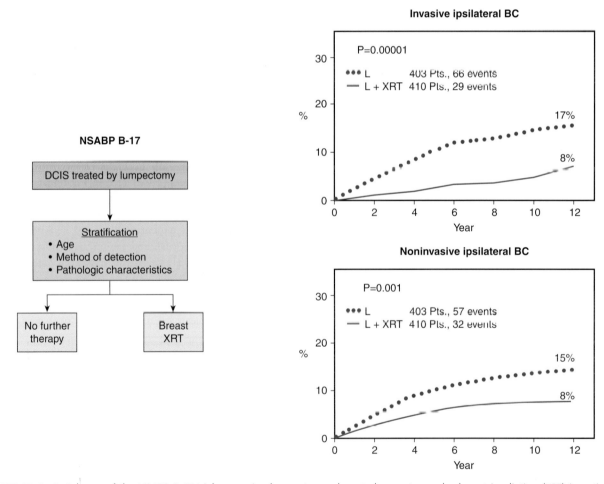

FIGURE 42-5 A. Schema of the NSABP B-17 trial comparing lumpectomy alone to lumpectomy plus breast irradiation (XRT) in patients with localized ductal carcinoma in situ (DCIS). **B.** Comparison of the 12-year cumulative incidence of invasive and noninvasive breast cancer recurrence between patients receiving lumpectomy alone (L) and those receiving lumpectomy plus breast radiotherapy (L+XRT). (BC, breast cancer.) *(Reproduced with permission from Mamounas EP. NSABP breast cancer clinical trials: recent results and future directions. Clin Med Res. 2003;1:309-326. Adapted from Fisher B, Land SR, Mamounas EP, et al. Prevention of invasive breast cancer in women with ductal carcinoma in situ: an update of the National Surgical Adjuvant Breast and Bowel Project experience. Semin Oncol. 2001;28:400-418.)*

8.0% (*p* = 0.001) (Fig. 42-5). More importantly, the cumulative incidence of invasive ipsilateral recurrence was also significantly reduced from 16.8% to 7.7% (*p* = 0.00001) (Fig. 42-5). No difference in overall survival has been observed between the 2 groups (86% vs 87%, *p* - 0.80), but over two-thirds of the deaths in this trial were not breast-cancer related. In a subset of 623 out of 814 evaluable patients from this trial, pathologic features were analyzed relative to their prognostic significance for ipsilateral breast cancer recurrence.[46] Only the presence of moderate/marked comedo necrosis was a statistically significant independent predictor of in-breast recurrence in both treatment groups. Moreover, breast irradiation markedly reduced the annual hazard rates for in-breast recurrence in all subgroups of patients.

NSABP B-24

Following completion of the B-17 trial, another randomized trial was conducted by the NSABP in patients with DCIS to evaluate the role of tamoxifen after lumpectomy and breast irradiation (NSABP B-24).[47,48] At that time, a large body of scientific evidence had accumulated demonstrating benefit from adjuvant tamoxifen in patients with resected early-stage invasive breast cancer.[49] In these patients, tamoxifen not only reduced the risk for systemic recurrence but also had a significant impact in reducing the rate of in-breast recurrence following lumpectomy

and breast irradiation.[50,51] More importantly, tamoxifen reduced the incidence of second primary breast cancers in the contralateral breast by about 40%.[49-55] The latter observation—along with preclinical evidence that tamoxifen inhibits both the initiation and promotion of tumors in experimental animals[56,57]—made tamoxifen an attractive agent for DCIS patients treated with lumpectomy and breast irradiation, for possibly reducing the rate of ipsilateral and contralateral invasive breast cancer events. Between 1991 and 1994, 1804 women with DCIS treated with lumpectomy were randomized to receive postoperative radiotherapy and either tamoxifen 20 mg daily for 5 years or placebo daily for 5 years (Fig. 42-6). In contrast to the B-17 trial, where lumpectomy margins were required to be free of DCIS for eligibility, in the B-24 trial patients were eligible whether the lumpectomy margins were free, involved, or unknown. As a result, about 75% of the patients in the B-24 trial had free lumpectomy margins, about 16% had involved margins, and in 10% the margins were unknown. Updated results after 7 years of follow-up continue to demonstrate, as previously reported,[48] that the addition of tamoxifen significantly improved DFS from 77.1% to 83.0% (*p* = 0.002). This improvement was mainly the result of a reduction in the incidence of invasive and noninvasive breast cancer events in the ipsilateral as well as in the contralateral breast. The cumulative incidence of all ipsilateral and contralateral breast cancer events was reduced by 39%, from 16.0 % in the placebo group to

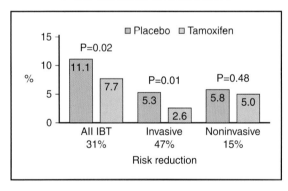

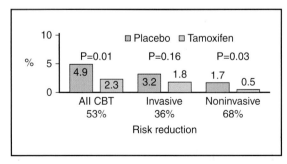

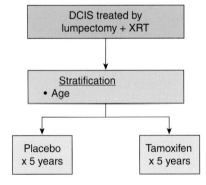

FIGURE 42-6 **A.** Schema of the NSABP B-24 trial comparing placebo with tamoxifen in patients with DCIS treated with lumpectomy plus breast radiotherapy (XRT). **B.** Comparison of the 7-year cumulative incidence of ipsilateral breast cancer events (IBT) and contralateral breast cancer events (CBT) between patients receiving placebo and those receiving tamoxifen. *(Reproduced with permission from Mamounas EP. NSABP breast cancer clinical trials: recent results and future directions.* Clin Med Res. *2003;1:309-326. Adapted from Fisher B, Land SR, Mamounas EP, et al. Prevention of invasive breast cancer in women with ductal carcinoma in situ: an update of the National Surgical Adjuvant Breast and Bowel Project experience.* Semin Oncol. *2001;28:400-418.)*

10.0% in the tamoxifen group (*p* = 0.0003).[47] Tamoxifen reduced the rate of all invasive breast cancer events by 45% (*p* = 0.0009) and the rate of noninvasive breast cancer events by 27% (*p* = 0.11). When the effect of tamoxifen was examined according to the location of the first event, the cumulative incidence of ipsilateral breast cancers was reduced by 31% (11.1% with tamoxifen vs 7.7% with placebo, *p* = 0.02) and the cumulative incidence of contralateral breast cancers was reduced by 47% (4.9% vs 2.3%, *p* = 0.010) (Fig. 42-6). Several patient and tumor characteristics were found to increase the rate of in-breast recurrence, such as age under 50, involved/unknown lumpectomy margins, presence of comedo necrosis, and DCIS presentation with clinical findings. The effect of tamoxifen in reducing in-breast recurrence was evident irrespective of age, margin status, or presence/absence of comedo necrosis. However, for women with clinically apparent DCIS at study entry, in-breast recurrence rates were similar between the tamoxifen and placebo groups although the number of patients in that category was small.

The results from the B-24 trial indicate a significant benefit from tamoxifen in patients with DCIS. When these results are viewed together with those demonstrating benefit from tamoxifen in women with prior invasive breast cancer[49-55] and in women with atypical hyperplasia and lobular carcinoma in situ (LCIS),[58] they support the use of tamoxifen in the entire spectrum of breast neoplasia. However, one outstanding question following disclosure of the B-24 results was whether the observed benefit from tamoxifen was limited to subsets of DCIS patients. Given the strong association between ER expression and tamoxifen benefit in patients with invasive breast cancer, presence of a similar association might also be expected in patients with DCIS. In 2002, Allred and associates presented data from the NSABP B-24 trial on tamoxifen benefit according to ER status of the primary DCIS tumor.[59] Of the 1804 patients participating in the trial, information on ER status was available in 628 patients (327 placebo, 301 tamoxifen). Seventy-seven percent of the patients had ER-positive tumors, and in these patients, the effectiveness of tamoxifen was clear (relative risk [RR] for all breast cancer events, 0.41; *p* = 0.0002). Significant reductions in breast cancer events were seen in both the ipsilateral and the contralateral breast. In patients with ER-negative tumors, little benefit was observed (RR for all breast cancer events, 0.80; *p* = 0.51), but the total number of events in this cohort was too small to rule out a small, clinically meaningful benefit. However, when these results are taken together with those evaluating the effect of tamoxifen in patients with invasive breast cancer and negative estrogen receptors, they are consistent with the observation that tamoxifen has no appreciable benefit in reducing rates of recurrence or rates of contralateral breast cancer in patients with ER-negative tumors. Furthermore, these results suggest that routine assessment of ER status should now be performed also in patients with DCIS to determine their candidacy for tamoxifen therapy.

NSABP B-35

In the 1990s significant enthusiasm developed with the demonstration of considerable activity and favorable toxicity profile with third-generation aromatase inhibitors in patients with hormone-responsive, advanced breast cancer.[60-66] As a result, several clinical trials have evaluated aromatase inhibitors as adjuvant therapy in patients with early-stage breast cancer. The first one to report results was the ATAC trial, which randomized more than 9000 early-stage breast cancer patients to receive anastrozole, tamoxifen, or the combination of anastrozole and tamoxifen, as adjuvant hormonal therapy.[67] Besides yielding provocative results regarding the activity of anastrozole in the adjuvant treatment of ER-positive postmenopausal breast cancer, this trial was the first to demonstrate that the risk of contralateral new primary breast cancers was significantly reduced with anastrozole when compared to tamoxifen (odds ratio 0.42, *p* = 0.007).[68] In addition, anastrozole demonstrated a more favorable side-effect profile when compared to tamoxifen (reduction in endometrial cancer, vaginal bleeding and discharge, cerebrovascular events, venous thromboembolic events, and hot flashes).[67] On the other hand, when compared to tamoxifen, anastrozole resulted in significantly more myoskeletal disorders and fractures, which may have significant implications for the long-term use of this drug in patients with DCIS. The efficacy and safety results from the ATAC trial were eventually confirmed in other similar large trials evaluating aromatase inhibitors in the adjuvant setting and provided ample rationale for the evaluation of aromatase inhibitors in patients with DCIS. These findings prompted the design and conduct of NSABP B-35, a phase III trial that randomized postmenopausal patients with localized, ER-positive and/or PgR-positive DCIS treated with lumpectomy plus breast irradiation to tamoxifen versus anastrozole for 5 years (Fig. 42-7). The primary aim of the trial is to evaluate the effectiveness of anastrozole compared to tamoxifen in preventing the subsequent occurrence of breast cancer (local, regional and distant recurrences, and contralateral breast cancer). In addition, the trial aims to ascertain the effects of anastrozole on patient symptoms and quality of life as compared to tamoxifen. This protocol has completed its accrual goal after accruing over 3100 patients and is currently awaiting maturation of follow-up.

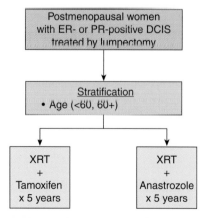

FIGURE 42-7 Schema of NSABP B-35 trial comparing tamoxifen with anastrozole in postmenopausal patients with localized DCIS treated with lumpectomy and breast irradiation (XRT).

NSABP B-43: Trastuzumab in HER-2 Positive DCIS

DCIS is more likely to overexpress HER-2 than is invasive cancer, and HER-2 overexpression is often associated with large-cell, comedo variety DCIS and more aggressive behavior.[69,70] Trastuzumab is more likely to be effective in DCIS because it intervenes earlier in the carcinogenic pathway where there are fewer alternative escapes, and HER-2–positive DCIS is more likely than invasive breast cancer to depend on a single pathway. About 45% of patients with ER-negative DCIS and about 20% of patients with ER-positive DCIS overexpress HER-2.[71] Preclinical data demonstrate that radiation enhances the anti- tumor effect of trastuzumab in tumors that overexpress the HER-2 oncogene.[72] Based on this rationale, along with the safety and efficacy data with adjuvant trastuzumab in several randomized trials ("Studies Evaluating Biologic Targeted Therapies in the Adjuvant Setting" section (p. 487)),[73,74] the NSABP developed protocol B-43, a phase III randomized trial to evaluate trastuzumab for patients with DCIS whose tumors overexpress HER2. Patients with HER-2–overexpressing DCIS treated with lumpectomy will be randomized to breast irradiation versus breast irradiation plus 2 doses of trastuzumab, starting on day 1 of breast irradiation and repeated once more 3 weeks later (Fig. 42-8). The primary end point of the study is the development of any breast cancer event. Secondary end points include in-breast recurrence and development of contralateral breast cancer. The NSABP B-43 trial opened 11/10/2008, with a goal of 2000 participants. As of September 2009, accrual is at 5.95%, with 119 patients.

ADJUVANT THERAPY TRIALS IN PATIENTS WITH NEGATIVE NODES

During the last 20 years the NSABP has also played a significant role in conducting randomized trials that lead to the acceptance of adjuvant chemotherapy and adjuvant hormonal therapy for the treatment of breast cancer patients with negative axillary nodes. Beginning in the early 1980s several important trials evaluated in a stepwise fashion the worth of chemotherapy and that of hormonal therapy in patients with ER-negative tumors (Fig. 42-9) as well as in those with ER-positive tumors (Fig. 42-10).

Studies in Patients with ER-Negative Tumors (NSABP B-13, B-19, B-23, B-36)

NSABP B-13

The NSABP B-13 trial randomized patients with negative nodes and negative estrogen receptors to surgery alone or surgery followed by 12 months of adjuvant chemotherapy with methotrexate

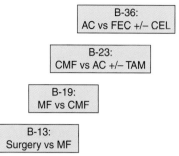

NSABP Node-negative, ER-negative trials*

FIGURE 42-9 NSABP adjuvant trials in node-negative breast cancer patients with ER-negative tumors evaluating, in a stepwise fashion, combination chemotherapy regimens, tamoxifen, and celecoxib. (*B-36 also includes patients with ER- or PR-positive tumors.) (AC, doxorubicin/cyclophosphamide; CEL, celecoxib; CMF, cyclophosphamide/methotrexate/5-fluorouracil; FEC, 5-fluorouracil/epirubicin/cyclophosphamide; MF, methotrexate/5-fluorouracil with leucovorin rescue; TAM, tamoxifen.)

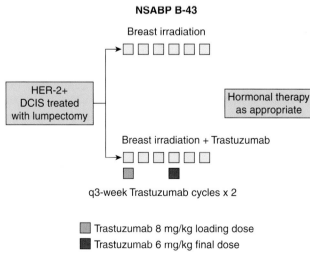

NSABP B-43

FIGURE 42-8 Schema of NSABP B-43 trial comparing breast irradiation alone with breast irradiation plus trastuzumab in lumpectomy-treated DCIS patients, whose tumors overexpress the HER-2 oncogene.

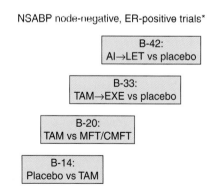

NSABP node-negative, ER-positive trials*

FIGURE 42-10 NSABP adjuvant trials in node-negative breast cancer patients with ER-positive tumors evaluating, in a stepwise fashion, tamoxifen, chemotherapy plus tamoxifen, exemestane, and letrozole (*B-33 and B-42 also include patients with node-positive tumors.) (AI, aromatase inhibitor; CMFT, cyclophosphamide/methotrexate/5-fluorouracil/tamoxifen; EXE, exemestane; LET, letrozole; MFT, methotrexate/5-fluorouracil/tamoxifen; TAM, tamoxifen.)

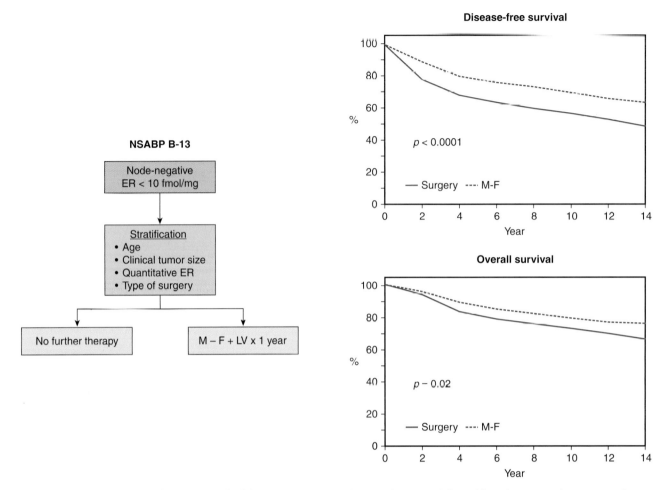

FIGURE 42-11 **A.** Schema of the NSABP B-13 trial comparing surgery alone with surgery followed by adjuvant methotrexate and 5-fluorouracil with leucovorin rescue (M – F + LV) in node-negative patients with estrogen receptor (ER)-negative tumors. **B.** Comparison of the 14-year disease-free and overall survival rates between the 2 groups. *(Reproduced with permission from Mamounas EP. NSABP breast cancer clinical trials: recent results and future directions.* Clin Med Res. *2003;1:309-326. Adapted from Fisher B, Jeong JH, Dignam J, et al. Findings from recent National Surgical Adjuvant Breast and Bowel Project studies of stage I breast cancer.* JNCI Monographs. *2001;30:62-66. Oxford University Press.)*

and sequentially administered 5-fluorouracil (5-Fu) (M-F) followed by leucovorin (Figs. 42-9 and 42-11). Findings through 14 years of follow-up[75] demonstrate that the improvements in disease-free and overall survival from M-F, previously reported after 5[76] and 0[77] years, have persisted ($p < 0.0001$ for the former and $p = 0.02$ for the latter) (Fig. 42-11). A statistically significant DFS was evident both for women less than 50 years of age ($p = 0.005$) as well as in those 50 years or more ($p = 0.001$). A statistically significant benefit in terms of survival was evident only in women 50 years of age or more ($p = 0.02$). For women less than 50 years of age, there was a nonsignificant trend toward improvement in overall survival with M-F ($p = 0.3$). However, there was no statistically significant evidence of an interaction between treatment group and age relative to overall survival ($p = 0.34$).

NSABP B-19

Following completion of the NSABP B-13, a subsequent trial in the same patient population (NSABP B-19) attempted to determine whether the alkylating agent cyclophosphamide contributed additional benefit when administered with

methotrexate and 5-FU (CMF regimen as developed by the Milan Group) (Figs. 42-9 and 42-12). Over a 6-month period, patients received either 6 courses of M-F or 6 courses of CMF. A total of 1095 patients were randomized. Through 8 years of follow-up,[75] just as first reported after 5 years,[77] the results continue to demonstrate a statistically significant disease-free and overall survival advantage with CMF over M-F ($p = 0.003$ and $p = 0.03$, respectively) (Fig. 42-12). Those advantages were most evident in women aged upto 50 years ($p = 0.0004$ and $p = 0.007$, respectively). In women aged more than 50 years, there was a small but nonsignificant advantage in both disease-free survival ($p = 0.2$) and overall survival ($p = 0.8$). As was also observed in the B-13 study, there was no evidence of a statistically significant interaction between treatment and age group relative to disease-free survival ($p = 0.22$) and overall survival ($p = 0.08$).

NSABP B-23

Following completion of the B-19 trial, the NSABP initiated protocol B-23, which attempted to determine whether tamoxifen

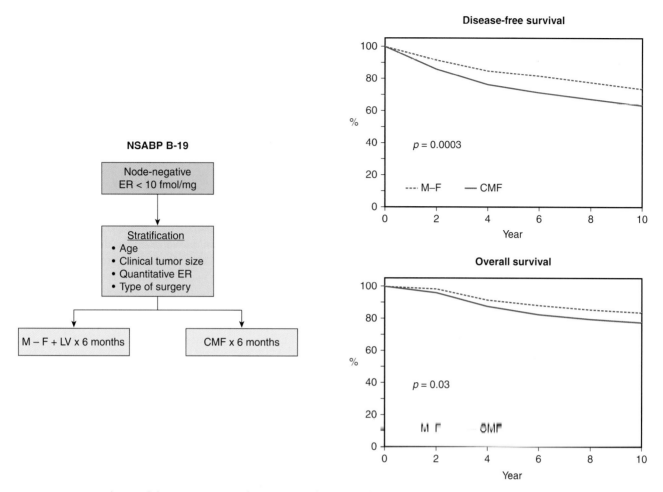

FIGURE 42-12 **A.** Schema of the NSABP B-19 trial comparing adjuvant methotrexate/5-fluorouracil/leucovorin (M – F + LV) with adjuvant cyclophosphamide/ methotrexate/5-fluorouracil (CMF) in node-negative patients with estrogen receptor (ER)-negative tumors. **B.** Comparison of the 8-year disease-free and overall survival rates between the 2 groups. *(Reproduced with permission from Mamounas EP. NSABP breast cancer clinical trials: recent results and future directions.* Clin Med Res. *2003;1:309-326. Adapted from Fisher B, Jeong JH, Dignam J, et al. Findings from recent National Surgical Adjuvant Breast and Bowel Project studies of stage I breast cancer.* JNCI Monographs. *2001;30:62-66. Oxford University Press.).*

has a role in patients with ER-negative tumors. In this study, patients with negative nodes and ER-negative tumors were randomized to 4 cycles of adjuvant doxorubicin/cyclophosphamide (AC) or 6 cycles of adjuvant CMF with or without tamoxifen (Fig. 42-9). The rationale for evaluating tamoxifen in patients with ER-negative tumors came both from preclinical and clinical observations. Results from several preclinical studies had demonstrated that tamoxifen acts not only through a blockade of the ER pathway but also by modulating the production of growth factors such as TGF-α and TGF-β, by increasing the levels of sex-hormone-binding globulin in the serum, by increasing natural killer cell counts, and by decreasing insulin-like growth factor. In addition, at the time of initiation of this study there was considerable clinical information suggesting that tamoxifen prolongs disease-free survival and survival irrespective of receptor status although the benefit in ER-negative tumors was of lesser magnitude.[78-81] Since that time, an increasing body of evidence has demonstrated that tamoxifen confers no significant advantage in patients with ER-negative tumors. The results of the B-23 trial confirmed these latter observations and demonstrated no significant

prolongation in DFS or OS with the addition of tamoxifen to chemotherapy (DFS: CMF, 83%; CMF + tamoxifen, 83%; AC, 83%; AC + tamoxifen, 82%; OS: CMF, 89%; CMF + tamoxifen, 89%; AC, 90%; AC + tamoxifen, 91%).[82] The results of the B-23 trial also confirmed (in the node-negative setting) the previous observation from the NSABP B-15 trial (in node-positive patients) that 4 cycles of AC were equivalent to 6 cycles of CMF in terms of disease-free and overall survival prolongation. One interesting observation in this trial was that tamoxifen did not confer a significant reduction in the incidence of contralateral breast cancer as it has been shown in patients with ER-positive tumors and negative nodes.[50,75] Explanation for this discrepancy was recently provided by a retrospective review of several NSABP trials, which found that there was significant concordance between the ER status of the primary breast cancer and that of contralateral breast cancer.[83] Thus, in about 80% of patients who initially present with an ER-negative primary and who develop contralateral breast cancer, the contralateral breast tumor is also ER-negative, making the potential chemopreventive effect of tamoxifen negligible.

NSABP B-36

One of the approaches utilized in order to improve the outcomes of CMF-treated node-negative breast cancer patients is the incorporation of doxorubicin into the chemotherapy regimen. As noted above, protocol B-23 demonstrated the equivalence between 6 cycles of CMF and 4 cycles of AC. However, several other trials have shown that 6 cycles of CAF/CEF/FAC or FEC are superior to 6 cycles of CMF.[84-87] These results suggest that cycle duration may be important in optimizing results with anthracycline-based regimens. Results from adjuvant trials evaluating 6 cycles of a dose-intense epirubicin-based regimen also suggested that the epirubicin-based regimens may be more effective than doxorubicin-based regimens.[88] The NIH Consensus Conference on Adjuvant Therapy of Breast Cancer held in November 2000 stressed the need for trials to address the issues of cycle duration with anthracycline-based chemotherapy.[89]

Moreover, an evolving body of preclinical and clinical literature had suggested that induction of cyclooxygenase 2 (COX-2) expression and the resultant increase in prostaglandins may contribute to the development of the malignant phenotype in breast cancer and other malignancies. Availability of well-tolerated, selective inhibitors of COX-2 provided an opportunity to evaluate COX-2 as a target for cancer treatment and prevention in women with node-negative breast cancer.

Thus, the NSABP B-36 trial (Fig. 42-9) was built on the experience from the previous NSABP trials, to evaluate chemotherapy in high-risk node-negative breast cancer patients. The trial randomizes women with node-negative breast cancer to either 4 cycles of AC or 6 cycles of FEC. The original design of the trial included a secondary randomization in a 2 × 2 factorial design to celecoxib versus placebo. However, the recent removal of rofecoxib from the market due to cardiovascular toxicities observed with COX-2 inhibitors resulted in modification of the B-36 trial and discontinuation of the randomization between celecoxib and placebo. The B-36 trial completed its accrual after accruing 2722 patients and is currently awaiting maturation of follow-up.

Studies in Patients with ER-Positive Tumors (NSABP B-14, B-20, B-33, B-42)

Parallel to the studies evaluating chemotherapy and tamoxifen in patients with node-negative, ER-negative breast cancer, the NSABP launched a series of trials that initially evaluated tamoxifen and the combination of tamoxifen plus chemotherapy in patients with node-negative, ER-positive disease and subsequently evaluated aromatase inhibitors as extended adjuvant therapy, either after 5 years of tamoxifen (B-33) or after 5 years of an aromatase inhibitor (B-42) in node-negative and node-positive patients with hormone-receptor-positive breast cancer (Fig. 42-10).

NSABP B-14

The NSABP B-14 trial randomized patients after surgery to 5 years of tamoxifen or 5 years of placebo (Figs. 42-10 and 42-13). Published results from this trial through 10 years of follow-up[51] continue to demonstrate a statistically significant disease-free survival benefit from tamoxifen (69% vs 57%, $p < 0.0001$). In addition, a significant survival advantage was demonstrated in this update (80% vs 76%, $p = 0.02$). The disease-free and overall survival advantage with tamoxifen was evident both in women < 50 as well as in those ≥ 50 years of age. Tamoxifen therapy continued to demonstrate a significant reduction in the rate of contralateral breast cancer (4.0% vs 5.8%, $p = 0.007$).

The significant advantage for disease-free and overall survival with tamoxifen has now persisted through 14 years of follow-up (Fig. 42-13).[75] In a most recent update[90] with 15 years of follow-up, the benefit from tamoxifen continues to be evident irrespective of age, menopausal status, or tumor estrogen-receptor concentration (hazard ratio [HR] for recurrence-free survival 0.58, 95% CI 0.50–0.67, $p < 0.0001$; HR for overall survival 0.80, 95% CI 0.71–0.91, $p = 0.0008$).

One of the most common questions asked while the NSABP B-14 trial was being conducted related to the optimal duration of tamoxifen administration. By design, patients were to receive 5 years of tamoxifen or 5 years of placebo. To answer the question of optimal tamoxifen duration beyond 5 years, patients randomized to tamoxifen who were alive and recurrence-free following 5 years of treatment were asked to be rerandomized to 5 additional years of tamoxifen or 5 years of placebo.[51] Originally reported results, through 4 years from rerandomization, demonstrated a significant disadvantage in disease-free survival (86% vs 92%, $p = 0.003$) and distant disease-free survival (90% vs 96%, $p = 0.01$) for patients who continued tamoxifen for more than 5 years versus those who discontinued the drug at 5 years.

Overall survival was 96% for those who discontinued tamoxifen compared with 94% for those who continued it ($p = 0.08$). Updated results, through 7 years from the time of rerandomization continue to demonstrate no additional benefit from the prolonged tamoxifen administration.[91] In fact, a slight advantage continues to exist for patients who discontinued tamoxifen after 5 years relative to those who continued to receive it (disease-free survival, 82% vs 78%, $p = 0.03$; relapse-free survival, 94% vs 92%, $p = 0.13$; overall survival, 94% vs 91%, $p = 0.07$, respectively). The lack of benefit from additional tamoxifen therapy was independent of age or other characteristics.

NSABP B-20

An important observation from the B-14 trial was that through 10 years of follow-up of tamoxifen-treated patients with ER-positive, node-negative breast cancer, the disease-free survival (69%) and overall survival (80%) were not as good as originally thought for this group of patients, who are generally considered to have a favorable prognosis.[51] These numbers further decreased after 14 years of follow-up,[75] with disease-free survival being around 60% and overall survival around 75%. Although a small proportion of the events included in the disease-free and overall survival analyses are non–breast-cancer related, these results underscore the need for further improvement of the outcome of these patients. Subsequent to the B-14 trial, the NSABP conducted protocol B-20 that evaluated the worth of adding chemotherapy to tamoxifen in patients with negative nodes and positive ER (Fig. 42-14). Between 1988 and 1993, 2363 patients were randomized to receive either tamoxifen for 5 years, or tamoxifen plus 6 cycles of sequential methotrexate and 5-Fu followed by leucovorin (MFT) or tamoxifen plus 6 cycles of cyclophosphamide, methotrexate, and 5-Fu (CMFT).

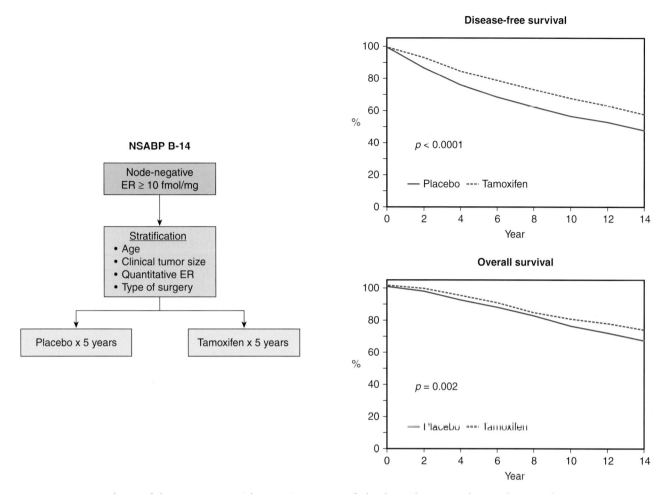

FIGURE 42-13   A. Schema of the NSABP B-14 trial comparing 5 years of placebo with 5 years of tamoxifen in node-negative, ER-positive patients. **B.** Comparison of 14-year disease-free and overall survival rates between the 2 groups. *(Reproduced with permission from Mamounas EP. NSABP breast cancer clinical trials: recent results and future directions. Clin Med Res. 2003;1:309-326. Adapted from Fisher B, Jeong JH, Dignam J, et al. Findings from recent National Surgical Adjuvant Breast and Bowel Project studies of stage I breast cancer. JNCI Monographs. 2001;30:62-66. Oxford University Press.)*

Through 5 years of follow-up, the combination of chemotherapy plus tamoxifen resulted in significantly improved disease-free survival over tamoxifen alone (90% for MFT vs 85% for tamoxifen, $p = 0.01$; 89% for CMFT vs 85% for tamoxifen, $p = 0.001$). A similar benefit was observed in overall survival (97% for MFT vs 94% for tamoxifen, $p = 0.05$; 96% for CMFT vs 94% for tamoxifen, $p = 0.03$).[92] The reduction in recurrence and mortality was greatest in patients aged 49 years or less. All subgroups of patients evaluated in this study benefited from chemotherapy. The results from the B-20 study were updated with 8 years of follow-up and continue to demonstrate a significant improvement in disease-free and overall survival with the addition of chemotherapy to tamoxifen when compared to tamoxifen alone (84% vs 77%, $p = 0.001$, for disease-free survival; 92% vs 88% for overall survival, $p = 0.018$) (Fig. 42-14).[75] The most recent update with 12 years of follow-up continues to demonstrate a significant improvement in disease-free survival and a borderline significant improvement in overall survival with the addition of chemotherapy.[90]

An important remaining question following the disclosure of the NSABP B-14 and NSABP B-20 trials was whether we can identify subgroups of these node-negative, ER-positive patients at low risk for recurrence when treated with tamoxifen

alone, which can be spared chemotherapy administration. In the past few years, genomic profiling of the primary breast tumor has shown considerable promise toward that goal. Using archival paraffin block material from the NSABP B-14 and NSABP B-20 trials, Genomic Health, in collaboration with the NSABP, developed and validated a reverse transcriptase polymerase chain reaction (RT-PCR)-based 21-gene assay (also know as 21-gene recurrence score or OncotypeDX) that predicts outcome and benefit from hormonal therapy and chemotherapy in these patients (Fig. 42-15).[93,94] This assay is currently commercially available for use in ER-positive, node-negative patients. According to the results of this assay, ER-positive, node-negative breast cancer patients with a low recurrence score have low risk of recurrence and receive little benefit from the addition of adjuvant chemotherapy to hormonal therapy. Those with a high recurrence score have a considerably high risk of recurrence and receive significant benefit from the addition of adjuvant chemotherapy to hormonal therapy and should be treated with both. A prospective randomized clinical trial (TAILORx) is currently being conducted to evaluate whether the addition of adjuvant chemotherapy to hormonal therapy is necessary for patients who have an intermediate recurrence score.

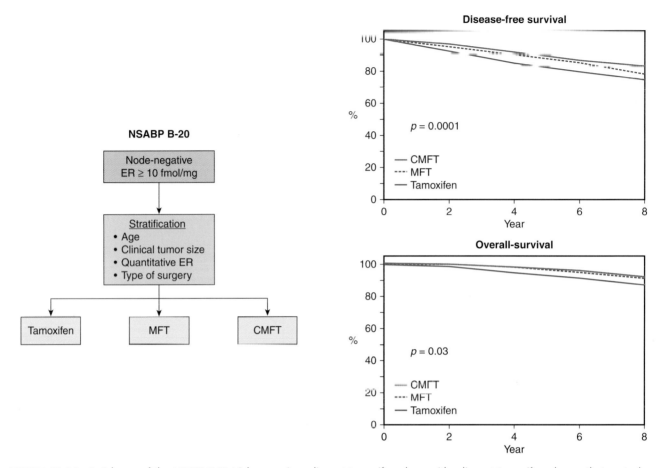

FIGURE 42-14 A. Schema of the NSABP B-20 trial comparing adjuvant tamoxifen alone with adjuvant tamoxifen plus methotrexate/5-fluorouracil plus leucovorin (MFT) and with tamoxifen plus cyclophosphamide/methotrexate/5-fluorouracil (CMFT) in node-negative patients with ER-positive tumors. **B.** Comparison of the 8-year disease-free and overall survival rates between the 3 groups of patients. *(Reproduced with permission from Mamounas EP. NSABP breast cancer clinical trials: recent results and future directions. Clin Med Res. 2003;1:309-326. Adapted from Fisher B, Jeong JH, Dignam J, et al. Findings from recent National Surgical Adjuvant Breast and Bowel Project studies of stage I breast cancer. JNCI Monographs. 2001;30:62-66. Oxford University Press.)*

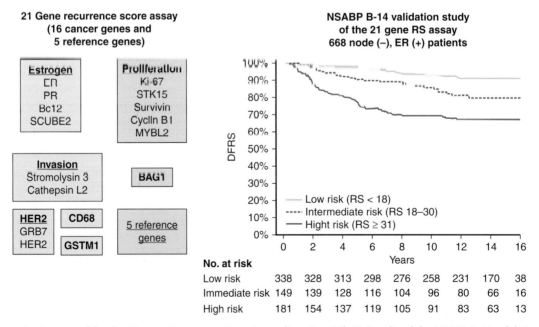

FIGURE 42-15 A. Gene panel for the 21-gene Recurrence Score Assay (OncotypeDX). **B.** Results of the NSABP B-14 validation study of the 21-gene Recurrence Score Assay. (DRFS, distant recurrence-free survival; ER, estrogen receptor; RS, recurrence score.) *(Adapted with permission from Paik S, Shack S, Tang J, et al. A multigene assay to predict recurrence of tamoxifen-treated, node-negative breast cancer. N Engl J Med. 2004;351:2817-2826. Copyright © 2004 Massachusetts Medical Society. All rights reserved.)*

NSABP B-33

The results from the NSABP B-14 trial demonstrating no additional benefit from continuing tamoxifen therapy for longer than 5 years,[91] as well as the appreciation of continued risk for recurrence in patients with hormone-receptor-positive breast cancer after 5 years of tamoxifen[95] led several investigators to consider additional adjuvant hormonal therapy interventions following completion of tamoxifen therapy. During the past several years, abundant information became available demonstrating substantial antitumor activity with the use of aromatase inhibitors in patients with advanced breast cancer who suffered a recurrence during or after tamoxifen therapy. Thus, attempting to further reduce the risk of subsequent recurrence in patients who remain disease free after completion of adjuvant tamoxifen by administering aromatase inhibitors became an important clinical research question. Based on the above rationale, the NSABP developed protocol B-33, a randomized trial comparing exemestane with placebo in postmenopausal patients who complete 5 years of tamoxifen and are recurrence-free (Fig. 42-16).[96] The primary aim of the trial was to determine whether exemestane will prolong DFS. Secondary aims were to determine whether exemestane will prolong OS, and to evaluate the effect of exemestane and that of tamoxifen withdrawal on fracture rate, bone mineral density, markers of bone turnover, levels of lipids and lipoproteins, and quality of life. Between May 2001 and October 2003, a total of 1598 women were randomized out of the 3000 required to complete the study. However, in October 2003, accrual to this study was terminated early per recommendation of the NSABP Data Monitoring Committee when results from a similar adjuvant trial (NCIC-CTG MA.17) became available demonstrating significant improvement with letrozole after 5 years of tamoxifen.[97] As a result of these findings, all patients in the NSABP B-33 trial were unblinded and 5 years of exemestane was offered to both groups at no cost. Despite the premature closure of the trial (50% of the target accrual) and the ensuing crossover to exemestane (about 50% of patients), original assignment to exemestane versus placebo resulted in borderline

improvement in disease-free survival and in a significant improvement in relapse-free survival of a similar magnitude to that seen in the NCIC MA.17 trial with letrozole.[98]

NSABP B-42

Aromatase inhibitors have demonstrated significant activity in the adjuvant setting either as up-front therapy, as sequential therapy after 2 to 3 years of adjuvant tamoxifen, or as extended adjuvant therapy after 5 years of tamoxifen.[99] As a result, aromatase inhibitors are increasingly utilized as adjuvant therapy in these 3 clinical situations. No data currently exist on the optimal duration of aromatase inhibitor therapy. The durations of therapy employed in the previously conducted trials were arbitrarily chosen from previous experience with tamoxifen or for purposes of study design (ie, in order to match the duration of tamoxifen). According to the experience with tamoxifen (as described previously), it is by no means intuitive that prolonging the use of adjuvant aromatase inhibitors would necessarily result in increased benefit when compared to shorter duration. Thus, there is a need to definitively address the question of aromatase inhibitor duration in a prospective randomized trial. The NSABP B-42 is a phase III, randomized, placebo-controlled, double-blind clinical trial that aims to determine whether prolonged adjuvant hormonal therapy with letrozole will improve disease-free survival in postmenopausal women with ER-positive and/or PgR-positive breast cancer who have completed 5 years of hormonal therapy with either 5 years of an aromatase inhibitor or up to 3 years of tamoxifen followed by an aromatase inhibitor (Fig. 42-17). The study will also determine whether prolonged letrozole therapy will improve survival, breast cancer–free survival, and time to distant recurrence. It will also examine whether prolonged letrozole

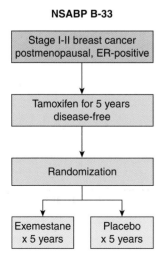

FIGURE 42-16 Schema of the NSABP B-33 trial evaluating adjuvant exemestane in postmenopausal patients who complete 5 years of tamoxifen and are recurrence free.

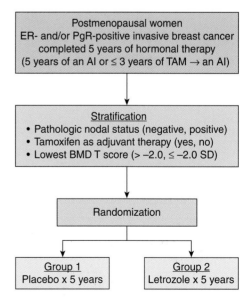

FIGURE 42-17 Schema of the NSABP B-42 trial evaluating extended adjuvant therapy with letrozole versus placebo in patients who are disease-free after completing 5 years of hormonal therapy consisting of either an aromatase inhibitor or tamoxifen followed by an aromatase inhibitor.

therapy will increase the incidence of osteoporotic-related fractures and arterial thrombotic events. Women eligible for the study must have had stage I, II, or IIIA breast cancer at the time of their original diagnosis and must be disease-free after completing 5 years of hormonal therapy consisting of an aromatase inhibitor or tamoxifen followed by an aromatase inhibitor. The sample size for the study is 3840 patients who will be accrued over a period of 5.25 years. The NSABP B-42 trial opened 8/14/2006, with a goal of 3840 participants. As of September 2009, accrual is at 82.40%, with 3164 patients.

ADJUVANT CHEMOTHERAPY TRIALS IN PATIENTS WITH POSITIVE NODES

Studies Evaluating Taxanes as Adjuvant Therapy in Node-Positive Breast Cancer

NSABP B-28

In the 1990s, the demonstration of significant antitumor activity with taxanes in patients with advanced breast cancer provided the rationale for evaluating these agents in the adjuvant setting.[40,41] Thus, in 1995 the NSABP initiated a randomized trial (NSABP B-28) to evaluate the worth of paclitaxel following standard dose AC chemotherapy in breast cancer patients with positive axillary nodes. Eligible patients were randomly assigned to receive 4 cycles of AC chemotherapy or 4 cycles of AC followed by 4 cycles of paclitaxel at 225 mg/m^2 given as a 3-hour infusion (Fig. 42-18). A total of 3060 patients were randomized. With a median follow-up of 64.6 months, a significant improvement in disease-free survival was observed in favor of the paclitaxel-containing arm (5-year DFS, 76% vs 72%, RR 0.83, p = 0.006). However, there was no significant difference in OS (5-year OS, 85% for both groups, RR 0.93, p = 0.46).[40] The results of the B-28 trial confirmed those previously reported by

CALGB from a trial of similar design (CALGB 9344)[41] and supported the sequential addition of a taxane after AC chemotherapy in patients with positive nodes.

NSABP B-30

The next logical step in the clinical development of taxanes as adjuvant treatment for breast cancer was to compare the sequential AC → taxane regimens (as administered in the first-generation adjuvant studies with taxanes) with combination regimens of taxanes with other active existing agents. Thus far, doxorubicin and docetaxel are among the most active agents against breast cancer. Combinations of doxorubicin with paclitaxel have demonstrated excellent response rates in phase II studies in patients with advanced breast cancer but have also been associated with a significant increase in cardiotoxicity.[100,101] Similar cardiotoxicity was not seen in phases I and II studies when docetaxel was used in combination with doxorubicin, although the increased efficacy was maintained.[102-105] Based on these studies, as well as phase III trials in patients with advanced breast cancer demonstrating increased efficacy with doxorubicin-docetaxel (AT) over AC[106] and with doxorubicin-docetaxel-cyclophosphamide (TAC) over 5-fluorouracil-doxorubicin-cyclophosphamide (FAC),[107] the NSABP B-30 study was designed to directly compare the sequential regimen of AC followed by docetaxel to the combination of doxorubicin plus docetaxel and to the triple combination of doxorubicin plus docetaxel plus cyclophosphamide (Fig. 42-19). This trial was initiated in 1999 and completed accrual in 2004 after accruing 5351 patients. Results from this trial were presented at the 2008 San Antonio Breast Cancer Symposium and are now in manuscript form.[108]

NSABP B-38

As noted earlier, results from large phase III trials conducted over the past decade have established the benefit of incorporating

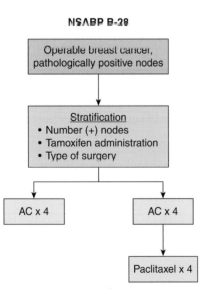

FIGURE 42-18 Schema of NSABP B-28 evaluating the sequential administration of paclitaxel after doxorubicin/cyclophosphamide (AC) in patients with resected node-positive breast cancer.

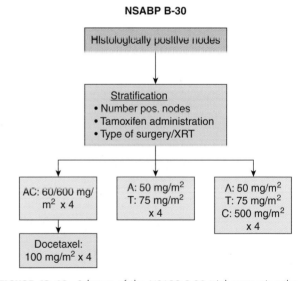

FIGURE 42-19 Schema of the NSABP B-30 trial comparing the sequential administration of doxorubicin/cyclophosphamide (AC) followed by docetaxel with the combination of doxorubicin (A) + docetaxel (T) and with the triple combination of doxorubicin (A) + docetaxel (T) + cyclophosphamide (C) in patients with resected node-positive breast cancer.

taxanes into anthracycline-based regimens as adjuvant treatment for node-positive breast cancer. The initial, first-generation trials (CALGB 9344 and NSABP B-28) evaluated sequential anthracycline-taxane regimens (AC → paclitaxel) and established their superiority over AC alone.[40,41] Following completion of CALGB-9344, the US Intergroup initiated and completed a second-generation taxane trial (CALGB 9741) that asked 2 questions in a 2 × 2 factorial design.[108] The first question was whether the concurrent AC followed by paclitaxel regimen (AC → T) was superior to the administration of each drug in a sequential, single-agent approach (A → T → C). The second question was whether shortening the interval between chemotherapy cycles to 2 weeks instead of the traditional 3 weeks (dose-dense therapy) will result in superior outcome without significantly affecting toxicity. Initial and subsequent results demonstrated improvement in both disease-free survival and overall survival with the dose-dense regimen compared to the traditional dosing interval, but no significant differences in outcome between the concurrent (AC → T) and the sequential (A → T → C) approach.[109] Because of the use of prophylactic filgrastim in order to administer the dose-dense therapy, no significant increase in hematologic toxicity was noted with the dose-dense regimens with the exception of red blood cell transfusions, which were given to 13% of patients treated on the AC → T dose-dense regimen. As a result of the increased efficacy without an overall increase in toxicity, dose-dense administration of the doxorubicin, cyclophosphamide, and paclitaxel regimen has become increasingly popular as adjuvant therapy in node-positive breast cancer. Another chemotherapy regimen that has been found to be of value as adjuvant treatment in patients with node-positive breast cancer is the triple combination of docetaxel, doxorubicin, and cyclophosphamide (TAC), which in BCIRG 001 significantly improved disease-free survival and overall survival compared to fluorouracil, doxorubicin, and cyclophosphamide (FAC).[110,111]

These results underscored the need to directly compare the effective TAC combination program (as in BCIRG 001) with an optimal sequential regimen such as the dose-dense AC → T regimen (as in CALGB 9741). Furthermore, although the TAC and AC → T dose-dense regimens have clearly improved outcomes, a substantial proportion of women treated with these regimens still developed disease recurrence. This reality provides a compelling reason to continue efforts to further improve therapy for node-positive breast cancer. One potential advantage of the dose-dense AC → T regimen is that its reported toxicity profile provides opportunity for incorporating a fourth chemotherapeutic agent into the program by adding it to the paclitaxel sequence. The antimetabolite gemcitabine has shown promise in combination with paclitaxel for the treatment of advanced breast cancer patients.[112-116] A phase III trial comparing paclitaxel alone with paclitaxel plus gemcitabine demonstrated improved response rates and time to progression with the combination in women with metastatic breast cancer previously treated with anthracyclines.[117] Updated results also demonstrated a significant improvement in overall survival with the combination regimen compared to paclitaxel alone.[118] These results demonstrate the potential for improvement of paclitaxel-containing adjuvant therapies with the addition of gemcitabine.

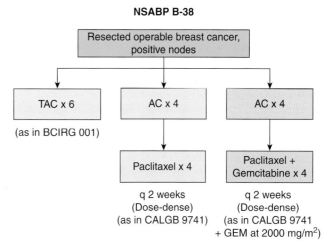

FIGURE 42-20 Schema of NSABP B-38 comparing docetaxel/doxorubicin/cyclophosphamide (TAC) with dose-dense doxorubicin/cyclophosphamide followed by dose-dense paclitaxel and with dose-dense AC followed by dose-dense paclitaxel plus gemcitabine in patients with resected node-positive breast cancer.

Thus, the NSABP B-38 trial was developed in order to compare the dose-dense AC → T regimen and the TAC regimen, and to further determine whether sequential dose-dense doxorubicin/cyclophosphamide followed by dose-dense paclitaxel/gemcitabine (AC → TG) can further improve the outcome compared to both TAC and dose dense AC → T (Fig. 42-20).[119] The primary end point for these comparisons is disease-free survival. Eligible patients for this trial have resected, operable breast cancer with positive axillary nodes. Between November 2004 and May 2007, a total of 4894 patients were randomized in the trial. Results are not available as of yet.

Studies Evaluating Biologic Targeted Therapies in the Adjuvant Setting

Despite considerable progress with adjuvant chemotherapy, there are still significant limitations with this approach both in terms of efficacy and, more importantly, in terms of toxicity. Thus, alternative adjuvant treatments that will increase the efficacy of therapy without significantly increasing side effects are highly desirable. During the past decade there has been an explosion in development of biological targeted therapies that hold promise of improving adjuvant therapy efficacy without significant increase in toxicity. Several approaches have been validated in the advanced-disease setting and have recently been evaluated in adjuvant trials. The evaluation of trastuzumab and bisphosphonates in NSABP adjuvant trials represent examples of how the evaluation of new molecular targeted therapies has been incorporated in the adjuvant setting.

NSABP Trials Evaluating Adjuvant Trastuzumab

NSABP B-31

During the 1990s a substantial amount of information accumulated in support of a significant role of HER-2 overexpression/

amplification in breast cancer both as a predictor of benefit from anthracycline-containing chemotherapy[73,119-123] and as a therapeutic target for antibody development.[124,125] As results from dose-intensification studies strongly suggested the existence of a "limit of cytoreduction," and as the overexpression of HER-2 indicated chemoresistance, it was hypothesized that targeting HER-2 with an inhibitory antibody such as trastuzumab (humanized monoclonal antibody against the extracellular domain of HER-2) might overcome resistance and augment the chemotherapy effect. In the advanced-disease setting, trastuzumab has activity as a single agent[124] and significantly increases the efficacy of chemotherapy in terms of response rates, time to progression, and overall survival.[125] However, this improvement was associated with a substantial increase in cardiac toxicity, particularly when an anthracycline-containing regimen was combined with trastuzumab. The NSABP B-31 trial was designed to evaluate the role of trastuzumab in the adjuvant setting. Results from the B-31 trial on the benefit of adjuvant trastuzumab in node-positive patients with HER-2–positive breast cancer represent one of the most exciting advances in the contemporary era of adjuvant clinical trials. The B-31 trial compared doxorubicin and cyclophosphamide followed by paclitaxel every 3 weeks with this same chemotherapy regimen plus 1 year of trastuzumab given concurrently with paclitaxel in node-positive, HER-2–positive patients. (Fig. 42-21) The trial was conducted in 2 parts. The primary aim of the first part was to evaluate the cardiac safety of the AC followed by paclitaxel plus trastuzumab regimen compared to the AC followed by paclitaxel regimen. The primary aim of the second part was to compare these 2 regimens in terms of efficacy. While the B-31 trial was being conducted, the North Central Cancer Treatment Group Trial N9831 conducted a similar trial that compared AC followed by weekly paclitaxel versus

the same chemotherapy plus trastuzumab either concurrently with paclitaxel or sequentially for 1 year. Besides node-positive patients, the N9831 trial also randomized 191 high risk/node-negative patients. The similarities between the 2 trials led to the decision to perform a joint analysis by combining the control arms and the concurrent trastuzumab arms from both trials. Interim analysis of the joined data set resulted in early disclosure of the results because of the magnitude of outcome difference in favor of adjuvant trastuzumab. The joined analysis revealed that with a median follow-up of 2 years, adjuvant trastuzumab reduced the risk of treatment failure by 52% (hazard ratio 0.48, $p < 0.0001$), and the risk of death by 33% ($p = 0.015$).[73] In the B-31 study, cardiac- related events occurred in 4.1% of the patients in the trastuzumab arm compared with 0.8% of the patients in the control arm. Cases of congestive heart failure were more common among older patients and among patients who had a decrease in ejection fraction following doxorubicin/paclitaxel chemotherapy.[126] The results of the joint analysis along with those from similar adjuvant trials conducted by other groups (HERA Trial, BCIRG 006 trial) established trastuzumab in combination with chemotherapy as an important treatment for patients with HER-2–positive early-stage breast cancer. Important biological correlative studies within all of these trials aim to discover markers that predict benefit from the addition of trastuzumab to chemotherapy such as phosphorylation status of HER-2, extracellular domain levels, autoantibodies, and array-based comparative genomic hybridization (CGH). A more recent update of the B-31/N9831 joint analysis was presented at the 2007 ASCO meeting.[127] With a median follow-up of 2.9 years, the benefit from the addition of trastuzumab remains. The 4-year DFS rate was 73.1% in the chemotherapy group and 85.9% in the chemotherapy plus trastuzumab group. The 4-year OS rates were 92.6% and 89.4%, respectively. The hazard ratio for adjuvant trastuzumab versus none was 0.49 ($p < 0.0001$, 95% CI 0.41–0.58) for DFS and 0.63 ($p = 0.0004$, 95% CI 0.49–0.81) for OS.[127]

NSABP B-44 /CIRG (TRIO) 011

The HER-2 proto-oncogene is amplified or overexpressed in 25% to 30% of breast cancers. HER-2 overexpression is associated with an increased rate of metastasis and decreased overall survival, but the mechanism(s) by which HER-2 overexpression mediates this aggressive phenotype remains unclear. It has been proposed that increased tumor angiogenesis, due to overexpression of pro-angiogenic factors such as vascular endothelial growth factor (VEGF), is one possible mechanism that could account, at least in part, for the poor prognosis of patients with breast carcinomas that overexpress HER-2. Blood vessels are not only required for tumors to grow beyond 1 to 2 mm³, but also to facilitate tumor metastasis.[128,129] VEGF is a central regulator of angiogenesis,[130,131] and disruption of a single VEGF allele in mice results in embryonic lethality.[132,133] Similar to HER-2, VEGF is an independent predictor of survival in patients diagnosed with breast and ovarian cancer.[134,135] Cancer cells with increased VEGF expression demonstrate both increased growth and increased metastatic potential.[136,137] VEGF protein expression is also influenced by oncogenes, such as v-Raf and v-Ha-Ras,

NSABP B-31

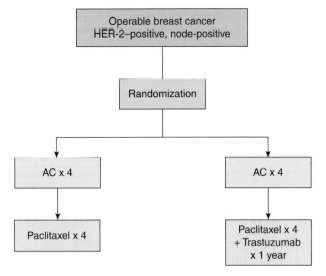

FIGURE 42-21 Schema of the NSABP B-31 study evaluating the effect of adjuvant trastuzumab in patients with node-positive, resected operable breast cancer, over-expressing the HER-2 oncogene.

genes that play a role in the HER-2 signaling pathway.[138] Preclinical data have demonstrated that stimulation of the HER-2 signaling pathway or inhibition with trastuzumab alters VEGF expression in cell lines that overexpress HER-2, indicating that VEGF is a downstream target of the receptor's signaling pathway. These data are further supported with results from clinical specimens[139] in which HER-2–positive breast cancers were significantly more likely to express high levels of VEGF than their HER-2–negative counterparts. Moreover, those women whose tumors contain both the HER-2 alteration and high levels of VEGF expression had the worst clinical outcome of any subgroup in this cohort. These observations provided the rationale for the simultaneous inhibition of the HER-2 and VEGF pathways leading to the conduct of a phase I and subsequently a phase II trial that demonstrated the safety and efficacy of the combination of trastuzumab plus bevacizumab in patients with HER-2–amplified locally recurrent, unresectable, or metastatic breast cancer.[140]

With the rationale just described, the NSABP and the Cancer International Research Group (CIRG) designed and implemented the NSABP B-44 trial (BETH), an international, multicenter, open-label, randomized phase III trial, which will determine the value of adding bevacizumab to the combination of chemotherapy plus trastuzumab in patients with resected node-positive or high-risk node-negative, HER-2–positive breast cancer (as determined by a central laboratory). This trial will determine if chemotherapy plus trastuzumab plus bevacizumab improves invasive disease-free survival (IDFS) relative to chemotherapy plus trastuzumab. Secondary aims include determining whether the addition of bevacizumab to chemotherapy plus trastuzumab improves DFS, OS, recurrence-free interval (RFI), and distant recurrence-free interval (DRFI). The benefit of adding bevacizumab for IDFS, DFS, OS, RFI, and DRFI will also be evaluated separately for each of the 2 chemotherapy regimens employed in the trial along with the cardiac and noncardiac toxicities of each of these regimens.

Patients in the BETH Trial are enrolled in 1 of 2 chemotherapy regimen cohorts. One cohort receives 6 cycles of docetaxel/carboplatin plus trastuzumab with or without bevacizumab (TCH → H or TCHB → HB); the other cohort receives 3 cycles of docetaxel plus trastuzumab given with or without bevacizumab followed by 3 cycles of FEC (TH → FEC → H or THB → FEC → HB). NSABP and CIRG investigators will only enroll patients in the TCH regimen cohort (Fig. 42-22). Additional investigators, referred to in the protocol as Independent Investigators, will enroll patients in either the TCH → H cohort or the TH → FEC → H regimen cohort depending on institutional preference. With both chemotherapy regimens, patients will continue trastuzumab with or without bevacizumab following chemotherapy to complete 1 year of targeted therapy. Following completion of chemotherapy, patients will also receive adjuvant radiotherapy and endocrine therapy as clinically indicated.

Patients will be given the option of allowing their tumor samples to be used for the BETH trial translational research. Also, patients will be asked to consent to the optional submission of serum and plasma samples during the study. LVEF assessments will be performed before study entry, at scheduled time-points during therapy, and at 15, 24, 36, and 60 months

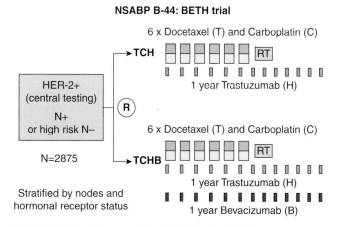

FIGURE 42-22 Schema of the NSABP B-44 (BETH) trial evaluating the effect of adding bevacizumab to adjuvant trastuzumab plus chemotherapy in resected operable breast cancer overexpressing the HER-2 oncogene.

following randomization. Accrual to this trial was initiated in 2008 and the target sample size is 2875 patients.

Studies Evaluating Bisphosphonates as Adjuvant Therapy

Bisphosphonates are emerging as a class of drugs with great potential for improving the outcome of breast cancer patients without adversely affecting their quality of life and without causing significant toxicity. Bisphosphonates act primarily by inhibiting osteoclast function with subsequent reduction in bone loss. Other mechanisms of action include a reduction in malignant cell adhesion to bone as well as decreased osteoblast-mediated osteoclast stimulation and adsorption to bone resorption surfaces, leading to protection against osteoclast action. Bisphosphonates have been found effective in patients with Paget disease, osteoporosis, and malignant bone disease, and they have been shown to reduce skeletal complications in patients with various malignancies. Phase III trials in patients with metastatic breast carcinoma involving bone have shown a reduction in skeletal complications when bisphosphonates are used in patients treated with either chemotherapy or hormonal therapy.[141] Patients with carcinoma of the breast who receive adjuvant chemotherapy have a higher rate of vertebral fracture than an age-matched population of patients who do not receive chemotherapy.[142] It has been hypothesized that the increased bone loss, particularly in premenopausal and perimenopausal women, is one of the causes of the propensity of breast cancer to metastasize to bone. One of the bisphosphonates—oral clodronate—has been shown to reduce the incidence of new bone metastases in patients with recurrent breast cancer. In addition it has been shown to reduce the incidence of bone relapse in patients with operable breast cancer who had cancer cells present in the bone marrow by immunohistochemistry.[143] This latter trial was randomized but used an open-label design. The trial also showed a reduction in the incidence of recurrence at sites other than bone, and—at the 7-year follow-up—a significant survival benefit for patients receiving clodronate. A mature analysis of a larger, placebo-controlled, randomized trial from the United Kingdom and Canada showed a significant reduction in the incidence of new bone metastases during the 2-year period in which clodronate was administered, but the difference lost its statistical significance with further follow-up when placebo/clodronate was stopped. This study further showed a nonsignificant reduction in the rate of nonskeletal metastases and a significant improvement in overall survival.[144] On the other hand, a smaller randomized Scandinavian study in 299 node-positive breast cancer patients showed that the addition of oral clodronate to adjuvant therapy did not reduce the rate of bone metastases. In addition, clodronate seemed to have a negative effect on disease-free survival by increasing the development of nonskeletal metastases.

NSABP B-34

Although the results of some of the early trials are encouraging, sufficient controversy remains relative to the value of bisphosphonates as adjuvant therapy, justifying the conduct of large confirmatory trials to test this important hypothesis. One such trial is the NSABP B-34 trial, a double-blinded, placebo-controlled randomized clinical trial evaluating oral clodronate as adjuvant therapy (Fig. 42-23). The primary aim of the trial was to determine whether oral clodronate administered for 3 years, either alone or in addition to other adjuvant therapies (ie, chemotherapy and/or hormonal therapy), would reduce the incidence of skeletal metastases and improve disease-free survival. Secondary aims were to determine whether the addition of adjuvant clodronate would improve overall survival, reduce the incidence of nonskeletal metastases, prevent skeletal events, improve patient quality of life, and reduce the rate of bone loss in a subgroup of patients. Between January 2001 and March 2004, a total of 3323 patients were accrued into this trial.

NSABP B-34

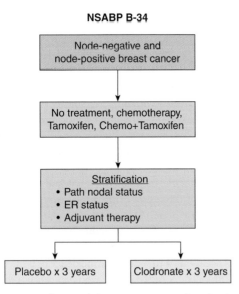

FIGURE 42-23 Schema of the NSABP B-34 trial evaluating adjuvant oral clodronate in patients with resected stage I and II operable breast cancer (Chemo, adjuvant chemotherapy; No Tx, no adjuvant therapy; Tam, adjuvant tamoxifen.)

Results from the trial are not available as of yet. Following completion of the B-34 trial, a second-generation trial was initiated under the leadership of Southwest Oncology Group (SWOG) comparing oral clodronate to more potent oral and parenteral bisphosphonates (ie, ibadronate and zoledronate).[145] The potential value of IV zoledronate in reducing breast cancer recurrence was recently shown in a clinical trial reported by the Austrian Breast and Colorectal Study Group, in premenopausal patients who were randomized to receive anastrozole or tamoxifen in addition to an LHRH analog.[146] Further confirmatory studies of IV zoledronate in postmenopausal patients have also been conducted and their results are eagerly awaited.

Neoadjuvant Chemotherapy Trials

The establishment of lumpectomy as the surgical treatment of choice for the majority of patients with operable breast cancer, and the demonstration of significant improvements in disease-free survival and overall survival with adjuvant systemic chemotherapy in patients with positive as well as negative axillary nodes, have offered clinical justification for considering the use of systemic chemotherapy prior to surgical resection (preoperative or neoadjuvant chemotherapy). In addition, several preclinical and clinical observations have provided biological rationale as to why such an intervention may have an advantage over the administration of chemotherapy in the conventional postoperative fashion[147-150] Although several single-institution, nonrandomized clinical series evaluated neoadjuvant chemotherapy in patients with operable breast cancer, before such treatment could become standard clinical practice it had to be evaluated in prospective randomized clinical trials.

NSABP B-18

In 1988, the NSABP initiated protocol B-18, a randomized trial in patients with operable breast cancer that compared preoperative versus postoperative administration of adjuvant chemotherapy (4 cycles of doxorubicin/cyclophosphamide) (Fig. 42-24).[151-154] The primary aim of the study was to determine whether preoperative chemotherapy will more effectively prolong disease-free survival and overall survival than the same chemotherapy given postoperatively. Secondary aims of the study included the evaluation of clinical and pathologic response of primary breast cancer to preoperative chemotherapy, the determination of the downstaging effect of preoperative chemotherapy in the axillary nodes, and the determination of whether preoperative chemotherapy increases the rate of breast-conserving surgery. In addition, the study attempted to determine whether primary breast cancer response to preoperative chemotherapy correlates with disease-free survival and overall survival.

Between October 1988 and April 1993, 1523 patients were accrued to the trial. Results on the effect of preoperative chemotherapy on tumor response[150,151] indicate that following administration of preoperative chemotherapy, 36% of patients obtained a clinical complete response and 43% of patients obtained a clinical partial response (cPR) for an overall response rate of 79%. More importantly, 13% of the patients achieved a pathologic complete response (pCR: absence of invasive tumor in the breast specimen following neoadjuvant chemotherapy).

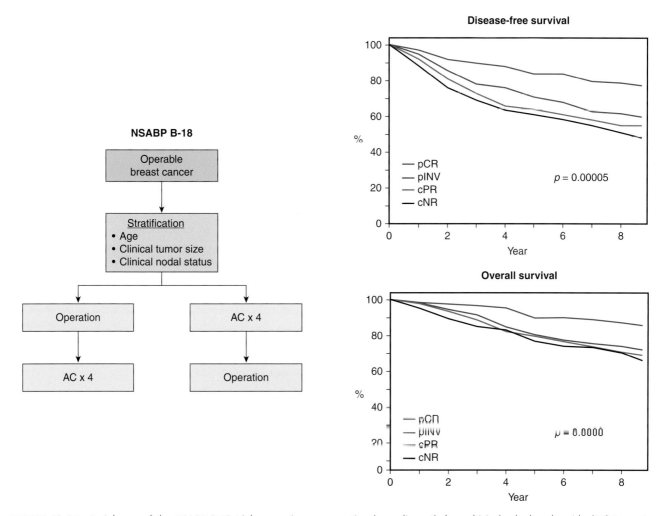

FIGURE 42-24   **A.** Schema of the NSABP B-18 trial comparing preoperative (neoadjuvant) doxorubicin/cyclophosphamide (AC) to postoperative (adjuvant) AC in patients with operable breast cancer. **B.** Comparison of the disease-free survival and overall survival according to clinical and pathologic breast tumor response. *(Reproduced with permission from Mamounas EP. NSABP breast cancer clinical trials: recent results and future directions. Clin Med Res. 2003;1:309-326. Reprinted with permission from Marshfield Clinic; adapted from Wolmark N, Wang J, Mamounas EP, et al. Preoperative chemotherapy in patients with operable breast cancer: nine-year results from National Surgical Adjuvant Breast and Bowel Project B-18. JNCI Monographs. 2001;30:96-102. Oxford University Press.)*

Administration of preoperative chemotherapy resulted in significant pathologic axillary lymph node down-staging in 37% of the patients presumed to be node-positive at the time of administration of preoperative chemotherapy. Patients receiving preoperative chemotherapy were significantly more likely to receive a lumpectomy than were patients receiving postoperative chemotherapy (67% vs 60%, *p* = 0.002). When the 2 treatment groups were compared in terms of outcome,[153] there was no difference in the disease-free survival, distant DFS, or OS between the 2 groups. There was evidence of significant correlation between pathologic response of primary breast tumors to preoperative chemotherapy and disease-free and overall survival. Patients achieving a pCR had a statistically significant improvement in disease-free survival and overall survival compared to those who had a clinical complete response (cCR) but residual invasive carcinoma in the breast specimen (pINV) or those who had a clinical partial response (cPR) or a clinical nonresponse (cNR) (Fig. 42-24). When the prognostic effect of pCR was examined after adjusting for other known clinical

prognostic factors such as clinical nodal status, clinical tumor size, and age, pCR remained a significant independent predictor for disease-free survival and a borderline significant predictor for overall survival. Recently the B-18 trial, with 9 years of follow-up, has continued to demonstrate equivalence between preoperative and postoperative chemotherapy and a significant correlation between pCR and outcome.[154] More recent results from B-18 with 16 years of follow-up continue to demonstrate no statistically significant differences in DFS and OS between the 2 groups. However, there are trends in favor of preoperative chemotherapy for DFS and OS in women less than 50 years old (HR = 0.85, *p* = 0.09 for DFS; HR = 0.81, *p* = 0.06 for OS). Disease-free survival conditional on being event-free for 5 years also demonstrated a strong trend in favor of the preoperative group (HR = 0.81, *p* = 0.053).[155]

The B-18 protocol also provided an opportunity to study patterns of locoregional failure as a function of preoperative versus postoperative systemic therapy. At 9 years the rate of ipsilateral breast tumor recurrence (IBTR) was slightly higher in

the preoperative group (10.7% vs 7.6%) although this difference was not statistically significant.[154] Risk of local recurrence
was somewhat higher in the subset of lumpectomy patients who
were down-staged to become BCT-eligible in comparison to the
BCT patients who were BCT candidates at presentation.[153]
However, this subset of down-staged BCT cases was predominantly comprised of T₃ tumors, and since local recurrence is an
indication of underlying tumor biology, it would be expected
that the more advanced stage lesions may have increased local
recurrence rates regardless of surgery type and treatment
sequence. Also, radiation boost doses were not consistently used
in the lumpectomy patients, and tamoxifen therapy was only
used in patients over 50 years of age. Both of these interventions,
if implemented uniformly, might have influenced local recurrence rates in down-staged tumors.

NSABP B-27

The results from the B-18 trial strengthened the biological and
clinical rationale for continuing to evaluate the role of neoadjuvant

chemotherapy in patients with operable breast cancer.[154,155,156]
The demonstration of significant antitumor activity with taxanes
in patients with advanced breast cancer provided the opportunity
to take the results from the NSABP B-18 trial a step further. In
1995 the NSABP implemented protocol B-27[42,43,157], a randomized trial that evaluated the worth of docetaxel when administered in the preoperative or the postoperative setting following 4
cycles of preoperative AC chemotherapy (Fig. 42-25).[156] The
main objective of the study was to determine whether the addition of 4 cycles of preoperative or postoperative docetaxel, following 4 cycles of preoperative AC, could more effectively
prolong disease-free survival and overall survival in patients with
operable breast cancer than 4 cycles of preoperative AC alone.
Secondary objectives were to determine whether the addition of
preoperative docetaxel following preoperative AC could increase
the rate of locoregional response, pCR, pathologic axillary
nodal down-staging, and breast-conserving surgery. Additional
secondary objectives were to determine whether any benefit
from the addition of postoperative docetaxel after preoperative

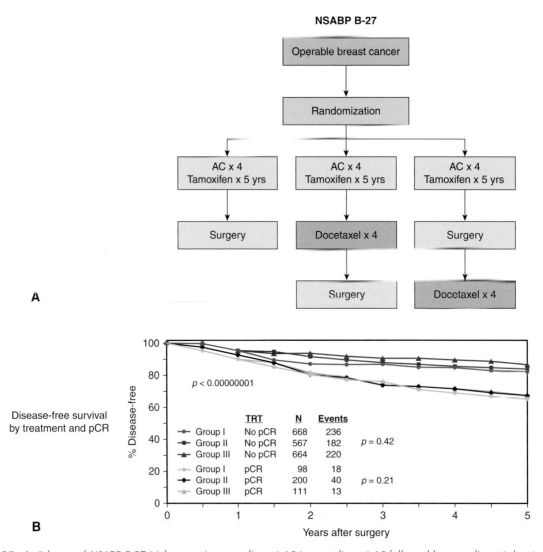

FIGURE 42-25 A. Schema of NSABP B-27 trial comparing neoadjuvant AC to neoadjuvant AC followed by neoadjuvant docetaxel and to neoadjuvant AC followed by adjuvant docetaxel in patients with operable breast cancer. **B.** Comparison of disease-free survival by treatment and pCR. (Tam, tamoxifen.)

AC might be limited to specific subgroups of patients, that is, those with residual positive nodes after preoperative AC. The trial opened in December 1995 and closed in December 2000, after accruing 2411 patients.

Although the addition of preoperative docetaxel to preoperative AC significantly increased the rates of pCR in the breast (26.1% vs 13.7%; $p < 0.001$) and significantly decreased the rates of pathologically positive nodes, it did not significantly increase further the rate of breast conservation.[42] Moreover, disease-free survival and overall survival were not significantly prolonged with the addition of preoperative or postoperative docetaxel after 5 years[43] and after 8 years of follow-up.[154] However, achievement of pCR remained a significant independent predictor of improved outcome, thus validating the use of this end point as a surrogate marker for the effectiveness of neoadjuvant chemotherapy (Fig. 42-24).

Incidentally, the B-27 protocol also provided a valuable opportunity to study the accuracy of lymphatic mapping and sentinel lymph node biopsy (SLNB) in women treated with neoadjuvant chemotherapy.[158] Although there was no specific protocol for lymphatic mapping as part of the study, 428 patients underwent SLNB followed by completion axillary lymph node dissection. At least 1 sentinel node could be identified in 89% of patients (90% with radiocolloid alone, 77% with blue dye alone, and 88% with the combination of both tracers). The false-negative rate was 11%, and this was comparable to the false-negative rate observed in multicenter studies of sentinel node biopsy before systemic therapy.

NSABP FUTURE DIRECTIONS WITH NEOADJUVANT CHEMOTHERAPY

The B-18 and B-27 trials, along with trials from other investigators, have established the value of pCR as a surrogate end point for disease-free survival and overall survival. As a result, the neoadjuvant setting provides the opportunity for the rapid evaluation of novel chemotherapy regimens (such as the combination of taxanes with other active chemotherapy agents) and for the introduction of novel biological targeted therapies (either alone or in combination with standard neoadjuvant chemotherapy regimens). An important component of such neoadjuvant trials is the incorporation of high-throughput technology in order to identify patients with tumors at high likelihood of achieving a pCR when treated with a certain neoadjuvant chemotherapy regimen (with or without the targeted therapy). Moreover, an important remaining question is whether there is a role for additional adjuvant therapies in patients who are found to have residual disease in the breast and/or axillary nodes following neoadjuvant chemotherapy. To address some of these questions, the NSABP has developed a new series of clinical trials evaluating novel taxane combinations with or without bevacizumab (for HER-2–negative patients) and with trastuzumab, lapatinib, or a combination of the 2 (for HER-2–positive patients). In addition, a new trial that is in the late stages of development will evaluate the small-molecule angiogenesis inhibitor sunitinib in patients who have residual disease after neoadjuvant chemotherapy.

NSABP B-40

The oral fluoropyrimidine capecitabine was rationally designed to provide prolonged exposure to 5-FU and to generate 5-FU preferentially in tumor tissue. Preclinical studies have demonstrated that administration of docetaxel or paclitaxel results in further upregulation of thymidine phosphorylase (TP) in tumor tissue.[159] This has been confirmed in women with primary breast cancer who were treated with preoperative docetaxel.[160] Coadministration of capecitabine and either docetaxel or paclitaxel in xenograft models resulted in synergistic antitumor activity, whereas, taxanes in combination with either 5-FU or uracil plus tegafur (UFT) demonstrated only additive efficacy.[159] A phase III comparison of capecitabine plus docetaxel versus docetaxel alone in patients with advanced or metastatic disease who either progressed while receiving anthracycline-containing therapy or relapsed after the completion of treatment showed an increase in objective response as well as significant prolongation in median time to progression and median overall survival for patients assigned to the combination.[161]

As mentioned earlier, gemcitabine is a nucleoside analog antimetabolite, which exhibits cell phase specificity, primarily killing cells undergoing DNA synthesis (S phase) and also blocking the progression of cells through the G1/S phase boundary. Multiple studies have established the efficacy of single-agent gemcitabine in patients with metastatic breast cancer.[112-115,162] Gemcitabine has also shown efficacy in combination with taxanes. Results from a phase III randomized trial comparing paclitaxel alone to paclitaxel with gemcitabine in patients with metastatic breast cancer who had received adjuvant anthracyclines demonstrated significant improvement in response rates, median time to progression, and median overall survival with the addition of gemcitabine to paclitaxel.[163] Finally, a phase III trial in 305 patients with anthracycline pretreated metastatic breast cancer has shown docetaxel/gemcitabine to have similar efficacy to docetaxel/capecitabine.[164]

Bevacizumab is a recombinant humanized monoclonal antibody against human vascular endothelial growth factor (VEGF). VEGF is a critical regulator of both normal and pathologic angiogenesis.[165] The biologic activity of VEGF is mediated by binding to 2 receptors on the surface of endothelial cells, namely Flt-1 and KDR. In breast cancer, bevacizumab has shown antitumor activity as a single agent as well as in combination with chemotherapy.[166-168] Results of ECOG (Eastern Cooperative Oncology Group) E2100 have demonstrated substantial activity of bevacizumab added to paclitaxel in the front-line treatment of metastatic breast cancer.[167] Neoadjuvant trials provide a unique opportunity for early correlation between potential molecular predictive factors and outcomes such as overall clinical response and complete pathologic response. Given the promise of bevacizumab, the NSABP felt that it is important to evaluate this agent in a large phase III neoadjuvant trial incorporating correlative science studies on tumor specimens.

NSABP B-40 evaluates the benefit of adding bevacizumab to the sequential docetaxel-based regimens (docetaxel alone, docetaxel/capecitabine, docetaxel/gemcitabine) in a 3 × 2 factorial design. Patients are randomized to 1 of the 3 chemotherapy regimens with a secondary randomization to receive bevacizumab or no bevacizumab. Bevacizumab 15 mg/kg every 3 weeks

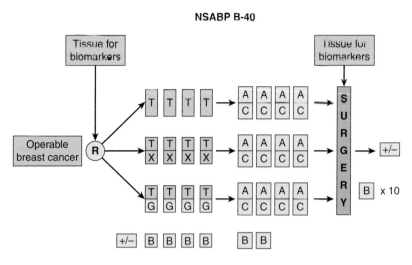

FIGURE 42-26 Schema of NSABP B-40 evaluating the effect on pCR of adding capecitabine or gemcitabine to docetaxel when administered before doxorubicin/cyclophosphamide (AC) with or without bevacizumab as neoadjuvant therapy in patients with palpable, operable breast cancer not overexpressing HER-2.

will be administered with the first 6 cycles of chemotherapy in the neoadjuvant setting and for 10 doses in the postoperative setting (Fig. 42-26).

The primary aims of the study are to determine whether adding capecitabine or gemcitabine to docetaxel followed by AC will increase the pCR rates in patients with palpable and operable HER-2–negative breast cancer and to determine whether the addition of bevacizumab to 3 docetaxel-based regimens followed by AC will increase pCR rates. Secondary aims include determination of whether pCR in the breast and axillary nodes, clinical overall response rates (cOR), and clinical complete response rates (cCR) can be increased by the additional therapies summarized in Figure 42-26 and the preceeding paragraph. Other secondary aims include determination of whether the addition of bevacizumab to the chemotherapy regimens will improve disease-free survival and/or increase surgical complication rates, toxicity, and adverse effects on cardiac function.

Pathology specimens will be collected and used to identify gene expression profiles that can predict pCR and to test a chemotherapy response assay as a predictor of pCR. The NSABP B-40 trial opened 11/20/2006, with a goal of 1200 participants. As of September 2009, accrual is at 71.08%, with 853 patients.

NSABP B-41

The identification of the HER-2 pathway and the development of anti–HER-2 therapies has introduced a new era in breast cancer therapy. Results from neoadjuvant and adjuvant trials evaluating trastuzumab in patients with early-stage and locally advanced breast cancer have demonstrated significant antitumor efficacy when trastuzumab is combined with standard chemotherapy regimens. In addition to monoclonal antibodies such

as trastuzumab, small-molecule tyrosine kinase inhibitors such as lapatinib have also shown significant antitumor activity in patients with advanced breast cancer, providing hope that these molecules will also be effective in the adjuvant and neoadjuvant settings. Lapatinib, an oral, small-molecule, dual tyrosine kinase inhibitor of HER-2 and epidermal growth factor receptor (EGFR),[169] has demonstrated non-cross-resistance with trastuzumab in preclinical studies[170] and activity in women with HER-2–positive, metastatic breast cancer progressing on trastuzumab.[171] Lapatinib binds to the intracellular domains of HER-2 and EGFR at the ATP-binding sites and prevents phosphorylation and activation of downstream signaling pathways. Results of a planned interim analysis of a phase III trial comparing the combination of lapatinib and capecitabine with capecitabine alone in women with progressive, locally advanced, or metastatic HER-2–positive breast cancer previously treated with an anthracycline, a taxane, and trastuzumab were recently disclosed. That trial demonstrated a significant improvement in median time to progression and overall response rates with the combination of lapatinib/capecitabine compared to capecitabine alone.[172] This improvement was achieved without an increase in serious toxicity. In addition, a large phase III trial of paclitaxel plus lapatinib compared to paclitaxel alone has also recently demonstrated improved response rates and time to progression with the combination but only in patients who overexpressed HER-2.[173] According to the results of these studies, it is appropriate to evaluate the safety and activity of paclitaxel plus lapatinib in the neoadjuvant setting. Furthermore, it will be important to evaluate whether the combination of trastuzumab and lapatinib is more effective than each of the agents alone. The combination of paclitaxel plus trastuzumab plus lapatinib is currently being compared to paclitaxel plus trastuzumab in the first-line metastatic breast cancer setting in a phase III trial.

The B-41 trial compares AC → weekly paclitaxel (WP) plus trastuzumab, versus AC → weekly paclitaxel plus trastuzumab plus lapatinib, versus AC → weekly paclitaxel plus lapatinib as neoadjuvant therapy for women with operable HER-2–positive breast cancer and explores molecular predictors of pCR for each of the regimens (Fig. 42-27). The primary end point of the trial is to determine whether the regimen of AC → WP plus trastuzumab plus lapatinib yields a greater rate of pCR (breast ± axillary nodes) than the regimen of AC → WP plus trastuzumab. In addition, the study examines whether the regimen of AC → WP plus lapatinib yields a greater rate of pCR than the regimen of AC → WP plus trastuzumab. Secondary aims include the determination of whether the regimen of AC → WP plus trastuzumab plus lapatinib yields a greater rate of pCR than the regimen of AC → WP plus lapatinib, and the comparison of cCR, clinical overall response, recurrence-free interval, overall survival, and cardiac toxicity rates among the 3 regimens along with molecular predictors of pCR with each of the regimens.

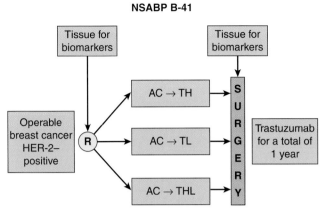

NSABP B-41

Endpoints: pCR, cardiac events, RFS, OS

FIGURE 42-27 Schema of NSABP B-41 evaluating trastuzumab, lapatinib, or the combination of trastuzumab plus lapatinib when given concurrently with paclitaxel following AC as neoadjuvant therapy in patients with palpable, operable breast cancer overexpressing HER-2.

The B-41 trial also provides an important opportunity to compare the cardiac effects of trastuzumab with trastuzumab plus lapatinib, as well as with lapatinib when the HER-2–targeting agents are administered with paclitaxel following AC. Since AC → WP plus trastuzumab has become one of the standard adjuvant regimens in the United States, it is important to evaluate the efficacy and safety of lapatinib in the context of that chemotherapy template. The cardiac monitoring program and mechanism used to assess cardiac events on B-31 and N9831 were effective in defining the symptomatic and asymptomatic effects of the chemotherapy regimen both with and without trastuzumab and will be utilized in this trial, with the exception that an 18-month left ventricular ejection fraction (LVEF) assessment will not be obtained.

Treatment of Patients with Residual Disease after Neoadjuvant Chemotherapy

Women with persistent disease in the breast or axilla after neoadjuvant chemotherapy have a poor prognosis.[43,153,154,174,175] Currently, there is no evidence for benefit from additional chemotherapy in these patients. In NSABP B-27, the pCR was doubled by the addition of neoadjuvant docetaxel to neoadjuvant AC and achieving a pCR was a significant predictor of overall survival (HR = 0.33, $p < 0.0001$). The pathologic nodal status after chemotherapy was also a significant prognostic factor for overall survival ($p < 0.0001$). There was a significant increase in the number of DFS events for the non-pCR group (n = 1899) versus the pCR group (n = 410) (674 vs 76, HR = 0.45, $p < 0.0001$). There was also a significant increase in the number of deaths in the non-pCR group versus the pCR group (420 vs 33, HR = 0.33, $p < 0.0001$).[43] In the Aberdeen neoadjuvant study,[176] patients with large operable and locally advanced breast cancer underwent 4 cycles of cyclophosphamide/vincristine/doxorubicin/prednisone (CVAP) chemotherapy. Patients

with a complete or partial response were then randomized to either 4 cycles of CVAP or 4 cycles of docetaxel (100 mg/m²). The addition of sequential docetaxel to CVAP neoadjuvant chemotherapy resulted in a significantly enhanced clinical response rate (94% vs 66%) and a substantially increased complete pathologic response rate (34% vs 16%, $p < 0.04$) when compared to patients receiving CVAP alone. Patients who did not have a clinical response after receiving CVAP chemotherapy went on to receive 4 cycles of docetaxel. In these patients, while the clinical response rate was 51%, pCR was only 2%. In the GEPARTRIO[177] study, patients with previously untreated, operable (T > 1.9 cm) or locally advanced breast cancer were treated with 2 cycles of neoadjuvant docetaxel/doxorubicin/cyclophosphamide (TAC) and if they responded clinically they continued to receive 4 additional cycles of TAC chemotherapy. Those who did not respond were randomized to either an additional 4 cycles of TAC or 4 cycles of vinorelbine/capecitabine. The pCR rate for patients who were responders and received 6 cycles of TAC was 23%. Nonresponders who received 6 cycles of TAC had a pCR (breast) of 6.6%, and nonresponders who received vinorelbine/capecitabine had a rate of 6.2%. From the above studies, it is evident that early clinical response to neoadjuvant chemotherapy predicts chemosensitivity to non-cross-resistant chemotherapy regimens but lack of early clinical response generally predicts chemotherapy resistance.

There are no available data to suggest benefit from additional "adjuvant" chemotherapy for women with persistent disease following neoadjuvant therapy with an anthracycline/taxane/cyclophosphamide regimen. Thus, novel targets need to be identified in order to develop new truly non-cross-resistant agents for the treatment of patients who have residual disease after neoadjuvant chemotherapy.

The NSABP is currently actively working toward the development of a clinical trial for this patient population.

NSABP BREAST CANCER CHEMOPREVENTION TRIALS

According to the American Cancer Society, an estimated 192,370 new cases of invasive breast cancer are expected to occur among women in the US during 2009. Improvements in the detection and treatment of this disease have resulted in decreasing rates of death over the past decade, but the fear of recurrence, the side effects and toxicities of treatment, and the costs, both financial and emotional, remain staggering. Epidemiologic data have documented a hormonally mediated basis for breast cancer. Both in vivo and in vitro laboratory studies have demonstrated that estrogen is a key factor in breast cancer initiation and promotion. Thus, it is not surprising that the first studies evaluating breast cancer chemoprevention have focused on methods to disrupt the actions of estrogen.

The selective estrogen receptor modulator (SERM) tamoxifen has been the most commonly prescribed hormonal breast cancer treatment in the world for many years. Randomized adjuvant trials that evaluated tamoxifen demonstrated a significant reduction in new primary breast cancers in the opposite breast of the women who received the drug. This observation led the NSABP to initiate Protocol P-1 in 1992.

NSABP P-1

P-1, also referred to as the Breast Cancer Prevention Trial (BCPT), is a large, multicenter chemoprevention trial designed to test the efficacy of tamoxifen in reducing the incidence of invasive breast cancer, fatal and nonfatal myocardial infarction, and specific fractures in healthy women at increased risk for breast cancer. Between July 1992 and September 1997, 13,388 women entered the trial and were assigned to receive either 5 years of tamoxifen or 5 years of placebo. To enter the trial the women had to be 35 years of age or older and they had to have an increased risk of developing breast cancer if they were younger than 60. All women 60 and older were risk eligible regardless of other risk factors. Those 35 or older with a histologic diagnosis of LCIS were also risk eligible for the study.

The results of the P-1 were announced in 1998, and with an average follow-up of almost 4 years, demonstrated that tamoxifen reduced the risk of developing an invasive breast cancer by 49%, a finding that was highly statistically significant. This reduction occurred primarily in ER-positive breast cancers.[58] Despite crossover to tamoxifen when the results of the study were announced, a recent update of the study at 7 years shows that the women who were originally randomized to tamoxifen continue to have a statistically significant reduction in invasive and noninvasive breast cancer.[178]

At 4 years, tamoxifen treatment in the BCPT did not alter the rate of ischemic heart disease but reduced the rate of fractures in the hip, spine, and radius. The rate of endometrial cancer was increased in the tamoxifen group (RR = 2.53), as was the risk of deep vein thrombosis (DVT), pulmonary emboli (PE), and stroke; these occurred predominantly in women 50 years and older. At 7 years, the risk of endometrial cancer with tamoxifen increased further (RR = 3.28). Relative risks of stroke and DVT were unchanged at 7 years, and the risk of PE was approximately 11% lower.

Several European trials with designs similar to that of P-1 have been conducted and have also demonstrated a reduction in breast cancer incidence among tamoxifen-treated patients.[179-181]

NSABP P-2

Raloxifene hydrochloride is also a SERM. In 1998 it was approved by the US FDA for the treatment and prevention of osteoporosis; one of the pivotal studies leading to that approval was the Multiple Outcomes of Raloxifene Evaluation (MORE) study, which included 7705 postmenopausal women.[182] The primary end point of the MORE study was bone fractures, but development of breast cancer was a secondary end point, and MORE showed that 4 years of raloxifene treatment appeared to reduce the risk of receptor-positive breast cancer by 72%. Like tamoxifen, raloxifene did increase the risk of thromboembolic events, but there was no apparent increase in endometrial cancer. A direct comparison of raloxifene and tamoxifen in a group of women at increased risk for breast cancer was a logical next step.

The NSABP P-2 or STAR trial (Study of Tamoxifen And Raloxifene) was a double-blinded, randomized clinical trial (Fig. 42-28) that entered 19,747 postmenopausal women who

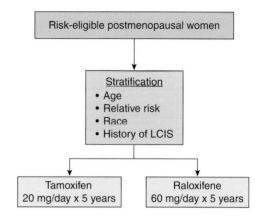

NSABP P-2: STAR trial

Risk-eligible postmenopausal women

Stratification
• Age
• Relative risk
• Race
• History of LCIS

Tamoxifen
20 mg/day x 5 years

Raloxifene
60 mg/day x 5 years

FIGURE 42-28 Schema of the NSABP P-2 (STAR) trial.

were at least 35 years of age and had a history of LCIS treated by local excision alone or a modified Gail score demonstrating a 5-year risk for invasive breast cancer of at least 1.66%.[183,184] Women in the study were assigned to receive either tamoxifen 20 mg per day plus a placebo, or raloxifene 60 mg per day plus a placebo, for 5 years. The primary end point of the study was the development of invasive breast cancer. Secondary end points included noninvasive breast cancer, uterine malignancy, DVT, PE, transient ischemic attack, cerebral vascular accident, cardiac disease, fractures, cataracts, quality of life, and death.

At the time of randomization, the mean predicted 5-year risk of developing breast cancer in the study population was 4.03%, and their projected lifetime risk to 80 years of age was 16%. More than 9% reported a personal history of LCIS treated by local excision prior to enrollment in the study, and 22.7% had a breast biopsy prior to enrollment that demonstrated atypical ductal or lobular hyperplasia.

With a mean follow-up time of 3.9 years, 163 of the women assigned to tamoxifen and 168 of those assigned to raloxifene had developed invasive breast cancer, demonstrating that there was no difference between the effect of tamoxifen and the effect of raloxifene on the incidence of invasive breast cancer. The rate per 1000 was 4.30 in the tamoxifen group and 4.41 in the raloxifene group (RR, 1.02; 95% CI 0.82–1.28). Using the Gail model scores of the women who entered the trial, we can estimate the number of invasive breast cancers that would have occurred in an untreated group and demonstrate that there was about a 47% reduction in incidence from treatment in the trial.[185]

Raloxifene did not appear to be as effective as tamoxifen in reducing the incidence of noninvasive breast cancer (LCIS or DCIS), although the difference did not reach statistical significance. There were 57 cases of noninvasive breast cancer among the women assigned to tamoxifen and 80 among women who took raloxifene (1.51 per 1000 women assigned to tamoxifen and 2.11 per 1,00 women assigned to raloxifene [RR, 1.40; 95% CI, 0.98–2.00]). The cumulative incidence through 6 years was 8.1 per 1000 in the tamoxifen group and 11.6 per 1000 in the raloxifene group ($p = 0.052$).

More uterine malignancies occurred in the tamoxifen-treated women than in those treated with raloxifene, but the difference was not statistically significant. There were 36 cases in the tamoxifen group and 23 cases in the raloxifene group. Uterine hyperplasia (with and without atypia) was less common in the raloxifene-treated group (14 cases raloxifene; 84 cases tamoxifen), and there were significantly fewer hysterectomies performed due to nonmalignant indications in the raloxifene group (221 tamoxifen; 87 raloxifene). No statistically significant differences were noted between the 2 treatment groups relative to the incidence of ischemic heart disease, TIA, stroke, or fractures (osteoporotic fractures or total fracture). Significantly fewer thromboembolic events (DVT or PE) occurred in the raloxifene group (141 in the tamoxifen group and 100 in the raloxifene group), demonstrating a 30% reduction in favor of the raloxifene-treated women. Mortality in the 2 groups was similar, with 101 deaths in those assigned to tamoxifen and 96 in those assigned to raloxifene. The distribution by cause of death did not differ by treatment.

The results of the STAR trial demonstrate that raloxifene is an effective alternative to tamoxifen for reducing the risk of invasive breast cancer in healthy postmenopausal women at increased risk for the disease. Raloxifene is also an attractive choice for these women because it has fewer serious side effects. However, raloxifene does not appear to be as effective as tamoxifen in preventing the development of noninvasive breast cancer, DCIS, or LCIS. It is interesting to note that women who entered STAR with a previous breast biopsy that demonstrated either atypical hyperplasia or LCIS benefited equally from tamoxifen and raloxifene in the reduction of risk of invasive breast cancer. This suggests that raloxifene may actually be as effective as tamoxifen in blocking the progression of premalignant or noninvasive disease to invasive breast cancer.

In summary, women at risk for breast cancer have the option of taking tamoxifen or raloxifene. However, tamoxifen, approved for this purpose in 1998, has been underutilized. Tamoxifen was well known to oncologists who had used it extensively to treat breast cancer patients with receptor-positive disease, but it was relatively unknown to primary care physicians who are the key providers of preventive health care. Tamoxifen was viewed as a "cancer drug," and media reports highlighting its toxicities proved to be a barrier to its use.

Raloxifene, on the other hand, has been utilized for more than a decade for the treatment and prevention of osteoporosis. Over 500,000 women in the United States are currently taking this drug for its benefits in bone, and on average, these women are older and have a lower breast cancer risk than do the women in the STAR trial. Most raloxifene prescriptions have been written by primary care providers. Thus, because these physicians are already familiar with this drug, barriers relative to its use for breast cancer chemoprevention may be lessened.

The ideal chemopreventative agent may still lie somewhere in the future, and significant work remains to be done before we arrive at that point. Tamoxifen and raloxifene reduce the risk of invasive breast cancer by 50%, an impressive benefit but one that leaves substantial room for improvement. The cancers that are prevented by SERMs are ER-positive. While these ER-positive tumors make up the majority of breast cancers that occur, ER-negative cancer is not rare. Although tamoxifen is approved for premenopausal women, raloxifene is not. Efforts

already underway in the laboratory and the clinic should help us address these gaps. However, at this point in time, raloxifene may offer the best chance for breast cancer prevention for many women.

SUMMARY

This chapter summarizes the results from several of the pivotal NSABP breast cancer clinical trials, which in a stepwise fashion have evaluated various locoregional and systemic therapy approaches in the management of patients with early-stage breast cancer. Results from these trials have contributed to the reduction in the extent of surgery for invasive and noninvasive breast cancer, to the establishment of breast irradiation as an effective method of controlling in-breast recurrence following lumpectomy, and more importantly, to significant improvements in disease-free and overall survival for patients with positive as well as for those with negative nodes with adjuvant systemic therapy. Newer trials that have recently completed accrual, are currently accruing patients, or are in the final stages of development, aim to further reduce the extent of surgical resection and the extent of breast irradiation with neoadjuvant chemotherapy, sentinel node biopsy, and partial breast irradiation. They also seek to optimize adjuvant chemotherapy and adjuvant hormonal therapy by evaluating newer taxane-based chemotherapy regimens, less cardiotoxic anthracyclines, and extended durations of aromatase inhibitors. Finally, several trials introduce novel molecular-targeted approaches to the adjuvant setting by evaluating novel angiogenesis inhibitors, anti–HER-2 therapies and bisphosphonates. It is hoped that these strategies will yield fruitful results that will further reduce morbidity from surgical and adjuvant therapy while maximizing patient outcomes. In addition, the work that the NSABP has completed in the field of chemoprevention has produced 2 therapies (tamoxifen and raloxifene) that have been shown to be effective in reducing breast cancer rates in women at increased risk.

NECESSARY FUTURE STUDIES TO ADVANCE THE FIELD

Despite considerable progress in the surgical and adjuvant treatment of breast cancer over the past 30 years, significant challenges remain. Future studies will need to focus on individualizing patient management, which will result in maximizing benefits while decreasing unnecessary side effects.

Future Directions in Breast Cancer Locoregional Therapy

Besides advancements in the field of surgery itself, advancements in many other disciplines involved in breast cancer management (such as radiology, genomics, molecular pathology, and radiation therapy) are expected to have a significant impact in the surgical management of the disease in the years to come.

As breast-conserving surgery and sentinel node biopsy are now well established, the next challenge would be to attempt to treat primary breast tumors without surgery.[186] Minimally invasive ablation of the primary breast tumor is possible by several different approaches such as percutaneous ablation, radiofrequency ablation, or cryoablation. With these methods, the primary tumor can be either removed without a formal surgical procedure (mammotome excision) or it can be eliminated through complete cell death.[186,187] Although the safety and efficacy of these new procedures has been shown in small pilot trials, before they can be widely adopted, randomized phase III trials have to show their equivalence or superiority compared to the standard surgical approach.

Developments in breast cancer imaging are taking place at a rapid pace. The utility of MRI in better defining the extent of the primary tumor, and in demonstrating additional incidental lesions in the vicinity of the primary tumor or in different quadrants, may redefine the most appropriate candidates for breast-conserving surgery. The increasing value of MRI in patients undergoing neoadjuvant chemotherapy and in those presenting with clinical adenopathy with a mammographically occult breast primary has been previously demonstrated.[188-190] Further improvements in MRI and other imaging modalities, such as PET scan, will undoubtedly have an increasing impact in the surgical management of primary breast tumors and axillary nodes.

Developments in genomics and molecular pathology will undoubtedly have a significant impact in the locoregional management of breast cancer in the years to come. Identification of sentinel node micrometastases by immunohistochemistry and sensitive molecular techniques has already become a reality. In the future, similar advances will need to take place in the management of primary breast tumors relative to margin assessment and relative to the classification of subsequent tumors in the ipsilateral breast as recurrences versus second primaries.

Significant developments in radiotherapy and the introduction of partial breast radiation and intraoperative radiation are already having a significant impact in the local management of the disease in the breast. In the next few years, it is expected that several randomized, phase III clinical trials comparing whole-breast radiation with partial-breast radiation will produce results. If the data from these trials are consistent with long-term efficacy and safety of the latter approach, the challenge for future studies will be to identify subgroups of patients who are most suitable for the use of partial breast radiation. The surgical oncologist is expected to play an increasingly important role in identifying those appropriate candidates and in adjusting the surgical approach to accommodate for the application of these new techniques.

With the development of more active neoadjuvant chemotherapy regimens (including biologicals), future studies should attempt to further individualize the extent of —or even the need for—surgical resection in the breast following complete clinical and radiologic response to neoadjuvant chemotherapy. Although previous studies of neoadjuvant chemotherapy followed by breast radiation and surgical resection have shown high rates of pCR (over 40%),[191,192] similar studies, in which breast irradiation was not followed by surgical resection, have shown high rates of ipsilateral breast tumor recurrence (IBTR)[193-195] Thus, if in future studies elimination of surgical resection is to be evaluated (either before or after breast radiation), one needs to at least attempt to demonstrate absence of residual tumor either by sensitive imaging studies or by percutaneous biopsy of the tumor bed area. Newer percutaneous tumor ablation techniques (such as radiofrequency ablation or cryoablation)[186] may become a substitute for surgical excision (either before or after breast radiation) in selected patients with complete clinical and radiologic response. However, before widespread adoption, the safety and efficacy of these newer techniques needs to be documented in large clinical trials.

Finally, genomic technology is starting to be utilized for identification of molecular signatures predictive of high likelihood of pCR in the breast.[196] This new technology could have a tremendous impact in the selection of appropriate candidates for exploring some of the preceeding questions.

Similar strategies need to be explored relative to the surgical management of the axilla. By identifying patients at high likelihood of having negative axillary nodes, sentinel node biopsy alone or even no axillary surgery may become appropriate options. For those patients at high likelihood of having residual positive nodes after neoadjuvant chemotherapy, or for those with a positive sentinel node, the most appropriate regional therapy strategy (surgery vs radiotherapy) is currently under investigation in randomized clinical trials.[197]

Future Directions in Breast Cancer Adjuvant/Neoadjuvant Therapy

With the recent explosion in the development of active, novel, biological therapies targeting important pathways in the cancer cell, the need to rationally optimize their clinical application has become paramount. We need to work diligently in identifying subgroups of patients who express a particular target in their tumor and who will benefit from a particular therapeutic intervention. In this way, we will not only lower the cost of delivering unnecessary therapy to patients who do not benefit from it, but—more importantly—we will likely improve outcomes considerably in those who do. Some examples of such individualization include the identification of the subgroups of HER-2–positive patients who benefit the most from adjuvant trastuzumab, the identification of patients with equivocal or low HER-2 expression who may also benefit from adjuvant trastuzumab, and the identification of subgroups of patients who may benefit the most from the addition of bevacizumab to adjuvant chemotherapy. Finally, new developments in pharmacogenomics hold considerable promise in our quest to determine whether effective drugs such as tamoxifen may be ineffective in subsets of patients because of poor metabolism to the active substance. Future research studies should explore similar associations with most of the active oncology drugs in our current armamentarium.

REFERENCES

1. Fisher B, Redmond C, Fisher ER, et al. Ten-year results of a randomized clinical trial comparing radical mastectomy and total mastectomy with or without radiation. *N Engl J Med.* 1985;312:674-681.
2. Fisher B, Redmond C, Poisson R, et al. Eight-year results of a randomized clinical trial comparing total mastectomy and lumpectomy with or without irradiation in the treatment of breast cancer. *N Engl J Med.* 1989;320:822-828.

3. Fisher B, Costantino J, Redmond C, et al. Lumpectomy compared with lumpectomy and radiation therapy for the treatment of intraductal breast cancer. *N Engl J Med.* 1993;328:1581-1586.

4. Veronesi U, Cascinelli N, Mariani L, et al. Twenty-year follow-up of a randomized study comparing breast-conserving surgery with radical mastectomy for early breast cancer. *N Engl J Med.* 2002;347:1227-1232.

5. Veronesi U, Saccozzi R, Del Vecchio M, et al. Comparing radical mastectomy with quadrantectomy, axillary dissection, and radiotherapy in patients with small cancers of the breast. *N Engl J Med.* 1981;305:6-11.

6. Fisher B, Jeong JH, Anderson S, et al. Twenty-five-year follow-up of a randomized trial comparing radical mastectomy, total mastectomy, and total mastectomy followed by irradiation. *N Engl J Med.* 2002;347:567-575.

7. Fisher B, Anderson S, Redmond CK, et al. Reanalysis and results after 12 years of follow-up in a randomized clinical trial comparing total mastectomy with lumpectomy with or without irradiation in the treatment of breast cancer. *N Engl J Med.* 1995;333:1456-1461.

8. Fisher B, Anderson S, Bryant J, et al. Twenty-year follow-up of a randomized trial comparing total mastectomy, lumpectomy, and lumpectomy plus irradiation for the treatment of invasive breast cancer. *N Engl J Med.* 2002;347:1233-1241.

9. NIH consensus conference. Treatment of early-stage breast cancer. *JAMA.* 1991;265:391-395.

10. Early Breast Cancer Trialists' Collaborative Group. Effects of radiotherapy and surgery in early breast cancer. An overview of the randomized trials. Early Breast Cancer Trialists' Collaborative Group. *N Engl J Med.* 1995;333:1444-1455.

11. Fisher B, Bryant J, Dignam JJ, et al. Tamoxifen, radiation therapy, or both for prevention of ipsilateral breast tumor recurrence after lumpectomy in women with invasive breast cancers of one centimeter or less. *J Clin Oncol.* 2002;20:4141-4149.

12. Overgaard M, Hansen PS, Overgaard J, et al. Postoperative radiotherapy in high-risk premenopausal women with breast cancer who receive adjuvant chemotherapy. Danish Breast Cancer Cooperative Group 82b Trial. *N Engl J Med.* 1997;337:919-955.

13. Ragaz J, Jackson SM, Le N, et al. Adjuvant radiotherapy and chemotherapy in node-positive premenopausal women with breast cancer. *N Engl J Med.* 1997;337:956-962.

14. Cox CE, Pendas S, Cox JM, et al. Guidelines for sentinel node biopsy and lymphatic mapping of patients with breast cancer. *Ann Surg.* 227:645-51; discussion 651-3, 1998.

15. Veronesi U, Paganelli G, Viale G, et al. Sentinel lymph node biopsy and axillary dissection in breast cancer: results in a large series. *J Natl Cancer Inst.* 1999;91:368-373.

16. Noguchi M, Motomura K, Imoto S, et al. A multicenter validation study of sentinel lymph node biopsy by the Japanese Breast Cancer Society. *Breast Cancer Res Treat.* 2000;63:31-40.

17. Motomura K, Inaji H, Komoike Y, et al. Combination technique is superior to dye alone in identification of the sentinel node in breast cancer patients. *J Surg Oncol.* 2001;76:95-99.

18. Nano MT, Kollias J, Farshid G, et al. Clinical impact of false-negative sentinel node biopsy in primary breast cancer. *Br J Surg.* 2002;89:1430-1434.

19. Procaccini E, Ruggiero R, Mansi L, et al. Modulation of the axillary lymph node dissection in breast cancer. *Ann Ital Chir.* 2003;74:21-28; discussion 28-29.

20. Giuliano AE, Kirgan DM, Guenther JM, et al. Lymphatic mapping and sentinel lymphadenectomy for breast cancer. *Ann Surg.* 1994;220:391-398; discussion 398-401.

21. Krag D, Weaver D, Ashikaga T, et al. The sentinel node in breast cancer—a multicenter validation study. *N Engl J Med.* 1998;339:941-946.

22. McMasters KM, Tuttle TM, Carlson DJ, et al. Sentinel lymph node biopsy for breast cancer: a suitable alternative to routine axillary dissection in multi-institutional practice when optimal technique is used. *J Clin Oncol.* 2000;18:2560-2566.

23. Tafra L, Lannin DR, Swanson MS, et al. Multicenter trial of sentinel node biopsy for breast cancer using both technetium sulfur colloid and isosulfan blue dye. *Ann Surg.* 2001;233:51-59.

24. Shivers S, Cox C, Leight G, et al. Final results of the Department of Defense multicenter breast lymphatic mapping trial. *Ann Surg Oncol.* 2002;9:248-255.

25. Krag DN, Weaver DL, Alex JC, et al. Surgical resection and radiolocalization of the sentinel lymph node in breast cancer using a gamma probe. *Surg Oncol.* 1993;2:335-359; discussion 340.

26. Giuliano AE, Haigh PI, Brennan MB, et al. Prospective observational study of sentinel lymphadenectomy without further axillary dissection in patients with sentinel node-negative breast cancer. *J Clin Oncol.* 2000;18:2553-2559.

27. Clarke D, Khonji NI, Mansel RE. Sentinel node biopsy in breast cancer: ALMANAC trial. *World J Surg.* 2001;25:819-822.

28. Harlow SP, Krag DN. Sentinel lymph node—why study it: implications of the B-32 study. *Semin Surg Oncol.* 2001;20:224-229.

29. Krag D. Why perform randomized clinical trials for sentinel node surgery for breast cancer? *Am J Surg.* 2001;182:411-413.

30. Wilke LG, Giuliano A. Sentinel lymph node biopsy in patients with early-stage breast cancer: status of the National Clinical Trials. *Surg Clin North Am.* 2003;83:901-910.

31. Veronesi U, Paganelli G, Viale G, et al. A randomized comparison of sentinel-node biopsy with routine axillary dissection in breast cancer. *N Engl J Med.* 2003;349:546-553.

32. Kim T, Giuliano AE, Lyman GH. Lymphatic mapping and sentinel lymph node biopsy in early-stage breast carcinoma: a meta-analysis. *Cancer.* 2006;106:4-16.

33. Wickerham DL, Costantino JP, Mamounas EP, et al. The landmark surgical trials of the National Surgical Adjuvant Breast and Bowel Project. *World J Surg.* 2006;30:1138-1146.

34. Julian T, Krag D, Brown A. Preliminary technical results of NSABP B-32, a randomized phase III clinical trial to compare sentinel node resection to conventional axillary dissection in clinically-node-negative breast cancer patients. Abstract 14. San Antonio Breast Cancer Symposium, 2004.

35. Krag DN, Anderson SJ, Julian TB, et al. Technical outcomes of sentinel-lymph-node resection and conventional axillary-lymph-node dissection in patients with clinically node-negative breast cancer: results from the NSABP B-32 randomised phase III trial. *Lancet Oncol.* 2007;8:881-888.

36. Julian TB, Mamounas EP. Partial breast irradiation: continuing the retreat from Halstedian breast cancer management. *Oncology Issues.* 2006;21:16-18.

37. Wapnir IL, Anderson SJ, Mamounas EP, et al. Prognosis after ipsilateral breast tumor recurrence and locoregional recurrences in five National Surgical Adjuvant Breast and Bowel Project node-positive adjuvant breast cancer trials. *J Clin Oncol.* 2006;21:2020-2037.

38. Halverson KJ, Perez CA, Kuske RR, et al. Locoregional recurrence of breast cancer: a retrospective comparison of irradiation alone versus irradiation and systemic therapy. *Am J Clin Oncol.* 1992;15:93-101.

39. Borner M, Bacchi M, Goldhirsch A, et al. First isolated locoregional recurrence following mastectomy for breast cancer: results of a phase III multicenter study comparing systemic treatment with observation after excision and radiation. Swiss Group for Clinical Cancer Research. *J Clin Oncol.* 1994;12:2071-2077.

40. Mamounas EP, Bryant J, Lembersky B, et al. Paclitaxel after doxorubicin-plus cyclophosphamide as adjuvant chemotherapy for node-positive breast cancer: results from NSABP B-28. *J Clin Oncol.* 2005;23:3686-3696.

41. Henderson IC, Berry DA, Demetri GD, et al. Improved outcomes from adding sequential paclitaxel but not from escalating doxorubicin dose in an adjuvant chemotherapy regimen for patients with node-positive primary breast cancer. *J Clin Oncol.* 2003;21:976-983.

42. Bear HD, Anderson S, Brown A, et al. The effect on tumor response of adding sequential preoperative docetaxel to preoperative doxorubicin and cyclophosphamide: preliminary results from National Surgical Adjuvant Breast and Bowel Project Protocol B-27. *J Clin Oncol.* 2003;21:4165-4174.

43. Bear HD, Anderson S, Smith RE, et al. Sequential preoperative or postoperative docetaxel added to preoperative doxorubicin plus cyclophosphamide for operable breast cancer: National Surgical Adjuvant Breast and Bowel Project Protocol B-27. *J Clin Oncol.* 2006;24:2019-2027.

44. Ries L, Eisner M, Kosary, CL, et al. *SEER Cancer Statistics Review, 1973–1999.* Bethesda, MD: National Cancer Institute; 2002.

45. Fisher B, Dignam J, Wolmark N, et al. Lumpectomy and radiation therapy for the treatment of intraductal breast cancer: findings from National Surgical Adjuvant Breast and Bowel Project B-17. *J Clin Oncol.* 1998;16:441-452.

46. Fisher ER, Dignam J, Tan-Chiu E, et al. Pathologic findings from the National Surgical Adjuvant Breast Project (NSABP) eight-year update of Protocol B-17: intraductal carcinoma. *Cancer.* 1999;86:429-438.

47. Fisher B, Land S, Mamounas E, et al. Prevention of invasive breast cancer in women with ductal carcinoma in situ: an update of the national surgical adjuvant breast and bowel project experience. *Semin Oncol.* 2001;28:400-418.

48. Fisher B, Dignam J, Wolmark N, et al. Tamoxifen in treatment of intraductal breast cancer: National Surgical Adjuvant Breast and Bowel Project B-24 randomised controlled trial. *Lancet.* 1999;353:1993-2000.

49. Early Breast Cancer Trialists' Collaborative Group. Tamoxifen for early breast cancer: an overview of the randomised trials. *Lancet.* 1998;351:1451-1467.

50. Fisher B, Costantino J, Redmond C, et al. A randomized clinical trial evaluating tamoxifen in the treatment of patients with node-negative breast cancer who have estrogen-receptor-positive tumors. *N Engl J Med.* 1989;320:479-484.

51. Fisher B, Dignam J, Bryant J, et al. Five versus more than five years of tamoxifen therapy for breast cancer patients with negative lymph nodes and estrogen receptor-positive tumors. *J Natl Cancer Inst.* 1996;88:1529-1542.

52. Baum M, Brinkley DM, Dossett JA, et al. Controlled trial of tamoxifen as a single adjuvant agent in the management of early breast cancer. "Nolvadex" Adjuvant Trial Organisation. *Br J Cancer.* 1988;57:608-611.

53. Adjuvant tamoxifen in the management of operable breast cancer: the Scottish Trial. Report from the Breast Cancer Trials Committee, Scottish Cancer Trials Office (MRC), Edinburgh. *Lancet.* 1987;2:171-175.

54. Rutqvist LE, Cedermark B, Glas U, et al. Contralateral primary tumors in breast cancer patients in a randomized trial of adjuvant tamoxifen therapy. *J Natl Cancer Inst.* 1991;83:1299-1306.

55. Cyclophosphamide and tamoxifen as adjuvant therapies in the management of breast cancer. CRC Adjuvant Breast Trial Working Party. *Br J Cancer.* 1988;57:604-607.

56. Jordan VC. Effect of tamoxifen (ICI 46,474) on initiation and growth of DMBA-induced rat mammary carcinomata. *Eur J Cancer.* 1976;12:419-424.

57. Jordan VC, Allen KE. Evaluation of the antitumour activity of the non-steroidal antioestrogen monohydroxytamoxifen in the DMBA-induced rat mammary carcinoma model. *Eur J Cancer.* 1980;16:239-251.

58. Fisher B, Costantino JP, Wickerham DL, et al. Tamoxifen for prevention of breast cancer: report of the National Surgical Adjuvant Breast and Bowel Project P-1 Study. *J Natl Cancer Inst.* 1998;90:1371-1388.

59. Allred C, Bryant J, Land S, et al. Estrogen receptor expression as a predictive marker of the effectiveness of tamoxifen in the treatment of DCIS: findings from NSABP Protocol B-24. *Br Ca Res Treat.* 2002;76:S36. Abstract 30.

60. Buzdar A, Douma J, Davidson N, et al. Phase III, multicenter, double-blind, randomized study of letrozole, an aromatase inhibitor, for advanced breast cancer versus megestrol acetate. *J Clin Oncol.* 2001;19:3357-3366.

61. Buzdar A, Jonat W, Howell A, et al. Anastrozole, a potent and selective aromatase inhibitor, versus megestrol acetate in postmenopausal women with advanced breast cancer: results of overview analysis of two phase III trials. Arimidex Study Group. *J Clin Oncol.* 1996;14:2000-2011.

62. Buzdar AU, Jonat W, Howell A, et al. Anastrozole versus megestrol acetate in the treatment of postmenopausal women with advanced breast carcinoma: results of a survival update based on a combined analysis of data from two mature phase III trials. Arimidex Study Group. *Cancer.* 1998;83:1142-1152.

63. Dombernowsky P, Smith I, Falkson G, et al. Letrozole, a new oral aromatase inhibitor for advanced breast cancer: double-blind randomized trial showing a dose effect and improved efficacy and tolerability compared with megestrol acetate. *J Clin Oncol.* 1998;16:453-461.

64. Kaufmann M, Bajetta E, Dirix LY, et al. Exemestane is superior to megestrol acetate after tamoxifen failure in postmenopausal women with advanced breast cancer: results of a phase III randomized double-blind trial. The Exemestane Study Group. *J Clin Oncol.* 2000;18:1399-1411.

65. Mouridsen H, Gershanovich M, Sun Y, et al. Superior efficacy of letrozole versus tamoxifen as first-line therapy for postmenopausal women with advanced breast cancer: results of a phase III study of the International Letrozole Breast Cancer Group. *J Clin Oncol.* 2001;19:2596-2606.

66. Nabholtz JM, Buzdar A, Pollak M, et al. Anastrozole is superior to tamoxifen as first-line therapy for advanced breast cancer in postmenopausal women: results of a North American multicenter randomized trial. Arimidex Study Group. *J Clin Oncol.* 2000;18:3758-3767.

67. The ATAC Trialists' Group. Anastrozole alone or in combination with tamoxifen versus tamoxifen alone for adjuvant treatment of postmenopausal women with early breast cancer: first results of the ATAC randomised trial. *Lancet.* 2002;359:2131-2139.

68. Julian T, Land S, Wolmark N. NSABP B-35: A clinical trial to compare anastrazole and tamoxifen for postmenopausal patients with ductal carcinoma in situ undergoing lumpectomy with radiation therapy. *Breast Dis Yearbook Q.* 2003;14:121-122.

69. Allred DC, Clark GM, Tandon AK, et al. HER-2/neu in node-negative breast cancer: prognostic significance of overexpression influenced by the presence of in situ carcinoma. *J Clin Oncol.* 1992;10:599-605.

70. van de Vijver MJ, Peterse JL, Mooi WJ, et al. Neu-protein overexpression in breast cancer. Association with comedo-type ductal carcinoma in situ and limited prognostic value in stage II breast cancer. *N Engl J Med.* 1988;319:1239-1245.

71. Claus EB, Chu P, Howe CL, et al. Pathobiologic findings in DCIS of the breast: morphologic features, angiogenesis, HER-2/neu and hormone receptors. *Exp Mol Pathol.* 2001;70:303-316.

72. Liang K, Lu Y, Jin W, et al. Sensitization of breast cancer cells to radiation by trastuzumab. *Mol Cancer Ther.* 2003;2.1113-1120.

73. Romond EH, Perez EA, Bryant J, et al. Trastuzumab plus adjuvant chemotherapy for operable HER2-positive breast cancer. *N Engl J Med.* 2005;353:1673-1684.

74. Slamon D, Eiermann W, Robert N, et al. Phase III randomized trial comparing doxorubicin and cylophosphamide followed by docetaxel (AC T) with doxorubacin and cyclophosphamide followed by docetaxel and trastuzumab (AC TH) with docetaxel, carboplatin and trastuzumab (TCH) in HER2 positive early breast cancer patients: BCIRG 006 study. *Breast Cancer Res Treat.* 2005;94:S5. Abstract 1.

75. Fisher B, Jeong JH, Dignam J, et al. Findings from recent National Surgical Adjuvant Breast and Bowel Project adjuvant studies in stage I breast cancer. *J Natl Cancer Inst Monogr.* 2001(30);62-66.

76. Fisher B, Redmond C, Dimitrov NV, et al. A randomized clinical trial evaluating sequential methotrexate and fluorouracil in the treatment of patients with node-negative breast cancer who have estrogen-receptor-negative tumors. *N Engl J Med.* 1989;320:473-478.

77. Fisher B, Dignam J, Mamounas EP, et al. Sequential methotrexate and fluorouracil for the treatment of node-negative breast cancer patients with estrogen receptor-negative tumors: eight-year results from National Surgical Adjuvant Breast and Bowel Project (NSABP) B-13 and first report of findings from NSABP B-19 comparing methotrexate and fluorouracil with conventional cyclophosphamide, methotrexate, and fluorouracil. *J Clin Oncol.* 1996;14:1982-1992.

78. Controlled trial of tamoxifen as single adjuvant agent in management of early breast cancer. Analysis at six years by Nolvadex Adjuvant Trial Organisation. *Lancet.* 1085;1:836-840.

79. Breast Cancer Trials Committee. Adjuvant tamoxifen in the management of operable breast cancer: the Scottish Trial. Report from the Breast Cancer Trials Committee, Scottish Cancer Trials Office (MRC), Edinburgh. *Lancet.* 1987;2:171-175.

80. Baum M, Brinkley DM, Dossett JA, et al. Improved survival among patients treated with adjuvant tamoxifen after mastectomy for early breast cancer. *Lancet.* 1983;2:450.

81. Bartlett K, Eremin O, Hutcheon A, et al. Adjuvant tamoxifen in the management of operable breast cancer: the Scottish Trial. Report from the Breast Cancer Trials Committee, Scottish Cancer Trials Office (MRC), Edinburgh. *Lancet.* 1987;2:171-175.

82. Fisher B, Anderson S, Tan-Chiu E, et al. Tamoxifen and chemotherapy for axillary node-negative, estrogen receptor-negative breast cancer: findings from National Surgical Adjuvant Breast and Bowel Project B-23. *J Clin Oncol.* 2001;19:931-942.

83. Swain S, Wilson J, Mamounas E, et al. Estrogen receptor (ER) status of primary breast cancer is predictive of ER status of contralateral breast cancer (CBC). *Proc Am Soc Clin Oncol.* 2002;21:38a. Abstract 150.

84. Levine MN, Bramwell VH, Pritchard KI, et al. Randomized trial of intensive cyclophosphamide, epirubicin, and fluorouracil chemotherapy compared with cyclophosphamide, methotrexate, and fluorouracil in premenopausal women with node-positive breast cancer. National Cancer Institute of Canada Clinical Trials Group. *J Clin Oncol.* 1998;16:2651-2658.

85. Levine MN, Pritchard KI, Bramwell VHC, et al. Randomized trial comparing cyclophosphamide, epirubicin, and fluorouracil with cyclophosphamide, methotrexate, and fluorouracil in premenopausal women with node-positive breast cancer: Update of National Cancer Institute of Canada Clinical Trials Group Trial MA5. *J Clin Oncol.* 2005;23:5166-5170.

86. Hutchins LF, Green SJ, Ravdin PM, et al. Randomized, controlled trial of cyclophosphamide, methotrexate, and fluorouracil versus cyclophosphamide, doxorubicin, and fluorouracil with and without tamoxifen for high-risk, node-negative breast cancer: treatment results of Intergroup Protocol INT-0102. *J Clin Oncol.* 2005;23:8313-8321.

87. Early Breast Cancer Trialists' Collaborative Group. Polychemotherapy for early breast cancer: an overview of the randomised trials. *Lancet.* 1998;352:930-942.

88. French Adjuvant Study Group. Benefit of a high-dose epirubicin regimen in adjuvant chemotherapy for node-positive breast cancer patients with poor prognostic factors: 5-year follow-up results of French Adjuvant Study Group 05 randomized trial. *J Clin Oncol.* 2001;19:602-611.

89. National Institutes of Health. Adjuvant Therapy for Breast Cancer. *NIH Consensus Statement.* 2000;17(4)1-35.

90. Fisher B, Jeong JH, Bryant J, et al. Treatment of lymph-node-negative, oestrogen-receptor-positive breast cancer: long-term findings from National Surgical Adjuvant Breast and Bowel Project randomised clinical trials. *Lancet.* 2004;364:858-868.

91. Fisher B, Dignam J, Bryant J, et al. Five versus more than five years of tamoxifen for lymph node-negative breast cancer: updated findings from the National Surgical Adjuvant Breast and Bowel Project B-14 randomized trial. *J Natl Cancer Inst.* 2001;93:684-690.

92. Fisher B, Dignam J, Wolmark N, et al. Tamoxifen and chemotherapy for lymph node-negative, estrogen receptor-positive breast cancer. *J Natl Cancer Inst.* 1997;89:1673-1682.

93. Paik S, Shak S, Tang G, et al. A multigene assay to predict recurrence of tamoxifen-treated, node-negative breast cancer. *N Engl J Med.* 2004;351:2817-2826.

94. Paik S, Shak S, Tang G, et al. Expression of the 21 genes in the Recurrence Score assay and tamoxifen clinical benefit in the NSABP study B-14 of node negative, estrogen receptor positive breast cancer. *J Clin Oncol.* 2005;23:6s. Abstract 510.

95. Saphner T, Tormey DC, Gray R. Annual hazard rates of recurrence for breast cancer after primary therapy. *J Clin Oncol.* 1996;14:2738-2746.

96. Mamounas EP. Adjuvant exemestane therapy after 5 years of tamoxifen: rationale for the NSABP B-33 trial. *Oncology (Huntingt).* 2001;15:35-39.

97. Goss PE, Ingle JN, Martino S, et al. A randomized trial of letrozole in postmenopausal women after five years of tamoxifen therapy for earlystage breast cancer. *N Engl J Med.* 2003;349:1793-1802.

98. Mamounas EP, Jeong JH, Wickerham DL, et al. Benefit from exemestane as extended adjuvant therapy after 5 years of adjuvant tamoxifen: intention-to-treat analysis of the National Surgical Adjuvant Breast and Bowel Project B-33 Trial. *J Clin Oncol.* 2008.

99. Mamounas EP, Lembersky B, Jeong JH, et al. NSABP B-42: a clinical trial to determine the efficacy of five years of letrozole compared with placebo in patients completing five years of hormonal therapy consisting of an aromatase inhibitor (AI) or tamoxifen followed by an AI in prolonging disease-free survival in postmenopausal women with hormone receptor-positive breast cancer. *Clin Breast Cancer.* 2006;7:416-421.

100. Gianni L, Munzone E, Capri G, et al. Paclitaxel by 3-hour infusion in combination with bolus doxorubicin in women with untreated metastatic breast cancer: high antitumor efficacy and cardiac effects in a dose-finding and sequence-finding study. *J Clin Oncol.* 1995;13:2688-2699.

101. Gehl J, Boesgaard M, Paaske T, et al. Combined doxorubicin and paclitaxel in advanced breast cancer: effective and cardiotoxic. *Ann Oncol.* 1996;7:687-693.

102. Dieras V. Docetaxel in combination with doxorubicin: a phase I dose-finding study. *Oncology (Huntingt).* 1997;11:17-20.

103. Misset JL, Dieras V, Gruia G, et al. Dose-finding study of docetaxel and doxorubicin in first-line treatment of patients with metastatic breast cancer. *Ann Oncol.* 1999;10:553-560.

104. Nabholtz JM, Mackey JR, Smylie M, et al. Phase II study of docetaxel, doxorubicin, and cyclophosphamide as first-line chemotherapy for metastatic breast cancer. *J Clin Oncol.* 2001;19:314-321.

105. Sparano JA, O'Neill A, Schaefer PL, et al. Phase II trial of doxorubicin and docetaxel plus granulocyte colony-stimulating factor in metastatic breast cancer: Eastern Cooperative Oncology Group Study E1196. *J Clin Oncol.* 2000;18:2369-2377.

106. Nabholtz JM, Falkson CI, Campos D. Doxorubicin and docetaxel (AT) is superior to standard doxorubicin and cyclophosphamide (AC) as 1st line CT for MBC: randomized phase III trial. *Breast Cancer Res Treat.* 1999;57:84. Abstract 485.

107. Mackey JR, Paterson A, Dirix LY, et al. Final results of the phase III randomized trial comparing doxetaxel (T), doxorubicin (A) and cyclophosphamide (C) to FAC as first line chemotherapy (CT) for patients (pts) with metastatic breast cancer (MBC). *Proc Am Soc Clin Oncol.* 2002;21:35a. Abstract 137.

108. Swain SM, Jeong J-H, Geyer CE, et al. NSABP B-30: definitive analysis of patient outcome from a randomized trial evaluating different schedules and combinations of adjuvant therapy containing doxorubicin, docetaxel and cyclophosphamide in women with operable, node-positive breast cancer. *SABCS.* 2008; HYPERLINK "http://www.abstracts2view.com/sabcs/view.php?nu=SABCS08L_1017&terms=" \t "_blank" Abstract 75.

109. Citron ML, Berry DA, Cirrincione C, et al. Randomized trial of dose-dense versus conventionally scheduled and sequential versus concurrent combination chemotherapy as postoperative adjuvant treatment of node-positive primary breast cancer: first report of Intergroup Trial C9741/Cancer and Leukemia Group B Trial 9741. *J Clin Oncol.* 2003;21:1431-1439.

110. Nabholtz JM, Pienkowski T, Mackey M, et al. Phase III trial comparing FAC (5-fluorouracil, doxorubicin, cyclophosphamide) with TAC (docetaxel, doxorubicin, cyclophosphamide) in the adjuvant treatment of node positive breast (BC) patients: interim analysis of the BCIRG 001 study. *Proc Am Soc Clin Oncol.* 2002;21:36a. Abstract 141.

111. Martin M, Pienkowski T, Mackey J, et al. Adjuvant docetaxel for node-positive breast cancer. *N Engl J Med.* 2005;352:2302-2313.

112. Blackstein M, Vogel CL, Ambinder R, et al. Gemcitabine as first-line therapy in patients with metastatic breast cancer: a phase II trial. *Oncology.* 2002;62:2-8.

113. Carmichael J, Possinger K, Phillip P, et al. Advanced breast cancer: a phase II trial with gemcitabine. *J Clin Oncol.* 1995;13:2731-2736.

114. Spielmann M, Llombart-Cussac A, Kalla S, et al. Single-agent gemcitabine is active in previously treated metastatic breast cancer. *Oncology.* 2001;60:303-307.

115. Brodowicz T, Kostler W, Moslinger R, et al. Single-agent gemcitabine as second and third-line treatment in metastatic breast cancer. *Breast.* 2000;9:338-342.

116. Murad AM, Guimaraes RC, Aragao BC, et al. Phase II trial of the use of paclitaxel and gemcitabine as a salvage treatment in metastatic breast cancer. *Am J Clin Oncol.* 2001;24:264-268.

117. O'Shaughnessy J, Nag S, Calderillo-Ruiz G, et al. Gemcitabine plus paclitaxel (GT) versus paclitaxel (T) as first-line treatment for anthracycline pre-treated metastatic breast cancer (MBC): Interim results of a global phase III study. *Proc Am Soc Clin Oncol.* 2003;22:7. Abstract 25.

118. Albain KS, Nag S, Calderillo Ruiz GC, et al. Global phase III study of gemcitabine plus paclitaxel (GT) vs paclitaxel (T) as frontline therapy for metastatic breast cancer (MBC): first report of overall survival. *Proc Am Soc Clin Oncol.* 2004;23:5. Abstract 510.

119. Mamounas EP, Geyer CE Jr., Swain SM. Rationale and clinical trial design for evaluating gemcitabine as neoadjuvant and adjuvant therapy for breast cancer. *Clin Breast Cancer.* 2004;4(suppl):S121-S126.

120. Thor AD, Berry DA, Budman DR, et al. erbB-2, p53, and efficacy of adjuvant therapy in lymph node-positive breast cancer. *J Natl Cancer Inst.* 1998;90:1346-1360.

121. Paik S, Bryant J, Park C, et al. erbB-2 and response to doxorubicin in patients with axillary lymph node-positive, hormone receptor-negative breast cancer. *J Natl Cancer Inst.* 1998;90:1361-1370.

122. Paik S, Bryant J, Tan-Chiu E, et al. HER2 and choice of adjuvant chemotherapy for invasive breast cancer: National Surgical Adjuvant Breast and Bowel Project Protocol B-15. *J Natl Cancer Inst.* 2000;92:1991-1998.

123. Ravdin PM, Green S, Albain KS, et al. Initial report of the SWOG biological correlative study of c-erb-2 expression as a predictor of outcome in a trial comparing adjuvant CAF T with tamoxifen (T) alone. *Proc Am Soc Clin Oncol.* 1998;17.

124. Cobleigh MA, Vogel CL, Tripathy D, et al. Efficacy and safety of Herceptin (humanized anti-Her2 antibody) as a single agent in 222 women with Her2 overexpression who relapsed following chemotherapy for metastatic breast cancer. *Proc Am Soc Clin Oncol.* 1998;17:97a. Abstract.

125. Slamon DJ, Leyland-Jones B, Shak S, et al. Use of chemotherapy plus a monoclonal antibody against HER2 for metastatic breast cancer that overexpresses HER2. *N Engl J Med.* 2001;344:783-792.

126. Tan-Chiu E, Yothers G, Romond E, et al. Assessment of cardiac dysfunction in a randomized trial comparing doxorubicin and cyclophosphamide followed by paclitaxel, with or without trastuzumab as adjuvant therapy in node-positive, human epidermal growth factor receptor 2-overexpressing breast cancer: NSABP B-31. *J Clin Oncol.* 2005;23:7811-7819.

127. Perez EA, Romond E, Suman VJ, et al. Updated results of the combined analysis of NCCTG N9831 and NSABP B-31 adjuvant chemotherapy with/without trastuzumab in patients with HER2-positive breast cancer. *Proc Am Soc Clin Oncol.* 25;2007. Abstract 512.

128. Folkman J. Tumor angiogenesis: therapeutic implications. *N Engl J Med.* 1971;285:1182-1186.

129. Folkman J. What is the evidence that tumors are angiogenesis dependent? *J Natl Cancer Inst.* 1990;82:4-6.

130. Yancopoulos GD, Davis S, Gale NW, et al. Vascular-specific growth factors and blood vessel formation. *Nature.* 2000;407:242-248.

131. Carmeliet P, Jain RK. Angiogenesis in cancer and other diseases. *Nature.* 2000;407:249-257.

132. Carmeliet P, Ferreira V, Breier G, et al. Abnormal blood vessel development and lethality in embryos lacking a single VEGF allele. *Nature.* 1996;380:435-439.

133. Ferrara N, Carver-Moore K, Chen H, et al. Heterozygous embryonic lethality induced by targeted inactivation of the VEGF gene. *Nature.* 1996;380:439-442.

134. Gasparini G. Prognostic value of vascular endothelial growth factor in breast cancer. *Oncologist.* 2000;5(suppl):37-44.

135. Shen GH, Ghazizadeh M, Kawanami O, et al. Prognostic significance of vascular endothelial growth factor expression in human ovarian carcinoma. *Br J Cancer.* 2000;83:196-203.

136. Potgens AJ, Lubsen NH, van Altena MC, et al. Vascular permeability factor expression influences tumor angiogenesis in human melanoma lines xenografted to nude mice. *Am J Pathol.* 1995;146:197-209.

137. Aonuma M, Saeki Y, Akimoto T, et al. Vascular endothelial growth factor overproduced by tumor cells acts predominantly as a potent angiogenic factor contributing to malignant progression. *Int J Exp Pathol.* 1999;80:271-281.

138. Grugel S, Finkenzeller G, Weindel K, et al. Both v-Ha-Ras and v-Raf stimulate expression of the vascular endothelial growth factor in NIH 3T3 cells. *J Biol Chem.* 1995;270:25915-25919.

139. Konecny GE, Meng YG, Untch M, et al. Association between HER-2/neu and vascular endothelial growth factor expression predicts clinical outcome in primary breast cancer patients. *Clin Cancer Res.* 2004;10:1706-1716.

140. Pegram MD, O'Callaghan C. Combining the anti-HER2 antibody trastuzumab with taxanes in breast cancer: results and trial considerations. *Clin Breast Cancer.* 2001;2(suppl):S15-S19.

141. Kanis JA, McCloskey EV, Powles T, et al. A high incidence of vertebral fracture in women with breast cancer. *Br J Cancer.* 1999;79:1179-1181.

142. Diel IJ, Solomayer EF, Costa SD, et al. Reduction in new metastases in breast cancer with adjuvant clodronate treatment. *N Engl J Med.* 1998;339:357-363.

143. Powles T, Paterson S, Kanis JA, et al. Randomized, placebo-controlled trial of clodronate in patients with primary operable breast cancer. *J Clin Oncol.* 2002;20:3219-3224.

144. Saarto T, Blomqvist C, Virkkunen P, et al. Adjuvant clodronate treatment does not reduce the frequency of skeletal metastases in node-positive breast cancer patients: 5-year results of a randomized controlled trial. *J Clin Oncol.* 2001;19:10-17.

145. Gralow J. Evolving role of bisphosphonates in women undergoing treatment for localized and advanced breast cancer. *Clin Breast Cancer.* 2005;5(suppl) S54-S62.

146. Gnant M, Mlineritsch B, Schippinger W, et al. Adjuvant ovarian suppression combined with tamoxifen or anastrozole, alone or in combination with zoledronic acid, in premenopausal women with hormone-responsive, stage I and II breast cancer: first efficacy results from ABCSG-12. *Proc Am Soc Clin Oncol.* 2008;26, May 20 Supp.

147. Skipper HE. Kinetics of mammary tumor cell growth and implications for therapy. *Cancer.* 1971;28:1479-1499.

148. Goldie JH, Coldman AJ. A mathematic model for relating the drug sensitivity of tumors to their spontaneous mutation rate. *Cancer Treat Rep.* 1979;63:1727-1733.

149. Gunduz N, Fisher B, Saffer EA. Effect of surgical removal on the growth and kinetics of residual tumor. *Cancer Res.* 1979;39:3861-3865.

150. Fisher B, Gunduz N, Saffer EA. Influence of the interval between primary tumor removal and chemotherapy on kinetics and growth of metastases. *Cancer Res.* 1983;43:1488-1492.

151. Fisher B, Rockette H, Robidoux A, et al. Effect of preoperative therapy for breast cancer (BC) on local-regional disease: first report of NSABP B-18. *Proc Am Soc Clin Oncol.* 1994;13:64. Abstract 57.

152. Fisher B, Brown A, Mamounas E, et al. Effect of preoperative chemotherapy on local-regional disease in women with operable breast cancer: findings from National Surgical Adjuvant Breast and Bowel Project B-18. *J Clin Oncol.* 1997;15:2483-2493.

153. Fisher B, Bryant J, Wolmark N, et al. Effect of preoperative chemotherapy on the outcome of women with operable breast cancer. *J Clin Oncol.* 1998;16:2672-2685.

154. Wolmark N, Wang J, Mamounas E, et al. Preoperative chemotherapy in patients with operable breast cancer: nine-year results from National Surgical Adjuvant Breast and Bowel Project B-18. *J Natl Cancer Inst Monogr.* 2001(30);96-102.

155. Rastogi P, Anderson SJ, Bear HD, et al. Preoperative chemotherapy: updates of National Surgical Adjuvant Breast and Bowel Project Protocols B-18 and B-27. *J Clin Oncol.* 2008;26:778-785.

156. Fisher B, Mamounas EP. Preoperative chemotherapy: a model for studying the biology and therapy of primary breast cancer. *J Clin Oncol.* 1995;13:537-540.

157. Mamounas EP. NSABP Protocol B-27. Preoperative doxorubicin plus cyclophosphamide followed by preoperative or postoperative docetaxel. *Oncology (Huntingt).* 1997;11:37-40.

158. Mamounas EP, Brown A, Anderson S, et al. Sentinel node biopsy after neoadjuvant chemotherapy in breast cancer: results from National Surgical Adjuvant Breast and Bowel Project Protocol B-27. *J Clin Oncol.* 2005;23:2694-2702.

159. Sawada N, Ishikawa T, Fukase Y, et al. Induction of thymidine phosphorylase activity and enhancement of capecitabine efficacy by taxol/taxotere in human cancer xenografts. *Clin Cancer Res.* 1998;4:1013-1019.

160. Kurosumi M, Tabei T, Suemasu K, et al. Enhancement of immunohistochemical reactivity for thymidine phosphorylase in breast carcinoma cells after administration of docetaxel as a neoadjuvant chemotherapy in advanced breast cancer patients. *Oncol Rep.* 2000;7:945-948.

161. O'Shaughnessy J, Miles D, Vukelja S, et al. Superior survival with capecitabine plus docetaxel combination therapy in anthracycline-pretreated patients with advanced breast cancer: phase III trial results. *J Clin Oncol.* 2002;20:2812-2823.

162. Possinger K, Kaufmann M, Coleman R, et al. Phase II study of gemcitabine as first-line chemotherapy in patients with advanced or metastatic breast cancer. *Anticancer Drugs.* 1999;10:155-162.

163. Kroep JR, Giaccone G, Voorn DA, et al. Gemcitabine and paclitaxel: pharmacokinetic and pharmacodynamic interactions in patients with non-small-cell lung cancer. *J Clin Oncol.* 1999;17:2190-2197.

164. Chan S, Romieu G, Huober J, et al. Gemcitabine plus docetaxel (GD) versus capecitabine plus docetaxel (CD) for anthracycline-pretreated metastatic breast cancer (MBC) patients (pts). *J Clin Oncol.* 2005;ASCO Ann Meet Proc.23(165),Part I of II, June 1 Supp.

165. Ferrara N, Davis-Smyth T. The biology of vascular endothelial growth factor. *Endocr Rev.* 1997;18:4-25.

166. Cobleigh MA, Langmuir VK, Sledge GW, et al. A phase I/II dose-escalation trial of bevacizumab in previously treated metastatic breast cancer. *Semin Oncol.* 2003;30:117-124.

167. Miller KD, Chap LI, Holmes FA, et al. Randomized phase III trial of capecitabine compared with bevacizumab plus capecitabine in patients with previously treated metastatic breast cancer. *J Clin Oncol.* 2005;23:792-799.

168. Miller MD, Wang M, Gralow J, et al. A randomized phase III trial of paclitaxel versus paclitaxel plus bevacizumab as first-line therapy for locally recurrent or metastatic breast cancer: a trial coordinated by the Eastern Cooperative Group (E2100). *Br Ca Res Treat.* 2005;94.S6. Abstract 3.

169. Rusnak DW, Lackey K, Affleck K, et al. The effects of the novel, reversible epidermal growth factor receptor/ErbB-2 tyrosine kinase inhibitor, GW2016, on the growth of human normal and tumor-derived cell lines in vitro and in vivo. *Mol Cancer Ther.* 2001;1:85-94.

170. Konecny GE, Pegram MD, Venkatesan N, et al. Activity of the dual kinase inhibitor lapatinib (GW572016) against HER-2-overexpressing and trastuzumab-treated breast cancer cells. *Cancer Res.* 2006;66:1630-1639.

171. Burris HA, 3rd, Hurwitz HI, Dees EC, et al. Phase I safety, pharmacokinetics, and clinical activity study of lapatinib (GW572016), a reversible dual inhibitor of epidermal growth factor receptor tyrosine kinases, in heavily pretreated patients with metastatic carcinomas. *J Clin Oncol.* 2005;23:5305-5313.

172. Geyer CE, Forster J, Lindquist D, et al. Lapatinib plus capecitabine for HER2-positive advanced breast cancer. *N Engl J Med.* 2006;355:2733-2743.

173. Di Leo A, Gomez H, Aziz Z, et al. Lapatinib (L) with paclitaxel compared to paclitaxel as first-line treatment for patients with metastatic breast cancer: A phase III randomized, double-blind study of 580 patients. *J Clin Oncol.* 2007; ASCO Ann Meet Proc. 23(165),1(25), June 20 Supp.

174. Gianni L, Baselga J, Eiermann W, et al. European Cooperative Trial in Operable Breast Cancer (ECTO): improved freedom from progression (FFP) from adding paclitaxel (T) to doxorubicin (A) followed by cyclophosphamide methotrexate and fluorouracil (CMF). *J Clin Oncol.* 2005;23:7s. Abstract 513.

175. Kuerer HM, Newman LA, Smith TL, et al. Clinical course of breast cancer patients with complete pathologic primary tumor and axillary lymph node response to doxorubicin-based neoadjuvant chemotherapy. *J Clin Oncol.* 1999;17:460-469.

176. Heys SD, Hutcheon AW, Sarkar TK, et al. Neoadjuvant docetaxel in breast cancer: 3-year survival results from the Aberdeen trial. *Clin Breast Cancer.* 2002;3(suppl):S69-S74.

177. von Minckwitz G, Blohmer JU, Loehr A, et al. Comparison of docetaxel/doxorubicin/cyclophosphamide (TAC) versus vinorelbine/capecitabine (NX) in patients non-responding to 2 cycles of neoadjuvant TAC chemotherapy—first results of the phase III GEPARTRIO-study by the German Breast Group. *Br Ca Res Treat.* 2005;94:S19. Abstract 38.

178. Fisher B, Costantino JP, Wickerham DL, et al. Tamoxifen for the prevention of breast cancer: current status of the National Surgical Adjuvant Breast and Bowel Project P-1 study. *J Natl Cancer Inst.* 2005;97:1652-1662.

179. IBIS Investigators. First results from the International Breast Cancer Intervention Study (IBIS-I): a randomised prevention trial. *Lancet.* 360:817-24, 2002.

180. Veronesi U, Maisonneuve P, Rotmensz N, et al. Italian randomized trial among women with hysterectomy: tamoxifen and hormone-dependent breast cancer in high-risk women. *J Natl Cancer Inst.* 2003;95:160-165.

181. Cuzick J, Powles T, Veronesi U, et al. Overview of the main outcomes in breast-cancer prevention trials. *Lancet.* 2003;361:296-300.

182. Cummings SR, Eckert S, Krueger KA, et al. The effect of raloxifene on risk of breast cancer in postmenopausal women: results from the MORE randomized trial. Multiple Outcomes of Raloxifene Evaluation. *JAMA.* 1999;281:2189-2197.

183. Vogel VG, Costantino JP, Wickerham DL, et al. Effects of tamoxifen vs raloxifene on the risk of developing invasive breast cancer and other disease outcomes: the NSABP Study of Tamoxifen and Raloxifene (STAR) P-2 trial. *JAMA.* 2006;295:2727-2741.

184. Land SR, Wickerham DL, Costantino JP, et al. Patient-reported symptoms and quality of life during treatment with tamoxifen or raloxifene for breast cancer prevention: the NSABP Study of Tamoxifen and Raloxifene (STAR) P-2 trial. *JAMA.* 2006;295:2742-2751.

185. Costantino JP, Gail MH, Pee D, et al. Validation studies for models projecting the risk of invasive and total breast cancer incidence. *J Natl Cancer Inst.* 1999;91:1541-1548.

186. Singletary SE. Minimally invasive surgery in breast cancer treatment. *Biomed Pharmacother.* 2001;55:510-514.

187. Sabel MS, Kaufman CS, Whitworth P, et al. Cryoablation of early-stage breast cancer: work-in-progress report of a multi-institutional trial. *Ann Surg Oncol.* 2004;11:542-549.

188. Orel SG, Weinstein SP, Schnall MD, et al. Breast MR imaging in patients with axillary node metastases and unknown primary malignancy. *Radiology.* 1999;212:543-549.

189. Henry-Tillman RS, Harms SE, Westbrook KC, et al. Role of breast magnetic resonance imaging in determining breast as a source of unknown metastatic lymphadenopathy. *Am J Surg* 1999;178:496-500.

190. Baker DR. Magnetic resonance imaging of occult breast cancer. *Clin Breast Cancer.* 2000;1:66-67.

191. Aryus B, Audretsch W, Gogolin F, et al. Remission rates following preoperative chemotherapy and radiation therapy in patients with breast cancer. *Strahlenther Onkol.* 2000;176:411-415.

192. Gerlach B, Audretsch W, Gogolin F, et al. Remission rates in breast cancer treated with preoperative chemotherapy and radiotherapy. *Strahlenther Onkol.* 2003;179:306-311.

193. Jacquillat C, Weil M, Baillet F, et al. Results of neoadjuvant chemotherapy and radiation therapy in the breast-conserving treatment of 250 patients with all stages of infiltrative breast cancer. *Cancer.* 1990;66:119-129.

194. Mauriac L, MacGrogan G, Avril A, et al. Neoadjuvant chemotherapy for operable breast carcinoma larger than 3 cm: a unicentre randomized trial with a 124-month median follow-up. Institut Bergonie Bordeaux Groupe Sein (IBBGS). *Ann Oncol.* 1999;10:47-52.

195. Scholl SM, Fourquet A, Asselain B, et al. Neoadjuvant versus adjuvant chemotherapy in premenopausal patients with tumours considered too large for breast conserving surgery: preliminary results of a randomised trial: S6. *Eur J Cancer.* 1994;30A:645-652.

196. Pusztai L, Ayers M, Simman FW, et al. Emerging science: prospective validation of gene expression profiling-based prediction of complete pathologic response to neoadjuvant paclitaxel/FAC chemotherapy in breast cancer. *Proc Am Soc Clin Oncol.* 2003;22:1. Abstract 1.

197. Hurkmans CW, Borger JH, Rutgers EJ, et al. Quality assurance of axillary radiotherapy in the EORTC AMAROS trial 10981/22023: the dummy run. *Radiother Oncol.* 2003;68:233-240.

CHAPTER 43

The Milan Cancer Institute's Landmark Clinical Trials

Umberto Veronesi
Stefano Zurrida

A 100 years ago, breast cancer struck 1 woman in 20. Since then, breast cancer incidence has increased steadily, not only because diagnostic modalities have become more sensitive and women and physicians are more aware of the disease, but because risk factors for the disease have become more pervasive. These include proliferation of the Western-style diet with its high proportion of animal fats, earlier menarche, delayed menopause, delayed first pregnancy, and decline of breastfeeding. These factors mainly affect developed countries but are increasingly evident in emerging countries, where, unfortunately, locally advanced breast cancers are usually diagnosed. At the end of the last century, 1 woman in 10 contracted breast cancer; now the figure is 1 in 8 in developed countries.[1]

Notwithstanding this alarming increase in breast cancer incidence (3 million new cases a year worldwide), we have seen a decrease in mortality for the disease in developed countries, and treatments have become much less aggressive, placing greater emphasis on the patient's quality of life.[2]

Italy, and the city of Milan with its 2 distinguished Cancer Institutes, has been at the forefront of breast cancer treatment and research for many years. The first pivotal clinical trials on less aggressive surgical approaches to the disease, which had a worldwide impact, were performed in the city. These trials marked the beginning of the shift in paradigm from maximum tolerated treatment to minimum effective treatment; from aggressive surgery and radiotherapy to targeted conservative treatments; from an anatomic concept of cancer spread toward a biologic concept. Today, breast cancer treatments are much more tolerable, personalized, and effective, encouraging women to present early for breast cancer screening so that the disease is diagnosed earlier and treatments are safer. More recently, the Milan Institutes have carried out important research in pharmacoprevention, results of which are now applied to populations of women most exposed to breast cancer risk factors.

This chapter traces the history of the landmark studies on breast cancer carried out in Milan over the last 40 years. These studies were initiated in the 1970s by our team at the National Cancer Institute and have continued at the European Institute of Oncology (Italian: Istituto Europeo di Oncologia [IEO]) of Milan.

THE HALSTED MASTECTOMY

Up to the end of the 19th century, breast cancer was considered invariably fatal. However, the American surgeon W.S. Halsted became convinced that breast cancer spread by direct extension into muscle and skin and through lymphatic ducts to regional lymph nodes, which held the cancer cells in check prior to widespread dissemination. If this were true, it meant that breast cancer was a mainly locoregional disease that could be cured definitively by timely and radical surgery.

In 1898, Halsted presented 76 mastectomized cases to the American Surgical Association[3] illustrating his thesis that breast cancer could be cured. Thereafter, radical mastectomy became the accepted treatment for breast cancer. In fact, in Western countries up to the 1970s, the Halsted mastectomy was the standard treatment even for small breast cancers. And although it undoubtedly saved the lives of many women, the treatment left an ugly scar, a depression beneath the clavicle, protruding ribs, and often required a skin graft.

TOWARD LESS AGGRESSIVE SURGERY

Two currents of thought developed slowly from Halsted's ideas. The first sought to convince ordinary people and physicians that if diagnosed early, breast cancer was curable; it implied the development of means to diagnose early disease and also wide dissemination of the message that early diagnosis was vital.

The second current of thought has been concerned with reducing the extent of surgical and subsequent treatment, and emerged as understanding of the natural history of breast cancer increased and the mode of its initial presentation changed. At the beginning of the century, breast cancer was usually diagnosed when locally advanced: when the mass was often large and the skin was involved and sometimes ulcerated. Today, small palpable lesions are the normal presentation, and thanks to mammography and other imaging techniques, preclinical nonpalpable lesions are increasingly identified.

As with many types of malignant tumor, surgeons became interested in the use of conservative surgery to treat small-size breast cancers in the 1970s. At that time, the disease came to be viewed as one generally involving only part of the breast and not necessarily affecting the whole gland.

THE GUY'S HOSPITAL STUDY

The first sporadic attempts to preserve the breast in an aesthetically acceptable way took place in the 1920s. Joseph Hirsch, a Frankfurt gynecologist, was probably the first to treat a substantial series of patients by simple breast resection followed by interstitial radiotherapy with encouraging results.[4] Numerous small-scale studies using limited surgery, and more extensive trials with radiotherapy, sought to find a substitute for the Halsted mastectomy. And although the overall trend of the results was encouraging, little notice was taken because the era of evidence-based medicine was at hand, and only a controlled, randomized study could provide convincing evidence as to whether conservative surgery could achieve an acceptable cure rate for breast cancer.

By the 1960s, it had become clear that very aggressive surgical and radiotherapeutic approaches (dissection of the internal mammary lymph nodes and high-dose radiotherapy to regional lymph nodes) were not effective. The first randomized controlled study of breast-conserving treatment was conducted at Guy's Hospital in the 1960s and early 1970s.[5] It compared the Halsted mastectomy plus radiotherapy at 32 Gy to the regional lymph nodes with a wide resection of the tumor followed by radiotherapy to the breast and supraclavicular, axillary, and internal mammary lymph nodes, again at the dose of 32 Gy. The results, published in 1972, revealed that the percentage of local recurrences was much higher in the group treated conservatively. However, almost 20% of these recurrences were in the axilla, whereas such recurrences were rare in the mastectomized group—as expected because the Halsted operation includes removal of all axillary lymph nodes. Initial results also indicated that survival was significantly inferior among the women treated by the conservative approach. However a long-term survival analysis, conducted later, showed that only in women with T1 tumors was the Halsted mastectomy superior to breast conservation.[6] This finding suggests that in most patients with tumor larger than 2 cm, occult metastases are already present in other body areas, so that the extent of local treatment in this group has little influence on long-term outcome. By contrast, for small tumors that were more often confined to the breast, the more radical local surgery was more likely to affect a cure.

An important aspect of the Guy's study is that the conservative treatment adopted would not be considered adequate today. First, because axillary dissection was not performed, even when there was clinical evidence of metastatic involvement, and second, because the radiotherapy dose (32 Gy) was too low to eradicate any residual local disease.

THE MILAN I, II, AND III TRIALS

The results of the Guy's study were not encouraging for breast conservation, and when, in 1968 we proposed a randomized trial study to compare Halsted mastectomy with a new conservative approach, the World Health Organization (WHO) Expert Committee in Geneva rejected our proposal. Fortunately, my perseverance and conviction that breast conservation should be further investigated won through against opposition, and the study was accepted by the WHO Committee in December 1969. The novelty of our approach was that the conservation procedure aimed to the radical, that is, to achieve effective locoregional control of the disease. It consisted of a wide local resection of the lesion (quadrantectomy), complete axillary dissection, and high-dose radiotherapy (50 Gy) to the breast (but not to the axilla) with an additional 10-Gy boost to the tumor bed. This treatment, called quadrantectomy plus axillary dissection and radiotherapy (QUART), was to prove so successful that it remains in widespread use today, although several modifications have evolved.

Following WHO approval, what was to be known as the Milan I trial began in 1973. Seven hundred and one patients with breast cancer were recruited. 349 were randomized to the standard treatment (Halsted mastectomy) and 352 were assigned to QUART. Eligible patients had infiltrating carcinoma up to 2 cm, without clinically suspect axillary lymph nodes (T1N0). Recruitment closed in 1980. The 2 groups of patients were closely comparable thanks to the strict randomization protocol. Patients were randomized in the operating room after excisional biopsy had confirmed the histology and size of the tumor. Patients were told of the 2 possible outcomes, breast removal or breast conservation, and only if they accepted these 2 possibilities were they admitted to the study. In the first 2 years, many patients refused to enter and specifically chose mastectomy, whereas in the final years of recruitment many patients refused mastectomy and were excluded because they chose quadrantectomy. Even among surgeons, attitudes changed over this period, and the scepticism that had been widespread gave way to enthusiasm as the initial results were published in the *New England Journal of Medicine* in 1981.[7]

The most recent analysis of the Milan I trial, after more than 20 years of follow-up[8] showed indistinguishable survival curves for the 2 study arms (Fig. 43-1). The latest data are that 28 of the patients (7.9%) treated conservatively and 8 (2.3%) in the Halsted group developed local recurrences. These events had no impact on survival.

The satisfyingly low rate of unfavorable events in the QUART group is in part attributable to the quality of the quadrantectomy operation. In developing this operation our aim had been to achieve secure local control. Earlier studies had

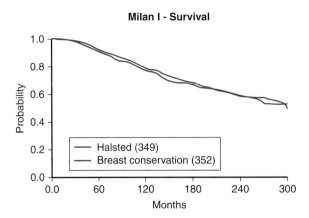

FIGURE 43-1 Long-term overall survival in the 2 arms of the Milan I trial.

indicated that intraductal spread was relatively frequent in breast cancer, and therefore it was necessary to excise the entire portion of the ductal tree (right up to the nipple) that was involved by the carcinoma. The ductal system of the breast is made up 10 to 15 relatively independent sets of branching ducts and lobules called lactiferous units, or mammary lobes. The term *quadrantectomy* seemed appropriate because the operation maintained the radicality that characterized mastectomy (removal of skin, subcutaneous tissue, gland, and fascia of the pectoralis muscle) but was limited to more or less 1 breast lobe. Furthermore, quadrantectomy indicates the position of the tumor to the surgeon.

Subsequent studies confirmed that local recurrence is often due to residual disease within the ductal system,[9] and Holland showed that invasive and in situ breast cancer was often limited to a single breast lobe and commented that breast cancer could be considered a "disease of the quadrant."[10]

Following analysis of the initial results of the Milan I trial, our group set about critically examining their experience. First, it was important to define a local failure. The practical attitude was adopted that any glandular, subcutaneous, or cutaneous lesion arising within 3 cm of the scar should be defined as local failure, and a neoplastic lesion within the same breast larger than 3 cm from the quadrantectomy or in a different breast quadrant was considered a second primary tumor. Next, it was important to determine whether the good results were mainly due to surgery or to radiotherapy. Thus we began a second randomized trial in 1985 to compare quadrantectomy with tumorectomy combined with complete axillary dissection and radiotherapy (TART). Tumorectomy removed the tumor mass with only a limited margin of surrounding tissue, so that the task of ensuring local control was entrusted mainly to radiotherapy (dose 46 Gy to the whole breast with 15 Gy to the tumor bed by interstitial ^{192}Ir). This second study (Milan II) concluded in December 1989, after recruiting 705 patients. Inclusion criteria were similar to those in Milan I except that tumor size could be up to 2.5 cm. As with Milan I, the comparability of the 2 groups was excellent. After 10 years of follow-up, the 2 groups differed significantly in terms of the frequency of local failures:

25 (9.3%) in the QUART group and 63 (23%) in the TART group, although overall survival was identical, again indicating that local failure is not a negative factor for survival. An additional finding of Milan II regarded the prognostic significance of the histopathologic entity known as extensive intraductal component (EIC). The presence of EIC was associated in both groups with increased risk of local failure; however, this risk was much higher in the TART than the QUART group. The reason for this was that when EIC was present, simple tumorectomy inevitably left residual local tumor. It was also shown that breast cancer with EIC is less radiosensitive. This finding had not emerged from the Milan I trial, in which only 3 local failures with EIC were observed, almost certainly because of the greater local extent of QUART. The conclusion of Milan II was that a wide resection such as quadrantectomy was necessary to reduce the risk of local failure to acceptable levels.[11]

But what of the role of radiotherapy within the QUART protocol? We started a new trial at the closure of Milan II designed to assess this. It was a randomized study that compared QUART with quadrantectomy plus axillary dissection *without* radiotherapy (QUAD). Five hundred and sixty-seven women were recruited between 1988 and 1989; 289 were randomized to QUART and 263 were randomized to QUAD.

The results showed a considerable difference in the rate of local failure between the 2 groups.[12] After a mean follow-up of 83 months, there were 50 local failures (19%) among QUAD women and 14 local failures (4.8%) in the QUART group. Another finding was that the local failure rate varied between pre- and postmenopausal patients. In patients less than 55 years of age, there were 41 of 167 local failures (24.5%), whereas in patients more than 55 years of age there were 11 of 160 local failures (10.3%). This may be explained by the fact that the postmenopausal breast atrophies: Adipose tissue predominates with remnant islands of fibroepithelial tissue while intraductal, lymphatic, and vascular connections—the natural pathways of tumor spread within the gland—are greatly reduced. It is therefore more likely that a simple but radical surgical excision will eradicate the disease without recourse to radiotherapy in postmenopausal women. The Milan III study also confirmed that the presence of EIC predicts local recurrence.[13,14] Overall survival did not differ between the 2 main study arms (Fig. 43-2).

PREOPERATIVE CHEMOTHERAPY

Although QUART proved to be a milestone in the treatment of breast cancer, both because it was the first conservative protocol to be scientifically validated and because it was a conservative treatment associated with a low incidence of local failure, new developments promised, on one hand, further reduction in the extent of surgery for breast cancer and, on the other, expansion of the indication for conservation to considerably larger tumors.

To expand the indication for conservation to large tumors, our idea was to employ neoadjuvant chemotherapy to reduce tumor size. The available data show that locally advanced breast cancer often responds well to neoadjuvant chemotherapy, so that breast conservation becomes possible in many of these women. Recent studies have shown that conservation is feasible

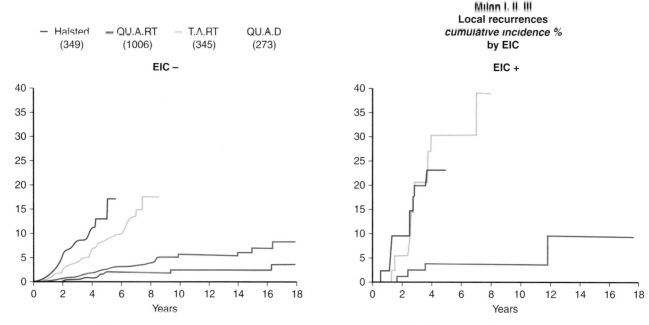

FIGURE 43-2 Cumulative incidence percentage of local recurrences by EIC status in the Milan I, II, and III trials.

after several cycles of preoperative chemotherapy in large-size breast cancer. In a study conducted by groups in Milan on 226 patients,[15] preoperative chemotherapy permitted conservative surgery in 90% of cases and did not depend on the chemotherapy regimen adopted. Nevertheless, this approach requires careful attention to several details. First, the extent of tumor regression must be carefully evaluated by the pathologist in the area of the involved breast. Second, microcalcifications, if present, must be identified prior to surgery and completely removed during the operation. Third, particular care must be taken with the cosmetic outcome, which, after all, is one reason why the patient undergoes the ordeal of primary chemotherapy. In rare cases the tumor does not respond to chemotherapy, and these must be identified quickly so mastectomy can be performed.

Endocrine-unresponsive disease and high proliferation rates (Ki67 expressed in 20% of tumor cells) are important predictors of complete pathologic response to 6 courses of primary chemotherapy. Disease-free survival is substantially longer for patients with endocrine-responsive disease than for patients who do not express steroid-hormone receptors, even though patients with endocrine-unresponsive disease are at least 4 times more likely to obtain a pathologic complete remission after primary chemotherapy.[16]

An important advantage of primary chemotherapy is that it probes the chemosensitivity of the tumor, providing information that is of great importance for further systemic treatments. The limiting factors of primary chemotherapy are (1) the fact that radical surgery must be postponed for 2 to 3 months while the tumor mass, although reduced in most cases, is still present and may contain actively proliferating cancer cells; (2) the biologic factors originally present in the primary carcinoma (estrogen receptor [ER], proliferation rate, grading, etc) may be modified by chemotherapy in an unpredictable way, sometimes

improving, sometimes worsening[17]; subsequently the disease may be understaged because chemotherapy alters these prognostic indices. To avoid understaging, sentinel node biopsy of the axilla may be performed before beginning chemotherapy.

AXILLARY DISSECTION AND SENTINEL NODE BIOPSY

Although axillary dissection was at one time an important staging procedure for breast cancer, patients were increasingly presenting with small carcinomas, and all too often axillary dissection revealed only healthy lymph nodes. Often too, axillary dissection was associated with postoperative sequelae such as chronic arm lymphedema, pain, and brachial plexopathy. We therefore turned our attention to the axilla, looking for ways to reduce axillary treatment. We studied the ability of sentinel node biopsy to predict axillary status and hence whether it was safe to forgo axillary dissection when the sentinel node was negative. After preliminary studies on radioactive dose and the best tracer substance to use to ensure migration within the lymphatic ducts but efficient retention by the lymph nodes, we recruited 376 consecutive breast cancer patients to a study in which we injected a small quantity of ^{99}Tc-labeled human albumin peritumorally. The next day, the sentinel node was identified and removed surgically (via a small incision) guided by the acoustic signals emitted by a handheld gamma ray–detecting probe. Total axillary dissection followed. The pathologic status of the sentinel node was compared with that of the whole axilla. A sentinel node was identified in 371 patients (98.7%) and correctly predicted the condition of the axilla in 359 (96.8%). Twelve false-negative cases were found among 203 negative sentinel nodes (6.7%).[18] Subsequently, the first major study in this area was conducted at the IEO. It randomized 516 patients and compared sentinel node biopsy plus immediate axillary dissection, with sentinel node biopsy plus axillary dissection only if the sentinel node was positive. After more than 5 years of follow-up, no differences between the arms that did and did not receive complete axillary dissection were found, either in terms of axillary recurrences or distant metastases.[19] Sentinel node biopsy using a radioactive tracer subsequently became part of the routine treatment of breast cancer patients at the IEO and has since been performed on more than 15,000 patients. The pathologic examination developed to examine the removed sentinel nodes is more exhaustive than normally performed on lymph nodes. This led to the more frequent discovery of metastases, with improved staging accuracy as a consequence. Another result of extensive pathologic examination of sentinel nodes is that micrometastases (<2 mm) and isolated tumor cells are found with greater frequency.[20] Current policy at the IEO is to perform complete axillary dissection whenever the sentinel node is macrometastatic. There are 2 main reasons for this. First, metastatic nodes in the axilla may grow and may be inoperable when discovered. Second, the prognosis depends on the number of involved axillary nodes and level of invasion. However, if the sentinel node contains micrometastasis only, it is not clear that complete axillary dissection is necessary. The ongoing trial of the International Breast Cancer Study Group (23-01) is designed to determine the prognostic significance of minimal (<2 mm) metastatic involvement of sentinel nodes in breast cancer; it randomizes patients with minimal involvement to total axillary dissection or no further axillary treatment.

INTERNAL MAMMARY NODE BIOPSY

Use of radioactive tracer to localize the sentinel nodes occasionally picks out lymph nodes in the internal mammary chain (IMC).[21] This lymphatic drainage pathway from the breast has been ignored in recent decades after randomized trials showed that IMC dissection did not improve survival.[22] Nevertheless, the long-term results of these trials did show that the metastatic status of the IMC was as important prognostically as axillary node status, and that the prognosis is very unfavorable if both axillary and IMC lymph nodes are involved. The IEO performed a study in which IMC status was explored in 182 breast cancer patients.[21] IMN involvement was found in 14 (7.7%) or 8.8% of the 160 patients in whom IMNs were found. According to the International Union Against Cancer staging classification, these cases migrated from N0 (4 cases) or N1 (10 cases) to N3. If internal mammary sampling had not been performed, they would have been understaged. The change of stage led to a modification of the postoperative treatment plan, with radiotherapy given to the IMC and systemic therapy also given in some cases.

RADIOGUIDED OCCULT LESION LOCALIZATION

Radioguided occult lesion localization (ROLL) is a sophisticated surgical technique developed at the IEO that employs radioactive tracer and a gamma ray detecting probe for the intraoperative localization and removal of nonpalpable breast lesions, which are detected with ever-increasing frequency thanks to the affirmation of mammographic screening and greater awareness by women of the dangers of breast cancer and the importance of early detection. ROLL involves injection of immobile radioactive tracer (as opposed to the mobile radiotracer used to identify sentinel nodes) into the nonpalpable lesion under mammographic or ultrasonographic control. The gamma probe is used intraoperatively to locate the lesion and guide its removal. ROLL is a simple and accurate technique that aids complete lesion excision but minimizes the amount of healthy tissue removed[23] (Fig. 43-3).

INTRAOPERATIVE RADIOTHERAPY

Because local breast cancer relapses occur mainly at the resection site, and relapses in other quadrants of the same breast are fairly rare, senologists at the IEO wondered whether it might be safe to restrict radiation to only a part of the breast. It became possible to test this idea with the development of partial irradiation techniques and technologies to deliver radiation intraoperatively.[24]

The IEO pioneered a technique called ELIOT, or electron intraoperative therapy. This is a method of delivering high-dose electron radiation intraoperatively to a very limited area—the part of the breast involved by the tumor (Fig. 43-4)—while sparing adjacent and underlying tissues. Since 1999 the IEO has used ELIOT on more than 2000 breast cancer patients. ELIOT is mainly used to give booster doses. A booster dose of 10 to 15 Gy given intraoperatively extends surgery by only 10 to 20 minutes yet reduces the length of the conventional radiotherapy course by 2 weeks, with improved patient well-being and reduced costs. However the technique as the only radiation treatment to the breast is still being investigated in a prospective randomized trial against conventional radiotherapy in women with early-stage breast cancer treated by conservative surgery.[25] ELIOT has several advantages over conventional radiotherapy to the residual breast. It costs less, solves the problem of difficult access to radiotherapy centers, and has a beneficial effect on patient quality of life. In addition, ELIOT does not irradiate the skin and contralateral breast, and irradiation of the lung and the heart is greatly reduced because of the surgical insertion of radiation shields under the breast. Another advantage of ELIOT is that it does not interfere with systemic therapy when this is indicated.

We began clinical research on ELIOT in 1999. The first task was to estimate the single dose of electrons biologically equivalent to standard fractionated radiotherapy for breast cancer. To do this, we used the linear-quadratic surviving fraction model, otherwise known as the multitarget surviving fraction model, which indicated that a single dose in the range of 20 to 22 Gy is equivalent to 58 to 60 Gy delivered in 2 Gy daily fractions, 5 days a week over 6 weeks (ie, the dose required to control microscopic residual disease after breast resection).

ELIOT is a promising feature in breast conservation; the reduction of the radiation field dramatically reduces the exposure of normal tissues, and the shortening of the radiation course from 5 to 6 weeks to one session is extremely positive in terms of patient quality of life. For this reason we included assessment of quality of life as a routine part of the ELIOT procedure.[26]

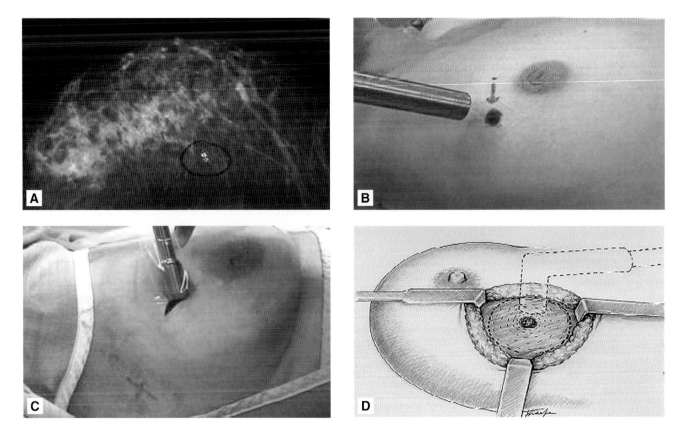

FIGURE 43-3 Stages in the radiologic and surgical procedure for radioguided occult lesion localization (ROLL). **A.** Mammography shows correct location of radio-opaque marker added with radiotracer. **B.** Gamma probe confirms correct position of cutaneous projection of lesion. **C.** and **D.** Gamma probe used to assist location and removal of occult lesion.

An interesting use of ELIOT is in nipple-sparing mastectomy (with breast reconstruction) in women who require mastectomy because their cancer is multicentric or has an EIC component. The surgical technique involves sparing of the skin and nipple-areola complex while the latter is treated intraoperatively with ELIOT to sterilize any involvement of this area.

PHARMACO-PREVENTION

To identify effective chemoprevention agents, it is in theory necessary to perform long and expensive studies on very large groups of patients to determine whether cancer risk is indeed reduced in the group taking the chemopreventive agent. One way around this—reducing study time, trial sample size and costs, and permitting the screening of many promising agents—is to study markers of cancer risk rather the development of cancer itself. Examples of such markers include levels of circulating proteins or their expression in tissue samples. Such markers can be used as intermediate end points (surrogate end-point biomarkers [SEBs]) to test investigational agents.

Several SEBs appear promising, including growth factors (eg, members of the insulin-like growth factor family), hormones (estradiol, estrone, estrone sulfate, dehydroepiandrosterone [DHEA], prolactin), atypical breast cells in cytologic samples, and mammographic density investigated using computerized techniques.

The synthetic retinoid fenretinide has shown promise as a cancer chemopreventative. In a randomized trial conducted by the National Cancer Institute in Milan to test its efficacy in preventing a second breast cancer in patients treated for first breast cancer, no difference in the frequency of second breast cancer in the treatment and placebo arms was found. However, a significantly reduced risk of second breast cancer was found in premenopausal women taking fenretinide, particularly the youngest women. The reduction in risk persisted at least 5 years after cessation of treatment.

In recent years, the Italian Tamoxifen Trial and 4 other chemoprevention studies have confirmed that tamoxifen is the most effective secondary chemopreventive currently available for women treated for breast cancer expressing ER-positive, the most common form of breast cancer.[27] The subsequent Tamoxifen Prevention Trial[28] conducted at the IEO showed that low-dose tamoxifen combined with anastrozole (aromatase inhibitor) does not reduce anastrozole bioavailability (unlike in other studies in which tamoxifen was used at standard dose) and has beneficial effects on markers of bone turnover like osteocalcin and C-telopeptide (particularly when given transdermally rather than orally), suggesting an overall beneficial effect in postmenopausal patients. Another important observation of the trial was that the protective effect of tamoxifen against breast cancer was more pronounced when combined with hormone replacement therapy (HRT), suggesting that the risk-benefit ratio

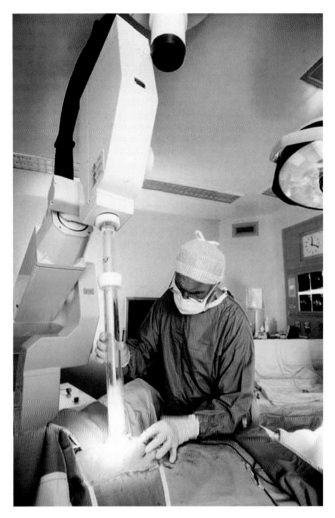

FIGURE 43-4 The linear accelerator used for electron intraoperative therapy (ELIOT).

of tamoxifen is particularly favorable in premenopausal women and HRT users, providing further justification for its wider use in breast cancer prevention. To confirm the benefits of the HRT/tamoxifen combination, the IEO is currently conducting the large national placebo-controlled HOT trial (hormone replacement therapy opposed by low-dose tamoxifen) in healthy postmenopausal HRT users who add low-dose (5 mg/day) tamoxifen for 5 years.

The IEO is also investigating other chemopreventive agents. In women with ER-positive intraepithelial neoplasia of the breast (a precancerous condition), the drug raloxifene (an ER inhibitor similar to tamoxifen) together with low-dose tamoxifen is being tested in premenopausal women, and exemestane plus celecoxib is being tested in postmenopausal women.

SUMMARY

Hundred years ago breast cancer struck 1 woman in 20. At the end of the last century, it struck 1 woman in 10. The current figure in developed countries is 1 in 8. Notwithstanding this alarming increase in breast cancer incidence, we have seen a decrease in mortality for the disease in developed countries while at the same time treatments have become much less aggressive, placing greater emphasis on patient quality of life.

Italy, and the city of Milan with its 2 distinguished Cancer Institutes, has been at the forefront of breast cancer treatment and research for many years. The early pivotal clinical trials on less aggressive surgical approaches to the disease were performed at the National Cancer Institute. These trials marked the beginning of the shift in paradigm from maximum tolerated treatment to minimum effective treatment; from aggressive surgery and radiotherapy to targeted conservative treatments; from an anatomic concept of cancer spread toward a biologic concept. This chapter traces the history of the landmark studies on breast cancer carried out in Milan over the last 40 years.

REFERENCES

1. Veronesi U, Boyle P. Breast cancer. In: Quah S, Heggenhougen K, eds. *International Encyclopedia of Public Health*. Vol. 1. Elsevier, San Diego Academic Press: 2008:348-357.
2. Stewart BW, Kleihues P, eds. *World Cancer Report*. WHO–OMS–IARC. Lyon, France: IARC Press: 2003.
3. Halsted WS. A clinical and histological study of adenocarcinoma of the breast. *Ann Surg*. 1898;28:557.
4. Hirsch J. Radiumchirurgia des brust Krebses. *Dtsch Med Wochenschr*. 1927; 43.1.119 1.121.
5. Atkins H, Hayward JL, Klugman DJ, Wayte AB. Treatment of early breast cancer: a report after 10 years of clinical trial. *Br Med J*. 1972;2:423-429.
6. Hayward J, Caleffi M. The significance of local control in the primary treatment of breast cancer. Lucy Wortham James clinical research award. *Arch Surg*. 1987;122(11):1244-1247.
7. Veronesi U, Saccozzi R, Del Vecchio M, et al. Comparing radical mastectomy with quadrantectomy, axillary dissection, and radiotherapy in patients with small cancers of the breast. *N Engl J Med*. 1981;305:6-11.
8. Veronesi U, Banfi A, Salvadori B, et al. Breast conservation is the treatment of choice in small breast cancer: long-term results of a randomized trial. *Eur. J. Cancer*. 1990;26:668-670.
9. Harris JR, Levene MB, Hellman S. The role of radiation therapy in the primary treatment of carcinoma of the breast. *Semin Oncol*. 1978;5(4):403-416.
10. Holland R, Connolly JL, Gelman R, et al. The presence of an extensive intraductal component following a limited excision correlates with prominent residual disease in the remainder of the breast. *J Clin Oncol*. 1990;8:113-118.
11. Veronesi U, Cascinelli N, Mariani L, et al. Twenty-year follow up of a randomized study comparing breast-conserving surgery with radical mastectomy for early breast cancer. *N Engl J Med* 2002;347:1227-1232.
12. Veronesi U, Luini A, Del Vecchio M, et al. Radiotherapy after breast-preserving surgery in women with localized cancer of the breast. *N Engl J. Med*. 1992;328:1587-1591.
13. Veronesi U, Luini A, Galimberti V, Zurrida S. Conservation approaches for the management of stage I/II carcinoma of the breast: Milan Cancer Institute trials. *World J Surg*. 1994;18(1):70-75.
14. Veronesi U, Salvadori B, Luini A, et al. Breast conservation is a safe method in patients with small cancer of the breast. Long-term results of three randomised trials on 1,973 patients. *Eur J Cancer*. 1995;31:1574-1579.
15. Veronesi U, Bonadonna G, Zurrida S, et al. Conservation surgery after primary chemotherapy in large carcinomas of the breast. *Ann Surg*. 1995;222(5):612-618.
16. Colleoni M, Viale G, Zahrieh D, et al. Chemotherapy is more effective in patients with breast cancer not expressing steroid hormone receptors: a study of preoperative treatment. *Clin Cancer Res*. 2004;10:6622–6628.
17. Daidone MG, Silvestrini R, Luisi A, et al. Changes in biological markers after primary chemotherapy for breast cancers. *Int J Cancer*. 1995;61:301-305.
18. Veronesi U, Paganelli G, Viale G, et al. Sentinel lymph node biopsy and axillary dissection in breast cancer: results in a large series. *J Natl Cancer Inst*. 1999;91(4):368-373.
19. Veronesi U, Paganelli G, Viale G, et al. A Randomized comparison of sentinel-node biopsy with routine axillary dissection in breast cancer. *N Engl J Med*. 2003;349:546-553.

20. Viale G, Maiorano E, Mazzarol G, et al. Histologic detection and clinical implications of micrometastases in axillary sentinel lymph nodes for patients with breast carcinoma. *Cancer.* 2001;92:1378–1384.

21. Galimberti V, Veronesi P, Arnone P, et al. Stage migration after biopsy of internal mammary chain lymph nodes in breast cancer patients. *Ann Surg Oncol.* 2002;9(9):924-928.

22. Veronesi U, Marubini E, Mariani L, et al. The dissection of internal mammary nodes does not improve the survival of breast cancer patients. 30-year results of a randomised trial. *Eur J Cancer.* 1999;35(9):1320-1325.

23. Luini A, Zurrida S, Paganelli G, et al. Comparison of radioguided excision with wire localization of occult breast lesions. *Br J Surg.* 1999;86:522–525.

24. Veronesi U, Orecchia R, Luini A, et al. A preliminary report of intraoperative radiotherapy (IORT) in limited-stage breast cancers that are conservatively treated. *Eur J Cancer.* 2001;37:2178-2183.

25. Veronesi U, Gatti G, Luini A, et al. Full-dose intraoperative radiotherapy with electrons during breast conserving surgery. *Arch Surg.* 2003;138:1253-1256.

26. Veronesi U, Orecchia R, Luini A, et al. Full dose intraoperative radiotherapy with electrons (ELIOT) during breast conserving surgery—experience with 1246 cases. *eCMS.* 2008;1:65.

27. Veronesi U, Maisonneuve P, Rotmensz N, et al. Tamoxifen for the prevention of breast cancer: late results of the Italian randomized tamoxifen prevention trial among women with hysterectomy. *J Natl Cancer Inst.* 2007;99:727-737.

28. Decensi A, Robertson C, Viale G, et al. A randomized trial of low-dose tamoxifen on breast cancer proliferation and blood estrogenic biomarkers. *J Natl Cancer Inst.* 2003;95:779-790.

CHAPTER 44

The ACOSOG Experience

Judy C. Boughey
Kelly K. Hunt

The American College of Surgeons Oncology Group (ACOSOG) was established primarily to evaluate the surgical management of patients with malignant solid tumors. The ACOSOG includes general and specialty surgeons, representatives of related oncologic disciplines, and allied health professionals in academic medical centers and community practices throughout the United States of America and abroad.

THE HISTORY OF THE ACOSOG

The ACOSOG is 1 of 10 cooperative groups funded by the National Cancer Institute (NCI) to develop and coordinate multi-institutional clinical trials and is the only cooperative group whose primary focus is the surgical management of patients with malignant solid tumors. The Cooperative Group Program was established in 1955 with an initial Congressional appropriation of $5 million. Continued growth has led to a progressive increase in funding, with an NCI appropriation of $154 million for the Cooperative Group Program in 2001. The plan to develop a new oncology cooperative group focused on surgical therapies originated in 1993. The American College of Surgeons (ACS) Board of Regents approved the concept and established a working committee of 7 surgical oncologists to devise a plan for the group's organization and structure. The committee's work was supported through a planning grant from the NCI and from funds appropriated by the ACS Board of Regents. Many individuals contributed to the effort, including surgical oncologists, radiation and medical oncologists, and biostatisticians.

After developing a set of clinical trials for a broad range of surgical specialties, a grant was submitted to the NCI, and a site visit was held at Washington University in St. Louis in June 1997. Upon the recommendation of the NCI subcommittee H, the grant was funded with an official start date of May 15, 1998. The ACOSOG was initially based at the American College of Surgeons administrative office in Chicago, Illinois, and was led by the group chair, Dr Samuel A. Wells. In January 2001, the ACOSOG moved its operations to the Duke University Medical Center. This move allowed the ACOSOG to form an association with the Duke Cancer Center and with the Statistics and Data Center based at Duke University. In addition, the ACOSOG formed an alliance with the Duke Clinical Research Institute, a well-established academic clinical research organization. After the ACOSOG grant was refunded in December 2004, Dr Wells passed the reigns to Drs Heidi Nelson and David Ota who currently share the Group Chair position. Dr David Ota, MD, FACS, oversees the ACOSOG Administrative Coordinating Center (ACC) at Duke University in Durham, North Carolina. Dr Heidi Nelson, MD, FACS, provides scientific leadership for the group and is based at the Mayo Clinic Cancer Center in Rochester, Minnesota. Dr Nelson recruited Dr Karla Ballman from the Mayo Clinic Cancer Center in Rochester, Minnesota, to lead the ACOSOG Statistics and Data Center (SDC). The ACOSOG SDC is currently based at the Mayo Clinic Cancer Center, Rochester, Minnesota, under the direction of Dr Karla Ballman. The Central Specimen Bank, funded by U24-CA114736-03 from the NIH, houses all of the biospecimens collected in the conduct of ACOSOG trials and is based at Washington University, St. Louis, Missouri, under the direction of Dr Mark Watson.

The ACOSOG is dedicated to developing clinical trials for patients with a cancer diagnosis and to conducting trials that are relevant to surgeons and the surgical management of solid tumors. The ACOSOG is strongly committed to educating surgeons in the regulations and conduct of clinical trials and to providing leadership in the cooperative group setting. The ACOSOG originally had a very broad portfolio with trials opened for patients with brain tumors, breast cancer, gastrointestinal malignancies, head and neck tumors, lung cancer, melanoma, prostate cancer, and soft tissue sarcomas. These trials were conducted by several disease site committees and working groups. More recently, the ACOSOG has sharpened its focus to four scientific committees (Basic Science, Breast, Gastrointestinal, and Thoracic). The Basic Science Committee, originally chaired by Dr Joseph Nevins of Duke University, has a major emphasis on genomics and proteomics. The committee leadership has recently been transitioned to Dr Elaine Mardis at Washington University in St. Louis, Missouri. The remaining scientific committees focus on the diseases with the greatest cancer burden in the United States: the Breast Committee, chaired by Dr Kelly K. Hunt from the MD Anderson Cancer Center in Houston, Texas; the Gastrointestinal Committee, co-chaired by Dr Mitchell C. Posner from the University of Chicago in Chicago, Illinois, and Dr Peter W. T. Pisters from the MD Anderson Cancer Center; and the Thoracic Committee, chaired by Dr Joe B. Putnam from Vanderbilt University in Nashville, Tennessee. Through this committee activity, ACOSOG has enrolled over 18,000 patients on phase II and III clinical trials and demonstrated that surgeons can conduct and complete multicenter trials within several disease sites. The activities of ACOSOG are also supported through the work of administrative committees including Audit, Constitution and Bylaws, Data Monitoring, Diagnostic Imaging, Education, Ethics, Membership, Nursing/CRA, Patient Advocates, Radiation Oncology, and Special Populations. A Peer-Review and Prioritization Committee was developed to ensure broad-based scientific review of concepts and protocols from each of the disease site committees prior to submission to the Cancer Therapy and Evaluation Program (CTEP) of the NCI.

The ACOSOG has renewed its NCI funding and is a cooperative group led by surgeons with strong multidisciplinary participation with the goal of improving the care of the surgical oncology patient through an innovative clinical research program. The scientific themes of the ACOSOG are

1. To test novel therapies that may increase response rates and cure rates and reduce morbidities and disabilities associated with cancer care
2. To conduct basic science studies in conjunction with clinical trials to better understand the biologic basis of diseases and treatments
3. To support individual members and investigator networks to accrue patients to trials and fulfill the scientific mission of the ACOSOG

ACOSOG MEMBERSHIP

The membership criteria of the ACOSOG are designed to encourage broad participation by general surgeons and subspecialty surgeons, as well as other physicians and allied health professionals in academic medical centers, community hospitals, and private practice settings. Patient registration on ACOSOG studies can only be performed by physicians. The membership model of ACOSOG was originally designed to be individual investigator–based in order to increase participation from community surgeons. The membership quickly burgeoned

to over 4100 members with 2167 surgeons, 1040 allied health professionals, 370 medical oncologists, and 273 radiation oncologists. The ACOSOG continues to support individual membership but is now building investigator networks within each of the disease sites (breast, gastrointestinal, and thoracic). These investigator networks are intended to facilitate the conduct of clinical trials and increase patient accrual while allowing the ACOSOG to fulfill its scientific mission. The trials run by the ACOSOG are relevant to both academic and community oriented surgeons and currently over 60% of enrollment on ACOSOG trials comes from surgeons in community practices who have incorporated clinical research into their daily practice. The ACOSOG leadership has endeavored to build on past successes, and to match the interests of the member networks in developing the clinical trials portfolio of the group. Membership interest based on accrual has indicated that the evolving scientific agenda should be focused on patients with malignancies of the breast, thoracic cavity, and gastrointestinal system.

THE ACOSOG BREAST COMMITTEE

The ACOSOG Breast Committee chair, Dr Kelly Hunt, is supported by 3 vice chairs, Dr Rache Simmons of the Weill Cornell Medical College, Dr Pat Whitworth of the Nashville Breast Center, and Dr Marilyn Leitch of the University of Texas Southwestern Medical Center. The Breast Committee has 3 aims, which are embodied within the research goals of the ACOSOG. The first is to improve cure rates and individualize care of patients through neoadjuvant therapies and molecular studies. The second is to increase prognostic accuracy for individual patients through investigations of novel biomarkers for risk stratification. And third, to improve the lives of our breast cancer patients through less invasive or less aggressive local-regional therapies, while not compromising the local-regional control that is so important in the long-term outcomes.

THE ACOSOG BREAST COMMITTEE TRIALS

Completed and Closed Trials

ACOSOG Z0010—A Prognostic Study of Sentinel Node and Bone Marrow Micrometastases In Women with Clinical T1 or T2 N0 M0 Breast Cancer

The Z0010 trial was designed to evaluate the incidence and impact of sentinel node and bone marrow micrometastases on patients with early-stage carcinoma of the breast treated with breast-conserving surgery and radiation therapy. The overall objective is to determine whether or not positivity in each compartment represents a different biological pathway and a different degree of prognostic significance. The study chair for Z0010 is Armando Giuliano, MD, of the John Wayne Cancer Institute in Santa Monica, California. This trial was activated in April 1999 with an accrual goal of 5300 patients. The trial was completed in May 2003 with a final accrual of 5539 patients. The ACOSOG was the only participating group in this trial.

Study Objectives. The primary objective of ACOSOG Z0010 was to estimate the prevalence and evaluate the prognostic significance of sentinel node micrometastases detected by immunohistochemistry (IHC), and to estimate the prevalence and evaluate the prognostic significance of bone marrow micrometastasis detected by immunocytochemistry (ICC). The secondary objectives were to evaluate the hazard rate for regional recurrence in women whose sentinel nodes are negative by hematoxylin and eosin (H&E) staining and to provide a mechanism for identifying women whose sentinel nodes contained metastases detected by H&E so that these women could be considered as candidates for ACOSOG Study Z0011.

Study Design. ACOSOG Z0010 was a phase II trial where all patients enrolled were planned for breast-conserving therapy (BCT) and sentinel lymph node dissection (SLND) (Fig. 44-1). Participants in the trial underwent bilateral anterior iliac crest bone marrow aspiration biopsies followed by segmental mastectomy and SLND. Bilateral bone marrow aspirates and sentinel lymph nodes found to be negative by H&E were submitted for ICC and IHC to the central lab. The results of the sentinel node and bone marrow micrometastasis studies were blinded to the individual investigators and decisions regarding the use of systemic therapy were left to the discretion of the treating clinician based on primary tumor factors. If a sentinel lymph node could not be identified during the SLND, a level I and II axillary lymph node dissection (ALND) was performed. Patients with negative sentinel lymph nodes, based on standard H&E sections, did not receive any specific axillary treatment (ALND or radiation). Patients with metastasis identified in the sentinel node(s) on H&E sections were eligible for registration and randomization on ACOSOG Z0011. Patients with a positive sentinel node who did not participate in Z0011 were treated with ALND. All patients received whole-breast radiation therapy.

Patients were followed at 6-month intervals for 5 years and then annually thereafter and assessed for local and regional recurrence, contralateral breast primary tumors, distant recurrence, and death. Special assessments for surgical side effects in the axilla and ipsilateral upper extremity were performed on all patients.

Eligibility Criteria. Eligible patients were female patients with clinical stage I or II (T1 or T2 N0 M0) invasive breast cancer amenable to treatment with breast-conserving surgery. Patients with prior ipsilateral axillary surgery, prepectoral breast implants, bilateral breast cancer, multicentric disease, or prior chemotherapy or hormonal therapy for the index breast cancer were excluded. Pregnant and lactating patients were also excluded from study participation.

Bone marrow aspiration was initially an optional procedure; however, this was later changed to a mandatory procedure for all study participants.

Surgeon Skills Verification. In order to enroll patients in this study, surgeons were required to have documented experience in performing SLND. Surgeons were allowed to participate in the Z0010 study after submitting documents demonstrating their experience in performing SLND with complete axillary lymph node dissection (ALND), by verifying training in the SLND technique through a surgical residency or fellowship training program, or through participation in an institution-wide validation study of SLND. Dr Lisa Newman, chair of the Special Populations Committee, obtained funding and initiated a project to educate surgeons working in underserved communities in the technology of sentinel node surgery who did not have training or access for this procedure to offer to their patients.

Initial Results of Z0010. From May 10, 1999 through May 30, 2003, 5539 patients were enrolled on Z0010 from 112 physician groups. Patient data eligibility review was conducted on the study population and revealed the ineligibility rate to be approximately 3%.

Surgeons from 126 different institutions participated in Z0010 with 48% academic, 20% teaching affiliated, and 29% community practice. Almost 75% of the patients were enrolled by 28% of the participating surgeons. Twenty-four percent of surgeons accrued 75% of minority patients. Female surgeons accrued 24% of patients and accounted for 30% of the study investigators. A survey of the participating surgeons revealed that 16% of respondents reported no prior experience with clinical trials.[1]

The median age of patients enrolled in Z0010 was 56 (range 23-95, see Table 44-1). A total of 3602 bone marrow specimens and 3729 sentinel node specimens were obtained and sent to the central lab for analysis. Immunocytochemistry (ICC) and immunohistochemistry (IHC) analyses of the bone marrow and lymph nodes, respectively, were performed on submission of the specimens to the central lab. Dr Richard Cote and his colleagues at the University of Southern California completed a review of all bone marrow and sentinel node specimens. In addition, a second external review of all positive bone marrow cases was completed by pathologists at the NCI.

The results of the primary endpoints of Z0010 are not yet evaluable as the clinical follow-up data continues to mature. However, we have been able to assess some

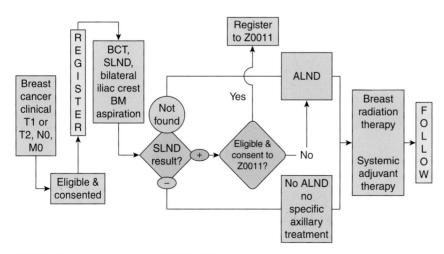

FIGURE 44-1 Schema of the ACOSOG Z0010 trial.

TABLE 44-1 Patient Demographics of ACOSOG Z0010 Participants, N = 5539

Age		
Median	56	
Minimum	23	
Maximum	95	
Race		
White	4808	86.8%
Hispanic	128	2.3%
Black	418	7.5%
Pacific Islander	10	0.2%
Asian	117	2.1%
American Indian/Alaska Native	4	0.1%
Other	33	0.6%

Summaries are based on available patient data.

of the secondary endpoints and have contributed to the published literature on the skill requirements and the surgical outcomes related to sentinel node surgery in breast cancer patients.

Participating surgeons were required to document 20 to 30 sentinel lymph node dissections performed with immediate completion axillary lymph node dissection, with a failure rate of less than 15%. Surgeons who completed a fellowship program or residency training program with training in SLND were exempt from the skill requirements as long as they had documentation of the surgical skill from their program director. At completion of patient accrual, 64.6% of participating surgeons qualified with 30 cases of SLND with ALND; 22.2% qualified with 20 cases of SLND with ALND; and 13.1% were exempted from the skills verification based on documentation from their training program. Surgeons used a combination of the blue dye and radiocolloid in 79.4% of cases, blue dye alone in 14.8% of cases, and radiocolloid alone in 5.7% of cases. Overall, surgeons achieved an SLN identification rate of 98.6% in the trial. The majority of patients had 1 (30%), 2 (34%), or 3 (19%) SLNs identified, with the average number of SLNs removed being 2.3. Patient factors that were associated with an increased likelihood of failure to identify an SLN included increasing body mass index (BMI) and increasing age ($p \leq$ .0001). The presence of nodal metastases, tumor stage, the number of positive lymph nodes, and the tumor histology were also assessed and were not found to be associated with a failure to identify an SLN. Surgeons with the highest patient accrual to Z0010 had the most success at identifying an SLN, and individual surgeon accrual of fewer than 50 patients was found to be associated with an increased failure rate ($p \leq$ .0001). The SLND technique, the specific surgeon skill qualification, and the type of institution where the procedure was performed were not associated with failure to identify an SLN.[2] These patient and surgeon related factors identified in the Z0010 trial that impacted the failure rate of identifying a SLN can be used in the preoperative counseling of patients with early-stage breast cancer.

The complication rate associated with SLND was very low and less than 1% of patients required hospitalization for management of postoperative complications. There were 1791 (32%) patients reported to have at least 1 surgical side effect following breast-conserving surgery and SLND. The surgical effects reported are shown in Table 44-2. There were 2 grade 4 adverse events reported during the conduct of the trial: 1 anaphylactic reaction to the blue dye and 1 hypoxic event which was thought to be possibly attributable to study intervention. The most common effect noted at 6 months of follow-up was axillary paresthesias; 8.6% (307 of 3573) of patients were noted to have axillary paresthesias with 92% reported as mild. Decreasing age and the use of radiocolloid alone were significantly associated with the incidence of paresthesias.

In comparison to the presurgical assessment, only 3.8% of patients (of 3071 assessed) had decreased range of motion of the ipsilateral upper extremity and 67% of these patients had a deficit that was <20. In multivariate analysis, use of radiocolloid alone for the mapping procedure was the only factor that was significantly associated with decreased range of motion. Arm measurements were taken at 10 cm proximal and distal to the medial epicondyle and were compared with the presurgical measurements and the contralateral upper extremity in order to assess lymphedema. A change in arm circumference of greater than 2 cm from the presurgical measurement and compared to the contralateral arm was defined as evidence of lymphedema. At 6 months following SLND, arm measurement data were available for 2904 patients and of these, 7% had lymphedema.[3] Factors identified on multivariate analysis that were significantly associated with the incidence of lymphedema included increasing age and increasing BMI.

TABLE 44-2 Surgical Effects Reported in ACOSOG Z0010 Participants, N = 5539

	Mild	Moderate	Severe
Allergic reaction	20 (<1%)	20 (<1%)	10 (<1%)
Axillary paresthesia	1249 (23%)	338 (6%)	50 (<1%)
Brachial plexus injury	76 (1%)	17 (<1%)	4 (0%)
Lymphedema	508 (9%)	102 (2%)	15 (<1%)
Pain/bruising from BM	253 (5%)	36 (<1%)	7 (<1%)
Maximum grade (per patient)	**1594 (29%)**	**455 (8%)**	**70 (<1%)**

For each patient the maximum grade per surgical effect is reported.

The primary objective of Z0010 was to estimate the prevalence and to evaluate the prognostic significance of sentinel node and bone marrow micrometastases detected by immunohistochemistry and immunocytochemistry. Twenty-four percent of patients had at least one positive SLN by H&E staining. The incidence of occult metastases within the bone marrow and sentinel nodes will be reported when the clinical data are mature enough to assess the primary endpoint. In the interim, laboratory studies using Z0010 specimens have been performed in order to examine occult metastases within these compartments. Evaluation of occult metastases in the bone marrow compartment has provided the first ever evidence of the existence of a putative stem cell–like phenotype within disseminated tumor cells in the bone marrow of patients with early-stage breast cancer (CD44+/CD24-low). The Cote lab used spectral imaging on bone marrow aspirates from Z0010 participants and evaluated the cells for hematoxylin, CD44, and cytokeratin. A total of 100 slides from clinical samples on 50 patients previously categorized as cytokeratin positive were analyzed. Of these samples, 100% of repeat cytokeratin-positive cases (47 patients) had cells with the CD44+/CD24-phenotype, suggesting putative breast cancer stem cells in the bone marrow. The mean prevalence of these cells in patients with a positive bone marrow was 72%, a substantially higher percentage than has been reported in primary tumors (<10%).[4] This is an important observation since stem cells are believed to be responsible for treatment failures in breast cancer patients. The identification of breast cancer stem cells in the bone marrow provides an opportunity for further characterization of these cells and ultimately an understanding of their resistance to standard therapies.

The prospective study of SLN surgery in early-stage breast cancer patients in Z0010 provides excellent short- and long-term data specific to the morbidities and disabilities associated with SLN surgery. Current results suggest low rates of local recurrence and modest rates of complications and 6-month disabilities. The data from clinical follow-up of the patients enrolled in Z0010 are under analysis for local, regional, and distant recurrence rates. It is anticipated that the presence of occult metastases in the sentinel nodes and the bone marrow will be highly prognostic in this early-stage breast cancer population. If this hypothesis is proved true when the clinical data are matched with the bone marrow and sentinel lymph node data, this would support the development of future trials using the results of bone marrow ICC and sentinel node IHC to stratify patients into high-, intermediate-, and low-risk groups.

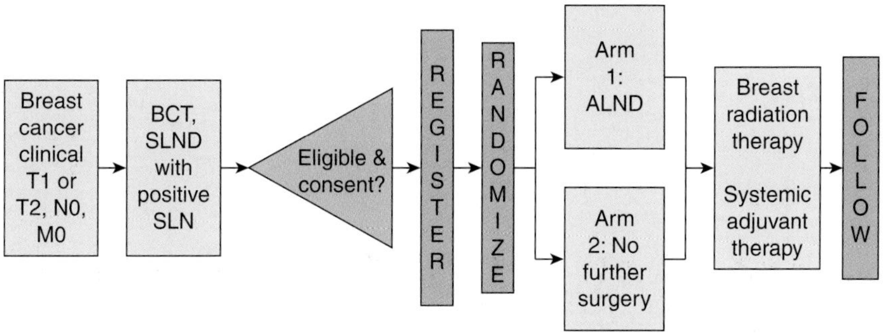

ACOSOG Z0011—A Randomized Trial of Axillary Node Dissection in Women with Clinical T1 or T2 N0 M0 Breast Cancer Who Have a Positive Sentinel Node

The Z0011 trial was designed to evaluate the impact of axillary dissection on the outcomes of patients with carcinoma of the breast and 1 or 2 positive sentinel lymph nodes. ACOSOG Z0011 was opened in May 1999, as a companion trial to ACOSOG Z0010 with Armando Giuliano, MD, serving as the study chair for both trials. This ACOSOG-led cooperative group trial was endorsed by the North Central Cancer Treatment Group (NCCTG) and the National Surgical Adjuvant Breast and Bowel Project (NSABP), and had participation from investigators enrolling through the Clinical Trials Support Unit (CTSU).

Objectives. The objectives of ACOSOG Z0011 include

1. To assess whether overall survival for patients with a positive SLN without completion ALND is equivalent to (or better) than that for patients with a positive SLN undergoing completion ALND
2. To quantify and compare the surgical morbidities associated with sentinel lymph node dissection (SLND) plus ALND versus SLND alone

Study Design. Women with clinical stage T1 or T2 N0 M0 breast cancer who underwent sentinel lymph node dissection (SLND) with breast-conserving therapy (BCT) and were found to have a sentinel node containing metastatic breast cancer, as documented on frozen section, touch prep, or permanent section evaluation by hematoxylin and eosin (H&E) staining, were eligible for this trial. The patients were randomized to 1 of 2 arms (see study schema in Fig. 44-2), where the interventions associated with these arms were

Arm 1: Completion axillary lymph node dissection (ALND)
Arm 2: No immediate additional axillary surgery or axillary-specific radiation

Women in both arms were to receive whole-breast radiation therapy, and systemic adjuvant therapy decisions were left to the discretion of the treating clinician. The Z0010 trial was intended to provide study participants for Z0011 by identifying women with positive SLNs; however, patients could participate in Z0011 without being registered to Z0010.

Special assessments for surgical side effects in the axilla and ipsilateral arm were performed within 30 days following the last study-related surgery, and at months 6 and 12 and then annually. Patients were monitored for local and regional recurrence (especially recurrence in the ipsilateral axilla), contralateral breast primary tumors, distant recurrence, and death.

FIGURE 44-2 Schema of ACOSOG Z0011 trial.

Eligibility Criteria. Eligible patients were female patients with invasive breast cancer with a tumor less than 5 cm in size, no palpable axillary lymph nodes, and no evidence of metastatic disease planned for breast-conserving therapy. Similar to Z0010, patients could have multifocal disease as long as the breast cancer could be resected with negative margins with a single lumpectomy. The sentinel lymph node containing metastatic breast cancer could be identified by frozen section, touch prep, or H&E staining on permanent section. Patients with metastatic breast cancer identified in the SLN by immunohistochemistry were not eligible for participation. Exclusion criteria included lactating women, those with prepectoral implants, prior treatment with chemotherapy or hormonal therapy for the index breast cancer, multicentric disease not amenable to a single lumpectomy, and prior ipsilateral axillary surgery. Patients found to have matted nodes or gross extranodal disease at the time of SLND, or patients with 3 or more positive SLN were excluded from participation.

Most patients were registered postoperatively following SLND and confirmation of metastatic breast cancer in a sentinel node by H&E staining on permanent section. An alternative mechanism was also provided for those sites that preferred to register patients preoperatively with intra-operative randomization based on the results of frozen section or touch prep assessment of the SLNs.

Initial Results of Z0011. ACOSOG Z0011 closed to patient accrual following a recommendation from the ACOSOG DMC on December 15, 2004, having accrued 891 patients over 5.6 years. Patient demographics are shown in Table 44-3. The early closure was due both to slow accrual and a lower than expected event rate in both arms. At interim analysis, there were 23 deaths with 868 patients remaining alive. The original study design assumed the hazard in the control arm was 1.3 times that in the ALND arm. Under that assumption, we expect that after 5 additional years of follow-up, a total of 134 deaths will have been observed and there would be 90% power to detect a hazard ratio of approximately 1.65 using a one-tailed test. This suggests that despite the fact that the trial was closed prior to the planned accrual of 1900 patients, there will still be power to assess a difference between the 2 arms if the hazard ratio is 1.7. The surgical effects and adverse events reported are shown in Tables 44-4 and 44-5.

Z0011 Surgical Morbidity. Although it seems intuitive that SLND would result in less morbidity than ALND, the ACOSOG Z0011 trial was the first prospective randomized trial in the United States to validate this hypothesis. The secondary objective of ACOSOG Z0011 was to quantify surgical morbidities associated with SLND plus ALND versus SLND alone. From May 1999 to December 2004, 891 patients were randomized to SLND plus ALND (n = 445) or SLND alone (n = 446). Information on wound infection, axillary seroma, paresthesias, brachial plexus injury, and lymphedema is available in 821 patients. Adverse surgical effects were reported in 70% (278 of 399) of patients after SLND plus ALND and 25% (103 of 411) after SLND alone ($p \leq .001$). SLND plus ALND resulted in more wound infections ($p \leq .0016$), seromas ($p \leq .0001$), and paresthesias ($p \leq .0001$) than did SLND alone. At 1 year of follow-up, lymphedema was subjectively reported by 13% (37 of 288) of patients following SLND plus ALND and only 2% (6 of 268) after SLND alone ($p \leq .0001$). There was no difference in lymphedema assessed by arm measurements ($p > .05$) at 30 days, 6 months, and 1 year between the 2 groups. Brachial plexus injuries occurred in less than 1% (8 of 821) of patients and these were all resolved by 6 months follow-up. The results from this prospective randomized trial confirmed the hypothesis that using SLND alone results in fewer postsurgical complications overall than using SLND plus ALND. We demonstrated that SLN dissection was associated

TABLE 44-3 Patient Demographics of Participants in the ACOSOG Z0011 Trial, N = 891				
	Arm 1 ALND N = 445		Arm 2 No ALND N = 446	
Age				
Median	56		54	
Minimum	24		25	
Maximum	92		90	
Race				
White	349	78.7%	366	82.7%
Hispanic	23	5.2%	19	4.3%
Black	48	10.8%	37	8.3%
Pacific Islander	1	0.2%	0	0.0%
Asian	6	1.3%	7	1.6%
American Indian/ Alaska Native	0	0.0%	0	0.0%
Other	3	0.7%	3	0.7%

Summaries are based on available patient data.

TABLE 44-4 Surgical Effects Reported in Participants in ACOSOG Z0011 (Data as of 21 Nov. 2005)

	Arm 1 ALND n = 445			Arm 2 No ALND n = 446		
	Mild	Mod.	Sev.	Mild	Mod.	Sev.
Allergic reaction	3 (<1%)	0 (0%)	1 (<1%)	5 (1%)	2 (<1%)	0 (0%)
Axillary paresthesia	178 (40%)	94 (21%)	10 (2%)	104 (23%)	22 (5%)	4 (1%)
Brachial plexus injury	15 (3%)	2 (<1%)	4 (1%)	4 (1%)	5 (1%)	0 (0%)
Lymphedema	65 (15%)	21 (5%)	7 (2%)	37 (8%)	3 (<1%)	2 (<1%)
Pain/bruising from BM	6 (1%)	4 (1%)	0 (0%)	8 (2%)	3 (<1%)	1 (<1%)
Maximum grade (per patient)	**177 (40%)**	**103 (23%)**	**18 (4%)**	**127 (29%)**	**26 (6%)**	**6 (1%)**

For each patient the maximum grade per surgical effect is reported.

with a lower rate of complications than axillary dissection; however, we could not confirm a difference in lymphedema rates at short-term follow-up based on objective measurements.[5] The long-term goal of ACOSOG Z0011 is to provide evidence to support replacing axillary lymph node dissection with sentinel lymph node dissection. It is hoped that surgical nodal staging can be replaced with molecular studies based on the primary tumor and systemic staging with bone marrow aspiration or other blood-based studies and the ACOSOG Z0011 trial is the first step toward that aim.

Timing of Completion Axillary Lymph Node Dissection. Patients with confirmed metastasis to the axillary sentinel lymph nodes usually undergo completion axillary lymph node dissection, either at the same time as the SLND or at a second procedure. Reasons for a delay include the failure to identify the SLN metastasis intraoperatively with frozen section or touch prep analysis and patient or surgeon preference. The impact of the timing of ALND on final pathologic staging results and postoperative complications in patients with positive SLNs has not been previously studied and we therefore

TABLE 44-5 Adverse Effects Reported in Participants from ACOSOG Z0011, N = 760

	Arm 1 ALND n = 378 Grade			Arm 2 No ALND n = 382 Grade		
	3	4	5	3	4	5
Cardiac general						
Thrombosis	0 (0 %)	0 (0 %)	0 (0 %)	1 (<1%)	0 (0 %)	0 (0 %)
Dermatology/skin						
Culture wound positive	1 (<1%)	0 (0 %)	0 (0 %)	0 (0 %)	0 (0 %)	0 (0 %)
Infection						
Catheter-related infection	1 (<1%)	0 (0 %)	0 (0 %)	0 (0 %)	0 (0 %)	0 (0 %)
Infection	1 (<1%)	0 (0 %)	0 (0 %)	1 (<1%)	0 (0 %)	0 (0 %)
Lymphatics						
Lymphatics—other	1 (<1%)	0 (0 %)	0 (0 %)	0 (0 %)	0 (0 %)	0 (0 %)
Musculoskeletal/soft tissue						
Musculoskeletal—other	1 (<1%)	0 (0 %)	0 (0 %)	0 (0 %)	0 (0 %)	0 (0 %)
Ocular/visual						
Cataract	1 (<1%)	0 (0 %)	0 (0 %)	0 (0 %)	0 (0 %)	0 (0 %)
Pain						
Headache	1 (<1%)	0 (0 %)	0 (0 %)	0 (0 %)	0 (0 %)	0 (0 %)
Syndromes						
Syndromes—other	1 (<1%)	0 (0 %)	0 (0 %)	0 (0 %)	0 (0 %)	0 (0 %)
Maximum grade (per patient)	**7 (1 %)**	**0 (0 %)**	**0 (0 %)**	**2 (<1%)**	**0 (0 %)**	**0 (0 %)**

Only those adverse events possibly, probably, or definitely related to study intervention are reported. For each patient the maximum grade per adverse event is reported.

used the results from the Z0010 and Z0011 trials to answer these questions. We performed a secondary analysis of 815 SLN-positive patients enrolled in Z0010 and Z0011 for factors including tumor size, grade, hormone receptor status, presence of lymphovascular invasion, and both the total number of lymph nodes recovered and the number of positive SLNs and non SLNs. There were a total of 799 evaluable patients with SLN metastasis that had immediate (n = 309) or delayed (n = 490) ALND. The median time to ALND in the delayed group was 19 days. The average number of SLNs (2.8 vs 2.6, p = .3) and axillary nodes removed (16.3 vs 17.3, p = .15) was similar between the 2 groups. When comparing patients with T1 tumors (n = 493), those in the immediate group had a greater number of positive axillary nodes (mean 2.5 vs 1.8, p = .006) and higher N stage (N2-3 14.5% vs 6.5%, p = .016) than those in the delayed group. Similar findings were noted in patients with T2 and T3 tumors (n = 306). Axillary paresthesias were more common in the immediate ALND group at 30 days (54% vs 37%, p < p.001) and 6 months (49% vs 41%, p = .04), but this difference had resolved by 1 year (36% vs 39%, p = .6). Axillary seromas occurred slightly more frequently in the immediate group (17% vs 12%, p = .05). A trend toward more lymphedema was reported in the delayed group at 6 months (13% vs 8%, p = .06), but was not observed at later time points. These data revealed that a delayed ALND after a finding of a positive SLN was associated with fewer positive non-SLNs and lower N stage compared to patients undergoing immediate ALND. Performing the axillary dissection either at the time of SLND or at a later time resulted in a similar rate of postoperative complications and similar numbers in terms of the total number of lymph nodes recovered. The reason for fewer positive nodes recovered after delayed ALND remains unclear but may due to the fact that larger metastases are likely to be detected intraoperatively by frozen section or touch prep and this would result in more immediate ALNDs. This supports the use of intraoperative evaluation of SLNs to facilitate immediate ALND when required.[6]

ACOSOG Z0011 demonstrated that higher rates of adverse surgical effects could be expected for patients undergoing SLN dissection plus axillary dissection versus those undergoing SLN dissection alone. Long-term follow-up data from Z0011, when mature, will report differences in regional failure rates between SLND alone and axillary dissection. Nested studies within Z0011 demonstrate that patients undergoing delayed ALND have fewer positive non-SLNs and lower N stage.

Open Trials

ACOSOG Z1031—A Randomized Phase III Trial Comparing 16 to 18 Weeks of Neoadjuvant Exemestane (25 mg daily), Letrozole (2.5 mg), or Anastrozole (1 mg) in Postmenopausal Women with Clinical Stage II and III Estrogen Receptor-Positive Breast Cancer

ACOSOG Z1031 is actively accruing patients with estrogen receptor (ER)–positive breast cancer for participation in this neoadjuvant treatment trial. The principal investigators are Matthew Ellis, MD, PhD, and John Olson, MD, PhD. This is a randomized phase III trial that is comparing 3 different aromatase inhibitors administered in the neoadjuvant setting to postmenopausal women with stage II or III, ER–positive breast cancer. The CALGB has endorsed the trial and it is open to other investigators through the CTSU mechanism.

Objectives. The primary objective of this study is to determine whether anastrozole, exemestane, or letrozole administered for 16 to 18 weeks as neoadjuvant endocrine treatment for postmenopausal patients with stage II or stage III ER–positive breast cancer should be chosen as the aromatase inhibitor of choice in a future study that will compare a neoadjuvant aromatase inhibitor treatment with neoadjuvant chemotherapy in this same patient population.

The secondary objectives are to compare the neoadjuvant treatment regimens relative to the rates of improvement in surgical outcome (for T4 a, b, c tumors: mastectomy with primary skin closure and negative surgical margins; for T3 tumors and T2 tumors classified as requiring mastectomy at baseline: breast-conserving surgery with negative final margins; for T2 tumors classified as potential candidates for breast conservation: wide excision at first attempt), to compare the radiological response rates (mammography and ultrasound by central radiological analysis) between the 3 aromatase inhibitors, and to compare the relative safety of the neoadjuvant treatment regimens in terms of reported adverse events.

Study Design. This is a randomized phase III trial with eligible patients randomized to 1 of 3 intervention arms as shown in the study schema (Fig. 44-3): 16 weeks of exemestane 25 mg daily; letrozole 2.5 mg daily; or anastrozole 1 mg daily. While receiving study drug, patients are assessed every 4 weeks for disease progression and study drug compliance. Response is measured clinically by physical examination of the primary tumor at monthly visits. An important aspect of the study is central radiologic review of the mammograms. Assessments are performed by the study radiologist, using bilinear measurements at the baseline and 16-week visit, to give a more accurate assessment of the radiologic response. At the completion of the 16- to 18-week course of study drug, patients are assessed for clinical and radiological disease response. If during the course of drug therapy the patient shows evidence of clinical progression and progression is confirmed radiologically, the patient may be taken off the study and either undergo surgery or be treated with chemotherapy as soon as possible without completing the 16-week course of the aromatase inhibitor. All patients will undergo resection of the primary tumor and assessment of the regional lymph nodes, as clinically indicated. Patients should continue to receive tamoxifen or anastrozole following completion of their surgical treatment. Patients are monitored every 6 months for evidence of local, regional, and distant recurrence.

Eligibility Criteria. Patients with T2-T4c, any N, M0 breast cancer by clinical staging are eligible for participation in this trial. The primary tumor must be palpable and measure at least 2 cm by caliper measurements in at least 1 dimension. Patients with metastatic disease are not eligible for participation.

Z1031 : A randomized phase III trial comparing 16 weeks of neoadjuvant Exemestane (25 mg daily), Letrozole (2.5 mg daily) or Anastrozole (1 mg daily), in postmenopausal women with clinical stage II or III estrogen receptor-positive breast cancer

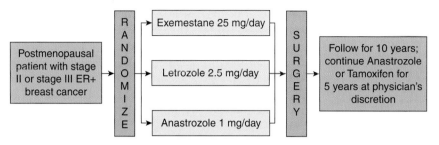

FIGURE 44-3 Schema of ACOSOG Z1031 trial.

Current Accrual Rates. The trial was activated in January 2006, and the first patient was registered in April 2006. The goal is for 375 patients to be registered in 3½ years. As of September 2008, 278 patients have been enrolled and the study is expected to meet accrual and close in May 2009. Accrual rates have been robust with a monthly average of 10 to 11 patients per month.

Rationale for Neoadjuvant Endocrine Therapy. Neoadjuvant therapy in breast cancer offers the opportunity to assess individual in vivo tumor response to the therapeutic agent rather than waiting for disease recurrence, as is the standard in adjuvant treatment trials. ACOSOG is well positioned to conduct such trials since the surgeon is generally the first point of contact for patients with a suspected or confirmed diagnosis of breast cancer. Tumor tissue can be obtained prior to the initiation of therapy and again following the treatment at the time of primary surgical intervention, and subjected to genomic and proteomic studies that can identify a pattern of resistance to the therapeutic agent. The rationale for performing this type of neoadjuvant trial in patients with ER–positive tumors is based on data demonstrating that endocrine therapy provides the greatest benefit in terms of reduction in risk of recurrence and death from breast cancer in postmenopausal women.[7] In support of the use of aromatase inhibitors, trials have demonstrated that aromatase inhibitors are superior to tamoxifen in postmenopausal women with hormone receptor–positive breast cancer.[8,9] Another factor is that neoadjuvant endocrine therapy can lead to significant shrinkage of the tumor, which can facilitate breast-conserving surgery in some patients and improved options for surgical management and local-regional control in others.[10] The use of aromatase inhibitors (AI) has both local-regional and systemic therapy benefits. If surgery is performed first and the AI is given in the adjuvant setting, it is only through long-term follow-up that we can determine the effectiveness of the agent in an individual patient. If it is given in the neoadjuvant or preoperative setting, the patient receives both local and systemic benefits and this provides an assessment of the effectiveness of this therapy by evaluating the response of the tumor with the potential to result in more surgical options and the potential for breast preservation. It has been shown that treatment with an aromatase inhibitor for only 3 or 4 months in the preoperative setting can convert a patient from mastectomy to breast-conserving surgery.

Correlative Science. Correlative science studies are an important component of the Z1031 trial and all patients are required to have a core biopsy performed prior to initiation of the AI therapy. Formalin-fixed core biopsies and OCT-embedded tumor, serum, and plasma are being collected and banked (CSB) for each patient at the Central Specimen Bank. The central theme of the primary tumor–based correlative science study is to develop an aromatase inhibitor response signature that can be translated into a widely applicable test that can identify patients with a high chance of responding to aromatase inhibitor therapy in either the adjuvant or neoadjuvant setting. Since the correlative science analysis will be conducted on patients from all 3 arms of the trial, the response signature that is developed will be broadly applicable and not agent specific. Primary tumor responses will be assessed and compared with baseline gene expression profiles and comparative genomic hybridization assays that will analyze the mutation status of genes known to be important in breast cancer. The patterns of gains and losses of DNA will be used to develop a multigene model for predicting response to endocrine therapy in postmenopausal women with ER-positive disease. There are several signatures that are available for assessing prognosis in these patients (Oncotype Dx, Mammaprint), and we will assess the ability of these existing signatures to predict response in comparison with the arrays we are performing. We also have the ability to perform these studies on the pretreatment and post-treatment specimens. The posttreatment specimens may actually provide us with the best information with respect to resistance to endocrine therapies. Additional biologic correlates are being investigated as well as proteomic studies of serum and plasma in each patient. It is anticipated that data from this trial will inform the design of the next generation of neoadjuvant trials comparing chemotherapy and endocrine therapy in this group.

ACOSOG Z1041—A Randomized Phase III Trial Comparing a Neoadjuvant Regimen of FEC-75 Followed by Paclitaxel plus Trastuzumab with a Neoadjuvant Regimen of Paclitaxel plus Trastuzumab Followed by FEC-75 plus Trastuzumab in Patients with HER-2–Positive Operable Breast Cancer

ACOSOG Z1041 is a neoadjuvant trial designed for patients with HER-2–positive breast cancer. The study chairs are Aman U. Buzdar, MD, and Peter D. Beitsch, MD. This trial was activated in July 2007, and is open to ACOSOG members and to other investigators through the CTSU mechanism. This is a randomized phase III trial targeting patients with HER-2–positive disease that is comparing a neoadjuvant chemotherapy regimen with concurrent trastuzumab and chemotherapy, versus the anthracycline-based combination chemotherapy alone followed by paclitaxel with concurrent trastuzumab. The patients will then undergo surgery, and the primary outcome that will be measured will be pathologic complete response rates.

Objectives. The primary objective is to compare the pathologic complete response rate (pCR) within the breast of a sequential regimen of concurrent weekly paclitaxel and trastuzumab, followed by continued trastuzumab administered concurrently with 5-flourouracil, epirubicin, and cyclophosphamide (FEC) (Arm 2), to the pCR rate of a sequential regimen of FEC alone followed by concurrent weekly paclitaxel and trastuzumab (Arm 1).

Secondary Objectives. There are several important secondary objectives in this trial. First, the cardiotoxicity of the 2 regimens will be compared to determine if there is a difference between the regimen with trastuzumab administered concurrently with FEC, compared with the cardiotoxicity of a sequential regimen of FEC followed by concurrent weekly paclitaxel and trastuzumab. The pCR rates in the breast and ipsilateral axilla will be compared between the 2 groups to determine whether the concurrent anthracycline and trastuzumab contributes significantly to the pCR rates. Additional endpoints include comparison of the clinical response rates (cRR) of the 2 regimens, the noncardiac toxicities of the 2 regimens, the breast conservation rates achieved with the 2 regimens evaluated in this study, and disease-free survival and overall survival at 5 years postrandomization.

Study Design. Z1041 is a randomized phase III trial enrolling patients with HER-2–positive operable breast cancer who will be randomized to 2 intervention arms:

Arm 1: Arm 1 will receive 4 cycles (12 weeks) of 5-flourouracil, epirubicin, and cyclophosphamide (FEC), followed by weekly paclitaxel for 12 weeks plus weekly administration of trastuzumab.

Arm 2: Arm 2 will receive weekly paclitaxel for 12 weeks plus weekly administration of trastuzumab, followed by 4 cycles (12 weeks) of FEC plus weekly administration of trastuzumab.

The study schema is shown in Figure 44-4

Upon completion of chemotherapy, patients in both arms will be assessed through clinical exam, radiological exam, and ultrasound for clinical response. Following this assessment, patients will receive the clinically indicated surgical resection of the tumor plus sentinel lymph node dissection (SLND) and/or axillary lymph node dissection (ALND). Breast and nodal tissue removed at the time of surgery will be assessed for pathological response. Patients will then receive trastuzumab 6 mg/kg IV every 3 weeks to complete 52 weeks of trastuzumab therapy plus radiation therapy, if indicated, in the adjuvant setting. Patients in both arms will be assessed for recurrence every 6 months for 2 years, and then at yearly intervals for 3 years. Patients with hormone receptor–positive tumors should receive endocrine therapy for 5 years.

The accrual goal for Z1041 is 275 patients and as of October 2008, 45 patients have been randomized on the trial.

Eligibility Criteria. Eligible patients are female patients with HER-2 overexpressing invasive breast cancer diagnosed by core needle biopsy that is amenable to surgical resection. Patients should have a tumor greater than 2 cm in size that is amenable to assessment by clinical or radiographic examination. Patients may not have had any surgical axillary staging procedure prior to study entry, however, fine needle aspiration of an axillary lymph node is allowed. Left ventricular ejection fraction measured by multiple gated acquisition scan must be greater than 55%. A recent amendment to the trial allows for registration of patients with N2b, N3, and T4 disease, as well as those with nodal disease without a measurable primary tumor. HER-2 positivity requires either fluorescent in situ hybridization (FISH) demonstrating gene amplification or immunohistochemistry (IHC) with a strongly positive (3+) staining intensity score. Patients with metastatic disease are excluded.

Rationale for the Z1041 Trial. The rationale for this trial is that trastuzumab has proven benefits in patients with HER-2–positive disease, and the addition of trastuzumab to standard chemotherapy markedly improves pathologic response rates. Z1041, designed to investigate the role of trastuzumab in the neoadjuvant setting, is a logical extension of several observations in advanced disease including the established benefits of neoadjuvant approaches, the effectiveness of trastuzumab in HER-2–positive breast cancer, and results from at least 1 single

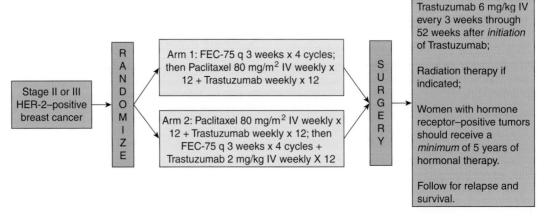

FIGURE 44-4 Schema of ACOSOG Z1041 trial.

institution experience demonstrating the success of this regimen in operable disease. Neoadjuvant chemotherapy is the established standard practice for patients with locally advanced breast cancer based on significant reductions in recurrences and deaths. In early-stage breast cancer, neoadjuvant therapy allows for higher rates of breast-conserving therapy without compromising local-regional control. A further advantage of neoadjuvant chemotherapy is that it provides a rapid in vivo method of evaluating the effectiveness of systemic therapy on the primary tumor and regional nodes. These facts considered, it is reasonable to assume that neoadjuvant approaches over time will facilitate the individual care of patients with operable breast cancer. Individualized treatments will favorably impact survival beyond current postoperative adjuvant approaches.

The rationale for testing trastuzumab as a targeted agent in early-stage breast cancer is based on the biology of the disease, the efficacy of trastuzumab in metastatic disease and the adjuvant setting, and promising results from a single institution study. Overexpression of the HER-2/neu proto-oncogene is identified in 25% to 30% of human breast cancers. Trastuzumab, a monoclonal antibody targeting the HER-2/neu receptor, has been extensively tested in patients overexpressing HER-2/neu with positive results in both the metastatic and the adjuvant setting. Initial results from several trials (Intergroup NCCTG N9831, NSABP B-31, BCIRG102, and HERA) suggest improved disease-free survival and it is FDA approved for the adjuvant therapy of patients with node-positive and high-risk node-negative HER-2–positive breast cancer. A single institution (MD Anderson Cancer Center) has taken this success to the next step and explored trastuzumab in the neoadjuvant setting, comparing 4 cycles of paclitaxel followed by 4 cycles of FEC, or the same chemotherapy with simultaneous weekly administration of trastuzumab for 24 weeks. The trial was stopped early by the Data Monitoring Committee due to markedly superior results for the group receiving chemotherapy plus trastuzumab. The pCR rates for chemotherapy plus trastuzumab were 65% compared to 26% for chemotherapy alone.

Z1041 will assess 2 different neoadjuvant regimens, 1 with concurrent anthracycline and trastuzumab therapy and 1 without concurrent anthracycline-trastuzumab therapy. This study will hopefully confirm the single institution rates of pCR attributed to neoadjuvant concurrent anthracyclines and trastuzumab, and further it will determine whether concurrent anthracyclines with trastuzumab are necessary to achieve the high pCR rates. Additional objectives will assess the cardiac safety of concurrent anthracycline and trastuzumab therapy as well as assess rates of breast conservation and disease-free survival.[11]

There have been additional patients treated with the MD Anderson regimen; and with longer follow-up, they have reported that there have been no recurrences to date in the patients who received trastuzumab plus chemotherapy, and cardiac safety with this regimen has been confirmed.[12] Subsequent to this, there have been several studies demonstrating similar findings, including a large trial from the NCI Milan, demonstrating that patients treated with trastuzumab plus chemotherapy have significantly higher pathologic complete response rates and that cardiac toxicity is 1% or less with concurrent trastuzumab and anthracycline therapy.[13]

Similar to the Z1031 trial, Z1041 will be measuring clinical, radiologic, and pathologic response rates, in addition to breast-conserving rates. This particular neoadjuvant regimen is of interest to breast cancer surgeons since such a high pathologic complete response rate should translate into improved breast-preservation rates for many of these patients.

Correlative Science. The Z1041 protocol is designed to evaluate the addition of trastuzumab to standard chemotherapy in the neoadjuvant setting for operable breast cancer. A number of laboratories are collaborating with the Basic Science Committee to provide correlative studies for Z1041 that address 4 specific aims. In the first aim, cell cycle regulatory proteins are examined as predictors of response to chemotherapy. Cyclin E has been shown to be deregulated in breast cancers and chemotherapeutic effects on the cell cycle raise the possibility that modulation of cyclin E may be a relevant target in predicting response to systemic therapy in breast cancer patients. The proposed studies in Z1041 will stringently identify the isoforms of cyclin E and test the hypothesis that cyclin E is a powerful independent predictor for response to chemotherapy, and examine molecular mechanisms by which cyclin E predicts responses. In the second aim, epigenetic changes are assessed as predictors of tumor response to neoadjuvant therapy. Methylation, the only postsynthetic modification of DNA that occurs in mammalian cells, is a process that contributes to the regulation of gene expression and carcinogenesis. There is growing evidence that individual methylation profiles of various cancers may have diagnostic, prognostic, and even therapeutic implications, such as the use of hypomethylating agents (such as 5-Aza-C), to potentially reverse these epigenetic changes.[14-16] Z1041 correlative studies will identify the DNA methylation patterns predictive of response to chemotherapy in this prospective study. In aim 3, gene expression signatures that predict response to neoadjuvant chemotherapy and can identify therapeutic options for resistant patients will be examined. The development of biomarkers as predictive and prognostic tools is central to oncology. Numerous studies have demonstrated the potential for the application of gene expression profiles to improving prognostic accuracy and therefore treatment efficacy for patients with cancer. Gene expression data also have the capacity to dissect the heterogeneity inherent in otherwise similar tumor samples, identifying patterns that can define the unique characteristics of individual tumors and predict individual patient outcomes.[17-21] In aim 4, investigators will use combined models incorporating gene expression, cyclin E, and DNA methylation data to develop predictors of tumor response to neoadjuvant therapy in patients with breast cancer. The proposed approach evaluates and uses multiple, related genomic patterns in combination with clinical factors, rather than a single genomic pattern to the exclusion of other informative factors. The plan is to refine and evolve the understanding of multiple forms of data relevant to moving genomic analysis through clinical trials to clinical practice using data from Z1041.

ACOSOG Z1072—A Phase II Trial Exploring the Success of Cryoablation Therapy in the Treatment of Invasive Breast Carcinoma

The primary objective is to determine the rate of complete tumor ablation in patients treated with cryoablation, with complete tumor ablation defined as no remaining invasive or in situ carcinoma present upon pathological examination of the targeted lesion and to evaluate the negative predictive value of magnetic resonance imaging (MRI) and intraoperative core biopsies in the postablation setting to determine residual in situ or invasive breast carcinoma. The study chair is Rache M. Simmons, MD. This is a phase II nonrandomized study that was activated in September 2008. Patients will undergo imaging by mammography, ultrasound, and breast MRI. Patients will be treated with cryoablation, followed by reimaging, and then surgery (as shown in the study schema in Fig. 44-5). Patients will be seen for one postoperative visit but will not have long-term follow-up. Z1072 is expected to accrue 99 patients. Investigator credentialing is required for the surgeon, radiologist, and participating pathologist.

The short-term and specific goals of Z1072 are to test the rate of complete tumor ablation and the ability to detect complete ablation using core biopsies and MRI. A broader goal includes the establishment of a timely investigative paradigm for primary ablative therapy of the breast. Just as breast cancer diagnosis has evolved from symptomatic detection to mammographic screening, breast cancer treatment has evolved from radical mastectomy to lumpectomy and sentinel lymph node dissection. The next phase of innovations will deliver the prospect of nonoperative, office-based interventions for diagnoses and treatment, specifically including primary tumor core biopsies, molecular and systemic risk profiling, and primary tumor ablation for early-stage breast cancer. There are limited data as well as investigational trials evaluating the use of molecular and systemic markers to replace the need for SLND in patients at low risk for axillary metastases. This is desirable as Z0010 demonstrated a defined morbidity associated with SLND. The Z1072 trial is the first investigational step toward eliminating the need for surgery for treatment of early-stage breast cancer. The success of these 2 strategies together would not only reduce surgical morbidities and enhance breast cosmesis, but would obviate the need for in-hospital breast cancer management. This vision of targeted therapy of the breast is in keeping with ACOSOG targeted strategies of breast cancer care.

The current clinical model and investigative framework for breast ablative therapy exists in the current office-based practice of cryoablation for benign fibroadenomas. In many centers, cryoablation of fibroadenomas is the preferred practice over surgical excision for several reasons, including the convenience of coupling the diagnostic and therapeutic approaches using a common office-based imaging system (ie, ultrasound, US). As such US-based cryoablation is available to all practitioners

equipped and certified in breast ultrasound. Furthermore, cryoablation is preferred by patients as it produces less pain, requiring less anesthesia. Cryoablation of fibroadenomas is also cosmetically advantageous and is associated with restoration of normal or near normal breast architecture on physical examination as well as by imaging with both ultrasound and mammography. The same advantages would be expected for primary cancer cryoablation. Finally, theoretical advantages for breast cancer treatment include the potential for enhancing immunologic responses. All things considered, US-guided cryoablation is a logical and reasonable starting place based on current office-based practices for benign breast conditions, and based on the widespread availability and defined certification process for breast ultrasound.

Since office-based US, breast US certification, and a clinical model for cryoablation in benign disease is established and in practice, it is anticipated that Z1072 would investigate the rate of complete ablation and the detection rate of complete ablation using histological evaluation of the resected specimen as the control as the first step toward treatment of malignancy. A second confirmatory trial would also be required.

Intergroup Participation. The ACOSOG Breast Committee has a number of collaborations with the Breast Cancer Intergroup of North America. We participated in the NSABP B-35 trial, which was recently completed. We are participating in the NSABPB-39/RTOG trial on partial breast irradiation for early-stage breast cancer patients. We have also endorsed and are actively participating in the TAILORx trial.

ECOG PACCT1—TAILORx: Program for the Clinical Cancer Test (PACCT-1) Trial Assigning Individualized Options for Treatment: The TAILORx Trial. ACOSOG Study Chair: John A. Olson, MD, PhD

Of the 137,000 women diagnosed annually with ER-positive, lymph node–negative breast cancer, roughly 80% to 85% of these women are adequately treated with surgery +/- irradiation and hormonal therapy. Adding chemotherapy decreases recurrence by approximately 25%. The absolute benefit is small (~3%-5% or less). The primary objectives of TAILORx is therefore to (1) determine whether adjuvant hormonal therapy is not inferior to adjuvant chemohormonal therapy in women whose tumors meet established clinical guidelines for adjuvant chemotherapy; and (2) create a tissue and specimen bank for patients enrolled in this trial, including formalin fixed paraffin embed-

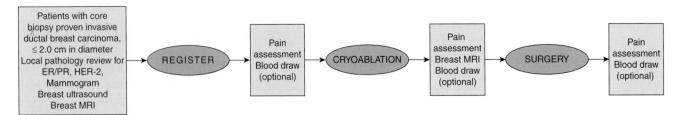

FIGURE 44-5 Schema of ACOSOG Z1072 trial.

ded tumor specimens, tissue microarrays, plasma, and DNA obtained from peripheral blood. Additional objectives include (1) to determine whether adjuvant hormonal therapy is sufficient treatment for women whose tumors meet established clinical guidelines for adjuvant chemotherapy; (2) to compare the outcomes projected at 10 years by adjuvant online with those made by the Genomic Health Oncotype DX test; (3) to estimate failure rates as a function of recurrence score separately in the chemotherapy and no chemotherapy groups; and (4) to determine the prognostic significance of the Oncotype DX recurrence score and of the individual RS gene groups. The TAILORx trial was activated on 4/7/06.

NSABP B-35: A Clinical Trial Comparing Anastrozole with Tamoxifen in Postmenopausal Patients with Ductal Carcinoma In Situ (DCIS) Undergoing Lumpectomy with Radiation Therapy. ACOSOG Study Chair: Pat W. Whitworth, MD

Despite treatment with lumpectomy and radiation therapy, up to 15% of patients with ductal carcinoma in situ will develop either ipsilateral recurrence (one-third of these will be invasive cancer) or contralateral cancer (6%). NSABP B-35 is designed to test tamoxifen versus anastrozole since tamoxifen, although effective, has been associated with serious adverse effects in older women and aromatase inhibitors are superior in post-menopausal women. The primary objectives of B-35 were to (1) compare the value of anastrozole versus tamoxifen, in terms of preventing recurrence (ie, local, regional, and distant recurrences and contralateral breast cancer), after lumpectomy and radiotherapy in postmenopausal women with ductal carcinoma in situ (DCIS); (2) compare subsequent disease occurrence, in terms of invasive breast cancer (local, regional, distant, or contralateral), ipsilateral and contralateral breast cancer (invasive and DCIS), and nonbreast second primary malignancies, in patients treated with these drugs; (3) compare quality of life and symptoms of patients treated with these drugs; (4) compare quality-adjusted survival time of patients treated with these drugs; (5) compare the occurrence of osteoporotic fractures in patients treated with these drugs; and (6) compare disease-free and overall survival of patients treated with these drugs. The B-35 trial was opened on 1/6/03 and activated on the CTSU menu on 1/14/03. The trial closed in June of 2006 after meeting accrual of 3104 patients of a planned 3000 patients. ACOSOG members Drs Pat Whitworth and Michael Grant were recognized by the CTSU for being 2 of the top CTSU accruers to the B-35 trial.

NSABP B-39/RTOG: A Randomized Phase III Study of Conventional Whole-Breast Irradiation (WBI) versus Partial Breast Irradiation (PBI) for Women with Stage 0, I, or II Breast Cancer. ACOSOG Study Chair: Henry M. Kuerer, MD, PhD

The primary aim of this phase III trial was designed to determine whether partial breast irradiation (PBI) limited to the region of the tumor bed following lumpectomy provides equivalent local tumor control in the breast compared to conventional whole breast irradiation (WBI) in the local management of early-stage breast cancer. Additional aims include (1) to compare overall survival, recurrence-free survival, and distant disease-free survival between women receiving PBI and women receiving WBI; (2) to determine whether PBI delivered on 5 treatment days over a period of 5 to 10 days can provide a comparable cosmetic result to WBI; (3) to determine if PBI produces less fatigue and treatment-related symptoms compared to WBI; (4) to determine if perceived convenience of care is greater for women receiving PBI compared to women receiving WBI; and (5) to compare acute and late toxicities between the radiation therapy regimens. The NSABP B-39 trial was activated on 3/22/05.

FUTURE PLANS FOR ACOSOG BREAST TRIALS

The Breast Committee shifted its activity from the SLN development trials to neoadjuvant approaches and we are now actively accruing to these trials and collecting quality tissues for the scientific endpoints. We are using targeted therapies to known predictive markers, such as the estrogen receptor and HER-2. We are combining this with genomic and proteomic approaches to identify resistant tumors to these targeted therapies. The Z1031 successor trial is planned to randomize patients to chemotherapy versus the best aromatase inhibitor, and the Z1041 trial will similarly identify the profile of tumors that would be predicted to be resistant to trastuzumab for alternate strategies with other targeted therapeutic approaches.

A long-term goal of the Breast Committee is to reduce or eliminate the need for surgery in the management of early-stage breast cancer. Results from Z0010 and Z0011 quantitate the short-term morbidities and long-term disabilities from sentinel lymph node dissection and axillary lymph node dissection. The possibility of providing a prognosis using methods other than SLND or ALND, such as bone marrow micrometastases or primary tumor microarray, are central to the scientific program of ACOSOG and should be reasonably achieved in the foreseeable future. Further, efforts to reduce the extensiveness of breast surgery include the up-front or neoadjuvant administration of aromatase inhibitors to facilitate less morbid and disfiguring surgical procedures. Along the same theme, the role of primary tumor cryoablation as an alternative to surgery will be investigated in Z1072, a phase II trial of primary tumor ablation in early-stage breast cancer. The long-term goal is to reduce or eliminate the need for excisional and disfiguring surgery.

HOW TO ENROLL IN AN ACOSOG TRIAL

For enrollment in an ACOSOG study, ACOSOG membership is required. See the ACOSOG Web site—www.acosog.org—for membership information. The membership criteria of the ACOSOG are designed to encourage broad participation by general and specialty surgeons, as well as other physicians and allied health professionals in the private practice community and at academic medical centers. Only physicians can enter patients on ACOSOG studies.

The ACOSOG needs your active participation and enrollment of patients into their ongoing trials. Future studies will further reduce the need for, and extent of, surgery using alternate nonsurgical methods of prognosticating, using neoadjuvant approaches to downsize, and exploring in-situ ablation techniques to reduce or eliminate the need for surgical excision.

SUMMARY

- Completing neoadjuvant endocrine therapy trial with robust accrual and tissue collection
- Initiating neoadjuvant treatment trial for patients with HER-2–positive disease
- Strengthening intergroup collaborations
- Exploring novel surgical approaches (cryoablation) for breast cancer patients, which may impact recurrence and quality of life
- Incorporating imaging to improve surgical outcomes
- Exploring adjuvant treatment strategies to reduce local and systemic recurrences

REFERENCES

1. Leitch AM, Beitsch PD, McCall LM, et al. Patterns of participation and successful patient recruitment to American College of Surgeons Oncology Group Z0010, a phase II trial for patients with early-stage breast cancer. *Am J Surg.* 2005;190:539-542.
2. Posther KE, McCall LM, Blumencranz PW, et al. Sentinel node skills verification and surgeon performance: data from a multicenter clinical trial for early-stage breast cancer. *Ann Surg.* 2005;242:593-599; discussion 599-602.
3. Wilke LG, McCall LM, Posther KE, et al. Surgical complications associated with sentinel lymph node biopsy: results from a prospective international cooperative group trial. *Ann Surg Oncol.* 2006;13:491-500.
4. Balic M, Lin H, Young L, et al. Most early disseminated cancer cells detected in bone marrow of breast cancer patients have a putative breast cancer stem cell phenotype. *Clin Cancer Res.* 2006;12:5615-5621.
5. Lucci A, McCall LM, Beitsch PD, et al. Surgical complications associated with sentinel lymph node dissection (SLND) plus axillary lymph node dissection compared with SLND alone in the American College of Surgeons Oncology Group Trial Z0011. *J Clin Oncol.* 2007;25:3657-3663.
6. Olson JA, Jr., McCall LM, Beitsch P, et al. Impact of immediate versus delayed axillary node dissection on surgical outcomes in breast cancer patients with positive sentinel nodes: results from American College of Surgeons Oncology Group trials Z0010 and Z0011. *J Clin Oncol.* 2008;26:3530-3535.
7. Early Breast Cancer Trialists' Collaborative Group (EBCTCG). Effects of chemotherapy and hormonal therapy for early breast cancer on recurrence and 15-year survival: an overview of the randomised trials. *Lancet.* 2005;365:1687-1717.
8. Wong ZW, Ellis MJ. First-line endocrine treatment of breast cancer: aromatase inhibitor or antioestrogen? *Br J Cancer.* 2004;90:20-25.
9. Baum M, Budzar AU, Cuzick J, et al. Anastrozole alone or in combination with tamoxifen versus tamoxifen alone for adjuvant treatment of postmenopausal women with early breast cancer: first results of the ATAC randomised trial. *Lancet.* 2002;359:2131-2139.
10. Dixon JM, Renshaw L, Bellamy C, et al. The effects of neoadjuvant anastrozole (Arimidex) on tumor volume in postmenopausal women with breast cancer: a randomized, double-blind, single-center study. *Clin Cancer Res.* 2000;6:2229-2235.
11. Buzdar AU, Ibrahim NK, Francis D, et al. Significantly higher pathologic complete remission rate after neoadjuvant therapy with trastuzumab, paclitaxel, and epirubicin chemotherapy: results of a randomized trial in human epidermal growth factor receptor 2-positive operable breast cancer. *J Clin Oncol.* 2005;23:3676-3685.
12. Buzdar AU, Valero V, Ibrahim NK, et al. Neoadjuvant therapy with paclitaxel followed by 5-fluorouracil, epirubicin, and cyclophosphamide chemotherapy and concurrent trastuzumab in human epidermal growth factor receptor 2-positive operable breast cancer: an update of the initial randomized study population and data of additional patients treated with the same regimen. *Clin Cancer Res.* 2007;13:228-233.
13. Gianni L, Semiglazov V, Manikas G, et al. Neoadjuvant trastuzumab in locally advanced breast cancer (NOAH): antitumour and safety analysis. *Journal of Clinical Oncology 2007 ASCO Annual Meeting Proceedings Part I.* 2007;25(18S) (June 20 supplement):532.
14. Buzdar AU, Singletary SE, Valero V, et al. Evaluation of paclitaxel in adjuvant chemotherapy for patients with operable breast cancer: preliminary data of a prospective randomized trial. *Clin Cancer Res.* 2002;8:1073-1079.
15. Buzdar AU, Hortobagyi GN, Asmar L, et al. Prospective randomized trial of paclitaxel alone versus 5-fluorouracil/doxorubicin/cyclophosphamide as induction therapy in patients with operable breast cancer. *Semin Oncol.* 1997;24:S17-31–S17-34.
16. Green MC, Buzdar AU, Smith T, et al. Weekly paclitaxel improves pathologic complete remission in operable breast cancer when compared with paclitaxel once every 3 weeks. *J Clin Oncol.* 2005;23:5983-5992.
17. West M, Blanchette C, Dressman H, et al. Predicting the clinical status of human breast cancer by using gene expression profiles. *Proc Natl Acad Sci. USA.* 2001;98:11462-11467.
18. Huang E, Cheng SH, Dressman H, et al. Gene expression predictors of breast cancer outcomes. *Lancet.* 2003;361:1590-1596.
19. Pittman J, Huang E, Dressman H, et al. Integrated modeling of clinical and gene expression information for personalized prediction of disease outcomes. *Proc Natl Acad Sci. USA.* 2004;101:8431-8436.
20. van't Veer LJ, Dai H, van de Vijver MJ, et al. Gene expression profiling predicts clinical outcome of breast cancer. *Nature.* 2002;415:530-536.
21. Potti A, Mukherjee S, Petersen R, et al. A genomic strategy to refine prognosis in early-stage non-small-cell lung cancer. *N Engl J Med.* 2006;355:570-580.

CHAPTER 45

The EORTC Experience: From DCIS to Locally Advanced Breast Cancer

Harry Bartelink
Philip Meijnen
Marieke Straver
Emiel Rutgers

The European Organization for Research and Treatment of Cancer (EORTC) Breast Group and the Radiotherapy Group successfully completed several clinical trials that included thousands of patients with the goal of improving outcomes by evaluating different approaches in the locoregional treatment of breast cancer. These trials addressed the need for and feasibility of alternative or more aggressive treatment regimens and new ways to predict therapeutic outcomes. For ductal carcinoma in situ (DCIS), the contribution of radiotherapy in achieving local control was examined. For stage I and II breast cancer, mastectomy was compared with breast-conserving therapy. This was followed by a trial in which 2 different dose levels of irradiation were tested (ie, is an extra boost dose required after whole-breast irradiation?). Reduction of morbidity is the aim of the After Mapping of the Axilla Radiotherapy or Surgery (AMAROS) trial comparing axillary lymph node dissection with axillary irradiation in patients with proven axillary metastases in the sentinel nodes. For locally advanced breast cancer, the contribution of hormonal therapy and chemotherapy was investigated. Finally, the possibility of predicting treatment outcomes and therefore individualizing treatment regimens is explored in ongoing trials incorporating genomic profiles. A selection of the EORTC breast cancer trials is presented in this overview, followed by some of the new studies and suggestions for future research.

COMPLETED TRIALS

The EORTC 10853 DCIS Trial: Whether or Not to Add Breast Radiotherapy After Local Excision

A randomized trial was conducted to investigate the role of breast radiotherapy after local excision of DCIS. We analyzed the efficacy of radiotherapy with 10 years of follow-up on both the overall risk of local recurrence (LR) and according to clinical, histologic, and treatment factors.

After microscopically complete local excision, women with DCIS were randomly assigned to no further treatment or radiotherapy (50 Gy whole-breast irradiation). One thousand and ten women with mostly (71%) mammographically detected DCIS were included. The median follow-up was 10.5 years.[1,2]

The 10-year LR-free rate was 74% in the group treated with local excision alone compared with 85% in the women treated by local excision plus radiotherapy (log-rank $p < 0.0001$; hazard ratio [HR] = 0.53). (Fig. 45-1A) The risk of DCIS and invasive LR was reduced by 48% ($p = 0.0011$) and 42% ($p = 0.0065$), respectively (Fig. 45-1B and 45-1C). Both groups had similar low risks of metastases and death. At multivariate analysis, factors significantly associated with an increased LR risk were young age (≤40 years; HR = 1.89), symptomatic detection (HR = 1.55), intermediately or poorly differentiated DCIS (as opposed

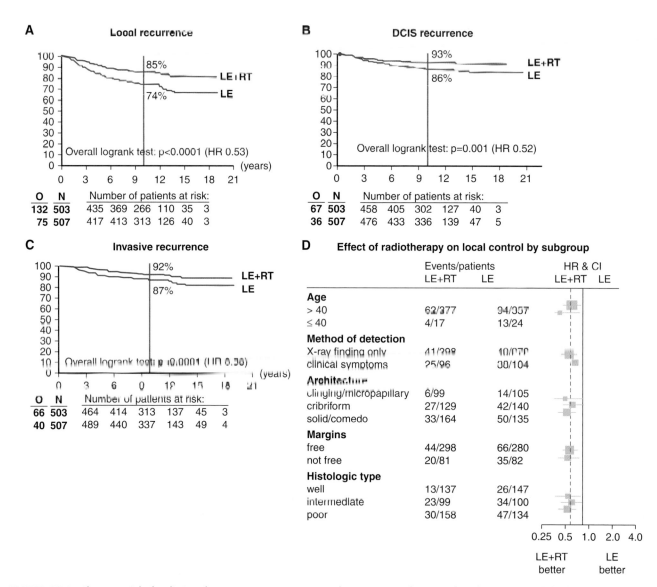

FIGURE 45-1 Phase III trial of radiation therapy versus no treatment for patients with in situ ductal carcinoma of the breast (EORTC 10853). Time to recurrence by treatment arm. **A.** All local recurrences. **B.** Ductal carcinoma in situ (DCIS) recurrences. **C.** Invasive recurrence. **D.** Effect of radiotherapy on local control by subgroup. (CI, 95% confidence interval; HR, hazard ratio; LE, local excision; N, number of patients; O, observed; RT, radiotherapy.) *[Reproduced, with permission, from Bijker N, Meijnen P, Peterse JL, et al. Breast-conserving treatment with or without radiotherapy in ductal carcinoma-in-situ: ten year results of European Organisation for Research and Treatment of Cancer randomized phase III trial 10853—a study by the EORTC Breast Cancer Cooperative Group and EORTC Radiotherapy Group. J Clin Oncol. 2006;24(21):3381-3387.]*

to well-differentiated DCIS; HR = 1.85 and HR = 1.61, respectively), cribriform or solid growth pattern (as opposed to clinging/micropapillary subtypes; HR = 2.39 and HR = 2.25, respectively), doubtful margins (HR = 1.84), and treatment by local excision alone (HR = 1.82). The effect of radiotherapy was homogeneous across all assessed risk factors (Fig. 45-1D).

We concluded that radiotherapy after local excision for DCIS reduced the risk of LR, with a 47% reduction at 10 years. All patient subgroups benefited from radiotherapy.

EORTC Trial 10801: Mastectomy Versus Breast-Conserving Therapy

Breast-conserving therapy (BCT) has been shown to be as effective as mastectomy in the treatment of tumors up to 2 cm. However, evidence of its efficacy, over the long term, in patients with tumors less than 2 cm was limited at that time. From May 1980 to May 1986, a randomized, multicenter trial comparing BCT with modified radical mastectomy for patients with tumors up to 5 cm was carried out.[3,4] In this analysis, we investigated whether the 2 treatments resulted in different overall survival, time to distant metastasis, or time to locoregional recurrence.

Of the 868 eligible breast cancer patients randomly assigned to the BCT arm or to the modified radical mastectomy arm, 80% had a tumor of 2.1 to 5 cm. BCT comprised lumpectomy with an attempted margin of 1 cm of healthy tissue and complete axillary clearance, followed by radiotherapy to the breast and a supplementary dose to the tumor bed. The median follow-up was 13.4 years. All *p* values are 2 sided.

At 10 years, there was no difference between the 2 groups in overall survival (66% for the mastectomy patients and 65% for the BCT patients; *p* = 0.11) or in distant metastasis-free rates (66% for the mastectomy patients and 61% for the BCT patients; *p* = 0.24). The rates of locoregional recurrence (occurring before or at the same time as distant metastasis) at 10 years did show a statistically significant difference (12% of the mastectomy and 20% of the BCT patients; *p* = 0.01) (Fig. 45-2).

We concluded that BCT and mastectomy resulted in similar survival rates in a trial in which the great majority of the patients had stage II breast cancer. However, a slightly higher local recurrence rate was seen in the BCT arm.

EORTC Trial 22881-10882: The Boost versus No Boost Irradiation After Whole-Breast Irradiation in Stage I and II Breast Cancer

The long-term impact of a boost radiation dose of 16 Gy was investigated in a randomized phase III trial with the following end points: local control, fibrosis, and overall survival for patients with stage I and II breast cancer who underwent breast-conserving therapy.[5,6]

A total of 5318 patients with microscopically complete excision followed by whole-breast irradiation of 50 Gy were randomly assigned to receive either a boost dose of 16 Gy (2661 patients) or no boost dose (2657 patients). At the time of the last analysis, median follow-up was 10.8 years.

The median age was 55 years. Local recurrence was reported as the first treatment failure in 278 patients with no boost versus 165 patients with boost; at 10 years, the cumulative incidence of local recurrence was 10.2% versus 6.2% for the no boost and the boost group, respectively (*p* < 0.0001). The HR of local recurrence was 0.59 (0.46 to 0.76) in favor of the boost, with no statistically significant interaction according to age (Fig. 45-3). The absolute risk reduction at 10 years according

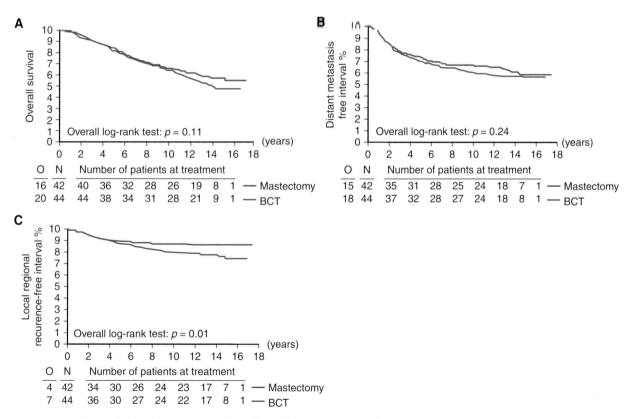

FIGURE 45-2 Randomized clinical trial to assess the value of breast-conserving therapy in stage I and stage II breast cancer (EORTC Trial 10801). Kaplan-Meier curves for **(A)** overall survival, **(B)** distant metastases-free survival, **(C)** locoregional recurrence-free survival in patients with a diagnosis of clinical stage I or II invasive carcinoma of the breast treated with either breast-conserving therapy (BCT) plus breast radiotherapy or with mastectomy. (N, number of patients; O, observed.) *[Reproduced with permission, from Van Dongen JA, Voogd AC, Fentiman IS, et al. Long-term results of a randomized trial comparing breast-conserving therapy with mastectomy: European Organization for Research and Treatment of Cancer 10801 trial. J Natl Cancer Inst. 2000;92(14):1143-1150.]*

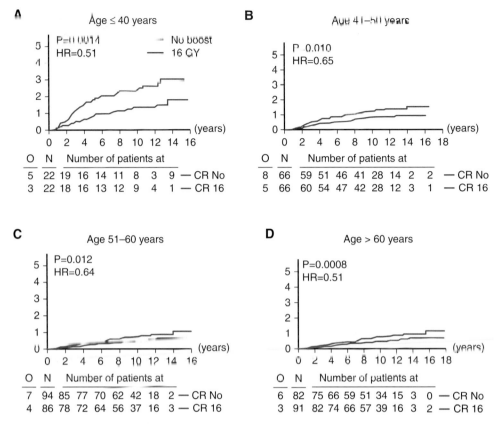

FIGURE 45-3 Phase III study in the conservative management of breast carcinoma by tumorectomy and radiotherapy: assessment of the role of a booster dose of radiotherapy (EORTC Trial 22881-10882): Cumulative incidence of ipsilateral breast cancer recurrence according to age. Age: **(A)** upto 40 years, **(B)** 41 to 50 years, **(C)** 51 to 60 years, and **(D)** more than 60 years. (HR, hazard ratio; N, number of patients at risk; O, occurrences.) *[Reproduced, with permission, from Bartelink H, Horiot JC, Poortmans PM, et al. Impact of a higher radiation dose on local control and survival in breast-conserving therapy of early breast cancer: 10-year results of the randomized boost versus no boost EORTC 22881-10882 trial. J Clin Oncol. 2007;25(22):3259-3265.]*

to age group was the largest in patients ≤40 years of age: 23.9% versus 13.5% (*p* < 0.0014). As a result, the number of salvage mastectomies has been reduced by 41%. Severe fibrosis was statistically significantly increased (*p* < 0.0001) in the boost group, with a 10-year rate of 4.4% versus 1.6% in the no boost group (*p* < 0.0001). Survival at 10 years was 82% in both arms (Fig. 45-3).

We concluded that a boost dose of 16 Gy led to improved local control in all age groups, but no difference in survival was observed.

EORTC Trial 10792: Treatment of Locally Advanced Breast Cancer with Radiotherapy Alone or in Combination with Hormonal and/or Chemotherapy

The long-term contribution of adjuvant chemotherapy (CT) and hormonal therapy (HT) was assessed in patients with locally advanced breast cancer in the EORTC Trial 10792 The impact of time of analysis was also evaluated on the results during accrual and up to 8 years after closure of this randomized phase III trial.[7,8]

Using a factorial design, 410 patients were randomized between radiotherapy (RT) alone, RT plus CT, RT plus HT, and RT plus HT plus CT. The results demonstrated that CT and HT each resulted in a significant prolongation of the time to locoregional tumor recurrence and to distant progression of disease, with the combined treatments providing the greatest therapeutic effect. At the time of trial closure, a significant improvement of survival was observed in patients who received CT (*p* = 0.004); however, with a longer follow-up duration, this effect disappeared (*p* > 0.05). HT did not initially appear to improve survival (*p* = 0.16); however, in the latest analysis with a long-term follow-up duration, a significant improvement of survival was seen (*p* = 0.02). A consistent 25% reduction in the HR of death was seen at all evaluations and since trial closure in patients who received HT. The best survival results were observed in patients who received RT, HT, and CT (*p* = 0.02), with a reduction of 35% in the HR of death (Fig. 45-4).

In summary, this study showed an improvement in survival attributable to HT in patients with locally advanced breast cancer. The greatest therapeutic effect was seen in the treatment group that received both CT and HT. The improvement obtained with HT became apparent only after long-term follow-up evaluation.

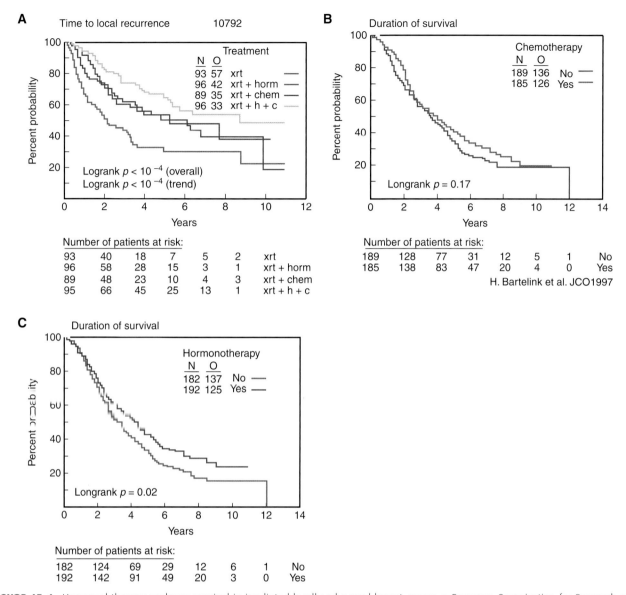

FIGURE 45-4 Hormonal therapy prolongs survival in irradiated locally advanced breast cancer: a European Organization for Research and Treatment of Cancer Randomized Phase III Trial (EORTC Trial 10792). **A.** Time to locoregional recurrence. **B.** Overall survival after yes or no adjuvant chemotherapy. **C.** Overall survival after yes or no adjuvant hormonal therapy. (C, chemotherapy; H, hormonal therapy; N, number of patients at risk; O, occurrences; XRT, radiotherapy.) [*Reproduced, with permission, from Bartelink H, Rubens RD, van der Schueren E, Sylvester R. Hormonal therapy prolongs survival in irradiated locally advanced breast cancer: European Organization for Research and Treatment of Cancer Randomized Phase III Trial. J Clin Oncol. 1997;15(1):207-215.*]

ONGOING TRIALS AND FUTURE DIRECTIONS

The AMAROS Trial: After Mapping of the Axilla Radiotherapy or Surgery of the Axilla

The AMAROS trial is a phase III study comparing axillary lymph node dissection (ALND) with axillary radiation therapy in patients with proven axillary metastasis by sentinel node biopsy (SNB). The main objective is to prove equivalent locoregional control and reduced morbidity for axillary radiation therapy. Additional aims of the study are to analyze technical results of the SNB procedure and to analyze the influence of the different treatment arms on adjuvant treatment decisions.

Patients with operable, unifocal invasive breast cancer (5 to 50 mm) and clinically negative lymph nodes are randomized between ALND and axillary radiation therapy. SNB is performed using the combined technique: radioactive tracer and blue dye. Before a participating institution was allowed to enter patients, it must have performed at least 30 SNB procedures followed by a complete ALND, and it must have been site visited as part of the surgical quality assurance. The identification rate had to be >90% and no more than 1 false-negative result should have been encountered. Quality of life and arm and shoulder function are evaluated yearly. In the ALND arm, at least a level 1 and 2 dissection is performed. The target area for the radiotherapy consists of all 3 levels and the medial supraclavicular fossa. The prescribed dose is 50 Gy in 25 fractions. Adjuvant systemic therapy and radiotherapy are given according to the institutional guidelines. The primary end point is axillary recurrence rate. Assuming a SNB-positive rate of 30%, 4766 patients need to be registered, which is expected to be realized by the end of 2009. Interim analysis of the first 2000 patients showed that the sentinel node identification rate was 97% (range per institute: 89% to 99%), 33% (n = 658) of the patients were SNB positive, 62% (n = 1245) were SNB negative, and 2% (n = 32) had other outcomes (nonaxillary, missing data). In the SNB positive group of 658 patients, the treatment noncompliance was 12%, 314 patients were correctly treated with ALND, and 277 patients were correctly treated with axillary radiation therapy. In the sentinel node positive group, 71% had 1 positive sentinel node. In the ALND arm, nodal involvement was seen in 1 to 3 lymph nodes in 83%, in 4 to 9 lymph nodes in 12%, and more than 9 lymph nodes in 5%. There were no significant differences between the ALND and axillary radiation therapy arm in the administration of adjuvant chemotherapy (both 58%) or adjuvant hormonal therapy (76% vs 71%, respectively). Of the patients treated with ALND, 6% received adjuvant axillary radiation therapy because more than 3 positive lymph nodes were found.

These interim results indicate that with a 97% detection rate in this prospective international multicenter study using the combination of radioactive tracer and blue dye, the sentinel node procedure is highly effective. Furthermore, this analysis shows that there are no major differences in prescribing adjuvant systemic therapy between the two treatment arms and assumes that the administration of adjuvant systemic therapy is mainly based on tumor and patient characteristics and SNB status alone.

Radiation Dose Intensity Study in Breast Cancer in Young Women: A Randomized Phase III Trial of Additional Dose to the Tumor Bed

The previously mentioned boost versus no boost trial showed that young age is an independent factor of LR after BCT. In patients less than 51 years of age, the rate of breast recurrence is decreased by 50% after a dose of 66 Gy to the tumor bed, compared with 50 Gy (no boost). The effect of increased radiation dose seems independent from the delivery of adjuvant systemic treatment. Because the LR for young patients is still quite high (>1% per year), a consecutive trial has been initiated in the Netherlands to investigate whether a higher boost dose will decrease the LR further. This trial will compare the effect of a low boost (16 Gy) versus a high boost (26 Gy) on LR and cosmesis, in patients less than 51 years of age. The second aim of this study is to investigate whether genetic and/or protein profiles can be determined that correlate with LR rate, lymph node metastases, distant metastases and survival, radiosensitivity, and age. Therefore, fresh-frozen tumor tissue and blood samples will be collected for designing mRNA and miRNA profiles. This trial plans to accrue 2400 patients, and it is expected that it will be completed in 2010.

The MINDACT Trial: Microarray in Node-Negative Disease May Avoid Chemotherapy

By using gene-expression profiling, the Netherlands Cancer Institute developed a 70-gene prognostic signature for node-negative breast cancer. The signature was developed as a dichotomous risk classification for the end point of distant metastasis within 5 years. The same group performed a first validation of this gene signature on 295 patients and confirmed that it outperforms all the traditional clinical prognostic factors and clearly separates patients to a group with an excellent prognosis at 10 years and to a group with a high risk of recurrence before 5 years. Furthermore, when compared with current commonly used risk classifications (ie, the St. Gallen guidelines and the National Institutes of Health [NIH] consensus), the 70-gene signature not only predicted those women who would have needed chemotherapy (as demonstrated by the onset of distant metastases within 5 years), but also women who could have been spared adjuvant chemotherapy, as seen from their excellent long-term outcome.[9-11]

The goal of the MINDACT trial is to prospectively validate the 70-gene prognosis signature, providing the level 1 evidence of its utility. This study aims to give us a definitive answer regarding the clinical relevance of the 70-gene signature, its performance compared with traditional prognostic factors, and, as a secondary aim, its ability to predict response to commonly prescribed adjuvant treatments. Using this new tool, MINDACT aims to better define patient prognosis and therefore to better select patients who need adjuvant chemotherapy; by doing so, it is expected that 10% to 20% of women who would normally receive adjuvant chemotherapy based on their clinicopathologic factors will be spared the inconvenience and morbidity of this therapy, without having any negative impact on their survival.

The primary objective of the trial is to confirm that the number of patients that can be safely spared adjuvant chemotherapy is significantly increased when the decision is based on the 70-gene signature rather than on clinicopathologic methods and the critical group of patients who have a high risk of recurrence according to the clinicopathologic criteria but a low risk according to the 70-gene prognosis signature is not undertreated. Because the 70-gene prognosis signature also outperforms traditional prognostic factors in predicting disease outcome in patients with 1 to 3 positive nodes, both patients with node-negative disease and those with 1 to 3 nodes positive are eligible for this trial.

All patients with operable breast cancer 0.5 to 5.0 cm in size 0 to 3 positive nodes are eligible. Before surgery, patients first consent that a part of their cancer is kept for research and microarray analysis. This is the registration phase of the trial. If, after surgery the patient is eligible for the study, consent is asked for the first randomization. Enrolled patients receive their clinical risk classification on the basis of Adjuvant Online! (high versus low clinical risk) and on the basis of the 70-gene signature (genomic high versus low risk). Patients who are concordant to clinical and genomic low-risk prognosis (and who have usually hormone-responsive tumors) are eligible for the hormonal therapy randomization: 7 years letrozole, 2.5 mg daily, versus 2 years tamoxifen, 20 mg daily, followed by 5 years of letrozole. Those patients who have concordant high-risk prognostic estimates will receive chemotherapy (and endocrine treatment if hormone receptor positive) and are eligible for the randomization between: anthracycline-based chemotherapy (including taxanes for node-positive patients) versus a non-anthracycline-containing regimen (docetaxel plus capecitabine). Primary end point is the breast cancer specific disease-free survival at 5 years in the discordant group clinically high/genomic low without chemotherapy (>93%).

The study started early 2007 and by September 2008, 1400 patients are registered and 550 enrolled. After enrollment of the first 800 patients, expected in December 2008, a thorough analysis will be performed on compliance, success of microarray analysis, and so on.

Notably, from all patients, complex 44 K gene arrays and RNA samples are available, allowing for research on predictive factors.

Power Trial: Positive Sentinel Node: Wait and See, Excision, or Radiotherapy

With the introduction of the SNB technique, the pathologic assessment of the sentinel node has increased. Immunohistochemical staining and multistep sectioning of lymph nodes have resulted in the detection of micrometastasis (0.2 to 2 mm) and (sub) micrometastasis (<0.2 mm). The prognostic impact of these sub-micrometastases and the appropriate treatment of these patients remain uncertain. Further nodal involvement in patients with micrometastases is seen in around 20%.[12] The overall false-negative rate of the SNB procedure is a median of 7%, and the axillary recurrence rate is 0.3% (67 of 14,959) after a median follow-up of 34 months.[13,14] These results assume that only 5% of the false-negative lymph node metastasis becomes clinically apparent. So, of the 100 patients with micrometastasis, 20 will have further nodal involvement and 1 will have an axillary recurrence. Because of this limited risk on clinically apparent recurrences, we hypothesized that patients with micrometastases in the sentinel node may be candidates for no further axillary treatment. The morbidity will be reduced by omitting unnecessary treatment and keeping sufficient regional control. The main objective of the trial is to prove less than 2% axillary recurrences at 3 years for patients with proven sub-micrometastases by SNB if axillary treatment is omitted. After finishing patient accrual in the AMAROS trial, this will become the new EORTC sentinel node trial.

SUMMARY

The trials of the EORTC Breast and Radiotherapy group have demonstrated that in patients with DCIS, radiotherapy reduced the ipsilateral breast recurrence rate with nearly a factor of 2 by giving whole-breast irradiation. For stage I and II invasive breast cancer, similar survival rates were observed after mastectomy or breast-conserving therapy. The ipsilateral breast recurrence rate after breast-conserving therapy could be reduced by

a factor of 2 if a boost dose of 16 Gy is given after whole-breast irradiation. This effect appeared to be independent of age. In patients with locally advanced breast cancer, it appeared that with longer follow-up, adjuvant hormonal therapy had a larger effect on survival than adjuvant chemotherapy.

In ongoing trials the possibility of a higher radiation dose in young women is being tested. Further, with the help of gene profiling, attempts are made to predict the sensitivity for adjuvant systemic therapy and radiotherapy to reach an individualized treatment prescription, which is independent from the well-known prognostic factors like grade, tumor size, and lymph node involvement. Finally, innovative investigations are also ongoing to potentially further reduce the toxicity of the treatment of the axilla following sentinel node biopsy.

REFERENCES

1. Julien JP, Bijker N, Fentiman IS, et al. Radiotherapy in breast-conserving treatment for ductal carcinoma in situ: first results of the EORTC randomised phase III trial 10853. *Lancet.* 2000;355(9203):528-533.
2. Bijker N, Meijnen P, Peterse JL, et al. Breast-conserving treatment with or without radiotherapy in ductal carcinoma-in-situ: ten-year results of European Organisation for Research and Treatment of Cancer randomized phase III trial 10853—a study by the EORTC Breast Cancer Cooperative Group and EORTC Radiotherapy Group. *J Clin Oncol.* 2006;24(21): 3381-3387.
3. van Dongen JA, Bartelink H, Fentiman IS, et al. Randomized clinical trial to assess the value of breast-conserving therapy in stage I and II breast cancer, EORTC 10801 trial. *J Natl Cancer Inst Monogr.* 1992;11:15-18.
4. Van Dongen JA, Voogd AC, Fentiman IS, et al. Long-term results of a randomized trial comparing breast-conserving therapy with mastectomy: European Organization for Research and Treatment of Cancer 10801 trial. *J Natl Cancer Inst.* 2000;92(14):1143-1150.
5. Bartelink H, Horiot JC, Poortmans P, et al. European Organization for Research and Treatment of Cancer Radiotherapy and Breast Cancer Groups. Recurrence rates after treatment of breast cancer with standard radiotherapy with or without additional radiation. *N Engl J Med.* 2001;345(19):1378-1387.
6. Bartelink H, Horiot JC, Poortmans PM, et al. Impact of a higher radiation dose on local control and survival in breast-conserving therapy of early breast cancer: 10-year results of the randomized boost versus no boost EORTC 22881-10882 trial. *J Clin Oncol.* 2007;25(22):3259-3265.
7. Rubens RD, Bartelink H, Engelsman E, et al. Locally advanced breast cancer: the contribution of cytotoxic and endocrine treatment to radiotherapy. An EORTC Breast Cancer Co-operative Group Trial (10792). *Eur J Cancer Clin Oncol.* 1989;25(4):667-678.
8. Bartelink H, Rubens RD, van der Schueren E, Sylvester R. Hormonal therapy prolongs survival in irradiated locally advanced breast cancer: a European Organization for Research and Treatment of Cancer Randomized Phase III Trial. *J Clin Oncol.* 1997;15(1):207-215.
9. Bogaerts J, Cardoso F, Buyse M, et al. TRANSBIG consortium. Gene signature evaluation as a prognostic tool: challenges in the design of the MINDACT trial. *Nat Clin Pract Oncol.* 2006;3(10):540-551.
10. Cardoso F, Van't Veer L, Rutgers E, et al. Clinical application of the 70-gene profile: the MINDACT trial. *J Clin Oncol.* 2008;26(5):729-735.
11. Mook S, Schmidt MK, Viale G, et al. On behalf of the TRANSBIG consortium. The 70-gene prognosis-signature predicts disease outcome in breast cancer patients with 1–3 positive lymph nodes in an independent validation study. *Breast Cancer Res Treat.* 2009;116(2):295-302.
12. Cserni G, Gregori D, Merletti F, et al. Meta-analysis of non-sentinel node metastases associated with micrometastatic sentinel nodes in breast cancer. *Br J Surg.* 2004;91:1245-1252.
13. Nieweg OE, Jansen L, Valdés Olmos RA, et al. Lymphatic mapping and sentinel lymph node biopsy in breast cancer. *Eur J Nucl Med.* 1999;26: S11-S16.
14. van der Ploeg IM, Nieweg OE, van Rijk MC, Valdes Olmos RA, Kroon BB. Axillary recurrence after a tumour-negative sentinel node biopsy in breast cancer patients: a systematic review and meta-analysis of the literature. *Eur J Surg Oncol.* 2008;34(12):1277-1284

CHAPTER 46

The UK Experience

Jayant S. Vaidya

The United Kingdom has one of the highest incidences of breast cancer (123 per 100,000 women were diagnosed with breast cancer in 2005) and has historically been home to pioneers of breast cancer treatments.

Without being exhaustive, the trials originating in the United Kingdom over the last century have contributed significantly to improving our understanding about breast cancer and changed practice worldwide. Many of these trials have a story behind them that illustrates how conceptual leaps essential for progress in medicine are taken. The current TARGIT (TARGeted Intraoperative radioTherapy) trial is a story that will be highlighted because it demonstrates the interweaving of various new concepts in the evolution of local treatment of breast cancer.

TRIALS TO REDUCE THE MORBIDITY OF SURGERY

Radical curative surgery for breast cancer was championed by William Halsted in North America and H. Sampson Handley and Gordon-Taylor in the United Kingdom and Europe. David Patey, working in the Middlesex Hospital in London, was one of the first to suggest in 1948 that removal of the pectoralis muscle was not necessary and that local treatment of breast cancer could be achieved without undue morbidity.[1] Several trials were conducted in the latter half of the 20th century including many from the United Kingdom. The number of patients in these trials was small and the concept of statistical power was ill understood. Consequently, although these trials of local therapy demonstrated how the benefit of radiotherapy was a clear reduction in local recurrence rate by two-thirds, most of these trials did not show any survival advantage, thus apparently supporting the Fisher hypothesis that local control does not in any way influence distant disease. This concept was challenged only because of 2 events—the amalgamation of all

trial data so the number of patients was adequate, and the longer follow-up that was almost necessitated by the continuing presence of the Early Breast Cancer Trialists' Collaborative Group (EBCTCG). It was the efforts of EBCTCG's review of randomized previously performed trials that has now conclusively demonstrated that local control influences distant disease, although the puzzle remains why this effect is only modest.

The psychological impact of breast cancer diagnosis and its treatment was long neglected and the studies in the United Kingdom were perhaps pioneering in terms of elucidating the psychological and social effects of a mastectomy compared with breast-conserving surgery, or more recently, axillary clearance compared with sentinel node biopsy.[2-4]

The low sensitivity of clinical examination or any other imaging modality to accurately screen out the negative axilla meant that many patients were having their uninvolved axillary tissue excised unnecessarily along with its posttraumatic morbidity such as lymphedema, numbness, and shoulder restriction. This was demonstrated with a high level of objective evidence by the Edinburgh group,[5] which also championed the concept of a formal 4-node axillary lymph node sampling. In their hands there was no false negative sample and the randomized trial confirmed that the procedure was safe and effective.[6-8] However, this procedure has not become popular, mainly because of the lack of standardization outside of the Edinburgh group, which is partly inherent in the nature of the procedure. Now it appears to have been overtaken by events, although adaptation to the blue dye–guided 4-node sample[9] appears to be an acceptable technique in those centers who do not have access to nuclear medicine services.

The elegant concept of the sentinel node—the existence of a "first" lymph node to drain lymph from the breast—was an anatomical boon to surgeons. It now appeared that at least in part, William Halsted and Handley were right in suggesting the systematic centrifugal march of cancer away from the breast. It was subsequently shown that in at least 90% to 95% of cases, breast cancer behaves in such a systematic manner that we can trace its path using a combination of a technetium labelled radiocolloid and a blue dye injected in the breast. Would it be safe to accept this 5% to 10% false-negative rate? A mathematical model suggests that the potential harm is unlikely to be clinically significant.[10] However, it is considered essential to test the safety of only removing this lymph node in a randomized trial. A randomized trial (N = 298) was launched in Cambridge in November 1999, and reported[11] that Sentinel Lymphy Node Biopsy (SLNB) in patients undergoing surgery for breast cancer results in a significant reduction in physical and psychological morbidity. The larger multicenter ALMANAC (Axillary Lymphatic Mapping Against Nodal Axillary Clearance) trial was launched in the United Kingdom (N = 1031, started in November 1999).[12-14] The unique nature of this trial was the audit phase[12] during which each center had to prove their ability to reliably detect the sentinel node. There have been associated techniques developed in the United Kingdom for needleless injection[15] of the radiocolloid as well as for intraoperative rapid diagnosis using touch imprint cytological diagnosis[16] and molecular biology techniques to detect the presence of cytokeratin-19 and mammaglobin mRNA.[17] These trials have resulted in 2 major changes in clinical practice: (1) that it is practically possible to avoid morbidity of axillary clearance using the technique of sentinel node biopsy and (2) establishment of a unique standardized training and accreditation program for a specific new procedure in surgical oncology. It is reasonable to deduce from the false-negative rate in the ALMANAC trial and mathematical modelling that the false negativity in the procedure is unlikely to be harmful. However, we should be aware that data on recurrence or ultimate survival are yet to come, and while learning the procedure patients should be properly consented with the information about its pros and cons. Reassuring results of these trials means that the local therapies are the least disruptive and women are able to lead a nearly normal life following treatment of breast cancer.

TRIALS OF HORMONE MANIPULATION

Breast cancer was one of the first to be recognized as having a hormonal influence (Table 46-1). Traditionally, the credit for this has been accorded to George Beatson after he wrote in the *Lancet* in 1896.[18,19] In 1876, young George Beatson (1848-1933) was asked to take medical charge of a man whose mind was affected, and went to reside with him at one of his estates in the west of Scotland. As his duties were not onerous, he had a good deal of leisure time to himself and decided that this was a good opportunity for writing his doctor of medicine thesis. He decided the subject to be lactation having observed the weaning of the lambs on a large adjoining sheep farm. At that time, lactation was thought to be controlled from the brain. His studies convinced him that this could not be the case. He also observed that in some countries castration of lactating cows was used to control lactation. He felt that the microscopic changes in the breast during lactation are only a shade different from that seen in a cancer.

Twenty years later, he was faced with a 33-year-old woman who had developed breast cancer during her pregnancy and lactation. After the first surgery the disease had quickly recurred on the chest wall. The only remedy that was being tried for such patients was thyroid extract to which this patient did not respond. Dr Beatson, having properly obtained the patient's consent, performed a bilateral oophorectomy that resulted in a long-lasting (4 years) response. In his second case he only had a partial response and in the last case described in the *Lancet* paper, he did not perform the operation because the patient was postmenopausal and he only gave her thyroid extract. As there was no response in her he concluded that thyroid extract does not have a beneficial effect, while oophorectomy was likely to be beneficial. It is remarkable that it was these 2 cases that inspired the conceptual leap that breast cancer is controlled in a nonneural manner by the ovaries. Stanley Boyd, an English surgeon, published his first 3 cases on October 2, 1897.[20] Importantly, he also used this technique as an adjuvant therapy. His working hypothesis was that "internal secretion of the ovaries in some cases favours the growth of the cancer"[20] and indicated that one-third of breast cancer patients clearly benefited from this approach.[21] His patients were included in the series of 99 cases reported in 1905.[22] The morbidity of the operation was the main stumbling block in the popularization of this approach and it took another 50 years before this concept was tested for the first time in a randomized trial, using nonsurgical methods.

The first trials to test the effectiveness of ovarian ablation either by radiotherapy or by chemical castration were initiated in the United Kingdom. The randomized trial (N = 189), testing

TABLE 46-1 The Evolution of Modern Day Hormonal Control of Breast Cancer

Agent	Initiation	Age Group	Mechanism
Surgical oopherectomy	1890s Beatson	Premenopausal	Complete removal of ovarian influence
Radiation to ovaries	1948 Christie	Premenopausal	Ablation of ovarian function by irradiation
Tamoxifen	1977 NATO	Pre- and postmenopausal	Competitive inhibition (poor agonist) of the ER receptor
Goserelin	1985 ZIPP	Premenopausal	Temporary chemical ovarian ablation with luteinizing hormone releasing hormone agonist
Anastrozole	1995 ATAC	Postmenopausal	Depleting the source of estrogen in postmenopausal women by inhibition of the aromatase enzyme

the role of ovarian ablation with radiotherapy, was initiated at the Christie Hospital in Manchester in 1948.[23,24] In this trial, 450 cGy radiotherapy was used for stopping the ovarian function and it was followed by many other ovarian ablation trials. In 1992, the Early Breast Cancer Trialists' Collaborative Group (EBCTCG) analyzed these ovarian suppression trials and demonstrated, contrary to the general opinion at the time, that ovarian suppression by any means improved survival from breast cancer.[25] The Cancer Research Campaign-Under 50s UK trial, testing the effectiveness of chemical ablation using goserelin, was started in 1987.[26] Goserelin is an agonist of the leutinizing hormone-releasing hormone (LHRH) and effectively blocks its effect, inducing an artificial temporary menopause. The ZIPP study (Zoladex in Premenopausal Patients) was born out of collaboration between the United Kingdom, Sweden, and Italy and compared in a 2×2 factorial design whether addition of goserelin improves disease-free and overall survival when added to standard adjuvant treatment including chemotherapy. The results were unequivocal. After a median follow-up of 5.5 years, ovarian suppression with goserelin for 2 years was well tolerated and improved disease-free survival (hazard ratio [HR] 0.80; 95% CI 0.69–0.92; $p = .002$) and overall survival (HR 0.81; 95% CI 0.67–0.99; $p = .038$) of premenopausal women.

ICI46474, which was to be later called tamoxifen, was developed by the ICI laboratories as an anti-estrogen contraceptive; it was a partial agonist of estrogen. The first presentation of its clinical effects on breast cancer was presented by Mary ("Moya") Patricia Cole,[27] from the Christie Hospital, Manchester. Professor Michael Baum used it in advanced disease and found that it was extremely well tolerated. Being quite convinced of the need to use an "adjuvant" therapy to reduce mortality from breast cancer, he felt that this could be an ideal drug for prolonged use and that it should be tested in a randomized trial. This led to the establishment of the multicenter Nolvadex Adjuvant Tamoxifen Organization (NATO) study (N = 1285) that began recruitment in November 1977. In those days, the general feeling was that hormone therapy merely delayed death without actually reducing mortality. The laboratory evidence that tamoxifen improved disease-free survival after breast cancer in laboratory mice was presented in 1982 at the Surgical Research Society meeting by Mr Alan Wilson.[28] The NATO trial was the first study to report a survival benefit from adjuvant tamoxifen in 1985.[29-32]

The Scottish adjuvant tamoxifen trial was started in 1978 and reported a similar benefit.[33] The effect of these United Kingdom trials was that tamoxifen was adapted as adjuvant treatment in the United Kingdom long before the rest of the world; consequently, the beginning of the fall in breast cancer mortality was first seen in the United Kingdom.

The data from the Scottish trial have been recently used to validate a new mathematical method of estimating what proportion of patients actually benefit from adjuvant therapy (the V-G equation).[34] By merely looking at the conventionally expressed results of a positive randomized clinical trial, it cannot be ascertained whether the additional benefit is distributed to all patients or limited to only a subgroup. We devised a new variance-guided equation to estimate the proportion (p) of the patients in whom a treatment is effective: $p = 1/(1 + [(v(T) -$

$v(C))/(s(T) - s(C))2])$, where v = variance; s = survival; T and C = logarithms of survival times of treated and control groups; variance = (number of events) $\times$ (standard error)^2. This equation was tested with the Scottish adjuvant tamoxifen trial (N = 1323). The trial included a significant number of patients with estrogen receptor (ER)–negative tumors who would not have derived any benefit from tamoxifen. Conveniently, 742 patients in this trial had their ER status ascertained and therefore could be used for validation. The new V-G equation independently predicted— only from the length of survival of individual patients—that 64% of patients in the Scottish trial benefited from tamoxifen, accurately predicting the proportion (60%–71%) of patients whose tumors were ER–positive. This vindication also supports a biologically plausible view that there is a subpopulation of patients among those treated who derive absolutely no benefit, while others may derive a variable amount of benefit. The equation can thus foretell the existence and frequency of a predictive factor (such as ER). Widely applicable to positive randomized clinical trials that have found an overall benefit from chemotherapy, hormone therapy, biologic therapy, or radiotherapy, this equation could suggest new biological and therapeutic insights and enable more precise patient consultation.

It should be noted that the NATO trialists did consider whether ER receptors were important predictors of response to tamoxifen. However, their data led them to conclude that it was probably not an important predictor.[35] They were also heretical and eventually right in trying to use it among premenopausal women because tamoxifen actually increased estrogen levels in these women. They did raise the possibility that a longer duration of treatment may further improve the results. The maturation of the latter idea through other trial results has resulted in 2 other United Kingdom–led trials: ATLAS (Adjuvant Tamoxifen—Longer Against Shorter) and aTTom (adjuvant Tamoxifen Treatment— offer more).

ATLAS is a multicenter international trial led from the Clinical Trial Service Unit and Epidemiological Studies, Oxford. It is testing whether continuation of tamoxifen for 10 years rather than stopping at 5 years provides any additional benefit, without significant harm. The recruitment closed in March 2005, after randomizing 15,252 patients. The preliminary results were presented at the San Antonio Breast Cancer Conference in December 2007 (Peto R, Davies C, on behalf of the ATLAS Collaboration. International randomized trial of 10 versus 5 years of adjuvant tamoxifen among 11 500 women—preliminary results. 30th San Antonio Breast Cancer Symposium: Abstract 48) and suggested a 12% reduction in recurrence, by continuing tamoxifen beyond 5 years. The aTTom results were presented in the ASCO meeting in Chicago in June 2008,[36] along with a meta-analysis of the 20,000 patients in such trials (ATLAS, aTTom, Scottish, ECOG, and the NSABP-14 trials). This suggested a 10% reduction (OR = 0.90, 95% CI 0.84–0.98, $p = .01$) in recurrence of breast cancer by taking 10 years of tamoxifen compared with 5 years. However, this needs to be balanced against the side effects and the current standard duration remains 5 years.

The preventive effect of tamoxifen was first suggested from the data in the CRC-2 trial.[37] This was a 2×2 factorial design trial that tested the benefit of tamoxifen and chemotherapy, alone or in combination. From these data it was spotted that while there was no difference between the chemotherapy arms, tamoxifen significantly reduced the risk of new contralateral breast cancer, prompting the concept of chemoprevention.[38]

Tamoxifen is a remarkably effective drug and has few side effects, and it was many years before an alternative emerged. Anastrozole is an inhibitor of the aromatase enzyme that is essential for peripheral conversion of androgens to estrogen and is responsible for the main source of estrogen in the postmenopausal woman. The ATAC trial was born, literally, on the back of an envelope (Fig. 46-1) during a discussion between Prof. Michael Baum, Prof. Jeffrey Tobias, and Prof. Mitch Dowsett. The ATAC trial compared anastrozole and tamoxifen, alone or in combination, as adjuvant treatment for breast cancer. This trial eventually became the largest adjuvant therapy trial in the world, with 9366 patients randomized into the 3 arms of the trial. The early analysis of the data showed that the patients in the combination arm did

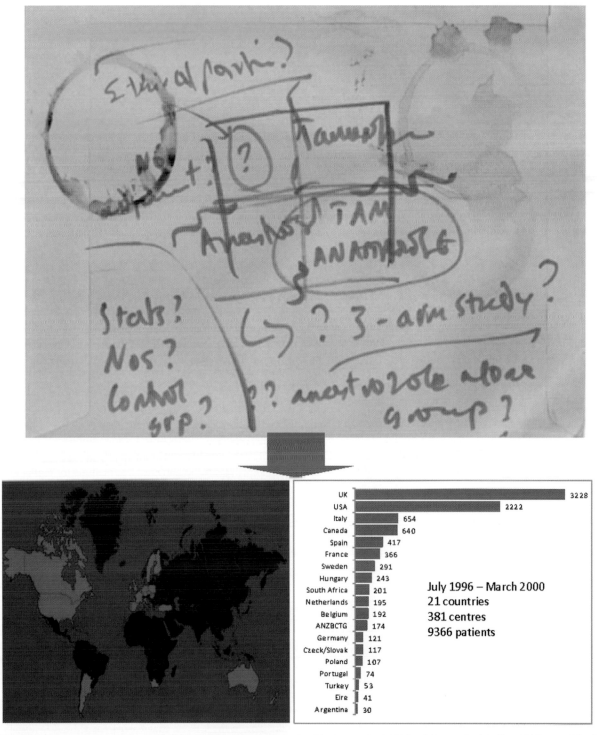

FIGURE 46-1 The envelope (*top*) on which the ATAC trial was conceived between Prof. Michael Baum, Prof. Jeffrey Tobias, and Prof. Mitch Dowsett (*Image courtesy Prof. Jeffrey Tobias*). This led to the largest adjuvant therapy trial that recruited in 21 countries (*bottom*).

not derive any additional benefit, while suffering from the side effects of both the drugs, so this arm has been unblinded and omitted from later analyses. The latest analysis at 100 months follow-up[39] confirmed that the use of anastrozole reduced the risk of relapse—local and distant—and the risk of contralateral breast cancer. However, there was no reduction in overall mortality and it has been suggested that in this aging population, the small difference in mortality may be overshadowed by competing causes of death.

There were several spinoffs from this trial. For example, the Impact study was one of the few studies that could demonstrate that the effectiveness of a drug during the perioperative window to change certain biological parameters (Ki-67 in this case) may predict the ultimate effectiveness of a drug.[40-43] Also, anastrozole was found to reduce the incidence of contralateral breast cancer, leading to the chemoprevention trial IBIS-II,[44-47] which is comparing anastrozole to placebo.

Older women have been perceived to have less aggressive disease and are frequently not fit enough to undergo surgery. This idea prompted many clinicians to use tamoxifen as the primary therapeutic measure and many observational studies yielded positive findings. These findings prompted 3 randomized trials (2 in the United Kingdom[48,49] and an EORTC trial[50]) with the belief that tamoxifen alone may be able to control the disease through a woman's natural lifespan. These trials did not show any survival benefit of surgery, although of course there was a clear benefit of local control. When the clear benefit of adjuvant tamoxifen was shown in the EBCTCG overview, 3 further trials were designed, again—1 European (Group for Research on Endocrine Therapy in the Elderly, GRETA[51]) and 2 in the United Kingdom: the Cancer Research Campaign (CRC)[52,53] and the Nottingham trial.[54] In the latest analysis of the CRC trial it was clearly shown that although tamoxifen is able to control the disease effectively for up to 3 years, breast cancer mortality, overall mortality, and local control are all better when surgery is added to the treatment schedule. This again added to the accumulating data challenging the idea that local control does not influence survival outcome. However, all these studies used 70 as an age cutoff. Even at the time of the trial initiation, the life expectancy at age 70 was 13 years. Tamoxifen alone was unlikely to have long-term control. Only 1 trial used ER receptor to select patients. However, the survival curves did not diverge for the first 3 years, despite having an unselected population in the CRC trial.

Today, we have a large number of older patients who are living longer with several comorbidities. We have drugs better than tamoxifen that are just as easy to use. In the NSABP P024 trial, the overall response rate was 55% for letrozole and 36% for tamoxifen ($p < .001$). Time to progression (in advanced disease) is longer for letrozole—about 1.5 times longer. At 80, the life expectancy is 89, and at 86 it is 92. Looking at it another way, on average, overall survival of women aged 80+ with breast cancer is 72% at 1 year and 58% at 5 years i.e., an estimated 65% at 3 years. Therefore, it is plausible that the hormonal treatment available today may provide good control for this period in a significant enough proportion of women to justify its use as the first-line treatment. This is the subject of the ESTEEM/PAINLESS trials that are hoping to start

recruitment soon. The recent data from the ABCSG-12 study provides support for the addition of zoledronic acid to the medical treatment arm as it may further extend the duration of control.

TRIALS OF CHEMOTHERAPY

Many of the early trials of chemotherapy, albeit not the first, were started in the United Kingdom. In fact, 10 of the 47 trials included in the 1995 overview were from the United Kingdom,[55] providing 21% of patients. More recently, the United Kingdom contributed significantly to the multicenter HERA trial,[56] which exemplified how a biological therapy is brought in successive steps from the bench to the bedside.

TRIALS OF RADIOTHERAPY

The UK trials (the St George's Hospital, Scottish, West Midlands, and the CRC) contributed to the evidence in the EBCTCG overview[57] that radiotherapy after breast-conserving surgery (BCS) was essential and that without it the risk of local recurrence as well as mortality was significantly increased by 29% and 17%, respectively. A note of caution was also published for the first time from the Kings/Cambridge trial. A 10-year analysis of this trial demonstrated a higher risk of death from other causes (cardiac and other cancers) in patients who received radiotherapy after a simple mastectomy on the left side.[58]

By the 1990s the clinical dogma created by the new evidence[59,60] was that BCS plus whole-breast fractioned radiotherapy is the gold standard of treatment. This approach, although "conservative" in name, is still "radical" in spirit—its intent is the same as that of the major extirpative surgery performed by William Halstead over 100 years ago,[61] while we are faced with the irony of offering radical local therapy to patients with smaller and smaller tumors. As we stand on these giants' shoulders, the next step—the real paradigm shift—to a local therapy truly localized to the tumor and its environs in selected patients might be easier.

The United Kingdom has been home to trials of partial breast irradiation. In the Christie hospital trial,[62] 708 patients were randomized to receive either the standard wide field (WF) radiotherapy or a limited field (LF) radiotherapy to the index quadrant. Overall, there was a higher recurrence rate in the latter (LF) arm. In the limited field arm, a constant size of radiotherapy field was used, irrespective of the tumor size, and this could have resulted in several instances of "geographical misses." More importantly, when the results were analyzed according to the type of the primary tumor, it was found that limited field radiotherapy was inadequate only in infiltrating lobular cancers or cancers with extensive intraductal component (EIC). In the 504 cases of infiltrating duct carcinoma, there was no significant difference in the local recurrence rates of the 2 arms.

There were also 2 smaller studies of patients given partial breast irradiation with interstitial implants from the Guy's Hospital and the Ninewells Hospital in Dundee, Scotland.[63] None of the patients in the Scottish series (N = 11) had recurred at the time of publication (median follow up 5.6 years), and in the Guy's Hospital series (N = 27)[64] a single continuous application of an iridium-192 implant delivering 55 Gy over 5 to 6 days replaced the standard radiotherapy regimen including whole breast radiotherapy plus tumor bed boost. The authors found a 20% increase in local recurrence compared with historical controls. However, as discussed in a letter in response to the study,[65] it was pointed out that the biologically effective dose (BED) was 20% lower than conventional radiotherapy and this almost completely explained the difference. In addition 12 out of the 27 patients were node positive and 15 out of the 27 had involved margins, putting these patients at high risk of local recurrence already.

Mastectomy rates around the world vary widely, being influenced by local culture, distance from radiotherapy facilities, the surgeon's choice, and the patient's preferences, not necessarily in that order. For example, within the ATAC trial, the mastectomy rates were 42% in the United Kingdom versus 51% in the United States. The perceived need for having a prolonged course of postoperative radiotherapy is a major barrier against wider acceptance of breast-conserving therapy for several reasons. It adds yet another tiresome 3- to 6-week course of radiotherapy, requiring daily hospital visits, for patients who may already have had a 6- to 9-month course of chemotherapy. The radiotherapy schedule is inconvenient for patients and contributes substantially to the unacceptable waiting lists experienced in many oncology departments worldwide. Many women are forced to choose mastectomy because they live too far away from a radiotherapy facility or have difficulty travelling to one. Even many patients treated with BCS may not receive optimal treatment because of living too far from a radiotherapy center. One study in the United States found that when the travel distance was less than 10 miles, 82% of patients received radiotherapy after BCS; when it was 50 to 75 miles, 69% received it; and when it was more than 100 miles, only 42% received it.[66] (The proportions of patients in these 3 groups receiving BCS including radiotherapy were 39%, 22%, and 14%, respectively.) Further, in countries with scarce radiotherapy resources, patients treated with BCS may wait a prolonged time before beginning radiotherapy. Another study[67] of 7800 patients suggests that delaying the initiation of conventional radiotherapy for 20 to 26 weeks after surgery was associated with decreased survival. The delay imposed by giving chemotherapy before radiotherapy might also increase the risk of local recurrence. When making decisions about which operation to choose, recurrence, radiation therapy, and quick recovery are the main factors women are concerned about.[68] Consequently, if radiation can be completed at the time of the surgery then 2 large concerns will be taken care of and perhaps fewer women will feel obliged to choose mastectomy just because they live far away from a radiotherapy facility[66] or to avoid prolonging their treatment.

It has been estimated that the externally delivered boost dose misses target volume in 24% to 88% of cases.[69,70] Thus, a large proportion of local recurrences could be attributed to this "geographical miss." This could be even more important today in the age of oncoplastic surgery when there is extensive remodelling of the breast performed to achieve a better cosmetic result.

In this situation, it is very difficult to delineate the tumor bed even with markers such as gold seeds. This can result either in complete missing of the target or a "precautionary" overtreatment by enlargement of the boost field. Delivering radiotherapy soon after tumor excision with the TARGIT approach, before remodelling occurs, could ensure that the radiotherapy (boost or alone) is delivered to the correct target.

A delay in delivery of radiotherapy, either because of a long waiting list or because chemotherapy is given first, may jeopardize its effectiveness,[67,71] though this has been difficult to substantiate. I believe that the really important delay may, however, be the one that occurs immediately after surgery. We have found that the tumor bed is a rich microenvironment that promotes proliferation, migration, and invasion.[72-74] Targeting this microenvironment at the right time could be crucially important. I would like to call missing this window of opportunity a "temporal miss" analogous to its spatial counterpart. Finally, whole-breast irradiation carries the risks of acute and long-term complications such as erythema, fatigue, prolonged discomfort, radiation pneumonitis, rib fracture, cardiovascular effects, and carcinogenesis that could compromise the long-term benefit from postoperative radiotherapy.[00,/5]

Recent molecular biology data provide more evidence for the concept of a field defect. The morphologically normal cells surrounding breast cancer demonstrate a loss of heterozygosity, which is often identical to that of the primary tumor.[76] In addition, aromatase activity in the index quadrant is higher than other quadrants[77] and via estrogen has the potential to stimulate mutagenesis, growth, and angiogenesis.[78,79] Patients with ipsilateral breast tumor recurrence (IBTR) have an increased risk of carrying the mutant p53 gene (23% vs 1%),[80] and young patients (<40 years) with IBTR have a disproportionately increased risk (40%) of carrying a deleterious BRCA1/2 gene mutation.[81] This suggests that local recurrence is probably related more to background genetic instability than to different tumor biology at a younger age. It appears that a dynamic interaction between the local factors (such as aromatase) present in the breast parenchyma, the systemic hormonal milieu, and genetic instability will determine the risk of local recurrence, in addition to the biology of the excised primary tumor.

The location of recurrence in the breast with respect to site of the primary tumor shows an interesting distribution. Between 80% and 100% of early breast recurrences occur in the quadrant that had the primary tumor, which is in contrast to the findings of 3-dimensional (3D) analysis of mastectomy specimens,[82] which reveals that 63% of breasts harbor occult cancer foci and 80% of these are situated remote from the index quadrant. It therefore appears that these widespread and occult multifocal/multicentric cancers in other quadrants of the breast remain dormant for a long time and have a low risk of causing clinical tumors. This is corroborated by the fact that although there is a high frequency (20% in young [median age 39] women and 33% in women between 50 and 55) of tumors found in breasts when analyzed in autopsy studies,[83] the frequency of clinical breast cancer in the population is considerably lower.

Arguably, in the EORTC study[84] only 56% of local recurrences are reported to have occurred in the original tumor bed. In fact, a further 27% recurred diffusely throughout the breast including the tumor bed, leaving 29% of recurrences outside the index quadrant. However, patients in this study received intensive mammographic follow-up, which may have unearthed subclinical occult tumors in other quadrants of unproven clinical significance.

Radiotherapy May Affect Both "the Seed" and "the Soil"

It is remarkable that most early local recurrence occurs in the index quadrant, whether or not radiotherapy is given[85-87] and irrespective of clear margins. Of the breast-conserving trials that have tested the effect of radiotherapy, patients in the NSABP-B06,[88] Ontario,[89] Swedish,[90] and Scottish[91] trials had less extensive surgery compared with the Milan III trial.[92] The recurrence rate in the control arm of the Milan III trial, in which the tumors were smaller and excision was considerably wider, was low (8.8% vs 24%-27% in other trials) albeit at the cost of cosmesis. Nevertheless, radiotherapy reduced it even further and at the same proportional rate as in other trials. If local recurrence were caused by residual disease only, then radiotherapy should have effected a much larger proportional reduction in those patients with positive margins or less extensive surgery; but radiotherapy is as effective in patients with negative margins, suggesting that radiotherapy may have an effect on the soil rather than the seed.[93]

Thus, radiotherapy may have a dual effect of inhibiting the growth of genetically unstable cells around the primary tumor and of making the whole breast tissue less conducive to growth.[93] This idea has been supported by translational research in patients undergoing intraoperative radiotherapy (IORT). A study performed at the Centro di Riferimento Oncologico, Aviano, Italy,[74] demonstrated for the first time that radiotherapy could be exerting its beneficial effect via an effect on the tumor microenvironment. We found that the wound fluid collected in the 24 hours following surgical local excision of cancer stimulates breast cancer cell lines to proliferate, migrate, and invade into Matrigel. On the other hand, the fluid collected from wounds that had received targeted IORT did not have such an effect. Thus, if radiotherapy is delivered immediately after the operation using the TARGIT approach, it could be superior to the conventional radiotherapy that suffers from what I call a "temporal miss."

There has been considerable evidence suggesting that surgery may perturb the hormonal milieu in a deleterious manner.[94-98] If IORT is able to locally change the composition of the wound fluid, which essentially derives from the peripheral serum, it is not completely inconceivable that there could be a measurable and important systemic effect of such a treatment. Alternatively, if the mechanism of action of these effects is elucidated with further studies, we may be able to replicate it with a systemic agent that can counter the ill effects of surgery.

Systemic therapies such as aromatase inhibitors or ovarian suppression may achieve a similar effect on the microenvironment through reduction of estrogen concentration in the breast and may have a synergistic effect with radiotherapy.[99] Thus, with increasing use of systemic therapy, IORT to the tissues surrounding the primary tumor might be all that is necessary and such an approach may solve many of the problems of postoperative radiotherapy discussed earlier and may allow many more women with breast cancer to conserve their breast.

Radiobiology of Intraoperative Radiotherapy

The main basis of IORT is that a single dose of IORT could have a biological effect on tissue that is equivalent to a full course of fractionated external beam radiotherapy (EBRT). This is therefore being tested in randomized trials. There is already some evidence suggesting the safety and effectiveness of a single dose of radiotherapy in achieving tumor cell kill.[93,100-102] The theoretical basis for calculation of the biological effects of a given dose of radiation is the linear-quadratic (LQ) model. This model is based on the different shapes of cell survival curves of acute- and late-reacting tissues. It is assumed that large single doses of radiation are more effective on late-responding tissues as compared to acute-reacting tissues. However, the LQ model is reliable for single doses up to 6 to 8 Gy only and may therefore not be appropriate for modelling the effects of higher single doses (~20 Gy), which are used in IORT or radiosurgery.

A detailed analysis of the radiobiological aspects specific to the Intrabeam system is available elsewhere.[103-105] As regards toxicity, the thickness of the chest wall should ensure that virtually no risk of pneumonitis is expected. The same is true for the heart. Since the dose to the heart and lungs during IORT is almost negligible, the mortality from cardiac ischemia that has been observed in some trials using conventional radiation therapy[75,106-108] should not be seen. The calculated low risk of toxicity is in good agreement with the available clinical data from patients treated with TARGIT.[101,109-112] The single-dose radiation using Intrabeam is administered over 25 to 35 minutes. Since normal tissues can repair their DNA within a few minutes, a large proportion of radiation-induced DNA damage is repaired in normal tissues during this long duration of IORT. On the other hand, cancer cells or precancerous cells with poor DNA-repair machinery are unable to do so. Thus, radiation using Intrabeam administered over 25 to 35 minutes would have a high therapeutic index, and would induce less normal tissue damage than similar doses given over 2 to 3 minutes[113,114] as used when electrons are employed (ELIOT trial).

We have developed a mathematical model[115,116] to estimate the effect of a single dose of radiotherapy as given with Intrabeam in the TARGIT trial. We hypothesized that the effectiveness of radiotherapy is influenced by the fact that breast cancers are surrounded by morphologically normal cells that already have loss of heterozygosity in critical genes.[76,117] These cells would be able to repair their DNA in response to fractionated radiotherapy just like normal cells. Continuing survival and subsequent transformation of these cells may be a large factor in development of local recurrence. This mathematical model is the first to offer an explanation for the observation that conventional radiotherapy is not effective in one-third of early breast cancer cases. This proportional reduction in recurrence by conventional radiotherapy (of 66%) is constant across tumor sizes and excision extents. However, when subjected to a single large dose of radiotherapy as in TARGIT, these cells would succumb and thus the source of local recurrence would be eliminated. Furthermore, the radiobiological effect of a single fraction of radiotherapy may actually be paradoxically higher at greater depth.[118]

Recent support from the results of the START trials[119,120] suggested that breast cancer tissue may be more sensitive to fraction size, and delivery in a small number of larger fractions could have a high therapeutic ratio, especially if the dose is being delivered accurately to the target tissues. Thus, the tissues immediately next to the Intrabeam applicator would have a high physical dose with low therapeutic ratio, and those away from the applicator would have lower physical dose but a high therapeutic ratio. This is an advantage of Intrabeam over the systems using electrons to deliver a uniform dose of radiation because its high (physical) dose region is small and it is expected that this would increase acute tumor effects while reducing normal tissue damage and long-term toxicity.

An early demonstration[121] of the immediate efficacy of the irradiation produced by Intrabeam in ablating tumor tissue was in a series of 3 breast cancer patients (T = 1–2.5 cm) who were treated in 1998 through 1999 with a PRS 400 (bare probe only, ie, without the applicators, but with the same Intrabeam machine that is used for IORT). These patients were too frail to have surgery. The tumor was localized on the Fisher Mammotest, a digital stereotactic prone mammography table. The tip of the probe was placed in the center of the tumor and radiation delivered for about 6 to 12 minutes. The tumors, ranging in size from 1 to 2.5 cm, were ablated with a single dose of radiotherapy as demonstrated on biopsy and serial contrast-enhanced magnetic resonance imaging (MRI)

An advantage of the TARGIT approach is that the tissues immediately next to the applicator would receive a high physical dose (with a low therapeutic ratio), and those further away from the applicator would receive a lower physical dose, but with a high therapeutic ratio.[118] This is an advantage of Intrabeam over the systems using electrons to deliver a uniform dose or radiation because its small high (physical) dose region would be expected to increase tumor cell killing while reducing normal tissue damage and long-term toxicity. In contrast, EBRT has a homogeneous dose distribution, and therefore the spatial distribution of the risk of recurrence depends only on the tumor cell density (which is highest close to the excision cavity). One may therefore expect that there is a "sphere of equivalence" around the excision cavity in which the risk of recurrence for IORT is equivalent to that obtained by EBRT.[122,123] The radius of this sphere depends on the applicator size and is about 15 mm for the most often used applicators.

As yet, there is no firmly established standardized IORT dose or dose rate for use in early breast cancer. IORT doses investigated for use in early breast cancer have ranged from 5 to 22 Gy using a variety of different IORT systems. The Intrabeam IORT system delivers a physical dose of 18 to 20 Gy administered to the tumor bed and about 5 to 7 Gy at a distance of 1.0 cm from the breast tumor cavity for a period of 20 to 25 minutes. Using their Novac 7 IORT technology, Veronesi et al have estimated that an external beam dose of 60 Gy delivered

in 30 fractions at 2 Gy per fraction is equivalent to a single IORT fraction of 20 to 22 Gy (using an α/β ratio of 10 Gy, typical for tumors and acute-reacting tissues). The doses delivered by other methods of partial breast irradiation such as intraoperative systems like Novac 7 have been criticized as being large,[124] and while that dose is uniform, the dose distribution delivered using the TARGIT approach theoretically approximates the geographical distribution of risk of recurrence within the breast.

There has been some discussion about the gap between IORT and EBRT when TARGIT is delivered as a boost. From the long-term data it appears that it is safe[110] and effective.[102] It also appears that the gap is necessary to avoid late toxicity[125] and we believe at least a 5- to 6-week gap could be the ideal.

Intraoperative Radiotherapy—an Elegant Method of Partial Breast Irradiation

Modern IORT devices derive benefit from miniaturization technology. No longer do we need to transport the patient to the purpose-built radiotherapy suite—the (mini) radiotherapy suite comes to the patient right in the operating room. The first device to be used for IORT was the Intrabeam (Photoelectron Corporation, Lexington, Massachusetts),[126,127] which is now manufactured by Carl Zeiss AG (Oberkochen, Germany). The 2 other systems of mobile linear accelerators are Mobetron System (Oncology Care Systems Group of Siemens Medical Systems, Intraop Medical Incorporated Santa Clara, California) and the Novac 7 System (Hitesys SPA, Italy). Some of the characteristics of these machines are shown in Table 46-2.[93]

The Intrabeam Machine and Surgical Technique (Fig. 46-2)

The story about the genesis of TARGIT may be worth recounting. In 1996 on my first day of working with Prof. Michael Baum in the Royal Marsden Hospital, I explained to him how my research[82,128] led me to believe that radiotherapy to the index quadrant alone may be adequate. Unknown to me, he had been approached by the manufacturer of the Photon Radiosurgery System about a new miniature radiotherapy device in the making. Professor Baum said to me, "You are at the right time at the right place." I started by writing up the rationale and preparing casts of breast tumor bed to inform us about what the shape of the radiotherapy applicators should be. The radiation oncologist who fully supported this heretical idea was Prof. Jeffrey Tobias. Eventually, after 2 long years, we treated the first pilot patient in July 1998 in an underground operation theatre, almost exactly 50 years after David Patey had promulgated the move from Halsted radical mastectomy to a less mutilating procedure, sparing the pectoralis muscles,[1] in the same Middlesex hospital on Mortimer Street in London. In 1999, I coined the acronym TARGIT as a short form for the procedure as well as the trial before submitting the trial for a review by Lancet.[126]

The Intrabeam machine contains a miniature electron gun and electron accelerator contained in an x-ray tube, which are powered by a 12-V power supply. "Soft" x-rays (50 kVp) are emitted from the point source. Tissue is kept at a distance from

TABLE 46-2 Some Characteristics of Intraoperative Radiotherapy Systems

Device	Randomized Trial	Radiation Type	Dose	Weight	Modification of Operating Room
Intrabeam Carl Zeiss AG, Germany	TARGIT	Soft x-rays at 50 kV	Physical dose of 20 Gy next to. the applicator (with a quick attenuation) over 25-30 minutes. Setting up time is about 10-12 minutes. In theory, the longer duration of treatment could improve therapeutic ratio and reduce late side effects such as fibrosis	1.8 Kg	Not required
Mobetron Intraop Med Inc, USA	—	Electrons at 4-12 MeV	20 Gy physical dose in 3-5 minutes. Setting up time is about 20 minutes.	1275 Kg	Necessary
Novac-7 Hitesys SPA, Italy	ELIOT	Electrons at 4-12 MeV	20 Gy physical dose in 3-5 minutes. Setting up time is about 20 minutes.	650 Kg	Necessary

Adapted from Vaidya JS, Tobias JS, Baum M, et al. Intraoperative radiotherapy for breast cancer. Lancet Oncol 2004;5(3):165-173, with permission.

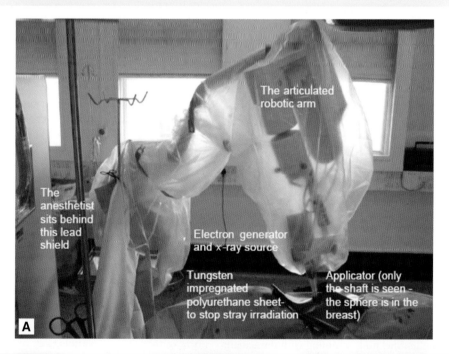

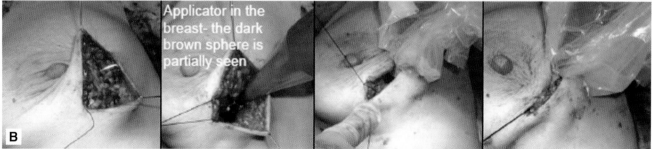

FIGURE 46-2   A. The Intrabeam system with the x-ray source in the wound and the electron generator and accelerator held by the articulated arm. **B.** These images demonstrate how the target breast tissue wraps around the applicator giving true conformal bracyhtherapy.

the source by spherical applicators to give a uniform dose. Various sizes of applicator spheres are available to suit the size of the surgical cavity. The precise dose rate depends on the diameter of the applicator and the energy of the beam, both of which may be varied to optimize the radiation treatment. For example, a dose of 18 to 20 Gy at applicator surface (ie, the tumor bed) can be delivered in about 25 to 35 minutes with a 3.5-cm applicator. The quick attenuation of the radiation minimizes the need for radiation protection to the operating personnel. Usually the operating team leaves the room, but the anesthetist (and anyone else interested in observing the procedure) sits behind a mobile lead shield, which prevents exposure. The technique has been previously described in detail,[129] and an operative video is available from the authors via the Internet (www.targit.org.uk).

In the operating room, wide local excision of the primary tumor is carried out in the usual manner, with a margin of normal breast tissue. After the lumpectomy, it is important to achieve complete hemostasis, because even a small amount of bleeding in the 20 to 25 minutes during which radiotherapy is being delivered can distort the cavity enough to considerably change the dosimetry. Different size applicators are tried until one is found that fits snugly within the cavity. A purse string suture needs to be skilfully placed: it must pass through the breast parenchyma and appose it to the applicator surface, but at the same time it must not bring the dermis too close to the applicator surface. It is important to protect the dermis, which should not be brought within 1 cm of the applicator surface. Fine prolene sutures can be used to slightly retract the skin edge away from the applicator. However, complete eversion of the skin or using self-retaining retractors will increase the separation from the applicator so much that it would jeopardize the radiation dose and risk undertreatment. For skin farther away from the edge that cannot be effectively retracted for fear of reducing the dose to target tissues, a customized piece of surgical gauze soaked in saline, 0.5 to 0.9 cm thick, can be inserted deep into the skin—this allows the dermis to be lifted off the applicator, while the breast tissue just deep to it still receives radiotherapy. If necessary, the chest wall and skin can be protected by radio-opaque tungsten-filled polyurethane material. These thin rubber-like sheets are supplied as caps that fit on the applicator or that can be cut to size from a larger flat sheet on the operating table so as to fit the area of pectoralis muscle that is exposed and does not need to be irradiated. These provide effective (95% shielding) protection to intrathoracic structures. In patients undergoing sentinel node sampling with immediate cytological or histological evaluation (so that complete axillary clearance can be carried out at the same sitting), TARGIT can often be delivered while the surgical team waits for this result without wasting operating room time. With this elegant approach the pliable breast tissue around the cavity of surgical excision wraps around the radiotherapy source (ie, the target is "conformed" to the source). This simple, effective technique avoids the unnecessarily complex techniques of using interstitial implantation of radioactive wires or the even more complex techniques necessary for conformal radiotherapy by external beams with multileaf collimators from a linear accelerator. It eliminates "geographical miss" and delivers radiotherapy at the earliest possible time after surgery. The quick attenuation of the

radiation dose protects normal tissues and allows the treatment to be carried out in unmodified operating theatres. Thus, in theory, the biological effect and cosmetic outcome could be improved.

The surgical part of the TARGIT technique is simple and does *not* require extensive dissection around the breast, separating it from the skin anteriorly and the chest wall posteriorly, which is necessary to give IORT with other devices such as the Novac 7 used in the ELIOT trial (Fig. 46-3). This means that it can be administered even under local anesthetic,[130] especially when it is being given as a second procedure a few days after the primary tumor is excised. This latter approach is useful when it is logistically easier and when the primary operation is not performed at a center equipped with the Intrabeam machine. We have found that about 10% of patients get additional EBRT and about 25% of patients are given TARGIT as a second procedure.

Results of Clinical Trials with Intrabeam System

Based on the hypothesis that index quadrant irradiation is sufficient, in July 1998 we introduced the technique of TARGIT[99,127,131,132] radiotherapy delivered as a single dose using low-energy x-rays, targeted to the peritumoral tissues from within the breast using the Intrabeam device.

In the pilot studies in the United Kingdom, the United States, Australia, Germany, and Italy testing the feasibility and safety of the technique, TARGIT was used as "boost" dose[101,102,133] and patients also received whole-breast EBRT. The median follow-up is 49 months, and the first patient was treated over 10 years ago. This was not a low-risk group. A third of the patients were younger than 51 years, 57% of cancers were between 1 and 2 cm (21% > 2 cm), 29% had a grade 3 tumor, and 29% were node positive. Among these 300 patients, 5 patients have had a local recurrence (5-year actuarial recurrence rate = 1.52% [SE = 0.76%]). This compares favorably with the recurrence rates seen in recent trials of radiotherapy (Table 46-3) despite having a cohort of patients with a worse prognosis. It appears that given as a boost, TARGIT yields very low recurrence rates.

TARGIT is already used as a standard option for the routine tumor bed boost in many centers and is in the 2008 German radiation oncology guidelines. While we recognize that TARGIT boost is at least equivalent to conventional EBRT boost, we believe that there is pathological, biological (geographical and temporal accuracy), mathematical-modelling, and clinical evidence to suggest that it may be superior. Hence, we have recently launched the TARGIT-boost trial aimed at ascertaining whether it yields a lower recurrence rate than EBRT in higher risk (especially young) patients who still suffer a significant (8% to 13%) local recurrence rate.

Some patients during this pilot phase and some patients later on, received TARGIT as the sole modality of radiotherapy.[100] The updated report of such patients who could not otherwise be given EBRT or entered in the TARGIT trial now includes 78 patients[134] with a median follow-up of 2 to 3 years and with excellent local control, giving us reassurance that an inferior result is unlikely. Over 1000 patients have been treated with the

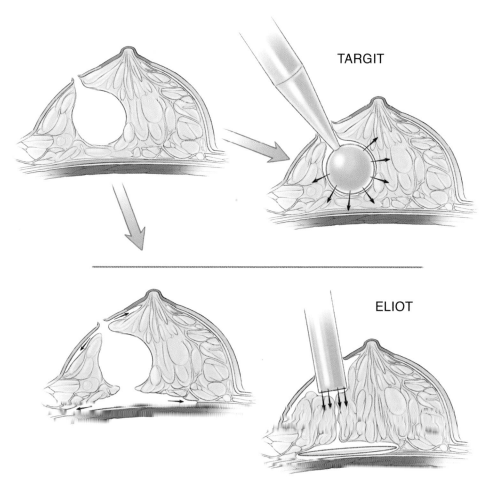

FIGURE 46-3 Difference between the TARGIT (TARGeted Intraoperative radioTherapy) and ELIOT (Electron Intraoperative Therapy) intra-operative radiotherapy techniques.

TARGIT technique. Apart from 2 patients treated early in these studies, wound healing has been excellent. The cosmetic outcome was assessed formally in available patients treated in the United Kingdom at a median follow-up of 42 months by a surgeon and a nurse not involved in the trial.[109] On a scale of 1 to 5 (with 5 being best), mean scores for appearance, texture, and comfort of the breast given by these observers were 3.5, 2.7, and 3.7, respectively. The corresponding scores given by the patient herself were 4, 3.1, and 3.5.

The first patient in the multicenter randomized trial TARGIT[93,124,132,136] using the Intrabeam system was randomized in March 2000 and the trial is now recruiting patients at 29 centers in the United Kingdom, Germany, Italy, Denmark, Poland, Norway, Switzerland, the United States, Canada, and Australia. Over 1850 patients have already been randomized.

In this trial, patients with invasive breast cancer, over the age of 45 and suitable for breast-conserving therapy, are enrolled prior to tumor excision to receive either IORT or conventional whole-breast radiotherapy. Patients with preoperative diagnosis of invasive lobular carcinoma are excluded because these are indicative of a higher risk of recurrence away from the tumor bed. The pragmatic design (Fig. 46-4) of the trial means that if factors such as lobular carcinoma, extensive intraductal compo-nent, and positive margins are found only postoperatively, then

TABLE 46-3 Comparison of TARGIT Boost Results with Recent Clinical Trial Data			
High-Risk Factors	**EORTC Boost**[135]	**START-B Trial**[120]	**TARGIT Boost**[101,102]
Young age	37% (≤50)	21% (<50)	32% (<50)
% >1 cm	75%	86%	78%
% Grade 3	N/A	23%	29%
% Node +	21%	23.6%	29%
Actuarial recurrence rate at 5 years	**4.3%**	**2.8%**	**1.52%**

whole-breast EBRT can be added safely without jeopardizing the trial analysis. In addition, each center can choose (at the outset) to give additional EBRT in patients in whom they feel it is needed (eg, those who are found to have multiple lymph node involvement or extensive lymphovascular invasion). We have found that such an addition of EBRT has occurred in 10% of the ~1300 patients randomized to date. This facility allows pragmatic management of patients with an equipoise that can be decided by every individual center before starting to recruit in the trial. Furthermore, the trial allows the radiotherapy to be delivered at a second procedure, after the final histopathology is available and eligibility criteria are satisfactorily met. Initially, at University College London we were exclusively delivering IORT at the time of the primary operation. Our Australian collaborators administered TARGIT as a second procedure for logistic reasons and found that it is indeed safe. At Dundee, Scotland, for example, both approaches are being used and this allows

recruitment of patients from another hospital that is part of the same NHS trust, but is situated some distance away in Perth.

It is well recognized as in every adjuvant situation that postoperative whole-breast radiotherapy is an overtreatment 60% to 70% of times since only 30% to 40% of patients will ever get a local recurrence after surgery alone. Our approach using IORT intends to refine the treatment of breast cancer patients by introducing a risk-adapted strategy—the elderly patient with a T1 low-grade tumor should perhaps be treated with a different kind of therapy such as TARGIT only, as compared to the young patient with a T2 high-grade tumor who would have a more accurate boost with TARGIT in addition to whole-breast radiotherapy. The TARGIT trial is testing exactly such a strategy. Hence, the TARGIT approach exemplifies a treatment tailored to the patient and her tumor. Delivering IORT with the Intrabeam prolongs the primary operation by 5 to 45 minutes (the shorter extra time when it is performed in conjunction with immediate

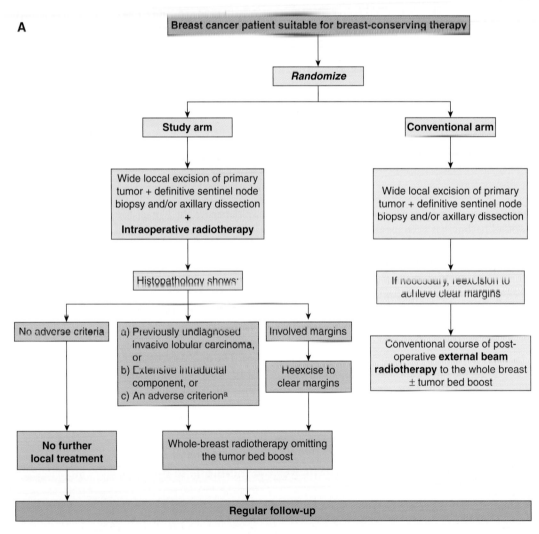

^{a}Decided by each center at the outset—such as grade III, node involvement, lymphovascular invasion, etc.
Adjuvant systemic therapy should be delivered as and when appropriate

FIGURE 46-4 Protocol for entry in the TARGIT trial. **A.** When the primary tumor has not yet been excised. **B.** When the primary tumor has already been excised.

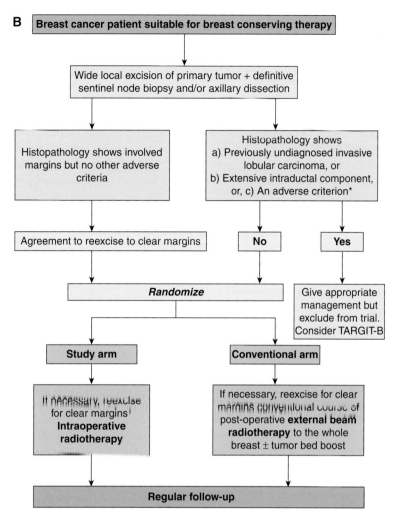

B | Breast cancer patient suitable for breast conserving therapy

Wide local excision of primary tumor + definitive sentinel node biopsy and/or axillary dissection

Histopathology shows involved margins but no other adverse criteria

Histopathology shows
a) Previously undiagnosed invasive lobular carcinoma, or
b) Extensive intraductal component, or, c) An adverse criterion*

Agreement to reexcise to clear margins

No   Yes

Randomize

Give appropriate management but exclude from trial. Consider TARGIT-B

Study arm   **Conventional arm**

If necessary, reexcise for clear margins†
Intraoperative radiotherapy

If necessary, reexcise for clear margins conventional course of post-operative **external beam radiotherapy** to the whole breast ± tumor bed boost

Regular follow-up

* Decided by each center at the outset—such as grade III, node involvement, lymphovascular invasion, etc.
† If reexcision does not achieve clear margins and IORT has already been delivered, then further reexcision to clear margins should be performed followed by EBRT (without boost). Adjuvant systemic therapy should be delivered as and when appropriate.

FIGURE 46-4 (*Continued*)

analysis of the sentinel lymph node). In addition, approximately 1 hour of a radiotherapy physicists' time is needed to prepare the device. External-beam radiotherapy requires about 9 man-hours of planning, 6 hours of radiotherapy room time, and 30 to 60 hours of patient time. If the cost of conventional radiotherapy were £2400, using the most conservative estimates, then considering only the 66% saving of man-hours this novel technique would save £1800 per patient. If we assume that 25% of the 27,000 breast cancer patients diagnosed every year in the United Kingdom might be treated by BCS and IORT instead of conventional EBRT, the yearly savings for the National Health Service would be £12,150,000. This does not include the substantial saving of expensive time on the linear accelerators, which would allow reduced waiting lists—and, most importantly, the saving of time, effort, and inconvenience for patients. Thus, unlike most other "new" treatments, this one may actually be less expensive than the current standard if it proves to be as effective in preventing local and regional breast cancer recurrences.

As I have reiterated before,[93,137] mere novelty and the convenience of this new technology should not submit or inhibit of its proper scientific assessment before it is used for standard care. Randomized clinical trials are essential to test this revolutionary approach. We believe that the future for local treatment of breast cancer could be tailored to the needs of the patient and the tumor. The patient, the surgeon, and the radiation oncologist will be able to choose from several well-tested approaches. This may mean not just wider availability of breast-conserving therapy, but also that small incremental benefits from targeted and tailored treatment may reduce morbidity and even mortality.

Conventional Radiotherapy Scheduling

The START trial was a multicenter trial in the United Kingdom that tested whether a 3-week schedule (15 fractions) was equivalent to the usual 5- to 6-week schedule (START-B). The results of the START-B trial[120] have demonstrated that a 3-week schedule is as good as the conventional longer one and has now supported the increasing popularity of a 3-week course of radiotherapy in the United Kingdom, although this has not been widely adopted elsewhere in the world. Furthermore, the START-A trial[119] also demonstrated that breast tissue is more sensitive to fractionation than previously thought, suggesting that fewer and larger fractions may well be the best way of treating breast cancer. Of course, this ultimately points to the single dose of radiotherapy, which by virtue of being delivered intraoperatively may still maintain its potential advantages in terms of avoiding geographical and temporal misses and reducing the duration from 15 to 20 postoperative fractions to a single intraoperative fraction of radiotherapy, while also retaining its promise of significantly improving the accessibility to breast-conserving surgery in remote areas around the world.

THE SCIENCE OF CLINICAL TRIALS AND THE OXFORD OVERVIEW

Pioneering work (from James Lind to Michael Baum) in the science and promulgation of randomized clinical trials has come from the United Kingdom. James Lind (fellow of the Royal College of Physicians of Edinburgh) is credited with the first modern randomized trial. He performed a trial[138,139] of 6 different treatments, randomly allocated to 2 patients of scurvy each (total 12 patients) and concluded that oranges and lemons were the best treatment, long before the existence of vitamin C was known. R. A. Fisher and A. B. Hill laid the foundation of a randomized clinical trial. Fisher[140] emphasized how randomization is essential to avoid bias in the design and analysis of experiments. Sir Austin Bradford Hill[141] proposed that random assignment of treatments is essential in clinical trials to avoid bias, leading to the first modern randomized trial of streptomycin for pulmonary tuberculosis.[142,143] In the last 60 years, since

the publication of this trial, over 150,000 trials have been published—and perhaps many are unpublished. To learn the truth, first one must learn the extent of uncertainty, and for this we need to collect all available evidence including those trials that were not published either because of unexpected, unpalatable results or for any other reason. This idea of analyzing many trials together was first conceived and illustrated by Prof. Sir Richard Peto in the Oxford overview of clinical trials of breast cancer.

In the 1980s several clinical trials had been published on the use of adjuvant chemotherapy for breast cancer. However, each of the trials was small and had a limited follow-up. Some demonstrated a strikingly positive effect while others showed no effect. This was most puzzling. It was suggested by Prof. Sir Richard Peto that all the trialists meet at Heathrow Airport (not on anyone's home ground) and exchange raw data. Each investigator presented their data on the first day, Sir Richard performed his new meta-analysis, collating all the raw data from 61 randomized trials among 28,896 women, and presented the most remarkable results under the chairmanship of Prof. Michael Baum, to demonstrate for the first time that polychemotherapy and tamoxifen reduce the 5-year mortality after breast cancer surgery.[144] This Early Breast Cancer Trialists' Collaborative Group has since been meeting every 5 years and producing compelling evidence that has changed treatment policies around the world. The latest overview[145] had 144,939 patients from 194 trials with only (estimated) 9% of all worldwide trials being unavailable. Examples of such changes are the following: that ovarian ablation, tamoxifen, and chemotherapy all reduce mortality from breast cancer (Fig. 46-5), that radiotherapy after mastectomy can improve both local relapse as well as survival, and that local control translates into improvement in overall survival by a factor of 1:4 (ie, if a local treatment effectively reduces local recurrence by an absolute value of 20% at 5 years, this translates into a 5% reduction in overall survival at 15 years[146] (Fig. 46-6).

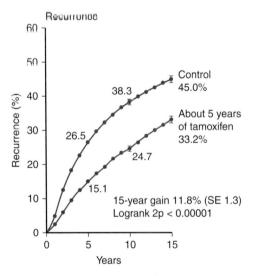

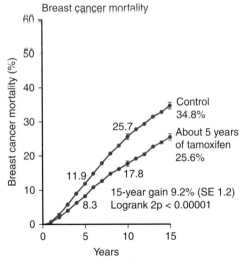

FIGURE 46-5 Five years of tamoxifen versus not in ER-positive (or ER-unknown) disease: 15-year probabilities of recurrence and of breast cancer mortality; 10,386 women. [*Reproduced, with permission, Clarke M, Collins R, Darby S, et al. from Early Breast Cancer Trialists' Collaborative Group. Effects of chemotherapy and hormonal therapy for early breast cancer on recurrence and 15-year survival: an overview of the randomized trials. Lancet. 2005;365(9472):1687-1717.*]

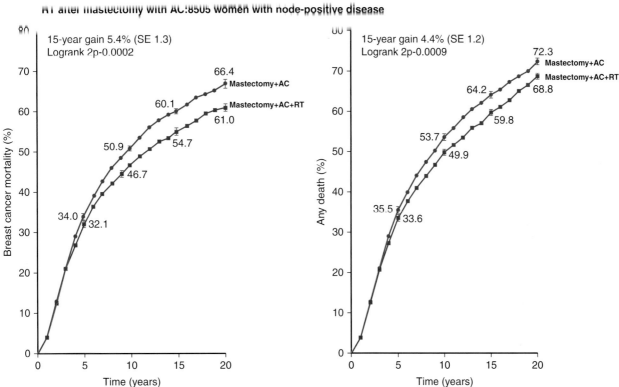

FIGURE 46-6 Effect of radiotherapy (RT) on breast cancer mortality and on all-cause mortality after breast-conserving surgery (BCS) or after mastectomy with axillary clearance (AC). Fifteen-year or 20-year probabilities, vertical lines indicate 1 SE above or below the 5-, 10-, and 15-year percentages. *[Reproduced, with permission, from Clarke M, Collins R, Darby S, et al. Early Breast Cancer Trialists' Collaborative Group (EBCTCG). Effects of radiotherapy and of differences in the extent of surgery for early breast cancer on local recurrence and 15-year survival: an overview of the randomised trials. Lancet. 2005;366(9503):2087-2106.]*

SUMMARY

Breast cancer could be called a pioneer among cancers in terms of stimulating new ideas—not only in terms of basic science but also in terms of breaking new conceptual grounds in the approach to new therapies for cancer. The UK experience has had a fair share in this evolution of paradigms (Fig. 46-7) in terms of its heretic ideas, pragmatic approach, and honest perseverance of the truth. This chapter focused on landmark and fundamental clinical trials of surgery for the breast and axillary lymph nodes; trials of systemic hormonal manipulation and chemotherapy; trials of radiotherapy; and the science of clinical trials including the Oxford Overview Analyses. Currently accruing open trials in Europe are listed in Table 46-4.

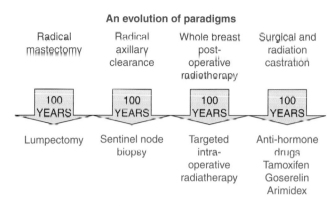

FIGURE 46-7 An evolution of breast cancer treatment paradigms.

TABLE 46-4 Currently Open and Accruing European Breast Cancer Trials

Acronym	Title	Design
ACTION	Adjuvant chemotherapy in older women	Interventional
ACU.FATIGUE	The effectiveness of acupuncture and self-acupuncture in managing cancer-related fatigue in breast cancer patients: a pragmatic randomized trial	Interventional
ALTTO	Adjuvant Lapatinib and/or Trastuzumab Treatment Optimization study: a randomized, multicenter, open-label, phase III study of adjuvant trastuzumab, their sequence and their combination in patients with HER2/ErbB2 positive primary breast cancer	Interventional
AMWELL-SL	An exploratory study to evaluate the use of acupuncture and moxibustion to promote well-being and improve quality of life in patients with secondary lymphedema	Interventional and observational
ATN-224	A Cancer Research UK randomized phase II trial of ATN-224 (copper binding agent) in combination with exemestane vs exemestane alone in post-menopausal women with recurrent or advanced, ER- and/or PR-positive breast cancer	Interventional
B-AHEAD	Randomized comparison of 3 weight control programs during adjuvant treatment for early breast cancer (Breast—Activity and Healthy Eating After Diagnosis)	Interventional
BBC Study	A national population-based study of treatment effect and endocrine, genetic, and cellular risk factors for contralateral primary breast cancer in women in Britain	Observational
BBC-NCRN cohort	British Breast Cancer Study—NCRN cohort	Observational
BEATRICE	An international multicenter open-label 2-arm phase III trial of adjuvant bevacizumab in triple negative breast cancer	Interventional
BETTER-CARE Study	Breast Cancer, Early Disease: Toxicity from Therapy with adjuvant Epirubicin Regimens: Cardiac Assessment and Risk Evaluation Study	Observational
BISMARK	Cost-effective use of BISphosphonates in metastatic bone disease—a comparison of bone MARKer directed zoledronic acid therapy to a standard schedule: The BISMARK Trial	Interventional
BRCA Trial	Breakthrough Breast Cancer and Cancer Research UK Genetic Breast Cancer Trial: A randomized phase II pilot trial of carbopatin compared to docetaxel for patients with metastatic genetic breast cancer	Interventional
BresDex	A decision explorer for women deciding about breast cancer treatments: BresDex	Interventional and observational

(Continued)

TABLE 46-4 Currently Open and Accruing European Breast Cancer Trials (*Continued*)

Acronym	Title	Design
DietCompLyf	The role of diet, complementary treatment, and lifestyle in breast cancer survival	Observational
Effect of lifestyle intervention	The effect of a lifestyle intervention on body weight, psychological health status, and risk factors associated with disease recurrence in women recovering from breast cancer treatment	Interventional
EMBRACE	Epidemiological study of familial breast cancer	Observational
EORTC 10981	After mapping of the axilla—Radiotherapy or Surgery: EORTC 10981-22023	Interventional
ESTEeM	Endocrine with or without Surgical Therapy for Elderly women with Mammary cancer	Interventional
Gem Carbo in breast	A phase II study of carboplatin in combination with gemcitabine as a dose dense schedule in patients with locally advanced or metastatic breast cancer that are resistant to anthracyclines and taxanes	Interventional
GENFABRCA	Genetic factors affecting breast cancer progression	Observational
GLACIER	A study to investigate the Genetics of LobulAr Carcinoma In situ in EuRope	Observational
HER-PCI	Prospective randomized clinical trial testing the role of prophylactic cranial radiotherapy in patients treated with trastuzumab (Herceptin) for metastatic breast cancer	Interventional
IBIS-II DCIS	IBIS-II DCIS: An international multicenter study of anastrozole vs tamoxifen in postmenopausal women with ductal carcinoma in situ (DCIS)	Interventional
IBIS-II Prevention	IBIS-II Prevention: An international multicenter study of anastrozole vs placebo in postmenopausal women at increased risk of breast cancer	Interventional
ICICLE	A study to Investigate the genetiCs of In situ Carcinoma of the ductaL subtypE	Observational
IMPORT LOW	Randomized trial testing intensity modulated and partial organ radiotherapy following breast conservation surgery for early breast cancer	Interventional
IMPORT HIGH	Randomized trial testing dose escalated intensity-modulated radiotherapy in women with higher than average local tumor recurrence risk after breast-conservation surgery and appropriate systemic therapy for early breast cancer	Interventional
Lapatinib Pre-surgical	Lapatinib pre-surgical phase II study in primary breast cancer	Interventional
Lymphedema after axillary node surgery	Identification of women at risk of developing arm swelling (lymphedema) after axillary node surgery	Interventional
MAPLE	A double-blind short term presurgical study to assess the Molecular Antiproliferative Predictors of Lapatinib's™ Effects in primary breast cancer	Interventional
MINDACT	Microarray In Node negative Disease may Avoid ChemoTherapy—A prospective, randomized study comparing the 70-gene expression signature with common clinical-pathological criteria in selecting patients for adjuvant chemotherapy in node negative breast cancer (EORTC Protocol 10041 and BIG 3-04)	Interventional
NeoExcel	Neoadjuvant trial of preoperative exemestane or letrozole +/- celecoxib in the treatment of ER-positive postmenopausal early breast cancer	Interventional
NEOcent	A neoadjuvant study of chemotherapy vs endocrine therapy in postmenopausal patients with primary breast cancer	Interventional
OPTION	Ovarian Protection Trial In Premenopausal Breast Cancer Patients	Interventional
PARP BRCA trial	A Cancer Research UK Phase II Proof of Principle Trial of the activity of the intravenous PARP-1 inhibitor, AG-014699, in known carriers of a BRCA1 or BRCA2 mutation with locally advanced or metastatic breast or advanced ovarian cancer	Interventional
Persephone	Duration of trastuzumab with chemotherapy in women with early stage breast cancer: 6 months vs 12	Interventional
PG-SNPS	The Pharmacogenetics of Early Breast Cancer Chemotherapy (sub-study)	Interventional
POETIC	Trial of Perioperative Endocrine Therapy—Individualizing Care	Interventional

(Continued)

TABLE 46-4 Currently Open and Accruing European Breast Cancer Trials (*Continued*)

Acronym	Title	Design
POSH	Prospective study of Outcomes of treatment in Hereditary vs Sporadic breast cancer	Observational
PRIME II	Postoperative Radiotherapy In Minimum-risk Elderly Phase II	Interventional
REACT	Randomized European Celecoxib Trial: A phase III multicenter double-blind randomized trial of celecoxib vs placebo in primary breast cancer patients	Interventional
RIB	A multicenter randomized trial of single dose Radiotherapy compared to Ibandronate for localized metastatic bone pain	Interventional
SEARCH	A population-based study of genetic predispositions and gene-environment interactions in breast cancer in East Anglia—A population-based study of genetic predisposition and gene-environment interactions in colorectal cancer—A population-based study of genetic predisposition and gene-environment interactions in endometrial cancer—A population-based study of genetic predisposition and gene-environment interactions in ovarian cancer	Observational
SoFEA	Study of Faslodex with or without concomitant Arimidex vs Exemestane following progression on nonsteroidal Aromatase inhibitors	Interventional
SOFT	Suppression of Ovarian Function Trial	Interventional
SUPREMO	Selective use of postmastectomy radiotherapy after mastectomy	Interventional
TACT Trial Long Term QL (sub-study)	TACT Trial Long-Term Quality of Life sub-study	Interventional
TACT2	Trial of Accelerated Adjuvant Chemotherapy with Capecitabine in Early Breast Cancer	Interventional and observational
TARGIT (A)	Targeted intraoperative radiotherapy vs standard postoperative radiotherapy	Interventional
TARGIT (B)	Targeted intraoperative radiotherapy boost vs standard external beam boost	Interventional
TEXT	Tamoxifen and Exemestane Trial	Interventional
TNT	Triple Negative Breast Cancer Trial: A randomized phase III trial of carboplatin compared to docetaxel for patients with metastatic or recurrent locally advanced ER-, PR-, and HER-2- breast cancer	Interventional
ZICE	A randomized, phase III, open-label, multicenter, parallel group clinical trial to evaluate and compare the efficacy, safety profile, and tolerability of oral ibandronate vs intravenous zoledronate in the treatment of breast cancer patients with bone metastases	Interventional
Zoledronate and letrozole study	Short term biological effects of zoledronate and letrozole on invasive breast cancer (preoperative study)	Interventional

REFERENCES

1. Patey DH, DYSON WH. The prognosis of carcinoma of the breast in relation to the type of operation performed. *Br J Cancer.* 1948;2(1):7-13.
2. Fallowfield LJ, Baum M, Maguire GP. Effects of breast conservation on psychological morbidity associated with diagnosis and treatment of early breast cancer. *Br Med J (Clin Res Ed).* 1986;293(6558):1331-1334.
3. Fallowfield LJ, Hall A, Maguire GP, Baum M. Psychological outcomes of different treatment policies in women with early breast cancer outside a clinical trial. *BMJ.* 1990;301(6752):575-580.
4. Fleissig A, Fallowfield LJ, Langridge CI, et al. Post-operative arm morbidity and quality of life. Results of the ALMANAC randomized trial comparing sentinel node biopsy with standard axillary treatment in the management of patients with early breast cancer. *Breast Cancer Res Treat.* 2006;95(3):279-293.
5. Aitken RJ, Gaze MN, Rodger A, Chetty U, Forrest AP. Arm morbidity within a trial of mastectomy and either nodal sample with selective radiotherapy or axillary clearance. *Br J Surg.* 1989;76(6):568-571.
6. Chetty U, Jack W, Prescott RJ, Tyler C, Rodger A. Management of the axilla in operable breast cancer treated by breast conservation: a randomized clinical trial. Edinburgh Breast Unit. *Br J Surg.* 2000;87(2):163-169.
7. Steele RJ, Forrest AP, Gibson T, Stewart HJ, Chetty U. The efficacy of lower axillary sampling in obtaining lymph node status in breast cancer: a controlled randomized trial. *Br J Surg.* 1985;72(5):368-369.
8. Forrest AP, Everington D, McDonald CC, et al. The Edinburgh randomized trial of axillary sampling or clearance after mastectomy. *Br J Surg.* 1995;82(11):1504-1508.
9. Chetty U, Chin PK, Soon PH, Jack W, Thomas JS. Combination blue dye sentinel lymph node biopsy and axillary node sampling: the Edinburgh experience. *Eur J Surg Oncol.* 2008;34(1):13-16.
10. Vaidya JS, Dewar JA, Brown DC, Thompson AM. A mathematical model for the effect of a false-negative sentinel node biopsy on breast cancer mortality: a tool for everyday use. *Breast Cancer Res.* 2005;7(5):225-227.
11. Purushotham AD, Upponi S, Klevesath MB, et al. Morbidity after sentinel lymph node biopsy in primary breast cancer: results from a randomized controlled trial. *J Clin Oncol.* 2005;23(19):4312-4321.

12. Clarke D, Newcombe RG, Mansel RE. The learning curve in sentinel node biopsy: the ALMANAC experience. *Ann Surg Oncol.* 2004;11 (3 Suppl):211S-215S.

13. Fleissig A, Fallowfield LJ, Langridge CI, et al. Post-operative arm morbidity and quality of life. Results of the ALMANAC randomized trial comparing sentinel node biopsy with standard axillary treatment in the management of patients with early breast cancer. *Breast Cancer Res Treat.* 2006;95(3):279-293.

14. Mansel RF, Fallowfield L, Kissin M, et al. Randomized multicenter trial of sentinel node biopsy versus standard axillary treatment in operable breast cancer: the ALMANAC Trial. *J Natl Cancer Inst.* 2006;98(9):599-609.

15. Hyde NC, Prvulovich E, Keshtgar MR. A needle free system for cervical lymphatic mapping and sentinel node biopsy in oral squamous cell carcinoma. *Oral Oncol.* 2002;38(8):797-799.

16. Chicken DW, Kocjan G, Falzon M, et al. Intraoperative touch imprint cytology for the diagnosis of sentinel lymph node metastases in breast cancer. *Br J Surg.* 2006;93(5):572-576.

17. Mansel RE, Goyal A, Douglas-Jones A, et al. Detection of breast cancer metastasis in sentinel lymph nodes using intra-operative real time GeneSearchtrade mark BLN Assay in the operating room: results of the Cardiff study. *Breast Cancer Res Treat.* 2009;115(3):595-600.

18. Beatson GT. On treatment of inoperable cases of carcinoma of the mamma: suggestions for a new method of treatment with illustrative cases. *Lancet.* 1896;2:104-107.

19. Beatson GT. On treatment of inoperable cases of carcinoma of the mamma: suggestions for a new method of treatment with illustrative cases. *Lancet.* 1896; 2:162-165.

20. Boyd S. On oophorectomy in the treatment of cancer. *Br Med J.* 1897;2:890-896.

21. Boyd S. On oophorectomy in cancer of the breast. *Br Med J.* 1900;2:1161-1167.

22. Lett H. An analysis of 99 cases of inoperable carcinoma of the breast treated by oophorectomy. Report of the Royal Medical and Chirurgical Society. *Lancet.* 1905;1122; 778.

23. Paterson R, Russell MH. Clinical trials in malignant disease: part II. Breast cancer; value of irradiation of the ovaries. *J Fac Radiol.* 1959;10: 130-133.

24. Early Breast Cancer Trialists' Collaborative Group. Ovarian ablation for early breast cancer. *Cochrane Database Syst Rev.* 2000;(2):CD000485.

25. Early Breast Cancer Trialists' Collaborative Group. Systemic treatment of early breast cancer by hormonal, cytotoxic, or immune therapy. 133 randomized trials involving 31,000 recurrences and 24,000 deaths among 75,000 women. *Lancet.* 1992;339(8784):1-15.

26. Baum M, Hackshaw A, Houghton J, et al. Adjuvant goserelin in premenopausal patients with early breast cancer: results from the ZIPP study. *Eur J Cancer.* 2006;42(7):895-904.

27. Cole MP, Jones CT, Todd ID. A new anti-estrogenic agent in late breast cancer. An early clinical appraisal of ICI46474. *Br J Cancer.* 1971;25(2): 270-275.

28. Wilson AJ, Tehrani F, Baum M. Adjuvant tamoxifen therapy for early breast cancer: an experimental study with reference to estrogen and progesterone receptors. *Br J Surg.* 1982;69(3):121-125.

29. Baum M, Brinkley DM, Dossett JA, et al. Improved survival among patients treated with adjuvant tamoxifen after mastectomy for early breast cancer. *Lancet.* 1983;2(8347):450.

30. Wilson AJ, Baum M, Brinkley DM, et al. Six-year results of a controlled trial of tamoxifen as single adjuvant agent in management of early breast cancer. *World J Surg.* 1985;9(5):756-764.

31. Baum M, Brinkley DM, Dossett JA, et al. Controlled trial of tamoxifen as single adjuvant agent in management of early breast cancer. Analysis at six years by Nolvadex Adjuvant Trial Organisation. *Lancet.* 1985;1(8433): 836-840.

32. Nolvadex Adjuvant Trial Organisation. Controlled trial of tamoxifen as adjuvant agent in management of early breast cancer. Interim analysis at four years by Nolvadex Adjuvant Trial Organisation. *Lancet.* 1983;1(8319): 257-261.

33. Forrest P, George WD, Preece P, et al. Adjuvant tamoxifen in the management of operable breast cancer: the Scottish Trial. Report from the Breast Cancer Trials Committee, Scottish Cancer Trials Office (MRC), Edinburgh. *Lancet.* 1987;2(8552):171-175.

34. Vaidya JS, Gadgil S. Estimation of the proportion of patients in whom an experimental treatment is effective in a positive randomized trial, using a novel variance-guided equation. *Eur J Cancer Suppl.* 2008;6(7):113-113 doi:10.1016/S1359-6349(08)70536-6.

35. Singh L, Wilson AJ, Baum M, et al. The relationship between histological grade, estrogen receptor status, events and survival at 8 years in the NATO ('Nolvadex') trial. *Br J Cancer.* 1988;57(6):612-614.

36. Gray RG, Rea DW, Handley K, et al. aTTom (adjuvant Tamoxifen—To offer more?): Randomized trial of 10 versus 5 years of adjuvant tamoxifen among 6,934 women with estrogen receptor-positive (ER+) or ER untested breast cancer—Preliminary results. *J Clin Oncol.* 2008;26 (May 20 Suppl):Abstr 513.

37. Baum M, Houghton J, Riley D. Results of the Cancer Research Campaign Adjuvant Trial for Perioperative Cyclophosphamide and Long-Term Tamoxifen in Early Breast Cancer reported at the tenth year of follow-up. Cancer Research Campaign Breast Cancer Trials Group. *Acta Oncol.* 1992;31(2):251-257.

38. Cuzick J, Baum M. Tamoxifen and contralateral breast cancer. *Lancet.* 1985;2(8449):282.

39. Forbes JF, Cuzick J, Buzdar A, et al. Effect of anastrozole and tamoxifen as adjuvant treatment for early-stage breast cancer: 100-month analysis of the ATAC trial. *Lancet Oncol.* 2008;9(1):45-53.

40. Ellis MJ, Tao Y, Luo J, et al. Outcome prediction for estrogen receptor-positive breast cancer based on postneoadjuvant endocrine therapy tumor characteristics. *J Natl Cancer Inst.* 2008;100(19):1380-1388.

41. Dowsett M, Smith IE, Ebbs SR, et al. Prognostic value of Ki67 expression after short-term presurgical endocrine therapy for primary breast cancer. *J Natl Cancer Inst.* 2007;99(2):167-170.

42. Smith IE, Dowsett M, Ebbs SR, et al. Neoadjuvant treatment of postmenopausal breast cancer with anastrozole, tamoxifen, or both in combination: the Immediate Preoperative Anastrozole, Tamoxifen, or Combined with Tamoxifen (IMPACT) multicenter double-blind randomized trial. *J Clin Oncol.* 2005;23(22):5108-5116.

43. Dowsett M, Smith IE, Ebbs SR, et al. Short-term changes in Ki-67 during neoadjuvant treatment of primary breast cancer with anastrozole or tamoxifen alone or combined correlate with recurrence-free survival. *Clin Cancer Res.* 2005;11(2 Pt 2):951s-958s.

44. Baum M. Has tamoxifen had its day? *Breast Cancer Res.* 2002;4(6):213-217.

45. Cuzick J. Aromatase inhibitors in prevention—data from the ATAC (arimidex, tamoxifen alone or in combination) trial and the design of IBIS-II (the second International Breast Cancer Intervention Study). *Recent Results Cancer Res.* 2003;163:96-103.

46. Jenkins VA, Ambroisine LM, Atkins L, et al. Effects of anastrozole on cognitive performance in postmenopausal women: a randomized, double-blind chemoprevention trial (IBIS II). *Lancet Oncol.* 2008;9(10): 913-914.

47. Cuzick J. IBIS II: a breast cancer prevention trial in postmenopausal women using the aromatase inhibitor anastrozole. *Expert Rev Anticancer Ther.* 2008;8(9):1377-1385.

48. Gazet JC, Ford HT, Coombes RC, et al. Prospective randomized trial of tamoxifen vs surgery in elderly patients with breast cancer. *Eur J Surg Oncol.* 1994;20(3):207-214.

49. Kenny FS, Robertson JFR, Ellis IO, Elston CW, Blamey RW. Long-term follow-up of elderly patients randomized to primary tamoxifen or wedge mastectomy as initial therapy for operable breast cancer. *Breast.* 1998;7:335-339.

50. Fentiman IS, Christiaens MR, Paridaens R, et al. Treatment of operable breast cancer in the elderly: a randomized clinical trial EORTC 10851 comparing tamoxifen alone with modified radical mastectomy. *Eur J Cancer.* 2003;39(3):309-316.

51. Mustacchi G, Ceccherini R, Milani S, et al. Tamoxifen alone versus adjuvant tamoxifen for operable breast cancer of the elderly: long-term results of the phase III randomized controlled multicenter GRETA trial. *Ann Oncol.* 2003;14(3):414-420.

52. Fennessy M, Bates T, MacRae K, et al. Late follow-up of a randomized trial of surgery plus tamoxifen versus tamoxifen alone in women aged over 70 years with operable breast cancer. *Br J Surg.* 2004;91(6):699-704.

53. Bates T, Fennessy M, Latteier J, et al. Surgery for early breast cancer improves survival in the elderly: result of a randomized trial of tamoxifen alone versus surgery plus tamoxifen. *Br J Surg.* 2001;88(41) (abstract).

54. Willsher PC, Robertson JFR, Jackson L, et al. Investigation of primary tamoxifen therapy for elderly patients with operable breast cancer. *Breast.* 1997;6:150-154.

55. Early Breast Cancer Trialists' Collaborative Group. Polychemotherapy for early breast cancer: an overview of the randomized trials. *Lancet.* 1998;352(9132):930-942.

56. Piccart-Gebhart MJ, Procter M, Leyland-Jones B, et al. Trastuzumab after adjuvant chemotherapy in HER2-positive breast cancer. *N Engl J Med.* 2005;353(16):1659-1672.

57. Early Breast Cancer Trialists' Collaborative Group. Effects of radiotherapy and of differences in the extent of surgery for early breast cancer on local recurrence and 15-year survival: an overview of the randomized trials. *Lancet.* 2005;366(9503):2087-2106.

58. Haybittle JL, Brinkley D, Houghton J, A'Hern RP, Baum M. Postoperative radiotherapy and late mortality: evidence from the Cancer Research Campaign trial for early breast cancer. *BMJ*. 1989;298(6688):1611-1614.

59. Early Breast Cancer Trialists' Collaborative Group. Effects of radiotherapy and surgery in early breast cancer. An overview of the randomized trials. *N Engl J Med*. 1995;333(22):1444-1455.

60. Early Breast Cancer Trialists' Collaborative Group. Favourable and unfavourable effects on long-term survival of radiotherapy for early breast cancer: an overview of the randomized trials. *Lancet*. 2000;355(9217):1757-1770.

61. Halsted WS. The results of operations for the cure of cancer of the breast performed at The Johns Hopkins Hospital from June 1889 to January 1894. *Johns Hopkins Hospital Reports*. 1894;4:297-350.

62. Ribeiro GG, Magee B, Swindell R, Harris M, Banerjee SS. The Christie Hospital breast conservation trial: an update at 8 years from inception. *Clin Oncol (R Coll Radiol)*. 1993;5(5):278-283.

63. Samuel LM, Dewar JA, Preece PE, Wood RAB. A pilot study of radical radiotherapy using a perioperative implant following wide local excision for carcinoma of the breast. *Breast*. 1999;8(2):95-97.

64. Fentiman IS, Poole C, Tong D, et al. Inadequacy of iridium implant as sole radiation treatment for operable breast cancer. *Eur J Cancer*. 1996;32A(4):608-611.

65. Dale RG, Jones B, Price P. Comments on inadequacy of iridium implant as sole radiation treatment for operable breast cancer, Fentiman et al, *Eur J Cancer*. 1996, 32A, pp 608-611. *Eur J Cancer*, 1997;33(10):1707-1708.

66. Athas WF, Adams-Cameron M, Hunt WC, Amir Fazli A, Key CR. Travel distance to radiation therapy and receipt of radiotherapy following breast conserving surgery. *J Natl Cancer Inst*. 2000;92(3):269-271.

67. Mikeljevic JS, Haward R, Johnston C, et al. Trends in postoperative radiotherapy delay and the effect on survival in breast cancer patients treated with conservation surgery. *Br J Cancer*. 2004;90(7):1343-1348.

68. Katz SJ, Lantz PM, Janz NK, et al. Patient involvement in surgery treatment decisions for breast cancer. *J Clin Oncol*. 2005;23(24):5526-5533.

69. Sedlmayer F, Rahim HB, Kogelnik HD, et al. Quality assurance in breast cancer brachytherapy: geographic miss in the interstitial boost treatment of the tumor bed. *Int J Radiat Oncol Biol Phys*. 1996;34(5):1133-1139.

70. Machtay M, Lanciano R, Hoffman J, Hanks GE. Inaccuracies in using the lumpectomy scar for planning electron boosts in primary breast carcinoma. *Int J Radiat Oncol Biol Phys*. 1994;30(1):43-48.

71. Wyatt RM, Beddoe AH, Dale RG. The effects of delays in radiotherapy treatment on tumor control. *Phys Med Biol*. 2003;48(2):139-155.

72. Massarut S, Baldassare G, Belleti B, et al. Intraoperative radiotherapy impairs breast cancer cell motility induced by surgical wound fluid. *J Clin Oncol*. 2006;24(18S):10611.

73. Baldassarre G, Belleti B, Vaidya JS, et al. Intraoperative radiotherapy (IORT) impairs surgical wound-stimulated breast cancer cell invasion. *J Clin Oncol*. 2007;25(18S):21139.

74. Belletti B, Vaidya JS, D'Andrea S, et al. Targeted intraoperative radiotherapy impairs the stimulation of breast cancer cell proliferation and invasion caused by surgical wounding. *Clin Cancer Res*. 2008;14(5):1325-1332.

75. Rutqvist LE, Johansson H. Mortality by laterality of the primary tumor among 55,000 breast cancer patients from the Swedish Cancer Registry. *Br J Cancer*. 1990;61(6):866-868.

76. Deng G, Lu Y, Zlotnikov G, Thor AD, Smith HS. Loss of heterozygosity in normal tissue adjacent to breast carcinomas. *Science*. 1996;274(5295):2057-2059.

77. O'Neill JS, Elton RA, Miller WR. Aromatase activity in adipose tissue from breast quadrants: a link with tumor site. *Br Med J (Clin Res Ed)*. 1988;296(6624):741-743.

78. Nakamura J, Savinov A, Lu Q, Brodie A. Estrogen regulates vascular endothelial growth/permeability factor expression in 7,12-dimethylbenz (a)anthracene-induced rat mammary tumors. *Endocrinology*. 1996;137(12):5589-5596.

79. Lu Q, Nakmura J, Savinov A, et al. Expression of aromatase protein and messenger ribonucleic acid in tumor epithelial cells and evidence of functional significance of locally produced estrogen in human breast cancers. *Endocrinology*. 1996;137(7):3061-3068.

80. Turner BC, Gumbs AA, Carbone CJ, et al. Mutant p53 protein overexpression in women with ipsilateral breast tumor recurrence following lumpectomy and radiation therapy. *Cancer*. 2000;88(5):1091-1098.

81. Turner BC, Harrold E, Matloff E, et al. BRCA1/BRCA2 germline mutations in locally recurrent breast cancer patients after lumpectomy and radiation therapy: implications for breast-conserving management in patients with BRCA1/BRCA2 mutations. *J Clin Oncol*. 1999;17(10):3017-3024.

82. Vaidya JS, Vyas JJ, Chinoy RF, et al. Multicentricity of breast cancer: whole-organ analysis and clinical implications. *Br J Cancer*. 1996;74(5):820-824.

83. Nielsen M, Thomsen JL, Primdahl S, Dyreborg U, Andersen JA. Breast cancer and atypia among young and middle-aged women: a study of 110 medicolegal autopsies. *Br J Cancer*. 1987;56(6):814-819.

84. Bartelink H, Horiot JC, Poortmans P, et al. Recurrence Rates after Treatment of Breast Cancer with Standard Radiotherapy with or without Additional Radiation. *N Engl J Med*. 2001;345(19):1378-1387.

85. Clark RM, Wilkinson RH, Mahoney LJ, Reid JG, MacDonald WD. Breast cancer: a 21 year experience with conservative surgery and radiation. *Int J Radiat Oncol Biol Phys*. 1982;8(6):967-979.

86. McCulloch PG, MacIntyre A. Effects of surgery on the generation of lymphokine-activated killer cells in patients with breast cancer. *Br J Surg*. 1993;80(8):1005-1007.

87. Clark RM, McCulloch PB, Levine MN, et al. Randomized clinical trial to assess the effectiveness of breast irradiation following lumpectomy and axillary dissection for node-negative breast cancer. *J Natl Cancer Inst*. 1992;84(9):683-689.

88. Fisher B, Anderson S, Redmond CK, et al. Reanalysis and results after 12 years of follow-up in a randomized clinical trial comparing total mastectomy with lumpectomy with or without irradiation in the treatment of breast cancer. *N Engl J Med*. 1995;333(22):1456-1461.

89. Clark RM, Whelan T, Levine M, et al. Randomized clinical trial of breast irradiation following lumpectomy and axillary dissection for node-negative breast cancer: an update. Ontario Clinical Oncology Group. *J Natl Cancer Inst*. 1996;88(22):1659-1664.

90. Liljegren G, Holmberg L, Bergh J, et al. 10-Year results after sector resection with or without postoperative radiotherapy for stage I breast cancer: a randomized trial. *J Clin Oncol*. 1999;17(9):2326-2333.

91. Forrest AP, Stewart HJ, Everington D, et al. Randomized controlled trial of conservation therapy for breast cancer: 6-year analysis of the Scottish trial. Scottish Cancer Trials Breast Group. *Lancet*. 1996;348(9029):708-713.

92. Veronesi U, Luini A, Del Vecchio M, et al. Radiotherapy after breast-preserving surgery in women with localized cancer of the breast. *N Engl J Med*. 1993;328(22):1587-1591.

93. Vaidya JS, Tobias JS, Baum M, et al. Intraoperative radiotherapy for breast cancer. *Lancet Oncol*. 2004;5(3):165-173.

94. Retsky MW, Demicheli R, Hrushesky WJ, Baum M, Gukas ID, Dormancy and surgery-driven escape from dormancy help explain some clinical features of breast cancer. *APMIS*. 2008;116(7-8):730-741.

95. Demicheli R, Retsky MW, Hrushesky WJ, Baum M. Tumor dormancy and surgery-driven interruption of dormancy in breast cancer: learning from failures. *Nat Clin Pract Oncol*. 2007;4(12):699-710.

96. Baum M. Commentary: false premises, false promises and false positives—the case against mammographic screening for breast cancer. *Int J Epidemiol*. 2004;33(1):66-67.

97. Baum M, Houghton J. Contribution of randomized controlled trials to understanding and management of early breast cancer. *BMJ*. 1999;319(7209):568-571.

98. Brown BO, Vaidya JS. Haematogenous dissemination of prostate epithelial cells during surgery does surgery disseminate or accelerate cancer? *Lancet*. 1996;347(8997):325-326.

99. Azria D, Larbouret C, Cunat S, et al. Letrozole sensitizes breast cancer cells to ionizing radiation. *Breast Cancer Res*. 2005;7(1):R156-R163.

100. Vaidya JS, Tobias JS, Baum M, et al. TARGeted Intraoperative radiotherapy (TARGIT): an innovative approach to partial-breast irradiation. *Semin Radiat Oncol*. 2005;15(2):84-91.

101. Vaidya JS, Baum M, Tobias JS, et al. Targeted intraoperative radiotherapy (TARGIT) yields very low recurrence rates when given as a boost. *Int J Rad Oncol Biol Phys*. 2006;66(5):1335-1338.

102. Vaidya JS, Baum M, Tobias JS, et al. Efficacy of targeted intraoperative radiotherapy (Targit) boost after breast conserving surgery: updated results. *J Clin Oncol*. 2008;26:abstr 565.

103. Brenner DJ, Leu CS, Beatty JF, Shefer RE. Clinical relative biological effectiveness of low-energy x-rays emitted by miniature x-ray devices. *Phys Med Biol*. 1999;44(2):323-333.

104. Herskind C, Steil V, Kraus-Tiefenbacher U, Wenz F. Radiobiological aspects of intraoperative radiotherapy (IORT) with isotropic low-energy x-rays for early-stage breast cancer. *Radiat Res*. 2005 Feb;163(2):208-15.

105. Vaidya JS. APBI with targeted intraoperative radiotherapy. In: Wazer DE, Vicini F, Arthur D, eds. *Accelerated Partial Breast Irradiation Techniques and Clinical Implementation*. 2nd ed. Springer Verlag; 2008.

106. Lind DS, Kontaridis MI, Edwards PD, et al. Nitric oxide contributes to adriamycin's antitumor effect. *J Surg Res*. 1997;69(2):283-287.

107. Bates T, Evans RG. Audit of brachial plexus neuropathy following radiotherapy. *Clin Oncol (R Coll Radiol)*. 1995;7(4):236.

108. Meinardi MT, Van Veldhuisen DJ, Gietema JA, et al. Prospective evaluation of early cardiac damage induced by epirubicin-containing adjuvant chemotherapy and locoregional radiotherapy in breast cancer patients. *J Clin Oncol.* 2001;19(10):2746-2753.

109. Vaidya JS, Wilson AJ, Houghton J, et al. Cosmetic outcome after targeted intraoperative radiotherapy (targit) for early breast cancer. *Breast Cancer Res Treat.* 2003;82(S180):1039.

110. Kraus-Tiefenbacher U, Bauer L, Scheda A, et al. Long-term toxicity of an intraoperative radiotherapy boost using low energy x-rays during breast-conserving surgery. *Int J Radiat Oncol Biol Phys.* 2006;66(2):377-381.

111. Kraus-Tiefenbacher U, Bauer L, Kehrer T, et al. Intraoperative radiotherapy (IORT) as a boost in patients with early-stage breast cancer—acute toxicity. *Onkologie.* 2006;29(3):77-82.

112. Joseph DJ, Bydder S, Jackson LR, et al. Prospective trial of intraoperative radiation treatment for breast cancer. *ANZ J Surg.* 2004;74(12):1043-1048.

113. Herskind C, Schalla S, Hahn EW, Hover KH, Wenz F. Influence of different dose rates on cell recovery and RBE at different spatial positions during protracted conformal radiotherapy. *Radiat Prot Dosimetry.* 2006;122(1-4):498-505.

114. Herskind C, Steil V, Kraus-Tiefenbacher U, Wenz F. Radiobiological aspects of intraoperative radiotherapy (IORT) with isotropic low-energy x-rays for early-stage breast cancer. *Radiat Res.* 2005;163(2):208-215.

115. Enderling H, Anderson AR, Chaplain MA, Munro AJ, Vaidya JS. Mathematical modelling of radiotherapy strategies for early breast cancer. *J Theor Biol.* 2006;241(1):158-171.

116. Enderling H, Chaplain MA, Anderson AR, Vaidya JS. A mathematical model of breast cancer development, local treatment and recurrence. *J Theor Biol.* 2007;246(2):245-259.

117. Deng G, Chen LC, Schott DR, et al. Loss of heterozygosity and p53 gene mutations in breast cancer. *Cancer Res.* 1994;54(2):499-505.

118. Astor MB, Hilaris BS, Gruerio A, Varricchione T, Smith D. Preclinical studies with the photon radiosurgery system (PRS). *Int J Radiat Oncol Biol Phys.* 2000;47(3):809-813.

119. Bentzen SM, Agrawal RK, Aird EG, et al. The UK Standardisation of Breast Radiotherapy (START) Trial A of radiotherapy hypofractionation for treatment of early breast cancer: a randomized trial. *Lancet Oncol.* 2008;9(4):331-341.

120. Bentzen SM, Agrawal RK, Aird EG, et al. The UK Standardisation of Breast Radiotherapy (START) Trial B of radiotherapy hypofractionation for treatment of early breast cancer: a randomized trial. *Lancet.* 2008;371(9618):1098-1107.

121. Vaidya JS, Hall-Craggs M, Baum M, et al. Percutaneous minimally invasive stereotactic primary radiotherapy for breast cancer. *Lancet Oncol.* 2002;3(4):252-253.

122. Herskind C, Griebel J, Kraus-Tiefenbacher U, Wenz F. Sphere of equivalence—a novel target volume concept for intraoperative radiotherapy using low-energy x-rays. *Int J Radiat Oncol Biol Phys.* 2008 Dec 1; 72(5): 1575-81.

123. Vaidya JS, Baldassarre G, Massarut S. Beneficial effects of intraoperative radiotherapy on tumor microenvironment could improve outcomes. *Int J Radiat Oncol Biol Phys.* 2009 Jul 1;74(3):976.

124. Pawlik TM, Kuerer HM. Accelerated partial breast irradiation as an alternative to whole breast irradiation in breast-conserving therapy for early-stage breast cancer. *Women's Health.* 2005;1(1):59-71.

125. Wenz F, Welzel G, Keller A, et al. Early initiation of external beam radiotherapy (EBRT) may increase the risk of long-term toxicity in patients undergoing intraoperative radiotherapy (IORT) as a boost for breast cancer. *Breast.* 2008;17(6):617-622.

126. Vaidya JS, Baum M, Tobias JS, Houghton J. Targeted Intraoperative Radiothearpy (TARGIT)-trial protocol. *Lancet.* 1999. Available at: http://www.thelancet.com/journals/lancet/misc/protocol/99PRT-47.

127. Vaidya JS, Baum M, Tobias JS, et al. Targeted intra-operative radiotherapy (Targit): an innovative method of treatment for early breast cancer. *Ann Oncol.* 2001;12(8):1075-1080.

128. Vaidya JS, Vyas JJ, Mittra I, Chinoy RF. Multicentricity and its influence on conservative breast cancer treatment strategy. HongKong International Cancer Congress 1995; Abstract 44.4.

129. Vaidya JS, Baum M, Tobias JS, Morgan S, D'Souza D. The novel technique of delivering targeted intraoperative radiotherapy (Targit) for early breast cancer. *Eur J Surg Oncol.* 2002;28(4):447-454.

130. Vaidya JS, Walton L, Dewar J. Single dose targeted intraoperative radiotherapy (TARGIT) for breast cancer can be delivered as a second procedure under local anaesthetic. *World J Surg Oncol.* 2006;4:2.

131. Vaidya JS, Baum M, Tobias JS, Morgan S, D'Souza D. The novel technique of delivering targeted intraoperative radiotherapy (Targit) for early breast cancer. *Eur J Surg Oncol.* 2002;28(4):447-454.

132. Vaidya JS. A novel approach for local treatment of early breast cancer. PhD Thesis, University of London 2002. Available at: http://www.jayantvaidya.org/.

133. Vaidya JS, Baum M, Tobias JS, et al. Targeted intraoperative radiotherapy (TARGIT) as a boost yields very low recurrence rates. *Breast Cancer Res Treat.* 2005;94:S180.

134. Keshtgar M, Tobias JS, Vaidya JS, et al. Breast cancer patients treated with intra-operative radiotherapy alone when conventional external beam radiation therapy was not possible. *Eur J Cancer Suppl.* 2008;6(7):146-147.

135. Bartelink H, Horiot JC, Poortmans PM, et al. Impact of a higher radiation dose on local control and survival in breast-conserving therapy of early breast cancer: 10-year results of the randomized boost versus no boost EORTC 22881-10882 trial. *J Clin Oncol.* 2007;25(22): 3259-3265.

136. Vaidya JS, Joseph D, Hilaris BS, et al. Targeted intraoperative radiotherapy for breast cancer: an international trial. Abstract Book of ESTRO-21, Prague. 2002;21:135.

137. Vaidya JS, Tobias J, Baum M, et al. Intraoperative radiotherapy: the debate continues. *Lancet Oncol.* 2004;5(6):339-340.

138. Lind J. *A Treatise of the Scurvy. In Three Parts. Containing an Inquiry into the Nature, Causes and Cure, of That Disease. Together with a Critical and Chronological View of What Has Been Published on the Subject.* Edinburgh, UK. Printed by Sands, Murray and Cochran for A Kincaid and A Donaldson; 1753.

139. Lind J. Nutrition classics. A treatise of the scurvy by James Lind, MDCCLIII. *Nutr Rev.* 1983;41(5):155-157.

140. Fisher RA. *The Design of Experiments.* London, UK: Oliver and Boyd; 1935.

141. Hill AB. The clinical trial. *N Engl J Med.* 1952;247(4):113-119.

142. Hill AB, MRCI. Streptomycin treatment of pulmonary tuberculosis. *Br Med J.* 1948;2(4582):769-782.

143. Daniels M, Hill AB. Chemotherapy of pulmonary tuberculosis in young adults; an analysis of the combined results of three Medical Research Council trials. *Br Med J.* 1952;1(4769):1162-1168.

144. Early Breast Cancer Trialists' Collaborative Group. Effects of adjuvant tamoxifen and of cytotoxic therapy on mortality in early breast cancer. An overview of 61 randomized trials among 28,896 women. Early Breast Cancer Trialists' Collaborative Group. *N Engl J Med.* 1988;319(26): 1681-1692.

145. Early Breast Cancer Trialists' Collaborative Group. Effects of chemotherapy and hormonal therapy for early breast cancer on recurrence and 15-year survival: an overview of the randomized trials. *Lancet.* 2005; 365(9472):1687-1717.

146. Clarke M, Collins R, Darby S, et al. Effects of radiotherapy and of differences in the extent of surgery for early breast cancer on local recurrence and 15-year survival: an overview of the randomised trials. *Lancet.* 2005;366(9503):2087-2106.

CHAPTER 47

The Austrian Breast and Colorectal Cancer Study Group Experience

Sebastian F. Schoppmann
Karl Thomanek
Michael Gnant
Raimund Jakesz

The Austrian Breast and Colorectal Cancer Study Group (ABCSG), formerly known as "Cooperative Studiengruppe Mammakarzinom," was established in 1984 as a cooperative institution conducting multicenter clinical trials in breast and colorectal cancer. Since its inception, more than 20,000 patients have been enrolled in some 30 prospective randomized phase III studies. The key scientific treatment issues studied until now in major clinical programs have been (1) adjuvant endocrine therapy for pre- and postmenopausal women, as well as the role of bisphosphonates, and (2) chemotherapy in the neoadjuvant setting. The goal of this chapter is to provide a brief synopsis of the high-impact trials carried out by the ABCSG with respect to breast surgical oncology and to examine their study results in a broader context.

ADJUVANT ENDOCRINE THERAPY IN PREMENOPAUSAL WOMEN

ABCSG Trial 5 (ABCSG-5) and Trial 12 (ABCSG-12) were clinical investigations exploring the efficacy of adjuvant endocrine treatment in premenopausal patients with early-stage breast cancer.

ABCSG-5

Aim and Background

When ABCSG-5 was initiated in 1990, the adjuvant treatment of premenopausal breast cancer patients was considered to be a domain of adjuvant chemotherapy. Yet the fact that premenopausal women responded significantly better to adjuvant chemotherapy than older patients raised the hypothesis that this effect could mainly be mediated through endocrine manipulation rather than being a direct effect of cytostatic action.[1] Supported by initial reports on 2 other modalities tamoxifen (TAM) and ovarian ablation[2,3]—ABCSG-5 was designed to compare the efficacy of combination endocrine treatment with standard chemotherapy.

Study Design

ABCSG-5 randomized patients to receive either 3 years of the luteinizing hormone-releasing hormone analog goserelin (GOS) plus 5 years of TAM or 6 cycles of cyclophosphamide, methotrexate, and fluorouracil (CMF; Table 47-1). The trial subjects were stratified according to their hormone receptor status, tumor stage and grading, number of involved nodes, and type of surgery.

Results of the Study

Results of the final analysis were published in 2002.[4] A total of 1034 assessable patients had completed a 60-month median follow-up period. By that time, 17.2% of patients in the endocrine treatment group and 20.8% of those undergoing chemotherapy had developed relapses. The data showed a significant difference in relapse-free survival (RFS; 81% vs 76%, $p = 0.037$; Fig. 47-1) and local RFS (95% vs 92%, $p = 0.015$) in favor of endocrine therapy. This translated into a 40% increase in the relative risk of

TABLE 47-1 ABCSG Trials of Endocrine Treatment in Hormone Receptor-Positive Premenopausal Patients with Stage I and II Breast Cancer

Criteria	ABCSG-5	ABCSG-12 (BMD Substudy)
Reference	Jakesz et al[4] (2002)	Gnant et al[9] (2008)
Regimen	TAM 20 mg/d, 5a + GOS 3.6 mg every 28 days, 3a vs CMF 600/40/600 × 6 every 4 weeks	TAM 20 mg/d, 3a + GOS 3.6 mg every 28 days, 3a ± ZA 4 mg every 6 months, 3a vs ANA 1 mg/d, 3a + GOS 3.6 mg every 28 days, 3a ± ZA 4 mg every 6 months, 3a
No. of assessable patients	1034	404
Characteristics	pT1-3, N±, G1-3,x	T1a-T4d, N±, G1-3,x
Primary end points	OS, RFS	Change in BMD
Recruitment period	December 1990 to June 1999	June 1999 to May 2006
Median follow-up (months)	60	48

BMD, bone mineral density; CMF, cyclophosphamide, methotrexate, and fluorouracil; GOS, goserelin; OS, overall survival; RFS, recurrence-free survival; TAM, tamoxifen; ZA, zoledronic acid.

experiencing a relapse for patients treated with CMF as compared with those receiving TAM plus GOS (relative risk = 1.4, 95% confidence interval [CI] 1.06–1.87). In summary, ABCSG-5 provided evidence that complete endocrine blockade with GOS and TAM is superior to standard chemotherapy in premenopausal women with hormone-responsive stage I and II breast cancer.

Brought into Context

The data generated with ABCSG-5 correlate well with those from other studies showing that adjuvant endocrine therapy with GOS, either alone or in combination with TAM, is at least as effective as CMF-based chemotherapy in this setting with regard to overall survival (OS) and disease-free survival (DFS).[5,6] These trials finally resulted in a recommendation to use adjuvant endocrine therapy as an alternative to chemotherapy in premenopausal women with hormone-responsive breast cancer in the framework of the consensus guidelines developed at the 2001 International Conference on the Adjuvant Therapy of Primary Breast Cancer in St Gallen.[7]

ABCSG-12

Aim and Background

The rationale for TAM as standard of care for more than 20 years is based on evidence that it reduces the risk of recurrence and improves survival in patients treated for 5 years.[3] However, it is also associated with an increased risk of endometrial cancer and vascular events. Deduced from the data generated with third-generation aromatase inhibitors (AIs) in the adjuvant postmenopausal setting, either as a replacement therapy for or as follow-up to TAM, ABCSG Trial 12 was the first study to investigate the combination of GOS with an AI in premenopausal women. Its objective was to assess the benefit of adjuvant treatment with the combination of GOS plus either TAM or anastrozole (ANA) on DFS and OS in premenopausal patients with hormone-responsive cancer. Due to the observed significant loss of bone mineral density (BMD) associated with AI therapy, a prospectively defined BMD subprotocol was initiated to evaluate the effect of concomitant zoledronic acid (ZA) on BMD.

Study Design

ABCSG-12 was launched in 1999 and finally enrolled a total of 1803 women. Following ovarian suppression with GOS,

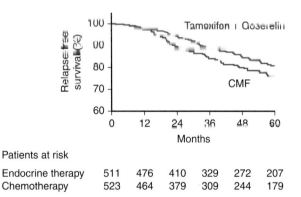

FIGURE 47-1 Kaplan-Meier estimates of relapse-free survival in the group assigned to endocrine therapy (tamoxifen and goserelin) and the group assigned to CMF. Differences were significant (p = 0.037, log-rank test). (*Reprinted with permission from Jakesz R, Hausmaninger H, Kubista E, et al. Randomized adjuvant trial of tamoxifen and goserelin versus cyclophosphamide, methotrexate, and fluorouracil: evidence for the superiority of treatment with endocrine blockade in premenopausal patients with hormone-responsive breast cancer—Austrian Breast and Colorectal Cancer Study Group Trial 5. J Clin Oncol. 2002;20:4621-4627.*)

patients were randomly assigned to 1 of 4 treatment groups and received either TAM ± ZA or ANA ± ZA together with GOS as basic therapy (Table 47-1). Within the bone substudy protocol, BMD was measured at 0, 6, 12, 36, and 60 months in 404 women.

Results of the Study

The first outcome results of ABCSG-12 were presented in the Highlights Plenary Session of the 2008 Annual Meeting of the American Society of Clinical Oncology (ASCO) in Chicago.[8] The full publication appeared in the New England Journal of Medicine in 2009[9], and data showed no significant difference in DFS between ANA and TAM. However, the addition of ZA to endocrine therapy, yielded a reduction of 36% in the risk of disease progression (hazard ratio [HR] = 0.64, 95% CI 0.46-0.91, p = 0.01) at 4 years of follow-up.[9] Mature data deriving from this clinical program thus demonstrate that ZA added to adjuvant endocrine therapy improves outcome in premenopausal patients with endocrine-responsive disease.

In addition, in its first published analysis (at 36 months' follow-up), the substudy assessing ZA for preventing BMD loss already showed a significant degree of loss in patients who received endocrine therapy alone (BMD: 17.3% vs 11.6%, $p < 0.001$) and maintenance in BMD in women who received endocrine therapy plus ZA (BMD 11.4%, $p = 0.001$) as compared to those not given ZA.[10] In the final analysis 2 years after completion of treatment (median follow-up: 48 months), patients not receiving ZA still had decreased BMD ($p = 0.001$, 2-sample t-test), while those receiving ZA had increased BMD ($p = 0.02$, 2-sample t-test) as compared to baseline (Figure 47-2).[11]

Brought into Context

In conclusion, ABCSG-12 showed that significant BMD loss caused by endocrine therapy for premenopausal women with

breast cancer can be effectively inhibited by the administration of ZA. Moreover, the survival data provide evidence that the antitumor activity of adjuvant ZA improves the outcome of premenopausal breast cancer patients beyond the effect of endocrine therapy.

ADJUVANT ENDOCRINE THERAPY IN POSTMENOPAUSAL WOMEN

The objective of the ABCSG-6, ABCSG-6a, and ABCSG-8 (± Arimidex-Nolvadex [ARNO] 95) trials was to evaluate the effect of combined adjuvant endocrine therapy (TAM plus AI) given simultaneously or sequentially for the treatment of endocrine-responsive breast cancer in postmenopausal patients.

n   ABCSG-6 and ABCSG-6a

Aim and Background

Adjuvant endocrine therapy after primary surgery for breast cancer has been shown to reduce the risk of recurrence and increase OS beyond the period of treatment for women with estrogen receptor–positive disease when ABCSG-6 was conducted.[12] Today, the substantial and persistent benefit from adjuvant TAM compared with no adjuvant treatment has been well demonstrated.[13] The intention driving ABCSG-6 was to answer the question whether the results of adjuvant TAM could be improved by the addition of other endocrine agents in an attempt to target TAM-resistant cell clones or perhaps to suppress the partially agonist action shown by TAM.[14] Aminoglutethimide (AG), one of the first AIs that became available for clinical use and shown to be effective in the treatment of postmenopausal women with advanced breast cancer, was used in this study. The follow-up ABCSG-6a trial was an extension of ABCSG-6 that aimed to investigate the efficacy of extended adjuvant therapy with ANA in patients who remained recurrence-free after 5 years of adjuvant TAM.

Study Designs

ABCSG-6 was launched in 1990 and assigned a total of 1986 assessable trial participants to receive either TAM alone for 5 years or TAM in combination with AG for the first 2 years of treatment. ABCSG-6a included 852 patients who had received 5 years of adjuvant TAM with or without AG and who were free of disease by the end of ABCSG-6. These trial participants were re-randomized to receive either 3 years of ANA or no further therapy (Table 47-2).

Results of the Studies

The analysis of 5-year DFS rates between the 2 groups in ABCSG-6 revealed no significant difference (83.6% vs 83.7%, p = 0.89).[15] Similarly, there was no significant difference in 5-year OS between the 2 groups (91.4% vs 91.2%, p = 0.74). In conclusion, this study showed that the application of AG given for 2 years in addition to TAM for 5 years failed to improve the outcomes of postmenopausal patients in this setting. The results of ABCSG-6a in turn demonstrated that women who

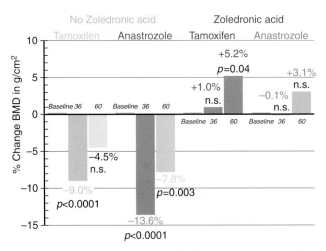

FIGURE 47-2 Percentage change in lumbar spine bone-mineral density from baseline to 36 and 60 months. Patients were randomly assigned to anastrozole or tamoxifen with or without zoledronic acid for 36 months and then no treatment from 36 to 60 months. (*Reprinted with permission from Gnant M, Mlineritsch B, Schippinger W, et al. Endocrine therapy plus zoledronic acid in premenopausal breast cancer. N Engl J Med. 2009;360:679-691.*)

TABLE 47-2 ABCSG Trials of Endocrine Treatment in Hormone Receptor–Positive Postmenopausal Patients with Stage I and II Breast Cancer

Criteria	ABCSG 6	ABCSG-6a	ABCSG-8 (+ ARNO 95)
Reference	Schmid et al[15] (2003)	Jakesz et al[16] (2007)	Jakesz et al[21] (2005)
Regimen	TAM 20 mg/d, 5a* + AG 500 mg/d, 2a† vs TAM 20 mg/d, 5a*	ANA 1 mg/d, 3a vs 0	TAM 20 mg/d, 2a‡ → ANA 1 mg/d, 3a vs TAM 20 mg/d, 5a‡
No. of assessable patients	1986	852	3224
Characteristics	pT1b–pT3a, N±, G1–3,x	pT1–pT3a, N±, G1–3,x	T1–3, N±, G1–3,x
Primary end points	OS, RFS	RFS	EFS
Recruitment period	December 1990 to December 1995	March 1996 to March 2001	January 1996 to June 2004
Median follow-up (months)	63.6	62.3	28

AG, aminoglutethimide; ANA, anastrozole; EFS, event free survival; OS, overall survival; RFS, recurrence-free survival; TAM, tamoxifen.

*TAM given at 40 mg/d for the first 2 years.

†AG loading dose at 250 mg/d for the first week, 375 mg/d for the second week.

‡TAM given at 20 to 30 mg/d in ARNO 95.

received 3 years of ANA as extended adjuvant therapy experienced statistically significantly fewer recurrences than women who did not.[16] The risk of recurrence was reduced by 38% (HR = 0.62, 95% CI 0.40–0.96, p = 0.031), yielding a recurrence rate of 11.8% for patients in the no-further-treatment arm at 10 years after surgery, compared with 7.1% for patients receiving adjuvant treatment with ANA (Fig. 47-3). However, there was no improvement in OS between the 2 study arms, with 55 deaths (11.7%) for the observation arm versus 40 deaths (10.3%) for the ANA arm (HR = 0.89, 95% CI 0.59–1.34, p = 0.570). The data from ABCSG-6a provide further evidence for the benefit of extending adjuvant endocrine therapy beyond 5 years with ANA as compared with no further treatment.

ABCSG-8

Aim and Background

The Arimidex, Tamoxifen, Alone or In Combination trial and other studies have demonstrated the improved efficacy and tolerability of ANA over TAM, and data today support the use of 5 years of ANA as adjuvant therapy for postmenopausal women with early breast cancer.[17] When ABCSG 8 was initiated in 1996, the antiestrogen TAM had been established, for more than 20 years, as the standard endocrine adjuvant therapy after surgery in this setting. Various studies had shown that TAM treatment beyond 5 years could not provide any further benefit.[18,19] Moreover, side effects originating mainly from the partially estrogenic activity of TAM, as well as concerns with possible TAM resistance, led to search for alternative endocrine therapies with increased efficacy and fewer long-term complications.[13,20] The aim of both ABCSG-8 and the Arimidex-Nolvadex (ARNO) 95 trial conducted by the German Adjuvant Breast Cancer Group—data of which were pooled for an analysis in 2005—was to assess whether switching to ANA after 2 years of TAM treatment is more effective then the standard 5 years of adjuvant TAM therapy.

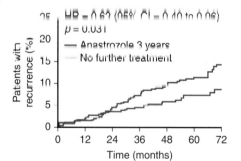

Number at risk:

Anastrozole	386	370	354	332	269	188	96
No further treatment	466	444	418	377	301	201	117

FIGURE 47-3 Kaplan-Meier estimates of recurrence rates in 852 women receiving anastrozole or no further treatment. CI = confidence interval; HR = hazard ratio. (*Reprinted with permission from Jakesz R, Greil R, Gnant M, et al. Extended adjuvant therapy with anastrozole among postmenopausal breast cancer patients: results from the randomized Austrian Breast and Colorectal Cancer Study Group Trial 6a. J Natl Cancer Inst. 2007;99:1845-1853.*)

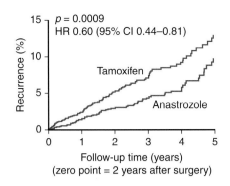

p = 0.0009
HR 0.60 (95% CI 0.44–0.81)

At risk:					
Tamoxifen	1217	858	593	343	176
Anastrozole	1243	874	623	375	178

Estimated percentage recurrence:					
Tamoxifen	2.52	5.37	7.30	9.40	13.16
Anastrozole	1.37	2.88	4.25	5.24	9.72

FIGURE 47-4 Kaplan-Meier estimates of event rates in 3224 women receiving anastrozole or tamoxifen after 2 years of tamoxifen. (*Reprinted with permission from Jakesz R, Jonat W, Gnant M, et al. Switching of postmenopausal women with endocrine-responsive early breast cancer to anastrozole after 2 years' adjuvant tamoxifen: combined results of ABCSG trial 8 and ARNO 95 trial. Lancet. 2005;366:455-462.*)

Study Designs

The combined analysis of ABCSG-8 (2262 patients) and ARNO 95 (962 patients) finally included 3224 postmenopausal women who had completed 2 years of adjuvant TAM (Table 47-2). Patients were randomized to either continue on TAM or to switch to ANA for 3 years.

Results of the Pooled Analysis

At a median follow-up of 28 months, event-free survival (EFS) was higher in patients who had been switched to ANA than those who continued on TAM.[21] The analysis showed a 40% decrease in risk for an event (HR = 0.60, 95% CI 0.44–0.81, *p* < 0.001), with 67 events in the ANA group and 110 events in the TAM group (Fig. 47-4). The EFS rate 3 years after switching was 92.7% for the TAM arm and 95.8% for the patients who had received ANA. A meta-analysis including these 2 studies and the Italian Tamoxifen Anastrozole (ITA) study (448 patients)—another trial with basically the same study design and inclusion criteria—showed that the described clinical benefit in terms of EFS for patients switched to ANA over those in the TAM group translated into a benefit in OS.[22] The final analysis of 4006 eligible patients showed that patients who were switched to ANA had fewer recurrences (92 vs 159) and deaths (66 vs 90) than those who had continued TAM therapy. Patients who had switched to ANA had significant improvements in EFS (HR = 0.55, 95% CI 0.42–0.71, *p* < 0.001), distant RFS (HR = 0.61, 95% CI 0.45–0.83; *p* = 0.002), and OS (HR = 0.71, 95% CI 0.52–0.98, *p* = 0.038) compared with those continuing on TAM therapy.

Brought into Context

The ABCSG-8 study and the combined analyses with the ARNO 95 and ITA trials provided evidence that patients who switch to ANA after 2 to 3 years of TAM have significantly fewer disease recurrences and significant advantages in terms of OS as compared with those who remained on TAM.

NEOADJUVANT CHEMOTHERAPY AND BREAST-CONSERVING SURGERY

Although broadly standardized criteria to determine response are currently lacking, achievement of pathologic complete response (pCR) is considered today to be strongly predictive of DFS and OS benefits. Identifying likely responders to specific therapies may aid in guiding treatment decisions and, wherever possible, may rule out exposure to potential toxicity, thus resulting in improved treatment outcomes. Neoadjuvant (preoperative) chemotherapy is the standard treatment approach for patients with early-stage breast cancer in which cytoreducing/downstaging the primary tumor facilitates breast-conserving surgery (BCS) and decreases the rate of local nodal metastasis.[23-25] The current ABCSG program of neoadjuvant chemotherapy investigations—ABCSG-7, ABCSG-14, and ABCSG-24—was initially influenced by the results gained with early ABCSG clinical trials in adjuvant CMF chemotherapy conducted from 1984 to 1991 and published between 1998 and 2003.[26-28]

ABCSG 7

Aim and Background

Accruing 398 assessable high-risk patients over the 1990s, ABCSG-7 aimed at investigating the long-term prognostic impact of pre- and postoperative chemotherapy with CMF versus exclusively postoperative chemotherapy. Although the study was limited to endocrine nonresponsive women originally, the protocol was amended in 1996 to also include randomization of endocrine-responsive breast cancer patients.

Study Design

In the framework of ABCSG-7, 3 cycles of preoperative CMF were randomly administered to 203 trial participants, and postoperative chemotherapy alone was given to 195 patients (Table 47-3). In the exclusively postoperative treatment arm, node-negative patients were given another 3 cycles of CMF, whereas node-positive patients received 3 cycles of epirubicin and cyclophosphamide.

Results of the Study

The overall response rate to preoperative chemotherapy was 56.2%.[29] Twelve patients (5.9%) experienced pCR. RFS was significantly improved in patients receiving postoperative chemotherapy only (HR = 0.7, CI 0.52–0.96, *p* = 0.024; Fig. 47-5). ABCSG-7 is the first prospective randomized trial to indicate a potential drawback in terms of RFS after preoperative chemotherapy.

Brought into Context

The authors of this study concluded that high-risk breast cancer patients draw an insufficient benefit from preoperative chemotherapy with CMF. This study was limited by the fact that patient selection was inhomogeneous, that the recruitment

TABLE 47-3 ABCSG Trials of Neoadjuvant Chemotherapy in Patients with Breast Cancer

Criteria	ABCSG 7	ABCSG 14	ABCSG 24
Reference	Taucher et al[29] (2007)	Steger et al[30] (2007)	Steger et al[33] (2006)
Regimen	preop CMF 600/40/600 × 3 every 28 days → postop CMF 600/40/600 × 3 every 28 days or EC 70/600 every 3 weeks* vs postop CMF 600/40/600 × 3 every 28 days → postop CMF 600/40/600 × 3 every 28 days or EC 70/600 every 3 weeks*	ED 75/75 × 6 every 21 days + G vs ED 75/75 × 3 every 21 days + G	ED 75/75 + CAP 1000 ± TRAST 6 mg/kg† × 6 every 21 days + G vs ED 75/75 ± TRAST 6 mg/kg† × 6 every 21 days + G
No. of assessable patients	398	288	188‡
Characteristics	cT1–3, N±	T1–4a-c, N±, HER2/neu±	T1–4a-c, N±, HER2/neu±
Stage	I–II	I–III	I–III
Primary end points	OS, RFS	pCR	pCR
Recruitment period	October 1991 to October 1999	June 1999 to December 2002	July 2004 to September 2008
Median follow-up (months)	108	NA	NA

CAP, capecitabine; CMF, cyclophosphamide, methotrexate, and fluorouracil; EC, epirubicin/cyclophosphamide; ED, epirubicin/docetaxel; G, granulocyte-colony stimulating factor; OS, overall survival; pCR, pathological complete response; preop, preoperative; postop, postoperative; RFS, recurrence-free survival; TRAST, trastuzumab.
*CMF was administered to lymph node–negative patients, and EC was administered to lymph node–positive patients.
†TRAST was administered to HER2 positive patients, loading dose cycle 1, 8 mg/kg.
‡Recruitment was completed in October 2008 with 536 patients.

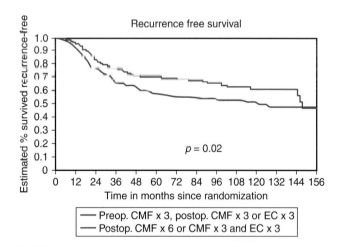

FIGURE 47-5 Recurrence-free survival in 398 patients receiving pre- and postoperative chemotherapy or postoperative chemotherapy alone. (*Reprinted with permission from Taucher S, Steger GG, Jakesz R, et al. The potential risk of neoadjuvant chemotherapy in breast cancer patients: results from a prospective randomized trial of the Austrian Breast and Colorectal Cancer Study Group (ABCSG-07). Breast Cancer Res Treat. 2007;112:309-316.*)

interval exceeded 9 years, and that the chemotherapy used was insufficient by today's standards. Moreover, the results could have been influenced by an imbalance in total chemotherapy given between the 2 groups as a result of nodal downstaging in the preoperative chemotherapy group. Still, the treatment effect in mainly hormone unresponsive patients was shown to be similar to that achieved with endocrine therapy in hormone-responsive patients. Delayed surgery and anthracycline-based chemotherapy are considered to result in shorter RFS but not OS.

ABCSG-14

Aim and Background

The subsequent trial in the ABCSG neoadjuvant treatment program was guided by the hypothesis that pCR to neoadjuvant chemotherapy may be a surrogate of longer OS—a beneficial effect that still remains to be fully established. Therefore, ABCSG-14 explored whether prolonging the number of cycles of neoadjuvant treatment from 3 to 6 could increase the rate of pCR. The rationale behind this strategy is that many patients would be undergoing surgery in the course of an ongoing partial response and that these responses could be translated into pCRs in the presence of prolonged chemotherapy.

Study Design

Patients presenting with biopsy-proven breast cancer were eligible for participation and were randomly assigned to receive either 3 or 6 cycles of epirubicin and docetaxel on day 1 and granulocyte colony-stimulating factor on days 3 through 10 (ED + G; Table 47-3). The primary end point of ABCSG-14 was the pCR rate in the final breast tumor sample (yT0 or yDCIS). Pathologic nodal status after surgery and the BCS rate were secondary end points. A total of 292 patients were accrued, and 288 women were assessable for efficacy and safety analyses.

Results of the Study

As compared with 3 cycles of ED + G—the standard of care at the time in Austria—6 cycles of chemotherapy resulted in a significantly higher pCR rate of 18.6% vs 7.7%, respectively ($p = 0.005$), a higher percentage of women with noninvolved axillary nodes (56.6% vs 42.8%, respectively; $p = 0.02$), as well as a trend toward an increase in BCS (75.9% versus 66.9%, respectively; $p = 0.10$).[30] Rates of adverse events were comparable, and no patients died on treatment. Within the group undergoing 6 cycles of chemotherapy, 76% were suitable for conservative surgery as compared with 67% of patients after 3 cycles, resulting in improved functional and cosmetic outcomes in a higher proportion of women.

Brought into Context

Although no data have been published from randomized trials directly comparable to ABCSG-14, several analyses suggest that a longer period of chemotherapy compares favorably with a shorter treatment.[31,32] In conclusion, ABCSG-14 demonstrated higher rates of pCR and axillary node negativity—with no excess of adverse events—by prolonging the number of neoadjuvant ED + G cycles from 3 to 6. Six cycles of ED + G are therefore currently considered the standard of neoadjuvant treatment for operable breast cancer when using this combination chemotherapy and have served as the basis for the concept guiding the current ABCSG Trial 24. This trial was designed to evaluate the additional impact of capecitabine on pCR within an ED ± trastuzumab treatment strategy (Table 47-3); a recent interim analysis showed no major safety concerns.[33]

■ Breast-Conserving Surgery

Aim and Background

As mentioned previously, the future of neoadjuvant therapy lies in tailoring treatment to individuals by identifying response predictors and developing novel agents. Survival rates in breast cancer patients have variously been shown to depend on stage and not on the extent of surgical breast tissue removal, as long as resection margins are free of tumor infiltration. The objective of a retrospective analysis carried out by the ABCSG in 2003 was to confirm evidence that BCS does not impair the prognosis in breast cancer patients as compared with mastectomy.[34]

Study Design

Six different ABCSG clinical trials accrued a total of 4259 women with hormone-responsive disease between 1984 and 1997.

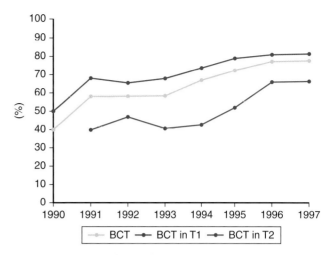

FIGURE 47-6 Surgical procedures in 1202 postmenopausal patients with lymph node metastases. (*Reprinted with permission from Jakesz R, Samonigg H, Gnant M, et al. Significant increase in breast conservation in 16 years of trials conducted by the Austrian Breast and Colorectal Cancer Study Group. Ann Surg. 2003;237:556-564.*)

From these patients, the authors selected and compared 3 groups (n = 3316) according to age, pathologic stage, and the surgical procedure used.

Results of the Study

During the time interval, the BCS rate in the premenopausal node-positive subgroup (n = 447) was highly significantly increased from 27.2% to 73.2% overall ($p < 0.001$). In the group of postmenopausal node-negative women (n = 1667), the BCS rate increased significantly from 40% to 77.3% ($p < 0.001$; Fig. 47-6).[34] Finally, with an overall BCS rate increasing from 22.5% to 56.8% in postmenopausal node-positive patients (n = 1202), those presenting with T1 tumors experienced a significant increase in BCS rates from 35.1% to 65.9% ($p < 0.001$). Over time, the death and local recurrence rates were stable or even decreased substantially in all subgroups.

Brought into Context

This analysis demonstrated significant increases in the rate of BCS procedures over a 16-year period, which in no way were counterbalanced by higher local recurrence or mortality rates. Within the context of this nonrandomized comparison, the ABSCG has thus demonstrated BCS to be a safe standard of care for T1 and increasingly for T2 breast tumors.

SUMMARY

In 2009, the ABCSG looks back on nearly a quarter century's theoretical and empirical evolution through various series of concepts in the treatment of early-stage breast cancer. In premenopausal hormone-responsive patients, the path has led from the use of higher- and lower-dose alkylation-antimetabolite chemotherapy to endocrine treatment strategies based on TAM and luteinizing hormone-releasing hormone, and to the important inclusion of AIs and bisphosphonates. In the postmenopausal hormone-responsive setting, the need to move on with the development of novel AIs has become clearer, as well as the superiority of switching treatment modalities with these agents. In the domain of neoadjuvant chemotherapy approaches, we have shown evidence for the substantial efficacy of anthracycline-taxane combination therapy and are looking forward to potential additional benefits by including antimetabolites and monoclonal antibodies (MAb).

Structured upon these insights, the current ABCSG portfolio includes investigations into extended nonsteroidal AIs, MAb, and estrogen receptor antagonist strategies for hormone-responsive postmenopausal patients, in addition to diverse protocols in tailored sequential chemotherapy and chemotherapy-MAb combinations. Pipeline projects in adjuvant and neoadjuvant chemotherapy will focus on combined and sequential treatments with bisphosphonates, MAb, and tyrosine kinase inhibitors.

Overall, in addition to the significant improvements in DFS and RFS rates achieved over the years in the framework of ABCSG clinical trials, we are fortunate to be able to offer DCIS to an increasing number of breast cancer patients in Austria, thus providing benefits both in terms of survival as well as quality of life.

REFERENCES

1. Polychemotherapy for early breast cancer: an overview of the randomised trials. Early Breast Cancer Trialists' Collaborative Group. *Lancet.* 1998;352: 930-942.
2. Tamoxifen for early breast cancer: an overview of the randomised trials. Early Breast Cancer Trialists' Collaborative Group. *Lancet.* 1998;351:1451-1467.
3. Chlebowski RT, Collyar DE, Somerfield MR, Pfister DG. American Society of Clinical Oncology technology assessment on breast cancer risk reduction strategies: tamoxifen and raloxifene. *J Clin Oncol.* 1999;17:1939-1955.
4. Jakesz R, Hausmaninger H, Kubista E, et al. Randomized adjuvant trial of tamoxifen and goserelin versus cyclophosphamide, methotrexate, and fluorouracil: evidence for the superiority of treatment with endocrine blockade in premenopausal patients with hormone-responsive breast cancer—Austrian Breast and Colorectal Cancer Study Group Trial 5. *J Clin Oncol.* 2002;20:4621-4627.
5. Castiglione-Gertsch M, O'Neill A, Price KN, et al. Adjuvant chemotherapy followed by goserelin versus either modality alone for premenopausal lymph node-negative breast cancer: a randomized trial. *J Natl Cancer Inst.* 2003;95:1833-1846.
6. Kaufmann M, Jonat W, Blamey R, et al. Survival analyses from the ZEBRA study: goserelin (Zoladex) versus CMF in premenopausal women with node-positive breast cancer. *Eur J Cancer* 2003;39:1711-1717.
7. Goldhirsch A, Glick JH, Gelber RD, et al. Meeting highlights: International Consensus Panel on the Treatment of Primary Breast Cancer. Seventh International Conference on Adjuvant Therapy of Primary Breast Cancer. *J Clin Oncol.* 2001;19:3817-3827.
8. Gnant M, Mlineritsch W, Schippinger W, et al. Adjuvant ovarian suppression combined with tamoxifen or anastrozole, alone or in combination with zoledronic acid, in premenopausal women with hormone-responsive, stage I and II breast cancer: first efficacy results from ABCSG-12. *J Clin Oncol.* 2008;26(suppl 1):15S.
9. Gnant M, Mlineritsch B, Schippinger W, et al. Endocrine therapy plus zoledronic acid in premenopausal breast cancer. *N Engl J Med.* 2009;360:679-691.
10. Gnant MFX, Mlineritsch B, Luschin-Ebengreuth G, et al. Zoledronic Acid effectively prevents cancer treatment-induced bone loss in premenopausal women receiving adjuvant endocrine therapy for hormone-responsive breast cancer: a report from the Austrian Breast and Colorectal Cancer Study Group. *J Clin Oncol.* 2007;25:820-828.
11. Gnant M, Mlineritsch B, Luschin-Ebengreuth G, et al. Adjuvant endocrine therapy plus zoledronic acid in premenopausal women with early-stage breast cancer: 5-year follow-up of the ABCSG-12 bone-mineral density substudy. *Lancet Oncol.* 2008;9:840-849.
12. Controlled trial of tamoxifen as adjuvant agent in management of early breast cancer. Interim analysis at four years by Nolvadex Adjuvant Trial Organisation. *Lancet.* 1983;1:257-261.
13. Effects of chemotherapy and hormonal therapy for early breast cancer on recurrence and 15-year survival: an overview of the randomised trials. *Lancet.* 2005;365:1687-1717.
14. Fornander T, Rutqvist LE, Cedermark B, et al. Adjuvant tamoxifen in early breast cancer: occurrence of new primary cancers. *Lancet.* 1989;1:117-120.
15. Schmid M, Jakesz R, Samonigg H, et al. Randomized trial of tamoxifen versus tamoxifen plus aminoglutethimide as adjuvant treatment in postmenopausal breast cancer patients with hormone receptor-positive disease: Austrian Breast and Colorectal Cancer Study Group Trial 6. *J Clin Oncol.* 2003;21:984-990.
16. Jakesz R, Greil R, Gnant M, et al. Extended adjuvant therapy with anastrozole among postmenopausal breast cancer patients: results from the randomized Austrian Breast and Colorectal Cancer Study Group Trial 6a. *J Natl Cancer Inst.* 2007;99:1845-1853.
17. Howell A, Cuzick J, Baum M, et al. Results of the ATAC (Arimidex, Tamoxifen, Alone or in Combination) trial after completion of 5 years' adjuvant treatment for breast cancer. *Lancet.* 2005;365:60-62.
18. Fisher B, Dignam J, Bryant J, et al. Five versus more than five years of tamoxifen therapy for breast cancer patients with negative lymph nodes and estrogen receptor-positive tumors. *J Natl Cancer Inst.* 1996;88:1529-1542.
19. Goldhirsch A, Wood WC, Gelber RD, et al. Meeting highlights: updated international expert consensus on the primary therapy of early breast cancer. *J Clin Oncol.* 2003;21:3357-3365.
20. Clarke R, Leonessa F, Welch JN, Skaar TC. Cellular and molecular pharmacology of antiestrogen action and resistance. *Pharmacol Rev.* 2001;53:25-71.
21. Jakesz R, Jonat W, Gnant M, et al. Switching of postmenopausal women with endocrine-responsive early breast cancer to anastrozole after 2 years' adjuvant tamoxifen: combined results of ABCSG trial 8 and ARNO 95 trial. *Lancet.* 2005;366:455-462.
22. Jonat W, Gnant M, Boccardo F, et al. Effectiveness of switching from adjuvant tamoxifen to anastrozole in postmenopausal women with hormone-sensitive early-stage breast cancer: a meta-analysis. *Lancet Oncol.* 2006;7:991-996.
23. Kaufmann M, von Minckwitz G, Bear HD, et al. Recommendations from an international expert panel on the use of neoadjuvant (primary) systemic treatment of operable breast cancer: new perspectives 2006. *Ann Oncol.* 2007;18:1927-1934.
24. Mamounas EP. Neoadjuvant chemotherapy for operable breast cancer: is this the future? *Clin Breast Cancer.* 2003;4(suppl 1):S10-S19.
25. Wolmark N, Wang J, Mamounas E, et al. Preoperative chemotherapy in patients with operable breast cancer: nine-year results from National Surgical Adjuvant Breast and Bowel Project B-18. *J Natl Cancer Inst Monogr.* 2001:96-102.
26. Jakesz R, Hausmaninger H, Haider K, et al. Randomized trial of low-dose chemotherapy added to tamoxifen in patients with receptor-positive and lymph node-positive breast cancer. *J Clin Oncol.* 1999;17:1701-1709.
27. Jakesz R, Samonigg H, Gnant M, et al. Very low-dose adjuvant chemotherapy in steroid receptor negative stage I breast cancer patients. Austrian Breast Cancer Study Group. *Eur J Cancer.* 1998;34:66-70.
28. Ploner F, Jakesz R, Hausmaninger H, et al. Randomised trial: one cycle of anthracycline-containing adjuvant chemotherapy compared with six cycles of CMF treatment in node-positive, hormone receptor-negative breast cancer patients. *Onkologie.* 2003;26:115-119.
29. Taucher S, Steger GG, Jakesz R, et al. The potential risk of neoadjuvant chemotherapy in breast cancer patients: results from a prospective randomized trial of the Austrian Breast and Colorectal Cancer Study Group (ABCSG-07). *Breast Cancer Res Treat.* 2007;112:309-316.
30. Steger GG, Galid A, Gnant M, et al. Pathologic complete response with six compared with three cycles of neoadjuvant epirubicin plus docetaxel and granulocyte colony-stimulating factor in operable breast cancer: Results of ABCSG-14. *J Clin Oncol.* 2007;25:2012-2018.
31. Therasse P, Mauriac L, Welnicka-Jaskiewicz M, et al. Final results of a randomized phase III trial comparing cyclophosphamide, epirubicin, and fluorouracil with a dose-intensified epirubicin and cyclophosphamide + filgrastim as neoadjuvant treatment in locally advanced breast cancer: an EORTC-NCIC-SAKK multicenter study. *J Clin Oncol.* 2003;21:843-850.
32. von Minckwitz G, Blohmer JU, Raab G, et al. In vivo chemosensitivity-adapted preoperative chemotherapy in patients with early-stage breast cancer: the GEPARTRIO pilot study. *Ann Oncol.* 2005;16:56-63.
33. Steger GG, Greil R, Samonig H, et al. An interim safety analysis of ABCSG-24: 6 cycles of docetaxel, epirubicin, and capecitabine + pegfilgrastim (DEC) vs 6 cycles of epirubicin + pegfilgrastim (DE) in the neoadjuvant treatment of operable breast cancer. *Breast Cancer Res Treat.* 2006;100(suppl 1):Poster Session III.
34. Jakesz R, Samonigg H, Gnant M, et al. Significant increase in breast conservation in 16 years of trials conducted by the Austrian Breast and Colorectal Cancer Study Group. *Ann Surg.* 2003;237:556-564.

CHAPTER 48

The German Experience: Primary Systemic Therapy with Cytotoxic Agents

Michael Untch
Gunter von Minckwitz

The success of preoperative, neoadjuvant chemotherapy for locally advanced and inflammatory breast cancer, combined with emerging data on the use of adjuvant chemotherapy, led to the evaluation of the primary systemic therapy (PST) (neoadjuvant) approach for women with primary operable breast cancer. Potential advantages of PST include increasing rates of breast conservation, reducing mortality with lower toxicity, and in vivo testing of sensitivity of cancer cells to the systemic therapy used.[1]

Both the German Breast Group (GBG), an academic research organization conducting clinical trials on breast cancer therapy, as well as the German Gynecological Oncology Working Group (Arbeitsgemeinschaft Gynäkologische Onkologie [AGO]) in the German Society for Gynecology and Obstetrics (Deutsche Gesellschaft für Gynäkologie und Geburtshilfe [DGGG]) and the German Cancer Society (Deutsche Krebsgesellschaft) have performed a comprehensive randomized clinical trial program evaluating the role of neoadjuvant chemotherapy for women with primary breast cancer.

CLOSED AND PUBLISHED STUDIES

GeparDo Study Program

GeparDo

After a dose-finding phase IIa study,[2] the first randomized study (GeparDo) of the GBG series of neoadjuvant trials investigated the effect of adding tamoxifen to a preoperative dose-dense doxorubicin and docetaxel regimen on the pathologic response in 250 women with primary operable breast cancer (tumor size ≥3 cm, N0–2, M0).[3] Patients were prospectively randomized to receive every 14 days a total of 4 cycles of doxorubicin, 50 mg/m², and docetaxel, 75 mg/m² (ADoc), with or without tamoxifen. Granulocyte colony-stimulating factor (G-CSF) was routinely given on days 5 to 10. Surgery followed 8 to 10 weeks after the start of treatment. The results showed that a dose-dense regimen of ADoc with G-CSF offers high compliance, moderate toxicity, and can achieve a pathologic complete response (pCR) rate of 9.7%; however, tamoxifen did not increase antitumor activity. A further 2.4% of patients showed only nonresidual disease in the surgically removed tissue.

GeparDuo

The phase III GeparDuo study randomized 913 patients with untreated operable breast cancer (T2–3, N0–2, M0) to 2 neoadjuvant chemotherapy regimens. The primary end point of the study was to compare the pCR rate in the breast and axillary nodes with the 8-week dose-dense combination regimen ADOC (doxorubicin, 50 mg/m², plus docetaxel, 75 mg/m², every 14 days for 4 cycles with filgrastim support), as studied in GeparDo, with that of a 24-week sequential schedule of AC followed by docetaxel (AC-DOC; doxorubicin, 60 mg/m², plus cyclophosphamide, 600 mg/m², every 21 days followed by docetaxel, 100 mg/m², every 21 days for 4 cycles each). All patients received tamoxifen simultaneously to chemotherapy irrespective of the hormone receptor content of the tumors.[4]

A pCR was achieved in 94 patients (10.6%), but the likelihood was significantly greater with AC-DOC (14.3%; n = 63) than with the ADOC regimen (7.0%; n = 31) (odds ratio, 2.22; 90% confidence interval [CI], 1.52 to 3.24; $p < 0.001$). Independent predictors of achieving a pCR included the use of sequential therapy, high tumor grade, and negative hormone receptor status. The clinical response rates detected by palpation and by imaging were significantly higher with AC-DOC (85.0% and 78.6%, respectively) than with ADOC (75.2% and 68.6%, respectively; both p values < 0.001). The rate of breast-conserving surgery was 63.4% for AC-DOC and 58.1% for ADOC (p = 0.05). GeparDuo demonstrated that the sequential preoperative regimen of 8 cycles of AC-DOC given over 24 weeks is more effective at inducing pCR than the preoperative regimen of 4 cycles of dose-dense ADOC given over 8 weeks.

GeparTrio

Women without an early clinical response to the first 2 to 4 cycles of chemotherapy have a low chance to obtain a pCR after completion of the chemotherapy schedule and have a significant risk of recurrent disease. Preceded by a pilot study on 278 patients,[5] the GeparTrio trial was the first prospective randomized phase III study to address the question of alternative regimen in those not early responding patients.[6] Of 2072 women enrolled in the GeparTrio study, 622 (29.8%) who did not respond to 2 initial cycles of TAC (docetaxel, 75 mg/m[2]; doxorubicin, 50 mg/m[2]; and cyclophosphamide, 500 mg/m[2]) with a decrease in tumor size by at least 50% were randomly assigned to switch to a better tolerated, non-cross-resistant regimen consisting of 4 cycles of vinorelbine, 25 mg/m[2], and capecitabine, 2000 mg/m[2] (NX; N = 301) or to continue with 4 additional cycles of TAC (N = 321). The use of a non-cross-resistant chemotherapy regimen was based on the hypothesis that cancer cells surviving a particular chemotherapy regimen ("resistant" cells) may be more sensitive to a different regimen.

Sonographic response rate was 50.5% for the TAC arm and 51.2% for the NX arm. The difference of 0.7% (95% CI = –7.1% to 8.5%) demonstrated noninferiority of NX (p = 0.008). Similar numbers of patients in both arms received breast-conserving surgery (184 [57.3%] in the TAC arm versus 180 [59.8%] in the NX arm) and had a pCR (5.3% versus 6.0%). Fewer patients in the NX arm than in the TAC arm had hematologic toxic effects, mucositis, infections, and nail changes, but more had hand-foot syndrome and sensory neuropathy. In conclusion, pCRs were low with both chemotherapy regimens. Among patients who did not respond to the initial neoadjuvant TAC treatment, similar efficacy but better tolerability was observed by switching to NX rather than continuing with TAC.

The GeparTrio-study also examined the benefit of an intensified neoadjuvant chemotherapy regimen consisting of 4 (n = 704) or 6 (n = 686) additional TAC cycles for those women who responded to 2 initial cycles of TAC (N = 1390).[7] Breast conservation was possible in 67.5% of the responding patients and in 57% of nonresponders. After 6 cycles of TAC, the pCR rate was 28.6% and after 8 cycles 33.2%. Interestingly, the pCR was 40% in patients with triple negative tumors (ER-, PR-, HER-2/neu–negative). In summary, patients receiving 8 TAC cycles had statistically significantly higher sonographic response rates but not pCR rates when compared with those receiving 6 TAC cycles. However, 8 TAC cycles showed more side effects. Therefore, 8 cycles of TAC cannot be recommended for the whole group of patients responding to 2 initial cycles of TAC.

AGO STUDY

A multicenter phase III trial of the AGO demonstrated the feasibility of a dose-dense, intensified biweekly protocol.[8] This study was designed to compare the frequency of breast-conserving surgery, the response rates, and the safety between 2 regimens containing epirubicin (E) and paclitaxel (T) given either as 6 cycles of single dose-dense, intensified, sequential chemotherapy (arm A) or in 4 cycles of standard combination dose (arm B), both as preoperative therapy for primary breast cancer. Patients with large primary tumors (T >3 cm) or inflammatory disease were randomly assigned to receive either 3 cycles of epirubicin, 150 mg/m[2], followed by 3 cycles of paclitaxel, 250 mg/m[2], every 2 weeks with G-CSF support or 4 cycles of combination epirubicin, 90 mg/m[2], and paclitaxel, 175 mg/m[2], every 3 weeks as preoperative therapy. Preliminary data from 475 of the total 631 enrolled patients demonstrated a significantly higher frequency of breast-conserving surgery (66% versus 55%, p = 0.016), pCR (18% versus 10%, p = 0.03), and negative axillary lymph nodes at surgery (51% versus 42%, p = 0.098) with the twice-weekly regimen.

Based on this evidence, the current German AGO guidelines recommend the neoadjuvant chemotherapy regimen AC–D (doxorubicin, cyclophosphamide, followed by docetaxel; Oxford/AGO 2 B, A +), DAC (docetaxel, doxorubicin, cyclophosphamide; Oxford/AGO 2 B, B +), and AP-CMF (doxorubicin, paclitaxel, cyclophosphamide, methotrexate, 5-fluorouracil; Oxford/AGO 2 B, B +) for their use in routine practice. Trastuzumab is recommended for women with HER-2–positive tumors.[9]

GEPARQUATTRO

The prospective, randomized, phase III trial GeparQuattro study conducted jointly by the AGO and GBG study groups is the largest neoadjuvant clinical trial in women with HER-2–positive breast cancer. A total of 1510 women received 4 cycles of EC (epirubicin, 90 mg/m[2]; cyclophosphamide, 600 mg/m[2]) and were then randomized to either 4 cycles of docetaxel (100 mg/m[2]) (arm A) or 4 cycles of docetaxel plus capecitabine (Doc 75 mg/m[2]/X 1800 mg/m[2]) (arm B) or 4 cycles of Doc (75 mg/m[2]) followed by 4 cycles of X (1800 mg/m[2]) (arm C) (Fig. 48-1). Women with HER-2–positive tumors (N = 456; HercepTest IHC 3+ or central FISH+) received trastuzumab, 6 mg/kg intravenously (IV), every 3 weeks concomitantly to cytotoxic treatment, starting with a loading dose of 8 mg/kg IV on day 1 of the first EC cycle. A total number of 8 (in the EC-Doc and EC-DocX arm) or 12 (in the EC-Doc-X arm) infusions will be given preoperatively. To minimize the cardiac risk, patients with any previous heart problems and/or an ejection fraction less than 55% were excluded.

The trial had 2 primary objectives: first, to analyze the effect of capecitabine, and second, to analyze the effect of trastuzumab by comparing patients with HER-2–positive tumors being treated with trastuzumab with patients with HER-2–negative tumors treated without trastuzumab.

The pCR (no invasive or noninvasive breast tumor at surgery, independent of the nodal status; primary end point), which was the primary end point of the study, could not be improved by adding capecitabine neither in combination nor in sequence to

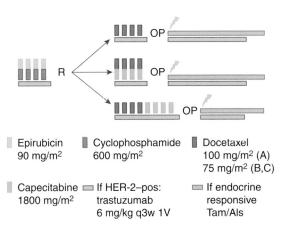

FIGURE 48-1 GeparQuattro study design.

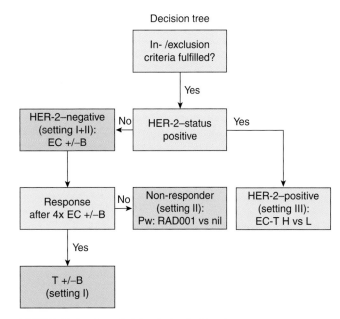

FIGURE 48-2 GeparQuinto study: decision tree.

the ECDoc (arm A: 22.3%, arm B: 19.5%, arm C: 22.3%) ($p = 0.560$ for with or without capecitabine; $p = 0.535$ for shorter versus longer). Breast conservation rate was 70.1%, 68.4%, and 65.3%, respectively. Treatment with capecitabine was associated with more diarrhea, stomatitis, mucositis, nail changes, and hand-foot syndrome but less leukopenia and edema.[10]

EC-Doc(X) was administered with trastuzumab in 445 patients with HER-2 positive tumors and without trastuzumab in 1050 patients with HER-2–negative tumors. The pCR rates at surgery were 31.7% with trastuzumab and 15.7% without trastuzumab ($p < 0.001$). Patients with no response to the first 4 cycles of EC showed a 5-fold higher pCR rate when treated with trastuzumab. Breast conservation rate was 63.1% and 64.7%, respectively ($p = 0.559$). Addition of trastuzumab to EC-T(X) did not increase hematologic, nonhematologic, or short-term cardiac toxicity, except febrile neutropenia. Thus, combining trastuzumab with anthracycline-taxane-based neoadjuvant chemotherapy doubles the pCR rate without clinically relevant early toxicity.[11]

NEW PST CONCEPTS

Ongoing or not yet published neoadjuvant trials integrate modern concepts of treatment like tumor targeting with new biologic agents or dose-intensified strategies to improve the outcome.

GeparQuinto

To improve the selection of patients according to their tumors' sensitivity to chemotherapy as well as implementing small molecules with specific mechanism of action, the prospective, randomized, open label, multicenter phase III GeparQuinto trial was initiated. Treatment for patients participating in the GeparQuinto study will be allocated according to the HER-2 status of the tumor as well as according to the sonographic response after the first 4 cycles of chemotherapy (Fig. 48-2). Experimental therapy with bevacizumab, an inhibitor of the vascular endothelial growth factor pathway targeting tumor neo-angiogenesis; lapatinib, an inhibitor of the EGFR- and HER-2–receptor tyrosine kinase (TK); and everolimus (RAD001), an inhibitor of the mammalian target of rapamycin molecule, a central controller of tumor cell growth and angiogenesis and

chemosensitizer, will be randomly added in distinct settings (Fig. 48-3). Primary end point is the comparison of the pCR rates of breast and lymph nodes in all three settings. Enrollment started in November 2007, and will go on until May 2010; proposed accrual are 2547 women.

TECHNO

The multicenter phase II study TECHNO (Taxol-Epirubicin-Cyclophosphamide-Herceptin Neoadjuvant) of the AGO evaluates preoperative 4 cycles of EC, 90/600 mg/m², every 3 weeks followed by 4 cycles of paclitaxel (P), 175 mg/ m², every 3 weeks with a trastuzumab (T) loading dose, 8 mg/kg, followed by 6 mg/kg every 3 weeks, followed by surgery and postoperative T every 3 weeks, 6 mg/kg, for 9 months in 217 patients with HER-2–positive breast cancer (IHC 3+ or fluorescent in situ hybridization positive confirmed by central pathology).[12] Radiotherapy and endocrine therapy were applied according to standard recommendations. In 119 analyzed patients, 37% achieved a histopathologic complete response, and 17% had only residual ductal carcinoma in situ in the breast. In 73% of the women, axillary nodes at surgery were histologically tumor free. Updated data will be available at the end of 2009.

Neo-ALTTO

The currently recruiting randomized, open-label multicenter phase III study Neo-ALTTO (Neoadjuvant Lapatinib and/or Trastuzumab Treatment Optimisation) is comparing the efficacy of neoadjuvant lapatinib, a novel orally active small molecule and dual TK inhibitor of both EGFR and HER-2, plus paclitaxel, versus trastuzumab plus paclitaxel, versus concomitant lapatinib and trastuzumab plus paclitaxel given as neoadjuvant treatment in HER-2 overexpressing and/or amplified primary breast cancer (Fig. 48-4). Patients will be randomized to receive

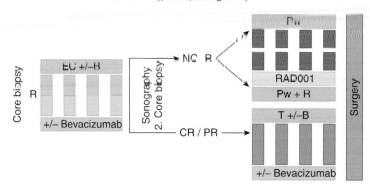

HER-2–negative (setting I + II)

E = Epirubicin (90 mg/m² : day 1 q day 21-4 cycles)
C = Cyclophosphamide (600 mg/m² : day 1 q day 21-4 cycles)
B = Bevacizumab (15 mg/kg IV: day 1 q day 21-8 cycles)

Pw = Paclitaxel, weekly (80 mg/m² : day 1 q day 8-12 wks)
R = RAD001 (5 mg daily)
T = Docetaxel (100 mg/m² : day 1 q day 21-4 cycles)

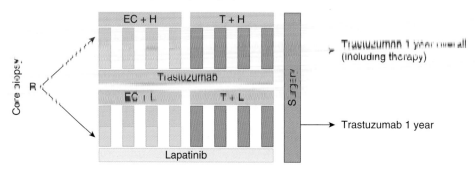

HER-2–positive (setting III)

E = Epirubicin (90 mg/m² : day 1 q day 21-4 cycles)
C = Cyclophosphamide (600 mg/m² : day 1 q day 21-4 cycles)
T = Docetaxel (100 mg/m² : day 1 q day 21-4 cycles)

H = Trastuzumab (8 mg/kg: LD/6 mg/kg: day 1 q day 21)
L = Lapatinib (1250 mg daily 24 wks,
    CAVE: Run-in phase cycles 1 and 5. 1000 mg daily)

FIGURE 48-3   GeparQuinto study: treatment in settings I, II, and III.

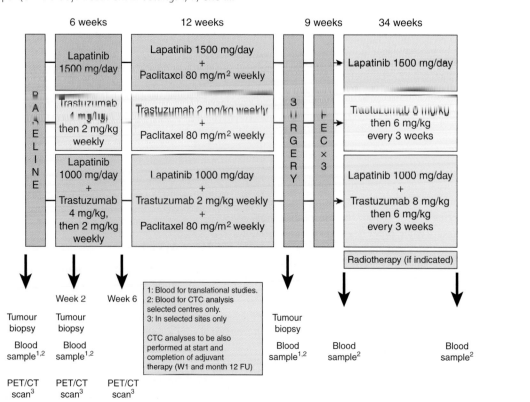

FIGURE 48-4   Neo-ALTTO study design.

either lapatinib, 1500 mg daily, trastuzumab, 4 mg/kg IV load, followed by 2 mg/kg IV weekly, or the lapatinib, 1000 mg daily, with trastuzumab, 4 mg/kg IV load, followed by 2 mg/kg IV weekly for a total of 6 weeks. After this biologic window, patients will continue on the same targeted therapy plus weekly paclitaxel, 80 mg/m^2, for a further 12 weeks, up to definitive surgery. After surgery, patients will receive 3 courses of adjuvant chemotherapy with FEC followed by the same targeted therapy as in the neoadjuvant setting for a further 34 weeks. The planned total duration of the anti-HER-2 therapy will be 1 year. The primary objective of this study is to evaluate and compare the rate of pCR at the time of surgery (18 weeks) in patients randomized to receive neoadjuvant lapatinib or trastuzumab or their combination plus paclitaxel. Estimated enrollment will be 450 patients. The study started in November 2007 and will be completed in May 2010.

PREPARE

The ongoing, not recruiting PREPARE (Preoperative Epirubicin Paclitaxel Aranesp) phase III study started in 2002 and was developed, conducted, and analyzed by the AGO and GBG. It was designed to evaluate the relapse-free survival time and overall survival of a sequential dose-dense and dose-intensified regimen of epirubicin, paclitaxel, and CMF compared with preoperative sequential administration of epirubicin and cyclophosphamide followed by paclitaxel in 733 women with primary breast cancer. Pegfilgrastim was used as a secondary preventive after febrile neutropenia in the standard arm of the study, or in exceptional cases also after severe febrile neutropenia necessitating postponement of the treatment by more than 1 week. In addition, the influence of darbepoetin alfa on the response rate and quality of life was investigated in both treatment arms. The pCR rate was higher in the $E_{dd} \rightarrow T_{dd} \rightarrow CMF$ group versus the EC$\rightarrow$T group (18.7% versus 13.2%, $p = 0.0425$). Patients with ductal cancers, tumor grade III, and negative hormone receptors achieved a higher pCR. Breast-conserving surgery rates were similar in the 2 arms ($E_{dd} \rightarrow T_{dd} \rightarrow CMF$, 65.3%; EC-T, 67.0%). Darbepoetin had no effects on pCR or breast conservation. Patients receiving darbepoetin maintained a mean hemoglobin level of 13.6 g/dL; patients without darbepoetin had a decreased level of 12.6 g/dL. No difference between the 2 chemotherapies or between with and without darbepoetin concerning hematologic toxicities was observed. Patients on $E_{dd} \rightarrow T_{dd} \rightarrow CMF$ had more grades 3 to 4 mucositis/stomatitis/proctitis, sensory neuropathy, and neurologic complaints.[13] Therefore, the dose-dense, dose-intensified chemotherapy $E_{dd} \rightarrow T_{dd} \rightarrow CMF$ is superior to EC$\rightarrow$T in terms of pCR, whereas darbepoetin alfa had no effect on tumor response.[16] Long-term follow-up will be available by the end of 2009.

SOFIA

The open-label, multicenter, single-arm, phase II study SOFIA (study of neoadjuvant epirubicin, cyclophosphamide [EC] plus sorafenib followed by paclitaxel [P] + sorafenib in women with previously untreated primary breast cancer) was initiated by the GBG to determine the efficacy and safety of sorafenib, a small molecular multikinase inhibitor targeting several serine/threonine and receptor TKs, in the neoadjuvant setting in patients with primary breast cancer. A total of 62 women will receive 4 cycles of EC (epirubicin, 90 mg/m^2 IV, on day 1 and cyclophosphamide, 600 mg/m^2 IV, on day 1) followed by 12 weeks of weekly paclitaxel (80 mg/m^2 IV) and sorafenib (400 mg twice daily).

SUMMARY

More than 7000 patients have participated in the collaborative neoadjuvant trials of the GBG and AGO. Based on the large body of evidence gained, PST can be offered as a standard option for patients with large, inoperable, or inflammatory disease but also for those with primary operable disease who are candidates for adjuvant systemic chemotherapy, irrespective of the size of the tumor.[1] PST increases the rate of breast-conserving surgeries and is associated with fewer positive axillary lymph nodes at the time of surgery. The preoperative addition of a taxane to preoperative AC results in a significant increase in the rate of CCR, pCR, and negative axillary nodes in patients with operable breast cancer. Trastuzumab is recommended for patients with HER-2–positive tumors. The concurrent use of the anti-HER-2 antibody with an anthracycline-containing regimen should only be given in clinical trials.[1]

REFERENCES

1. Kaufmann M, von Minckwitz G, Bear HD, et al. Recommendations from an international expert panel on the use of neoadjuvant (primary) systemic treatment of operable breast cancer: new perspectives 2006. *Ann Oncol.* 2007;18:1927-1930.
2. von Minckwitz G, Costa SD, Eiermann W, et al. Maximized reduction of primary breast tumor size using preoperative chemotherapy with doxorubicin and docetaxel. *J Clin Oncol.* 1999;17:1999-2005.
3. von Minckwitz G, Costa SD, Raab G, et al. Dose-dense doxorubicin, docetaxel, and granulocyte colony-stimulating factor support with or without tamoxifen as preoperative therapy in patients with operable carcinoma of the breast: a randomized, controlled, open phase IIb study. *J Clin Oncol.* 2001;19:3506-3515.
4. Von Minckwitz G, Raab G, Caputo A, et al. Doxorubicin with cyclophosphamide followed by docetaxel every 21 days compared with doxorubicin and docetaxel every 14 days as preoperative treatment in operable breast cancer: the GEPARDUO study of the German Breast Group. *J Clin Oncol.* 2005;23:2676-2685.
5. von Minckwitz G, Blohmer JU, Raab G, et al. In vivo chemosensitivity-adapted preoperative chemotherapy in patients with early-stage breast cancer: the GEPARTRIO pilot study. *Ann Oncol.* 2005;16(1):56-63.
6. Von Minckwitz G, Kümmel S, Vogel P, et al. For the German Breast Group. Neoadjuvant vinorelbine-capecitabine versus docetaxel-doxorubicin-cyclophosphamide in early nonresponsive breast cancer: phase III randomized GeparTrio trial. *J Natl Cancer Inst.* 2008;100:542-551.
7. von Minckwitz G, Kümmel S, Vogel P, et al. For the German Breast Group. Intensified neoadjuvant chemotherapy in early-responding breast cancer: phase III randomized GeparTrio study. *J Natl Cancer Inst.* 2008;100:552-562.
8. Untch M, Konecny G, Ditsch N, et al. Dose-dense sequential epirubicin-paclitaxel as preoperative treatment of breast cancer: results of a randomised AGO study. *J Clin Oncol.* 2009;27:2938-2945.
9. Arbeitsgemeinschaft Gynäkologische Onkologie. Guidelines primary systemic therapy. Guideline Breast Version 2008. Available at: http://www.ago-online.org/download/g_mamma_08_1_1_c_04_primary_systemic_therapy.pdf. Accessed December 12, 2008.
10. von Minckwitz G, Rezai M, Loibl S, et al. Capecitabine given concomitantly or in sequence to EC$\rightarrow$Docetaxel as neoadjuvant treatment for early breast cancer. A GBG/AGO intergroup-study. SABCS 2008. Abstract 79.

11. Untch M. Neoadjuvant treatment of HER2 overexpressing primary breast cancer with trastuzumab given concomitantly to epirubicin/cyclophosphamide followed by docetaxel + capecitabine. First analysis of efficacy and safety of the GBG/AGO multicenter intergroup study "GeparQuattro" EBCC-6 2008. Abstract 0450.

12. Untch M, Stoeckl D, Konecny G, et al. A multicenter phase II study of preoperative epirubicin, cyclophosphamide (EC) followed by paclitaxel (P) plus trastuzumab (T) in HER2 positive primary breast cancer. SABCS 2005. Abstract 1064.

13. Untch M, Fasching PA, Stöckl D, et al. PREPARE trial. A randomized phase III trial comparing preoperative dose dense, dose intensified chemotherapy with epirubicin, paclitaxel and CMF with standard dosed epirubicin/cyclophosphamide followed by paclitaxel ± darbepoetin alfa in primary breast cancer: a preplanned interim analysis of efficacy at surgery. ASCO 2008. *J Clin Oncol.* 2008, 26 (suppl), Abstract 517.

CHAPTER 49

The Eastern Cooperative Oncology Group (ECOG) Experience

Lawrence J. Solin

The Eastern Cooperative Oncology Group (ECOG) has contributed a number of important research findings to the literature that are worthy of study by surgical oncologists. Large randomized trials have been performed by ECOG in conjunction with other cooperative groups, and pilot studies have been conducted within the confines of ECOG member institutions. Although many of the ECOG studies have focused on systemic treatment, a number of studies have generated information that is directly related to and of great significance for the local regional management of breast cancer. The current chapter reviews selected ECOG studies and discusses their implications for current surgical oncology practice.

DUCTAL CARCINOMA IN SITU

Ductal carcinoma in situ (DCIS; intraductal carcinoma) is a non-obligate precursor of invasive carcinoma of the breast. Newly diagnosed DCIS is typically detected on routine screening mammography, most commonly from suspicious microcalcifications. Patients with such findings are frequently interested in breast conservation treatment, either with or without definitive radiation. Multiple prospective randomized trials have demonstrated that the addition of radiation treatment after lumpectomy (excision) significantly reduces the risk of local recurrence.[1-7] This reduction in risk is approximately 50% for local recurrence, as well as for the subset of invasive local recurrence. This risk reduction can be further improved by the addition of adjuvant tamoxifen for hormone receptor–positive DCIS tumors, although a statistically significant benefit of tamoxifen was found in only 1 of 2 randomized clinical studies.[2,3,6,8,9]

Notwithstanding the substantial improvement in local recurrence associated with adjuvant radiation treatment, efforts continue to attempt to identify a subset of patients with favorable DCIS who are at a sufficiently low risk of local recurrence that the omission of radiation is reasonable. A substantial fraction of patients are treated in the United States using excision alone, without radiation treatment. Although retrospective studies have suggested the possibility of omitting radiation treatment in favorable patients, no prospective trial has definitively identified such a subset of patients.

In the early 1990s, ECOG developed E5194, a registration trial for presumably favorable DCIS lesions for treatment using excision alone without radiation. At the time of study development, a number of different criteria for selecting patients with DCIS for treatment using excision alone had been proposed in various retrospective institutional studies. Thus, although recognizing there was (and is) no uniformly accepted set of criteria for selecting favorable-risk patients for omission of radiation treatment after lumpectomy, the guidelines for entry into the ECOG protocol are reasonably similar to many, if not most, retrospective studies.

Selection criteria for enrollment into E5194 study were either (1) low- or intermediate-grade DCIS, ≤2.5 cm in size, or (2) high-grade DCIS, ≤1.0 cm in size. All patients were required to have pathologically confirmed negative margins of excision, with either a minimum negative margin width of at least 3 mm or no tumor on reexcision. Complete processing of the lumpectomy specimen was required. A central pathology review was performed, although eligibility for protocol entry was based on the original institutional pathology findings. A postbiopsy mammogram was required to confirm removal of all suspicious microcalcifications, if present on preoperative mammography. Patients entered into E5194 after 2000 were allowed the option to take adjuvant tamoxifen.

The findings from the ECOG E5194 study have been reported.[10] The patients entered into the trial were heavily weighted toward more favorable characteristics, as evidenced by a minimum negative margin width of ≥10 mm or no tumor in the reexcision for 48.5% of the lower-risk group (low or intermediate grade) and 53.3% of the higher-risk group (high grade), as well a median tumor size of 6 mm in the lower-risk group and 5 mm in the higher-risk group. With a median follow-up of 6.2 years, the 5-year rate of ipsilateral local recurrence for the 565 eligible patients in the lower-risk group was 6.1% (95% confidence interval [CI] of 4.1% to 8.2%), and the 7-year rate was 10.5% (95% CI, 7.5% to 13.6%). With a median follow-up of 6.7 years, the 5-year rate of local recurrence for 105 patients in the higher-risk group was 15.3% (95% CI, 8.2% to 22.5%), and the 7-year rate was 18.0% (95% CI, 10.2% to 25.9%).

The data from this study suggest that the higher-risk group is not suitable for treatment using excision alone, without radiation treatment. For the lower-risk group, the 5- and 7-year results need to be interpreted cautiously in view of the relatively short follow-up period and the increasing risk of local recurrence beyond 5 years, albeit with wide CIs. The shapes of the local recurrence curves in the E5194 study are similar to the findings from a collaborative multi-institutional study of 260 patients treated with lumpectomy plus radiation treatment.[11] In this latter study, higher-risk lesions were compared to lower-risk lesions on the basis of pathologic findings (comedo subtype plus nuclear grade 3 versus other, respectively). There was an early rise for the higher-risk group compared with the lower-risk group at 5 years (12% versus 3%, respectively) with the 2 curves approaching each other at 10 years (18% versus 15%, respectively, $p = 0.15$), similar to the E5194 study. Thus additional follow-up for patients in E5194 will be needed to determine the long-term rate of local recurrence in the lower-risk group and whether this rate of local recurrence will be acceptable to patients and physicians in clinical practice.

POSTMASTECTOMY RADIATION TREATMENT

Historical guidelines for the recommendation to deliver postmastectomy radiation treatment include 4 or more positive axillary lymph nodes or pathologic tumor size more than 5 cm.[12,13] However, the value of postmastectomy radiation treatment for the subset of patients with 1 to 3 positive axillary lymph nodes and pathologic T1 to T2 tumors remains an area of controversy. No prospective randomized trial data directly address this large and important subset of node-positive breast cancer patients, although indirect data come from subset analyses of prospective randomized trials.

In the Danish Breast Cancer Group (DBCG) and British Columbia randomized trials of postmastectomy radiation treatment, significant improvement for both local control and survival was demonstrated for the subset of patients with 1 to 3 positive axillary lymph nodes, as well as for the subset of patients with 4 or more positive axillary lymph nodes.[14,15] Some studies, including the DBCG and British Columbia randomized studies, have been criticized for having a very high baseline risk of local regional recurrence for the groups of patients without postmastectomy radiation treatment, which, in turn, suggests

that the value of postmastectomy radiation treatment may have been overestimated by compensating for inadequate surgery. To attempt to correct for this potential bias, subset analysis from the DBCG 82 b&c trials was limited to patients with a minimum of 8 lymph nodes evaluated (ie, likely to have had adequate surgery).[15]

In the Oxford overview of randomized clinical trials, mathematical modeling of the data demonstrated that the value of adding postmastectomy radiation treatment to reduce local regional recurrence was directly proportional to the baseline risk of local regional recurrence without radiation.[16] For the patient with a given risk of local regional recurrence (without radiation treatment), the addition of radiation treatment reduced the risk of local regional recurrence by approximately two-thirds with a further reduction of approximately a quarter for breast cancer mortality. Thus the absolute improvements for local regional recurrence and breast cancer mortality can be calculated for an individual patient or patient subset by determining the baseline risk of local regional recurrence after mastectomy without radiation treatment.

The prospective, randomized Intergroup trial S9927 had previously been opened under the leadership of the Southwest Oncology Group (SWOG) specifically to test the value of postmastectomy radiation treatment for the subset of patients with 1 to 3 positive axillary lymph nodes and pathologic T1 to T2 tumors.[17] However, this randomized trial closed prematurely because of inadequate patient accrual.

With the background described, ECOG analyzed the results for patients treated with mastectomy plus adjuvant CMF (cyclophosphamide, methotrexate, and 5-fluorouracil) chemotherapy, with or without tamoxifen.[18] Analysis was limited to 2016 patients who had not undergone postmastectomy radiation treatment. The goal of this study was to determine the risk of local regional failure at 10 years without postmastectomy radiation treatment, both for the overall group of patients and for clinically relevant subsets of patients. The median follow-up for patients without recurrence was 12.1 years (range = 0.07 to 19.1 years). The median number of lymph nodes evaluated was 15, and 79% of the patients had more than 10 lymph nodes evaluated.

The ECOG analysis demonstrated that the 10-year risk of local regional failure (with or without simultaneous distant failure) at 10 years was 12.9% for patients with 1 to 3 positive axillary lymph nodes, and 28.7% for patients with 4 or more positive lymph nodes.[18] Tumor size, number of involved lymph nodes, estrogen receptor status, and number of examined lymph nodes correlated with the risk of local regional failure on multivariate analysis.

One of the important aspects of the ECOG study was the detailed analysis of the risk of local regional recurrence by narrowly defined subsets of patients (Table 49-1). The value of the table is to facilitate clinical decision making by estimating the baseline risk of local regional failure (without radiation) for an individual patient, in particular, with a pathologic T1 to T2 tumor and 1 to 3 positive axillary lymph nodes. In contrast, most other studies have combined these patients into a single subset, which renders decision making difficult, if not impossible, for individual patients.

Woodward et al from the MD Anderson Cancer Center (MDACC) reported 1031 patients treated with a mastectomy and doxorubicin-based chemotherapy, but without postmastectomy

TABLE 49-1 Ten-Year Cumulative Incidence of Local Regional Failure According to Narrow Combinations of Pathologic Tumor Size and Number of Involved Axillary Lymph Nodes

No. of Involved Lymph Nodes	Type of Relapse	PATHOLOGIC TUMOR SIZE (cm)					
		≤1.0 (%)	1.1-2.0 (%)	2.1-3.0 (%)	3.1-4.0 (%)	4.1-5.0 (%)	≥5.1 (%)
1	ILRF	3.3	6.1	4.3	10.4	3.0	27.3
	LRF ± DF	3.3	10.6	2.1	10.4	6.2	27.3
2	ILRF	4.2	11.2	4.4	18.4	5.6	23.1
	LRF ± DF	8.2	14.4	12.3	20.4	14.0	30.8
3	ILRF	20.0	14.2	3.2	5.5	4.3	18.2
	LRF ± DF	20.0	17.5	10.9	8.3	13.6	36.4
4	ILRF	6.2	10.1	11.5	17.5	21.1	22.2
	LRF ± DF	18.8	16.8	21.7	26.0	36.8	33.3
5-6	ILRF	10.5	13.8	13.3	14.3	11.1	23.5
	LRF ± DF	21.5	22.6	23.4	24.5	22.3	47.1
7-9	ILRF	12.5	26.2	14.5	16.2	24.5	23.8
	LRF ± DF	12.5	33.4	30.3	32.4	32.5	41.3
≥10	ILRF	19.5	13.6	15.0	24.3	24.7	5.9
	LRF ± DF	39.0	30.4	30.9	35.8	35.4	31.1

DF, distant failure; ILRF, isolated local-regional failure; LRF, local-regional failure.

Modified and reproduced with permission from Recht A, Gray R, Davidson NE, et al. Locoregional failure 10 years after mastectomy and adjuvant chemotherapy with or without tamoxifen without irradiation: experience of the Eastern Cooperation Oncology Group. *J Clin Oncol.* 1999;17:1689-1700.

radiation treatment,[19] The data for local regional recurrence in the MDACC study were similar to the ECOG study, notwithstanding the difference of doxorubicin-based chemotherapy in the MDACC study compared to CMF-based chemotherapy in the ECOG study.

TRASTUZUMAB (HERCEPTIN)

Trastuzumab (Herceptin) has become a standard adjuvant treatment for HER-2 positive patients based on prospective randomized trial data. However, radiation treatment for left-sided breast cancers and trastuzumab have each been associated with cardiac toxicity. Thus the potential exists for an increased risk of cardiac toxicity for patients with left-sided breast cancer receiving both trastuzumab and radiation treatment.

The 3-arm randomized Intergroup trial N9831 demonstrated the value of adding adjuvant trastuzumab to adjuvant systemic chemotherapy consisting of doxorubicin (Adriamycin) plus cyclophosphamide (AC), followed by paclitaxel.[20] To evaluate for the potential interaction, if any, of trastuzumab with radiation on toxicity for left sided breast cancer patients, Halyard et al reported an analysis of 1503 irradiated patients from the N9831 study.[21] The median follow-up after treatment was 3.7 years. Given the limited follow-up, late toxicity could not be assessed.

Comparing irradiated patients with left-sided versus right-sided primary tumors, Halyard et al found no difference in the cumulative incidence of cardiac events, pneumonitis, dyspnea, cough, dysphagia, neutropenia, or acute skin reaction. Leukopenia was noted to be increased in the patients treated with trastuzumab. No increase in congestive heart failure or other cardiac events was seen for patients with left-sided breast cancer compared with patients with right-sided breast cancer, all of whom had received radiation treatment. Although there was no evidence of an interaction or increase in acute toxicity for patients treated with trastuzumab plus left-sided radiation, longer follow-up will be needed to evaluate for late complications. Because detailed radiation treatment parameters were not required for protocol study, an in-depth analysis of the effect of radiation treatment parameters relative to potential normal tissues at risk, particularly cardiac structures, could not be performed.

Although the protocol specifications excluded radiation treatment to the internal mammary nodes (IMNs), 44 patients nonetheless received IMN radiation treatment. The number of patients who underwent IMN radiation was small, but there did not appear to be an increase in the frequency of cardiac events or pneumonitis. Given the small number of patients, these results for IMN radiation should be interpreted with caution.

OVARIAN ABLATION

Ovarian ablation is a well known, effective adjuvant therapy for premenopausal breast cancer patients. In the Intergroup randomized clinical trial E3193, premenopausal patients with early-stage breast carcinoma were randomized to tamoxifen versus tamoxifen plus ovarian ablation. In this trial, a subset of 22 patients underwent radiation ovarian ablation.[22] The radiation treatment was delivered to the pelvis using 2 Gy per fraction to a total of 20 Gy in 10 fractions. Twenty of the 22 patients were able to be evaluated with adequate follow up information, and 15 (75%) achieved successful ovarian ablation with radiation treatment. With a median follow-up of 54 months, no grade 3 or grade 4 complications from radiation treatment were observed. These results demonstrate that pelvic radiation treatment is an effective and safe method of ovarian ablation for premenopausal patients, and a potential alternative to medical or surgical ovarian ablation.

CURRENT AND FUTURE STUDIES

Bevacizumab (Avastin)

Bevacizumab (Avastin) is an antiangiogenic agent with clinical activity for patients with breast carcinoma. Bevacizumab is an antibody directed against vascular endothelial growth factor (VEGF) and inhibits the growth of human tumor cells based on its antiangiogenic properties.

In a report of 722 patients with metastatic disease, Miller et al analyzed a randomized clinical trial of paclitaxel plus bevacizumab versus paclitaxel alone.[23] The addition of bevacizumab significantly prolonged progression-free survival (median 11.8 months versus 5.9 months, respectively; $p < 0.001$). However, there was no difference in overall survival between the 2 groups (median 26.7 months versus 25.2 months, respectively; $p = 0.16$).

The most successful clinical application of an antiangiogenic agent is likely to be for patients with micrometastatic disease with growing tumor cells. In the adjuvant setting, micrometastatic disease may be associated with nascent vascular formation. Therefore, a prospective randomized trial of bevacizumab in the adjuvant setting is warranted.

ECOG has developed an ongoing prospective randomized clinical trial, E5103, to test the value of bevacizumab in the adjuvant setting for lymph node positive or high-risk lymph node negative patients.[24] Figure 49-1 shows the schema for E5103. This trial is designed to evaluate both the potential benefit and the duration of adjuvant bevacizumab. The primary end point is disease-free survival, and secondary end points include overall survival and toxicity.

Statistical considerations include an accrual goal of 4950 patients in the three arms, randomized in a 1:2:2 fashion. Accrual is planned over approximately 2.1 years. A total of 3351 patients had been entered into the study as of September 5, 2009.

PACCT-1 (Program for the Assessment of Clinical Cancer Tests) TAILORx (Trial Assigning Individualized Options for Treatment) Trial

The Oncotype DX recurrence score is based on a 21-gene panel. This recurrence score has been developed to predict the risk of distant recurrence and the value of adjuvant systemic chemotherapy based on retrospective analyses from randomized studies. The recurrence score assay is valid not only for prognosis but also for prediction of benefit from adjuvant systemic chemotherapy, and possibly also for prediction of risk of local regional recurrence.

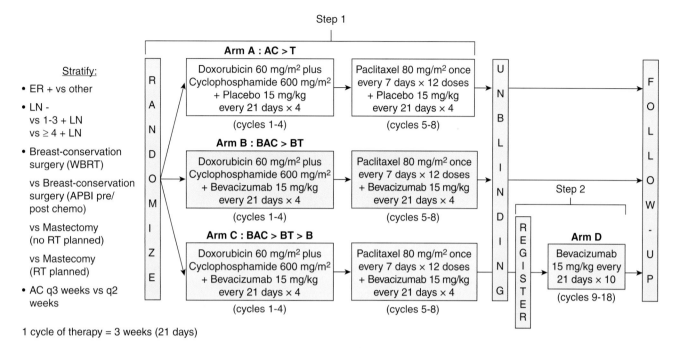

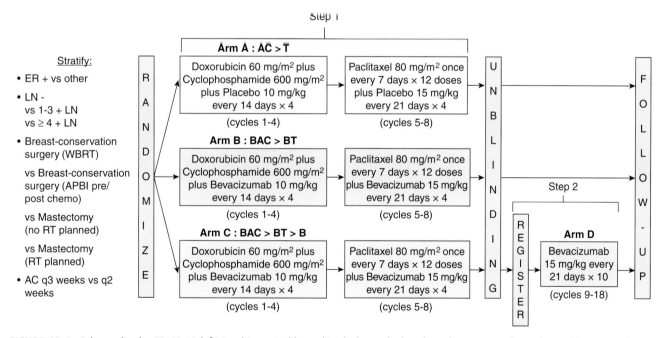

FIGURE 49-1 Schema for the E5103 trial. [AC, Adriamycin (doxorubicin) plus cyclophosphamide; APBI, accelerated partial breast irradiation; ER, estrogen receptor; LN, lymph node; PR, progesterone receptor; RT, radiation treatment; WBRT, whole-breast radiation treatment.]

The ongoing PACCT-1 (Program for the Assessment of Clinical Cancer Tests) TAILORx (Trial Assigning Individualized Options for Treatment) trial was developed to determine whether the Oncotype DX recurrence score can be used in a prospective fashion to guide individual decision making regarding

adjuvant systemic chemotherapy.[25] The schema for the PACCT-1 TAILORx trial is shown in Figure 49-2. In this trial, node-negative, hormone receptor–positive tumors undergo testing using the Oncotype DX assay. Patients with tumors in the low-risk group (recurrence score <11) are assigned to adjuvant hormonal

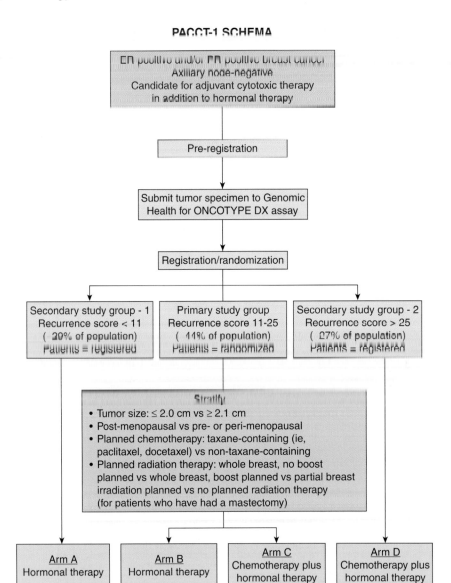

FIGURE 49-2 Schema for the PACCT-1 TAILORx trial. (ER, estrogen receptor; PR, progesterone receptor.)

therapy, and patients with tumors in the high-risk group (recurrence score >25) are assigned to adjuvant systemic chemotherapy plus hormonal therapy. Patients with tumors in the intermediate-risk group (recurrence score of 11 to 25) are randomized to receive adjuvant hormonal therapy with versus without adjuvant systemic chemotherapy. The primary end points are disease-free survival, distant recurrence-free interval, recurrence-free interval, and overall survival.

Statistical considerations include an accrual goal of 10,046 patients. Stratification factors include tumor size, menopausal status, planned type of chemotherapy, and planned type of radiation treatment. A total of 7649 patients had been entered into study as of September 5, 2009.

for patient-specific subgroups. ECOG clinical trials have substantially advanced the clinical practice and the science of treating breast carcinoma. A number of these studies have had an impact on local regional management in various clinically relevant settings. Future directions in adjuvant systemic therapy trials include the testing of bevacizumab to evaluate the role of this antiangiogenic factor. The PACCT-1 TAILORx trial uses a genomic-based recurrence score assay to evaluate and test the value of tailored adjuvant systemic chemotherapy. In collaboration with other cooperative groups, ECOG has contributed valuable data for optimizing the local regional treatment of breast carcinoma, with the long-term goal of increasingly tailored patient treatment.

SUMMARY

As a major participant and member of the Intergroup, ECOG has the goal of developing and conducting prospective randomized clinical trials that will lead to increasingly tailored treatments

REFERENCES

1. Fisher B, Dignam J, Wolmark N, et al. Lumpectomy and radiation therapy for the treatment of intraductal breast cancer: findings from National Surgical Adjuvant Breast and Bowel Project B-17. *J Clin Oncol.* 1998;16: 441-452.

2. Fisher B, Land S, Mamounas E, et al. Prevention of invasive breast cancer in women with ductal carcinoma in situ: an update of the National Surgical Adjuvant Breast and Bowel Project experience. *Semin Oncol.* 2001;28:400-418.

3. Wapnir I, Dignam J, Julian TB, et al. Long-term outcomes after invasive breast tumor recurrence (IBTR) in women with DCIS in NSABP B-17 and B-24. *Proc Am Soc Clin Oncol.* 2007;25:7s. Abstract 520.

4. Bijker N, Meijnen P, Peterse JL, et al. Breast-conserving treatment with or without radiotherapy in ductal carcinoma-in-situ: ten-year results of European Organisation for Research and Treatment of Cancer randomized phase III trial 10853—a study by the EORTC Breast Cancer Cooperative Group and EORTC Radiotherapy Group. *J Clin Oncol.* 2006;24:3381-3387.

5. Bijker N, Peterse JL, Duchateau L, et al. Risk factors for recurrence and metastasis after breast-conserving therapy for ductal carcinoma-in-situ: analysis of European Organization for Research and Treatment of Cancer Trial 10853. *J Clin Oncol.* 2001;19:2263-2271.

6. Houghton J, George WD, Cuzick J, et al. Radiotherapy and tamoxifen in women with completely excised ductal carcinoma in situ of the breast in the UK, Australia, and New Zealand: randomised controlled trial. *Lancet.* 2003;362:95-102.

7. Holmberg L, Garmo H, Granstrand B, et al. Absolute risk reductions for local recurrence after postoperative radiotherapy after sector resection for ductal carcinoma in situ of the breast. *J Clin Oncol.* 2008;26:1247-1252.

8. Fisher B, Dignam J, Wolmark N, et al. Tamoxifen in treatment of intraductal breast cancer: National Surgical Adjuvant Breast and Bowel Project B-24 randomised controlled trial. *Lancet.* 1999;353:1993-2000.

9. Allred DC, Bryant J, Land S, et al. Estrogen receptor expression as a predictive marker of the effectiveness of tamoxifen in the treatment of DCIS: findings from NSABP protocol B-24. *Breast Cancer Res Treat.* 2002;76 (suppl 1):S36. Abstract.

10. Hughes LL, Wang M, Page DL, et al. Local excision alone without irradiation for ductal carcinoma in situ of the breast: a trial of the Eastern Cooperative Oncology Group. *J Clin Oncol.* in press

11. Solin LJ, Kurtz J, Fourquet A, et al. Fifteen-year results of breast-conserving surgery and definitive breast irradiation for the treatment of ductal carcinoma in situ of the breast. *J Clin Oncol.* 1996;14:754-763.

12. Recht A, Edge SB, Solin LJ, et al. Postmastectomy radiotherapy: clinical practice guidelines of the American Society of Clinical Oncology. *J Clin Oncol.* 2001;19:1539-1569.

13. Marks LB, Zeng J, Prosnitz LR. One to three versus four or more positive nodes and postmastectomy radiotherapy: time to end the debate [editorial]. *J Clin Oncol.* 2008;26:2075-2077.

14. Ragaz J, Olivotto IA, Spinelli JJ, et al. Locoregional radiation therapy in patients with high-risk breast cancer receiving adjuvant chemotherapy: 20-year results of the British Columbia randomized trial. *J Natl Cancer Inst.* 2005;97:116-126.

15. Overgaard M, Nielsen HM, Overgaard J. Is the benefit of postmastectomy irradiation limited to patients with four or more positive notes, as recommended in international consensus reports? A subgroup analysis or the DBCG 82 b&c randomized trials. *Radiother Oncol.* 2007;82:247-253.

16. Clarke M, Collins R, Darby S, et al. Effects of radiotherapy and of differences in the extent of surgery for early breast cancer on local recurrence and 15-year survival: an overview of the randomised trials. *Lancet.* 2005;366:2087-2106.

17. Randomized trial of post-mastectomy radiotherapy in stage II breast cancer in women with one to three positive axillary nodes, phase III. Available at: https://swog.org/visitors/ViewProtocolDetails.asp?ProtocolID=1807. Accessed November 24, 2008.

18. Recht A, Gray R, Davidson NE, et al. Locoregional failure 10 years after mastectomy and adjuvant chemotherapy with or without tamoxifen without irradiation: experience of the Eastern Cooperation Oncology Group. *J Clin Oncol.* 1999;17:1689-1700.

19. Woodward WA, Strom EA, Tucker SL, et al. Locoregional recurrence after doxorubicin-based chemotherapy and postmastectomy: implications for breast cancer patients with early-stage disease and predictors for recurrence after postmastectomy radiation. *Int J Radiat Oncol Biol Phys.* 2003;57:336-344.

20. Romond EH, Perez EA, Bryant J, et al. Trastuzumab plus adjuvant chemotherapy for operable HER2-positive breast cancer. *N Engl J Med.* 2005;353:1673-1684.

21. Halyard MY, Pisansky TM, Dueck A, et al. Radiotherapy and adjuvant trastuzumab in operable breast cancer: tolerability and adverse event data from North Central Cancer Treatment Group phase III trial N9831. *J Clin Oncol.* 2009;27(16):2638-2644.

22. Hughes LL, Gray RJ, Solin LJ, et al. Efficacy of radiotherapy for ovarian ablation: results of a breast intergroup study. *Cancer.* 2004;101:969-972.

23. Miller K, Wang M, Gralow J, et al. Paclitaxel plus bevacizumab versus paclitaxel alone for metastatic breast cancer. *N Engl J Med.* 2007;357:2666-2676.

24. Doxorubicin, cyclophosphamide, and paclitaxel with or without bevacizumab in treating patients with lymph node-positive and high-risk, lymph node-negative breast cancer. Available at: http://www.cancer.gov/search/ViewClinicalTrials.aspx?cdrid=528930&version=Patient. Accessed November 24, 2008.

25. Phase III Randomized Study of Adjuvant Combination Chemotherapy and Hormonal Therapy Versus Adjuvant Hormonal Therapy in Women with Previously Resected Axillary Node-Negative Breast Cancer with Various Levels of Risk for Recurrence (TAILORx Trial) (ECOG-PACCT-1). Available at: http://www.cancer.gov/clinicaltrials/ft-ECOG-PACCT-1. Accessed November 24, 2008.

CHAPTER 50

The Cancer and Leukemia Group B Trials

Amanda J. Wheeler
Barbara L. Smith
Kevin Hughes

The Cancer and Leukemia Group B (CALGB) was founded in 1956 and is now "a national network including 26 university medical centers, over 225 participating community hospitals and more than 3,000 oncology specialists who collaborate in clinical research studies aimed at reducing the morbidity and mortality from cancer, relating the biological characteristics of cancer to clinical outcomes and developing new strategies for the early detection and prevention of cancer."[1]

CALGB investigators have designed and conducted a number of pivotal clinical trials addressing treatment of breast cancer. CALGB is a member of the Breast Cancer Intergroup of North America where it regularly leads and participates in Intergroup trials. This chapter highlights trials led by the CALGB.

CALGB trials have addressed systemic therapy questions in breast cancer patients including optimum total dose of drug, schedule of drug delivery and dose density, combination versus sequential administration of different agents, as well as assessment of different agents. Many CALGB trials incorporate a factorial design in which patients are randomized into 2 or more arms for the first portion of treatment and then undergo a second randomization to 2 or more different arms for the second part of treatment. This approach allows testing of multiple hypotheses within the same trial.

CALGB has consistently had a strong correlative science program with companion laboratory studies that collect tissue, blood, and data from patients on trial to address mechanism of response, predictors of response, and other questions. For example, a correlative science study assessed different methods for assessment of HER-2 overexpression, and demonstrated fluorescence in situ hybridization (FISH) was a reliable method for measuring HER-2 expression.

ADJUVANT CHEMOTHERAPY IN EARLY STAGE BREAST CANCER

A series of CALGB trials addressed questions of total dose of chemotherapy, dose density of chemotherapy delivery, and administration of agents sequentially versus in combination for early stage breast cancer.

By 1985, the NIH Consensus Conference concluded that the use of chemotherapy in node-positive premenopausal women was standard of care, while the efficacy of chemotherapy in node-positive postmenopausal women was unclear, although some studies suggested a benefit.[2] Building on this basic belief, the CALGB worked to further clarify the role of adjuvant chemotherapy.

CALGB 8541: Dose and Dose Intensity of Adjuvant Chemotherapy for Stage II, Node-Positive Breast Carcinoma

CALGB 8541 addressed 2 main questions regarding CAF chemotherapy in both pre- and postmenopausal women with node-positive breast cancer. The impact of dose of drug administered per cycle was assessed using 3 different doses. The impact of dose density versus duration of treatment was also addressed as 2 of the arms administered the same total amount of drug, one over 6 cycles and the other in only 4 cycles with a higher dose per cycle.

Patients were randomized to 1 of 3 regimens of cyclophosphamide, doxorubicin, and fluorouracil (CAF):

Group 1 (high dose) 600/60/600 mg/m^2 IV every 28 days for 4 cycles

Group 2 (moderate dose) 400/40/400 mg/m² IV every 28 days for 6 cycles

Group 3 (low dose) 300/30/300 mg/m² IV every 28 days for 4 cycles

The trial enrolled 1572 patients, making it one of the largest prospective trials performed at that time. After a median follow-up of 3.4 years, Wood et al reported that increasing the dose of doxorubicin from 30 to 60 mg/m² improved disease-free and overall survival with acceptable toxicity.[3]

This study was significant because it was one of the first to show a difference in survival resulting from the use of different doses of chemotherapy over varying time intervals. It helped define the concept of a threshold effect for breast cancer chemotherapy (ie, that doses below a critical level show significantly reduced efficacy). Whereas both the moderate- and high-dose regimens delivered the same cumulative dose, there was a trend favoring the high-intensity regimen. This observation would lead to a later trial (CALGB 9741) directly assessing the impact of dose density.

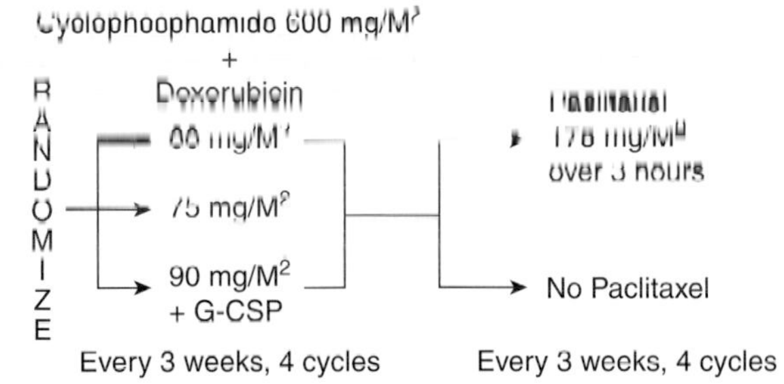

FIGURE 50-1 CALGB 9344 protocol schema; 3 × 2 factorial design. After completion of chemotherapy, radiation therapy was administered if patient was treated with lumpectomy or at discretion of physician if patient was treated with mastectomy, and tamoxifen 20 mg/d was administered for 5 years if the tumor was receptor positive. (*Reproduced, with permission, from Henderson IC. Improved outcomes from adding sequential paclitaxel but not from escalating doxorubicin dose in an adjuvant chemotherapy regimen for patients with node-positive primary breast cancer.* J Clin Oncol. 2003;21:976-983.)

CALGB 9344/Intergroup 0148: Adjuvant High-Dose versus Standard Dose AC with and without Paclitaxel in Node-Positive Breast Cancer

The novel mechanism of action of paclitaxel, its lack of cross-resistance with anthracyclines, and its manageable toxicity led to interest in incorporating it into adjuvant chemotherapy regimens. This led to several studies of its use in the treatment of early breast cancer.

CALGB 9344/INT0148 enrolled 3121 patients with node-positive breast cancer between 1994 and 1999 into a 3 × 2 factorial design trial comparing different doses of doxorubicin plus cyclophosphamide with or without the addition of paclitaxel. Patients were randomized to a control arm of the most effective doxorubicin dose from CALGB 8541 (60 mg/m²), versus even higher doses (75 or 90 mg/m²) administered with cyclophosphamide (600 mg/m²) for 4 cycles. Patients then underwent a second randomization to an additional 4 cycles of paclitaxel (175 mg/m²) versus observation (Fig. 50-1). This trial design allowed comparison of the impact of the use of paclitaxel or not on 3 different doses of doxorubicin with cyclophosphamide.

After completion of chemotherapy, radiation therapy to the breast was administered if the patient was treated with lumpectomy or at the discretion of the investigator if the patient was treated with mastectomy (Fig. 50-2). Tamoxifen (20 mg PO daily) was administered for 5 years if the tumor was hormone-receptor positive.

The addition of paclitaxel was shown to improve both disease-free and overall survival.[4] At 5 years, 70% of women who received paclitaxel were disease-free, compared with 65% of women who did not. Overall survival was 80% in the paclitaxel group versus 77% in the no-paclitaxel group. There was no benefit seen with doses of doxorubicin above 60 mg/m². A subset analysis based on estrogen receptor status showed significant benefit from the addition of paclitaxel to those women whose tumors lacked estrogen receptors, although this correlation of benefit with estrogen receptor status was not confirmed by a similar NSABP trial.[5]

This trial also demonstrated that the increased time between surgery and radiotherapy resulting from delivery of additional cycles of paclitaxel after doxorubicin and cyclophosphamide did not adversely impact local control.[6] In fact, the addition of paclitaxel afforded better local control than doxorubicin and cyclophosphamide alone in patients treated with breast-conserving therapy.

CALGB 9741/Intergroup C9741: A Randomized Trial of Dose Dense versus Conventionally Scheduled and Sequential versus Concurrent Combination Chemotherapy as Postoperative Adjuvant Treatment of Node-Positive Primary Breast Cancer

Some models of tumor killing by chemotherapy agents suggest that more frequent administration of chemotherapy treatments will result in greater tumor cell killing by reducing the time during which the tumor is allowed to proliferate between chemotherapy doses.[7]

CALGB 9741 addressed this hypothesis by assessing frequency of chemotherapy administration, termed dose density, and the impact of delivering chemotherapy agents sequentially versus in combination. The same total drug doses were delivered in 4 different patterns as outlined below.

One thousand nine hundred and seventy-three women with node-positive primary breast cancer were assigned to 1 of 4 treatment regimens using doxorubicin (A), paclitaxel (T),

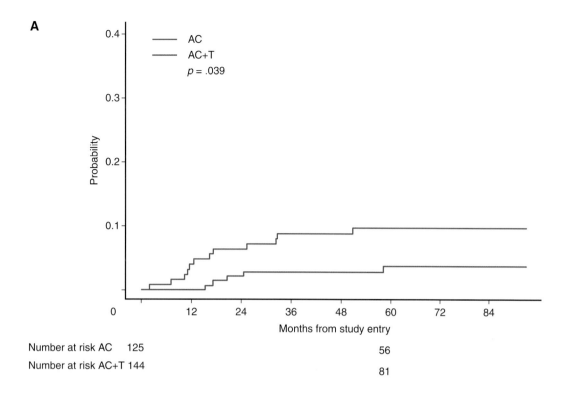

Number at risk AC   125   56
Number at risk AC+T 144   81

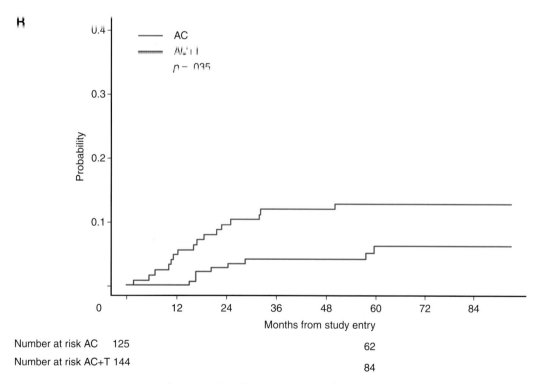

Number at risk AC   125   62
Number at risk AC+T 144   84

FIGURE 50-2   CALGB 9344. Breast-conserving therapy with radiotherapy. **A.** Cumulative incidence of isolated locoregional recurrence; **B.** cumulative incidence of locoregional recurrence as any component of failure. AC, doxorubicin plus cyclophosphamide; AC+T, AC plus paclitaxel. *(Reproduced, with permission, from Sartor CI, et al. Effect of addition of adjuvant paclitaxel on radiotherapy delivery and locoregional control of node-positive breast cancer: Cancer and Leukemia Group B 9344. J Clin Oncol. 2005;23:30-40.)*

and cyclophosphamide (C) following surgery. Regimens administered at 3-week intervals were termed "conventional" and those administered at 2-week intervals "dose dense." Patients in the dose-dense arms all received growth factor support to prevent treatment-limiting neutropenia.

Conventional with sequential administration of A→T→C at 3-week intervals

Dose-dense with sequential administration of A→T→C at 2-week intervals

Conventional with concurrent administration of A+C→T at 3-week intervals

Dose-dense with concurrent administration of A+C→T at 2-week intervals

Results showed that the 2 dose-dense regimens provided significantly higher disease-free survival than those regimens using conventional dosing.[8] There was no difference in efficacy between sequential and concurrent dose-dense regimens. Disease-free survival was 82% after 4 years for patients on the dose-dense regimens, compared to 75% for those who received conventional therapy (p = .010). This difference corresponded to a 26% overall reduction in the risk of cancer recurrence. These results predict that increasing dose density will improve therapeutic results and that sequential chemotherapy that maintains dose density would preserve efficacy while reducing toxicity.

CALGB 9082: Randomized Comparison of High-Dose Chemotherapy with Stem-Cell Support versus Intermediate-Dose Chemotherapy after Surgery and Adjuvant Chemotherapy in Women with High-Risk Primary Breast Cancer

CALGB 8541 demonstrated that increasing the dose of chemotherapy delivered, especially if the total dose was delivered in a shorter time, improved survival in node-positive breast cancer patients.[3] This led to the hypothesis that even higher doses of chemotherapy would result in even higher survival rates. However, bone marrow toxicity limited the maximum dose of chemotherapy that could be safely delivered. Advances in bone marrow and stem cell transplantation applied to other malignancies led to application of this approach to patients with high-risk breast cancers.

Based on this result, CALGB 9082 compared the efficacy of high-dose cyclophosphamide, cisplatin, and carmustine (HD CPB) chemotherapy with autologous stem cell transplantation with that of intermediate-dose CPB chemotherapy with G-CSF support. Randomization occurred after 4 cycles of CAF with restaging between the third and fourth cycle. Eligible patients included 785 women aged 22 to 66 years with stage IIA, IIB, or IIIA breast cancer involving 10 or more axillary lymph nodes (Fig. 50-3).

At a median follow-up of 7.3 years the transplant arm experienced higher complication rates and had no improvement in overall survival relative to the standard chemotherapy arm (p = .75).[9] These data, combined with data from other cooperative group trials, led to abandonment of autologous stem cell transplantation in breast cancer patients.

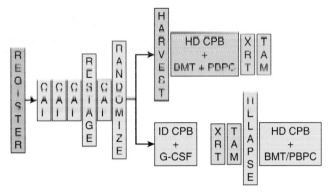

FIGURE 50-3 CALGB 9082 trial design. Patients were randomly assigned after 4 cycles of cyclophosphamide, doxorubicin, and fluorouracil (CAF) chemotherapy to receive high-dose cyclophosphamide, cisplatin, and carmustine (HD CPB) with bone marrow (BMT) and peripheral-blood progenitor cell (PBPC) support or intermediate-dose CPB (ID CPB) with granulocyte-stimulating factor support (G-CSF). (XRT, radiation therapy; TAM, tamoxifen.) [Reproduced, with permission, from Peters WP, et al. Prospective, randomized comparison of high-dose chemotherapy with stem cell support versus intermediate-dose chemotherapy after surgery and adjuvant chemotherapy in women with high-risk primary breast cancer: a report of CALGB 9082, SWOG 9114, and NCIC MA-13. J Clin Oncol. 2005;23(10):2191-2200.]

IMPACT OF HER-2 OVEREXPRESSION ON BREAST CANCER TREATMENT

By the 1990s it was recognized that HER-2 overexpression in breast cancer was associated with a poor prognosis. Using archival material from CALGB 8541, CALGB investigators launched one of the first studies examining the relationship between HER-2 overexpression and response to different systemic therapy regimens in patients with node-positive breast cancer.

The first of these studies correlated HER-2 expression levels with response to chemotherapy in 442 patients in CALGB 8541.[10] In the 114 patients (29%) with more than 50% increase in HER-2 expression, overall and disease-free survival was significantly improved in patients receiving higher doses of chemotherapy. There was no relationship between dose and overall or disease-free survival seen in patients with a low HER-2 expression in the primary tumor (Fig. 50-4).

A companion study CALGB 8869 further analyzed 992 tumors from CALGB 8541 for HER-2 (ErbB-2) expression with the hypothesis that there was a "plausible interaction between HER-2 expression and doxorubicin dose response."[11] This analysis confirmed that higher doses of adjuvant CAF chemotherapy were associated with improved overall and disease-free survival in patients with HER-2 overexpressing tumors. Additional analysis with 11-year follow-up confirmed these conclusions.[12] These results led to the hypothesis that HER-2 overexpressing tumors were relatively resistant to standard chemotherapy regimens and highlighted the need to identify targeted therapies for this group of tumors.

There continued to be controversy regarding the best laboratory method to assess HER-2 expression levels in breast cancers. Dressler and colleagues compared HER-2 evaluation using

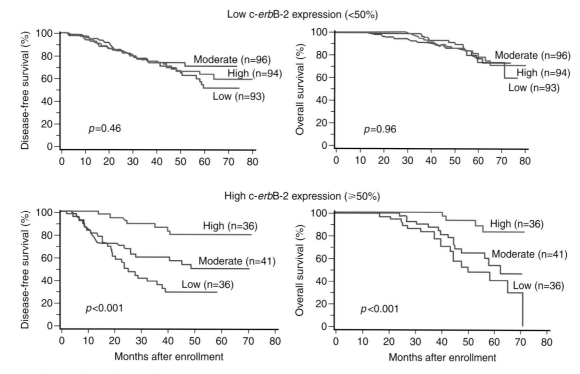

FIGURE 50-4 Disease-free and overall survival according to treatment group (high-, moderate-, or low-dose chemotherapy) and level of c-erbB-2 expression. (Reproduced, with permission, from Muss HB, et al. C-erbB-2 expression and response to adjuvant therapy in women with node positive early breast cancer. N Engl J Med. 1994;330:1260-1266.)

FISH and immunohistochemistry (IHC) in the same 992 patient cohort studies in CALGB 8869.[13] FISH determination of HER-2 status was found to be a reliable method to predict clinical outcome following adjuvant doxorubicin-based therapy for stage II breast cancer patients. FISH has now become a standard approach for assessing HER-2 status, particularly for cases found to have intermediate levels of HER-2 expression by IHC analysis.

HER-2 expression levels were also correlated with benefit from paclitaxel in node-positive breast cancer in CALGB 9344. HER-2 expression was assessed by IHC in tumors from 1500 patients in CALGB 9344. The addition of paclitaxel to doxorubicin and cyclophosphamide was beneficial in tumors showing overexpression of HER-2, but showed no additional benefit in estrogen receptor–positive patients without HER-2 overexpression.[14] It was concluded that paclitaxel could safely be omitted in patients with HER-2-negative, estrogen receptor–positive, node-positive breast cancer (Fig. 50-5).

ASSESSING THE IMPACT OF RADIATION THERAPY AFTER LUMPECTOMY IN THE ELDERLY

CALGB 9343: Comparison of Lumpectomy Plus Tamoxifen with and without Radiotherapy in Women 70 Years of Age or Older Who Have Clinical Stage I, Estrogen Receptor–Positive Breast Carcinoma

Breast cancer often has a more indolent course in elderly women. In addition, decreased life expectancy resulting from age and comorbid conditions shortens the time during which older women are at risk for recurrence. CALGB trial 9343 examined the contribution of radiation after lumpectomy in women age 70 and older with estrogen receptor–positive breast cancers 2 cm or smaller in size. Patients were required to have a clinically negative axilla, and clear margins on the lumpectomy specimen were required. Surgical staging of the axilla was optional.

Patients were randomized to lumpectomy plus tamoxifen and radiation or lumpectomy plus tamoxifen alone. All received tamoxifen 20 mg daily for 5 years and those randomized to radiation underwent whole-breast irradiation with tangential fields. With a median follow-up of 8.2 years, the benefit of radiation was found to be minimal.[15,16] Although breast cancer recurrences were more frequent in those who did not receive radiation than in those receiving radiation (Fig. 50-6), there was no significant difference in mastectomy rate (9/319 vs 4/317, respectively) or in overall survival (Fig. 50-7).

This study also assessed axillary recurrence rates among elderly women who did not undergo axillary dissection. Of the 200 women in the tamoxifen and radiation group there were no recurrences in the axilla as compared to 4 (2%) recurrences in the axilla in the tamoxifen alone group out of 203 women. It was concluded that lumpectomy followed by tamoxifen, without radiation, is a reasonable treatment option for women 70 and older with small, estrogen receptor–positive breast cancers.

Tumor markers were evaluated in this elderly breast cancer population in a correlative science companion trial. These tumors had generally favorable patterns of marker expression with only 9% (23/354) p53 positive and only 7% showing

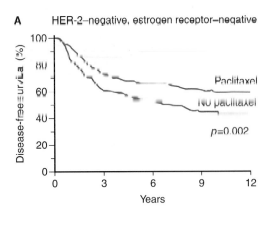

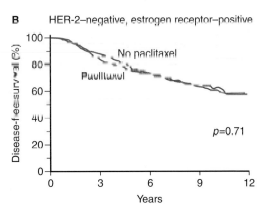

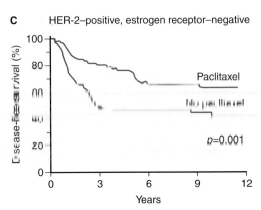

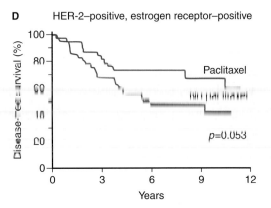

FIGURE 50-5   Disease-free survival among patients treated with or without paclitaxel according to estrogen receptor status and HER-2 expression. *[Reproduced, with permission, from Hayes DF, et al. HER2 and response to paclitaxel in node-positive breast cancer. N Engl J Med. 2007;357(15):1496-1506.]*

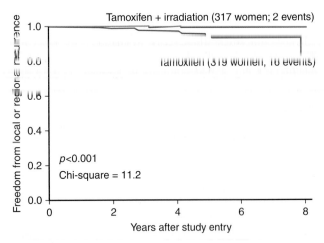

FIGURE 50-6   CALGB 9343: comparison of lumpectomy plus tamoxifen with and without radiotherapy in women 70 years of age or older who have clinical stage I estrogen receptor–positive breast carcinoma. Time to first local or regional recurrence. *(Courtesy of Dr Kevin Hughes.)*

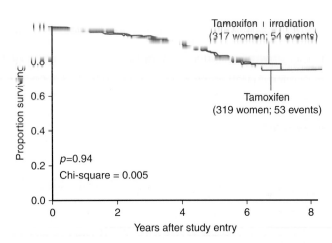

FIGURE 50-7   CALGB 9343: comparison of lumpectomy plus tamoxifen with and without radiotherapy in women 70 years of age or older who have clinical stage I, estrogen receptor–positive breast carcinoma. Overall survival. *(Courtesy of Dr Kevin Hughes.)*

HER-2 overexpression. Among tumors overexpressing HER-2 protein, most did not demonstrate gene amplification.[17]

FUTURE DIRECTIONS

SOFT (CALGB 40401) is a phase III trial (led by IBCSG) evaluating the role of ovarian suppression and the role of exemestane as adjuvant therapies for premenopausal women with endocrine-responsive breast cancer. With a greater understanding of molecular profiling, the TAILORX trial (led by ECOG) is looking at assigning individualized options for treatment. CALGB has commenced a contrast-enhanced breast magnetic resonance imaging (MRI) trial with correlative science studies to characterize tumor response in patients undergoing neoadjuvant treatment for locally advanced breast cancer. New trials by CALGB will continue to impact the surgical oncologist's practice by changing treatment paradigms.

SUMMARY

Over the past 50 years the efforts of the CALGB clinical trials have impacted adjuvant chemotherapy protocols, established targeted molecular markers, and defined subset populations for adjuvant treatment. The armamentarium in the treatment of early stage breast cancer continues to evolve as a result of randomized trials and correlative science projects set forth by the CALGB in collaboration with other cooperative groups.

REFERENCES

1. The Cancer and Leukemia Group B: Welcome to the Cancer and Leukemia Group B Web site. Available at: http://www.calgb.org/. Accessed December 15, 2008.
2. National Institutes of Health Consensus Development Conference Statement: Adjuvant Chemotherapy for Breast Cancer. *CA-A Cancer Journal for Clinicians.* 1985; September 9-11.
3. Wood WC, Budman DR, Korzun AH, et al. Dose and dose intensity of adjuvant chemotherapy for stage II, node-positive carcinoma. *N Engl J Med.* 1994;330:1253-1259.
4. Henderson IC, Berry DA, Demetri GD, et al. Improved outcomes from adding sequential paclitaxel but not from escalating doxorubicin dose in an adjuvant chemotherapy regimen for patients with node-positive primary breast cancer. *J Clin Oncol.* 2003;21:976-983.
5. Mamounas EP, Bryant J, Lembersky B, et al. Paclitaxel after doxorubicin plus cyclophosphamide as adjuvant chemotherapy for node-positive breast cancer: results from NSABP B-28. *J Clin Oncol.* 2005;23:3686-3696.
6. Sartor CI, Peterson BL, Woolf S, et al. Effect of addition of adjuvant paclitaxel on radiotherapy delivery and locoregional control of node-positive breast cancer: Cancer and Leukemia Group B 9344. *J Clin Oncol.* 2005;23:30-40.
7. Norton L. Theoretical concepts and the emerging role of taxanes in adjuvant therapy. *Oncologist.* 2001;6(suppl):30-35.
8. Citron ML, Berry DA, Cirrincione C, et al. Randomized trial of dose-dense versus conventionally scheduled and sequential versus concurrent combination chemotherapy as postoperative adjuvant treatment of node-positive primary breast cancer: first report of Intergroup Trial C9741/Cancer and Leukemia Group B Trial 974. *J Clin Oncol.* 2003;21:1431-1439.
9. Peters WP, Rosner GL, Vredenburgh JJ, et al. Prospective, randomized comparison of high-dose chemotherapy after surgery and adjuvant chemotherapy in women with high-risk primary breast cancer: a report of CALBG 9082, SWOG 9114, and NCIC MA-13. *J Clin Oncol.* 2005;23:2191-2200.
10. Muss HB, Thor AD, Berry DA, et al. c-erbB-2 expression and response to adjuvant therapy in women with node-positive early breast cancer. *N Engl J Med.* 1994;330:1260-1266.
11. Thor AD, Berry DA, Budman DR, et al. ErbB-2, p53 and efficacy of adjuvant therapy in lymph node-positive breast cancer. *J Natl Cancer Inst.* 1998;90:1346-1360.
12. DiGiovanna MP, Stern DF, Edgerton S, et al. Influence of activation state of ErbB-2 (HER-2) on response to adjuvant cyclophosphamide, doxorubicin, and fluorouracil for stage II, node-positive breast cancer: study 8541 from the Cancer and Leukemia Group B. *J Clin Oncol.* 2008;26(14):2364-2372.
13. Dressler LG, Berry DA, Broadwater G, et al. Comparison of HER2 status by fluorescence in situ hybridization and immunohistochemistry to predict benefit from dose escalation of adjuvant doxorubicin-based therapy in node-positive breast cancer patients. *J Clin Oncol.* 2005;23:4287-4297.
14. Hayes DF, Thor AD, Dressler LG, et al. HER2 and response to paclitaxel in node-positive breast cancer. *N Engl J Med.* 2007;357(15):1496-1506.
15. Hughes KS, Schnaper LA, Berry D, et al. Lumpectomy plus tamoxifen with or without irradiatioin in women 70 years of age or older with early breast cancer. *N Engl J Med.* 2004;351:971-977.
16. Hughes KS, Schnaper LA, Berry D, et al. Lumpectomy plus tamoxifen with or without irradiation in women 70 years of age or older with early breast cancer: a report of further followup. San Antonio Breast Cancer Symposium, 2006 [online]. Available at: http://www.abstracts2view.com/sabcs06/view.php?nu=SABCS06L_433. Accessed December 4, 2008.
17. Dressler LG, Berry DA, Broadwater G et al. Comparison of HER2 status by fluorescence in situ hybridization (FISH) and immunohistochemistry (IHC) to predict benefit from dose escalation of adjuvant doxorubicin-based therapy in node positive breast cancer patients: CALGB 8869 a laboratory companion to CALGB 8541. *J Clin Oncol.* 2005;23(19):4287-4297.

CHAPTER 51

The RTOG Experience

Beryl McCormick
Julia White

The RTOG Cooperative Group celebrated its 40-year anniversary this year. However, the present Working Group is much younger, established in 1994 to focus on local-regional breast cancer issues involving radiation therapy questions. This chapter discusses those initiatives.

RTOG 95-17: PARTIAL BREAST RADIATION TRIAL

The concept of partial breast irradiation (PBI) was brought to the attention of the RTOG by Dr Robert Kuske, at one of the first meetings of the group. The idea was not new; Fentiman and colleagues had published a pilot study exploring the use of a small iridium 192 implant for breast cancer treatment in 1991. The local failure rate was higher than that of standard whole breast radiation, and the cosmetic outcome was inferior.[1]

However, both Kuske at the Ochsner Clinic and Vicini at William Beaumont Hospital pursued the idea of treating less than the whole breast after lumpectomy, utilizing low-dose-rate (LDR) and then high-dose-rate (HDR) brachytherapy when it became available. Based on their early, positive results,[2,3] the RTOG Breast Group began to design the first cooperative group PBI trial, RTOG 95-17. This phase I/II trial specifically targeted small lesions (3 cm or less) with invasive ductal histology (IDC) only. Invasive lobular carcinoma was specifically excluded, as were patients with an extensive intraductal component to their IDC. This decision was made to exclude carcinomas characterized by microscopic extension beyond their clinically or radiographically apparent borders. In addition to the lumpectomy, an axillary node dissection was required, reflecting the surgical standard of the time. Women were eligible for entry in the trial with up to 3 nodes involved, although no extra capsular extension was allowed.

For women with an indication for systemic chemotherapy, the order of treatment was radiation first, followed by chemotherapy, with at least a 2 week interval from the completion of the radiation. The original accrual goal was 46 HDR cases and 46 LDR cases.

RTOG 95-17: Accrual and Results

The study opened in 1997 and completed accrual in 2000; 100 women were accrued, with just 1 excluded from analysis because she underwent a sentinel node biopsy only. Reflecting changing trends in brachytherapy, 66 cases were accrued to the HDR arm and 33 to the LDR arm. Of interest, only 11 RTOG institutions placed cases on this protocol, reflecting the high level of skill required of the oncologist to perform these implants.

This study set a high standard for quality assurance (QA), requiring a credentialing process for each participating center before enrolling cases. In addition, each case was "rapidly reviewed" by the principal investigator within 24 hours of catheter placement. For 8 patients, this led to revisions in their implant dosimetry prior to treatment. The success of the quality assurance program is evidenced by 96% of cases meeting specified requirements and only minor variation in the other 4% on final analysis.[4] This plan formed the foundation for quality assurance in the large phase III RTOG 0413/NSABP B-39 trial that was to follow.

The 99 cases in this study included stage I-II breast cancer patients (88% T1 tumors, 20% N1 axilla) and with predominantly estrogen receptor–positive disease (75%). Median age of women in this study was 62 years; 45% were between the ages 50 and 69, 35% were 70 years or above, and just 21% were below 50 years. Tamoxifen was the most commonly used systemic agent, prescribed alone or in combination with chemotherapy in

55% of the patients. Analysis of this study demonstrated acceptable acute toxicity with 4% grade 3 to 4 toxicity occurring during treatment, 10% ≥ grade 3 toxicity at any point during follow-up and 4% ≥ grade 3 toxicity at last follow-up.[5] The excellent/good cosmetic rate for 66 HDR patients at 2 years was 78% as reported by radiation oncologists, and 86% as reported by the patients.[6] With a median follow-up time of 7 years, there have been 6 in-breast failures for a 5-year rate of 4% and 4 regional nodal failures for a 5-year rate of 3%.[7]

PBI with MammoSite Brachytherapy

Another brachytherapy technique for PBI was industry developed based on the principles of multicatheter PBI used in RTOG 95-17 with the goal of simplifying the technology to improve utilization. The MammoSite device is a single catheter with an inflatable balloon at the distal end that expands to fill the surgical cavity after placement. There are 2 channels in the catheter: one for balloon inflation with sterile normal saline and the second to carry a small radioactive source into the device after it is in position in the breast following a lumpectomy. An initial multi-institutional phase I-II study evaluating the feasibility and safety of the device treated 43 women with stage I breast cancer with invasive ductal histology only, between 2000 and 2001. The 5-year follow-up of the study has demonstrated excellent local control, and acceptable toxicity and cosmetic outcome.[8]

MammoSite was approved by the FDA in May 2002, and because of its relative simplicity to use, was met with great popularity across the United States. It is estimated that more than 2500 balloons were placed by late 2003.[9] The original manufacturer of the device, Proxima Therapeutics, did initiate a registry for its use, which was taken over by the American Society of Breast Surgeons in late 2003. Its first report documented placement of the device in 1403 women enrolled in the study, from May 2002 through July 2004.[10]

PBI WITH EXTERNAL BEAM: RTOG 0319

In 2000, Vicini and colleagues at William Beaumont Hospital initiated a phase I/II study to explore an external beam method of doing PBI. Using 4 or 5 non-coplanar beams, and with additional margin around the planned target volume to accommodate breathing motion, the group reported on results with their first 9 patients in 2003. The initial dose in the study was 34 Gy in 10 fractions, delivered BID. However, in brachytherapy the dose prescribed is generally the minimum dose covering the target; the external beam technique resulted in a very uniform dose throughout the target. Based on radiobiology modelling, to estimate the equivalent dose to most of the target with external beam PBI compared to brachytherapy, the total dose was increased to 38.5 Gy.[11]

This study was rapidly embraced by the RTOG Breast Group, as a possible means of expanding its role in investigating PBI, but using a technology familiar to all RTOG members, not just those select few with the technical skills required to perform breast brachytherapy. Under Dr Vicini's leadership,

RTOG 0319 was conceived using similar entry criteria as 95-17. The most significant aspect of this trial is that a treatment planning computed tomography (CT) simulation was required, with contouring of both target and normal structures and a QA program for pretreatment documentation of dose delivery to the target and avoidance of normal tissues. This represents the first use of CT-based conformal radiation for breast cancer in a cooperative group clinical trial.

In just 9 months, 31 centers were credentialed for participation in the study, and accrual of 58 women was reached. Analysis of the first 42 patients in the study demonstrated both feasibility and reproducibility of this technique on a large scale across many centers.[12] Other endpoints such as local control and cosmetic outcome will require longer follow-up.

THE PHASE III RTOG 0413/NSABP B-39 TRIAL

In an effort to gather support for a phase III trial comparing PBI to the standard of care, whole-breast external beam radiation, the NCI hosted a meeting between the NSABP and RTOG leadership to facilitate the collaboration in designing and carrying out such a trial. The group leadership agreed to co-lead this study, with RTOG taking the lead in quality assurance, and the NSABP in patient data management.

A phase III trial (NSABP B39/RTOG 0413) randomizing stage 0 to II breast cancer patients who have undergone lumpectomy to whole-breast irradiation (WBI) versus PBI with multicatheter brachytherapy, MammoSite, or 3-dimensional (3D) conformal external beam PBI opened in March 2005. Eligibility criteria for this trial were more permissive than the ones used in either RTOG 95-17 or RTOG 0319, with the goal of evaluating whether PBI was not inferior to WBI in all patient groups technically feasible to undergo PBI after lumpectomy with any of the 3 methods under study. Eligibility includes women more than 18 years of age with tumors less than 3 cm in size with negative resection margins after lumpectomy, and noninvasive and all invasive histology, including those with infiltrating lobular disease or an extensive intraductal component. Patients with up to 3 positive axillary nodes are also eligible. Radiation dose prescription for multicatheter and 3D conformal external beam PBI methods was adopted from RTOG 95-17 and RTOG 0319, respectively. MammoSite PBI radiation dose prescription was based on the initial industry-sponsored multi-institutional trial evaluating safety and feasibility of the device. For all 3 PBI methods, defined CT volumes for targets were established and required to be contoured on all CT scans. Radiation dose specifications for acceptable target volume coverage and limits for avoidance of normal tissue volumes were defined for all 3 PBI methods.

Activation of this trial required establishment of a rigorous radiation QA process in collaboration with the Advanced Technology Consortium (ATC) to ensure that each of the CT-based PBI methods delivered dose accurately to protocol-specified target volumes and met normal tissue dose constraints. Institutions were first credentialed for each PBI method used, prior to enrolling patients in the trial. The first patient on each PBI method is rapidly reviewed (72 hours) by the ATC and one of the study investigators, and the patient cannot be treated until the case is approved. The next 4 cases of each PBI method are reviewed in a timely manner within a week of treatment. After the first 5 reviews and a summary review, the institution's subsequent cases for each BPI method are then randomly reviewed. The PBI QA is Web based, allowing study investigators to remotely review cases.

The WBI on this trial was based on prior RTOG and NSABP studies, but for the first time in a cooperative group trial for breast cancer, a CT scan for radiation treatment planning was recommended and guidance for its use outlined in the protocol. RTOG implemented a large Web-based database for documentation of WBI QA.

In the phase III NSABP B-39/RTOG 0413 clinical trial, quality-of-life (QOL) endpoints may become the primary focus if local control proves equivalent in the 2 arms. This study is comparing QOL issues related to cosmesis, fatigue, treatment-related symptoms, and perceived convenience of care between 980 women receiving PBI and WBI based on their receipt of chemotherapy. The Breast Cancer Treatment Outcome Scale (BCTOS) is used to assess cosmetic results using patient self-reports in addition to patient and physician scoring of the cosmetic appearance of the breast. Other QOL scales used for this trial include a Convenience of Care scale and the MOS SF-36 Vitality Scale to assess fatigue. An RTOG Web-based database for cosmetic photos was established to support the QOL objectives.

DCIS: THE RTOG 9804 TRIAL

The indications for and benefits from radiation following a breast-conserving procedure for ductal carcinoma in situ (DCIS) have been demonstrated in several large phase III trials, including the NSABP B-17 trial (see NSABP chapter), the similar EORTC trial 10853 (see EORTC chapter), and the more recent SweDCIS trial.[13,14] In all these trials, the addition of radiation to surgery alone resulted in decreased risk of local failure of approximately 50% or greater. Yet despite these consistent results, the use of radiation for DCIS remains controversial for many surgeons in the so-called low-risk group of patients.

The RTOG addressed this issue with trial 9804, designed to study radiation versus none after wide local excision, in patients specifically in the low-risk group. For the trial, this low-risk group was defined as women with unicentric disease found by mammogram only, or those incidentally found at surgery, of low or intermediate nuclear grade, and with necrosis in less than one-third of the ducts examined. Size was 2.5 cm or less, as defined on imaging if possible, and minimal margin width for trial entry was 3 mm. Patients were stratified by age, size of lesion, and final margin width (ie, 3-9 mm, 10 mm or more, or negative reexcision). Tamoxifen for 5 years was prescribed for all women in the original version, but made optional several years into the study.

Accrual was planned for 1800 women; the study was closed in 2007, with just over 600 women randomized over almost 10 years. This patient group will be analyzed when all women in the study have completed treatment, including the 5 years of hormone therapy.

CALGB TRIAL 9343

After the Breast Intergroup was organized, support for the open CALGB/ECOG trial comparing whole-breast radiation plus tamoxifen for 5 years to tamoxifen alone, for women 70 years of age or older, was sought. The RTOG opened that study as RTOG 9702, with strong support from its membership, contributing over one-third of the women in the study by the time the study reached accrual. Details of the study and its results are presented in the CALGB chapter.

FUTURE DIRECTIONS

The RTOG Breast Cancer Working Group's goal is to maximize local-regional control by designing trials that evaluate the benefits of new radiation technology, seek to reduce treatment-related toxicity, optimize radiation based on chemotherapy response, and establish biomarkers for radiation response with translational models. Also, the Breast Cancer Working Group will continue to support Intergroup phase III trials evaluating novel systemic therapies in breast cancer that include radiation as a treatment component.

There has been unparalleled technological advancement for planning and delivery of radiation therapy in recent years. Planning systems use 3D conformal radiation therapy (CRT) and intensity modulated radiation therapy (IMRT) for maximizing target coverage and minimizing inclusion of normal tissues. Image-guided treatment delivery with ultrasound and CT are now practiced daily in many radiation oncology facilities. These newer radiation technologies were integral to the successful development of PBI after lumpectomy for early-stage breast cancer. The RTOG 0319 trial represents the first use, in a clinical cooperative trial, of CT volume-based radiation treatment planning, defined limits for target doses and normal tissue constraints, as well as dose-volume analysis (DVA) for the treatment of breast cancer. All of these technical radiation delivery parameters were subsequently developed for each of the 3 PBI methods used on the RTOG 0413/NSABP B-39 phase III trial that is presently accruing.

Dosimetry studies have demonstrated that IMRT can minimize the dose heterogeneity for breast irradiation.[15,16] One randomized trial has reported reduced grade III acute skin reactions from WBI delivered with IMRT when compared to 2-dimesional delivery methods.[17] Currently, there are no guidelines for the use of IMRT for breast irradiation such as the optimal number of treatment segments or QA methods. In addition, there is no consistent method for using CT-based volumes for WBI, including how to define on CT the targeted breast, the definition of the margin to be used around the lumpectomy cavity, or the lung and heart volumes as dose-limiting structures. In the future the RTOG Breast Working Group plans to evaluate whether improved targeting with CT-based volumes and reduced dose heterogeneity with IMRT or 3D CRT methods can improve the therapeutic ratio for WBI.

Using CT-based volumes and IMRT or 3D CRT, an accelerated WBI method is feasible that can differentially deliver a higher total dose to the lumpectomy cavity plus margin while irradiating the remainder of the breast over 18 to 22 total treatments.[18]

The reduced number of treatment visits could potentially lessen the burden of care on the patient, assist in improving breast-conservation rates, and decrease the impact of increased health care costs associated with implementing IMRT. This study is under development for the group.

The RTOG Breast Working Group is committed to developing CT-based conformal radiation therapy methods for regional nodal disease both postmastectomy and with breast conservation in appropriate patients. A Breast Cancer Atlas for CT anatomical volumes for regional nodes, including supraclavicular, axillary, and internal mammary; as well as breast, chest wall, and normal tissues at risk; heart; and lung has been developed by a subcommittee.[19] Doses for each target volume are being established along with maximum and minimum dose-volume tolerances for lung and heart. Once established, this information will be incorporated into clinical trials so that quality assurance can be instituted that reviews dose-volume analyses (DVA) to determine the reproducibility of dosing the target organs, cancer control related to dose volume, and toxicity associated with dose volume of normal tissue irradiated. The neoadjuvant approach to clinical stage III breast cancer represents a unique opportunity for incorporating and evaluating new conformal radiation therapy methods and identifying markers for radiation response.

Radiosurgery is the delivery of a highly conformal large radiation dose to a localized tumor by a stereotactic approach. This allows for ablative doses to be delivered to localized tumors and creates a steep gradient dose fall-off that provides sparing of immediately adjacent normal tissue. Stereotactic body radiation therapy (SBRT) has been used successfully in treatment of bone, lung, and liver metastases in separate trials reporting in-field local control rates of 80% to 90% at 1 to 2 years.[20] Most studies for SBRT for metastatic cancer have focused on technical dose delivery and outcome to an anatomical metastatic site (eg, spine, liver) and breast cancer patients were among many different primary disease sites. The Breast Working Group aims to establish if this technology can impact the progression free survival of oligometastatic breast cancer and to determine if biological markers can be identified that can predict for response.

SUMMARY

The RTOG Breast Cancer Working Group was established in 1994 to focus on local-regional breast cancer issues involving radiation therapy questions. Most recently the RTOG has been studying the role of radiation for DCIS, partial breast radiation, and accelerated partial breast radiation using various methods. The RTOG Breast Cancer Working Group's goals for future studies are to maximize local-regional control by designing trials that evaluate the benefits of new radiation technology and trials that seek to reduce treatment-related toxicity, optimize radiation based on chemotherapy response, and establish biomarkers for radiation response with translational models. The RTOG Breast Cancer Working Group will continue to support Intergroup phase III trials evaluating novel systemic therapies in breast cancer that include radiation as a treatment component.

REFERENCES

1. Perihan T, Pablo C, Tong Li, et al. Iridium implant plus external radiotherapy for operable breast cancer. A pilot study. *Eur J Cancer*. 1991;27:447-450.
2. King T, Bolton J, Kuske R, et al. Long-term results of wide-field brachytherapy as the sole method of radiation therapy after segmental mastectomy for Tis,1,2 breast cancer. *Am J Surg*. 2000;180:299-304.
3. Vicini F, Baglan K, Kestin L, et al. Accelerated treatment of breast cancer. *J Clin Oncol*. 2001;19:1993-2001.
4. Ibbott G, Hanson W, O'Meara E, et al. Dose specification and quality assurance of Radiation Therapy Oncology Group protocol 95-17: a cooperative group study of iridium 192 breast implant as sole therapy. *Int J Radiat Oncol Biol Phys*. 2007;69:1572-1578.
5. Kuske R, Winter K, Arthur D, et al. Phase II trial of brachytherapy alone after lumpectomy for select breast cancer: toxicity analysis of RTOG 95-17. *Int J Radiat Oncol Biol Phys*. 2006;65(1):45-51.
6. Rabinovitch R, Winter K, Taylor M, et al. Mature toxicity and cosmesis outcomes from RTOG 95-17: a phase I/II trial to evaluate brachytherapy as the sole method of radiation therapy for stage I and II breast carcinoma. San Antonio Breast Cancer Conference, December, 2007.
7. Arthur D, Winter K, Kuske R, et al. A phase II trial of brachytherapy alone following lumpectomy for select breast cancer: tumor control and survival outcomes of RTOG 95-17. *Int J Radiat Oncol Biol Phys*. 2008;72(2):467-473.
8. Benitez PR, Keisch ME, Vicini F, et al. Five-year results: the initial clinical trial of MammoSite balloon brachytherapy for partial breast irradiation in early-stage breast cancer. *Am J Surg*. 2007;194(4):456-462.
9. Arthur D. Accelerated partial breast irradiation: a change in treatment paradigm for early stage breast cancer. *J Surg Oncol*. 2003;84:185-191.
10. Vicini F, Beitsch P, Quiet C, et al. First analysis of patient demographics, technical reproducibility, cosmesis, and early toxicity. *Cancer*. 2005;104(6):1138-1148.
11. Baglan K, Sharpe M, Jaffray D, et al. Accelerated partial breast irradiation using 3D conformal radiation therapy (3D-CRT). *Int J Radiat Oncol Biol Phys*. 2003;55(2):302-311.
12. Vicini F, Winter K, Straube W, et al. A phase I/II trial to evaluate three-dimensional conformal radiation therapy confined to the region of the lumpectomy cavity for stage I/II breast cancer: initial report of feasibility and reproducibility of radiation therapy oncology group (RTOG) study 0319. *Int J Radiat Oncol Biol Phys*. 2005;63(5):1531-1537.
13. Bijker N, Meijnen P, Peterse J, et al. Breast-conserving treatment with or without radiotherapy in ductal carcinoma in site: ten-year results of European Organization for research and treatment of cancer randomized phase III trial 10853—a study by the EORTC Breast Cancer Cooperative Group and EORTC Radiotherapy Group. *J Clin Oncol*. 2006;24(21):3381-3387.
14. Emdin S, Granstrand B, Ringberg A, et al. SweDCIS: radiotherapy after sector resection for ductal carcinoma in situ of the breast. Results of a randomized trial in a population offered mammography screening. *Acta Oncologica*. 2006;45:536-543.
15. Kestin L, Sharpe M, Frazier R, et al. Intensity modulation to improve dose uniformity with tangential breast radiotherapy: initial clinical experience. *Int J Radiat Oncol Biol Phys*. 2000;48:1559-1568.
16. Ahunbay E, Chen G, Thatcher S, et al. Direct aperture optimization based intensity modulated radiotherapy for whole breast irradiation. *Int J Radiat Oncol Biol Phys*. 2007;67:1248-1258.
17. Donovan E, Bleakley N, Denholm E, et al. Randomized trial of standard 2D radiotherapy (RT) versus intensity modulated radiotherapy (IMRT) in patients prescribed breast radiotherapy. *Radiother Oncol*. 2007;82:254-264.
18. Freedman G, Anderson P, Goldstein L, et al. Four-week course of radiation for breast cancer suing hypofractionated intensity modulated radiation therapy with an incorporated boost. *Int J Radiat Oncol Biol Phys*. 2007;68:347-353.
19. Li XA, Tai A, Arthur D, et al. Variability of target and normal structure delineation for breast cancer radiotherapy: an RTOG multi-institutional and multi-observer study. *Int J Radiat Oncol Biol Phys*. 2009;73:944-51.
20. Milano M, Zhang H, Metcalfe S, et al. Oligometastatic breast cancer treated with curative-intent stereotactic body radiation therapy. *Breast Cancer Res Treat*. 2009;115:601-608.

OPERATIVE MANAGEMENT

Anthony Lucci

Tari King

CHAPTER 52

Paravertebral Block as an Anesthetic Technique in Patients Undergoing Breast Cancer Surgery

Farzin Goravanchi
Ronald Parris

It has been well documented that a paravertebral block (PVB) reduces the stress response in patients with breast cancer, and PVB has been used in various surgical procedures and for the management of chronic pain.[1] PVB is a form of regional anesthesia and was first performed by Hugo Sellheim of Leipzig, Germany in 1905 as a replacement for spinal anesthesia.[2] The literature describes PVB being used in the thoracic and lumbar regions in a unilateral and bilateral fashion. PVB may be used for multiple surgical procedures, including, but not limited to, thoracotomy, laparoscopic or open cholecystectomy, colectomy, gastrectomy, abdominal and inguinal hernia repairs, appendectomy, transurethral prostatectomy, hip replacement, and total knee replacement.[3] At The University of Texas MD Anderson Cancer Center, we primarily use PVB for breast cancer–related surgeries, including mastectomies, axillary dissections, and breast reconstruction.

ANATOMY

The thoracic paravertebral space is the space on each side of the vertebrae. For breast surgery, we use the T1 through T6 paravertebral spaces. Anterolaterally, the space is formed by parietal pleura; medially, the space is formed by the vertebral body, intervertebral disk, and intervertebral foramen; and posteriorly, the space is formed by the superior costotransverse ligament. The intercostal space is lateral to the paravertebral space and contains the intercostal nerve, and the epidural space is medial to it. In the paravertebral space, the spinal nerves are not covered by the fascial sheath.[4]

INDICATIONS/PATIENT SELECTION

PVB is used for unilateral and bilateral breast surgery, as well as postmastectomy breast reconstruction. To be candidates for undergoing PVB, patients have to meet certain minimum requirements. First, the surgical field should not exceed the area being covered by the block. Second, the anesthesiologist, the surgeon, and the patient should agree on the necessity of the block. The patient's anatomy should be compatible with the block, as discussed below. We also routinely perform PVB in patients who are undergoing bilateral mastectomies with breast tissue expander placements (Figs. 52-1 and 52-2).

NEEDLE PLACEMENT

In an attempt to be time efficient, placement of the PVB is performed in the preoperative holding area.[4] During the actual placement of the paravertebral block, the patient is fully monitored (oxygen saturation as measured by pulse oximetry, electrocardiogram, noninvasive blood pressure with supplemental oxygen) with resuscitation and intubation equipment immediately available if necessary.[4] At MD Anderson Cancer Center, we routinely block the Thoracic 1 (T1) through Thoracic 6 (T6) paravertebral spaces for many of our breast surgical procedures (eg, modified radical mastectomy, total mastectomy, axillary dissections, cosmetic breast surgical procedure such as tissue expanders, breast augmentation with implants, and mastopexy). Most of the patients who undergo PVB also receive a general anesthetic during surgery. The PVB is primarily used for postoperative pain control.

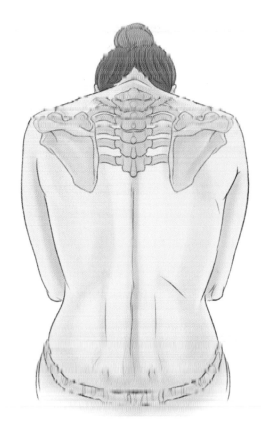

FIGURE 52-1 Patient positioning for the block.

Patients who undergo PVB are placed in the sitting position and sedated with midazolam 2 mg administered intravenously (IV), fentanyl 50 to 100 µg IV, and a titrated dose of propofol.[5] All patients receive promethazine 6 mg IV and famotidine 20 mg IV before actual placement of the PVB. The literature suggests that placement of the PVB can occur in the lateral decubitus position and the side being blocked in the elevated aspect of the patient.[11]

PVB is generally performed with the patient in the sitting position; the patient's neck should be flexed, shoulders dropped forward, and back arched, and the patients' chin should rest on the chest, with the patient slightly leaning forward.[4] The needle entry point is found by observing the midline of the superior aspect of the thoracic spinous processes (T1-T6), measuring 2.5 cm unilateral or bilaterally, and marking the point of entry, which should overlie the inferior aspect of the transverse process.[7] The patient's back is cleaned and prepped in the usual sterile fashion with povidone-iodine or chlorhexidine gluconate and then anesthetized with a local anesthetic at the needle entry site in a unilateral or bilateral manner. Ropivacaine 1% (2-3 mL) is injected subcutaneously along the line where the injections should be made.[8] The amount of sedation required to place the PVB is one that requires the patient to be cooperative and the airway maintained without assistance.[5]

The transverse process should be expected to be contacted 2 to 4 cm beyond the point at which the needle penetrates the skin.[5] Knowledge of the approximate depth from the skin to the paravertebral space is required for safe and effective placement of the PVB.[9] The approximate median depth of the skin to the paravertebral space is 33 mm in the T1 to T6 dermatome levels.[6] It has been well documented that a patient's body mass index (BMI) influences the distance between the skin and paravertebral space.[6] Thus the greater the BMI, the greater the distance from the skin to the paravertebral space.

Using a 22-gauge 10-cm Tuohy spinal needle attached with extension tubing to the syringe containing the local anesthetic, the needle is incrementally advanced approximately 1 mm anteriorly and is perpendicular to the back in all planes until the transverse process is contacted.[5] The needle is then withdrawn from the transverse process and walked off in a caudal fashion.[5] Once all contact from the transverse process is lost, the needle is then advanced approximately 1 cm to the paravertebral space.[5,9] If the needle is inserted at the appropriate depth and the transverse process is not contacted, then the needle is probably between 2 transverse processes.[4] Advancing the needle to a deeper depth is not recommended; instead, the needle should be withdrawn and redirected in a cephalad or caudal fashion until the transverse process is located.[4] If the angle is too extreme while attempting to walk off the transverse process in a caudal fashion, the needle is probably contacting the transverse process in the superior aspect instead of the desired inferior aspect.[4] In this situation, there are 2 recommended options. One option is to withdraw the needle back to the skin and reinsert the needle approximately 0.5 to 1.0 cm inferiorly to locate the paravertebral space.[4] Another option is to walk off the transverse

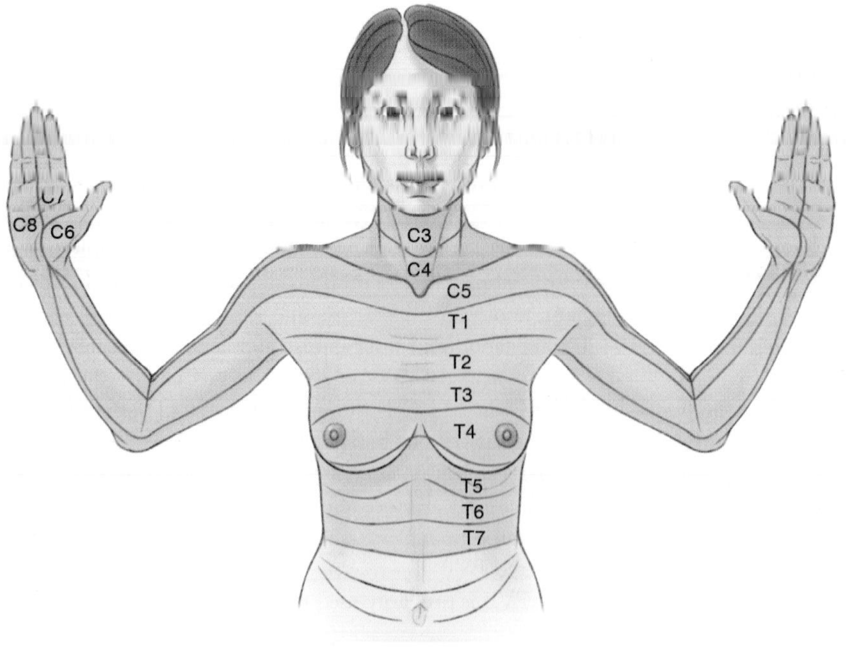

FIGURE 52-2 Dermatomes.

process in a cephalad fashion, remaining cognizant of the fact that the nerve root is being blocked 1 level higher than originally intended.[4] If the 22-gauge Tuohy needle advances beyond the appropriate depth, it may contact bone, which is probably the rib, because the ribs are anterior to the transverse process. Once again, the needle should be withdrawn to find the desired superficial contact of bone, and this should be the transverse process.[4]

When the Tuohy needle passes through the costotransverse ligament, it causes a "popping" sound, and a loss of resistance is felt. However, relying on the popping sound is not always pathognomonic for locating the paravertebral space when one has successfully walked off the transverse process.

The needle should never be redirected medially because of the increased risk of the needle passing into the intervertebral foramina and resulting in an epidural or spinal anesthetic or a spinal cord injury.[8] Medial needle insertion is identical to the paramedial approach for an epidural or spinal block[8] (Fig. 52-3).

INTEROPERATIVE MANAGEMENT

The breast surgical procedure can be managed in several different ways:

1. PVB with no further sedation. This technique can be used for patients who are pregnant or who have multiple comorbidities and are, therefore, not candidates for further anesthesia.

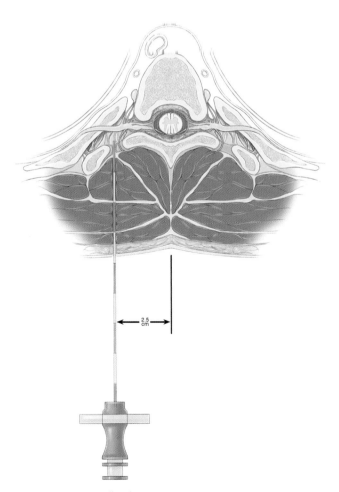

FIGURE 52-3 Needle placement.

2. PVB with intravenous sedation. This technique can be used for most patients.
3. PVB with general anesthesia. Most patients at MD Anderson receive a light general anesthesia with a laryngeal mask airway (LMA). In addition, LMA with spontaneous respiration has been used, because LMA is less invasive for the airway than endotracheal tube and there are fewer requirements for intraoperative narcotics secondary to the endotracheal tube. Most patients require approximately 50 μg of fentanyl intraoperatively; this amount includes the fentanyl used for sedation for the block in the holding area.

POSTOPERATIVE MANAGEMENT

The postanesthesia care unit (PACU) nursing management of patients undergoing a PVB does not require additional nursing skills.[2] Postoperatively, PVB provides high-quality pain relief and minimizes the need for opioids postoperatively.[2] The anesthetic complications of postoperative nausea and vomiting (PONV) have been present in 20% to 50% of patients.[10] The incidence is higher among female patients, patients with postoperative pain, and patients undergoing general anesthesia. The incidence of PONV has been less in patients who received a PVB than in those who underwent general anesthesia.[11,12] Patients who received a PVB are also discharged earlier than patients who underwent general anesthesia alone.[13] However, PONV prolongs the patient discharge time from the PACU and potentially requires hospitalization. By incorporating a PVB, the PACU narcotic use is decreased, so that patients can undergo ambulatory surgery.[13]

HOSPITAL UTILIZATION: DURATION OF HOSPITAL STAY AND COST OF PVB

At times of managed care and cost confinement, we have used PVB as a means of cost reduction in our practice. Patients who have PVB and undergo mastectomy or axillary dissection may be discharged home earlier than patients who do not have PVB performed.[14] A previous study reported a 75% to 78% cost reduction in patients who underwent ambulatory breast cancer surgery as compared with patients who were discharged 2 to 3 days postoperatively.[14] This reduction in cost was because of elimination of the hospital room fee, materials, and pharmacy charges.[14] The material cost of performing a PVB, including pharmaceuticals, needle, prep solution, and gloves, is approximately $49 at our institution.

In our practice, PVB has not prolonged operating room, postoperative care unit, or PACU utilization time, nor does PVB require expensive equipment. With this technique, patients can be discharged the same day as their procedure for a shorter overall hospital stay. If the patient is discharged the same day, there is no need for the surgical team to make rounds the next day. Our follow-up data show patients are satisfied with being able to return home earlier; this may also give patients a sense of control over their disease process and activity level, and a decreased sense of sickness.[14] With decreased time spent in the hospital, there is also a decreased chance of acquiring a nosocomial infection or distribution of the wrong medication, which could also prove to be very costly.

CONTRAINDICATION

PVB is contraindicated in patients who refuse to have the procedure or those who have coagulopathy. Local sepsis or tumor involvement in the paravertebral space also precludes patients from undergoing PVB. In addition, patients with scoliosis, chest deformity, or certain neuropathy, those who are psychologically unsuitable, or those who have undergone prior operations that have altered the anatomy of the paravertebral space should not undergo PVB. Alteration of the anatomy around the paravertebral space could potentially cause penetration of the needle and the local anesthesia into the pleura, intervertebral foramen, or the subarachnoid space.

Patients who are morbidly obese (BMI > 35) or patients with a very thin anatomy also have a relative contraindication to PVB. First, it is technically difficult to feel the anatomy or place a PVB correctly in morbidly obese patients. In addition, morbidly obese patients may not be ideal candidates for LMA and spontaneous ventilation. There is higher risk of aspiration with an LMA in these patients, and it may be more difficult for the patients to breathe spontaneously in the supine position. Second, thin patients have a narrow paravertebral space and therefore a higher chance of developing complications, such as pneumothorax, epidural spread of the block, or subarachnoid block.

RISKS

Pleural Puncture/Pneumothorax

Given the close proximity of the paravertebral space and the parietal pleura, the 2 major complications most associated with PVB are pleural puncture and pneumothorax.[4] Although popular through the 1930s, PVB lost favor by the 1950s and 1960s and practically disappeared from the literature,[2] which was likely due to the risk of a pneumothorax during the procedure.[15] In the late 1970s, there appeared to be a renewed interest in PVB, and a subsequent reappearance in the literature,[2,15] as lower incidences of pneumothorax were cited.[15] It was documented that the actual risks of pleural puncture and pneumothorax were 0.8% to 1.1% and 0.5%, respectively,[3,9] and that the incidences of pleural puncture and pneumothorax were rare when the procedure was performed by an experienced anesthesiologist.[3] The literature suggests that patients who develop a pleural puncture rarely develop a symptomatic pneumothorax.[1] One should suspect a pleural puncture if aspiration of air occurs during the procedure or if there is little to no resistance upon injecting the local anesthetic.[9]

In our practice, we rarely provide positive pressure ventilation because of the risk of developing a tension pneumothorax. Consequently, there is an 8-fold increase in plural puncture and pneumothorax when the PVB is bilateral instead of unilateral[3,9]; however, the incidence of pneumothorax is still relatively low. At MD Anderson, our incidence of pneumothorax has been 0.15% in patients with multiple injections (T1-T6) in either bilateral or unilateral PVBs. Other risks associated with PVB are spinal anesthesia, epidural anesthetic hypotension, local anesthetic toxicity, hematoma, pain at the site of skin puncture, and failed block.[9]

Epidural and Spinal Spread

Because of the location of the central neuroaxial structures (dural cuff and intervertebral foramina), medial needle placement of the PVB can result in an accidental spinal or epidural blockade.[4] A unilateral paravertebral block in which the local anesthesia spreads into the epidural space or in which the dural cuff is accidentally punctured may cause the patient to have bilateral symptoms of an epidural or spinal anesthetic, respectively.[3] Naja and colleagues[3] suggest that the signs of epidural and spinal spread occur in about 1% of patients. One of the reasons for the lower rate of spinal or epidural block in our practice has been because of the lower volume injected at each level.

Hypotension

Hypotension may occur during the placement of a PVB, in which a unilateral block may be associated with the spread of local anesthetic into the epidural space.[2] Hypotension associated with a bilateral PVB may be due to the inhibition of the cardiac accelerator fibers.[10] The incidence of hypotension is thought to be approximately 4% to 5%, which makes this the second most common complication.[3] Hypotension occurs more frequently when clonidine is used as an adjunct to the local solution.[16]

Vascular Puncture

The literature suggests that the most common risk associated with PVB is accidental vascular puncture, which occurs in approximately 6.8% of the patients.[3] This is evident by the aspiration of blood through the needle before injection of a local anesthetic.[3] The use of vascular markers, such as epinephrine 1:400,000, is a safeguard when there is a false negative for intervascular injections. Epinephrine also plays a role in decreasing systemic vascular absorption of the local anesthetic, and therefore the risk of toxicity is rare.[3,4] The incidence of vascular puncture doubles when a bilateral PVB is performed.[3,9] In our practice, the incidence of vascular puncture has been lower than 0.1%.

Failed Block

A failed block has been defined as a pain score more than 5 of 10, with 10 being the worst pain score, and patients requiring excessive postoperative opioids in the PACU.[3] It can be associated with anatomical variations of the nerve in the lateral aspect of the paravertebral space.[17] Naja and colleagues have stated that the failure rate is actually as low as 6.1% to 10.0% in experienced hands.[1,3] The reason for this discrepancy in failure rates is associated with the technique that is used to place the block.[3] Lower failure rates may be due to the use of a peripheral nerve stimulator, and higher failure rates may be due to more conventional placement of the PVB.[3]

Other Minor Risks

Published literature suggests that some patients have complained of localized discomfort at the site of injection (approximately 1.3%), for which therapy with oral analgesics was sufficient.[3] There have also been reports of hematoma at the site of injection (approximately 2.4%), which has been treated with external compression.[3] In our practice, the patients who most commonly have reported postoperative pain at the site of the injection have been muscular female or male patients who have larger paraspinal muscles at the injection site. This pain is caused by the physical tear of the muscle fibers by the block needle, but this pain usually dissipates within a couple of days.

FUTURE STUDIES

Currently, there is a prospective study being conducted at MD Anderson examining the long-term effects of PVB in patients with breast cancer. Factors studied include possible beneficial effects of PVB on recurrence rates in breast cancer patients, as well as decreases in the costs associated with long-term patient care. There is still room for improvement in techniques and solutions used to optimize PVB and minimize side effects. Future studies should focus on the use of newer medications that could provide long-lasting analgesia with few side effects.

SUMMARY

PVB is a safe and effective technique to add to any anesthetic practice. PVB provides good analgesia, reduces PONV, and reduces the need for postoperative narcotics. Finally, PVB provides patients with the choice to be discharged from the hospital earlier than if they had received general anesthesia, which may result in a decrease in hospital and patient costs.

REFERENCES

1. Lonnqvist PA, MacKenzie J, Soni AK. Paravertebral blockade. *Anaesthesia.* 1995;50:813-815.
2. Richardson J, Lonnqvist PA. Thoracic paravertebral block. *Br J Anaesth.* 1998;81:230-238.
3. Naja Z, Lonnqvist PA. Somatic paravertebral nerve blockade. *Anaesthesia.* 2001;56:1181-1201.
4. Klein SM, Steele SM, Greengrass RA. A clinical overview of paravertebral blockade. *Internet J Anesthesiol.* 1999;3:1.
5. Klein SM, Bergh A, Steele SM, et al. Thoracic paravertebral block for breast surgery. *Anesth Analg.* 2000;90:1402-1405.
6. Naja MZ, Gustafsson AC, Ziade MF, et al. Distance between the skin and the thoracic paravertebral space. *Anaesthesia.* 2005;60:680-684.
7. Greengrass RA. Regional anesthesia for ambulatory surgery. *Anesthesiol Clin North Am.* 2000;18:341-353.
8. Hedzic A, Vloka JD. Continuous thoracic paravertebral block. Available at: www.nysora.com/peripheral_nerve_blocks/classic_block_techniques/3070-continuous_thoracic_paravertebral_block.html. 2006.
9. Bockenmair CC, Steele SM, Nielsen KC, et al. Bilateral continuous paravertebral catheters for reduction mammoplasty. *Acta Anaesthesiol Scand.* 2002;46:1042-1045.
10. Hirsch J. Impact of postoperative nausea and vomiting in the surgical setting. *Anesthesia.* 1994;49:30-33.
11. Metter S, Kitz D, Yuong M, et al. Nausea and vomiting after outpatient laparoscopy: incidence, impact on recovery room stay and cost. *Anest Analg.* 1987;66:S116.
12. Miguel R, Rothschiller J, Majchrzak J. Breast surgery is a high risk procedure for development of nausea and vomiting. *Anesthesiology.* 1994;78:A1095.
13. Coveney L, Weltz C, Greengrass R, Iglehart D, Leigh O, Steele S, et al. Use of paravertebral block anesthesia in the surgical management of breast cancer. *Ann Surg.* 1998;227:496-501.
14. McManus S, top D, Hopkins C. Advantages of outpatient breast surgery. *Am Surg.* 1994;60:967-970.
15. Boezaart AP, Raw RM. Continuous thoracic paravertebral block for major breast surgery. *Reg Anesth Pain Med.* 2006;31(5):470-476.
16. Eisenach J, De Kock M, Klimscha W. Alpha sub 2-adrenergic agonists for regional anesthesia: A clinical review of clonidine (1984–1995). *Anesthesiology.* 1996;85:655-674.
17. Eason MJ, Wyatt R. Paravertebral thoracic block: a reappraisal. *Anesthesia.* 1979;34:638-642.

CHAPTER 53

Excisional Breast Biopsy

Leslie Montgomery

The excisional breast biopsy (EBB) is defined as a surgical procedure in which an indeterminate lesion or calcifications are removed from the breast. In addition to establishing a tissue diagnosis, the secondary goal is complete removal of the lesion or calcifications in question.

INDICATIONS

The traditional method of obtaining a tissue diagnosis of a palpable breast mass is the EBB. If the practitioner feels a suspicious mass, then the next appropriate step is to obtain diagnostic imaging in the form of a bilateral mammogram and a unilateral ultrasound directed at the suspicious lesion. The ultrasound will distinguish a simple cyst from a complex cyst or solid mass in addition to further characterization of any solid lesion. The bilateral mammogram will effectively screen the contralateral breast and provide comparison in the parenchymal tissue pattern between both breasts.

If the imaging is noncontributory but the practitioner is still concerned about the palpable mass, the option of fine-needle aspiration, percutaneous core biopsy (PCB), or an EBB should be considered. At any time, the patient may opt for EBB rather than observation or PCB.

If an indeterminate solid lesion or calcifications are identified by mammogram or ultrasound, an image-guided PCB is the preferred approach for tissue diagnosis. If the practitioner cannot perform an image-guided PCB personally or does not have a local radiologist who can perform a PCB, then image-guided localization and EBB are indicated.

A radial scar has a very distinct mammographic pattern, characterized by a spiculated density, often with a radiolucent center. An EBB is usually the most efficient means of making the diagnosis of radial scar because a benign result obtained by PCB would be considered discordant with the suspicious imaging characteristics, and an EBB would ultimately be recommended. In addition, occult malignancy has been reported in 4% of patients diagnosed with radial scar by PCB who subsequently underwent EBB.[1] A patient who presents with pathologic nipple discharge and has a retroareolar lesion seen by mammogram, ultrasound, or ductogram should also undergo an EBB because the lesion often represents a papillary lesion. The diagnosis of a papillary lesion on PCB should prompt an EBB for definitive diagnosis to rule out a papillary carcinoma, and therefore PCB is often not helpful in establishing a benign diagnosis.

Once a PCB has been performed (either directed by palpation or image-guided), the tissue diagnosis may prompt an EBB. EBB is indicated if the PCB results reveal lobular carcinoma in situ (particularly if the lobular carcinoma in situ is associated with necrosis or calcifications), atypical ductal hyperplasia, atypical lobular hyperplasia, columnar cell lesion with atypia, radial scar, or a papillary lesion. The concern regarding these diagnoses obtained by PCB is that an *error in sampling* by the radiologist or an *error in interpretation* by the pathologist may have occurred, which can produce a false-negative diagnosis. The diagnosis of columnar cell lesion with atypia is concerning because of the high association of this lesion with tubular carcinoma. Approximately 80% of patients with tubular carcinoma have associated columnar cell lesions with atypia.[2,3]

Table 53-1 summarizes recent literature regarding the incidence of carcinoma diagnosed by EBB after atypical results at PCB. These studies are limited by small numbers, retrospective design, a variety of PCB indications, bias regarding which patients were chosen for EBB, and limited discussion regarding satisfaction by the radiologist that the lesion in question was accurately sampled at PCB. Nevertheless, the frequent finding of carcinoma at excision after a PCB diagnosis of atypia warrants consideration.

TABLE 53-1 PCB False-Negative Rate by Histology

PCB Pathology	Malignant EBB Pathology (%)
LCIS	13-25[4,7]
ADH	31-33[5]
ALH	16-25[5-7]
Papillary lesion	5-33[9,11]

ADH, atypical ductal hyperplasia; ALH, atypical lobular hyperplasia; EBB, excisional breast biopsy; LCIS, lobular carcinoma in situ; PCB, percutaneous core biopsy.

Any benign diagnosis that is obtained by PCB must be confirmed as a *concordant* result by the physician who performed the biopsy. Only the physician who performed the biopsy can determine that the lesion was sampled appropriately during the procedure and that a benign diagnosis is a reasonable result. Depending on the level of suspicion by the physician who performed the biopsy, a benign result may be considered *discordant* with the imaging characteristics, and an EBB is then indicated. For this reason, the clinician should confirm concordance with the radiologist before conveying PCB results to the patient.

There are many situations in which a PCB is not technically feasible, and therefore an EBB is the only means of obtaining a tissue diagnosis of an image-detected indeterminate lesion. Patients with lesions that are too superficial or immediately retroareolar cannot undergo a PCB due to the possibility that the core needle may inadvertently exit the skin after passing through the superficial lesion. The possibility of the core biopsy needle passing into and out of ("through and through") the breast during the PCB procedure is also a concern in patients undergoing a biopsy that requires breast compression (mammogram or magnetic resonance imaging [MRI]–guided) when the breast itself compresses substantially. The compression of the breast is often noted on the diagnostic mammogram, and a breast that compresses to less than 30 mm can make a PCB very challenging, if not impossible.

Posterior lesions may not be accessible for stereotactic biopsy due to limitations in patient positioning on the stereotactic table. In addition, inadvertent injury to the pectoralis major, intercostal muscles, ribs, or pleura is possible during PCB of extreme posterior lesions in thin women and should be avoided. Care must be taken in performing a PCB in a woman with retroglandular breast augmentation as the core needle can easily damage an implant. The radiologist may decide that the lesion is too close to the implant to perform a PCB safely and request an EBB for tissue diagnosis. Occasionally, PCB will be attempted but deemed unsuccessful by the radiologist due to inadequate sampling. This situation can occur in patients with extremely dense breast tissue or in patients with very faint indeterminate calcifications that are not well visualized during the stereotactic procedure.

Finally, patient compliance and patient habitus may make a PCB unfeasible. An EBB is necessary for a patient who cannot cooperate during a PCB procedure for any number of reasons (ie, anxiety, pain, mental disability). Patients with severe kyphosis or pectus excavatum may find it difficult to be positioned appropriately in the prone position for a stereotactic or MRI-guided PCB. These patients may require an EBB in the supine position for diagnosis.

OPERATIVE TECHNIQUE

The goal of an EBB is simply to provide an accurate tissue diagnosis with a good cosmetic result. Extensive tissue removal is not appropriate in the situation in which the procedure is being performed for diagnosis.

The presence and location of any palpable breast mass should be confirmed by both the patient and the surgeon in the upright and supine positions and carefully marked. The patient should confirm the mass before receiving any sedation. The incision should be planned within the lines of minimal skin tension. For central lesions, a periareolar incision provides an excellent cosmetic result (Fig. 53-1). For peripheral lesions, options include a curvilinear or transverse incision, depending on the contour of the patient's breast and the natural skin creases (Langer lines). Whenever possible, care should also be taken to plan the biopsy incision within the boundaries of potential incisions for skin-sparing mastectomy should that procedure be required for definitive treatment in the future. Alternatively, a peripheral EBB requires placement of the incision far from the nipple-areolar complex so the remaining skin bridge between the EBB incision (which requires reexcision if malignant) and the nipple-areolar complex excision during a skin-sparing mastectomy is viable. Skin should not be removed during EBB, because a malignant diagnosis has not been established and skin excision significantly diminishes the cosmetic result. For nonpalpable lesions that have undergone preoperative needle localization, it is important to remember that the location of the wire as it protrudes from the skin may be remote from the actual lesion, and careful examination of the localization mammograms and incision planning are required to avoid

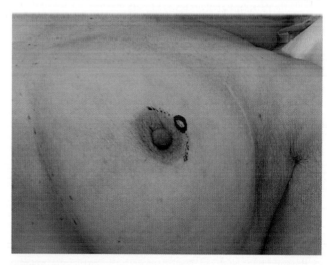

FIGURE 53-1 Periareolar incision placement. *(© MSKCC 2008)*

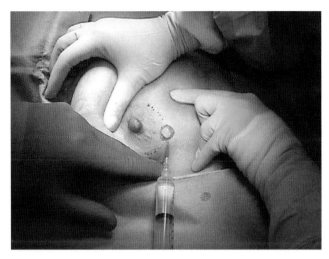

FIGURE 53-2   Injection of 1% lidocaine without epinephrine into the subcutaneous and deep tissues of the breast. *(© MSKCC 2008)*

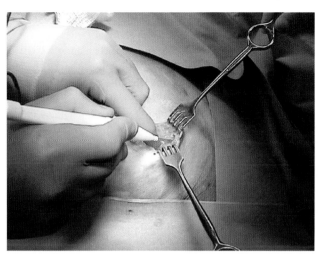

FIGURE 53-3   Retraction of skin and division of deep tissues with electrocautery. *(© MSKCC 2008)*

excessive tunneling and tissue removal. The incision should be placed in close proximity to the lesion in question, which is not necessarily where the localization wire enters the breast.

Most EBBs can be performed with sedation and local anesthetic. An effective and short-acting combination that is often used at Memorial Sloan-Kettering Cancer Center is a combination of propofol and midazolam for sedation and fentanyl for pain control. Once sedated, the patient is prepped and draped in the usual sterile fashion. One percent lidocaine without epinephrine is injected into the subcutaneous and deep tissues (Fig. 53-2). Lidocaine *without* epinephrine is used in order to confirm proper hemostasis at the conclusion of the case. It is important to clearly document the location of any palpable lesion with respect to the incision before the injection of lidocaine, as the injection may cause distortion of the breast tissues and may mask subtle breast abnormalities. Intraoperative antibiotics are not necessary for a diagnostic EBB.

The incision is made sharply through the dermis, and hemostasis is achieved at the skin edges with careful electrocautery. The skin is retracted and the deep tissues are divided using electrocautery (Fig. 53-3). Raising flaps is only necessary if the mass is superficial. Lesions located deep within the breast parenchyma should be approached by incising the breast tissue superficial to the mass without raising flaps. For superficial lesions, skin flaps can be elevated using electrocautery or sharp dissection. If possible, the subcutaneous fat should be preserved to maintain cosmesis.

It is often helpful to grasp the breast tissue overlying the lesion with a tenaculum clamp. The clamp facilitates excision of the mass by elevating the surrounding breast tissue, and when placed parallel to the incision, the clamp assists with orientation of the mass with respect to the surrounding tissue. It is important to note that the mass itself is not grasped with the clamp, as this risks tumor disruption (Fig. 53-4).

The mass in question is sharply excised with a rim of normal tissue surrounding the abnormality. An extensive surgical excision is not required for diagnosis of a palpable mass; however, if the biopsy is being performed for a highly suspicious lesion,

it is wise to take a margin of at least 0.5 to 1.0 cm of normal tissue around the lesion. It is considered an error in surgical technique if the lesion is transected during EBB. Care should be taken to protect the skin edges if a small incision has been made, since a No. 10 blade has a very high cutting surface and can damage the skin edges during dissection. A No. 15 blade is more appropriate in this setting. In general, it is preferable to avoid electrocautery for the excision, as it makes pathologic assessment of the margins more difficult.

The specimen is carefully delivered from the wound cavity in the anatomic orientation. The specimen is removed as a single piece of tissue and should not be transected unless the pathologist is informed.

The specimen is oriented with marking sutures (or clips) after complete excision. One protocol is to place a 2–0 silk suture at the lateral margin of the specimen, cut long; and another 2–0 silk suture is placed at the superior margin of the

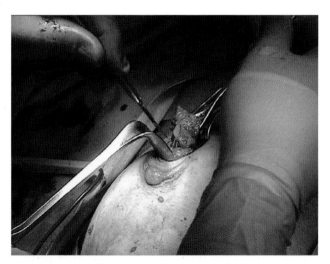

FIGURE 53-4   The breast tissue overlying the lesion is grasped with a tenaculum clamp. *(© MSKCC 2008)*

specimen, cut short (long-lateral, short-superior, or LL/SS). Alternatively, small hemoclips can be placed for orientation. The protocol at Memorial Sloan-Kettering Cancer Center is to place 1 clip on the superior margin and 2 clips on the lateral margin. The advantage to clip orientation is that the surgeon can identify whether a radiographic lesion is close to the lateral or superior margin on the specimen radiograph. Orientating markers should be placed on all lesions removed from the breast, regardless of the level of suspicion, and gross inspection of the specimen should be performed in the operating room to identify "close" margins. Even with palpable lesions, a specimen radiograph may be helpful in identifying close margins. Additional tissue can be excised from any questionable or close area and identified as the new margin for the pathologist. Any EBB that is based on localization of calcifications or a biopsy clip must have a radiograph of the specimen to document the presence of the radiographic marker or calcifications in question. If the EBB was performed for a palpable mass, the surgeon should carefully palpate the specimen and confirm the presence of the mass in question. The specimen is sent to pathology fresh for inked margins.

The wound is then further inspected, both visually and by direct palpation, for evidence of pathology. If a suspicious area is identified, it should be excised as well. If the posterior aspect of the biopsy cavity abuts the pectoralis major muscle, note this in the operative dictation, as this may influence final margin status.

Hemostasis is obtained using electrocautery and must be meticulous. The development of a postoperative hematoma may complicate reexcision of a positive margin or delay adjuvant therapy. Injection of long-acting local anesthetic, such as bupivacaine, may be used at the periphery of the cavity to assist with postoperative pain control.

Reapproximation of breast tissue ("oncoplastic surgery") is left to the discretion of the surgeon. Attempts to reconstruct underlying breast tissue when the patient is supine on the operating table with the breast in a laterally pendulous position may result in peculiar distortion when the patient assumes the upright position, particularly in the upper half of the breast. Drainage of the cavity is not necessary and not advisable.

Incisions are usually closed in 2 layers, with a 3-0 braided (polyglactin 910) subcutaneous interrupted suture and a 4-0 monofilament (poliglecaprone 25) subcuticular continuous running suture. Circumareolar incisions can be closed with single-layer 4-0 monofilament (poliglecaprone 25) subcuticular interrupted suture (Fig. 53-5). Steri-Strips or Dermabond is used as the final skin approximation.

The patient is awakened in the operating room and returned to the recovery room. She is usually ready for discharge within 1 to 3 hours after the biopsy procedure. Patients are typically given narcotics for pain control. It is recommended they use an ice pack intermittently for the first 24 hours while awake and keep their dressing in place and dry for the first 48 hours. The patient removes the dressing after 48 hours, and she may shower normally from that point on. The patient often sees the surgeon on postoperative day 7 to 10, and the Steri-Strips are removed at that time. Patients are instructed to wear a good supportive bra during the postoperative period while awake to minimize breast movement and discomfort. Postoperative oral antibiotics are not required.

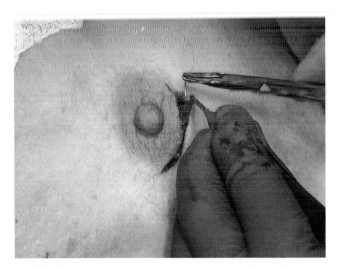

FIGURE 53-5 Closure of circumareolar incision with single-layer 4-0 monofilament (poliglecaprone 25) subcuticular interrupted suture.

POSTOPERATIVE ASSESSMENT

At the postoperative visit, the surgeon must reconcile a benign pathology report with the initial patient presentation. If the EBB was performed for calcifications, then calcifications must be documented on the pathology report. If calcifications cannot be identified in the specimen submitted to pathology, then a postexcision mammogram should be performed to assess the accurate removal of the calcifications in question. If the EBB was performed after a PCB that revealed an atypical lesion, then previous biopsy site changes must be documented on the pathology report. If the EBB was performed for a highly suspicious, spiculated solid mass, then the pathology report must provide an explanation for such concerning preoperative imaging. Ultimately, the surgeon is responsible for assuring concordance with the radiologist between the radiographic presentation and any benign pathology report.

SUMMARY

An EBB is performed to provide an accurate tissue diagnosis of an indeterminate breast lesion when a PCB is not available, not appropriate, or not conclusive. It is important to remember that the majority of EBBs produce benign results, and that cosmetic deformity or an unsightly scar should be minimized whenever possible. It is ultimately the responsibility of the surgeon to confirm that the lesion in question has been excised and that the pathology obtained is concordant with the level of clinical suspicion.

REFERENCES

1. Douglas-Jones AG, Denson JL, Cox AC, Harries IB, Stevens G. Radial scar lesions of the breast diagnosed by needle core biopsy: analysis of cases containing occult malignancy. *J Clin Pathol.* 2007;60:295-298.
2. Abdel-Fatah TM, Powe DG, Hodi Z, et al. High frequency of coexistence of columnar cell lesions, lobular neoplasia, and low grade ductal carcinoma

in situ with invasive tubular carcinoma and invasive lobular carcinoma. *Am J Surg Pathol.* 2007;31:417-426.

3. Brandt SM, Young GQ, Hoda SA. The "Rosen Triad": tubular carcinoma, lobular carcinoma in situ, and columnar cell lesions. *Adv Anat Pathol.* 2008;15:140-146.

4. Liberman L, Sama M, Susnik B, et al. Lobular carcinoma in situ at percutaneous breast biopsy: surgical biopsy findings. *AJR Am J Roentgenol.* 1999;173:291-299.

5. Margenthaler JA, Duke D, Monsees BS, et al. Correlation between core biopsy and excisional biopsy in breast high-risk lesions. *Am J Surg.* 2006;192:534-537.

6. Elsheikh TM, Silverman JF. Follow-up surgical excision is indicated when breast core needle biopsies show atypical lobular hyperplasia or lobular carcinoma in situ: a correlative study of 33 patients with review of the literature. *Am J Surg Pathol.* 2005;29:534-543.

7. Brem, RF, Lechner, MC, Jackman RJ, et al. Lobular neoplasia at percutaneous breast biopsy: variables associated with carcinoma at surgical excision. *AJR Am J Roentgenol.* 2008;190:637-641.

8. Philpotts LE, Shaheen NA, Jain KS, Carter D, Lee CH. Uncommon high-risk lesions of the breast diagnosed at stereotactic core-needle biopsy: clinical importance. *Radiology.* 2000;216:831-837.

9. Valdes EK, Tartter PI, Genelus-Dominique E, et al. Significance of papillary lesions at percutaneous breast biopsy. *Ann Surg Oncol.* 2006;13:480-482.

10. Mercado CL, Hamele-Bena D, Oken SH, Singer CI, Cangiarella J. Papillary lesions at percutaneous core-needle biopsy. *Radiology.* 2006;238:801-808.

11. Liberman L, Tornos C, Huzjan R, et al. Is surgical excision warranted after benign, concordant diagnosis of papilloma at percutaneous breast biopsy? *AJR Am J Roentgenol.* 2006;186:1328-1324.

CHAPTER 54

Tissue Marking and Processing

Amanda L. Kong
Alexandra Shaye Brown

An essential component to any surgical procedure is the documentation and labeling of the surgical specimen. Correct orientation of the specimen allows the pathologist to properly evaluate resection margins and correlate gross findings with the clinical history. It also allows for optimal oncologic outcomes, as the pathologist can notify the surgeon if additional tissue needs to be excised to achieve negative margins. In the case of breast-conservation therapy, it may also lead to improved cosmetic results with the removal of only the necessary tissue to achieve negative margins. The ultimate importance of labeling surgical resection specimens pertains to patient safety, as errors may lead to incorrect diagnosis and treatment.

In 1998, the American College of Radiology, the American College of Surgeons, the College of American Pathologists and the Society of Surgical Oncology published a report on consensus standards for diagnosis and management of invasive breast cancer. This report was a follow-up to their previously published report in 1992 establishing the initial consensus standards for breast-conservation treatment.[1] The recommendations from the 1998 report stated that the surgeon must orient the specimen with the use of sutures, clips, multicolored indelible ink, or another suitable technique. It was noted that the specimen should not be sectioned before submission to the pathologist, and that any uncertainty regarding the proper orientation of the specimen should be clearly indicated to the pathologist by the surgeon. In terms of pathologic evaluation, the group stated that the specimen should be submitted with appropriate clinical history and specification of anatomic site, including laterality (left or right breast) and quadrant (upper-outer, lower-inner, etc). The surgeon should also orient the specimen (eg, superior, medial, lateral) with markers or sutures, as well as document the type of surgical specimen (lumpectomy, total mastectomy, etc).[1,2]

As a follow-up to the 1992 report, White et al[3] disseminated a study-specific questionnaire to 842 hospitals, yielding a total of 16,643 patients throughout the United States to determine whether practice patterns for patients with breast carcinoma who underwent breast-conservation therapy were consistent with the standards established 2 years before Winchester et al.[2] Poor compliance was noted with the labeling of lumpectomy specimens with the affected quadrant and proper spatial orientation. Furthermore, orientation of the specimen with suture or markers was noted for only 67% of cases.[3]

There remains a paucity of literature examining the outcomes of specimen identification errors. Makary et al[4] chose to address this issue by prospectively examining errors that occurred in the "pre-analytical phase," which they defined as the interval when the transfer of information from physician to nurse during a procedure takes place, with subsequent specimen labeling, packaging, and transport. In a total of 21,351 surgical specimens, 91 (4.3 of 1000) surgical specimen identification errors were identified. Procedures involving the breast were the most common type to involve an identification error (11 of 91). The authors noted, however, that the extent of patient harm was unknown. In addition, they noted the potential for significant costs to the institution and distrust from the community.[4]

Currently, there is a lack of standardization for labeling specimens across institutions. Efforts are underway to improve consistency in specimen labeling and marking. The new Joint Commission on Accreditation of Healthcare Organization National Patient Safety Goals requires the labeling of specimens with at least 2 patient identifiers and that the specimen containers are labeled in the presence of the patient, with a preoperative verification step occurring in the presence of a physician.[5] Several groups have implemented using methods such as radio-opaque threads,[6,7] radio-opaque clips, metal clips, and/or silk suture for marking specimens. When used correctly, silk suture remains the standard, cost-efficient manner for orienting specimens.

PROCEDURE

Segmental and total mastectomy specimens both require marking to orient the pathologist regarding how the specimen resided in situ. There are several dimensions to each specimen, including the following designated margins: superior (12 o'clock position), inferior (6 o'clock position), medial (3 o'clock position on the right breast, 9 o'clock position on the left breast), lateral (3 o'clock position on the left breast, 9 o'clock position on the right breast), anterior (toward the skin), and posterior (toward the chest wall). By convention, we traditionally only mark the superior and lateral margins.

The optimal time to mark the specimen is before its complete removal from the body (Fig. 54-1). Before the dissection is completed (ie, removed from the chest wall or posteriorly), a 2–0 silk suture is used to mark the specimen and to orient it correctly for the pathologist. By convention, we view the breast en face as a clock face. In the 12 o'clock position, halfway between the most anterior and the most posterior portions of the specimen, we place a single silk suture. We cut both ends of the suture equally short to designate "short superior, 12 o'clock" to mark the superior margin. We place a second single silk suture in the 9 o'clock position, halfway between the most anterior and the most posterior portions of the specimen, and leave both ends equally long. This suture is designated "long lateral, 9 o'clock" to mark the lateral margin (Fig. 54-2).

By marking the specimen in situ, one is able to correctly mark the orientation, eliminating any confusion in orientation once the specimen is removed. This technique is particularly important when performing a segmental mastectomy or skin-sparing mastectomy, where once the specimen is removed, it is difficult to determine the proper orientation of the specimen because of its similar appearance in all aspects. Some surgeons choose not to orient the specimen when performing a modified radical mastectomy, as the axillary nodal basin is always located in the upper-outer quadrant of the breast. However, sutures

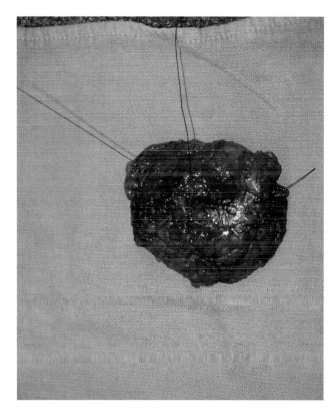

FIGURE 54-2 The long suture marks the lateral (9 o'clock) position, whereas the short suture designates the superior (12 o'clock) position. All marking sutures should be placed while the tissue is still in situ, even with the localization wire in place (as shown in this photo).

should still be placed to properly orient the specimen for the pathologist to avoid any error or confusion (Fig. 54-3).

In lumpectomy specimens, we designate the posterior margin, in addition to marking the superior and lateral margins, by inking it with a marking pen (Fig. 54-4). The purpose of inking

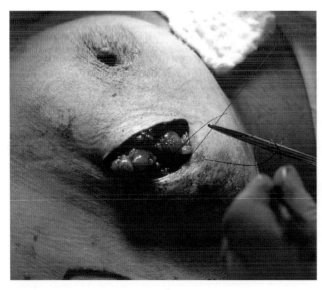

FIGURE 54-1 Tissue orientation and marking performed with the specimen in situ. Here a short suture designates "superior" 12 o'clock position for the pathologist.

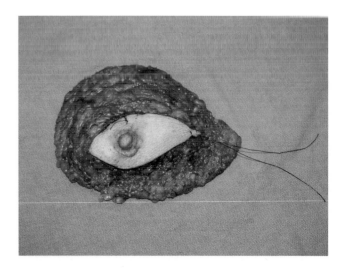

FIGURE 54-3 Orientation of a mastectomy specimen. Again, the short suture designates superior (12 o'clock) and the long suture marks the lateral position (9 o'clock). Mastectomy specimens should be oriented to avoid any possible error during gross specimen evaluation, inking, and sectioning.

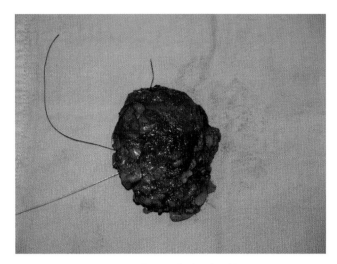

FIGURE 54-4 Orientation of a needle-localized lumpectomy specimen with "short superior" and "long lateral" sutures in place. Purple pen ink is applied by the surgeon to the deep margin during removal to maintain optimal 3-dimensional orientation before formal inking and pathologic sectioning.

this posterior margin is that when the specimen is received by pathology and placed on the processing board, the specimen is no longer in its original orientation. It is a challenge to the pathologist or technician to determine how the original specimen rested in situ. After the posterior margin is marked with ink, the pathologist is able to determine the true posterior margin as the specimen rested in situ, differentiating it from the lateral, medial, superior, and inferior margins.

It is important to annotate these margin designations on the pathology form before sending the specimen to pathology from the operating room. Laterality, marking sutures, or any orienting clips should be noted on the pathology form. In addition, the quadrant from which a segmental mastectomy has been removed should be noted, as well as whether the specimen requires immediate processing for margin status (ie, frozen section), gross evaluation, specimen mammogram, or permanent processing. It is also necessary to provide a brief clinical history for the patient, with information including the age of the patient, clinical size and location of the tumor, and treatment history.

Repeating this information verbally with the circulating nurse or assistant after it is recorded on the pathology form, before the specimen being sent to pathology, is essential to decrease chances for mislabeling. Correct labeling of the container with the specimen should also be confirmed. If there are any questions regarding the orientation of the specimen once it is received by pathology, or if the surgeon would like the pathologist to examine a certain aspect of the specimen in detail, the surgeon should communicate with the pathologist directly, either by telephone or in person.

When margins require reexcision, the process of labeling these additional margins is also essential to achieve an optimal oncologic outcome while obtaining the best cosmetic result. The margin should first be labeled with its location and be designated as a secondary margin (ie, additional superior margin). On the aspect of the specimen that is the new true margin (ie, the side that is further away from the prior segmental mastectomy cavity), clips or ink should be placed throughout, delineating the accurate extent of the new specimen margin.

The importance of labeling margins and its effect on oncologic outcomes has been well established in the literature. Luu et al[8] examined 235 patients who were candidates for breast-conservation therapy. Of these patients, 132 (56%) of 235 had "unsatisfactory" margins, defined as microscopic involvement with tumor, or the margin was close at initial excisional biopsy, and the surgeon opted for reexcision. On multiple logistic regression, 1 factor associated with a satisfactory margin was the orientation of specimen margins by the surgeon ($p = 0.027$). The authors also found that patients with unsatisfactory margins were 67 times more likely to undergo mastectomy than patients with satisfactory margins after adjusting for other significant factors.[8]

SUMMARY

Ensuring the correct orientation and labeling of specimens is an essential part of the surgical procedure. Mislabeling and providing insufficient clinical information may lead to incorrect diagnoses or treatment. It is important to include clinical history, specimen name, laterality, quadrant (if applicable), type of processing, and designation of margins on the pathology requisition form. Regardless of whether sutures or clips are used to mark the specimen, the significance of these markers should be clearly stated on the pathology form. The labeling of the specimen container and pathology requisition form should be verified with the surgeon before the specimen is sent to pathology. Finally, if there are any questions about the specimen, there should be clear, direct communication between the pathologist and the surgeon.

REFERENCES

1. Winchester, DP, Cox JD. Standards for breast-conservation treatment. *CA Cancer J Clin.* 1992;42:134-162.
2. Winchester DP, Cox JD. Standards for diagnosis and management of invasive breast carcinoma. *CA Cancer J Clin.* 1998;48:83-107.
3. White J, Morrow M, Moughan J, et al. Compliance with breast-conservation standards for patients with early-stage breast carcinoma. *Cancer.* 2003;97:893-904.
4. Makary M, Epstein J, Pronovost P, et al. Surgical specimen identification errors: a new measure of quality in surgical care. *Surgery.* 2007;141:450-455.
5. The Joint Commission: 2008 National Patient Safety Goals. Available at: http://www.jointcommission.org/PatientSafety/NationalPatientSafetyGoals/. Accessed November 18, 2008.
6. Mercky J, Weitbruch D, Moyses B, et al. Breast specimen lumpectomy orientation: which technique is the best? *Eur J Surg Oncol.* 2006;32:1249.
7. Vaidya JS, Wilson AJ, Choudhury R. Orientation of a breast specimen with radio-opaque thread: a novel solution. *Eur J Surg Oncol.* 2004;30:460-461.
8. Luu HH, Otis CN, Reed WP Jr, et al. The unsatisfactory margin in breast cancer surgery. *Am J Surg.* 1999;178:362-366.

CHAPTER 55

Needle Localization and Radioguided Occult Lesion Localization Techniques

Simonetta Monti
Julia Rodriguez-Fernandez
Helio Rubens De Oliveira Filho

In parallel with the increasing use of mammographic screening and ultrasonography, nonpalpable breast lesions have been diagnosed with increasing frequency over the past 2 decades and at present constitute approximately 20% of all breast lesions.[1]

Nonpalpable lesions are a challenge to breast surgeons, because they must be precisely localized preoperatively and subsequently excised with clear margins and without excessive removal of breast tissue if the excision is merely diagnostic. Microcalcifications often found by screening mammography are frequently an early sign of neoplastic proliferation and must also be completely excised, an intervention that can forestall the development of infiltrating breast carcinoma.[2] There are various methods for localizing these lesions: hooked wires, carbon particles, cutaneous markers, and large-molecular-weight colloids labeled with radioisotope.[2] All are in current use. Needle localization is the most widely and frequently used method.[3-5] The aim is to obtain accurate lesion localization and simultaneous surgical removal of the lesion with adequate margins.

NEEDLE LOCALIZATION

Needle localization was first introduced in 1965 and became popular mainly thanks to refinement by Kopans and colleagues.[6,7]

Needle Localization Procedure

A guide needle containing a stainless steel wire (Kopans wire) hooked at its distal end is inserted into the lesion under ultrasonic, mammographic, or magnetic resonance imaging (MRI) guidance. Ideally the guide needle should pass through the lesion and extend approximately 1 cm beyond. The wire must be long enough to protrude from the skin after insertion and withdrawal of the guide needle.[8] Lesions revealed by ultrasound are best localized under ultrasonic control.[9,10] Similarly, lesions detected only by MRI can now be localized using MRI guidance, and these procedures are becoming more refined.[11] Once the correct position of the wire has been confirmed, the guide needle is carefully withdrawn. At this point, the hook in the wire reforms and anchors it in the tissue.[8] More than 1 needle can be inserted into a single breast, for example to mark an extensive lesion by delimiting its borders. After localization, a 2-view mammogram (craniocaudal [CC] and mediolateral oblique [MLO]) is performed and sent to the operating room with the patient to document the location of the lesion and aid the surgeon with incision planning. The location of the target lesion within the breast is determined by estimating the distance from the nipple in both views; the CC view is used to determine whether the lesion lies medial or lateral to the nipple, and the MLO view is used to determine whether the lesion lies superior or inferior to the nipple. The depth of the lesion is also noted. Using the localization films in this manner allows the surgeon to estimate the location of the lesion in 3 dimensions and to place the surgical incision over the lesion itself, avoiding unnecessary dissection or tunneling through the breast if the entry site of the wire is in another quadrant of the breast.

Once proper incision placement is determined and the procedure is underway, the surgeon follows the wire down to the lesion site and removes the lesion together with the wire.[8] If the incision has been placed away from the entry site of the wire, a superficial flap is raised at the level of the breast parenchyma to bring the wire into the field of the dissection, and the wire is then traced down to the site of the lesion. The removed specimen is marked with radiopaque clips or threads to define its orientation. Specimen radiography is performed if the needle localization procedure was performed for microcalcifications or if preoperative diagnosis was obtained with image-guided biopsy with clip placement. In the former case, the specimen x-ray serves to document that the targeted microcalcifications have been removed, and in the latter case, to document that the biopsy clip is contained within the specimen. Radiopaque clip marking of the specimen and placement onto a Plexiglas support, with the posterior margin placed accurately onto the Plexiglas surface, makes it possible to assess the distance of the lesion from the margins, and if clinically indicated, additional tissue may be excised. Needle localization can also be performed on breasts subjected to augmentation: the technique of Ecklund is used, and rates of lesion removal are close to 100%.[12]

Complications of Needle Localization

The most common complications in order of occurrence are displacement of the wire from the breast, patient discomfort and pain, incorrect wire positioning, pneumothorax (rare), and wire migration to lung or abdomen (very rare).[10]

Another complication is that the wire occasionally breaks so that residual fragment of wire may be left within the breast.[13-15]

RADIOGUIDED OCCULT LESION LOCALIZATION

In 1996, the European Institute of Oncology, Milan, developed a new method for localizing occult lesions, called radioguided occult lesion localization (ROLL), the idea for which came from experience with radiocolloid injected close to the breast lesion (typically intradermally) to identify the sentinel node. The radioactive particles travel within the lymphatic ducts to be taken up by sentinel lymph nodes, usually in the axilla. It was noticed that some radioactivity always remained at the injection site, and the idea developed that, if the particles were too large to pass into the lymphatic system, all would remain at the injection site. Further, if this material were injected directly into a nonpalpable lesion, the radioactivity would remain there and serve as a beacon during surgical removal.

Studies showed that macroaggregate human albumin colloid, the particles of which have a larger average diameter than the microaggregate used in sentinel node biopsy, were practically immobile. After technetium 99m (^{99m}Tc) has been chemically bound to the particles, they could be injected directly into the occult lesion under stereotactic mammographic or ultrasonic control. In the operating room, a gamma ray–detecting probe locates the lesion and has proven invaluable in guiding its complete removal.[16,17] After a pilot phase during which the quantity of radioactivity to be injected was optimized, ROLL became the method of choice for locating nonpalpable lesions at the European Institute of Oncology. It is effective, easily reproducible, and has a short learning curve.[18]

ROLL Injection Technique

Twenty-four hours before the operation, human albumin macroaggregate (particle size 10-150 nm in diameter; Macrotec, Sorin Biomedica, Saluggia, Italy) labeled with 3.7 MBq of ^{99m}Tc in 0.2 mL of saline is injected directly into the lesion under ultrasonic or mammographic control (Fig. 55-1).

For lesions detected ultrasonically, the radiotracer is injected under the guidance of a linear probe attached to a needle biopsy device, which is inserted into the breast manually. The needle tip is positioned at the center of the lesion, as shown by a change of echogenicity at the lesion site. Radiotracer is then injected, followed by an additional minimal quantity of saline to flush the needle and help avoid dispersing the radioactivity. For lesions visible by ultrasound and mammography, injection under ultrasonic control is preferred.

For microcalcifications or other anomalies revealed only mammographically, mammographic equipment attached to a computerized stereotactic system is used to guide injection. Again a small quantity of pure saline (0.2 mL) is injected, and this is followed by a minimum quantity of radiopaque contrast medium via the same needle. The needle is then removed, and a standard orthogonal mammogram is taken a few minutes later to verify exact correspondence between the lesion and injected radiotracer/radiopaque material (Fig. 55-2). If a lesion has been completely removed by preoperative mammotome biopsy, the clip is located by mammography and the radiotracer injected at the clip site under stereotactic guidance.

Lateral and anterior scintigraphic images are taken after a few minutes and 5 hours later. The lateral image is obtained with the patient prone using a polystyrene block to hold the breast in position and a flexible wire cobalt source to outline the breast contour (Fig. 55-3). The anterior image is obtained with the patient standing, after placing a cobalt 57 point source on the nipple as landmark. The scintigraphic images are assessed for the presence of radioactive contamination. When the hotspot appears as a small, well-delimited area, the patient is referred for surgery. If the skin is contaminated with radioactivity, it is carefully cleaned and the scan repeated. The current success rate at our institute is 98.8%. Reasons for unsuccessful tracer localization include contamination of the needle track, skin contamination, and intraductal dissemination of the tracer. As with any new technology, the success rate has improved since the initial evaluation published 1998.[16]

The Probe

The hand held gamma ray–detecting probe used for radioguided surgery consists of a metal cylinder approximately 15 to 20 cm long and approximately 1.5 cm in diameter gloved in a transparent sterile sheath. It is connected to a device that transduces the signal into an audio signal and digital display. The intensity and frequency of the audio signal is directly proportional to number of counts detected. Newer probes are wireless (Bluetooth) and may be more convenient to use.

ROLL Surgical Technique

Use of the probe allows the surgeon to immediately locate the skin projection of the radioactive hotspot and hence decide the most appropriate incision (often based on aesthetic considerations), irrespective of the injection site. In our experience, this is a major advantage over determining the location of the lesion mammographically with the needle localization technique.

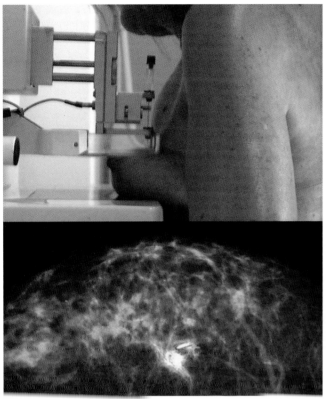
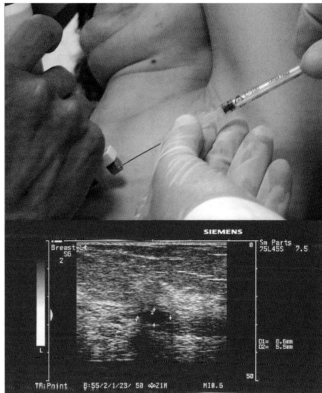

FIGURE 55-1 Paraintra-arterial injection under stereotactic control (*left*) and ultrasonic control (*right*).

During surgery, the probe is used to guide lesion removal. Once removed, the probe is used to confirm that the radioactivity is completely within the excised specimen and, importantly, that no radioactivity remains in the excision site.

The margins of the removed specimen containing the lesion are oriented, usually on 3 points, with radiopaque clips or surgical thread. If the lesion is only visible mammographically (for example, microcalcifications or post-mammotome clips), the specimen is x-rayed intraoperatively to verify that all has been removed by comparison with the preoperative x-ray. If necessary, the excision is enlarged and more material removed. If the lesion is a small, nonpalpable nodule, intraoperative frozen-section examination can confirm lesion retrieval. If clinically indicated, intraoperative histologic examination may be performed to establish the diagnosis, and in the setting of malignancy, the procedure can be converted to a therapeutic resection.

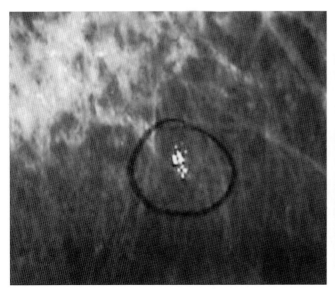
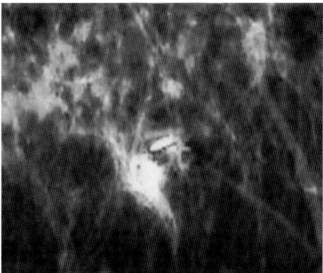

FIGURE 55-2 Injection of radiopaque contrast medium into the cluster of microcalcifications after injection of radiotracer.

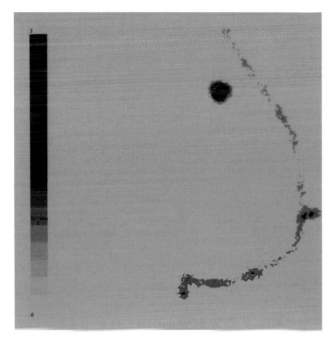

FIGURE 55-3   Scintigraphic lateral view after injection of radiotracer.

Contraindications for ROLL

ROLL is not indicated for the localization of extensive microcalcifications. In such cases, traditional needle localization or placement of a cutaneous marker indicating the area including the microcalcifications can be used. ROLL is also contraindicated for multifocal or large, multicentric lesions. Two ROLL procedures should not be performed in the same breast because it is not easy to clearly distinguish the 2 sites of radioactivity using the gamma probe. If more than 1 nonpalpable lesion is present, 1 can be localized by ROLL and additional lesions can be localized by another method, generally needle localization. A retroareolar lesion is also a relative contraindication for ROLL because the radiotracer may be injected intraductally, increasing the risk of tracer spread away from the target site.

Complications of ROLL

The most common complication is movement or dissemination of the injected radioactivity away from point of injection. When this happens, the localization is a failure and another technique, such as needle localization, must be used. The half-life of ^{99m}Tc is only approximately 24 hours.

INDICATIONS FOR NEEDLE LOCALIZATION AND ROLL

Both needle localization and ROLL are indicated for suspicious nonpalpable breast lesions revealed by mammography, ultrasound, or MRI[9,11] that require surgical biopsy or excision and so must be localized before the operation to facilitate accurate surgical removal. The 2 techniques therefore have largely overlapping indications, and the choice between these 2 localizing methods is largely determined by institutional expertise. Both techniques require a multidisciplinary team consisting of a radiologist, pathologist, and surgeon. The ROLL technique also requires the addition of a nuclear medicine physician.

Needle localization has been suggested as good for lesions in breasts with a high proportion of glandular tissue, because there is low probability of needle movement after positioning. ROLL is also easily performed for lesions in highly glandular breasts and may be preferable as some have reported difficulty placing localizing wires in dense breast tissue.[19] Our experience is that ROLL is easier than needle localization, and once the technique has been learned, surgeons prefer this approach. In the few circumstances when ROLL is contraindicated (see above), needle localization is probably the best alternative. Several studies comparing the 2 techniques have concluded that both are effective, yet ROLL is easier, less painful for the patient, allows more precise planning of the cutaneous incision and hence better aesthetic outcomes, fewer postoperative symptoms, and smaller excision volumes.[19,22]

DISCUSSION

Needle localization is widely used to find the lesion when conservative surgery is indicated. However, its role in the diagnosis of impalpable lesions should be reconsidered, because less invasive procedures produce equally good results.[23]

A major advantage of ROLL compared with needle localization is that it and allows the surgeon to choose the most direct or most convenient surgical access route to the lesion with greater precision. This has aesthetic implications, as well as shortening surgery time. The probe can be used at any time during the operation to check lesion position and ensure that the removed specimen completely contains the hotspot centered within nonradioactive active tissue (Figs. 55-4 and 55-5). Removal of additional tissue for residual radioactivity is rarely necessary.

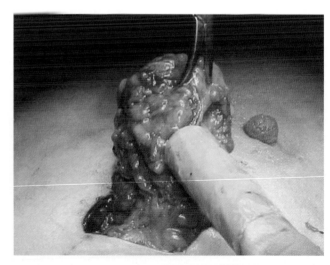

FIGURE 55-4   Use of gamma probe to check that radioactivity is confined to the center of the specimen.

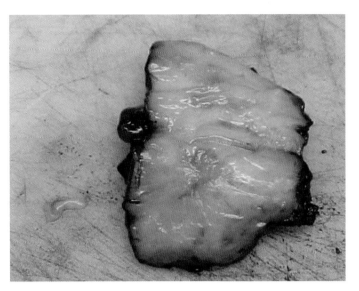
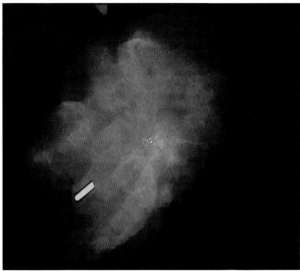

FIGURE 55-5 Left nodule centered within the specimen x-ray confirms presence of microcalcifications.

ROLL does not require special radioprotection measures. Studies have demonstrated that ROLL is safe for patients, radiologists, surgeons, and operating room and ward nurses. The doses absorbed by the surgeon's hands after 100 operations is 0.45 mGy, and the mean effective dose is 0.09 mSv (approximately 1% of the annual dose limit for the general population). Absorbed doses to all hospital personnel involved in the procedure are low compared with the recommended annual limits established by the International Commission on Radiological Protection and smaller than those arising from other radiologic examinations.[24]

The ROLL procedure is characterized by low cost of radioactive tracer and other consumable materials. However, the probe is expensive, and its high cost does not appear justified if only used for ROLL, especially as other localization methods are cheaper. However, such probes are increasingly used in various types of radioguided surgery, the most common being sentinel lymph node biopsy for breast cancer and melanoma. The application of the sentinel node technique to gynecologic malignancies and thoracic malignancies may also increase the utility of such probes.

FUTURE DIRECTIONS

At present, nonpalpable breast lesions constitute approximately 20% of all breast lesions.[1] This proportion is certain to increase in the future. ROLL is the newest localization method, and because it is easier and quicker for the surgeon, less painful for the patient, and associated with better aesthetic outcomes, is likely to grow in popularity. Although needle localization is an effective technique and will continue to be used, particularly when ROLL is unsuitable (ie, for very extensive microcalcifications and multifocal or multicentric lesions), it is likely that it will give way to ROLL, as the use of radioactive tracers and other modern technologies becomes ever more widespread in oncology.

SUMMARY

As women have become increasingly aware of breast cancer, and mammographic screening has come into widespread use, the incidence of nonpalpable breast lesions has markedly increased [1] and this trend is likely to continue. The challenge for surgeons is obtaining accurate preoperative localization to guide excision. Various methods of occult lesion localization are available. The most commonly used procedures are needle localization and ROLL. Needle localization involves insertion of a guide needle containing a stainless steel wire into the lesion under mammographic-stereotactic, ultrasonic, or MRI guidance. During surgery, the wire is followed along its length to the lesion, which is removed together with the wire. In the ROLL procedure, radiotracer is injected into the lesion under stereotactic, ultrasonic, or MRI guidance 24 hours before surgery. During surgery, a gamma probe is used to locate the lesion and guide its surgical removal. The ROLL method requires the addition of a nuclear medicine physician to the multidisciplinary team.

REFERENCES

1. Tubiana M, Holland R, Kopans DB, et al. Commission of the European Communities "Europe Against Cancer" Programme. European School of Oncology Advisory Report. Management of non-palpable and small lesions found in mass breast screening. *Eur J Cancer*. 1994;30A:538-547.
2. Homer MJ. Breast imaging: pitfalls, controversies, and some practical thoughts. *Radiol Clin North Am*. 1985;23:459-472.
3. Silverstein MJ, Gamagami P, Rosser RJ, et al. Hooked-wire directed breast biopsy and overpenetrated mammography. *Cancer*. 1987;59:715-722.
4. Lannin DR, Grube B, Black DS, Ponn T. Breast tattoos for planning surgery following neoadjuvant chemotherapy. *Am J Surg*. 2007;194:518:20.
5. Haid A, Knauner M, Dunzinger S, et al. Intra-operative sonography: a valuable aid during breast-conserving surgery for occult breast cancer. *Ann Surg Oncol*. 2007;14:3090-3101.
6. Besic N, Zgajnar J, Hocevar M, et al. Breast biopsy with wire localization: factors influencing complete excision of nonpalpable carcinoma. *Eur Radiol*. 2002;12:2684-2689.
7. Kopans DB, deLuca S. A modified needle-hookwire technique to simplify preoperative localization of occult breast lesions. *Radiology*. 1980;134:781.

8. Gossmann A, Bangard C, Warm M, et al. Real-time MR-guided wire localization of breast lesions by using an open 1.0-T imager: initial experience. *Radiology.* 2008;247:535-542.

9. Robertson CL, Kopans DB, McCarthy KA, Hart NE. Nonpalpable lesions in the augmented breast: preoperative localization. *Radiology.* 1989;173:873-874.

10. Banitalebi H, Skaane P. Migration of the breast biopsy localization wire to the pulmonary hilus. *Acta Radiol.* 2005;46:28-31.

11. Kopans DB, Meyer JE, Lindfors KK, Bucchianeri SS. Breast sonography to guide cyst aspiration and wire localization of occult solid lesions. *AJR Am J Roentgenol.* 1984;143:489-492.

12. Vuorela AL, Ahonen A. Preoperative stereotactic hookwire localization of nonpalpable breast lesions with and without the use of a further stereotactic check film. *Anticancer Res.* 2000;20:1277-1279.

13. Liberman L, Kaplan J, Van Zee KJ, et al. Bracketing wires for preoperative breast needle localization. *AJR Am J Roentgenol.* 2001;177:565-572.

14. Silverstein MJ, Gamagami P, Rosser RJ, et al. Hooked-wire-directed breast biopsy and overpenetrated mammography. *Cancer.* 1987;59:715-722.

15. Homer MJ. Nonpalpable breast lesion localization using a curved-end retractable wire. *Radiology.* 1985;157:259-260.

16. Luini A, Zurrida S, Galimberti V, et al. Radioguided surgery of occult breast lesions. *Eur J Cancer.* 1998;34:204-205.

17. Luini A, Zurrida S, Paganelli G, et al. Comparison of radioguided excision with wire localization of occult breast lesions. *Br J Surg.* 1999;86:522-525,526.

18. Gennari R, Galimberti V, De Cicco C, et al. Use of technetium 99m-labeled colloid albumin for preoperative and intraoperative localization of nonpalpable breast lesions. *J Am Surg.* 2000;190;692-699

19. Nadeem R, Chagla LS, Harris O, et al. Occult breast lesions: a comparison between radioguided occult lesion localization (ROLL) vs. wire guided lumpectomy (WGL). *Breast.* 2005;14:283-289.

20. Rampaul RS, Bagnall M, Burrel H, et al. Randomized trial comparing radioisotope occult lesion localization and wire-guided excision for biopsy of occult breast lesions. *Br J Surg.* 2004;91:1575-1577.

21. Medina-Franco H, Abarca-Perez L, Garcia-Alvarez M, et al. Radioguided occult localization (ROLL) versus wire-guided lumpectomy for nonpalpable breast lesions: a randomized prospective evaluation. *J Surg Oncol.* 2008;97:108-111.

22. Moreno M, Wiltgen JE, Bodanese B, et al. Radioguided breast surgery for occult lesion localization-correlation between two methods. *J Exp Clin Cancer Res.* 2008;27:29.

23. Teh W, Singhal H: Breast, Needle localization. Available at: http://www.emedicine.com/radio/topic911.htm. Accessed July 4, 2008.

24. Cremonesi M, Ferrari M, Sacco, et al. Radiation protection in radioguided surgery of breast cancer. *Nucl Med Commun.* 1999;20:919-924.

CHAPTER 56

Mammographic and Intraoperative Ultrasound Guidance

Richard E. Fine

INDICATIONS FOR LOCALIZATION

An increasing number of nonpalpable breast lesions are identified due to screening mammography and breast magnetic resonance imaging (MRI). After appropriate diagnostic imaging workup, many of these image-detected abnormalities require a biopsy for pathologic confirmation. The positive predictive value of mammography (the number of cancers diagnosed per number of biopsies recommended) historically has ranged from 15% to 35%.[1] Fortunately, a substantial number of these lesions are initially evaluated with percutaneous image-guided breast biopsy, providing a less costly, less invasive method to obtain an accurate diagnosis without sacrificing accuracy. After a benign diagnosis is obtained with a minimally invasive image-guided biopsy, no further workup is recommended, and the patient is placed in an established follow-up protocol. The goal of reserving open surgical biopsy for definitive clinical management and eliminating it for the sole purpose of diagnosis is increasingly being accomplished.

Even with the advent of image-guided needle biopsy, there is still a need for localization and excision of nonpalpable (and some palpable) lesions. Despite the potential advantage of image-guided percutaneous breast biopsy, some patients are only satisfied with complete surgical removal of their mammographic abnormality. Other patients may not have access to facilities with equipment for stereotactic procedures because of their insurance plans or locale. There are also certain patient characteristics, such as obesity or arthritic conditions and certain lesion types and locations (diffuse calcifications/posterior near the chest wall) that make image-guided biopsy with stereotactic guidance difficult or inappropriate. Excision is also indicated after an image-guided percutaneous breast biopsy if the diagnosis is malignant or high risk (such as atypical lobular or ductal

hyperplasia) or if there is discordance between the radiographic impression and the pathologic result.[7,8] Attention to judgment is crucial in any image-guided breast biopsy program. If the procedure was technically unsatisfactory, the imaging was less than ideal, or poor quality tissue cores were obtained, the physician should not hesitate to recommend a surgical excision. Moreover, because most of these abnormalities are nonpalpable, a localization procedure would be necessary, which traditionally was performed with mammography guidance but increasingly is accomplished with intraoperative ultrasound.

ADVANTAGES/DISADVANTAGES OF MAMMOGRAPHIC VERSUS INTRAOPERATIVE ULTRASOUND LOCALIZATION

Open surgical biopsy with preoperative wire localization has several drawbacks. The failure of removing the targeted lesion has been reported as high as 22%.[4,5] The ability to accomplish a successful biopsy of a nonpalpable breast abnormality may be limited by substandard preoperative wire placement in radiology; dislodgement, migration, or transaction of the wire either pre- or intraoperatively; the failure of the surgeon to excise the lesion accurately; or the failure to obtain a specimen radiograph to confirm that the lesion was adequately removed. Finally, it may be difficult for the pathologist to identify a very small lesion accurately within a large volume of excised tissue.[4-6]

Patients report high anxiety with the wire placement procedure with episodes of syncope in 9% to 20% of patients who are awake and usually upright.[4-6] Many patients report that the localization was the most difficult part of their perioperative experience. From the surgeon's perspective, scheduling early morning cases is limited by the ability to schedule the localization procedure in the radiology department, and there may be delays in the surgery schedule because of complicated or difficult localizations. Dislodgement or transection of the localization wire is another disadvantage of preoperative needle-wire localization, which could lead to an increased miss rate at the time of surgical excision.[4,6] In addition, the clip marker placed at the time of a successful stereotactic breast biopsy, where image evidence of the lesion has been removed, can migrate as much as 1 cm on average and as much as 2 cm up to 20% of the time.[7] These difficulties have led to the use of preoperative and intraoperative ultrasound localization as a replacement for the traditional preoperative localization with mammogram guidance.[8-11]

MAMMOGRAPHIC NEEDLE-WIRE LOCALIZATION

Technique

Preoperative wire localization for surgical excision is usually performed with orthogonal mammography in the radiology department.[6,12-14] The needle-wire combination is guided into the breast through the fenestrated compression paddle alongside or through the target lesion, parallel to the chest wall, using the approach with the shortest skin-to-lesion distance. The patient's breast is then compressed in the corollary view, and the alphanumeric grid is used to adjust the depth of the needle-wire combination before the needle is withdrawn to engage the tip or barb of the wire.[14] At this point, craniocaudad and straight mediolateral mammograms can be taken with the localization wire in place. It is helpful if the radiology technologist places "BB" skin markers on the nipple and at the point where the wire enters the skin. This allows the surgeon viewing the localization mammograms in the operating room to judge the distance the wire travels from the skin to the lesion. The key to a successful excision after an accurate wire placement is to view the craniocaudad mammogram and determine if the tip of the wire is lateral or medial to the lesion. In addition, viewing the mediolateral film determines if the lesion is above or below the wire tip. The nipple and entry site markers help determine how far above/below and medial/lateral the lesion is to the nipple, and by triangulating the depth from the entry marker, the position of the incision is chosen. The incision, therefore, does not need to extend from the wire entry site to the lesion but can be made in a cosmetic fashion on the skin more directly above the lesion.

Stereotactic Mammography-Guided Localization

Preoperative wire localization can also be performed with stereotactic guidance.[15] Using the same stereotactic principles for a stereotactic-guided percutaneous breast biopsy, the position of the lesion can be accurately calculated using the stereotactic table software. A needle holder placed on the stereotactic table guides the wire of choice to the target lesion. With this technique, it is sometimes difficult to choose the skin entrance site to have the smallest skin-to-lesion distance. Regardless of the technique used to place a localization wire, it is helpful if it is not greater than 5 to 10 mm from the lesion to limit potential errors in excision and improve accuracy.

INTRAOPERATIVE ULTRASOUND LOCALIZATION

Overview

Schwartz et al first described the use of intraoperative ultrasound for localization and excision in 1988.[16] Wilson et al, in 1998, described using ultrasound in radiology to localize the lesion by marking the skin and reporting the depth of the target for the surgeon.[17] Since that time, there have been numerous reports on using intraoperative ultrasound for the successful excision of partially palpable and nonpalpable breast abnormalities along with obtaining adequate margins when excising malignant lesions.[8-11,18,19]

Intraoperative ultrasound is a valuable tool for the breast surgeon. Ultrasound can be used to aid in the excision of palpable and nonpalpable lesions with or without placement of a wire for localization during the procedure. For the vaguely palpable lesion, especially one that has been confirmed by a prior image-guided biopsy to be malignant, ultrasound can give the surgeon information about the size and depth of the lesion and help in decision making regarding incision placement and how much tissue to remove. The use of intraoperative ultrasound for localization can allow for earlier start times in the operating room and avoid delays in radiology. Because the surgeon can directly visualize the lesion in the position the patient will be in during removal of the lesion, incision placement is more accurate and placed appropriately close to the lesion with a greater chance for an improved cosmetic result.[10,11] Intraoperative use of ultrasound is associated with a higher free margin rate, less tissue removal, and immediate confirmation of removal of the lesion.[10,18]

Intraoperative Ultrasound Localization with Wire Placement

The operating surgeon can perform wire localization using ultrasound guidance immediately before surgery after the patient is placed on the operating table, eliminating a trip to radiology preoperatively. With intraoperative ultrasound wire placement for localization, the patient is supine and is either sedated or under general anesthesia, eliminating additional pain, anxiety, or syncope. The wire placement can be performed before the patient is prepped and draped. After the surgeon scrubs and the patient is prepped, the wire is placed using a sterile technique with an ultrasound transducer cover, sterile gel packets, and localization wires. When the operating surgeon places the wire personally, there is much more control over the skin entrance site and the direction of the wire. The surgeon gains information about the depth of the lesion and is better able to visualize the location of the wire tip. This allows wire placement in accordance with the location and direction of the planned incision.

Wire Placement Technique

With the appropriate sterile prep and/or draping, ultrasound imaging is performed to visualize the target lesion. Imaging is optimized with equipment designed for high resolution, near-field imaging, using a linear array transducer with a minimum 7.5-MHz frequency. If the wire is placed prior to the patient being prepped and the surgeon having scrubbed, the transducer does not require a sterile sleeve or cover, and the skin may be simply prepped with an alcohol wipe. When using an ultrasound transducer cover for wire placement under sterile conditions, it is important to place ultrasound gel on the inside of the sleeve to create an acoustic coupling between the transducer and the sleeve. Individual packets of sterile gel are available to use on the skin, or sterile Betadine gel may be used for acoustic coupling. If the patient is not under general anesthesia, local anesthetic can be directed under real-time visualization to eliminate the concern of obscuring the target lesion that may be experienced with mammogram guidance.

Multiple localization wires—Hawkins (Boston Scientific; Watertown, Massachusetts), Bard (CR Bard, Inc; Covington, Georgia), or Kopans (Cook; Bloomington, Indiana)—that previously were used only for mammographic localization are available and easily inserted under ultrasound guidance, and the choice is physician preference.[20] The Hawkins FlexStrand wire offers the advantage of easily bringing the wire into the excision cavity without causing a cumbersome bend in the wire, and the cabling of the wire make accidental transection more difficult. The Bard wire is preferred by some for its ability to be retracted back into the placement needle after it has been engaged to allow for readjustment of location. Regardless of wire type, the needle-wire combination is inserted at the proximal edge of the ultrasound transducer. As the localization needle-wire is advanced toward the target lesion, alignment is maintained within the narrow ultrasound scan plane, which follows the long axis of the transducer. The angle of insertion is determined by triangulating between the depth of the lesion as seen on the ultrasound monitor and the length of the transducer footplate (Fig. 56-1). Once guided through the target to the distal side, the needle is withdrawn, engaging the wire hook to minimize the chance that it will become dislodged during dissection. By placing a wire with intraoperative ultrasound guidance, the insertion site is usually no more than a few centimeters (based on the length of the transducer footplate) from the center of the proposed incision site, directly over the targeted lesion. Once the incision is made, the wire can be brought into the confines of the excision cavity and its direction and depth of placement used to guide an appropriate excision.

INTRAOPERATIVE LOCALIZATION OF NONPALPABLE LESIONS WITHOUT A WIRE

For the vaguely palpable lesion or the nonpalpable lesion, intraoperative ultrasound localization can be successfully performed without the use of any localization device or wire. Pararno et al compared intraoperative ultrasound excision in 15 patients with a matched group of 15 patients who underwent preoperative wire localization in the radiology department.[9] All of the lesions were successfully excised, leading to the conclusion reported that ultrasound-guided localization and excision was effective, feasible, and by eliminating a trip to the radiology department, it allowed the entire procedure to be performed in the operating room.

In 1999, Snider and Morrison reported on 44 cancers equally divided between preoperative wire localization and intraoperative ultrasound localization. Excision was 100% successful in both groups, and there was no difference in the rate or width of uninvolved margins. However, there was a significant decrease in excision volume when intraoperative ultrasound was used to guide excision.[8]

Technique for Localization Without a Wire

An intercept technique can be used where the lesion is visualized and centered on the ultrasound screen. The skin is marked at each end of the ultrasound transducer with a marking pen. A line is drawn between the 2 points. The transducer is then turned 90°; the lesion is again visualized in the center of the ultrasound monitor, and the skin is marked at either end of the probe. Another line is drawn connecting these 2 points. The point where the 2 lines intersect represents the point on the skin that lies directly above the center of the visualized target.[10] Figure 56-2 shows a similar technique that involves drawing a line along the length of the transducer on each side at perpendicular angles creating a box overlying the target.[20] For a larger tumor, ultrasound can also be used to map out the perimeter of the tumor in all directions. This is accomplished by first localizing the target to the center of the ultrasound monitor. The transducer is then moved in a superior direction, perpendicular to the long axis of the footplate and marking the skin when the target is no longer visualized. The transducer is then moved in the opposite direction to mark the most inferior point where the target is seen. These 2 steps are repeated in the medial and lateral direction (Fig. 56-3). Mapping out the limits of the target on the skin are especially helpful when the size of the ultrasound transducer prevents placing it within the excision cavity. If the transducer has a small enough footplate to be placed inside, the dissection can be monitored under real-time ultrasound. The "in line of site" technique, similar to that illustrated for using the gamma detection device in sentinel lymph node biopsy, has been described.[11] After using ultrasound to localize the target position and making an incision, the transducer is placed in the wound and the lesion is again visualized. The transducer is angled to determine a 1-cm margin in 4 directions (superior, inferior, medial, and lateral). Dissection is carried out toward the pectoral muscle along this "line of site." The ultrasound transducer is then angled perpendicular to the lesion and parallel to the muscle to determine the deep margin. The lesion is then excised in a "boxlike fashion." Confirmation of excision and adequate margin is accomplished with ultrasound of the specimen. The specimen ultrasound may be performed in a basin with saline, assessing the superficial, deep, superior, and inferior margins with the transducer in a single position and then rotating it 90° to visualize the medial and lateral margins.[8] The specimen can also be examined ex vivo using sterile ultrasound gel to determine the width of the margins (Fig. 56-4).

CONVERTING AN ULTRASOUND-INVISIBLE LESION TO AN ULTRASOUND-VISIBLE STATUS

The target for intraoperative ultrasound localization includes nonpalpable, partially palpable, and even palpable abnormalities. Most of these have had preoperative percutaneous image-guided

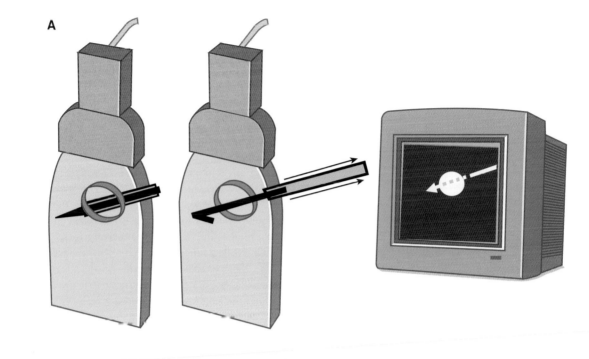

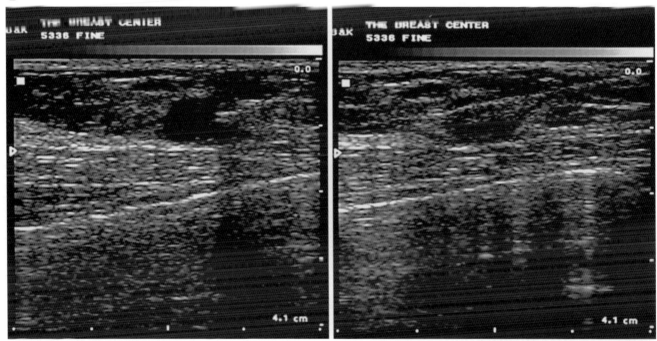

FIGURE 56-1 **A.** The needle-wire combination is inserted at the proximal edge of the ultrasound transducer and advanced toward the target lesion, maintaining alignment within the narrow ultrasound scan plane, which follows the long axis of the transducer. Once guided through the target to the distal side, the needle is withdrawn, engaging the wire hook to minimize the chance that it will become dislodged during dissection. **B.** The angle of insertion is determined by triangulating between the depth of the lesion as seen on the ultrasound monitor and the length of the transducer footplate.

needle biopsies of an ultrasound-visible lesion and require excision for a malignant or high-risk pathology or because of discordance between the radiographic imaging impression and the pathology diagnosis. However, many lesions (microcalcifications) that require definitive excision are not visible by ultrasound. The advantages of intraoperative ultrasound localization over preoperative wire localization have been expanded to the lesions that are traditionally considered ultrasound invisible by converting them into ultrasound-visible status.[20,21] Markers are now available that can be placed at the time of image-guided biopsy, such as a stereotactic guided needle biopsy for microcalcifications.[21,22] These markers are made with an absorbable

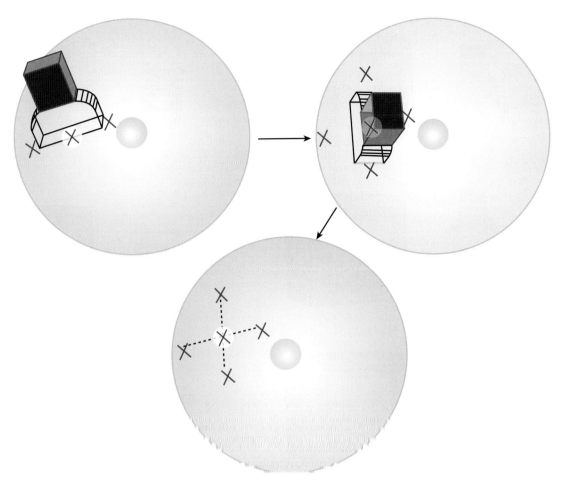

FIGURE 56-2 Intercept technique. The lesion is visualized and centered on the ultrasound screen. The skin is marked at each end of the ultrasound transducer with a marking pen. A line is drawn between the 2 points. The transducer is then turned 90°, and the process is repeated. The point where the 2 lines intersect represents the point on the skin that lies directly above the center of the visualized target.

echogenic material, similar to VICRYL (Ethicon, Inc; Somerville, NJ), which is visible with ultrasound and may remain so for several weeks.[22] In addition, a metallic portion provides longer-term visibility (after absorption of the echogenic marker) for localization with either a mammographic or stereotactic localization technique or a more permanent marking to monitor the position of an image-guided target that does not require excision. The type of marker, how it was placed, and the length of time that has elapsed between marker placement and surgery may affect the ability to image the marker successfully and guide an intraoperative excision. It is therefore important to have the patient have a preoperative ultrasound evaluation a couple of days before the planned excision to verify the marker visibility. Often if the marking clip is not clearly visible, a small biopsy cavity or hematoma can serve as the imaging target. In fact, Smith et al described using the resultant hematoma in the cavity from a vacuum-assisted stereotactic biopsy to guide excision successfully in 20 patients up to 56 days after the biopsy.[23] Another technique involves injecting the patient's blood into

the cavity created with a vacuum-assisted biopsy device, to establish a clearly localizable target without the use of any marker. This may also be used in localizing lesions detected only by MRI.[24]

INTRAOPERATIVE ULTRASOUND LOCALIZATION TO GUIDE SURGICAL EXCISION OF NONPALPABLE BREAST CARCINOMA: MARGIN ASSESSMENT WITHOUT WIRE LOCALIZATION

Increased screening with high-quality mammography has led to a greater number of nonpalpable breast carcinomas usually diagnosed with image-guided biopsy. When the patient chooses breast-conserving surgery, the goal is complete excision with specimen margins that are free of tumor on pathology evaluation. The advantages of intraoperative ultrasound localization provide a better opportunity for accuracy of tumor localization, with a more appropriately placed incision and the ability to

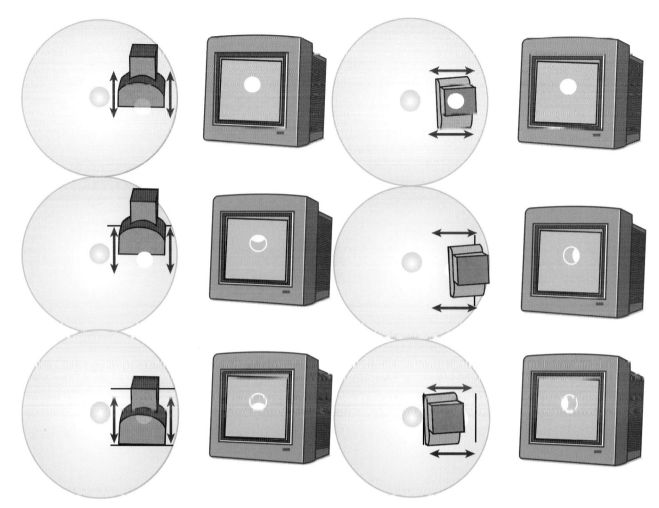

FIGURE 56-3 Mapping out the perimeter of the tumor in all directions. After localizing the target to the center of the ultrasound monitor, the transducer is then moved in a superior direction, perpendicular to the long axis of the footplate and marking the skin when the target is no longer visualized. The transducer is then moved in the opposite direction to mark the most inferior point where the target is seen. These 2 steps are then repeated in the medial and lateral direction.

monitor the excision during surgery, real-time, to ensure adequate excision. The excised lumpectomy specimen may be evaluated intraoperatively on the operating table to confirm the presence of the tumor and judge the adequacy of the margins. Rahusen et al performed a feasibility study in 1999 for the accuracy of obtaining margins with ultrasound-guided lumpectomy.[25] Of the 19 patients who underwent ultrasound localization, 17 (89%) had adequate margins compared with only 17 of the 43 patients (42%) that were excised with wire localization. Harlow et al described this technique in the first 65 cancers using intraoperative ultrasound guidance, without a localization wire, for the excision of nonpalpable breast cancers.[10] Overall success rate of achieving negative margins was 97% (63 of 65 cancers). A second operation (reexcision) was performed in 3 patients (4.8%), 2 for positive margins and 1 for a margin less than 1 mm. After the first excision, the mean closest margin was 0.8 cm. Intraoperative localization was feasible for nonpalpable lesions and gives results in terms of pathologic

margins that are comparable with those achieved by standard needle-wire-guided excisions. Smith et al also evaluated the ability of intraoperative ultrasound to obtain adequate lumpectomy margins and decrease the rate of reexcision requiring another surgery.[11] Eighty-one patients underwent intraoperative ultrasound excision excisions with an attempt to achieve 1-cm margins. All localizations were successful, and 24 of 25 malignant lesions had a 1-cm or larger margin. Improving the ability of the surgeon to assess the adequacy of margins at the time of excision can even be accomplished using intraoperative ultrasound with palpable cancers where digital manipulation and visual inspection were traditionally used to guide excision.[19] Moore randomized 51 patients with biopsy-proven T1 and T2 palpable breast carcinoma to ultrasound-guided surgery (27 patients) and wire localization surgery (24 patients). Intraoperative ultrasound provided clear resection margins in 26 of 27 patients (97%) with a mean margin width of 7.7 mm. Only 14 of 24 patients (71%) had negative margins with a mean width of 4.8 mm.

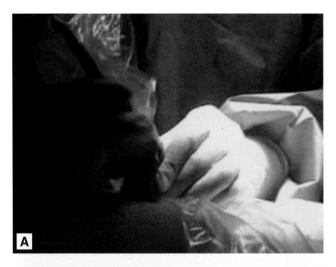

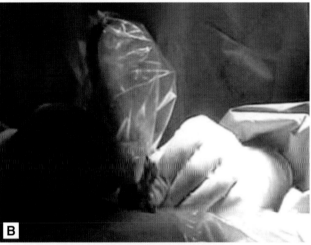

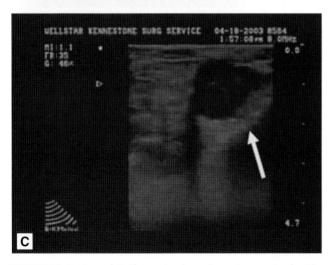

FIGURE 56-4 **A.** and **B.** The excised specimen is examined with the ultrasound transducer and sterile coupling gel, and then the specimen is rotated to view each of 6 margins. **C.** The width of the margin is judged to be adequate *(white arrow pointing at the deep margin),* and if too narrow, reexcision of additional margin is obtained.

INTRAOPERATIVE ULTRASOUND-GUIDED LUMPECTOMY: FUTURE DIRECTIONS

The use of image-guided technology has revolutionized the detection of an increasing number of nonpalpable breast abnormalities by providing a technique that is minimally invasive and reduces the volume of tissue removed. In an attempt to obtain adequate margins while reducing the volume of tissue removed, several technologies are being explored to further the advantages and value of ultrasound-guided surgery. Some provide the advantage of creating a palpable entity from a nonpalpable abnormality to facilitate excision; others provide a method of performing an ultrasound-guided excision in situ. Cryofreezing and radiofrequency involved in both diagnostic and therapeutic devices are being adapted as an adjunct to lumpectomy using intraoperative ultrasound for sonographically visualized, nonpalpable breast cancers.

Cryo-Assisted Lumpectomy

The Visica cryoprobe (Sanarus Medical; Pleasanton, California) is inserted under ultrasound guidance into the center of the target lesion. The center position is confirmed with a cross-sectional 90° ultrasound scan. The argon gas generates an ice ball that is easily visualized with ultrasound, and under real time its growth can be monitored until it encompasses the tumor along with a predetermined margin of uninvolved breast tissue. Surgical resection is facilitated by the palpation of the ice ball and the manipulation and traction of the cryoprobe (a ball-on-a-stick effect)[20] (Fig. 56-5). A pilot study in 24 patients, all successfully localized, showed that with an ice ball providing a greater than 6-mm frozen margin, the reexcision rate was only 5.6%.[26] The cryofreezing did not interfere with pathologic margin evaluation but did affect the accuracy of ancillary studies such as ER, PR, and HER-2, but these can be obtained from the diagnostic core biopsy. This pilot was followed by a multicenter, prospective, randomized trial in 310 patients comparing cryo-assisted lumpectomy (CAL) with localization using needle-wire placement under mammogram or ultrasound guidance.[27] The positive margin rate did not differ significantly between the 2 groups (28% in the cryo group versus 31% in the control group). However, CAL did decrease the excision volume from 66 to 47 mL. Further clinical evaluation is needed because the control group did not allow the use of intraoperative ultrasound to guide the excision beyond needle-wire placement.

Electrosurgical Flexible Cutting Loop Assisted Lumpectomy

Despite the many advantages of intraoperative ultrasound localization and excision, the surgeon can still experience certain difficulties related to the surgical resection. It can be challenging to determine the level of dissection for the deep margin, especially when the ultrasound transducer cannot be placed in the incision. The potential to decrease the incision size and reduce the volume of excision while obtaining adequate margin could be achieved if the dissection around the tumor, including

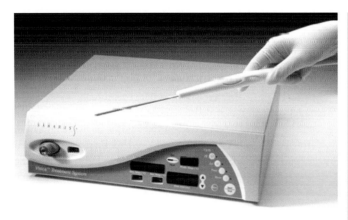
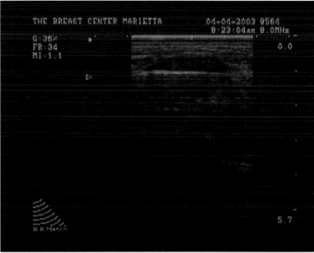
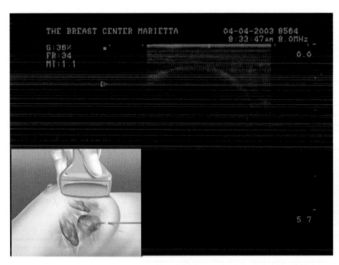
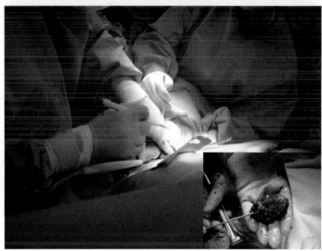

FIGURE 56-5 The Visica cryoprobe is inserted under ultrasound guidance into the center of the target lesion. The argon gas generates an ice ball that is easily visualized with ultrasound until its growth encompasses the tumor along with a predetermined margin of uninvolved breast tissue. Surgical resection is facilitated by the palpation of the ice ball, and manipulation and traction of the cryoprobe (a ball-on-a-stick effect).

the deep margin, is accomplished under real-time imaging prior to making the incision. The Phantom Electrosurgical Flexible Cutting Loop (Rubicor Medical, Inc; Redwood City, California) is a minimally invasive device with a radiofrequency cutting loop that can be used by surgeons to perform an ultrasound-guided excision or lumpectomy. The distal end of the device consists of a bladed introducer and a 30-mm radiofrequency-activated cutting loop that can be deployed to a height of 25 mm. The handle of the device has a thumb control for deploying and retracting the cutting loop. The power cable is connected to a standard Valleylab (Boulder, Colorado) electrosurgical pencil. The Phantom is guided under the tumor with ultrasound from a small lateral "stab" incision. While in a cross-sectional scanning view, the radiofrequency-activated loop can be visualized while it is extended and then rotated around the circumference of the lesion with a margin of normal tissue and then retracted to a closed position, completing the dissection. The Phantom device is removed from the breast. An incision is made directly over the tumor, and the subcutaneous tissue is divided straight down to the newly created lumpectomy cavity. The specimen is lifted out of the cavity, immediately oriented, and then scanned with ultrasound to confirm excision and judge the adequacy of the margin (Figs. 56-6 and 56-7). Additional margins can be excised if needed, and the uniform cavity wall optimizes the easy of reexcision.

A prospective analysis involving 4 centers was conducted to examine the efficacy of the Phantom device when used under ultrasound guidance.[28] Surgical procedures were performed between April 10, 2007, and September 12, 2007, at 4 centers in the United States. Seventy-nine patients were evaluated as requiring surgical excision of a breast lesion. Fifty-nine of 79 lesions were demonstrated to be malignant; of these, 51 cases (86.4%) had noninvolved final margins resulting in a reexcision rate (second operation) of 13.6%. Average cancer diameter was 1.5 cm (range: 0.4-3.2 cm) with an average specimen size of 21.3 cm^3 (range: 1.2-52.0 cm^3) compared with the average

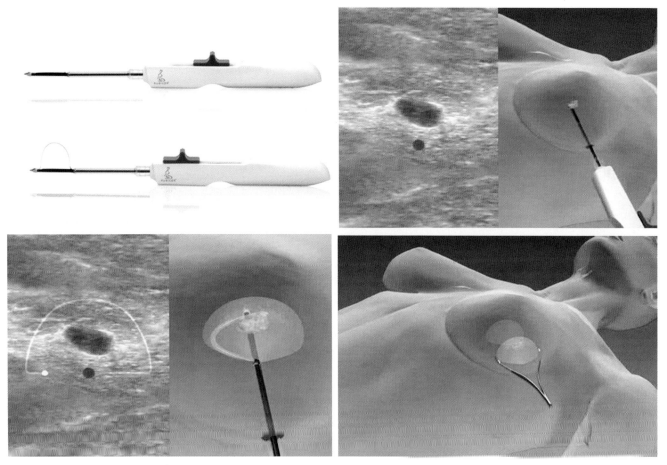

FIGURE 56-6   A. The Phantom Electrosurgical Flexible Cutting Loop. The device consists of a bladed introducer and a 30-mm radiofrequency-activated cutting loop that can be deployed to a height of 25 mm with a thumb control. **B.** The Phantom is guided under the tumor with ultrasound from a small lateral "stab" incision. **C.** The radiofrequency-activated loop is visualized while it is extended and then rotated around the circumference of the lesion with a margin of normal tissue and then retracted to a closed position, completing the dissection. An incision is made directly over the tumor, and the specimen is lifted out of the cavity.

specimen size of 60 to 100 cm^3 in the literature. The incision size for specimen removal was 3.5 cm (range: 2.0-6.0 cm). The in situ resection allows the incision for specimen removal to be smaller, and real-time circumferential dissection with the target lesion held in place by the surrounding breast tissue removes a smaller volume of tissue with the potential for improved cosmetic result and decreased surgical time. The results demonstrate improved efficiency, decrease in volume of excision, smaller incision size, and very low need for reoperation secondary to involved margins with the use of the Phantom device for real-time, ultrasound-guided lumpectomy.

SUMMARY

Intraoperative ultrasound is a useful technology for localizations of nonpalpable as well as palpable lesions with and without localization devices. By eliminating preoperative needle-wire localization in the radiology department, there are no scheduling conflicts or delays. The potential advantages for patients include streamlining their care during a stressful time and avoiding an uncomfortable procedure with risk of syncope. The surgeon can place the surgical incision more accurately, preserving cancer principles with a direct approach to the tumor. The use of intraoperative ultrasound has also improved the ability to obtain adequate margins during cancer surgery and can be used to assess the excised specimen immediately for confirmation of successful tumor removal and margin status immediately after lumpectomy.

With continued screening with high-quality mammography and MRI in high-risk individuals, there will be an increasing number of early-stage breast cancers diagnosed that are amenable to breast-conserving surgery. The focus in diagnosis and treatment continues to be a minimally invasive approach. New technology may further improve on the advantages of intraoperative ultrasound to lower reexcision rates for positive margins while decreasing the volume of tissue removed and improve the cosmetic result without sacrificing survival outcomes.

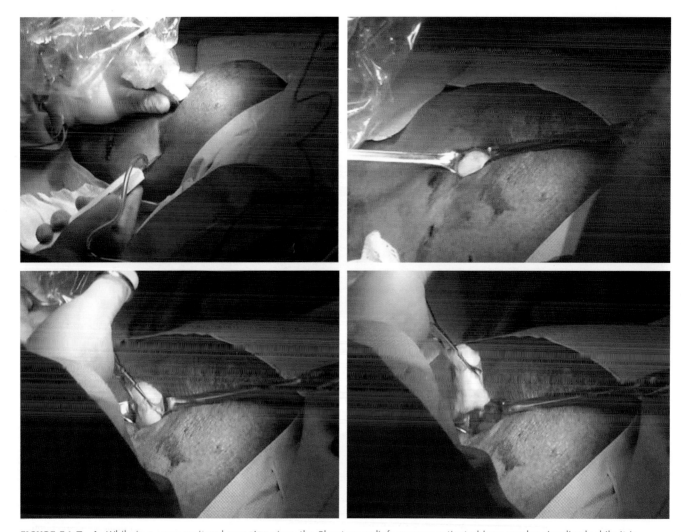

FIGURE 56-7   A. While in a cross-sectional scanning view, the Phantom radiofrequency-activated loop can be visualized while it is extended and then rotated around the circumference of the lesion with a margin of normal tissue. **B.** An incision is made directly over the tumor, and the subcutaneous tissue is divided straight down to the newly created lumpectomy cavity. **C.** and **D.** The specimen is lifted out of the cavity.

REFERENCES

1. Kopans DB. The positive predictive value of mammography. *AJR Am J Roentgenol.* 1992;158:521-526.
2. Libernam L, Cohen MA, Dershaw DD, et al. Atypical ductal hyperplasia diagnosed at stereotaxic core biopsy of breast lesions: an indication for surgical biopsy. *AJR Am J Roentgenol.* 1995;164:111-113.
3. Jackman RJ, Nowels KWW, Shepard MJ, et al. Stereotaxic large-core needle biopsy of 450 non-palpable breast lesions with surgical correlation in lesions with cancer or atypical hyyerplasia. *Radiology.* 1994;193:91-95.
4. Rissanen TJ, Makarainen SI, Mattilla AI, et al. Wire localization biopsy of breast lesions: a review of 425 cancers found in screening or clinical mammography. *Clin Radiol.* 1993;27:14-22.
5. Norton LW, Zeligman BE, Pearlman MD. Accuracy and cost of needle localization breast biopsy. *Arch Surg.* 1988;123:947-950.
6. Homer MJ, Smith TJ, Safaii H. Prebiopsy needle localization: methods, problems, and expected results. *Radiol Clin North Am.* 1992;30:139-153.
7. Kass R, Kumar G, Klimberg VS, et al. Clip migration. *Am J Surg.* 2002;184(4):325-331.
8. Snider HC Jr, Morrison DG. Intraoperative ultrasound localization of nonpalpable breast lesions. *Ann Surg Oncol.* 1999;6(3):308-314.
9. Paramo JC, Landeros M, McPhee MD, et al. Intraoperative ultrasound-guided excision of nonpalpable breast lesions. *Breast J.* 1999;5(6):389-394.
10. Harlow SP, Krag DN, Ames SE, et al. Intraoperative ultrasound localization to guide surgical excision of nonpalpable breast carcinoma. *J Am Coll Surg.* 1999;189(3):241-246.
11. Smith LF, Rubio IT, Henry Tillman R, et al. Intraoperative ultrasound-guided breast biopsy. *Am J Surg.* 2000;180(6):419-423.
12. Feig SA. Localization of clinically occult breast lesions. *Radiol Clin North Am.* 1983;21:155.
13. Homer MJ, Smith TJ, Marchant DJ. Outpatient needle localization and biopsy for nonpalpable breast lesions. *JAMA.* 1984;252:2452-2454.
14. Kopans DB, Meyer JE, Lindfors KK, et al. Spring-hookwire breast lesion localizer: use with rigid compression mammographic systems. *Radiology.* 1985;157:537-538.
15. Fine RE, Boyd BA. Stereotactic breast biopsy: a practical approach. *Am Surg.* 1996;62:96-102.
16. Schwartz GF, Goldberg BB, Riften MD, et al. Ultrasonography: an alternative to x-ray guided needle localization of non-palpable breast masses. *Surgery.* 1988;104:870.
17. Wilson M, Boggis CR, Mansel RE, et al. Non-invasive ultrasound localization of impalpable breast lesions. *Clin Radiol.* 1993;47:337-338.
18. Henry-Tillman R, Johnson AT, Smith LF, et al. Intraoperative ultrasound and other techniques to achieve negative margins. *Semin Surg Oncol.* 2001;20(3):206-213.
19. Moore MM, Whitney LA, Cerilli L, et al. Intraoperative ultrasound is associated with clear lumpectomy margins for palpable infiltrating ductal breast cancer. *Ann Surg.* 2001;233:761-768.

20. Fine RE, Staren ED. Updates in breast ultrasound. *Surg Clin N Am.* 2004;84:1001-1034.
21. Whaler D, Adamczyk D, Jensen E. Sonographically guided needle localization after stereotactic breast biopsy. *AJR Am J Roentgenol.* 2003;180:352-354.
22. Lechner M, Day D, Kusnick C, et al. Ultrasound visibility of a new breast biopsy marker on serial evaluation. *Radiology.* 2002;223(suppl):115.
23. Smith LF, Henry-Tillman R, Rubio IT, et al. Intraoperative localization after stereotactic breast biopsy without a needle. *Am J Surg.* 2001;182:584-589.
24. Smith LF, Henry-Tillman RS, Harms S, et al. Hematoma-directed ultrasound-guided breast biopsy. *Ann Surg.* 2000;180(6):434-438.
25. Rahusen FD, Taets Van Amerongen AH, Van Diest PJ, et al. Ultrasound-guided lumpectomy of nonpalpable breast cancers: a feasibility study looking at the accuracy of obtained margins. *J Surg Oncol.* 1999;72:72-76.
26. Tafra L, Smith SJ, Woodward JE, et al. Pilot trial of cryoprobe-assisted breast-conserving surgery for small ultrasound-visible cancers. *Ann Surg Oncol.* 2003;10(9):1018-1024.
27. Tafra L, Fine R, Whitworth P, et al. Prospective randomized study comparing cryo-assisted and needle-wire localization of ultrasound visible breast tumors. *Am J Surg.* 2006:192(4):462-470.
28. Fine RE, Schwalke, MA, Pellicane, JV, et al. A novel ultrasound-guided electrosurgical loop device for intra-operative excision of breast lesions; an improvement in surgical technique. Poster presented at: American Society of Breast Surgeons; 2008.

CHAPTER 57

Central Duct Exploration for Nipple Discharge

Lisa M. Sclafani

Nipple discharge affects 5% to 30% of women during their lifetime. Surgery is rarely indicated. Many benign conditions cause nipple discharges including duct ectasia, cystic disease, papillomas, infection, and abnormal production of prolactin. In addition, many medications can produce discharge. Discharges are usually categorized as physiologic or pathologic, depending on their color, frequency, and the involvement of single or multiple ducts. Those discharges that are bilateral, creamy or greenish in color, draining from multiple ducts, non-spontaneous, and associated with an otherwise normal physical exam and mammogram are rarely due to cancer or papillomas and do not require surgery except rarely for relief of symptoms. Clinical characteristics that suggest a pathologic discharge are unilateral discharge through a single duct; the presence of a bloody, clear, or serous discharge; discharge that is spontaneous; and those associated with a mass. Pathologic discharges usually require surgery to rule out a malignant cause, although cancer as a cause of nipple discharge is unusual.[1-3] In a series of 204 patients presenting to a multidisciplinary group with nipple discharge, only 7 (3%) were found to have cancer or 9% of those ultimately referred for surgery.[2] In a group of 82 patients referred to a surgical clinic with pathologic nipple discharge (spontaneous red or serous discharge from a single duct), 4 were found to have cancer (5%). Advanced age has been seen to be a predictor of cancer in women with nipple discharge.[1,2]

PREOPERATIVE EVALUATION

A patient presenting with a pathologic nipple discharge for evaluation should have a mammogram and physical examination.

Physical Examination

A physical exam should include the usual palpation of the breast as well as looking for trigger points that elicit the discharge. This trigger point is often used to decide on location for the circumareolar incision. The nipple is carefully inspected for adenomas in the nipple as well as excoriations or skin changes that can lead to blood on the surface of the nipple. Excoriations from trauma, eczema, fungal rashes, and Paget disease can lead to blood staining of the bra, which patients can mistake for a nipple discharge.

The nipple discharge should be elicited to confirm the color, volume, and whether a single or multiple ducts are involved. The color should be distinguished by placing it on a white surface like gauze as the green-black discharge of duct ectasia is often mistaken for blood and these 2 discharges are treated differently. Yellow or green discharge from multiple ducts is usually a sign of duct ectasia and rarely requires surgery. The absence of blood on a guaiac card does not eliminate the possibility of a pathologic discharge,[4] but its strong presence demands further evaluation. Any palpable mass should be needle biopsied. A nearby cyst can discharge into the nipple causing a serous discharge, and aspiration can halt the discharge. Similarly, infectious processes may discharge into the nipple and signs of infection should be treated with antibiotics and the patient reevaluated after the infection is cleared. Follow-up of these patients for recurrence of symptoms is essential, however, because an underlying cause like an obstructing papilloma or cancer may be present and usually will cause recurrence of the discharge. Sonogram may be helpful in these cases to identify an obstructing lesion.

Mammography

Mass lesions, suspicious calcifications, or dilated retroareolar ducts may be seen on mammography in a patient with nipple discharge. Masses and calcifications can be stereotactically biopsied with a clip placed for preoperative localization and excision if atypia, papilloma, or cancer is seen. However, it is important to ensure that the abnormality identified is the cause of the discharge and not an incidental finding. Obviously, size and proximity to the nipple are important in making this decision.

If both physical exam and mammogram are found to be normal, various approaches have been suggested as preoperative evaluation.

Sonography

Many investigators use routine retroareolar sonography in conjunction with mammography for preoperative evaluation.[2,5,6] The ability of ultrasound to visualize the causative lesion ranges from 26% to 69%[2,5-7] and is clearly operator dependent. Rissanen et al reported on 52 patients with bloody or serous discharge who underwent both galactography and sonography prior to surgery.[5] In 69% of patients, an intraductal lesion was seen on sonography, identifying 65% of papillomas but only 1 of 5 malignant lesions. Dilated ducts were seen in 3 of 5 cases with malignant lesions, and in 1 the sonogram was normal. Sonography identified 3 tumors not identified by galactography. Gray et al reported on 204 patients presenting to a multispecialty group practice with true nipple discharge.[7] Sonography was performed in 142 patients and a mass was identified in 30 (21%). Among 7 patients (3%) ultimately diagnosed with cancer, 6 had a preoperative sonogram, 5 of which identified the malignancy preoperatively. However, sonography had a low specificity in this series as in others. In a study from MD Anderson, 64 patients with pathologic discharge undergoing surgery had a sonogram; 13 sonograms showed a suspicious mass and 18 showed duct ectasia.[8] Among 19 patients ultimately found to have cancer, the sonogram was abnormal in 12; 7 showed suspicious masses and 5 showed duct ectasia. While there are false-negative sonograms in all series, sonography is inexpensive, noninvasive, and widely available, and if a lesion is found, it can be percutaneously biopsied or sonographically localized the day of surgery. Vargas et al recommend percutaneous biopsy of any lesion found sonographically and surgical duct excision for those with no imaging findings.[6]

Role of Preoperative Ductography

Ductography, a radiologic examination, has the potential to pinpoint the offending lesion in the major duct that is causing the discharge, thereby aiding in diagnosis, limiting the extent of surgical resection, and making it more likely the pathologic lesion will be removed.[8,9] The discharging duct is cannulated with a small (30-gauge) catheter, and at this point the duct can be aspirated or lavaged to obtain a cytologic specimen. The duct is then injected with water-soluble contrast until the patient experiences discomfort or the contrast flow is reversed. Mammograms are then taken in craniocaudal (cc) and lateral views and any other views as necessary to demonstrate the intraductal pathology.[10] Cutoff of the duct, filling defects, or duct ectasia are considered abnormal (Figs. 57-1 and 57-2). Repeating the ductogram on the day of surgery, with injection of methylene blue dye and in conjunction with preoperative wire localization, may allow for a limited surgical duct excision and

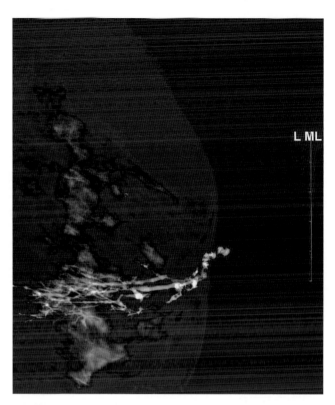

FIGURE 57-1 Ductogram showing multiple filling defects due to extensive intraductal cancer. The defects were needle localized the day of surgery ensuring removal of the entire lesion.

preservation of a patient's ability to breast feed, while ensuring that the responsible lesion is removed.

Possible difficulties encountered during ductography may be that the discharge is not able to be produced at the time of the exam, the occasional inability to cannulate the offending duct because of small size, the cannulation of the wrong duct, perforation of the duct with extravasation of contrast, or the introduction of air bubbles that can mimic intraductal lesions.

In a review of duct excisions at Memorial Sloan-Kettering Cancer Center, Van Zee et al reported on 46 duct excisions of which 21 had preoperative ductography.[9] Sixteen of these excisions were performed with preoperative ductography repeated the morning of surgery, with methylene blue in most, and in 4 with lesions distant from the nipple a localizing wire was placed. In these 21 duct excisions, a papilloma or cancer was found in 17 (81%) patients. This is in contrast to the 30 patients who did not undergo preoperative ductography and whose surgery was performed as a total duct excision without guidance. In this group, papillomas or cancer was found in 13 (43%), duct ectasia in an additional 7 (23%), and no cause for the discharge was found in 10 (33%) patients.

In a similar evaluation of all patients undergoing ductography at Baylor between 1995 and 1998, Lamont et al reported on 35 patients of which abnormalities were detected in 30.[11] Twenty-seven of the 30 had excision, either by total duct excision (14/27), focused duct excision (12/27), or mammotome (1/27). All patients were found to have a pathologic cause for the discharge; 20 patients were found to have a papilloma, 1 of

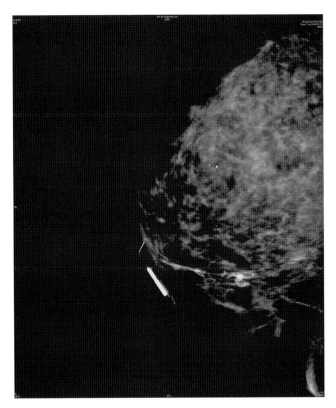

FIGURE 57-2 Intraductal filling lesion due to a papilloma 4.5 cm from the nipple, which may have been missed in a standard total duct excision.

clear. In a review of 1948 cytologic smears from 1530 patients over a 20-year period, Gupta et al found malignant cytology in 67 (4%) patients, 2 of which were found to be a false-positive result when excision revealed a fibroadenoma in 1 and florid gynecomastia in the other.[13] When cytology was read as suspicious for malignancy, carcinoma was found in 18 of 22 patients. In the 229 cases read as suspicious for a papillary lesion, 53 underwent surgery and a papilloma was found in 41. No other pathology was found in the remaining 12 patients. No patients with a benign cytology were found to have cancer on follow-up but the method of follow-up in this series in not clear. Of note, 492 smears (32%) were read as inadequate for interpretation. In a smaller series from Pritt, 466 cytology samples from 395 patients with nipple discharge were reviewed.[13] Only 45 of the 98 cases with abnormal cytology had pathologic follow-up. A finding of atypia (n = 29) corresponded to a papilloma in 24 cases, papillary hyperplasia in 2, moderate epithelial hyperplasia in 7 cases, and duct ectasia in 3. Some had more than 1 diagnosis. Two cases with normal cytology had surgery and an intraductal papilloma was found in both. Of the 13 cases with cancer, 11 had suspicious or malignant cytology, but there were 2 false negatives. In addition, there was 1 false-positive malignant cytology. In a similar study of 351 cases of nipple cytology by Dinkel et al, cytology had a sensitivity of 31% and a specificity of 97% for malignancy, but 11 false negatives and 4 false positives were seen.[14] Sauter et al found 50% of patients with cancer had abnormal cytology, but the cytology was positive for cancer in their series of 49 patients with discharge undergoing surgery.[4] Most authors conclude that discharge cytology has limitations including both false negatives and false positives, making cytology unreliable in determining whether surgery should be performed. For this reason, we have largely abandoned nipple discharge cytology as a diagnostic preoperative tool.

Nipple aspiration cytology, often as an adjunct to galactography or ductoscopy, may hold more promise.[15] In comparing discharge cytology and aspiration cytology, Baitchev et al showed half as many nondiagnostic cytologies in the aspiration group compared to the discharge group (11% vs 22%).[16] Among cases with cancer diagnosed following surgery for abnormal discharge, 9/16 had suspicious or malignant discharge cytology compared to 12/16 with suspicious or malignant aspiration cytology. However, there was also 1 cancer patient with a false-negative cytology by both methods. In a study of women who were undergoing surgery for an abnormal imaging study, palpable mass, or abnormal discharge, aspiration cytology was performed by Sauter et al in conjunction with ductoscopic examination in 88 patients.[17] Thirty-three percent of cytologies were nondiagnostic. Four of 5 aspirates called malignant were found in patients with cancer and 1 was in a patient with a papilloma. Only 5 of 37 patients with cancer had suspicious or malignant cytology, but this may reflect the patient population chosen because many of these patients did not have discharge as the indication for surgery. Brushings taken through the microendoscope may also improve accuracy as shown by Beechey-Newman et al.[18] Overall, the role of aspiration cytology in patients with nipple discharge is still unclear but deserves further investigation. Its role in studying the microenvironment of the ductal system is also being explored.[19]

whom also had ductal carcinoma in situ; and 7 had duct ectasia. Among 5 patients with normal ductograms, 2 had surgery, 1 was found to have a papilloma, and 1 had duct ectasia. The other 3 were followed and none of these was found to develop cancer; the follow-up period was not stated in this paper. In a study of 42 patients with pathologic discharge in whom 21 had ductograms, 14 were reported as abnormal.[12] Twenty percent of ductograms showed a lesion greater than 3 cm from the nipple. Six of 14 abnormal ductograms showed multiple lesions, some of which were localized by needle preoperatively. In these cases, ductography was instrumental in removing lesions that might have not been included in a total duct excision without localization. On the other hand, 4 patients with normal ductograms had papillomas found at surgery. This may be due to injecting the wrong duct, a pitfall of ductography. The authors conclude that a normal ductogram does not preclude a duct excision. In a study of 94 patients undergoing surgery for pathologic discharge, Cabioglu et al demonstrated that with the exception of an abnormal mammography or sonography to guide excision, a ductography-guided operation had a higher likelihood of finding a pathologic correlate for the nipple discharge compared to lacrimal probe guidance or central duct excision.[8]

Nipple Discharge Cytology and Intraductal Aspiration Cytology

Nipple fluid is often sent for cytologic examination but its utility in differentiating benign from malignant conditions is not

MICRODOCHECTOMY

Excision of the duct causing the abnormal discharge, thereby determining its cause, is the primary aim of microdochectomy. It is both diagnostic and therapeutic. The major advantage of microdochectomy compared to total duct excision is removal of a smaller volume of breast tissue[20] and possible preservation of the ability to breast-feed. The identification of the discharging duct can be performed by multiple techniques, including the use of lacrimal probes inserted into the discharging duct intraoperatively, injection of methylene blue dye, transillumination with a ductoscope placed into the discharging duct, or preoperative wire localization in patients with an abnormal mammogram, sonogram, or ductogram. These localizing procedures enable a smaller amount of tissue to be removed and, as previously stated, may make it more likely that the pathologic cause of the discharge will be identified and removed.[9,21,22] Vargas et al reported a series of 63 patients who underwent lacrimal duct probe localization and microdochectomy for nipple discharge with otherwise normal exam, mammogram, and sonogram.[6] All patients had a pathologic diagnosis, although duct ectasia and fibrocystic changes were felt to be responsible for 92% of cases. After a median follow-up of 18 months, no patient has had recurrence of symptoms, and 1 patient was diagnosed with cancer associated with a new mammographic finding. Other authors report similar results.[9,21]

Microdochectomy is usually performed under local anesthesia with intravenous sedation. A circumareolar incision is made near the discharging duct or as localized by the previously noted techniques.[23] The discharging duct is identified and divided close to the nipple insertion and followed down into the underlying breast tissue for at least 5 to 6 cm, until the point of abnormality is included or until the duct is no longer dilated (Fig. 57-3). The injection of methylene blue, use of lacrimal probes, or needle localization of the intraductal abnormality may facilitate this dissection. The specimen is oriented for the pathologist and sent fresh for margins in the event cancer is found. The underlying tissue is reapproximated and the skin closed with subcuticular closure.

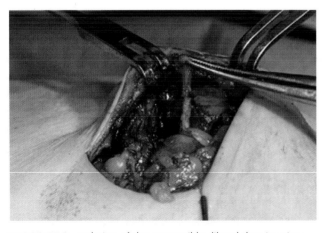

FIGURE 57-3 Isolation of the responsible dilated duct in microdochectomy.

TOTAL DUCT EXCISION

Not all patients are able to have pre- or intraoperative visualization or localization of the discharging duct and may not be able to undergo a microdochectomy. Cannulation of the offending duct may be technically difficult, ductoscopy is not widely available, and preoperative ductography may have been unsuccessful due to small duct size or inability to reproduce discharge, or may have been normal or limited by air bubbles or technical expertise. In such cases, total duct excision will ensure removal and diagnosis of most lesions,[20] prevent recurrence of symptoms from multiple lesions, and generally provides good cosmetic results. In addition, total duct excision is the operation of choice for chronic subareolar infections. However, inability to breast-feed is a result and should be discussed with all patients of childbearing age. Loss of nipple sensation and nipple necrosis has been variously reported in patients undergoing microdochectomy or total duct excision. In a series of 87 consecutive patients undergoing total duct excision, Chapman et al reported an 18% incidence of wound breakdown or infection; however, 6 of the 16 infections were in women with a history of previous infection. Similarly, the rate of nipple necrosis was 13%, but with the exception of 1 case, they were all limited to the tip of the nipple only.[24] This rate was 29% for smokers and 4% for nonsmokers. Two thirds of patients reported loss of nipple sensation, but 71% of patients said it improved with time. Likewise, two thirds of patients reported maintenance of erectile function of the nipple. Cosmetic outcome was obtained from a patient questionnaire by Dixon et al in 100 patients undergoing total duct excision, principally performed for periductal mastitis and duct ectasia.[25] Ninety-four percent of patients reported excellent or good cosmetic outcome, and 86% reported that the nipple looked normal and was fully everted. Thirty percent of patients reported decreased nipple sensation. Loss of sensation was correlated with previous complaints of pain, recurrent infections, and cigarette smoking. Patients with these risk factors should be told of the possibility of loss of nipple sensation.

The technique for total duct excision is similar to microdochectomy and can also be performed under local anesthesia with or without intravenous sedation. Circumareolar incision is made in the area of the discharging duct, the nipple is raised as a full thickness graft, and the major ducts are transected close to the nipple (Fig. 57-4). A cone of tissue extending at least 5 cm into the breast is removed, encompassing the dilated ducts, and the specimen is oriented for the pathologist. In most cases, the underlying defect will require closure with interrupted absorbable sutures. Rarely is it necessary to place a subcutaneous stitch at the base of the nipple to evert it, but nipple eversion should be ensured before the subcuticular sutures are placed to close the skin. Preoperative antibiotics are only used in cases with a history of previous infection.

MINIMALLY INVASIVE TECHNIQUES

Some authors have advocated stereotactic or ultrasound-guided mammotomy as definitive treatment for pathologic discharges. Govindarajulu et al[26] describe a method of sonographically identifying the dilated duct and using a percutaneously placed

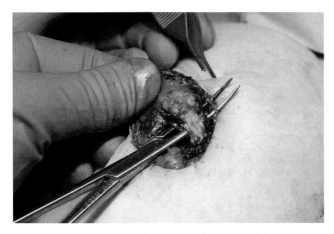

FIGURE 57-4 Transection of the major ducts in total duct excision.

mammotome, either resecting the mass, if one has been identified, or in the absence of a mass, resecting the entire dilated duct. Of 81 procedures performed, cancer was found in 4, papilloma in 33, periductal mastitis in 25, and benign hyperplasia in 19 patients. In 4 patients, symptoms recurred and duct excision was performed identifying a papilloma in 2 cases and benign duct ectasia in 2 cases.

Resection of lesions found by ductography and confirmed on ultrasound using the mammotome to completely remove the lesion was performed by Torres-Tabanera et al in 45 patients.[26,27] Mean ultrasound size was 8 mm and excision was considered complete in 91% of patients. However, nipple discharge continued in 6 patients originally felt to have been completely resected. Two of these were surgically resected and 4 were reresected percutaneously. All cases had benign pathology. Since other investigators have shown underreporting of cancer in patients whose core biopsies showed papillary lesions, longer follow-up of patients treated in this fashion is necessary before this method can be routinely advocated for benign papillary lesions.[28-30] Similarly, biopsy and resection of intraductal lesions through the ductoscope has been proposed but is still investigational.[15,31,32]

FUTURE DIRECTIONS AND STUDIES

The aim of the preoperative evaluation for nipple discharge using various imaging and minimally invasive techniques has been to identify cancers or high-risk lesions that require excision and possibly limit the extent of surgery when it is performed, leading to lower morbidities. False-negative studies have been reported for all preoperative techniques including mammography, cytology, ductography, and sonography; therefore, no single technique is reliable enough to eliminate a surgical procedure. The search for more reliable techniques, like ductoscopy, will be addressed in Chapter 58 by Dr Kim Julian, and require further investigation and study. Ductoscopy has been shown to find more peripheral lesions and multiple lesions but is not widely available.[22] In addition, the exact role of magnetic resonance imaging (MRI) in patients with nipple discharge is

not clear and requires further investigation.[33] Follow-up of patients undergoing less invasive techniques (mammotomy, image-guided microdochectomy, and excision via ductoscopy) is necessary to quantitate the rates of symptom recurrence and complications, including loss of nipple sensation and inability to breast-feed, and, of course, to follow patients for the subsequent development of breast cancer.

SUMMARY

Pathologic discharge from the nipple is one that is persistent, from a single duct, spontaneous, and is bloody, clear, or serous. The most common cause is a papilloma or other benign condition, but cancer can be responsible for 3% to 9% of cases of pathologic discharge, even with a normal mammogram and physical exam. The correct preoperative workup is controversial, but authors have found mammography, sonography, ductography, and more recently ductoscopy of some utility. Cytology is rarely helpful and the absence of blood or suspicious cells in the nipple discharge does not preclude the necessity for surgery. Localization of the abnormality intraoperatively improves the likelihood of finding the pathologic cause. The choice of microdochectomy versus total duct excision is dependent on the ability to localize the abnormality preoperatively or intraoperatively. Further research is necessary to determine the best preoperative workup and to determine if surgery can be avoided in some cases. In addition, the use of newer technologies such as percutaneous mammotomy and ductoscopy are anxiously awaited.

REFERENCES

1. Lau S, Kuchenmeister I, Stachs A, et al. Pathologic nipple discharge: surgery is imperative in postmenopausal women. *Ann Surg Oncol.* 2005;12(7):546-551.
2. Gray RJ, Pockaj BA, Karstaedt PJ. Navigating murky waters: a modern treatment algorithm for nipple discharge. *Am J Surg.* 2007;194(6):850-854; discussion 854-855.
3. Dillon MF, Mohd Nazri SR, Nasir S, et al. The role of major duct excision and microdochectomy in the detection of breast carcinoma. *BMC Cancer.* 2006;6:164.
4. Sauter ER, Schlatter L, Lininger J, Hewett JE. The association of bloody nipple discharge with breast pathology. *Surgery.* 2004;136(4):780-785.
5. Rissanen T, Reinikainen H, Apaja-Sarkkinen M. Breast sonography in localizing the cause of nipple discharge: comparison with galactography in 52 patients. *J Ultrasound Med.* 2007;26(8):1031-1039.
6. Vargas HI, Vargas MP, Eldrageely K, Gonzalez KD, Khalkhali I. Outcomes of clinical and surgical assessment of women with pathological nipple discharge. *Am Surg.* 2006;72(2):124-128.
7. Adepoju LJ, Chun J, El-Tamer M, et al. The value of clinical characteristics and breast-imaging studies in predicting a histopathologic diagnosis of cancer or high-risk lesion in patients with spontaneous nipple discharge. *Am J Surg.* 2005;190(4):644-646.
8. Cabioglu N, Hunt KK, Singletary SE, et al. Surgical decision making and factors determining a diagnosis of breast carcinoma in women presenting with nipple discharge. *J Am Coll Surg.* 2003;196(3):354-364.
9. Van Zee KJ, Ortega Perez G, Minnard E, Cohen MA. Preoperative galactography increases the diagnostic yield of major duct excision for nipple discharge. *Cancer.* 1998;82(10):1874-1880.
10. Slawson SH, Johnson BA. Ductography: how to and what if? *Radiographics.* 2001;21(1):133-150.
11. Lamont JP, Dultz RP, Kuhn JA, Grant MD, Jones RC. Galactography in patients with nipple discharge. *Proc (Bayl Univ Med Cent).* 2000;13(3):214-216.
12. Dawes LG, Bowen C, Venta LA, Morrow M. Ductography for nipple discharge: no replacement for ductal excision. *Surgery.* 1998;124(4):685-691.

13. Gupta RK, Gaskell D, Dowle CS, et al. The role of nipple discharge cytology in the diagnosis of breast disease: a study of 1948 nipple discharge smears from 1530 patients. *Cytopathology.* 2004;15(6):326-330.

14. Dinkel HP, Gassel AM, Muller T, et al. Galactography and exfoliative cytology in women with abnormal nipple discharge. *Obstet Gynecol.* 2001;97(4):625-629.

15. Shen KW, Wu J, Lu JS, et al. Fiberoptic ductoscopy for breast cancer patients with nipple discharge. *Surg Endosc.* 2001;15(11):1340-1345.

16. Baitchev G, Gortchev G, Todorova A, et al. Intraductal aspiration cytology and galactography for nipple discharge. *Int Surg.* 2003;88(2):83-86.

17. Sauter ER, Ehya H, Schlatter L, MacGibbon B. Ductoscopic cytology to detect breast cancer. *Cancer J.* 2004;10(1):33-41; discussion 15-36.

18. Beechey-Newman N, Kulkarni D, Kothari A, et al. Breast duct microendoscopy in nipple discharge: microbrush improves cytology. *Surg Endosc.* 2005;19(12):1648-1651.

19. Lang JE, Kuerer HM. Breast ductal secretions: clinical features, potential uses, and possible applications. *Cancer Control.* 2007;14(4):350-359.

20. Sharma R, Dietz J, Wright H, et al. Comparative analysis of minimally invasive microductectomy versus major duct excision in patients with pathologic nipple discharge. *Surgery.* 2005;138(4):591-596; discussion 596-597.

21. Moncrief RM, Nayar R, Diaz LK, et al. A comparison of ductoscopy-guided and conventional surgical excision in women with spontaneous nipple discharge. *Ann Surg.* 2005;241(4):575-581.

22. Dietz JR, Crowe JP, Grundfest S, Arrigain S, Kim JA. Directed duct excision by using mammary ductoscopy in patients with pathologic nipple discharge. *Surgery.* 2002;132(4):582-587; discussion 587-588.

23. Lanitis S, Filippakis G, Thomas J, et al. Microdochectomy for single-duct pathologic nipple discharge and normal or benign imaging and cytology. *Breast.* 2008;17(3):309-313.

24. Chapman D, Britton TB, Purushotham A, Wishart G. Post-operative complications following subarcolar duct clearance. *Cancer Nursing Practice.* 2006;5:36-39

25. Dixon JM, Kohlhardt SR, Dillon P. Total duct excision. *Breast J.* 1998;7:216-219.

26. Govindarajulu S, Narreddy SR, Shere MH, et al. Sonographically guided mammotome excision of ducts in the diagnosis and management of single duct nipple discharge. *Eur J Surg Oncol.* 2006;32(7):725-728.

27. Torres-Tabanera M, Alonso-Bartolome P, Vega-Bolivar A, et al. Percutaneous microductectomy with a directional vacuum-assisted system guided by ultrasonography for the treatment of breast discharge: experience in 63 cases. *Acta Radiol.* 2008;49(3):271-276.

28. Liberman L, Bracero N, Vuolo MA, et al. Percutaneous large-core biopsy of papillary breast lesions. *AJR Am J Roentgenol.* 1999;172(2):331-337.

29. Rosen EL, Bentley RC, Baker JA, Soo MS. Imaging-guided core needle biopsy of papillary lesions of the breast. *AJR Am J Roentgenol.* 2002;179(5):1185-1192.

30. Masood S, Loya A, Khalbuss W. Is core needle biopsy superior to fine-needle aspiration biopsy in the diagnosis of papillary breast lesions? *Diagn Cytopathol.* 2003;28(6):329-334.

31. Okazaki A, Hirata K, Okazaki M, Svane G, Azavedo E. Nipple discharge disorders: current diagnostic management and the role of fiber-ductoscopy. *Eur Radiol.* 1999;9(4):583-590.

32. Louie LD, Crowe JP, Dawson AE, et al. Identification of breast cancer in patients with pathologic nipple discharge: does ductoscopy predict malignancy? *Am J Surg.* 2006;192(4):530-533.

33. Morrogh M, Morris EA, Liberman L, Borgen PI, King TA. The predictive value of ductography and magnetic resonance imaging in the management of nipple discharge. *Ann Surg Oncol.* 2007;14(12):3369-3377.

CHAPTER 58

Endoscopy for Nipple Discharge

Julian Kim

FIBEROPTIC ENDOSCOPES FOR EVALUATION OF THE BREAST DUCTAL ANATOMY

The development of microendoscopes for visualization of mammary ductal anatomy has progressed rapidly over the past 2 decades. The first published reports of mammary ductoscopy appeared in 1991 authored by Okazaki et al as well as Makita et al in which the endoscopy was performed with essentially a bare fiberoptic cord with no working channel for insufflation or aspiration.[1,2] Subsequently, Susan Love published a small series of breast endoscopy in 9 patients with a diagnosis of ductal carcinoma in situ at the time of mastectomy.[3] Again, using an early generation instrument, they encountered difficulties with insufflation of the ducts and navigation of ductal branches due to rigidity of the scope. As technology improved, a number of semiflexible microendoscopes emerged, which allowed insufflation via a working channel that was formed by a sheath that surrounded the fiberoptic core. Reports of the feasibility of visualization and navigation to the level of the terminal ductal lobular units were generated initially in human mastectomy specimens and subsequently in patients under local anesthesia.[4,5] These technologic developments resulted in visualization of submillimeter intraductal lesions and access into the terminal human mammary ducts, which has spawned a new era of intraductal approaches to diagnosis and treatment of breast diseases.

ANATOMY OF THE BREAST DUCTAL SYSTEM

The anatomy and pathophysiology of the human mammary ductal system is still an area of active research investigation. Murine transgenic models continue to provide insight into the checkpoints and proliferative mechanisms that are critical to development of the mature mammary ductal system. Interestingly, injection molds of human mastectomy specimens date back to the early anatomists such as Sir Astley Paston Cooper, who published his illustrations in the treatise *On the Anatomy of the Breast* in 1840. A modern counterpart to these anatomic studies has been published by JJ Going which elegantly details the fine arborization of ductal systems that are overlapping but not communicating (Fig. 58-1).[6] This pattern of complex arborization has been confirmed in patients undergoing galactography as well. In total, these studies illustrate the anatomic challenges that face investigators who have plans to survey and sample the human mammary ductal system.

PATHOLOGIC NIPPLE DISCHARGE

Pathologic nipple discharge (PND) has been subjected to a wide variety of definitions that illustrate one source of variation in comparing patients enrolled in clinical trials at different institutions. One critical defining feature is to differentiate pathologic nipple discharge from physiologic nipple discharge. In the instance of physiologic nipple discharge the consensus is that this is due to hormonal or endocrine stimulation of the breast glandular tissue resulting in bilateral, multiduct discharge. By contrast, pathologic nipple discharge is easiest to diagnose when it is unilateral, uniductal, spontaneously elicited, and bloody. However, if pathologic nipple discharge is defined by the presence of intraductal pathology on subsequent duct excision (both benign and malignant), then there are instances where clear discharge, nonspontaneous discharge, bilateral discharge, and multiduct discharge can all be associated with pathologic findings.[7] One such study, which carefully evaluated the characteristics of the nipple discharge (milky, sticky, purulent, bloody, etc), of 586 patients who underwent duct excision demonstrated benign findings in over 70% (intraductal papillomata 48%, and fibrocystic changes 33%). As a general rule, most authors agree that although intraductal papilloma is

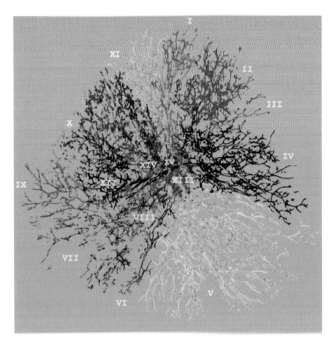

FIGURE 58-1 Reconstruction of human mammary ductal system. A human mastectomy specimen was injected with artificial materials of different colors to form a cast of the human mammary ductal system. Each color represents a different ductal system. Note the tremendous branching and the overlap of ductal systems which do not communicate. *[Reproduced, with permission, from Going JJ, Moffat DF. Escaping from flatland: clinical and biological aspects of human mammary duct anatomy in three dimensions. J Pathol. 2004;203(1):538-544.]*

by far the most common etiology for PND, the character of the discharge cannot always predict the absence of malignancy.

Evaluation of PND

Patients who present with pathologic nipple discharge undergo routine breast physical exam as well as mammography as part of their complete evaluation. Patients who have abnormal findings on any of these tests typically will then undergo either further imaging or biopsy of the imaged or palpable abnormality. In patients with PND who have no palpable breast mass or mammographic abnormality, a variety of diagnostic tests have been analyzed for sensitivity and specificity. Cytology of nipple discharge has notoriously yielded variable sensitivity and specificity, with individual studies demonstrating poor predictive values.[8] Galactography in general demonstrates a higher sensitivity in finding intraductal abnormalities but suffers from poor specificity due to the nonspecific nature of "filling defects."[9] Other modalities currently under investigation include magnetic resonance enhanced galactography as well as molecular testing of nipple discharge cellular samples.[10,11] Currently, there is no sufficient evidence that any diagnostic test or combination of preoperative tests can conclusively predict the lack of malignancy in patients with PND. This background provides the rationale for investigation of the use of modalities that visualize the ductal system in real time such as mammary ductoscopy to improve the diagnostic accuracy of duct excision for PND.

Published Series Evaluating the Role of Ductoscopy in the Evaluation of PND

There are several studies that have evaluated the utility of mammary ductoscopy in the evaluation and treatment of patients with PND. To date, there have been no prospective, randomized clinical trials comparing the sensitivity and specificity of mammary ductoscopy to alternative modalities such as major duct excision or mammary galactography. However, in total the results of mammary ductoscopy in over 1000 patients with PND have been published, and these studies provide the best available evidence as to whether ductoscopy provides patient benefit.

Two endpoints that are frequently measured in the observational studies of ductoscopy are the diagnostic accuracy of the procedure in defining the source of the PND as well as the identification of clinically occult malignancy. Several large studies have demonstrated the utility of mammary ductoscopy in identifying intraductal pathology in patients with PND.[5,12-14] Initial reports of mammary ductoscopy using a fiberoptic flexible scope demonstrated a fairly low proportion of patients (92 of 259 or 36%) where an intraductal papillary lesion was visualized.[17] However, subsequent reports demonstrated visualization of intraductal abnormalities in over 90% of patients with PND.[5,13] The increased identification of intraductal lesions was likely contributed by several factors including improvement of scope optics, better patient selection for single-duct defined nipple discharge, surgeon progression along the learning curve, and a loosening of the criteria for visualization of abnormalities with included categories such as "wall thickening" and intraductal "debris" as well as "stricture." Dietz et al compared the ductoscopy findings with those identified during preoperative galactography and suggested a higher rate of visualization of intraductal pathology with ductoscopy as compared to galactography (90% vs 76%, respectively).[5] In addition, in that particular study ductoscopy was able to identify additional papillary lesions downstream from the initial papilloma identified by galactography, which could have theoretically been left behind without a ductoscopy-directed excision. Other subsequent studies have demonstrated similar results, suggesting that the use of intraoperative ductoscopy might negate the need for preoperative galactography. Dooley et al reported the feasibility of office ductoscopy to determine which patients with pathologic nipple discharge should undergo duct excision.[15] Conceptually, this approach merits further study, although the author does admit that poor sensitivity and specificity of ductal brushing and cytology and lack of intraductal biopsy is a limiting factor in terms of being able to reassure patients that they do not have malignancy.[16]

Although the use of ductal washing cytology is beyond the scope of this chapter, one noteworthy study that nicely correlated ductal cytology using a catheter-based system demonstrated a very low sensitivity (17%) for detection of malignant or atypical cells in patients with known cancer.[17] However, as demonstrated by Sauter et al, the sensitivity and specificity of ductoscopy in combination with ductal washing cytology through the ductoscopy and image analysis could increase the sensitivity to identify malignancy to 92% with 60% specificity.[18] The contrast between these studies as well as findings from other studies suggest that the cytologic yield from ductoscopy washings may be superior to that of nipple aspiration or ductal lavage catheters, and thus ductoscopy may prove to be a useful tool for obtaining representative cytology samples from deep within the ductal system for research purposes.

Ductoscopy as a Method of Identifying Occult Malignancy in Patients with PND

As mentioned previously, most studies to date have demonstrated that preoperative assessment of patients with PND using nipple discharge cytology, hemoccult testing, or routine mammography fail to predict the presence of malignancy in a significant proportion of patients.[19,20] Table 58-1 demonstrates cumulative results of several published series of large case series with respect to the identification rate of occult malignancy. The indications for performing duct excision as well as the method of ductoscopy varies among the studies cited and may explain the wide variance in identification of occult malignancy rates from 2% to over 24%, but overall the mean of over 600 patients is approximately 5%. Interestingly, several case series of the identification of occult malignancy in patients with PND undergoing duct excision without mammary ductoscopy also cite detection rates ranging from 9% to 13%.[19,21,22] This brings into question whether the use of mammary ductoscopy increases the detection of occult malignancies beyond that identified by routine duct excision. Dietz et al performed a comparative analysis of 95 patients who underwent mammary ductoscopy during ductal excision to 140 patients who underwent routine major duct excision.[23] Although the study was not randomized, the 2 groups were comparable in terms of factors that could increase the risk of the presence of breast cancer such as atypical cytology on preoperative nipple aspirate cytology, presence of abnormality on mammogram or preoperative galactography, and percentage of patients with a final diagnosis of atypical ductal hyperplasia. In reviewing the final pathology, the percentage of patients who had cancer visualized by ductoscopy was lower than that of patients who had a major duct excision (3% vs 9%). The volume of tissue removed in the ductoscopy group was also less than that removed during routine duct excision, and the authors concluded that the higher identification rate of occult malignancy could have simply reflected a better tissue sampling when ductoscopy was not used.

Another challenge of identification of malignancy during ductoscopy is the lack of morphologic features that consistently correspond with a final pathology report of malignancy. Figure 58-2 demonstrates several ductoscopic images from both a benign papillomata as well as papillary ductal carcinoma in situ, which are essentially indistinguishable from morphologic appearance. Louie et al reviewed operative reports of 14 patients who had a final diagnosis of malignancy out of 188 who underwent ductoscopy for pathologic nipple discharge.[24] Although duct wall irregularities or intraluminal growths were identified by ductoscopy in 8(57%) out of 14 patients who had a final diagnosis of malignancy, there were no consistent morphologic features that were mentioned within the operative reports, which suggested that malignancy was suspected. One factor that might contribute to the low predictive value of ductoscopy for malignancy is the observation that careful analysis of mastectomy specimens demonstrate that infiltrating cancers have no significant intraductal component and may actually obliterate the ductal orifice, making ductoscopic visualization difficult.[25] Badve et al examined 801 mastectomy specimens and observed that most nipples have from 15 to 20 ductal orifices and found a lack of intraductal components in 17% of cases of infiltrating ductal carcinoma.[25] Detailed studies by Going et al confirm the complexity of the human mammary ductal system, which consists of 10 to 12 ductal systems that can be intertwined but not communicating.[6,26,27] These anatomic studies support the idea that despite complete ductoscopic evaluation of one or more than 1 ductal system, the percentage of total ductal epithelium surveyed using ductoscopy would be quite low. More importantly, the anatomic relationships between ductal systems that are intertwined but not communicating may provide another explanation why occult cancers are being identified in duct excision specimens when ductoscopy failed to visualize any specific intraductal abnormality.

FUTURE DIRECTIONS

Microbiopsies

Many experts and critics alike would agree that the single technology advance that would clarify the sensitivity and specificity reporting of mammary ductoscopy would be to develop instruments that would allow biopsy of the visualized intraductal abnormality. One of the difficulties in developing such instrumentation is the extremely small size of a scope diameter of less than 1 mm. The ideal microbiopsy instrument would allow the scope to remain in place before, during, and after the biopsy to ensure that what was visualized was truly what was sampled for histologic confirmation. This would allow for classification of morphologic features that are associated with benign and malignant disease and improve overall diagnostic accuracy.

Hunerbein et al have been the leaders in the area of intraductal biopsy and have reported on a vacuum-assisted intraductal biopsy device that was technically successful in all but one of 38 patients with PND.[28] The intraductal biopsy results were then confirmed by the histology on the duct excision resection specimen in all cases. The further application and

TABLE 58-1 Incidence Rates of Occult Cancer Identified in Patients with PND Who Underwent Mammary Ductoscopy and Duct Excision

Author	# Patients	# Cancer	% CA
Dietz[5]	119	5	4
Dooley[15]	26	2	7
Sauter[18]	40	2	5
Shen[12]	415	11	2.5
Makita[2]	22	5	24
Okazaki[1]	24	4	16
Total	646	29	4.5

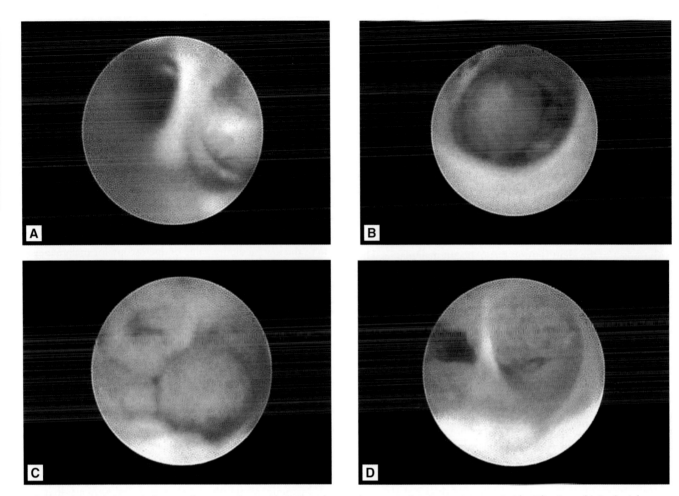

FIGURE 58-2 Ductoscopic images from a patient with PND and normal preoperative mammogram. **A.** Identification of intraductal hemorrhage. **B.** Visualization of a benign-appearing papillary lesion. **C.** Additional papillary lesion identified downstream with intraductal growth. **D.** Clear evidence of intraductal growth involving subsegmental branches. The patient had excision of the duct which demonstrated ductal carcinoma in situ, micropapillary type.

development of intraductal biopsy techniques will certainly advance the understanding of the true utility of mammary ductoscopy in these patients.

Ductoscopic Washings and Analysis of Cellular Samples

As mentioned previously, several studies have suggested that mammary ductoscopy may provide improved ductal cellular samples as compared to nipple aspiration, analysis of nipple discharge, or ductal lavage specimens derived from catheter-based systems. The ability to access cellular samples either once or repeatedly during therapy may provide important information for determining breast cancer risk, early detection of breast cancer, or response of biomarkers during chemoprevention or treatment. The use of molecular studies such as DNA methylation status or chromosomal abnormalities using fluorescence in situ hybridization have demonstrated improved diagnostic accuracy for detection of malignant cells on ductal lavage specimens as compared to routine cytology.[29,30] Further development of

novel preventive or therapeutic drugs which target specific biochemical pathways may benefit from ductoscopy-derived cell samples to look for changes in biomarkers as an indicator of efficacy.

Using Intraductal Localization to Guide the Use of Ablative or Intraductal Therapies

Finally, mammary ductoscopy provides access deep into the mammary ductal system to components of the individual ductal system, which may harbor premalignant or malignant pathology. Development of ablative technologies such as radiofrequency ablation probes may allow for ablation of intraductal lesions following histologic confirmation that could spare patients surgery. A likely clinical scenario would be a patient who has an office ductoscopy for pathologic nipple discharge and an intraductal biopsy that demonstrates a benign papilloma. A subsequent office ductoscopy could be performed and the lesion ablated, such that the symptoms of nipple discharge are resolved, the patient and surgeon have histologic confirmation of the etiology of the symptoms, and the patient avoids the complications associated with duct excision. The use of ductoscopy in this setting could provide improvement to patient care and possibly reduce overall medical costs in patients with PND and provide a compelling area of future study.

In addition, Murata et al have performed preclinical studies on the use of intraductal chemotherapy to ablate ductal epithelium in murine models.[31] Intraductal administration of pegylated liposomal adriamycin (Doxil) in transgenic mice and rats resulted in ablation of ductal epithelium, prevention of spontaneous tumor formation, and therapeutic efficacy of established mammary tumors. This exciting work has heralded a novel line of investigation into intraductal administration of prevention and therapy agents. Mammary ductoscopy may provide a vehicle for targeted administration as well as repeated assessment and ductal epithelial sampling as translation into human clinical trials moves forward.

NECESSARY FUTURE STUDIES

Are Randomized Studies Necessary?

The current medical environment has emphasized not only evidence-based decision making but also an awareness of how physicians practice within a medical system—the competency of "systems-based practice." The introduction of technology that does not add demonstrable patient benefit is no longer acceptable in a medical environment where resources are limited and medical care is not being distributed to all of those who need it. Thus, although a prospective, randomized trial of the use of mammary ductoscopy in patients with pathologic nipple discharge may provide the best level of evidence in determining whether removal of additional papillomas or identification of occult carcinoma truly improves patient outcome, the number of patients required in such studies based upon currently reported single-arm observational studies is probably not justified. However, prospective multicenter databases with long-term patient follow-up have been useful in advancement of other technologies such as partial breast radiation devices, and a similar approach may at least document the diagnostic and therapeutic efficacy of mammary ductoscopy in a broad population of patients with PND.[33]

Defining the Benefits of Ductoscopy

The purpose of this chapter was to outline the data presented on the use of mammary ductoscopy in patients with pathologic nipple discharge. Studies have been performed on the use of ductoscopy specifically in patients with known breast cancer to assess the extent of disease, and this is presented in the ensuing chapter. However, based upon current evidence, there are several *possible* benefits of mammary ductoscopy in patients with PND. These include

1. Better diagnostic accuracy than preoperative galactography in identifying intraductal pathology
2. Identification of additional intraductal pathology not visualized by preoperative galactography
3. Identification of occult malignancy

4. Use of office ductoscopy to identify patients who should go on to duct excision
5. Research tools to obtain cellular samples from individual ductal systems for analysis

Determination of whether these benefits can be realized will be enhanced by development of the instruments mentioned in the Future Directions section above, including molecular testing of cytology samples as well as development of intraductal biopsy and ablation tools.

SUMMARY

Mammary ductoscopy is a procedure that has broadened the horizon of intraductal diagnosis and therapy. The development of microendoscopes has allowed physicians to visualize submicroscopic abnormalities within the mammary ductal system that are arguably years prior to identification by routine imaging such as mammography. The utility of this fascinating technology is still an area of debate, but the mounting evidence certainly suggests that ductoscopy will play an important role in the management of patients with breast diseases in the future.

REFERENCES

1. Okazaki A, Okazaki M, Asaishi K, et al. Fiberoptic ductoscopy of the breast: a new diagnostic procedure for nipple discharge. *Jpn J Clin Oncol.* 1991;21(3):188-193.
2. Makita M, Sakamoto G, Akiyama F, et al. Duct endoscopy and endoscopic biopsy in the evaluation of nipple discharge. *Breast Cancer Res Treat.* 1991;18(3):179-187.
3. Love SM, Barsky SH. Breast-duct endoscopy to study stages of cancerous breast disease. *Lancet.* 1996;348(9033):997-999.
4. Dietz JR, Kim JA, Malycky JL, Levy L, Crowe J. Feasibility and technical considerations of mammary ductoscopy in human mastectomy specimens. *Breast J.* 2000;6(3):161-165.
5. Dietz JR, Crowe JP, Grundfest S, Arrigain S, Kim JA. Directed duct excision by using mammary ductoscopy in patients with pathologic nipple discharge. *Surgery.* 2002;132(4):582-587; discussion 587-588.
6. Going JJ, Moffat DF. Escaping from flatland: clinical and biological aspects of human mammary duct anatomy in three dimensions. *J Pathol.* 2004;203(1):538-544.
7. Leis HP Jr. Management of nipple discharge. *World J Surg.* 1989;13(6):736-742.
8. Takeda T, Matsui A, Sato Y, et al. Nipple discharge cytology in mass screening for breast cancer. *Acta Cytol.* 1990;34(2):161-164.
9. Tabar L, Dean PB, Pentek Z. Galactography: the diagnostic procedure of choice for nipple discharge. *Radiology.* 1983;149(1):31-38.
10. Yoshimoto M, Kasumi F, Iwase T, et al. Magnetic resonance galactography for a patient with nipple discharge. *Breast Cancer Res Treat.* 1997;42(1):87-90.
11. Nakahara H, Namba K, Watanabe R, et al. A comparison of MR imaging, galactography and ultrasonography in patients with nipple discharge. *Breast Cancer.* 2003;10(4):320-329.
12. Shen KW, Wu J, Lu JS, et al. Fiberoptic ductoscopy for patients with nipple discharge. *Cancer.* 2000;89(7):1512-1519.
13. Matsunaga T, Ohta D, Misaka T, et al. Mammary ductoscopy for diagnosis and treatment of intraductal lesions of the breast. *Breast Cancer.* 2001;8(3):213-221.
14. Yamamoto D, Shoji T, Kawanishi H, et al. A utility of ductography and fiberoptic ductoscopy for patients with nipple discharge. *Breast Cancer Res Treat.* 2001;70(2):103-108.
15. Dooley WC, Francescatti D, Clark L, Webber G. Office-based breast ductoscopy for diagnosis. *Am J Surg.* 2004;188(4):415-418.
16. Dooley WC. The future prospect: ductoscopy-directed brushing and biopsy. *Clin Lab Med.* 2005;25(4):845-850, ix.
17. Khan SA, Wiley EL, Rodriguez N, et al. Ductal lavage findings in women with known breast cancer undergoing mastectomy. *J Natl Cancer Inst.* 2004;96(20):1510-1517.

18. Sauter ER, Ehya H, Klein Szanto AJ, Wagner Mann C, MacGibbon B. Fiberoptic ductoscopy findings in women with and without spontaneous nipple discharge. *Cancer*. 2005;103(5):914-921.

19. Simmons R, Adamovich T, Brennan M, et al. Nonsurgical evaluation of pathologic nipple discharge. *Ann Surg Oncol*. 2003;10(2):113-116.

20. Funovics MA, Philipp MO, Lackner B, et al. Galactography: method of choice in pathologic nipple discharge? *Eur Radiol*. 2003;13(1):94-99.

21. Lau S, Küchenmeister I, Stachs A, et al. Pathologic nipple discharge: surgery is imperative in postmenopausal women. *Ann Surg Oncol*. 2005;12(7):546-551.

22. Lanitis S, Filippakis G, Thomas J, et al. Microdochectomy for single-duct pathologic nipple discharge and normal or benign imaging and cytology. *Breast*. 2008;17(3):309-313.

23. Sharma R, Dietz J, Wright H, et al. Comparative analysis of minimally invasive microductectomy versus major duct excision in patients with pathologic nipple discharge. *Surgery*. 2005;138(4):591-596; discussion 596-597.

24. Louie LD, Crowe JP, Dawson AE, et al. Identification of breast cancer in patients with pathologic nipple discharge: does ductoscopy predict malignancy? *Am J Surg*. 2006;192(4):530-533.

25. Badve S, Wiley E, Rodriguez N. Assessment of utility of ductal lavage and ductoscopy in breast cancer-a retrospective analysis of mastectomy specimens. *Mod Pathol*. 2003;16(3):206-209.

26. Going JJ, Mohun TJ. Human breast duct anatomy, the "sick lobe" hypothesis and intraductal approaches to breast cancer. *Breast Cancer Res Treat*. 2006;97(3):285-291.

27. Moffat DF, Going JJ. Three dimensional anatomy of complete duct systems in human breast: pathological and developmental implications. *J Clin Pathol*. 1996;49(1):48-52.

28. Hunerbein M, Raubach M, Gebauer B, Schneider W, Schlag PM. Ductoscopy and intraductal vacuum assisted biopsy in women with pathologic nipple discharge. *Breast Cancer Res Treat*. 2006;99(3):301-307.

29. Evron E, Dooley WC, Umbricht CB, et al. Detection of breast cancer cells in ductal lavage fluid by methylation-specific PCR. *Lancet*. 2001;357(9265): 1335-1336.

30. King BL, Tsai SC, Gryga ME, et al. Detection of chromosomal instability in paired breast surgery and ductal lavage specimens by interphase fluorescence in situ hybridization. *Clin Cancer Res*. 2003;9(4):1509-1516.

31. Murata S, Kominsky SL, Vali M, et al. Ductal access for prevention and therapy of mammary tumors. *Cancer Res*. 2006;66(2):638-645.

32. Leach DC. The ACGME competencies: substance or form? Accreditation Council for Graduate Medical Education. *J Am Coll Surg*. 2001;192(3): 396-398.

33. Zannis V, Beitsch P, Vicini F, et al. Descriptions and outcomes of insertion techniques of a breast brachytherapy balloon catheter in 1403 patients enrolled in the American Society of Breast Surgeons MammoSite breast brachytherapy registry trial. *Am J Surg*. 2005;190(4):530-538.

CHAPTER 59

Intraductal Therapy

Robert J. Goulet, Jr.
Theodore N. Tsangaris
Susan M. Love

The epithelium of the breast ductal system is the site of origin for nearly all breast cancers.[1,2] The intraductal environment and the significance of the secretions produced within the human mammary gland have been debated for centuries. The recognition of the role of carcinogens in the production of malignancies led to a renewed interest in the ductal anatomy and physiology in the 20th century. Today, the combination of technological enhancement providing direct and indirect access to the luminal milieu and advances in cellular methodology that hold the promise of reliable diagnostic and predictive markers of breast cancer are driving investigators to pursue a ductal approach to breast cancer diagnosis and therapy that will be preemptive and accurate with less toxicity and breast disfigurement.

The identification of high-risk individuals through statistical screening (ie, Gail and Claus models), histologic or cytologic identification of proliferative breast lesions (ie, atypical ductal or lobular hyperplasia and lobular carcinoma in situ), and recognition of genetic abnormalities (ie, BRCA1 and BRCA2) have resulted in an established paradigm for the management of high-risk individuals. Increased surveillance, chemoprevention, and breast extirpation are designed to either diagnose the disease at a treatable stage or prevent it entirely. If a malignancy is diagnosed, then a multidisciplinary approach, using some combination of local therapy with surgical intervention and radiation therapy and systemic therapy with cytotoxic chemotherapy, hormonal therapy, or targeted therapy is today's standard. Despite dramatic advances, local therapy often results in alterations in the appearance of the breast, and the adverse events associated with systemic therapy remain discouraging.

In defining an ideal intraductal therapy, one seeks an approach that addresses all the tissue at risk, the mammary duct epithelium. Second, the technique for ductal access must be reliable and reproducible, for therapy as well as follow-up.

Finally, the agents used intraluminally must exert their effect at a local level without systemic side effects or impact on the consistency or appearance of the breast. This is the challenge facing intraductal investigators. In this chapter, we review recent literature related to the breast ductal anatomy, the preclinical trials evaluating the efficacy of intraducal therapy, and the results of early clinical trials evaluating intraductal therapy.

DUCTAL ANATOMY

The anatomy of the breast ductal system has been the subject of much debate. At issue are questions regarding the number of ductal orifices on the surface of the nipple and the distribution of the arborizing ductal network. The literature divides into those that note 15 to 20 ducts and those that report 6 to 9. This discrepancy can be explained in part by the technique used for the study. Those reports that based their observation on cannulating intact nipples or imaging intact lactating or nonlactating breasts all report 6 to 9 functional ductal orifices.[3-7] On the other hand, the studies that transected the nipple and described the ductal cross-sections concur on 15 to 20 ducts in the subareolar location.[8-11] It is likely that some of the differences come from early bifurcations and trifurcations of the ductal network, as noted in ductoscopic examinations,[12] whereas others may relate to additional subareolar structures that have yet to be characterized. These questions were addressed in an article evaluating the median number of ducts in the nipple, the volume of the complete duct system or lobes, and modeling of the collecting ducts in the nipple by using a digital 3-dimensional system.[13,14] The authors described 3 distinct nipple duct populations that included ducts that maintained a wide communication with the surface of the nipple (type A), ducts that tapered to a minute lumen at their origin (type B), and a group of ducts that arose at the base of the nipple. Seven type A ducts were noted. These results and those of several other careful analyses suggest that further research is necessary to fully characterize this area of the breast.

PRECLINICAL STUDIES

Early work in prevention of mammary cancer in a chemically induced tumor model evaluated the impact of intraductal viral transduction of breast epithelial cells and subsequent intraductal therapy with gancyclovir.[15] The authors postulated that the rapidly dividing epithelial cells in the terminal end buds of the glands were susceptible to chemical carcinogens, and therefore elimination of these cells should reduce malignant transformation. Although greater than 90% of the cells in question were eliminated, the remaining cells had a higher incidence of tumor formation.

The efficacy of triweekly intraductal administration of paclitaxel was contrasted with intraperitoneal treatment of rats with chemically induced mammary cancer.[16] The animals were assessed for tumor burden, total number of mammary tumors, apoptosis, and microvessel density. None of the animals treated intraductally developed complications associated with paclitaxel. The intraductally treated animals had significantly reduced tumor burden with increased apoptosis and decreased microvessel density, suggesting an advantage to locally administered therapy with less toxicity.

A more recent study has taken a more comprehensive look at intraductal administration of hormonal and chemotherapeutic agents in the prevention and treatment of breast cancer. Sukumar et al[17] used a chemically induced tumor model and an HER-2/neu transgenic spontaneous tumor model. They began by demonstrating they could access the glandular elements of the mouse and rat breasts. Unlike humans, mice and rats have a solitary duct that drains the breast tissue. Excellent distribution of the experimental agents was confirmed. They then evaluated the pharmacology of the intraductally versus intravenously administered pegylated liposomal doxorubicin (PLD) using high-powered liquid chromatography. The peak serum concentrations differed by a factor of 10 when the routes were compared. No myelosuppression was noted in the animals treated with intraductal PLD. They then showed that intraductally administered 4-hydroxytamoxifen, the active metabolite of tamoxifen, was highly effective in preventing chemically induced breast tumors. This effect was comparable to subcutaneously administered tamoxifen. The intraductal administration of PLD reduced the size of established spontaneous tumors in transgenic mice. The therapeutic response had variable durability, but 4 of 10 tumors remained in regression throughout the study. With respect to prevention, intraductal PLD resulted in significant reduction of spontaneous development after intraductal therapy when compared with glands that went untreated or received placebo. This study provided comprehensive evidence that translational studies evaluating intraductally administered agents for the prevention and treatment of breast cancer were necessary and appropriate.

These studies raise a host of concerns that must be addressed in clinical trials. Is the accessibility of the human breast ductal system a reliable and reproducible route for the administration of intraductal agents? Is therapy through a single ductal orifice sufficient, or should therapy be administered through the entire ductal system? What are the pharmacokinetics and toxicity of chemotherapeutic agents administered through the human lactiferous duct? Will intraductal therapy result in unanticipated beneficial effects, such as tumor autoimmunity?

CLINICAL STUDIES

The study that provided proof that the concept of intraductal distribution of chemotherapeutic agents was possible in the human breast came in 2004 when intraductal nanoparticles containing epirubicin, a naturally florescent drug, were administered to mastectomized breasts from women undergoing treatment for breast cancer.[18] The primary goal of the study was to confirm that agents introduced into the human lactiferous duct would be distributed throughout the entire drainage system. Secondarily the authors were interested in the utility of nanoparticles as a vehicle for delivery of the medication. There are several advantages to this approach. First, nanoparticles provide controlled delivery of an agent in a predesigned manner. The release of the drug can be programmed to be constant or cyclic, with the release of the agent determined by the constituents of the nanoparticles or by external factors. A commercially available microcatheter was used to access the ducts.

Women undergoing mastectomy for the treatment of early-stage breast cancer were recruited. These included women over the age of 18 years, who were not pregnant, without inflammatory breast cancer, periareolar surgery, or previous radiation therapy to the involved breast. The nanoparticles were composed of poly (lactic-co-glycolic) acid copolymer. After mastectomy, the ducts were accessed ex vivo with a microcatheter, and the epirubicin containing nanoparticles were instilled. A vital dye was also infused to help identify the treated duct. The duct was dissected from the specimen, and the tumor-bearing portion of the breast was sent for pathologic evaluation. The treated ducts were step-sectioned at 1- to 2-cm intervals and evaluated by hematoxylin and eosin technique and fluorescent microscopy. Success was defined as the presence of intact nanoparticles within the ductal lumen of the distal one-third of the duct.

The study showed that 61.5% of the ducts had fluorescent nanoparticles in the terminal duct lobular units (Fig. 59-1). The study showed for the first time that chemotherapy of the human lactiferous ductal system was possible using epirubicin-containing nanoparticles. Comparable to previous rodent studies, the complex human lactiferous duct could be accessed for drug delivery to the most remote extents of the glands. The reliability of this approach and the pharmacology of intraductally administered chemotherapy remained to be addressed.

The first in-woman instillation of a chemotherapeutic agent into a woman's breast was done in Eureka, California, in a woman scheduled for a prophylactic mastectomy. This outpatient procedure instilled 10 mL of PLD into 1 duct under local anesthesia without complications. The woman underwent a planned prophylactic mastectomy 3 months later without incident.[19]

Based on observations in preclinical studies that PLD decreased tumor volume, eradicated premalignant disease, and

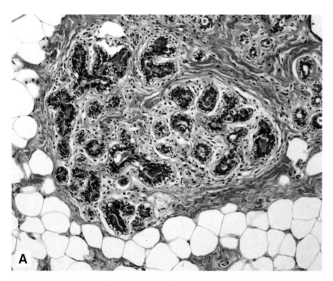
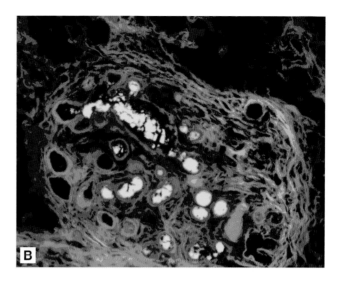

FIGURE 59-1 Terminal duct lobular unit. **A.** H&E. **B.** Fluorescent microscopy showing epirubicin containing nanoparticles.

prevented the development of new epithelial lesions, the breast group at Johns Hopkins conducted a phase I trial assessing the feasibility and safety of intraductally administered PLD in women with breast cancer.[20] In this clinical study, women 18 years and older with a diagnosis of in situ or invasive breast cancer were enrolled. Patients with inflammatory breast cancer or prior surgical procedures that might have altered the ductal anatomy were excluded. The investigators sought to determine the maximum-tolerated dose of PLD administered to a single human lactiferous duct, in vivo, before mastectomy. The pharmacokinetics of intraductally administered PLD were evaluated, including the determination of serial concentrations of doxorubicin and doxorubicinol, a metabolite of doxorubicin, in plasma and tissue. The dose of PLD was escalated from 2 mg to a maximum dose of 10 mg, which was administered on day 0 of the trial, with samples taken for pharmacokinetic studies on days 1, 2, 8, and the day of surgery. All patients were monitored for adverse drug reactions.

Three patients were available for evaluation at each of the doses of PLD. The patients reported minimal discomfort with the procedure, both before and after the administration of the PLD. At 2- and 5-mg doses, serum concentrations of doxorubicin peaked at 4 hours at 18.3 to 28.5 nmol/L, with no detectable metabolites. At the 10-mg dose, the serum levels peaked at 24 hours after administration at 481 nmol/L and remained detectable at day 8, with only a transient appearance of doxorubicinol at 24 hours. Tissue concentration displayed levels directly related to the dose of PLD administered. No doxorubicin or doxorubicinol was detected in the contralateral breast at any dose.

The authors concluded that PLD could be administered to women intraductally. Intraductal PLD was associated with a dose-dependent increase in both systemic and local exposure to doxorubicin and doxorubicinol. No inflammatory or morphologic changes were noted in the mastectomy specimen.

A second phase I trial was conducted by investigators from the United States and China. This was a dose-escalation study of 2 drugs: PLD and carboplatin. Again, chemotherapeutic agents were administered intraductally in women awaiting mastectomy for the treatment of in situ and invasive breast cancer.[21] In this study, multiple ducts (5-8 per patient) were accessed, and selected agents were infused (Fig. 59-2). For carboplatin, the doses ranged from 60 to 300 mg per breast, and for PLD, the doses ranged from 10 to 50 mg per breast. The individual ductal doses varied based on the number of ducts cannulated. Histopathology of the treated ducts was done in each patient. The end points of the study included local and systemic tolerability of the drug, histopathology changes, and the pharmacokinetics of the administered drugs.

The only local adverse event that the authors encountered was mild pain on instillation of the drugs. With respect to the pharmacokinetics of carboplatin, rapid absorption was noted, with peak serum concentrations, equivalent to those of the intravenously administered agent, within 30 minutes of intraductal

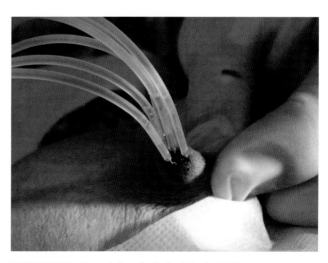

FIGURE 59-2 Cannulating ducts for intraductal therapy.

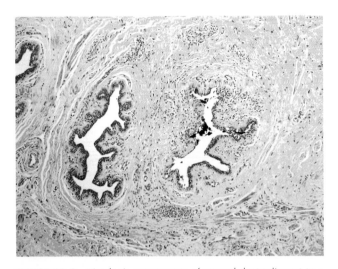

FIGURE 59-3 Histologic appearance of normal duct adjacent to a duct treated with 20 mg of PLD.

administration. For PLD, the absorption was much slower, with peak levels noted on day 3. No drug metabolites were detected. The maximum drug concentration in the serum was 20% of that expected with an equivalent intravenously administered dose.

Adverse events noted with the patients receiving the high dose and 1 of the patients receiving the mid dose of carboplatin was mild nausea and vomiting. For PLD, the patients treated with the high dose (50 mg/breast) experienced erythema and tenderness of the area around the nipple, beginning hours after intraductal administration of the agent and lasting 2 to 3 days. On histologic evaluation of the specimen, carboplatin demonstrated a dose-dependent stripping of the epithelial layer of the ducts, which was incomplete. A similar but less intense response was noted in patients treated with PLD (Fig. 59-3). The clinical significance of the epithelial remnants remains to be determined. The PLD treated patients had evidence of local inflammation with eosinophilic infiltration and hyperemia.

The authors concluded that the local delivery of chemo therapeutic agents into multiple ductal systems simultaneously is feasible and safe, with a greater potential to increase the local exposure to therapeutic agents with less systemic toxicity. It appeared that PLD has a better distribution profile when administered via multiple ducts.

At the time of this writing, 1 neoadjuvant ductal carcinoma in situ study was underway.

SUMMARY

Preclinical and early clinical evaluations of intraductal breast cancer prevention and therapy have been very encouraging. Obviously much work remains in identifying the optimum chemotherapeutic agents and techniques of administration; however, the potential of this approach includes aromatase inhibitors as well as targeted therapy using nanotechnology. The interest in intraductal treatment and prevention of breast cancer is sure to increase as indicators of tumor development and surrogate markers of treatment efficacy become available.

REFERENCES

1. Tavassoli FA. *Pathology of the Breast.* 2nd ed. Stamford, CT: Appleton & Lange: 1999:59.
2. Wellings SR, Jensen HM, Marcum RG. An atlas of subgross pathology of the human breast with special reference to possible precancerous lesions. *J Natl Cancer Inst.* 1975;55:231-273.
3. Cooper A. *The Anatomy and Diseases of the Breast.* Philadelphia, PA: Lea and Blanchard: 1845.
4. Teboul M. Halliwell. *Atlas of Ultrasound and Ductal Echography of the Breast.* Oxford, UK: Blackwell Science: 1995.
5. Ramsay DT, Kent JC, Hartmann RA, Hartmann PE. Anatomy of the lactating human breast redefined with ultrasound imaging. *J Anat.* 2005;206:525-534.
6. Sartorious OW, Smith HS, Norris P, Benedict D, Friesen L. Cytologic evaluation of breast fluid in the detection of breast disease. *J Natl Cancer Inst.* 1977;59:1073-1080.
7. Love SM, Barsky SH. Anatomy of the nipple and breast ducts revisited. *Cancer.* 2004;101:1947-1957.
8. Moffat DF, Going JJ. Three-dimensional anatomy of complete duct systems in human breast: pathological and developmental implications. *J Clin Pathol.* 1996;49:48-52.
9. Ohtake T, Kimijima I, Fukushima T, et al. Computer-assisted complete three-dimensional reconstruction of the mammary ductal/lobular systems: implications of ductal anastomoses for breast conserving surgery. *Cancer.* 2001;91:2263-2272.
10. Taneri F, Kurukahvecioglu O, Akyurek N, et al. Microanatomy of milk ducts in the nipple. *Eur Surg Res.* 2006;38:545-549.
11. Rusby JE, Brachtel EF, Michaelson JS, Koerner FC, Smith BL. Breast duct anatomy in the human nipple: three dimensional patterns and clinical implications. *Breast Cancer Res Treat.* 2007;106:171-179.
12. Dietz JR, Kim JA, Malycky JL, Levy, Corwe J. Feasibility and technical considerations of mammary ductoscopy in human mastectomy specimens. *Breast J.* 2000;6:161-165.
13. Going J, Moffat DF. Escaping from Flatland: clinical and biological aspects of human mammary duct anatomy in three dimensions. *J Pathol.* 2004;203:538-544.
14. Going J, Moffat DF. Human breast duct anatomy, the "sick lobe" hypothesis and intraductal approaches to breast cancer. *Breast Cancer Res Treat.* 2006;97:285-291.
15. Sivaraman I, Gay J, Hilsenbeck SG, et al. Effect of selective ablation of proliferating mammary epithelial cells on MNU induced rat mammary tumorigenesis. *Breast Cancer Res Treat.* 2002;73:75-83.
16. Okugawa H, Yamamoto D, Uemura Y, et al. Effect of periductal paclitaxel exposure on the development of MNU induced mammary carcinoma in female S-D rats. *Brest Cancer Res Treat.* 2005;91:29-34.
17. Murata S, Kominsky SL, Vail M, et al. Ductal access for prevention and therapy of mammary tumors. *Cancer Res.* 2006;66:638-645.
18. Goulet RJ, Badve S, Brannon-Pepas L, et al. Pilot trial assessing the feasibility of intra-ductal delivery of epirubicin (epi)-containing nanoparticles (NP) via InDuct@ Breast Microcatheter (IDBM). *Proc Am Soc Clin Oncol.* 2004;22:828a. Abstract.
19. King B, Love SM, Rochman S, Kim J. The fourth international symposium on the intraductal approach to breast cancer, Santa Barbara, California, 10-13 March 2005. *Breast Cancer Res.* 2005;7:198-204.
20. Stearns V, Singh B, Tsangaris T, et al. A prospective randomized pilot study to evaluate predictors of response in serial core biopsies to single agent neoadjuvant doxorubicin or paclitaxel for patients with locally advanced breast cancer. *Clin Cancer Res.* 2003;6:4610-4617.
21. Love SM, Zhang B, Zhang W, et al. Local drug delivery to the breast: A Phase I study of breast intraductal cytotoxic agent administration prior to mastectomy. *AACR Meeting Abstracts.* 2008;LB-245.

CHAPTER 60

Cryoablation of Fibroadenomas

Pat W. Whitworth
Jaime Lewis

Breast masses occur frequently, as evidenced by more than 1.3 million excisional biopsies performed on American women yearly.[1,2] Approximately 80% of these procedures are for benign lesions, most commonly fibroadenomas.[1-4] Although it has been repeatedly stated that one-third to one-half of fibroadenomas will regress within 5 years of diagnosis, the data on the natural history of fibroadenomas varies.[5-8] Fibroadenomas may occur at any age, but are most likely to occur in the second and third decades of life and are the most common breast masses in women under 30 years of age.[2,9-11] Up to 10% of women will develop a fibroadenoma during their lifetime, and the majority will choose to undergo a procedure to remove the mass.[2,4] Fibroadenomas account for 30% to 75% of all breast biopsies, more than 500,000 annually, and 75% of breast biopsies in women younger than 20 years.[3,9,10]

Fibroadenomas have typical characteristics on physical exam, mammography, and ultrasound.[9] On physical exam, a fibroadenoma is a painless, spherical, smooth, and mobile mass (historically termed a "breast mouse" by European surgeons) with highly circumscribed margins, typically 1 to 3 cm in diameter.[2,3,9] Ultrasound characteristics are typical of a benign mass and include a smooth, well-defined lesion that is iso- or mildly hypoechoic. It may be surrounded by a thin, echogenic pseudocapsule.[12,13] On mammography, fibroadenomas are again seen as smooth round or oval masses that may contain course calcifications; multiple lesions may be noted.[12,13] Fibroadenomas may be multiple in up to 15% to 20% of patients, especially dark-skinned individuals.[2,10,12] The differential diagnosis for these lesions includes fast-growing juvenile fibroadenoma, phyllodes tumor, and colloid and medullary carcinomas.[2] Most lesions require biopsy at some point. Others may be monitored without biopsy if they meet strict criteria, such as those described by Stavros and colleagues.[14] Image-guided large-core needle biopsy is the method of choice, as the sample provides better differentiation of benign from malignant masses and fibroadenoma from phyllodes tumor.[2]

Acceptable management includes observation, excisional biopsy, and newer, minimally invasive alternatives. Adolescents may be safely observed for a period of time after physical exam reveals an apparently benign mass. Older women and those with persisting or enlarging masses should have histologic confirmation.[3] Although a period of observation is acceptable for teenage patients, there are several valid reasons to support treating some benign lesions more aggressively. Large lesions may become symptomatic, causing feelings of heaviness, asymmetry, pain, or discomfort.[9] Infrequently, benign masses may increase in size during pregnancy or during use of hormonal contraception or other types of hormonal therapy.[10] Emotional distress created by the frequent follow-up required when patients attempt nonoperative therapy causes many to choose alternative approaches.[1,3,9] In addition, benign masses may impair physical examination and mammographic evaluation due to mass effect.[2]

For many years, excisional biopsy has been the definitive treatment for all breast lesions. The financial burden placed on the health care system for serial office visits and/or operating suite utilization, as well as the morbidity, cosmetic alteration due to scarring, and patient discomfort caused by surgical excision, have stimulated the search for alternative therapies.[2,4,9] Recently, several minimally invasive approaches have been considered, including percutaneous excision and thermal ablation. Thermal ablation includes radiofrequency ablation, microwave therapy, high-intensity focused ultrasound, laser ablation, and cryoablation.[3,4] Percutaneous excision may be performed using vacuum-assisted core biopsy devices.[9] This technique may be performed in an office setting. The primary limitations of vacuum-assisted percutaneous excisions include incomplete excision and recurrence of tumor. Complete excision of all imaged evidence of a given lesion requires skill and may leave histologic remnants, which can occasionally regrow in younger patients. Approximately 30% of patients have some residual visible abnormality, as is also the case with open excision, especially in patients with larger tumors.[9,15] Prior studies have suggested that residual tumor may give rise to recurrence necessitating a second procedure, but there are few long-term follow-up data to support this assumption.[2,10]

CRYOABLATION TECHNIQUE

Cryoablation works to achieve tissue necrosis by alternately freezing and thawing the targeted tissue.[2,4] Injury is caused by intracellular ice formation, osmotic imbalances, and resultant membrane rupture.[2,4] Damage to endothelial cells of the microcirculation causes ischemia, leading to indirect injury of the lesion.[2,4]

Cryoablation, developed in the late 1990s, is an attractive, minimally invasive therapy for many patients. Experience with this technique reveals that it is a cost-effective approach. Because cold acts as a natural anesthetic, it requires only local anesthesia for probe insertion, can be performed in an office setting without sedation, and is a relatively simple procedure.[2,4] It has low morbidity and cosmetic benefits compared with surgical excision, as it does not require tissue removal and leaves minimal skin scarring.[10] To minimize unnecessary concern and disappointment, patients and their treating physicians, including breast imagers, must be properly counseled and educated regarding the expected parenchymal changes that may be detected on physical and radiologic exams for 12 to 36 months after the procedure.

INDICATIONS/INCLUSION CRITERIA

Masses suitable for cryoablative therapy include those detected by physical exam and, in certain patients, by imaging and biopsy consistent with a fibroadenoma.[3] The mass must be visible by ultrasound. Before performing cryoablation, it is necessary to obtain adequate tissue for histologic diagnosis, as biopsy interpretation cannot be performed after this procedure due to coagulation necrosis in the lesion.[3]

The primary limitation of cryoablation is a persistent palpable mass or scar created by the intended tissue injury associated with the procedure. Patients undergoing cryoablation, including those with nonpalpable masses before the procedure, must be willing to accept the development of a temporarily (12 to 36 months) palpable mass after the procedure.[10] Several studies have provided the following results: 50% will have a palpable mass at 6 months, up to 35% will have a palpable mass after 12 months, and 16% will still have a palpable mass at an average of 2.6 years of follow-up.[2,5,10] Larger lesions have a greater likelihood of remaining palpable for a longer period of time or indefinitely.[2,10]

Two studies have focused on long-term results. Nurko et al[10] presented data from 444 fibroadenomas treated by cryoablation. The palpability of these lesions over time is presented in Table 60-1. At 12 months, visibility of the lesions by ultrasound was 27% in those 2 cm or smaller and 32% in those greater than 2 cm, and no recurrences were seen. Patient satisfaction was rated at 91% and 88% at 6 and 12 months of follow-up, respectively.

TABLE 60-1 Palpability of Fibroadenomas Treated by Cryoablation[10]

| | % OF PATIENTS | | |
	Registration	6 Months	12 Months
All patients	73	48	31
≤ 2 cm at registration (n = 329)	65	35	24
> 2 cm at registration (n = 151)	91	77	49

Data updated by personal communication, February 2007.

A second, smaller study published by Kaufman et al[1] followed 32 women for 2 to 3 years after cryoablation of breast fibroadenomas. At the time of registration, 84% of these women had palpable lesions. At a mean follow-up period of 2.6 years, palpability of lesions was 16% overall, 6% in those with lesions 2 cm or smaller, and 27% with larger lesions. No regrowth of lesions was noted. Ninety-seven percent of patients were satisfied with the procedure and results.

Though studies have not focused on other lesions, cryoablation may be considered for benign diagnoses other than fibroadenoma.[3] In our opinion, though, the ideal candidate for a cryoablation procedure is one with a palpable fibroadenoma who desires lesion destruction without tissue loss and also understands the implications of a slowly resolving palpable mass.

RELATIVE AND ABSOLUTE CONTRAINDICATIONS/EXCLUSION CRITERIA

Until results of clinical trials of cryoablation for small breast cancers are available, patients presenting with anything other than a completely benign neoplasm, including atypical hyperplasia and malignancy, should not be treated with cryoablation, but should undergo open resection.[3]

Proximity to skin is not a contraindication to cryoablation as saline may be injected between the skin and forming ice ball for skin protection.[5] Patients with multiple lesions may have them treated in the same setting.[3]

TECHNIQUES

The cryoablation procedure may be performed in the office setting under local anesthesia. Sterile technique should be maintained throughout the procedure. The equipment used to perform the cryoablation procedure is available as the Visica 2 Treatment System (Sanarus Medical; Pleasanton, California). The main components of the system include a cryoablation probe, computerized console, and liquid nitrogen as the cryogen for freezing the tumor. In order to perform this procedure, one must also be facile with the use of ultrasound, as its use allows visualization of the entire procedure.[16]

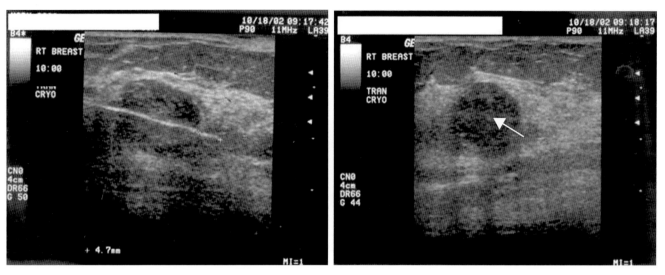

FIGURE 60-1 Cryoablation probe placement visualized with ultrasound. Proper placement of the cryoablation probe as seen on longitudinal *(left)* and transverse *(right)* views.

Under ultrasound guidance, a probe is inserted into the lesion through a 3-mm skin incision made in a cosmetically and technically appropriate location. The first-generation probe (2.4 mm in diameter, 11.5 cm in length, and with a pointed tip) formed an oblong ice ball in the tissue during use as it became cold along its entire length.[3] It therefore required meticulous observation and measures to protect skin. Second-generation probes have a proximal insulated portion, improving skin protection, and a distal active freezing zone, which forms more spherical ice balls.[3] They also have a trocar tip and are available in 2 lengths. The smaller V2 ICE Probe SL is 2.4 mm in diameter, with a 3.5-cm distal active freezing zone, best used for lesions 2 cm or smaller. The larger V2 ICE Probe, useful for lesions larger than 2 cm, is 3.4 mm in diameter and has a 4.5-cm

distal active freezing zone. The probe must be inserted to a length at least 0.5 cm longer than its distal active freezing zone.

The length of the ice ball along the length of the probe is always larger than the diameter of the ice ball perpendicular to the probe, therefore, the probe should be placed directly through the longest axis of the lesion.[3] To ensure the accuracy of probe placement both transversely and longitudinally through the lesion (Fig. 60-1) and to monitor ice ball formation within the fibroadenoma, ultrasound visualization must be performed throughout the procedure.[10] If the ice ball comes in close proximity to the skin, sterile saline must be available to inject between the skin and the forming ice ball (Fig. 60-2). In addition, the skin must be carefully observed during the procedure for any changes associated with thermal injury.

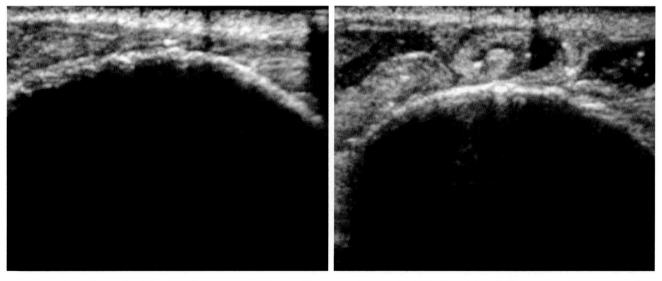

FIGURE 60-2 Before saline injection, there is a 3-mm interval between the growing ice ball and skin *(left)*. After a subcutaneous saline injection, there is a 5-mm interval *(right)*.

TABLE 60-2 Current Trials of Cryoablation Therapy

Title	Phase	Sponsor	Protocol ID	Open
Sequential Administration of Cryoablation and Cyclophosphamide for Advanced Solid Epithelial Cancer	Not specified	National Cancer Institute	JHOC-J0685	June 2007
A Phase II Trial Exploring the Success of Cryoablation Therapy in the Treatment of Invasive Breast Carcinoma	Phase II	National Cancer Institute	ACOSOG-Z1072	January 2009

The cryoablation probe uses liquid nitrogen to cool the probe and surrounding tissue to subzero temperatures. Suggested ablation times based on the size of the lesion are provided with the equipment, but these times may be tailored according to clinical judgment and ultrasound monitoring during the procedure. A few additional millimeters of ice ball formation beyond the limits of the fibroadenoma are desirable, as the outer few millimeters of ice are not lethal.[3] After the freeze cycle, an electrical component warms the probe to facilitate its removal. After removal of the probe, compression must be held until hemostasis is achieved.

AVOIDING COMPLICATIONS

After cryoablation of fibroadenomas, most complications are minor, and no serious adverse events have been noted.[1-3,5,10] Periprocedural edema and swelling are common and expected effects. Although ecchymosis may occur in 41%, distinct hematoma formation occurs in only 4% of patients, similar to the historical frequency associated with surgical incision.[5] Minor infections have been reported in less than 2% of patients.[5]

Pain and tenderness are generally rated less than with surgical excision, though symptoms may be chronic after cryoablation in a small number of patients.[2,5] Most pain after cryoablation is rated as minor (78%), requiring only over-the-counter analgesics; the remainder of patients require a short course of narcotics.[5]

Tape blisters have been noted to occur due to procedural edema in combination with tight compression dressings and may result in depigmentation in a small percentage of patients.[3,5] Thermal injury from inadvertent cryoprobe contact with the skin at the insertion site or inadequate depth of insertion has been noted.[3] Significant skin necrosis has not been reported.[5]

Another possible complication results from patient or physician dissatisfaction with the procedure. This can be minimized by adequately preparing patients and physicians, including breast imagers, before the procedure. If patients and physicians are not properly counseled to expect slow resolution of a palpable fibroadenoma with 12 to 36 months of disorganization of tissues on ultrasound, unnecessary removal may be requested.

POSTPROCEDURAL MANAGEMENT

Although there are no specific postprocedural guidelines, treating physicians must be aware of postprocedural tissue changes before reabsorption. Residual debris on follow-up ultrasound may appear similar to a surgical scar or a malignant lesion, appearing as an ill-defined, irregular, hypoechoic mass without shadowing.[2] It is important to communicate these possible findings with any radiologist performing future exams. Minimal findings have been noted on mammography; however, none have been reported to adversely affect interpretation, though it should be noted that some patients will develop benign macrocalcifications and/or nonspecific asymmetric density.[2,3] With 3- to 5-year follow up data available, patients and physicians appear to be pleased, with levels of satisfaction more than 90% at 1 year.[5]

CURRENT AND FUTURE CLINICAL TRIALS

Future studies of fibroadenoma treatment should be directed at determining any advantage cryoablation therapy may have over percutaneous excision in terms of reducing the risk of recurrence, for young women in particular.

Two trials are currently ongoing in the use of cryotherapy for breast cancer (Table 60-2). The first, from Johns Hopkins Oncology Center (JHOC-J0685), is a pilot study looking at the radiologic and/or tumor marker response of epithelial tumors (including breast cancer) to cryotherapy of lesions followed by cyclophosphamide administration. The second trial, from the American College of Surgeons Oncology Group (ACOSOG-Z1072), recently started accruing patients. The primary objective of this study is to determine the rate of complete tumor ablation by cryotherapy in patients with invasive ductal carcinoma.

SUMMARY

Fibroadenomas are a frequent cause of breast masses in women, and the majority of women with fibroadenomas will choose to have them removed. For patients with masses that are consistent with the diagnosis of fibroadenoma by physical exam, imaging, and histologic confirmation, cryoablation therapy is a safe and effective alternative to watchful waiting or open excision. Current and future clinical studies will further define any advantage of cryoablation therapy over excision, as well its role in the treatment of breast cancer.

REFERENCES

1. Kaufman CS, Bachman B, Littrup PJ, et al. Cryoablation treatment of benign breast lesions with 12-month follow-up. *Am J Surg.* 2004;188: 340-348.
2. Kaufman CS, Littrup PJ, Freeman-Gibb LA, et al. Office-based cryoablation of breast fibroadenomas with long-term follow-up. *Breast J.* 2005; 11:344 350.
3. Caleffi M, Filho D, Borghetti K, et al. Cryoablation of benign breast tumors: evolution of technique and technology. *Breast.* 2004;13:397-407.
4. Whitworth P, Rewcastle JC. Cryoablation and cryolocalization in the management of breast disease. *J Surg Oncol.* 2005;90:1-9.
5. Edwards MJ, Broadwater R, Tafra L, et al. Progressive adoption of cryoablative therapy for breast fibroadenoma in community practice. *Am J Surg.* 2004;188:221-224.
6. Wilkinson S, Anderson T, Rifkind E, Chetty U, Forrest A. Fibroadenoma of the breast: a follow-up of conservative management. *Br J Surg.* 1989;76:390-391.
7. Cant P, Madden M, Coleman M, Dent D. Non-operative management of breast masses diagnosed as fibroadenoma. *Br J Surg.* 1995;82:792-794.
8. Dixon J, Dobie V, Lamb J, Walsh J, Chetty U. Assessment of the acceptability of conservative management of fibroadenoma of the breast. *Br J Surg.* 1996;83:264-265.
9. Fine R, Whitworth P, Kim JA, et al. Low-risk palpable breast masses removed using a vacuum-assisted hand-held device. *Am J Surg.* 2003;186:362-367.
10. Nurko J, Mabry CD, Whitworth P, et al. Interim results from the FibroAdenoma Cryoablation Treatment Registry. *Am J Surg.* 2005;190: 647-651.
11. Alle K, Moss J, Vencgas R, Khalkhali I, Klein S. Conservative management of fibroadenoma of the breast. *Br J Surg.* 1996;83:992-993.
12. Greenberg R, Skornick Y, Kaplan O. Management of breast fibroadenomas. *J Gen Intern Med.* 1998;13:640-645.
13. James JJ, Robin A, Wilson M, Evans J. Women's imaging: the breast. In: Adam A, Dixon AK, Grainger RG, Allison DJ, eds. *Grainger & Allison's Diagnostic Radiology.* 5th ed. Philadelphia, PA: Elsevier: 2008:1173-1200.
14. Dennis MA, Parker SH, Klaus AJ, et al. Breast biopsy avoidance: The value of normal mammograms and normal sonograms in the setting of a palpable lump. *Radiology.* 2001;219:186-191.
15. Sperber F, Blank A, Metser U, et al. Diagnosis and treatment of breast fibroadenomas by ultrasound-guided vacuum-assisted biopsy. *Arch Surg.* 2003;138:796-800.
16. Nurko J, Edwards MJ. Image-guided breast surgery. *Am J Surg.* 2005;190:221-227.

CHAPTER 61

Breast-Conserving Surgery

Mary Morrogh
Vittorio Zanini
Lea Regolo
Bettina Ballardini
Lisa Wiechmann
Virgilio Sacchini

From radical mastectomy to breast-conserving surgery (BCS), the last 35 years have witnessed a fascinating evolution in the role of surgery in the treatment of breast cancer. For almost a century, Halsted's mastectomy was the treatment of choice for all stages of breast cancer. However, multiple prospective, randomized trials with more than 20 years' follow-up have since documented that breast-conserving operations followed by whole-breast irradiation offers survival outcomes equivalent to mastectomy in appropriately selected patients.

Breast-conserving surgery is defined as the complete removal of the tumor with a concentric margin of surrounding healthy tissue with maintenance of acceptable cosmesis, and should be followed by radiation therapy to achieve an acceptably low rate of local recurrence. Appropriate selection of patients, adequate surgery, and breast irradiation are important components of successful breast-conserving therapy (BCT). Surgical evaluation of the axillary lymph nodes should be performed in patients undergoing BCT for invasive carcinoma, but the status of the axilla does not influence the decision on BCS. Incorporating oncoplastic techniques may be considered to optimize cosmetic outcome in select patients.

GENERAL PRINCIPLES

Six modern, prospective, randomized trials have demonstrated that breast-conserving therapy (lumpectomy followed by radiation) offers survival rates equivalent to mastectomy (Table 61-1)[1-7]; however, when negative margins are not achieved or when radiation therapy is not pursued, breast conservation is associated with higher rates of local recurrence (Tables 61-1 and 61-2).[1,2,8-14] Until recently, the impact of local recurrence on survival remained unclear. In 2005, the Early Breast Cancer Trialists' Collaborative Group (EBCTCG) published the results of a large meta-analysis combining all individual patient data for 42,080 women who collectively took part in 78 treatment comparisons (more vs less surgery, more surgery vs radiotherapy, radiotherapy vs none) to determine the impact of local recurrence on survival. Specifically, among 10 breast-conservation trials included in the EBCTCG analysis (7311 women), postoperative radiation treatment (XRT) was associated with a statistically significant reduction in local recurrence in each individual trial. Furthermore, postoperative XRT was associated with an overall absolute reduction in local recurrence of 19% at 5 years, an absolute reduction in breast cancer–specific mortality of 5.4% at 15 years, and similar reductions in 15-year overall mortality. They concluded that optimal locoregional control does confer a quantifiable survival benefit in early-stage breast cancer and as such the importance of local control is no longer a matter of debate.[15]

Patient Selection

For BCT to be successful, 3 conditions must be met: It must be possible to (1) achieve negative surgical margins while maintaining cosmesis of the breast, (2) safely deliver radiation therapy, and (3) promptly detect local recurrence. Careful patient selection is important to ensure a low rate of local recurrence as well as acceptable cosmetic outcome. Contraindications to BCT are listed in Table 61-3.

TABLE 61-1 Prospective, Randomized Trials Comparing Mastectomy and Axillary Dissection to Breast-Conservation Therapy

Clinical Trial	Dates	N	TNM	Margin Status	XRT Boost	Follow Up (Years)	LOCAL RECURRENCE (%)		OVERALL SURVIVAL (%)	
							Mx	BCT&XRT	Mx	BCT&XRT
NSABP B06[1]	1976-1984	1217	≤4 cm N0N1 M0	Tumor free	Yes	20	10.2	14.3	47.2	46.2
EORTC[5]	1980-1986	874	≤5 cm N0N1 M0	1 cm	Yes	8	10	15	64	66
Danish Breast Cancer Group[4]	1983-1987	859	Any size N0N1 M0	Grossly free	Yes	6	4	3	82	79
National Tumour Institute, Milan[2,3]	1973-1980	701	≤2cm N0N1 M0	Wide free	Yes	20	2.3	8.8	41.2	41.7
National Cancer Institute, US[5]	1979-1987	247	≤5 cm N0N1 M0	Grossly free	Yes	10	10	18	75	77
Institute Gustave-Roussy France[6,7]	1972-79	179	≤2cm N0N1 M0	2cm	Yes	14.5	11	11.4	65	72

TABLE 61-2 Prospective, Randomized Trials Comparing Local Recurrence Rates after BCS with and without Postoperative XRT

	Median Follow-Up (yr)	Local Recurrence with XRT (%)	Local Recurrence without XRT (%)
NSABP B-06[1]	12.5	10	35
Veronesi et al[2]	9.1	5.8	23.5
Renton et al[8]	6.1	13	35
Clark et al[9]	7.6	11.3	35.2
Forrest et al[10]	5.7	5.8	24.5
Liljegren et al[11]	8.8	8.5	24
Malmstrom et al[12]	7	4.4	13.3
Holli et al[13]	6.7	7.5	18.1
NSABP B-21[14]	7.2	9.3	16.5

Patient factors, such as young age, have been associated with an increased risk for local failure after BCT or after mastectomy. However, the EBCTCG found that the absolute effects of radiotherapy after breast-conserving surgery (generally with axillary clearance) for node-negative disease were greater in women less than 50 years old compared to women more than 50 years old; therefore, young age alone should not preclude breast conservation. A number of tumor factors, such as size and involvement of axillary lymph nodes, that are strong predictors of the risk for distant recurrence are not associated with the risk for recurrence in the breast. Histologic tumor type also is not a risk factor, and studies have shown that recurrence rates after excision of infiltrating lobular carcinoma to negative margins do not differ from those after excision of infiltrating ductal tumors. Most studies also indicate that histologic grade is not predictive of recurrence. Some studies have identified lymphatic invasion at the primary tumor site as a risk factor, but this has also been shown to be a risk factor for local recurrence after mastectomy.

For the older patient, controversy exists as to whether or not XRT can be safely omitted after breast conservation.[16] In 2004, the Cancer and Leukemia Group B (CALGB) reported that women more than 70 years of age with estrogen receptor–positive cancers of smaller than 2 cm treated with lumpectomy and tamoxifen without XRT experienced a 3% increase in the risk of local recurrence.[17] Yet, this increase in local recurrence did not translate into a decrease in time to distant metastases or overall survival. The EBCTCG also failed to demonstrate a statistically significant improvement in breast cancer–specific mortality or overall mortality for women more than 70 years old undergoing conservative surgery plus radiotherapy versus surgery alone at 15 years (2.8% vs 2.9%, and 30.4% vs 28.9%, respectively).[15] These data suggest that individualizing the decision about XRT in older women based on tumor characteristics and physiologic age rather than chronologic age should be considered.

A family history of breast cancer does not increase local failure rates. The introduction of specialized surveillance for women with a strong family history of breast cancer or a known BRCA mutation has increased the likelihood that breast cancer will be detected at a stage suitable for breast conservation. In women with mutations of BRCA1 or BRCA2, the risk of new second primary cancers is increased in both breasts, but the risk of local failure does not seem to be elevated.[18] A recently published case-control series evaluated the outcome of BCT and estimated the 10-year in breast tumor recurrence (IBTR) risk to be equivalent between sporadic controls and mutation carriers (9% vs 12%, hazard ratio = 1.37; $p = .19$). However, on multivariate analysis, mutation status was an independent predictor of recurrence in women *with* intact ovaries (hazard ratio = .99, $p = .04$).[19] Other studies reporting an increased risk of IBTR in mutation carriers have median follow-up times greater than 7 years,

TABLE 61-3 Contraindications to Breast-Conserving Surgery

Absolute contraindications
- Multicentric disease
- Diffuse malignant-appearing microcalcifications
- Persistent positive margins after reasonable attempts to conserve the breast
- Need to deliver radiation during pregnancy
- Previous irradiation

Relative contraindications
- History of scleroderma
- Active systemic lupus erythematosus
- Unfavorable tumor size to breast size ratio

suggesting that these events are new second primary cancers. Although these findings sound a cautionary note for young mutation carriers considering BCT (especially those with intact ovaries), mutation status alone is not an absolute contraindication to BCT.[20-23]

Patients with a history of autoimmune diseases such as scleroderma, systemic or discoid lupus, and dermatomyositis may have increased sensitivity to radiation resulting in abnormal fibrosis, which may compromise the cosmetic outcome. Such conditions are not absolute contraindications to BCT, but rather are dealt with in a case-by-case manner. Whether other connective tissue diseases are associated with an increased risk of acute or late skin complications is controversial. A history of mantle radiation for Hodgkin disease may interfere with the conventional radiation therapy for overlapping of the radiation fields. Again, feasibility of BCT should be evaluated in a case-by-case manner with the consideration of a possible increase risk of second primary and contralateral cancers.[24]

There is no definite tumor size limitation to BCS as long as excision with clear margins can be achieved with acceptable cosmesis (favorable breast size to tumor size ratio). In an effort to increase the number of patients eligible for breast conservation, the use of neoadjuvant chemotherapy to shrink the primary tumor before surgical therapy has been studied.[25] In a large randomized trial, National Surgical Adjuvant Breast and Bowel Project (NSABP) protocol B-18, 1523 patients with tumors of any size were randomized to receive 4 cycles of doxorubicin (A) and cyclophosphamide (C), either preoperatively or postoperatively.[26] All patients over age 50 received tamoxifen. A reduction in tumor diameter of 50% was noted clinically in 80% of the patients, and in 37%, no tumor could be felt after chemotherapy. Only one-fourth of the patients thought to be complete responders, however, had no tumor identified microscopically after surgery, and the rate of breast conservation increased by only 8%, from 60% to 68%. In a subsequent study, the addition of docetaxel to AC treatment preoperatively increased the clinical complete response rate from 40.1% to 63.6% ($p < .001$) and the pathologic complete response rate from 13.7% to 26.1% ($p < .001$).[27] Despite this increase in response rate, the use of BCT did not differ between patients receiving preoperative AC and those receiving AC plus docetaxel (Taxotere). This is probably because of the inability of the physical examination and imaging studies to reliably predict the degree of pathologic response. To date, neoadjuvant therapy has not been shown to improve survival in comparison with therapy given postoperatively.

Multicentricity (ie, 2 separate cancers in different quadrants of the same breast) is an important contraindication to BCS. It has been suggested that if 2 lesions are close enough then they can be excised through a single incision as a single specimen with clear margins and acceptable cosmesis, the BCT may be considered. Historically, it was believed that extensive intraductal component (EIC) was associated with an increase risk of IBTR; however, subsequent data has shown that when EIC-positive tumors are excised to negative margins, local recurrence rates are comparable to those seen in EIC-negative tumors.[28] As such, no particular volume of ductal carcinoma in situ (DCIS) within the primary lesion should preclude BCS.

Operative Techniques

Breast cancer treatment is becoming more conservative in each of its multiple aspects, including medical therapy, radiation therapy, and breast surgery. The goal of this conservative approach is to combine optimal oncologic outcome with optimal cosmetic outcome. The majority of women with T1 and small T2 (smaller than 3 cm) cancers are suitable candidates for breast conservation. With oncoplastic surgery, larger tumors can be treated by BCT if the primary tumor can be excised adequately with clear margins and acceptable cosmesis. By combining sound principles of surgical oncology with those of plastic surgery, oncoplastic surgery can extend breast-conservation possibilities and is gaining acceptance as a useful tool in breast surgical oncology.

The surgical term "breast-conserving therapy" encompasses a range of procedures including quadrantectomy (segmentectomy), lumpectomy (tumorectomy, tylectomy), partial mastectomy, and many other definitions found in the literature. The quadrantectomy, first described by Veronesi et al, is an en bloc resection of the breast parenchyma, the overlying skin, and the underlying pectoralis fascia. It is typically performed through a long radial incision and removes a larger volume of breast tissue than other approaches, typically incorporating at least a 2-cm margin of normal tissue around the lesion (Fig 61-1A, B).[29] The anatomic basis of the quadrantectomy is that the ductal system of the breast is made up of 10 to 15 relatively independent sets of radially branching ducts and lobules. The pathologic basis is that the intraductal spread of cancer cells occurs relatively frequently along the ductal unit and, therefore, it is necessary to excise the entire portion of the ductal tree harboring the cancer. These concepts are supported by pathologic studies that demonstrate that breast cancer, both invasive and in situ carcinoma, is often limited to a single quadrant of the breast,[30] and by the observation that DCIS often presents as microcalcifications extending along ducts of the breast. Once the specimen is removed, to obtain a better cosmetic result the breast parenchyma may be detached from the overlying skin and/or the underlying fascia of the pectoralis major over a distance of 1 cm (Fig. 61-1C). Mobilizing the breast in the deep and superficial plane facilitates reapproximation of the breast parenchyma and minimizes retraction or distortion of the breast (Figs. 61-1C, D).

In the lumpectomy, the excision is less generous with respect to quadrantectomy. The volume of breast tissue removed is usually 1 cm surrounding the palpable or nonpalpable cancer.[31] The skin incision should be placed directly over the tumor whenever possible (Fig. 61-2A); this approach minimizes "tunneling" through uninvolved tissue planes, maximizes exposure, and thereby improves the odds of an adequate tumor excision with negative margins at the first operation. The incision should be of adequate size to allow complete tumor excision under direct vision; small incisions made with the goal of optimal cosmesis too often result in piecemeal tumor excision requiring reoperation to achieve adequate margins. An adequate skin incision is made, going just deep to the dermis. Skin flaps are then elevated in all the anatomical direction for about 1 cm, facilitating the exposure of the specimen (Fig. 61-2B). The excision is then carried out with the purpose of having 1-cm grossly free margins around the tumor (Fig. 61-2C). Closing the breast tissue in lay-

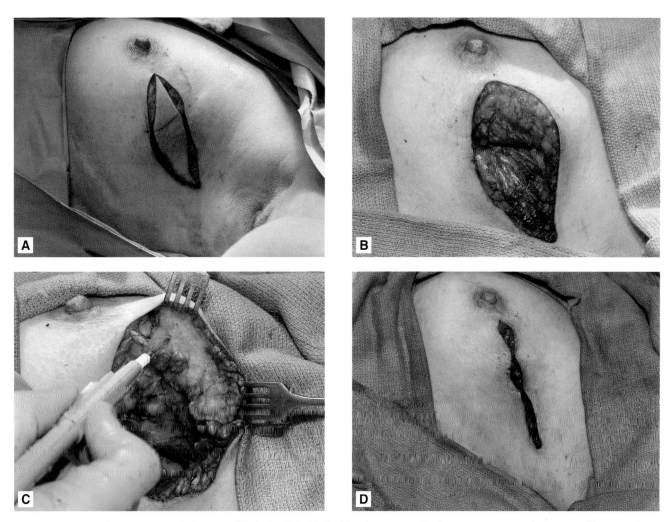

FIGURE 61-1 Quadrantectomy technique. **A.** Elliptical radial skin incision for a cancer in the outer-upper quadrant. **B.** En bloc resection of the breast parenchyma, the skin ellipse, and the pectoralis fascia. **C.** The breast parenchyma may be detached from the overlying skin and/or the underlying fascia of the pectoralis major and then reapproximated. **D.** After the reapproximation of the breast parenchyma the skin is sutured.

ers is controversial. It may cause retraction and dimpling of breast tissue and skin, but, if possible, it minimizes seroma formation and speeds healing. The skin is then sutured in layers with a running subcuticular monofilament suture.

Management of Margins

The first goal of breast conservation is to excise an adequate amount of tissue to minimize risk of local recurrence. Margin status correlates with local failure and as such is an important predictor of residual disease after BCS. However, the appropriate extent of surgical resection needed to minimize this risk remains controversial and there is a lack of consensus regarding optimal method of margin assessment. This represents one of the ongoing "great debates" in breast cancer management.

For palpable lesions, gross inspection of the specimen at the time of removal permits identification of positive or close margins and immediate reexcision, if appropriate. This will decrease the need to return to the operating room for reexcision.[32] Immediate margin assessment with cytologic touch prep analysis

can identify the presence of tumor at the cut margin; however, this method cannot identify close margins and does not guarantee the absence of microscopic tumor on permanent sections. Precise marking and inking of the specimen allows for accurate orientation for the pathologist; however, a degree of tissue manipulation during specimen radiography and pathologic processing is inevitable.[33] All methods of margin assessment have varying technical or practical limitations, which in turn carry important clinical implications. For example, although shaved margins are associated with greater rates of "positive margins" compared with perpendicular-inked margins, the rates of residual disease upon reexcision are comparable between techniques.[34]

The NSABP defines a positive margin as the presence of tumor at the inked margin, and a negative margin as the absence of tumor at the inked margin. Negative margins have lower rates of local failure compared to those that have involved margins. In one series, the local control rate was 100% among patients with negative margins versus 78% for those without negative margins.[35] In practice, positive or unknown histologic

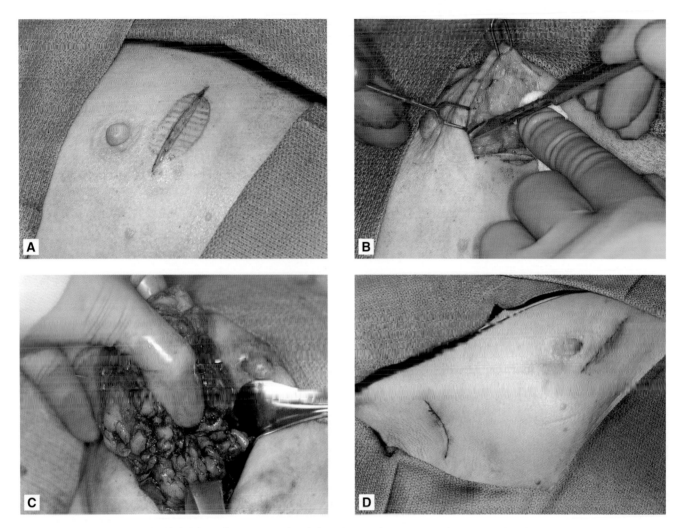

FIGURE 61-2 Lumpectomy technique. **A.** Skin incision placed directly over the tumor. **B.** Elevation of the skin flaps in all the anatomical directions. **C.** The specimen with the cancer is handled, retracted, and freed. **D.** Skin closure.

margins should prompt reexcision, since such patients are at higher risk for local recurrence even with XRT. For those with positive margins who undergo reexcision, residual disease will be found in approximately 50% of cases, with rates varying depending on histologic subtype. In one series, residual cancer was detected in 67% of invasive tumors with associated DCIS, 50% of infiltrating lobular carcinomas, and 35% of infiltrating ductal carcinomas without associated DCIS.[36]

Other factors reported to be associated with a higher likelihood of reexcision include younger age, detection by physical exam only, smaller tumor size, and the presence of EIC. In one series, among 2770 patients undergoing BCS, 60% of patients underwent reexcision. Reexcision was more common among patients less than 40 years of age and with DCIS or lobular carcinoma in situ (LCIS) on final histology. Among those undergoing reexcision, the number of reexcisions performed did not predict for local recurrence.[37] Other studies have also demonstrated that negative margins can be achieved in as many as 95% of cases that undergo reexcision.[38] As such, for patients with positive margins, reexcision should be performed to achieve negative margins. The number of excisions required does not

affect local failure rates; however, multiple excisions may affect cosmetic outcome.

Less clear are cases where the margin is reported as "close." Over the last decade, efforts have been made to classify margin status based on the distance of the tumor cells from the inked margin (< 1 mm, < 2 mm, etc). Subset analysis of breast-conservation trials looking at local recurrence rates based on varying definitions of negative margin (Table 61-1) have failed to support that excision of additional tissue results in decreased rates of local recurrence. Institutional policies vary both in terms of the definition of a "close" margin and XRT practice patterns based on proximity of cancer cells to the margin edge. Studies reporting higher rates of local recurrence among patients with "close" margins are limited and discordant in their findings.[39]

While data consistently show that positive margins carry a greater risk of local recurrence,[40,41] a negative margin does not guarantee the absence of residual disease.[30] However, it is believed that the residual disease burden in patients with negative margins is small enough to be controlled adequately with XRT. Finally, there is renewed interest in the finding of LCIS at the margin. Although studies examining this question have had discordant results, it appears unlikely that LCIS at or close to the margin leads to greater risks of local failure.[42-44] As long as final margins are negative for invasive carcinoma or DCIS, patients with LCIS should receive postoperative XRT and adjuvant therapy in the same manner as those without LCIS, and remain appropriate candidates for breast conservation.[45]

ONCOPLASTIC SURGERY

Oncoplastic surgery cannot be described as a specific technique or procedure. Instead, it should be thought of as the joining of old plastic surgery principles with a new concept of oncologic surgery. We have moved away from a surgical philosophy that once aimed to remove as much as possible, to a more modern philosophy that aims to remove "as much as needed, as little as possible," and that conserves breast tissue as a result. The goal of oncoplastic surgery is to follow standard oncologic principles while ensuring an acceptable cosmetic outcome to patients.[46-52] Oncoplastic techniques may allow for a greater extent of resection with simultaneous reconstruction of the residual defect.[53] Oncoplastic techniques are used to remodel both the affected tumor-bearing breast and the nonaffected breast with the goal of achieving symmetry.[54]

Oncoplastic surgery is based on 4 fundamental principles:

1. Appropriate removal of tumor in alignment with oncologic standards
2. Breast reconstruction to correct breast tissue defects
3. Immediate reconstruction with plastic surgery techniques
4. Correction of contralateral breast asymmetry

Indications for Oncoplastic Surgery

Oncoplastic techniques may be used when the necessary oncologic procedure results in significant breast deformity.[55] Although 90% of patients treated with BCS rate their cosmetic outcome as excellent or good, cosmetically poor outcomes such as extensive scarring, breast deformity, and asymmetry are a reality for some. Unsatisfactory results are often due to poor patient selection, poor surgical planning (ie, unfavorable incision placement, greater breast resection than expected due to intraoperative findings), and/or postradiation changes. Surgical correction of severe cosmetic defects may be complex and require extensive tissue resection, including mastectomy with autologous or heterologous reconstruction. These procedures may difficult for the breast-conservation patient to accept.

Breast cosmetic defects following resection are difficult to classify. This is partly due to the differing contributory factors such as incision type and location, size and shape of the breast, tumor location, size of defect, extent of skin resection, and use of radiation therapy. The morphologic classification described below was proposed in 1987 to characterize breast deformities that follow surgery in the setting of breast conservation, and is currently used to plan surgical correction in oncologically related breast deformity cases.[56] This classification identifies 4 deformity subtypes as follows:

Type I: Distortion and displacement of the nipple-areolar complex (NAC)
Type II: Insufficient skin, subcutaneous tissue, or both

Type III: Breast retraction
Type IV: Severe deformity secondary to radiation therapy

Such deformities most frequently occur when (1) volume loss is 20% or more of total breast volume; (2) the tumor is located in the inferior or medial quadrants, or in the retroareolar region of the breast; (3) axillary dissection is undertaken through the incision used for partial lumpectomy; and/or (4) the surgeon fails to mobilize the breast parenchyma.

Another indication for oncoplastic surgery is when women with significant breast hypertrophy request breast-reduction surgery at the same time as their cancer surgery.

BCS employing oncoplastic principles is contraindicated when mastectomy is necessary to achieve microscopically tumor-free margins. This may be due to large tumor size, extensive malignant calcifications, or the presence of multicentric disease.

Selection of Technique

Breast remodeling can be obtained by techniques that use autologous tissues other than breast tissue, or by mobilizing breast tissue after resection. In the first case, flaps are used to reconstitute missing tissue volume. The most frequently used flap is the latissimus dorsi myocutaneous flap. This flap is also conveniently used as a second option to correct a poor cosmetic outcome deriving from BCT (conservative resection plus radiation) and only rarely requires correction of the contralateral breast for symmetry. In patients for whom breast remodeling is done by mobilizing breast tissue within the resected breast, parenchymal flaps are used to "fill in" the defect. The most commonly used oncoplastic techniques that use mobilization of residual mammary tissue are the *superior* and *inferior pedicle vertical mammaplasty* techniques. A third technique that should be mentioned is remodeling the breast after removal of the central breast region, including the NAC.

Preoperative planning is the most important part of surgery. By using diagrams representing the different volume displacement techniques, the surgeon can resect an appropriate amount of normal and tumor-bearing tissue, thereby satisfying the principles of good oncologic resection and good cosmesis. If the breast is divided via a horizontal plane that traverses the nipple, tumors that arise in the superior, inferior, or central quadrants can be treated with the following different oncoplastic techniques:

1. Simple *glandular remodelling* if the amount of tissue removed is not excessive
2. The *superior pedicle vertical mammaplasty technique* with vertical or "inverted T" incision if the tumor is in the inferior quadrants
3. The *inferior pedicle vertical mammaplasty technique* with vertical or "inverted T" incision if the tumor is in the superior quadrants
4. The *round block* or *Grisotti* technique for centrally located tumors

The initial designs are the same, independent of whether a superior or inferior pedicle approach is used to reconstruct the breast tissue defect, and are dependent on tumor location. In this initial phase, the surgeon draws the lines that not only observe the general mastoplasty principles, but also concurrently take into consideration how much breast tissue needs to be removed to adequately resect the tumor with good margins. As a result, even medial or lateral tumors located near the imaginary horizontal line that traverses the nipple can be included in the preparatory designs for inferior or superior pedicle reconstructive mastoplasties. In these cases, the designs can be rotated to match patients' needs or, based on the incision lines created for traditional mastoplasties, the surgeon can approach the tumor by creating subcutaneous tunnels. Once the incision has been made according to the previously described mastoplasty techniques, oncologic resection can be performed based on tumor location by creating rotational flaps with breast parenchyma. By reconstructing the defect, the surgeon can avoid the cosmetic deformities that are commonly observed with traditional surgical breast conservation.

Marking the Patient

Preoperative marking is an important phase in the preparation of the patient for surgery. The following description is commonly used for inferior or superior pedicle reconstructive mastoplasties. An important instrument used by plastic surgeons in this phase is a metal "keyhole" that marks the areola and the direction of the inferior incisions in reduction mammoplasty patients. As indicated by the name, the metal keyhole resembles exactly that, with an arcuate superior portion and 2 straight, inferior portions (resembling arms). The length of the arcuate portion is usually 12.56 cm, which corresponds to a circle with a 4-cm diameter. The length can be increased up to 16 cm depending on the desired size of the areola (Fig. 61-3).

Figure 61-4 depicts the patient markings commonly used for inferior or superior pedicle reconstructive mastoplasties. With the patient in the sitting or standing position, the surgeon marks the landmarks, including the sternal notch (point A), a line extending from the sternal notch to the umbilicus, the inframammary creases, and the line running from the midclavicular portion to the nipple to the inframammary fold, indicating the vertical axis of the breast. Next, the surgeon marks point B, the new location of the nipple. This point is identified by measuring 18 to 23 cm from point A to the vertical axis of the breast. By moving 2 cm cephalad from point B along the breast axis, the surgeon identifies point C, the new superior margin of the areola. By positioning the "Wise Pattern" with the most superior point placed at point C, the surgeon can identify points D and E, which correspond to the most lateral and medial points of the new areola. The surgeon then moves the breast medially and laterally and marks 2 lines that connect points D and E to the previously marked breast axis. Using moderate traction to distend the skin, points F and G, representing the inferior margin of the nipple and the inframammary fold, are drawn along the line representing the breast axis and drawn 5 to 6 cm apart. This distance varies from between 4.5 and 5 cm in small breasts to 6 to 7 cm in larger ones. Next, the surgeon draws point L, which represents the intersection of the line representing the breast axis and the inframammary fold, and which is located 8 to 10 cm from the sternum. Finally, by connecting points L and F, and L and G, the length of the incision within the fold can be determined. At this point,

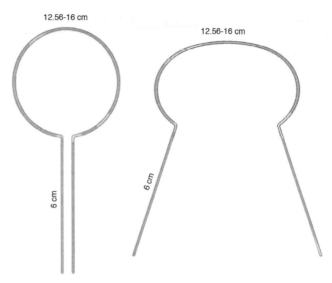

FIGURE 61-3 A metal "keyhole" marks the areola and the direction of the inferior incisions for reduction mammoplasty. The length of the arcuate portion is usually 12.56 cm, which corresponds to a circle with a 4 cm diameter. The length can be increased up to 16 cm depending on the desired size of the areola.

preoperative patient marking has now been completed. The surgeon will now, depending on tumor location, proceed with the incisions based on the inferior or superior pedicle reconstructive approaches.

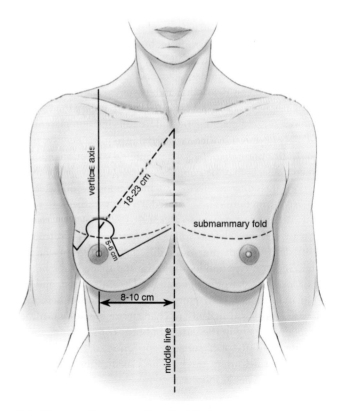

FIGURE 61-4 Patient markings for inferior or superior pedicle reconstructive mastoplasty.

Tumors Located in the Inferior Quadrant: The Superior Pedicle Approach/Inverted T Incision

Once preoperative patient marking has been completed, the surgeon proceeds with a circumareolar incision based on the new areolar size (diameter: 4 cm). After de-epithelializing the area between the areola and the marked surface, the surgeon extends the incision along the lateral and medial arms and along the inframammary crease. Starting from the crease, breast tissue is elevated off the muscle fascia inferiorly to superiorly up to the superior pole of the breast. At this point, the breast tissue resembles a broad blanket lifted off the thoracic wall. By using the nondominant hand to retract the breast tissue, the surgeon can, depending on tumor location, resect different portions of tissue in the inferior, lateral, and medial quadrants (Fig. 61 5).

If caution is used, the surgeon can resect different portions of tissue in the superior quadrants as well, as long as a tongue of tissue (approximately 2-cm deep) below the NAC is left to ensure adequate blood flow. If the tumor is not located in the area included within the markings, the resection area will be prepared by creating subcutaneous tunnels. By lifting the breast off the chest wall superiorly and laterally, the axillary region can be accessed subcutaneously, and sentinel lymph node biopsy or even axillary lymph node dissection can be performed.

The technique described here allows surgeons to preserve unaffected quadrants and reconstruct the tissue defect using rotational or advancement local flaps. After completing hemostasis, reconstruction of the breast parenchyma can be undertaken,

with the first suture approximating the superior apex of the areola with point C.

Tumors Located in the Inferior Quadrants: Superior Pedicle Approach/Vertical Incision

This technique is a variation on the previously described procedure and is also based on the use of the superior pedicle approach. It is used when the tumor is located in the lower outer quadrant up to the outer limit of the areola.

Preoperative patient marking begins with the determination of the new position of the areola and nipple, using the Wise Pattern described, and marking points D and E as described earlier. The inferior part of the marking resembles a "comma" that extends to the inframammary crease and gently turns toward the lateral portion of the breast. In drawing these lines, the vertical and lateral segments of points F and G converge toward the axis of the breast and end in a rounded fashion (Fig. 61-6). Depending on the location of the tumor in the inferior quadrants, the axis of the metal Wise Pattern keyhole can be rotated to best encompass the resection segment.

The procedure is similar to the one previously described. The first step is de-epithelializing the skin based on the preoperative markings. Next, the surgeon makes full-thickness incisions in the medial and lateral de-epithelialized areas, starting from points D and E, until the muscle fascia is identified. The breast tissue is

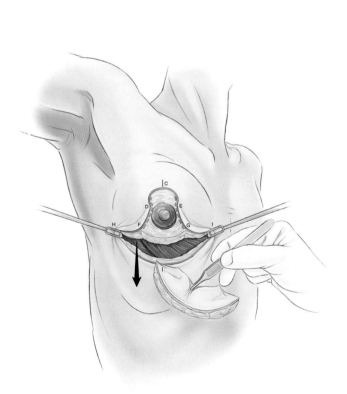

FIGURE 61-5 The superior pedicle approach/inverted T incision. This approach is suitable for tumors located in the inferior quadrants of the breast.

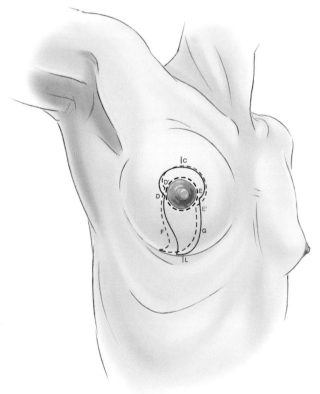

FIGURE 61-6 The superior pedicle approach/vertical incision. This approach is preferable when the tumor is located in the lower-outer quadrant up to the outer limit of the areola.

lifted off the chest wall inferiorly to superiorly. When using this technique, access to the axilla via a subcutaneous tunnel is simplified. Removal of breast tissue mostly involves the inferior pole and is done in accordance with tumor location and size. This surgical approach avoids distorting the NAC, which would otherwise be shifted laterally, and also preserves the contour of the breast.

Tumors Located in the Superior Quadrants: Inferior Pedicle Approach/Inverted T Incision Approach

Preoperative patient marking for the inferior pedicle approach is similar to the technique using the "keyhole" as described above (Fig. 61-4). It is completed by marking the inferior pedicle itself. With the patient in the supine position, a tongue of tissue extending laterally and medially to the vertical axis of the breast and measuring 6 to 8 cm in width is marked (Fig. 61-7). The surgeon first carries the incision circumferentially along the arcuate portion of the marked arcuate line (4 cm), and the inferior flap included within the marked area is de-epithelialized. Next, a full-thickness incision is carried out on the lateral aspects of the flap down to the muscle fascia, taking particular care not to devascularize the base of the flap. The breast parenchyma is then lifted off of the chest wall, thus obtaining a glandular flap resembling a "horseshoe" and encompassing the

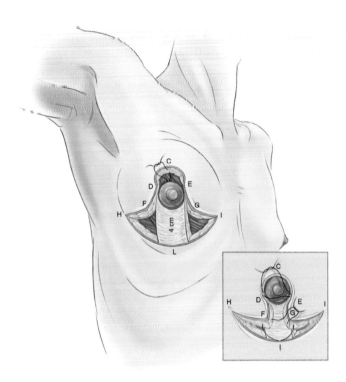

FIGURE 61-8 Reapproximation of the breast parenchyma. Points L-F-G are brought together as the first step, followed by points D-E.

internal, external, and superior quadrants. Next, the involved breast tissue is removed by full-thickness excision of points H-F-D-C-E-G-I. If the tumor is located within the horseshoe, it can be removed en bloc. If needed, subcutaneous tunneling can be used to resect other areas of the breast depending on tumor location. Once complete hemostasis is achieved, reapproximation of the breast parenchyma is undertaken. The suturing of points L-F-G, and subsequently points D-E, is followed by skin closure as previously described (Fig. 61-8).

The inferior pedicle/inverted T incision technique is one of the most useful oncoplastic techniques because it allows for resection of large tumors, including those greater than 3 cm in diameter, in medium- to large-breasted women. It is ideal for tumors located in the superior quadrants, does not lead to alteration of breast contour, and at times even improves breast contour. This is made possible by the fact that in designing and creating the flap, large portions of the superior breast parenchyma can be mobilized and rotated up to 90° to 120° to replace any defect created by the oncologic procedure. Each of these oncoplastic techniques allows for large resections with good oncologic margins without deforming the breast.

Tumors Located in the Central Breast: the Round Block or Grisotti Technique

When tumors are located in the retro-areolar region, the NAC cannot be preserved, and the surgeon must proceed with a central quadrantectomy with removal of the NAC. Breast reconstruction in this case is performed using the Grisotti technique,[57]

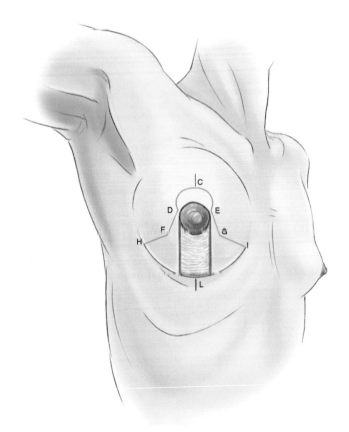

FIGURE 61-7 The inferior pedicle approach/inverted T incision. This approach is suitable for tumors located in the superior quadrants of the breast.

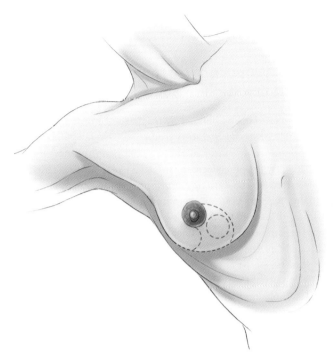

FIGURE 61-9 The Grisotti technique for breast reconstruction following central quadrantectomy with removal of the NAC.

by which a dermoglandular flap is raised from the inferolateral breast margin to replace the defect formed by the excision (Fig. 61-9). This flap includes a portion of breast tissue that extends inferiorly and laterally from the inferior aspect of the excision cavity to the inframammary crease. This flap is de-epithelialized, with the exception of a circular area in the superomedial aspect of the flap itself, which will reconstruct the new areola.

After de-epithelializing the area that is to represent the superficial aspect of the flap, breast tissue is incised medially

down to the thoracic wall, and the incision is carried laterally until it encounters the inframammary crease. Next, the breast parenchyma, including the flap and the lateral portion of the breast parenchyma, is lifted off the chest wall. The flap, including the area with preserved skin coverage, is then advanced and rotated to replace the tissue removed with the excision. The flap is vascularized via its lateral aspect. Nipple reconstruction and/or tattooing, and potential correction of contralateral asymmetries are carried out at a later date.

BREAST-CONSERVING SURGERY FOLLOWING NEOADJUVANT CHEMOTHERAPY

The primary role of neoadjuvant chemotherapy is to improve operability of large, locally advanced tumors. Tumor response may be concentric or multicentric/irregular. With concentric regression of a unifocal breast tumor, breast conservation may be feasible. However, with multicentric or irregular regression, excision of the entire area originally occupied by the tumor is required and may preclude conservation therapy. Careful assessment of tumor response with physical examination and repeat imaging studies (mammography [MG], magnetic resonance imaging [MRI], ultrasonography [US]) after neoadjuvant chemotherapy are critical to guide locoregional treatment recommendations.[58] Between 50% and 90% of women with noninflammatory LABC who do not qualify for BCS at the time of initial presentation can be successfully treated with breast-conserving techniques after neoadjuvant chemotherapy.[59-61] Progression of local disease during neoadjuvant chemotherapy is reported in less than 5% of patients,[62] Contraindications to BCS after neoadjuvant therapy are presented in Table 61-4.[63,64]

If patients are potential BCS patients, the primary tumor should be localized before starting neoadjuvant chemotherapy so that the tumor bed is identifiable in the setting of a complete clinical response. This can be accomplished by inserting a radioopaque clip into the central portion of the tumor under

---

TABLE 61-4 Contraindications to Breast-Conserving Surgery after Neoadjuvant Chemotherapy

Absolute contraindications
- Progression of disease on treatment
- No response to chemotherapy
- Inflammatory or extensive T4 lesions
- Poor cosmetic outcome
- Multicentric disease
- Excisional biopsy reveals extensive residual tumor or islands of tumor throughout the specimen or positive margins
- Extensive microcalcifications associated with an EIC documented to persist postchemotherapy
- Small breast where excision of residual nidus produces an unacceptable cosmetic outcome

Relative contraindications
- History of scleroderma
- Active systemic lupus erythematosus
- Unfavorable tumor size to breast size ratio

ultrasound guidance for subsequent needle localization prior to surgery. In addition, it is recommended that a core biopsy of the tumor be performed prior to starting neoadjuvant chemotherapy so that full pathologic assessment, hormone receptor status, and HER-2 status can be obtained. Surgery is usually performed 2 to 4 weeks after the last cycle of chemotherapy. Resection should aim to achieve a complete resection with negative margins. Neoadjuvant therapy may increase the risk for surgical and radiation-related complications, but this is a theoretical concern and not proven.[65]

Compared to women who are eligible for BCS at the time of diagnosis or who undergo mastectomy after neoadjuvant chemotherapy, local failure rates may be higher for some women who require downstaging to be eligible for breast conservation.[66-68] However, long-term follow-up from the NSABP B-18 randomized pivotal landmark study of preoperative chemotherapy versus postoperative chemotherapy for operable breast cancer did not demonstrate a significantly increased rate of local recurrence for women receiving preoperative chemotherapy compared with those receiving postoperative chemotherapy. The increased rates of local failure among patients undergoing BCS after neoadjuvant chemotherapy are likely explained by the nonuniform pathological response and discordance between a cCR and complete pathological (pCR) response. For example, Veronesi et al reported on 226 patients with tumors larger than 3 cm who underwent neoadjuvant chemotherapy with various chemotherapy regimens followed by surgery. In this series, final pathology showed residual multifocal disease in 16%, and pCR was evident in only 3.5%.[69] In a retrospective study by Clouth et al of 101 patients with LABC undergoing neoadjuvant therapy, 25% achieved a cCR; however, 36% of these patients had an incomplete pathologic response with multicentric disease in 89%.[70] A prognostic index to estimate the likelihood of an in-breast or locoregional tumor recurrence has been suggested from a series of 340 patients undergoing BCT after neoadjuvant chemotherapy for noninflammatory LABC. One point was assigned for each unfavorable characteristic: (1) residual pathologic tumor size larger than 2 cm, (2) multifocal residual disease, (3) lymphovascular space invasion, (4) clinical N2 or N3 disease. Five-year rates of recurrence-free survival were 97% for patients with upto 1 point compared with 82% for patients with 3 to 4 points. Corresponding rates of locoregional recurrence-free survival were 94% and 58%, respectively.[71]

There are no studies specifically addressing the role of oncoplastic BCS in LABC after neoadjuvant therapy. Individual case series have shown that these techniques can be used in the resection of large operable tumors.[72] In general, these techniques involve breast reshaping or volume replacement and frequently include contralateral surgery. They allow for large excisions, including overlying skin where appropriate, thereby potentially reducing the incidence of margin involvement and hence local recurrence without compromising the cosmetic outcome.[73] However, careful assessment of treatment response with preoperative imaging studies should be considered to avoid extensive skin and tissue rearrangement in patients who have a high likelihood of requiring mastectomy for definitive treatment.

Management of the axilla for patients undergoing BCS after neoadjuvant chemotherapy is discussed in detail elsewhere.

LOCAL RECURRENCE FOLLOWING BREAST-CONSERVING SURGERY

A local recurrence is defined as reappearance of cancer in the ipsilateral conserved breast. A regional recurrence refers to the (re)appearance of tumor in the regional lymph nodes (ipsilateral axillary, supraclavicular, infraclavicular, and/or internal mammary). In the current era of improved overall survival for patients with breast cancer, more patients are living with the disease, thus over time more isolated locoregional recurrences may become apparent.[74] Local recurrence rates may also be impacted by the increasing use of neoadjuvant chemotherapy to allow for breast conservation, as well as the increasing popularity of partial breast irradiation. Furthermore, the use of sentinel lymph node biopsy rather than axillary lymph node dissection to stage the axilla may not only impact the incidence of regional recurrence, but also the approach to the patient with an isolated locoregional recurrence.

Aggressive multimodality treatment has the potential to provide long-term disease control for many patients who develop an isolated locoregional recurrence after BCT. Multidisciplinary evaluation and management of these cases appears to improve patient outcome and overall satisfaction.[75]

Incidence

Approximately 10% to 15% of patients undergoing BCT for operable breast cancer will develop a locoregional recurrence within 10 years (Table 61-1). This risk is only slightly higher than that of a locoregional recurrence following mastectomy (5%-10%). Recurrences tend to occur later after BCT than after mastectomy (median 3-4 years vs 2-3 years, respectively).[18,76,77] The time to recurrence may be even longer after BCT in patients who receive adjuvant hormonal and/or chemotherapy.

Many IBTRs after BCT are detected by mammography alone. The finding of disease in an ipsilateral preserved breast can represent either a local recurrence of the initial cancer or a second primary tumor. As the interval from initial diagnosis lengthens, disease is more likely to present in other quadrants of the breast and as such may be new primary tumors.[78] The distinction between true recurrences versus a new primary is generally made on clinical grounds (ie, histologic subtype, location, mammographic appearance).[79] In the future, molecular classification may provide a more reliable means of distinguishing between local recurrences and new primaries. The distinction is important, as a local recurrence will carry a worse prognosis then an ipsilateral new primary.

Local recurrence after BCT may be either invasive or in situ cancer. For patients who were initially treated for invasive disease, more than 80% of locoregional recurrences are invasive; the remainder are noninvasive (intraductal) lesions. Approximately 75% are isolated to the breast and clinically solitary; 5% to 15% present with a simultaneous regional node recurrence, and another 5% to 15% may present with synchronous distant disease. For patients initially treated for in situ cancer (DCIS), approximately 50% will recur with DCIS and 50% with invasive disease.[67,80]

Risk Factors for Local Recurrence

As discussed previously, failure to achieve optimal local control (ie, suboptimal excision, omission of XRT) after BCS is the principle risk factor for local recurrence. Other risk factors for local recurrence after BCT include (1) the presence of an EIC within the tumor in individuals who do *not* have negative resection margins or who do *not* have extensive remaining residual suspicious microcalcifications, (2) younger patient age, and (3) negative hormone receptor status. In addition, tumors with inherently aggressive biology are more likely to fail locally; indeed the local recurrence may represent the first site of metastatic disease. Whether an inherited susceptibility to breast cancer increases the risk of a local recurrence is controversial.[81]

Patients who present with an invasive local recurrence after BCT should have complete restaging to rule out distant metastases. The risk of a systemic disease ranges from 20% to 40% at 5 years, and 24% to 64% at 10 years.[82] Clinical predictors of poor prognosis in patients with IBTR include invasive disease, tumor size, skin involvement, nodal involvement, and hormone receptor–negative disease. In addition short time interval between initial BCT and local recurrence appears predictive of poor biology.[3,83]

Surgical Management

Mastectomy is considered the standard approach for an IBTR after BCT. Immediate reconstruction can be carried out as long as there is no skin involvement. Most series report an operability rate of at least 85%, where the remaining 15% are considered inoperable due to the extensive local disease (skin involvement, large fixed tumors), inoperable nodal disease, or simultaneous distant metastases. Patients with skin involvement have a poor prognosis and are treated with systemic therapy prior to locoregional therapy.[84-87] The risk of subsequent chest wall recurrence following mastectomy in patients with an invasive IBTR after BCT is approximately 10%.[10,67,68,88,89] Five-year relapse-free survival rates range from 60% to 79%.

There are limited data evaluating the benefit of chest wall or regional nodal irradiation after mastectomy in this setting. Irradiation of the regional nodes may be considered if the patient did not undergo regional nodal irradiation at the time of BCT or if they have extensive disease (tumor size larger than 5 cm, more than 4 to 5 positive nodes) at the time of mastectomy. Reirradiation of the chest wall is not standard practice. In the uncommon situation of a local recurrence in a patient who underwent lumpectomy alone without whole-breast irradiation, repeat BCS followed by XRT can be considered.

For patients who underwent initial BCS with whole-breast XRT, repeat conserving surgery comes with high rates (up to 35%) of a second IBTR as repeat irradiation is not generally recommended. Limited small series suggest that catheter-based interstitial brachytherapy or limited external beam partial breast reirradiation may be feasible in select women who previously underwent whole-breast XRT with acceptable morbidity rates and cosmesis. However, repeat BCT with limited field re-irradiation is not considered a standard treatment option at most institutions and this approach requires further prospective study.[44,68,89-92]

Axillary evaluation of the patient with an IBTR should begin with a thorough physical examination and ultrasound of the axilla. Fine-needle aspiration (FNA) biopsy should be performed for any clinically suspicious lymph nodes. In the pre–sentinel lymph node (SLN) biopsy era, up to 27% of patients with prior axillary lymph node dissection (ALND) were found to have axillary disease at the time of local recurrence.[67,93,94] The incidence of nodal involvement associated with an IBTR in women who have had a prior negative SLN biopsy is unknown. For patients presenting with an IBTR without prior ALND or SLN biopsy, axillary staging with lymphatic mapping and SLN biopsy is reasonable as long as there is no clinical or radiographic evidence of axillary disease. For patients who have undergone previous SLN biopsy, repeat SLN may also be feasible.[95-98] There is no consensus on the optimal management of the axilla in patients who have already undergone ALND. The utility of SLN biopsy in this setting is being evaluated[99]; however, the utility of the technique is often limited as the SLN frequently maps to the contralateral axilla or is not identified.[100] Exploration of the axilla at the time of mastectomy, resecting any areas of obvious adenopathy, is a common approach.

FUTURE DIRECTIONS

- In the current era of molecular classification of tumors, advances in the genomic or molecular subclassification of tumors might identify differences in local recurrence risk among patients with breast cancer, which could be useful in a clinical setting. Future research models investigating and developing clinical algorithms for personalized treatment may guide surgical decisions regarding eligibility for BCS and risks/utility of reexcision for positive or close margins.
- Evolving techniques of "minimally invasive oncoplasty" have been proposed, but remain experimental. For example, an increasing amount of clinical evidence supports the therapeutic potential of mesenchymal stem cells for ischemic tissue revascularization and restoration of function. Preclinical and clinical studies highlight the potential role of adipose stem cells. An interesting application of adipose stem cells in is the treatment of radiation-induced deformities of the breast. The chronic ischemic state that underlies this injury represents a challenge for the oncoplastic surgeon. Traditionally, this degree of tissue damage is thought to be a prerequisite for surgical excision followed by reconstruction with distant flaps. The ability to graft fat from one area of the body to another has the potential to conserve damaged tissues.

NECESSARY STUDIES

- Although neoadjuvant chemotherapy is effective in reducing tumor burden and facilitating surgical therapy, no survival advantage has been demonstrated for the use of preoperative (as opposed to postoperative) chemotherapy in randomized trials. Future neoadjuvant trials with newer targeted agents may increase rates of breast conservation as well as survival.

- Controlled trials are needed to establish whether all patients with a pathologic complete response to neoadjuvant chemotherapy require both XRT and surgery.

- In the absence of distant disease, complete mastectomy is the standard treatment for patients presenting with local recurrence after BCS. Small experiences with further attempts at breast preservation by using excision alone or repeated irradiation of small areas of the breast after surgical excision have been reported, but larger numbers of patients and longer follow-up periods are needed to determine the role of these therapies.[90]

SUMMARY

For appropriately selected patients, BCT is a safe and acceptable alternative to mastectomy. Optimal local control with margin negative surgery and postoperative XRT are critical elements to minimize local relapse and mortality from breast cancer. In general, patients with positive margins should undergo reexcision. Incorporating oncoplastic surgical techniques should be considered to optimize cosmetic outcome in appropriate cases, such as those requiring a large volume excision. Neoadjuvant chemotherapy to downstage the primary tumor can improve eligibility for breast conservation therapy. Potential candidates for neoadjuvant therapy should have the tumor bed marked and full pathologic assessment of the tumor completed prior to initiation of chemotherapy. Careful assessment of tumor response after neoadjuvant chemotherapy with physical examination and repeat imaging studies should be used to guide locoregional treatment recommendations.

Risk factors for local recurrence include (1) suboptimal local control (ie, positive margins, omission of XRT), (2) younger age, and (3) negative hormone receptor status. Future studies may identify distinct genomic signatures predictive of local recurrence following BCT. For patients with an isolated IBTR, mastectomy is the surgical treatment of choice. Five-year relapse free survival rates range from 60% to 79% after the procedure, and further chest wall recurrences are uncommon.

REFERENCES

1. Fisher B, Anderson S, Bryant J, et al. Twenty-year follow-up of a randomized trial comparing total mastectomy, lumpectomy, and lumpectomy plus irradiation for the treatment of invasive breast cancer. *N Engl J Med.* 2002;347(16):1233-1241.
2. Veronesi U, Cascinelli N, Mariani L, et al. Twenty-year follow-up of a randomized study comparing breast-conserving surgery with radical mastectomy for early breast cancer. *N Engl J Med.* 2002;347(16):1227-1232.
3. Van Dongen JA, Bartelink H, Fentiman I, et al. Randomized clinical trial to assess the value of breast-conserving therapy in stage I and II breast cancer, EORTC 10801 trial. *J Natl Cancer Inst Monogr.* 1992;(11):15-18.
4. Blichert-Toft M, Nielsen M, Düring M, et al. Long-term results of breast conserving surgery vs. mastectomy for early stage invasive breast cancer: 20-year follow-up of the Danish randomized DBCG-82TM protocol. *Acta Oncol.* 2008;47(4):672-681.
5. Jacobson JA, Danforth DN, Cowan KH, et al. Ten-year results of a comparison of conservation with mastectomy in the treatment of stage I and II breast cancer. *N Engl J Med.* 1995;332(14):907-911.
6. Sarrazin D, Lê M, Rouëssé J, et al. Conservative treatment versus mastectomy in breast cancer tumors with macroscopic diameter of 20 millimeters or less. The experience of the Institut Gustave Roussy. *Cancer.* 1984;53(5):1209-1213.
7. Sarrazin D, Le MG, Arriagada R, et al. Ten-year results of a randomized trial comparing a conservative treatment to mastectomy in early breast cancer. *Radiother Oncol.* 1989;14(3):177-184.
8. Renton S, Gazet J, Ford H, et al. The importance of the resection margin in conservative surgery for breast cancer. *Eur J Surg Oncol.* 1996;22:17-22.
9. Clark R, Whelan T, Levine M, et al. Randomized clinical trial of breast irradiation following lumpectomy and axillary dissection for node negative breast cancer: an update. *J Natl Cancer Inst.* 1996;88:1659-1664.
10. Forrest A, Stewart H, Everington D, et al. Randomised controlled trial of conservation therapy for breast cancer: 6-year analysis of the Scottish trial. Scottish Cancer Trials Breast Group. *Lancet.* 1996;348:708-713.
11. Liljegren G, Holmberg L, Bergh J, et al. Ten-year results after sector resection with or without postoperative radiotherapy for stage I breast cancer: a randomized trial. *J Clin Oncol.* 1999;17:2326-2333.
12. Malmstrom P, Holmberg L, Anderson H, et al. Breast conservation surgery, with and without radiotherapy, in women with lymph node-negative breast cancer: a randomised clinical trial in a population with access to public mammography screening. *Eur J Cancer.* 2003;39:1690-1697.
13. Holli K, Saaristo R, Isola J, et al. Lumpectomy with or without postoperative radiotherapy for breast cancer with favourable prognostic features: results of a randomized study. *Br J Cancer.* 2001;84:164-169.
14. Fisher B, Bryant J, Dignam J, et al. Tamoxifen, radiation therapy, or both for prevention of ipsilateral breast tumor recurrence after lumpectomy in women with invasive breast cancers of one centimeter or less. *J Clin Oncol.* 2002;20:4141-4149.
15. Early Breast Cancer Trialists' Collaborative Group, Clarke M, Collins R, Darby S, et al. (Early Breast Cancer Trialists' Collaborative Group) (EBCTCG): Effects of radiotherapy and of differences in the extent of surgery for early breast cancer on local recurrence and 15-year survival: an overview of the randomised trials. *Lancet.* 2005;366(9503):2087-2106.
16. Ferretti G, Mandala M, Bria E, et al. Lumpectomy and tamoxifen alone without additional radiotherapy for women 70 years of age or older with estrogen receptor-positive breast cancer. *Breast Cancer Res Treat.* 2005;90(3):319.
17. Hughes KS, Schnaper LA, Berry D, et al. (Cancer and Leukemia Group B; Radiation Therapy Oncology Group; Eastern Cooperative Oncology Group): Lumpectomy plus tamoxifen with or without irradiation in women 70 years of age or older with early breast cancer. *N Engl J Med.* 2004;351(10):971-977.
18. Haffty BG, Harrold E, Khan AJ, et al. Outcome of conservatively managed early-onset breast cancer by BRCA1/2 status. *Lancet.* 2002;359:1471-1477.
19. Pierce LJ, Levin AM, Rebbeck TR, et al. Ten-year multi-institutional results of breast-conserving surgery and radiotherapy in BRCA1/2-associated stage I/II breast cancer. *J Clin Oncol.* 2006;24(16):2437-2443.
20. Verhoog LC, Brekelmans CTM, Seynaeve C, et al. Survival and tumour characteristics of breast-cancer patients with germline mutations of BRCA1. *Lancet.* 1998;351:316-321.
21. Haffty B, Harrold E, Khan A, et al. Outcome of conservatively managed early-onset breast cancer by BRCA1/2 status. *Lancet.* 2002;359:1471-1477.
22. Robson M, Levin D, Federici M, et al. Breast-conservation therapy for invasive breast cancer in Ashkenazi women with BRCA gene founder mutations. *J Natl Cancer Inst.* 1999;91:2112-2117.
23. Eccles D, Simmonds P, Goddard J, et al. Familial breast cancer: an investigation into the outcome of treatment for early stage disease. *Familial Cancer.* 2001;1:65-72.
24. Deutsch M, Gerszten K, Bloomer WD, et al. Lumpectomy and breast irradiation for breast cancer arising after previous radiotherapy for Hodgkin's disease or lymphoma. *Am J Clin Oncol.* 2001;24(1):33-34.
25. Bonadonna G, Veronesi U, Brambilla C, et al. Primary chemotherapy to avoid mastectomy in tumors with diameters of three centimeters or more. *J Natl Cancer Inst.* 1990;82:1539-1545.
26. Fisher B, Bryant J, Wolmark N, et al. Effect of preoperative chemotherapy on the outcome of women with operable breast cancer. *J Clin Oncol.* 1998;16:2672-2685.
27. Bear H, Anderson S, Brown A, et al. The effect on tumor response of adding sequential preoperative docetaxel to preoperative doxorubicin and cyclophosphamide: preliminary results from National Surgical Adjuvant Breast and Bowel Project B-27. *J Clin Oncol.* 2003;22:4165-4174.
28. Schnitt SJ, Abner A, Gelman R, et al. The relationship between microscopic margins of resection and the risk of local recurrence in patients with breast cancer treated with breast-conserving surgery and radiation therapy. *Cancer.* 1994;74(6):1746-1751.

29. Sacchini V. Quadrantectomy and sentinel node biopsy. In: TA King, PI Borgen. *Atlas of Procedures in Breast Cancer Surgery* (Chapter 8). London, UK and New York, NY: Taylor and Francis: 2002:71-77.

30. Holland R, Veling SH, Mravunac ML, et al. Radiotherapy histologic multifocality of Tis, T1–2 breast carcinomas. Implications for clinical trials of breast-conserving surgery. *Cancer.* 1985;56: 979–990.

31. Cody H. Breast-conservation therapy. In: TA King, PI Borgen. *Atlas of Procedures in Breast Cancer Surgery* (Chapter 9). London, UK and New York, NY: Taylor and Francis: 2002:41-55.

32. Cabioglu N, Hunt KK, Sahin AA, et al. Role for intraoperative margin assessment in patients undergoing breast-conserving surgery. *Ann Surg Oncol.* 2007;14(4):1458-1471.

33. Graham RA, Homer MJ, Katz J, et al. The pancake phenomenon contributes to the inaccuracy of margin assessment in patients with breast cancer. *Am J Surg.* 2002;184(2):89-93.

34. Wright MJ, Park J, Fey JV, et al. Perpendicular inked versus tangential shaved margins in breast-conserving surgery: does the method matter? *J Am Coll Surg.* 2007;204(4):541-549.

35. Smitt M, Nowels K, Zdeblick M, et al. The importance of the lumpectomy surgical margin status in long-terms results of breast conservation. *Cancer.* 1995;76:259-267.

36. Schmidt-Ullrich RK, Wazer DE, DiPetrillo T, et al. Breast conservation therapy for early stage breast carcinoma with outstanding 10-year locoregional control rates: a case for aggressive therapy to the tumor bearing quadrant. *Int J Radiat Oncol Biol Phys.* 1993;27(3):545-552.

37. O'Sullivan MJ, Li T, Freedman G, Morrow M. The effect of multiple reexcisions on the risk of local recurrence after breast conserving surgery. *Ann Surg Oncol.* 2007;14(11):3133-3140.

38. Kearney TJ, Morrow M. Effect of reexcision on the success of breast-conserving surgery. *Ann Surg Oncol.* 1995;2(4):303-307.

39. Taghian A, Mohiuddin M, Jagsi R, et al. Current perceptions regarding surgical margin status after breast-conserving therapy: results of a survey. *Ann Surg.* 2005;241(4):629-639

40. Luini A, Rososchansky J, Gatti G, et al. The surgical margin status after breast-conserving surgery. discussion of an open issue. *Breast Cancer Res Treat.* 2009;113(3):397-402.

41. Singletary SE. Surgical margins in patients with early-stage breast cancer treated with breast conservation therapy. *Am J Surg.* 2002;184(5):383-393.

42. Ben-David MA, Kleer CG, Paramagul C, et al. Is lobular carcinoma in situ as a component of breast carcinoma a risk factor for local failure after breast-conserving therapy? Results of a matched pair analysis. *Cancer.* 2006;106:28-34.

43. Sasson AR, Fowble B, Hanlon AL, et al. Lobular carcinoma in situ increases the risk of local recurrence in selected patients with stages I and II breast carcinoma treated with conservative surgery and radiation. *Cancer.* 2001;91:1862-1869.

44. Abner AL, Connolly JL, Recht A, et al. The relation between the presence and extent of lobular carcinoma in situ and the risk of local recurrence for patients with infiltrating carcinoma of the breast treated with conservative surgery and radiation therapy. *Cancer.* 2000;88:1072-1077.

45. Ciocca RM, Li T, Freedman GM, Morrow M. Presence of lobular carcinoma in situ does not increase local recurrence in patients treated with breast-conserving therapy. *Ann Surg Oncol.* 2008;15(8):2263-2271.

46. Munhoz AM, Aldrighi CM, Aldrighi JM. Is necessary the participation of the surgeon plastic in the programming of the surgery conservative of the breast neoplasm? *Rev Assoc Med Bras.* 2005;51(1):5-6.

47. Baildam AD. Oncoplastic surgery of the breast. *Br J Surg.* 2002;89:532-533.

48. Anderson BO, Masetti R, Silverstein MJ. Oncoplastic approaches to partial mastectomy: an overview of volume-displacement techniques. *Lancet Oncol.* 2005;6:145-157.

49. Munhoz AM, Montag E, Arruda EG, et al. The role of the lateral thoracodorsal fasciocutaneous flap in immediate conservative breast surgery reconstruction. *Plast Reconstr Surg.* 2006;117(6):1699-1710.

50. Munhoz AM, Montag E, Fels KW, et al. Outcome analysis of breast-conservation surgery and immediate latissimus dorsi flap reconstruction in patients with T1 to T2 breast cancer. *Plast Reconstr Surg.* 2005;116(3):741-752.

51. Munhoz AM, Montag E, Arruda EG, et al. Critical analysis of reduction mammaplasty techniques in combination with conservative breast surgery for early breast cancer treatment. *Plast Reconstr Surg.* 2006;117(4):1091-1103; discussion 1104-1107.

52. Fedorcik GG, Sachs R, Goldfarb MA. Oncologic and aesthetic results following breast-conserving therapy with 0.5 cm margins in 100 consecutive patients. *Breast J.* 2006;12:208-211.

53. Petit JY, Rietjens M, Garusi C, et al. Integration of plastic surgery in the course of breast-conserving surgery for cancer to improve cosmetic results and radicality of tumor excision. *Recent Results Cancer Res.* 1998;152:202-211.

54. Slavin SA. Reconstruction of the breast conservation patient. In: Spear SL, ed. *Surgery of the Breast: Principles and Art.* Philadelphia, PA: Lippincott-Raven Publishers: 1998:221-238.

55. Audretsch WP. Reconstruction of the Lippincott-Raven Publishers:1998: 155-196.

56. Berrino P, Campora E, Santi P. Postquadrantectomy breast deformities: classification and techniques of surgical correction. *Plast Reconstr Surg.* 1987;79:(4)567-572.

57. Petit J, Garusi C, Greuse M, et al. One hundred and eleven cases of breast conservation treatment with simultaneous reconstruction at the European Institute of Oncology (Milan). *Tumori.* 2002;88(1):41-47.

58. Chuthapisith S, Eremin JM, Eremin O. Predicting response to neoadjuvant chemotherapy in breast cancer: molecular imaging, systemic biomarkers and the cancer metabolome. *Oncol Rep.* 2008;20(4):699-703.

59. Fisher B, Brown A, Mamounas E, et al. Effect of preoperative chemotherapy on local-regional disease in women with operable breast cancer: findings from National Surgical Adjuvant Breast and Bowel Project B-18. *J Clin Oncol.* 1997;15:2483-2493.

60. van der Hage JA, van de Velde CJ, Julien JP, et al. Preoperative chemotherapy in primary operable breast cancer: results from the European Organization for Research and Treatment of Cancer trial 10902. *J Clin Oncol.* 2001;19:4224-4237.

61. Bonadonna G, Valagussa P, Brambilla C, et al. Primary chemotherapy in operable breast cancer: eight-year experienceat the Milan Cancer Institute. *J Clin Oncol.* 1998;16:93-100.

62. Fisher B, Bryant J, Wolmark N, et al. Effect of preoperative chemotherapy on the outcome of women with operable breast cancer. *J Clin Oncol.* 1998;16:2672-2685.

63. Singletary SE, McNeese MD, Hortobagyi GN, et al. Feasibility of breast-conservation surgery after induction chemotherapy for locally advanced breast carcinoma. *Cancer.* 1992;69(11):2849-2852.

64. Chen AM, Meric-Bernstam F, Hunt KK, et al. Breast conservation after neoadjuvant chemotherapy. *Cancer.* 2005;103(4):689-695.

65. Graham MV, Perez CA, Kuske RR, et al. Locally advanced (noninflammatory) carcinoma of the breast: results and comparison of various treatment modalities. *Int J Radiat Oncol Biol Phys.* 1991;21(2):311-318.

66. Fisher B, Bryant J, Wolmark N, et al. Effect of preoperative chemotherapy on the outcome of women with operable breast cancer. *J Clin Oncol.* 1998;16(8):2672-2685.

67. Danforth DN Jr, Zujewski J, O'Shaughnessy J, et al. Selection of local therapy after neoadjuvant chemotherapy in patients with stage IIIA,B breast cancer. *Ann Surg Oncol.* 1998;5(2):150-158.

68. Rouzier R, Extra JM, Carton M, et al. Primary chemotherapy for operable breast cancer: incidence and prognostic significance of ipsilateral breast tumor recurrence after breast-conserving surgery. *J Clin Oncol.* 2001;19(18):3828-3835.

69. Veronesi U, Bonadonna G, Zurrida S, et al. Conservation surgery after primary chemotherapy in large carcinomas of the breast. *Ann Surg.* 1995;222:612-618.

70. Clouth B, Chandrasekharan S, Inwang R, et al. The surgical management of patients who achieve a complete pathological response after primary chemotherapy for locally advanced breast cancer. *Eur J Surg Oncol.* 2007; 33:961-966.

71. Makris A, Powles TJ, Ashley SE, et al. Reduction in the requirements for mastectomy in a randomized trial of neoadjuvant chemoendocrine therapy in primary breast cancer. *Ann Oncol.* 1998;9(11):1179-1184.

72. Khanna M, Mark R, Silverstein M, et al. Breast conservation management of breast tumours 4 cm or larger. *Arch Surg.* 1992;127:1038-1043.

73. Asgeirsson KS, McCulley SJ, Pinder SE, Macmillan RD. Size of invasive breast cancer and risk of local recurrence after breast conservation therapy. *Eur J Cancer.* 2003;39(17):2462-2469.

74. Berry DA, Cronin KA, Plevritis SK, et al. Effect of screening and adjuvant therapy on mortality from breast cancer. *N Engl J Med.* 2005;353(17):1784-1792.

75. Newman EA, Guest AB, Helvie MA, et al. Changes in surgical management resulting from case review at a breast cancer multidisciplinary tumor board. *Cancer.* 2006;107(10):2346-2351.

76. van Tienhoven G, Voogd AC, Peterse JL, et al. Prognosis after treatment for loco-regional recurrence after mastectomy or breast conserving therapy in two randomised trials (EORTC 10801 and DBCG-82TM). EORTC Breast Cancer Cooperative Group and the Danish Breast Cancer Cooperative Group. *Eur J Cancer.* 1999;35(1):32-38.

77. Voogd AC, van Oost FJ, Rutgers EJ, et al. Long-term prognosis of patients with local recurrence after conservative surgery and radiotherapy for early breast cancer. *Eur J Cancer.* 2005;41(17):2637-2644.

78. Alpert TE, Lannin DR, Haffty BG, et al. Ipsilateral breast tumor recurrence after breast conservation therapy: outcomes of salvage mastectomy

vs. salvage breast-conserving surgery and prognostic factors for salvage breast preservation. *Int J Radiat Oncol Biol Phys.* 2005;63(3):845-851.

79. Huang E, Buchholz TA, Meric F, et al. Classifying local disease recurrences after breast conservation therapy based on location and histology: new primary tumors have more favorable outcomes than true local disease recurrences. *Cancer.* 2002;95(10):2059-2067.

80. Dalberg K, Mattsson A, Sandelin K, et al. Outcome of treatment for ipsilateral breast tumor recurrence in early-stage breast cancer. *Breast Cancer Res Treat.* 1998;49(1):69-78.

81. Wapnir IL, Anderson SJ, Mamounas EP, et al. Prognosis after ipsilateral breast tumor recurrence and locoregional recurrences in five National Surgical Adjuvant Breast and Bowel Project node-positive adjuvant breast cancer trials. *J Clin Oncol.* 2006;24(13):2028-3207.

82. Meric F, Mirza NQ, Vlastos G, et al. Positive surgical margins and ipsilateral breast tumor recurrence predict disease-specific survival after breast-conserving therapy. *Cancer.* 2003;97(4):926-933.

83. Huang EH, Tucker SL, Strom EA, et al. Postmastectomy radiation improves local-regional control and survival for selected patients with locally advanced breast cancer treated with neoadjuvant chemotherapy and mastectomy. *J Clin Oncol.* 2004;22(23):4691-4699.

84. Fowble B, Solin LJ, Schultz DJ, et al. Breast recurrence following conservative surgery and radiation: patterns of failure, prognosis, and pathologic findings from mastectomy specimens with implications for treatment. *Int J Radiat Oncol Biol Phys.* 1990;19(4):833-842.

85. Kurtz JM, Jacquemier J, Brandone H, et al. Inoperable recurrence after breast-conserving surgical treatment and radiotherapy. *Surg Gynecol Obstet.* 1991;172(5):357-361.

86. Recht A, Schnitt SJ, Connolly JL, et al. Prognosis following local or regional recurrence after conservative surgery and radiotherapy for early stage breast carcinoma. *Am J Radiat Oncol Biol Phys.* 1989;17(1):3-9.

87. Huston TL, Simmons RM. Inflammatory local recurrence after breast conservation therapy for noninflammatory breast cancer. *Am J Clin Oncol.* 2005;28(4):431-432.

88. Shen J, Hunt KK, Mirza NQ, et al. Predictors of systemic recurrence and disease-specific survival after ipsilateral breast tumor recurrence. *Cancer.* 2005;104(3):479-490.

89. Ring A, Webb A, Ashley S, et al. Is surgery necessary after complete clinical remission following neoadjuvant chemotherapy for early breast cancer? *J Clin Oncol.* 2003;21(24):4540-4545.

90. Kuerer HM, Arthur DW, Haffty BG, et al. Repeat breast-conserving surgery for in-breast local breast carcinoma recurrence: the potential role of partial breast irradiation. *Cancer.* 2004;100(11):2269-2280.

91. Santiago RJ, Harris EE, Qin L, et al. Similar long-term results of breast-conservation treatment for stage I and II invasive lobular carcinoma compared with invasive ductal carcinoma of the breast. *Cancer.* 2005;103:2447-2454.

92. McGuire SE, Gonzalez-Angulo AM. Postmastectomy radiation improves the outcome of patients with locally advanced breast cancer who achieve a pathologic complete response to neoadjuvant chemotherapy. *Int J Radiat Oncol Biol Phys.* 2007;68(4):1004-1009.

93. Abner AL, Recht A, Eberlein T, et al. Prognosis following salvage mastectomy for recurrence in the breast after conservative surgery and radiation therapy for early-stage breast cancer. *J Clin Oncol.* 1993;11(1):44-48.

94. Meijer-van Gelder ME, Look MP, Bolt-de Vries J, et al. Breast-conserving therapy: proteases as risk factors in relation to survival after local relapse. *J Clin Oncol.* 1999;17(5):1449-1457.

95. Port ER, Garcia-Etienne CA, Park J, et al. Reoperative sentinel lymph node biopsy: a new frontier in the management of ipsilateral breast tumor recurrence. *Ann Surg Oncol.* 2007;14(8):2209-2214.

96. Cox CE, Furman BT, Kiluk JV, et al. Use of reoperative sentinel lymph node biopsy in breast cancer patients. *J Am Coll Surg.* 2008;207(1):57-61.

97. Intra M, Trifirò G, Viale G, et al. Second biopsy of axillary sentinel lymph node for reappearing breast cancer after previous sentinel lymph node biopsy. *Ann Surg Oncol.* 2005;12(11):895-899.

98. Boughey JC, Ross MI, Babiera GV, et al. Sentinel lymph node surgery in locally recurrent breast cancer. *Clin Breast Cancer.* 2006;7(3):248-253.

99. Newman LA. Lymphatic mapping and sentinel lymph node biopsy for locally recurrent breast cancer: new clues to understanding the biology of these small relapses. *Ann Surg Oncol.* 2007;14:2182.

100. Newman EA, Cimmino VM, Sabel MS, et al. Lymphatic mapping and sentinel lymph node biopsy for patients with local recurrence after breast-conservation therapy. *Ann Surg Oncol.* 2006;13(1):52-57.

CHAPTER 62

Sentinel Lymph Node Biopsy

Jennifer R. Garreau
Armando E. Giuliano

The sentinel node (SN) concept as currently applied to breast cancer and melanoma is predated by the idea that a single lymph node can reflect the tumor status of an entire lymphatic basin. Famous examples include the Virchow node (left supraclavicular node to which gastric cancer spreads), the Sister Mary Joseph node (an umbilical lymph node that represents metastatic intra-abdominal spread), the Delphian node of the thyroid, and the Cloquet node of the groin.[1] The concept of the SN technique as first described by Cabanas in 1977 for use in squamous cell carcinoma of the penis was based on detailed penile lymphangiographic studies that demonstrated consistent drainage of the penile lymphatics into a node located near the saphenous/femoral vein junction.[2] When this so-called SN was negative for tumor, metastasis to other ilioinguinal lymph nodes did not occur. Cabanas therefore postulated that the status of the SN could be used to decide whether or not regional lymphatic clearance was necessary. Although multiple studies have since found that a fixed-location SN is an unreliable indicator of nodal status in penile cancer, this work paved the way for mapping the SN in patients with solid cancers that drain via the lymphatics.

Sentinel node biopsy (SNB) for melanoma was first described in 1992 by Morton and colleagues.[3] They defined the SN as the first draining node of a tumor. If nodal spread has occurred, it will target the SN before other lymph nodes. Therefore, if the SN is tumor negative, the other nodes should be negative as well. These investigators showed that when a vital blue dye is injected around the site of the primary melanoma, the SN is the first blue-staining node in the lymphatic basin and therefore the first nodal site of lymphatic drainage from a primary cutaneous melanoma. After identification and removal of the SN, Morton et al performed a completion lymph node dissection for that nodal basin.[3] They found that the pathologic status of

the SN was a highly accurate predictor of the pathologic status of the entire nodal basin. These findings suggested that melanoma could be accurately staged with procedures that were far less extensive than complete nodal dissections.

The status of the axilla is the most important prognostic factor in breast cancer. Before the development of SNB, an axillary lymph node dissection (ALND) was required to stage the axilla. This procedure can be associated with significant morbidity, including nerve damage or lymphedema. In an effort to spare patients from these potential complications, attempts were made to develop a less invasive technique for identification of positive nodes in the axilla. Giuliano and colleagues[4] successfully adapted SNB for breast cancer and began a pilot study in 1991. This study was reported in 1994 after 174 lymphatic mapping procedures were performed using a vital dye injected at the primary breast cancer site. SNs were identified in 114 (65.5%) of 174 procedures and accurately predicted axillary nodal status in 109 (95.6%) of 114 cases. On the basis of these results, they concluded that intraoperative lymphatic mapping could accurately identify the SN and that this technique could enhance staging accuracy while potentially avoiding the need for ALND. SNB has also been performed using radiolabeled colloid and/or blue dye and is now considered the standard of care for staging of the axilla in breast cancer.

INDICATIONS AND CONTRAINDICATIONS

SNB can successfully stage the axilla after any type of diagnostic biopsy and regardless of the size and location of the primary tumor. SNB can be used in males with breast cancer,[5] in elderly and/or obese patients, and in patients with multicentric breast cancer.

TABLE 62-1 Absolute Contraindications to Sentinel Node Biopsy

Use of dye in patient with history of dye allergy
Use of dye in pregnancy
Inflammatory breast cancer

Contraindications

There are few absolute contraindications to SNB for patients with clinically node-negative breast cancer. These include allergy to tracers used for lymphatic mapping, dye in pregnancy, and inflammatory breast cancer (Table 62-1).

Pregnancy

Use of blue dye for lymphatic mapping is contraindicated by pregnancy because the ability of the dye to enter the fetal circulation and its potential effects on the fetus are not completely understood. However, radiolabeled colloids can be safely used in pregnant patients.[6] Some centers do offer lymphoscintigraphy and SNB for these women; however, most surgeons prefer routine (elective) ALND if the patient is pregnant.[7] Alternatively, if a patient is close to term, it is sometimes possible to wait until after the patient delivers and then perform SNB.

Inflammatory Breast Cancer

In patients with inflammatory breast cancer, the lymphatic channels are occluded and may not follow a normal drainage pattern due to the typically extensive lymphatic involvement. There are currently insufficient data to support performing SNB in patients with inflammatory breast cancer, and it should not be performed.

Areas of Controversy

A few controversies regarding the proper use of SNB still exist. These areas of controversy will be discussed below (Table 62-2).

Ductal Carcinoma In Situ

The incidence of ductal carcinoma in situ (DCIS) has increased since introduction of routine screening mammography; DCIS is now found in 15% to 20% of all screening mammograms.[8,9] Even though the neoplastic cells in DCIS have not extended through the basement membrane, 5% to 15% of patients with

TABLE 62-2 Areas of Controversy for Use of Sentinel Node Biopsy

Ductal carcinoma in situ
Clinically positive axilla
Prior axillary surgery
Prophylactic mastectomy
Neoadjuvant chemotherapy

DCIS will have tumor-positive SNs, and 10% to 20% will subsequently be found to have invasive cancer.[10-13] However, not all patients with DCIS need SNB. We recommend SNB for patients whose DCIS is large (larger than 4 cm), palpable, extensive, high-grade, or requires mastectomy.

Clinically Positive Axilla

Although ALND is the standard of care in patients with clinically palpable axillary disease, approximately 30% of patients with clinically positive axillae will have histologically tumor-negative axillary nodes.[14,15] Preoperative axillary ultrasound and ultrasound-guided fine-needle aspiration (FNA) are useful in this situation.[16] Patients with positive FNA results can undergo ALND, whereas patients with negative FNA results can undergo SNB, with ALND if an SN contains tumor. However, all clinically palpable or suspicious nodes should be removed at the time of surgery, regardless of uptake of the mapping agent.

Prior Axillary Surgery

It was previously thought that prior axillary surgery disrupted the normal lymphatic drainage pattern, thereby removing SNB as an option for these patients. Recent studies have shown that reoperative SNB is possible and is dependent on the number of lymph nodes removed.[17] It will become progressively more common to see patients with local recurrence after prior axillary surgery. Although we do not believe that prior axillary surgery is an absolute contraindication to SNB, the possibility of lymphatic disruption mandates use of lymphoscintigraphy in addition to dye-directed lymphatic mapping.

Prophylactic Mastectomy

Prophylactic mastectomy is an accepted form of treatment for women who have a strong family history of breast cancer or are carriers of BRCA1 and BRCA2 genetic mutations. The reported risk of occult breast cancer in a mastectomy specimen is approximately 5%.[18] Once the breast is removed, the ability to perform an SNB is lost. Therefore, if an invasive cancer is identified in the mastectomy specimen, axillary staging can only be accomplished with an ALND. Performing SNB at the time of prophylactic mastectomy spares the patient an additional operation for ALND if invasive cancer is later identified in the mastectomy specimen. A study by Dupont et al[19] evaluated patients who underwent prophylactic mastectomy for either lobular carcinoma in situ or BRCA1/2 genetic mutations: 2 of 57 patients had metastatic nodal disease in the absence of carcinoma in the breast and then underwent a complete axillary node dissection. Additionally, 2 patients had invasive breast cancer with negative SNs and were spared an ALND. Therefore, 7% (4 of 57) of patients in this study had a change in their surgical management as a result of these findings.[19] SNB should be offered to all women undergoing prophylactic mastectomy who have an increased risk for invasive breast carcinoma, although it is often not helpful.

Neoadjuvant Chemotherapy

Neoadjuvant chemotherapy (NAC) can downstage large or locally advanced breast cancers, thereby allowing breast-conserving surgery. The exact timing and optimal use of SNB in this setting continues to be a matter of debate. Those in favor of SNB before NAC argue that axillary staging is critical to determine which patients will subsequently need an ALND or axillary radiation.[7] It is thought that NAC results in excessive fibrosis of the tumor-involved lymphatics and that obstruction of these lymphatic channels with cellular debris or tumor emboli may lead to inaccurate lymphatic mapping.[20] A retrospective study of the National Surgical Adjuvant Breast and Bowel Project (NSABP) B-27 NAC trial demonstrated that the overall rate of SN identification was 84.8%. The SN identification rate was 90% with a radiocolloid mapping agent, 77% with blue dye, and 88% with both agents. The false-negative rate (FNR) was 14% with blue dye, 5% with radiocolloid, and 9.3% with both agents.[21] A recent meta-analysis by Xing et al[22] found that the SN identification rate after NAC was 90% and the FNR was 12%. These results are inferior to those usually seen for SNB and suggest that SNB performed after NAC is not always reliable. An American Society of Clinical Oncology (ASCO) panel from 2005 has concluded that there are insufficient data to suggest appropriate timing of SNB for patients receiving NAC.[23] Furthermore, there is no evidence that a tumor-negative SNB specimen after NAC eliminates the need to treat the axilla. At our institution, we commonly perform SNB before NAC because we believe this more accurately stages the axilla, and those patients who are SN negative can avoid axillary treatment.

PREOPERATIVE LYMPHOSCINTIGRAPHY

Preoperative lymphoscintigraphy can identify the lymphatic drainage basin and approximate the location of the SN(s). It is very helpful in patients with melanoma because skin lesions, particularly those on the trunk or the head/neck, may have multiple possible drainage patterns. However, preoperative lymphoscintigraphy is not routine for SN localization in patients with breast cancer. Although it can identify internal mammary SNs, the clinical importance of nonaxillary SNs remains controversial.[24] Borgstein et al[25] reported that the use of an intraoperative gamma probe was superior to preoperative lymphoscintigraphy in identifying radioactive nodes. Intraoperative use of a handheld gamma probe is sufficient for identification of radioactive SNs, but preoperative lymphoscintigraphy may be performed, especially if extra-axillary SNs are sought.

RADIOLABELED COLLOID VERSUS BLUE DYE

The technique of SNB has been described using radiolabeled colloid, blue dye, or a combination of the two. Krag et al[26] first described the use of a radioisotope and a handheld gamma probe to identify the SN in 1993. The SN was identified in 18 of 22 patients in this study, for an identification rate of 82%. In 1994, Giuliano et al[4] reported his experience using 1% isosulfan blue in 172 patients with T1 to T3 breast cancers. This group reported an identification rate of 65.5% (114 of 174), and the nodal status was accurately predicted in 109 of 114 cases (95.6%). Sentinel nodes identified in the last 87 procedures

were 100% predictive. Albertini et al[27] in 1996 reported an identification rate of 92% using a combination of both of these techniques. A recent meta-analysis evaluating these 3 techniques reviewed 69 studies and over 8000 patients who underwent SNB. This study found that the success rate for SN identification was 89.2% with radioisotope alone, 83.1% with blue dye alone, and 91.9% when both techniques were used. The FNRs were 8.8%, 10.9%, and 7.0%, respectively.[28] This suggests that the combination technique is the most accurate and reliable in inexperienced hands. Finally, in 1999, Morrow et al[29] reported the only randomized trial comparing blue dye with radiolabeled colloid. Patients with clinical T1 or T2 tumors and negative axilla were randomized to SNB with blue dye (n = 50) or blue dye plus radiolabeled colloid (n = 42). The SN predicted the status of the axilla in 96% of cases. There was no difference in the SN identification rate between the 2 groups (88% for blue dye alone, 86% for blue dye plus radiolabeled colloid). These authors concluded that there was no advantage to using blue dye plus radiolabeled colloid over blue dye alone, even for surgeons learning the technique. At our institution, we use blue dye alone, unless the patient has had prior axillary surgery, has a contraindication to dye (eg, allergy or pregnancy), or we seek extra-axillary SNs. However, the technique used should be determined by the training and experience of the surgeon.

TYPES OF RADIOISOTOPE AND BLUE DYE

In the United States, technetium sulfur colloid and isosulfan blue dye (Lymphazurin 1%, United States Surgical, a division of Tyco Healthcare Group LP, Norwalk, CT) are the most widely used agents for lymphatic mapping.[20] Isosulfan blue dye has the disadvantage of being associated with a 1% to 3% incidence of allergic and anaphylactic reactions such as urticaria, rash, blue hives, pruritus, and hypotension.[30,31] The American College of Surgeons Oncology Group Z0010 study, a prospective multicenter trial designed to evaluate the prognostic significance of micrometastases in SNs, reported anaphylaxis in 0.1% of patients (5 of 4975) in whom isosulfan blue dye was used.[32] Methylene blue is equivalent to isosulfan blue, is less expensive, and has a lower risk of allergic reactions. However, it can cause skin and nipple necrosis when injected intradermally and as such, it must be used in a 1:2 dilution.[33,34]

SITE OF INJECTION

When initially described by Giuliano et al,[4] blue dye was injected in a peritumoral fashion, or if the primary tumor had been excised, it was injected into the wall of the biopsy cavity and surrounding breast parenchyma. In 1997, Veronesi et al[35] reported that subdermal injection of radioisotope resulted in an identification rate of 98.2% and an FNR of 4.7%. It is now known that because the breast and its overlying skin have the same axillary lymphatic drainage pattern, the mapping agent can be injected at intradermal, subdermal, periareolar, or subareolar sites.[36] Subareolar injection is expeditious and accurate for multicentric and unicentric disease.[37] However, subareolar and dermal injections of blue dye can cause persistent discoloration of the breast that can last for several months,[20] and this method cannot evaluate for nonaxillary nodes. Several studies have reported high identification and concordance rates for subareolar injection of blue dye and/or radioisotope.[38-40] A study by Rodier et al[41] in 2007 using both blue dye and radioisotope found that periareolar injection was equivalent to peritumoral injection in SN detection. Multiple other studies have supported the finding that identification rates using subareolar and peritumoral injection are similar.[39,42,43] Therefore, surgeons should use the technique that is most familiar to them.

NUMBER OF SENTINEL NODES REMOVED DURING SN BIOPSY

Most surgeons remove 1 to 3 nodes during SNB.[20] If a radiolabeled tracer is used, the number of "hot" nodes identified will depend on the timing of injection, the concentration of radiolabeled colloid, and the definition of hot. Various definitions exist and include the following: the hottest node, 10 × background, 3 × background, and all nodes with counts more than 10% of the hottest SN. Chung et al[44] recently evaluated the use of the 10% rule to define the SN when using radiolabeled colloid. The 10% rule was first described by Martin and McMasters in 2000[45] and dictates that all SNs with counts more than 10% of the most radioactive node be removed. To evaluate this, Chung and colleagues retrospectively reviewed a prospective SN database from Memorial Sloan-Kettering Cancer Center that included 6519 patients. They found that the 10% rule identified 98.3% of positive nodes in patients with multiple SNs and concluded that this is a reliable guideline for SNB.

Multiple studies have demonstrated that removal of 2 to 3 nodes identifies 93% to 99% of node-positive patients, and removal of 4 nodes identifies 100% of node-positive patients.[46-48] The Axillary Lymphatic Mapping Against Nodal Axillary Clearance (ALMANAC) Trialists group found that 99.6% of node-positive patients were identified by removing no more than 4 SNs. The FNR was 10% when 1 SN was removed and 1% when 2 or more SNs were removed.[49] These studies suggest that removal of more than 4 SNs is unnecessary.

INTRAOPERATIVE MAPPING

After induction of general anesthesia or sedation with local anesthesia, 5 mL of isosulfan blue dye, or dilute methylene blue, is injected into the parenchyma around the tumor or into the subareolar region, depending on the technique most familiar to the surgeon (Fig. 62-1). The breast is then massaged for 5 minutes to push the dye along the afferent lymphatics to the axilla. A transverse incision of approximately 3 cm is made just below the hair-bearing region of the axilla (Fig. 62-2A). The incision is carried through the subcutaneous tissue and the axillary fascia (Fig. 62-2B). Blunt dissection is then performed until a blue-stained lymphatic tract is identified. The dye-filled lymphatic tract is then traced to the first blue-stained node (Fig. 62-3). If possible, the tract is also followed proximally to the tail of the breast to ensure that the identified lymph node

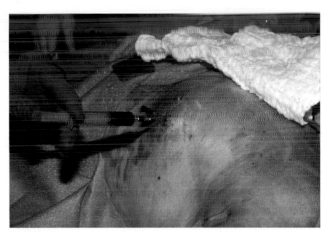

FIGURE 62-1 Wire-localized peritumoral injection.

is the most proximal lymph node and thus the SN. At this point, the SN is excised. During this dissection, care should be taken to grasp the tissue around the node rather than the node itself. The key in identifying the SN is to identify and follow

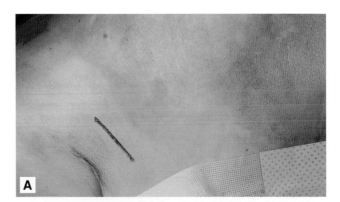

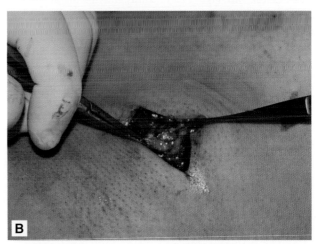

FIGURE 62-2 **A.** The planned site of the axillary incision for sentinel node biopsy procedure can be seen at the inferior edge of the hair-bearing area of the axilla. **B.** The incision is carried through the subcutaneous tissue and the axillary fascia. In this case, a blue node was identified immediately below the axillary fascia, as shown in this picture.

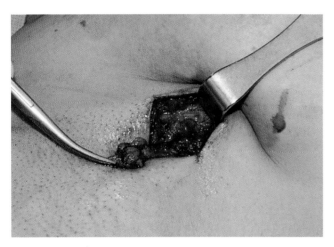

FIGURE 62-3 A blue-stained lymphatic tract is identified leading to the sentinel node. In this case, 2 lymphatic tracts can be easily seen.

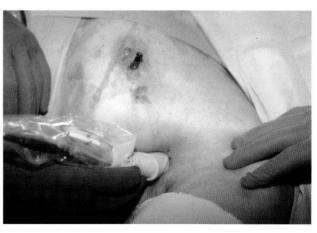

FIGURE 62-5 When radiolabeled colloid is used, a probe is placed in the axillary region to identify the area of greatest radio-activity. This facilitates placement of the axillary incision. The probe is also intermittently placed in the axillary field during the operation so that dissection is in the direction of greatest radioactivity.

the dye-filled lymphatic tract to the node itself as opposed to looking directly for the SN. This is why the technique was originally termed "lymphatic mapping."

If a radioactive tracer is used, the timing of injection may vary from several hours before the procedure to the day prior. At our institution, tracer is usually injected the morning of surgery and lymphoscintigraphy is performed (Fig. 62-4). Intraoperatively, a handheld gamma probe is used to identify a "hot spot" or the area of maximal radioactivity on the skin

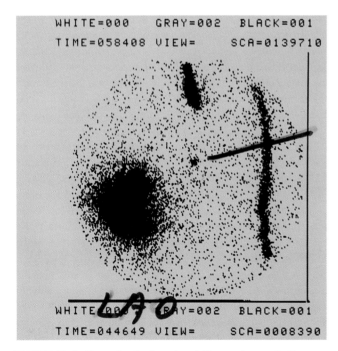

```
WHITE=000    GRAY=002    BLACK=001
TIME=058408  VIEW=        SCA=0139710
```

```
WHITE=000    GRAY=002    BLACK=001
TIME=044649  VIEW=        SCA=0008390
```

FIGURE 62-4 Example of a lymphoscintigram demonstrating drainage to a single sentinel node in the ipsilateral axilla. The line points to the area of maximal uptake in the axilla, which corresponds to the sentinel node.

overlying the axilla. The hot spot can then be used to guide the placement for the axillary incision (Fig. 62-5). Dissection is also facilitated by intermittently placing the probe in the axillary field and dissecting in the direction of greatest radioactivity. If blue dye is used in conjunction with the radiolabeled colloid, the SN should be both hot and blue. All blue, hot, or suspicious-appearing nodes are excised.

HISTOPATHOLOGIC ANALYSIS

The identification of an SN allows for more focused histopathologic evaluation of nodes that may potentially harbor metastatic disease. This may be accomplished intraoperatively using touch-prep or frozen-section analysis or with permanent section analysis, including hematoxylin and eosin (H&E) staining and immunohistochemistry (IHC). Intraoperative analysis of the SN allows ALND to be performed at the same operation should metastatic disease be identified in the SN. Imprint cytology has been shown to be rapid and effective with 88% sensitivity for macrometastases (larger than 2 mm), but only 22% for micrometastases (0.2-2 mm).[50] Frozen-section analysis does have better sensitivity than imprint cytology, but is associated with tissue destruction, interference with subsequent pathologic analysis, and incomplete sections.[20] A skilled cytopathologist is necessary for touch-prep analysis.

Focused histopathologic analysis of the SN with IHC and multilevel sectioning facilitates the detection of micrometastases (0.2-2 mm) and isolated tumor cells (ITCs) or clusters (smaller than 0.2 mm). This allows for possible upstaging in approximately 10% of patients who have negative SNs by H&E analysis but are found to have micrometastases.[51] The clinical significance of micrometastases remains controversial, and the ASCO 2005 guidelines do not recommend routine use of IHC analysis for the evaluation of SNs in breast cancer.[23]

At our institution, we do not perform frozen section, but prefer permanent section analysis. The reasons for this are severalfold. One is to avoid intraoperative false negatives, which can cause significant psychological trauma to the patient. Permanent section analysis also allows for a more in-depth discussion with the patient about ALND should this become necessary. Finally, this decreases the stress for the patient at the time of surgery, as she may be anxious about what will actually happen during the operation (ie, will she wake up to find that she has had an axillary dissection).

ACCURACY AND FEASIBILITY OF SNB

Several studies have demonstrated the safety and efficacy of SNB. Giuliano et al[52] prospectively evaluated the safety and efficacy of SNB in 122 women with primary invasive breast cancers 4 cm or smaller and no axillary lymphadenopathy. Lymphatic mapping and SNB were performed using a vital blue dye. Completion ALND was performed at the time of SNB if no SN was identified or if a frozen section of this node contained tumor cells. SNB was successful in 124 (99%) of 125 procedures. Twenty (35%) of 58 patients who underwent ALND developed axillary complications, including seroma (n = 9), wound infection (n = 3), hematoma (n = 4) and chronic lymph edema (n = 1). However, only 2 (3%) of 67 patients who underwent SNB without ALND developed local axillary wound complications (1 superficial cellulitis, 1 seroma). No lymph edema was seen in the SN-only group. Veronesi et al[53] randomly assigned 516 patients with primary breast cancers 2 cm or smaller to SNB followed by ALND or to SNB followed by ALND only if the SN was positive. Comparison of SNB and ALND specimens from the same patients showed that SN-based assessment of the nodal basin's tumor status had an overall accuracy of 96.9%, sensitivity of 91.2%, specificity of 100%, and FNR of 8.8%. Patients who underwent SNB without ALND had less pain and numbness, as well as better arm mobility.

The long-term morbidity of SNB versus ALND was recently evaluated by Crane-Okada et al.[54] In this study, 192 female breast cancer survivors who remained disease free for at least 3 years after ALND or SNB with breast-conserving surgery completed a questionnaire and a brief neurosensory physical exam. ALND was associated with a significantly greater late likelihood of subjective arm numbness and arm or hand swelling.

NEED FOR COMPLETION ALND?

In 40% to 60% of SN-positive cases, the SN is the only positive node. Because most of these patients will receive chemotherapy regardless of the status of the remaining nodes, is a completion ALND necessary? Should these patients be subjected to potential operative morbidity without further prognostic, therapeutic, or diagnostic benefit? The Memorial Sloan-Kettering Cancer Center (MSKCC) has evaluated the incidence of axillary recurrence after a tumor-positive SNB without ALND. At a median follow-up of 31 months, the axillary recurrence rate was 0.35% with ALND versus 1.4% without ALND.[55] Other studies have demonstrated no axillary recurrence after 28 to 32 months of follow-up in this subset of patients.[56-58] These results suggest that there is a select group of patients who may not

need ALND. However, this group cannot be reliably identified. Currently, ALND is preferred if a positive SN is identified.

A recent meta-analysis found that if the SN had micrometastases, 15% of non-SNs also were tumor positive; by contrast, if the SN contained ITCs, only 10% of non-SNs were involved.[59] Several studies of patients who did not undergo ALND for SN micrometastases reported no axillary recurrence after 30 to 42 months of follow-up.[56,57,60] The American College of Surgeons Oncology Group (ACOSOG) Z0011 trial was a phase III, controlled, multicenter trial that randomized patients with SN metastases to ALND versus no further surgery. The primary aims of this study were to evaluate overall survival, disease-free survival, locoregional control, and morbidity.[61,62] Unfortunately, the trial was closed in 2004 due to poor accrual rates with more than 900 patients.

FUTURE DIRECTIONS

Clinical Significance of Micrometastases

Several ongoing clinical trials are evaluating the impact of SN micrometastases on survival, locoregional control, and morbidity. These trials include the European Organization for Research and Treatment of Cancer (EORTC) 10981-22023 AMAROS trial, the International Breast Cancer Study Group (IBCSG) 23-01 trial, the NSABP B-32 trial, and the ACOSOG Z0010 trial.

AMAROS is an acronym for After Mapping of the Axilla: Radiotherapy or Surgery. This phase III EORTC trial enrolls patients with operable invasive breast cancer less than 3 cm (T1–T2) and clinically normal regional nodes. All patients undergo SNB; those with positive SNs are randomly assigned to completion ALND or axillary radiotherapy.[63] The main objective of this trial is to compare locoregional control in the 2 treatment arms. A second objective is to determine whether adequate axillary control can be obtained without ALND in patients with a negative SN. The first interim analysis evaluated the first 2000 patients enrolled with unifocal breast cancer (5-30 mm) and clinically negative lymph nodes.[64] Results indicated no major differences in adjuvant systemic therapy between the 2 treatment arms.

The IBCSG trial will randomly assign 1960 patients with T1 or T2 breast cancers and SN micrometastases to completion ALND or no further surgery. The goal is to determine whether ALND is necessary for patients with micrometastatic disease.[65]

The NSABP B-32 trial began in 1999 and has completed accrual. In this randomized trial, patients with early breast cancer undergo SNB followed either by routine ALND or by ALND only for SN metastases. The goal of this trial is to determine whether SNB can achieve the same therapeutic goals as conventional ALND with less morbidity. A secondary aim for this trial is to determine whether patients with IHC-detected micrometastases have worse survival as compared with patients with negative axillary lymph nodes, assessed by both H&E and IHC analysis. The reported overall accuracy of SN resections was 97.1%, with an FNR of 9.8%.[66] The results regarding survival in patients with micrometastases have yet to be published.

The ACOSOG Z0010 trial began in 1999.[61] This trial enrolled patients with clinical T1 or T2, N0, M0 breast cancer who were candidates for breast-conserving therapy. At the time of breast-conserving therapy, patients underwent bilateral iliac crest bone marrow aspirations and SNB. One of the objectives of this trial is to estimate the prevalence and to evaluate the prognostic significance of SN micrometastases detected by IHC. More than 5000 patients have been enrolled, and the study is now closed to patient entry.

Because the results of these studies are still unknown, the ASCO guidelines currently recommend ALND for patients with SN micrometastases.[23] However, routine ALND is not recommended for patients with SN ITCs, because the clinical relevance of these cells has not been established.

Predictive Models for Non–Sentinel Node Metastases

There are several pathologic features associated with non-SN metastases. These include pathologic tumor size larger than 2 cm, lymphovascular invasion, multifocality, SN macrometastasis (larger than 2 mm), extranodal spread, and more than 1 disease-positive node.[67-69] A nomogram from MSKCC to estimate the risk of non-SN metastasis is based on nuclear grade, lymphovascular invasion, multifocality, estrogen receptor status, number of negative SNs, number of positive SNs, pathologic size, and method of detection of SN metastases (ie, IHC, H&E, frozen). This nomogram may indicate the probability of additional metastases and was able to predict non-SN metastases in a prospective evaluation of 373 patients.[70] However, although this nomogram has been validated at MSKCC and at several other institutions, it should only be considered a tool for estimating risk of non-SN metastasis when a positive sentinel node is identified. An ALND still needs to be performed when a tumor-positive SN is identified.[68,71,72]

Molecular Analysis of SN

Current intraoperative frozen-section analysis of SNs is known to have high false-negative rates. Molecular analysis may be more sensitive, but until recently has not been rapid enough for intraoperative use. The GeneSearch Breast Lymph Node (BLN) Assay is a real-time reverse-transcriptase polymerase chain reaction assay that detects nodal metastases greater than 0.2 mm. The BLN assay measures the expression of breast or epithelial cell-specific mammaglobin and cytokeratin 19. Elevated levels of these markers indicate the presence of metastases greater than 0.2 mm. In 2008, Julian et al[73] reported a validation study of the assay in 416 patients. Alternating sections from each SN were processed for permanent-section histology and the BLN assay. The sensitivity of the BLN assay was 97.9% for macrometastases (n = 94) and 56.5% for micrometastases (n = 23). The BLN assay had higher sensitivity (95.6%) and negative predictive value (98.2%) than frozen-section evaluation (sensitivity, 85.6%; negative-predictive value, 94.5%) in 319 patients who had both frozen-section H&E results and BLN assay results. Time for the assay ranged from 36 to 46 minutes for 1 to 3 nodes. This study concluded that the BLN assay allowed for rapid evaluation of 50% of each SN and was more sensitive than current frozen-section technology. Further evaluation of this technology is underway.

SUMMARY

Since its introduction in 1994, the SNB technique has revolutionized the treatment of clinically node-negative breast cancer patients and has now become the preferred treatment for staging the axilla. The indications for SNB continue to evolve. Currently, SNB without further nodal dissection is safe and acceptable for patients with tumor-negative SNs. However, the management of tumor-positive SNs remains ALND. Studies evaluating long-term outcomes after SNB will provide important information that may influence decisions about locoregional treatment in the future.

REFERENCES

1. Mabry H, Giuliano AE. Sentinel node mapping for breast cancer: progress to date and prospects for the future. *Surg Oncol Clin N Am.* 2007;16:55-70.
2. Cabanas RM. An approach for the treatment of penile carcinoma. *Cancer.* 1977;39:456-466.
3. Morton DL, Wen DR, Wong JH, et al. Technical details of intraoperative lymphatic mapping for early stage melanoma. *Arch Surg.* 1992;127:392-399.
4. Giuliano AE, Kirgan DM, Guenther JM, et al. Lymphatic mapping and sentinel lymphadenectomy for breast cancer. *Ann Surg.* 1994;220:391-398; discussion 398-401.
5. Rusby JE, Smith BL, Dominguez FJ, et al. Sentinel lymph node biopsy in men with breast cancer: a report of 31 consecutive procedures and review of the literature. *Clin Breast Cancer.* 2006;7:406-410.
6. Gentilini O, Cremonesi M, Trifiro G, et al. Safety of sentinel node biopsy in pregnant patients with breast cancer. *Ann Oncol.* 2004;15:1348-1351.
7. Amersi F, Hansen NM. The benefits and limitations of sentinel lymph node biopsy. *Curr Treat Options Oncol.* 2006;7:141-151.
8. Ernster VL, Barclay J. Increases in ductal carcinoma in situ (DCIS) of the breast in relation to mammography: a dilemma. *J Natl Cancer Inst Monogr.* 1997;151-156.
9. Ernster VL, Ballard-Barbash R, Barlow WE, et al. Detection of ductal carcinoma in situ in women undergoing screening mammography. *J Natl Cancer Inst.* 2002;94:1546-1554.
10. Wilkie C, White L, Dupont E, et al. An update of sentinel lymph node mapping in patients with ductal carcinoma in situ. *Am J Surg.* 2005;190:563-566.
11. Kell MR, Morrow M. An adequate margin of excision in ductal carcinoma in situ. *BMJ.* 2005;331:789-790.
12. Solin LJ, Fourquet A, Vicini FA, et al. Long-term outcome after breast-conservation treatment with radiation for mammographically detected ductal carcinoma in situ of the breast. *Cancer.* 2005;103:1137-1146.
13. Morrow M, Strom EA, Bassett LW, et al. Standard for the management of ductal carcinoma in situ of the breast (DCIS). *CA Cancer J Clin.* 2002;52:256-276.
14. Fisher B, Wolmark N, Bauer M, et al. The accuracy of clinical nodal staging and of limited axillary dissection as a determinant of histologic nodal status in carcinoma of the breast. *Surg Gynecol Obstet.* 1981;152:765-772.
15. Specht MC, Fey JV, Borgen PI, et al. Is the clinically positive axilla in breast cancer really a contraindication to sentinel lymph node biopsy? *J Am Coll Surg.* 2005;200:10-14.
16. Krishnamurthy S, Sneige N, Bedi DG, et al. Role of ultrasound-guided fine-needle aspiration of indeterminate and suspicious axillary lymph nodes in the initial staging of breast carcinoma. *Cancer.* 2002;95:982-988.
17. Port ER, Fey J, Gemignani ML, et al. Reoperative sentinel lymph node biopsy: a new option for patients with primary or locally recurrent breast carcinoma. *J Am Coll Surg.* 2002;195:167-172.

18. Hartmann LC, Schaid DJ, Woods JE, et al. Efficacy of bilateral prophylactic mastectomy in women with a family history of breast cancer. *N Engl J Med*. 1999;340:77-84.

19. Dupont EL, Kuhn MA, McCann C, et al. The role of sentinel lymph node biopsy in women undergoing prophylactic mastectomy. *Am J Surg*. 2000;180:274-277.

20. Samphao S, Eremin JM, El-Sheemy M, et al. Management of the axilla in women with breast cancer: current clinical practice and a new selective-targeted approach. *Ann Surg Oncol*. 2008;15:1282-1296.

21. Mamounas EP. Sentinel lymph node biopsy after neoadjuvant systemic therapy. *Surg Clin North Am*. 2003;83:931-942.

22. Xing Y, Foy M, Cox DD, et al. Meta-analysis of sentinel lymph node biopsy after preoperative chemotherapy in patients with breast cancer. *Br J Surg*. 2006;93:539-546.

23. Lyman GH, Giuliano AE, Somerfield MR, et al. American Society of Clinical Oncology guideline recommendations for sentinel lymph node biopsy in early-stage breast cancer. *J Clin Oncol*. 2005;23:7703-7720.

24. Kawase K, Gayed IW, Hunt KK, et al. Use of lymphoscintigraphy defines lymphatic drainage patterns before sentinel lymph node biopsy for breast cancer. *J Am Coll Surg*. 2006;203:64-72.

25. Borgstein PJ, Pijpers R, Comans EF, et al. Sentinel lymph node biopsy in breast cancer: guidelines and pitfalls of lymphoscintigraphy and gamma probe detection. *J Am Coll Surg*. 1998;186:275-283.

26. Krag DN, Weaver DL, Alex JC, et al. Surgical resection and radiolocalization of the sentinel lymph node in breast cancer using a gamma probe. *Surg Oncol*. 1993;2:335-339, discussion 340.

27. Albertini JJ, Lyman GH, Cox C, et al. Lymphatic mapping and sentinel node biopsy in the patient with breast cancer. *JAMA*. 1996;276:1818-1822.

28. Kim T, Giuliano AE, Lyman GH. Lymphatic mapping and sentinel lymph node biopsy in early-stage breast carcinoma: a metaanalysis. *Cancer*. 2006;106:4-16.

29. Morrow M, Rademaker AW, Bethke KP, et al. Learning sentinel node biopsy: results of a prospective randomized trial of two techniques. *Surgery*. 1999;126:714-720; discussion 720-722.

30. Lyew MA, Gamblin TC, Ayoub M. Systemic anaphylaxis associated with intramammary isosulfan blue injection used for sentinel node detection under general anesthesia. *Anesthesiology*. 2000;93:1145-1146.

31. Kuerer HM, Wayne JD, Ross MI. Anaphylaxis during breast cancer lymphatic mapping. *Surgery*. 2001;129:119-120.

32. Wilke LG, McCall LM, Posther KE, et al. Surgical complications associated with sentinel lymph node biopsy: results from a prospective international cooperative group trial. *Ann Surg Oncol*. 2006;13:491-500.

33. Blessing WD, Stolier AJ, Teng SC, et al. A comparison of methylene blue and lymphazurin in breast cancer sentinel node mapping. *Am J Surg*. 2002;184:341-345.

34. Thevarajah S, Huston TL, Simmons RM. A comparison of the adverse reactions associated with isosulfan blue versus methylene blue dye in sentinel lymph node biopsy for breast cancer. *Am J Surg*. 2005;189:236-239.

35. Veronesi U, Paganelli G, Galimberti V, et al. Sentinel-node biopsy to avoid axillary dissection in breast cancer with clinically negative lymph-nodes. *Lancet*. 1997;349:1864-1867.

36. Rubio IT, Klimberg VS. Techniques of sentinel lymph node biopsy. *Semin Surg Oncol*. 2001;20:214-223.

37. Layeeque R, Henry Tillman R, Korourian S, et al. Subareolar sentinel node biopsy for multiple breast cancers. *Am J Surg*. 2003;186:730-735, discussion 735-736.

38. Kern KA. Sentinel lymph node mapping in breast cancer using subareolar injection of blue dye. *J Am Coll Surg*. 1999;189:539-545.

39. Klimberg VS, Rubio IT, Henry R, et al. Subareolar versus peritumoral injection for location of the sentinel lymph node. *Ann Surg*. 1999;229:860-864; discussion 864-865.

40. Kern KA. Concordance and validation study of sentinel lymph node biopsy for breast cancer using subareolar injection of blue dye and technetium 99m sulfur colloid. *J Am Coll Surg*. 2002;195:467-475.

41. Rodier JF, Velten M, Wilt W, et al. Prospective multicentric randomized study comparing periareolar and peritumoral injection of radiotracer and blue dye for the detection of sentinel lymph node in breast sparing procedures: FRANSENODE trial. *J Clin Oncol*. 2007;25:3664-3669.

42. Reitsamer R, Peintinger F, Rettenbacher L, et al. Subareolar subcutaneous injection of blue dye versus peritumoral injection of technetium-labeled human albumin to identify sentinel lymph nodes in breast cancer patients. *World J Surg*. 2003;27:1291-1294.

43. Bauer TW, Spitz FR, Callans LS, et al. Subareolar and peritumoral injection identify similar sentinel nodes for breast cancer. *Ann Surg Oncol*. 2002;9:169-176.

44. Chung A, Yu J, Stempel M, et al. Is the "10% rule" equally valid for all subsets of sentinel-node-positive breast cancer patients? *Ann Surg Oncol*. 2008;15:2728-2733.

45. Martin RC 2nd, Edwards MJ, Wong SL, et al. Practical guidelines for optimal gamma probe detection of sentinel lymph nodes in breast cancer: results of a multi-institutional study. For the University of Louisville Breast Cancer Study Group. *Surgery*. 2000;128:139-144.

46. McCarter MD, Yeung H, Fey J, et al. The breast cancer patient with multiple sentinel nodes: when to stop? *J Am Coll Surg*. 2001;192:692-697.

47. Duncan M, Cech A, Wechter D, et al. Criteria for establishing the adequacy of a sentinel lymphadenectomy. *Am J Surg*. 2004;187:639-642; discussion 642.

48. Zakaria S, Degnim AC, Kleer CG, et al. Sentinel lymph node biopsy for breast cancer: how many nodes are enough? *J Surg Oncol*. 2007;96:554-559.

49. Goyal A, Newcombe RG, Mansel RE. Clinical relevance of multiple sentinel nodes in patients with breast cancer. *Br J Surg*. 2005;92:438-442.

50. Tew K, Irwig L, Matthews A, et al. Meta-analysis of sentinel node imprint cytology in breast cancer. *Br J Surg*. 2005;92:1068-1080.

51. Schreiber RH, Pendas S, Ku NN, et al. Microstaging of breast cancer patients using cytokeratin staining of the sentinel lymph node. *Ann Surg Oncol*. 1999;6:95-101.

52. Giuliano AE, Haigh PI, Brennan MB, et al. Prospective observational study of sentinel lymphadenectomy without further axillary dissection in patients with sentinel node-negative breast cancer. *J Clin Oncol*. 2000;18:2553-2559.

53. Veronesi U, Paganelli G, Viale G, et al. A randomized comparison of sentinel-node biopsy with routine axillary dissection in breast cancer. *N Engl J Med*. 2003;349:546-553.

54. Crane-Okada R, Wascher RA, Flashoff D, et al. Long-term morbidity of sentinel node biopsy versus complete axillary dissection for unilateral breast cancer. *Ann Surg Oncol*. 2008;14:1996-2005.

55. Naik AM, Fey J, Gemignani ML, et al. The risk of axillary relapse after sentinel lymph node biopsy for breast cancer is comparable with that of axillary lymph node dissection: a follow-up study of 4008 procedures. *Ann Surg*. 2004;240:462-468; discussion 468-471.

56. Hwang RF, Gonzalez-Angulo AM, Yi M, et al. Low locoregional failure rates in selected breast cancer patients with tumor-positive sentinel lymph nodes who do not undergo completion axillary dissection. *Cancer*. 2007;110:723-730.

57. Guenther JM, Hansen NM, DiFronzo LA, et al. Axillary dissection is not required for all patients with breast cancer and positive sentinel nodes. *Arch Surg*. 2003;138:52-56.

58. Fant JS, Grant MD, Knox SM, et al. Preliminary outcome analysis in patients with breast cancer and a positive sentinel lymph node who declined axillary dissection. *Ann Surg Oncol*. 2003;10:126-130.

59. Cserni G, Gregori D, Merletti F, et al. Meta-analysis of non-sentinel node metastases associated with micrometastatic sentinel nodes in breast cancer. *Br J Surg*. 2004;91:1245-1252.

60. Langer I, Marti WR, Guller U, et al. Axillary recurrence rate in breast cancer patients with negative sentinel lymph node (SLN) or SLN micrometastases: prospective analysis of 150 patients after SLN biopsy. *Ann Surg*. 2005;241:152-158.

61. White RL Jr, Wilke LG. Update on the NSABP and ACOSOG breast cancer sentinel node trials. *Am Surg*. 2004;70:420-424.

62. Lucci A, McCall LM, Beitsch PD, et al. Surgical complications associated with sentinel lymph node dissection (SLND) plus axillary lymph node dissection compared with SLND alone in the American College of Surgeons Oncology Group Trial Z0011. *J Clin Oncol*. 2007;25:3657-3663.

63. Rutgers EJ, Meijnen P, Bonnefoi H. Clinical trials update of the European Organization for Research and Treatment of Cancer Breast Cancer Group. *Breast Cancer Res*. 2004;6:165-169.

64. Straver ME, Tienhoven G, van de Velde CJ, et al. Patterns of care in the EORTC AMAROS sentinel node trial. Presented at the 2008 American Society of Clinical Oncology Breast Cancer Symposium, Washington, DC, September 5-7, 2008. Abstract.

65. Galimberti V. International Breast Cancer Study Group Trial of sentinel node biopsy. *J Clin Oncol*. 2006;24:210-211.

66. Krag DN, Anderson SJ, Julian TB, et al. Technical outcomes of sentinel-lymph-node resection and conventional axillary-lymph-node dissection in patients with clinically node-negative breast cancer: results from the NSABP B-32 randomised phase III trial. *Lancet Oncol*. 2007;8:881-888.

67. Degnim AC, Griffith KA, Sabel MS, et al. Clinicopathologic features of metastasis in nonsentinel lymph nodes of breast carcinoma patients. *Cancer*. 2003;98:2307-2315.

68. Ponzone R, Maggiorotto F, Mariani L, et al. Comparison of two models for the prediction of nonsentinel node metastases in breast cancer. *Am J Surg*. 2007;193:686-692.

69. Turner RR, Chu KU, Qi K, et al. Pathologic features associated with non-sentinel lymph node metastases in patients with metastatic breast carcinoma in a sentinel lymph node. *Cancer.* 2000;89:574-581.

70. Van Zee KJ, Manasseh DM, Bevilacqua JL, et al. A nomogram for predicting the likelihood of additional nodal metastases in breast cancer patients with a positive sentinel node biopsy. *Ann Surg Oncol.* 2003;10:1140-1151.

71. Lambert LA, Ayers GD, Hwang RF, et al. Validation of a breast cancer nomogram for predicting nonsentinel lymph node metastases after a positive sentinel node biopsy. *Ann Surg Oncol.* 2006;13:310-320.

72. Smidt ML, Kuster DM, van der Wilt GJ, et al. Can the Memorial Sloan-Kettering Cancer Center nomogram predict the likelihood of nonsentinel lymph node metastases in breast cancer patients in the Netherlands? *Ann Surg Oncol.* 2005;12:1066-1072.

73. Julian TB, Blumencranz P, Deck K, et al. Novel intraoperative molecular test for sentinel lymph node metastases in patients with early-stage breast cancer. *J Clin Oncol.* 2008;26:3338-3345.

CHAPTER 63

Axillary Lymph Node Dissection

Heather B. Neuman
Kimberly J. Van Zee

The status of the axillary lymph nodes is the most significant known predictive of long-term survival in patients with breast cancer. Axillary lymph node dissection (ALND) is an effective staging procedure and provides durable local control with a low rate of recurrence (NSABP B-4).[1] Furthermore, although ALND has never been associated with an improvement in overall survival in individual randomized controlled trials (RCT), a meta-analysis of trials comparing ALND with observation suggests that a benefit exists.[2]

INDICATIONS/CONTRAINDICATIONS

ALND has been the traditional means of staging the axilla in patients with breast cancer. However, since the advent of sentinel lymph node mapping, ALND is no longer the preferred staging procedure in patients with small, clinically node-negative breast cancer.[3,4] The role of ALND in current practice is limited to women with locally advanced breast cancer and a subset of women with early breast cancer: in patients with clinically or radiologically apparent nodal disease at the time of presentation, in patients in whom a sentinel lymph node cannot be identified at the time of mapping, and in patients who have undergone a sentinel lymph node biopsy and were found to have an involved lymph node. The ACOSOG Z0011 trial was designed to study whether ALND after identification of a positive sentinel lymph node is associated with a survival benefit compared with observation alone.[5] Its recent closure due to slow accrual ensures that ALND will continue to play a significant role in the management of patients with breast cancer.

Few absolute contraindications to ALND exist. Relative contraindications include comorbidities prohibiting general anesthesia or operative procedures (ie, coagulopathy), preexisting lymphedema, or shoulder immobility.

ANATOMY OF THE AXILLA

Boundaries

The axilla is a pyramidal-shaped space existing between the upper arm and thoracic chest wall and is bounded by the following structures: superiorly by the axillary vein; anteriorly by the pectoralis major and minor (encased within the clavipectoral fascia); posteriorly by the subscapularis, teres major, and scapular insert of the latissimus dorsi muscle; laterally by the latissimus dorsi muscle; and medially by the serratus anterior muscle and chest wall (Fig. 63-1). The apex of the triangle (the highest point of the axillary dissection) is the costoclavicular ligament or Halsted ligament.

Axillary Contents: Pertinent Neurovascular Structures (Fig. 63-2)

The long thoracic nerve arises from C5-7 and passes inferiorly on the lateral surface of the serratus anterior muscle, which it innervates. It is most commonly found within 1 cm of the chest wall, superficial to the investing fascia of serratus anterior muscle. Injury to the long thoracic nerve results in a "winged" scapula.

The thoracodorsal nerve arises from C6-8 and travels inferolaterally on the posterior axillary wall to supply the latissimus dorsi muscle. No obvious deficits are noticeable after transection of the thoracodorsal nerve.

The intercostobrachial nerve is the lateral cutaneous branch of the second intercostal nerve combined with the medial cutaneous nerve of the arm. It travels transversely across the axilla after emerging from the second intercostal space. The intercostobrachial nerve supplies sensory innervation to the skin of the axilla and upper medial arm. It is trauma to this nerve that results in the commonly experienced sensory morbidity after axillary surgery.[6-8]

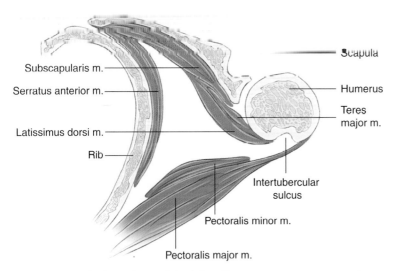

FIGURE 63-1 The boundaries of the left axilla on cross-section. m, Muscle. *(Reproduced, with permission, from Petrek JA, Blackwood MM. Axillary dissection: current practice and technique.* Curr Prob Surg. *1995;32:285.)*

The medial pectoral nerve arises from C8 and T1 (medial cord of the brachial plexus) and enters the deep surface of the pectoralis minor muscle to supply the pectoralis minor and the lateral aspect of pectoralis major. It can often be identified sweeping around the lateral aspect of the pectoralis minor. Division of the medial pectoral nerve may result in muscle atrophy.

The lateral pectoral nerve arises from C5-7 (lateral cord of the brachial plexus) and supplies the pectoralis major muscle. It is seen medial to the pectoralis minor muscle as well as the

medial pectoral nerve. Injury to this nerve would result in significant atrophy of the pectoralis major muscle.

The axillary artery originates medial to the pectoralis minor and crosses the axilla transversely. The second portion of the axillary artery, defined as posterior to the pectoralis minor, has 2 branches often identified during the course of an ALND, the thoracoacromial and long thoracic artery. Distal to these branches is the origination of the thoracodorsal artery, which is joined inferiorly by the thoracodorsal nerve. Axillary venous branches parallel the arterial anatomy.

Axillary Lymph Node Levels

By convention, the axillary lymph nodes are described in 3 levels, defined by the relationship to the pectoralis minor muscle. The level I nodes are found lateral to pectoralis minor. Level II is located posterior and level III medial to pectoralis minor on chest wall. Additional lymph nodes (called Rotter nodes) can be identified in the interpectoral (or Rotter) space, which is the space between the pectoralis major and minor muscles.

Important Congenital Anomalies

Langer arch is one of the more common congenital anomalies observed during an ALND and occurs in 5% of patients. It results from aberrant fibers of the latissimus dorsi muscle extending anteriorly and medially toward the pectoralis major muscle. Presence of a Langer arch may distort the typical axillary anatomy, and failure to recognize its presence may result in residual nodal tissue being left medial to the true latissimus dorsi insertion (the lateral border of the dissection). When identified, a Langer arch is handled by severing the aberrant muscle fibers at the level of lateral axillary vein.

The axillary vein may exist as a bifid or trifid vein. Early recognition and avoiding ligating structures traveling transversely in the axilla until the axillary vein is clearly delineated allows avoidance of injury.

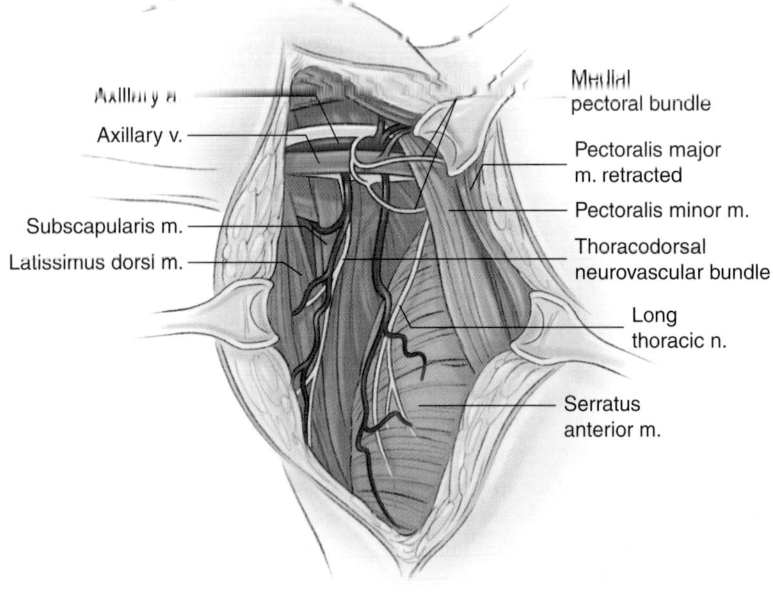

OPERATIVE MANAGEMENT

Preoperative Workup

Preoperative workup includes the standard preoperative clearance, including laboratory tests, chest radiograph, and electrocardiogram when indicated.

Positioning, Prepping, and Draping

The patient is positioned supine on the operating table with the operative arm extended onto an arm board at 90° (Fig. 63-3). A U-shaped "ether

FIGURE 63-2 Axillary contents—pertinent neurovascular structures.

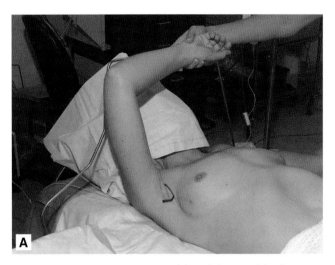
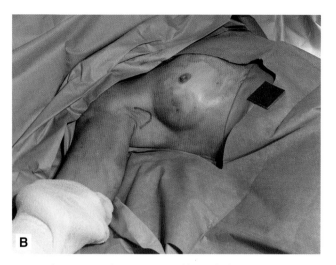

FIGURE 63-3 Patient positioning **(A)** and draping **(B).** The patient is positioned supine on the operating table with the operative arm extended onto an arm board at 90°; a U-shaped "ether screen" can be used to facilitate positioning of the arm anterior to the patient during the procedure. In cases where a mastectomy is being performed, the ALND is often performed through the mastectomy incision. In other circumstances, we prefer a curvilinear incision, placed just within or at the inferior margin of the hairline. © 2008 MSKCC

screen" can be attached to the operating table prior to draping to allow positioning of the arm anterior to the patient during the procedure; positioning of the arm at a 90° angle above the table allows the pectoralis muscles to relax and provides better access into the medial aspects of the axilla. After induction of general anesthesia, a circumferential prep of the upper extremity, ipsilateral shoulder, and chest wall is performed. The arm board is draped with a Mayo stand cover, and the arm is covered with a free drape. Careful positioning to ensure that the arm is not abducted superiorly past 90° is critical to avoid placing stretch on the brachial plexus with a resultant plexopathy. The first assistant generally stands above the arm at the patient's head.

Preoperative Antibiotics

A single dose of a preoperative antibiotic with coverage of skin flora is administered prior to incision.

Incision Planning

Several options are available for the axillary incision, based on the breast surgery planned and the body habitus. In cases where a mastectomy is being performed, the ALND is often performed through the mastectomy incision. In other circumstances, we prefer a curvilinear incision, placed just within or at the inferior margin of the hairline (Fig. 63-3); the incision should extend within the curve of the axilla from the pectoralis major to the medial border of the latissimus dorsi. This incision will be hidden when the woman is standing upright with her arms to her side and is most cosmetically acceptable because it will not be visible when wearing sleeveless tops. Furthermore, the curve provides a longer incision and therefore better exposure than a straight incision extending from the pectoral fold to the latissimus muscle.

Creation of Skin Flaps

After incision of the skin with a scalpel, skin flaps are created. Laterally to the anterior border of latissimus, medially to the lateral aspect of the pectoralis muscle, superiorly to the approximate level of the axillary vein, and inferiorly to the fourth or fifth rib. Skin hooks, rakes, or Adair clamps are employed to facilitate retraction by the assisting surgeon. The operating surgeon applies countertension by retracting on the axillary fat with a laparotomy pad, and electrocautery is used to create flaps. The medial skin flaps will be naturally thinner if a concurrent mastectomy is performed to ensure complete removal of all breast tissue. However, flaps superiorly and laterally should be thicker because the primary goal of an ALND is to remove nodal tissue and not subcutaneous fat; no lymph nodes are present within the axilla superficial to axillary fascia.

Definition of Axillary Boundaries

After skin flaps have been circumferentially raised, the next step is to define the boundaries of the axilla. The lateral boundary is the latissimus dorsi muscle. When identifying the latissimus dorsi muscle, care should be taken to not dissect too superficially because one can easily pass the muscle posteriorly and may disrupt more sensory nerves. Similarly, dissection too medially can result in disruption of the serratus anterior fascia and potential injury to the long thoracic nerve. Medially, the lateral border of the pectoralis major and minor muscles are identified and delineated by incising the clavipectoral fascia. The medial pectoral bundle will be observed because it sweeps either laterally around or through pectoralis minor muscle and should be preserved if possible. The inferior border of the dissection should be inferior to the end of the axillary tail of the breast, typically the fourth or fifth rib, to ensure level I lymph nodes are not left behind. When defining the medial and inferior borders of the axilla, one should be aware of the position of the long thoracic nerve. In general, dissection can be performed anterior to the intercostobrachial nerve without danger of injury to the long thoracic nerve. Additionally, at the level of the fourth or fifth rib, the long thoracic nerve will have already entered the serratus anterior muscle.

Dissection of the Axillary Vein

At this point the axillary vein is approached. Most often when performing an ALND for breast cancer, a lateral approach to the axillary vein is performed. To identify the axillary vein, the latissimus dorsi muscle can be followed superiorly until it becomes tendinous; at this level, it passes posterior to the axillary vein prior to its insertion on the humerus. This marks the lateral boundary of the dissection. The axillary vein may also be identified medially. The medial position of the axillary vein can be estimated by extending an imaginary line in a horizontal course from the groove between the biceps and triceps muscle (when the arm is abducted) toward the medial pectoral bundle; the axillary vein will be found along this line.

Traditional teaching is that lymphedema risk is minimized if the lymphatic tissue on the superior aspect of the vein is preserved. Therefore, the inferior aspect of the axillary vein is skeletonized of lymphatic and fatty tissue, with care being taken to avoid including superior tissue as the specimen is retracted inferiorly. All inferiorly coursing superficial branches from the axillary vein are ligated, either with clips or ties, and sharply divided. The thoracoepigastric vein is the only named superficial branch on the axillary vein and should not be mistaken for the thoracodorsal vein, which enters more posteriorly.

Dissection of Level II and III Lymph Nodes

A Richardson retractor is used to retract the pectoralis major and minor muscles medially to allow access to the level II and III lymph nodes (Fig. 63-4). At this time, repositioning the

arm into a 90° angle anterior to the patient will facilitate the dissection. The medial pectoral nerve will be visualized where it emerges just lateral to pectoralis minor. Lymphatic tissue on the chest wall is retracted inferolaterally as the dissection is continued along the inferior aspect of the axillary vein, clipping or tying any tissue of substance. At this time, the interpectoral (Rotter) space can be palpated and any identified nodes removed.

If necessary when mobilizing the level III nodes, the pectoralis minor muscle can be divided from its insertion on the coracoid process. If the pectoralis minor muscle is transected, great care should be taken to achieve hemostasis; small vessels within the muscle can retract and bleed later. To facilitate hemostasis, the superior portion of the pectoralis minor muscle at the level of the axillary vein can be clamped with a Kocher clamp and then the muscle divided inferior to the clamp with electrocautery. The Kocher clamp prevents retraction of vessels until hemostasis has been confirmed. When combined with a total mastectomy, the division of the pectoralis minor muscle has been labeled a "Patey" modified radical mastectomy, as compared with an "Auchincloss" modified radical mastectomy in which the pectoralis minor muscle is preserved. After level II and III lymph node tissue has been freed from the inferior aspect of the axillary vein, this tissue can be swept laterally into level I of the axilla, preparing the way for exposure of the long thoracic nerve.

Completion of Dissection

The long thoracic nerve lies approximately 1 cm from the chest wall, deep in the axilla and superficial to the investing fascia of the serratus anterior muscle. Often it can be palpated as a "piano string" in the fatty tissue. Care should be taken to avoid dissecting the nerve away from the chest wall. Once identified, a blunt spread in a plane superficial and parallel to the nerve can dissect the nerve from the surrounding axillary tissue and place it back against the chest wall. The tissue lateral and

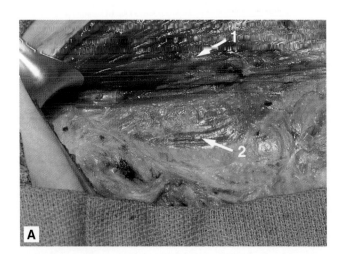
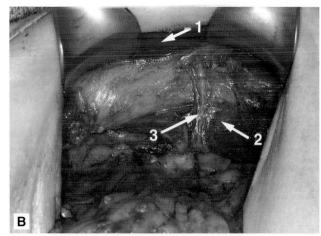

FIGURE 63-4 Relationship of the pectoralis major and minor muscles with the medial pectoral bundle. **A.** The lateral border of the pectoralis major (1) and minor (2) muscles is delineated by incising the clavipectoral fascia. **B.** A Richardson retractor is used to retract the pectoralis major and minor muscles medially. The medial pectoral nerve (3) will be visualized where it emerges just lateral to the pectoralis minor. 1, pectoralis major muscle; 2, pectoralis minor muscle; 3, medial pectoral bundle. (© 2008 MSKCC)

inferior to the long thoracic nerve can be divided with careful protection of the nerve by the surgeon's finger.

At this point, the thoracodorsal neurovascular bundle is identified just lateral to the long thoracic nerve and deep to the thoracoepigastric vein. The remaining axillary tissue between the thoracodorsal and long thoracic nerves is then removed. With gentle inferior traction, a Kelly clamp can be carefully placed onto the residual tissue, after clear visualization of both nerves, and ligated. By sweeping bluntly with a sponge from superior to inferior, the axillary tissue anterior to the subscapularis muscle can then be cleared. Prior to this maneuver, ensure that the long thoracic nerve has been mobilized back to the chest wall and is separate from the axillary tissue (Fig. 63-5).

The lateral aspect of the thoracodorsal neurovascular bundle is then skeletonized. Small branches must be ligated or clipped. This is continued caudad until the nerve and vessels are seen to enter the latissimus dorsi muscle. A branch of the artery and vein turn medially to join the chest wall near the long thoracic nerve; these vessels can be preserved. The axillary specimen is then freed from the latissimus dorsi with electrocautery, and the specimen is passed from the table.

At the completion of the dissection, if clips were not used in the dissection of level II and III nodes, clips should be placed to mark the highest level of dissection (to assist in any necessary radiation treatment planning). Hemostasis is confirmed and a single closed suction drain placed. Skin closure with absorbable sutures is performed.

EXTENT OF DISSECTION

For most women, a dissection of the level I and II lymph nodes alone will provide accurate axillary staging. Fewer than 1% of women have metastases to level III lymph nodes without involvement of level II.[9] Additionally, level III nodes are likely to be negative if the overall burden of disease in the axilla is low. Positive level III axillary nodes are found in only 2% of women with <3 positive axillary nodes and in 19% of women with 4 to 8 positive axillary nodes[9]; similarly, the probability of positive disease in the Rotter space is low. Therefore, a level I and II axillary dissection alone can be considered sufficient for most women unless the axillary nodal burden of disease is high or grossly palpable nodes in level III or Rotter space are present.

POSTOPERATIVE MANAGEMENT

We place an axillary drain at the time of surgery, which remains in place until the output from the drain is <30 to 50 mL/24 hours. At our institution, we encourage range-of-motion activity starting on the first postoperative day.

Guidelines for the prevention of lymphedema in limbs at risk have been formulated (Table 63-1).[10] Currently, little evidence-based literature addressing the prevention of postoperative lymphedema exists, and guideline recommendations are based on expert consensus. In the absence of data supporting or contradicting these recommendations, patient education regarding behavior following an ALND should follow these guidelines.

Historically, avoidance of overuse of the at-risk extremity has been recommended. Two recent studies, one, a retrospective study of breast cancer survivors[11] and the other, a RCT of weight training after axillary surgery,[12] did not demonstrate an association between extremity use and lymphedema development. A recommendation for gradual build-up of activity with careful monitoring of the extremity seems reasonable given the findings of these new studies.

ADEQUACY OF DISSECTION

The National Comprehensive Cancer Network guidelines recommend a level I and II lymph node dissection in all breast cancer patients requiring ALND and that a minimum of 10 lymph nodes be harvested.[13] This recommendation was originally derived from a mathematical model developed by Kiricuta and Tausch in 1992,[14] in which they demonstrated that a minimum of 10 axillary lymph nodes must be examined and found to be negative to ensure with 90% certainty that the remainder of the axilla is node negative. This recommendation has since been supported by a number of institutional studies.[15-17] Note that although harvesting 10 lymph nodes is

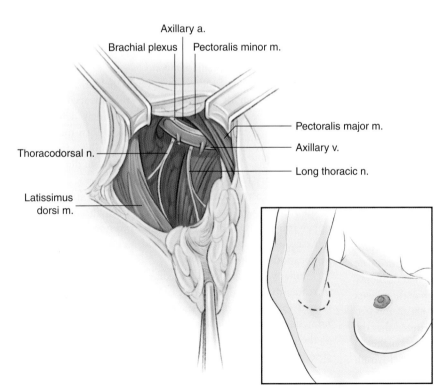

FIGURE 63-5 Identification of thoracodorsal nerve and long thoracic nerve. The remaining axillary tissue between the nerves is removed and axillary tissue swept inferiorly. For purposes of illustration, the contents of the axillary sheath are shown. *(Reproduced, with permission, from Petrek JA, Blackwood MM. Axillary dissection: current practice and technique.* Curr Prob Surg. *1995;32:285.)*

TABLE 63-1 Lymphedema Risk-Reduction Practices

I. Skin care: avoid trauma/infection to reduce infection risk
- Keep extremity clean and dry
- Pay attention to nail care; do not cut cuticles
- If possible, avoid punctures such as injections or blood draws
- Wear gloves while doing activity that may cause skin injury (dishes, gardening, etc.)

II. Activity/lifestyle
- Gradually build up the duration and intensity of any activity or exercise
- Monitor the extremity before and after activity for any change in size, shape, texture, soreness, heaviness, or firmness
- Maintain optimal weight

III. Avoid limb constriction
- If possible, avoid having blood pressure taken in at-risk limb

IV. Compression garments
- Support the at-risk limb during strenuous activity
- Consider wearing a well-fitting compression garment for air travel

V. Extremes of temperature
- Avoid exposure to extreme cold
- Avoid prolonged exposure to heat (particularly hot tubs or saunas)

considered a minimum standard, the median number of lymph nodes removed in a standard ALND is significantly higher (2 recent RCT evaluating sentinel lymph node biopsy versus ALND in breast cancer identified a median 15 [range: 1 to 42][4] and median 16 [range: 1 to 56] nodes[5]).

An incomplete ALND (ie, partial level I) can result in <10 lymph nodes being examined. However, sampling of <10 nodes may not always be indicative of poor surgical technique. A number of studies have suggested that the use of neoadjuvant chemotherapy[18-20] and increasing age[21-23] may be associated with a lower lymph node retrieval. Additionally, surgeon experience and hospital affiliation may play a role.[22,23]

COMPLICATIONS

Since the advent of sentinel lymph node biopsy, a number of prospective and RCTs have been performed comparing immediate morbidity and long-term outcomes of sentinel lymph node biopsy versus ALND.[3-8,24-28] These studies provide us with accurate data on complications and sequelae of ALND in the era of modern surgical techniques (Table 63-2). It should be recognized that the dissection may be more difficult and complication rates higher in patients with previous axillary surgery (including sentinel lymph node biopsy) or who have undergone axillary radiation.

Neurovascular Injuries

The best operative technique to avoid injury to neurovascular structures in the axilla is direct visualization and identification of all relevant structures.

Injury to the long-thoracic nerve occurs infrequently during ALND (<1%). Injury (either by transection, traction, or thermal trauma) results in a winged scapula and is cosmetically unacceptable. Recognition of a transection injury at the time of surgery may allow immediate repair.

The thoracodorsal nerve innervates the latissimus dorsi muscle. Although division of this nerve and accompanying vascular bundle results in no obvious neurologic defect, division would prevent the use of the latissimus dorsi muscle as a future reconstructive flap. In the case of bulky adenopathy, sacrifice of the thoracodorsal neurovascular bundle is sometimes necessary for complete resection of disease.

The intercostobrachial nerve is often divided in the course of an ALND as it crosses transversely from the axilla to the upper arm. Division of this nerve results in numbness and paresthesias on the inner upper arm and may have quality of life implications for women.[6-8]

Similarly, division of the medial pectoral nerve occurs not infrequently during the course of an ALND. Although defects related to division of the medial pectoral nerve may not be immediately noticeable, injury to the nerve may lead to atrophy of the lateral aspect of pectoralis major muscle and result in a cosmetic defect over the long term.

Hematoma

The incidence of postoperative hematoma in the literature is reported at 2% to 10%,[29] although recent prospective trials have reported much lower incidences (0% to 2%).[24,25] The incidence has decreased with the introduction of electrocautery for dissection.

TABLE 63-2 Complications After Axillary Lymph Node Dissection

	Year	Study Design	N	Postoperative Time Reported	Infection	Seroma	Hematoma	Lymphedema (Objective)	Lymphedema (Subjective)	Axillary Sensations (Objective)	Axillary Sensations (Subjective)
Baron et al[7]	2007	Prospective	187	60 mo							55%
Langer et al[25]	2007	Prospective	210	29.5 mo (median)	2.9%	7.6%	0.05%	19.1%			37.7%
Crane-Okada et al[24]	2008	Prospective	68	79.7 mo (mean)	2.9%	8.8%	1.4%	12.3%	30.9%	42.6%	83.1%
McLaughlin et al[27,28]	2008	Prospective	936	60 mo (median)				16%	27%		
Veronesi et al[3]	2003	RCT	100	24 mo				12%			68%
Purushotham et al[8]	2005	RCT	155	12 mo		21%				65%*	
ALMANAC[4]	2006	RCT	405	>12 mo	15%				13%	31%	31%
ACOSOG Z0011[5]	2007	RCT	399	12 mo	8%	14%		11%	13%		39%
Sentinella/GIVOM[26]	2007	RCT	341	24 mo				8%			15%

*Percent ever experiencing during the year after surgery.

TABLE 63-3 Randomized Controlled Trials of the Role of Antibiotics in Breast Surgery

	Year	N	Type of Surgery	Timing of Antibiotic Administration	Follow-up	Infection Rate Without Antibiotics	With antibiotics	p Value
Platt et al[71]	1990	606	Lumpectomy, mastectomy, reduction mammoplasty (40% ALND)	90 min prior to procedure	4-6 wk	12.2%	6.6%	RR = 0.51* (CI, 0.28-0.89)
Wagman et al[72]	1990	118	Partial or total mastectomy (95% ALND)	Preoperative and 6 doses postoperative	30 d	8.5%	5.1%	0.72
Bold et al[73]	1998	92	ALND for breast cancer or melanoma	60 min prior to procedure	4 wk	13.3%	5.7%	0.08
Gupta et al[74]	2000	334	Partial or total mastectomy (axillary clearance in majority)	Prior to incision	10-14 d	18.8%	17.7%	0.79
Tejirian et al[30] (meta-analysis)	2006	1307	Breast surgery	Variable	Variable			RR = 0.60* (CI, 0.45-0.31)

*Favoring antibiotics. ALND, axillary lymph node dissection; CI, confidence interval; RR, relative risk.

If possible, aspirin-containing products, nonsteroidal anti-inflammatory drugs, platelet inhibitors such as clopidogrel (Plavix), and anticoagulation should be discontinued at least 1 week prior to surgery. Additionally, over-the-counter supplements, such as gingko biloba, garlic, ginseng, and vitamin E, may interfere with hemostasis and should be avoided. Postoperatively, the use of a supportive brassiere anecdotally decreases the incidence of ecchymosis and clinically evident hematoma.[29]

Wound Infection

In a recent audit of breast surgery in the prospectively collected National Surgical Quality Improvement Program database, the reported incidence of postoperative wound infections was 3.6%.[30] Higher infection rates have been observed when an ALND is included as part of the procedure,[31] with wound infections after ALND reported in 2.9% to 15% of women in recent trials.[4,5,24,25] Additionally, reoperative surgery has been associated with a higher risk of infection.[32] In one study, reoperative surgery was defined broadly to include a prior breast needle biopsy as well as a prior sentinel lymph node biopsy. Although the outcomes after repeat axillary surgery (ie, sentinel lymph node followed by delayed completion ALND) were not reported separately in this study, it is reasonable to conclude that patients undergoing a delayed completion ALND may be at higher risk of postoperative infection than those patients undergoing sentinel lymph node biopsy and ALND in a single procedure. A secondary analysis of the ALMANAC trial[4] compared patients undergoing immediate versus delayed completion ALND after a positive sentinel node. Although no difference in postoperative infection was observed (12% vs 15%; $p = 0.53$), the use of preoperative antibiotics in this trial was not explicitly described, and therefore conclusions regarding the risk of postoperative infection in this setting cannot be definitively made from this study.[33] The majority of postoperative infections resolve with treatment with intravenous or oral antibiotics. If a seroma or abscess is present, drainage should be performed.

The role of preoperative antibiotics in breast surgery is uncertain. Multiple RCTs have been performed and reach disparate conclusions (Table 63-3). A recent meta-analysis of the RCTs of preoperative antibiotics versus placebo in patients undergoing breast surgery was performed by Tejirian et al. In their analysis, the use of preoperative antibiotics was associated with a reduction in infection (relative risk = 0.60; confidence interval [CI] 0.45 to 0.81), and the authors concluded that preoperative antibiotics are beneficial in the prevention of infection.[30] Given that patients undergoing axillary procedures, especially those who have had a previous sentinel lymph node biopsy, may be at higher risk of developing a postoperative infection, the use of preoperative antibiotics in all patients undergoing ALND appears indicated.

Seroma

Some degree of seroma is present in nearly 100% of patients after an ALND and may be considered a consequence of surgery more than a complication. However, the presence of a prolonged seroma may extend recovery and delay initiation of adjuvant therapy. Additionally, as the duration of seroma increases, so does the risk of infection. A variety of techniques for seroma prevention have been attempted with variable results.[34] The evidence suggests that the use of electrocautery for dissection, as opposed to sharp dissection, increases the rate of seroma formation. Surgical techniques aimed at decreasing seroma rates, including operative closure of the dead space after axillary dissection and the use of fibrin sealants, have not consistently been effective.[34] Similarly, the use of postoperative compression dressings do not appear to result in a decrease in seromas and is associated with poor patient compliance.[35]

The impact of axillary drains on the rate of seroma formation has been extensively studied in RCTs.[34] Studies addressing the relative merits of drain versus no drain,[36-38] active versus passive suction,[39,40] high- versus low-pressure suction,[41-43] single versus multiple drains,[44] and early versus late drain removal[45-47] have all been performed. Although the studies are far from definitive, they suggest that the use of a single, closed, low-pressure suction drain may lead to a decrease in seroma.[34] Increased duration of drain use is associated with a higher incidence of infection but does not lead to a difference in seroma formation.

Finally, it has been hypothesized that early postoperative shoulder mobility increases the incidence of seroma formation. In a meta-analysis of 12 RCTs comparing early versus delayed shoulder mobilization after ALND, a statistically significant difference in drainage volume was not observed ($p = 0.12$).[48] However, the combined mean drainage volume was 175 mL lower in the delayed mobilization group ($p = 0.12$), lending some support to a program of delayed arm exercise of 5 to 12 days. The potential benefit of delay in range-of-motion (ROM) exercises on seroma formation must be balanced against the potential negative impact on shoulder morbidity.

Brachial Plexus Neuropathy

Brachial plexus neuropathy most commonly occurs as a result of patient positioning. Located superior to the axillary vessels, the brachial plexus is protected from most direct dissection injuries; however, care must be taken to avoid dissection superior to the axillary vein. Rarely, a component of the brachial plexus drapes inferiorly to the level of the axillary vein and is vulnerable. It is important, therefore, to identify all nerve structures encountered during an ALND prior to transection. Almost all brachial plexus neuropathy due to positioning resolve completely over time with conservative management.

Lymphedema

Lymphedema is one of the most commonly discussed and difficult to define complications observed after ALND. Incidence of lymphedema varies dramatically (6% to 70%) across the literature based on study design, patient population, method of measurement of lymphedema, and length of follow-up.[11,27,28,49,50] Additionally, differences in rates of lymphedema are observed when comparing patient self-report with objective measurement, with patients both under- and overreporting symptoms of lymphedema when compared to their objective measurements.[11,27,28] Clinical symptoms related to lymphedema may be more apparent in patients whose surgery was ipsilateral to their dominant arm, in young patients, or in thin patients. Lymphedema rates seem to increase most rapidly in the first few years postsurgery, with 70% to 80% of women that ultimately develop lymphedema becoming symptomatic during this time period; however, clinically significant lymphedema may develop as long as 20 years after surgery.[11,50]

Studies have correlated rates of lymphedema with the number of nodes removed during the ALND.[27,50-52] Although the number of positive nodes identified has been associated with higher rates of lymphedema in some studies,[50,51] this has not been consistently observed.[53,54] Lymphedema may also be more common in the obese[27,28,52,55] or in women who gain a significant amount of weight postoperatively (over a period of years).[11] Finally, a history of postoperative infection or injury to the ipsilateral arm,[11,27,28,52,55] and axillary radiation[50,54] may increase rates of lymphedema formation.

There are limited treatment options for lymphedema, with the most effective treatment being good prevention (see previous discussion of postoperative management). Good skin care and protection of the skin minimizes the risk of infection in the at-risk extremity. Techniques to facilitate lymphatic drainage within the arm, such as manual lymphatic drainage or massage, are sometimes beneficial. If a reduction in arm volume is observed as a result of these treatments, techniques can be taught to the patient or family for continued management long term. Compression therapy, through compression bandages, compression garments, or pneumatic compression pumps, may also play a role. No medication or surgical intervention has been shown to be effective.[49]

Decreased Range of Motion

Decreased ROM is observed early after ALND, due to self-restriction secondary to pain with movement. However, most limitations resolve over the first 3 to 6 postoperative months as pain resolves, and development of a frozen shoulder is only rarely seen. Physical therapy and ROM exercises can play a critical role in increasing ROM in those with residual limitations.

FUTURE DIRECTIONS

Endoscopic Axillary Surgery

Although the acceptance of sentinel lymph node biopsy as the primary axillary staging technique has decreased the number of patients requiring ALND, there are still a significant number of patients who undergo ALND annually. In an attempt to decrease the morbidity of ALND, minimally invasive endoscopic ALND has been introduced. To date, few prospective studies and little long-term data are available assessing outcomes in patients undergoing endoscopic axillary surgery.[56-58] Available trials have found lower numbers of harvested lymph nodes in endoscopic ALND specimen when compared with the open procedure,[56,59] and studies in which a backup open ALND was performed after the endoscopic procedure identified

"missed" nodes and incomplete axillary clearance.[60,61] The only published long-term outcomes of endoscopic axillary surgery are from Langer et al,[57] who reported a prospective study of 52 patients (median follow-up: 61.9 months). In their study, 8 patients (15%) developed an axillary seroma requiring drainage and 1 patient (2%) suffered a nerve injury resulting in a winged scapula. Two patients (4%) developed port-site metastases at 24 and 29 months postoperative. At last follow-up, minimal functional restrictions were present, and 3 patients (6%) developed lymphedema. Therefore, at the present time, the risk of missed axillary nodes and port-site metastases, accompanied by at best a marginal benefit in morbidity, suggests that endoscopic surgery cannot be considered an acceptable option for definitive axillary clearance.

Seroma Minimization

Postoperative seroma remains a common sequelae of ALND and may prolong recovery and delay treatment. Although no current techniques have been consistently demonstrated to prevent seroma development, new technology continues to emerge that may prove efficacious in minimization of seroma. Continued exploration and application of technological advances in prevention of postoperative seroma is relevant.

Axillary Reverse Mapping

Recent anatomic studies demonstrate that the lymphatic drainage of the arm is unique from that in the breast.[62] Although traditional teaching suggests that avoidance of circumferential dissection of the axillary vein will protect the lymphatic drainage of the arm, the true location of the upper extremity lymphatics is unknown. The goal of axillary reverse mapping (ARM), first described by Thompson et al,[63] is to identify the upper extremity lymphatics and potentially preserve them during an ALND, thus decreasing the risk of postoperative lymphedema. The initial pilot study consisted of 18 patients who underwent ALND after ARM.[63] In 11 of 18 cases, blue lymphatics draining the arm were identified and there was significant variation in the location of the blue lymphatics relative to the axillary vein. The blue ARM nodes were sampled in the first 7 cases and found to be negative for breast cancer. In a second study recently published from France, 23 patients underwent ALND after ARM.[64] In this study, ARM nodes were initially identified by the blue lymphatics and preserved during the ALND. After completing the ALND, these nodes were then harvested and separately analyzed in pathology. In 2 of the 23 patients, ARM failed to map the upper extremity lymphatics. In the remaining 21 patients, 18 had no evidence of disease in the ARM nodes. All 3 patients with involved ARM nodes had significant nodal involvement in the axilla (>10 positive nodes).

These studies demonstrate the potential feasibility of ARM in identifying the lymphatics draining the upper arm and suggest that these lymphatics may be able to be preserved during an ALND. Further study to confirm these findings, and to determine ease of teaching this technique to other surgeons, reproducibility of results, and long-term oncologic outcomes, is necessary.

Patient-Tailored Therapy

Therapy tailored to individual patients is becoming more frequent, with increasing knowledge of prognostic molecular markers. Although the status of the ALND currently remains the most significant factor predictive of breast cancer survival, an increased understanding of the molecular mechanisms of cancer development and progression may decrease the prognostic value of the axillary lymph nodes. This may influence which patients will benefit from an ALND.

In addition, mathematical models to more accurately predict for an individual the risk of sentinel node metastases and the risk of additional nodal metastases in the setting of a positive sentinel node have been created. These nomograms are being increasingly used to direct patient clinical discussions and tailor surgical treatment.[65,66]

NECESSARY FUTURE STUDIES

1. Are outcomes after sentinel lymph node biopsy and ALND equivalent? Is ALND after a negative sentinel lymph node necessary?

   Sentinel lymph node biopsy has become the standard of care for axillary staging in breast cancer. However, the long-term outcomes of patients undergoing observation after a negative sentinel lymph node biopsy are unknown. Specifically, the equivalency of observation alone versus ALND after a negative sentinel lymph node biopsy has not been demonstrated to date in RCTs.

   NSABP-B32 is a RCT designed to answer the question of whether sentinel lymph node biopsy is equivalent to ALND with regard to regional control, disease-free survival, and overall survival.[67] Additionally, comparative morbidity between the 2 procedures will be assessed. Patients with clinically node negative, "operable" breast cancer were randomized to undergo sentinel lymph node biopsy followed by immediate ALND versus sentinel lymph node biopsy with ALND only if the sentinel node is positive. The trial opened in 1999 and closed to accrual in 2004; follow-up is continuing.

2. Can radiotherapy replace surgery for local control of the axilla in breast cancer?

   ALND provides important prognostic staging information and durable local control in the axilla. Sentinel lymph node biopsy alone can determine if positive nodes exist in the axilla with at least 90% certainty, and in current treatment algorithms, most adjuvant treatment recommendations can be determined based on the presence of a single positive axillary node. In this context, the question of whether radiotherapy versus surgery is associated with lower morbidity and better local control of the axilla is relevant. Additionally, the impact of axillary radiotherapy on the morbidity of future ALND if clinical recurrence occurs is a pertinent consideration.

   The EORTC AMAROS (After Mapping of the Axilla: Radiotherapy or Surgery) trial is a RCT in which patients with a positive sentinel node are randomized to axillary radiation versus a completion ALND.[68] The primary end point of the study is axillary recurrence, with secondary end points of disease-free survival, overall survival, quality of life, and shoulder function. Initial study eligibility included patients with small (0.5 to 3.0 cm), clinically node-negative breast cancer. Although the initial study accrual goal was reached in 2008, study accrual has been continued due to low sentinel lymph node positivity rates, noncompliance with treatment randomization, and lower than expected event rates. Eligibility has been expanded to include tumors up to 5 cm in size (excluding those who receive neoadjuvant therapy) and multifocal tumors. Accrual will continue for 2 additional years, with expected interim analyses addressing patterns of care and technical aspects of the sentinel lymph node biopsy.

3. Is ALND after a positive sentinel lymph node necessary?

   Although ALND provides good local control and prognostic information, it is a potentially morbid procedure with only a small impact on survival.[2] Additionally, only those patients with positive axillary nodes will theoretically benefit from the ALND. The sentinel lymph node is found to be the only involved axillary node in approximately 50% of patients with a clinically negative axilla.[65] As a result, the necessity of ALND in all patients with a positive sentinel lymph node has been questioned.

   The ACOSOG Z0011 trial was designed to study whether ALND after identification of a positive sentinel lymph node is associated with a survival benefit. This trial was recently closed due to slow accrual, but the question remains a prominent one. Although previous studies indicate that only 50% of patients will have additional axillary disease beyond the sentinel lymph node, this data is based on routine pathologic examination of the ALND specimen, and micrometastases may therefore be present that were not identified. Nomograms and other models may help in predicting the likelihood that patients will have additional positive axillary nodes beyond the sentinel node; however, these models are unable to predict with certainty for a given patient.[65] For women with residual (even micrometastatic) disease in the axilla that is not surgically removed, there may be local control and even survival ramifications.[2,69,70] Therefore, the necessity of ALND after a positive sentinel lymph node remains a critical question to be addressed in future studies.

SUMMARY

In the era of modern therapy, ALND continues to play an important role in staging and local control of the axilla. Although sentinel lymph node biopsy has diminished the number of patients in whom an ALND is indicated, clear indications for ALND still exist. Further study on the impact of ALND on survival in the current era will define the future role of ALND in the treatment of breast cancer.

REFERENCES

1. Fisher B, Jeong JH, Anderson S, et al. Twenty-five-year follow-up of a randomized trial comparing radical mastectomy, total mastectomy, and total mastectomy followed by irradiation. *N Engl J Med.* 2002;347(8): 567-575.

2. Orr RK. The impact of prophylactic axillary node dissection on breast cancer survival—a Bayesian meta-analysis. *Ann Surg Oncol.* 1999;6(1):109-116.

3. Veronesi U, Paganelli G, Viale G, et al. A randomized comparison of sentinel node biopsy with routine axillary dissection in breast cancer. *N Engl J Med.* 2003;349(6):546-553.

4. Mansel RE, Fallowfield L, Kissin M, et al. Randomized multicenter trial of sentinel node biopsy versus standard axillary treatment in operable breast cancer: the ALMANAC Trial. *J Natl Cancer Inst.* 2006;98(9):599-609.

5. Lucci A, McCall LM, Beitsch PD, et al. Surgical complications associated with sentinel lymph node dissection (SLND) plus axillary lymph node dissection compared with SLND alone in the American College of Surgeons Oncology Group Trial Z0011. *J Clin Oncol.* 2007;25(24):3657-3663.

6. Temple LK, Baron R, Cody HS III, et al. Sensory morbidity after sentinel lymph node biopsy and axillary dissection: a prospective study of 233 women. *Ann Surg Oncol.* 2002;9(7):654-662.

7. Baron RH, Fey JV, Borgen PI, et al. Eighteen sensations after breast cancer surgery: a 5-year comparison of sentinel lymph node biopsy and axillary lymph node dissection. *Ann Surg Oncol.* 2007;14(5):1653-1661.

8. Purushotham AD, Upponi S, Klevesath MB, et al. Morbidity after sentinel lymph node biopsy in primary breast cancer: results from a randomized controlled trial. *J Clin Oncol.* 2005;23(19):4312-4321.

9. Rosen PP, Lesser ML, Kinne DW, Beattie EJ. Discontinuous or "skip" metastases in breast carcinoma. Analysis of 1228 axillary dissections. *Ann Surg.* 1983;197(3):276-283.

10. National Lymphedema Network Medical Advisory Committee. Position statement of the National Lymphedema Network. *Lymphedema Risk Reduction Practices.* 2008. Available at: http://www.lymphnet.org/pdfDocs/nlnriskreduction.pdf

11. Petrek JA, Senie RT, Peters M, Rosen PP. Lymphedema in a cohort of breast carcinoma survivors 20 years after diagnosis. *Cancer.* 2001;92(6):1368-1377.

12. Ahmed RL, Thomas W, Yee D, Schmitz KH. Randomized controlled trial of weight training and lymphedema in breast cancer survivors. *J Clin Oncol.* 2006;24(18):2765-2772.

13. *The NCCN GUIDELINE NAME Clinical Practice Guidelines in Oncology, Breast Cancer (Version 2.2008).* © 2006 National Comprehensive Cancer Network, Inc. Available at: http://www.nccn.org. Accessed August 12, 2008.

14. Kiricuta CI, Tausch J. A mathematical model of axillary lymph node involvement based on 1446 complete axillary dissections in patients with breast carcinoma. *Cancer.* 1992;69(10):2496-2501.

15. Axelsson CK, Mouridsen HT, Zedeler K. Axillary dissection of level I and II lymph nodes is important in breast cancer classification. The Danish Breast Cancer Cooperative Group (DBCG). *Eur J Cancer.* 1992;28A(8-9):1415-1418.

16. Somner JE, Dixon JM, Thomas JS. Node retrieval in axillary lymph node dissections: recommendations for minimum numbers to be confident about node negative status. *J Clin Pathol.* 2004;57(8):845-848.

17. Schaapveld M, de Vries EG, van der Graaf WT, et al. The prognostic effect of the number of histologically examined axillary lymph nodes in breast cancer: stage migration or age association? *Ann Surg Oncol.* 2006;13(4):465-474.

18. Neuman H, Carey LA, Ollila DW, et al. Axillary lymph node count is lower after neoadjuvant chemotherapy. *Am J Surg.* 2006;191(6):827-832.

19. Belanger J, Soucy G, Sideris L, et al. Neoadjuvant chemotherapy in invasive breast cancer results in a lower axillary lymph node count. *J Am Coll Surg.* 2008;206(4):704-708.

20. Baslaim MM, Al Malik OA, Al-Sobhi SS, et al. Decreased axillary lymph node retrieval in patients after neoadjuvant chemotherapy. *Am J Surg.* 2002;184(4):299-301.

21. Schaapveld M, Otter R, de Vries EG, et al. Variability in axillary lymph node dissection for breast cancer. *J Surg Oncol.* 2004;87(1):4-12.

22. Petrik DW, McCready DR, Sawka CA, Goel V. Association between extent of axillary lymph node dissection and patient, tumor, surgeon, and hospital factors in patients with early breast cancer. *J Surg Oncol.* 2003;82(2):84-90.

23. Chagpar AB, Scoggins CR, Martin RC II, et al. Factors determining adequacy of axillary node dissection in breast cancer patients. *Breast J.* 2007;13(3):233-237.

24. Crane-Okada R, Wascher RA, Elashoff D, Giuliano AE. Long-term morbidity of sentinel node biopsy versus complete axillary dissection for unilateral breast cancer. *Ann Surg Oncol.* 2008;15(7):1996-2005.

25. Langer I, Guller U, Berclaz G, et al. Morbidity of sentinel lymph node biopsy (SLN) alone versus SLN and completion axillary lymph node dissection after breast cancer surgery: a prospective Swiss multicenter study on 659 patients. *Ann Surg.* 2007;245(3):452-461.

26. Del Bianco P, Zavagno G, Burelli P, et al. Morbidity comparison of sentinel lymph node biopsy versus conventional axillary lymph node dissection for breast cancer patients: results of the Sentinella-GIVOM Italian randomised clinical trial. *Eur J Surg Oncol.* 2008;34(5):508-513.

27. McLaughlin S, Wright M, Morris K, et al. Prevalence of lymphedema in 936 women with breast cancer 5 years after sentinel lymph node biopsy or axillary dissection: I. Objective measurements. *J Clin Oncol.* 2008;26(32):5213-5219.

28. McLaughlin S, Wright M, Morris K, et al. Prevalence of lymphedema in 936 women with breast cancer 5 years after sentinel lymph node biopsy or axillary dissection: II. Patient perceptions and precautionary behaviors. *J Clin Oncol.* 2008;26(32):5220-5226.

29. Vitug AF, Newman LA. Complications in breast surgery. *Surg Clin North Am.* 2007;87(2):431-451.

30. Tejirian T, DiFronzo LA, Haigh PI. Antibiotic prophylaxis for preventing wound infection after breast surgery: a systematic review and metaanalysis. *J Am Coll Surg.* 2006;203(5):729-734.

31. Witt A, Yavuz D, Walchetseder C, Strohmer H, Kubista E. Preoperative core needle biopsy as an independent risk factor for wound infection after breast surgery. *Obstet Gynecol.* 2003;101(4):745-750.

32. Tran CL, Langer S, Broderick-Villa G, DiFronzo LA. Does reoperation predispose to postoperative wound infection in women undergoing operation for breast cancer? *Am Surg.* 2003;69(10):852-856.

33. Goyal A, Newcombe RG, Chhabra A, Mansel RE. Morbidity in breast cancer patients with sentinel node metastases undergoing delayed axillary lymph node dissection (ALND) compared with immediate ALND. *Ann Surg Oncol.* 2008;15(1):262-267.

34. Agrawal A, Ayantunde AA, Cheung KL. Concepts of seroma formation and prevention in breast cancer surgery. *ANZ J Surg.* 2006;76(12):1088-1095.

35. O'Hea BJ, Ho MN, Petrek JA. External compression dressing versus standard dressing after axillary lymphadenectomy. *Am J Surg.* 1999;177(6):450-453.

36. Cameron AE, Ebbs SR, Wylie F, Baum M. Suction drainage of the axilla: a prospective randomized trial. *Br J Surg.* 1988;75(12):1211.

37. Jain PK, Sowdi R, Anderson AD, MacFie J. Randomized clinical trial investigating the use of drains and fibrin sealant following surgery for breast cancer. *Br J Surg.* 2004;91(1):54-60.

38. Zavotsky J, Jones RC, Brennan MB, Giuliano AE. Evaluation of axillary lymphadenectomy without axillary drainage for patients undergoing breast-conserving therapy. *Ann Surg Oncol.* 1998;5(3):227-231.

39. Morris AM. A controlled trial of closed wound suction. *Br J Surg.* 1973;60(5):357-359.

40. Whitfield PC, Rainsbury RM. Suction versus siphon drainage after axillary surgery for breast cancer: a prospective randomized trial. *Br J Surg.* 1994;81(4):547.

41. Bonnema J, van Geel AN, Ligtenstein DA, Schmitz PI, Wiggers T. A prospective randomized trial of high versus low vacuum drainage after axillary dissection for breast cancer. *Am J Surg.* 1997;173(2):76-79.

42. van Heurn LW, Brink PR. Prospective randomized trial of high versus low vacuum drainage after axillary lymphadenectomy. *Br J Surg.* 1995;82(7):931-932.

43. Chintamani, Singhal V, Singh J, Bansal A, Saxena S. Half versus full vacuum suction drainage after modified radical mastectomy for breast cancer—a prospective randomized clinical trial [ISRCTN24484328]. *BMC Cancer* 2005;5:11

44. Petrek JA, Peters MM, Cirrincione C, Thaler HT. A prospective randomized trial of single versus multiple drains in the axilla after lymphadenectomy. *Surg Gynecol Obstet.* 1992;175(5):405-409.

45. Gupta R, Pate K, Varshney S, Goddard J, Royle GT. A comparison of 5 day and 8-day drainage following mastectomy and axillary clearance. *Eur J Surg Oncol.* 2001;27(1):26-30.

46. Dalberg K, Johansson H, Signomklao T, et al. A randomised study of axillary drainage and pectoral fascia preservation after mastectomy for breast cancer. *Eur J Surg Oncol.* 2004;30(6):602-609.

47. Parikh HK, Badwe RA, Ash CM, et al. Early drain removal following modified radical mastectomy: a randomized trial. *J Surg Oncol.* 1992;51(4):266-269.

48. Shamley DR, Barker K, Simonite V, Beardshaw A. Delayed versus immediate exercises following surgery for breast cancer: a systematic review. *Breast Cancer Res Treat.* 2005;90(3):263-271.

49. Harris SR, Hugi MR, Olivotto IA, Levine M. Clinical practice guidelines for the care and treatment of breast cancer: 11. Lymphedema. *CMAJ.* 2001;164(2):191-199.

50. Herd-Smith A, Russo A, Muraca MG, Del Turco MR, Cardona G. Prognostic factors for lymphedema after primary treatment of breast carcinoma. *Cancer.* 2001;92(7):1783-1787.

51. Kiel KD, Rademacker AW. Early-stage breast cancer: arm edema after wide excision and breast irradiation. *Radiology.* 1996;198(1):279-283.

52. Paskett ED, Naughton MJ, McCoy TP, Case LD, Abbott JM. The epidemiology of arm and hand swelling in premenopausal breast cancer survivors. *Cancer Epidemiol Biomarkers Prev.* 2007;16(4):775-782.

53. Purushotham AD, Bennett Britton TM, Klevesath MB, et al. Lymph node status and breast cancer-related lymphedema. *Ann Surg.* 2007;246(1): 42-45.

54. Coen JJ, Taghian AG, Kachnic LA, Assaad SI, Powell SN. Risk of lymphedema after regional nodal irradiation with breast conservation therapy. *Int J Radiat Oncol Biol Phys.* 2003;55(5):1209-1215.

55. Soran A, D'Angelo G, Begovic M, et al. Breast cancer-related lymphedema—what are the significant predictors and how they affect the severity of lymphedema? *Breast J.* 2006;12(6):536-543.

56. Salvat J, Knopf JF, Ayoubi JM, et al. Endoscopic exploration and lymph node sampling of the axilla. Preliminary findings of a randomized pilot study comparing clinical and anatomo-pathologic results of endoscopic axillary lymph node sampling with traditional surgical treatment. *Eur J Obstet Gynecol Reprod Biol.* 1996;70(2):165-173.

57. Langer I, Kocher T, Guller U, et al. Long-term outcomes of breast cancer patients after endoscopic axillary lymph node dissection: a prospective analysis of 52 patients. *Breast Cancer Res Treat.* 2005;90(1):85-91.

58. de Wilde RL, Schmidt EH, Hesseling M, et al. Comparison of classic and endoscopic lymphadenectomy for staging breast cancer. *J Am Assoc Gynecol Laparosc.* 2003;10(1):75-79.

59. Kuehn T, Santjohanser C, Grab D, et al. Endoscopic axillary surgery in breast cancer. *Br J Surg.* 2001;88(5):698-703.

60. Malur S, Bechler J, Schneider A. Endoscopic axillary lymphadenectomy without prior liposuction in 100 patients with invasive breast cancer. *Surg Laparosc Endosc Percutan Tech.* 2001;11(1):38-41; discussion 42.

61. Hussein O, El-Nahhas W, El-Saed A, Denewer A. Video-assisted axillary surgery for cancer: non-randomized comparison with conventional techniques. *Breast.* 2007;16(5):513-519.

62. Suami H, Taylor GI, Pan WR. The lymphatic territories of the upper limb: anatomical study and clinical implications. *Plast Reconstr Surg.* 2007;119(6):1813-1822.

63. Thompson M, Korourian S, Henry-Tillman R, et al. Axillary reverse mapping (ARM): a new concept to identify and enhance lymphatic preservation. *Ann Surg Oncol.* 2007;14(6):1890-1895.

64. Nos C, Kaufmann G, Clough KB, et al. Combined axillary reverse mapping (ARM) technique for breast cancer patients requiring axillary dissection. *Ann Surg Oncol.* 2008;15(9):2550-2555.

65. Van Zee KJ, Manasseh DM, Bevilacqua JL, et al. A nomogram for predicting the likelihood of additional nodal metastases in breast cancer patients with a positive sentinel node biopsy. *Ann Surg Oncol.* 2003;10(10):1140-1151.

66. Bevilacqua JL, Kattan MW, Fey JV, et al. Doctor, what are my chances of having a positive sentinel node? A validated nomogram for risk estimation. *J Clin Oncol.* 2007;25(24):3670-3679.

67. Krag DN, Julian TB, Harlow SP, et al. NSABP-32: Phase III, randomized trial comparing axillary resection with sentinel lymph node dissection: a description of the trial. *Ann Surg Oncol.* 2004;11(3 suppl):208S-210S.

68. Rutgers EJ, Meijnen P, Bonnefoi H. Clinical trials update of the European Organization for Research and Treatment of Cancer Breast Cancer Group. *Breast Cancer Res.* 2004;6(4):165-169.

69. Park J, Fey JV, Naik AM, et al. A declining rate of completion axillary dissection in sentinel lymph node-positive breast cancer patients is associated with the use of a multivariate nomogram. *Ann Surg.* 2007;245(3):462-468.

70. Clarke M, Collins R, Darby S, et al. Effects of radiotherapy and of differences in the extent of surgery for early breast cancer on local recurrence and 15-year survival: an overview of the randomised trials. *Lancet.* 2005;366(9503):2087-2106.

71. Platt R, Zaleznik DF, Hopkins CC, et al. Perioperative antibiotic prophylaxis for herniorrhaphy and breast surgery. *N Engl J Med.* 1990;322(3):153-160.

72. Wagman LD, Tegtmeier B, Beatty JD, et al. A prospective, randomized double-blind study of the use of antibiotics at the time of mastectomy. *Surg Gynecol Obstet.* 1990;170(1):12-16.

73. Bold RJ, Mansfield PF, Berger DH, et al. Prospective, randomized, double-blind study of prophylactic antibiotics in axillary lymph node dissection. *Am J Surg.* 1998;176(3):239-243.

74. Gupta R, Sinnett D, Carpenter R, Preece PE, Royle GT. Antibiotic prophylaxis for post-operative wound infection in clean elective breast surgery. *Eur J Surg Oncol.* 2000;26(4):363-366.

CHAPTER 64

Modified Radical Mastectomy and Techniques for Avoiding Skin Necrosis

Roshni Rao
A. Marilyn Leitch

Modified radical mastectomy (MRM) involves complete removal of the breast along with the overlying skin and all axillary contents. It has been, and continues to be, a critical component of breast cancer surgery. Although partial mastectomy followed by radiation therapy is an accepted form of therapy, recent studies indicate that the rates of mastectomy in the United States are actually rising.[1] It is therefore critical for the practicing surgeon to be familiar with the surgical techniques available for performing mastectomy and reducing postoperative complications.

This chapter describes the performance of total mastectomy using Bovie electrocautery (Bovie Medical Corp; St. Petersburg, Florida), tumescent techniques, and harmonic dissection.

PATIENT AND SURGEON POSITIONING

For performance of MRM, patients are placed in a supine position with the ipsilateral arm extended. The patient is shifted to a position as close to the edge of the operating table as safe to facilitate access and visualization. A small roll, typically either a rolled-up operative towel or sheet, can be placed longitudinally just posterior, and medial to, the latissimus muscle. In heavy patients, this can assist in palpating and dissecting the medial aspect of the latissimus muscle. Additional blankets should be placed under the extended arm to ensure the shoulder is at a level, neutral position rather than falling posteriorly. The arm should be prepped circumferentially and draped into the field with either a surgical stockinette or towels, which can be wrapped around the arm. A 6- to 8-cm length of the upper arm and the axillary area remains exposed. This ensures mobility of the arm if needed for access to the axilla and minimizes exposed skin. The surgeon should stand inferior to the extended arm. The assistant can stand either superior to the arm or on the contralateral side.

GENERAL PRINCIPLES

The incision for an MRM should be oriented in a fashion to remove skin overlying the tumor, and, if reconstruction is not planned, a large enough skin ellipse should be removed to allow for a flat chest wall at closure. The avoidance of skin flap redundancy reduces seroma formation and skin edge necrosis. Longer skin flaps will have more complications related to inadequate blood supply. Generally, an elliptical incision incorporating the nipple areolar complex is appropriate (Fig. 64-1). If a prior needle or surgical biopsy has been performed, the biopsy site should be encompassed within the skin ellipse. The incision should include 1.0- to 2.0-cm margins away from the tumor or the previous biopsy incision. For a very superficial tumor, it is prudent to take a wider skin margin to avoid a positive anterior soft tissue margin. The flaps are elevated superiorly to the clavicle and lateral deltopectoral groove, medially to the sternal border, laterally to the latissimus dorsi muscle, and inferiorly to the upper edge of the rectus sheath (Fig. 64-2). The breast in an MRM should be removed en bloc with the axillary contents. The incision should extend far enough laterally to allow adequate exposure for axillary dissection. For details on axillary lymph node dissection, see Chapter 63.

TECHNIQUES FOR RAISING FLAPS

Electrocautery for Elevation of Skin Flaps

The use of electrocautery for elevation of the mastectomy skin flaps results in less blood loss than scalpel dissection. In the era of scalpel dissection, blood transfusion during mastectomy was common. Comparative studies of scalpel versus electrocautery

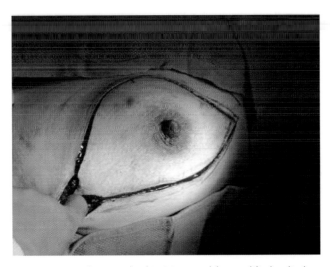

FIGURE 64-1 Photograph of incision used for modified radical mastectomy. Wide skin paddle will be excised to allow for closure of the chest wall with minimum skin redundancy.

dissection reveal a statistically significant reduction in blood loss with electrocautery.[1,4] With electrocautery dissection, transfusion is infrequent.

The mastectomy incision is made with the knife through the skin and dermis to allow the skin edges to separate. The skin edges are then grasped with skin hooks or Lahey clamps to provide traction during the flap elevation. The cautery is set on the lowest level that allows transection of the tissues with the least fat necrosis. With the coagulation setting, there is better control of bleeding; the cutting mode vaporizes cells and is less effective with coagulation. The goals in flap elevation are to leave some subcutaneous fat on the skin flap and to avoid leaving breast tissue. The subcutaneous fat is incised just anterior to the superficial fascia. A thinner patient generally has thinner flaps than a heavier patient who has more subcutaneous fat. In

the thin patient, there may be only 2 to 3 mm of fat on the skin flap. It is critical to preserve the subcutaneous vascular plexus. Recent anatomic studies indicate significant interdigitation of fat with the breast parenchymal tissue. It is therefore important to remain in the plane of the subcutaneous fat and avoid deeper dissection into the fat interdigitating with the glandular tissue.[5] This error is more likely to occur in the patient with thicker subcutaneous fat or a fatty replaced breast. With upward retraction on the skin edges, the tip of the cautery is used to incise the fat along the full length of the skin incision, maintaining a broad front of dissection. The dissection is performed under direct vision so that the thickness of the flap and the nature of the tissue transected can be visualized. The cautery is applied in a smooth sweeping fashion medial to lateral and lateral to medial. The opposite hand is used to retract the breast in the direction opposite the skin flap. During the dissection of the flap, it is important to advance the retracting hand to apply traction close to the point of the tissue transection with the cautery. Inadequate retraction results in uneven flaps and more difficulty incising the tissue. As the extent of dissection proceeds farther from the skin edge, it is usually necessary to replace the skin hooks with long lighted retractors. The shorter Bovie electrocautery tip can be replaced with a longer tip to facilitate the dissection at the extreme edges of the flap elevation. As with all techniques of flap dissection, it is important to avoid excessive skin traction that may compromise blood supply to the flap. With this technique, it is important not to get too close to the skin with the cautery, which can result in thermal injury. This is most likely to occur while using the cautery to coagulate small vessels. The visualization of the white dermal tissue during flap elevation should prompt the surgeon to re-establish the plane of dissection in the subcutaneous tissue. The skin edges are covered with moist laparotomy pads to protect the skin edges during retraction for removal of the breast from the pectoral muscle. During the subsequent breast removal, the surgeon and assistants must be mindful of the skin flaps and apply retraction as gently as possible.

Tumescent Technique

Tumescent mastectomy has been described under local anesthesia[6] with the use of specialty tumescent infiltration trocars[7] or with scissors.[8] The scissors technique uses equipment readily available in the operating room and we therefore prefer it. The use of sharp dissection rather than electrocautery minimizes collateral damage and may reduce mastectomy skin flap necrosis rates, a complication present in up to 30% of patients.[9] Figure 64-3 shows the specialty equipment necessary for the performance of total mastectomy with the tumescent technique. Extremely sharp scissors are needed, such as Jarit Supercuts (Jarit; Hawthorne, New York), which are typically used for surgical facelifts. Scissors with a slight degree of curvature assist in following the contour of the breast and staying in the appropriate plane. Freeman facelift retractors (Anthony Products Inc.; Indianapolis, Indiana) are used to retract the skin. Double skin hooks may also be used for retraction. Additionally, a 60-mL syringe and a 22-G spinal needle are used for infiltration of the tumescent solution. Tumescent solution should include

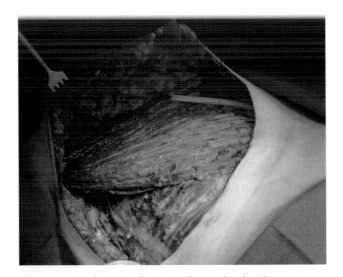

FIGURE 64-2 Elevation of superior flap to the clavicle.

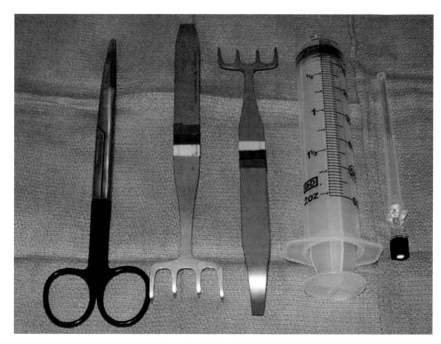

FIGURE 64-3 Instruments required for tumescent mastectomy with scissors techniques.

normal saline, lidocaine, and epinephrine. A combination of 1% lidocaine with epinephrine (20 mL) is readily available in the operating room and may be mixed with 60 mL of injectable normal saline. Alternatively, using 1 amp (1:100,000) of epinephrine with 20 mL of lidocaine and 1 L of injectable normal saline provides increased volume and may provide better hemostasis.

Step 1

After the incision is made, a small lip of tissue is raised just below the dermal layer across the entire incision (Fig. 64-4). To minimize collateral damage, electrocautery is typically set on cutting current. Tension with the contralateral hand is key in visualizing the appropriate plane.

Step 2

Tumescent solution is infiltrated using the 60-mL syringe and the 22-G spinal needle. The needle is insinuated just below the dermal layer (Fig. 64-5) to the hub of the needle. Once in place, the needle is slowly retracted backward, and it is at this point that the solution is infiltrated. A wheal should not be visualized during infiltration. The needle is typically palpable just beneath the skin along the course of infiltration. This ensures that the solution is just below the fascia but above the breast parenchyma.

Step 3

The skin is then retracted by the assistant using either Freeman retractors or skin hooks (Fig. 64-6A). The assistant should apply retraction in a direction toward the operator rather than directly upward, which assists the surgeon in being able to look directly down the line of dissection. The nondominant hand of the operator is placed against the mastectomy skin flap to be raised. Initially, small snips are taken across the length of the flap to be raised, just below the dermal layer. Once this is completed, the scissors are opened to a distance of approximately 1 to 1.5 cm and placed into position just between the breast fascia and the breast parenchyma (Fig. 64-6B). Then, in a smooth motion, the scissors essentially slide between the 2 layers. Due to the infiltration of the tumescent, the correct plane has already been

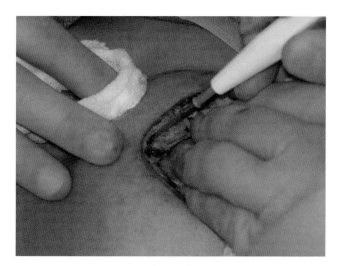

FIGURE 64-4 Retraction by the nondominant hand of the surgeon facilitates the creation of an edge of tissue just deep to the dermal layer. This was created with electrocautery on cutting current.

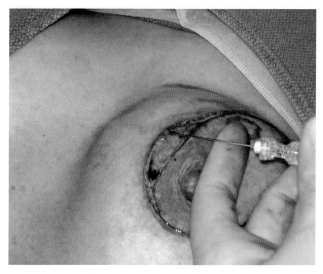

FIGURE 64-5 Infiltration of tumescent solution using a flexile 22-G spinal needle.

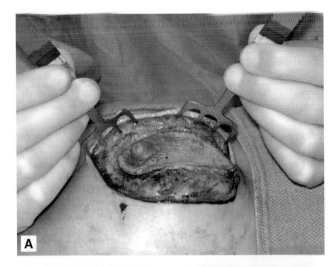

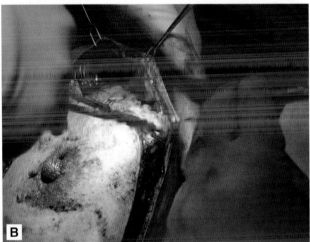

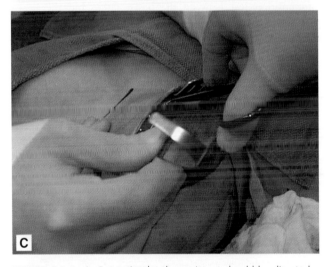

FIGURE 64-6 **A.** Retraction by the assistant should be directed toward the surgeon to facilitate exposure and dissection of the correct plane. **B.** Small snips are taken with the scissors to initially create the flap for dissection. **C.** Scissors are passed through the plane in one smooth motion.

elevated and the scissors will slide with minimal to no resistance (Fig. 64-6C). If resistance is encountered, the operator is likely in the wrong plane, and adjustments either more superficially or deeper should be made. Each flap should be infiltrated and then immediately raised, as opposed to injecting all flaps and then raising. This maximizes the hemostatic properties of the tumescent solution.

Ultrasonic Dissection

Ultrasonic dissection uses a high-power ultrasound transducer that oscillates longitudinally. High temperatures along with cavitation and coagulation occur at the interface between the blade and the tissues, which allows for sealing of vascular and lymphatic structures as well as the ability to divide tissues.[10] Ultrasonic dissection avoids thermal injury or smoke generation, and normal temperatures are achieved at a 3-mm area of distance away from the blade, thereby minimizing collateral damage. With the introduction of the Harmonic Focus (Johnson & Johnson; New Jersey), ultrasonic dissection has been increasingly used in breast surgery. Previous studies indicate decreased acute blood loss,[11-13] a relatively easy learning curve, and decreased drainage, although there are also data that report no difference in blood loss and seroma formation.[14]

MRM using ultrasonic dissection allows the surgeon to minimize the use of clips and ties. The Harmonic Focus is a single-use instrument, and the individual surgeon in conjunction with the operating room administration will have to analyze the cost-benefit ratio.

The Harmonic Focus is used in the same fashion as an electrocautery and has been approved to seal lymphatics. After the incision is made, the skin is retracted, and flaps are raised using the ultrasonic shears (Fig. 64-7).

Previous studies have also reported the use of bipolar scissors or radiofrequency coagulation as an alternative to electrocautery. Bipolar scissors may offer an advantage in decreasing blood loss when compared with scalpel technique[15]; however, it did not appear to be effective in reducing skin necrosis rates.[16]

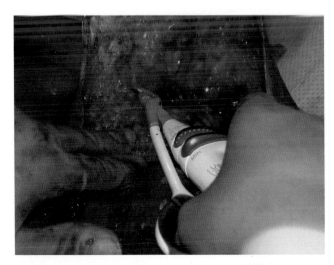

FIGURE 64-7 Ultrasonic dissection using the Harmonic Focus.

REMOVAL OF THE BREAST

The posterior border of the MRM is the pectoralis fascia. All breast tissue above this should be removed when mastectomy is performed. Preservation of the pectoralis fascia does not appear to compromise survival or increase recurrence, and it may facilitate reconstruction.[17,18] Separation of the breast from its posterior attachments proceeds from the superior-most aspect of the dissection, at the level of the clavicle. Using electrocautery, dissection is performed in a lateral to medial fashion following the muscle fibers of the pectoralis muscle to minimize damage to the muscle (Fig. 64-8). Care is taken to identify the medial perforating branches of the internal mammary vessels. These may be divided and suture ligated. These are in varying locations but can be readily visualized during careful dissection along the lateral border of the sternum. Dissection is carried down to 2 to 3 cm below the inframammary fold. The breast should be oriented with marking sutures at the completion of dissection and sent for pathologic evaluation.

CLOSURE

Irrigation

After dissection is complete, the wound should be copiously irrigated. In vitro studies have revealed increased tumor lysis and decreased rates of laparoscopic port site tumor seeding with irrigation.[19,20] Irrigation with water or normal saline, however, does not appear to prevent tumor bed recurrence when in vitro melanoma models are studied.[21] There have been no prospective studies regarding breast cancer and irrigation. Retrospective studies in colorectal cancer patients, however, do support the use of irrigation to decrease recurrence.[22] There are no data demonstrating in vivo superiority of one irrigation fluid over another, and the choice depends on the surgeon.

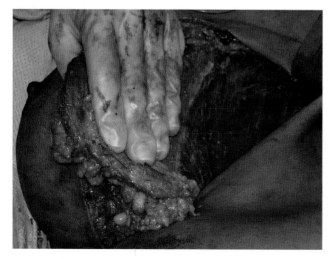

FIGURE 64-8 Fibers of the pectoralis major muscle and its overlying fascia are identified; in this case the fascia is being removed, leaving only muscle behind.

Drains

Due to the risk of seroma formation, closed suction drains should be placed prior to closure of an MRM. Drains should be sutured to the skin using a sturdy (2–0 or 3–0) monofilament suture. Alternatively, some centers perform a layered closure known as "axillary padding" and omit drain placement,[23-25] although this technique has not become popular in the United States.

Drains may be removed on an outpatient basis when drainage is less than 30 mL per day. Early drain removal has been found to increase the incidence of seroma formation.[26]

As a routine, 2 drains are placed: one on the chest wall and the other in the axilla. Randomized trials of 1 drain versus 2 have not demonstrated an advantage with the additional drain.[27,28]

Skin Closure

If at the end of the removal of the breast, the skin edges appear traumatized or hemorrhagic, consider trimming the skin back 5 to 10 mm. Closure is performed in 2 layers. Initially an interrupted, buried, deep dermal layer using absorbable polyglactin suture (Vicryl, Ethicon; Somerville, New Jersey) is placed. Recently, INSORB (Incisive Surgical; Plymouth, Minnesota), an absorbable suture stapler, has also become available and may facilitate rapid closure of the deep dermal layer. The skin edges are then approximated using a running, subcuticular absorbable 4–0 monofilament suture. A skin stapler is also used by some surgeons for closure of the skin. Care should be taken to remove these staples within 5 to 7 days to prevent "train tracks" at the incision site. Due to this concern, and the potential psychological trauma associated with staple removal from the location where a breast was, the authors prefer a subcuticular suture closure. The use of tissue adhesive to approximate the skin has also been reported to decrease overall operative costs and improve patient cosmetic satisfaction.[29]

Dressings

Steri-strips (3M; St. Paul, Minnesota) can be placed over the incision. These can be oriented full length and parallel with the incision site to prevent pulling the incision apart during removal, or they can be cut into short strips and oriented perpendicularly for distribution of tension on skin incision over a wider area. There is no advantage to compression dressing placement at the wound site.[30] The wound may be dressed with 4 × 4 gauze and either tape or Tegaderm (3M; St. Paul). Based on the lack of data supporting one dressing over another, patient comfort and surgeon preference dictate mastectomy bra application and choice of dressing.

SUMMARY

Modified radical mastectomy continues to be an important part of breast cancer surgery. Alternatives to the use of electrocautery to raise mastectomy skin flaps include dissection with the tumescent technique, ultrasonic dissection, and bipolar scissors. Small prospective randomized trials do not clearly support one technique over another. It is useful to become familiar with all techniques and then use the one that generates the best outcomes for the individual surgeon.

REFERENCES

1. Tuttle TM, Habermann EB, Grund EH, et al. Increasing use of contralateral prophylactic mastectomy for breast cancer patients: a trend toward more aggressive surgical treatment. *J Clin Oncol.* 2007;25(33):5203-5209.

2. Kakos GS, James AG. The use of cautery in "bloodless" radical mastectomy. *Cancer.* 1970;26:666-668.

3. Miller E, Paull DE, Morrissey K, et al. Scalpel versus electrocautery in modified radical mastectomy. *Am Surg.* 1988;54:284-286.

4. Porter KA, O'Connor S, Rimm E, et al. Electrocautery as a factor in seroma formation following mastectomy. *Am J Surg.* 1998;176:8-11.

5. Nickell WB, Skelton J. Breast fat and fallacies: more than 100 years of anatomical fantasy. *J Hum Lact.* 2005;21(2):126-130.

6. Carlson GW. Total mastectomy under local anesthesia: the tumescent technique. *Breast J.* 2005;11(2):100-102.

7. Staradub VL, Morrow M. Modified radical mastectomy with knife technique. *Arch Surg.* 2002;137(1):105-110.

8. Shoher A, Hekier R, Lucci A Jr. Mastectomy performed with scissors following tumescent solution injection. *J Surg Oncol.* 2003;83(3):191-193.

9. Margulies AG, Hochberg J, Kepple J. Total skin-sparing mastectomy without preservation of the nipple-areola complex. *Am J Surg.* 2005;190(6):907-912.

10. Kock C, Frierich T, Metternich F, et al. Determination of temperature elevation in tissue during the application of the harmonic scalpel. *Ultrasound Med Biol.* 2003;29(2):301-309.

11. Adwani A, Ebbs SR. Ultracision reduces acute blood loss but not seroma formation after mastectomy and axillary dissection: a pilot study. *Int J Clin Pract.* 2006;60(5):562-564.

12. Deo SV, Shukla NK. Modified radical mastectomy using harmonic scalpel. *J Surg Oncol.* 2000;74(3):204-207.

13. Deo SV, Shukla NK, Asthana S, et al. A comparative study of modified radical mastectomy using harmonic scalpel and electrocautery. *Singapore Med J.* 2002;43(5):226-228.

14. Galatius H, Okholm M, Hoffmann J. Mastectomy using ultrasonic dissection: effect on seroma formation. *Breast.* 2003;12(5):338-341.

15. Rodd CD, Velchuru VR, Holly-Archer F, et al. Randomized clinical trial comparing two mastectomy techniques. *World J Surg.* 2007;31(6):1164-1168.

16. Meretoja TJ, von Smitten KA, Kuokkanen HO. Complications of skin-sparing mastectomy followed by immediate breast reconstruction. *Ann Plast Surg.* 2008;60(1):24-28.

17. Dalberg K, Johansson H, Signomklao T. A randomized study of axillary drainage and pectoral fascia preservation after mastectomy for breast cancer. *Eur J Surg Oncol.* 2004;30(6):602-609.

18. Sandelin K, Wickman M, Billgren AM. Oncological outcome after immediate breast reconstruction for invasive breast cancer: a long-term study. *Breast.* 2004;13(3):210-218.

19. Park KG, Chetty U, Scott W, et al. The activity of locally applied cytotoxics to breast cancer cells in vitro. *Ann R Coll Surg Engl.* 1991;73(2):96-99.

20. Ost MC, Patel KP, Rastinehad AR, et al. Pneumoperitoneum with carbon dioxide inhibits macrophage tumor necrosis factor-alpha secretion: source of transitional-cell carcinoma port-site metastasis, with prophylactic irrigation strategies to decrease laparoscopic oncologic risks. *J Endourol.* 2008;22(1):105-112.

21. Sweitzer KL, Nathanson SD, Nelson LT, et al. Irrigation does not dislodge or destroy tumor cells adherent to the tumor bed. *J Surg Oncol.* 1993;53(3):184-190.

22. Constantinides VA, Cheetham D, Nichols RJ, et al. Is rectal washout effective for preventing localized recurrence after anterior resection for rectal cancer? *Dis Colon Rectum.* 2008;51(9):1339-1344.

23. Classe JM, Berchery D, Campion L, et al. Randomized clinical trial comparing axillary padding with closed suction drainage for the axillary wound after lymphadenectomy for breast cancer. *Br J Surg.* 2006;93(7):820-824.

24. Classe JM, Dupre PF, Francois T, et al. Axillary padding as an alternative to closed suction drainage for ambulatory axillary lymphadenectomy: a prospective cohort of 207 patients with early breast cancer. *Arch Surg.* 2002;137(2):169-172.

25. Garnier JM, Hamy A, Classe JM, et al. A new approach to the axilla: functional axillary lymphadenectomy and padding. *J Gynecol Obstet Biol Reprod (Paris).* 1993;22(3):237-242.

26. Barton A, Blitz M, Callahan D, et al. Early removal of postmastectomy drains is not beneficial: results from a halted randomized controlled trial. *Am J Surg.* 2006;191(5):652-656.

27. Puttawibul P, Sangthong B, Maipang T, et al. Mastectomy without drain at pectoral area: a randomized controlled trial. *J Med Assoc Thai.* 2003;86(4):325-331.

28. Terrell GS, Singer JA. Axillary versus combined axillary and pectoral drainage after modified radical mastectomy. *Surg Gynecol Obstet.* 1992;175(5):437-440.

29. Gennari R, Rotmensz N, Ballardini B, et al. A prospective, randomized, controlled clinical trial of tissue adhesive (2-octylcyanoacrylate) versus standard wound closure in breast surgery. *Surgery.* 2004;136(3):593-599.

30. O'Hea BJ, Ho MN, Petrek JA. External compression dressing versus standard dressing after axillary lymphadenectomy. *Am J Surg.* 1999;177(6):450-453.

CHAPTER 65

The Concept of Prophylactic Mastectomy

Isabelle Bedrosian

PRIMARY PROPHYLAXIS IN BRCA MUTATION CARRIERS

The discovery of the BRCA1 and BRCA2 mutation identifies a group of nearly homogeneous patients at substantially increased risk of breast cancer. The risk of breast cancer by age 70 in BRCA1 mutation carriers is estimated to range from 44% to 78% and for BRCA2 mutation carriers from 31% to 56%.[1,2] Bilateral prophylactic mastectomy (BPM) is thus an important consideration for this population. Alternative approaches that have been investigated include frequent surveillance that includes the use of breast magnetic resonance imaging (MRI) and chemoprevention using tamoxifen.

Meijers-Heijboer and colleagues compared breast cancer related outcomes among BRCA1/2 mutation carriers who opted for BPM and compared this with those who chose to undergo surveillance.[3] Many of the patients who underwent surveillance also had regular MRI of the breast. Among the 76 women who underwent BPM, no cases of breast cancer were identified after 2.9 years of follow-up. In contrast, 8 of 63 women who opted for a surveillance approach were diagnosed with breast cancer during this follow-up period. Importantly, among these 8 women, 1 death from breast cancer was also reported. Thus the authors estimated that the 5-year risk of breast cancer in the surveillance group was 12% with BPM reducing this risk by 66% to 100% (Fig. 65-1). In addition, although more women who underwent BPM also underwent prophylactic oophorectomy, the benefits of BPM in reducing breast cancer events was still significant even after controlling for this difference. Although data from this cohort suggested substantial benefit to BPM, the number of patients in the study as well as the follow-up was small, with a resulting wide estimate of risk reduction conferred by BPM. Thus this study leaves open the possibility that BPM in BRCA1/2 mutation carriers may confer less of an advantage than estimated by these initial findings.

Breast cancer related outcomes in a larger population of BRCA1/2 mutation carriers was reported by the PROSE study group.[4] In this multicenter study, 483 women with deleterious BRCA1 or BRCA2 mutations were followed for a mean of 6.4 years. Of the 105 women who elected to undergo BPM, 2 cases of breast cancer (1.9%) were reported compared with 184 of 378 (48.7%) age-matched controls who did not undergo BPM. BPM thus afforded a 90% relative reduction in breast cancer risk, and this relative risk (RR) reduction increased to 95% when adjusted for prophylactic oophorectomy. More importantly, the absolute risk reduction seen with BPM was 46.8%. However, despite this dramatic difference, the PROSE study group did not provide survival outcomes between the 2 groups. Because women who undergo prophylactic mastectomy have a small but real risk of breast cancer as seen in the PROSE study and women in surveillance programs generally present with early-stage, highly curable cancer,[5] it is possible that the breast cancer specific survival between the 2 groups would be less dramatic than the differences in breast cancer incidence.

Given the lack of survival data, Schrag and colleagues used a decision analysis model to predict the effects of prophylactic surgery on life expectancy among women with BRCA1 and BRCA2 mutations.[6] They demonstrate substantial gains in life expectancy with prophylactic surgery, with the benefit maximized when intervention is carried out at earlier ages. Thus they estimated that a 30-year-old patient with a BRCA1 or BRCA2 mutation stands to gain 2.9 to 5.3 years of life with BPM (Fig. 65-2). Additional gains in life expectancy are also seen with the use of prophylactic oophorectomy, with little loss of this benefit if oophorectomy was delayed to the age of 40. These gains in life expectancy are on par with and in some cases exceed the benefits seen with other prophylactic medical interventions such as smoking cessation.

Data regarding efficacy of chemoprevention in the BRCA1/2 population are limited to subgroup analyses from large multicenter

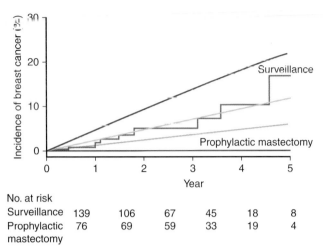

FIGURE 65-1 Actuarial incidence of breast cancer among women with a BRCA1 or BRCA2. Mutation after prophylactic mastectomy or during surveillance. The surveillance group includes data obtained before prophylactic mastectomy in 76 of the 139 women. The dashed line represents the probability of breast cancer during surveillance, and the dotted lines represent the 95% confidence interval. Values were calculated with the use of an exponential model in which the hazard rate was assumed to be constant. [Reproduced, with permission, from Meijers Heijboer H, van Geel B, van Putten WL, et al. Breast cancer after prophylactic bilateral mastectomy in women with a BRCA1 or BRCA2 mutation. N Engl J Med. 2001;345(3):159-164.]

trials. Analysis of 288 breast cancer cases in the NSABP-P1 demonstrated that 8 patients were BRCA1 and 11 patients were BRCA2 mutation carriers. Of the 8 women with BRCA1 mutations who developed breast cancer, 5 had been randomized to tamoxifen and 3 to placebo (RR = 1.67; 95% confidence interval [CI], 0.032 to 10.7). Of the 11 women with BRCA2 mutations who developed breast cancer, 3 had received tamoxifen and 8 received placebo (RR = 0.38; 95%CI, 0.06 to 1.56). Although the risk reduction achieved with tamoxifen in the BRCA2 population was similar to that of the non-BRCA population, this reduction in breast cancer events in the BRCA2 cohort was not statistically significant given the small sample size. As noted in this study and several others, patients with BRCA1 mutations tend to predominantly develop estrogen receptor (ER)-negative tumors; thus there would be little expectation of achieving meaningful risk reduction among BRCA1 mutation carriers. However, the proportion of ER-positive cancers is higher in BRCA2 mutation carriers, and thus theoretically this population would derive benefit from antiestrogens as a prevention strategy. Nonetheless given the limited data, tamoxifen for chemoprevention is not widely used as a risk-reducing strategy among BRCA1/2 mutation carriers.

SECONDARY PROPHYLAXIS IN BRCA MUTATION CARRIERS

With development of an index cancer, women with BRCA mutations have substantial risk of a second contralateral breast cancer event. However, the role of routine contralateral mastectomy in this setting has not been established, and the data available in the literature are conflicting.

Metcalfe and colleagues followed 491 BRCA1/2 patients with stage I and stage II breast cancer and examined the effects of surgical and medical interventions on the risk of contralateral breast cancer. They found that women who do not undergo oophorectomy or receive antiestrogen therapy, have a 43.4% (BRCA1) and 34.6% (BRCA2) actuarial risk of a contralateral breast cancer 10 years following an initial cancer diagnosis.[8] These risks were reduced following oophorectomy or tamoxifen

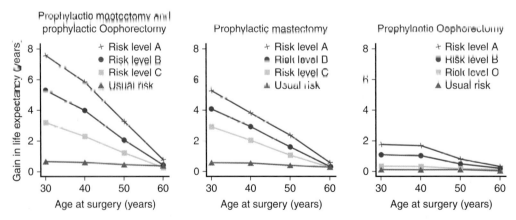

FIGURE 65-2 Gains in life expectancy among women with BRCA1 or BRCA2 mutations, according to age, cumulative risk of cancer, and type of prophylactic surgery. The graph shows the gains expected for 30-year-old women treated according to 3 prophylactic-surgery strategies, as compared with a strategy of no prophylactic surgery, according to age at the time of surgery for each of 4 levels of risk: the usual risk in the general population, risk level A (40% risk of breast cancer and 5% risk of ovarian cancer by the age of 70 years), risk level B (60% risk of breast cancer and 20% risk of ovarian cancer), and risk level C (85% risk of breast cancer and 40% risk of ovarian cancer). [Reproduced, with permission, from Schrag D, Kuntz KM, Garber JE, Weeks JC. Decision analysis—effects of prophylactic mastectomy and oophorectomy on life expectancy among women with BRCA1 or BRCA2 mutations. N Engl J Med. 1997;336(20): 1465-1471.]

therapy to 18.8% in BRCA1 patients and 13.1% in BRCA2 patients. However, the greatest reduction in contralateral breast cancer events was seen among women who underwent contralateral prophylactic mastectomy (CPM). Only 1 cancer (0.7%) was seen at an average of 9.2 years of follow-up among the 146 women who had CPM compared with 97 (28.8%) contralateral breast cancer cases among the 336 women who did not undergo CPM. Although these data show striking outcomes with CPM, a number of important limitations to the study are also noted. Most important among these was the lack of ER data on a significant number of the patient population, and similarly the relative distribution of ER status between CPM and no CPM groups was not known. In addition, a survival analysis to see whether the increased risk of death from index cancer was offset by the potential survival benefit afforded by preventing a contralateral breast cancer was not evaluated.

Survival end points were the focus of another report of CPM among BRCA1/2 mutation carriers.[9] One hundred and forty-eight women with a history of stage I to IIIa breast cancer were followed for a mean of 3.5 years. Among this group, 79 women underwent CPM. The use of CPM also strongly correlated with the use of bilateral prophylactic oophorectomy (BPO). Although patients undergoing CPM had substantial reduction in contralateral breast cancer risk, after adjusting for BPO, no overall survival benefit was seen for those who had CPM. Additional analyses in this cohort demonstrated that the survival benefit was associated with BPO, rather than CPM, thus suggesting that the greater risk to survival among BRCA1/2 mutation carriers is from ovarian cancer rather than breast cancer. It is not clear whether with longer follow-up CPM would also be associated with improved survival.

Lastly, decision analysis using Markov modeling has also been applied to this setting to determine benefits in life expectancy from a number of different prophylactic interventions, including CPM, tamoxifen, and BPO.[10] Maximal benefit in life expectancy was seen among women with high penetrance mutations, with early-stage breast cancer diagnosed early in life. The maximum gains in life expectancy were seen for a 30-year-old with early-stage breast cancer and ranged from 1.3 years for tamoxifen therapy to 2.1 years for CPM. These gains in life expectancy are substantially less than those anticipated for a 30-year-old woman who is a BRCA1/2 carrier without a breast cancer diagnosis who undergoes BPM. These differences speak to the need to additionally factor in prognosis from the index carcinoma when counseling BRCA1/2 mutation carriers who have already developed breast cancer. Thus the complex interplay between age, stage at diagnosis, and its subsequent impact on survival as well as mutation penetrance and probability of a contralateral breast cancer event all need to be carefully considered when counseling BRCA1/2 mutation carriers regarding CPM.

PRIMARY PROPHYLAXIS IN NON-BRCA MUTATION CARRIERS

Women who are not BRCA1/2 mutation carriers yet are felt to be at increased risk due to family history or a history of lobular carcinoma in situ (LCIS) or atypical ductal hyperplasia (ADH) at biopsy represent a very heterogeneous population of patients who may be considered for prophylactic mastectomy. Assessing future risk of cancer in this population has proven to be especially problematic, and differing definitions have been used when examining the effect of prophylactic mastectomy in this population.

The Mayo Clinic was among the first to report on the impact of BPM in reducing breast cancer events among a large group of women without a personal history of breast cancer. Hartmann and colleagues investigated the outcomes of 639 women treated with BPM over a 30-year period.[11] These women were stratified by family history into high and moderate personal risk for developing breast cancer. Their outcomes were compared with sisters who did not undergo prophylactic surgery as well as to predicted breast cancer events based on the Gail model. In all women undergoing BPM, the procedure resulted in a 90% relative reduction in risk of breast cancer. In absolute terms, the reduction in risk of breast cancer for the high-risk group was 16.1% and it was 7.9% for the moderate-risk group. They also estimated that BPM reduced the risk of death by at least 80%, corresponding to an absolute risk reduction of 2.4% to 4%.

To place these findings into perspective, Hamm et al estimated the number of patients needed to treat in order for one patient to derive benefit from BPM either through a prevention of a breast cancer event or a prevention of a breast cancer associated death.[12] They estimated that for the high-risk group, 6 women will undergo BPM to prevent 1 case of breast cancer and 25 women will have to undergo BPM to prevent 1 breast cancer–related death (Table 65-1). For the moderate risk group, 13 women would need to be treated to prevent 1 breast cancer and 42 women would need to be treated to prevent 1 breast cancer death. Thus most women without a documented BRCA1/2 mutation will derive no benefit from prophylactic surgery. This analysis highlights the challenges of identifying women truly at highest risk for a breast cancer event and thus minimizing the number of cases where no oncologic benefit would be derived from BPM.

Alternatives to surgery for the primary prevention of breast cancer in the non-BRCA population have also been studied. One important trial that opened the doors to chemoprevention was the Breast Cancer Prevention Trial conducted by the National Surgical Adjuvant Breast and Bowel Project.[13] This study randomized 13,388 women more than 35 years of age to receive either tamoxifen or placebo for 5 years. Increased risk was defined using the Gail model with an estimated 5-year risk of at least 1.7% or a personal history of LCIS. Overall, tamoxifen decreased the incidence of invasive breast cancer by 50% (Fig. 65-3) with an even greater reduction (86%) seen in subgroups of women with a personal history of ADH. The reduction was seen in ER-positive breast cancer events with no difference in ER-negative breast cancer events between the 2 arms. Although subsequent trials have not all confirmed the findings of the BCPT, overall meta-analysis confirms the efficacy of tamoxifen in the prevention setting.[14]

Despite its demonstrated efficacy in reducing breast cancer, tamoxifen has not gained widespread acceptance as a prevention agent, likely due to its associated side effects and risks. Raloxifene, a second-generation selective ER modulator with a somewhat different side-effect profile, has recently been confirmed as another chemoprevention option, albeit limited to

TABLE 65-1 Relative Risk Reduction and Number Needed to Treat for the Outcomes for Breast Cancer and Death in High- and Moderate-Risk Women Who Underwent Prophylactic Mastectomy[*]

Risk and Outcomes	Outcome Rate without Mastectomy	Outcome Rate with Mastectomy	Absolute Risk Reduction	Relative Risk Reduction	Number Needed to Treat
High					
Breast cancer	0.175	0.014	0.161	0.920	6
Death	0.049	0.009	0.040	0.816	25
Moderate					
Breast cancer	0.088	0.009	0.079	0.898	13
Death	0.024	0.000	0.024	1.000	42

[*]The outcome rate is the proportion of women with the indicated outcome, on the basis of the data reported by Hartmann et al. The absolute risk reduction is calculated as the outcome rate without treatment minus the outcome rate with the treatment, the relative risk reduction is calculated as the absolute risk reduction divided by the outcome rate without treatment, and the number needed to treat is calculated as 1 divided by the absolute risk reduction. [Reproduced, with permission, from Hamm RM, Lawler F, Scheid D. Prophylactic mastectomy in women with a high risk of breast cancer. *N Engl J Med.* 1999;340(23):1837-1838.]

postmenopausal women. Starting in 1999, more than 19,000 postmenopausal women accrued to the Study of Tamoxifen and Raloxifene trial were randomized to receive either tamoxifen or raloxifene for 5 years.[15] The results of this study showed equivalence between the 2 agents in preventing invasive breast cancer events, although raloxifene was less effective than tamoxifen in preventing LCIS and ductal carcinoma in situ.

SECONDARY PROPHYLAXIS IN NON-BRCA MUTATION CARRIERS

Women with an index breast cancer are at increased risk for a second, contralateral malignancy. For most women without a substantial family history and without a BRCA mutation, this risk is estimated to be approximately 0.7% to 1% per year.[16-18] For women who are ER positive, this risk can be substantially mitigated through the use of adjuvant antiestrogen therapy. As with all studies on the efficacy of prophylactic mastectomy, CPM in this setting has been shown to reduce the risk of contralateral breast cancer by 90%.[19-22] However, again, because the risk of a second primary breast cancer remains small for the majority of women with an index breast cancer, it is likely that most women undergoing CPM will be overtreated. Furthermore, the benefit of CPM in reducing breast cancer deaths remains understudied.

To identify groups of patients at higher risk for a contralateral breast cancer event, Goldflam and colleagues examined the primary tumor characteristics of women who underwent CPM to identify predictors of high-risk lesions or occult malignancy in the contralateral breast.[21] They found that patients with an index invasive lobular carcinoma (ILC), those with ER-progesterone (PR)-positive tumors, ipsilateral breast high- to moderate-risk lesions as well as less than 60 years at diagnosis predicted unfavorable contralateral breast histology. Thus clinical and histologic features in the index breast may help stratify women at higher than average risk for a contralateral breast cancer who thus stand to derive greater benefit from CPM. It is important to remember that this study did not compare long-term outcomes between the CPM and non-CPM cohort and that in a substantial number of ER-positive patients, the use of adjuvant antiestrogen therapy would likely offset the adverse features noted in the contralateral breast and thus lower contralateral breast cancer risk.

Although ILC is commonly believed to increase the probability of contralateral breast cancer, recent data would suggest otherwise. In a study comparing patients with early-stage invasive ductal cancer with those with early-stage invasive lobular cancer, no differences in contralateral breast cancer risk were noted after mean follow-up more than 10 years.[23] Babiera et al examined survival outcomes in patients with ILC comparing those who underwent CPM to those that did not.[22] After

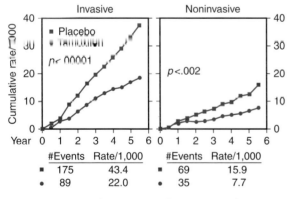

FIGURE 65-3 Cumulative rates of invasive and noninvasive breast cancers occurring in participants receiving placebo or tamoxifen. The *p*-values are 2 sided. [Reproduced, with permission, from Fisher B, Costantino JP, Wickerham DL, et al. Tamoxifen for prevention of breast cancer: report of the National Surgical Adjuvant Breast and Bowel Project P-1 Study. J Natl Cancer Inst. 1998;90(18):1371-1388.]

68 months of follow-up, 3 contralateral breast cancer events were noted in the surveillance group and no differences were noted in breast cancer–specific survival between the 2 groups. One reason for these findings in recent series may be the propensity of ILC tumors to be ER positive, and thus these patients would derive significant chemoprevention benefit with the use of adjuvant hormonal therapy.

Patients with a personal history of breast cancer coupled with a significant family history, even if no BRCA mutation is identified, likely have a greater risk for breast cancer than those without such a family history. McDonnell et al examined the efficacy of CPM in 745 breast cancer patients without BRCA1/2 mutation but with a positive family history stratified as parent/child, sibling, or second-degree relative diagnosed with breast cancer.[20] The probability of contralateral breast cancer was further adjusted to account for the potential effects of adjuvant chemotherapy and tamoxifen. Adjustments were also made for menopausal status at diagnosis of primary breast cancer. Median follow-up was 10 years. As expected, CPM reduced the probability of contralateral breast cancer by 95%, although the absolute risk reduction was greater among premenopausal women compared with postmenopausal patients (25.5% versus 13.5% at 10 years, respectively). Survival end points were not measured in this study.

Few studies have investigated the impact of CPM on survival. In a retrospective analysis, Peralta et al reported that among women undergoing CPM, 15-year disease-free survival was 55% compared with 28% for those who did not undergo CPM.[19] Rates of recurrence and overall survival were similar between the 2 groups. This suggests that the differences in disease-free survival were due largely to differences in incidence of contralateral breast cancer, and although CPM effectively prevented the development of contralateral disease this was offset by the risk of death from the index cancer. There was, however, a trend toward improved disease-specific survival in the subgroup of patients with early-stage breast cancer treated with CPM (stage 0 to 2; $p = 0.06$).

Herrinton et al examined the impact of CPM on reducing deaths from breast cancer.[24] They compared the outcomes of 1072 women who underwent CPM with a representative subgroup of 317 women (from a larger database of 55,328 patients) who did not undergo CPM. They found that CPM was associated with a 43% relative reduction in death from breast cancer. Breast cancer specific mortality was 8% in the CPM group compared with 12% in the no-CPM group.[24] However, overall survival was also improved among women who underwent CPM, thereby raising the possibility that the improvement noted in breast cancer specific survival was a reflection of patient selection bias rather than a true effect of CPM. These findings thus require confirmation in other large patient cohorts.

AESTHETIC SATISFACTION AND PSYCHOSOCIAL OUTCOMES AFTER PROPHYLACTIC SURGERY

Multiple studies have addressed patient satisfaction and psychosocial outcomes following prophylactic surgery. Almost all studies show that a small proportion of women who undergo either CPM or BPM are dissatisfied with the cosmetic outcome.[25]

Despite this, studies on psychosocial outcomes and quality of life demonstrate that women who choose to undergo prophylactic mastectomy fare as well on these parameters as women at similar risk for breast cancer who opt not to undergo surgical prophylaxis.[26-28] These outcomes hold true for both BRCA1/2 and non-BRCA1/2 mutation carriers, and in both BPM and CPM populations. These data underscore the personalized nature of the decision to undertake radical surgical intervention.

FUTURE DIRECTIONS

Unlike most areas of oncology, prophylactic efforts are unlikely to be subjected to randomized clinical trials. Undergoing prophylactic mastectomy is a personal issue and, even aside from the ethical concerns in randomizing women to such surgery, it is doubtful that any trial randomizing to a surgical prophylaxis arm would be able to accrue effectively. Thus, in the absence of such studies, other approaches are needed to address the challenges of taking care of women who seek prophylactic measures. Such approaches include use of large registries to provide sufficient sample size and thus sufficient statistical power to be able to determine survival benefits of prophylactic intervention. In addition, for women who are not carriers of known breast cancer risk genes, greater research is needed to improve risk stratification beyond the currently available clinical variables of family history and personal history of breast cancer and breast disease. In this regard, research into early molecular changes within the histologically nonneoplastic breast that may be indicative of cellular transformation or identification of single nucleotide polymorphisms in DNA extracted from blood that associate with significant increase in breast cancer risk would be invaluable. Through these multiple avenues, it is hoped that our current broad guidelines for prophylactic mastectomy, which result in substantial overtreatment, can be narrowed to limit such radical therapy only to those women who are highly likely to benefit.

SUMMARY

Preventing breast cancer through surgical means has been recognized for several decades. In the last 10 years, medical strategies have also been developed that reduce future risk of breast cancer. Despite the availability of the means to reduce breast cancer, significant controversy exists regarding the extent to which these strategies should be implemented. Foremost among the challenges in this area is the heterogeneity of patients at increased risk for breast cancer. This heterogeneity, coupled with significant limitations in predicting future breast cancer risk, a lack of data directly comparing medical with surgical prophylaxis, as well as a paucity of studies evaluating survival end points, underscores the need to counsel women extensively prior to selecting whether and which prophylactic measure to undertake.

REFERENCES

1. Chen S, Parmigiani G. Meta-analysis of BRCA1 and BRCA2 penetrance. *J Clin Oncol.* 2007;25(11):1329-1333.
2. Antoniou A, Pharoah PD, Narod S, et al. Average risks of breast and ovarian cancer associated with BRCA1 or BRCA2 mutations detected in case

series unselected for family history: a combined analysis of 22 studies. *Am J Hum Genet* 2003;72(5):1117-1130.

3. Meijers-Heijboer H, van Geel B, van Putten WL, et al. Breast cancer after prophylactic bilateral mastectomy in women with a BRCA1 or BRCA2 mutation. *N Engl J Med.* 2001;345(3):159-164.

4. Rebbeck TR, Friebel T, Lynch HT, et al. Bilateral prophylactic mastectomy reduces breast cancer risk in BRCA1 and BRCA2 mutation carriers: the PROSE Study Group. *J Clin Oncol.* 2004;22(6):1055-1062.

5. Scheuer L, Kauff N, Robson M, et al. Outcome of preventive surgery and screening for breast and ovarian cancer in BRCA mutation carriers. *J Clin Oncol.* 2002;20(5):1260-1268.

6. Schrag D, Kuntz KM, Garber JE, Weeks JC. Decision analysis—effects of prophylactic mastectomy and oophorectomy on life expectancy among women with BRCA1 or BRCA2 mutations. *N Engl J Med.* 1997;336(20):1465-1471.

7. King MC, Wieand S, Hale K, et al. Tamoxifen and breast cancer incidence among women with inherited mutations in BRCA1 and BRCA2: National Surgical Adjuvant Breast and Bowel Project (NSABP-P1) Breast Cancer Prevention Trial. *JAMA.* 2001;286(18):2251-2256.

8. Metcalfe K, Lynch HT, Ghadirian P, et al. Contralateral breast cancer in BRCA1 and BRCA2 mutation carriers. *J Clin Oncol.* 2004;22(12):2328-2335.

9. van Sprundel TC, Schmidt MK, Rookus MA, et al. Risk reduction of contralateral breast cancer and survival after contralateral prophylactic mastectomy in BRCA1 or BRCA2 mutation carriers. *Br J Cancer.* 2005;93(3):287-292.

10. Schrag D, Kuntz KM, Garber JE, Weeks JC. Life expectancy gains from cancer prevention strategies for women with breast cancer and BRCA1 or BRCA2 mutations. *JAMA.* 2000;283(5):617-624.

11. Hartmann LC, Schaid DJ, Woods JE, et al. Efficacy of bilateral prophylactic mastectomy in women with a family history of breast cancer. *N Engl J Med.* 1999;340(2):77-84.

12. Hamm RM, Lawler F, Scheid D. Prophylactic mastectomy in women with a high risk of breast cancer. *N Engl J Med.* 1999;340(23):1837-1838; author reply 1839.

13. Fisher B, Costantino JP, Wickerham DL, et al. Tamoxifen for prevention of breast cancer: report of the National Surgical Adjuvant Breast and Bowel Project P-1 Study. *J Natl Cancer Inst.* 1998;90(18):1371-1388.

14. Cuzick J, Powles T, Veronesi U, et al. Overview of the main outcomes in breast-cancer prevention trials. *Lancet.* 2003;361(9354):296-300.

15. Vogel VG, Costantino JP, Wickerham DL, et al. Effects of tamoxifen vs raloxifene on the risk of developing invasive breast cancer and other disease outcomes: the NSABP Study of Tamoxifen and Raloxifene (STAR) P-2 trial. *JAMA.* 2006;295(23):2727-2741.

16. McCredie JA, Inch WR, Alderson M. Consecutive primary carcinomas of the breast. *Cancer.* 1975;35(5):1472-1477.

17. Healey EA, Cook EF, Orav EJ, et al. Contralateral breast cancer: clinical characteristics and impact on prognosis. *J Clin Oncol* 1993;11(8):1545-1552.

18. Fisher ER, Fisher B, Sass R, Wickerham L. Pathologic findings from the National Surgical Adjuvant Breast Project (Protocol No. 4). XI. Bilateral breast cancer. *Cancer.* 1984;54(12):3002-3011.

19. Peralta EA, Ellenhorn JD, Wagman LD, et al. Contralateral prophylactic mastectomy improves the outcome of selected patients undergoing mastectomy for breast cancer. *Am J Surg.* 2000;180(6):439-445.

20. McDonnell SK, Schaid DJ, Myers JL, et al. Efficacy of contralateral prophylactic mastectomy in women with a personal and family history of breast cancer. *J Clin Oncol.* 2001;19(19):3938-3943.

21. Goldflam K, Hunt KK, Gershenwald JE, et al. Contralateral prophylactic mastectomy. Predictors of significant histologic findings. *Cancer.* 2004;101(9):1977-1986.

22. Babiera GV, Lowy AM, Davidson BS, Singletary SE. The role of contralateral prophylactic mastectomy in invasive lobular carcinoma. *Breast J.* 1997;3(1):2-6.

23. Vo TN, Meric-Bernstam F, Yi M, et al. Outcomes of breast-conservation therapy for invasive lobular carcinoma are equivalent to those for invasive ductal carcinoma. *Am J Surg.* 2006;192(4):552-555.

24. Herrinton LJ, Barlow WE, Yu O, et al. Efficacy of prophylactic mastectomy in women with unilateral breast cancer: a cancer research network project. *J Clin Oncol.* 2005;23(19):4275-4286.

25. Isern AE, Tengrup I, Loman N, et al. Aesthetic outcome, patient satisfaction, and health-related quality of life in women at high risk undergoing prophylactic mastectomy and immediate breast reconstruction. *J Plast Reconstr Aesthet Surg.* 2008;61(10):1177-1187.

26. Geiger AM, West CN, Nekhlyudov L, et al. Contentment with quality of life among breast cancer survivors with and without contralateral prophylactic mastectomy. *J Clin Oncol.* 2006;24(9):1350-1356.

27. Geiger AM, Nekhlyudov L, Herrinton LJ, et al. Quality of life after bilateral prophylactic mastectomy. *Ann Surg Oncol.* 2007;14(2):686-694.

28. Tercyak KP, Peshkin BN, Brogan BM, et al. Quality of life after contralateral prophylactic mastectomy in newly diagnosed high-risk breast cancer patients who underwent BRCA1/2 gene testing. *J Clin Oncol.* 2007;25(3):285-291.

CHAPTER 66

Skin-Sparing Mastectomy

Judy C. Boughey
Kari M. Rosenkranz

Women with breast cancer and those who are at increased risk of developing breast cancer may consider mastectomy as an option for treatment or a step toward risk reduction. Historically, mastectomy in the absence of breast reconstruction was associated with a significant change in body image. For this reason, breast conservation therapy emerged as an oncologically safe and emotionally less impacting option for the surgical treatment of breast cancer. Following the reporting of pivotal trials from Milan and the National Surgical Adjuvant Breast and Bowel Project (NSABP) in the 1970s and 1980s, breast-conservation rates rose dramatically. In recent years, however, mastectomy rates are increasing. This is thought to be at least in part due to improvements in cosmetic outcomes after mastectomy.

Initially the Halsted radical mastectomy, which resected en bloc the breast, regional lymph nodes, and underlying pectoralis muscles, left a severely disfigured chest wall and resulted in significant morbidity. Adoption of the modified radical mastectomy (MRM) technique allowed preservation of the pectoralis major and minor muscles, and internal mammary and supraclavicular nodal basins, resulting in significantly less disfigurement and reducing morbidity. The goal of mastectomy is to remove all breast tissue; data suggest that approximately 95% of breast tissue is resected in a traditional simple or modified radical mastectomy. The anatomical boundaries of the breast are the clavicle superiorly, the inframammary fold inferiorly, the sternum medially, and the mid-axillary line laterally. Sufficient skin overlying the chest wall is preserved at the time of a simple mastectomy in order to allow coverage of the chest wall and primary closure of the incision.

Since the skin is not part of the glandular breast tissue itself but rather an envelope around the breast tissue, the idea of preserving the skin envelope led to the development of skin-sparing mastectomy (SSM). Skin-sparing mastectomy was first described by Toth and Lappert in the literature in 1991.[1] I describes the procedure of mastectomy, either simple or modified radical, with a minimum amount of skin excision. The surgical skin excision must (1) include the nipple areolar complex (NAC), (2) include the biopsy site, and (3) allow for access to the axilla for possible dissection. Also incorporated into the SSM definition are preservation of both the inframammary fold and any uninvolved skin. Early SSM excised an ellipse of skin encompassing the NAC and some of the surrounding skin medially and laterally, but preserved more of the skin overlying the breast than conventional mastectomy. This incision afforded wide access to the boundaries of the breast, and resulted in removal of a similar amount of breast tissue and a similar long horizontal incision, but preserved more of the skin envelope for immediate reconstruction. As the technique evolved, smaller and smaller incisions provided appropriate access to the breast tissue and maximal skin preservation. Currently, most surgeons utilize a circumareolar incision that resects the NAC while preserving the entirety of the breast envelope.

ONCOLOGIC SAFETY

With the advent of SSM, investigators appropriately questioned whether preservation of the skin envelope results in higher risk of local-regional recurrence. If SSM is not performed meticulously, and additional breast tissue is left on the skin flaps, the risk for local recurrence could be higher due to technically inadequate surgery. Multiple studies have evaluated the question of recurrence and established the oncological safety of the SSM approach. In patients matched for stage and length of followup (41-72 months), studies have shown favorable or equivalent rates of local recurrence with 3.9% to 9.5% recurrence in simple mastectomies compared to 0% to 7.0% in SSM (Table 66-1). Similarly, Slavin et al[2] reported an 11.7% (14/120) locoregional recurrence rate after non-SSM with

TABLE 66-1 Local Recurrence Rate in Published Studies after Skin-Sparing Mastectomy (SSM) Compared with Non–Skin-Sparing Mastectomy (NSSM)

Study	Institution	F/U	N (SSM)	LR in SSM (%)	N (NSSM)	LR in NSSM (%)	p-Value
Carlson (1997)[17]	Emory	41	327	4.8	188	9.5	NS
Kroll (1999)[25]	MDACC	72	114	7.0	40	7.5	NS
Rivadeneira (2000)[26]	Cornell	49	71	5.6	127	3.9	NS
Gerber (2003)[6]	Munich	59	112	5.4	134	8.2	NS
Newman (1998)[4]	MDACC	50	437	6.2			
Carlson (2003)[27]	Emory	65	565	5.5			
Toth (1999)[28]	California Pacific	57	50	0			

immediate flap reconstruction with a median follow-up of 5.4 years. No patients with stage 0 or I breast cancer in this study recurred. No studies have demonstrated that the timing of reconstruction compromises the primary surgical resection, alters survival, or interferes with the detection and treatment of tumor recurrence. Based on the data from these studies, immediate reconstruction has gained acceptance and popularity.

The main advantage of SSM is the preservation of the skin envelope, which maintains the natural breast contour for the reconstruction to fill. Additionally, the shorter incision results in decreased scarring and improved cosmesis. The cosmetic outcome from a SSM with immediate reconstruction is better in women with a smaller body habitus than obese women. This is mainly due to the ability of the reconstruction to fill the natural skin envelope. Nipple-sparing mastectomy is the latest advancement in technique to preserve more tissue and improve cosmesis (see Chapter 67). Patient selection for SSM is important. Patients with inflammatory breast cancer are not candidates for SSM. Similarly, in cases of locally advanced breast cancers with skin involvement, a skin-sparing approach is not recommended. Neoadjuvant chemotherapy can convert a locally advanced breast cancer with skin involvement into a candidate for SSM if the skin changes completely resolve. However, if residual skin changes remain, SSM is not advised. Intraoperative analysis of margins is important for a skin-sparing approach and if the tumor extends close to the anterior margin, the overlying skin is often resected. Close margin does not, however, necessarily require conversion to a total mastectomy. Often, the skin in the area overlying the tumor can be resected either as an extension of the NAC incision or via a separate incision directly over the tumor.

Smoking is a relative contraindication to SSM. Most breast surgeons and plastic surgeons will not perform a SSM with immediate reconstruction on a patient who is actively smoking. This is due to the effect of smoke on small vessels and the associated increased risk of necrosis of the skin flaps and vasoconstriction of the myocutaneous flaps. The skin envelope of the native breast loses the blood supply from the underlying breast after SSM, and therefore the viability of the skin is dependent on the medial perforators. The larger the breast and the longer the skin flap, the higher the risk of skin necrosis. Surgeons vary in the minimum acceptable period of smoking cessation prior to surgery. Some surgeons will operate as few as 2 weeks smoke-free

whereas others require 6 weeks. Nicotine levels in the urine can be checked to confirm smoking cessation.

Patients not interested in any form of immediate reconstruction should undergo simple mastectomy with the goal of resecting enough skin to create a flat chest wall. This optimizes healing and allows the best fit for an external prosthesis. The advantage of the skin sparing technique is for the immediate reconstruction and, therefore, if reconstruction is not planned excess skin should be removed rather than preserved for potential delayed reconstruction. Skin-sparing mastectomy may be utilized in conjunction with autogenous tissue or implant-based reconstructions. These techniques provide superior cosmesis compared to a conventional mastectomy and compared to delayed reconstruction.

Patients who are likely to require postmastectomy radiation should consider the complications associated with radiation of a reconstructed breast before proceeding with SSM with reconstruction. Women with larger tumors (>5 cm), close margins, and positive lymph nodes may be considered for postmastectomy radiation and this can affect the outcome from SSM.

SURVEILLANCE AND SSM

As most recurrences will occur in skin of the chest wall, the ability to detect local recurrence is not impaired following SSM. Due to an absence of breast tissue, routine screening mammogram is not indicated for annual surveillance. Any recurrence is usually superficial and detected by physical examination. When any new palpable abnormality is detected, complete workup with mammogram, ultrasound, and magnetic resonance imaging (MRI) as indicated with biopsy of the lesion is recommended to rule out local recurrence.

INCISIONS

The final appearance of the reconstructed breast is greatly dependent on the relative amounts of skin and breast tissue excised at the time of the mastectomy and on the exact location of the skin incision. A complete mastectomy may be performed using modified skin incisions to avoid the sacrifice of unnecessary breast skin. The type of skin-sparing incision used varies based on the exact location of the tumor and the size of the breast, but it always includes the NAC and the biopsy site.

Input from the plastic surgeon regarding orientation and extent of skin incisions for SSM with immediate reconstruction is important, especially when a nonstandard incision is required in order to resect any additional skin due to concern of involvement with tumor.[1]

INTRAOPERATIVE MARGIN EVALUATION

Careful intraoperative evaluation of the mastectomy specimen is an important component to minimize the risk of positive margins following SSM. Intraoperative inking of margins with frozen section analysis of any close margins to fully evaluate all areas of concern is recommended. Resection of additional skin should be performed as necessary. At MD Anderson Cancer Center (MDACC), mammography of serial sections of the mastectomy specimen is performed if calcifications are present to assess for calcifications approaching a margin. At the Mayo Clinic, intraoperative frozen section of the mastectomy specimen with margin evaluation is routinely performed. Close margins mandate additional margin resection inclusive of overlying skin if necessary. Often if there is clinical concern preoperatively about an area of skin, preoperative imaging with MRI or ultrasound can help evaluate whether skin resection is required. Additionally, any areas of concern clinically can be marked with a marking pen prior to incision and if pathology reveals close margins in this area, the skin is clearly marked allowing accurate resection of the correct area of overlying skin. At Portsmouth-Tidewater Medical Center an alternative approach has been pioneered for transverse rectus abdominis muscle reconstruction (TRAM) reconstruction. In these women, a staged approach allows for the final inset of the TRAM 4 to 5 days following mastectomy. This allows final pathologic review prior to decisive closure. Nonviable mastectomy skin is replaced with redundant TRAM skin and reexcision of close or positive margins is based on final pathology. Although margins should be cleared surgically, postmastectomy radiation should be considered if postoperative margins are microscopically positive and not resected.

Because chest wall recurrence is the most frequent site of local failure after mastectomy, concerns over inadequate skin excision resulting in increased risk of local recurrence have been addressed. Slavin et al evaluated 51 patients with stage 0 to II breast cancer. Thirty-two SSMs were performed with a 5 mm margin of skin around the border of the NAC, and a total of 114 biopsies were taken from the remaining native skin flap edges. Histology revealed no evidence of breast ducts in the remaining tissue. Over a median follow-up of 45 months the local recurrence rate was 2%.[3]

Data from MDACC reported on 437 SSMs in 372 patients with T1 or T2 breast cancers. At a median follow-up of 50 months, 23 patients (6.2%) had experienced a local recurrence. The median time to recurrence was 25 months with a median size of the recurrence being 1 cm. Twenty-two of the 23 patients presented with a palpable skin mass (96%). The nonpalpable recurrence was detected on a chest x-ray. In 22 of 23 (96%) patients the histology was consistent with the primary tumor.[4]

Barton et al compared 27 SSMs to 28 conventional mastectomies and took multiple chest wall biopsies. They found equivalent amounts of residual glandular breast tissue remaining on the anterior chest walls of 27 patients who had undergone SSM compared to 28 patients following conventional mastectomy, based on multiple chest wall biopsies. Mammary tissue was identified in 5% of all biopsies. The amount of residual breast tissue in both standard mastectomy and skin-sparing mastectomy was approximately 0.2% of the preoperative breast tissue volume.[5]

Gerber et al compared MRM to SSM with and without preservation of the NAC. No significant difference was seen between SSM with resection of the NAC and MRM in terms of local recurrence rates, distant recurrence rates, and death rates.[6]

PATIENT SELECTION

Breast-conservation therapy remains an excellent option for the majority of women undergoing treatment for breast cancer. Nearly 50% of women diagnosed with breast cancer, however, continue to undergo mastectomy for definitive surgical therapy. Reasons for mastectomy include patient preference, multicentric disease, extensive ductal carcinoma in situ, history of prior breast irradiation, large tumor to breast size ratio, pre-existent comorbid conditions which include the possibility of adjuvant radiation therapy, and inflammatory breast cancer. For most of these women who request or require mastectomy, SSM with immediate breast reconstruction provides a reasonable clinical option.

The oncologic safety and satisfactory cosmesis of SSM with immediate reconstruction in early-stage (0, I, and IIB) breast cancer have been well documented in several retrospective studies as outlined above. Immediate reconstruction affords a psychological benefit to women confronted with mastectomy and minimizes the number of surgical procedures necessary to complete breast reconstruction.[7] Women with early-stage breast cancer should therefore be counseled preoperatively about the option of SSM with immediate reconstruction.

Patient selection for SSM in women with stage IIB and III breast cancer is more controversial. Inflammatory breast cancer and/or extensive skin involvement of primary tumor remain contraindications to SSM. Recent studies have begun to address the prudence of SSM with immediate reconstruction in women with locally advanced cancers. Theoretical concerns linger with respect to a potential delay in the initiation of adjuvant chemotherapy in patients experiencing surgical complications. Increasing numbers of women with locally advanced cancers are undergoing neoadjuvant chemotherapy. The completion of chemotherapy prior to definitive surgery obviates a potential postoperative delay in adjuvant systemic therapy delivery. For women treated with adjuvant chemotherapy, several retrospective studies have negated the concern regarding a delay in systemic treatment. Multiple authors have failed to demonstrate a statistically significant difference in the length of time from surgery to systemic therapy in women undergoing breast conservation, mastectomy without reconstruction, or SSM with immediate reconstruction.[8,9]

The issue of chest wall irradiation is more controversial in terms of patient selection for SSM. Danish and Canadian studies have conclusively illustrated a survival benefit following chest wall irradiation in women with tumors larger than 5 cm and/or 4 or more lymph nodes.[10-12] The role of chest wall irradiation in women with 1 to 3 positive nodes is being further elucidated but is not currently standard therapy.[13] As recommendations for postmastectomy chest wall irradiation evolve, particularly in younger women and potentially in the 1 to 3 node group, the number of women being recommended to undergo this therapy may significantly increase.[14] The question of whether these women are appropriate candidates for SSM with immediate reconstruction remains controversial and will be further addressed later in this chapter.

TECHNIQUE

The overriding goal of SSM is preservation of the natural breast envelope in order to facilitate a natural appearance of the reconstructed breast. Various incisions and a myriad of techniques are used to achieve this goal. Nipple-areolar sparing techniques will be discussed in Chapter 67 a separate chapter. In women undergoing excision of the NAC, incisions should be designed to minimize scarring and maximizing skin preservation. Most commonly, a circumareolar incision is utilized (Figs. 66-1, 66-2, and 66-3). For larger-breasted women, a lateral extension facilitates extirpation of the underlying breast tissue. When implants are placed, a horizontal ellipse facilitates implant or expander placement. Alternatively, breast reduction or mastopexy incisions may be used to address issues of contralateral symmetry and enlarge the area of dissection to minimize flap tension during retraction. Contralateral procedures are sometimes performed simultaneously or, alternatively, procedures for symmetry may be performed at a later date to match irradiated reconstructions. Most authors also recommend excision of biopsy scars at the time of mastectomy, although data regarding recurrence in the absence of excision are scant.[15,16] Sentinel node mapping and excision are generally performed through

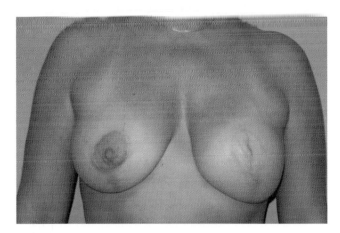

FIGURE 66-2 Immediate appearance following left TRAM and right reduction mammoplasty for symmetry.

the incisions described earlier. For women requiring completion axillary dissection, a separate axillary incision facilitates adequate dissection while minimizing stretch trauma to the mastectomy flaps. In women with smaller breasts, axillary dissection may alternatively be completed through the lateral extension of a periareolar incision. Some centers proceed with sentinel node biopsy in a prior surgery so that definitive axillary surgery is complete at the time of reconstruction.

Once an incision is made, skin flaps are elevated in an avascular plane just anterior to the superficial layer of the superficial fascia of the breast. Thickness of flaps varies with patient habitus; generally, women with minimal subcutaneous fat will have flaps 2 to 3 mm thick. The skin is gently retracted and dissection is undertaken in a circumferential manner (Fig. 66-4). Several instruments including the cut feature of electrocautery, harmonic scalpel, knife, or scissor may be used to carry out the dissection. Trauma to the flaps with heat coagulation or aggressive traction increases the risk of flap necrosis. Dissection is performed using the defined landmarks of the breast as in a

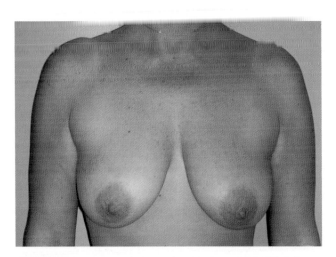

FIGURE 66-1 Preoperative appearance of a patient with left invasive ductal carcinoma.

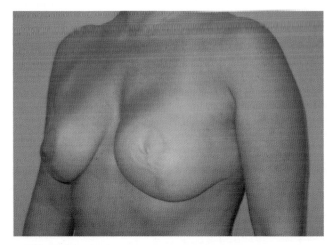

FIGURE 66-3 Appearance of same patient 18 months postoperatively.

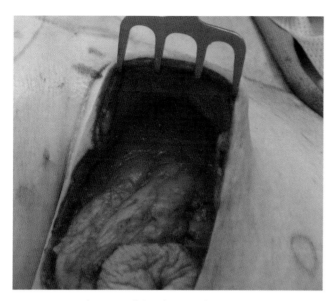

FIGURE 66-4 Elevation of the skin envelope in an avascular plane just anterior to the superficial layer of the superficial fascia of the breast.

standard simple mastectomy. The breast tissue is mobilized laterally to the border of the latissimus dorsi, medially to the sternal border, inferiorly to the inframammary fold, and superiorly to the clavicular border. Particular care should be taken to avoid disruption of the inframammary fold to maximize cosmesis following reconstruction. The fascia of the pectoralis major is included in the specimen as the deep margin. Regardless of mastectomy technique, some glandular tissue persists. Studies demonstrate equivalent amounts of residual glandular tissue when comparing MRM to SSM.[5]

COMPLICATIONS

Incidence of complications following SSM and reconstruction approaches 40%. Many of these complications are specific to the reconstructive technique utilized including implant loss, donor site infection or seroma, ventral hernia, and poor wound healing. The most common complication of SSM is native flap necrosis. The risk ranges from 8% to 24%[17-20] and smokers and diabetic patients harbor an increased risk.[17,21] Avoidance of unnecessarily thin flaps and minimizing the trauma to the subdermal vascular plexus with aggressive flap traction decrease the risk of flap ischemia. Less common complications include hematoma, cellulitis, and seroma formation. Diabetes, smoking, increased body mass index, and previous history of irradiation have all been linked to increased risk of complication following SSM.[20,21]

RADIATION AND SKIN-SPARING MASTECTOMY

As described above, the timing of radiation in the setting of breast reconstruction remains controversial. Radiation has a clear negative impact on the cosmesis of SSM with breast reconstruction. Major complication rates are also significantly impacted regardless of whether radiation precedes or follows reconstruction. Most importantly, however, is the oncologic question: Is the quality of radiation negatively affected by the presence of a reconstructed breast mound? Motwani et al concluded that 52% of radiation plans were altered due to the presence of an immediately reconstructed breast.[22] Other authors have formulated opposing beliefs concluding that SSM with immediate reconstruction in locally advanced breast cancer does not compromise adjuvant radiation planning and results in equivalent overall survival and local recurrence rates.[23] Prospective studies are required to better understand the issues involving radiation therapy following SSM. Until that time, we recommend the cautious use of SSM in women for whom radiation will likely be recommended. A discussion regarding the potential risks may steer women toward delayed reconstruction.

Predicting which women will be recommended postmastectomy irradiation is becoming increasingly difficult as indications are evolving. From this unpredictability, the concept of the delayed immediate SSM has evolved.[24] In this novel approach, SSM is performed with placement of a temporary tissue expander. In women for whom postmastectomy radiation is ultimately recommended, the expander is inflated until the time of radiation. The expander is then deflated to allow radiation fields to target the flattened chest wall obviating the interference of a breast mound and the subsequent compromise of delivery. Once radiation is complete, the expander is exchanged for a permanent reconstruction. Given the risk of fibrosis, capsular contracture, and infection with the placement of an implant in an irradiated field, autologous reconstruction is preferred.

RECURRENCE AND SKIN-SPARING MASTECTOMY

Retrospective studies have evaluated the risk of recurrence following SSM versus non-SSM. No statistically significant difference has been illustrated as detailed above. Data show that the presence of a reconstructed breast mound does not lead to delay in diagnosis of chest wall recurrence. The majority of recurrences present within the skin and are detected on clinical exam. Treatment includes excision with negative margins with the possible addition of radiation or chemotherapy. Rarely does local recurrence mandate complete removal of the reconstructed tissue unless multiple foci of disease are encountered or the patient expresses her preference for such treatment.

FUTURE DIRECTIONS

Multiple studies have demonstrated the oncologic safety, acceptable major complication rate, and good to excellent patient satisfaction associated with SSM. Many data, however, are retrospective. Prospective studies are required to address current issues of controversy including the timing of chest wall irradiation in women undergoing SSM with reconstruction, and the wisdom of immediate reconstruction in women with locally advanced cancers. New surgical devices may lead to lower complication rates, in particular, decreased incidence of native flap necrosis.

SUMMARY

Skin-sparing mastectomy is an oncologically safe, psychologically beneficial option for women undergoing mastectomy for risk reduction or for treatment of breast cancer. SSM is technically more demanding and has a significant complication rate, which can be minimized with attentiveness to surgical technique. Currently, we offer SSM to all women undergoing mastectomy for stage 0, I, and IIA breast cancer. We support the cautious use of SSM in women with locally advanced cancers following discussion with a multidisciplinary tumor board. Where possible, we encourage neoadjuvant chemotherapy to negate the possibility of a delay in initiation of systemic therapy in the event that surgical complications are encountered. In women for whom chest wall irradiation is predicted preoperatively, we support a discussion regarding risks and benefits of immediate versus delayed reconstruction. Particularly in the case of delayed reconstruction following chest wall irradiation, we encourage the use of autologous rather than implant reconstruction due to the high risk of major complications following implant reconstruction.

REFERENCES

1. Toth BA, Lappert P. Modified skin incisions for mastectomy: the need for plastic surgical input in preoperative planning. *Plast Reconstr Surg.* 1991;87:1048-1053.
2. Slavin SA, Love SM, Goldwyn RM. Recurrent breast cancer following immediate reconstruction with myocutaneous flaps. *Plast Reconstr Surg.* 1994;93:1191-1204; discussion 1205-1207.
3. Slavin SA, Schnitt SJ, Duda RB, et al. Skin-sparing mastectomy and immediate reconstruction: oncologic risks and aesthetic results in patients with early-stage breast cancer. *Plast Reconstr Surg.* 1998;102:49-62.
4. Newman LA, Kuerer HM, Hunt KK, et al. Presentation, treatment, and outcome of local recurrence afterskin-sparing mastectomy and immediate breast reconstruction. *Ann Surg Oncol.* 1998;5:620-626.
5. Barton FE Jr, English JM, Kingsley WB, et al. Glandular excision in total glandular mastectomy and modified radical mastectomy: a comparison. *Plast Reconstr Surg.* 1991;88:389-392; discussion 393-394.
6. Gerber B, Krause A, Reimer T, et al. Skin-sparing mastectomy with conservation of the nipple-areola complex and autologous reconstruction is an oncologically safe procedure. *Ann Surg.* 2003;238:120-127.
7. Schain WG, Wellisch DK, Pashan RO, et al. The sooner the better: a study of psychological factors in women undergoing immediate versus delayed breast reconstruction. *Am J Psychiatry.* 1985;142:40-46.
8. Mortenson MM, Schneider PD, Khatri VP, et al. Immediate breast reconstruction after mastectomy increases wound complications: however, initiation of adjuvant chemotherapy is not delayed. *Arch Surg.* 2004;139:988-991.
9. Giny S, Bourgier H, Miooum MC, et al. Immediate reconstruction after neoadjuvant chemotherapy: effect on adjuvant treatment starting and survival. *Ann Surg Oncol.* 2005;12:161-166.
10. Overgaard M, Jensen MB, Overgaard J, et al. Postoperative radiotherapy in high-risk postmenopausal breast-cancer patients given adjuvant tamoxifen: Danish Breast Cancer Cooperative Group DBCG 82c randomised trial. *Lancet.* 1999;353:1641-1648.
11. Early Breast Cancer Trialists' Collaborative Group. Favourable and unfavourable effects on long-term survival of radiotherapy for early breast cancer: an overview of the randomised trials. *Lancet.* 2000;355:1757-1770.
12. Ragaz J, Olivotto IA, Spinelli JJ, et al. Locoregional radiation therapy in patients with high-risk breast cancer receiving adjuvant chemotherapy: 20-year results of the British Columbia randomized trial. *J Natl Cancer Inst.* 2005;97:116-126.
13. Recht A, Edge SB. Evidence-based indications for postmastectomy irradiation. *Surg Clin North Am.* 2003;83:995-1013.
14. Truong PT, Olivotto IA, Whelan TJ, et al. Clinical practice guidelines for the care and treatment of breast cancer: 16. Locoregional post-mastectomy radiotherapy. *CMAJ.* 2004;170:1263-1273.
15. Uriburu JL, Vuoto HD, Cogorno L, et al. Local recurrence of breast cancer after skin-sparing mastectomy following core needle biopsy: case reports and review of the literature. *Breast J.* 2006;12:194-198.
16. Chao C, Torosian MH, Boraas MC, et al. Local recurrence of breast cancer in the stereotactic core needle biopsy site: case reports and review of the literature. *Breast J.* 2001;7:124-127.
17. Carlson GW, Bostwick J 3rd, Styblo TM, et al. Skin-sparing mastectomy. Oncologic and reconstructive considerations. *Ann Surg.* 1997;225:570-575; discussion 575-578.
18. Pinsolle V, Grinfeder C, Mathoulin Pelissier S, et al. Complications analysis of 266 immediate breast reconstructions. *J Plast Reconstr Aesthet Surg.* 2006;59:1017-1024.
19. Wijayanayagam A, Kumar AS, Foster RD, et al. Optimizing the total skin-sparing mastectomy. *Arch Surg.* 2008;143:38-45; discussion 45.
20. Hultman CS, Daiza S. Skin-sparing mastectomy flap complications after breast reconstruction: review of incidence, management, and outcome. *Ann Plast Surg.* 2003;50:249-255; discussion 255.
21. Chang DW, Reece GP, Wang B, et al. Effect of smoking on complications in patients undergoing free TRAM flap breast reconstruction. *Plast Reconstr Surg.* 2000;105:2374-2380.
22. Motwani SB, Strom EA, Schechter NR, et al. The impact of immediate breast reconstruction on the technical delivery of postmastectomy radiotherapy. *Int J Radiat Oncol Biol Phys.* 2006;66:76-82.
23. Downes KJ, Glatt BS, Kanchwala SK, et al. Skin-sparing mastectomy and immediate reconstruction is an acceptable treatment option for patients with high-risk breast carcinoma. *Cancer.* 2005;103:906-913.
24. Kronowitz SJ, Robb GL. Breast reconstruction with postmastectomy radiation therapy: current issues. *Plast Reconstr Surg.* 2004;114:950-960.
25. Kroll SS, Khoo A, Singletary SE, et al. Local recurrence risk after skin-sparing and conventional mastectomy: a 6-year follow up. *Plast Reconstr Surg.* 1999;104:421-425.
26. Rivadeneira DE, Simmons RM, Fish SK, et al. Skin-sparing mastectomy with immediate breast reconstruction: a critical analysis of local recurrence. *Cancer J.* 2000;6:331-335.
27. Carlson GW, Styblo TM, Lyles RH, et al. Local recurrence after skin-sparing mastectomy: tumor biology or surgical conservatism? *Ann Surg Oncol.* 2003;10:108-112.
28. Toth BA, Forley BG, Calabria R. Retrospective study of the skin-sparing mastectomy in breast reconstruction. *Plast Reconstr Surg.* 1999;104:77-84.

CHAPTER 67

Nipple- and Areola-Sparing Mastectomy

Meredith Kato
Rache M. Simmons

It is hard to believe that we are only a generation away from the widespread use of the Halstead radical mastectomy. Indeed, breast surgery, as in other areas of surgery, has moved away from more invasive procedures toward minimally invasive techniques. This, coupled with the desire for improved cosmetic outcomes, has been the driving force behind innovation in breast surgery over the last 30 years. The success of the skin-sparing mastectomy (SSM) has emboldened surgeons to consider procedures that preserve the nipple and areola as well. Despite the fact that nipple and areola reconstructions generally have excellent satisfaction rates, the nipple remains the cornerstone of breast identity, and evidence of the psychological importance of the nipple-areola complex (NAC) abounds.[1] Furthermore, preserving the nipple has the potential to salvage nipple sensation. There is a growing body of evidence on nipple-sparing (NSM) and areola-sparing (ASM) mastectomies. Nevertheless, the topic remains controversial amid concerns about oncologic safety, and there is consensus for neither selection criteria nor technique.

The NSM was first described by Freeman in 1962, who called it the subcutaneous mastectomy. The procedure involved removal of the breast through a submammary or thoracomammary incision while preserving NAC and was recommended for recurrent chronic or subacute mastitis.[2] The surgery was plagued by complications, especially flap necrosis, and was eventually abandoned.[3] Of note, patients who had the surgery, which removed the breast tissue from an inferior incision, reported a delayed return of sensation to the nipple with permanent loss in many. In 1978, Freeman went on to describe an areola-sparing procedure, called a total glandular mastectomy, for patients with noninvasive cancers.[4] A year later Randall et al described an "apple coring" technique for a subcutaneous mastectomy in an effort to improve oncologic safety while preserving as much of the NAC as possible.[5] Despite these early efforts, the procedure was abandoned in the proceeding decades amid concerns for oncologic safety.

ANATOMY

Central to the debate over the oncologic safety of the NSM is the anatomy of the NAC and the risk of cancer developing in remaining tissue following surgery. Anatomic studies of the areola date back to Morgagni's work in the 1719. The first thorough description was undertaken by Montgomery in 1837. He described the raised areolar prominences that bear his name and established that lactiferous ducts indeed empty into the areola. In 1980, Smith et al looked at serial sections of Montgomery's tubercles from 12 mastectomy specimens. They found that the tubercles were associated with lactiferous ducts 97% of the time.[6] Of note, they found focal atypia in 2 of the tubercles and ductal carcinoma in situ (DCIS) in 1. In 1992, Schnitt et al looked at 8 mastectomy specimens performed for invasive carcinoma.[7] They found mammary ducts in the areola of all 8 cases and carcinoma in 2 of them.

Obviously, the nipple contains the ducts draining the breast parenchyma and this ductal tissue is vulnerable to neoplastic transformation, but recent work has made our understanding more sophisticated. Stolier and Wang looked at nipple cross sections from mastectomy specimens. They found that 9% of mastectomy specimens contained terminal duct lobular units, the origin of most cancers.[8] Rusby et al also did nipple cross sections from mastectomy specimens and subjected them to 3-dimensional reconstructions (Fig. 67-1).[9] They found that ducts were arranged in a central bundle surrounded by a duct-free rim of tissue. Some of the ducts originated in the areola, but these were morphologically different from ducts forming the central duct bundle, tending to be narrower and without crenellations.

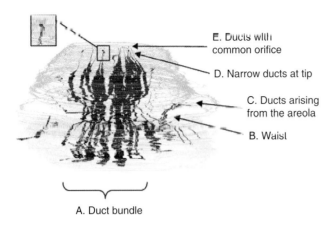

FIGURE 67-1 Three-dimensional reconstruction of the nipple. Skin in tan, cut edge in yellow, and ducts in purple. **A.** Ducts in a central bundle. **B.** Bundle narrows to a waist just beneath the skin. **C.** Some ducts originate in the areola or partway up the nipple. **D.** Most ducts narrow as they approach the tip of the nipple. **E.** Many of the ducts originate from a few clefts. *[Reproduced, with permission, from Rusby JE, Brachtel EF, Michaelson JS, et al. Breast duct anatomy in the human nipple: three-dimensional patterns and clinical implications. Breast Cancer Res Treat. 2007;106(2):171-185.]*

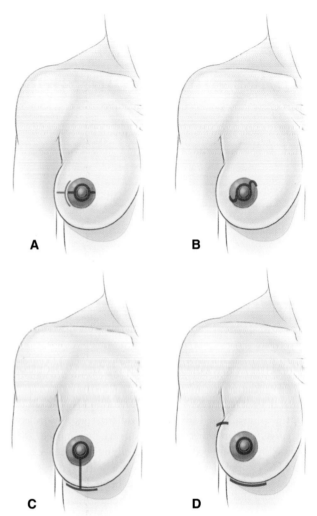

FIGURE 67-2 Schematic representation of incisions used for ASM (small purple line indicates line of incision). **A.** Linear intra-areola incision with extra-areola extension. **B.** S-shaped intra-areola incision. **C.** Inverted-T inframammary crease incision. **D.** Triple incision with inframammary crease, peri-nipple, and axillary incisions. *[Reproduced from Simmons RM, Hollenbeck ST, Latrenta GS. Areola-sparing mastectomy with immediate breast reconstruction. Ann Plast Surg. 2003;51(6):547-551.]*

They also noted that position of a duct within a nipple did not predict where it terminated in the breast parenchyma. Sections from additional specimens demonstrated that leaving a 2-mm rim of tissue in the nipple papilla excised 96% of the ducts while still leaving 50% of the blood supply.[10]

Erectile function and sensation of the NAC is dependent upon preservation of the nerve supply. The majority of the nerve supply comes from T4; nerves travel along the chest wall and move medially toward the nipple. There is a secondary supply that originates from the medial T3, emerges lateral to the sternum, and travels to the skin via the lower inner corner of the NAC.[11]

AREOLA-SPARING MASTECTOMY

Risk of Malignancy in the Areola

While few have looked at the anatomy of the areola as a separate entity, even fewer have attempted to identify the risk of cancer of the areola apart from that of the nipple. Simmons et al undertook a retrospective analysis of 217 mastectomy specimens looking for malignant involvement of the nipple, areola, or both by serial sectioning.[12] They found that the areola was only involved in 2 of 217 patients (0.9%) and both specimens had large (>5 cm), centrally located tumors. Similar results were published by Banerjee et al, who found areolar involvement in 2 of 219 (0.9%) mastectomy patients.[13] Paget disease isolated to the areola is extremely rare, but has been described in the literature.[14]

Areola-Sparing Mastectomy

Based on the results of their pathologic analysis of mastectomy specimens, Simmons et al performed ASMs on women for DCIS

and small peripheral infiltrating carcinomas, and for prophylactic mastectomy.[15] Patients with inflammatory carcinoma, invasive cancer directly beneath the nipple, and locally advanced disease were excluded. One of 4 incisions was used in all cases: tennis racquet, s-shaped, inverted T inframammary crease, or a triple incision (Fig. 67-2). The choice of incision was based upon size of the breast and areola, whether or not a reduction mammoplasty was performed on the opposite breast, and surgeon preference. The procedure resected the nipple, any previous biopsy scar, and all breast parenchyma leaving the areola and a maximum amount of skin for reconstruction immediately to follow. Sentinel node biopsies were performed for patients with carcinoma. A touch prep cytologic evaluation[16] of the underside of the areolar flaps was performed on 2 patients with DCIS and microinvasion resulting in negative cytology. Obviously, any gross extension of tumor into the areola or positive touch prep cytology required conversion to a SSM. The flaps were assessed

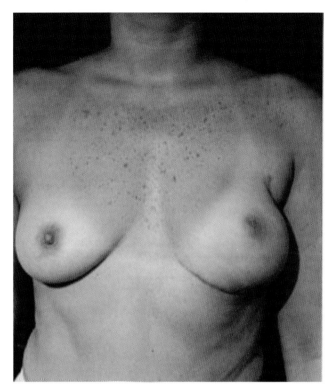

FIGURE 67-3   Cosmetic outcomes for ASM. [Reproduced, with permission, from Simmons RM, Hollenbeck ST, Latenta GS. Areola-sparing mastectomy with immediate breast reconstruction. Ann Plast Surg. 2003;51(6):547-551.]

for viability and converted to a SSM if perfusion to the areola was compromised. There were good cosmetic results with no instances of flap necrosis (Fig. 67-3).

Simmons et al published 2-year follow-up on 12 of these patients receiving 17 ASMs with immediate reconstructions.[17] Of all the procedures performed, 4 were for DCIS; 3 were for peripherally located, infiltrating carcinomas less than 2 cm; and 10 were for prophylaxis. Patients were followed for complications and recurrence. Ten patients underwent sentinel node biopsy and none were positive. All patients had negative histologic margins. None of the patients had chemotherapy of radiation. Two patients with DCIS and microinvasion underwent intraoperative subareolar touch-prep cytological evaluation with negative results. There was only 1 postoperative complication—a wound infection which resolved with oral antibiotics. With a median of 24 months follow-up, there were no recurrences.

Though the data generated by Simmons et al are compelling, they lack the power to generate a consensus among practitioners. Key to success when performing ASM is patient selection. Simmons et al currently recommend an ASM for prophylaxis, DCIS, and small, peripherally located infiltrating carcinoma, but not for inflammatory carcinoma, invasive cancer directly beneath or involving the NAC, or locally advanced disease. There is no consensus in the literature; additional studies and further follow-up are needed to establish the ASM as the standard of care for a select patient population.

NIPPLE-SPARING MASTECTOMY

The NSM has long been a temptation for the breast surgeon, with presumed psychological, cosmetic, and functional improvements over the skin-sparing mastectom. These benefits must be carefully weighed against the oncologic safety of the procedure. The topic is hotly debated and a review of the literature is a worthy exercise.

Risk of Cancer in the Nipple

Interest in the risk of malignancy, specifically of the NAC, dates back at least 30 years. Several groups in the 1970s and 1980s looked at serial sections of mastectomy specimens to look for the presence of disease in the NAC. Pathologic evaluation of the NACs revealed involvement in anywhere from 8% to 58%.[18] Most of the studies examined nipple sections of consecutive mastectomy specimens and did not exclude patients with clinically evident involvement of the NAC. However, Morimoto et al did exclude patients with tumor directly below the NAC and those with clinically abnormal nipples. They still found nipple involvement in 31% after looking at 141 specimens.[19] It is tempting, given the increased surveillance and earlier intervention, to question the applicability of these results to today's mastectomy patients. However, more recent studies do not indicate that the risk of nipple involvement at the time of surgery is any less than it was 30 years ago.

Several groups have looked at this question more recently. Laronga et al investigated 286 consecutive mastectomy specimens finding NAC involvement in 5.6%. They found that the only correlate with NAC involvement was tumor location; subareolar and multicentric cancers were more likely to involve the nipple.[20] Simmons et al found malignant nipple involvement in 10.6% of patients (23/217). The only variable that reliably predicted nipple involvement was the location of the tumor in the breast. Central, diffuse, or retroareolar tumors had nipple involvement 27.3% of the time compared to only 6.4% of peripherally located tumors.[12] Banerjee et al looked at 219 mastectomy specimens and revealed nipple involvement in 19%. They too found that tumor location was the most important predictor. Schecter et al found a rate of 42% of NAC involvement. This number dropped only to 29% when they excluded clinically evident nipple involvement at the time of surgery. They found that tumor distance from the NAC, tumor size, and pathologic stage helped to predict NAC involvement. However, in contrast to many other studies, location of tumor in the breast did not correlate with NAC involvement.[21]

While studies attempting to quantify the risk of nipple involvement reveal widely varying results, most report numbers that are beyond a comfort zone of oncologic safety. Nonetheless, many groups have assessed outcomes after NSM.

Outcomes Following NSM

Several groups performing NSMs for prophylaxis and cancer have reported their outcomes. Total recurrence rates range from 0% to 44% and nipple recurrence from 0% to 12% (Table 67-1). Gerber et al conducted a prospective study comparing NSM, SSM, and modified radial mastectomy (MRM) outcomes over

TABLE 67-1 Comparison of Recurrence Rates for NSM

Author	Year	NSM: DCIS or Cancer	NSM: Prophylaxis	Total Recurrence (Local and Distant Metastasis)	Nipple Recurrence	Follow-Up in Months
Bishop[35]	1990	24	0	7 (29%)	3(12%)	3.8 (mean)
Cheung[30]	1997	134	0	19 (14%)	6 (4.4%)	30 (min)
Hartmann[27]	1999	0	179	7 (3.9%)*	1 (0.56%)*	168 (median)
Gerber[22]	2003	61	0	17 (28%)	1 (1.6%)	59 (mean)
Margulies[40]	2005	26	5	0	0	7.9 (mean)
Caruso[39]	2006	50	0	6 (12%)	1 (2%)	66 (mean)
Sacchini[29]	2006	68	55	5 (4%)	0	25 (median)
Benediktsson[23]	2007	216	0	96 (44%)	Not reported	156 (median)
Denewer[28]	2007	41	0	0	0	7.9 (median)
Petit[26]	2008	579	0	27 (4.7%)	0	19 (median)

*New cancers, not recurrences.

a mean of 59 months. While they did have 1 nipple recurrence (1.6%) in the NSM group, overall there were nonsignificant differences in local recurrence, distant metastasis, and overall survival.[22] Benediktsson et al recently published long term follow-up for NSM.[23] Of 216 patients receiving NSM, 52 (24%) of them had a locoregional recurrence and 44 (20%) of them developed distant metastasis. However, due to the long follow-up (median 13 years), not all of the patients received today's standard of care. When patients receiving postoperative radiotherapy were stratified out, the locoregional recurrence rate dropped to 5.9% for premenopausal women and 10.3% for postmenopausal patients.

Petit et al described a novel technique adding intraoperative radiotherapy to NSM and followed over 1000 patients receiving this treatment for an average of 20 months.[24,25] They observed 14 (1.4%) loco-regional recurrences, 36 (3.6%) patients with distant metastasis, and 4 (0.4%) deaths. Of note, no recurrences were noted in the NAC even for patients with close or positive margins on final pathology.[26]

The risk of de novo cancer in the nipple is particularly pertinent for candidates for NSM. Hartmann et al conducted a study to follow high-risk women after a prophylaxic NSM. Of 573 moderate- and high-risk patients who underwent an NSM, only 7 went on to develop cancer (3.9%) including 1 who developed a new cancer in the nipple (0.2%). There was no significant difference between the groups receiving a total mastectomy and those receiving an NSM, though statistical power was low.[27]

Cosmetic Outcome and Functionality Following NSM

The potential benefits of the NSM have long been described, but seldom quantified, in the literature. Improved cosmetic outcomes and improved functionality are frequently cited as reasons to pursue NSM in appropriately selected patients. Several groups have looked at cosmetic outcomes of NSM and reported excellent aesthetic results in over 75% of patients.[22,28-30] Only Gerber et al conducted a head-to-head comparison

between NSM and SSM from the perspective of both the surgeon and the patient. Patients reported similar results from both groups. Eighty-two percent of NSM patients reported an excellent result compared to 78.4% of SSM patients. The surgeons saw greater differences; only 53.8% of SSM results were judged to be excellent in the SSM, compared to 73.8% of the NSM group (Fig. 67-4). In general, the available literature demonstrates that patients are very satisfied with the aesthetic[31] outcome of SSM and that the improvement provided by NSM is marginal at best.

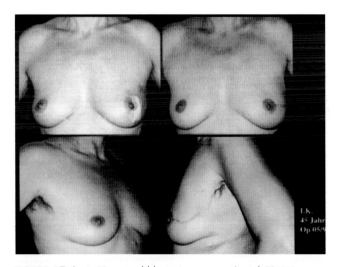

FIGURE 67-4 A 40-year-old breast cancer patient (pT2, N1, M0, R0) after an NSM with a latissimus dorsi flap reconstruction 6 months post-op. [Reproduced, with permission, from Gerber B, Krause A, Reimer T, et al. Skin-sparing mastectomy with conservation of the nipple-areola complex and autologous reconstruction is an oncologically safe procedure. Ann Surg. 2003;238(1):120-127.]

Another central argument for NSM is improved functional outcomes.[32] Retaining not only the NAC, but also some of its nerve supply, has the potential to maintain sensation and erectile function of the nipple. Few of the studies address this crucial point, none of them with systematic, objective measurement. Denewer and Farouk found that 90% of NSM patients retained some sensation in the nipple and 68.2% found it to be the same as before NSM.[28] Gerber et al had similar results, with 75.4% reporting some sensation in the nipple.[22] In contrast, Petit et al found return of sensation in only 33% of patients undergoing NSM with intraoperative radiotherapy.[25]

No group has measured the psychological benefit of retaining the nipple. It is intuitive that amputation results in a sense of mutilation in patients, but the benefit of keeping the nipple has not been measured.

Technical Considerations of NSM

The NSM entails the removal of as much breast parenchyma as possible while preserving the nipple and areola complex. There are at least 4 incisions used for NSM (Fig. 67-5).[28,29,33-35] Choice of incision is determined by the location of any previous biopsy scars and surgeon preference. Central to the technical success of the procedure is the preservation of the blood supply to the NAC. Consequently, some breast tissue must be left behind to insure viability.[36] To counter this, some groups core out the major ducts from within the lumen of the nipple and send it as a separate pathological specimen.[29,37] The dreaded complication associated with this procedure is NAC necrosis, occurring when too much of the underlying tissue is removed and the blood supply is compromised. Rates depend on the surgeon and vary from 0% to 20%.[29,33,34,37,38]

All surgeons remove the NAC if there is evidence of malignant involvement. Most groups employ intraoperative frozen section to identify residual tumor either at the areolar margin or the nipple core.[22,23,25,37,39]

SUMMARY

ASM and NSM remain controversial procedures, as available data do not allow consensus among practitioners. While the literature supports the practice of ASM in carefully selected patients, the studies are too few and underpowered. The excellent cosmetic outcome and oncologic safety of the ASM notwithstanding, the bulk of current research still focuses on saving the nipple.

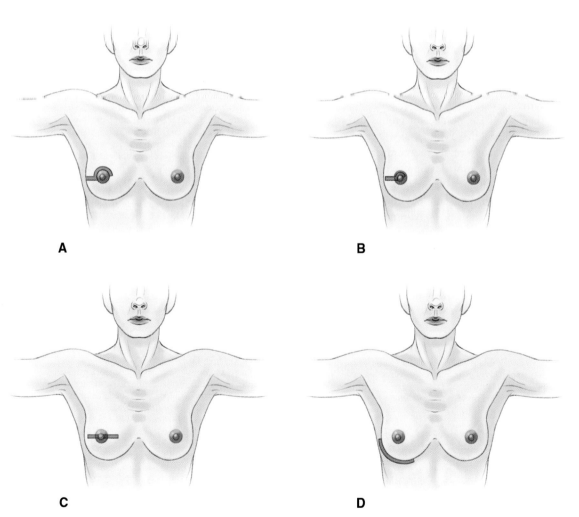

A   **B**

C   **D**

FIGURE 67-5 Incisions used for NSM. *[Reproduced from Chung AP, Sacchini V. Nipple-sparing mastectomy: where are we now? Surg Oncol. 2008;17(4):261-266.]*

TABLE 67-2 Areas of Further Research

Additional pathologic studies looking at the risk of cancer in the areola

Long-term, prospective studies for oncologic outcomes of ASM and NSM

Comparison of aesthetic outcome between NSM and SSM

Functionality assessments following NSM

The available data suggest that cancer in the nipple is not a rare event, ranging from 8% to 58% of pathologic specimens. However, outcomes data, including long-term follow-up of NSM, show that recurrence in the nipple is low, probably less than 5%. At the very core of the issue is the question, "How much risk is too much?" or, alternatively, "How little benefit is too little benefit?"

There is powerful motivation among patients and practitioners to save the nipple. Unfortunately, results supporting NSM to maximize cosmetic outcome and functionality are mixed. Objective measurements, especially those from patients, reveal a similar level of satisfaction in NSM patients and SSM patients. Preservation of sensation to the nipple is seldom reported, but is a crucial factor in determining the risk to benefit ratio. Currently, postoperative sensation varies widely among surgeons who report on it. Psychological factors, such as retention of breast identity and decreased sense of mutilation, have not been measured, but these benefits are easy to understand from the patient's perspective.

Currently, there are a fair number of groups investigating this issue, but it is doubtful that a consensus will emerge among practitioners. In sharp contrast to the comparison between SSM and MRM, where the cosmetic improvement was vast and the oncologic risk was comparable, the differences between NSM and SSM are much more subtle. Still, further research will help clarify the issue (Table 67-2). Ultimately, the application of the NSM to individual patients will depend upon the patient's tolerance for risk, her personal desire to save the nipple, and her practitioner's comfort level with the procedure. As with any surgical procedure, good communication between a patient and her doctor will lead to the best outcomes.

REFERENCES

1. Wellisch DK, Schain WS, Noone RB, Little JW 3rd. The psychological contribution of nipple addition in breast reconstruction. *Plast Reconstr Surg.* 1987;80(5):699-704.
2. Freeman BS. Subcutaneous mastectomy for benign breast lesions with immediate or delayed prosthetic replacement. *Plast Reconstr Surg Transplant Bull.* 1962;30:676-682.
3. Freeman BS. Complications of subcutaneous mastectomy with prosthetic replacement, immediate or delayed. *South Med J.* 1967;60(12):1277-1280.
4. Freeman BS, Wiemer DR. Total glandular mastectomy. Modifications of the subcutaneous mastectomy for use in premalignant disease of the breast. *Plast Reconstr Surg.* 1978;62(2):167-172.
5. Randall P, Dabb R, Loc N. "Apple coring" the nipple in subcutaneous mastectomy. *Plast Reconstr Surg.* 1979;64(6):800-803.
6. Smith DM Jr, Peters TG, Donegan WL. Montgomery's areolar tubercle. A light microscopic study. *Arch Pathol Lab Med.* 1982;106(2):60-63.

7. Schnitt SJ, Goldwyn RM, Slavin SA. Mammary ducts in the areola: implications for patients undergoing reconstructive surgery of the breast. *Plast Reconstr Surg.* 1993;92(7):1290-1293.
8. Stolier AJ, Wang J. Terminal duct lobular units are scarce in the nipple: implications for prophylactic nipple-sparing mastectomy: terminal duct lobular units in the nipple. *Ann Surg Oncol.* 2008;15(2):438-442.
9. Rusby JE, Brachtel EF, Michaelson JS, et al. Breast duct anatomy in the human nipple: three-dimensional patterns and clinical implications. *Breast Cancer Res Treat.* 2007;106(2):171-179.
10. Rusby JE, Brachtel EF, Taghian A, et al. George Peters Award. Microscopic anatomy within the nipple: implications for nipple-sparing mastectomy. *Am J Surg.* 2007;194(4):433-437.
11. Laronga C. Quality of life with skin-sparing mastectomy: sensation in the nipple-areola complex. *J Support Oncol.* 2006;4(5):234-235.
12. Simmons RM, Brennan M, Christos P, et al. Analysis of nipple/areolar involvement with mastectomy: can the areola be preserved? *Ann Surg Oncol.* 2002;9(2):165-168.
13. Banerjee A, Gupta S, Bhattacharya N. Preservation of nipple-areola complex in breast cancer—a clinicopathological assessment. *J Plast Reconstr Aesthet Surg.* 2008;61(10):1195-1198.
14. van der Putte SC, Toonstra J, Hennipman A. Mammary Paget's disease confined to the areola and associated with multifocal Toker cell hyperplasia. *Am J Dermatopathol.* 1995;17(5):487-493.
15. Simmons RM, Hollenbeck ST, Latrenta GS. Areola-sparing mastectomy with immediate breast reconstruction. *Ann Plast Surg.* 2003;51(6):547-551.
16. Klimberg VS, Westbrook KC, Korourian S. Use of touch preps for diagnosis and evaluation of surgical margins in breast cancer. *Ann Surg Oncol.* 1998;5(3):220-226.
17. Simmons RM, Hollenbeck ST, Latrenta GS. Two-year follow-up of areola-sparing mastectomy with immediate reconstruction. *Am J Surg.* 2004;188(4):403-406.
18. Garcia-Etienne CA, Borgen PI. Update on the indications for nipple-sparing mastectomy. *J Support Oncol.* 2006;4(5):225-230.
19. Morimoto T, Komaki K, Inui K, et al. Involvement of nipple and areola in early breast cancer. *Cancer.* 1985;55(10):2459-2463.
20. Laronga C, Kemp B, Johnston D, et al. The incidence of occult nipple-areola complex involvement in breast cancer patients receiving a skin-sparing mastectomy. *Ann Surg Oncol.* 1999;6(6):609-613.
21. Schecter AK, Freeman MB, Giri D, et al. Applicability of the nipple-areola complex-sparing mastectomy: a prediction model using mammography to estimate risk of nipple-areola complex involvement in breast cancer patients. *Ann Plast Surg.* 2006;56(5):498-504; discussion 504.
22. Gerber B, Krause A, Reimer T, et al. Skin-sparing mastectomy with conservation of the nipple-areola complex and autologous reconstruction is an oncologically safe procedure. *Ann Surg.* 2003;238(1):120-127.
23. Benediktsson KP, Perbeck L. Survival in breast cancer after nipple-sparing subcutaneous mastectomy and immediate reconstruction with implants: a prospective trial with 13 years median follow-up in 216 patients. *Eur J Surg Oncol.* 2008;34(2):143-148.
24. Petit JY, Veronesi U, Luini A, et al. When mastectomy becomes inevitable: the nipple-sparing approach. *Breast.* 2005;14(6):527-531.
25. Petit JY, Veronesi U, Orecchia R, et al. Nipple-sparing mastectomy in association with intra operative radiotherapy (ELIOT): a new type of mastectomy for breast cancer treatment. *Breast Cancer Res Treat.* 2006;96(1):47-51.
26. Petit JY, Veronesi U, Rey P, et al. Nipple sparing mastectomy with nipple areola intraoperative radiotherapy: one thousand and one cases of a five years experience at the European institute of oncology of Milan (EIO). *Breast Cancer Res Treat.* 2009;117:333-338.
27. Hartmann LC, Schaid DJ, Woods JE, et al. Efficacy of bilateral prophylactic mastectomy in women with a family history of breast cancer. *N Engl J Med.* 1999;340(2):77-84.
28. Denewer A, Farouk O. Can nipple-sparing mastectomy and immediate breast reconstruction with modified extended latissimus dorsi muscular flap improve the cosmetic and functional outcome among patients with breast carcinoma? *World J Surg.* 2007;31(6):1169-1177.
29. Sacchini V, Pinotti JA, Barros AC, et al. Nipple-sparing mastectomy for breast cancer and risk reduction: oncologic or technical problem? *J Am Coll Surg.* 2006;203(5):704-714.
30. Cheung KL, Blamey RW, Robertson JF, et al. Subcutaneous mastectomy for primary breast cancer and ductal carcinoma in situ. *Eur J Surg Oncol.* 1997 Aug;23(4):343-7.
31. Salhab M, Al Sarakbi W, Joseph A, et al. Skin-sparing mastectomy and immediate breast reconstruction: patient satisfaction and clinical outcome. *Int J Clin Oncol.* 2006;11(1):51-54.
32. Opatt D, Morrow M. The dual role of nipple preservation. *J Support Oncol.* 2006;4(5):233-234.

33. Stolier AJ, Sullivan SK, Dellacroce FJ. Technical considerations in nipple-sparing mastectomy: 82 consecutive cases without necrosis. *Ann Surg Oncol.* 2008;15(5):1341-1347.

34. Wijayanayagam A, Kumar AS, Foster RD, Esserman LJ. Optimizing the total skin-sparing mastectomy. *Arch Surg.* 2008;143(1):38-45; discussion 45.

35. Bishop CC, Singh S, Nash AG. Mastectomy and breast reconstruction preserving the nipple. *Ann R Coll Surg Engl.* 1990;72(2):87-89.

36. Vlajcic Z, Rado Z, Stanec S, Stanec Z. Nipple-areola complex preservation. *Plast Reconstr Surg.* 2006;118(6):1493-1495.

37. Crowe JP Jr, Kim JA, Yetman R, et al. Nipple-sparing mastectomy: technique and results of 54 procedures. *Arch Surg.* 2004;139(2):148-150.

38. Komorowski AL, Zanini V, Regolo L, et al. Necrotic complications after nipple- and areola-sparing mastectomy. *World J Surg.* 2006;30(8):1410-1413.

39. Caruso F, Ferrara M, Castiglione G, et al. Nipple sparing subcutaneous mastectomy: sixty-six months follow-up. *Eur J Surg Oncol.* 2006;32(9):937-940.

40. Margulies AG, Hochberg J, Kepple J, et al. Total skin-sparing mastectomy without preservation of the nipple-areola complex. *Am J Surg.* 2005;190(6):907-912.

CHAPTER 68

Radical and Extended Radical Mastectomy

Regina M. Fearmonti
Elisabeth K. Beahm

Halsted advocated radical mastectomy (RM) to achieve locoregional control for breast cancer at the end of the 19th century, stemming from his theory of the sequential progression of breast cancer metastases from the primary tumor to regional lymphatics and on to distant sites.[1] The RM and extended radical mastectomy (ERM) embodied the theory of aggressive local control, and emerged as mainstays of surgical treatment for breast cancer (Fig. 68-1). Nonetheless, as early as 1912, Murphy and other proponents of pectoralis muscle preservation began to challenge these techniques with modified radical mastectomy (MRM) and total mastectomy. They demonstrated adequate local control without the associated cosmetic and functional morbidities.[2] Patey and Dyson later modified the Halsted technique for resection of small (T1 and T2) breast cancers, advocating level I, II, and III axillary dissection, preserving pectoralis major, and removing only the pectoralis minor muscle.[3,4] Neoadjuvant chemotherapy further served to lessen the surgical approach required by greatly facilitating resectability. The criteria for breast cancer inoperability published by Haagensen and Stout were established before the wide acceptance and advances in chemotherapy and modern radiation techniques.[5] Accordingly, criteria for the role of surgery in locally advanced breast cancer (LABC) are evolving, yet still remain largely reserved for palliation, comfort, hygiene, and wound management.[6]

RADICAL MASTECTOMY

The Halsted RM involves removal of all breast tissue, the pectoralis major and minor muscles, and level I, II, and III axillary and supraclavicular lymph node dissections. Since Haagensen and Stout's 1943 publication detailing the bleak results (5-year local recurrence and survival rates of 46% and 6%, respectively) achieved with RM as sole treatment for LABC, other studies emerged comparing less aggressive surgical approaches and radiotherapy, alone and in combination with surgery, to RM for the treatment of LABC.[5] Baker and associates compared the results of MRM to RM in patients with operable breast cancer, citing no statistically significant differences in 5-year survival or incidence of local or regional recurrence between the 2 surgical modalities.[7] Patients with stage III disease, however, demonstrated statistically significant higher incidences of axillary and chest wall recurrences when treated with MRM versus RM, leaving the authors to conclude that MRM is appropriate for early-stage breast cancer only. Likewise, MRM sparing the pectoralis major muscle using the Patey technique was demonstrated to yield as many axillary lymph nodes as RM. This suggested that MRM was comparable to RM and sufficient for locoregional control and prognostic determination for early-stage breast cancer.[8]

While surgical therapy appears imperative to effective management of LABC, RM does not appear to improve outcome. Neither therapeutic doses of chest wall radiation alone[9,10] or in conjunction with radical surgery[11,12] yielded vast improvements in control of disease. Publication of the results of the National Surgical Adjuvant Breast and Bowel Project (NSABP) B-04—a prospective study detailing 25-year follow-up data for primary breast cancer patients randomized to treatment with RM, total mastectomy, or total mastectomy with adjuvant radiation—revealed no benefit for RM over less radical surgical treatments.[13] Indications for RM were becoming increasingly select. The application of neoadjuvant chemotherapy to patients with LABC in the decade that followed demonstrated that it in fact enhanced surgical resectability, making more radical surgery for breast cancer of historical interest only.[14-16]

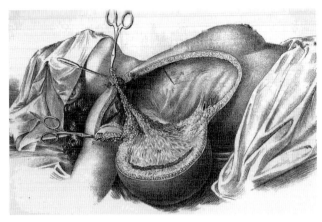

FIGURE 68-1 Halsted radical mastectomy. From initial description of the surgical procedure as reported in 1894. *(Reproduced with permission from Halsted W. The results of operations for the cure of cancer of the breast performed at the Johns Hopkins Hospital from June 1889 to January 1894. Ann Surg. 1894;5:497-555.)*

Radical mastectomy, along with radiotherapy and chemotherapy, remains a key component of the multimodal approach to some locally advanced (T3/T4 tumors and N2/N3 disease) and recurrent breast cancers. At present time, optimal control of LABC is achieved through neoadjuvant chemotherapy, followed by surgery and radiotherapy. Surgical treatment of the intact primary stage IV breast cancer is recommended for palliation—specifically, in cases of hemorrhage, ulceration, infection, and for local wound management. Data are emerging in support of radical surgical resection of the intact primary tumor as part of a multimodal approach for patients with stage IV breast cancer and stable metastatic disease.[17-20] Clinical studies to date suggest that resection of the intact primary may yield a survival advantage, yet the magnitude of this advantage in relation to morbidity remains to be determined in a prospective randomized control trial.

Operative Technique

The technique for RM is comparable to that of MRM. RM is traditionally performed via an obliquely oriented, elliptical incision beginning at the lateral border of the sternum that is directed toward the axilla. Most critically, RM must include en bloc resection of all breast parenchyma, the nipple-areolar complex, pectoralis major and minor, and complete en bloc axillary lymphadenectomy (levels I, II, and III). This is performed with a wide skin margin that encompasses the entire skin envelope and beyond to ensure complete tumor extirpation. The design of the skin incision should incorporate previous biopsy scars and the primary neoplasm en bloc with margins that are at least 3 to 4 cm from the superior and inferior edges of the tumor. The resultant extent of dissection results in an increased morbidity compared to MRM with minimally or poor overall aesthetic result, and often significant issues in wound breakdown and healing.

EXTENDED RADICAL MASTECTOMY

The ERM evolved to include internal mammary (IM) node dissection based upon the Halstedian principle that more extensive surgical extirpation is warranted to ensure eradication of the primary tumor. Prompted by increasing evidence of frequent IM node involvement in breast cancer, the suggestion the IM nodal involvement was associated with a poorer prognosis, and retrospective comparisons suggesting improved survival from ERM, a multinational randomized trial comparing Halsted mastectomy versus ERM was initiated in 1963.[21] Overall results were first reported in 1976 and updated in 1983 and showed that ERM did not improve overall survival.[22] This trial, however, was underpowered and computed tomography (CT) scans were not used to stage these patients. In addition, systemic therapy was not used, further reducing the power of this study to detect a potentially clinically significant survival difference from improved locoregional control. Subsequent updates separately by the French and Italian cohorts continued to show no survival improvement with ERM for the overall cohort.[23] Other studies concluded that ERM versus Halsted RM or total mastectomy with postoperative radiation yielded no survival advantage.[25,26]

The incidence of isolated metastases to IM lymph nodes (that is, without concomitant axillary nodal metastases) has been demonstrated to be quite low.[27] Studies of ERM specimens have been used in attempts to identify those patients where IM nodal biopsy may be indicated, not for IM node dissection, but rather to identify those patients who may benefit from adjuvant chemotherapy and radiation to the IM nodal chain.[28] Improved surgical techniques over the last few years have induced thoracic surgeons to more frequently perform sternal resections even in apparently extreme situations. These aggressive resections are not without morbidity. Prospective study evaluating quality of life of patients and risk-benefit analysis with sternal involvement and the morbidity associated with radiation-induced osteoradionecrosis of the chest wall has led surgical oncologists to adopt a more conservative approach to these cases.

Operative Technique

Extended radical mastectomy involves a MRM or RM with complete (levels I, II, and III) axillary lymphadenectomy in addition to IM node dissection. The IM dissection is performed en bloc and includes IM vessels and lymph nodes from the first to the fourth intercostal space, with resection of the corresponding portion of the pleura. This often involves a subtotal, if not total, sternectomy to gain access to the IM nodes and varying degrees of resection of adjacent ribs.

Sternectomy

Sternal involvement may occur either from direct invasion by enlarged IM lymph nodes or from hematogenous spread, presenting as a sternal metastasis. In patients with breast cancer, the presence of either sternal involvement or an isolated sternal metastasis is relatively uncommon, with reported incidences of 5.2% and 1.9% to 2.4%, respectively.[29] In contrast to vertebral lesions, which tend to result in multicentric bony disease from spread through the paravertebral (Batson) plexus, some sternal lesions have been observed to remain solitary and localized to the sternum with time, likely due to the absence of a well-developed vascular network around the sternum.[30] This microenvironment is quite different from that created by the paravertebral venous plexus and may explain why the resection of a single metastatic lesion in the sternum can potentially be curative. The limited vascular supply also explains the relatively high rate of osteoarthritis and nonhealing sternal wounds, a consideration in reconstructive approaches. Sternectomy for isolated breast cancer recurrence remains a controversial issue, with retrospective case series composing the bulk of the literature. When performed in conjunction with parasternal and mediastinal lymphadenectomy, sternectomy along with node dissection has been shown to provide additional prognostic information before commencing endocrine or chemotherapy.[30] Surgery has been mainly used with palliative intent after the failure of radiotherapy, but improvement in survival following sternectomy for isolated breast cancer recurrence has been reported.[31]

An isolated sternal metastasis should be approached with caution, as it is more likely to herald systemic disease than to be truly solitary. A full metastatic workup is mandated, as is a multimodality treatment approach. Surgical resection should be reserved for palliation or for instances in which the other treatment modalities are not possible.

Preoperative MRI or bone scintigraphy should be reviewed to assess for involvement of the manubrium. Likewise, intraoperative specimen analysis should be conducted to assess for microscopic invasion of tumor beyond the sternomanubrial joint.

The surgical resection begins with a vertical elliptical incision centered on the mass. Mobilization is then begun first on one side of the sternum, with exposure and resection of the adjacent ribs. The sternum is approached from the periphery, reserving any critical point of bone attachment to the heart and great vessels for the final steps of the operation. Both IM vessels are identified, dissected out, and preserved (if possible) or ligated before sternal division. A bone saw is then used to transect the sternum at its upper free margin.

Bony resection margins are controversial, many authors recommend leaving 3 to 4 cm of free tissue around the tumor or the irradiated tissue,[32] while others advocate removing at least 4 cm of free tissue en bloc with the resection specimen throughout the thickness of the involved bone (manubrium, body, or the entire sternum) and the anterior tracts of the bilaterally corresponding ribs, as well as 1 uninvolved rib above and below the lesion, including the related intercostal space.[33-35]

Partial (subtotal) sternectomy is advocated in cases of tumors localized to the sternal manubrium, inferior sternal tract, or involving the lateral portion of the bone. If partial sternectomy is deemed feasible, a surgical margin of at least 2 cm should be preserved with radical resection including a 3- to 4-cm margin macroscopically free of disease at both the cutaneous and deep-tissue levels.[32] If involved with tumor, underlying lung and mediastinal structures are removed en bloc. Total sternectomy is advised in cases of manubrial, mediosternal or sternomanubrial joint involvement. In both cases, the IM veins

and arteries should be spared when possible for targets in free or pedicled tissue reconstruction.

Brachial Plexus Involvement

Locoregional recurrence or metastatic involvement of the brachial plexus is a condition that is often associated with LABC. In the last 25 years, safer and more refined plastic surgical approaches have been developed that provide options to treat even complex recurrent disease. Known as metastatic plexopathy, tumor infiltration of surrounding nerves is often a disabling accompaniment of LABC and may involve any of the peripheral nerve plexuses. Brachial plexopathy most commonly occurs in carcinoma of the breast and lung and is typically is associated with severe unrelenting pain as the cardinal clinical feature. Weakness and focal sensory disturbances occur in the distribution of plexus involvement. Surgical exploration and neurolysis should be performed as soon as possible after the appearance of neurologic deficits to halt the development of neural ischemia and degeneration.

Treatment is palliative and includes radiotherapy to the tumor mass and chemotherapy. In selected patients, however, subtotal surgical resection of the tumor may be warranted, with a team consisting of a surgical oncologist, neurosurgeon, and plastic surgeon. At the time of surgery, if the tumor is found to encroach upon the brachial plexus, sharp dissection should be applied with fields included, to allow intraoperative nerve and electrical stimulation of the brachial plexus and its motor branches to the shoulder and upper extremity.

Brachial plexus syndromes in patients with breast cancer can ensue from various mechanisms including metastatic involvement, radiation injury, soft-tissue changes due to surgery or radiation, ischemia, idiopathic causes, or any combination of these.[36,37] Clinical history, neurologic examination, EMG, and imaging studies aid in both diagnosis and management. Thorough neurologic examination during assessment of patients with LABC is essential to rule out central nervous system involvement (brain or spinal cord metastases) and tailor adjuvant radiotherapy and chemotherapy accordingly. Likewise, neurotoxic effects from chemotherapeutic agents should be assessed frequently. The response to therapy is modest and generally short lived. Significant radiation-induced brachial plexopathy is often seen for 1 to 2 years post treatment. This is often severe, progressive, and defies surgical treatment. Efforts should be made to provide adequate pain control, to maximize remaining neurologic function, and to prevent complications of immobility produced by neuromuscular dysfunction.

Axillary and Subclavian Vessels

Lesions of the subclavian artery can be managed surgically in a number of ways including carotid-brachial bypass, subclavian-brachial bypass, axillary-brachial bypass, and direct transthoracic revascularization with aorto-innominate bypass. The relative safety and efficacy of extrathoracic repair of brachiocephalic and subclavian occlusive disease was confirmed in early studies by Debakey and Crawford.[38] When there is dense sclerosis of the axillary fossa, tunneling a vascular graft through this fibrotic tissue may be hazardous to both the axillary vein and the brachial plexus. This may also lead to an increased rate of graft failure caused by compression from scar tissue. Recent studies have emerged detailing success with retrohumeral tunneling of a reversed vein graft from the right common carotid artery to the right brachial artery to avoid the previously operated and irradiated field.[39] Prior studies have revealed 2 basic principles of upper extremity revascularization: the more proximal the bypass is located, the greater the long-term patency, and the use of the common carotid artery as a donor vessel is safe.[40]

Choice of optimal conduit remains somewhat controversial, with excellent long-term patency rates achieved for both expanded polytetrafluoroethylene (PTFE) and reversed greater saphenous vein grafts in the proximal brachial position.[41] Optimal conduit choice is a question that requires future prospective consideration. The issue of graft compression also requires constant patient awareness and minor lifestyle changes, such as wearing a strapless brassiere and carrying one's handbag on the contralateral shoulder.

CHEST WALL RECONSTRUCTION

Postoperative morbidity and mortality associated with chest wall resection have been reported to range from 8% to 27% in various series.[30] Stability and dynamic elasticity of the thorax are required to support the mechanics of normal respiratory function. Extirpation of a locally advanced or recurrent breast cancer often involves resection of ribs, sternum, adjacent chest wall musculature, lung, pericardium, and thymus. Chest wall reconstruction thus often requires recreation of both skeletal and soft-tissue components. Reconstruction following simple or MRM involves both immediate and delayed reconstructive options; reconstruction following RM or ERM, however, presents unique challenges, as the aims are not only aesthetic but functional. When skin graft is utilized for closure following a RM for LABC, the appearance of the graft is unaesthetic and less stable compared with more complex reconstructive methods (Fig. 68-2). Respiratory disturbance after resection of the anterior chest wall is a major problem, and different techniques of chest wall reconstruction have been described. A reconstructed chest wall should prevent paradoxical movement of the thorax, protect underlying mediastinal structures, and be immunologically inert as well as translucent on chest radiograph. The anatomic site and size of the defect must also be taken into consideration when choosing the materials and technique. Figure 68-3 describes the reconstructive ladder of increasingly complex approaches that can be applied to the reconstruction of chest wall defects.

Skin Graft

A skin graft may be an appropriate reconstructive option for defects limited to the skin and subcutaneous tissues. Placed over a greater omental flap, a split-thickness skin graft can be used to resurface the chest wall.[42] Likewise, skin grafts may also

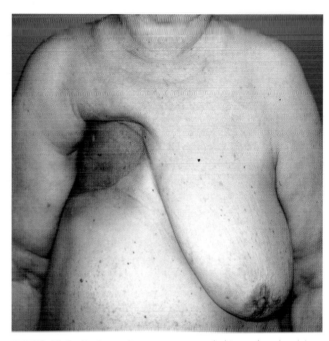

FIGURE 68-2 Postoperative appearance of skin graft utilized for closure of radical defect. Locally advanced breast cancer in high-risk patients with multiple medical comorbidities as managed with a skin graft. The unaesthetic appearance of a graft as well as the less stable nature of the grafts can be noted.

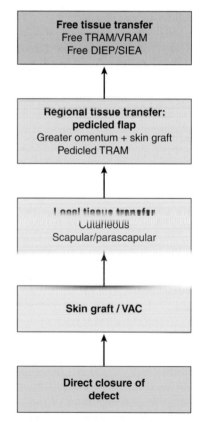

FIGURE 68-3 Reconstructive ladder for chest wall defects demonstrating increasing complexity. (DIEP, deep inferior epigastric artery perforator; IGAP, inferior gluteal artery perforator; SGAP, superior gluteal artery perforator; SIEA, superficial inferior epigastric artery perforator; TRAM, transverse rectus abdominis myocutaneous; VAC, vacuum-assisted closure; VRAM, vertical rectus abdominis myocutaneous.)

be used to assist with primary donor site closure after harvesting myocutaneous flaps for chest wall coverage.

The process of engraftment involves revascularization of the skin graft, as the graft initially has no vascular connection and survives via plasma imbibition. The process of revascularization commences approximately 48 hours after graft placement, but graft take may be compromised in a radiated wound bed. This process can be hastened with use of the vacuum-assisted closure (VAC) device (Kinetic Concepts Inc, San Antonio, Texas), which is placed at the time of the initial operation, left in place over the skin graft for 5 days, and then removed at the bedside.[43,44] The VAC not only protects the graft in the wound bed but provides a means to improve the adherence of skin grafts in compromised tissues, thus expediting wound closure. Disadvantages of using a skin graft include its propensity to contract and provide a far less aesthetic and durable form of coverage than a vascularized flap.

Skeletal Reconstruction

Various techniques have been used to restore chest wall stability and recreate the chest wall scaffold with the aim of limiting flap movement and consequent paradoxical respiration. The need for a skeletal reconstruction depends on the size and site of the resection; that is, skeletal reconstruction is necessary in cases of removal of the sternum and the anterior and lateral tracts of the ribs, but it may not be necessary for the repair of posterior wall defects entirely covered by the scapula or if the defect can be stabilized by the action of adjacent muscles. While traditionally all sternal defects with greater than 2 adjacent ribs were deemed necessary for rigid stabilization these considerations are evolving. Many authors believe that defects of the sternal and posterior walls need to be stabilized less frequently than anterior or lateral defects.[45] Options include the use of autogenous bone grafts, autogenous fascia lata grafts, and numerous synthetic materials, alone or in various combinations.

Synthetic Materials

A spectrum of prosthetic materials may be used for chest wall reconstruction, including metal plates, stainless steel mesh, absorbable mesh (Vicryl mesh, Johnson & Johnson, New Brunswick, New Jersey), nonabsorbable polypropylene mesh (Marlex mesh, Chevron Phillips Chemical, Woodlands, Texas; Prolene mesh, Ethicon, Somerville, New Jersey), and nonporous prosthetic mesh (Gore-Tex mesh; W L. Gore & Associates, Newark, Delaware). The use of synthetic materials is often necessary when reconstructing locally advanced or locally recurrent cancers involving the chest wall (Fig. 68-4). Rigid prosthetic materials, both permanent and absorbable, while less commonly used, may be needed in larger defects (resin plates, methylmethacrylate, and hydroxyapatites combined with tricalcium phosphate).

Prosthetic mesh is easy to handle and can be sutured under tension, thus improving the stability of the thoracic wall.

Gore-Tex has the advantage of being impermeable to air and liquids, but it is very expensive. More importantly, Gor-Tex does not allow for tissue penetration and has a greatly increased rate of seroma formation and infection even late postoperatively

and is accordingly less feasible in reconstructive application; porous mesh initially allows passage of fluid through the prostheses, and then tissue ingrowth favors their incorporation into neighboring structures. Vicryl mesh, as it is absorbable, is usually only considered a temporary measure. While a foreign body, vicryl allows tissue ingrowth, making significant complications rare. Polypropylene meshes are the most widely used because of their resistance, manageability, and tolerability over time. Marlex and Prolene are both polypropylene and inert; the difference is that the former has a double and the latter a single layer: when Prolene is extended, it remains rigid in all directions, whereas Marlex is rigid in only one direction. After a total sternectomy or a broad resection including the lateral portion of the thoracic wall and more than 4 ribs, a sandwiched polypropylene and methacrylate mesh offers the best results in terms of stability, intrathoracic organ protection, and pulmonary expansion, but with the utilization of methacrylate the incidence of seroma and complications increase. Accordingly, some authors prefer using prostheses or simple muscle flaps without rigid supports.[33,34,45]

When the inferior part of the sternum is resected, use of a rigid prosthesis has been advocated to prevent paradoxical movement of the thorax. In contrast, when only the manubrium is resected, soft mesh can be used.[46] In patients who have undergone previous mastectomy, there is little subcutaneous tissue remaining over the chest wall. Likewise, radiotherapy has been demonstrated to impair wound healing with resultant skin ulceration, especially with a foreign body or prosthetic material. This has become a challenge for reconstruction. While placement of a Prolene mesh over the surface of the methylmethacrylate has been suggested to aid in skin incorporation with a rigid nonporous foreign body in several studies citing increased success of methylmethacrylate covered on adjacent sites with Prolene mesh, it must be remembered that adequate soft-tissue cover is imperative to insure successful application of such.[47,48] In addition, while Gore-Tex mesh has been utilized to cover the heart or in diaphragmatic repairs in cases of broad pericardial and adjacent resections, it must be remembered that these materials remain a foreign body and that they must have adequate soft-tissue coverage or even in the late postoperative course, exposure or compromise of these tissues can result in severe infectious complications that may compromise the patient's health and minimally require removal of the prosthetic material.

Accordingly, the role of newer prosthetic materials that are biocompatible so called bioprosthetic materials that become completely incorporated into the local healing wound are encouraging. These newer prosthetic materials may stem from either human cadaveric dermis (eg, Alloderm, Lifecell, Houston, Texas) or bovine or porcine material (eg, Stratus, Lifecell, Houston, Texas). These materials have been utilized successfully for abdominal wall reconstruction and have found a role increasingly in chest wall applications as well. Currently, however, long-term rigidity and the overall strength of these materials is unclear, as well as the potential for some long-term reabsorbtion. However, these appear to be encouraging materials in application for general truck reconstruction. The utilization for bone grafts and other biological materials in a nonvascularized

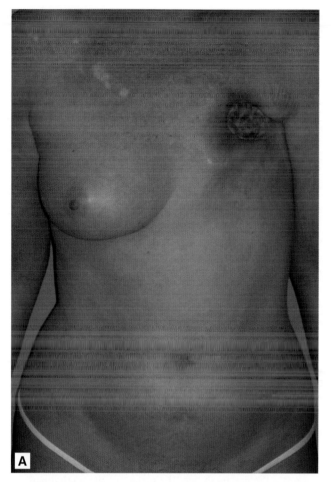
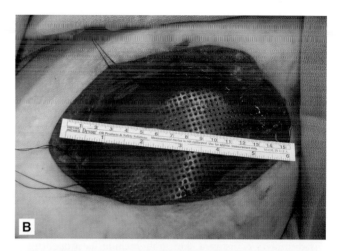
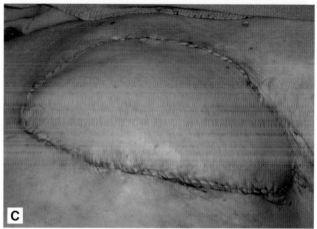

FIGURE 68-4 Locally recurrent breast cancer with erosion into the chest wall **(A)**. Reconstruction of the chest wall with a prosthetic mesh **(B)** and subsequent rectus abdominis myocutaneous flap **(C)** are noted.

setting has not demonstrated any improved efficacy in terms of incorporation or infectious complications compared to synthetic materials, and accordingly, due to their more expensive nature and more limited source and volume available for reconstruction, have not played a role even in more recent applications of chest wall deformity reconstruction. It is important to remember that the combination of prosthetic materials with their easy availability but potential for infection and delayed incorporation is most efficaciously employed with the combination of adequate soft-tissue coverage, and this usually involves the application of a muscle or myocutaneous flap in the setting of prior radiation in order to minimize the potential for wound-related complications.

SOFT-TISSUE RECONSTRUCTION

Well-vascularized soft-tissue coverage is also essential for restoration of normal respiratory dynamics, in addition to protection from infection and proper wound healing. When the surrounding skin and soft tissue are also involved and their

vascularization is compromised by previous radiotherapy, it is necessary to provide broad surface coverage of the chest wall defect, and this requires careful planning. Myocutaneous flaps have largely now replaced skin flaps and contralateral breast transposition for the reconstruction of the soft-tissue layer due to their reliability. The excellent vascularity of and ability to incorporate over irregular surfaces have resulted in myocutaneous flaps becoming the mainstay of reconstructive options in LABC. This is particularly important in cases of breast cancer relapses and radiation necrosis because the surrounding tissue has usually been damaged by the previous treatments. Depending on the circumstances, various types of myocutaneous flaps can be used alone or in combination.

Fasciocutaneous and Local Flaps

Cutaneous flaps may be random or axial, the latter defined by their vascular supply. Axial flaps are based on a defined blood vessel; most commonly in the chest they are based on perforating branches of the IM and intercostal vessels. These flaps have the advantage of not having a functional downside, that is, there is no muscle compromise at their harvest, and can be effective in smaller defects or in conjunction with larger distant flaps. The success of local flaps is generally considered to be dependent on the vascularity and health of the surrounding tissues. Local flaps can be considered if there has not been compromise of these tissues by prior radiation, surgery, or tobacco use. Any of these foreseen risk factors in the setting of a critical reconstructive venture, such as that of a chest wall over a prosthetic, would suggest the use of an axial pattern fasciocutaneous flap or a myocutaneous flap far more preferentially. The most common utilization of axial fasciocutaneous flaps in the chest wall includes those based on the IM vessels, the so-called intercostal flaps, which can be also used as intercostal perforator flaps. These bring only a small amount of tissue, leave a fairly significant deformity in the inframammary folder from which they are harvested, but were the mainstay of local chest wall flaps for a number of years. Scapular and parascapular flaps, which are based on the circumflex scapular vessels, are robust and can be transferred as a pedicled flap for posterior chest wall defects or as a free flap for anterior chest wall defects. Parascapular flaps have the advantage of not connoting any functional deformity, and have a highly versatile skin paddle, with the ability to harvest bone. However, as they are posterior based and the majority of defects in LABC are anterior, this rules out an intraoperative position change and accordingly these are less often utilized due to the logistics and time constraints of these flaps.

Omental Flaps

The highly vascularized greater omentum, which hangs from the greater curvature of the stomach, has been used for chest wall reconstruction for almost 30 years. The omentum has been used primarily as a pedicled flap covered by a skin graft to repair extensive thoracic defects caused by radionecrosis or following the resection of an LABC.[42,49,50] The omentum has also been used for breast reconstruction, most recently via endoscopic techniques.[51] Although either the right or left gastroepiploic artery may be used to supply the omental flap, the right gastroepiploic artery (a branch of the gastroduodenal artery) is the main pedicle and affords a 5- to 10-cm greater arc of rotation. The omentum is relatively easy to harvest, is very well vascularized, and may provide a large flap. There are, however, some drawbacks to the use of this flap. Neither the thickness nor surface area of the available greater omental apron is possible to predict preoperatively, as it does not directly correlate with the patient's morphologic characteristics. The omentum has an irregular surface; this may result in difficulties with fixation to the chest wall, retraction from the edges of the defect and instability of overlying skin graft. Harvest of the omental flap previously required a laparotomy, which held potential for a host of intraabdominal complications. Reports of laparoscopic flap harvesting procedures have demonstrated decreased postoperative complication rates and donor site morbidity.[52] Pedicled omentoplasty with meshed skin graft and VAC therapy has shown encouraging results for reconstruction of full-thickness chest wall defects.[53]

Latissimus Dorsi Myocutaneous Flap

The latissimus dorsi myocutaneous flap has been one of the most commonly utilized flaps for chest wall reconstruction for advanced breast cancer due to its ease of harvest and reliability (Fig. 68-5). Proximity of the flap to the chest is conducive to transfer as a pedicle flap, although the long vascular pedicle will permit microsurgical transfer if necessary. The latissimus dorsi myocutaneous flap is based on the dominant thoracodorsal system, which provides the vascular basis of a pedicled latissimus flap used to reconstruct the chest wall. Its arc of rotation can be increased by releasing its humeral insertion or transection of the vascular branches to the serratus muscle, thus permitting the flap to reach the midline of the chest. This flap generally has a robust blood supply, though flap vascularity may have been compromised by prior surgery or radiotherapy. Although prior irradiation to the axilla is not a contraindication to latissimus flap transfer, when prior division of the thoracodorsal pedicle is combined with radiation to the wound bed, the incidence of flap loss is increased.[54] Intraoperative strategy to minimize this complication is to carefully evaluate the vascular pedicle of the flap, which is traditionally based on the dominate thoracodorsal system but also can be transferred based on the accompanying serratus anterior muscle vascular branches as well. In many situations of transfer for a locally advanced chest wall defects, both vascular sources can be kept in tact with an arch of rotation that is suitable, thus maximizing the vascularity of the flap. The latissimus flap has remained a mainstay of reconstructive surgery in the chest wall due to its reliability and location, which permits its transfer as a pedicled flap. The defect size of the skin paddle is limited by the ability to achieve primary closure of the defect after flap harvest, and this tends to be a width of 8 to 10 cm maximally. Dehiscence and complications of the back wound are highly problematic, and skin grafts on the back do not fare well, although if necessary can be secured with use of a vacuum-assisted closure device. The general disadvantages of the latissimus flap include the seromas accumulation in the donor site, the thickened back scar donor site, and some occasional reports of weakness of the shoulder in the overhead position, although this is a rare. In general, this flap remains a first choice for moderate-sized defects of the chest wall.

Pectoralis Major Flap

The pectoralis major flap is based on the thoracoacromial vessels, which supply the dominant vascular supply to this flap. The flap can also be utilized secondarily as a turnover based on the medial vascular supply stemming from the IM vessels. This is less favorable due to the bulkiness that occurs and the loss of rotation when it is moved along its sternal borders. Additionally, this area is often compromised in a resection for locally advanced cancer. The pectoralis major flap is well suited to defects of the anterior and superior chest, and with release laterally and along the clavicle it can provide excellent coverage to across the midline. This flap is most applicable for smaller defects and it must be remembered that there will be some functional compromise. While this flap has been used extensively

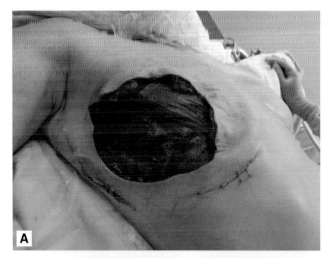

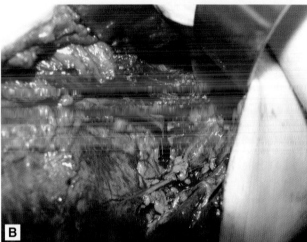

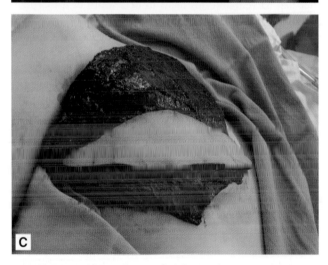

FIGURE 68-5 A large chest wall defect with intact pectoralis major and serratus muscle noted in the defect **(A)**. The thoraco-dorsal vessels are identified in the dissection with a microsurgical clip and noted on the nerve which will be transected to avoid unnecessary postoperative motion **(B)**. A large latissimus flap is brought forth and sutured into place **(C)**.

for sternal and chest wall reconstruction, it is most reliable as a muscle-only flap. The skin paddle, while it may be incorporated, does not connote the same reliability.[55-57]

External Oblique Flap

In cases in which the latissimus dorsi and rectus abdominis myocutaneous flaps are not suitable, the external oblique myocutaneous flap is an alternate method of reconstruction for LABC. The external oblique muscle is a large muscle that takes origin from the 6th to the 12th ribs and receives segmental blood supply from the lateral cutaneous branches of the inferior 8 posterior intercostal vessels. Flap territory is large, extending from the midline of the abdomen to the anterior axillary line, enabling it to easily cover defects measuring up to 300 cm². The flap is elevated medially, with dissection between the internal and external oblique muscles, progressing laterally to the posterior midline with preservation of the perforating vessels, and rotated superiorly into the defect. Proponents of this flap cite straightforward flap harvest that obviates the need to intraoperatively reposition the patient, maintenance of abdominal wall integrity by sparing the rectus abdominis, and reliable closure of large defects. Likewise, operative time is minimal, generally requiring about 2 hours, and complications are few, with superficial necrosis being the most frequently reported. Several successful series of the external oblique flap for chest wall reconstruction have been reported.[58-60] The segmental blood supply to the muscle, however, limits the useful arc of rotation. Although an extended modification to increase the flap reach has been reported, extensive dissection to facilitate flap rotation may compromise these segmental vascular pedicles. Hernia formation is also a concern. These considerations have limited the use of the external oblique flaps for chest wall reconstruction.

Rectus Abdominis Transposition and Free Flaps

Rectus abdominis myocutaneous flaps are the workhorse flaps in reconstructive surgery because of their ease of elevation, reliability, and the large size that may be harvested with partial primary closure of the donor site.[61] The rectus abdominis muscle is supplied primarily by the deep inferior and deep superior epigastric arteries, which communicate at the periumbilical watershed area. The deep inferior epigastric artery, the dominant blood supply to the muscle, is the most suitable pedicle for microvascular anastomosis. The deep superior epigastric artery (a branch of the IM artery) provides the vascular basis for superiorly based rectus flaps. The muscle also receives direct vascular contributions from posterior perforating intercostal and IM vessels. Because the rectus abdominis flap may be based on either of these vessels, numerous flap configurations are possible.

Vertical Rectus Abdominis Myocutaneous Flap

The vertical rectus abdominis myocutaneous (VRAM) flap is simple and quick to harvest and has the most robust vascularity of all the rectus abdominis flap configurations because the skin paddle is positioned directly over the muscle, where it is richly supplied by perforating vessels.[62,63] The drawbacks of the VRAM include a less aesthetic donor site and a smaller available skin paddle in comparison to the TRAM flap. Nonetheless, often 15 cm or more of skin may be harvested with a VRAM flap because of the generalized skin laxity in an older population. Patients should be advised of a resultant off-center abdominal scar and umbilicus following reconstruction with a VRAM flap.

Pedicled Transverse Rectus Abdominis Myocutaneous Flap

The single-pedicle transverse rectus abdominis myocutaneous (TRAM) flap, with a transversely oriented skin island, is the most common flap used for autologous postmastectomy breast reconstruction.[64] It is suited for patients desiring autologous breast reconstruction from an abdominal donor site and patients with an inadequate skin envelope and/or ptotic contralateral breast to which they desire to achieve symmetry. The transverse orientation permits harvest of a generous skin paddle, and the donor scar, although long, is well hidden by undergarments. If the flap is placed low on the rectus muscle, it has a long axis of rotation allowing the skin paddle to rotate quite far laterally or high into the axilla.

The single-pedicle superior-based TRAM flap is hindered by the less robust nature of its blood supply because a large part of the skin paddle does not lie directly over the muscle. As such, the flap is dependent on the integrity of a small number of perforating vessels, vascular anastomoses between the superior and inferior epigastric vessels, and periumbilical vascular interconnections, which provide for blood flow from one vascular pedicle across both sides of the abdomen. In addition, pedicled TRAM flaps may be problematic in chest wall reconstruction because of harvest of the IM vessels, which form the dominant vascular pedicle to the flap. Although superior-based rectus flaps have been successfully based solely on the costal marginal (eighth intercostal) vessels, this is a less well-vascularized configuration, and in this situation a free-tissue transfer is preferable.[65] As such, if the defect is small or the chest wall is intact, the superior-based pedicled TRAM flap may be a reasonable choice. In patients who smoke, are diabetic, or have multiple abdominal scars, however, circulation may be inadequate and may severely limit the size and viability of the flap. Accordingly, alternatives to the single-pedicle TRAM flap, such as the double-pedicle, "supercharged," "turbocharged," and free TRAM flaps, have been used as means to enhance flap vascularity.

Free-Tissue Transfer

The free rectus flap (either TRAM or VRAM) is based solely on the deep inferior epigastric vessels and necessitates microvascular anastomoses to reestablish blood supply to the flap.[66] During chest wall resections, a variety of recipient vessels are usually available for anastomoses. As a smaller amount of muscle is harvested, the proximal portions of the IM vessels are most commonly used as recipient vessels as well as those of the

thoracoacromial trunk or thoracodorsal vessels. Other alternatives including utilization of neck vessels with turned down vein grafts are possible, but are less commonly employed. Early studies suggested that free flaps compared to pedicled flaps are mostly efficacious in respect to the vascularity of the tissue that is transferred, with early studies suggesting a lower incidence of postoperative pain, hernia, and bulge, and a quicker recovery.[67] However, the aspect of donor site morbidity, which is significant in flap harvest at the rectus territory, is more efficacious if these flaps are harvested as a muscle sparing or perforator type approach where less than all the muscle is utilized for transfer. This has suggested, especially in bilateral cases of improved donor site morbidity, the consensus among plastic surgeons in this regard is not complete. Additionally in the setting of LABC, the potential for a higher incidence of flap loss rate or complication with a muscle-sparing or perforator-type variant of rectus abdominis flap is often not deemed prudent, especially in severe cases, and accordingly individual practitioners will use their judgment on the best approach due to the size of the defect, the degree of prosthetic material utilized, and other clinical factors that may dictate whether a full muscle or a muscle-sparing or perforator-type rectus-based flap should be utilized. Criticisms of the need for microsurgical transfer in chest wall reconstruction have focused largely on the less reliable nature of the flap due to concerns of anastomotic patency. In experienced hands, the free flap success rate is well over 95%, but in less experienced hands consideration for utilizing a pedicled flap (with enhanced vascularity from microsurgical anastomosis of the inferior vascular pedicle to either the mammary or thoracodorsal vessels or by utilizing the superior pedicle in a supercharged or turbocharged configuration) may be a more appropriate option. While the free-tissue or pedicled transfer of the rectus abdominis flap is associated with a significant recovery, classically 4 to 6 weeks, the stability and reliability as far as the quality of coverage has in the long term been the most efficacious.

Deep and Superficial Inferior Epigastric Artery Perforator Flaps

Concerns stemming from abdominal donor site morbidity following TRAM reconstruction have prompted the increased use of perforator flaps for breast reconstruction.[68-72] Perforator flaps represent the most recent evolution of autologous flap reconstructions and theoretically permit transfer of tissue from numerous donor sites to almost any distant site with suitable recipient vessels for microsurgical anastomosis.

The deep inferior epigastric perforator (DIEP) flap, like the free TRAM flap, employs the inferior epigastric artery for its vascular supply. Microvascular anastomoses are performed to either the IM or thoracodorsal vessels. As the inferior epigastric artery is the dominant artery supplying the lower abdominal wall, this flap enables transfer of a sizeable amount of tissue with minimal fat necrosis and is thus suited for patients who smoke or have risks factors of morbid obesity or diabetes.[73] These flaps are also associated with less abdominal wall morbidity, as perforator vessels from the inferior epigastric artery can de dissected free without sacrificing muscle or fascia. The superficial inferior epigastric artery (SIEA) flap, with blood supply derived from the superficial inferior epigastric artery (from the common femoral artery), can be harvested without an abdominal wall incision and thus also preserves abdominal wall integrity. The superficial inferior epigastric artery is only present in approximately half of the population, however, which limits the applicability of the SIEA flap.[72]

A recent retrospective study comparing reconstructive outcomes of the DIEP to the pedicled TRAM flap for postmastectomy breast reconstructions cites shorter hospital stays (4 vs 5 days), longer operative times (5.5 vs 4.5 hours), lower fat necrosis rates (17.7% vs 58.5%), and lower incidences of abdominal wall hernias (1% vs 16%) with the DIEP flap (all $p < 0.001$).[74] Prospective studies are needed to validate these observed outcomes.

In summary, while the perforator flaps usually tolerate radiation well, sparing the flap the damaging effects of radiation, combined with the ability to subsequently excise the irradiated chest wall skin, make reconstruction following radiation the more favorable option as it produces a superior aesthetic result. Absolute contraindications specific to perforator flaps include history of previous suction assisted lipectomy of the donor site, donor site surgery (eg, prior abdominoplasty in the case of a DIEP flap), or smoking within 1 month before surgery, with need for postoperative radiation constituting a relative contraindication.

In the reconstruction of full-thickness chest wall defects as often result from treatment for locally advanced and extensive local recurrence of breast cancer, our group does not routinely employ perforator flaps because of the profound implications of flap loss in this setting. This is especially true in the face of prior radiotherapy, which appears to increase the risk of fat necrosis.[75] The variability of flap anatomy, harvest techniques and reconstructive needs essentially precludes a controlled prospective study and hinders definitive conclusions regarding the true perfusion of perforator flaps compared to muscle sparing or full muscle flaps in the setting of both chest wall and breast reconstruction. This area continues to be a focus of study in the plastic surgery literature.[76] Table 68-1 summarizes the characteristics and utility of the various local and regional muscle, myocutaneous, and fasciocutaneous flaps.

FUTURE DIRECTIONS

Data are emerging in support of radical surgical resection of the intact primary tumor as part of a multimodal approach for patients with stage IV breast cancer and stable metastatic disease.[17-20] Clinical studies to date suggest that resection of the intact primary may yield a survival advantage, yet the magnitude of this advantage in relation to morbidity remains to be determined in a prospective randomized controlled trial.

Likewise, sternectomy for isolated breast cancer recurrence remains a controversial issue, with retrospective case series composing the bulk of the literature. A greater understanding of oncologic diseases as a whole, prospective studies evaluating quality of life of patients with sternal involvement, and the morbidity associated with radiation-induced osteoradionecrosis of the chest wall have led surgical oncologists to adopt a more resolute attitude in terms of therapeutic options. Prospective studies analyzing effects of sternectomy on quality of life are

TABLE 68-1 Flaps for Coverage of Chest Wall Defects

Muscle	Flap Type	Blood Supply	Coverage Capability
Trapezius	Muscle/myocutaneous	Transverse cervical a., v. Posterior intercostals a., v. Occipital a., v.	Posterior-superior CW
Periscapular	Fasciocutaneous	Circumflex scapular a., venae comitantes	Shoulder, axilla, lateral CW
Latissimus dorsi	Muscle/myocutaneous	Thoracodorsal a., v. Posterior intercostals and lumbar a., v.	Superior aspect posterior CW Anterior midline CW Reverse flap, contralateral Posterior CW
Pectoralis major	Muscle/myocutaneous	Thoracromial a., venae comitantes Intercostal branches from IMA	Midline sternal defects
Serratus anterior	Muscle/myocutaneous/fascial	Lateral thoracic and thoracodorsal br.	Anterior and posterior CW Intrathoracic cavitary defects
External oblique	Muscle/myocutaneous	Lateral cutaneous br. inferior intercostals and venae comitantes	Anterior CW
Rectus abdominis	Muscle/myocutaneous	Superior and inferior epigastric a., v. Intercostal a. and venae comitantes	Anterior CW

a., artery; br., branch(es); CW, chest wall; IMA, internal mammary artery; v., vein.

lacking and would be of great utility in treating this difficult patient population.

Lastly, with regard to reconstruction of chest wall defects, variability in flap anatomy, harvest techniques, and reconstructive needs essentially precludes a controlled prospective study and hinders definitive conclusions regarding the true perfusion of perforator flaps compared to muscle-sparing or full-muscle flaps in the setting of both chest wall and breast reconstruction. This area continues to be a focus of study in the plastic surgery literature, and as new techniques emerge to aid in the visualization of flap perfusion, patients' reconstructive needs can be better individualized.

SUMMARY

The resurgence of a more aggressive breast cancer surgery in the era of better systemic therapies and more conformal radiotherapy is discussed within the historical context of the Halsted and ERM in relationship to current indications and potential patient morbidity. Options for reconstruction of both soft-tissue and skeletal chest wall defects have been described in relation to the resultant defects that may occur. The decision to undertake a major and potentially highly morbid surgical procedure is complicated when the patient's life expectancy may be extremely limited, as in most cases of LABC or extensive local regional recurrences. Surgical palliation should be considered in the framework of a multimodal approach to the treatment of solitary bone metastases that includes radiotherapy, chemotherapy, and hormonal therapy. A breast cancer relapse or metastasis exclusively localized to the thoracic wall has a better prognosis in the absence of metastases to the mediastinal lymph nodes and the IM chain. Mediastinal lymph node involvement increases the likelihood of disease progression. In such cases when local control cannot be obtained by means of radiotherapy or chemotherapy, surgery can still be considered with the aim of symptom palliation. Surgery can be considered with good results when there is a long disease-free interval (more than 24 months) or when there is a single sternal metastasis. The multidisciplinary treatment team must carefully weigh the risks and potential benefits of a highly complex but technically feasible operation against the long-term goals and expectations of the patient.

REFERENCES

1. Halsted W. The results of operations for the cure of cancer of the breast performed at the Johns Hopkins Hospital from June 1889 to January 1894. *Ann Surg.* 1894;5:497-555.
2. Murphy J. Carcinoma of the breast. *Surg Clin.* 1912;1:779.
3. Patey D, Dyson W. The prognosis of carcinoma of the breast in relation to the type of operation performed. *Br J Cancer.* 1948;2:7.
4. Patey D. A review of 146 cases of carcinoma of the breast operated on between 1930 and 1943. *Br J Cancer.* 1967;21:260.
5. Haagensen C, Stout A. Carcinoma of the breast. II. Criteria of operability. *Ann Surg.* 1943;118: 859.
6. Kuerer HM, Beahm EK, Swisher SG, et al. Surgery for inoperable breast cancer. *Am J Surg.* 2002;183:160-161.
7. Baker R, Montague A, Childs J. A comparison of modified radical mastectomy to radical mastectomy in the treatment of operable breast cancer. *Ann Surg.* 1979;189:553.
8. Nemoto T, Dao TL. Is modified radical mastectomy adequate for axillary lymph node dissection? *Ann Surg.* 1975;182:722-723.
9. Harris JR, Sawicka J, Gelman R, et al. Management of locally advanced carcinoma of the breast by primary radiation therapy. *Int J Radiat Oncol Biol Phys.* 1983;9:345-349.
10. Rao DV, Bedwinek J, Perez C, et al. Prognostic indicators in stage III and localized stage IV breast cancer. *Cancer.* 1982;50:2037-2043.
11. Townsend CM Jr., Abston S, Rish JC. Surgical adjuvant treatment of locally advanced breast cancer. *Ann Surg.* 1985;201:604-610.
12. Montague ED, Fletcher GH. Local regional effectiveness of surgery and radiation therapy in the treatment of breast cancer. *Cancer.* 1985;55:2266-2272.
13. Fisher B, et al. Twenty-five year follow-up of a randomized trial comparing radical mastectomy, total mastectomy, and total mastectomy followed by irradiation. *N Engl J Med.* 2002;347:567-574.
14. De Lena M, Varini M, Zucali R, et al. Multimodal treatment for locally advanced breast cancer. Result of chemotherapy-radiotherapy versus chemotherapy-surgery. *Cancer Clin Trials.* 1981;4:229-236.
15. Papaioannou A, Lissaios B, Vasilaros S, et al. Pre- and postoperative chemoendocrine treatment with or without postoperative radiotherapy for locally advanced breast cancer. *Cancer.* 1983;51:1284-1290.
16. Perloff M, Lesnick GJ, Korzun A, et al. Combination chemotherapy with mastectomy or radiotherapy for stage III breast carcinoma: a Cancer and Leukemia Group B study. *J Clin Oncol.* 1988;6:261-269.
17. Khan SA, Stewart AK, Morrow M. Does aggressive local therapy improve survival in metastatic breast cancer? *Surgery.* 2002;132:620-626.
18. Carmichael AR, Anderson ED, Chetty U, et al. Does local surgery have a role in the management of stage IV breast cancer? *Eur J Surg Oncol.* 2003;29:17-19.
19. Rapiti E, Verkooijen HM, Vlastos G, et al. Complete excision of primary breast tumor improves survival of patients with metastatic breast cancer at diagnosis. *J Clin Oncol.* 2006;24:2743-2749.
20. Babiera GV, Rao R, Feng L, et al. Effect of primary tumor extirpation in breast cancer patients who present with stage IV disease and an intact primary tumor. *Ann Surg Oncol.* 2006;13:776-782.
21. Lacour J, Bucalossi P, Cacers E, et al. Radical mastectomy versus radical mastectomy plus internal mammary dissection: five-year results of an international cooperative study. *Cancer.* 1976;37:206-214.
22. Lacour J, Le M, Caceres E, et al. Radical mastectomy versus radical mastectomy plus internal mammary dissection: ten year results of an international cooperative trial in breast cancer. *Cancer.* 1983;51:1941-1943.
23. Lacour J, Le MG, Hill C, et al. Is it useful to remove internal mammary nodes in operable breast cancer? *Eur J Surg Oncol.* 1987;13:309-314.
24. Veronesi U, Valagussa P. Inefficacy of internal mammary nodes dissection in breast cancer surgery. *Cancer.* 1981;47:170-175.
25. Veronesi U, Marubini E, Mariani L, et al. The dissection of internal mammary nodes does not improve the survival of breast cancer patients: 30-year results of a randomized trial. *Eur J Cancer.* 1999;35:1320-1325.
26. Johansen H, Kaae S, Schiodt T. Simple mastectomy with postoperative irradiation versus extended radical mastectomy in breast cancer. *Acta Oncol.* 1990;29:709-715.
27. Urban J, Marjani M. Significance of internal mammary lymph node metastases in breast cancer. *Am J Roentgenol Radium Ther Nucl Med.* 1971;111:130-136.
28. Morrow M, Foster R. Staging of breast cancer, a new rationale for internal mammary node biopsy. *Arch Surg.* 1981;116:748-751.
29. Ohtake E, Murata H, Maruno H. Bone scintigraphy in patients with breast cancer: malignant involvement of the sternum. *Radiat Med.* 1994;12: 25-28.
30. Noguchi S, Miyauchi K, Nishizawa Y, et al. Results of surgical treatment for sternal metastasis of breast cancer. *Cancer.* 1988;62:1397-1401.
31. Lequaglie C, Massone PB, Giudice G, et al. Gold standard for sternectomies and plastic reconstructions after resections for primary or secondary sternal neoplasms. *Ann Surg Oncol.* 2002;9:472-479.
32. McCormack PM, Bains MS, Burt ME, et al. Local recurrent mammary carcinoma failing multimodality therapy: a solution. *Arch Surg.* 1989;124:158-161.
33. Martini N, Huvos AG, Burt ME, et al. Predictors of survival in malignant tumors of the sternum. *J Thorac Cardiovasc Surg.* 1996;111:96-106.
34. Pairolero PC, Arnold PG. Chest wall tumors: experience with 100 consecutive patients. *J Thorac Cardiovasc Surg.* 1985;90:367-372.
35. Perry RR, Venzon D, Roth JA, Pass HI. Survival after surgical resection for high-grade chest wall sarcomas. *Ann Thorac Surg.* 1990;49:363-369.
36. Kori S, Foley KM, Posner JB. Brachial plexus lesions in patients with cancer: 100 cases. *Neurology.* 1981;31:45-50.
37. Olsen NK, Pfeiffer P, Johannsen L, et al. Radiation-induced brachial plexopathy: neurological follow-up in 161 recurrence-free breast cancer patients. *Int J Radiat Oncol Biol Phys.* 1993;26:43-49.

38. Crawford ES, Debakey ME, Morris GL, Howell SF. Surgical treatment of occlusion of the innominate, common carotid and subclavian arteries: a 10-year experience. *Surgery*. 1969;65(1)-31.

39. Marone L, Nigri G, LaMuraglia GM. A novel technique of upper extremity revascularization: the retrohumeral approach. *J Vasc Surg*. 2002;35:1277-1279.

40. Jain KM, Simoni EJ, Munn JS, Madson DL. Long-term follow-up of bypasses to the brachial artery across the shoulder joint. *Am J Surg*. 1996,172.127-129.

41. Mesh CL, McCarthy WJ, Pearce WH, et al. Upper extremity bypass grafting a 15 year experience. *Arch Surg*. 1993;128:795-802.

42. Arnold PG, Witzke DJ, Irons GB, Woods JE. Use of omental transposition flaps for soft-tissue reconstruction. *Ann Plast Surg*. 1983;11:508.

43. Argenta LC, Morykwas MJ. Vacuum-assisted closure: a new method for wound control and treatment: clinical experience. *Ann Plast Surg*. 1997;38:563.

44. Morykwas MJ, Argenta LC, Shelton-Brown EI, McGuirt W. Vacuum-assisted closure: a new method for wound control and treatment: animal studies and basic foundation. *Ann Plast Surg*. 1997;38:553.

45. Avital S, Cohen M, Skornik Y, et al. Solitary sternal breast cancer metastases treated by sternectomy and muscle flap reconstruction. *Eur J Surg*. 2000;166:92-94.

46. Brower ST, Weinberg H, Tartter PI, et al. Chest wall resection for locally recurrent breast cancer: indications, technique and results. *J Surg Oncol*. 1992;49:189-195.

47. Lequaglie C, Massone PB, Giudice G, et al. Gold standard for sternectomies and plastic reconstructions after resections for primary or secondary sternal neoplasms. *Ann Surg Oncol*. 2002;9:472-479.

48. McCormack PM. Use of prosthetic materials in chest wall reconstruction. Assets and liabilities. *Surg Clin North Am*. 1989;69:965-976.

49. Deleure T. L'emploi du grand épiploon dans la chirurgie du sein cancéreux. *Ann Med*. 1908;2:1-18.

50. Kiricuta I, Popescu V. Le traitement de la radionécrose de la main par plastie avec épiploon greffé à l'aide d'autotransplants de peau libre. *Ann Chir Plast*. 1974;19:243.

51. Cothier-Savey I, Tamtawi B, Dohnt F, et al. Immediate breast reconstruction using a laparoscopically harvested omental flap. *Plast Reconstr Surg*. 2001;107:1156.

52. Hultman CS, Carlson GW, Losken A. Utility of the omentum in the reconstruction of complex extraperitoneal wounds and defects: donor-site complications in 135 patients from 1975 to 2000. *Ann Surg*. 2002;235:782-795.

53. Ferron G, Garrido I, Martel P, et al. Combined laparoscopically harvested omental flap with meshed skin grafts and vacuum-assisted closure for reconstruction of complex chest wall defects. *Ann Plast Surg*. 2007;58:150-155.

54. Salmon RJ, Razaboni R, Soussaline M. The use of the latissimus dorsi musculocutaneous flap following recurrence of cancer in irradiated breasts. *Br J Plast Surg*. 1988;41:41.

55. Arnold PG, Pairolero PC. Chest-wall reconstruction: an account of 500 consecutive patients. *Plast Reconstr Surg*. 1996;98:804.

56. Larson DL, McMurtrey MJ. Musculocutaneous flap reconstruction of chest-wall defects: an experience with 50 patients. *Plast Reconstr Surg*. 1984;73:734.

57. Rivas B, Carrillo J, Escobar G. Reconstructive management of advanced breast cancer. *Ann Plast Surg*. 2001;47:234.

58. Hugo NE, Kammerer V, Marks T. Reconstruction of an extensive chest wall defect using an external oblique myocutaneous flap following resection of an advanced breast carcinoma: report of a case. *Br J Cancer*. 2006;13:364-368.

59. Bogossian N, Chaglassian T, Rosenberg PH, et al. External oblique myocutaneous flap coverage of large chest-wall defects following resection of breast tumors. *Plast Reconstr Surg*. 1996;97:97.

60. Moschella F, Cordova A. A new extended external oblique musculocutaneous flap for reconstruction of large chest-wall defects. *Plast Reconstr Surg*. 1999;103:1378.

61. Mathes SJ, Bostwick J III. A rectus abdominis myocutaneous flap to reconstruct abdominal wall defects. *Br J Plast Surg*. 1977;30:282.

62. Cormack GC, Lamberty GH. *The Arterial Anatomy of Skin Flaps*. New York: Churchill Livingstone; 1986.

63. Robbins TH. Rectus abdominis myocutaneous flap for breast reconstruction. *Aust NZ J Surg*. 1979;49:527.

64. Hartrampf CR, Scheflan M, Black PW. Breast reconstruction with a transverse abdominal island flap. *Plast Reconstr Surg*. 1982;69:216.

65. Paletta CE, Vogler G, Freedman B. Viability of the rectus abdominis muscle following internal mammary artery ligation. *Plast Reconstr Surg*. 1993;92:234.

66. Grotting JC, Urist MM, Maddox WA, et al. Conventional TRAM flap versus free microsurgical TRAM flap for immediate breast reconstruction. *Plast Reconstr Surg*. 1989;83:842.

67. Schusterman MA, Kroll SS, Miller MJ. The free TRAM flap for breast reconstruction: a single center's experience with 211 consecutive cases. *Ann Plast Surg*. 1994;32:234.

68. Blondeel PN, et al. The fate of the oblique abdominal muscles after free TRAM flap surgery. *Br J Plast Surg*. 1997;50:315.

69. Blondeel PN, et al. The donor site morbidity of free DIEP flaps and free TRAM flaps for breast reconstruction. *Br J Plast Surg*. 1997;50:322.

70. Kaplan JL, Allen RJ. Cost-based comparison between perforator flaps and TRAM flaps for breast reconstruction. *Plast Reconstr Surg*. 2000;105:943.

71. Koshima I, Soeda S. Inferior epigastric artery skin flap without rectus abdominis muscle. *Br J Plast Surg*. 1989;42:645.

72. Granzow JW, Levine JL, Chiu ES, et al. Breast reconstruction with perforator flaps. *Plast Reconstr Surg*. 2007;120;1-12.

73. Moran SL, Serletti JM. Outcome comparison between free and pedicled TRAM flap breast reconstruction in the obese patient. *Plast Reconstr Surg*. 2001;108:1954-1960.

74. Garvey PB, Buchel EW, Pockaj BA, et al. DIEP and pedicled TRAM flaps: a comparison of outcomes. *Plast Reconstr Surg*. 2006;117:1711-1719.

75. Williams KJ, et al. The effects of radiation treatment after TRAM flap breast reconstruction. *Plast Reconstr Surg*. 1997;100:1153.

76. Williams KJ, et al. The effects of radiation treatment after TRAM flap breast reconstruction. *Plast Reconstr Surg*. 1997;100:1153.

CHAPTER 69

Management of Local Recurrence after Mastectomy

Anees B. Chagpar

EPIDEMIOLOGY OF CHEST WALL RECURRENCE

Incidence

Although mastectomy is associated with excellent local control in most breast cancer patients, chest wall recurrence (CWR) after mastectomy has been noted in up to a third of cases. Jatoi et al found that breast-conserving surgery was associated with a greater odds of locoregional recurrence than mastectomy in a pooled analysis of randomized controlled trials (pooled odds ratio [OR]: 1.561; 95% confidence interval [CI]: 1.289-1.890), locoregional recurrence still occurred in 8.5% of mastectomy patients.[1] CWR rates of up to 40% have been reported depending on primary tumor characteristics and initial treatment.[2] Even with the addition of adjuvant systemic therapy, CWR remains a significant issue in a considerable proportion of patients (Table 69-1).

Prevention

A number of studies have demonstrated that the addition of postmastectomy radiation therapy (PMRT) may reduce the rate of CWR by up to 70%.[3] Although the British Columbia[4] and Denmark studies[5,6] were criticized for a variety of reasons, the American Society of Clinical Oncology[7] and the American Society of Therapeutic Radiology and Oncology[8] have both issued guidelines recommending PMRT in patients with tumors larger than 5 cm or with 4 or more positive lymph nodes. Although PMRT is not recommended for node-negative patients with tumors smaller than 5 cm, PMRT remains controversial in the 1 to 3 positive-node group. The finding of the Early Breast Cancer Trialists' Collaborative Group (EBCTCG) that a 20% reduction in 5-year local recurrence risk results in a 5% absolute reduction in 15-year breast cancer mortality may prompt more widespread use of PMRT in these patients.[3]

Diagnosis

The diagnosis of CWR, clinical as a breast cancer recurrence in the skin, subcutaneous tissue, muscle, or underlying bone after mastectomy, requires a high index of suspicion. Many CWRs occur within 2 to 3 years after mastectomy, but some have been found more than 10 years later. Careful surveillance of the chest wall after mastectomy is therefore required. Although some CWR present as large fungating masses, most are subtle, often presenting with an asymptomatic nodule in the skin or a slight erythematous rash. More than half of all CWR present as a solitary nodule in the skin; the remainder present as multiple nodules or diffuse disease encompassing the chest wall.[9] In 23 to 70% of cases, the recurrence involves the previous mastectomy scar.[10-12] Because CWRs may be mistaken for foreign body granuloma, fat necrosis, or radiation-induced injury,[13] histologic confirmation is required and can be obtained with a punch biopsy.

PROGNOSTIC STRATIFICATION

The finding of a CWR is accompanied by the presence of distant metastases in up to a third of patients.[13] Patients who present with an isolated CWR, however, will not uniformly have a grim prognosis. A number of factors are associated with improved prognosis in these patients, and a variety of prognostic tools are available to assist clinicians in predicting survival in these patients.[10,14,15]

In a study of 130 patients with isolated CWR, investigators from the University of Texas MD Anderson Cancer Center found that initial node-negative status, time to CWR more than 24 months, and treatment with radiation therapy for the CWR were independent predictors of improved disease-free and overall survival.[15] Patients with all 3 favorable features had

TABLE 69-1 Incidence of Chest Wall Recurrence after Mastectomy and Adjuvant Chemotherapy

Study	N	Follow-up	Incidence of CWR
NSABP B-12[26]	1093	5.3 y	9%
Ludwig I and II[27]	818	6 y	15%
Danish[28]	737	5 y	28%
NSABP B-11[26]	697	5.3 y	22%
NCCGTC/Mayo[29]	564	8 y	20%
ECOG 5177[30]	553	7.7 y	28%

CWR, chest wall recurrence.

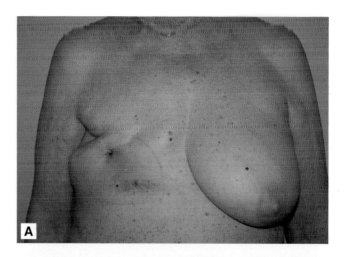

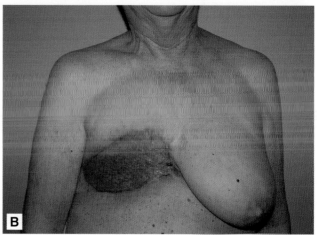

FIGURE 69-1 A. Chest wall recurrence presenting as multiple skin nodules and **B.** postoperative resection with skin graft coverage. *(Photos courtesy of Dr T. McCurry, University of Louisville)*

a median overall survival of 141 months (10-year actuarial survival: 75.4%), those with 1 or 2 favorable features had a median overall survival of 54 months (10-year actuarial survival: 25.1%), and those without any favorable features had a median overall survival of 16 months (10-year actuarial survival: 0%).[16] These data suggest that patients presenting with CWR are a heterogeneous population, and aggressive management using a multidisciplinary approach is warranted in a subset of patients for whom a good prognosis may be anticipated.

Fodor et al similarly found that patients who were initially node negative and who developed a CWR more than 24 months from their initial mastectomy had a better 10-year cause-specific survival.[16] In addition, they found that if the recurrence was operable and was a single lesion in the scar, prognosis was improved.

SURGICAL THERAPY

Chest Wall Recurrence Following Conventional Mastectomy

Surgical resection of CWR is an important aspect of the management of patients with CWR because it provides excellent local control in patients with resectable disease. Surgery is particularly useful in patients who have previously had radiation therapy or those in whom radiation therapy is ill advised.

For patients with isolated recurrences involving only the skin or the surgical scar, resection of the CWR is often straightforward. Resection with primary closure is generally feasible and provides excellent local control. With more extensive disease, coverage with either a skin graft (Fig. 69-1) or autologous flap (Fig. 69-2) may be needed. Preoperative consultation with a plastic surgeon should be obtained as part of a multidisciplinary approach. The goal of resection should be the attainment of clear margin. Although there is no consensus on what constitutes a "clear margin," wide resection is generally recommended.

For patients with CWR extending to underlying bony elements, the utility of resection of ribs and sternum remains controversial. Such extensive resections are often associated with significant morbidity, although some authors have reported reasonable long-term results of full-thickness resections in selected patients (Table 69-2).

Chest Wall Recurrence Following Mastectomy with Reconstruction

With increased use of skin-sparing mastectomy and immediate reconstruction, there has been some concern regarding the incidence, detection, and management of CWR in this setting. In terms of incidence of CWR, no evidence indicates there is any difference in the local recurrence rates following skin-sparing mastectomy versus conventional mastectomy (Table 69-3). Furthermore, the incidence of CWR does not vary with the type of reconstruction.[17]

Langstein et al have demonstrated that the most (72%) CWRs following skin-sparing mastectomy with reconstruction occur under the skin and are easily palpable on clinical examination.[17] Although the length of time between mastectomy and finding CWR may be slightly longer in patients who have had reconstruction, the prognosis between these patients and those who develop a CWR after a conventional mastectomy is not significantly different.[18]

The management of a CWR in patients with a reconstructed breast does not necessarily mandate a take-down of the reconstruction.[18,19] In patients who have had transverse

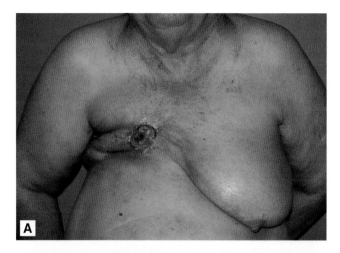

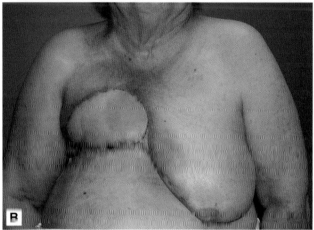

FIGURE 69-2 A. Obvious solitary ulcerated chest wall recurrence and **B.** postoperative resection with latissimus dorsi flap closure. *(Photos courtesy of The University of Texas MD Anderson Cancer Center)*

rectus abdominus musculocutaneous (TRAM) or latissimus flap reconstruction, the CWR can often be resected with local flap rearrangement to preserve the breast mound (Fig. 69-3). In patients who have had implant-based reconstruction, however, removal of the implant is often warranted to facilitate subsequent radiation therapy.

TABLE 69-2 Survival Following Full-Thickness Chest Wall Resection

Study	N	5-Year Survival (%)
Downey et al[31]	38	15
Santillan et al[32]	28	18
Snyder et al[33]	24	29
Shah and Urban[34]	52	41
Friedel et al[38]	63	46
Faneyte et al[36]	44	47
Miyauchi et al[37]	23	48
Palmeijer et al[38]	22	71

ADJUVANT THERAPY

Radiation Therapy

Radiation therapy, when used to treat a CWR, has been found to be an independent factor leading to improved prognosis.[15] In general, large field radiotherapy encompassing the entire chest wall is preferable to less extensive radiation. In a study of 224 patients with CWR, Halverson et al found that the 5- and 10-year disease-free survival of patients treated with large field radiation was 75% and 63%, respectively, compared with 36% and 18% when smaller fields were used.[20] Subsequent supraclavicular metastases were also significantly reduced with the use of radiation therapy (16% vs 6% without radiation therapy).[20] For recurrences that were completely excised, good local control could be achieved using doses ranging from 4500 to 7000 cGy.[20]

For patients who have previously been treated with radiation therapy to the chest wall, data were previously sparse in terms of the value of reirradiation. A recent multi-institutional study of reirradiation in the setting of CWR reviewed 81 patients presenting with a local recurrence after a median of 60-Gy radiation.[21] Thirty-one of these patients had originally had a mastectomy with PMRT and subsequently presented with a CWR. This study found that a second course of radiation at the time of the local recurrence (median: 48 Gy) was not associated with significant grade 4 to 5 toxicity and was associated with a 57% overall complete response rate. Factors correlating with an improved 1-year disease-free survival included longer interval from initial radiation therapy, greater dose of radiation therapy at the time of recurrence, and use of concurrent chemotherapy.

Systemic Therapy

Given that CWR often signifies aggressive disease and is frequently accompanied by distant metastases, systemic therapy is generally part of the multidisciplinary management of these patients. Although local control is generally the purview of surgery and radiation therapy, some studies have found a trend (albeit not statistically significant) toward improved survival using systemic chemotherapy after adequate resection and radiation therapy.[11] In patients with an estrogen receptor (ER)-positive CWR, the use of hormonal therapy has also been associated with an improved prognosis.[20] In a multicenter trial in which ER-positive patients with isolated CWR were randomized to tamoxifen or placebo after complete local excision and radiation therapy, Borner et al found a significant reduction in second local failures at 5 years.[22] Overall survival, however, was not significantly changed.[22] Given the potential usefulness of hormonal therapy and the fact that the ER status is the same as the original tumor in only 75 to 85% of cases, the hormone receptor status of the CWR should be ascertained.

Other Treatment Modalities

Hyperthermia in conjunction with radiation therapy has been evaluated by a number of studies. Although there was no significant difference in terms of complete response rates between radiation therapy alone and that combined with hyperthermia

TABLE 69-3 Local Recurrence Rates after Skin-Sparing Mastectomy versus Conventional Mastectomy

Study	Follow-up (mo)	N	LR (%) Skin-Sparing Mastectomy	LR (%) Conventional Mastectomy
Murphy et al[39]	75	1444	1.3	0.7
Newman et al[40]	50	874	6.2	7.4
Carlson et al[41]	41	271	4.8	9.5
Simmons et al[42]	16	231	3.9	3.2
Rivadeneira et al[43]	49	198	5.6	3.9
Kroll et al[44]	72	154	7.0	7.5

LR, local recurrence.

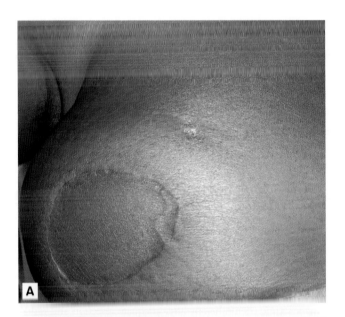

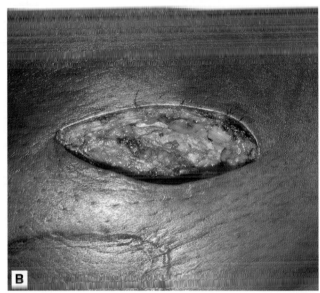

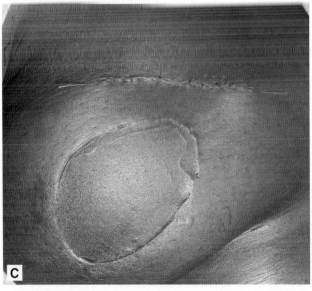

FIGURE 69-3   A. Solitary chest wall recurrence (CWR) in patient with previous transverse rectus abdominis musculocutaneous (TRAM) flap, **B.** resection of CWR, and **C.** postoperative resection with local tissue rearrangement. *(Photos courtesy of Jason D. Sciarretta.)*

in 4 studies, 2 other trials found a benefit to the addition of hyperthermia.[13] A meta-analysis showed a benefit to hyperthermia with complete response rate of 59% versus 41% in patients treated with radiation therapy alone (OR: 2.3; 95% CI: 1.4-3.8; $p = 0.007$).[23] This benefit was particularly noted in those who had undergone previous radiation therapy and seemed to be maintained in follow-up. These findings have been echoed by a prospective randomized controlled trial of hyperthermia and radiation therapy for superficial tumors.[24] In this study of 109 patients, 70 of whom had CWRs, the complete response rate for hyperthermia and radiation was 66% versus 42% for radiation therapy alone. Again, previously irradiated patients had the greatest benefit (68.2% vs 23.5%).

Other modalities that have been tried in the treatment of CWR include photodynamic therapy and intra-arterial chemotherapy.[13] Both of these, however, result in transient responses. Some investigators have found that injection of interferon into the recurrence (with or without concomitant radiation therapy) yields reasonable results, but these studies are few.[13]

FUTURE DIRECTIONS/NECESSARY FUTURE STUDIES

Further study is needed to delineate optimal management of these patients. Although surgery is often needed for optimal local control, little is known about the feasibility and potential benefit of lymph node evaluation in these patients. Sentinel node biopsy has been shown to be feasible in the setting of recurrent breast cancer, albeit with altered drainage pathways, and some authors have now begun investigating the feasibility of sentinel node biopsy following mastectomy.[25] How this will affect the management of patients with CWR remains unclear.

In terms of radiation therapy, there continues to be controversy regarding reirradiation of the chest wall and the incorporation of hyperthermia. Further studies will help elucidate when these modalities should be used, and further whether concomitant chemotherapy should be used as a radiosensitizing agent.

The issue of whether cytotoxic chemotherapy is needed in patients with a resected CWR is the subject of the ongoing Breast International Group (BIG) 1-02, the International Breast Cancer Study Group (IBCSG) 27-02, and the National Surgical Adjuvant Breast and Bowel Project (NSABP) B-27 Study. This trial will randomize 977 patients with locally recurrent breast cancer to receive chemotherapy or no chemotherapy; radiation therapy, trastuzumab, and hormonal therapy will be given as appropriate. Although this study will not answer the question of "optimal" chemotherapy because the regimen of cytotoxic therapy is left to the treating physician, it will answer the more fundamental question of whether cytotoxic chemotherapy is truly beneficial in these patients.

As more tailored approaches to systemic therapy emerge, with newer biological agents, chemotherapy for CWR will also evolve. Further studies to evaluate the potential utility of genomic profiles of CWR in estimating the usefulness of chemotherapeutic agents will be an important area of research. Potentially, by understanding the molecular and genomic basis of CWR, optimal therapeutic regimens may be fashioned.

Finally, there must continue to be a focus on prevention. Although the current guidelines for PMRT recommend treatment of patients with tumors larger than 5 cm or those with 4 or more positive nodes, there remains controversy as to how to manage patients with 1 to 3 positive nodes. This is the subject of the ongoing Medical Research Council (MRC) Selective Use of Postoperative Radiotherapy After Mastectomy (SUPREMO) trial. Although this study will answer an important question, as we move forward, biological markers of tumor aggressiveness and radiosensitivity may be found that may help tailor therapy even further.

Novel treatments for CWR, including cryotherapy, radiofrequency ablation, laser and microwave therapy, will also continue to be explored as we try to move toward less aggressive but more effective management of CWR.

SUMMARY

CWR following mastectomy is a challenging clinical problem that requires a multidisciplinary approach. Although it has frequently been believed that CWR is a harbinger of a poor prognosis, and in general, many of these patients present with metastatic disease, this is a heterogeneous population. Patients who develop their CWR more than 2 years from their original mastectomy, and who originally were node negative, have a reasonable long-term survival, particularly if they can be treated aggressively with surgery, radiation, and systemic therapy.

REFERENCES

1. Jatoi I, Proschan MA. Randomized trials of breast-conserving therapy versus mastectomy for primary breast cancer: a pooled analysis of updated results. *Am J Clin Oncol.* 2005;28(3):289-294.
2. Chagpar A, Kuerer HM, Hunt KK, Strom EA, Buchholz TA. Outcome of treatment for breast cancer patients with chest wall recurrence according to initial stage: implications for post-mastectomy radiation therapy. *Int J Radiat Oncol Biol Phys.* 2003;57(1):128-135.
3. Clarke M, Collins R, Darby S, et al. Effects of radiotherapy and of differences in the extent of surgery for early breast cancer on local recurrence and 15-year survival: an overview of the randomised trials. *Lancet.* 2005;366(9503):2087-2106.
4. Ragaz J, Jackson SM, Le N, et al. Adjuvant radiotherapy and chemotherapy in node-positive premenopausal women with breast cancer. *N Engl J Med.* 1997;337(14):956-962.
5. Overgaard M, Hansen PS, Overgaard J, et al. Postoperative radiotherapy in high-risk premenopausal women with breast cancer who receive adjuvant chemotherapy. Danish Breast Cancer Cooperative Group 82b Trial. *N Engl J Med.* 1997;337(14):949-955.
6. Overgaard M, Jensen MB, Overgaard J, et al. Postoperative radiotherapy in high-risk postmenopausal breast-cancer patients given adjuvant tamoxifen: Danish Breast Cancer Cooperative Group DBCG 82c randomised trial. *Lancet.* 1999;353(9165):1641-1648.
7. Recht A, Edge SB, Solin LJ, et al. Postmastectomy radiotherapy: clinical practice guidelines of the American Society of Clinical Oncology. *J Clin Oncol.* 2001;19(5):1539-1569.
8. Harris JR, Halpin-Murphy P, McNeese M, et al. Consensus statement on postmastectomy radiation therapy. *Int J Radiat Oncol Biol Phys.* 1999;44(5):989-990.
9. Freedman GM, Fowble BL. Local recurrence after mastectomy or breast-conserving surgery and radiation. *Oncology (Williston Park).* 2000;14(11):1561-1581.
10. Willner J, Kiricuta IC, Kolbl O. Locoregional recurrence of breast cancer following mastectomy: always a fatal event? Results of univariate and multivariate analysis. *Int J Radiat Oncol Biol Phys.* 1997;37(4):853-863.
11. Schwaibold F, Fowble BL, Solin LJ, Schultz DJ, Goodman RL. The results of radiation therapy for isolated local regional recurrence after mastectomy. *Int J Radiat Oncol Biol Phys.* 1991;21(2):299-310.

12. Donegan WL, Perez-Mesa CM, Watson FR. A biostatistical study of locally recurrent breast carcinoma. *Surg Gynecol Obstet*. 1966;122(3):529-540.

13. Recht A, Come S, Troyan SL, Sadowsky N. Management of recurrent breast cancer. In: Harris JR, Lippman ME, Morrow M, Osborne C.K., eds. *Diseases of the Breast*. 2nd ed. Philadelphia, PA: Lippincott Williams & Wilkins: 2000:731-748.

14. Kamby C, Sengelov L. Pattern of dissemination and survival following isolated locoregional recurrence of breast cancer. A prospective study with more than 10 years of follow up. *Breast Cancer Res Treat*. 1997;45(2):181-192.

15. Chagpar A, Meric-Bernstam F, Hunt KK, et al. Chest wall recurrence after mastectomy does not always portend a dismal outcome. *Ann Surg Oncol*. 2003;10(6):628-634.

16. Fodor J, Major T, Polgar C, et al. Prognosis of patients with local recurrence after mastectomy or conservative surgery for early-stage invasive breast cancer. *Breast*. 2008;17(3):302-308.

17. Langstein HN, Cheng MH, Singletary SE, et al. Breast cancer recurrence after immediate reconstruction: patterns and significance. *Plast Reconstr Surg*. 2003;111(2):712-720.

18. Chagpar A, Langstein HN, Kronowitz SJ, et al. Treatment and outcome of patients with chest wall recurrence after mastectomy and breast reconstruction. *Am J Surg*. 2004;187(2):164-169.

19. Howard MA, Polo K, Pusic AL, et al. Breast cancer local recurrence after mastectomy and TRAM flap reconstruction: incidence and treatment options. *Plast Reconstr Surg*. 2006;117(5):1381-1386.

20. Halverson KJ, Perez CA, Kuske RR, et al. Isolated local-regional recurrence of breast cancer following mastectomy: radiotherapeutic management. *Int J Radiat Oncol Biol Phys*. 1990;19(4):851-858.

21. Wahl AO, Rademaker A, Kiel KD, et al. Multi-institutional review of repeat irradiation of chest wall and breast for recurrent breast cancer. *Int J Radiat Oncol Biol Phys*. 2008;70(2):477-484.

22. Borner M, Bacchi M, Goldhirsch A, et al. First isolated locoregional recurrence following mastectomy for breast cancer: results of a phase III multicenter study comparing systemic treatment with observation after excision and radiation. Swiss Group for Clinical Cancer Research. *J Clin Oncol*. 1994;12(10):2071-2077.

23. Vernon CC, Hand JW, Field SB, et al. Radiotherapy with or without hyperthermia in the treatment of superficial localized breast cancer: results from five randomized controlled trials. International Collaborative Hyperthermia Group. *Int J Radiat Oncol Biol Phys*.1996;35(4):731-744.

24. Jones EL, Oleson JR, Prosnitz LR, et al. Randomized trial of hyperthermia and radiation for superficial tumors. *J Clin Oncol*. 2005;23(13):3079-3085.

25. Intra M, Veronesi P, Gentilini OD, et al. Sentinel lymph node biopsy is feasible even after total mastectomy. *J Surg Oncol*. 2007;95(2):175-179.

26. Fisher B, Redmond C, Wickerham DL, et al. Doxorubicin-containing regimens for the treatment of stage II breast cancer: The National Surgical Adjuvant Breast and Bowel Project experience. *J Clin Oncol*. 1989;7(5):572-582.

27. Goldhirsch A, Gelber RD, Castiglione M. Relapse of breast cancer after adjuvant treatment in premenopausal and perimenopausal women: patterns and prognoses. *J Clin Oncol*. 1988;6(1):89-97.

28. Overgaard M, Christensen JJ, Johansen H, et al. Evaluation of radiotherapy in high-risk breast cancer patients: report from the Danish Breast Cancer Cooperative Group (DBCG 82) Trial. *Int J Radiat Oncol Biol Phys*. 1990;19(5):1121-1124.

29. Pisansky TM, Ingle JN, Schaid DJ, et al. Patterns of tumor relapse following mastectomy and adjuvant systemic therapy in patients with axillary lymph node-positive breast cancer. Impact of clinical, histopathologic, and flow cytometric factors. *Cancer*. 1993;72(4):1247-1260.

30. Tormey DC, Gray R, Gilchrist K, et al. Adjuvant chemohormonal therapy with cyclophosphamide, methotrexate, 5-fluorouracil, and prednisone (CMFP) or CMFP plus tamoxifen compared with CMF for premenopausal breast cancer patients. An Eastern Cooperative Oncology Group trial. *Cancer*. 1990;65(2):200-206.

31. Downey RJ, Rusch V, Hsu FI, et al. Chest wall resection for locally recurrent breast cancer: is it worthwhile? *J Thorac Cardiovasc Surg*. 2000;119(3):420-428.

32. Santillan AA, Kiluk JV, Cox JM, et al. Outcomes of locoregional recurrence after surgical chest wall resection and reconstruction for breast cancer. *Ann Surg Oncol*. 2008;15(5):1322-1329.

33. Snyder AF, Farrow GM, Masson JK, Payne WS. Chest-wall resection for locally recurrent breast cancer. *Arch Surg*. 1968;97(2):246-253.

34. Shah JP, Urban JA. Full thickness chest wall resection for recurrent breast carcinoma involving the bony chest wall. *Cancer* 1975;35(3):567-573.

35. Friedel G, Kuipers T, Dippon J, et al. Full-thickness resection with myocutaneous flap reconstruction for locally recurrent breast cancer. *Ann Thorac Surg*. 2008;85(6):1894-1900.

36. Faneyte IF, Rutgers EJ, Zoetmulder FA. Chest wall resection in the treatment of locally recurrent breast carcinoma: indications and outcome for 44 patients. *Cancer*. 1997;80(5):886-891.

37. Miyauchi H, Hirata T, Teruya T, et al. Surgical treatment for chest wall recurrence of breast cancer. *Nippon Geka Gakkai Zasshi* 1997;78(6):1059-1062.

38. Dahlstrom CD, Smith RJ, McOmbill DP, et al. Full-thickness chest wall resection for recurrent breast carcinoma: an institutional review and meta-analysis. *Am Surg*. 2005;71(9):711-715.

39. Murphy RX Jr, Wahhab S, Rovito PF, et al. Impact of immediate reconstruction on the local recurrence of breast cancer after mastectomy. *Ann Plast Surg*. 2003;50(4):333-338.

40. Newman LA, Kuerer HM, Hunt KK, et al. Presentation, treatment, and outcome of local recurrence after skin-sparing mastectomy and immediate breast reconstruction. *Ann Surg Oncol*. 1998;5(7):620-626.

41. Carlson GW, Bostwick J III, Styblo TM, et al. Skin-sparing mastectomy. Oncologic and reconstructive considerations. *Ann Surg*. 1997;225(5):570-575.

42. Simmons RM, Fish SK, Gayle L, et al. Local and distant recurrence rates in skin-sparing mastectomies compared with non-skin-sparing mastectomies. *Ann Surg Oncol*. 1999;6(7):676-681.

43. Rivadeneira DE, Simmons RM, Fish SK, et al. Skin-sparing mastectomy with immediate breast reconstruction: a critical analysis of local recurrence. *Cancer J*. 2000;6(5):331-335.

44. Kroll SS, Khoo A, Singletary SE, et al. Local recurrence risk after skin-sparing and conventional mastectomy: a 6-year follow-up. *Plast Reconstr Surg*. 1999;104(2):421-425.

CHAPTER 70

Surgery for Gynecomastia

Sarah McLaughlin
Hiram S. Cody

Gynecomastia (GM) is a benign proliferation of the glandular component of the male breast caused by an increase in the ratio of estrogens to androgens. It presents as a palpable, concentric, and often painful subareolar mass and may be unilateral or bilateral. Although the finding of breast enlargement may be embarrassing or distressing to the patient, surgery for GM is rarely indicated, and cancer is present in less than 1% of patients. Gynecomastia is common. Two historical case series report 57% of healthy older men have GM, which increases to nearly 70% in hospitalized older men.[1,2] Further, autopsy series found GM in 40% to 55% of unselected cases.[3]

ETIOLOGY

Gynecomastia occurs physiologically with 3 natural peaks—in the neonatal period, puberty, and senescence. During the neonatal period, 60% to 90% of infants have transient breast enlargement due to maternal estrogen influence. By puberty, 50% to 75% of boys experience breast enlargement as estrogen concentrations peak earlier than the nearly 30-fold increase in testosterone concentrations.[4] Most GM related to puberty spontaneously regresses within 2 years. Finally, as men age, free testosterone levels decline and obesity becomes more prevalent, increasing relative estrogen concentrations and therefore the incidence of GM.

Although GM is often physiologic, it may be idiopathic or associated with more serious disease, congenital syndromes, and/or medications (Tables 70-1 and 70-2).[5] All result in either an increase in estrogen, decrease in androgen, or a deficit in androgen receptors. Nearly 75% of men seeking evaluation have idiopathic GM, persistent GM after puberty, or drug-induced GM.[6]

DIAGNOSIS

The etiology of GM is frequently ascertained simply by comprehensive clinical evaluation, including history and physical examination. Attention must be given to a complete review of systems and medication evaluation. Frequently in long standing GM no further evaluation is necessary. Gynecomastia of recent onset typically presents as a tender, smooth, mobile, rubbery mass centrally within the breast with a normal appearance to the overlying skin, nipple, and areola. In contrast, breast cancers are hard, ill-defined masses, and they may be associated with skin flattening or retraction. Nipple bleeding or discharge may be present in up to 10% of men with breast cancer.[7] Gynecomastia can be unilateral or bilateral, and although unilateral GM must be differentiated from breast cancer, the overwhelming proportion of unilateral breast masses in men are benign. However, the physical findings of GM and early breast cancer may be quite similar, and any persistent breast mass of recent onset requires further evaluation.

GRADING SCALE

Many classification systems categorize GM with only slight variation in definition.[8-10] Only Rohrich[10] attempts to quantify breast tissue volumes preoperatively. None is used routinely in practice, and none is standardized in published literature. Practically, the most useful grading scale may be one that incorporates breast size, shape, and the anatomic findings that will affect surgical decision making. Although identification of breast enlargement is important for diagnosis, features such as nipple location in reference to the inframammary fold, degree of breast ptosis, and quantity of

TABLE 70-1 Pathologic Causes of Gynecomastia

Pathologic	
Androgen insensitivity syndromes	
Congenital syndromes	Klinefelter syndrome
Genetic mutation in aromatase gene	
Neurologic disease	Spinal cord injury
Primary or secondary gonadal failure	
Starvation and refeeding	
Systemic illness	Liver or renal failure
Thyroid disease	
True hermaphroditism	
Tumors	Adrenal, colon, lung, liver, pituitary, prostate, testicular (Leydig, Sertoli, and germ cell)

TABLE 70-2 Pharmacologic Causes of Gynecomastia

Drugs	
Angiotensin-converting enzyme inhibitors	
Amiodarone	
Anabolic steroids or testosterone replacement	
Androgen receptor blockers	Flutamide, finasteride
Calcium channel blockers	
Cytotoxic chemotherapeutics	Vincristine, methotrexate
Gonadotrophin-releasing hormone agents	
Estrogen containing cream or cosmetics	
H2 antagonists and proton pump inhibitors	
Isoniazid	
Ketoconazole	
Marijuana and heroin	
Metronidazole	
Phytoestrogens: soy products, beer	
Spironolactone	
Theophylline	
Tricyclic antidepressants	

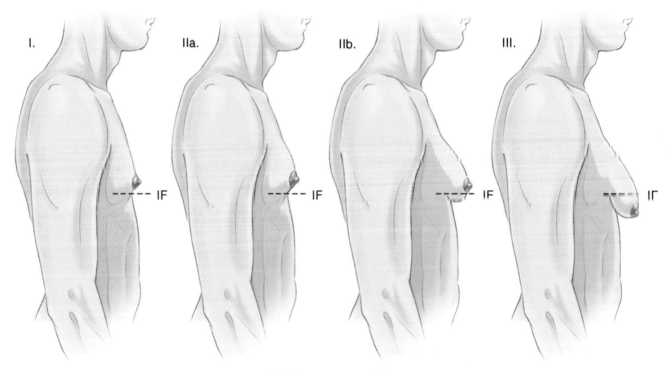

IF=Inframammary fold

FIGURE 70-1 Line drawing illustration of the grades of gynecomastia. Grade I: profile view of a breast bud with prominence only in the retroareolar location. Grade IIA: profile view with larger prominence in retroareolar location. Grade IIB: same as IIA but also with visible inframammary fold. Grade III: larger than IIB, visible inframammary fold, and ptosis with nipple at or below the inframammary fold.

skin redundancy are important considerations when determining the appropriate surgical procedure for these patients. In general, the grades of GM are as follows[9] (Fig. 70-1):

Grade I: small visible breast enlargement without skin redundancy
Grade IIA: moderate breast enlargement without skin redundancy
Grade IIB: moderate breast enlargement with skin redundancy
Grade III: marked breast enlargement with skin redundancy and ptosis

HISTOLOGY

Gynecomastia can be classified into 2 histologic types based on morphologic features: the florid type and fibrous type. The florid type exhibits epithelial cell hyperplasia, stromal edema, and increased cellularity. This proliferative phase is composed of ≥2 cell layers often with fingerlike projections extending into the ductal lumen. The fibrotic type of GM is characterized by dense fibrous, acellular stroma, atrophic glands, and scattered ducts with a minimal degree of proliferative activity.

ROLE FOR IMAGING

Mammography is reasonable in most men under evaluation for GM surgery, and particularly if there is any suspicion of cancer. In the setting of a known tissue diagnosis, mammography has a sensitivity of 90% and a specificity of 92%, respectively,[11] but it is limited by a positive predictive value of 55%. In the setting of clinical symptoms, the benefit is less clear. Among 190 men with breast symptoms (tenderness, mass, tender mass, nipple sensitivity, nonspecific breast enlargement) 203 of 212 mammograms (96%) demonstrated benign findings.[12] The authors concluded that mammography adds little to the initial comprehensive male breast evaluation. As in women, mammography in men can be falsely negative and should not be taken as reassurance in the setting of a dominant breast mass.[13,14] The role of ultrasound in the evaluation of GM is less clear because findings include a hypoechoic mass with irregular margins in up to 80% of benign GM cases.[13] No evidence supports the use of magnetic resonance imaging in the evaluation of GM.

Fine-needle aspiration of male breast masses can be helpful, with a reported negative predictive value greater than 95% and a positive predictive value of 100%.[15] However, this technique requires an experienced cytopathologist and can be associated with a high rate of unsatisfactory (acellular) specimens, especially when the GM has a prominent component of stromal fibrosis.[16]

INDICATIONS FOR SURGERY

Although patients with physiologic GM frequently seek evaluation, few seek additional treatment when reassured that symptoms are transient and usually regress.[4] Most patients with nonphysiologic GM usually require no treatment. Most resolve spontaneously within a few months or with the removal of precipitating factors. Specific treatment is indicated only when symptoms of breast enlargement are persistently painful, embarrassing, or distressing to the patient and negatively affect his overall quality of life. There is little role for medical treatment, which is only effective during the early proliferative phase before the development of stromal hyalinization and fibrosis.[17] Surgical treatment of GM aims to reduce breast size, alleviate symptoms, and restore the chest contour. The most commonly employed techniques are local excision, liposuction, or subcutaneous mastectomy. Techniques such as breast reduction, mastopexy, and free nipple grafting or revision can be added as primary or secondary procedures depending on degree of skin redundancy and nipple location.

GENERAL PRINCIPLES

When possible, incisions should be either circumareolar or in a remote lateral position for the best cosmetic results. Extension of the incision within the pigmented areola may result in a white line as it scars, whereas those placed on the skin may result in a hypertrophic scar in 5% to 10% of cases.[18] Surgical markings should be made preoperatively with the patient awake in the upright position because the exact position of the areolar border may be difficult to find especially after the injection of tumescent solutions or local anesthetics containing epinephrine.

LOCAL EXCISION

Correction of grade I GM is usually a simple procedure. Local excision of the retroareolar tissue through a circumareolar incision is well tolerated and can be performed under local anesthesia. The major problem with this technique is nipple retraction, which is prevented by limiting the extent of excision and by approximating the tissue layers deep to the nipple. Overall satisfaction after local excision is high.[19]

LIPOSUCTION

Liposuction is a significant advance in the treatment of GM. It removes parenchymal tissue and fat[20,21]; it allows more cosmetic incisions; it helps contour the chest wall, and it permits rapid and precise tissue removal. Low grades of GM are best treated with liposuction alone, and contemporary techniques of ultrasound-assisted liposuction are more effective in fibrous GM.[10] Liposuction and surgical excision are easily combined in the same operation, or each method can be used in a delayed surgical procedure to correct the deficiencies of the other.

Preoperative surgical markings should include both the incision site and a topographical map outlining areas of breast enlargement (Fig. 70-2). The patient is placed supine, anesthetized, and infiltrated with a tumescent solution (lidocaine, epinephrine, and saline) to distend the breast tissues and facilitate suctioning in dense tissue areas. The tumescent solution gives local anesthesia and enhances postoperative pain control, but most patients are more comfortable under general anesthesia or monitored anesthesia care with intravenous sedation.

Possible incision sites include the inframammary crease medially, the anterior axillary line (or axillary fold) laterally, and the areolar border centrally. In general, larger suction cannulas (4-8 mm) are suitable for removal of fatty breast tissue in the subcutaneous plane laterally, and smaller cannulas (2.4 mm) are more effective for the glandular or fibrous component of the

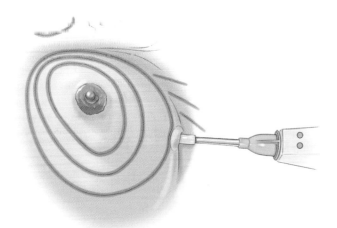

FIGURE 70-2 Line drawing illustration of a topographical map drawn prior to liposuction treatment of gynecomastia (GM). Supine patient with grade IIA or IIB GM and 3 concentric rings around the nipple and areolar complex spreading outward from the nipple showing different elevation levels (decreasing) away from the nipple and areola.

breast suction begins centrally, using the left hand to pinch the breast tissue up and off the pectoralis muscle, and removing tissue in sequential concentric rings as diagrammed by the preoperative topographical map. The initial passes of the cannula may be resistant, but this diminishes with persistence. Dissection of the glandular component in the subdermal plane may promote skin contraction and thereby eliminate the need for skin excision.[22,23] Finally, power-assisted liposuction contours the chest wall, feathering the remaining breast tissue and blending each concentric ring. If small nodules of dense parenchyma remain after suctioning, these can be removed through the liposuction incision using a pull-through technique or through a small circumareolar counterincision.[22] Illustrative pre- and postoperative photos of liposuction for GM are found in Figures 70-3 and 70-4.

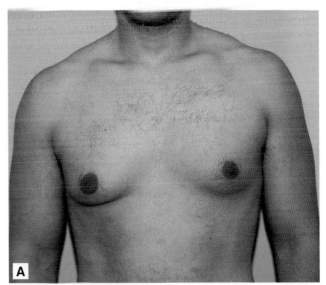

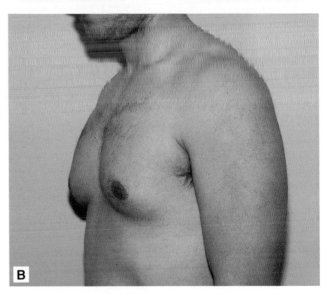

FIGURES 70-3 Persistent pubertal GM treated with liposuction alone. Preoperative **(A)** front view, **(B)** oblique view.

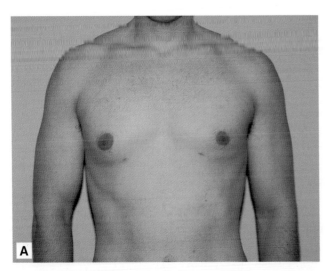

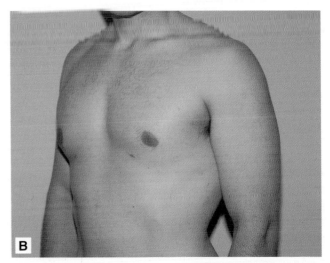

FIGURE 70-4 Persistent pubertal GM treated with liposuction alone. Six-month postoperative **(A)** front view, **(B)** oblique view.

Overall patient satisfaction with cosmetic outcome after liposuction treatment for GM is high. Hodgson et al reported a patient satisfaction score of 9.1 of 10 and a self-confidence score after surgery of 8.9 of 10.[23] Complications of aggressive dissection in the subareolar location may include a central "saucer" deformity or nipple necrosis. Surgical complications aside, the major limitations of liposuction include the failure to remove glandular breast tissue and the inability to perform pathologic analysis of the resected tissue.

SUBCUTANEOUS MASTECTOMY

Despite the growing popularity of liposuction, subcutaneous mastectomy retains a significant role in GM surgery. In a recent 10-year analysis, subcutaneous mastectomy was the only surgical intervention performed in 56% of patients, and it was combined with liposuction or mastopexy in an additional 35% of patients.[18] Subcutaneous mastectomy is particularly suited for high-grade GM because it allows correction of skin redundancy and histologic analysis of resected tissue.[19,24-26] Although local or regional anesthetic options (such as paravertebral blocks) are feasible, subcutaneous mastectomy is usually best done under general anesthesia.

A circumareolar incision is suitable for most patients having subcutaneous mastectomy and allows a radial extension if needed, but an intramammary approach has been reported as well.[19] Skin-reducing approaches include the complete circumareolar incision or the horizontal ellipse method. The complete circumareolar incision incorporates deepithelialization of circumareolar tissue allowing for skin and deep tissue reduction,[26,27] and the horizontal ellipse method allows nipple and areolar complex repositioning by taking advantage of breast reduction principles.[28] All incorporate the removal of the majority of glandular and fatty breast tissue leaving only a small amount of remnant breast tissue along the mastectomy flaps (8-10 mm). Skin-sparing incisions are appropriate when little ptosis and skin redundancy are minimal (Figs. 70-5 and 70-6). In grade II GM, the

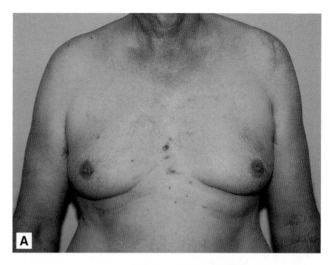

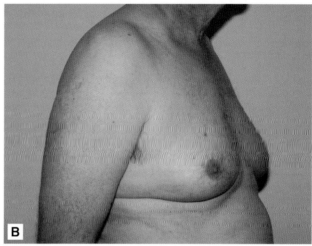

FIGURES 70-5 Gynecomastia treated by skin-sparing subcutaneous mastectomy. Preoperative **(A)** front view, **(B)** oblique view.

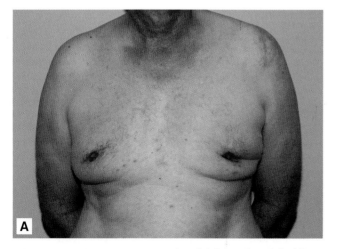

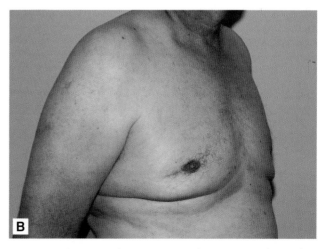

FIGURE 70-6 One year postoperative, **(A)** front view, **(B)** oblique view. Postoperative views demonstrate good cosmetic result in right breast with nipple and areolar retraction of left breast **(A).**

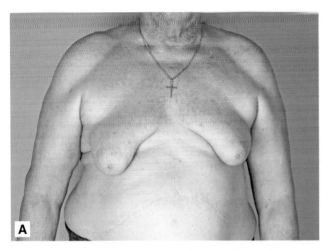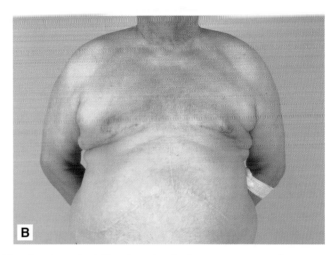

FIGURE 70-7 Severe gynecomastia due to end-stage liver disease. After liver transplantation, breast reduction was necessary for correction. **A.** Preoperative, **B.** 6 weeks postoperative.

addition of liposuction to subcutaneous mastectomy can improve chest wall contouring,[29] but for severe high grade GM, techniques that incorporate skin reduction and nipple repositioning are often necessary.

True breast reduction is rarely done, and only when the nipple is more than 1 cm below the inframammary fold.[27] These patients are often obese, or have recently had significant weight loss, where standard subcutaneous mastectomy will leave redundant skin and unacceptable scars. Possible incisions include the transverse, vertical, and periareolar. Some maintain the blood supply of the nipple-areolar complex (NAC) vascularity on a central pedicle; others employ free grafting of the NAC (Fig. 70-7).[30-32] Regardless of incision chosen, a second-stage procedure may be required for scar correction.

NEW SURGICAL APPROACHES

To decrease the sensory morbidity of standard surgical approaches, some advocate endoscopic management of GM.[33] This method claims to allow dissection and en bloc excision under direct visualization through a lateral incision, but disadvantages include a difficult learning curve, long operative time, and sparse outcome data.

POSTOPERATIVE MANAGEMENT

Closed suction drains are placed after subcutaneous mastectomy or reduction mammoplasty and removed when 24-hour output is less than 30 mL. Patients are wrapped with an elastic compressive garment and instructed to wear it for 2 to 4 weeks postoperatively; this technique is anecdotally believed to limit early postoperative complications (seroma or hematoma) while enhancing skin retraction.[27] Patients are encouraged to return to regular activities within 48 hours of surgery.

RISKS AND COMPLICATIONS

Complications after liposuction alone appear to be minimal; several studies report no early postoperative hematoma, seroma,

infection, or thermal injury.[23,34] Late complications after liposuction alone include a residual mass in 10%, persistent hypoesthesia in 3%, and undercorrection of the deformity in 4%.[33] Nipple necrosis is infrequent.

The most common complication of subcutaneous mastectomy is hyperesthesia of the nipple, affecting 70% of patients in one series.[18] This is transient but may persist in 6% to 14% of patients, and especially in those with periareolar incisions[18,19] Wound infection, hematoma, and seroma each occur in 5% to 15%; hematoma is more common with smaller incisions.[19,26] In one series, postoperative complications were associated with larger specimen sizes.[26] Other complications include nipple necrosis or epidermolysis occurring in 7%, areolar retraction in nearly 30% (Fig. 70-6), skin redundancy or "dog ears" in 6% to 10%, and hypertrophic scars in 3% to 14% of patients.[18,19,26]

FUTURE DIRECTIONS

Most patients with GM do not require surgery, and there may be a growing role for medical management. In patient populations at risk for GM, such as prostate cancer patients treated with bicalutamide or flutamide, randomized trials have demonstrated that the addition of tamoxifen decreases breast symptoms from 9% to 8% without affecting disease control or prostate-specific antigen (PSA) suppression.[35,36] The addition of antiestrogen therapies may induce androgen production by blocking the negative feedback of estrogens,[37] and in theory, excess aromatization of androgens to estrogens may cause GM. However, in a randomized trial, the aromatase inhibitor anastrozole was no more effective than placebo in decreasing breast symptoms.[38] Finally, prophylactic breast irradiation can prevent GM in prostate cancer patients before androgen suppression, but the possibility of treatment-associated cardiac toxicity has not been ruled out.[36,39,40]

Regarding surgery, the convergence of open and minimally invasive techniques will continue. Gynecomastia is a benign condition, and future advances should therefore focus on optimizing cosmesis and minimizing morbidity. No current guidelines or standardized treatment algorithm exist or are considered practical in the United States. The United Kingdom has attempted to establish uniform treatment guidelines in 2006 (allowing surgery only if more than 200 g of tissue can be removed per side) but because only 3 of 48 patients treated between 2003 and 2006 in the United Kingdom would have met these criteria,[41] it appears that the indication for surgery in GM will remain in large part subjective.

NECESSARY FUTURE STUDIES

It is unlikely that a large surgical trial will ever be performed to determine the best surgical approach because the anatomy of each patient and surgeon experience will uniquely influence outcomes. Future studies should focus on the best combination of hormonal therapy for patients with GM due to medically treated prostate cancer and include accurate endocrinologic and clinical follow up. Additionally, more study into the pathophysiology of GM and the role of aromatase inhibitors is needed.

SUMMARY

Gynecomastia is common. A thorough history and physical examination is usually sufficient for diagnosis and determination of etiology. Gynecomastia typically regresses within 2 years of puberty, with observation, or after the offending drug is removed or pathologic process is treated. Although medical options are available for early GM, persistent GM that is embarrassing or distressing to the patient can be effectively treated with liposuction or a variety of surgical options removing glandular breast tissue. Cosmetic results and patient satisfaction after surgery are high.

REFERENCES

1. Nuttall FQ. Gynecomastia as a physical finding in normal men. *J Clin Endocrinol Metab.* 1979;48(2):338-340.
2. Niewoehner CB, Nuttal FQ. Gynecomastia in a hospitalized male population. *Am J Med.* 1984;77(4):633-638.
3. Andersen JA, Gram JB. Male breast at autopsy. *Acta Pathol Microbiol Immunol Scand [A].* 1982;90(3):191-197.
4. Niewoehner CB, Schorer AE. Gynaecomastia and breast cancer in men. *BMJ.* 2008;336(7646):709-713.
5. Braunstein GD. Clinical practice. Gynecomastia. *N Engl J Med.* 2007;357(12):1229-1237.
6. Braunstein GD. Gynecomastia. *N Engl J Med.* Feb 18, 1993;328(7):490-495.
7. Giordano SH, Buzdar AU, Hortobagyi GN. Breast cancer in men. *Ann Intern Med.* 2002;137(8):678-687.
8. Nydick M, Bustos J, Dale JH Jr, Rawson RW. Gynecomastia in adolescent boys. *JAMA.* 1961;178:449-454.
9. Simon BE, Hoffman S, Kahn S. Classification and surgical correction of gynecomastia. *Plast Reconstr Surg.* 1973;51(1):48-52.
10. Rohrich RJ, Ha RY, Kenkel JM, Adams WP Jr. Classification and management of gynecomastia: defining the role of ultrasound-assisted liposuction. *Plast Reconstr Surg.* 2003;111(2):909-923; discussion 924-925.
11. Evans GF, Anthony T, Turnage RH, et al. The diagnostic accuracy of mammography in the evaluation of male breast disease. *Am J Surg.* 2001;181(2):96-100.
12. Hines SL, Tan WW, Yasrebi M, DePeri ER, Perez EA. The role of mammography in male patients with breast symptoms. *Mayo Clin Proc.* 2007;82(3):297-300.
13. Gunhan-Bilgen I, Bozkaya H, Ustun EE, Memis A. Male breast disease: clinical, mammographic, and ultrasonographic features. *Eur J Radiol.* 2002;43(3):246-255.
14. Dershaw DD, Borgen PI, Deutch BM, Liberman L. Mammographic findings in men with breast cancer. *AJR Am J Roentgenol.* 1993;160(2):267-270.
15. Westenend PJ, Jobse C. Evaluation of fine-needle aspiration cytology of breast masses in males. *Cancer.* 2002;96(2):101-104.
16. Siddiqui MT, Zakowski MF, Ashfaq R, Ali SZ. Breast masses in males: multi-institutional experience on fine-needle aspiration. *Diagn Cytopathol.* 2002;26(2):87-91.
17. Bannayan GA, Hajdu SI. Gynecomastia: clinicopathologic study of 351 cases. *Am J Clin Pathol.* 1972;57(4):431-437.
18. Handschin AE, Bietry D, Husler R, Banic A, Constantinescu M. Surgical management of gynecomastia—a 10-year analysis. *World J Surg.* 2008;32(1):38-44.
19. Colombo-Benkmann M, Buse B, Stern J, Herfarth C. Indications for and results of surgical therapy for male gynecomastia. *Am J Surg.* 1999;178(1):60-63.
20. Rosenberg GJ. Gynecomastia: suction lipectomy as a contemporary solution. *Plast Reconstr Surg.* 1987;80(3):379-386.
21. Becker H. Subdermal liposuction to enhance skin contraction: a preliminary report. *Ann Plast Surg.* 1992;28(5):479-484.
22. Lista F, Ahmad J. Power-assisted liposuction and the pull-through technique for the treatment of gynecomastia. *Plast Reconstr Surg.* 2008;121(3):740-747.
23. Hodgson EL, Fruhstorfer BH, Malata CM. Ultrasonic liposuction in the treatment of gynecomastia. *Plast Reconstr Surg.* 2005;116(2):646-653; discussion 654-655.
24. Tashkandi M, Al-Qattan MM, Hassanain JM, Hawary MB, Sultan M. The surgical management of high-grade gynecomastia. *Ann Plast Surg.* 2004;53(1):17-20; discussion 21.
25. Cordova A, Moschella F. Algorithm for clinical evaluation and surgical treatment of gynaecomastia. *J Plast Reconstr Aesthet Surg.* 2008;61(1):41-49.
26. Steele SR, Martin MI, Place RJ. Gynecomastia: complications of the subcutaneous mastectomy. *Am Surg.* 2002;68(2):210-213.
27. Persichetti P, Berloco M, Casadei RM, et al. Gynecomastia and the complete circumareolar approach in the surgical management of skin redundancy. *Plast Reconstr Surg.* 2001;107(4):948-954.
28. Gheita A. Gynecomastia: the horizontal ellipse method for its correction. *Aesthetic Plast Surg.* 2008;32(5)795-801.
29. Esme DL, Beekman WH, Hage JJ, Nipshagen MD. Combined use of ultrasonic-assisted liposuction and semicircular periareolar incision for the treatment of gynecomastia. *Ann Plast Surg.* 2007;59(6):629-634.
30. Hamilton S, Gault D. The tuberous male breast. *Br J Plast Surg.* 2003;56(3):295-300.
31. Lejour M. Vertical mammaplasty and liposuction of the breast. *Plast Reconstr Surg.* 1994;94(1):100-114.
32. Fruhstorfer BH, Malata CM. A systematic approach to the surgical treatment of gynaecomastia. *Br J Plast Surg.* 2003;56(3):237-246.
33. Zhu J, Huang J. Surgical management of gynecomastia under endoscope. *J Laparoendosc Adv Surg Tech A.* 2008;18(3):433-437.
34. Boni R. Tumescent power liposuction in the treatment of the enlarged male breast. *Dermatology.* 2006;213(2):140-143.
35. Fradet Y, Egerdie B, Andersen M, et al. Tamoxifen as prophylaxis for prevention of gynaecomastia and breast pain associated with bicalutamide 150 mg monotherapy in patients with prostate cancer: a randomised, placebo-controlled, dose-response study. *Eur Urol.* 2007;52(1):106-114.
36. Perdona S, Autorino R, De Placido S, et al. Efficacy of tamoxifen and radiotherapy for prevention and treatment of gynaecomastia and breast pain caused by bicalutamide in prostate cancer: a randomised controlled trial. *Lancet Oncol.* 2005;6(5):295-300.
37. Gikas P, Mokbel K. Management of gynaecomastia: an update. *Int J Clin Pract.* 2007;61(7):1209-1215.
38. Plourde PV, Reiter EO, Jou HC, et al. Safety and efficacy of anastrozole for the treatment of pubertal gynecomastia: a randomized, double-blind, placebo-controlled trial. *J Clin Endocrinol Metab.* 2004;89(9):4428-4433.
39. Tyrrell CJ, Payne H, Tammela TL, et al. Prophylactic breast irradiation with a single dose of electron beam radiotherapy (10 Gy) significantly reduces the incidence of bicalutamide-induced gynecomastia. *Int J Radiat Oncol Biol Phys.* 2004;60(2):476-483.
40. Nieder C, Pawinski A, Andratschke NH, Molls M. Can prophylactic breast irradiation contribute to cardiac toxicity in patients with prostate cancer receiving androgen suppressing drugs? *Radiat Oncol.* 2008;3:2.
41. Shamsian N, Jones L, Ghosh S. Gynaecomastia: Are surgical guidelines realistic? *BMJ.* 2008;336(7648):790.

CHAPTER 71

Central Venous Access in Breast Oncology Patients

April Spencer
Ervin B. Brown

Since April 2005 the senior author, (Erwin B. Brown) has placed more than 1600 ports at the University of Texas MD Anderson Cancer Center for breast cancer patients, using ultrasound guidance. Although the routine use of ultrasound guidance is not required, the National Institute of Clinical Excellence advocates the use of 2 dimensional ultrasound when obtaining venous access in elective cases.[1]

Central venous access can be divided into 2 types of access: (1) implanted central venous catheters, including chest ports (using jugular or subclavian vein) and arm ports (eg, Passport), and (2) nonimplanted central venous access, including peripherally inserted central catheter (PICC) lines, subclavian catheters, and tunneled catheters without implanted subcutaneous ports. Currently, arm ports are not being inserted at MD Anderson Cancer Center. Central venous access can be achieved using various puncture sites, but the most common are the internal jugular veins, the subclavian veins, and the upper limb veins for PICCs. Femoral veins are seldom used, but may be necessary in selective situations. The choice of access route depends on multiple factors, including the reason for central venous catheter insertion, the anticipated duration of access, the intact venous sites available, and the skills of the operator. The internal jugular vein is preferred over the subclavian vein for implanted ports at our institution, compared with the cannulation of the subclavian vein.

IMPLANTED PORT VENOUS ACCESS SYSTEM

Preparation

A dedicated central venous access team is essential for central venous access in breast oncology patients. Adequate sedation facilitates safe and efficient central venous access in this patient population. This can be achieved by using conscious or unconscious sedation. Our institution's preferred method of sedation is unconscious sedation or general anesthesia. A basic preoperative health evaluation should be performed, including history, current medications (including herbals), allergies, and physical exam. Cardiac and respiratory evaluations should also be conducted. At the start of the procedure, all essential staff and equipment should be in place. Control of personnel traffic is vital.

Technique

A knowledge of the surface anatomical landmarks is essential (Fig. 71-1A). The patient should be prepared and draped in the standard sterile fashion for surgical vascular access and then placed in Trendelenburg position. Using a sterile marker, the proposed infraclavicular skin incision should be outlined parallel to the clavicle. The subcutaneous tunnel should be outlined from the wire entrance site to the proposed infraclavicular incision (Fig. 71-1B). The ideal location for the reservoir is thought to be along the anteromedial aspect of the second rib. This high medial position keeps the port away from the breast tissue and reduces the risk of inadvertent retraction of the catheter.

The internal jugular and subclavian veins should be visualized with ultrasound. Our preference is the Site-Rite ultrasound (Bard Access Systems; Salt Lake City, Utah) with its needle guides. The veins are then confirmed to be compressible and patent. The internal jugular is preferably used at our institution. Using 1% local anesthetic (eg, lidocaine) a skin wheal is created at the point of percutaneous access. A Micro-Introducer Kit (Vascular Solutions; Minneapolis, Minnesota) is used to access the jugular vein. Under ultrasound guidance, a 21-gauge needle is used to percutaneously access the internal jugular vein. This needle allows safe access into the venous system with a 0.018-in diameter guidewire, versus the 0.035-in J-wire and

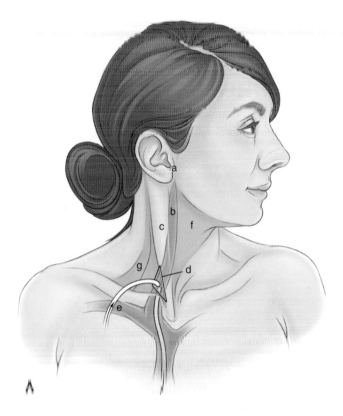

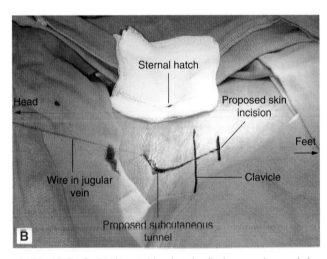

FIGURE 71-1 A. Anatomical landmarks. Surface anatomy of the internal jugular vein: a, intertragic notch; b, internal jugular vein; c, sternocleidomastoid; d, internal jugular vein between sternal and clavicular heads of sternocleidomastoid; e, subclavian vein passing under the clavicle; f, anterior triangle of the neck; and g, posterior triangle of the neck. The red triangle shows the area where intravenous access is obtained. **B.** Premarking the infraclavicular skin incision. The proposed infraclavicular skin incision should be outlined parallel to the clavicle. The subcutaneous tunnel should be outlined from the wire entrance site to the proposed infraclavicular incision. The ideal location for the reservoir is thought to be along the anteromedial aspect of the second rib. This high medial position keeps the port away from the breast tissue and prevents inadvertent retraction of the catheter

19-gauge needle included with most venous access catheters. In breast surgical oncology patients, a micropuncture needle system is ideal, as it facilitates the safe puncture of veins in patients with coagulopathy. The use of ultrasound avoids attempting to access thrombosed veins and decreases the risk of arterial puncture. The glide wire is then threaded through the needle. Once the wire has been negotiated into the central circulation, its location should then be checked under fluoroscopy and confirmed to be in an appropriate position in the superior vena cava and devoid of kinks. Additional local anesthesia is injected in the infraclavicular region at the port site and along the proposed subcutaneous tunnel.

Next, the premarked infraclavicular incision should be made, and the incision should be carefully deepened to the pectoralis fascia. A pocket is then bluntly created at the level of the pectoralis fascia to accommodate the port. A small skin incision is made at the wire entrance site. A 4-French introducer is then passed over the wire. The J-wire is then threaded through the introducer, which is then removed. The position of the J-wire should be checked under fluoroscopy. Using mosquito forceps, any subcutaneous tissue around the J-wire should be gently freed from around the J-wire. The appropriate-sized introducer should then be passed gently over the J-wire, being certain that the J-wire moves freely within the introducer as it is being inserted (Fig. 71-2).

The wire and vein dilator are removed, and the catheter is threaded through the peel-away introducer. The sheath is then peeled away, leaving the catheter in situ (Fig. 71-3). Pinching the peel-away sheath during the introduction of the catheter through this sheath is important to decrease the complication of air embolism. Placing the patient in the Trendelenburg position before the start of the procedure can also minimize the risk of air embolus. If an air embolism does occur, the patient should be immediately positioned in the left lateral decubitus position so that the air can remain in the right heart chambers

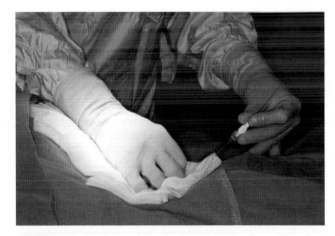

FIGURE 71-2 Introducer insertion. The introducer is threaded over the J-wire, which dilates the tissue. Removal of the vein dilator and J-wire leaves the peel-away sheath within the vein for subsequent introduction of the catheter.

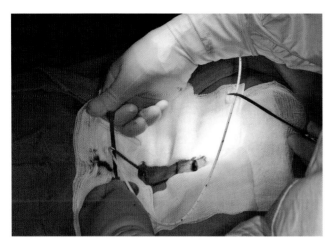

FIGURE 71-3 Sheath peel-away. The peel-away sheath can then be introduced into the central circulation for final placement of the catheter. Pinching the peel-away sheath during the introduction of the catheter through this sheath is important in preventing the complication of an air embolism.

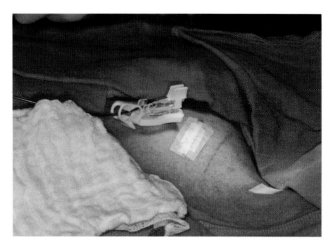

FIGURE 71-4 Accessing the port. The port should then be accessed with a Gripper needle. There should be excellent blood return from the catheter system.

until it can be syringe aspirated. Life support measures should then be initiated as clinically appropriate.

A tunneler is passed between the cervical incision and the infraclavicular incision. The catheter is then attached to the tunneler and is drawn from the cervical incision to the infraclavicular incision through the subcutaneous tunnel. Care should be used to avoid kinking or twisting the catheter. The catheter is advanced or withdrawn under fluoroscopic guidance until the tip of the catheter is in optimal position in the distal superior vena cava or the region of the cavoatrial junction. The catheter is trimmed to the appropriate length and is attached to the port with the locking device. The port is then positioned within the pocket and sutured to the underlying pectoralis fascia with nonabsorbable monofilament sutures to prevent it from twisting or rotating within the pocket. The catheter should then be checked again under fluoroscopy to confirm satisfactory position. There should be a gentle curve in the catheter at its apex in the neck. The pocket is then irrigated with normal saline and exquisite hemostasis should be achieved.

The infraclavicular incision should then be closed with absorbable sutures. The cervical incision should be closed with a subcuticular suture. The skin around both incisions should be prepped after closure with ChloraPrep (Cardinal Health Skin Prep Solutions; El Paso, Texas). Steri-strips (3M; St. Paul, Minnesota) should then be applied. The port should then be accessed with a ¾- or 1-in Gripper needle. There should be excellent blood return from the catheter system (Fig. 71-4). Once this is confirmed, the catheter system should be flushed with heparinized saline. The heparinized saline should flush freely (Fig. 71-5). Sterile dressings are then applied.

When the subclavian vein is chosen as the catheter entrance site, the subclavian vein is accessed under ultrasound guidance with the 21-gauge needle. The wire is passed through the needle, and its position is confirmed with fluoroscopy. The skin incision is outlined with the marking pen parallel to the clavicle

and removed upon the wire. The 6 French introducer is passed over the wire, and a J-wire is threaded through the introducer, which is then removed. The skin incision is made, and the pocket is created at the level of the pectoralis fascia. The peel-away introducer is passed over the J-wire. The catheter is threaded through the introducer, which is then peeled away, leaving the catheter in situ. The catheter is advanced out under fluoroscopic guidance until the tip of the catheter is in the distal superior vena cava or region of the cavoatrial junction. The catheter is trimmed to the appropriate length and attached to the port with the locking device. The port is positioned within the pocket and sutured to the pectoralis fascia with 2 nonabsorbable monofilament sutures. The incision is then closed, as with the internal jugular port.

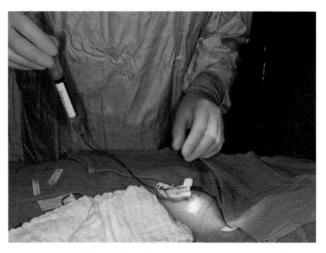

FIGURE 71-5 Flushing the catheter system. Once proper placement is confirmed, the catheter system should be flushed with heparinized saline. The heparinized saline should flush freely.

ARM PORTS

Peripherally inserted central venous catheters with implanted subcutaneous port (Passport) are available, but are not currently being implanted at MD Anderson Cancer Center. There are some patients who present with arm ports placed at outside institutions.

PICC LINES

Peripherally inserted central venous catheters (PICC) lines are inserted by nurses on the infusion therapy service at MD Anderson Cancer Center. Peripherally inserted central venous catheters lines may be inserted with or without ultrasound guidance. Most PICC lines are currently being inserted with ultrasound guidance. However, non–image-guided PICC lines can be placed into visible superficial veins that are large enough to accommodate 3 to 5 French catheters. If superficial access sites have been used, or if advancing the catheter into the central circulation is difficult, central lines are traditionally used. In general, PICC lines offer temporary access until an indwelling catheter can be placed. With no complications, the average catheter patency rate is 30.58 days.[3] Non–image-guided placement of PICC lines can result in catheter tip malpositioning (eg, placement of the tip into the internal jugular vein or contralateral brachiocephalic vein).[4] Subsequent repositioning is required. The upper arm is currently the preferred site of insertion of PICC lines. Sedation has been used more frequently and has been associated with a higher insertion success rate and lower phlebitis rate. PICC lines are available with single or dual lumens. Power PICC lines that can be used for pressure injection for computed tomography scans and magnetic resonance imaging exams are available.

TECHNIQUE OF SUBCLAVIAN CATHETER INSERTION USING ANATOMIC LANDMARKS

At MD Anderson Cancer Center, subclavian catheters are inserted in a special out-patient line clinic. Catheters vary in size from 7 to 12 French. Large-bore pheresis catheters are used for stem cell collection. The patient is placed supine with arms toward the side and head turned away from the implanting clinician. ChloraPrep is used as skin preparation. Maximum sterile barrier is used. The patient is placed in Trendelenburg position. The sternal notch and acromion are palpated. The site for needle insertion is chosen midway between the sternal notch and acromion below the curve of the clavicle. Using a 22-gauge needle, 1% lidocaine is injected at the needle entrance site. The needle is then advanced toward the clavicle and directed a finger breadth above the sternal notch, keeping the needle and the barrel of the syringe in the horizontal plane. As the needle touches the clavicle, additional local anesthesia is injected. The 18-gauge needle is then inserted and advanced horizontally toward the clavicle, again directing it 1 finger breadth above the clavicle. The needle is then marched down under the clavicle and again advanced along toward a point 1 finger breadth above the sternal notch. The entrance of the needle into the subclavian vein is confirmed by blood return. The J-wire is threaded through the needle, which is then removed over the J-wire. A vein dilator is passed over the J-wire. The catheter is then threaded over the J-wire, which is removed. The catheter is flushed with heparinized saline. The catheter is secured with 3–0 silk sutures.

TECHNIQUE OF SUBCLAVIAN CATHETER INSERTION USING ULTRASOUND GUIDANCE

The patient is placed supine with arms toward the side and head turned away from the implanting clinician. ChloraPrep is used as skin preparation. Maximum sterile barrier is used. The patient is placed in Trendelenburg position. The subclavian vein is visualized with the Site-Rite ultrasound. The ultrasound probe is placed vertically just below the clavicle. The compressibility of the vein is confirmed with gentle pressure. The appropriate-depth needle guide is chosen. The needle entrance site is anesthetized with 1% lidocaine local anesthesia. The 21-gauge needle is advanced along the needle guide and into the vein under ultrasound guidance. Once blood return has been confirmed, the needle is disconnected from the guide, and a wire is passed through the needle. A 4-French introducer is passed over the wire. The J-wire is threaded through the introducer, which is then removed. The vein dilator is threaded over the wire. The catheter is threaded over the J-wire, which is then removed. The catheter is flushed with heparinized saline. The catheter is secured with 3–0 silk sutures.

POTENTIAL COMPLICATIONS

Although experienced operators using the ultrasound-guided central venous access method can achieve relatively high success rates with few complications, in the literature, failure rates for initial central venous catheter insertion have been reported to be as high as 35%.[5] Complications associated with venous access devices may be categorized as early (30 days postprocedure) or late (after 30 days postprocedure). Early complications include procedural complications directly related to catheter placement, such as arterial puncture or injury, pneumothorax, air embolism, arrhythmia, catheter malpositioning, venous rupture, and catheter transection that results in its migration. The rates of most complications can be significantly reduced with the aid of imaging guidance during catheter placement. Late complications of venous access devices include catheter-related infection, catheter occlusions, venous thrombosis, fibrin sheathing, and catheter fracture and migration. For brevity sake, only the more common complications will be discussed.

▪ Early Complications

Pneumothorax

Pneumothorax may occur during central venipuncture.[6] With the increasing frequency of use of ultrasound guidance, this complication is low; its incidence was reported as 0.1% in a recent series.[7] This complication can be minimized if, while inserting the needles for subclavian catheters using anatomic landmarks, the needles are kept parallel to the ground while being advanced beneath the clavicle. When accessing the subclavian or jugular vein with ultrasound guidance, one must maintain awareness of the depth of the needle insertion. If the pneumothorax is small, it may be managed with observation. If the size warrants, or if the size of the pneumothorax enlarges with observation, a tube thoracostomy is indicated. A small pig-tail catheter inserted in interventional radiology is usually sufficient to allow expansion of the lung.

Arrhythmias

No matter how judicious the operator is in manipulating the wires and catheters, arrhythmias occur because of the unavoidable contact with the walls of the right side of the heart.[8] Several cardiac rhythms may be observed; atrial ectopic beats and atrial tachycardia and ventricular ectopic beats and ventricular tachycardia may occur. Fluoroscopic guidance makes manipulation of the wires and catheter more precise. Any rhythm abnormality should be corrected by immediately changing the position of the catheter or guidewire. Sustained arrhythmias may require treatment with intravenous medications, which may include esmolol, lidocaine, or adenosine.[1]

Air Embolism

The complication of air embolism and its intervention was discussed earlier in the chapter.

Late Complications

Infection

Infection is one of the more frequently encountered complications in the immune-compromised population of breast oncology patients. Catheter-related infections present in 1 of 3 ways: (1) tunnel or pocket infection—this often requires removal of the catheter and concurrent antibiotic treatment, (2) exit-site infections, which can typically be managed with oral or intravenous antibiotics, and (3) catheter-related sepsis. Catheter-related sepsis always warrants prompt port removal and intravenous antibiotics specific to catheter tip culture results. An incidence of 1.4 infections per 1000 catheter days has been reported.[9] The most common organisms are *Staphylococcus epidermis* (incidence 25%-50%), *Staphylococcus aureus* (incidence 25%), and *Candida albicans* (5%-10% incidence).[10] The most critical factor in preventing surgical infection is meticulous attention to sterile technique. Tissues should be handled gently. Hemostasis should be complete. Wound closure should be precise. The use of prophylactic antibiotics is controversial. Nursing staff should be educated on proper port access, including using alternate infusion sites over the port. If the access site were the face of a clock, infusion nurses should be instructed to access a different hour for each chemotherapy infusion.

Thrombosis

Catheter occlusions are commonly related to the formation of a thrombus within the lumen, the formation of a fibrin sheath around the catheter end, the malpositioning of a catheter tip against the vessel wall or within a small branch vessel, or the presence of thrombosis or stenosis in the native vein. Venous thrombosis is very common in breast oncology patients, as they often are in a hypercoagulable state and have constant venous irritation from the presence of the catheter and stasis of blood in the vein occupied by the catheter. This complication is unpredictable and difficult to avoid. Currently, less than 10% of patients with central venous catheters receive any systemic prophylaxis. Although its general use is not recommended, low-dose warfarin may be a low-risk treatment option in select oncology patients (those with adequate nutrition and hepatic function). Additional studies are needed to validate the use of prophylactic low-dose warfarin. Catheter thrombosis is one of the most common complications.[11] This is manifested clinically by failure of the port to tolerate infusion without resistance or the failure of adequate volume return during aspiration. This complication is best evaluated radiographically. If kinking or twisting of the catheter is absent, then thrombosis is assumed. Prevention involves flushing the catheter sufficiently with heparin, adherence to sterility (as infection results in thrombosis), and adhering to proper positioning of the catheter during the initial insertion. The superior vena cava right atrial junction is ideal, and the accuracy of placement is increased when done under fluoroscopy. Intraluminal catheter thrombosis may be treated with thrombolytic agents such as tissue-type plasminogen activator (tPA) (eg, alteplase [Activase]; Genentech, Inc.; South San Francisco, California) or reteplase (Retavase; Centocor, Inc.; Malvern, Pennsylvania).[11,12] The entire lumen of the catheter is filled with approximately 2 mg of tPA diluted in the appropriate volume to fill the catheter. This is left in place for 30 to 60 minutes. Care must be taken to infuse just enough solution so that it fills only the lumen of the catheter and to prevent systemic administration of the thrombolytic agent. The procedure may result in clearing the thrombus within or around the tip of the catheter. If this fails, short infusions of tPA through the catheter, as described by Savader et al (2.5 mg over 3 hours), may be used.[13] If such an infusion is used, the patient must be appropriately monitored in the hospital, because this treatment entails exposing the patient to systemic thrombolytic therapy. After the appropriate time, the thrombolytic agent is aspirated. This can be repeated twice if needed, to establish patency. This treatment, although highly successful, has a high recurrence rate. If catheter thrombolysis fails, occluded nonimplanted catheters can often be replaced with a new catheter by using a guidewire. When placing tunneled catheters, the authors make a small cut down over the previous access site, then cut and remove the catheter over a stiff angled glidewire (Boston Scientific; Washington, DC), and finally create a new tunnel to minimize the risk of infection. However, replacement of the catheter over 1 or 2 stiff glidewires has been described and is routinely used in many centers.[14]

Fibrin Sheathing

Fibrin deposition is inevitable. It occurs regardless of the insertion technique, catheter material used, and port maintenance regime. Interestingly, although most clinicians consider "fibrin" to be the extraluminal material responsible for catheter occlusion, experimental studies have proven this material is cellular collagen tissue covered by endothelium, which migrates from the injured endoluminal wall. Physiologically it can encircle the catheter shaft and tip and eventually occlude the catheter at its tip. Clinically, fluid can be freely infused, but aspiration is halted. Treatment may involve several different maneuvers. The traditional treatment option is catheter replacement. However, the patient can be referred to interventional radiology for removing the fibrin sheath. A fibrin sheath may be managed by a transcatheter approach with nonimplanted catheters. A guidewire can be advanced through the catheter and used to create a hole in the fibrin sheath. Unfortunately, this usually results in the creation of only a small hole that can easily become re-occluded. In addition, many catheters have side holes that remain covered by the fibrin sheath. An angled guidewire can be placed through the catheter and used to clear each hole under fluoroscopy, but this procedure is cumbersome and may create small holes that are prone to reocclusion.[15] A ureteral brush can be inserted in the lumen of the catheter to release the fibrin deposits with rotating motions. A better approach is to attempt to remove the entire fibrin sheath. Usually, this is performed via a femoral venous approach. An appropriately sized loop snare, such as an Amplatz Goose Neck Snare (available in 5- to 35-mm diameters; Microvena; White Bear Lake, Minnesota), is advanced through the IVC and used to capture the catheter.[16] This snare, once placed around the catheter, is moved up around the proximal portion of the catheter. Then, the snare is tightened over the catheter and pulled back across the distal end of the catheter to dislodge the fibrin sheath.

Catheter Fracture/Migration

Catheter fractures can occur along the intravascular or extravascular portions of the catheter. Common causes include excessively vigorous exercise or hyperextension of the upper neck and body, overzealous flushing and testing of the catheter, and pinch-off. When the subcutaneous extravascular course of the catheter is between the clavicle and first rib, pinch-off syndrome may result.[17] The catheter can become occluded, and with repeated trauma, it can fracture. Fracture of a catheter may result in extravasation or other malfunction of the catheter. Complete fracture or transaction of the catheter may result in embolization of the distal fragment.[18] The catheter fragment can become lodged in the heart, resulting in cardiac arrhythmias or possible cardiac perforation, or embolization to the pulmonary artery. If recognized early, the interventional radiologist can usually capture the catheter fragments and successfully remove them. If the fragments within the central vasculature remain unrecognized, thrombus formation and fibrosis around the catheter can result in catheter attachment to the vessel wall. The risk of catheter pinch-off when inserting a subclavian catheter using anatomic landmarks can be decreased by avoiding too medial of an entry into the subclavian vein. The use of ultrasound guidance for the initial venipuncture decreases the potential for pinch-off as the venous entrance site positioned further laterally. Pinch-off syndrome can be eliminated by using the jugular venous approach. Malposition may occur as a late complication, when a previously appropriately positioned catheter/tip becomes malpositioned. Too generous of tunnel size, inadequate securing of port to fascia, and excessive Valsalva may lead to malposition of a catheter. Frequent

coughing and emesis is common in breast oncology patients. Palliation of these symptoms may help to avoid this complication. The tip of an intact catheter can migrate into the opposite brachiocephalic vein, jugular vein, or azygos veins. Interventional radiologists play an important role in repositioning misplaced catheters. With tunneled catheters that have migrated, a snare can be passed up from a femoral venous approach to redirect the catheter into the appropriate location. Occasionally, a catheter can be buckled down into the superior vena cava by advancing a guidewire through it, allowing the catheter to flip into the superior vena cava.

FUTURE DIRECTIONS

Obtaining traditional central venous access has been achieved by using surface anatomical landmarks and their palpable association with its companion artery to enter the central vein. This method may be insufficient in many breast oncology patients. Coagulopathy, postradiation fibrosis, surgical scarring, hyperdynamic circulation secondary to metastatic disease or chemotherapy induced heart failure (anthracyclines, trastuzumab), and the patient's body habitus may limit the use of surface landmarks in obtaining safe access, even in routinely used vessels such as the internal jugular and subclavian vein.[19] Hind et al[20] performed a meta-analysis reviewing the use of ultrasound for central venous catheter placement and advocated its routine use. Venous access under ultrasonographic and fluoroscopic guidance has the added advantage of significantly decreasing the rate of immediate complications, such as inadvertent arterial puncture, pneumothorax, and catheter tip malpositioning. Ultrasonographic evaluation also allows better planning of the access, and ultimately, it may decrease the procedure time.[21,22]

SUMMARY

Procedures to establish long-term venous access is in increasing demand as better systemic therapies for breast cancer are being developed. The placement of indwelling central venous catheter should be performed by a dedicated team. A complete understanding of the challenging anatomy and physiology unique to this patient population is of paramount importance in achieving central venous access in a safe, comfortable, and efficient manner. Even with the most experienced physicians, complications from the placement and presence of indwelling venous access devices do occur. However, using ultrasound guidance to obtain central venous access is an invaluable tool in reducing the early complications of this procedure. In the future, the use of 2-dimensional ultrasound guidance method may become the standard of care in breast surgical oncology patients.

REFERENCES

1. National Institute for Health and Clinical Excellence: Central Venous Catheters—Ultrasound Localizing Devices. The Clinical Effectiveness and Cost Effectiveness of Ultrasonic Locating Devices for the Placement of Central Venous Lines. Available at: http://www.nice.org.uk/guidance/TA49. Accessed September 2002.

2. Haskal ZJ, Leen VH, Thomas-Hawkins C, et al. Transvenous removal of fibrin sheaths from tunneled hemodialysis catheters. *J Vasc Interv Radiol.* 1996;7:513-517.
3. Chu FSK, Cheng VCC, Law MWM, et al. Efficacy and complications in peripherally inserted central catheter insertion: a study using 4-Fr non-valved catheters and a single infusate. *Australas Radiol.* 2007;51:453-457.
4. Rockall AG, Harris A, Whetton CW, et al. Stripping of failing hemodialysis catheters using the Ampltaz gooseneck snare. *Clin Radiol.* 1997;52:616-620.
5. Andris DA, Krzywda EA. Catheter pinch-off syndrome: recognition and management. *J Intraven Nurs.* 1997;20:233-237.
6. Coles CE, Whitear WP, Le Vay JH. Spontaneous fracture and embolization of a central venous catheter: prevention and early detection. *Clin Oncol (R Coll Radiol).* 1998;10:412-414.
7. Xiang DZ, Verbeken EK, Van Lommel ATL, et al. Composition and formation of the sleeve enveloping a central venous catheter. *J Vasc Surg.* 1998;28:260-271.
8. Gordon AC, Saliken JC, Johns D, et al. US-guided puncture of the internal jugular vein: complications and anatomic considerations. *J Vasc Interv Radiol.* 1998;9:333-338.
9. Mauro MA, Jaques PF. Radiologic placement of long-term central venous catheters: a review. *J Vasc Interv Radiol.* 1993;4:127-137.
10. Docktor BL, Sadler DJ, Gray RR, et al. Radiologic placement of tunneled central catheters. *AJR Am J Roentgenol.* 1999;173:457-460.
11. Owens CA, Yaghmai B, Warner D. Complications of central venous catheterization. *Semin Intervent Radiol.* 1998;15:341-355.
12. Denny DF Jr. Placement and management of long-term central venous access catheters and ports. *AJR Am J Roentgenol.* 1993;161:385-393.
13. Ahmad I, Ray CE Jr. Radiologic placement of venous access ports. *Semin Intervent Radiol.* 1998; 15:259-272.
14. Lokich JJ, Bothe A Jr, Benotti P, et al. Complications and management of implanted venous access catheters. *J Clin Oncol.* 1985;3:710-717.
15. Davis SN, Vermeulen L, Banton J. Activity and dosage of alteplase dilution for clearing occlusions of venous-access devices. *Am J Health Syst Pharm.* 2000;57:1039-1045.
16. Semba CP, Bakal CW, Calis KA, et al. Alteplase as an alternative to urokinase. Advisory Panel on Catheter-Directed Thrombolytic Therapy. *J Vasc Interv Radiol.* 2000;11:279-287.
17. Savader SJ, Ehrman KO, Porter DJ. Treatment of hemodialysis catheter-associated fibrin sheaths by rt-PA infusion: critical analysis of 124 procedures. *J Vasc Interv Radiol.* 2001;12:711-715.
18. Garofalo RS, Zaleski GX, Lorenze JM, et al. Exchange of poorly functioning tunneled permanent hemodialysis catheters. *AJR Am J Roentgenol.* 1999;173:155-158.
19. Wyles S, Browne G, Gui G. Pitfalls in Portacath location using the landmark technique: case report. *Int Semin Surg Oncol.* 2007;4:13.
20. Hind D, Calvert N, McWilliams R, et al. Ultrasonic locating devices for central venous cannulation: meta-analysis. *BMJ.* 2003;327:361.
21. Lyon SM, Given M, Marshall NL. Interventional radiology in the provision and maintenance of long-term central venous access. *J Med Imaging Radiat Oncol.* 2008;52:10-17.
22. Ishizuka M, Nagata H, Takagi K, Kubota K. External jugular venous catheterization with a Groshong catheter for central venous access. *J Surg Oncol.* 2008;98:67-69.

CHAPTER 72

Surgery in Patients with Stage IV Metastatic Breast Cancer

Jane E. Méndez
S. Eva Singletary
Gildy V. Babiera

Historically, women who present with stage IV metastatic breast cancer (MBC), even those with an intact primary tumor, are not offered surgical treatment. Instead, the recommended primary treatment approach is systemic therapy. However, improved breast cancer screening and imaging technology have presented a different dilemma: patients with MBC may have oligometastatic or stable metastatic disease with an operable intact primary tumor, suggesting that surgery may be effective. Furthermore, over the past 25 years, multimodality treatments for new and advanced breast cancers have resulted in improved median survival times for patients with MBC.[1] Therefore, for patients with MBC, it is time to reevaluate the role of *resection* of the intact primary tumor and the role of metastasectomy in patients without an intact primary tumor.

RESECTION OF THE INTACT PRIMARY TUMOR IN PATIENTS WITH MBC

It is generally accepted that mastectomy does not confer a survival advantage after metastases have developed.[2] Surgical treatment of intact primary tumors in patients with MBC has generally been reserved for palliation, such as treatment of bleeding, tumor ulceration, infection, or hygienic conditions. A salvage, or "toilet," mastectomy is generally performed as a last resort, with no intent for cure. However, multiple national databases and single-institution studies in the past 8 years have reexamined the role of resection of intact primary tumors for patients with MBC to clarify its role in the care of breast cancer patients (Table 72-1).[3-8]

Retrospective studies addressing the role of resection of the intact primary tumor for patients with MBC have shown an association with improved survival and metastatic disease-free survival (DFS). The best results have been observed in patients with negative surgical margins and only bone metastases.[6,8] However, in several of the studies, the data are limited on the tumor characteristics that are associated with prognosis and on the use of adjuvant therapy, such as chemotherapy, hormonal therapy, and radiation therapy. This lack of information and the confounding effects of the multimodality therapies used in breast cancer treatment make it difficult to interpret the results and discern the value of surgical intervention. Furthermore, given the retrospective nature of these studies, there is little information about the clinical criteria used in deciding which patients underwent surgery and which did not.

In order to design a clinical trial many important questions regarding surgery in patients with MBC still remain unanswered: When is the best time to resect the intact primary tumor from these patients? What are the effects of systemic chemotherapy and local radiation therapy? What is the role of axillary surgery? What criteria should be used to decide whether resection of the intact primary tumor should be performed?

Unfortunately, to date, only 1 study has addressed the question of the best time to resect the intact primary tumor in patients with MBC. Rao et al performed a retrospective review of all patients with breast cancer who were treated at the University of Texas MD Anderson Cancer Center between 1997 and 2002 and who presented with an intact primary tumor and synchronous metastatic disease.[9] A multivariate analysis revealed that patients who had only 1 site of metastasis ($p = .024$) and negative margins upon resection of the primary tumor ($p = .013$) and who were white ($p = .004$) had longer progression-free survival (PFS) times than other patients.

TABLE 72-1 Retrospective Studies on Resection of the Intact Primary Tumor in Patients with Metastatic Breast Cancer

Investigator	Study Period	Type of Study	Number of Patients Who Underwent Resection	Number of Patients Who Did Not Undergo Resection	Primary End Point	Results
Khan et al[3]	2002	NCDB	6861	9162	Time to death	No surgery: NA Surgery with negative margins: HR = 0.61, $p < .0137$ Surgery with positive margins: HR = 0.75, $p < .1035$
Rapiti et al[4]	2006	Geneva Cancer Registry	127	173	5-year breast cancer–specific survival	No surgery: NA Surgery with negative margins: HR = 0.6, $p = .5$ Surgery with positive margins: HR = 1.3.
Babiera et al[5]	2006	Single institution	82	142	1. Overall survival 2. Metastatic PFS	No surgery: NA Surgery: PFS, HR = 0.54, $p < .007$ OS: HR = 0.5, $p < .12$
Fields et al[6]	2007	Single institution	187	222	Overall survival	No surgery: NA Surgery: HR = 0.53, $p < .0001$ Median survival = surgery 31.9 months vs no surgery 15.4 months
Gnerlich et al[7]	2007	SEER program data	4578	5156	Overall survival	Median survival = surgery 36 months vs no surgery 21 months, $p < .001$
Blanchard et al[8]	2008	Single institution	242	153	Overall survival	Median survival = surgery 27.1 months vs no surgery 16.8 months, $p < .0001$

HR, hazard ratio; NA, not applicable; NCDB, National Cancer Data Base; OS, overall survival; PFS, progression-free survival; SEER, Surveillance, Epidemiology, and End Results.

Interestingly, further analysis revealed that non-Caucasian patients more often underwent resection for palliative indications than for curative intent, which could explain these patients' worse outcomes. Patients who underwent surgery 3.0 to 8.9 months or later after diagnosis had longer metastatic PFS. Rao et al concluded that surgical extirpation of the primary tumor in patients with MBC was associated with longer metastatic PFS when performed more than 3 months after diagnosis. However, it was not clear whether the longer metastatic PFS resulted from the surgery or was a reflection of the added benefit of systemic chemotherapy.

Because of the limitations associated with retrospective studies, and the fact that these are the only types of studies that have been performed to determine the value of resection of an intact primary tumor in patients with MBC, the most important question still remains unanswered: Does resection of an intact primary breast tumor really improve survival in patients with MBC?[10] Or do these results reflect a selection bias? To conclusively answer this question, a prospective, randomized clinical trial needs to be conducted. Fortunately, 2 prospective trials on local therapy in patients with MBC have already been initiated outside of the United States.[11] One trial started in February 2005 in India (NCT00193778), and the second trial started in November 2007 in Turkey (NCT00557986). The trial in India is being conducted at the Tata Memorial Hospital and is randomizing patients who responded to 6 cycles of chemotherapy into 2 groups: surgery and no surgery. The Turkish trial is randomizing patients to surgery or no surgery before receiving any systemic therapy. In the meantime, until data are available from these prospective trials, surgery may be considered for select stage IV patients with oligometastatic or stable metastatic disease with an operable intact primary tumor.

METASTASECTOMY IN THE TREATMENT OF SELECTED PATIENTS WITH MBC

Breast cancer most commonly metastasizes to bone, followed by the lungs, brain, and liver.[12] Up until now, the treatment focus for MBC has been on palliative care rather than cure. However, a more aggressive and potentially curative treatment approach may be adequate for patients with MBC limited to a solitary metastasis or to multiple metastases at a single organ site.[13] In selected patients with MBC with a controlled primary tumor (typically those treated previously), a long disease-free period, and good performance status, resection of the distant metastatic sites (metastasectomy) might be a viable option. The main goal of metastasectomy would be improved quality of life and prolonged DFS in these patients, although, as noted, cure may also be possible.

BONE METASTASIS

The most common first site of breast cancer metastases is bone. Patients with only bone metastases have been reported to have a more favorable prognosis and a more "indolent" course[14] than patients with bone metastases and additional visceral metastases. In addition, patients with solitary bone metastases have a 59% chance of being alive after 5 years.[15,16] Bone metastases have been reported to occur more frequently in certain types of breast cancers. Recent data have shown that luminal A breast cancers are more likely to metastasize to bone than basal-type cancers.[17]

Treating bone metastases is crucial, as bone metastases may result in considerable skeletal-related morbidity from bone pain, fractures, spinal cord compression, or hypercalcemia. In weight-bearing bones, bone metastases can lead to problems of mobility. In addition, spinal cord compression can occur and can be an acute life-threatening complication.[13] Usually, the first treatment option for bone metastases on bones that are not at risk of fracturing is either endocrine- or chemotherapy-based systemic therapy. The incidence of bone metastases is increasing as patients with breast cancer are living longer.[18]

Surgery is most frequently used for treating long bone metastases and femoral fractures.[19] The goals of relieving pain and restoring mobility may be accomplished by a variety of surgical techniques. Prophylactic surgical fixation for lytic lesions has been recommended for lesions of the cortex that are larger than 2.5 cm in size, lesions involving more than 50% of the bone diameter, or lesions that are painful despite prior radiation therapy. In addition, Weber et al advocates using adjuvant radiation therapy for all patients with surgically treated bone metastases.[18] For these patients, the standard radiation dose used is 30 Gy, with few side effects seen.[20] Postoperative radiation therapy should start 10 to 14 days after surgery to allow wound healing. Epidural spinal cord compression is an oncologic emergency often heralded by increasing pain in a patient with known vertebral metastases. Early diagnosis is the key to maintaining neurologic function because once neurologic deficiencies are present, surgery is rarely performed and functional improvement is unlikely.[21]

Sternal bone metastases should be considered to be in a different category than vertebral bone metastases. Since the sternum lacks communication with the paravertebral venous plexus, through which cancer cells spread easily to other bones, sternal metastases seem to remain solitary for a longer time.[22] Noguchi et al studied 9 patients with solitary sternal metastases from breast carcinoma who were treated aggressively with partial or total resection of the sternum. The median survival time in all 9 patients was 30 months. The prognosis of the patients who also had mediastinal or parasternal lymph node metastases was poor, and all of these patients died because of a second relapse within 30 months. The prognosis of patients without mediastinal or parasternal lymph node metastasis was quite favorable (3 of them survived more than 6 years). From their study, they concluded that sternectomy should be indicated for the solitary sternal metastasis when no evidence of systemic spread is noted since it can improve the quality of life and occasionally may result in long-term survival. In addition, improvements in surgical techniques, especially by means of myocutaneous flaps and prosthetic materials, have resulted in safe, successful sternectomies and simultaneous reconstructions.[23]

PULMONARY METASTASIS

Isolated pulmonary metastases have been reported to occur in 10% to 20% of all women with breast cancer.[24] Approximately 3% of all women with breast cancer develop a solitary pulmonary lesion detectable by chest radiography, of which 33% to 40% will be breast cancer metastases.[25,26] Considering the low morbidity and mortality rates associated with pulmonary metastasectomy, it can be considered in selected patients with pulmonary metastases from breast cancer.

Friedel et al identified 467 patients with pulmonary metastases from breast cancer from the International Registry of Lung Metastasis and evaluated the long-term survival and prognostic factors in these patients.[27] In 84% of the patients, a complete resection was possible, with 5-, 10-, and 15-year survival rates of 38%, 22%, and 20%, respectively. The positive prognostic factors were a disease-free interval of more than 36 months, with 5-, 10-, and 15-year survival rates of 45%, 26%, and 21%, respectively. Solitary pulmonary metastases were associated with a survival rate of 44% after 5 years and 23% after both 10 and 15 years, but this was not statistically different when compared with the outcomes associated with completely resected multiple pulmonary metastases. In addition, there were no significant differences in outcome between the types of resection performed (wedge or segmental resection, lobectomy, or pneumonectomy) in patients who underwent a complete resection.

For patients with breast cancer and pulmonary metastases, the prognostic factors statistically associated with longer survival include the number of metastases, a disease-free interval of more than 12 months, and complete resection of all disease.[28,29] Yoshimoto et al[30] showed that resecting pulmonary metastases may prolong the survival times in certain subgroups of patients to a greater extent than administering systemic therapy alone. Furthermore, the survival times were significantly longer for patients who initially presented with clinical stage I disease at the time of surgery than for those with stage II to IV disease.[30]

As part of the metastatic workup, it is important to differentiate between a metastatic pulmonary lesion and primary lung cancer. Early histologic identification of the tumor is critical for appropriate treatment strategies to be implemented as proper aggressive evaluation can affect what type of treatment the patient receives and impact the patients' survival times.[31] Rena et al studied the role of surgery, including video-assisted thoracoscopic surgery, in the diagnosis and treatment of a solitary pulmonary nodule in patients who had undergone previous surgery for breast cancer.[32] The histology of the solitary pulmonary nodules was primary lung cancer in 38 patients, pulmonary breast cancer metastasis in 27 patients, and a benign entity in 14 patients. Rena et al concluded that video-assisted thoracoscopic surgery is a good procedure for the diagnostic management and pathologic confirmation of peripheral solitary pulmonary nodules to determine the appropriate surgical treatment.

HEPATIC METASTASIS

The liver is an uncommon site for solitary first metastasis in breast cancer, with only 3% to 9% of patients affected. However, breast cancer hepatic metastases are found in 55% to 75% of autopsies performed on patients who died of breast cancer,[33] suggesting that they ultimately form in most patients with advanced disease. In fact, Cutler et al found that hepatic metastases usually occur at later stages of disseminated disease and carry a very poor prognosis, with a median survival of 6 months.[34] Even with systemic chemotherapy, the median survival time is approximately 19 months for patients with MBC to the liver only or with limited disease elsewhere.[35] Hormonal therapy is generally of limited use because most hepatic metastases are hormone receptor negative. At this point, surgery has been proposed as a potential therapeutic tool for patients with isolated hepatic metastasis.[13]

In one study, Vlastos et al studied the long-term survival of 31 patients with breast cancer with metastases limited to the liver who underwent hepatic resection at MD Anderson Cancer Center.[36] The hepatic metastases had developed after a median of 22 months from initial diagnosis. Solitary hepatic metastases were found in 20 patients, and multiple hepatic metastases were found in 11 patients. Major hepatic resections (3 or more segments resected) were performed in 14 patients, and minor resections (less than 3 segments resected) with or without radiofrequency ablation were performed in 17 patients. The median size of the largest hepatic metastasis was 2.9 cm. A total of 87% of the patients received either pre- or postoperative systemic therapy, with a median survival of 63 months. The overall 2- and 5-year survival rates were 86% and 61%, respectively, while the 2- and 5-year DFS rates were 39% and 31%, respectively. Vlastos et al were unable to identify any treatment- or patient-specific variables associated with the survival rates. They concluded from their results that in selected patients with hepatic metastases from breast cancer, an aggressive surgical approach was associated with a favorable long-term survival and that hepatic resection should be considered as a component of the multimodality treatment of breast cancer in these patients.

In another study, Adam et al offered hepatic resection to all patients with hepatic metastases provided that curative resection was feasible and extrahepatic disease was controlled with medical and/or surgical therapy.[37] The outcomes of 85 consecutive patients with hepatic metastases treated from 1984 to 2004 were reviewed. Solitary hepatic metastases were found in 38% of the patients, and multiple (more than 3) hepatic metastases were found in 31%. Of note, extrahepatic metastases had been treated prior to hepatic resection or were synchronously present in 27 (32%) patients. After a median follow-up of 38 months, the median survival time was 32 months and the 5-year survival rate was 37%, and the median DFS time was 20 months and the 5-year DFS rate was 21%. The variables associated with a poor survival were failure to respond to preoperative chemotherapy, an R2 resection, and the absence of a repeat hepatectomy. Patients who underwent a repeat hepatectomy had a higher 5-year overall survival rate (81%) than patients with unresectable hepatic recurrences and patients with fulminant extrahepatic metastatic disease. In addition, Adam et al determined that the disease-free interval was not an independent prognostic factor. Of note, the median survival times were longer in the group of patients treated from 1994 to 2004 than in those treated from 1983 to 1993. These longer survival times might reflect the effects of improved diagnostic technology, surgical techniques, and the use of systemic therapy. Adam et al concluded that favorable outcomes were achievable even in patients with controlled extrahepatic disease, indicating that surgery should be considered more frequently in the multidisciplinary care of patients with hepatic metastases.

However, patient selection and operative criteria for hepatic resection are still controversial. The important criteria seem to be that patients have less than 4 hepatic metastases, no extrahepatic disease, and demonstrated disease regression or stability with systemic therapy before resection.[37] At a minimum, a patient should have a normal performance status and normal hepatic function tests.[13] Pocard and Selzner agreed that the size and number of hepatic metastases was an important factor.[38] Patients in whom hepatic metastases were found more than 1 year after resection of the primary cancer had significantly better outcomes than those with early (less than 1 year after resection of the primary cancer) metastatic disease. The type of hepatic resection, the lymph node status at the time of the primary cancer resection, and the use of neoadjuvant high-dose chemotherapy had no significant impact on patient survival in this study.[38] Furthermore, Martinez et al showed that survival was longer in patients with an estrogen receptor–positive primary tumor and hepatic metastases, HER-2/neu-positive hepatic metastases, 2 or fewer hepatic metastases, and age more than 50 years at the time of metastasectomy.[39]

In terms of when to perform a hepatic resection, the preference is for patients to receive chemotherapy prior to undergoing hepatic resection.[36] In addition, before considering hepatic resection, an extensive preoperative staging evaluation is recommended. For example, diagnostic laparoscopy is recommended to avoid a nontherapeutic laparotomy if extrahepatic disease based on preoperative imaging is suggested. In addition, the use of intraoperative ultrasonography has become very useful in assessing resectability. Hepatic resection is preferable if metastases can be safely removed with a negative surgical margin. Radiofrequency ablation should be reserved for those patients with tumors not amenable to a safe resection or used as an adjunct to resection.[37]

BRAIN METASTASIS

Multiple and solitary brain metastases are diagnosed in 10% to 20% of patients with MBC.[40-43] Parenchymal brain lesions from breast carcinoma are usually diagnosed in end-stage metastatic disease, but they may also appear as the first instance of relapse. For example, breast cancer is the most common solid tumor to metastasize to the leptomeninges.[44] However, solitary brain metastases are uncommon. Historically, the mean 1-year survival rate of patients with brain metastases has been only 20%,[45] and most patients with brain metastases die as a result of uncontrolled progression of extracerebral systemic disease.[46]

There is a growing body of evidence suggesting that the incidence of central nervous system metastases is increasing in patients with breast cancer.[47] This is most likely due to the improved antitumor effects of newer chemotherapy regimens and targeted therapies for nonbrain metastases that do not cross the blood-brain barrier, allowing subsequent development of brain metastases. The most widely accepted risk factors for the development of brain metastases are young patient age and estrogen receptor–negative primary tumors. While young patients develop aggressive disease, the tropism of the brain suggests that inherent biological differences might be operative.[44,48] Metastasis to other sites, such as liver, lungs, or bone, also strongly predicted the development of brain metastasis. Finally, HER-2/neu overexpression was recognized to be a potential risk factor in 2 studies.[44,47]

Chemotherapy is of limited use in the treatment of most brain metastases, which may be due to, in part, the limitations of drug delivery imposed by the blood-brain barrier. Radiation therapy, especially whole-brain radiation therapy (WBRT), is a mainstay, especially for patients with multiple (more than 3) lesions. For patients with fewer lesions, resection followed by WBRT has been shown to extend survival and to minimize neurological debility and death.[44] Resection is useful in cases where few lesions are present, their location is favorable for resection, and a rapid amelioration of the symptoms is needed.[49] In properly selected patients with brain metastases, stereotactic-guided radiosurgery (eg, Gamma Knife surgery) with WBRT confers a survival advantage over WBRT alone. Stereotactic-guided radiosurgery is recommended for lesions 3 cm or smaller in diameter. In addition, stereotactic-guided radiosurgery is the treatment of choice for lesions that are located in the deep cortical structures and cerebellar nuclei and cannot be safely resected.[50] WBRT is commonly recommended after the complete resection of brain metastases to help eradicate undiagnosed micrometastases.

Wrónski et al analyzed their experience with resection of brain metastases from patients with breast carcinoma (N = 70) at Memorial Sloan-Kettering Cancer Center.[50] The 1-, 2-, 3-, and 5-year survival rates were 55.3%, 25.7%, 18.6%, and 7.0%, respectively. Meningeal carcinomatosis was diagnosed in 16 patients, whose median survival time was significantly shorter than that of patients without meningeal carcinomatosis. Patients with a positive hormone receptor status had significantly longer survival times after craniotomy than patients with a negative hormone receptor status (21.9 months vs 12.5 months). A trend toward longer survival times was noted for patients aged 50 years or less and for patients with lesions 3 cm or smaller in diameter. Interestingly, there was no difference in survival between the patients with multiple brain metastases and those with a single lesion. Furthermore, patients who underwent external WBRT had longer survival times than patients who did not undergo WBRT. Based on their results, Wrónski et al recommended that patients with solitary brain metastases or 2 or 3 accessible metastases from breast cancer be considered for focal treatment, such as resection or stereotactic-guided radiosurgery followed by WBRT.

In another study, Lee et al retrospectively analyzed the overall survival times of 198 breast cancer patients with brain metastases.[51] In this study, 7 (3.6%) patients underwent resection of solitary brain metastases, 22 (11%) patients underwent Gamma Knife surgery, 3 (1.5%) patients underwent intrathecal chemotherapy, and 9 (4.6%) patients received no treatment. The median overall survival time was 5.6 months for all of the patients, and 23.1% of the patients survived for more than 1 year. The median overall survival time was 5.4 months for patients treated with WBRT, 14.9 months for patients treated with surgery or Gamma Knife surgery only, and 2.1 months for patients who received no treatment ($p < .001$). The performance status, number of brain metastases, and treatment modalities and whether patients underwent systemic chemotherapy after the development of brain metastases were significantly associated with survival. Lee et al concluded that patients with a solitary brain metastases and good performance status should undergo aggressive treatment. In addition, the characteristics of the primary breast tumor did not affect survival after brain metastasis.

SUMMARY

Over the years, breast cancer treatment has improved, resulting in increased median DFS times for patients with MBC.[1] In selected patients with an intact primary tumor and solitary metastases or multiple lesions at a single organ site, the existing data support the idea that surgery with the intent of improving outcome should be considered. However, randomized, prospective clinical trials are still lacking, and until these are performed, surgery for this group of patients will remain controversial. Finally, selected patients who present with stage IV disease after resection of the intact primary tumor may be considered for resection of the distant metastasis with the hopes of lengthening DFS times. Unfortunately, because of the relatively rare presentation of this clinical situation, randomized, prospective trials will most likely never be performed. Thus, it would be beneficial for national cancer registries to track these patients and their outcomes.

REFERENCES

1. Giordano SH, Buzdar AU, Smith TL, et al. Is breast cancer survival improving? *Cancer*. 2004;100(1):44-52.
2. Lang JE, Babiera GV. Locoregional resection in stage IV breast cancer: Tumor biology, molecular and clinical perspectives. *Surg Clin N Am*. 2007;87(2):527-538.

3. Khan UA, Stewart AK, Morrow M. Does aggressive local therapy improve survival in metastatic breast cancer? *Surgery*. 2002;132(4):620-626.

4. Rapiti E, Verkooijen HM, Vlastos G, et al. Complete excision of primary breast tumor improves survival of patients with metastatic breast cancer at diagnosis. *J Clin Oncol*. 2006;24(18):2743-2749.

5. Babiera GV, Rao R, Feng L, et al. Effect of primary tumor extirpation in breast cancer patients who present with stage IV disease and an intact primary. *Ann Surg Oncol*. 2006;13(6):776-782.

6. Fields RC, Jeffe D, Trinkaus K, et al. Surgical resection of the primary tumor is associated with increased long-term survival in patients with stage IV breast cancer after controlling for site of metastasis. *Ann Surg Oncol*. 2007;14(12):3345-3351.

7. Gnerlich J, Jeffe DB, Deshpande AD, et al. Surgical removal of the primary tumor increases overall survival in patients with metastatic breast cancer: analysis of the 1988–2003 SEER data. *Ann Surg Oncol*. 2007;14(8):2187-2194.

8. Blanchard DK, Shetty PB, Hilsebeck SG, Elledge RM. Association of surgery with improved survival in stage IV breast cancer patients. *Ann Surg Oncol*. 2008;247(5):732-738.

9. Rao R, Feng L, Kuerer HM, et al. Timing of surgical intervention for the intact primary in stage IV breast cancer patients. *Ann Surg Oncol*. 2008;15(6):1696-1702.

10. Khan SA. Does resection of an intact breast primary improve survival in metastatic breast cancer? *Oncology*. 2007;21(8):924-931.

11. Fitzal F. Local therapy in stage IV breast cancer patients. *Ann Surg Oncol*. 2008;15(9):2618.

12. Patanaphan V, Salazar OM, Risco R. Breast cancer: metastatic patterns and their prognosis. *South Med J*. 1988;81(9):1109-1112.

13. Singletary SE, Walsh G, Vaurhey JN, et al. A role for curative surgery in the treatment of selected patients with metastatic breast cancer. *Oncologist*. 2003;8(3):241-251.

14. Sherry MM, Greco FA, Johnson DH, et al. Metastatic breast cancer confined to the skeletal system: an indolent disease. *Am J Med*. 1986;81:381-385.

15. Dürr HR, Müller PE, Lenz T, et al. Surgical bone metastases in patients with breast cancer. *Clin Orthop Relat Res*. 2002;396:191-196.

16. Coleman RE, Rubens RD. The clinical course of bone metastses from breast cancer. *Br J Cancer*. 1987;55:61-66.

17. Smid M, Wang Y, Zhang Y, et al. Subtypes of breast cancer show preferential site of relapse. *Cancer Res*. 2008;68(9):3108-3114.

18. Weber KL, Randall RL, Grossman S, et al. Management of lower-extremity bone metastasis. *J Bone Joint Surg Am*. 2006;88A(suppl 4):11-19.

19. Beals RK, Lawton GD, Snell W. Prophylactic internal fixation of secondary neoplastic deposits in long bones. *Cancer*. 1971;28:1350-1354.

20. Rose CM, Kagan AR. The final report of the expert panel for radiation oncology bone metastasis work group of the American College of Radiology. *Int J Radiat Oncol Biol Phys*. 1998;40:1117-1124.

21. Sorensen PS, Borgesen SE, Rohde K, et al. Metastatic spinal cord compression: results of treatment and survival. *Cancer*. 1990;65:1502-1508.

22. Noguchi S, Miyauchi K, Nishizawa Y, et al. Results of surgical treatment for sternal metastasis of breast cancer. *Cancer*. 1988;62:1397-1401.

23. Incarbone M, Nava M, Lequaglie C, et al. Sternal resection for primary or secondary tumors. *J Thorac Cardiovasc Surg*. 1997;114(1):93-99.

24. Planchard D, Soria JC, Michiels S, et al. Uncertain benefit from surgery in patients with lung metastases from breast carcinoma. *Cancer*. 2004;100(1):28-35.

25. Casey JJ, Stempel BG, Scanlon EF, et al. The solitary pulmonary nodule in the patient with breast cancer. *Surgery*. 1994;96(4):801-805.

26. McDonald M, Deschamps C, Ilstrup DM, et al. Pulmonary resection for metastatic breast cancer. *Ann Thorac Surg*. 1994;58:1599-1602.

27. Friedel G, Pastorino U, Ginsberg RJ, et al. Results of lung metastasectomy from breast cancer: prognostic criteria on the basis of 467 cases of the international registry of lung metastases. *Eur J Cardiothorac Surg*. 2002;22:335-344.

28. Lanza LA, Natarajan G, Roth GA, et al. Long-term survival after resection of pulmonary metastases from carcinoma of the breast. *Ann Thorac Surg*. 1992;54(2):244-247.

29. Staren ES, Salermo C, Rongione A, et al. Pulmonary resection for metastatic breast cancer. *Arch Surg*. 1992;127:1282-1284.

30. Yoshimoto M, Tada K, Nishimura S, et al. Favourable long-term results after surgical removal of lung metastases of breast cancer. *Breast Cancer Res Treat*. 2008;110:485-491.

31. Chang EY, Johnson W, Karamlou K, et al. The evaluation and treatment implications of isolated pulmonary nodules in patients with a recent history of breast cancer. *Am J Surg*. 2006;191(5):641-645.

32. Rena O, Papalia E, Ruffini E, et al. The role of surgery in the management of solitary pulmonary nodule in breast cancer patients. *Eur J Surg Oncol*. 2007;33(5):546-550.

33. Schneebaum S, Walker MJ, Young D, et al. The regional treatment of liver metastases from breast cancer. *J Surg Oncol*. 1994;55:26-32.

34. Cutler SJ, Asire AJ, Taylor SG. Classification of patients with disseminated cancer of the breast. *Cancer*. 1969;24:861-869.

35. Atalay G, Biganzoli L, Renard F, et al. Clinical outcome of breast cancer patients with liver metastases in the anthracycline-taxane era. *Breast Cancer Res Treat*. 2002;76(suppl 1):S47.

36. Vlastos G, Smith D, Singletary E, et al. Long-term survival after an aggressive surgical approach in patients with breast cancer hepatic metastases. *Ann Surg Oncol*. 2004;11(9):869-874.

37. Adam R, Aloia T, Bralet MP, et al. Is liver resection justified for patients with hepatic metastases from breast cancer? *Ann Surg*. 2006;244(6):897-907.

38. Selzner M, Morse MA, Myers WC, et al. Liver metastases from breast cancer: long-term survival after curative resection. *Surgery*. 2000;127(4):383-389.

39. Martinez SR, Young SE, Giuliano AE, et al. The utility of estrogen receptor, progesterone receptor, and HER2/neu status in predicting survival in patients undergoing hepatic resection for breast cancer metastases. *Am J Surg*. 2006;191(2):281-283.

40. Pieper DR, Hess KR, Sawaya RE. Role of surgery in the treatment of brain metastases in patients with breast cancer. *Ann Surg Oncol*. 1997;4(6):481-490.

41. Boogerd W, Hart AAM, Tjahja IS. Treatment and outcome of brain metastasis as first site of distant metastasis from breast cancer. *J Neurooncol*. 1997;35:161-167.

42. Fernandez-Vicioso E, Suh JH, Kupelian PA, et al. Analysis of prognostic factors for patients with single brain metastases treated with stereotactic surgery. *Radiat Oncol Invest*. 1997;5:31-37.

43. DiStefanoA, Yap HY, Hortobagyi GN, et al. The natural history of breast cancer patients with brain metastases. *Cancer*. 1979;44:19134-19138.

44. Palmieri D, Smith QR, Lockman PR, et al. Brain metastases of breast cancer. *Breast Dis*. 2006–2007;26:139-147.

45. Evans A, James J, Comford E, et al. Brain metastases from breast cancer: identification of a high risk group. *Clin Oncol*. 2004;16:345-349.

46. Šimonová G, Lišák R, Novotny J, et al. Solitary brain metastases treated with the Leksell gamma knife: prognostic factors for patients. *Radiother Oncol*. 2000;57:207-213.

47. Altundag K, Bondy ML, Mirza NQ, et al. Clinicopathologic characteristics and prognostic factors in 420 metastatic breast cancer patients with central nervous system metastases. *Cancer*. 2007;110(12):2640-2647.

48. Crivellari D, Pagani O, Veronesi A, et al. International Breast Cancer Study Group. High incidence of central nervous system involvement in patients with metastatic or locally advanced breast cancer treated with epirubicin and docetaxel. *Ann Oncol*. 2001;12:353-356.

49. Patchell R, Tibbs P, Walsh J, et al. A randomized trial of surgery in the treatment of single metastases to the brain. *N Engl J Med*. 1990;322:494-500.

50. Wrónski M, Arbit E, McCormick B. Surgical treatment of 70 patients with brain metastases from breast carcinoma. *Cancer*. 1997;80(9):1746-1754.

51. Lee SS, Ahn JH, Kim MK, et al. Brain metastases in breast cancer: prognostic factors and management. *Breast Cancer Res Treat*. 2008;111:523-530.

SECTION 6
PLASTIC AND BREAST RECONSTRUCTION

Steven J. Kronowitz

CHAPTER 73

The Epidemiology of Breast Reconstruction in North America

Amy K. Alderman
Rachel Streu
Edwin G. Wilkins

After years of lobbying by women's health advocates and amidst much fanfare, the 1998 Federal Breast Cancer Reconstruction Law (also referred to as the Women's Health and Cancer Rights Act of 1998, or WHCRA) was signed into law by President Bill Clinton.[1] Passage of this legislation marked the culmination of intensive lobbying efforts by breast cancer survivors, clinicians, researchers, and policymakers to ensure coverage of breast reconstruction following mastectomy by health care payers. In the 2 decades prior to the passage of the WHCRA, a growing body of research demonstrated significant psychosocial and quality-of-life benefits for those receiving breast reconstruction.[2-4] Largely as a consequence of these studies, provider and patient perceptions evolved away from viewing breast reconstruction as a "cosmetic" procedure. Instead, health care professionals and consumers concluded that the creation of a new breast following mastectomy was a reconstructive operation and, for many women, an important element in breast cancer recovery. Despite changing attitudes, some health care payers had failed to include breast reconstruction among their covered benefits, steadfastly maintaining that these operations were cosmetic in nature. With enactment of the WHCRA, this barrier was removed. The law mandated that health plans include breast and nipple reconstruction as well as contralateral breast symmetry procedures among their benefits afforded to mastectomy patients.

The WHCRA was a significant milestone in several respects. It was a tangible sign that breast cancer had become a prominent issue in health care policy and that breast cancer advocacy had evolved into a potent lobbying force on the national political scene. The new law also signaled that breast reconstruction had become widely recognized as an important element in breast cancer treatment and rehabilitation. Finally, the WHCRA demonstrated the power of consumers to impact health care policy on a national level.

Currently, the WHCRA has been the law of the land for 10 years. The following is a discussion of the effects of this federal mandate, along with other factors, on breast reconstruction practice patterns.

WHAT DO WE KNOW ABOUT BREAST RECONSTRUCTION RATES IN THE UNITED STATES?

Measuring the current rate of breast reconstruction may seem like a straightforward proposition. In fact, determining recent rates of postmastectomy reconstruction in the United States presents a daunting challenge, largely due to the fragmented nature of clinical databases in this country. While many other developed countries have nationalized health care systems with comprehensive patient databases, the US system, with its hodgepodge of public and private payers, does not currently possess a single data clearinghouse for the entire patient population. Researchers seeking to evaluate national trends for health care utilization are forced to rely on databases that include only segments of the treatment population. Thus, the generalizability of the results of these studies is severely limited. For example, the Medicare database contains a nationwide sample of patients, but is largely restricted to those over 65 years of age. Since breast reconstruction is relatively uncommon in the elderly, using Medicare data to study reconstruction rates for the general population would not be appropriate. Medicaid databases are similarly flawed, as they are mainly limited to patients within a narrow socioeconomic spectrum.

Our best estimates for the utilization of breast reconstruction have been obtained through analyses of the Surveillance, Epidemiology and End Results (SEER) database, which was created by the National Cancer Institute.[5] The SEER program is currently the most comprehensive source for national cancer incidence and outcome data in the United States. Although the program covers only 26.2% of the US population,[6] the 18 regional registries that contribute data provide a fairly representative sample of the nation as a whole (Fig. 73-1). Inclusion of diverse socioeconomic, geographic, ethnic, and age groups greatly enhances the generalizability of the sample to the general US population.[7]

To date, most published studies on breast reconstruction utilization have relied upon the SEER program. While the SEER database mainly includes patient-specific information on breast cancer staging, treatment, and outcomes, the registry also records basic details on mastectomy reconstruction. The database tracks reconstructions performed at the time of mastectomy (immediate procedures) or within 4 months following mastectomy (early delayed procedures).[8] Delayed reconstructions carried out later than 4 months after mastectomy are not recorded, a deficiency that constitutes the database's premier limitation in analyzing breast reconstruction rates. However, information identifying the types of reconstruction performed (eg, implant versus autogenous tissue) is included.

Two published reports have used the SEER program to analyze rates of breast reconstruction. The first study, published in 2000 by Polednak, analyzed SEER data from 1988 through 1995, and demonstrated overall rates for mastectomy patients receiving reconstruction to rise from 4.3% in 1988 to 10.8% in 1995. Polednak also examined regional and socioeconomic variations in these rates. Geographic region was a statistically significant predictor for breast reconstruction in all age categories. Over the entire study period, the registry with the largest proportion of women undergoing reconstruction was Atlanta (16.0%), while the lowest was Hawaii (3.3%). Income level also had a significant effect on reconstruction rates, with the 2 lowest income quintiles having less likelihood of receiving reconstruction.

In a more recent study (2003), our group evaluated patients from the 1998 SEER database.[9] Within the immediate to early delayed period, the overall reconstruction rate for the 10,406 women with mastectomy was 15.4%. Among all reconstructions, 41.8% used autogenous tissue (muscle flaps), 24.0% were tissue expander/implant, and 11.5% utilized combined flap/implant procedures. Several sociodemographic variables were found to be significantly associated with the use of breast reconstruction (Table 73-1). Compared with women ages 45 to 54 years, those 35 to 44 years were significantly more likely to receive reconstruction (odds ratio [OR] = 1.52, $p < 0.001$). Those 55 to 64, 65 to 74, and 75 years and older were significantly less likely to undergo reconstruction (OR = 0.42, $p < 0.001$; OR = 0.16, $p < 0.001$; and OR = 0.29, $p < 0.001$, respectively). In addition to patient age, ethnicity also had a

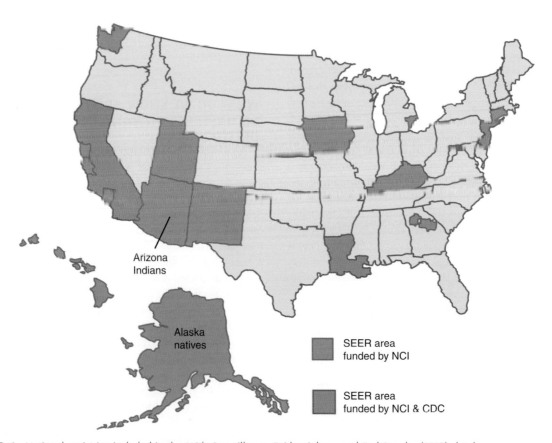

FIGURE 73-1 National registries included in the NCI's Surveillance, Epidemiology, and End Results (SEER) database.

TABLE 73-1 Multivariate Analysis of Predictors of Immediate and Early Delayed Breast Reconstruction in the 1998 SEER[a] Population (N = 10,404)

Independent Variables	Adjusted OR[b]	95% CI	p Value
Age (years)			
< 35	1.24	0.86, 1.79	0.246
35-44	1.52	1.28, 1.80	< 0.001
45-54[d]	—	—	
55-64	0.42	0.35, 0.49	< 0.001
65-74	0.16	0.13, 0.19	< 0.001
> 75	0.04	0.03, 0.06	< 0.001
Race			
African American	0.51	0.40, 0.65	< 0.001
Hispanic	0.47	0.36, 0.62	< 0.001
Asian/other	0.30	0.23, 0.40	< 0.001
Caucasian[d]	—	—	
Marital status[c]	0.91	0.80, 1.04	0.18
Registry			
San Francisco[d]	—	—	
Connecticut	0.37	0.28, 0.51	< 0.001
Metro Detroit	1.36	1.08, 1.71	0.009
Hawaii	0.56	0.34, 0.91	0.020
Iowa	0.47	0.36, 0.62	< 0.001
New Mexico	0.76	0.53, 1.09	0.134
Seattle (Puget Sound)	0.77	0.15, 0.77	< 0.001
Utah	0.75	0.54, 1.04	0.087
Metro Atlanta	2.49	1.90, 3.27	< 0.001
San Jose-Monterey	1.05	0.80, 1.39	0.713
Los Angeles	0.84	0.66, 1.05	0.125
Stage of disease			
In situ	2.44	2.03, 2.94	< 0.001
Stage I	1.25	1.07, 1.45	0.005
Stage II[d]	—	—	
Stage III	0.63	0.49, 0.83	0.001
Stage IV	0.61	0.37, 1.01	0.056
Adjuvant radiotherapy[e]	0.71	0.58, 0.86	0.001

[a]SEER; Surveillance, Epidimiology, and End Results database.
[b]Odds ratio.
[c]Married patients comprise the reference group.
[d]Reference group.
[e]Patients who received radiotherapy comprised the reference group.

significant effect on the likelihood of postmastectomy reconstruction in the SEER population. Compared with Caucasian women, African American, Hispanic, and Asian-American women were significantly less likely to receive breast reconstruction (OR = 0.48, p < 0.001; OR = 0.45, p < 0.001; and OR = 0.29, p < 0.001, respectively).[9]

Our analysis also found large regional variation in rates of postmastectomy breast reconstruction (Table 73-2).[9] While the Atlanta registry reported the highest rate (33.6%), Hawaii recorded the lowest (7.6%). Thus, the proportion of mastectomy patients receiving reconstruction showed a 4-fold variation

among the regions. Controlling for potential confounding variables (patient age, race, disease stage, marital status, and use of adjuvant radiotherapy), regression analysis found that 6 of 10 regions had significantly different rates of reconstruction compared with the reference rate (San Francisco) (Table 73-1). Choice of procedure type also showed considerable regional variation; for example, 83.2% of reconstructions in Atlanta used autogenous tissue, compared with 53.5% in San Jose-Monterey and 53.5% in Iowa (Table 73-2).

Evidence of low utilization of breast reconstruction also was reported by Polednak in a statewide study using the Connecticut

TABLE 73-2 Patterns of Use of Breast Reconstruction Across SEER Registries in 1998 (N = 1243)

SEER Registry	Immediate & Early Delayed Reconstruction (%)[a]	Autogenous Tissue Reconstruction (%)	Total
Metro Atlanta	33.6	82.3	643
Metro Detroit	22.9	69.9	1332
San Jose-Monterey	17.2	53.5	727
Utah	17.1	73.7	461
San Francisco	16.7	69.5	1226
New Mexico	14.4	65.4	446
Los Angeles	13.6	65.0	2024
Seattle (Puget Sound)	11.6	83.6	907
Connecticut	9.2	70.5	963
Iowa	8.8	53.7	1310
Hawaii	7.6	66.7	367

[a]Reconstruction at the time of the mastectomy or within 4 months of the mastectomy. The rate is calculated by dividing the number of patients who underwent reconstruction by the total number of mastectomy-treated breast cancer patients in that registry.

Office of Health Care Access and Connecticut Tumor Registry databases.[10] In this study Polednak analyzed reconstruction rates for mastectomy patients diagnosed between 1992 and 1996 and reported an overall rate of 12.5% for the entire study period, ranging from 8.8% in 1992 to 15.6% in 1996. As in his earlier SEER study, he also found that economic status was a significant predictor of reconstruction. In 2 of 3 age categories analyzed, low-income patients were significantly less likely to receive reconstruction.

WHAT ARE THE CURRENT TRENDS IN BREAST RECONSTRUCTION RATES?

Based on a review of the SEER data described in the preceding section, it appears that breast reconstruction experienced slow but steady growth in the United States from 1990 through 1998. This trend likely reflected increasing awareness and acceptance of postmastectomy reconstruction by patients, providers, and payers. With passage of the WHCRA in 1998, it would seem reasonable to expect that the trend would continue or even accelerate, due in part to the law's removal of financial barriers to reconstruction for many women.

While determining current trends for breast reconstruction with complete accuracy remains elusive, it is possible to draw some conclusions based on available, but (as we discussed earlier) imperfect databases. To date, the SEER program provides reconstruction data up to the end of the year 2000. Overall reconstruction rates for the 11 registries were 16.8% for 1999 and 18.0% for 2000. The distribution of procedure types also showed minor changes compared with 1998: for 1999, 55.7% of patients received autogenous tissue reconstructions, 27.0% underwent expander/implant techniques, and 17.3% had combined flap/implant procedures. In the year 2000, the rates were 54.9%, 29.3%, and 15.7%, respectively.

The American Society of Plastic Surgeons also provides data on trends in breast reconstruction.[11] Information is self-reported by plastic surgeons across the country. Although these statistics may be subject to sampling error, the ASPS database still represents one of the more comprehensive and up-to-date sources of information on reconstructive procedures. According to these data, a large increase in the number of breast reconstructions occurred between 1992 and 1998 (from 29,607 to 69,683 cases). Between 1998 and 2001, there was an additional rise in case volume to 81,089. However, for 2002, the total declined to 73,026.

In summary, the case volume for postmastectomy reconstruction remains relatively low compared with the number of women still undergoing mastectomies each year in the United States. Despite the passage of the WHCRA in 1998, breast reconstruction utilization continues to rise at an extremely modest rate of slightly more than 1% per year, roughly the same rate seen during the decade prior to 1990. These findings raise a variety of health care delivery and policy issues, some of which we will address in the paragraphs to follow.

WHAT IMPACT DID THE WHCRA HAVE ON USE OF BREAST RECONSTRUCTION?

Our group used the SEER database to evaluate changes in use of breast reconstruction with the passage of the WHCRA.[12] Between 1998 and 2002, the annual rate of reconstruction did not change significantly ($p = 0.68$ for trend) and 51,184 (16.5%) patients underwent breast reconstruction within 4 months of the mastectomy.[12] Wide geographical variations in reconstruction rates persisted in the period after WHCRA passage (Table 73-3). In 2000 to 2002, adjusted regional rates varied more than 7-fold, from 4.5% in Alaska to 34.7% in Atlanta. Compared with rates prior to the passage of the WHCRA, some fluctuation in regional reconstruction rates

TABLE 73-3 Use of Breast Reconstruction Across SEER Registries Before and After the Passage of the WHCRA

| | ADJUSTED PERCENTAGE RECEIVING BREAST RECONSTRUCTION[a] | | |
SEER Registry	Pre-WHCRA (1998) (N = 10,684[b])	Post-WHCRA (2000-2002) (N = 40,500[b])	p Value[c]
San Francisco % (N)	17.2 (212)	14.4 (720)	0.02
Connecticut % (N)	11.1 (106)	17.7 (580)	<0.01
Metro Detroit % (N)	22.9 (316)	24.1 (1068)	0.11
Hawaii % (N)	7.2 (28)	8.1 (108)	0.57
Iowa % (N)	8.9 (116)	11.4 (510)	0.02
New Mexico % (N)	14.8 (68)	22.3 (376)	<0.01
Seattle % (N)	11.9 (114)	10.0 (474)	<0.01
Utah % (N)	17.0 (79)	17.9 (330)	0.94
Metro Atlanta % (N)	35.3 (241)	34.7 (1015)	0.68
Alaska % (N)	15.4 (4)	4.5 (6)	0.10
San Jose-Monterey % (N)	17.7 (127)	18.6 (496)	0.54
Los Angeles % (N)	13.6 (281)	13.4 (1052)	0.43
Rural Georgia % (N)	12.5 (4)	13.2 (19)	0.94
Total % (N)[d]	15.9 (1696)	16.8 (6754)	0.23

SEER, Surveillance, Epidemiology and End Results database; WHCRA, Women's Health and Cancer Rights Act.
[a]Adjusted for patient age, marital status, race, stage of disease, and use of adjuvant radiotherapy.
[b]SEER population of mastectomy patients for the pre and post-WHCRA time periods.
[c]Comparison of pre-WHCRA and post-WHCRA using χ^2-test; 1999 data was excluded since this was a transition year.
[d]SEER population receiving breast reconstruction for the pre- and post-WHCRA time periods.

occurred, although no significant change took place across the total sample population. Similarly, the WHCRA did not eliminate disparities in the use of breast reconstruction among racial and ethnic subgroups (Fig. 73-2). Compared to Caucasians, black patients were considerably less likely to undergo breast reconstruction (adjusted OR, 0.54; 95% confidence interval [CI], 0.49-0.65), as were Hispanic patients (OR 0.48, 95% CI 0.42-0.55) and Asian patients (OR 0.36, 95% CI 0.31-0.42). These data suggest that the WHCRA has had little impact on the overall use of postmastectomy breast reconstruction or reduced variations in use across geographical regions and racial subgroups.

WHY ARE BREAST RECONSTRUCTION RATES SO LOW?

Given the extensive efforts by patient advocates and providers over the past 20 years to promote postmastectomy breast reconstruction, the low utilization and small rate of increase reported for this procedure are disappointing. When considering these results, it is tempting to focus on the weaknesses of existing research and to simply maintain that breast reconstruction is under-reported. This may be the case with the SEER database, because it does not track reconstructions performed more than 4 months following mastectomy. The ASPS database indicates that 39% to 42% of reconstructions performed by its members are immediate,[11] leading one to speculate that SEER data may overlook a substantial proportion of reconstructions performed in the delayed setting. However, even if the "true" rate (including both immediate and delayed reconstructions) is twice that reported in the SEER analyses, only about 1 in 3 mastectomy patients are receiving reconstruction. In reality, this estimate is probably overly generous: Polednak's study of the Connecticut

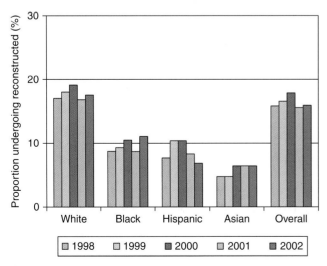

FIGURE 73-2 Trends in the proportion of women undergoing postmastectomy breast reconstruction from 1998 to 2002, overall and by racial/ethnic group.

databases for 1992 to 1996 included both immediate and delayed procedures and still reported reconstruction rates in the range of 9% to 15%.[10]

The reason for the low utilization reported for breast reconstruction may be attributable to many factors. Perhaps the vast majority of mastectomy patients simply do not want reconstruction. In a single center, single plastic surgeon retrospective study, Finlayson and coworkers found that only 21% of women undergoing mastectomy chose immediate or delayed reconstruction, despite the opportunity for preoperative consultation with a plastic surgeon and receiving what the authors describe as "specific preoperative counseling about postmastectomy breast reconstruction."[13] Given the questionable generalizability of these findings and the lack of additional studies, which address the issue of patient preference, we can only speculate about the "right" rate for reconstruction (ie, the rate at which well-informed patients, with access to appropriate care, would choose breast reconstruction). Despite knowing little about preferences for reconstruction among mastectomy patients, wide variations in rates of reconstruction across demographic variables such as locality, race, and income level suggest that barriers to reconstruction still exist, regardless of federal mandates. For example, both Polednak and our group have observed 4 to 5 fold variations in regional rates of breast reconstruction.[8,9] While it is not inconceivable that patient preferences play a major role in accounting for these differences, it also seems unlikely that women in Atlanta are 3 times more likely to want reconstruction than women in Los Angeles (controlling for age, race, and disease stage).[9] A more likely etiology for this variation is a series of flaws in our health care system that continue to limit patients' access to reconstruction (and to other health care resources).

WHAT BARRIERS REMAIN FOR WOMEN SEEKING BREAST RECONSTRUCTION?

Due to a paucity of research on utilization of postmastectomy reconstruction, we can only speculate about the potential barriers that still exist for women seeking these procedures. However, based on what little we do know, several factors appear to limit access: (1) ongoing financial barriers, (2) race-based inequalities in health care, (3) lack of patient knowledge about options for reconstruction, and (4) geographic variations in access to reconstructive services. We will examine each of these issues in the following paragraphs.

Financial Barriers

As noted earlier, the WHCRA mandated coverage of postmastectomy reconstruction by all health care payers as of January 1, 1999. As patients and plastic surgeons have discovered in the last decade, the WHCRA is unfortunately riddled with loopholes. The act overlooks the 47 million Americans who lack health care coverage of any kind, leaving uninsured women to either pay out of pocket for reconstruction or forego an important quality of life-enhancing procedure. And, due to the lack of provisions addressing payer compliance and enforceable penalties for infractions, health care payers remain on the "honor system" to fund reconstruction for their mastectomy

patients. And physicians are complaining that third-party payers, in particular health maintenance organizations, are refusing to cover postmastectomy reconstruction despite federal legislation and patient advocacy letters.[14]

Another weakness in the WHCRA is its failure to address physician reimbursement. While the law mandates that payers include breast reconstruction as a covered benefit, uniform rates of physician reimbursement are not specified. To assess the impact of this oversight, a discussion group of 15 plastic surgeons from 6 states was initiated by the last author in December 2003. All practice types and levels of experience were represented. After a presentation on current rates of reconstruction, participants were queried about barriers to breast reconstruction observed in their geographic areas. Overwhelmingly, reimbursement was the most common factor identified by the practitioners. The majority of the group did not participate in health care plans for breast reconstruction. Among those declining managed care and third-party plans for reconstruction, the primary reason given was inadequate reimbursement. As a method of coping with low reimbursement, some of the surgeons still participating in health care plans tended to choose less time-consuming options, such as tissue expanders, rather than more complex autogenous tissue procedures. The experiences relayed by these surgeons are probably not atypical. Furthermore, in its 2002 member survey, the American Society of Plastic Surgeons found that the issue with the greatest impact on members' practices was declining reimbursement.[15]

Race-Based Inequalities in Care

While teasing out the etiologies for disparity in our health delivery system is a monumental task, disparities in the utilization of health care resources between racial/ethnic minorities and Caucasians have been well documented in many areas of medicine. Compared to Caucasians, African Americans often receive less medical care, receive less aggressive treatment interventions, and are diagnosed at later stages of disease.[16-18] The SEER data echoes this trend, as race was a significant predictor of postmastectomy reconstruction.[9,12] Compared with Caucasians, the odds of reconstruction for African American and Hispanic women were approximately half as likely and for Asian woman were approximately one-third as likely.

Since the classic Whitehall study of the 1960s, the disturbing relationship between social class and health status haunts our society.[19] Financial status could partially explain the lower rates of reconstruction in the minority populations. One could also postulate that financial status affects the type of reconstruction a woman chooses. Expander-implant techniques may be less popular in a financially disadvantaged group due to concerns regarding transportation and time away from work. The provision of mandated insurance coverage for reconstruction only removes one small fraction of the financial barriers faced by women in lower socioeconomic classes. Other financial burdens, such as child care, transportation, and lack of sick leave from employers, limit "non–life-saving" health provisions such as reconstruction.

Financial barriers cannot account for all of the discrepancies found in the delivery of postmastectomy breast reconstruction. The cultural value of women's breasts may differ across ethnicities.

In our experience, Asian women often receive similar health care services as Caucasians, but Asian women in the SEER database were significantly less likely to receive breast reconstruction compared to Caucasians.[9] In addition, each subculture of our society has varying levels of trust in the health care system, which impacts health care choices. Perhaps born out of the Tuskegee syphilis experiments, the African American culture has historically been distrustful of the traditional health care system. This inherent distrust in the health care system may explain the lower likelihood of breast reconstruction in African Americans compared to Caucasians.

Inadequate Knowledge about Breast Reconstruction

Imperfect information can also act as a barrier to health care. Although the WHCRA requires payer coverage, it does not mandate public knowledge or referral to plastic surgeons for all mastectomy patients. Thus, the postmastectomy patient may not be aware that (1) breast reconstruction is a safe option, (2) this procedure is covered by insurance, or (3) the benefits of reconstruction extend beyond aesthetics.

Either the treating physician or the media generally provide information regarding reconstructive options. Historically, the health care profession has had marginal success in preventing unbiased health care choices in patients. Breast cancer is no exception. The option of breast-conserving therapy has not always been provided to women by their physicians, which

triggered governmental intervention. Physicians were mandated to provide information on both mastectomy and breast-conserving treatment options.[20] A population-based study of breast cancer patients by Morrow and associates suggests that patients have inadequate knowledge about reconstruction, with only 11.2% of women correctly answering 3 basic knowledge questions about postmastectomy reconstruction.[21] African American compared to Caucasian women were significantly more likely to report inadequate information as a reason for not pursing breast reconstruction.[21]

Referring physicians may also be biased against postmastectomy reconstruction. The option for reconstruction may not be presented to all patients or may be provided with cultural biases to different patient populations. An underlying cultural assumption is that breast reconstruction is for the young and sexually active.[22] These factors may very well influence some physicians' referral patterns for reconstructive surgery and may contribute to the significantly lower rates of postmastectomy reconstruction in older women, as previously discussed. A population-based study by our group observed that almost half of general surgeons (44%) referred less than 25% of women to a plastic surgeon prior to the mastectomy.[14] High-referral surgeons were more likely to be women, to have a high clinical breast surgery volume, and to work in cancer centers (Table 73-4),[14] whereas low-referral surgeons were more likely to perceive that patient finances and availability of reconstructive services diminished opportunities for reconstruction (Table 73-5). On the other hand, women may know that reconstruction is available but

TABLE 73-4 Multivariate Analysis of Correlates of a High Referral General Surgeon (refers more than 75% of breast cancer patients to plastic surgery for reconstruction)

Independent Variable	Adjusted Odds Ratio (95% CI)	p Value
SEER registry[a]	1.50 (0.81, 2.76)	0.20
Years in practice[b]	0.99 (0.96, 1.02)	0.40
Female[c]	2.30 (1.09, 4.84)	0.03
Clinical breast volume		
Low[d]	1.0	—
Medium	2.98 (1.30, 6.82)	0.01
High	4.08 (1.76, 9.42)	< 0.01
F test: $\chi^2 = 10.9$ ($p < 0.01$)		
Hospital setting		
Community hospital[d]	1.0	—
Teaching hospital	1.73 (0.89, 3.36)	0.10
Cancer center	2.41 (1.16, 5.04)	0.01
F test: $\chi^2 = 5.6$ ($p = 0.05$)		

[a]Detroit is the reference group.
[b]Continuous variable.
[c]Men are the reference group.
[d]Reference group.

TABLE 73-5 Surgeons' Perceptions of Why Women Do Not Choose Breast Reconstruction by Surgeon Referral Practice to Plastic Surgery for Breast Reconstruction

	RESPONDED VERY COMMON,[a] N (%)				
	All Surgeons (N =342[b]) (%)	Low-Referral Surgeon[c] (N = 152) (%)	Moderate-Referral Surgeon[c] (N = 109)(%)	High-Referral) Surgeon[c] (N = 81)(%)	p Value[d]
"Patient Desire"					
No desire for more surgery	64	62	70	60	0.32
Not important	57	58	58	53	0.67
Require too much time	39	30	51	40	< 0.01
"Patient Concern"					
Concerned about cancer surveillance	25	24	30	19	0.19
Concerned about the look or feel of the reconstruction	15	16	17	9	0.21
"Access Barriers"					
Concerned about cost	46	58	47	22	< 0.001
Not enough knowledge about reconstruction	22	32	16	12	< 0.001
Unavailability of plastic surgery	19	30	13	8	< 0.001
"Patient Priorities"					
Focused on breast cancer treatment, not reconstruction	21	31	13	12	< 0.001

[a]Responded 4 or 5 on 5-point Likert scale, from very uncommon to very common.
[b]23 surgeons had missing data on referral practice.
[c]Low-referral surgeon has less than 25% of breast cancer patients referred to plastic surgeon prior to mastectomy; moderate-referral surgeon refers 25% to 75% of patients; high-referral surgeon refers more than 75% of patients.
[d]χ^2 evaluating differences in responses by referral practice.

may not be aware that it is a financially viable option. Breast cancer patients may also have the misperception that breast reconstruction is not covered by insurance.

Outcomes research on postmastectomy reconstruction is inundated with data supporting the psychosocial benefits of these procedures. Women who choose postmastectomy reconstruction have significantly improved emotional health, general mental health, social functioning, and body image postoperatively.[2-4] The effects of reconstruction extend beyond "cosmetics," but awareness of these benefits may be limited outside of the plastic surgery community.

Geographic Variations in Access to Reconstruction

The geographic variation in breast reconstruction rates noted earlier is hardly unique to this procedure. As early as 1986, Chassin and coworkers observed at least 3-fold differences in the rates of 67 out of 123 medical and surgical procedures studied among Medicare beneficiaries in 13 large service areas across the United States.[23] More recently, Birkmeyer and colleagues reported up to 10-fold variations across regions in the rates of 11 common surgical procedures in the 1995 Medicare population.[24] Speculation over potential etiologies for these variations is widespread in the current health services literature ranging from ethnic and socioeconomic differences across regions[25] to variations in the practice patterns of physicians.[24] Providers may disagree about the effectiveness of health care interventions, including breast reconstruction. Chassin theorizes that geographic differences in the use of health care may be attributable to variations in the prevalence of physicians who are "enthusiasts" for particular interventions.[26] In the case of breast reconstruction, areas with higher rates may be populated with physicians who are knowledgeable about reconstruction and who actively promote this operation among their mastectomy patients. If this is so, efforts to educate providers, particularly oncologists and primary care physicians, about the benefits of reconstruction might encourage more practitioners to consider this procedure as an option for their patients.

Variation in the availability of local plastic surgeons may also account for some of regional differences in breast reconstruction rates. The relationship between the number of surgeons who perform a particular procedure and the number of these operations carried out in a geographic location has been examined previously for other types of surgery. For example, Leape and coworkers found that regional rates for carotid endarterectomy were in part linked to the number of surgeons performing the operation in the area.[27] Similarly, the relatively low rates of breast reconstruction observed in our study of the SEER regions may be attributable (in part) to the limited availability of plastic surgeons (or of those offering breast reconstruction) in some communities.

SUMMARY

The overall use of postmastectomy breast reconstruction is low and characterized by wide geographical and racial disparities in use. A large proportion of these variations represent inadequate referrals to plastic surgeons, limited patient knowledge of reconstructive options, and financial barriers to reconstructive services. In an effort to confront these obstacles to reconstruction, we need to continue development of nationwide cancer treatment databases (such as SEER) that capture clinical information on large and diverse populations of patients. This will greatly enhance the generalizability of research findings, allowing investigators to evaluate utilization and the impact of care on a wide variety of demographic groups. Better understanding of breast reconstruction utilization will require not only database research, but will also necessitate survey research to study the decision-making processes of patients and providers making reconstructive choices. This information will help us determine (in the words of health services researcher Jack Wennberg) "what rate is right?"[24] In addition, plastic surgeons must partner with patient-advocates and health care policy-makers to remedy systemic flaws which block access to reconstruction. Strengthening the WHCRA, educating our patients and colleagues, and addressing infrastructure and manpower needs all may contribute to

achieving the "right" rate of breast reconstruction on a national scale. In the years to come, we certainly have our work cut out for us.

REFERENCES

1. http://www.cms.hhs.gov/HealthInsReformforConsume/06_TheWomen's HealthandCancerRightsAct.asp. Accessed August 5, 2008.
2. Dean C, Chetty U, Forrest AP. Effects of immediate breast reconstruction on psychosocial morbidity after mastectomy. *Lancet*. 1983;320:459-462.
3. Schain WS. Breast reconstruction. Update of psychosocial and pragmatic concerns. *Cancer*. 1991;68(suppl):1170-1175.
4. Cederna PS, Yates WR, Chang P, et al. Postmastectomy reconstruction: comparative analysis of the psychosocial, functional, and cosmetic effects of transverse rectus abdominis musculocutaneous versus breast implant reconstruction. *Ann Plast Surg*. 1995;35:458-468.
5. http://seer.cancer.gov/. Accessed August 5, 2008.
6. http://seer.cancer.gov/registries/data.html. Accessed August 5, 2008.
7. http://seer.cancer.gov/registries/. Accessed August 5, 2008.
8. Polednak A. Geographic variation in postmastectomy breast reconstruction rates. *Plast Reconstr Surg*. 2000;106:298-301.
9. Alderman AK, McMahon L, Wilkins EG. The national utilization of immediate and early delayed breast reconstruction & the impact of sociodemographic factors. *Plast Reconstr Surg*. 2003;11:695-703.
10. Polednak AP. How frequent is postmastectomy breast reconstructive surgery? A study linking two statewide databases. *Plast Reconstr Surg*. 2001;108:73-77.
11. *2002 Plastic Surgery Statistics*. Arlington Heights, IL: American Society of Plastic and Reconstructive Surgeons, 2003.
12. Alderman AK, Wei Y, Birkmeyer JD. Use of breast reconstruction after mastectomy following the Women's Health and Cancer Rights Act. *JAMA*. 2006;295:387-388.
13. Finlayson CA, MacDermott TA, Arya J. Can specific preoperative counseling increase the likelihood a woman will choose postmastectomy breast reconstruction? *Am J Surg*. 2001;182:649-653.
14. Alderman AK, Hawley ST, Waljee J, et al. Correlates of referral practices of general surgeons to plastic surgeons for mastectomy reconstruction. *Cancer*. 2007;109:1715-1720.
15. www.plasticsurgery.org. Accessed July 4, 2003.
16. Amey CH, Miller MK, Albrecht SL. The role of race and residence in determining stage at diagnosis of breast cancer. *J Rural Health*. 1997;13:99-108.
17. Mitchell JB, Khandker RK. Black-white treatment differences in acute myocardial infarction. *Health Care Financ Rev*. 1995;17:61-70.
18. Hargraves JL, Cunningham PJ, Hughes RG. Racial and ethnic differences in access to medical care in managed care plans. *Health Serv Res*. 2001;36:853-868.
19. Marmot MG, Shipley MJ, Rose G. Inequalities in death—specific explanations of a general pattern? *Lancet*. 1984;1:1003-1006.
20. Nattinger AB, Hoffman RG, Shapiro R, et al. The effect of legislative requirements on the use of breast-conserving surgery. *N Engl J Med*. 1996;335:1035 1040.
21. Morrow M, Mujahid M, Lantz PM, et al. Correlates of breast reconstruction. Results from a population-based study. *Cancer*. 2005;104:2340-2346.
22. Tereskerz PM, Pearson RD, Jagger J. Infected physicians and invasive procedures: national policy and legal reality. *Milbank Q*. 1999;77:511-529, iii.
23. Chassin MR, Brook RH, Park RE, et al. Variations in the use of medical and surgical services by the Medicare population. *N Engl J Med*. 1986;314:285-290.
24. Birkmeyer JD, Sharp SM, Finlayson SR, et al. Variation profiles of common surgical procedures. *Surgery*. 1998;124:917-923.
25. Carlisle DM, Valdez RB, Shapiro MF, Brook RH. Geographic variation in rates of selected surgical procedures within Los Angeles County. *Health Serv Res*. 1995;30:27-42.
26. Chassin MR. Explaining geographic variations. The enthusiasm hypothesis. *Med Care*. 1993;31(suppl):YS37-YS44.
27. Leape LL, Park RE, Solomon DH, et al. Relation between surgeons' practice volumes and geographic variation in the rate of carotid endarterectomy. *N Engl J Med*. 1989;321:653-657.

CHAPTER 74

Oncologic Considerations for Breast Reconstruction

Grant W. Carlson

Fifteen percent of women treated for breast cancer with total mastectomy receive immediate or early breast reconstruction.[1,2] The percentage is higher in young women and those treated in tertiary care medical centers. Immediate breast reconstruction (IBR) has several advantages.[3,4] It can prevent some of the negative psychological and emotional sequelae seen with mastectomy. The aesthetic results of immediate reconstruction are superior to those seen after delayed reconstruction. IBR also reduces hospital costs by reducing the number of procedures and length of hospitalization. IBR has the potential to impact the treatment of breast cancer. It could affect the delivery of adjuvant therapy and the detection and treatment of recurrent disease. Chemotherapy and radiation therapy could also impact the complication rates of reconstruction. The oncologic considerations of breast reconstruction are outlined in this chapter.

LOCAL RECURRENCE AFTER SKIN-SPARING MASTECTOMY

Skin sparing mastectomy (SSM) has markedly improved the aesthetic results of IBR (Fig. 74-1). Preservation of the native skin envelope and the inframammary fold reduces the amount of tissue necessary for reconstruction.[5] Breast symmetry can often be achieved without operating on the contralateral breast, and the periareolar incisions are inconspicuous in clothes.

There have been concerns that the skin and inframammary fold preservation reduce the effectiveness of total mastectomy. Despite these concerns, there is a large body of evidence that the local recurrences (LRs) after SSM are comparable to non-SSM.[6-8] Care must be taken, however, in patients with superficial cancers or diffuse ductal carcinoma in situ (DCIS) to assure adequate surgical margins. The follow-up of patients after SSM to detect LRs is discussed in the next section.

POSTRECONSTRUCTION IMAGING

The role of postreconstruction imaging after the treatment of breast cancer remains controversial. There is a paucity of data that addresses the issue and there no established guidelines.[9] The incidence of LR of breast cancer is related to tumor stage. Most LRs after total mastectomy are in the skin and subcutaneous tissue and are readily detected by physical examination.[10] A flap or implant could potentially delay the discovery of chest wall recurrences.

Systemic relapse is not inevitable following LR, especially after the treatment of DCIS.[11,12] This argues that early detection of LRs may have a potential survival impact. All forms of mastectomy leave residual breast tissue. The differences are in terms of the microscopic breast tissue left behind in the skin and inframammary fold, which are largely preserved after SSM. Torresan et al evaluated residual glandular tissue in the skin flaps that would have been preserved after SSM.[13] They found that 60% contained residual glandular tissue, and it correlated with skin flap thickness.

The completeness of mastectomy is important in the treatment of DCIS because most cases of recurrence represent unexcised residual disease. Several authors have reported LR of DCIS treated by SSM and IBR.[11,14,15] They found that the majority of LRs were invasive carcinomas. This suggests that postreconstruction mammography can have a role in the early detection of recurrences prior to the development of invasive carcinoma. Physical examination of implant reconstruction is relatively easy. There is minimal soft tissue covering the implant except along the inframammary fold and in the axillary tail. Deep chest wall recurrences are extremely unlikely because the implants are placed in the submuscular plane. Conventional mammographic evaluation has limited utility because the implants obscure soft tissue visualization. Magnetic resonance

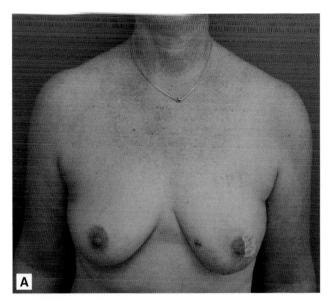
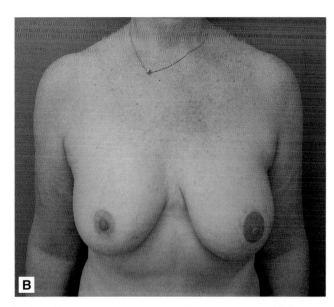

FIGURE 74-1 A. Preoperative photograph. **B.** Postoperative photograph after skin-sparing mastectomy and transverse rectus abdominis musculocutaneous flap reconstruction.

imaging (MRI), which has been used extensively to evaluate the integrity of silicone gel implants, may have a role in the selective surveillance after implant reconstruction.[16-19]

The sensitivity of physical examination of autologous reconstruction is lower than that seen with implant reconstruction. Deep chest wall recurrences often avoid detection until symptoms develop. Autologous reconstruction causes less impairment of mammographic tissue visualization.[20] Benign mammographic findings after transverse rectus abdominis musculocutaneous (TRAM) flap reconstruction include fat necrosis, lipid cysts, calcifications, lymph nodes, and epidermal inclusion cysts (Fig. 74-2).[21] Breast cancer recurrences in autologous tissue reconstruction are mammographically similar to that of primary tumors (Fig. 74-3).[22,23] Proponents of surveillance mammography believe that screening breast cancer patients with autologous reconstructions can detect nonpalpable recurrences before clinical examination.

Helvie et al evaluated surveillance mammography in 113 patients after TRAM flap reconstruction.[24] Six patients underwent biopsy for suspicious mammographic findings, and 2 LRs were detected. Two patients in the study group went on to develop recurrences that were detected by physical examination. There was one false-negative mammogram resulting in a sensitivity of 67% and specificity of 98% for surveillance mammography after TRAM flap reconstruction.

There is a paucity of data regarding the efficacy of MRI of the breast following autogenous breast reconstruction.[25,26] Breast MRI has been shown to clearly delineate autogenous flaps from residual mammary adipose tissue. The absence of contrast medium uptake during breast MRI precludes recurrent carcinoma to a high probability. Fat necrosis in a TRAM flap will show early postoperative contrast enhancement, but this resolves within 6 to 12 months. Rieber et al evaluated MRI of

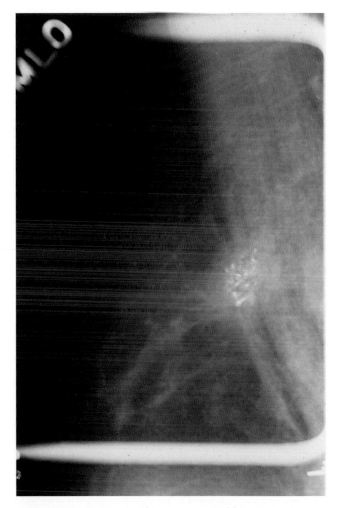

FIGURE 74-2 Mammographic appearance of fat necrosis in a transverse rectus abdominis musculocutaneous flap reconstruction.

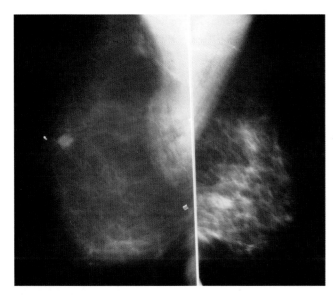

FIGURE 74-3 Mammographic appearance of local recurrence in transverse rectus abdominis musculocutaneous flap (*L*), opposite breast (*R*).

the breast in the follow-up of 41e patients who had undergone autogenous tissue breast reconstruction.[27] MRI was able to distinguish flaps from surrounding residual breast tissue in all cases. It excluded disease recurrence in 4 patients with suspicious mammographic or sonographic findings. It returned false-positive findings in 3 cases.

The potential indications for postreconstruction imaging include patients with close surgical margins and patients with diffuse DCIS treated by SSM. Its routine use after autologous reconstruction after SSM for invasive carcinoma warrants further study. The low detection rate and specificity does not justify the routine use of MRI in the follow-up of patients postreconstruction. MRI is most useful in patients with abnormal findings on physical examination or mammography and ultrasound. It is also helpful to delineate the extent of local disease recurrence.

BREAST RECONSTRUCTION AND ADJUVANT THERAPY

There are concerns that IBR may delay the administration of adjuvant chemotherapy. A survey of 376 consultant breast surgeons in the United Kingdom and Ireland found that the majority (57%) preferred delayed reconstruction because of these concerns.[28] Breast reconstruction does have a high complication rate especially in patients who are obese, smoke tobacco, or have a history of chest wall irradiation. Alderman et al performed a multi-institutional study of complication rates after tissue expander or TRAM flap reconstruction.[29] They reported a 52% complication rate, with major complications occurring in 30% of patients.

It seems logical that the high complication rate of IBR could potentially delay the administration of adjuvant therapy. Studies comparing onset of chemotherapy after IBR and control group treated with mastectomy alone have failed to show significant differences.[30-32] Wound complications after IBR must be treated

aggressively to remove necrotic, potentially infected tissue. Patients with clean, open wounds can receive chemotherapy with minimal compromise in wound healing. These patients must be followed closely to detect early signs of infection.

Patients with locally advanced, stage III breast cancer are generally treated with chemotherapy followed by total mastectomy and adjuvant radiation. The 5-year survival is 50% to 80%, and patients with a poor response to chemotherapy have an especially bad prognosis. It may be preferable to delay reconstruction until after mastectomy and adjuvant radiation in these patients. This avoids the potential problems with radiation delivery and the adverse effects of postmastectomy radiation therapy on immediate reconstruction. These issues are discussed in detail in another chapter.

Neoadjuvant chemotherapy has not been shown to increase the complication rate of IBR. Deutsch et al reported a 55% complication rate in 31 patients after immediate TRAM flap reconstruction who received neoadjuvant chemotherapy.[33] Six percent had a delay in resumption of chemotherapy because of complications. Sultan et al found a 14% complication rate in 21 patients who received neoadjuvant chemotherapy and underwent IBR.[34] The mean interval between surgery and resumption of chemotherapy was 19 days, and there was no delay in any patients.

TREATMENT OF LOCAL RECURRENCE AFTER BREAST RECONSTRUCTION

Surgical options following LR after breast reconstruction depend on the location and number of metastatic deposits and previous treatment. Imaging of the reconstructed breast and body scans are necessary to delineate the extent of tumor involvement (Fig. 74-4). Isolated LRs can be treated with removal of as much reconstructed tissue as necessary to achieve negative margins. Adjuvant chest wall radiation is usually administered (Fig. 74-5).

In cases of implant reconstruction, it may be necessary to remove a portion of the implant capsule necessitating implant removal in most cases. Howard et al reviewed 16 cases of LR after TRAM flap reconstruction.[35] Eight recurrences occurred in the skin and were detected on physical examination. Eight recurrences occurred in the chest wall and were symptomatic, detected on physical examination or diagnostic imaging. Twelve were believed amenable to surgical resection, and 3 required removal of the entire TRAM flap.

ONCOLOGIC CONSIDERATIONS IN PARTIAL MASTECTOMY RECONSTRUCTION

Oncoplastic surgery combines the principles of oncologic surgery (breast-conserving therapy) and plastic surgery (breast reconstruction). It has the potential for better tumor-free margins and enhancement of the cosmetic outcome.[36] Reconstruction can be performed via parenchymal rearrangement or volume replacement with local or distant flaps.[37,38]

Studies suggest these techniques are associated with low LR, but the long-term oncologic safety of these procedures is not

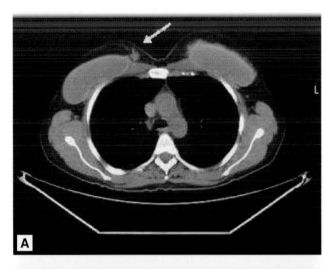

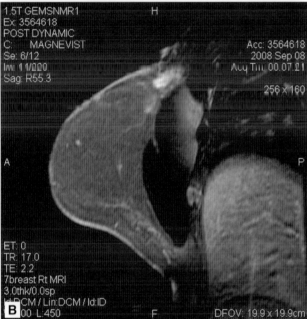

FIGURE 74-4   A. Positron emission tomography computed tomography scan showing local recurrence after transverse rectus abdominis musculocutaneous flap/implant reconstruction. **B.** Breast magnetic resonance imaging scan of same patient showing contrast enhancement of local recurrence.

clearly defined.[39] Young patients, especially those with diffuse high-grade DCIS; do not appear to be good candidates because of the increase in margin involvement and LR. Follow-up mammographic evaluation does not appear to be significantly impacted by oncoplastic reconstruction.

SENTINEL LYMPH NODE BIOPSY AND BREAST RECONSTRUCTION

Sentinel lymph node (SLN) biopsy has replaced axillary dissection as the standard of care for axillary node sampling. The sensitivity of intraoperative pathologic SLN analysis is 68% to 91%.[40-42] It is related to the size of the metastatic deposits, which is related to tumor size. False-negative intraoperative

diagnoses of SLN metastases present unique problems in breast cancer patients after IBR. The standard of care for patients with tumor-positive SLNs is a complete axillary lymph node dissection. This procedure can be technically demanding if a latissimus dorsi flap reconstruction has been performed or the thoracodorsal vessels have been used for microvascular reconstruction.[43] Fortunately, the internal mammary vessels have become the vessels of choice for microsurgical breast reconstruction. They are easier to access and permit early postoperative arm mobilization without risk of injury to the flap vascular pedicle. Vessel location facilitates placement, and the latissimus dorsi muscle blood supply is preserved if salvage surgery is necessary. Internal mammary lymph nodes can sometimes be encountered at the time of vessel dissection.[44] Involvement of these lymph nodes has prognostic significance and should be biopsied when they are discovered.

The indications for postmastectomy radiation therapy are based on the risk of locoregional recurrence as well as the potential morbidity of heart, lung, and blood vessel irradiation. Large tumor size, locally advanced cancer, and ≥4 metastatic lymph nodes have been indications for postmastectomy adjuvant radiation. Recent data have shown a survival advantages for any patient with node-positive breast cancer treated by total mastectomy.[45,46] These studies have been criticized for having low number of lymph nodes removed at axillary dissection, outdated chemotherapy, and a high regional recurrence rate in the control group not receiving radiation. Despite these concerns, many centers have adopted a policy of treating all node-positive patients with postmastectomy radiation. Radiation has a deleterious effect on all forms of breast reconstruction, and the SLN status could have a significant impact on the decision to perform IBR. A few studies have suggested SLN biopsy prior to mastectomy and IBR.[47-49] This could facilitate decision making regarding IBR and avoid a second operation in cases of false-negative SLN biopsies. McGuire et al found that SLN biopsy before mastectomy and IBR changed the operative strategy in 62% of patients.[50]

CONTRALATERAL PROPHYLACTIC MASTECTOMY

More women are choosing to have a contralateral prophylactic mastectomy (CPM) at the time of treatment of their unilateral breast cancer. Tuttle et al used Surveillance Epidemiology and End Results Program (SEER) data to evaluate the treatment of unilateral breast cancer from 1998 to 2003.[51] They found the rate of CPM in women undergoing total mastectomy more than doubled in the 6-year period. Contralateral prophylactic mastectomy at the time of total mastectomy and IBR has 2 main advantages: it reduces the risk of developing a new cancer and it facilitates breast reconstruction.

Women with unilateral breast cancer have an increased risk of developing a second cancer in the contralateral breast. The annual incidence of new breast cancer has been reported to be 0.7% to 1.8%.[52-54] Adjuvant hormonal therapy has been shown to reduce this risk. Despite the high incidence of cancer development, most patients will not experience a survival benefit from a CPM. The risk of systemic metastases from the index

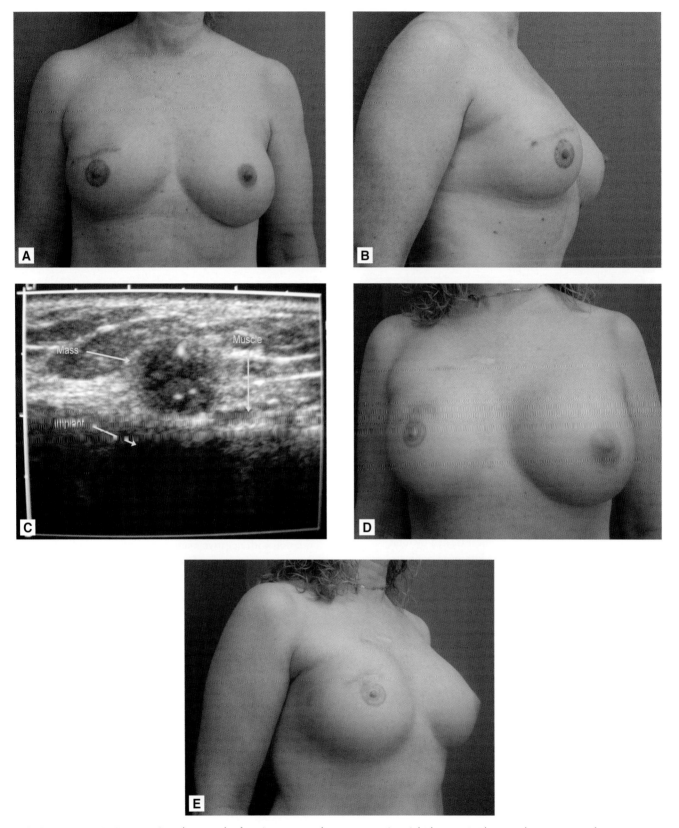

FIGURE 74-5   A, B. Preoperative photograph after tissue expander reconstruction right breast. **C.** Ultrasound appearance of LR.
D, E. Appearance after local excision and adjuvant radiation therapy.

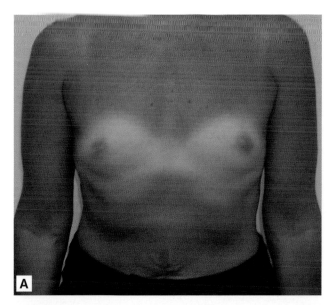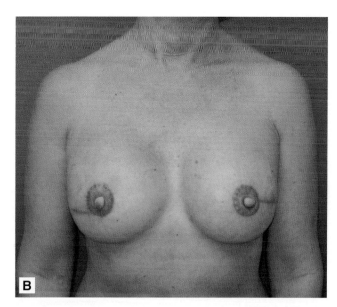

FIGURE 74-6 A. Preoperative photograph. **B.** Postoperative photograph after bilateral skin-sparing mastectomies and tissue expander reconstruction.

cancer exceeds the risk of contralateral cancers, which tend to be lower in stage.

The Society of Surgical Oncology updated their position statement on prophylactic mastectomy in 2007.[55] It detailed potential indications in patients with current or previous diagnosis of breast cancer to include the following:

1. Patients at high risk of contralateral breast cancer (BRCA mutation, strong family history)
2. Patients with mammographically dense breasts or those with diffuse indeterminate microcalcifications
3. Patients with unilateral breast cancer treated by total mastectomy and IBR who desire improved symmetry or have a desire for bilateral reconstruction

A CPM and bilateral reconstruction is especially useful in cases of implant-based reconstruction (Fig. 74-6). The contralateral breast frequently requires remedial surgery to achieve symmetry with an implant reconstructed breast. Clough et al found that the cosmetic outcome of unilateral implant reconstruction deteriorated with time.[56] They attributed this asymmetry largely to ptosis of the native breast seen with aging. Bilateral reconstruction would prevent this asymmetry development.

Most women are satisfied with their decision to undergo CPM.[57] The most common reasons for regret appear to be poor cosmetic outcome and a diminished sense of sexuality.[58]

FUTURE DIRECTIONS

1. The use of breast MRI to follow the contralateral breast in women treated for breast cancer will provide much needed data about postreconstruction imaging.
2. More data are needed to determine the safety of oncoplastic surgery of the breast. This will define which patients are appropriate candidates and who should be treated with mastectomy and immediate reconstruction.

SUMMARY

1. Postreconstruction imaging may allow early detection of LRs of breast cancer. Patients with close surgical margins and those with diffuse DCIS treated by SSM are potential candidates.
2. Careful patient selection is necessary to avoid many of the complications of breast reconstruction. A delay in the administration of adjuvant chemotherapy has never been shown after IBR.
3. Isolated LRs after breast reconstruction are treated with excision with negative margins and adjuvant radiation. This may necessitate removal of the breast implant in some cases.
4. Oncoplastic surgery has the potential for larger tumor resection margins and improved cosmetic outcome. The long-term oncologic safety of these procedures is not clearly defined.
5. False-negative intraoperative diagnoses of SLN metastases present problems after IBR. Axillary dissection can be difficult after latissimus flap reconstruction or if the thoracodorsal vessels were used for microvascular reconstruction. The use of the internal mammary vessels has eliminated many of the problems seen with SLN biopsy.
6. CPM facilitates implant-based reconstruction. It reduces the risk of new breast cancer but has negligible impact on survival.

REFERENCES

1. Alderman AK, McMahon L Jr, Wilkins EG. The national utilization of immediate and early delayed breast reconstruction and the effect of sociodemographic factors. *Plast Reconstr Surg.* 2003;111(2):695-703; discussion 704-705.
2. Polednak AP. How frequent is postmastectomy breast reconstructive surgery? A study linking two statewide databases. *Plast Reconstr Surg.* 2001;108(1):73-77.
3. DeBono R, Thompson A, Stevenson JH. Immediate versus delayed free TRAM breast reconstruction: an analysis of perioperative factors and complications. *Br J Plast Surg.* 2002;55(2):111-116.

4. Schain WS, Wellisch DK, Pasnau RO, et al. The sooner the better: a study of psychological factors in women undergoing immediate versus delayed breast reconstruction. *Am J Psychiatry.* 1985;142(1):40-46.

5. Carlson GW. Skin sparing mastectomy: anatomic and technical considerations. *Am Surg.* 1996;62(2).151-155.

6. Carlson GW, Bostwick J III, Styblo TM, et al. Skin-sparing mastectomy. Oncologic and reconstructive considerations. *Ann Surg.* 1997;225(5):570-575; discussion 575-578.

7. Kroll SS, Khoo A, Singletary SE, et al. Local recurrence risk after skin-sparing and conventional mastectomy: a 6-year follow-up. *Plast Reconstr Surg.* 1999;104(2): 421-425.

8. Simmons RM, Fish SK, Gayle L, et al. Local and distant recurrence rates in skin-sparing mastectomies compared with non-skin-sparing mastectomies. *Ann Surg Oncol.* 1999;6(7):676-581.

9. Barnsley GP, Grunfeld E, Coyle D, et al. Surveillance mammography following the treatment of primary breast cancer with breast reconstruction: a systematic review. *Plast Reconstr Surg.* 2007;120(5):1125-1132.

10. Langstein HN, Cheng MH, Singletary SE, et al. Breast cancer recurrence after immediate reconstruction: patterns and significance. *Plast Reconstr Surg.* 2003;111(2):712-720; discussion 721-722.

11. Carlson GW, Page A, Johnson E, et al. Local recurrence of ductal carcinoma in situ after skin-sparing mastectomy. *J Am Coll Surg.* 2007;204(5):1074-1078; discussion 1078-1080.

12. Carlson GW, Styblo TM, Lyles RH, et al. Local recurrence after skin-sparing mastectomy: tumor biology or surgical conservatism? *Ann Surg Oncol.* 2003;10(2):108-112.

13. Torresan RZ, dos Santos CC, Okamura H, et al. Evaluation of residual glandular tissue after skin-sparing mastectomies. *Ann Surg Oncol.* 2005;12(12):1037-1044.

14. Rubio IT, Mirza N, Sahin AA, et al. Role of specimen radiography in patients treated with skin sparing mastectomy for ductal carcinoma in situ of the breast. *Ann Surg Oncol.* 2000;7(7):544-548.

15. Slavin SA, Love SM, Goldwyn RM. Recurrent breast cancer following immediate reconstruction with myocutaneous flaps. *Plast Reconstr Surg.* 1994;93(6):1191-1204; discussion 1205-1207.

16. Done D, Aspelin P, Liberg D, et al. Contrast enhanced MR imaging of the breast in patients with breast implants after cancer surgery. *Acta Radiol.* 1995;36(2):111-116.

17. Gorczyca DP, Sinha S, Ahn CY, et al. Silicone breast implants in vivo: MR imaging. *Radiology.* 1992;185(2):407-410.

18. Harms SE, Flamig DP, Evans WP, et al. MR imaging of the breast: current status and future potential. *AJR Am J Roentgenol.* 1994;163(5):1039-1047.

19. Heywang SH, Hilbertz T, Beck R, et al. Gd-DTPA enhanced MR imaging of the breast in patients with postoperative scarring and silicon implants. *J Comput Assist Tomogr.* 1990;14(3):348-356.

20. Lindbichler F, Hoflehner H, Schmidt F, et al. Comparison of mammographic image quality in various methods of reconstructive breast surgery. *Eur Radiol.* 1996.6(6): 925-928.

21. Hogge JP, Robinson RE, Magnant CM, et al. The mammographic spectrum of fat necrosis of the breast. *Radiographics.* 1995;15(6):1347-1356.

22. Eidelman Y, Liebling RW, Buchbinder S, et al. Mammography in the evaluation of masses in breasts reconstructed with TRAM flaps. *Ann Plast Surg.* 1998;41(3):229-233.

23. Helvie MA, Wilson TE, Roubidoux MA, et al. Mammographic appearance of recurrent breast carcinoma in six patients with TRAM flap breast reconstructions. *Radiology.* 1998;209(3):711-715.

24. Helvie MA, Bailey JE, Roubidoux MA, et al. Mammographic screening of TRAM flap breast reconstructions for detection of nonpalpable recurrent cancer. *Radiology* 2002;224(1):211-216.

25. Ahn CY, Narayanan K, Gorczyca DP, et al. Evaluation of autogenous tissue breast reconstruction using MRI. *Plast Reconstr Surg.* 1995;95(1):70-76.

26. Kurtz B, Audretsch W, Rezai M, et al. Initial experiences with MR-mammography in after-care following surgical flap treatment of breast carcinoma [in German]. *Rofo Fortschr Geb Rontgenstr Neuen Bildgeb Verfahr.* 1996;164(4):295-300.

27. Rieber A, Schramm K, Helms G, et al. Breast-conserving surgery and autogenous tissue reconstruction in patients with breast cancer: efficacy of MRI of the breast in the detection of recurrent disease. *Eur Radiol.* 2003;13(4):780-787.

28. Callaghan CJ, Couto E, Kerin MJ, et al. Breast reconstruction in the United Kingdom and Ireland. *Br J Surg.* 2002;89(3):335-340.

29. Alderman AK, Wilkins EG, Kim HM, et al. Complications in postmastectomy breast reconstruction: two-year results of the Michigan Breast Reconstruction Outcome Study. *Plast Reconstr Surg.* 2002;109(7):2265-2274.

30. Allweis TM, Boisvert ME, Otero SE, et al. Immediate reconstruction after mastectomy for breast cancer does not prolong the time to starting adjuvant chemotherapy. *Am J Surg.* 2002;183(3):218-221.

31. Caffo O, Cazzolli D, Scalet A, et al. Concurrent adjuvant chemotherapy and immediate breast reconstruction with skin expanders after mastectomy for breast cancer. *Breast Cancer Res Treat.* 2000;60(3):267-275.

32. Taylor CW, Horgan, K, Dodwell, D. Oncological aspects of breast reconstruction. *Breast.* 2005;14(2):118-130.

33. Deutsch MF, Smith M, Wang B, et al. Immediate breast reconstruction with the TRAM flap after neoadjuvant therapy. *Ann Plast Surg.* 1999;42(3):240-244.

34. Sultan MR, Smith ML, Estabrook A, et al. Immediate breast reconstruction in patients with locally advanced disease. *Ann Plast Surg.* 1997;38(4):345-349; discussion 350-351.

35. Howard MA, Polo K, Pusic AL, et al. Breast cancer local recurrence after mastectomy and TRAM flap reconstruction: incidence and treatment options. *Plast Reconstr Surg.* 2006;117(5):1381-1386.

36. Clough KB, Thomas SS, Fitoussi AD, et al. Reconstruction after conservative treatment for breast cancer: cosmetic sequelae classification revisited. *Plast Reconstr Surg.* 2004;114(7):1743-1753.

37. Clough KB, Kroll SS, Audretsch W. An approach to the repair of partial mastectomy defects. *Plast Reconstr Surg.* 1999;104(2):409-420.

38. Kat CC, Darcy CM, O'Donoghue JM, et al. The use of the latissimus dorsi musculocutaneous flap for immediate correction of the deformity resulting from breast conservation surgery. *Br J Plast Surg.*1999;52(2):99–103.

39. Asgeirsson KS, Rasheed T, McCulley SJ, et al. Oncological and cosmetic outcomes of oncoplastic breast conserving surgery. *Eur J Surg Oncol.* 2005;31(8):817-823.

40. Chao C, Wong SL, Ackermann D, et al. Utility of intraoperative frozen section analysis of sentinel lymph nodes in breast cancer. *Am J Surg.* 2001;182(6):609-615.

41. Dupont EL, Kuhn MA, McCann C, et al. The role of sentinel lymph node biopsy in women undergoing prophylactic mastectomy. *Am J Surg.*2000;180(4):274-277.

42. Khalifa K, Pereira B, Thomas VA, et al. The accuracy of intraoperative frozen section analysis of the sentinel lymph nodes during breast cancer surgery. *Int J Fertil Womens Med.* 2004;49(5):208-211.

43. Kronowitz SJ, Chang DW, Robb GL, et al. Implications of axillary sentinel lymph node biopsy in immediate autologous breast reconstruction. *Plast Reconstr Surg.* 2002;109(6):1888-1896.

44. Hofer SO, Rakhorst HA, Mureau MA, et al. Pathological internal mammary lymph nodes in secondary and tertiary deep inferior epigastric perforator flap breast reconstructions. *Ann Plast Surg.* 2005;55(6):583-586.

45. Nielsen HM, Overgaard M, Grau C, et al. Study of failure pattern among high-risk breast cancer patients with or without postmastectomy radiotherapy in addition to adjuvant systemic therapy: long-term results from the Danish Breast Cancer Cooperative Group DBCG 82 b and c randomized studies. *J Clin Oncol.* 2006;24(15): 2268-2275.

46. Ragaz J, Olivotto IA, Spinelli JJ, et al. Locoregional radiation therapy in patients with high-risk breast cancer receiving adjuvant chemotherapy: 20-year results of the British Columbia randomized trial. *J Natl Cancer Inst.* 2005;97(2):116-126.

47. Brady B, Fant J, Jones R, et al. Sentinel lymph node biopsy followed by delayed mastectomy and reconstruction. *Am J Surg.* 2003;185(2): 114-117.

48. Klauber-Demore N, Calvo BF, Hultman CS, et al. Staged sentinel lymph node biopsy before mastectomy facilitates surgical planning for breast cancer patients. *Am J Surg.* 2005;190(4):595-597.

49. Schrenk P, Woelfl S, Bogner S, et al. The use of sentinel node biopsy in breast cancer patients undergoing skin sparing mastectomy and immediate autologous reconstruction. *Plast Reconstr Surg.* 2005;116(5):1278-1286.

50. McGuire K, Rosenberg AL, Showalter S, et al. Timing of sentinel lymph node biopsy and reconstruction for patients undergoing mastectomy. *Ann Plast Surg.* 2007;59(4): 359-363.

51. Tuttle TM, Habermann EB, Grund EH, et al. Increasing use of contralateral prophylactic mastectomy for breast cancer patients: a trend toward more aggressive surgical treatment. *J Clin Oncol.* 2007;25(33):5203-5209.

52. Hankey BF, Curtis RE, Naughton MD, et al. A retrospective cohort analysis of second breast cancer risk for primary breast cancer patients with an assessment of the effect of radiation therapy. *J Natl Cancer Inst.* 1983;70(5):797-804.

53. Peralta EA, Ellenhorn JD, Wagman LD, et al. Contralateral prophylactic mastectomy improves the outcome of selected patients undergoing mastectomy for breast cancer. *Am J Surg.* 2000;180(6):439-445.

54. Rosen PP, Groshen S, Kinne DW, et al. Contralateral breast carcinoma: an assessment of risk and prognosis in stage I (T1N0M0) and stage II (T1N1M0) patients with 20-year follow-up. *Surgery.* 1989;106(5):904-910.

55. Giuliano AE, Boolbol S, Degnim A, et al. Society of Surgical Oncology position statement on prophylactic mastectomy. Approved by the Society of Surgical Oncology Executive Council, March 2007. *Ann Surg Oncol.* 2007;14(9):2425-2427.

56. Clough KB, O'Donoghue JM, Fitoussi AD, et al. Prospective evaluation of late cosmetic results following breast reconstruction: I. Implant reconstruction. *Plast Reconstr Surg.* 2001;107(7):1702-1709.

57. Frost MH, Slezak JM, Tran NV, et al. Satisfaction after contralateral prophylactic mastectomy: the significance of mastectomy type, reconstructive complications, and body appearance. *J Clin Oncol.* 2005;23(31):7849-7856.

58. Montgomery LL, Tran KN, Heelan MC, et al. Issues of regret in women with contralateral prophylactic mastectomies. *Ann Surg Oncol.* 1999;6(6):546-552.

CHAPTER 75

Considerations and Strategies for the Timing of Breast Reconstruction

Steven J. Kronowitz

Postmastectomy radiation therapy (PMRT) can improve survival and locoregional control in patients with invasive breast cancer. The optimal timing and technique of breast reconstruction in patients requiring PMRT is controversial. The purpose of this chapter is to examine the most recent literature on breast reconstruction in patients receiving PMRT to help breast reconstructive surgeons make the best treatment decisions.

IMPLANT-BASED BREAST RECONSTRUCTION IN PATIENTS RECEIVING PMRT

With an increasing number of patients receiving PMRT, the decision of whether to offer implant-based or autologous tissue breast reconstruction has never been so relevant. Recent studies indicate that implant-based breast reconstruction in patients receiving PMRT is problematic.

Outcomes of Implant-Based Reconstruction with Modern Radiation Delivery Techniques

Studies evaluating the outcomes of 2-stage breast reconstruction, with placement of a tissue expander followed by placement of a permanent breast implant after PMRT, consistently reveal high rates of acute and chronic complications and poor aesthetic outcomes.[1] Capsular contracture that results from PMRT not only distorts the appearance of the breast, but also causes chronic chest wall pain and tightness that can be crippling. Many surgeons attribute the poor outcomes with implant-based breast reconstruction to older, less precise techniques of radiation delivery. However, even with modern radiation delivery techniques, complication rates with implant-based reconstruction are high.

Ascherman and colleagues[2] recently evaluated the complications and aesthetic outcomes of 104 patients who underwent 2-stage implant-based reconstruction. Twenty-seven patients also underwent radiation therapy, either before mastectomy (patients who were undergoing salvage mastectomy after lumpectomy and radiation therapy) or after mastectomy. In all 27 of these patients, radiation therapy was completed before the tissue expander was exchanged for a permanent breast implant or before the expander port was removed. Despite use of the latest prosthetic materials and modern radiation delivery techniques, the overall complication rates for the irradiated and nonirradiated breasts were 40.7% and 16.7%, respectively ($p \leq$ 0.01). Complications that resulted in removal or replacement of the prosthesis occurred in 18.5% of the irradiated and only 4.2% of the nonirradiated breasts ($p \leq 0.025$). In addition, the extrusion rate was higher for implants in irradiated breasts (14.8% vs 0%; $p \leq 0.001$). Breast symmetry scores were significantly higher in the patients who did not receive radiation therapy ($p < 0.01$). Despite the retrospective study design, these findings are important because they represent the experience of a single surgeon who evaluated patients treated using the latest prosthetic devices with total submuscular coverage and modern radiation therapy techniques.

In another recent study, Benediktsson and Perbeck[3] used applanation tonometry to prospectively evaluate rates of capsular contracture around saline-filled, textured implants in 107 patients who underwent mastectomy with immediate breast reconstruction. Twenty-four of the patients received PMRT. Radiation was delivered using a modern, 3-beam technique with a combination of photons and electrons, and reconstruction was accomplished using the latest prosthetic devices. The rate of capsular contracture was significantly higher for irradiated breasts than for nonirradiated breasts (41.7% vs 14.5%;

$p = 0.01$). The difference in contracture rates was not evident during the first 6 months, but was highly significant thereafter, even 5 years later.

In 2006, Behranwala and colleagues[4] published results from a series of 136 breast reconstructions with a median follow-up of 4 years: 62 reconstructions were performed with submuscular implants alone and 74 with a latissimus dorsi flap plus an implant. Forty-four reconstructed breasts received PMRT. Capsule formation was detected in 14.1% of the nonirradiated reconstructed breasts and 38.6% of the irradiated reconstructed breasts. On univariate analysis, PMRT was the only variable related to capsule formation ($p < 0.001$). Significant differences in geometric measurements of the breasts and worse photographic assessments were seen in the group that received PMRT. Pain that persisted for 2 years or more after surgery was present in 27% of breasts with capsular contracture and less than 1% of breasts without capsular contracture.

Impact of Performing the Tissue Expander–Permanent Implant Exchange before Rather than after Radiation Therapy

In a departure from the standard approach of exchanging the tissue expander for the permanent breast implant after PMRT, Cordeiro and colleagues[5] have been exchanging the expander for the implant before PMRT. Whereas Ascherman and colleagues[2] had to remove or replace the implant in 18.5% of the irradiated patients who had the permanent implant placed after PMRT, Cordeiro and colleagues[5] had to remove or replace the implant in only 11.1% of 81 patients. In addition, their technique resulted in acceptable aesthetic outcomes in most patients.

Although placing the permanent implant before PMRT should decrease the occurrence of acute wound healing problems (ie, wound dehiscence, infection, and implant exposure), there is no known pathophysiologic explanation for the relatively low frequency (5.9%) of severe (Baker classification, grade 4) capsular contracture described in Cordeiro and colleagues' study. In fact, the literature is replete with studies showing much higher rates of severe capsular contracture—in the range of 16% to 68%—when the permanent breast implant is in situ during the delivery of PMRT.[1,4]

Another consideration with the approach of Cordeiro and colleagues[5] is that it is not generally feasible in patients who undergo neoadjuvant chemotherapy, in whom PMRT is usually started within 4 weeks after mastectomy, leaving inadequate time for postoperative expansion and exchange of the expander for the permanent implant. This issue is important because many medical centers are increasing their use of neoadjuvant chemotherapy in patients with locally advanced breast cancer, even in patients with lesser degrees of local and regional disease, and many of the patients who are either known or suspected preoperatively to require PMRT are the same patients who may benefit from neoadjuvant chemotherapy.

In another, more recent study from the Memorial Sloan-Kettering group,[6] the authors further evaluated their approach of exchanging the expander for the implant before PMRT in 12 patients (only 10 patients were available for follow-up) who

underwent bilateral mastectomy and required PMRT in only 1 of the reconstructed breasts. When the authors compared the degree of capsular contracture (Baker classification) between the irradiated and contralateral nonirradiated breast, they found no difference in 4 patients, a single-grade difference in 5 patients, and a 2-grade difference in 1 patient. This series was too small and the median follow-up period (23.5 months) too short to permit any significant conclusions, especially considering that capsular contracture sometimes does not occur until 5 or more years[3] after reconstruction and that it may progress over time. However, a statistically significant comparative analysis should be possible as the authors' experience increases and more patients with longer follow-up are available for study. Another potential concern with this study is the authors' suggestion that the contralateral breast was an ideal control. In patients with bilateral implant-based reconstruction, the contralateral breast often receives radiation scatter in its medial aspects because of treatment of the medial aspect of the involved breast and/or the internal mammary nodes.[7] Therefore, in a patient who undergoes bilateral implant-based breast reconstruction and PMRT of 1 breast, the contralateral breast may also be at increased risk for capsular contracture.

Current Role of Reconstruction with a Latissimus Dorsi Flap plus a Breast Implant in Breast Cancer Patients Who Receive PMRT

In a study reported by Evans and colleagues[8] that examined the outcomes of patients who underwent breast reconstruction with an implant and an autologous tissue flap, the authors found that the addition of the tissue flap—either a transverse rectus abdominis myocutaneous (TRAM) flap or a latissimus dorsi myocutaneous flap—did not appear to offer protection against capsular contracture, a common complication of PMRT. The authors advocated breast reconstruction with autologous tissue alone in patients who have undergone or are about to undergo PMRT.

In 2007, Spear and colleagues[9] published a retrospective review of the role of the latissimus dorsi flap with an implant in reconstruction of previously irradiated breasts. The authors concluded that in patients with unsatisfactory outcomes after 2-stage implant-based reconstruction as a result of the adverse effects of PMRT, the aesthetic outcome can be improved by adding a latissimus dorsi flap, generally to the inferior pole of the breast.

Immediate Implant-Based Breast Reconstruction Can Compromise the Design of the Radiation Treatment Fields

Not only can PMRT adversely affect the aesthetic outcome of immediate implant-based breast reconstruction, but there is increasing evidence that such reconstructions may interfere with the delivery of PMRT (Fig. 75-1).[7,10-16] This interference can occur with a breast implant, a fully inflated tissue expander in situ on the chest wall, or even a partially deflated expander. The sloping contour of a reconstructed breast results in an imprecise geometric match of the medial and lateral radiation fields, which can lead to underdosing of the chest wall, especially centrally underneath the breast prosthesis and near the internal mammary

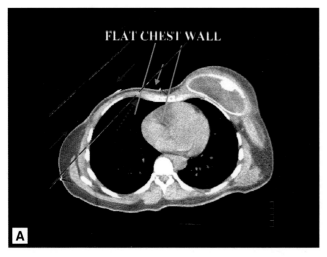
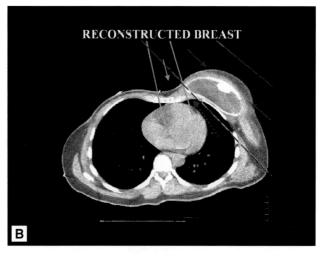

FIGURE 75-1 Potential problems with radiation delivery after breast reconstruction. **A.** Typical approach for chest wall irradiation. The medial chest wall and internal mammary nodes are treated with an anterior electron beam field that is geometrically matched to 2 lateral chest wall electron beams. The medial chest wall beam has a rapid dose fall-off after the chest wall and lung interface (*orange arrow*) and when combined with the lateral photon fields (*red arrows*) treats a small volume of lung. The flat chest wall surface allows for a relatively precise junction of the fields (*blue arrow*). **B.** The sloping contour of a reconstructed breast leads to an imprecise geometric match of the medial and lateral radiation fields, which can lead to underdosing of areas of the chest wall (*blue arrow*) and a nonuniform dose distribution (*red arrows*). A second consequence of the sloping contour is that the thickness of the chest wall across the width of the electron beam field becomes nonuniform. The electron beam field falls off as a function of tissue thickness, so that nonuniformity can also lead to an inhomogeneous dose distribution within the treatment field *(Reproduced with permission from Buchholz TA, Strom EA, Perkins GH, et al. Controversies regarding the use of radiation after mastectomy in breast cancer. Oncologist. 2002;7:539-546.)*

nodes.[15] The sloping contour also leads to nonuniform thickness of the chest wall across the width of the electron beam field, which can lead to a nonhomogeneous dose within the treatment field because the electron beam dose falls off as a function of tissue thickness.[15] Chest wall treatment in patients who have undergone reconstruction must be accomplished using traditional, 2-beam tangential fields alone rather than modern, 3-beam technique.[7,15,16] Unfortunately, it is not feasible to reconstruct the medial and apical breast to result in more favorable geometry for radiation treatment because of the higher density of flap tissues from the abdomen and gluteal regions.

Although recent studies[17,18] have found that the metallic port within a tissue expander does not result in significant scatter, which could lead to "hot" or "cold" spots that alter the homogenous treatment of the chest wall, the problem of the beam geometry and whether it allows treatment of all necessary tissue regions without increased damage to the heart or lungs remains a concern. On the other hand, some radiation oncologists believe that the effect of a breast implant or inflated tissue expander is negligible.[19]

In 2005, Schechter and colleagues[7] at the University of Texas MD Anderson Cancer Center found that immediate breast reconstructions may limit treatment planning for PMRT. They retrospectively reviewed the records of 152 patients treated with PMRT, 17 of whom underwent immediate breast reconstruction and had expanders, flaps, and/or implants in place at the time of PMRT. The authors evaluated the impact of various reconstructive techniques on the ability to treat the breadth of the chest wall, treat the internal mammary nodes within the first 3 interspaces, avoid the lung, and avoid the heart (Table 75-1). They found that completely deflated expanders resulted in no compromise, a partially deflated expander prevented treatment of the internal mammary nodes, and fully inflated expanders

moderately or severely compromised treatment of the internal mammary nodes and chest wall.

AUTOLOGOUS TISSUE BREAST RECONSTRUCTION IN PATIENTS RECEIVING PMRT

Although the consensus in the literature is that autologous tissue is preferable to breast implants within an irradiated operative field, even autologous tissue reconstructions can be adversely affected by PMRT.[20-23] Some studies, mainly those conducted by radiation oncologists, have found acceptable outcomes with TRAM flap reconstruction and PMRT, even when the flap is transferred before radiation delivery.[24] However, until less destructive methods of radiation delivery can be implemented and proven effective, delayed reconstruction may be the best option in patients known at the time of mastectomy to require PMRT.

Timing of Flap Transfer in Relation to PMRT

Unfortunately, the evaluation of complication rates and aesthetic outcomes in patients undergoing autologous tissue reconstruction before or after PMRT is extremely difficult because of significant variations in the administration of systemic therapy, the duration of follow-up, and the techniques of radiation delivery and breast reconstruction. Furthermore, few new studies evaluating this issue have emerged in recent years, probably because of decreased use of immediate reconstruction in patients who may require PMRT.

In 2001, investigators at MD Anderson Cancer Center published a retrospective study[21] comparing complication rates in 32 patients who underwent immediate TRAM flap reconstruction

TABLE 75-1 Impact of Immediate Reconstruction on Choice of Postmastectomy Irradiation Technique*

Laterality	Immediate Reconstruction Technique	Postmastectomy Irradiation Technique	Avoidance of Heart	Avoidance of Lung	Treatment of Ipsilateral Internal Mammary Region	Treatment of Chest Wall Breadth	Comments
R	TRAM	TANGENTS	1	1	0	½	
R	TRAM	TANGENTS	1	1	0	½	
R	TRAM	TANGENTS	1	1	0	½	Bilateral reconstruction
R	TRAM	TANGENTS	1	1	0	½	Bilateral reconstruction
R	EXPANDER FI	TANGENTS	1	1	0	½	
R	EXPANDER PD	TANGENTS	1	1	0	1	
R	EXPANDER CD	TANGENTS + IMC e−	1	1	1	1	
L	LATISSIMUS (Dbl)	TANGENTS	1	1	0	½	Bilateral reconstruction
L	LATISS + SALINE	TANGENTS	1	1	0	0	
L	TRAM	PD TANGENTS	1	½	½	½	
L	TRAM	PD TANGENTS	½	½	1	1	
L	TRAM	PD TANGENTS	1	½	1	½	
L	TRAM	PD TANGENTS	1	½	1	1	
L	TRAM	PD TANGENTS	1	1	0	0	
L	EXPANDER FI	PD TANGENTS	1	1	½	½	Bilateral reconstruction
L	LATISS + EXP CD	TANGENTS + IMC e−	1	1	1	1	
L	TRAM	TANGENTS + IMC e−	1	1	1	1	
L	TRAM	TANGENTS + IMC e−	1	1	1	1	

*Scoring: 1 = no compromise, ½ = moderately compromised, 0 = severely compromised.
Reprinted from Schechter NR, Strom EA, Perkins GH et al. Immediate breast reconstruction can impact postmastectomy irradiation. *Am J Clin Oncol.* 2005;28:485-494 with permission.

before PMRT and 70 patients who underwent PMRT before TRAM flap reconstruction. The mean follow-up times after the end of treatment for the immediate and delayed reconstruction groups were 3 and 5 years, respectively. The incidence of early flap complications (vessel thrombosis and partial or total flap loss) did not differ significantly between the 2 groups. However, the incidence of late complications (fat necrosis, flap volume loss, and flap contracture) was significantly higher in the immediate reconstruction group (87.5% vs 8.6%; $p < 0.001$). Furthermore, 28% of the patients with immediate reconstruction required an additional flap to correct a distorted contour resulting from flap shrinkage and severe flap contracture after PMRT.

In a study published in 2002, Rogers and Allen[22] evaluated the effects of PMRT on breasts reconstructed with a deep inferior epigastric perforator (DIEP) flap. A matched-pairs analysis was performed of 30 patients who underwent PMRT after reconstruction and 30 patients who did not. Patients who underwent PMRT had higher incidences of fat necrosis in the DIEP flap (23.3% vs 0%; $p = 0.006$), fibrosis and shrinkage (56.7% vs 0%; $p < 0.001$), and flap contracture (16.7% vs 0%; $p = 0.023$).

In a study published in 2005, Spear and colleagues[23] evaluated the effects of PMRT before or after pedicled TRAM flap breast reconstruction. They found that patients who had PMRT after reconstruction had worse aesthetic outcomes, symmetry, and contractures. The authors recommended that pedicled TRAM flap reconstruction be postponed until after PMRT.

Immediate Autologous Tissue Breast Reconstruction Can Compromise the Design of the Radiation Treatment Fields

Just as the presence of a breast reconstructed with an implant affects the delivery of radiation therapy (see the section "Immediate Implant-Based Breast Reconstruction Can Compromise the Design of the Radiation Treatment Fields" earlier in this chapter), so does the presence of a breast reconstructed with autologous tissue. In patients who undergo immediate autologous tissue breast reconstruction, the treatment plan must usually be compromised to safely deliver PMRT. A recent study from MD Anderson showed that whereas a native breast tends to drape flatly on the chest wall with the patient in the supine position, a breast reconstructed with autologous tissue has greater medial fullness, owing to the higher density of the adipose tissue from the abdomen and buttocks.[7] Irradiation of the internal mammary chain is challenging if reconstruction causes a steep angulation between the breast mound and the central chest wall, adversely affecting electron dosimetry and radiation toxicity.[7] Omitting the electrons and treating with "partially" deep tangential fields can allow for coverage of the first 3 intercostal spaces, but at the expense of increased pulmonary damage. In these circumstances, the opposite breast is also difficult to avoid, especially if it was also reconstructed.[15] Also, with PMRT delivered after an immediate reconstruction, it is not possible to adequately cover the breadth of the chest wall, the single most important target for PMRT.[25,26]

In the study by Schechter and colleagues,[7] a latissimus dorsi flap plus breast implant reconstruction severely compromised treatment of the internal mammary nodes and chest wall. The authors also found that some TRAM flaps compromised the treatment of the internal mammary nodes and chest wall and/or made it impossible to avoid the heart and lungs in patients with left-sided breast cancers.

In another study from MD Anderson,[16] 52% of patients who underwent immediate breast reconstruction with a TRAM flap and were subsequently found to require PMRT had compromises to their treatment plans (18% of which were considered major), compared with 7% of patients in a control group who did not have reconstruction. Among the major findings:

- Immediate reconstruction substantially compromised treatment of the internal mammary nodes and made it less possible to use a modern, 3-beam technique with a separate medial electron beam to treat this region.
- In patients with right-sided reconstructions, the chest wall and internal mammary chains were treated with deeper tangential beams (traditional, 2-beam tangential beam technique) at the expense of irradiation of more lung parenchyma.
- In patients with left-sided reconstructions (accounting for 67% of the compromised treatment plans), the heart and lung were spared at the expense of suboptimal coverage of the chest wall and internal mammary nodes.
- Sixty-five percent of patients with compromised internal mammary node coverage also had compromised coverage of the chest wall and suboptimal sparing of lung and epicardial heart structures (including the left anterior descending branch). Thus even if the internal mammary nodes had not been treated, these patients' plans would not have been optimal.

Regardless of whether one treats the internal mammary nodes, immediate breast reconstruction can adversely affect the delivery of PMRT.

STRATEGIES FOR THE MASTECTOMY PATIENT WHO MAY OR WILL NEED RADIATION TREATMENT

Delayed-Immediate Reconstruction in Patients Who Might Require Postmastectomy Radiation Therapy

Studies of autologous tissue reconstruction indicate that reconstruction should be delayed in patients who are known at mastectomy to require PMRT.[8,21-23,27] However, because recommendations regarding PMRT are often based on pathologic analysis of the mastectomy specimen, the need for PMRT is not always known at the time of mastectomy. Today, almost all patients with invasive breast cancer may be found to require PMRT after review of the permanent pathology specimens because many decisions regarding PMRT are made after mastectomy, at the time of review of the permanent sections, because it's hard to tell at the time of mastectomy and sentinel lymph node biopsy whether lymph node micrometastases are present.[28] In addition, the increasing use of fine-needle aspiration and stereotactic core biopsy techniques instead of open excisional biopsy techniques to make the diagnosis of breast cancer has limited the ability to accurately assess the amount of invasive tumor within the breast parenchyma until after mastectomy and review of the permanent sections.

One option is to always delay breast reconstruction until after completion of PMRT. In fact, many major medical centers are increasingly using this approach. However, this denies patients who ultimately do *not* require PMRT the aesthetic benefits available with immediate reconstruction. Until we can reliably predict the need for PMRT, decrease its adverse effects through more targeted therapy, and ensure optimal radiation delivery after immediate breast reconstruction, delayed-immediate reconstruction may be the best option to maintain the balance between optimal aesthetic outcomes and effective radiation delivery.

In this approach, which has been described in detail elsewhere,[11-14] a subpectoral tissue expander is placed at the time of mastectomy to preserve the initial shape and thickness of the breast skin flaps and the dimensions of the breast skin envelope until the final pathology results are available (Fig. 75-2).[11-14] An acellular dermal matrix may also be placed at the time of the expander. However, anecdotal evidence from surgeons performing delayed-immediate reconstruction suggests that acellular dermal matrices may play a role in the occurrence of persistent infection after PMRT because of the inability of intravascular antibiotic to penetrate the nonvascular dermal matrix at this stage of healing. In patients found not to require PMRT, preservation of the breast skin envelope enables the plastic surgeon to achieve aesthetic outcomes (Fig. 75-3)[11-14]

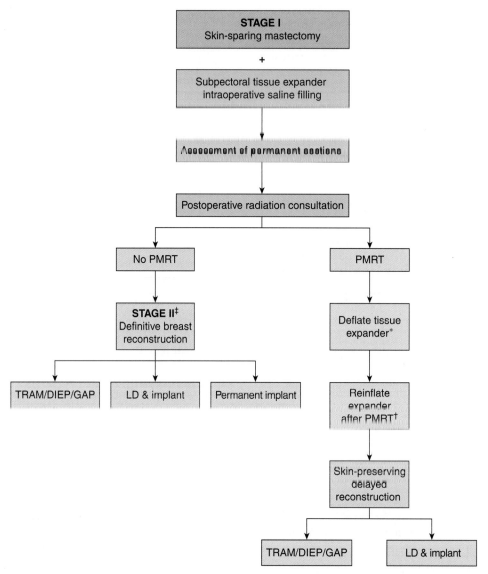

FIGURE 75-2 Schema for delayed-immediate breast reconstruction. *After the completion of chemotherapy but before the initiation of radiation therapy. If patient had neoadjuvant chemotherapy, leave expander inflated during the 4- to 6-week period before the initiation of radiation therapy. †Allow several weeks for skin desquamation to resolve. Results regarding expander reinflation are pending. ‡Usually performed 2 weeks after mastectomy and stage I of delayed-immediate reconstruction to prevent a delay of chemotherapy. If patient had neoadjuvant chemotherapy, definitive reconstruction may be delayed longer than 2 weeks. Note: Figure shows procedure for patients with unilateral breast cancer not treated with prophylactic contralateral mastectomy and for patients with bilateral breast cancer. In patients with unilateral breast cancer who elect prophylactic contralateral mastectomy, contralateral mastectomy and immediate reconstruction are performed at the time of definitive reconstruction of the breast with cancer. (DIEP, deep inferior epigastric perforator flap; GAP, gluteal artery perforator flap; LD, latissimus dorsi myocutaneous flap, TRAM, transverse rectus abdominis myocutaneous flap.) *(Reproduced with permission from Kronowitz SJ, Hunt KK, Kuerer HM, et al. Delayed-immediate breast reconstruction.* Plast Reconstr Surg. *2004;113:1617-1628.)*

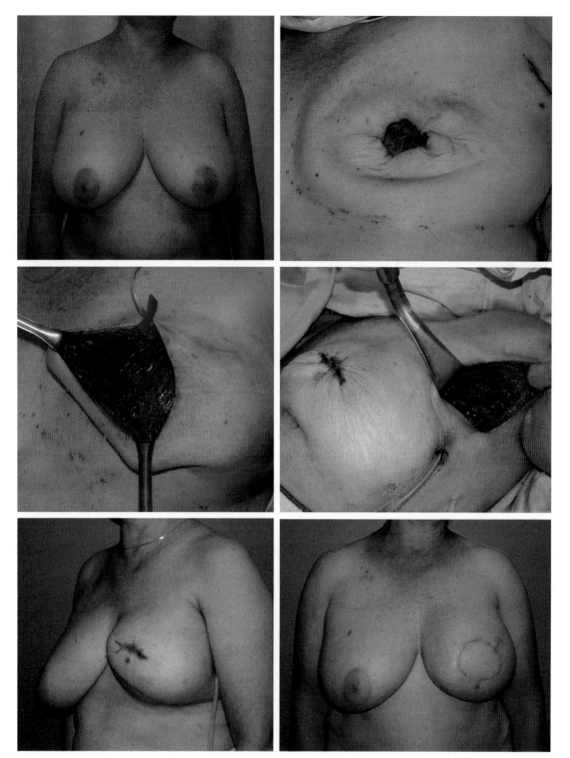

FIGURE 75-3 Delayed-immediate breast reconstruction in a 55-year-old woman with stage II (T2 multifocal N0M0) left breast cancer who was subsequently found to not require PMRT. *(Above, left)* Preoperative view after neoadjuvant chemotherapy. *(Above, right)* A periareolar mastectomy incision is preferred with delayed immediate reconstruction. *(Center, left)* A periareolar incision avoids the need for use of the serratus anterior muscle (required with a racquet-handle mastectomy incision) and allows for the use of the pectoralis major muscle alone to provide muscle coverage around the mastectomy incision in the event that mastectomy skin necrosis occurs. *(Center, right)* Intraoperative view during complete axillary lymph node dissection performed 10 days after mastectomy because of a positive sentinel lymph node on permanent pathology that was negative on intraoperative assessment using imprint cytology. If this patient had undergone an immediate autologous breast reconstruction with an axillary-based blood supply, the vascular pedicle could have been injured and the flap could have suffered an ischemic injury during complete axillary dissection. Another important benefit of delayed-immediate reconstruction is that the expander can remain inflated, preserving the breast skin envelope during a subsequent completion node dissection and serving as a "bridge" until all pathologic analysis is completed and a final decision is rendered regarding the need for PMRT. *(Below, left)* Four weeks after a left skin-sparing total mastectomy with axillary sentinel lymph node biopsy and subpectoral placement of a textured saline tissue expander expanded intraoperatively to the saline-fill volume of 700 mL. *(Below, right)* Six months after microvascular transverse rectus abdominis myocutaneous flap reconstruction. Although the patient underwent a subsequent right vertical mastopexy for symmetry, this image is shown to illustrate the outcome of delayed-immediate reconstruction in patients not requiring PMRT before any revision procedures.

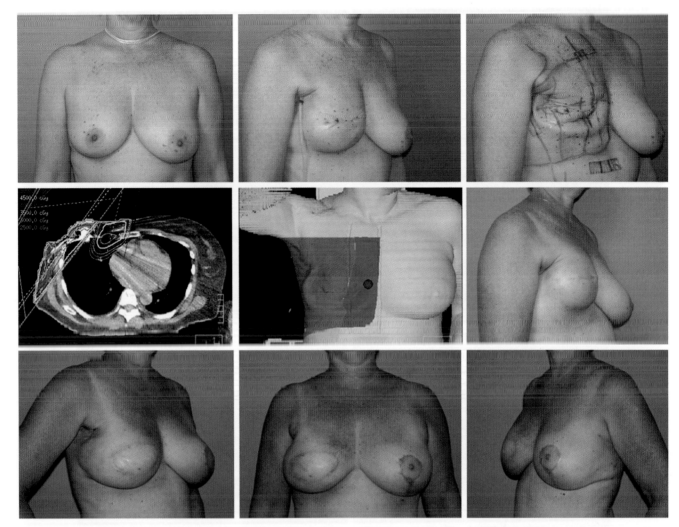

FIGURE 75-4 "Skin-preserving" delayed microvascular transverse rectus abdominis myocutaneous flap reconstruction in a 52-year-old woman with a clinical stage II [T2N1 (1 biopsy-proven positive axillary lymph node) M0] right breast cancer who was found after stage I of delayed-immediate reconstruction to require postmastectomy radiation therapy (PMRT). (*Above, left*) Preoperative view after neoadjuvant chemotherapy. (*Above, center*) Postoperative view 3 weeks after right skin-sparing modified radical mastectomy and stage I of delayed-immediate reconstruction with placement of a subpectoral textured saline tissue expander with an intraoperative saline-fill volume of 600 mL. The permanent pathology after review of the mastectomy specimen upstaged the disease to stage III (T2N2M0). (*Above, right*) Before the start of PMRT, the patient underwent complete deflation of the expander, with removal of 600 mL, in an office setting. Complete deflation of the expander before PMRT allows for treatment of the internal mammary lymph nodes without excessive injury to the heart and lungs and avoids nonuniform radiation dose distribution. (*Center, left and center*) Three-dimensional plan for the design of the radiation treatment fields performed using computed tomography (axial and 3-dimensional image). Despite the 600-ml fill volume used in this patient, deflation created a relatively flat chest wall surface for radiation delivery. (*Center, right*) Two weeks after the completion of PMRT, the tissue expander was reinflated to a volume of 600 mL. Seven months after completion of PMRT, the patient underwent a skin-preserving delayed breast reconstruction with removal of the tissue expander and placement of a microvascular transverse rectus abdominis myocutaneous flap. (*Below*) Postoperative views 22 months after definitive breast reconstruction. Six months after the skin-preserving delayed breast reconstruction, a left vertical mastopexy was performed to achieve symmetry.

similar to those obtainable with immediate breast reconstruction. In patients who do require PMRT, the tissue expander can be deflated before the start of PMRT to create a flat chest wall surface and permit modern, 3-beam radiation delivery, and the expander can be reinflated after PMRT to permit "skin-preserving" delayed reconstruction. Expander reinflation is usually begun 2 weeks after completion of PMRT, at which time the expander is reinflated to at least 50% of the predeflation volume. Delayed reconstruction is usually performed 3 months after completion of PMRT (Fig. 75-4).

Placement of the fully inflated expander allows for more precise positioning of the expander on the chest wall. Placement of an inflated expander also avoids the need for skin expansion and stretching of already thin mastectomy skin flaps, which can adversely affect the safety (expander exposure) and aesthetic outcome (telangiectasia formation) of breast reconstruction.

Expanded breast skin also tends not to tolerate PMRT because of dermal tears that result from the expansion process, which can enhance dermal scarring and subsequently result in skin contracture from PMRT; however, maintenance of the initial thickness of breast flaps after mastectomy, as in delayed-immediate reconstruction, results in better tolerance of the inflammatory effects of PMRT because the normal architecture of the dermis is preserved.

Whether to deflate the expander or leave it inflated during PMRT has been controversial. At MD Anderson, our radiation oncologists prefer that we deflate the tissue expander to improve the geometry of the chest wall for radiation delivery. It is unclear whether expander deflation adversely affects the aesthetic outcome of skin-preserving delayed reconstruction. Deflation may actually enhance the aesthetic outcome because the breast skin may tolerate the effects of radiation better when the skin is not stretched.

Delayed-Delayed Breast Reconstruction in Patients with Planned Postmastectomy Radiation Therapy

The inability to preserve the breast skin for delayed reconstruction after postmastectomy radiation therapy (PMRT) results in loss of the opportunity for the best possible aesthetic outcome. There is increasing evidence that neoadjuvant chemotherapy and PMRT plus skin-preserving mastectomy in patients with locally advanced breast cancer (LABC) results in favorable long-term control and survival rates. The upfront use of chemotherapy may also provide for less aggressive surgical resection with the opportunity to preserve the breast skin and improve the cosmetic outcomes, even in patients with LABC. The majority of patients with LABC do not often have tumor involving the breast skin, but much of the skin is usually resected in an elliptical fashion by the breast surgeon to avoid skin redundancy because no immediate intervention at skin preservation has been planned.

In 2003, at MD Anderson Cancer Center, we implemented a new skin-preserving approach to delayed breast reconstruction for patients with LABC who are known preoperatively to require PMRT (Fig. 75-5). The purpose of this skin-preserving approach, so-called delayed-delayed breast reconstruction is to improve the aesthetic outcomes, decrease the complications rates, and reduce the psychological disadvantages associated with standard delayed breast reconstruction after PMRT.

At MD Anderson Cancer Center, patients with clinical stage IIB and III are evaluated preoperatively by a multidisciplinary breast cancer team that includes a radiation oncologist to determine their eligibility for delayed-delayed breast reconstruction. Patients who are deemed to be eligible for this skin-preserving approach to delayed breast reconstruction (minimal or no need to resect breast skin at mastectomy) and who desire breast reconstruction are considered candidates for delayed-delayed breast reconstruction. Patients who undergo delayed-delayed breast reconstruction undergo neoadjuvant chemotherapy to reduce the morbidity of the extirpative resection (minimize need to resect breast skin) and to theoretically decrease any subclinical involvement of the dermal lymphatics located

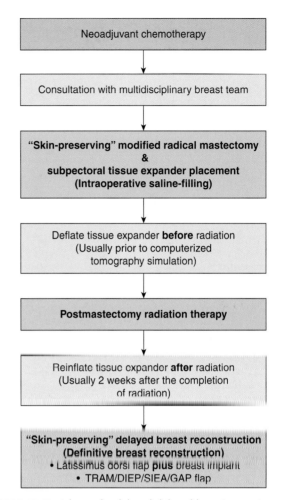

FIGURE 75-5 Schema for delayed-delayed breast reconstruction. Patients who undergo delayed-delayed breast reconstruction undergo neoadjuvant chemotherapy to decrease the morbidity of mastectomy, including decreasing the need to resect breast skin and to treat any subclinical involvement of the dermal lymphatics that may increase the propensity for recurrence after mastectomy, despite the use of postmastectomy radiation therapy (PMRT). At MD Anderson, patients with clinical stage IIB and III are evaluated preoperatively by a multidisciplinary breast cancer team to determine their eligibility for delayed-delayed breast reconstruction, which includes the minimal need to resect breast skin at mastectomy. Most patients with locally advanced breast cancer do not have skin involvement, but the skin is usually resected anyway, in an elliptical fashion by the breast surgeon to avoid skin redundancy because no immediate intervention at skin preservation has been planned. Patients then proceed to a skin-preserving mastectomy with immediate placement of a fully inflated tissue expander that preserves the shape and dimensions of the breast skin envelope. Before the computerized tomography simulation for planning the radiation delivery, the expander is deflated in an office-based setting to create a flat wall surface for radiation delivery. Several weeks after the completion of radiation therapy and resolution of any radiation-induced skin desquamation, the expander is reinflated over several office visits to the predeflation saline-fill volume. Approximately 3 months after completion of PMRT along with the subsequent reinflation of the expander, the tissue expander is removed and definitive reconstruction is performed using the preserved breast skin envelope, usually along with an autologous tissue flap. (DIEP, deep inferior epigastric perforator flap; GAP, gluteal artery perforator flap; TRAM, transverse rectus abdominis myocutaneous flap.)

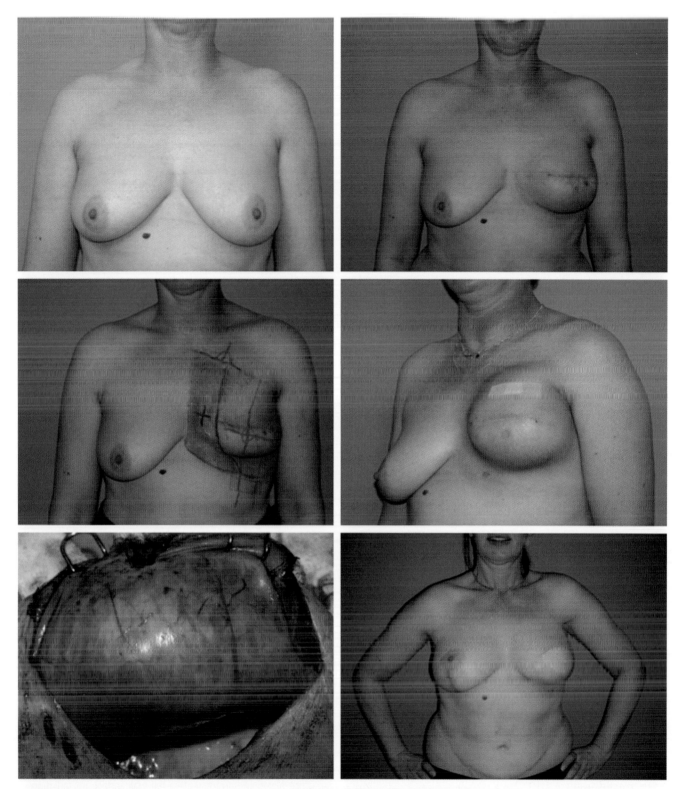

FIGURE 75-6 Delayed-delayed breast reconstruction in a 45-year old female who presented with a T2N3M0 left breast cancer who was known preoperatively to require postmastectomy radiation therapy (PMRT). (*Above, left*) Preoperative view after neoadjuvant chemo-therapy. (*Above, right*) Several weeks after stage I (subpectoral tissue expander at the time of mastectomy) with an intraoperative saline fill volume of 500 mL. (*Center, left*) The tissue expander was deflated in clinic to result in a flat chest wall surface for the delivery of external beam irradiation just before the start of PMRT. (*Center, right*) Seventeen days after PMRT, the patient was reinflated over 8 weeks to the predeflation volume of 500 mL. (*Below, left*) After removal of the expander, the remaining scar capsule layer is an ideal vascularized recipient for the nonradiated flap to revascularize the preserved breast skin. (*Below, right*) Sixteen months after removal of the tissue expander along with a skin-preserving delayed reconstruction with a deep inferior epigastric perforator (DIEP) flap and 22 months after PMRT with no evidence of contracture. The patient also underwent a right vertical mastopexy for symmetry.

within the breast skin that may increase the propensity for recurrence, despite the use of PMRT. Patients then proceed to a skin-preserving mastectomy with immediate placement of a fully inflated tissue expander that preserves the shape and dimensions of the breast skin envelope. Immediate expander placement with complete saline-filling also immediately initiates the formation of a scar capsule around the expander (especially important in patients who undergo neoadjuvant therapy who will be ready for PMRT 4 to 6 weeks after mastectomy), which creates a large-potential internal capsule-lined space that is formed before deflation (required for PMRT) of the expander and the initiation of PMRT. Creation of the internal scar capsule-lined potential space before expander deflation for PMRT maintains this space throughout PMRT, despite the inflammatory effects of PMRT, and allows for the ease of reinflation after the completion of PMRT. Before the computerized tomography simulation for planning the radiation delivery, the expander is deflated in an office-based setting to create a flat wall surface for radiation delivery. Several weeks after the completion of radiation therapy and resolution of any radiation-induced skin desquamation, the expander is reinflated over several office visits to the predeflation saline-fill volume. Approximately 3 months after completion of PMRT along with the subsequent reinflation of the expander, the tissue expander is removed and definitive reconstruction is performed usually with an autologous tissue flap (Fig. 75-6).

FUTURE DIRECTIONS

Currently, the greatest risk to the future of immediate breast reconstruction is that the need for PMRT cannot be reliably determined in all patients before or at the time of mastectomy because recommendations for radiation therapy are often based on pathologic analysis of sections obtained from the mastectomy specimen. Although delaying breast reconstruction in all patients may avoid the compromising situation of immediate reconstruction's being performed in a patient subsequently found (after pathologic review of the mastectomy specimen) to require PMRT, routinely delaying reconstruction also denies patients who ultimately do not require PMRT the potential benefits of immediate reconstruction. Until we can reliably predict the need for PMRT, decrease its adverse effects through more targeted therapy, and ensure optimal radiation delivery after immediate breast reconstruction, delayed-immediate reconstruction may be the best option to maintain the balance between optimal aesthetic outcomes and effective radiation delivery. Unfortunately, many major medical centers are increasing the use of delayed reconstruction. If new strategies such as delayed-immediate reconstruction are not adopted, patients may be denied one of the most significant advances in breast reconstruction—skin-sparing mastectomy—and more patients may have to awaken from mastectomy without a breast and with the prospect of less optimal outcomes.

SUMMARY

The optimal timing and technique of breast reconstruction in patients who may require PMRT is controversial. To help surgeons make the best decisions, we reviewed the recent literature on this topic. Even with the latest prosthetic materials and modern radiation delivery techniques, the complication rate for implant-based breast reconstruction in patients undergoing PMRT is greater than 40%, and the extrusion rate is 15%. Modified sequencing of 2-stage implant reconstruction such that the expander is exchanged for the permanent implant before PMRT results in higher rates of capsular contracture and is not generally feasible after neoadjuvant chemotherapy. Current evidence suggests that PMRT also adversely affects autologous tissue reconstruction. Even with modern radiation delivery techniques, immediate implant-based or autologous tissue breast reconstruction can distort the chest wall and limit the ability to treat the targeted tissues without excessive exposure of the heart and lungs. In patients for whom PMRT appears likely but may not be required, delayed-immediate reconstruction, in which tissue expanders are placed at mastectomy, avoids the difficulties associated with radiation delivery after immediate reconstruction and preserves the opportunity for the aesthetic benefits of skin-sparing mastectomy. In patients who will receive or have already received PMRT, the optimal approach is delayed autologous tissue reconstruction after PMRT. If PMRT appears likely but may not be required, delayed-immediate reconstruction may be considered.

REFERENCES

1. Spear SL, Onyewu C. Staged breast reconstruction with saline-filled implants in the irradiated breast: recent trends and therapeutic implications. *Plast Reconstr Surg.* 2000;105:930-942.
2. Ascherman JA, Hanasono MW, Newman MI, et al. Implant reconstruction in breast cancer patients with radiation therapy. *Plast Reconstr Surg.* 2006;117:359-365.
3. Benediktsson K, Perbeck L. Capsular contracture around saline-filled and textured subcutaneously placed implants in irradiated and non-irradiated breast cancer patients: five years of monitoring of a prospective trial. *J Plast Reconstr Aesthet Surg.* 2006;59:27-34.
4. Behranwala KA, Dua RS, Ross GM, et al. The influence of radiotherapy on capsule formation and aesthetic outcome after immediate breast reconstruction using biodimensional anatomical expander implants. *J Plast Reconstr Aesthet Surg.* 2006;59:1043-1051.
5. Cordeiro PG, Pusic AL, Disa JJ, et al. Irradiation after immediate tissue expander/implant breast reconstruction: outcomes, complications, aesthetic results, and satisfaction among 156 patients. *Plast Reconstr Surg.* 2004;113:877-881.
6. McCarthy CM, Pusic AL, Disa JJ, et al. Unilateral postoperative chest wall radiotherapy in bilateral tissue expander/implant reconstruction patients: a prospective outcomes analysis. *Plast Reconstr Surg.* 2005;116:1642-1647.
7. Schechter NR, Strom EA, Perkins GH, et al. Immediate breast reconstruction can impact postmastectomy irradiation. *Am J Clin Oncol.* 2005;28:485-494.
8. Evans GR, Schusterman MA, Kroll SS, et al. Reconstruction and the radiated breast: is there a role for implants? *Plast Reconstr Surg.* 1995;96:1111-1115.
9. Spear SL, Boehmler JH, Taylor NS, et al. The role of the latissimus dorsi flap in reconstruction of the irradiated breast. *Plast Reconstr Surg.* 2007;119:1-9.
10. Woodward W, Strom EA, Tucker SL, et al. Locoregional recurrence after doxorubicin-based chemotherapy and postmastectomy radiation: implications for patients with early stage disease and predictors for recurrence after radiation. *Int J Radiat Oncol Biol Phys.* 2003;57:336-344.
11. Kronowitz SJ, Robb GL. Breast reconstruction with postmastectomy radiation therapy: current issues. *Plast Reconstr Surg.* 2004;114:950-960.
12. Kronowitz SJ. Immediate versus delayed reconstruction. *Clin Plast Surg.* 2007;34:39-50.
13. Kronowitz SJ, Kuerer HM. Advances and surgical decision-making for breast reconstruction. *Cancer.* 2006;107:893-907.

14. Kronowitz SJ, Hunt KK, Kuerer HM, et al. Delayed-immediate breast reconstruction. *Plast Reconstr Surg.* 2004;113:1617-1628.

15. Buchholz TA, Strom EA, Perkins GH, et al. Controversies regarding the use of radiation after mastectomy in breast cancer. *Oncologist.* 2002;7:539-546.

16. Motwani SB, Strom EA, Schechter NR, et al. The impact of immediate breast reconstruction on the technical delivery of postmastectomy radiotherapy. *Int J Radiat Oncol Biol Phys.* 2006;66:76-82.

17. Damast S, Beal K, Ballangrud A, et al. Do metallic ports in tissue expanders affect postmastectomy radiation therapy? *Int J Radiat Oncol Biol Phys.* 2006;66:305-310.

18. Moni J, Graves-Ditman M, Cederna P, et al. Dosimetry around metallic ports in tissue expanders in patients receiving postmastectomy radiation therapy: an ex vivo evaluation. *Med Dosim.* 2004;29:49-54.

19. Jackson WB, Goldson AL, Staud C. Postoperative irradiation following immediate breast reconstruction using a temporary tissue expander. *J Natl Med Assoc.* 1994;86:538-542.

20. Williams JK, Carlson GW, Bostwick J III, et al. The effects of radiation treatment after TRAM flap breast reconstruction. *Plast Reconstr Surg.* 1997;100:1153-1160.

21. Tran NV, Chang DW, Gupta A, et al. Comparison of immediate and delayed TRAM flap breast reconstruction in patients receiving postmastectomy radiation therapy. *Plast Reconstr Surg.* 2001;108:78-82.

22. Rogers NE, Allen RJ. Radiation effects on breast reconstruction with the deep inferior epigastric perforator flap. *Plast Reconstr Surg.* 2002;109:1919-1924.

23. Spear SL, Ducic I, Low M, et al. The effect of radiation therapy on pedicled TRAM flap breast reconstruction: outcomes and implications. *Plast Reconstr Surg.* 2005;115:84-95.

24. Chawla AK, Kachnic LA, Taghian AG, et al. Radiotherapy and breast reconstruction: complications and cosmesis with TRAM versus tissue expander/implant. *Int J Radiat Oncol Biol Phys.* 2002;54:520-526.

25. Katz A, Strom EA, Buchholz TA, et al. Locoregional recurrence patterns after mastectomy and doxorubicin-based chemotherapy: implications for postoperative irradiation. *J Clin Oncol.* 2000;18:2817-2827.

26. Recht A, Gray R, Davidson NE, et al. Locoregional failure ten years after mastectomy and adjuvant chemotherapy with or without tamoxifen without irradiation: experience of the Eastern Cooperative Oncology Group. *J Clin Oncol.* 1999;17:1689-1700.

27. Kroll SS, Schusterman MA, Reece GP, et al. Breast reconstruction with myocutaneous flaps in previously irradiated patients. *Plast Reconstr Surg.* 1994;93:460-469.

28. Kronowitz SJ, Chang DW, Robb GL, et al. Implications of axillary sentinel lymph node biopsy in immediate autologous breast reconstruction. *Plast Reconstr Surg.* 2002;109:1888-1896.

CHAPTER 76

Partial Breast Reconstruction Using Local Tissue

Albert Losken

Breast conservation therapy (BCT) is a popular treatment option for women with breast cancer, and that trend continues to rise.[1] This is in part driven by equivalent survival rates and by preservation of body image, quality of life, and reduced psychological morbidity with breast-sparing surgery.[2,3] However, there remains an innate conflict between the goals of oncology and cosmesis, with the former being to eliminate all locoregional disease, and the latter relying on preservation of as much breast tissue as possible for optimal aesthetic outcome. The wider the margin of resection, the lower the risk of local recurrence,[4,5] and it often becomes a dilemma for the surgeon to meet both these end points. Breast shape becomes compromised and significant contour deformities, breast asymmetry, and poor aesthetic outcomes are not uncommon. Up to 30% of women will have a residual deformity that may require surgical correction,[6] the correction of which is often difficult.[7]

In order to support the complex nature of the ever-expanding criteria for breast conservation, there has been a surge of reconstructive techniques for the partial mastectomy defect prior to breast irradiation, often referred to as the oncoplastic approach. This approach is intended to improve outcomes from both an oncologic as well as a cosmetic standpoint by combining the principles of oncology and plastic surgery.

OPTIONS AVAILABLE FOR RECONSTRUCTING THE PARTIAL MASTECTOMY DEFECT

The 2 main options available include (1) volume displacement techniques using parenchymal remodeling (volume shrinkage) and (2) volume replacement techniques using local or distant tissue (volume preserving). The decision is usually based on tumor characteristics (size and location), breast characteristics (size and shape), and patient desires. Large- or moderate-sized breasts, or ptotic breasts with sufficient parenchyma remaining

following resection are amenable to reshaping procedures. When additional tissue (volume and skin) is required to maintain the desired breast size or shape (ie, smaller or nonptotic breasts), volume replacement procedures are required. The focus of this chapter is volume displacement (parenchymal modeling) techniques using local breast tissue.

VOLUME DISPLACEMENT TECHNIQUES

Breast reshaping procedures all essentially rely on advancement, rotation, or transposition of a large area of breast to fill a small- or moderate-sized defect. This absorbs the volume loss over a larger area. In its simplest form, it entails mobilizing the breast plate from the area immediately around the defect in a *breast flap advancement technique* as proposed by Anderson et al.[8]

Other local breast options include *dermatoglandular flaps* to fill small defects that might otherwise have caused an unfavorable result due to skin or parenchymal deficiency being inadequately reconstructed.

The use of *reduction or mastopexy techniques* to reconstruct the partial mastectomy defect prior to breast irradiation has recently become more popular, and will be discussed in detail below. This approach initially became popular in Europe for reconstructing quadrantectomy defects in the lower pole.[9] In the United States, the popularity likely evolved out of frustration in the management of breast cancer patients with macromastia.[10-13] Plastic surgeons are all familiar with these techniques, making the incorporation of this approach into their reconstructive practice an easy addition. Women with large pendulous breasts are often more difficult to reconstruct following total mastectomy due to body habitus and the inherent difficulty associated with skin envelope reduction and other morbidities. They are often deemed poor candidates for reconstruction and associated with increased complications and unfavorable cosmetic results (Fig. 76-1).

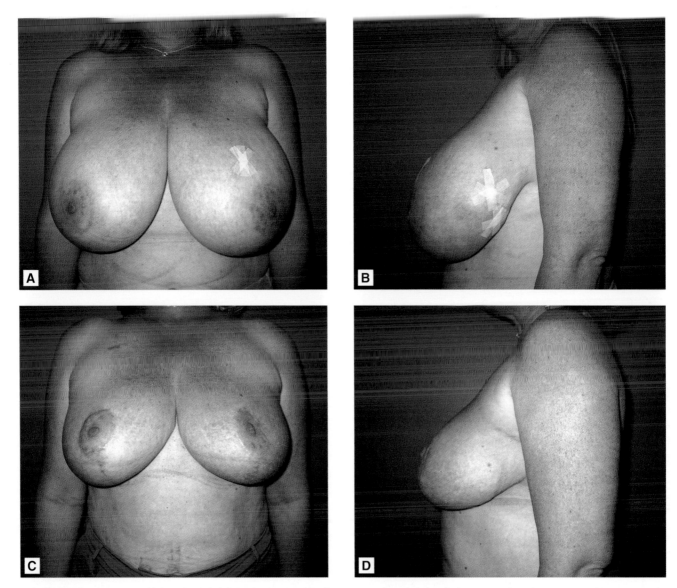

FIGURE 76-1 A 46-year-old female with bilateral macromastia (bra size 36G) with left-sided invasive ductal carcinoma. She expressed an interest in breast preservation and it was felt that given her large breasts she would be a better candidate with a simultaneous breast reduction. Skin-sparing mastectomy and reconstruction would be difficult given her breast size and body habitus. She had a left partial mastectomy (225 g) from the lateral quadrant with clear margins. A simultaneous superomedial breast reduction was performed removing an additional tissue g from the left breast and 1205 g from the right side. She is shown 6 months following radiation therapy with preservation of shape and symmetry.

Macromastia was initially felt to be a relative contraindication to BCT with poor cosmetic results, greater radiation fibrosis, and less effective radiation therapy.[14-17] On the other hand, women with macromastia and large pendulous breasts are often overweight, and total breast reconstruction is more challenging, being associated with higher complication rates and less favorable cosmetic outcomes. The addition of reduction mammaplasty techniques was therefore welcomed by the patient, the resective surgeon, and the reconstructive surgeon. It allows women with macromastia to be candidates for breast conservation without having to accept significant deformities; it allows the resective surgeon to remove a generous amount without having to worry about a residual deformity; and it makes breast reconstruction more predictable in an otherwise difficult patient population.

Women with large tumor to breast ratios and women with small to moderate breasts who have insufficient residual breast tissue for rearrangement require partial reconstruction using nonbreast local or distant flaps.

INDICATIONS

The indications for partial breast reconstruction using local tissue are numerous. The 2 main reasons to reconstruct partial mastectomy defects are (1) to increase the indications for BCT, making breast conservation practical in patients who otherwise might require a mastectomy, and (2) to minimize the potential for a poor aesthetic result.

Women with large pendulous breasts who are felt by the surgeon to be poor candidates for BCT alone benefit from the oncoplastic reduction techniques, minimizing the potential for a poor cosmetic result and allowing them to be candidates for breast conservation. The ideal patient is one whose tumor can be widely excised within the reduction specimen, and for whom a smaller breast is viewed as a positive outcome. Older women with macromastia are well suited for this approach compared to mastectomy and reconstruction. Another indication for the oncoplastic reduction technique is when the surgeon anticipates a large defect, or is concerned about being able to achieve clear margins in women with moderate to large breasts (Fig. 76-2). The potential for an unfavorable result exists in this situation regardless of breast size or tumor location. Other indications are patient driven, in those women who desire breast conservation, or who desire smaller breasts due to their limitations caused by symptomatic macromastia. As we become more comfortable with these techniques the indications will become more liberal. Essentially anyone with large breasts amenable to breast conservation is a candidate for this procedure. However, the importance of stringent patient selection criteria cannot be overstated, and is required to ensure minimal cosmetic outcomes as well as oncological safety.

Partial mastectomy defects in the central or lateral location, or high tumor to breast ratios (more than 20%) will often benefit from reconstruction. Mastopexy techniques that reposition the nipple will often allow preservation of shape and symmetry in ptotic or even asymmetric breasts when used in combination with lumpectomy.

CONTRAINDICATIONS

Contraindications include patients who are not good candidates for breast conservation, a history of prior irradiation, or situations when there is insufficient residual breast tissue following resection to allow reshaping. Similar selection criteria are used when deciding on elective breast reduction procedures and need to be taken into consideration. Patients with multiple medical comorbidities or active smokers are not ideal candidates for additional elective surgery, and the risks will often outweigh the benefits in these situations.

TIMING

The general trend is to reconstruct the partial mastectomy defect prior to breast irradiation with the benefits of not operating on an irradiated, scarred, and contracted breast where the lack of elasticity makes reconstruction more difficult. Reconstruction prior to radiation therapy is considered *immediate reconstruction*. There are situations where poor results are encountered years following radiation therapy, which then require *delayed reconstruction*. Similar techniques are employed in delayed reconstruction, more often requiring flaps such as the latissimus dorsi myocutaneous flap, and are associated with

higher complication rates (42% vs 26%) and worse cosmetic outcome.[7] The main concern with immediate reconstruction is the potential for positive margins. *Delayed-immediate reconstruction* is another alternative where the reconstruction is delayed a week until final margin status has been determined. This gives the benefit of immediate reconstruction with the luxury of negative margins, however, at the expense of a second procedure.

MARGINS

One of the most important variables in ensuring a safe oncologic outcome is patient selection and how it relates to margin status. Positive margins on final are potentially complicated by altered architecture if parenchymal rearrangement has already been performed. The options for managing positive margins include reexcision or completion mastectomy and reconstruction. The extent of the disease in these situations, especially given the previous generous oncoplastic resection, will often dictate that completion mastectomy is a more appropriate treatment plan. If reexcision is performed, this needs to be done with the reconstructive surgeon. Fortunately the incidence of positive margins using this approach is felt to be less given the more generous resections. We have demonstrated specimen weight over 200 g in oncoplastic resections, compared to about 50 g for nononcoplastic procedures (Fig. 76-1).[10,18] The incidence of positive margins is less in oncoplastic resections.[19] When completion mastectomy and reconstruction is required, the disadvantages of the reduction procedure are minimal. The benefits of this approach are that (1) no reconstruction options (ie, flaps) have been used; (2) the contralateral symmetry procedure has already been performed; (3) skin envelope has been reduced; and (4) it is now easier to reconstruct a smaller reduced breast than a large ptotic one.

One way to avoid positive margins is to delay reconstruction a few weeks until confirmation of margin status has been obtained (delayed-immediate reconstruction). Most series report a positive margin rate of about 5% to 10%, and rather than perform an unnecessary second procedure 90% to 95% of the time, we need to minimize the incidence of positive margins. *Preoperative breast imaging* (ie, magnetic resonance imaging [MRI], ultrasound, or mammography) is helpful in determining the extent of the disease guiding the necessary resection and should be employed judiciously when indicated. An imaging study showed that tumor size was underestimated 14% by mammography and 18% by ultrasound, whereas MRI showed no difference when compared to the pathological specimen.[20] *Separate cavity margins* sent at the time of lumpectomy significantly reduce the need for reexcision. Cao et al demonstrated that final margin status was negative in 60% of patients with positive margins on initial resection.[21] Additional intraoperative confirmatory procedures include radiography of the specimen and intraoperative frozen sections for invasive cancer. *Patient selection* is another important consideration. A recent series has demonstrated a higher rate of positive margins in women under the age of 40 years old with extensive ductal carcinoma in situ (DCIS), suggesting delayed immediate reconstruction in

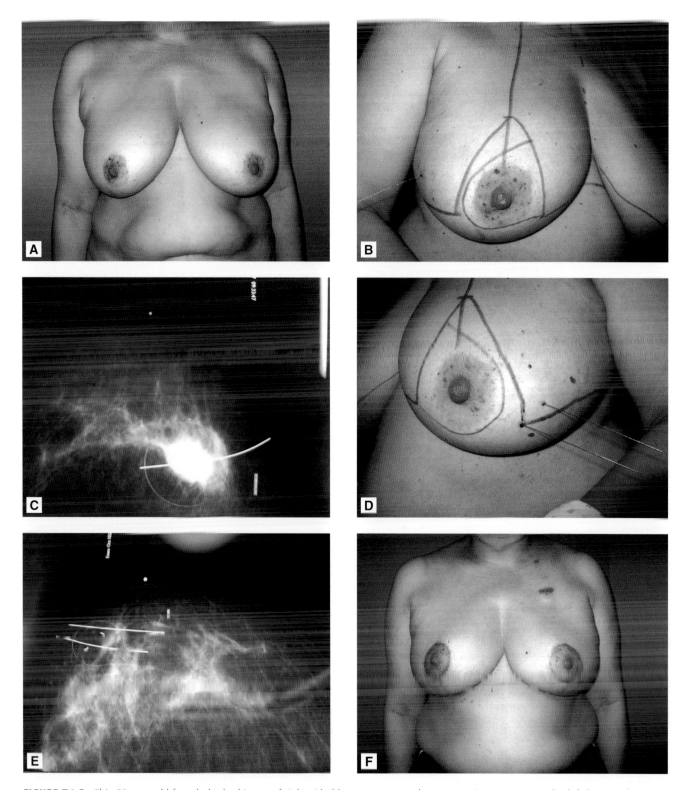

FIGURE 76-2 This 53-year-old female had a history of right-sided breast cancer and some suspicious areas on the left breast. She underwent a right lateral partial mastectomy (200 g) and an additional 80 g with her simultaneous superomedial breast reduction. On the left side her biopsy was negative for carcinoma with the specimen weight 90 g, and an additional 250 g from that side.

those situations.[10] Other patients with potentially difficult margin issues include those with prior chemotherapy, infiltrating lobular carcinoma, and multicentric disease. In these patients, and in any other patient where there is intraoperative concern regarding margin status, the reconstruction should be delayed until margin status has been confirmed.

OPERATIVE APPROACH

If *preoperative planning* is being performed by a 2-team approach, then it is crucial that communication exists between the teams. They should review the radiographic imaging together, and discuss the anticipated defect location and defect size. This will assist with determination of the most appropriate glandular pedicle required to maintain nipple viability and reshape the mound. A backup plan is important as occasionally the defect is different from that anticipated, and an alternative approach is required. The patient is marked preoperatively on both sides, outlining the breast boundaries. If a Wise Pattern is drawn, vertical limbs are slightly longer than normal, and the angle is smaller (to ensure minimal tension on the incisions and reduce the potential for healing problems). If radiographically placed wires are being used for the lumpectomy, these should be examined and films reviewed. The combined team should discuss possible access incisions on the mound for tumor resection. Poorly placed incisions could interfere with viability of skin flaps and worsen results.

Tumor resection is performed with oncoplastic principles in mind, to provide the most aesthetic scars and ones that will complement local tissue reconstruction and not violate potential options. When reduction techniques are being used, the resection is performed within Wise Patterns if possible, with attention to blood supply and nipple viability. The specimen is weighed to assist with determination of resection goals on the contralateral side. Intraoperative margin assessment could include radiographic imaging, macroscopic assessment, frozen section, or touch cytology. Once separate cavity samples are sent to pathology, the cavity is clipped for postoperative surveillance and guidance for radiation boosts to the tumor bed if required.

Partial mastectomy *reconstruction* is initiated by examining the defect in terms of size and location. It is important to examine the remaining breast tissue, and determine where it is in relation to the defect, the nipple, and the breast mound.

Advancement and Dermatoglandular Flaps

Nipple position is typically preserved. Flaps are mobilized of the chest wall in a full thickness fashion. When advancement flaps are being used, the dissection is over the pectoralis muscle and essentially involves a full-thickness segment of breast fibroglandular tissue advanced to fill the dead space. These procedures are indicated for small- to medium-sized breasts and upper pole defects where the resection does not lead to any significant volume alteration that might cause breast asymmetry. A contralateral symmetry procedure is typically not required. Dermatoglandular flaps also involve skin and parenchyma, and are rotated in to fill the central or lateral defect. They are elevated in a full thickness fashion and often are lifted off the chest wall to adequately rotate without unnecessary tension on the

nipple or residual breast mound (Fig. 76-3). The orientation of these flaps is such that incisions are within aesthetic units and breast shape is preserved. Once again, for smaller defects, a contralateral symmetry procedure is often not required.

Reduction Techniques

Reduction techniques require meticulous preoperative planning and coordinating with the various services. Intraoperative decisions are equally important. The first decision is *how to keep the nipple alive*. Typically the shortest pedicle will maximize nipple viability and allow additional glandular manipulation without worrying about nipple compromise. Many options exist for nipple pedicles, and most surgeons have a favorite. For example, if the superomedial pedicle is your procedure of choice for standard breast reductions, then this technique could be employed for most oncoplastic defects if the patient is a candidate, as long as the defect location is not medial to the nipple. As a general rule, if the pedicle points to or can be rotated into the defect, it can be used. Occasionally, it is not possible to preserve the nipple, either because of the size of the breasts or the location of the tumor. Options include amputation and free nipple graft, or nipple reconstruction at a later date.

Once a decision has been made on nipple preservation, the pedicle is then delineated and dissected with the cautery unit enough to allow rotation into the proposed nipple position. *The second decision then is how to fill the dead space.* At this point glandular resection has not yet been performed. If the defect is removed as part of a reduction specimen, and is adequately filled through glandular displacement with the pedicle and/or remaining glandular tissue, then autoaugmentation is not required. If it is felt that additional glandular flaps are required to fill the dead space, as determined above, then a decision is made based on what tissue is available and where it is in relation to the nipple pedicle. If the defect can be filled by rotating an extended portion of the original nipple pedicle this is often the technique of choice. Once it has been determined how to fill the dead space and reshape a breast mound, the *excess dermatoglandular tissue can then be resected.* The weight of the specimen is then added to this additional resection, calculating a total weight for that side. This is useful in trying to keep the ipsilateral breast larger. The *breast mound shaping* is then performed using the glandular pedicles and remaining breast tissue. Glandular shaping is performed using resorbable sutures where necessary, and the skin is then redraped over the mound. Drains are used if the defect is in communication with the axillary dissection.

Skin Pattern

The Wise Pattern markings are more versatile and allow easy access to tumor location anywhere within the breast mound. It also gives more options to reconstruct the defect using glandular flaps. If it is unclear whether glandular flaps will be required to reconstruct the defect, the standard Wise flaps can be elevated about 1-in thick up to the chest wall without resecting any additional breast tissue or skin. Numerous options will then exist for either primary or secondary pedicles to keep the nipple alive or fill the defect with the skin flaps then re-draped over the mound to complete the reconstruction. The vertical type reduction or

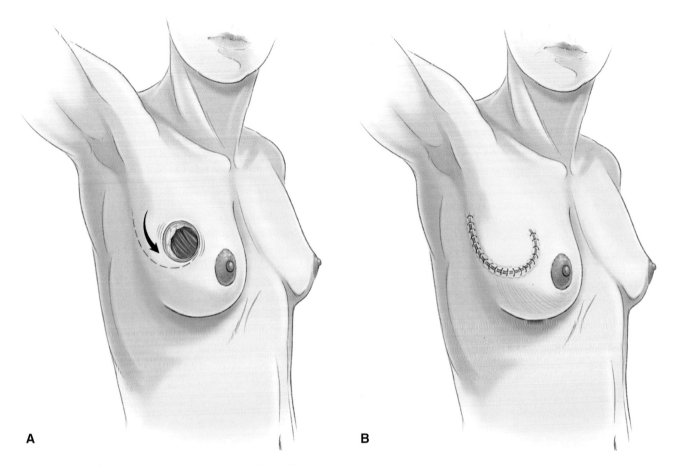

A   **B**

FIGURE 76-3 A lateral pole defect in a patient with small breasts being reconstructed using local fasciocutaneous flaps.

mastopexy is useful for smaller breasts, when the defect is easily accessed through this approach.

Contralateral Breast

Management of the contralateral breast is typically performed using a similar technique to that used on the ipsilateral side to maximize symmetry. If an inferior pedicle was used on the involved breasts, an inferior pedicle is often chosen on the contralateral side. Since the ipsilateral side involves a volume loss procedure (partial mastectomy), glandular resection is always required on the opposite breast, even if a mastopexy technique was used for partial breast reconstruction. The contralateral side is purposely kept about 10% smaller than the ipsilateral breasts to allow for anticipated radiation fibrosis (Fig. 76-4). My preference is to

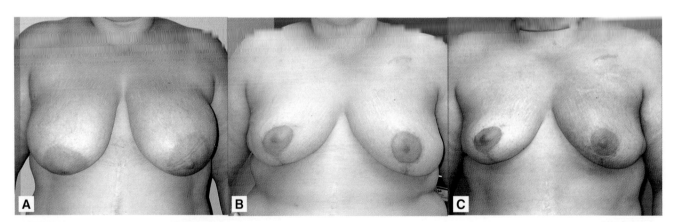

A   **B**   **C**

FIGURE 76-4 A 49-year-old woman with a left stage I ductal carcinoma in the inner quadrant **(A)** who underwent a 195-g resection with immediate reduction reconstruction removing 502 g (including lumpectomy) from the left breast and 536 g from the right. The left breast is larger immediately postoperatively **(B)** with improvement at 2 years following radiation therapy **(C)**. *[Reproduced, with permission, from Losken A, Styblo IM, Carlson GW, Jones G, Amerson B. Management algorithm and outcome evaluation of partial mastectomy defects treated using reduction or mastopexy techniques. Ann Plast Surg. 2007;59(3):235.]*

perform the contralateral procedure at the time of resection. If minor changes in shape and size of the contralateral side are required years after radiation therapy these "fine tuning" procedures are easier and more predictable than doing the full reduction at that time, which might then require additional revisions to maximize symmetry. Other options include doing the opposite breast following breast irradiation which then would commit a second procedure in everyone, which is often unnecessary since the contralateral revision rate when done simultaneously is only about 5% to 10%. It is important that the contralateral breast tissue be sent to pathology given the 2% to 5% incidence of synchronous breast cancer being diagnosed on that side in women with breast cancer.[10,11]

Reconstruction by Defect Location

Lower quadrant tumors in women with larger breasts are ideally suited for the oncoplastic reduction or mastopexy approach. Quadrantectomy type resections are possible, removing skin and parenchyma from this location, reshaping the breast using a superior or superomedial pedicle. Lower pole tumors in moderate-sized breasts can be excised along with skin as needed in the usual vertical pattern utilizing a superior pedicle followed by plication of the vertical pillars, and vertical reduction on the contralateral side (Fig. 76-5). *Upper quadrant tumors* can be filled as long as the defect is under the skin. Autoaugmentation techniques have become popular to fill the

dead space and maintain shape. Inferior, medial, or central pedicles allow for safe excisions in the upper half of the breast without impairing nipple viability (Fig. 76-6). When skin is resected in the upper half of the breast, such remodeling techniques are not possible.

Lateral or upper-outer quadrant defects allow parenchymal remodeling using the superomedial pedicle or inferior pedicle (Fig. 76-1). Upper-outer quadrant defects can be more difficult to reconstruct when insufficient residual breast tissue is present in that location to fill the defect. In women with medium-sized ptotic breasts and moderate volume void in the upper-outer quadrant, the superomedial pedicle can be extended down to the inframammary fold as an autoaugmentated pedicle. This can then be rotated to fill a lateral volume void. The vertical pillars are then plicated in the usual fashion to maintain shape.

Medial defects are often reconstructed using inferior lateral or central type pedicles (Fig. 76-7). When the defect is above the proposed Wise Pattern markings, the remaining breast parenchyma below the markings is preserved and used to fill the defect. Any contour irregularities in the medial quadrant significantly affect shape and need to be avoided.

Central tumors have in the past been considered relative contraindications to BCT; however, with the oncoplastic approach in women with macromastia the tumor and nipple areolar complex can be widely excised and reconstructed using a variety of techniques.[22,23] The mound can be remodeled in the inverted T-closure pattern, similar to formal amputation

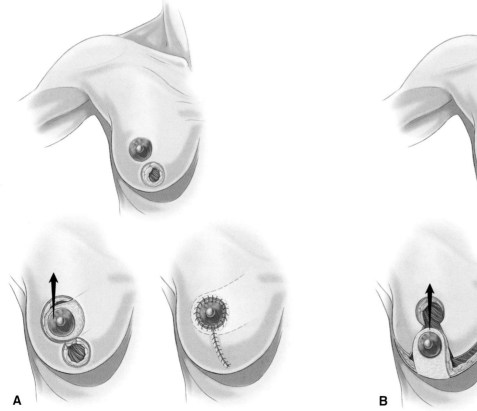
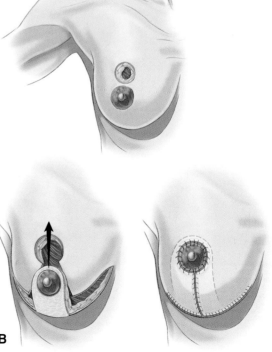

FIGURE 76-5 A. Illustration demonstrating a lower pole defect being reconstructed using a superomedial mastopexy type approach. **B.** Illustration demonstrating an upper pole defect being reconstructed using an inferior pedicle reduction technique.

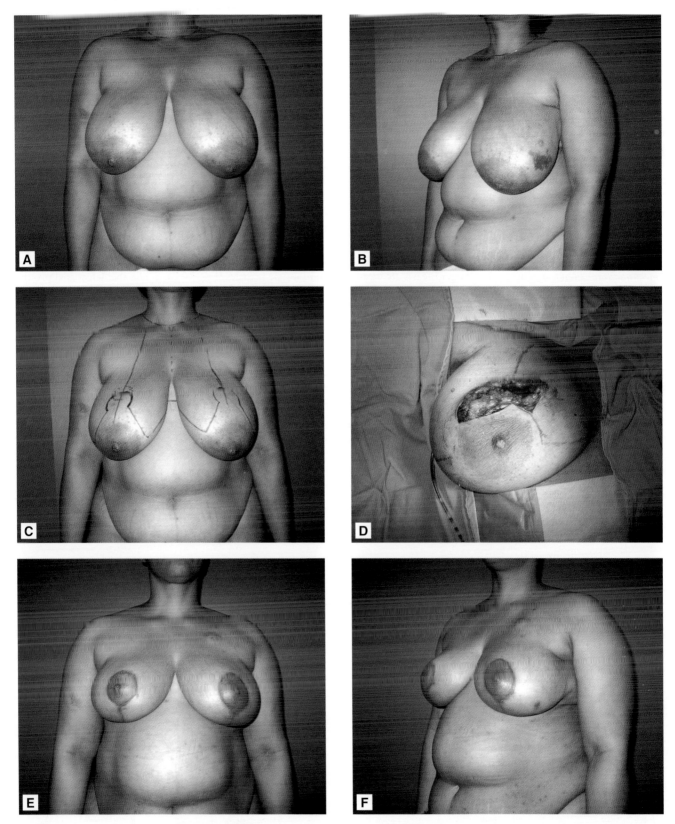

FIGURE 76-6 A 40-year-old female with an upper pole breast cancer relatively close to the skin who desired breast conservation. She had a 125-g resection including skin and parenchyma from above the nipple-areola complex. Once confirmation of margin status was achieved, she underwent a bilateral breast reduction utilizing the inferior pedicle with a total of 475 g on the right (including specimen) and 525 g on the left. Her shape and symmetry are preserved despite a generous resection.

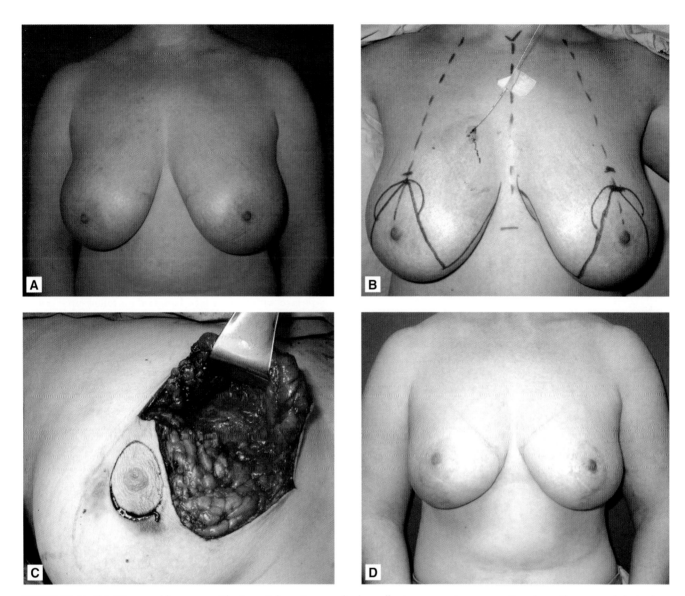

FIGURE 76-7 This 33-year-old woman with stage III breast cancer had excellent response to preoperative chemotherapy and desired breast conservation. In order to minimize the potential for a poor cosmetic result with a defect in the upper pole, she underwent a right wire-guided lumpectomy (100 g) with simultaneous bilateral breast reduction (total volumes 250 g left and 150 g right). The nipple was moved based on an inferiorly based dermatoglandular pedicle. Her result is shown at 1 year following completion of right breast radiation therapy.

reduction techniques. The nipple is then reconstructed later using the reconstruction technique of choice. When the nipple is spared, it can be replaced as a free nipple graft following reconstruction of the mound. Another option if the tumor is located more superiorly or lateral is to perform a central elliptical excision of skin, nipple, and parenchyma, and mirror image contralateral reduction for symmetry. A third option includes creation of a skin island on a dermatoglandular pedicle to rotate into the central defect to allow for shape preservation and nipple reconstruction. The breast is marked preoperatively for an inverted T or a vertical approach depending on breast size, and the skin island is brought in from inferior or medial.

OPERATIVE SEQUENCE

1. Decision to proceed with the oncoplastic approach to breast conservation, team discussion
   a. Immediate
   b. Delayed immediate
2. Preoperative marking
3. Wire placement in breast imaging if necessary
4. Another team discussion (resective and reconstructive surgeon)
5. Tumor excision with or without lymph node sampling
6. Mammographic confirmation with frozen sections if appropriate

7. Separate cavity sampling
8. Clip cavity for orientation
9. Evaluation of the deformity (size and location), and residual breast tissue
10. Intraoperative reconstructive goals
    a. Preserve nipple viability if possible, and position on the mound
    b. Elimination of dead space
    c. Resect excess breast parenchyma and skin
    d. Reshape breast to preserve shape
    e. Contralateral procedure for symmetry if necessary

OUTCOME

Local recurrence is an important outcome measure; however, longer-term studies are required before any definitive conclusions can be made regarding tumor recurrence and survival. It has been proposed that local recurrence would be less given the ability to widely excise the tumor. Studies on partial breast reconstruction are typically small, often lack oncological outcomes, and long-term results are not available.[18] This review of the literature found that on intermediate follow-up (up to 4.5 years), local recurrence rates varied from 0% to 1.8 % per year, and cosmetic failure rates varied from 0% to 18%. Clough et al demonstrated an actuarial 5-year local recurrence rate using this technique of 9.4%.[18] Another series of 70 patients who underwent oncoplastic surgery for breast cancer demonstrated an actuarial 5-year local recurrence rate of 8.5%.[25]

Postoperative *surveillance* is also important in this patient population, and in order for this approach to be deemed safe we need to demonstrate that it does not interfere with our ability to detect recurrence. One concern has been that the additional surgery and tissue rearrangement of breast tissue could potentially alter the architecture and influence the pattern of recurrence or ability to accurately screen. Surgical clips at the tumor margin will identify the tumor bed to assist with radiation boosts, postoperative surveillance, and reexploration if necessary. We have recently compared mammographic changes and surveillance in women with BCT alone versus those with oncoplastic reductions and found no interference in the accuracy of postsurveillance.[26] The other question we had was whether the combined procedure delayed the concept of mammographic stabilization, or reduced the sensitivity of this screening tool. There was a slight trend toward longer times to mammographic stabilization in the study group (21.2 months for BCT vs 25.6 months for oncoplastic, *p* = .23), which is expected given the additional scarring, inflammation, and parenchymal alteration associated with the reconstruction. This time to mammographic stability in the oncoplastic group demonstrated a 95% confidence interval between 20 and 30 months. Parenchymal density was similar in both groups suggesting that the sensitivity of mammography was not affected. This suggests longer than 6-months screening is necessary in these patients, possibly until about 2.5 to 3 years. Additional tissue sampling (fine-needle aspiration [FNA], core biopsy, etc) is often required given the nature of these combined procedures, and the importance of ruling out tumor recurrence. These issues all need to

be discussed with the patient preoperatively, as well as with the multidisciplinary team.

Local *wound healing complications* include delayed healing, skin necrosis, infection, and wound dehiscence; however, these are usually minimal and do not delay the initiation of neoadjuvant therapy. Most series have demonstrated excellent patient and surgeon satisfaction with the cosmetic results using these techniques; however, longer-term outcomes will be interesting especially given the persistent effects of radiation with time. Breast shape is typically preserved with time; however, some radiation fibrosis can be encountered. In these situations it is relatively easy to further reduce the contralateral breast than to reconstruct a radiated deformity.

Another important outcome measure is *patient satisfaction*. A limited group of women in our series report an acceptable aesthetic result in 95% of cases at 6 months follow-up. Although this is relatively short follow-up, patients are generally pleased with their results. Longer-term follow-up is crucial especially given the effects of radiation therapy on breast shape with time. Other series have reported favorable aesthetic results and patient satisfaction with this approach.

FUTURE DIRECTIONS

The oncoplastic approach to the management of women with early-stage breast cancer is relatively new, and most reports in the literature are small series reviews with relatively short follow-up. It will be interesting in the future to analyze these patients on a long-term basis, possibly even with multi-institutional studies, to evaluate outcomes from a cosmetic and oncologic basis. This will invariable allow us to provide more effective treatment algorithms and further refine our patient selection and surgical techniques, and ultimately improve patient satisfaction. Technological advances in breast imaging and radiation therapy (partial breast) are likely in the future and will also contribute to streamlining the process. There remains no clear consensus regarding training and organization, whether a 2-team or a single-surgeon approach. Future directions in board status, accreditation, and training curriculum will become evident as the popularity and demand for this approach continues. Despite these organizational differences, the ultimate goals are the same, which is why our cumulative efforts will continue to make advances and ultimately improve outcomes for women with breast cancer.

SUMMARY

The immediate reconstruction of partial mastectomy defects using local breast tissue is both safe and effective in appropriately selected patients. Its popularity will likely continue to increase given the increased demand for breast conservation and the decreased tolerance for poor cosmetic results. These techniques are often the preferred approach given their relative simplicity, predictability, and lack of a donor site, especially in women with macromastia, where mastectomy and reconstruction is often more difficult, with higher morbidity and worse cosmetic results. More stringent patient selection and attention to tumor resection will minimize the incidence of positive margins and improve outcome. This approach broadens the indications for BCT, preserves symmetry and shape, and maintains patients' satisfaction while maintaining successful oncological outcome and cancer surveillance.

REFERENCES

1. NCI Breast Cancer Database, 2007.
2. Fisher B, Anderson S, Bryant J, et al. Twenty-year follow up of a randomized trial comparing total mastectomy, lumpectomy, and lumpectomy plus irradiation of the treatment of invasive breast cancer. *N Eng J Med.* 2002;347:1233-1241.
3. Veronesi U, Casinelly N, Mariani L, et al. Twenty-year follow-up of a randomized study comparing breast conserving surgery with radical mastectomy for early breast cancer. *N Eng J Med.* 2002;347:1227-1232.
4. Silverstein MJ, Lagios MD, Groshen S, et al. The influence of margin width on local control of ductal carcinoma in situ of the breast. *N Engl J Med.* 1999;340:1455-1461.
5. Veronesi U, Volteranni F, Luini A, et al. Quadrantectomy versus lumpectomy for small size breast cancer. *Eur J Cancer.* 1990;26:671-673.
6. Clough KB, Cuminet J, Fitoussi A, et al. Cosmetic sequalae after conservative treatment for breast cancer: classification and results of surgical correction. *Ann Plast Surg.* 1998;41:471-481.
7. Kronowitz SJ, Feledy JA, Hunt KK, et al. Determining the optimal approach to breast reconstruction after partial mastectomy. *Plast Reconstr Surg.* 2006;117(1):1-11.
8. Anderson BO, Masetti R, Silverstein MJ. Oncoplastic approaches to partial mastectomy: an overview of volume replacement techniques. *Lancet Oncol.* 2005;6(3):145-157.
9. Clough KB, Nos C, Salmon RJ, Soussaline M, et al. Conservative treatment of breast cancer by mammaplasty and irradiation: a new approach to lower quadrant tumors. *Plast Reconstr Surg.* 1995;96(2):363-370.
10. Losken A, Styblo TM, Carlson GW, Jones G, Amerson B. Management algorithm and outcome evaluation of partial mastectomy defects treated using reduction or mastopexy techniques. *Ann Plast Surg.* 2007;(59)3:235.
11. Munhoz AM, Montag E, Arruda EG, et al. Critical analysis of reduction mammaplasty techniques in combination with conservative breast surgery for early breast cancer treatment. *Plast Reconstr Surg.* 2006;117(4):1091-1103.
12. Spear SL, Burke JB, Forman D, et al. Experience with reduction mammaplasty following breast conservation surgery and radiation therapy. *Plast Reconstr Surg.* 1998;102(6):1913-1916.
13. Kronowitz SJ, Hunt KK, Kuerer HM, et al. Practical guidelines for repair of partial mastectomy defects using the breast reduction technique in patients undergoing breast conservation therapy. *Plast Reconstr Surg.* 2007;120(7):1755.
14. Gray JR, McCormick B, Cox L, et al. Primary breast irradiation in large-breasted or heavy women: analysis of cosmetic outcome. *Int J Radiat Oncology Biol Phys.* 1991;21:347-354.
15. Zierhut D, Flentje M, Frank C, et al. Conservative treatment of breast cancer: modified irradiation technique for women with large breasts. *Radiother Oncol.* 1994;31:256-261.
16. Brierly JD, Paterson ICM, Lallemand RC, Rostom AY. The influence of breast size on late radiation reaction following excision and radiotherapy for early breast cancer. *Clin Oncol.* 1991;3:6-9.
17. Clark K, Le MG, Sarrazin D, et al. Analysis of locoregional relapse in patients with early breast cancer treated by excision and radiotherapy: experience of the Institute Gustave-Roussy. *Int J Radiat Oncol Biol Phys.* 1985;11:137-145.
18. Clough KB, Lewis JS, Couturaud B, et al. Oncoplastic techniques allow extensive resections for breast-conserving therapy of breast cancer. *Ann Surg.* 2003;237(1):26-34.
19. Kaur N, Petit JY, Rietjens M, Maffini F, et al. Comparative study of surgical margins in oncoplastic surgery and quadrantectomy in breast cancer. *Ann Surg Oncol.* 2005;12(7):539-545.
20. Boetes C, Mus RD, Holland R, et al. Breast tumors: comparative accuracy of MR imaging relative to mammography and US for demonstrating extent. *Radiology.* 1995;197:743-747.
21. Cao, D, Lin C, Woo SH, et al. Separate cavity margin sampling at the time of initial breast lumpectomy significantly reduces the need for re-excision. *Am J Surg Pathol.* 2005;29(12):1625-1632.
22. Chung TL, Schnaper L, Silverman R, et al. A novel reconstructive technique following central lumpectomy. *Plast Reconstr Surg.* 2006;118(1):23-27.
23. McCulley SJ, Dourani P, Macmillan RD. Therapeutic mammaplasty for centrally located breast tumors. *Plast Reconstr Surg.* 2006;117(2):366-373.
24. Asgeursson KS, Rasheed T, McCulley SJ, Macmillan RD. Oncological and cosmetic outcomes of oncoplastic breast conserving surgery. *Eur J Surg Oncol.* 2005;31(8):817-823.
25. Cothier-Savey I, Otmezguine Y, Calitchi E, et al. Value of reduction mammoplasty in the conservative treatment of breast neoplasm. Apropos of 70 cases. *Ann Chir Plast Esthet.* 1996;41:346-353.
26. Losken A, Schaefer TG, Newell M, Styblo TM. The impact of partial breast reconstruction using reduction techniques on postoperative cancer surveillance. *Plast Reconstr Surg.* 2009;124(1):9-17.

CHAPTER 77

Immediate Repair of Partial Mastectomy Defects Using Perforator Flaps

Moustapha Hamdi
Filip Stillaert

The reconstructive approach to breast defects is challenging, as the resultant glandular tissue deficiency not only needs to be replaced or reconstructed following the "tissue-like" principle but also necessitates a contour deformity restoration. Conservative breast surgery with postoperative irradiation has replaced modified radical mastectomy as the preferred treatment for early invasive breast cancer. Breast-conservation surgery with quadrantectomy or lumpectomy procedures creates primary or delayed secondary (postradiation) defects of the conical breast shape with or without involvement, and subsequent repositioning, of the nipple–areola complex (NAC).

The objective in breast-conservation surgery is to establish disease-free surgical margins while the reconstructive part will tend to preserve as much glandular tissue as possible allowing primary, tension-free closure with an acceptable aesthetic appearance and satisfying breast symmetry. When primary closure without tissue distortion is not feasible, mobilization of adjacent or locoregional tissue is warranted.

Up to 30% of patients are dissatisfied with the aesthetic result after partial mastectomy with irradiation.[1] Distortion, retraction, and mammary volume changes together with NAC repositioning extenuating asymmetry all have a profound impact on the aesthetic appearance of the breast. Therefore, we prefer to perform immediate reconstruction whenever it is indicated and feasible, as operating on irradiated breasts has high complication rates with frequently poor esthetic results. During immediate reconstruction, the breast can be manipulated prior to radiation. This potentially decreases complications and improves the outcome. As for any conservative breast therapy, tumors up to 3 cm in diameter are generally considered safe for quadrantectomy associated with postoperative radiotherapy.

On the other hand, any immediate partial reconstruction should be delayed if the surgeon is uncertain about the margins or tumor extension despite the preoperative radiologic assessment. A delayed immediate reconstruction can still be performed within a few days after the definitive margins become known.[2]

CLINICAL APPROACH

The combination of wide glandular breast tissue excision with subsequent immediate reconstruction has been considered a decisive stage in the evolution of breast cancer surgery. This approach allows not only wider tumor resection to obtain safer margins but is also advantageous in handling the healthy resultant glandular tissue to achieve better aesthetic outcomes. However, if there is any doubt about the margins of resection or tumor extension, the procedure should be delayed and the delayed stage can still be done a few days later when the definitive margins are known. Many surgeons have suggested incorporating a reduction mammaplasty procedure during the tumor resection in hypertrophic breasts.[3-7]

The size and location of the breast defect and the ratio of breast volume to resection volume are fundamental determinants to choose the methods of reconstruction. One of the relative contraindications for rearranging the breast parenchyma is a large tumor to breast ratio, with smaller breasts requiring different, more challenging reconstruction approaches. An extensive resection in a smaller breast necessitates the recruitment of nonglandular tissue, and different flaps are available to fill the tissue deficiency.

SURGICAL TECHNIQUES

Displacement Techniques

If the defect involves less than 30% volume deficiency in a relatively moderate to large breast, rearrangement surgery using dermoglandular or glandular flaps based on breast tissue can be performed as long as a tension-free closure can be obtained and the final outcome will be aesthetically acceptable.[1,3,8-10] Skin rotation flaps or lateral thoracic axial skin flaps can be used for small lateral defects, but most of those flaps become unavailable when axillary lymph node dissection is part of the oncologic procedure.

Replacement Techniques

The versatility of the pedicled perforator flaps available around the mammary gland is definitely an advantage to obtain acceptable results. Defects involving up to 30% of the breast volume are usually considered for reconstruction with pedicled flaps as well are defects involving an unacceptable aesthetic outcome with breast asymmetry. Our algorithm to recruit distant tissue for partial breast reconstruction is to turn first to pedicled flaps and then to free flaps with completion mastectomy if pedicled flaps are insufficient, unavailable, or potentially compromised due to previous surgery.

Free tissue transfer for immediate partial breast reconstruction is not recommended because it eliminates the use of the flap for a local recurrence or a new tumor in the contralateral breast. It is, as mentioned before, better to complete the mastectomy followed by the autologous reconstruction.

Perforator Flaps

The *thoracodorsal, intercostal,* or *superior epigastric pedicle* axes can be used to elevate perforator flaps based on the desired location within the breast. The flaps can be raised in the axillary and back region as well as from the anterior thoracic and upper abdominal areas.

Depending on the tumor location and the extent of the resultant defect, a variety of pedicled perforator flaps are available (Fig. 77-1). The most commonly used pedicled perforator flaps used to reconstruct considerable breast defects are described next.

The *thoracodorsal artery perforator* (TDAP) flap, suitable for *superior* defects, is based on the perforators from the descending or the horizontal branches of the thoracodorsal vessels (Fig. 77-1).[1,11]

Intercostal artery perforator (ICAP) flaps are nourished through the perforators arising from the costal groove. The lateral intercostal artery perforator (LICAP) flap is suitable to restore defects in the lateral quadrant or small defects in the medial quadrant.[12] The flap provides a short pedicle, but the flap can be rotated 180 degrees without torsion of the perforator. The LICAP flap is a good alternative to the TDAP flap for lateral and inferior breast defects. The anterior intercostal artery perforator (AICAP) flap is supplied by perforators originating from the muscular segment. The AICAP, on the other hand, is an option to reconstruct defects in the medial quadrant.

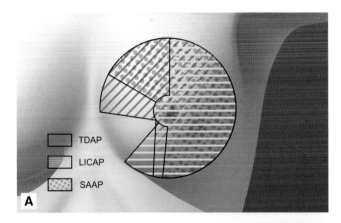

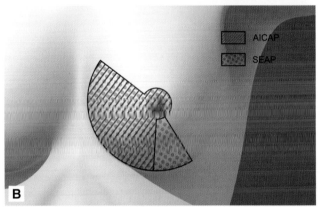

FIGURE 77-1 Indications of pedicled perforator flaps depending on the location of the breast defect.

The *serratus anterior artery perforator* (SAAP) flap is based on the connection between the serratus branch of the thoracodorsal artery and the intercostal perforators. However, these perforators can be found in only 21% of the cases, as shown by our anatomic study.[12]

The *superior epigastric artery perforator* (SEAP) flap is based on perforators originating from the superficial or the deep branch of the superior epigastric artery. This flap can be used to reconstruct tissue deficiencies in the medial quadrant.[13]

Latissimus Dorsi Flaps

The latissimus dorsi (LD) myocutaneous flap has an excellent blood supply and provides enough bulk tissue for filling glandular defects and pliable skin to substitute for skin deficiencies. However, the donor-site morbidity consists of seroma formation and the presence of conspicuous scars on the back with loss of some back muscular function.[14] Avoiding a scar on the back can be achieved by harvesting the LD without a skin paddle through the lateral breast incision used for the oncologic excision or approaching the defect using a mini-LD flap.[15]

OPERATIVE TECHNIQUE

Perforator Mapping

The perforator will determine the flap viability, and careful preoperative mapping of those perforators will influence the flap design and its location. This mapping reduces the operating time and complication rate significantly while giving the surgeon a reference point of how to design the flap to address the defect. Perforators are tracked using a Doppler ultrasound device. Perforators in the thoracodorsal region are sought out in a region 8 to 10 cm below the axillary crease and within 5 cm of the anterior border of the LD muscle.[16,17] To avoid the background signal from the main thoracodorsal pedicle, the patient is positioned for perforator mapping in the same position as for the surgical procedure, which is a lateral position with 90 degrees of shoulder abduction and 90 degrees of elbow flexion.

When the signal is heard in front of the anterior border of the LD muscle, a direct perforator (a septal perforator) of the thoracodorsal pedicle can be expected. This direct perforator can be found in 55% of the cases, which makes the dissection easier and quicker, but the disadvantage is a shorter pedicle and the flap may not be able to reach more distant defects.[16,17] This septal perforator arises from the thoracodorsal vessels at a high level and it may be damaged by axillary lymph node surgery. Therefore, it is mandatory to check the vascular course of this perforator before committing to raise the flap based on it.

Mapping of an *intercostal* or *superior epigastric perforator* is done on the patient in supine position.

Recently, it has become possible to obtain a real-time image of the perforator using multidetector CT (MD-CT). This method shows the anatomic course of the perforator with the location of the pedicle and an assessment of its diameter.[18]

Flap Marking

As for the TDAP flap, the anterior border of the LD muscle is palpated and marked with the patient in an upright position. The patient is then asked to lie down on her lateral side similar to the intraoperative position. The width of the TDAP flap is determined on one hand depending on the expected defect and on the other hand by the possibility for primary donor site closure. The excess of skin-fat of the back is determined by the pinch test. The average flap size is 20 × 8 cm (range of length, 16-25 cm; range of width, 6-10 cm). The flap paddle is oriented parallel to the skin lines. The island can also be horizontally designed according to the wishes of the patient (Fig. 77-2). It is always extended over the anterior

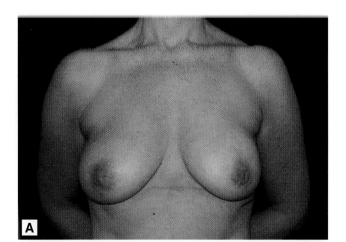
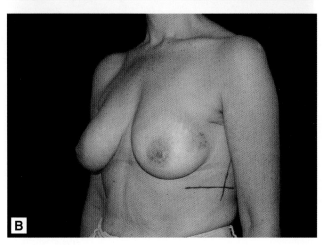
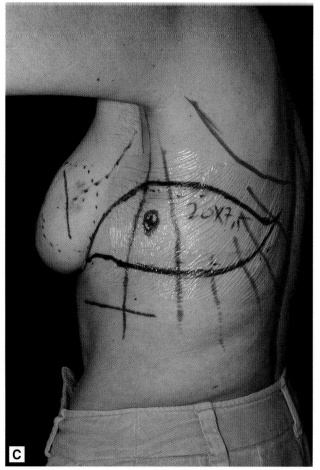

FIGURE 77-2 A 49-year-old patient with a ductal carcinoma in the superolateral quadrant of the left breast. The patient was a good candidate for quadrantectomy with axillary dissection and immediate partial breast reconstruction with a TDAP flap. **A, B.** Preoperative views. **C.** Flap markings. The perforator was mapped preoperatively using a multidetector row CT (MDCT) scan study.

border of the LD muscle in order to include the premuscular perforators, if they can be found. The length of the skin paddle depends on the location of the defect. When the defect is located on the lateral or superolateral quadrants, the skin paddle is designed over the lateral thoracic area. The proximal edge of the flap reaches the inframammary fold. For more medially located defects the skin paddle is designed more distally toward the back.

Flap Dissection

The Thoracodorsal Artery Perforator (TDAP) Flap

The elevation of a TDAP flap is carried out after completion of the oncologic resection (Fig. 77-3A).[17] The patient is then repositioned into lateral decubitus with the arm abducted 90 degrees and the skin and subcutaneous tissues are incised unveiling the muscle fascia. Flap dissection is done under loupe magnification. Flap elevation proceeds from distal to proximal and from medial to lateral in a suprafascial level until the preoperatively marked perforator or an alternative good caliber perforator is encountered. After assessing the pulsatile and morphologic (diameter of more than 0.5 mm) characteristics of the perforator, a decision is made to elevate a perforator flap (Fig. 77-3B). The muscle is split among its muscle fibers, the perforator freed from the surrounding tissue, and side branches clipped or coagulated using a micro-bipolar device to ensure complete hemostasis and obtain a good intraoperative view (Fig. 77-3C). Nerve branches are preserved and the perforator is dissected more proximally until reaching its origin from the main pedicle in order to provide a long pedicle (Fig. 77-3D). After completion of an atraumatic vessel dissection the skin paddle can be further raised from the LD muscle (Fig. 77-3E, F). The skin paddle is tunneled into the breast area, taking care not to damage the perforator during this maneuver (Fig. 77-3G). The flap is secured onto the anterior axillary line with a few stitches and the donor site closed on a suction drain. In the final stage of the procedure the patient is turned into a supine position for the final

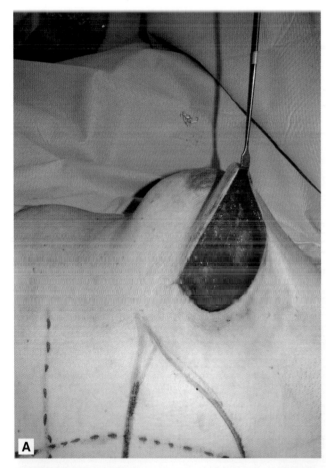
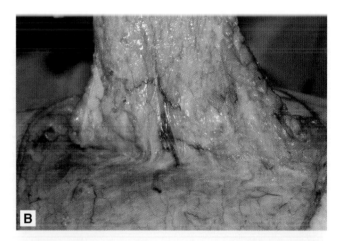
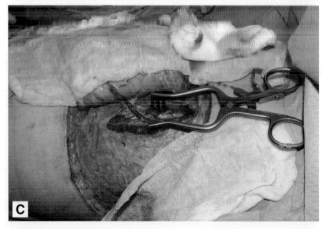

FIGURE 77-3 Surgical technique of the TDAP flap. **A.** The quadrantectomy is performed. **B.** The flap is harvested with a posterior approach until the marked perforator is found. **C.** The LD muscle is split and the perforator is freed. **D.** The perforator is dissected through the split LD muscle until the main pedicle. The thoracodorsal nerve is spared. **E.** When the pedicle is completely dissected and the tunnel under the anterior border of the muscle is made, the posterior side of the perforator is then freed from the muscle fibers. **F.** The skin paddle, which was based on one perforator, is totally dissected from the LD muscle. **G.** The skin paddle is passed under the anterior strip of the LD muscle towards the breast defect. **H.** The patient is repositioned into supine position for flap shaping.

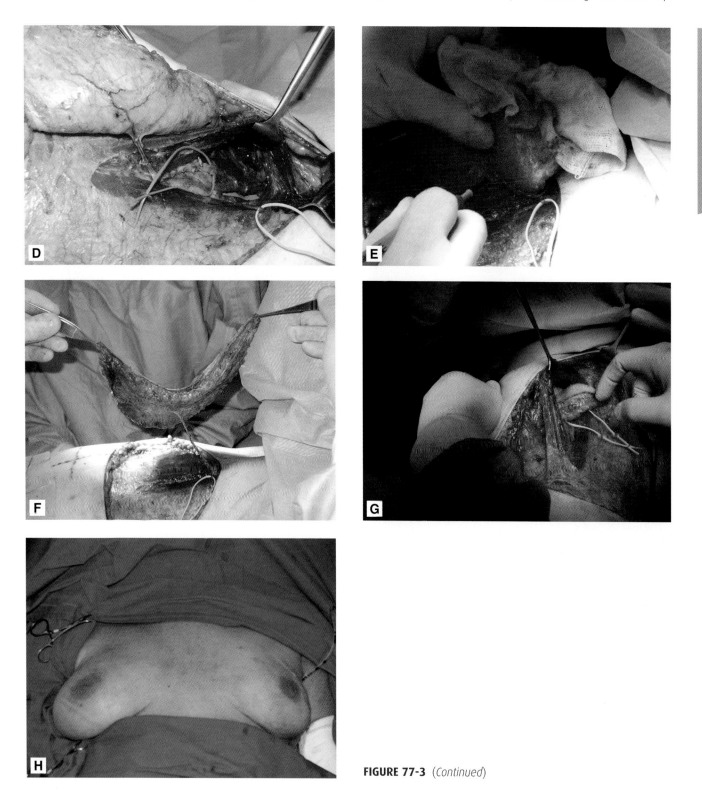

FIGURE 77-3 (Continued)

shaping of the flap (Fig. 77-3H). The latter can either be folded to obtain an acceptable breast contour or discarded from excess tissue. Nevertheless, an overcorrection is always performed. The flap is de-epithelialized depending on the defect and the skin paddle is left only when breast skin was removed with the tumor. The flap is positioned without kinking of the perforator and anchored to the pectoralis fascia. Another suction drain is left between the flap and the breast skin. The scars heal inconspicuously after radiotherapy (Fig. 77-4). When breast skin should be excised with the tumor, a skin paddle is left on the breast and the rest of the TDAP flap is de-epithelialized and buried under the breast skin (Fig. 77-5).

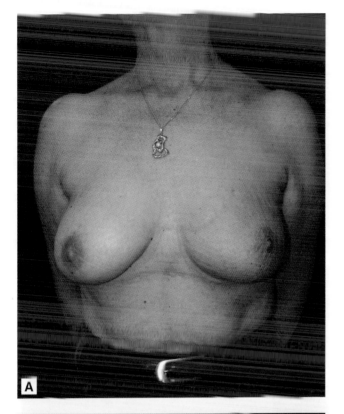

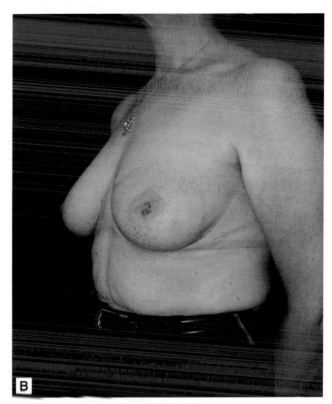

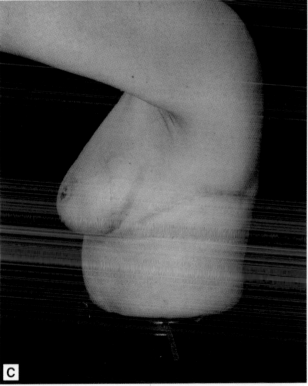

FIGURE 77-4 The results at 1 year postoperatively.

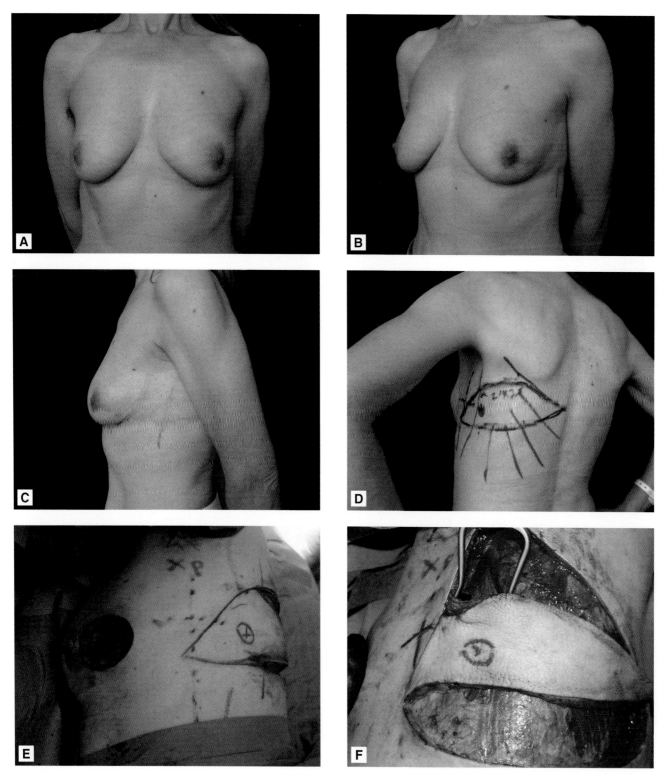

FIGURE 77-5 A case of 53-year-old patient with an invasive ductal carcinoma in the lateral quadrant of the left breast. The tumor was close to the breast skin, and therefore a large resection with the breast skin was planned. Due to the moderate size of the breast, immediate partial breast reconstruction was offered to the patient as an alternative to the mastectomy. **A-C.** Preoperative views. **D.** TDAP flap markings with the marked perforator using the MDCT. **E.** The tumorectomy with the covered breast skin is done. **F, G.** TDAP flap dissection. The perforator is found exactly at the marked point by the MDCT. **H.** The TDAP is partially de-epithelialized to fill the defect. **I, J.** The results at 1 year postoperatively. **K, L.** The donor site of the TDAP flap.

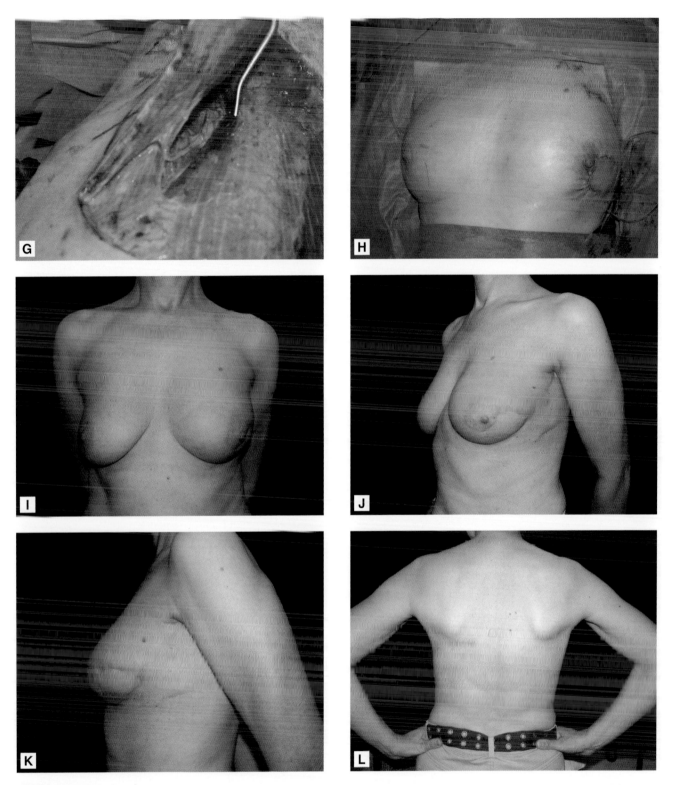

FIGURE 77-5 (*Continued*)

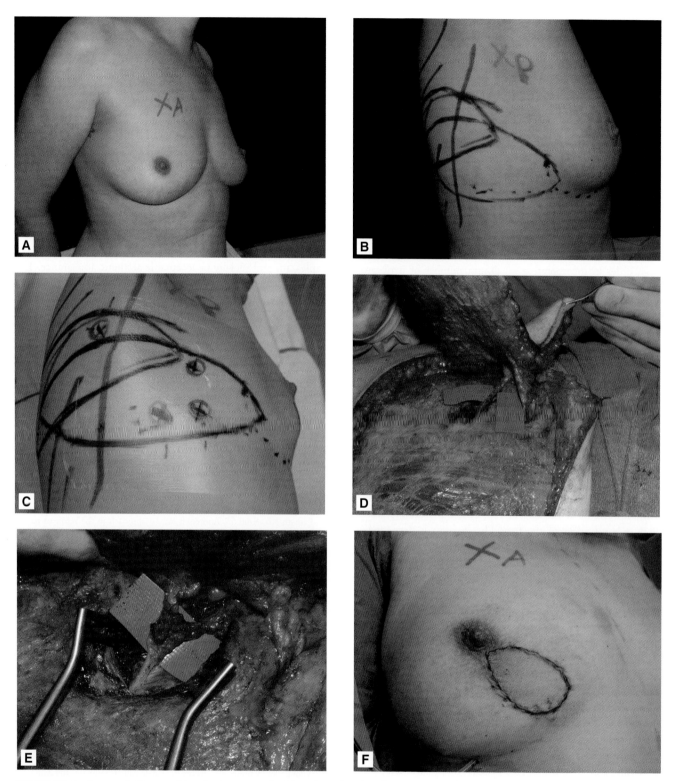

FIGURE 77-6 A case of 47-year-old patient presented with an invasive ductal carcinoma at the junction of the inferior quadrant of the right breast. An immediate breast reconstruction was planned using a LICAP pedicle flap. **A, B.** Preoperative views. The LICAP flap was planned at the level of the inframammary fold. **C.** Three perforators are located using a unidirectional Doppler. The lower 2 are expected to arise from the same intercostal space. **D.** Intraoperative view shows the posterior and anterior branch of the fifth intercostal perforator in front of the anterior border of the LD muscle. **E.** The 2 branches are dissected and the serratus anterior strip in between is sectioned. The flap is based on the 2 branches. **F.** The breast defect is covered by the flap, which was de-epithelialized and folded up.

The Muscle-Sparing–Thoracodorsal Artery Perforator (MS-TDAP) Flap

The muscle-sparing thoracodorsal artery perforator (MS-TDAP) is used in those cases where small-sized pulsatile perforators are found intraoperatively.[17] MS-TDAP I is used to harvest the flap with a 2-cm LD muscle piece. In this case, the perforators will be "deroofed" within the split LD muscle. This requires including the muscle under direct visualization of the perforators in order not to damage them during harvesting of the muscular segment. This technique can also be used when the flap is planned to reach a more medial defect in the breast. By keeping the perforator attached to the muscle segment, safer flap inset can be obtained without direct traction on the perforator.

If the perforators are very tiny and nonpulsating, then the flap should be converted to a muscle-sparing flap type II (MS-TDAP II) in order to incorporate a maximum number of perforators within the flap. The nerve that innervates the rest of the LD muscle is always preserved. In these specific cases, the (MS-TDAP I or II) flap enables the surgeon a safer harvesting of the flap.

The Lateral Intercostal Artery Perforator Flap

The *LICAP flap* is designed in a similar way to the TDAP flap.[12] Our anatomic study[12] showed the largest perforators to be used for breast surgery are located between the fourth and the sixth intercostal spaces. Their distance to the anterior border of the LD muscle ranges from 0.8 to 3 cm. Therefore, the LICAP flap is more suitable to approach defects in the lateral and inferior quadrants. The flap is designed over the lateral thoracic region at the level of the inframammary fold.

A posterior incision is made first with an anterior extension at the lower end of the flap to explore the perforators and to allow easy elevation of the flap. The incision is deepened to expose the LD muscle. It is safer to include the muscle fascia in the flap to avoid an accidental injury of the posterior branches of the pedicle. After visualization of the anterior border of the LD muscle, the smaller posterior branch of the lateral cutaneous branch is identified. This branch is followed to find the bigger anterior branch. The dissection proceeds by elevating the slip of origin of the serratus muscle and retracting the LD muscle belly. A pedicle length of 3 to 5 cm is adequate to reach a defect over the lateral or superior part of the breast. The LICAP flap can reach the interior quadrant if it was planned at the level of the inframammary fold (at the fifth to sixth intercostal space) as shown in Figure 77-6. The flap can easily be folded on itself to fill a breast defect for partial breast reconstruction after a quadrantectomy.

Raising a *SAAP* flap can *only* be performed when the vascular connection between the serratus branch and an intercostal perforator is found intraoperatively. The flap can reach the superior and inferior lateral quadrants. Defects in the inferomedial quadrants are difficult to reach with pedicled perforator flaps based on the thoracodorsal pedicle.

In selected cases, the *AICAP* or *SEAP* flaps are valuable options. The flap is designed over the inframammary region with the patient in supine position. Flap width is estimated by the pinch test (up to 6 cm).

The concept of using pedicled perforator flaps is based on a proven reduction in donor site morbidity together with a shorter postoperative recovery and less pain at the donor site.[19] On the other hand, LD muscle preservation has an obvious benefit that results in less contour deformity of the donor site than LD harvest. We conducted a functional study to evaluate shoulder strength, range of motion, and the thickness of LD muscle after harvesting a pedicled TDAP flap. Our study clearly showed that LD muscle strength was not affected by harvesting a pedicled TDAP flap for breast reconstruction.[20]

SUMMARY

Defects of the mammary gland consist not only of tissue volume deficiencies but also alter the shape of the breast into an unpleasant and socially unacceptable aesthetic appearance. The reconstruction of those defects needs to be approached with the tissue-like principle substituting the breast parenchyma and skin deficiencies to approximate the native or natural appearance. Several potential pedicled flaps are available adjacent to the breast gland and their choice will depend on the location and the extent of the defect. In cases where the resection volume to breast volume ratio is disturbed, free flaps might be a better option to obtain aesthetically more acceptable results.

REFERENCES

1. Hamdi M, Wolfli J, Van Landuyt K. Partial mastectomy reconstruction. *Clin Plast Surg.* 2007;34:51-62.
2. Kronowitz SJ, Feledy JA, Hunt KK, et al. Determining the optimal approach to breast reconstruction after partial mastectomy. *Plast Reconstr Surg.* 2006;117:1-11.
3. Clough KB, Kroll SS, Audretsch W. An approach to the repair of partial mastectomy defects. *Plast Reconstr Surg.* 1999;104:409-420.
4. Spear SL, Pelletiere CV, Wolfe AJ, et al. Experience with reduction mammaplasty combined with breast conservation therapy in the treatment of breast cancer. *Plast Reconstr Surg.* 2003;111:1102-1109.
5. Munhoz AM, Montag E, Arruda EG, et al. Critical analysis of reduction mammaplasty techniques in combination with conservative breast surgery for early breast cancer treatment. *Plast Reconstr Surg.* 2006;117:1091-1093; discussion 1104-1107.
6. Petit JY, Garusi C, Greuze M, et al. One hundred and eleven cases of breast conservation treatment with simultaneous reconstruction at the European Institute of Oncology (Milan). *Tumori.* 2002;88:41-47.
7. Losken A, Styblo TM, Carlson GW, et al. Management algorithm and outcome evaluation of partial mastectomy defects treated using reduction or mastopexy techniques. *Ann Plast Surg.* 2007;59:235-242.
8. Berrino P, Campora E, Leone S, et al. Correction of type II breast deformities following conservative cancer surgery. *Plast Reconstr Surg.* 1992;90:846-853.
9. Berrino P, Campora E, Santi P. Postquadrantectomy breast deformities: classification and techniques of surgical correction. *Plast Reconstr Surg.* 1987;79:567-572.
10. Clough KB, Cuminet J, Fitoussi A, et al. Cosmetic sequelae after conservative treatment for breast cancer: classification and results of surgical correction. *Ann Plast Surg.* 1998;41:471-481.
11. Hamdi M, Van Landuyt K, Monstrey S, et al. Pedicled perforator flaps in breast reconstruction: a new concept. *Br J Plast Surg.* 2004;57:531-539.
12. Hamdi M, Spano A, Van Landuyt K, et al. The lateral intercostal artery perforators: anatomical study and clinical application in breast surgery. *Plast Reconstr Surg.* 2008;121:389-396.
13. Hamdi M, Van Landuyt K, Ulens S, et al. Clinical applications of the superior epigastric artery perforator (SEAP) flap: anatomical studies and preoperative perforator mapping with multidetector CT. *J Plast Reconstr Aesthet Surg.* 2009 Sep;62(9):1127-1134.

14. Randolph LC, Barone J, Angelats J, et al. Prediction of postoperative seroma after latissimus dorsi breast reconstruction. *Plast Reconstr Surg.* 2005;116:1287-1290.

15. Rainsbury RM. Breast-sparing reconstruction with latissimus dorsi mini-flaps. *Eur J Surg Oncol.* 2002;28:891-895. Review.

16. Guerra AB, Metzinger SE, Lund KM, et al. The thoracodorsal artery perforator flap: clinical experience and anatomic study with emphasis on harvest techniques. *Plast Reconstr Surg.* 2004;114:32-41; discussion 42-43.

17. Hamdi M, Van Landuyt K, Hijjawi JB, et al. Surgical technique in pedicled thoracodorsal artery perforator flaps: a clinical experience with 99 patients. *Plast Reconstr Surg.* 2008;121:1632-1641.

18. Masia J, Clavero JA, Larranaga JR, et al. Multidetector-row computed tomography in the planning of abdominal perforator flaps. *J Plast Reconstr Aesthet Surg.* 2006;59:594-599.

19. Kroll S, Sharma S, Koutz C, et al. Postoperative morphine requirements of free TRAM and DIEP flaps. *Plast Reconstr Surg.* 2001;107:338-341.

20. Hamdi M, Decorte T, Demuynck M, et al. Shoulder function after harvesting a thoracodorsal artery perforator flap. *Plast Reconstr Surg.* 2008;122: 1111-1117.

CHAPTER 78

Correction of Partial Breast Deformities with the Lipomodeling Technique

Emmanuel Delay

Moderate sequelae of conservative treatment of breast cancer are a real challenge for the surgeon.[1] No technique yet gave entirely satisfactory results. The only options offered to patients, such as musculocutaneous latissimus dorsi flaps,[2,3] were often disabling and disproportionate to the breast deformity.[1] But a few years after treatment of their cancer, patients are very eager for surgical correction of their deformity to erase or attenuate the visible signs of their disease. It was therefore important to seek a solution that would correct these sequelae and help these patients to regain better self-esteem and to reintegrate their breast in their body image.

We had obtained very good results with fat transfer in the face, and so in 1998 we proposed fat transfer for breast improvement after reconstruction. We first introduced this approach after autologous latissimus dorsi flap reconstruction.[4,5] Finding that fat transfer was effective and innocuous, we proposed using it to correct therapeutic sequelae of the breast. We carried out a radiological study on reconstructed breasts that had undergone lipomodeling, and this showed no deleterious effects on breast imaging.[6]

This chapter presents the information that should be given to the patients and the precautions that should be taken before carrying out this procedure, the surgical technique, the results that may be expected, the advantages and drawbacks of the technique, the potential radiological appearance after lipomodeling, and lastly the possible medicolegal aspects if local recurrence of cancer occurs coincidentally with lipomodeling.

JUSTIFICATION OF THIS SURGICAL APPROACH

The use of fat transfer in breast surgery is not a new concept.[7] More recently, and from the early days of modern liposuction, Illouz[8] and Tournier[9] suggested using the fat obtained from liposuction for moderate breast augmentations. Bircoll[10] presented a similar approach and drew attention to the advantages of this technique in a paper published in February 1987 in the *Journal of Plastic and Reconstructive Surgery*[10]: simplicity, absence of residual scarring, early return to normal activity, elimination of the need for implants and also their complications, with an additional secondary advantage in the areas of fat harvesting. Then in April 1987 he published[11] a report of a patient who had undergone bilateral fat transfer after unilateral reconstruction with a transverse rectus abdominis muscle flap (improvement of the reconstructed breast and restoration of symmetry). These 2 papers at once prompted considerable extremely virulent opposition.[12-16] His detractors underlined the fact that fat injections in a native breast could produce microcalcifications and cysts, making a cancer difficult to detect. Although Bircoll stressed in his replies[17,18] that the calcifications after fat transfer differ from neoplastic calcifications by their location and their radiological appearance, and that breast reduction surgery also generates microcalcifications, the debate started unfavorably, and in 1987, the American Society of Plastic and Reconstructive Surgeons (ASPRS) ruled as follows: "The committee is unanimous in deploring the use of autologous fat injection in breast augmentation. Much of the injected fat will not survive, and the known physiological response to necrosis of this tissue is scarring and calcification. As a result, detection of early breast carcinoma through xerography and mammography will become difficult and the presence of disease may go undiscovered." These affirmations were made without any previous scientific studies and were based on the opinion of the committee members of the ASPRS. Since then, in spite of the lack of more intensive references, and although it was recognized at the time that any breast surgery could potentially generate oily cysts and/or mammographic changes, injection of fat in the breasts had become a powerful taboo that no one officially attempted to breach. Ironically, in 1987, a retrospective study of mammographic changes after breast reduction[19] published in the same journal reported that calcifications were found in 50% of cases at 2 years, and the authors stressed that in the majority it was possible to differentiate them from cancerous changes. In spite of this very high incidence and once again the risk of interference with detection of a breast cancer, of course no discussion took place on abandoning breast reductions.

In 1998, the aims of our research on fat transfer in the breast were to improve the technique so as to reduce fat necrosis and to attack the powerful taboo that for some 10 years had halted research, evaluation, and publications on this topic. In fact, because we had observed that fat transfer was extremely effective in the face, in aesthetic surgery, and in treatment of facial sequelae after injury or cancer treatments (a technique that we used notably after the publications of Coleman[20,21]), we thought of applying this technique to breast reconstruction, and we decided it should be one of our areas of research. First of all, we applied fat transfers to breast reconstructions with an autologous latissimus dorsi flap.[22] This technique of autologous breast reconstruction had in fact been developed in our unit of plastic and reconstructive surgery.[22] It restored satisfactory breast volume in 70% of cases, but in 30% the volume was insufficient and either the opposite breast had to be reduced or an implant had to be used. This meant that the procedure was no longer purely autologous, and it was accompanied by the drawbacks of implants (less natural shape and consistency, need for implant replacement). So we then started to use fat transfers in breasts reconstructed with autologous latissimus dorsi flaps, where the risk of local recurrence was considered very low. The protocol was initially offered to voluntary patients who agreed to undergo strict surveillance. Then, as we found that this technique was extremely effective and that tolerance was excellent, we extended its indications to most patients who had breast reconstruction with autologous latissimus dorsi flaps and who wished for optimal shape and consistency and as natural a décolleté as possible. In parallel, we carried out a mammographic, ultrasound, and magnetic resonance imaging (MRI) study[0] that showed that the effect on breast imaging was far from unacceptable. We then progressively extended the indications of lipomodeling to the various situations of breast reconstruction, then to breast and thoracic deformities, to sequelae of conservative treatment, and more recently to cosmetic breast surgery. The first presentations to the Société Française de Chirurgie Plastique et Reconstructrice[23] and the International Confederation[24] gave rise to sometimes acid comments, reviving the antagonisms of 1987. These were countered point by point. Then as the presentations continued, the opposition of the scientific community lessened as one congress followed another, and fat transfers are now accepted as part of the therapeutic armamentarium for breast reconstruction. Our efforts toward systematic scientific evaluation led to the request that our team write the chapter on the subject in the American reference work on plastic surgery of the breast.[4]

PATIENT INFORMATION

During the preoperative visit, the patient's details and the history of her disease are recorded and her expectations are assessed. Each patient is given precise, detailed information both orally and in written form (a specific information sheet) that comprehensively explains the modalities of the procedure, its advantages, drawbacks, and possible complications. We particularly emphasize that fat loss is normal during the early months, that the procedure may possibly have to be repeated if the patient has major sequelae, and that the result may alter if she gains or loses weight. Patients are also informed of the postoperative bruising, which can be impressive at the donor site, and of residual scarring, even if this is minimal.

During meticulous clinical examination, the conserved breast is compared with the opposite breast, and the areas that require correction are identified and marked with the patient standing. The symmetry of the breasts is assessed, their overall volume and fullness, the position of the nipple-areola complex, the severity of loss of substance and volume, and depressed or retractile scars if any. The quantity of fat to be harvested and transferred is also assessed, as well as the need for any complementary measures such as restoration of symmetry, tattooing, and/or a nipple graft. The adipose areas where the fat will be harvested are identified. Abdominal fat is most often used because harvesting in this area does not require a change in the patient's position during the procedure. The second site is the trochanteric region (saddlebags), often combined with harvesting from the inside of the knees and the back of the thighs. It is important that the patient's weight be stable at the time of the procedure because the transferred fat retains the memory of its origins, and if the patient loses weight after lipomodeling, she will lose some of the benefit of the procedure.

As part of the protocol, all patients undergo full imaging, including mammography, ultrasound, and MRI, before as well as 1 year after the procedure. The risk of local recurrence is clearly explained to the patient, as well as the risk that a cancer may occur coincidentally with lipomodeling. It is also explained that in the event of recurrence, mastectomy with immediate reconstruction will be performed.[0]

SURGICAL TECHNIQUE

The lipomodeling technique used in the sequelae of conservative treatment is derived from that used in breast reconstruction.[2,3] It aims to transfer fat from an area with excess adipose tissue to the conserved breast that presents a deformity or is lacking in volume. The procedure is carried out in the surgical suite under general anesthesia. Conventional prophylactic antibiotics are usually given perioperatively.

The patient is installed and draped so that she can be moved from a supine to a semisitting position if fat is harvested from abdominal and suprailiac deposits. If fat is harvested from the trochanteric or subgluteal area or the inside of the thighs, the patient is placed in a prone position and then turned over and entirely redraped for the reinjection.

Fat is harvested with a blunt 3-mm cannula (Fig. 78-1A) after preliminary infiltration of serum with adrenaline.

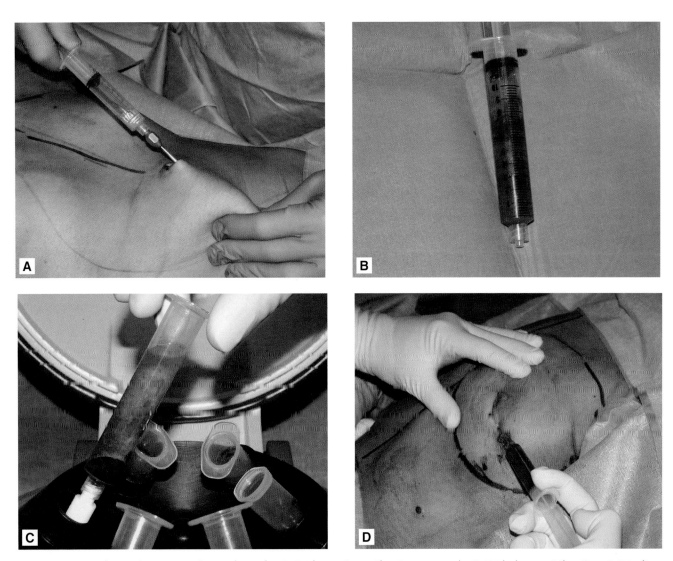

FIGURE 78-1   Fat harvesting, preparation, and transfer. **A.** Fat harvesting with a 3-mm cannula. **B.** Fat before centrifugation. **C.** Fat after centrifugation. **D.** Technique of fat transfer.

The incisions are made according to the harvesting area, with a No. 15 blade. Abdominal fat is harvested through 4 cardinal incisions around the navel. In the flanks, a suprailiac incision is made on each side. For the gluteal and trochanteric regions, the incisions lie in the subgluteal folds. We use 10-mL Luer Lock syringes.

With the finger, the operator makes a moderate, gradual depression that creates a differential of a few cubic centimeters between the aspirated fat and the piston to minimize damage to the adipocytes (Fig. 78-1A).

Both deep and superficial fat are harvested. At the end of the procedure, the harvesting site is often recontoured by liposuction for a better cosmetic result. When harvesting is completed, the same cannula is used to inject 7.5 mg Naropin (ropivacaine hydrochloride) with an equal volume of normal saline to alleviate postoperative pain during the first 24 hours.

The incisions are closed by separate stitches using rapidly absorbed suture material (Vicryl Rapide 3–0).

As harvesting continues, the instrument nurse prepares the syringes for centrifugation. They are sealed with a plastic cap, the piston is withdrawn, and they are placed in the centrifuge in batches of 6 for 3 minutes at 3000 revolutions per minute. After purification, the fat separates into 3 layers (Figs. 78-1B, C):

A top layer of oil resulting from cell lysis (chylomicrons and triglycerides)

A bottom layer of blood residues

A middle layer of purified adipocytes (this is the valuable part that will be used for transfer)

After preparation of the fat, several punctate incisions are made with the bevel of a pink trocar to create a cross-work of tunnels for the transfer of fatty tissue. The fat is then reimplanted in its new site using special disposable fine 1.5-mm cannulas (Fig. 78-1D). Deep tunnels must be made in all planes, from the ribs to the skin, following the preoperative markings and forming a 3-dimensional honeycomb. The fat

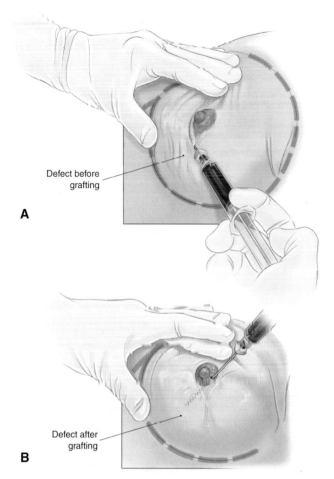

Defect before grafting

A

Defect after grafting

B

FIGURE 78-2   Lipomodeling technique.

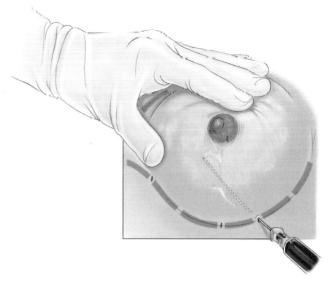

FIGURE 78-3   Fat transfer in small quantities: the "fat spaghetti" principle.

must be reinjected while the cannula is withdrawn. Care must be taken to avoid using too much pressure (Fig. 78-2), and the fat should be injected in small quantities as if it were spaghetti (Fig. 78-3). This is because of the risk that necrotic cysts will form if too great a volume of fat is injected (centripetal revascularization does not allow survival of large-sized fragments, which become the site of central necrosis with liquefaction and cyst formation).

If possible, volume should be overcorrected. As about 30% of fat is reabsorbed, 140% of the desired volume should be transferred. But very often after conservative treatment, overcorrection is not possible because the tissue receiving the fat is fibrotic. It is advisable not to attempt to continue but to program a second session. During the second session, because of the antifibrotic effect of the fat, larger quantities can often be transferred. At the end of the procedure, the lipomodeled area is covered with a dry dressing, taking care to avoid compression. A compressive Elastoplast dressing is applied to the harvesting sites.

POSTOPERATIVE CARE

The patient leaves the unit on the same day or the day after the procedure, with class 1 analgesics. The dry dressing on the

breast is changed every 72 hours by a private nurse or by the patient herself. The compressive dressing on the harvesting sites is kept in place for 5 days; then these areas are left exposed to the air. Major bruising of the harvesting site is common, and this is generally the most painful area in the immediate postoperative period. The breast is also swollen, but bruising is less marked. At the harvesting site, bruising clears in 3 weeks, sometimes leaving some firmer nodular areas that return to normal in the months after the procedure, and more rapidly if the patient massages them.

The breast attains its definitive volume 4 months after the procedure, but from the first month it is supple and soft to the touch. This technique enables made-to-measure corrections of the sequelae of conservative treatment. If correction is not sufficient, 1 or even 2 further sessions can be carried out after an interval of 3 to 4 months.

RESULTS

To date, our team has treated 70 patients according to this protocol. Last year, the results were assessed in 42 patients who had undergone lipomodeling for the sequelae of conservative treatment between May 2002 and March 2007.[7] Their mean age was 50.7 years at the time of treatment, with a range of 35 to 64 years, and their mean body mass index was 21.8.

Fifty-four procedures were carried out in 42 patients, a mean of 1.3 per patient; 22% of patients required a second procedure, and only 1 patient required a third (2.4%).

During the first session of lipomodeling, a mean of 274 mL of fat was harvested (minimum 120 mL; maximum 480 mL). After centrifugation, the mean volume of fat recovered was 187 mL (71.2% of the volume centrifuged, with 28.8% lost during the process). The mean quantity reinjected was 166 mL, with a range of 76 to 302 mL. The results were assessed by 2 surgeons by clinical examination and from the photographic records of

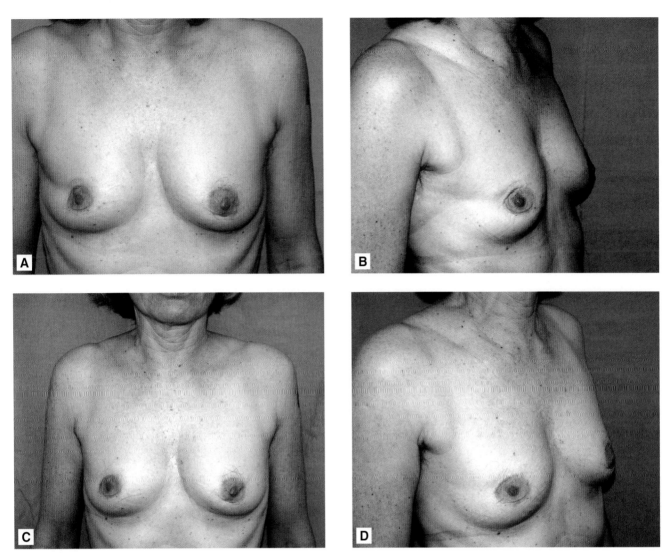

FIGURE 78-4 Correction of a moderate deformity of the outer quadrants of the right breast. Transfer of 140 mL of fat. Result at 12 months. **A.** Preoperative frontal view. **B.** Preoperative three-quarter view. **C.** Postoperative frontal view. **D.** Postoperative three-quarter view.

each patient before and after the procedure, and 93% were considered good or very good (Fig. 78-4). These results can be judged from the photographs (Fig. 78-5) but are even more striking on clinical examination. Ninety percent of patients were satisfied or very satisfied.

THE ADVANTAGES OF LIPOMODELING

These advantages are seen in better perspective if we remember that until the advent of lipomodeling, there was no technique that satisfactorily corrected moderate morphologic deformities after conservative treatment of breast cancer. Previous techniques led to complications, involved major surgery, or carried major constraints in view of the limited deformity of the breast. So before the advent of lipomodeling, therapeutic abstention was the advice most often given to patients with moderate aesthetic sequelae of the breast.[1]

Few Contraindications

There are no contraindications as such, and the method merely has limitations in very slim patients who have no adequate adipose areas yielding sufficient fat for a satisfactory result. A quantity of fat equal to twice the desired final volume is needed to compensate for losses through centrifugation and through resorption in the early months. Sufficient adipose areas must be available for fat harvesting, allowing for an average of 30% loss during centrifugation and 30% in the early months by resorption. However, fat can be harvested several times from a single area if the reserves allow it.

Autologous Tissue

The fatty tissue is autologous, and there is no immunologic rejection. An implant with its risks and disadvantages is not needed. Unlike an implant, it is also living tissue with resistance to infection.

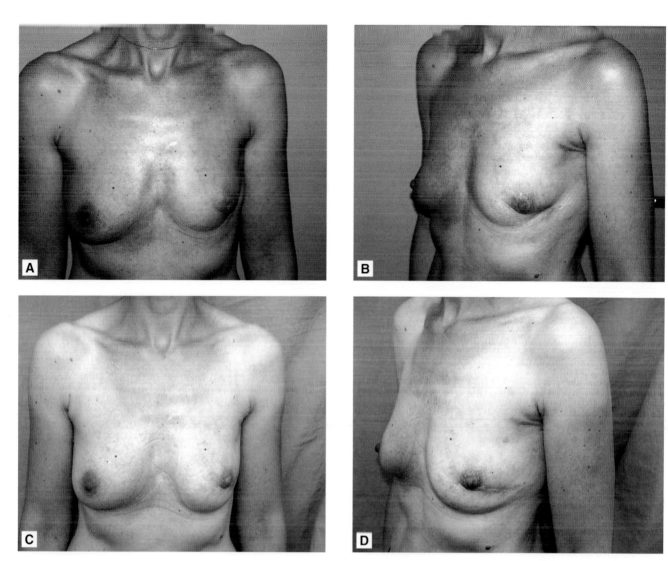

FIGURE 78-5 Correction of a major deformity of the lower quadrants of the left breast. Two sessions of lipomodeling with transfer of 170 mL and 150 mL of fat were carried out at an interval of 8 months. Result 12 months after the second procedure. **A.** Preoperative frontal view. **B.** Preoperative three-quarter view. **C.** Postoperative frontal view. **D.** Postoperative three-quarter view.

Reproducibility of the Method

Fat harvesting and reinjection is a concept that is clear and easily understood by the patients. However, a learning curve applies to the natural history, the quality of the results, and the rate of fat necrosis. The technique must be precise, carried out meticulously and with care; but with specific training, it can be easily put into practice by an experienced plastic surgeon. Once the learning curve is over, the technique is easily reproducible. In addition, because there are few postoperative constraints, repeat sessions if required are well accepted by the patients.

Low Cost

This sophisticated technique does not require a major investment. The costs are limited to those of the disposable cannulas and syringes, and the purchase of a centrifuge for sterile preparation of the fat. Compared with certain treatments used in other areas of cancerology, these costs are very acceptable in view of the services rendered to the patients and to their strong demand.

Relatively Noninvasive

Fat is harvested and reinjected through small incisions that need little postoperative care. Scarring is limited, and the patient can rapidly resume normal activities. The complications and constraints of lipomodeling thus appear much less irksome than those of conventional breast surgery.

Few Complications

True complications are rare or even exceptional. In the short term, we observed no hematoma. This is a potential complication of any surgical act but is more than exceptional in breast lipomodeling. In 850 such procedures that we have carried out, all indications taken into account, we have never met with this complication.

The risk of pneumothorax is exceptional, and we have not encountered it in this series of corrections of deformities due to the sequelae of conservative treatment. In 850 lipomodeling procedures of the breast and thorax, this complication occurred only once. This was in a patient who had undergone lipomodeling after breast reconstruction with an autologous latissimus dorsi flap after mastectomy. Fat had been injected perpendicular to the thoracic wall because of a marked lack of projection. The diagnosis was suggested by 2 episodes of oxygen desaturation (one during the procedure and the second in the recovery room) and was confirmed by lung radiograph. The pneumothorax required the insertion of a pleural drain but did not affect the result of the lipomodeling in any way. Following this experience, we practice and advise the practice of injections parallel to the thoracic wall. If areolar projection needs improvement, this must be achieved through 2 incisions in the inframammary fold.

Fat embolism, a risk that has been described in theory and highlighted by detractors of lipomodeling, could occur in the event of intravascular injection of fat under considerable pressure. Embolism is prevented by the use of cannulas with lateral openings and by strict adherence to the principle of injecting only while withdrawing the cannula. No embolism occurred in the present indication or in my personal series of 850 cases of lipomodeling of the breast and thorax, all indications taken together, carried out by the same operator.

Finally, the main short-term risk is infection. It is prevented by strictly aseptic conditions and by flash antibiotic prophylaxis during the procedure. Infection may develop in the breast, with the skin becoming red. The suture in the transfer area must be removed. A cloudy effusion of fat may develop, but this problem can be fully resolved by topical treatment and antibiotics, together with the application of ice. In our series, 2 patients had an infection that was rapidly arrested by this method and did not impair the final result.

Local infection may also develop around the navel, shown by redness of the surrounding skin. It can be treated without difficulty by antibiotics and local application of ice.

The long-term complications are the risk of fat necrosis and unevenness at the harvesting site. Focal clinical fat necrosis may appear if too much fat has been injected at the same spot. It then forms a firm nodule corresponding to a radiolucent image on mammography and an oily cyst on ultrasound. These may sometimes resolve if drained. Drainage yields a thick, yellowish, acellular fluid. Nodules of fat necrosis are mainly seen in the early days of the practitioner's learning curve, and their incidence decreases as experience increases, if the principle of the 3-dimensional network is respected and if the receiving tissues are not oversaturated.

Unevenness at the donor site may result from irregular harvesting of the fat deposit. This is why harvesting is sometimes completed by liposuction to refine the result and to increase patient satisfaction. Experience in liposuction is valuable here to reduce the risk of this complication and also to give the patient the best possible cosmetic result. For this reason, we believe this procedure should preferably be performed by experienced plastic surgeons who have already completed their learning curve in liposuction and lipomodeling (starting with breast reconstruction).

Adaptable Volume

The volume harvested and reinjected is calculated according to the deficiency to be filled, ensuring that each patient has "made-to-measure" correction of her sequelae. The limiting factors are the donor tissue (quantity of fat available at a given site) and the receiving site (volume of fat that can be accepted). If the volume of fat that can be accepted is limited, several sessions should be planned from the very beginning.

Natural Result

If all goes well, the consistency and warmth to the touch of the reconstructed breast are the same as those of the opposite breast. The breast follows the patient's movements more naturally and it ages similarly to the opposite breast, unlike reconstruction using implants. Our results have shown that the size and shape of the breasts are durable and natural in appearance. Injected in a 3-dimensional network, the transplanted fat gives a texture and suppleness that no other surgery can provide.

Stable Results

If the patient's weight remains constant, the result is maintained; if she gains weight, the reconstructed breast may become larger. In our experience, stable results are obtained at 4 months. Our research on repair surgery of the breast has made us aware of the public health problem represented by the increasing number of patients with a breast neoplasm (46,000 new cases of breast cancer each year in France). We have therefore chosen to use reliable, reproducible techniques of reconstruction. Our work indicates that lipomodeling fulfils the criteria of reliability and reproducibility and that it vouchsafes cosmetic and morphologic results of quality.

Secondary Advantage

An improved silhouette is a secondary advantage of the aspiration of fat deposits, in particular if aspirations are repeated. This may well play a nonnegligible role in the very high patient satisfaction rate observed in our study. Because this surgery aims to improve the quality of life of our patients, this additional advantage may be a further argument for the use of this technique, rather than a criticism.

Improved Skin Trophicity

We have observed an improvement in the suppleness, color, and elasticity of the skin that is particularly appreciable in irradiated tissue. Several works have demonstrated the benefits to the skin of fat transfer, probably through the introduction of stem cells of fatty origin.[7]

THE DRAWBACKS OF LIPOMODELING

Repeat Sessions

It should be borne in mind from the very beginning that if the deformity is significant, repeat sessions will be required if the initial correction is inadequate due to poor evaluation of the deficiency, rapid saturation of the tissues with fat, or marked resorption. If tissue has been irradiated, its lack of elasticity limits the amount of fat that can be injected. Repeat sessions are sometimes planned from the start if the volume to be corrected is significant. In this case, the patient must be clearly informed of the need for complementary sessions, which in practice are performed at intervals of 3 to 4 months. However, this drawback is generally well tolerated, especially because the secondary advantages are increased if the patient has numerous unaesthetic fat deposits.

Results Dependent on Experience

A learning curve applies to the cosmetic results. It is difficult to judge at once how much overcorrection is required, and it is often underestimated during the first procedures performed. Only 70% of the volume harvested is in fact recovered as pure fat after centrifugation, and it is considered that 30% of this volume will be resorbed. This means that if we wish to obtain an increase of 100 mL, 140 mL must be available after centrifugation and so 200 mL must be harvested.[4] This demands considerable and time-consuming labor, and it may hamper the surgeon in the early stages of experience.

Laborious, Time-Consuming Harvesting

Manual aspiration with a syringe is known to be less damaging to the adipocytes than mechanical aspiration.[4,20] But harvesting is long and laborious, and so the team must be well organized. In particular, an instrument nurse should be in charge of fat preparation and centrifugation so that the rest of the team can continue with the procedure. When fat is harvested from trochanteric deposits, the patient's position has to be changed during the procedure, which further lengthens the operating time. For this reason the abdominal region is the first choice for harvesting if there are sufficient fat deposits.

Pain

Pain in the breast is not very severe, but it can be quite intense at the harvesting site. We advocate infiltration of diluted Naropin in the harvesting tunnels using the harvesting cannula. For the duration of the procedure, ordinary class 1 analgesics such as paracetamol are usually sufficient.

Edema and Bruising

Edema and bruising are frequent at both the donor and the receiving sites, due to local trauma caused by tunneling for harvesting or reinjection. Bruising persists for about 2 to 3 weeks depending on the patient.

The morphologic result at the donor site is obtained in 3 to 4 months, the time necessary for resorption of edema. On the breast, some bruises resolve in about 2 weeks, and the edema caused by the procedure resolves in about 1 month. Volume is stable after about 3 to 4 months. When the fat harvested is oily (a very high percentage of oil after centrifugation), resorption may be greater, up to 50%, and may last longer, up to 5 or 6 months. It is noteworthy that the fat is usually very oily in overweight patients. This is why we usually ask patients to reach a stable weight and to lose weight if necessary before the procedure.

RADIOLOGICAL APPEARANCE AFTER LIPOMODELING OF THE SEQUELAE OF CONSERVATIVE TREATMENT

It is important to be familiar with radiological appearance because potential microcalcifications and fat nodules were the major criticism raised against fat transfer. Moreover, as we have seen, these virulent criticisms led to the abandon of fat transfers in the breast at the end of the 1980s and to the halting of research studies and of publications on the subject. Transfers were suspected of interfering with the diagnosis of a potential breast cancer. However, over the last 20 years radiological techniques have considerably improved, enabling much more precise diagnosis of the breast parenchyma and of any abnormalities. In addition, the development of small-gauge and large-gauge needle core biopsies since 1990 provides a histologic result that is as reliable as a surgical biopsy, using a percutaneous technique under local anesthesia. In most cases, these biopsies give a definitive diagnosis without the drawbacks of surgery and can easily be proposed if any breast abnormality is considered suspicious. With our team of radiologists, we have taken particular care to define precisely all images that may be encountered after lipomodeling for the sequelae of conservative treatment of breast cancer.[26]

Images Resulting from Lipomodeling

Microcalcifications

The formation of microcalcifications can be considered as a normal consequence of lipomodeling because it concerned 20% of our patients at 1 year, but it is also a normal and frequent effect of any breast surgery.[27,28] Moreover, in our series we observed that conservative treatment had also resulted in 20% of microcalcifications before lipomodeling (reflected in a total of 40% of microcalcifications at the end of treatment at 1 year).

The frequency of microcalcifications after lipomodeling is thus similar to that developing after conservative treatment. As in many types of breast surgery other than lipomodeling, these calcifications have no diagnostic or therapeutic consequences. Radiologically, microcalcifications following breast surgery or adipocyte transfer are benign in appearance. In the literature, there are few or no systematic studies of the formation of calcifications after lipomodeling, but it has been shown that calcifications may be found in 50% of cases 2 years after breast reduction.[27] Also, in this indication, the development of these calcifications has never been accused of interfering with the diagnosis of cancer. Calcifications on fatty necrosis are in most cases easily recognizable, classified as benign and dystrophic, very different from the suspect microcalcifications of recurrence. Our team has carried out 3 studies evaluating the radiological impact of lipomodeling. The first study concerned lipomodeling of breasts reconstructed with latissimus dorsi flaps,[6] the second concerned breasts after conservative treatment,[26] and the third, breast deformities treated by lipomodeling. All

3 studies concluded there was no harmful impact on the surveillance and radiological diagnosis of a breast abnormality. In the same spirit, we organized on May 12, 2007, in Lyons, France, a day symposium on breast imaging and plastic surgery. The radiological experts who were present unanimously maintained that fat transfer, properly performed, had no deleterious effect on breast imaging. Some even emphasized that "fat is the ally of the radiologist" because of its radiolucent nature that improves contrast and makes abnormalities easier to recognize.

Fat Necrosis

Focal fat necrosis may develop. but if the technique of transfer by reinjecting fat without forming a fatty pool is respected, and if the tissues are not oversaturated, it can be avoided.[4] We consider that clinical fat necrosis generally corresponds to a lack of experience (the principles of the 3-dimensional network and avoidance of oversaturation were not respected).

The radiological presentation is much more frequent, and it is variable: Generally, oily cysts are seen (57% in our series), and their diagnosis is evident whether by mammography or ultrasound: round, regular microcalcifications with a radiolucent center classified ACR 2 (19% in our series), which are not suspicious and are readily distinguishable from those that accompany a recurrence. More rarely, we have observed the formation of a mixed, complex cystic image with a fluid and semisolid component (19%), but here again the diagnosis of fat necrosis was made without difficulty. Radiologists with a particular interest in mammography are familiar with these images because it must not be forgotten that fat necrosis, like microcalcifications, appears after all types of breast surgery: biopsy, conservative treatment, breast reduction,[27] breast reconstruction,[28] or liposuction. It was noteworthy that in our series 15% of patients already presented images of fat necrosis on ultrasound and 20% on mammography, after conservative treatment and before lipomodeling. Overall, after lipomodeling, 76% of patients presented images of fat necrosis visible on ultrasound, of which most (57%) were simple oily cysts, whose diagnosis was never in doubt. In our experience, the risk lies in the fact that unfamiliarity with the subject may lead to a suspicious image being wrongly attributed to a consequence of lipomodeling and also that a recurrence may pass unrecognized. However, it is easy to make the diagnosis of benignity or malignancy, whether by mammography,[28] ultrasound,[29] or MRI.[30]

If there is the slightest doubt, certainty must be established by histologic diagnosis obtained by small-gauge or large-gauge needle core biopsy. It must be stressed here that an expert opinion should not be sought: If there is any doubt, certainty must be obtained by histology.

The percentage of images induced by lipomodeling may appear high. It is, however, comparable with that obtained after conservative treatment by oncoplastic surgery (primary mammoplasty and radiotherapy) for primary treatment of breast cancers, a technique that is now advocated by numerous leading teams in breast cancer surgery. Imaging investigations must therefore be interpreted with discernment, putting them in perspective and comparing them with the results of oncoplastic surgery, which has the same objectives: to offer at term the best possible results of conservative treatment. So it appears that lipomodeling carried out for correction of the sequelae of conservative treatment does not generate an image that leads to confusion with breast cancer. Nor does it hinder the diagnosis of a possible local recurrence or of a new cancer.

Protocol for Radiological Follow-Up

Surveillance of the treated breast is primarily clinical. At the present time, there is no reference radiological protocol for breasts reconstructed by lipomodeling. According to the results obtained, mammography appears to be indispensable because it is the most efficient modality for the diagnosis of microcalcifications. Ultrasound is also necessary because it is the best technique for detecting images of fat necrosis. In contrast, MRI seems to us to be of little value unless recurrence is suspected.[26]

Images of fat necrosis, notably microcalcifications, continue to appear after 1 year. It seems opportune to continue mammographic and ultrasound surveillance, generally yearly, according to the recommendations of the radiologist in charge of the patient's follow-up.[26]

MEDICOLEGAL ASPECTS

Recurrence of Cancer

The local recurrence rate after conservative treatment is 1.5% per year, or 5% to 10% of patients at 5 years.[25] In this indication we are working with patients who have had a breast deformity, which may perhaps introduce a recruitment bias (notably larger tumorectomy), and we have been surprised at the frequency of potentially sensitive coincident occurrence of cancer progression.[31] Very fortunately, thanks to our knowledge of cancerology and the fact that we work as a multidisciplinary team, we have been able to avoid situations that could lead to medicolegal complexities. The rate of local recurrences after conservative treatment followed by lipomodeling is probably the same as without lipomodeling, although no study has as yet precisely evaluated this rate. Large series and prolonged follow-up are necessary for such investigation. The incidence of development of a cancerous lesion coinciding with performance of lipomodeling, or above all after lipomodeling, is thus potentially spontaneously high. Yet the patient who seeks advice for correction of the sequelae of conservative treatment often considers herself more or less cured of her cancer. Before lipomodeling is carried out, the patient must be informed that she is at risk of local recurrence, whether she decides for or against lipomodeling. She must also be made aware of the importance of breast-imaging investigations before lipomodeling in reducing the risk that fat transfer may coincide with the presence of a breast cancer. Moreover, she must make a firm commitment to have breast imaging at 1 year, 2 years, and even 3 years, according to the recommendations of the specialist radiologist who follows the patient.

Moreover, the patient must be informed that if the tumor recurs after conservative treatment, total mastectomy must be done, generally accompanied by immediate breast reconstruction with a flap.[31]

Risk of Cancer Dissemination by Lipomodeling

Tumor cell dissemination is frequent during small-gauge needle core biopsies. Studies have evaluated the rate at about 30%.[32,33] Tissue migration in axillary lymph nodes has even been observed but without clinical or prognostic significance.[34] The risk of displacement is essentially related to tumor type and to the interval between biopsy and surgical excision, whereas factors such as the volume or grade of the invasive carcinomas or carcinomas in situ and the presence of lymph node invasion have no significant impact on tumor migration.[32] It is, in fact, mixed and invasive lobular carcinomas that have the highest migration rate, followed by invasive ductal carcinomas and lastly carcinomas in situ.[32]

It is important to stress that the frequency of the displacements observed is inversely related to the interval between biopsy and surgical excision, and if excision is later it is even possible that no tumor cell may be found.[36] These observations suggest that the displaced breast tumor cells are fragile and do not survive mechanical displacement, unlike the cells of a sarcoma or an ovarian cancer, which can give rise to secondary localizations at trocar entry points.

It has also been shown that tumor biopsy technique has no influence on recurrence rate.[35,36] The literature clearly indicates that these mechanical cell migrations are not at the origin of recurrence. However, it should be emphasized that the dissemination of tumor cells may lead to mistaken conclusions in the interpretation of histologic results: overestimation of the size of a small invasive carcinoma, erroneous diagnosis of invasive carcinoma if the disseminated cells of a carcinoma in situ are interpreted as stromal invasion, or even erroneous diagnosis of lymph node invasion.

By analogy with biopsy, if lipomodeling is carried out when a small cancer has gone undetected in preoperative investigations, we may legitimately consider that here also the tumor cells will not survive the mechanical displacement potentially generated by lipomodeling. Dissemination of neoplastic disease during lipomodeling is thus unlikely because breast cancer cells are very fragile.[31]

Training of Specialist Radiologists and Experts

Errors of interpretation with regard to the causal relationship between breast cancer and lipomodeling of breasts with sequelae of conservative treatment are potentially easily committed if the expert draws too rapid a conclusion, or if his or her knowledge of the subject is not up to date, or if he or she takes account of conventional but mistaken notions hostile to this technique. We believe the core of this question lies in the level of knowledge and training of experts and radiologists specialized in breast imaging. For these reasons, we organized in Lyons, France, on May 12, 2007, a day symposium on breast imaging after plastic surgery (Breast Imaging and Plastic Surgery) that focused particularly on imaging after lipomodeling and was attended by radiologists with a specific interest in this topic. It seems to us essential that those who are faced with diagnosing recurrence of breast cancer are trained to be thoroughly familiar with the signs and symptoms of breasts after lipomodeling. It is also essential that if breast cancer is diagnosed, their attitude should be appropriate and should foster no ambiguity with regard to lipomodeling and the genesis of breast cancers. Similarly, with this enlightened perspective, experts in plastic surgery and in cancerology should be able to put forward reasoned scientific arguments (because questions will not fail to be raised in the future in view of the frequency of this coincident occurrence, and also of the distress and feeling of injustice experienced by the patients confronted by these difficult situations) showing that the occurrence of a new breast cancer or a recurrence of cancer is not imputable to lipomodeling. We believe these last points are important because fat transfer still has its detractors, who could by an antagonistic, ill-considered or ungenerous remark worsen what is already a difficult situation (a new breast cancer or a recurrence of breast cancer) by compounding misfortune upon misfortune, and so encourage unjustified allegations causing distress and anxiety to the patients and the physicians involved.

We consider these points should be made clear before extensive development of this very promising technique that brings considerable improvement to our patients, but which is also a potential source of conflict because of the frequency of possible coincident occurrence of breast lipomodeling and breast cancer.

Conclusion

Repair surgery after conservative treatment is delicate and difficult because of radiation sequelae and also because of the wide range of postsurgical deformities affecting both the skin and the gland itself. The results of partial reconstructions for sequelae of conservative treatment are often disappointing, and their treatment may sometimes raise problems that are more difficult to solve than those of mastectomy. Lipomodeling appears to us to be a simple technique, although a learning curve is necessary to avoid the formation of fatty nodules. It achieves breasts with very good contour and suppleness while avoiding the use of an implant or sacrifice of muscle. The amounts of fat transferred must be appropriate in the receiving tissue. If the deformity is significant or the receiving tissue is thin, it is preferable to carry out several sessions. Stable results are obtained after the fat injection of the early months, if the patient maintains a constant weight. Complications are rare, mainly infectious in nature, and rapidly resolved. Radiological images of calcifications or fat necrosis frequently occur after lipomodeling. They are similar to those induced by any other type of breast surgery, notably by the initial conservative treatment. For a radiologist experienced in breast imaging, they do not lead to confusion with possible images of a breast cancer recurrence. If there is the slightest doubt, any suspicious image must undergo percutaneous small-gauge or large-gauge needle core biopsy.

Lastly, the lipomodeling technique as we have presented it here represents a considerable advance in the therapeutic armamentarium for moderate sequelae of conservative treatment. The restored breast has a contour and suppleness that no other surgical technique had yet been able to offer. Radiological studies have shown that radiological surveillance is still possible after this procedure. However, this method can only be envisaged as part of a multidisciplinary approach. The radiologist who carries out the preoperative imaging investigation must agree with the principle of the procedure, as must the surgical oncologist following the patient for her cancer. The opinion of each of those involved must be respected. This attitude and this sharing of responsibility enable all those involved to work in the same direction, making it possible to avoid inappropriate comment if local recurrence does develop, as is always a possibility after conservative treatment, with or without lipomodeling.

SUMMARY

The sequelae of conservative treatment of breast cancer are difficult to treat. Lipomodeling offers a new treatment option, consisting of transferring to the deformed breast fatty tissue that has been meticulously harvested and prepared. We consider lipomodeling a technique whose concept is simple but that requires a learning curve to avoid the formation of necrotic fat nodules. It yields very good results regarding contour and suppleness of the breast while avoiding the need to use an implant or to sacrifice muscle. Stable results are obtained after the normal fat resorption in the early months, if the patient maintains a constant weight. Radiological images of calcifications or fat necrosis are a frequent occurrence after lipomodeling and are similar to those induced by any type of breast surgery, notably the initial conservative treatment.

Although this technique appears to represent a considerable advance in the therapeutic armamentarium for moderate sequelae of conservative treatment, we consider it as only part of a multidisciplinary approach. The radiologist who carries out preoperative investigation must be in agreement with the principle of the procedure, as must the cancerologist following the patient for her cancer. The opinion of all those involved must be respected. Such an approach and sharing of responsibility allow all those involved to work together to limit the potential medicolegal complexities in the event of further progression of cancer.

REFERENCES

1. Delay E, Gosset J, Toussoun G, Delaporte T, Delbaere M. Post-treatment sequelae after breast cancer conservative surgery [in French]. *Ann Chir Plast Esthet*. 2008;53:135-152.
2. Delay E, Bobin JY, Rivoire M. Reconstructions partielles esthétiques des déformations majeures du sein et des rechutes intramammaires après traitement conservateur. In: Mole B, ed. *Actualités de chirurgie esthétique*. Paris, France: Masson: 1993:41-55.
3. Bobin JY, Delay E, Rivoire M. Reconstruction of severe breast deformities following conservative cancer surgery and radiation therapy with a latissimus dorsi myocutaneous flap. In: Szabo Z, Kerstein MD, Lewis JE, eds. *Surgical Technology International III. International Developments in Surgery and Surgical Research*. San Francisco, CA: Universal Medical Press: 1994:523-528.
4. Delay E. Lipomodeling of the reconstructed breast. In: Spear SL, ed. *Surgery of the Breast: Principles and Art*. 2nd ed. Philadelphia, PA: Lippincott Williams & Wilkins: 2006:930-946.
5. Delay E, Delaporte T, Sinna R. Breast implant alternatives [in French] *Ann Chir Plast Esthet*. 2005;50:652-672.
6. Pierrefeu-Lagrange AC, Delay E, Guerin N, Chekaroua K, Delaporte T. Radiological evaluation of breasts reconstructed with lipomodeling [in French]. *Ann Chir Plast Esthet*. 2006;51:18-28.
7. Delay E, Gosset J, Toussoun G, Delaporte T, Delbaere M. Efficacy of lipomodeling for the management of sequelae of breast cancer conservative treatment [in French]. *Ann Chir Plast Esthet*. 2008;53:153-168.
8. Illouz YG. Present results of fat injection. Aesthetic Plast Surg 1988; 12: 175-81.
9. Fournier PF. The breast fill. In: Fournier PF, ed. *Liposculpture: The syringe Technique*. Paris, France: Arnette Blackwell: 1991:357-367.
10. Bircoll M. Cosmetic breast augmentation utilizing autologous fat and liposuction techniques. *Plast Reconstr Surg*. 1987;79:267-271.
11. Bircoll M, Novack BH. Autologous fat transplantation employing liposuction techniques. *Ann Plast Surg*. 1987;18:327-329.
12. Hartrampf CR Jr, Bennett GK. Autologous fat from liposuction for breast augmentation [letter]. *Plast Reconstr Surg*. 1987;80:646.
13. Ettelson CD. Fat autografting [letter]. *Plast Reconstr Surg*. 1987;80:646.
14. Linder RM. Fat autografting [letter]. *Plast Reconstr Surg*. 1987;80:646.
15. Oustehout DK. Breast augmentation by autologous fat injection [letter]. *Plast Reconstr Surg*. 1987;80:868.
16. Gradinger GP. Breast augmentation by autologous fat injection [letter]. *Plast Reconstr Surg*. 1987;80:868.
17. Bircoll M. Reply [letter]. *Plast Reconstr Surg*. 1987;80:647.
18. Bircoll M. Autologous fat transplantation to the breast. *Plast Reconstr Surg*. 1988;82:361-362.
19. Brown FE, Sargent SK, Cohen SR, Morain WD. Mammographic changes following reduction mammaplasty. *Plast Reconstr Surg*. 1987;80:691-698.
20. Coleman SR. Long-term survival of fat transplants: controlled demonstrations. *Aesthetic Plast Surg*. 1995;19:421-425.
21. Coleman SR. Facial recontouring with lipostructure. *Clin Plast Surg*. 1997;24:347-367.
22. Delay E, Gounot N, Bouillot A, Zlatoff P, Rivoire M. Autologous latissimus breast reconstruction: a 3-year clinical experience with 100 patients. *Plast Reconstr Surg* 1998;102;1461-78.
23. Delay E, Delaporte T, Jorquera F, El Berbeni N, Vasseur C. Lipomodeling of the breast after reconstruction by latissimus dorsi flap without prosthesis implantation [in French]. Paper presented at: 46th Congress of the Société Française de Chirurgie Plastique, Esthétique et Reconstructice, Paris, France; October 17-19, 2001.
24. Delay E, Chekaroua K, Mojallal A, Garson S. Lipomodeling of the autologous latissimus reconstructed breast. Paper presented at: 13th International Congress of the International Confederation for Plastic Reconstructive and Aesthetic Surgery; Sydney, Australia; August 10-15, 2003. Abstract in *ANZ J Surg*. 2003;73:A170.
25. Mauriac L, Luporsi E, Cutuli B, et al. Summary version of the Standards, Options and Recommendations for non metastatic breast cancer. *Br J Cancer*. 2003;89(suppl 1):S17-31.
26. Gosset J, Guerin N, Toussoun G, Delaporte T, Delay E. Radiological evaluation after lipomodelling for correction of breast conservative treatment sequelae [in French]. *Ann Chir Plast Esthet*. 2008;53:178-189.
27. Brown FE, Sargent SK, Cohen SR, Morain WD. Mammographic changes following reduction mammaplasty. *Plast Reconstr Surg*. 1987;80:691-698.
28. Hogge JP, Robinson RE, Magnant CM, Zuurbier RA. The mammographic spectrum of fat necrosis of the breast. *Radiographics*. 1995;15:1347-1356.
29. Soo MS, Rosen EL, Baker JA, Vo TT, Boyd BA. Negative predictive value of sonography with mammography in patients with palpable breast lesions. *AJR Am J Roentgenol*. 2001;177:1167-1170.
30. Kinoshita T, Yashiro N, Yoshigi J, Ihara N, Narita M. Fat necrosis of breast: a potential pitfall in breast MRI. *Clin Imaging*. 2002;26:250-253.
31. Gosset J, Flageul G, Toussoun G, Guérin N, Tourasse C, Delay E. Lipomodeling for correction of breast conservative treatment sequelae. Medicolegal aspects. Expert opinion on five problematic clinical cases [in French]. *Ann Chir Plast Esthet*. 2008;53:190-198.
32. Diaz LK, Wiley EL, Venta LA. Are malignant cells displaced by large-gauge needle core biopsy of the breast? *AJR Am J Roentgenol*. 1999;173:1303-1313.
33. Youngson BJ, Liberman L, Rosen PP. Displacement of carcinomatous epithelium in surgical breast specimens following stereotaxic core biopsy. *Am J Clin Pathol*. 1995;103:598-602.
34. Carter BA, Jensen RA, Simpson JF, Page DL. Benign transport of breast epithelium into axillary lymph nodes after biopsy. *Am J Clin Pathol*. 2000;113:259-265.
35. Liberman L, Vuolo M, Dershaw DD, et al. Epithelial displacement after stereotactic 11-gauge directional vacuum-assisted breast biopsy. *AJR Am J Roentgenol*. 1999;172:677-681.
36. King TA, Hayes DH, Cederbom GJ, et al. Biopsy technique has no impact on local recurrence after breast-conserving therapy. *Breast J*. 2001;7:19-24.

CHAPTER 79

Implant-Based Reconstruction

Peter Cordeiro
Colleen McCarthy

Autogenous tissue reconstruction is generally thought to produce the most natural looking and feeling breast(s). Although the permanency of these results and lack of dependancy on a permanent prosthesis is also advantageous, the relative magnitude of these procedures is great. Many women will instead opt for a prosthetic reconstruction, choosing a less invasive operative procedure with a faster recovery and the capability of achieving excellent results. In fact, of the nearly 60,000 women in the United States who had postmastectomy reconstruction in 2007, the majority (approximately 70%) elected to pursue implant-based, postmastectomy reconstruction.[1]

RECONSTRUCTIVE OPTIONS

Current options for implant-based reconstruction include the following: (1) single-stage implant reconstruction with either a standard or an adjustable, permanent prosthesis; (2) 2-stage tissue expander/implant reconstruction; and (3) combined implant/autogenous tissue reconstruction.

Single-Stage Reconstruction

Immediate, single-stage breast reconstruction with a standard implant is best suited to the occasional patient who has a small, nonptotic breast and adequate skin at the mastectomy site, which will allow for immediate placement of a permanent implant. Selection criteria for single-stage, adjustable implant reconstruction is similar, yet it is the preferred technique when the ability to adjust the volume of the device postoperatively is desired. In small-breasted women where the skin deficiency is minimal, the implant can be partially filled at the time of reconstruction and gradually inflated to the desired volume postoperatively. In addition, disadvantages of this technique include the placement of a remote port and the need for its subsequent

removal. Finally, many suggest that the aesthetic outcomes tend not be as good as 2-stage reconstruction and/or revisional procedures are often necessitated. Consequently, this approach is not used for a majority of implant-based reconstructions.[1]

Two-Stage Expander/Implant Reconstruction

Although satisfactory results can be obtained with single-stage reconstruction, in the vast majority of patients, a more reliable approach involves 2-stage expander/implant reconstruction.[2] Tissue expansion is used when there is insufficient tissue after mastectomy to create the desired size and shape of a breast in a single stage. A tissue expander is placed in a submuscular pocket at the primary procedure. In the early postoperative period, the tissue expander is serially inflated with saline as a weekly office-based procedure. Once the expansions are completed (6-8 weeks), the tissues are allowed to relax and adjust to the new position for another 1 to 2 months (or until after adjuvant chemotherapy is completed). Exchange of the temporary expander for a permanent implant occurs at a subsequent operation. At the time of the secondary procedure, access to the implant pocket allows for release of capsular contracture, adjustment of the inframammary fold, and selection of the optimum-shaped and optimum-sized implant, which, in turn, maximizes the aesthetic result. Thus the 2-stage technique of tissue expander/implant reconstruction has become the most common approach to implant-based reconstruction.[1,3,4]

Combined Tissue/Autogenous Tissue Reconstruction

Many patients who undergo postmastectomy reconstruction are candidates for tissue expander/implant reconstruction. However, the absence of an adequate skin envelope is an absolute contraindication to expander/implant reconstruction alone. A large skin resection at the time of mastectomy, due to previous biopsies or locally advanced disease, may preclude the primary coverage of a tissue expander. In patients without the volume of soft tissue required to permit a tension-free closure over an expander, autogenous tissue (most commonly the ipsilateral latissimus dorsi myocutaneous flap) can provide additional soft tissue.[5] The combination of a latissimus dorsi flap and tissue expansion may also be appropriate in cases in which the remaining mastectomy skin is of insufficient quality to tolerate any tissue expansion. This is typically the case in the insetting of delayed reconstruction after mastectomy and postoperative radiation therapy.[6] The addition of autogenous tissue to implant reconstruction increases the length and complexity of the procedure, and addition of a donor site can increase the morbidity. Thus the combined autogenous tissue and tissue/implant reconstruction is generally reserved for a highly select patient population.

TIMING OF RECONSTRUCTION

Immediate postmastectomy reconstruction is currently considered the standard of care in breast reconstruction. Immediate reconstruction is assumed to be advantageous, as studies have shown that women who undergo immediate reconstruction have less psychological distress about the loss of a breast and have a better overall quality of life when compared with delayed procedures.[7] Technically, reconstruction is facilitated in the immediate setting because of the pliability of the native skin envelope and the delineation of the natural inframammary fold. In addition, immediate reconstruction has proven to be cost-effective and is less inconvenient for the patient.

The increasing use of postoperative radiotherapy for earlier-stage breast cancers has, however, challenged this thinking. Adjuvant radiotherapy has been shown to increase the risk of postoperative complications.[8-12] Given this data, whether or not to perform immediate reconstruction for patients in whom radiation therapy is planned remains controversial. Similarly, for those who may be unable to decide about reconstruction while adjusting to their cancer diagnosis, delayed expander/implant reconstruction remains an option.

In patients for whom the postoperative administration of adjuvant radiotherapy is likely, a decision to undergo expander/implant reconstruction may be delayed. In the setting of delayed expander/implant reconstruction, placing a prosthesis beneath healed, viable mastectomy flaps eliminates the concern for flap necrosis and expander exposure. However, the amount of skin is often greatly reduced because it comes from non–skin-sparing mastectomies. Therefore, expansion may be more uncomfortable and achieve less volume, making achievement of ptosis difficult.

In the situation where a tissue expander is already in place and the need for radiation therapy becomes evident only after final primary tumor and nodal pathology is available, proceeding with implant reconstruction is still a viable option. In this scenario, patients undergo expansion during chemotherapy, undergo the exchange procedure approximately 4 weeks after chemotherapy, and start radiation therapy as soon as 4 weeks after the exchange procedure. Patients who undergo reconstruction

using this approach have been found to closely have higher rate of capsular contracture; however, a successful reconstruction is still achieved greater than 90% of the time, and patient satisfaction remains high.[3,4]

The immediate insertion of a tissue expander as a first stage followed by removal and implant placement or removal and autogenous flap reconstruction is an alternative approach offered by some.[13] Stage 1 of this 2-stage approach consists of skin-sparing mastectomy with insertion of a tissue expander until the results of the permanent pathology are known. After review of permanent sections, patients who do not require radiation undergo stage 2 of the "delayed-immediate" reconstruction. Those patients who do require radiotherapy undergo deflation of the tissue expander, receipt of radiotherapy, and delayed reconstruction with autogenous tissue alone or combined autogenous tissue–implant reconstruction. Proponents of this approach suggest that patients who require postmastectomy radiation can avoid the aesthetic problems associated with the receipt of radiotherapy after immediate reconstruction. Future larger-scale evaluation of this approach is needed (see Areas of Uncertainty).

INDICATIONS AND CONTRAINDICATIONS

Most patients who undergo a mastectomy will be candidates for tissue expander/implant reconstruction. The most favorable results will be achieved, however, in patients who have a moderate breast volume (500 g or less) and mild to moderate ptosis. Patients with large or markedly ptotic breasts will generally require some type of matching procedure in order to obtain symmetry with a prosthetic reconstruction (Figs. 79-1 and 79-2). Tissue expander/implant reconstruction requires less operative time than does autologous reconstruction; therefore, it may be well suited for patients with comorbidities that preclude long procedures. Patients who undergo bilateral mastectomies may also be well suited to expander/implant reconstruction. Bilateral implant reconstructions can generally produce very favorable results, due to the fact that both breast contour and degree of ptosis are symmetrical.[3]

Relative contraindications to expander/implant reconstruction include smoking, obesity, and hypertension.[14,15] These comorbid conditions have been shown to contribute to increased local wound complications and are associated with an increased risk of reconstructive failure. It is important to note, however, that the overall incidence of complications after tissue expander/implant reconstruction in patients with these identifiable risk factors remains acceptably low. Thus patients who have these factors, such as obesity, should not be discouraged from undergoing expander/implant reconstruction; instead, these patients should be informed about the risks and benefits of the procedure as they pertain to themselves as individuals.

Previous chest wall irradiation and/or postmastectomy radiotherapy are also considered by many to be a relative contraindication for implant-based breast reconstruction. Earlier breast cancers are being increasingly treated with adjuvant chemotherapy and radiotherapy in an attempt to increase survival. It has been shown that chemotherapy does not increase the risk of postoperative complications after expander/implant reconstruction.[16,17] The possible implications of adjuvant radiotherapy

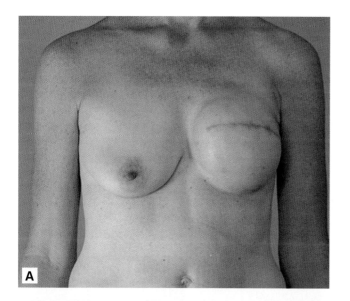

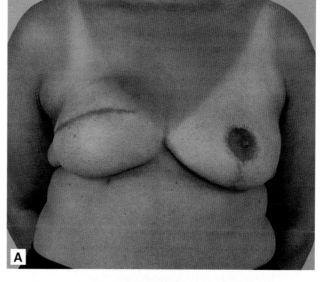

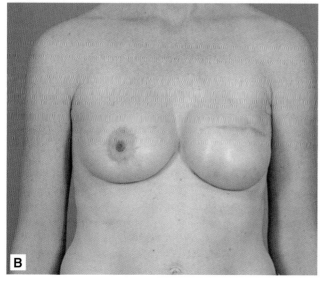

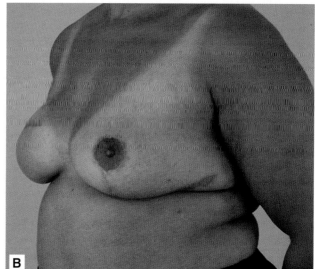

FIGURE 79-1 Immediate tissue expander/implant reconstruction left breast. **A.** Overexpansion of left breast completed. **B.** Exchange procedure performed left. Contralateral augmentation/mastopexy performed right for symmetry.

FIGURE 79-2 Immediate tissue expander/implant reconstruction right breast. Reduction mammoplasty performed left breast for symmetry. **A.** Anteroposterior view. **B.** Right oblique view. Note degree of ptosis achieved in right reconstructed breast.

on the outcomes after breast reconstruction are, however, both profound and controversial. Not only is tissue expansion difficult in previously irradiated tissues, but the risks of infection, expander exposure, and subsequent extrusion are increased.[18,19] Patients should be offered tissue expander/implant reconstruction only after a preoperative assessment determines the skin quality to be favorable and the presumed ability to perform a skin-sparing mastectomy. In this setting, a relative excess of skin is necessitated in order to permit a tension-free closure over an expander.

Studies have also shown that patients who receive postoperative radiotherapy have a significantly higher incidence of capsular contracture than controls.[4,12] Although some view postmastectomy radiation as an absolute contraindication to implant/expander reconstruction because of poor cosmesis and increased complications, others have demonstrated that

outcomes may vary with respect to differences in timing and dosing of radiation. Cordeiro et al[12] recently published their findings from a large consecutive series of patients who were uniformly treated with radiation 4 weeks after the exchange procedure. Although complication and contracture rates were increased in the tissue/expander group compared with controls, patient ratings of reconstructive success and satisfaction ultimately remained high, confirming similar conclusions made by Krueger et al.[11]

ADVANTAGES AND DISADVANTAGES

Postmastectomy implant reconstruction has the distinct advantage of combining a lesser operative procedure with the capability of achieving excellent results in well-selected patients. Donor-site morbidity is eliminated with the use of a prosthetic device, and in general, no new scars are introduced. Where necessary, tissue expansion provides skin with similar qualities of texture and color compared with that of the contralateral breast.

Patients who undergo tissue expander/implant breast reconstruction will, however, experience varying degrees of discomfort and chest wall asymmetry during the expansion phase. In addition, patients must make more frequent office visits for percutaneous expansion. Finally, the ultimate aesthetic result achieved with implant reconstruction is limited because the shape of the final breast mound is more rounded in appearance, there is limited projection of the lower pole of the breast, and minimal to no ptosis. Thus unless the patient has a contralateral breast that has the appearance of an implant, modification procedures to the other breast (augmentation mammoplasty, mastopexy, and reduction mammoplasty) become necessary in order to improve breast symmetry.

By contrast, in patients who undergo unilateral reconstruction, long-term aesthetic results may deteriorate over time. Clough et al,[20] by evaluating photographic evidence of reconstruction patients, determined that in those who demonstrated deterioration in their aesthetic result over time, late asymmetry was produced by the failure of both breasts to undergo symmetrical ptosis with aging. However, although these outcomes are important, they are relatively crude indicators of success in the realm of reconstructive breast surgery. Further inquiry into the identification of factors that ultimately influence patient satisfaction is needed so that a high level of satisfaction after not only tissue expander/implant reconstruction, but other reconstructive modalities is ensured (see Areas of Uncertainty).

APPROACH TO 2-STAGE TISSUE EXPANDER/ IMPLANT RECONSTRUCTION

Creating a Submuscular versus Subpectoral Pocket

In the setting of immediate implant reconstruction, both infectious complications and wound healing problems can have negative consequences. Not only can these outcomes necessitate the explantation of a permanent prosthesis, delaying the reconstructive process, but more importantly, they can delay the administration of adjuvant therapy for breast cancer. By placing an expander in a completely submuscular position, the risk of expander exposure and contamination in the setting of mastectomy flap necrosis is minimized. In addition, lateral displacement of the expander is prevented, as the lateral limits of the expander pocket are defined by the extent to which the serratus muscle/fascia is elevated rather than by the lateral limits of the mastectomy cavity. Intraoperatively, the lateral border of the pectoralis muscle is raised using electrocautery. Care is taken not to elevate the medial insertion of the muscle from the sternum. At the inferior aspect of the lateral pectoralis dissection, the anterior rectus sheath is elevated in continuity with the pectoralis muscle to allow for placement of the expander just below the level of the inframammary fold. Laterally, the serratus muscle and fascia are also elevated to permit total muscle coverage of the expander (Fig. 79-3).

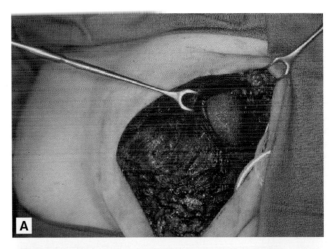

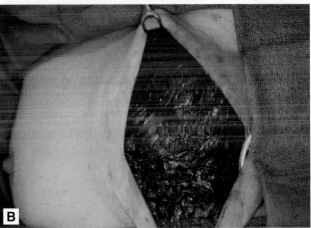

FIGURE 79-3 Immediate tissue expander placement left breast. **A.** Textured tissue expander placed in a complete submuscular pocket. **B.** Suture of the lateral pectoral border to the serratus anterior muscle/fascia complete.

Conversely, placement of the expander in a traditional subpectoral pocket allows for muscle coverage of the superiomedial portion only. In this setting, the inferolateral portion of the device sits directly underneath the subcutaneous tissue. Not only is the risk of expander exposure/extrusion higher in the setting of mastectomy flap complications, but the risk of lateral displacement of the tissue expander is greater. Some who believe that the elevation of the serratus anterior muscle/fascia adds significant morbidity have advocated for the use of the tissue substitute, AlloDerm (LifeCell; Branchburg, New Jersey).[21,22] By reconstructing the inferolateral expander pocket using AlloDerm, the need to elevate muscle/fascia inferolaterally is eliminated. It is important to note, however, that at the present time, the safety and effectiveness of AlloDerm in the setting of implant-based reconstruction remains untested in clinical trials (see Areas of Uncertainty).

Selecting an Expander

Intraoperatively, the mastectomy weight is recorded and the width of the expander pocket is then measured. An appropriate expander is then selected on the basis of its base dimensions and volume capability. Generally, the authors prefer to use textured, anatomic expanders. It is theorized that textured implants reduce the amount of device migration, whereas anatomical implants preferentially expand the lower pole of the breast. Low, medium, and full/tall height expanders are available for use. Which expander is chosen depends first on the patient's body habitus. For example, for a taller woman with a narrow chest, a full height expander is selected. Conversely, for a shorter woman with a wider chest, a medium height expander will be used. In the author's practice, low-height expanders are rarely chosen.

Tissue Expansion

After wound closure, intraoperative expansion is performed to tissue tolerance. Up to 50% of the tissue expander volume is generally placed, thus filling the submuscular cavity and preventing skin contracture. Perioperative antibiotics are routinely administered, and 2 closed-suction drains are placed in the mastectomy pocket. In the absence of skin flap necrosis or infection, postoperative expansions generally begin 10 to 14 days after surgery. The final expander volume is usually 20% greater than the recommended volume of the expander. This overexpansion ultimately creates a looser skin envelope and a greater potential for ptosis.

Exchange Procedure

At the second stage, a full circumferential capsulotomy is performed, and the inframammary fold is recreated. Along with the capsulotomy, the inferomedial border of the pectoralis muscle and the inframammary fold are released (Fig. 79-4). By fully releasing this skin/muscle envelope, the degree of projection is increased. The area of the fold is then advanced and approximated to the anterior chest wall with interrupted, permanent sutures (Fig. 79-4B), thereby enabling precise positioning of the inframammary fold and the creation of breast ptosis. The operating table is routinely placed in an upright sitting position and symmetry evaluated throughout the procedure. Various implant sizers are tested, and the final prosthesis is selected.

Choosing a Permanent Implant

Currently, both saline and silicone gel implants are available for use. Although saline-filled implants may still offer the greatest

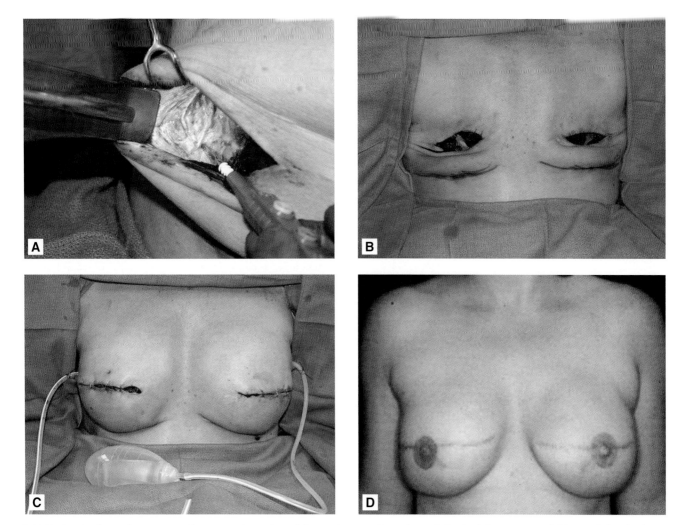

FIGURE 79-4 The exchange procedure. **A.** A circumferential capsulectomy is performed. **B.** The inframammary folds are defined using heavy silk sutures. **C.** Permanent implants are placed. **D.** Postoperatively, excellent breast contour and symmetry is achieved.

peace of mind for some patients in terms of safety implant palpability and rippling is more likely. Saline implants also tend to feel firmer to the touch and provide less natural upper-pole fullness. By contrast, the use of silicone gel implants generally allows for a softer, more natural-feeling breast. Issues of silicone safety have been carefully investigated.[23-28] To date, there is no definitive evidence linking breast implants to cancer, immunologic diseases, neurologic problems, or other systemic diseases. The potential risk to patients remains the possibility that in the event of a disruption in the integrity of the implant shell, silicone gel can theoretically leak into the surrounding tissues. To date, however, possible side effects of local silicone leak have not been well defined. At the present time, the US Food and Drug Administration (FDA) is stipulating that routine magnetic resonance imaging (MRI) is necessary to accurately identify silicone implant rupture and recommends that all patients with silicone implants undergo MRI at 3 years after implantation and every 2 years thereafter (see Areas of Uncertainty).

COMPLICATIONS

Prosthetic breast reconstruction is a relatively simple technique that is generally well tolerated. Complications are typically centered on the breast, with few systemic health implications and minimal overall patient morbidity. Thus implant reconstruction can often be performed on patients who might not be suitable candidates for the more complex and lengthy autologous procedures.

Early complications after expander insertion are significantly more common than after the exchange procedure.[3] Such complications include the development of a hematoma, seroma, infection, skin flap necrosis, and/or implant exposure/extrusion. Early aggressive treatment of breast cellulitis is warranted. Antibiotics are typically administered intravenously until obvious signs of improvement are seen. For those in whom the periprosthetic infection does not respond to antibiotic therapy, however, the premature removal of the expander (or implant) is necessitated. Similarly, the exposure of a temporary expander or implant typically requires removal. In the rare case, it may be possible to salvage an exposed expander. In the absence of any signs of infection, an exposed expander may be removed and exchanged after copious irrigation of the expander pocket. It may be prudent to remove some of the volume of the device to minimize wound tension. After the premature removal of a prosthetic device, the authors generally wait 3 to 6 months after explantation before initiating delayed reconstruction, when possible.

Late complications include palpable and/or visible rippling of the implant, particularly at the superomedial or inferolateral aspect of the reconstructed breast. This is especially noticeably in slender women, those with thin mastectomy flaps, and/or those with a saline device. Surgical options to correct rippling are limited. For those with saline implants, changing the device to a silicone cohesive gel implant may ameliorate the problem. Alternatively, changing to a new saline implant with an increased fill volume may partially correct the rippling. Other late complications include the development of an implant leak or deflation and capsular contracture[28] (Fig. 79-5). Although

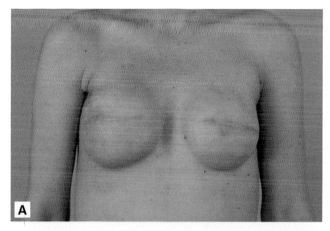

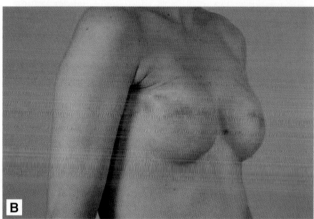

FIGURE 79-5 Bilateral tissue expander/implant reconstruction. Postmastectomy radiation received right breast. Grade 3 capsular contracture right breast. Grade 2 capsular contracture left. **A.** Anteroposterior view. **B.** Left oblique view.

capsular contracture occurs to some extent around all implants, in some women, the degree of contracture will increase in severity over time. In patients with significant capsular contracture resulting in size or shape distortions and/or other pain symptomatology, a then multi-partial capsulotomy or capsulectomy may be indicated.

BREAST CANCER RECURRENCE AFTER IMPLANT RECONSTRUCTION

Strong evidence exists that suggests that postmastectomy implant reconstruction is safe in the setting of invasive breast cancer. For example, researchers have demonstrated that there is no difference in the incidence of locoregional recurrence in breast cancer patients who undergo immediate, tissue expander/implant reconstruction compared with those patients who undergo mastectomy alone. Similarly, it has been shown that prosthetic breast reconstruction does not hinder or delay the detection of locoregional breast cancer recurrence.[29]

Although there are reliable screening tools for primary breast cancer, however, surveillance of the reconstructed breast for recurrence remains somewhat controversial. At our institution, mammography is not part of the routine follow-up of patients who have undergone mastectomy and reconstruction. Physical examination and directed imaging studies are instead the standard of care. Although computed tomography, MRI, and ultrasound have been shown to be effective modalities in the detection of recurrence, their use as initial screening tools has not yet been defined.[29]

AREAS OF UNCERTAINTY AND NECESSARY FUTURE STUDIES

Evaluating Patient-Reported Outcomes

Traditional assessments of outcome in plastic surgery have considered mortality, morbidity, and physiologic function. Although these are important issues, they are relatively crude indicators of success in the realm of reconstructive breast surgery. Moving forward, outcomes research must examine not only morbidity and mortality, but also *patient perceptions of the results of surgery*.[30] The assessment of patient experience is especially important in reconstructive breast surgery, as the overriding goal of surgery is to satisfy the patient with respect to her body image, physical well-being, and perception of the aesthetic result.[31] Rigorous measurement of satisfaction and quality of life are thus integral to any outcome analysis.

Thus, as part of any future outcome assessment, studies should include an evaluation of the effectiveness of an intervention from a patient perspective. By quantifying patient satisfaction and quality of life after reconstructive breast surgery, for example, we will ultimately improve patient care and support patient advocacy, future cost-effectiveness analyses, and patient education.

Radiation Therapy and Implant-Based Reconstruction

The cohort of patients who are currently receiving adjuvant radiation in addition to mastectomy and adjuvant chemotherapy continues to increase in number. Consensus regarding the optimal approach to postmastectomy implant-based reconstruction in this setting remains undefined. Controversy exists regarding the optimal timing and modality of reconstruction with respect to the timing and administration of radiation. Clinical outcomes research that evaluates the oncologic safety, the development of complications, and patients' perception of outcome can be used to guide us toward defining the best approach to these complex clinical problems.

FDA Recommendations

The FDA currently recommends that routine MRI is necessary to accurately identify silicone gel implant rupture and recommends that all patients with silicone implants undergo MRI at 3 years after implantation and every 2 years thereafter. The FDA's recommendation seems to reflect a belief that mass MRI screening of asymptomatic women may ultimately reduce patient morbidity due to implant rupture, yet this phenomenon has clearly not been demonstrated. Instead, this approach exposes patients unnecessarily to the risks of the screening test (including cost) and, potentially, to the risks of the unnecessary treatment.[32]

Although the detection of silent silicone implant ruptures may prove to be prudent, there is no conclusive evidence at this time to show that using MRI screening of asymptomatic women leads to a reduction in patient morbidity. In fact, when MRI screening is examined critically from the standpoint of the principles of screening, evidence from prospective studies to support its use in this setting is lacking and raises more questions than answers. For example, does the morbidity from silicone implant rupture warrant mass screening? Does the natural history of rupture justify regular MRI screening? Does the removal or exchange of an asymptomatic implant rupture substantiate the decision to screen all asymptomatic individuals?

In general, proof of benefit from a screening test ideally comes from randomized studies that demonstrate that the application of the test results in a significant decrease in patient morbidity. Thus, moving forward, our specialty should look to provide evidence that either supports or refutes the routine use of MRI as a screening tool for silent implant rupture. Until the time when that evidence is available, the responsibility for choosing one path or another should be shared by both the patient and her surgeon. For different women, underlying beliefs and values will sway decision making in different directions. Engaging women in the process of shared decision making may help women make decisions more consistent with their risk comfort level and their values.

AlloDerm in Tissue Expander/Implant Reconstruction

AlloDerm is an acellular, cryopreserved, dermal matrix lacking antigenic stimuli. Previous case series have demonstrated the feasibility of implantable AlloDerm in immediate postmastectomy reconstruction.[21,22] Proponents suggest that the use of an implantable dermal matrix affords multiple advantages when compared with traditional techniques. First, by using AlloDerm in the creation of the inferolateral expander pocket, elevation of the serratus fascia/musculature is avoided. It is hypothesized that the pain and sensory morbidity experienced due to the surgical disruption and subsequent expansion of the lateral intercostal nerves is therefore minimized. Second, because of the pliability of the acellular dermal matrix, it is suggested that the reconstructive process can be expedited by maximizing expansion volumes and thus minimizing the number of expansions required. Third, it is theorized that by facilitating expansion in the lower pole of the breast, a breast with greater ptosis and more natural contours can be created.

Although these hypotheses may make intuitive sense, it is important to note that at the present time, these hypotheses remain untested in clinical trials and are, at best, based on anecdotal evidence and/or expert opinion. The high cost of AlloDerm and the current lack of scientific data regarding its efficacy underscore the need to objectively evaluate its use. Thus future blinded, randomized controlled trials are necessary to elucidate the purported benefits of AlloDerm in the setting of implant-based reconstruction. By randomly allocating patients to different treatment groups, the risk that systematic differences exist between patients can be minimized. Similarly, by "blinding" patients and evaluators, preconceived views about an intervention cannot systematically bias the assessment of outcomes. By performing such a trial, the most unbiased, impartial evidence unmasking either the efficacy or lack the efficacy of AlloDerm in this setting can be elucidated.

SUMMARY

Contemporary techniques provide numerous options for postmastectomy reconstruction. Implant-based reconstruction has the capability of achieving excellent results in well-selected patients. Compared with autogenous tissue reconstruction, implant reconstruction is a less invasive procedure with a quicker convalescence. Ultimately, individualized selection of a reconstructive technique for each patient will be a predominant factor in achieving a reconstructive success. Future clinical research will continue to advance the field of postmastectomy reconstruction.

REFERENCES

1. American Society of Plastic Surgery. American Society of Plastic Surgery Web Site. Available at: http://www.plasticsurgery.org. Accessed 2008.
2. Pusic AL, Cordeiro PG. An accelerated approach to tissue expansion for breast reconstruction: experience with intraoperative and rapid postoperative expansion in 370 reconstructions. *Plast Reconstr Surg.* 2003;111:1871-1875.
3. Cordeiro PG, McCarthy CM. A single surgeon's 12-year experience with tissue expander/implant breast reconstruction; part I, A prospective analysis of early complications. *Plast Reconstr Surg.* 2006;118:825-831.
4. Cordeiro PG, McCarthy CM. A single surgeon's 12-year experience with tissue expander/implant breast reconstruction. part II. An analysis of long-term complications, aesthetic outcomes, and patient satisfaction. *Plast Reconstr Surg.* 2006;118: 832-839.
5. Hammond DC. Postmastectomy reconstruction of the breast using the latissimus dorsi musculocutaneous flap. *Cancer J.* 2008;14:248-252.
6. Disa JJ, McCarthy CM, Mehrara BJ, Pusic AL, Cordeiro PG. Immediate latissimus dorsi/prosthetic breast reconstruction following salvage mastectomy after failed lumpectomy/irradiation. *Plast Reconstr Surg* 2008;121:159e-164e.
7. Al Ghazal SK, Sully L, Fallowfield L, Blamey RW. The psychological impact of immediate rather than delayed breast reconstruction. *Eur J Surg Oncol* 2000;26:17-19.
8. McCormick B, Wright J, Cordeiro P. Breast reconstruction combined with radiation therapy: long-term risks and factors related to decision making. *Cancer J.* 2008;14:264-268.
9. Spear SL, Onyewu C. Staged breast reconstruction with saline-filled implants in the irradiated breast: recent trends and therapeutic implications. *Plast Reconstr Surg.* 2000;105:930-942.
10. McCarthy CM, Pusic AL, Disa JJ, et al. Unilateral postoperative chest wall radiotherapy in bilateral tissue expander/implant reconstruction patients: a prospective outcomes analysis. *Plast Reconstr Surg.* 2005;116:1642-1647.
11. Krueger EA, Wilkins EG, Strawderman M, et al. Complications and patient satisfaction following expander/implant breast reconstruction with and without radiotherapy. *Int J Radiat Oncol Biol Phys.* 2001;49:713-721.
12. Cordeiro PG, Pusic AL, Disa JJ, et al. Irradiation after immediate tissue expander/implant breast reconstruction: outcomes, complications, aesthetic results, and satisfaction among 156 patients. *Plast Reconstr Surg.* 2004;113:877-881.
13. Kronowitz SJ. Immediate versus delayed reconstruction. *Clin Plast Surg.* 2007;34:39-50.
14. McCarthy CM, Mehrara BJ, Riedel E, et al. Predicting complications following expander/implant breast reconstruction: an outcomes analysis based on preoperative clinical risk. *Plast Reconstr Surg.* 2008;121:1886-1892.
15. Goodwin SJ, McCarthy CM, Pusic AL, et al. Complications in smokers after postmastectomy tissue expander/implant breast reconstruction. *Ann Plast Surg.* 2005;55:16-19; discussion 19-20.
16. Nahabedian MY, Tsangaris T, Momen B, et al. Infectious complications following breast reconstruction with expanders and implants. *Plast Reconstr Surg.* 2003;112:467-476.
17. Vandeweyer E, Deraemaecker R, Nogaret JM, et al. Immediate breast reconstruction with implants and adjuvant chemotherapy: a good option? *Acta chirurgica Belgica.* 2003;103:98-101.
18. Forman DL, Chiu J, Restifo RJ, et al. Breast reconstruction in previously irradiated patients using tissue expanders and implants: a potentially unfavorable result. *Ann Plast Surg.* 1998;40:360-363.
19. Percec I, Bucky LP. Successful prosthetic breast reconstruction after radiation therapy. *Ann Plast Surg.* 2008;60:527-531.
20. Clough KB, O'Donoghue JM, Fitoussi AD, et al. Prospective evaluation of late cosmetic results following breast reconstruction: I. Implant reconstruction. *Plast Reconstr Surg* 2001;107:1702-1709.
21. Breuing KH, Colwell AS. Inferolateral AlloDerm hammock for implant coverage in breast reconstruction. *Ann Plast Surg.* 2007;59:250-255.
22. Bindingnavele V, Gaon M, Ota KS, Kulber DA, Lee DJ. Use of acellular cadaveric dermis and tissue expansion in postmastectomy breast reconstruction. *J Plast Reconstr Aesthet Surg.* 2007;60:1214-1218.
23. Deapen D, Hamilton A, Bernstein L, et al. Breast cancer stage at diagnosis and survival among patients with prior breast implants. *Plast Reconstr Surg.* 2000;105:535-540.
24. Deapen DM, Bernstein L, Brody GS. Are breast implants anticarcinogenic? A 14-year follow-up of the Los Angeles Study. *Plast Reconstr Surg.* 1997;99:1346-1353.
25. Karlson EW, Hankinson SE, Liang MH, et al. Association of silicone breast implants with immunologic abnormalities: a prospective study. *Am J Med.* 1999;106:11-19.
26. Sanchez-Guerrero J, Colditz GA, Karlson EW, et al. Silicone breast implants and the risk of connective-tissue diseases and symptoms. *N Engl J Med.* 1995;332:1666-1670.
27. Gaubitz M, Jackisch C, Domschke W, et al. Silicone breast implants: correlation between implant ruptures, magnetic resonance spectroscopically estimated silicone presence in the liver, antibody status and clinical symptoms. *Rheumatology (Oxford)* 2002;41:129-135; discussion 123-124.
28. Brown SL, Pennello G, Berg WA, et al. Silicone gel breast implant rupture, extracapsular silicone, and health status in a population of women. *J Rheumatol* 2001;28:996-1003.
29. McCarthy CM, Pusic AL, Sclafani L, et al. Breast cancer recurrence following prosthetic, postmastectomy reconstruction: incidence, detection, and treatment. *Plast Reconstr Surg.* 2008;121:381-388.
30. Cano SJ, Browne JP, Lamping DL. Patient-based measures of outcome in plastic surgery: current approaches and future directions. *Br J Plast Surg.* 2004;57:1-11.
31. Reaby LL, Hort LK, Vandervord J, Pruzinsky T. Body image, self-concept, and self-esteem in women who had a mastectomy and either wore an external breast prosthesis or had breast reconstruction and women who had not experienced mastectomy. Collaboration of plastic surgeon and medical psychotherapist. *Health Care Women Int.* 1994;15:361-375.
32. McCarthy CM, Pusic AL, Kerrigan CL. Silicone breast implants and magnetic resonance imaging screening for rupture: do U.S. Food and Drug Administration recommendations reflect an evidence-based practice approach to patient care? *Plast Reconstr Surg.* 2008;121:1127-1234.

CHAPTER 80

Breast Reconstruction with the Autogenous Latissimus Flap

Barbara Persons
Beth Collins
Christoph Papp
John McCraw

With the increasing use of skin-sparing mastectomies, oncoplastic procedures, and immediate reconstructions, the autogenous latissimus breast reconstruction has experienced a resurgence of interest. The "autogenous latissimus flap" refers to self-derived composite of muscle, fat, and skin. This concept is based on the ability of the latissimus muscle to "carry" fat on its surface. This composite of fat and muscle is extremely helpful in several ways. It adds volume, which may be adequate to replace the breast shape without using an implant. It is also an ideal local tissue replacement for oncoplastic procedures and the correction of irradiation fibrosis. The autogenous latissimus flap further serves as a "backup" flap for microvascular and TRAM flap breast reconstructions, when there is partial or complete flap loss. Finally, the autogenous latissimus flap can be used to create an aesthetic breast both with and without an implant. The latissimus muscle is an "expendable" muscle, in the sense that its loss of function is seldom noticed. The primary concern about functional loss is in the motion of "pushing off" with a ski pole.[1]

HISTORY

Iginio Tansini, a professor of surgery at the University of Padua in Padua, Italy (Fig. 80-1), described the first latissimus musculocutaneous flap in 1896.[2] He used the island latissimus flap to reconstruct the radical mastectomy defect with "like" tissue (Fig. 80-2). "Besides healing the wound … the flap is of considerable thickness and succeeds in providing an even better repair to the loss of matter, substituting the latissimus dorsi muscle for the pectoralis major muscle."[3] Tansini's contribution of the concept of the "island" latissimus flap, which "carried" the overlying skin, was a new concept. His goal was to repair the radical mastectomy defect by replacing both the lost skin and the pectoralis muscle. This "Tansini Method of Mastectomy" included radical removal and replacement of most of the breast skin and the pectoralis major muscle, and replacing the lost tissue with the latissimus dorsi musculocutaneous flap.[3] In Europe this became the most common method of obtaining a healed wound in the radical mastectomy defect during the first 2 decades of the 20th century.

In his grand tour of Europe in 1920, as America's first professor of surgery and most eminent surgeon, William S. Halsted objected to the use of a flap reconstruction at the time of mastectomy because of his fear that the latissimus flap might obscure diagnosis of breast cancer recurrences. Halsted advocated the use of skin grafts or secondary epithelialization for mastectomy defects, rather than a flap, so that recurrences could be recognized promptly. As he said in his 1907 paper, probably in reference to Tansini, "I should not care to say beware of the man with the plastic operation …. But to attempt to close the breast wound more less regularly by any plastic method is hazardous, and in my opinion to be vigorously discountenanced."[4] The Halsted method of radical mastectomy prevailed, and the flap reconstruction method of Tansini was abandoned by 1920. The surgical world was not ready for modern flaps.[5]

In the 1970s Nevin Olivari in Cologne, John McCraw in San Antonio, and Wolfgang Muhlbauer in Munich independently described the latissimus myocutaneous flap for chest wall reconstruction.[6-8] Schneider, Hill, and Brown from Atlanta first described the "standard" latissimus-implant breast reconstruction,

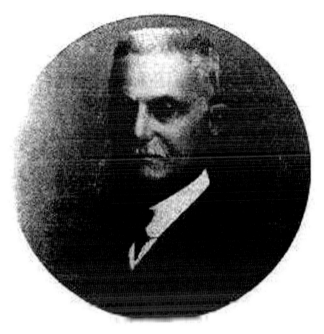

FIGURE 80-1 Iginio Tansini, Professor of Surgery, Parma, Italy. *(From Athena rassegna mensile di biologia clinical terapia. Anno VII. 1930, 1.55.)*

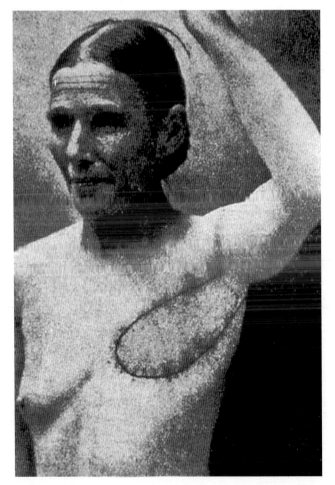

FIGURE 80-2 Tansini's latissimus island flap, 1906. *[From Tansini I. Sopra il mio nuovo processo di amputazione della mamella. Riforma Medica (Palermo, Napoli). 1906;12:757.]*

and Bostwick, Vasconez, and Jurkiewicz first described the use of the latissimus reconstruction method for the radical mastectomy deformity.[9,10] In 1985 Christoph Papp of Austria described the "autogenous" latissimus flap, which "carried" fat on the surface of the latissimus muscle, in order to recreate the contour of the breast without an implant. Papp and McCraw later reported an extensive combined experience, in which they also modified the standard latissimus flap design to include adipose tissue, and coined the term "autogenous latissimus" flap.[11] Many authors have reported success with this autogenous or "extended" myocutaneous flap, which eliminates the need for an implant, and can permit a totally autogenous reconstruction. This flap is particularly applicable to both small and large oncoplastic partial mastectomy defects, as well as Poland deformity.[12,13]

Advances in the application of the latissimus flap technique over the past 2 decades have demonstrated the utility of this reconstruction in primary and salvage flap breast reconstructions, both with and without an expander or permanent implant.[14] Endoscopic technology can also facilitate the dissection in the axilla and, in some cases, allow shorter incisions for flap harvest. It is now recognized that the skin-sparing mastectomy with immediate reconstruction is oncologically sound. In practice the result of the reconstruction is more dependent on the type of mastectomy, rather than the type of flap. The quality of the result of the autogenous latissimus reconstruction is primarily dependent upon the type of mastectomy, so the more deforming the mastectomy, the more compromised is the reconstructive effort. Good or excellent results can be predictably achieved with skin-sparing mastectomies. If a radical mastectomy or a comparably deforming Patey mastectomy is done, good results are seldom possible.[15]

INDICATIONS

The original (1977) latissimus myocutaneous flap incorporates a large implant, in order to provide both shape and volume.[16,17] The latissimus muscle is primarily used to provide coverage for the implant, and the skin paddle is inset transversely into the modified mastectomy scar. As a better method of breast shaping, the transverse rectus abdominis myocutaneous (TRAM) flap was introduced in 1982 as a completely autogenous reconstruction, which usually did not require an implant for volume replacement.[18] By 1985 the autogenous latissimus reconstruction became a good choice for reconstruction, because an implant was usually not needed to provide the breast shape. This offered a new method for reconstruction of the partial mastectomy, the bilateral mastectomy, the Poland chest wall deformity, or in reconstruction of small breasts.[19-21]

Today, one of the most frequent indications for using the autogenous latissimus breast reconstruction is as an alternative to the TRAM flap, when patients are either too thin, too obese, or because the supplying vessels have been injured by irradiation or previous abdominal surgery. Patients may choose to have the autogenous latissimus reconstruction because of the predictable results, limited discomfort, and the shorter recovery time compared to the TRAM flap breast reconstruction.[22]

Patients may choose not to have the TRAM flap reconstruction because they want to avoid abdominal surgery, scars, and possible abdominal wall weakness. Also, many active women, such as women with busy jobs or mothers with young children, may wish to avoid the longer recovery required for TRAM flap reconstruction. The latissimus flap is an option when free tissue transfer is not feasible because of patient anatomy, surgeon's choice, or lack of institutional resources. It also provides a good alternative to the free tissue transfer options, such as the muscle-sparing TRAM flap or the deep inferior epigastric perforator (DIEP) free flaps, when skin replacement is not a major issue. Finally, the latissimus flap is useful as a "salvage" or backup flap after failed implant or TRAM reconstructions, or after failed lumpectomy. It is the first line of defense for the treatment of radiation injuries, since it supplies soft tissue coverage as well as new vascularization to the neck, chest, and breast.

CONTRAINDICATIONS

Despite the utility of the latissimus in breast reconstruction, certain patients may not be candidates for this method. Previous axillary dissection with radiation may not permit safe dissection of the pedicle, or it may increase the risk of vascular insufficiency or vascular injury. Previous division of the thoracodorsal vascular pedicle in a mastectomy can represent an absolute contraindication. Other relative contraindications include patient refusal of an implant when it is needed for volume and projection, and patient desire to avoid any surgery on the back. The need for postoperative irradiation may also influence the timing of the reconstruction or affect the decision to use an implant. Most patients who elect to have latissimus flap reconstruction can return to such pursuits as golf and tennis, and approximately 80% of patients note no change in shoulder mobility and strength.[23] Patients with shoulder arthritis, or professional athletes who need full shoulder function, are not good candidates for the latissimus breast reconstruction.

FLAP COMPARISONS

The latissimus dorsi breast reconstruction provides a predictable method of supplying vascularized muscle and skin to the breast area in a single operative procedure. A relative disadvantage includes the need for an implant to augment the breast volume, but in patients who have adequate fat on the surface of the latissimus muscle, an implant is seldom required. When you can "pinch an inch," usually 600 mL of fat can be transposed with the muscle, which can provide symmetry with the opposite breast without an implant. Even in very thin patients with small breasts, 200 to 300 mL of volume can be transferred from the back to the breast. The TRAM flap, by comparison, provides more skin replacement, which may be needed in the case of very deforming mastectomies. The deep inferior epigastric artery perforator (DIEP) flap, which was introduced as a method of breast reconstruction by Koshima and Soeda in 1989, is popular with patients because it provides abdominal skin and fat without harming the rectus abdominis muscle.[24] DIEP free flaps offer predictably excellent results, but it is necessary to have specially trained surgeons and a most sophisticated operative team.

ANATOMY

Vascular Pattern

The latissimus dorsi muscle has a dual blood supply from both the thoracodorsal branch of the subscapular artery and the posterior paraspinous perforators. The dominant vascular supply to the muscle is via the thoracodorsal artery and vein, which are usually 2 mm in diameter (Fig. 80-3). The axillary artery gives off the subscapular artery high in the axilla, and the thoracodorsal artery branches off the subscapular artery. The serratus branch splits from the thoracodorsal artery to course on the surface of the serratus anterior muscle. The serratus branch exits from the thoracodorsal artery approximately 10 cm below the subscapular artery. The serratus branch must be carefully identified, so that the thoracodorsal artery is not mistakenly divided during the dissection. The thoracodorsal artery passes near the lateral border of the latissimus muscle, approximately 2 to 3 cm inside the lateral border of the muscle. Within the muscle the thoracodorsal artery splits into 2 terminal vessels. This parallel blood supply makes it possible to split the latissimus

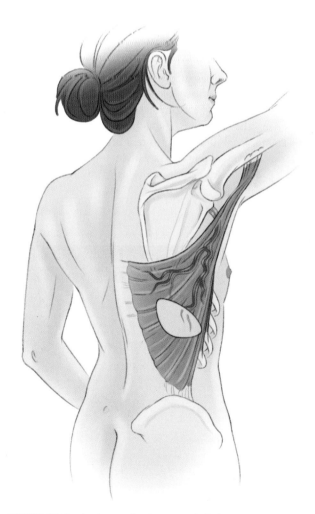

FIGURE 80-3 Anatomy of autogenous latissimus myocutaneous flap showing the thoracodorsal artery and vein, which is the main pedicle vessel to the latissimus muscle along with the serratus branch. The position of the skin paddle is also shown.

longitudinally into medial and lateral segments, which can be moved independently for small defects. The skin overlying the latissimus muscle is supplied by numerous muscular perforating vessels, which exit the surface of the muscle to supply the overlying fat and skin.

Nerves—Motor and Sensory

The motor nerve is the thoracodorsal nerve. The sensory innervation is from the dorsal cutaneous rami and includes the dorsal cutaneous rami 6 through 12. To test the thoracodorsal nerve function the surgeon supports the abducted arm while palpating the latissimus muscle and instructs the patient to push down while holding the arm up.

SURGICAL TECHNIQUE

Marking

Preoperatively, the latissimus muscle is outlined using a surgical marker with the patient in a standing position. The tip of the scapula is marked to define the superior margin of the latissimus muscle. Next, the anterior and inferior borders are identified by tensing the muscle, and are marked. A "crescent"-shaped skin paddle is designed on the surface of the latissimus muscle for skin replacement. This is done in a transverse orientation, so that the resulting closure will fall in a good skin line, which can be hidden by the bra strap (Fig. 80-4). A longitudinal orientation in the mid-axillary line or an oblique orientation of the skin island can also be used, but the scar is less favorable. In most patients the skin paddle should not exceed 8 cm in width in the craniocaudal dimension, so that primary closure of the donor site can be accomplished without significant tension. The skin paddle length may be as long as 25 cm if needed. The

vertical height of the flap should be measured in order to estimate arc over which the flap can be transposed onto the anterior chest.

Positioning and Preparation

During flap dissection, the patient should be placed in the lateral decubitus position supported by a beanbag with the arm draped free. Sequential compression devices are used for deep venous thrombosis prophylaxis. No Foley catheter is used because it is unnecessary in such a short procedure, which has almost no blood loss. It is also an unneeded source of infection. An endoscope should be available for visualization of the margins of the donor site and for dissection of the axillary vessels.

Combining the Mastectomy and Flap Elevation

The procedure is usually begun in the supine position for the mastectomy, and the patient is then turned into the lateral decubitus position with the arm draped free. In the bilateral reconstruction the patient is placed in a standard prone position. Care is taken to pad the patient's face and protect the airway. The arms are placed on arm boards with the hands above the head and the elbows bent in the "stick-up" position. The hips and knees should be carefully padded to protect pressure points.

The oncologic surgeon performs the mastectomy and axillary node dissection with the patient in the supine position. If the patient needs a sentinel lymph node biopsy, this is performed prior to mastectomy and reconstruction. The anterior border of the latissimus muscle is then identified from the mastectomy incision. The skin paddle is incised, and a layer of fat is left on the surface of the muscle. The thoracodorsal pedicle is

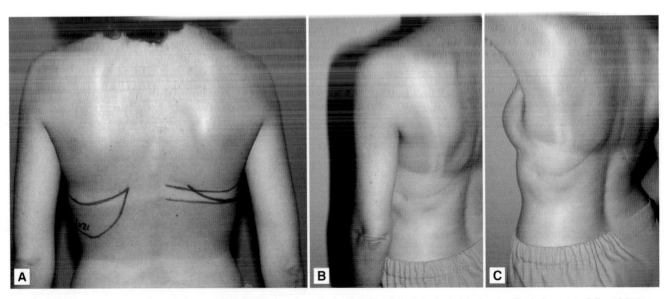

FIGURE 80-4 The crescent shaped skin paddles are outlined on the back **(A)**. While it is desirable for the final closure to fall within a thin bra line, the closures usually fall slightly below the bra line. The postoperative views **(B, C)** demonstrate the expected good scar, which is primarily the result of a closure in a favorable skin line.

identified about 2 cm from the lateral border of the muscle. Dissection in the loose areolar plane between the latissimus and serratus muscles is continued up to the tip of the scapula. At this point the latissimus muscle is freed and the vascular pedicle is protected cephalad to this dissection. A separate transverse axillary incision may also be used to facilitate transposition of the flap and dissection of the pedicle. The mastectomy incision is then temporarily closed prior to turning the patient.

Details of the Flap Dissection

Prior to turning the patient, the anterior border of the latissimus muscle is located from the mastectomy site and a tunnel is made for passage of muscle from the back to the chest. The thoracodorsal vessels are isolated 2 cm behind the anterior border of the latissimus muscle, and the long thoracic nerve is identified as it traverses along the chest wall to enter the serratus anterior muscle. Once the patient is turned, the skin paddle ellipse, which was previously marked on the back, is circumscribed with a scalpel. This incision is carried down and fanned out creating a cone of fat to the fat layer just superficial to the latissimus dorsi fascia. At this point the skin and subcutaneous ellipse may be temporarily tacked down to the fascia with several sutures from the dermis to the fascia to protect the skin paddle. The skin flaps overlying the surface of the latissimus muscle are then raised in the subcutaneous plane, leaving 1 to 2 cm of fat on the surface of the muscle. The dissection is extended posteriorly in this plane to the thoracolumbar fascia overlying the lower 6 vertebrae and the dissection is continued superficial to the latissimus muscular fascia toward the tip of the scapula. When lifting the posterior border of the muscle, care is taken to stay in the plane between the serratus and latissimus muscles near the tip of the scapula. Perforators are encountered in 2 rows on the undersurface of the latissimus muscle: one row of paraspinous perforators 5 cm from the spine and one row 10 cm from the spine. These must be divided as the undersurface of the muscle is elevated. The deep surface of the latissimus dorsi muscle is then dissected in a caudal direction away from the serratus muscle and the chest wall, until the origin is reached about 5 to 7 cm above the iliac crest. The insertion of the serratus muscle is identified at the tip of the scapula, and the upper border of the latissimus muscle is freed from these attachments. The latissimus muscle is then separated from the teres major muscle at the lateral border of the scapula. Once the latissimus has been detached from its origin, the muscle can be completely raised from inferior to superior to the level of the axilla. The final dissection is done to protect the island thoracodorsal vessels from harm.

Identifying and Dissecting the Pedicle

The serratus artery is identified running obliquely on the surface of the serratus muscle. It must be separated from the thoracodorsal artery and divided under direct vision if required to gain additional mobilization of the flap. If this is done incorrectly, the thoracodorsal artery can be ligated by mistake. The thoracodorsal pedicle is first visualized 5 to 10 cm caudal to the axilla. It is then further defined and followed from the latissimus muscle toward the axilla. A 30-degree, 5-mm endoscope or a lighted retractor may be used to complete the upper dissection and the latissimus tendon. The thoracodorsal vessels are freed from the surrounding axillary fascia, both from the axillary incision and the back incision. Superiorly, the tendinous insertion into the bicipital groove of the humerus is identified and divided under direct vision. This maneuver improves the anterior flap mobility and decreases the chance for a "muscle tug." After all superior attachments are divided, the flap is passed through the axillary passage into the breast that was created at the beginning of the procedure. Care is taken to avoid kinking the pedicle as it is passed from the back through the axilla into the breast defect.

Back Closure

Once the pedicle has been passed into the mastectomy defect, hemostasis is confirmed. Dependent drains are placed anteriorly and posteriorly. The wounds are closed in 3 layers. Scarpa fascia may be quilted down to the chest wall to prevent seroma formation. The skin flaps are closed with deep dermal sutures and subcuticular sutures. Inset of the latissimus flap is then performed after the patient is turned to the supine position.

Aesthetic Considerations of Flap Inset

The flap inset involves 3 areas of 3-dimensional reconstruction. This can be broken down into the footprint of the breast, the breast mound, and the skin envelope. The *footprint* is much like the shadow of a balloon on the ground and represents the 2-dimensional area of the reconstruction. The *breast mound* provides projection and shape. The flap is positioned with its attached fat to emulate the original or desired breast mound. The *skin envelope* creates the necessary cover. The skin cover is just as important as the mound in creating a good shape. In the case of a skin-sparing mastectomy, the good skin cover almost ensures a good shape. While in the case of a Patey mastectomy, the excessive removal of skin virtually ensures a poor shape of the reconstructed breast.

Latissimus Flap Inset

The pedicle is examined to ensure that it lays flat in its tunnel with no pressure or torsion. The skin paddle perfusion is clinically assessed. A pocket may be developed in a subpectoral plane for placement of a tissue expander or permanent implant. The latissimus muscle is then anchored to the chest wall, starting at the sternal margin and ending at the inframammary fold. Aesthetic principles of breast shaping are used to create an appearance that is both appropriate for the reconstructed breast and symmetrical with the opposite breast. A tissue expander can be placed at this time if needed for volume. The nipple can also be created at this time to make the latissimus reconstruction a single-stage procedure.

Second-Stage Procedures

Second-stage procedures are usually expected, and are needed to refine the shape and create a nipple-areolar complex. The basic shape of the breast is created in the first stage, and can suffice as the final result if a nipple and areola were created during the first stage and no implant is desired. If a tissue expander is used, it is inflated every 2 weeks to the desired volume, usually inflating by 50 to 100 mL per session. Overexpansion of the tissue expander, compared with the final implant, creates some ptosis that helps with matching the reconstructed breast with the opposite breast. In the second stage the nipple is created with a fishtail flap, or some form of double "wrapping" flap. The nipple reconstruction may be performed in the office. Alternatively, nipple reconstruction may be performed in the operating room if a permanent implant is to be placed or if a reduction mammaplasty or mastopexy is to be performed on the contralateral breast. Any final adjustments are made to achieve optimal symmetry and shape. This may include small revisions or excess fullness in the axilla of the reconstructed breast. If the areola is not created as an autogenous fishtail flap, the areola is tattooed to match the contralateral areola. Nipple reduction may be required on the contralateral breast, and this is achieved by excising a circumferential ring of epidermis from the wall of the nipple then closing it to create a less prominent nipple.

CASE EXAMPLES

Case 1: This case involves a 32-year-old woman with stage I invasive breast cancer. She underwent a skin-sparing mastectomy of the left breast with immediate latissimus reconstruction. Pre- and postoperative views at 6 years show adequate symmetry of the reconstructed left breast compared to the native right breast (Fig. 80-5). Side views of both right breast and left autogenous latissimus breast reconstruction illustrate the aesthetic concepts of matching the footprints of the breast, the breast mound, and the skin envelope (Fig. 80-6). The donor site on the back at 5 1/2 years is excellent (Fig. 80-7). Notice that the donor scar may be hidden in the bra line.

Case 2: This patient is a 34-year-old woman with ductal carcinoma in situ (DCIS) and is 1 of 5 sisters with breast cancer. Following bilateral skin-sparing mastectomies, she underwent bilateral autogenous latissimus dorsi flap breast reconstruction with 200 mL saline implants that were needed for volume in this thin patient. This was followed by a fishtail nipple reconstruction and areola tattooing. There is some ptosis related to the saline implants (Fig. 80-8).

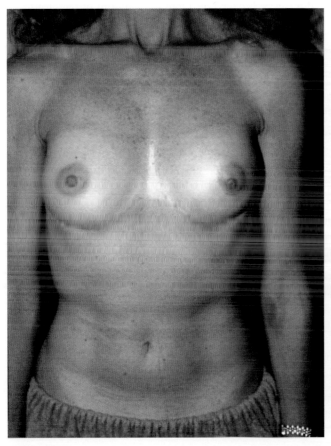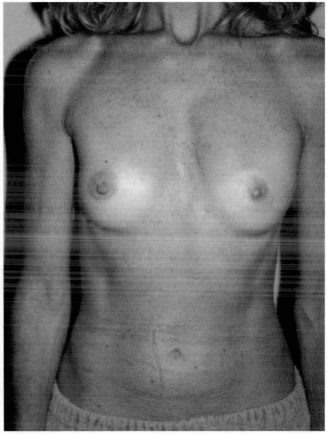

FIGURE 80-5 Preoperative and postoperative views of the left immediate, skin sparing autogenous latissimus breast reconstruction at 6 yeers. A saline was used initially, but deflated at 5 1/2 years. It was removed and not replaced. Symmetry was good at 6 years, primarily because 250 grams of fat were left on the surface of the latissimus muscle in this thin patient, and because the right breast volume has decreased with age.

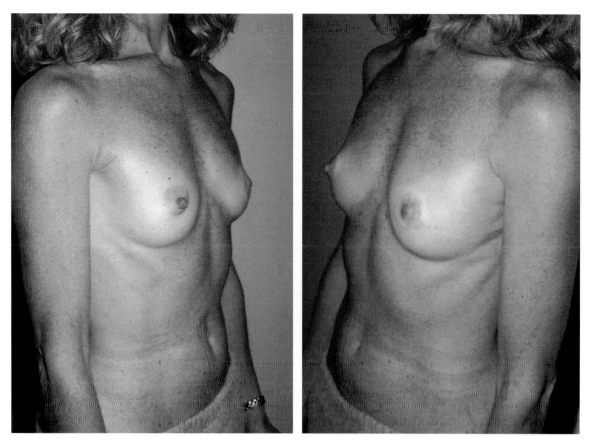

FIGURE 80-6 The oblique views demonstrate the excellent recreation of the anterior axillary fold, as well as upper "fill" and projection which are comparable to the normal right breast.

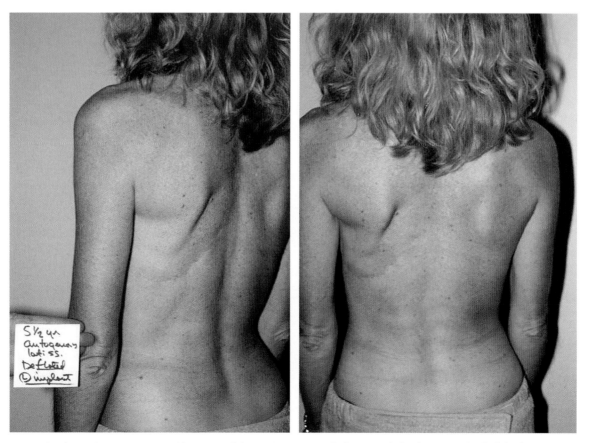

FIGURE 80-7 The donor site scars are good because of their orientation with the normal skin lines. Removal of the latissimus muscle has uncovered the tip of the scapula, but there is no winging of the scapula.

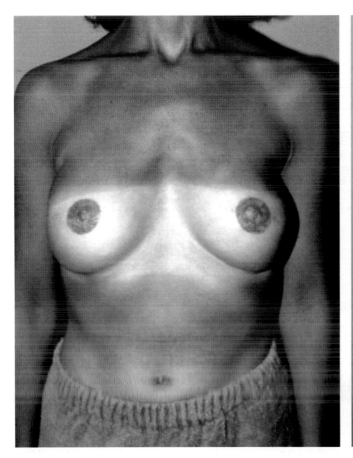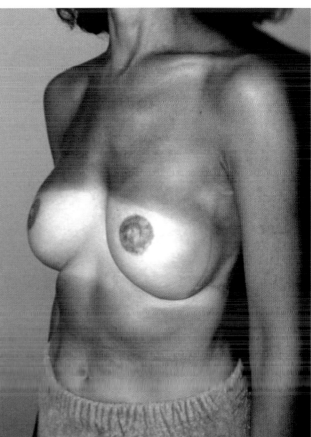

FIGURE 80-8 Five year followup of the bilateral autogenous breast reconstruction, including a 200cc saline implant. The implants are completely soft, but slightly ptotic. The autogenous latissimus flap contributes 200-300 grams of volume of fat per flap. This volume is helpful in re-creating the anterior axillary fold and the upper "fill," and the transposed fat reduces the need for a large implant. A fishtail nipple reconstruction and areolar tattooing were done, once the shape of the breast was definitive.

SUMMARY

The autogenous latissimus dorsi flap continues to play a central role in breast reconstruction and is a reliable option for many women. Exceptional aesthetic and functional results can be achieved with relatively rapid recovery. The autogenous latissimus muscle flap can be used without an implant to create a natural looking breast with symmetrical volume. It is an excellent alternative to the TRAM flap in high risk patients, and it can be used to reconstruct a wide range of defects. For partial mastectomy defects it is a viable option that can be performed as an immediate or delayed reconstruction.[27] The latissimus is a logical reconstruction for Poland syndrome, using a mirror image muscle from the back to correct the pectoralis defect on the anterior chest.[28] A total autologous reconstruction with skin-sparing mastectomy can be performed as single-stage procedure and completely rehabilitate the patient. The value of this combined procedure is inestimable and should be routinely offered to breast cancer patients.[29] The future will hold forth with several new materials, including better drains, new allodermal sheets or implant modifiers, absorbable skin and dermal sutures, or manufactured matrix materials for tissue replacement and revascularization. The improvement of endoscopic plastic surgery techniques

and even robotic surgery will facilitate the performance of these procedures, using smaller incisions with less trauma and better control.[30] This eliminates all incisions except the skin paddle and the mastectomy incisions. With 3-dimensional planning, the nipple areola reconstruction can be performed simultaneously with the flap procedure in a single stage.[31] Finally, fat grafting and tissue engineering will become routine and be commonly used for breast shaping and vascular in-growth. Today's methods will seem antique at some point, but they have allowed us to accomplish more in the past 30 years than has been accomplished in all of our previous surgical history.

REFERENCES

1. Fraulin FO, Louie G, Zorrilla L, Tilley W. Functional evaluation of the shoulder following latissimus dorsi muscle transfer. *Ann Plast Surg.* 1995;35(4):349-355.
2. Tansini I. Nuovo processo per l'amputazione della mammaella per cancre. *Reforma Medica.* 1896;12(3).
3. Tansini I. Sopra il mio nuovo processo di amputazione della mamella. *Riforma Medica (Palermo, Napoli).* 1906;12:757.
4. Halsted WS. I. The results of radical operations for the cure of carcinoma of the breast. *Ann Surg.* 1907;46(1):1-19.
5. Maxwell GP. Iginio Tansini and the origin of the latissimus dorsi musculocutaneous flap. *Plast Reconstr Surg.* 1980;65(5):686-692.

6. Olivari N. Use of thirty latissimus dorsi flaps. *Plast Reconstr Surg.* 1979;64(5):654-661.

7. Davis WM, McCraw JB, Carraway JH. Use of a direct, transverse, thoracoabdominal flap to close difficult wounds of the thorax and upper extremity. *Plast Reconstr Surg.* 1977;60(4):526-533.

8. McCraw JB, Penix JO, Baker JW. Repair of major defects of the chest wall and spine with the latissimus dorsi myocutaneous flap. *Plast Reconstr Surg.* 1978;62(2):197-206.

9. Papp C, McCraw JB. Autogenous latissimus breast reconstruction. *Clin Plast Surg.* 1998;25(2):261-266.

10. Olivari N. The latissimus flap. *Br J Plast Surg.* 1976;29(2):126-128.

11. McCraw JB, Papp C, Edwards A, McMellin A. The autogenous latissimus breast reconstruction. *Clin Plast Surg.* 1994;21(2):279-288.

12. Hernanz F, Regano S, Redondo-Figuero C, et al. Oncoplastic breast-conserving surgery: analysis of quadrantectomy and immediate reconstruction with latissimus dorsi flap. *World J Surg.* 2007;31(10):1934-1940.

13. Missana MC, Pomel C. Endoscopic latissimus dorsi flap harvesting. *Am J Surg.* 2007;194(2):164-169.

14. Disa JJ, McCarthy CM, Mehrara BJ, Pusic AL, Cordeiro PG. Immediate latissimus dorsi/prosthetic breast reconstruction following salvage mastectomy after failed lumpectomy/irradiation. *Plast Reconstr Surg.* 2008;121(4):159e-164e.

15. Patey DH, Dyson WH. The prognosis of carcinoma of the breast in relation to the type of operation performed. *Br J Cancer.* 1948;2(1):7-13.

16. McCraw JB, Dibbell DG. Experimental definition of independent myocutaneous vascular territories. *Plast Reconstr Surg.* 1977;60(2):212-220.

17. McCraw JB, Dibbell DG, Carraway JH. Clinical definition of independent myocutaneous vascular territories. *Plast Reconstr Surg.* 1977;60(3):341-352.

18. Hartrampf CR, Scheflan M, Black PW. Breast reconstruction with a transverse abdominal island flap. *Plast Reconstr Surg.* 1982;69(2):216-225.

19. Amuroso PI, Angelara J. Latissimus dorsi myocutaneous flap in Poland syndrome. *Ann Plast Surg.* 1984;13(4):362-390.

20. Mojallal A, Shipkov C, Braye F. Breast reconstruction in Poland anomaly with endoscopically-assisted latissimus dorsi muscle flap and autologous fat tissue transfer: a case report and review of the literature. *Folia Med (Plovdiv).* 2008;50(1):63-69.

21. Wechselberger G, Schoeller T, Otto A, Papp C. Extending the role of breast-conserving surgery by immediate volume replacement. *Br J Surg.* 1997;84(8):1172-1173.

22. McCraw JB, Maxwell GP, Horton CE. Reconstruction of the breast following mastectomy. *Acta Chir Belg.* 1980;79(2):131-133.

23. Clough KB, Louis-Sylvestre C, Fitoussi A, Couturaud B, Nos C. Donor site sequelae after autologous breast reconstruction with an extended latissimus dorsi flap. *Plast Reconstr Surg.* 2002;109(6):1904-1911.

24. Koshima I, Soeda S. Inferior epigastric artery skin flaps without rectus abdominis muscle. *Br J Plast Surg.* 1989;42(6):645-648.

25. Barnett GR, Gianoutsos MP. The latissimus dorsi added fat flap for natural tissue breast reconstruction: report of 15 cases. *Plast Reconstr Surg.* 1996;97(1):63-70.

26. Germann G, Steinau HU. Breast reconstruction with the extended latissimus dorsi flap. *Plast Reconstr Surg.* 1996;97(3):519-526.

27. Losken A, Schaefer TG, Carlson GW, et al. Immediate endoscopic latissimus dorsi flap: risk or benefit in reconstructing partial mastectomy defects. *Ann Plast Surg.* 2004;53(1):1-5.

28. Hester TR Jr, Bostwick J 3rd. Poland's syndrome: correction with latissimus muscle transposition. *Plast Reconstr Surg.* 1982;69(2):226-233.

29. de la Torre JI, Fix RJ, Gardner PM, Vasconez LO. Reconstruction with the latissimus dorsi flap after skin-sparing mastectomy. *Ann Plast Surg.* 2001;46(3):229-233.

30. Monticciolo DL, Ross D, Bostwick J 3rd, Eaves F, Styblo T. Autologous breast reconstruction with endoscopic latissimus dorsi musculosubcutaneous flaps in patients choosing breast-conserving therapy: mammographic appearance. *AJR Am J Roentgenol.* 1996;167(2):385-389.

31. Hammond DC, Khuthaila D, Kim J. The skate flap purse-string technique for nipple areola complex reconstruction. *Plast Reconstr Surg.* 2007;129(2):399-406.

CHAPTER 81

Total Breast Reconstruction Using Autologous Tissue: TRAM, DIEP, and SIEA Flaps

Maurice Y. Nahabedian
Ketan Patel

The role of autologous tissue for total breast reconstruction after mastectomy has had a significant impact in cancer management. Breast reconstruction using autologous tissue or prosthetic devices will provide emotional, psychological, and physical benefits in the majority of women. An advantage of autologous reconstruction is that it will last forever, improve over time, and remain soft and supple. Aesthetic and functional outcomes are generally excellent, and patient satisfaction is high.

When considering autologous reconstruction, one of the decisions is to select the appropriate donor site. Although there are several potential donor sites available, the anterior abdominal wall is most commonly used. This is because the adipocutaneous component of the abdomen is ideal for creating and shaping a new breast. It was Carl Hartrampf's initial description of the pedicle transverse rectus abdominis musculocutaneous (TRAM) flap in 1982 that changed the nature of autologous breast reconstruction and provided a foundation for many of the techniques currently available.[1] Since then, the methods by which the skin, fat, and muscle of the anterior abdominal wall are transplanted have evolved such that donor site morbidities have declined without compromising the aesthetic outcomes of the breast. As microvascular techniques developed, the free TRAM was introduced and allowed for the transplantation of greater quantities of skin and fat with less sacrifice of the rectus abdominis muscle.[2] An advantage of the free TRAM was its improved vascularity based on the perfusion characteristics of the deep inferior epigastric artery and vein. Further refinements in microvascular surgery resulted in the concept of perforator flaps for breast reconstruction.[3] With these flaps, the adipocutaneous component of a flap was transplanted without sacrifice of the donor site musculature. The principle abdominal perforator

flaps include the deep inferior epigastric artery flap (DIEP) and the superficial inferior epigastric artery flap (SIEA).[2,4] Thus the abdominal wall is the source of 4 flaps that include the pedicle TRAM, free TRAM, DIEP, and SIEA.

This chapter will focus on the various abdominal flaps that are currently used for total breast reconstruction after mastectomy. Emphasis will be placed on patient selection, flap selection, and operative techniques. The perspective will be based on the authors' personal experience with more than 900 breast reconstructions using the abdomen as the donor site.

PATIENT SELECTION

It is becoming increasingly appreciated that proper patient selection and good outcomes are intimately related.[5] Although many women interested in breast reconstruction may be candidates for autologous reconstruction, not all will be. Candidacy may be precluded for reasons such as medical comorbidities, extremes of body habitus, previous abdominal surgery, lack of interest, or a desire for a quick and simple procedure. That said, approximately 70% of my practice consists of women who have breast reconstruction using autologous tissues. This is in contrast to national trends in which approximately 75% of women have breast reconstruction using prosthetic devices.[6] This demographic difference can be partially explained based on the phenomenon of "surgeon selection" that is becoming more prevalent as reconstructive surgeons super specialize in a particular operation. Some surgeons are recognized for their expertise using autologous flaps and microsurgical techniques, whereas others are recognized for their expertise using prosthetic devices. Both methods have the potential for excellent outcomes.

When evaluating a patient for autologous breast reconstruction, several factors should be considered that are related to specific characteristics of the patient and breast. These include breast volume and contour, body habitus, donor site considerations, medical comorbidities, tumor characteristics, patient preference, and the potential for adjuvant therapies. The abdomen has been the donor site of choice for most women for a variety of reasons but is primarily related to tissue availability and quantity as well as breast aesthetics. In general, the most important physical finding is a sufficient quantity of skin and fat in order to reconstruct the desired breast volume. Although a woman may be slender with a paucity of abdominal fat, she may still be a candidate for an abdominal flap if the breast volume requirement is low. In women who are overweight or obese and have a large volume requirement, an abdominal flap can still be performed; however, the flap should be tailored to sustain its perfusion requirement and to minimize the incidence of fat necrosis.[7,8] The abdomen is usually not considered when there are abdominal scars that will preclude incorporating zones of tissue that would be needed for the reconstruction or when the patient is morbidly obese.

The topic of complications is discussed and reviewed with all patients considering total autologous reconstruction. Known complications include bleeding, infection, scar, flap failure, abdominal bulge or hernia, delayed healing, deep venous thrombosis, and further surgery. Success of an operation is dependent upon a variety of factors; however, flap survival is usually the primary concern. Personal success with the DIEP, free TRAM, and pedicle TRAM has been 98%. The risk of an abdominal bulge has ranged from 4% to 6% after a DIEP flap, 5% to 10% after a free TRAM flap, and 10% to 15% after a pedicle TRAM.[9-11] A postoperative bulge or hernia is not usually observed after an SIEA flap because the fascia and muscle are not violated. Secondary operations of the anterior abdominal wall have been performed in approximately 20% of women.[12] These have included elective procedures in 10% (scar revision, recontouring, and liposuction) and necessary procedures in 10% (bulge repair, hematoma evacuation, neuroma excision, debridement, and wound closure).

FLAP SELECTION

As previously mentioned, the abdomen is the preferred donor site for the majority of breast reconstruction procedures. It can be reasonably stated that the complexity of raising a given abdominal flap is directly related to the degree in which the abdomen musculature and anterior sheath are preserved. The SIEA flap does not violate the anterior rectus sheath or rectus abdominis muscle (Fig. 81-1) However, the superficial inferior epigastric vessels are present in roughly 60% of patients and suitable for microvascular anastomosis in approximately 30%. The DIEP flap requires an anterior rectus sheath incision and a myotomy in order to dissect out the perforator (Fig. 81-2). No muscle is removed. The blood supply is derived from the deep inferior epigastric artery and vein, which is present in all women and usually the dominant vascular system. The free TRAM by definition will include a segment of the rectus

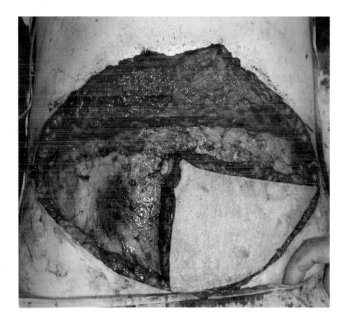

FIGURE 81-1   Intraoperative image of a hemi SIEA flap. There is no incision in the anterior rectus sheath.

abdominis muscle and the anterior rectus sheath (Fig. 81-3). This flap is preferred for very large volume breast reconstruction or when the abdominal perforators are deemed inadequate. The pedicle TRAM usually results in sacrifice of the entire rectus abdominis muscle, although lateral preservation is sometimes possible (Fig. 81-4). A classification for the various types of muscle sparing has been established (Table 81-1).[10]

The frequency and incidence for each particular flap is variable and dependent upon the skill and experience of the reconstructive surgeon. In this author's practice, a DIEP flap is performed in 80% of women, a free TRAM in 15%, and a pedicle TRAM or SIEA flap in the remaining 5%. The factors responsible for this are based on body habitus, quality of the

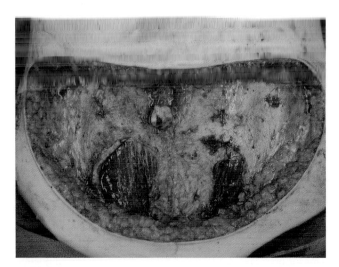

FIGURE 81-2   Intraoperative image of a bilateral DIEP flap demonstrating an incision in the anterior rectus sheath and a small myotomy in the rectus abdominis muscle.

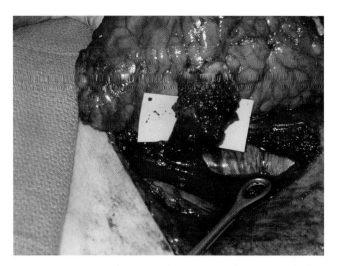

FIGURE 81-3 A muscle-sparing free TRAM is demonstrated. The central segment of the rectus abdominis muscle is harvested, leaving the medial and lateral segments intact.

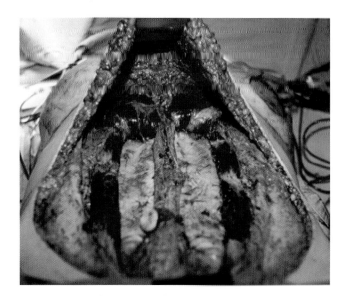

FIGURE 81-4 A bilateral muscle-sparing pedicle TRAM is depicted. The lateral segment of the rectus abdominis muscle is preserved.

TABLE 81-1 Classification of Muscle-Sparing (MS) Abdominal Flaps

Muscle-Sparing Technique	Definition (Rectus Abdominis)
MS-0	Full width, partial length
MS-1	Preservation of lateral segment
MS-2	Preservation of lateral and medial segment
MS-3 (DIEP)	Preservation of entire muscle

perforators, integrity of the deep inferior epigastric artery and vein, and the presence and caliber of the superficial inferior epigastric vessels.[13] If the perforators are suitable and the volume requirements are acceptable, then a DIEP flap is usually performed. In the event that the perforators are deemed inadequate, a muscle-sparing free TRAM is usually performed. If the inferior epigastric vessels have been previously ligated, a pedicle TRAM flap is considered. Some women are averse to the total harvest of the rectus abdominis muscle. In these women, an alternative donor site or prosthetic reconstruction will be considered. If the SIEA and SIEV are of suitable caliber, then it is considered. A limitation of the SIEA flap is that the angiosome is usually limited to the ipsilateral flap; therefore, inclusion of zone 3 will more likely than not result in fat necrosis.[14,15] Thus the SIEA flap is ideal for women having unilateral or bilateral breast reconstruction in which only a hemi flap is used. The aesthetic outcomes of the breast are similar regardless of the flap used, assuming that patient and flap selection has been appropriate.

One of the principle decisions for the microvascular surgeon is whether to perform a muscle-sparing free TRAM, DIEP, or SIEA flap.[13,16-19] This decision is ultimately made based on the presence and quality of the perforating vessels supplying the adipocutaneous component of the anterior abdominal wall.[17,20-22] The anatomic details of these blood vessels can be assessed preoperatively and/or intraoperatively. Preoperative assessment is best achieved using computed tomography (CT) angiography.[23,24] With this technique, the location and caliber of the perforating vessel or vessels can be adequately determined. This technique has proven to be effective for many surgeons. The advantage of preoperative CT angiography is that the "guesswork" regarding whether a perforator is present or suitable is essentially eliminated, and the harvesting of a DIEP flap can be more reliably executed. In addition, the CT angiogram can alert the surgeon regarding the subfascial course of the perforator. Although not routinely performed in these authors' practice, the benefits of preoperative imaging to facilitate perforator selection are appreciated.

Intraoperative assessment is equally effective in identifying the abdominal wall perforating vessels. Reliance on intraoperative assessment requires more experience because of the variability associated with perforator location, caliber, and number. The "Gent" consensus described the 5 most common perforator types, some of which are not suitable to adequately perfuse a flap.[25] In general, for a perforator flap to be successfully harvested and transferred, a single perforating artery and vein of at least 1.5 mm in diameter is recommended. These vessels are usually located in the periumbillical region. If a dominant perforator arising from the deep system is not identified, it may be because the superficial inferior epigastric system is the more dominant.[26] In this situation, one can consider performing an SIEA flap or a muscle-sparing free TRAM. The MS-2 muscle-sparing free TRAM is the authors' preferred flap. With this flap, a small central segment of the rectus abdominis muscle and anterior rectus sheath (2-4 cm) is harvested, incorporating several small (smaller than 1.5 mm) vessels. The authors' current algorithm for the selection of a DIEP or muscle-sparing free TRAM is depicted (Table 81-2).

TABLE 81-2 Current Algorithm for the DIEP and Muscle-Sparing Free TRAM Flaps

Factor	Free TRAM	DIEP
Breast Volume Requirements		
< 1000 g	+	+ +
> 1000 g	+ +	+
Abdominal Fat		
Mild to Moderate	+	+ +
Severe	+ +	+
Perforators > 1.5 mm		
0	+	No
> 1	+	+ +
Bilateral	+	+ +

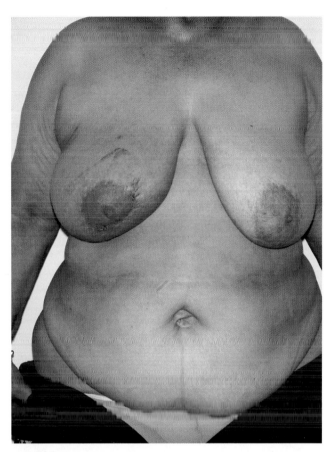

FIGURE 81-5 Preoperative image of a woman with right breast cancer.

OPERATIVE TECHNIQUE: TIPS AND TRAPS

As previously mentioned, the anterior abdominal wall is the source of 4 flaps. Although the adipocutaneous component of each flap is the same, the technique for harvesting each flap is different and associated with various degrees of complexity. The following section will highlight some of the tips and traps for successful harvest of these flaps.

Pedicle TRAM flap

Of the 4 flaps, the pedicle TRAM is the only flap that does not require microvascular techniques. In general, the pedicle TRAM is performed in women with mild to moderate lipodystrophy of the abdominal wall. In women with a body mass index greater than 30 or in a women with a history of tobacco use, a surgical delay procedure is considered to optimize flap perfusion and minimize the incidence of fat necrosis, partial flap loss, and delayed healing. It is well-known that the pedicle TRAM flap usually requires harvest of the entire rectus abdominis muscle. However, it is important to appreciate that the purpose of the rectus abdominis muscle is that of a carrier for the superior epigastric artery and vein. It is not a significant source of breast volume except perhaps in women who are thin with small volume requirements. When a pedicle TRAM flap is performed, it is this authors' preference to use the ipsilateral flap rather than the contralateral flap. This will reduce the incidence of epigastric fullness that is associated with the contralateral flaps.

When harvesting a pedicle TRAM flap, the decision regarding total versus partial muscle sacrifice is based on the intramuscular course of the inferior and superior epigastric artery and vein, the width of the rectus abdominis muscle, the width and location of the fascial island containing the perforating branches from the source vessel, and whether the reconstruction is unilateral or bilateral. A Doppler probe or manual palpation of the epigastric artery and vein can be used to determine the location of the vessels. When the main source vessel courses under the fascial island and the quantity of lateral muscle is adequate, then the central two-thirds of the muscle is harvested,

preserving the lateral segment (Fig. 81-4). It is important to preserve as much of the lateral intercostal innervations and vascularity to the remaining segment of muscle to retain some degree of function. An example of a woman after pedicle TRAM flap reconstruction is depicted (Figs. 81-5 and 81-6).

Free Tissue Transfer

The learning curve associated with microvascular breast reconstruction is one that is long and arduous. Mastery of microvascular surgery requires time, patience, technical ability, and thorough knowledge of the regional vascular anatomy. It is my personal opinion that approximately 100 flaps are necessary in order to feel comfortable with these operations and to perform them in a predictable and reproducible manner. Once that level of confidence is achieved, microvascular breast reconstruction can be performed safely and effectively.

DIEP Flap

Performance of a DIEP flap is facilitated by proper perforator selection and dissection. The selected perforator should be ideally located near the center of the flap in order to obtain equidistant perfusion (Fig. 81-7). A single perforator with a diameter of at least 1.5 mm is preferred (Fig. 81-8). When several perforators are available that meet this criteria, sequential

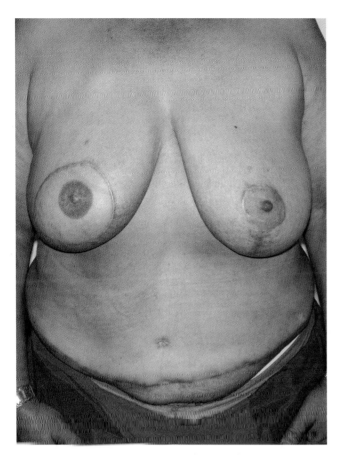

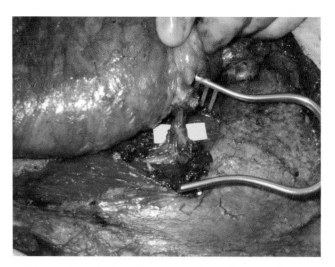

FIGURE 81-8 A single perforator DIEP flap is depicted. The perforator diameter is approximately 2 mm. A short myotomy is performed, exposing the base of the perforator and the inferior epigastric artery and vein.

FIGURE 81-6 Postoperative image after a unilateral pedicle TRAM flap and a contralateral mastopexy at 1-year follow-up.

tissue on the contralateral side (zone 3) to optimize perfusion (Fig. 81-9). A personal observation has been that not all women will have a dominant perforator (Fig. 81-10). In the absence of a perforator with a diameter of greater than 1.5 mm, a muscle-sparing free TRAM is usually performed, incorporating a small central segment of the rectus abdominis muscle.

Dissection of a DIEP flap requires few surgical instruments and includes a fine-tip mosquito clamp, Weitlaner retractors, fine scissors, tissue forceps, and a low-setting electrocautery device (Fig. 81-11). When initiating the dissection, including a small cuff of the anterior rectus sheath (1-2 mm) around the perforator is recommended, especially if the perforator is piercing the anterior rectus sheath at a tendinous inscription. During the dissection, it is imperative to preserve the lateral intercostal nerves as they pierce the rectus abdominis muscle at the junction

occlusion can be performed to assist with the selection process. Multiple perforators can be considered when they are aligned in series or in close proximity (Fig. 81-9). It should be remembered that multiple myotomies can impact muscle function. Medial row perforators are preferred when the flap will include

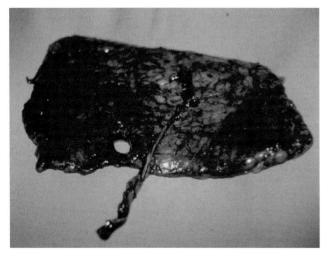

FIGURE 81-7 Typical appearance of a DIEP flap. There is no muscle harvested. The pedicle length can be up to 13 cm in length.

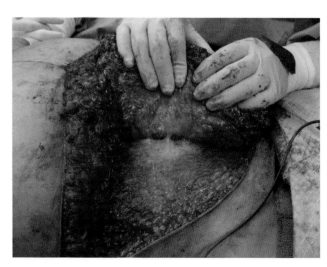

FIGURE 81-9 Intraoperative image of 3 medial row perforators that are all of suitable caliber.

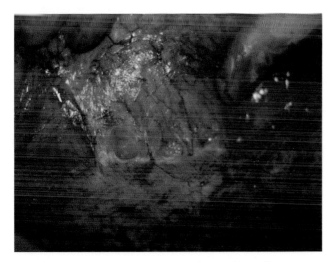

FIGURE 81-10 Intraoperative image of several lateral row perforators that are small caliber and not generally dissected out for a DIEP flap. Despite this image, large perforators with a caliber of 1.5 mm or more can be seen in the lateral row.

of the lateral and central longitudinal segments. Failure to do so will more likely than not result in abdominal weakness and may exacerbate an abdominal bulge. Motor nerve branches are frequently encountered during the dissection that cross the perforator or the source vessel. These are sharply divided and not clipped or cauterized. Whether or not to coapt the severed motor nerve is controversial. Some advocate using a micro suture for coaptation; however, it is these authors' preference to allow the transected end to neurotize into the adjacent muscle. The intramuscular dissection proceeds to the point that the perforator or inferior epigastric vessel becomes submuscular. At that point, the dissection progresses in the submuscular plane and continues from the lateral edge of the muscle toward the iliac vessels. It is recommended to continue the dissection until

the vessel diameter approaches 2.5 to 3 mm. This usually provides a pedicle length of 10 to 13 cm (Fig. 81-7).

Throughout the dissection of a DIEP flap, it is recommended to assess the perfusion from the peripheral edges of the flap. One can also use a handheld Doppler probe to listen for the arterial and venous signals. When a unilateral reconstruction is planned, it is wise to preserve the contralateral perforators in the event that a "lifeboat" is necessary. When a bilateral reconstruction is planned, it is advised to proceed cautiously when isolating and dissecting the perforators, because a contralateral lifeboat will not be available. When in doubt about the quality of the perforators, a muscle-sparing free TRAM flap is considered.

The recipient vessels of choice for the DIEP flap and all free flaps used for breast reconstruction are the internal mammary artery and vein.[27] These are used for all delayed reconstructions and most immediate reconstruction. The thoracodorsal artery and vein are used when an axillary lymph node dissection has been performed and the vessels are exposed. The internal mammary artery and vein are exposed at either the third or fourth interspace. The cartilaginous segment of the rib is excised. At this level, the diameter of the internal mammary vein is 2.5 to 3.5 mm and the internal mammary artery is 2.5 to 3 mm. An example of a woman after DIEP flap reconstruction is demonstrated (Figs. 81-12 and 81-13).

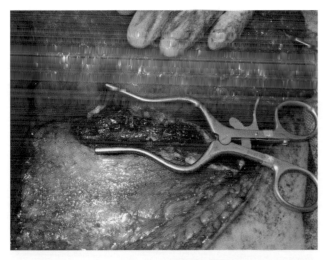

FIGURE 81-11 The dissection of a perforator requires a Weitlaner retractor for exposure. The 3 perforators are visualized attached to the source vessel.

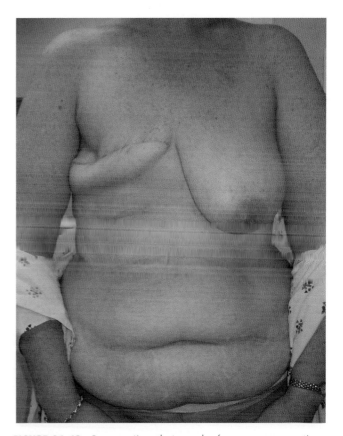

FIGURE 81-12 Preoperative photograph of a woman presenting for delayed reconstruction after mastectomy.

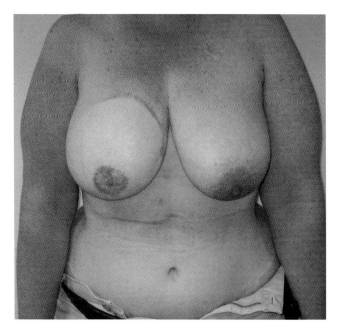

FIGURE 81-13 Postoperative photograph after autologous breast reconstruction with a 3-perforator DIEP flap. Excellent volume and contour symmetry are observed at 2-year follow-up.

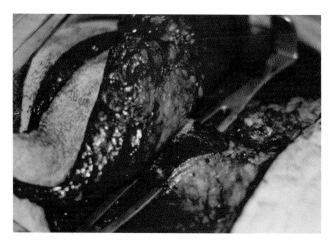

FIGURE 81-14 The rectus abdominis muscle is exposed and undermined when a pedicle TRAM flap is performed. This maneuver facilitates palpation of the inferior epigastric artery to determine its intramuscular course and to minimize injury.

Free TRAM

The free TRAM flap is a reliable flap that provides excellent aesthetic and functional outcomes. Although many microsurgeons will perform this flap as their primary flap, it is these authors' practice to use it when perforator diameter is less than 1.5 mm or in the event that the flap volume requirements exceed 1000 g. The advantage of the free TRAM compared with the DIEP is that multiple small or large caliber perforators can be included in the flap that may minimize the incidence of fat necrosis, vascular compromise, and partial or total flap failure. A muscle-sparing free TRAM (MS-1 or MS-2) is performed in order to maintain continuity of the rectus abdominis muscle. Once a network of perforators is visualized, an anterior sheath outline is delineated and incised. In contrast to the DIEP flap dissection, the anterior rectus sheath is elevated off the rectus abdominis muscle medially and laterally. The muscle is then undermined and the location of the inferior epigastric artery is visualized and palpated (Fig. 81-14) This maneuver will facilitate the dissection of the free TRAM and minimize injury to the perforators or pedicle. The rectus abdominis muscle is divided using a fine-tip mosquito clamp and a low-setting electrocautery device. When the perforators are located in the central segment of the rectus abdominis muscle, an MS-2 free TRAM is harvested (Fig. 81-15). When the perforators are predominately over the medial or lateral aspect of the muscle, an MS-1 free TRAM is harvested. It is important to preserve as many lateral intercostal motor innervations as possible to maintain function of the rectus abdominis muscle. An example of a woman after a bilateral MS-2 free TRAM flap is depicted (Figs. 81-16 and 81-17).

SIEA Flaps

Given that the SIEA flap can be performed in 30% of women, it is recommended to first visualize the superficial inferior epigastric artery and vein. Should the SIEA/V have a palpable pulse and be deemed useable, then it can be dissected to its origin. Should the SIEA/V be deemed not useable, then the vein can be preserved in the event that a secondary anastomosis is needed to augment venous flow.

The SIEA flap is technically easier to harvest when compared with the DIEP or muscle-sparing free TRAM flap. It is essentially an adipocutaneous flap that is perfused by a direct perforator, that is, the perforator does not course through a muscle. After visualization of the superficial inferior epigastric

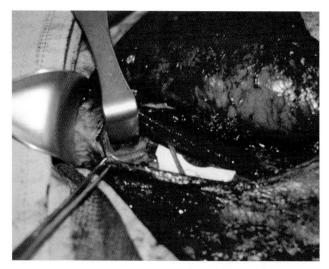

FIGURE 81-15 The central segment of the rectus abdominis muscle is harvested while maintaining the continuity of the rectus abdominis muscle. The lateral innervation of the muscle is preserved to maintain contractility of the muscle.

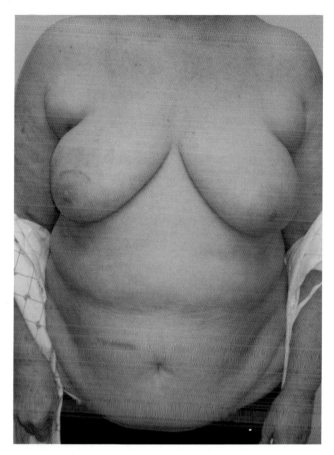

FIGURE 81-16 Preoperative photograph of a woman with right breast cancer.

artery and vein and the decision to proceed with this flap, it is wise to at least visualize the system of deep perforators. After their isolation, the perforators should be sequentially occluded to ensure that the perfusion from the SIEA/V is adequate. If it is, then the SIEA flap can be safely performed. Despite the gains in abdominal wall function, I remain somewhat skeptical

about its benefit. Concerns include the smaller-caliber vessels, the limited angiosomal territories, the increased incidence of fat necrosis, and the higher rate of redo arterial and venous anastomoses.[16] My personal philosophy is that the key to predictable and reproducible outcomes in "microvascular" surgery is to make it as "macrovascular" as possible.

SUMMARY

As microvascular surgeons continue to expand upon the armamentarium of autologous tissue options for breast reconstruction, outcomes will continue to improve. The goal with all types of reconstructive breast surgery is no longer to create just a breast mound but to create a breast with natural shape, volume, contour, and symmetry. Patient expectations after mastectomy and reconstruction have increased, and we as reconstructive plastic surgeons should continue to strive for excellence. Total breast reconstruction using the anterior abdominal wall as the donor site continues to evolve and provide women with excellent aesthetic and functional outcomes.

REFERENCES

1. Hartrampf CR, Scheflan M, Black PW. Breast reconstruction with a transverse abdominal island flap. *Plast Reconstr Surg.* 1982;69:216-225.
2. Grotting JC, Urist MM, Maddox WA, Vasconez LO. Conventional TRAM flap versus free microsurgical TRAM flap for immediate breast reconstruction. *Plast Reconstr Surg.* 1989:83:828-841.
3. Koshima I, Soeda S. Inferior epigastric artery skin flaps without rectus abdominis muscle. *Brit J Plast Surg.* 1989;42:645-648.
4. Allen RJ, Treece P. Deep inferior epigastric perforator flap for breast reconstruction. *Ann Plast Surg.* 1994;32:32-38.
5. Nahabedian MY, Momen B, Galdino G, Manson PN. Breast reconstruction with the free TRAM or DIEP flap: patient selection, choice of flap, and outcome. *Plast Reconstr Surg.* 2002;110:466-475.
6. American Society of Plastic Surgeons. ASPS Procedural Statistics: 2007 Reconstructive Breast Surgery. Arlington Heights, Ill: American Society of Plastic Surgeons: 2008.
7. Garvey PB, Buchel EW, Pockaj BA, Gray RJ, Samson TD. The deep inferior epigastric perforator flap in overweight and obese patients. *Plast Reconstr Surg.* 2005;115:447-457.
8. Chang DW, Wang B, Robb GL, et al. Effect of obesity on flap and donor site complications in free TRAM flap breast reconstruction. *Plast Reconstr Surg.* 2000;105:1640-1648.
9. Nahabedian MY, Dooley W, Singh N, Manson PN. Contour abnormalities of the abdomen following breast reconstruction with abdominal flaps: the role of muscle preservation. *Plast Reconstr Surg.* 2002;109:91-101.
10. Nahabedian MY, Manson PN. Contour abnormalities of the abdomen following TRAM flap breast reconstruction: A multifactorial analysis. *Plast Reconstr Surg.* 2002;105:81-97.
11. Nahabedian MY, Momen B. Lower abdominal bulge after DIEP flap breast reconstruction. *Ann Plast Surg.* 2005;54:124-129.
12. Nahabedian MY. Secondary operations of the anterior abdominal wall following microvascular breast reconstruction with the TRAM and DIEP flaps. *Plast Reconstr Surg.* 2007;120:365-372.
13. Nahabedian MY, Momen B, Tsangaris T. Breast reconstruction with the muscle sparing (MS-2) free TRAM and the DIEP flap: is there a difference? *Plast Reconstr Surg.* 2005;115:436-444.
14. Holm C, Mayr M, Hofter E, Ninkivic M. The versatility of the SIEA flap: a clinical assessment of the vascular territory of the superficial epigastric inferior artery. *J Plast Reconstr Aesthet Surg.* 2007;60:946-951.
15. Chevray PM. Brest reconstruction with superficial inferior epigastric artery flaps: a prospective comparison with TRAM and DIEP flaps. *Plast Reconstr Surg.* 2004;114:1077-1083.
16. Selber J, Vega S, Sonnad S, Serletti J. Comparing the SIEA and muscle sparing free TRAM: is the rate of flap loss worth the gains in abdominal wall function? Proceedings of the 86th Annual Meeting of the American Association of Plastic Surgeons, Coeur d' Alene, Idaho, May 19-22, 2007.

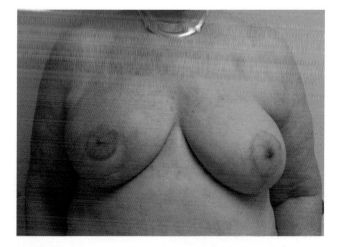

FIGURE 81-17 Postoperative photograph of a woman after an MS-2 free TRAM flap at 3-year follow up.

17. Lindsey JT. Integrating the DIEP and muscle-sparing (MS-2) free TRAM techniques optimizes surgical outcomes: presentation of an algorithm for microsurgical breast reconstruction based on perforator anatomy. *Plast Reconstr Surg.* 2007;119:18-27.

18. Bajaj AK, Chevray PM, Chang DW. Comparison of donor-site complications and functional outcomes in free muscle-sparing TRAM flap and free DIEP flap breast reconstruction. *Plast Reconstr Surg.* 2006;117:737-746.

19. Schaverien A, Perks S, McCulley J. Comparison of outcomes and donor-site morbidity in unilateral free TRAM versus DIEP flap breast reconstruction. *J Plast Reconstr Aesthet Surg.* 2007;60:1219-1224.

20. Rozen WM, Ashton MW, Pan WR, Taylor GI. Raising perforator flaps for breast reconstruction: the intramuscular anatomy of the deep inferior epigastric artery. *Plast Reconstr Surg.* 2007;120:1443-1449.

21. Rozen WM, Palmer KP, Suami H, et al. The DIEA branching pattern and its relationship to perforators: the importance of preoperative computed tomographic angiography for DIEA perforator flaps. *Plast Reconstr Surg.* 2008;121:367-373.

22. Munhoz AM, Ishida LH, Sturtz GP, et al. Importance of lateral row perforator vessels in deep inferior epigastric perforator flap harvesting. *Plast Reconstr Surg.* 2004;113:517-524.

23. Rosson GD, Williams CG, Fishman EK, Singh NK. 3D CT angiography of abdominal wall vascular perforators to plan DIEAP flaps. *Microsurgery.* 2007;27:641-646.

24. Alonso-Burgos A, Garcia-Totor E, Bastarrika G, et al. Preoperative planning of deep inferior epigastric artery perforator flap reconstruction with multislice-CT angiography: imaging findings and initial experience. *J Plast Reconstr Aesthet Surg.* 2006;59:585-593.

25. Blondeel PN, Van Landuyt KHI, Monstrey SJM, et al. The "Gent" consensus on perforator flap terminology: preliminary definitions. *Plast Reconstr Surg.* 2003;112:1378-1383.

26. Blondeel PN, Arnstein M, Verstraete K, et al. Venous congestion and blood flow in free transverse rectus abdominis myocutaneous and deep inferior epigastric perforator flaps. *Plast Reconstr Surg.* 2000;106:1295-1299.

27. Nahabedian MY. The internal mammary artery and vein as recipient vessels for microvascular breast reconstruction: are we burning a future bridge? *Ann Plast Surg.* 2004;53:311-316.

SYSTEMIC THERAPY OF BREAST CANCER

Lisa Carey

David W. Ollila

CHAPTER 82

General NCCN Guidelines

P. K. Morrow
Richard Theriault

In 2008, an estimated 184,450 new cases of breast cancer will occur in the United States.[1] In the same year, it is estimated that almost 41,000 women will die of breast cancer. These numbers demonstrate the impact of breast cancer among American women, but they cannot begin to address the diversity and complexity of the treatment of this malignancy. As research and advances in the care of the breast cancer patient occur, the need for greater understanding of the tenets and principles of clinical decision-making in the treatment of breast cancer increases.

In 1995, the National Comprehensive Cancer Network (NCCN) was developed in order to respond to the challenges of treating the most common cancers through clinical practice guidelines that delineated treatment through nonbiased, methodical algorithms. Based upon the Institute of Medicine's definition, which described guidelines as "systematically developed statements to assist practitioner and patient decisions about appropriate health care for specific clinical circumstances," the NCCN established a guideline program that proceeds as follows: comprehensive literature review by NCCN staff, development of prototype guidelines, review by site-specific panels, further analysis and clarification of guidelines, assessment by each NCCN member institution, collation of institutional review suggestions and issues, appraisal of the complete version of the guidelines by the NCCN Guidelines Steering Committee, and final approval by the NCCN Board of Directors. The guidelines are subsequently reviewed annually by the panel chair and 3 other multidisciplinary members to determine if further revisions are necessary. This chapter discusses the guidelines set forth by the NCCN regarding the treatment of primary invasive breast cancer (Figs. 82-1 to 82-4).

STRATIFICATION OF RISK

The Early Breast Cancer Trialists' Collaborative Group (EBCTCG) has demonstrated that the use of an anthracycline-containing chemotherapy and 5 years of tamoxifen may decrease mortality from breast cancer by more than 50% in women under 50 years of age, and by slightly less than 50% in women aged 50 to 69 years.[2] Thus, for patients under the age of 70 years, adjuvant therapy demonstrates significant benefit. To assist in risk stratification for this diverse population, Adjuvant! Online, a prospectively validated Web-based tool, may be utilized to estimate the benefit of adjuvant chemotherapy and endocrine therapy upon 10-year disease-free survival (DFS) and overall survival (OS) in patients with HER-2-negative breast cancer.[3,4] This program incorporates the patient's age, comorbidities, tumor size, tumor grade, number of positive lymph nodes, and estrogen receptor (ER) status in order to calculate these values.

Preoperative (Neoadjuvant) Chemotherapy

The NSABP B-18 trial demonstrated that the administration of chemotherapy in the neoadjuvant setting did not improve DFS or OS when compared to adjuvant administration.[5] However, the use of neoadjuvant chemotherapy may offer certain advantages. Specifically, patients with pathologic complete response (pCR) following neoadjuvant chemotherapy have been found to have improved DFS and OS,[6,7] and neoadjuvant chemotherapy is associated with a higher rate of successful breast-conserving therapy than adjuvant therapy.[5] However, given the equivalency of benefit in the neoadjuvant and adjuvant settings, the chemotherapeutic regimens that are recommended in the adjuvant setting are appropriate for consideration in the neoadjuvant setting.

Adjuvant Chemotherapy

The EBCTCG's overview demonstrated that the use of polychemotherapy significantly reduced the risk of recurrence and

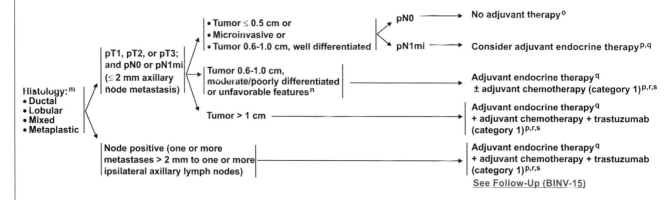

NCCN® Practice Guidelines in Oncology – v.2.2008 | **Invasive Breast Cancer**

SYSTEMIC ADJUVANT TREATMENT - HORMONE RECEPTOR POSITIVE - HER2 POSITIVE DISEASE[b]

[b] See Principles of HER2 Testing (BINV-A).
[m] Mixed lobular and ductal carcinoma as well as metaplastic carcinoma should be graded based on the ductal component and treated based on this grading. The metaplastic or mixed component does not alter prognosis.
[n] Unfavorable features: angiolymphatic invasion, high nuclear grade, or high histologic grade.
[o] If ER-positive consider endocrine therapy for risk reduction and to diminish the small risk of disease recurrence.
[p] Evidence supports that the magnitude of benefit from surgical or radiation ovarian ablation in premenopausal women with hormone receptor-positive breast cancer is similar to that achieved with CMF alone. Early evidence suggests similar benefits from ovarian suppression (ie, LHRH agonist) as from ovarian ablation. The combination of ovarian ablation/suppression plus tamoxifen therapy may be superior to suppression alone. The benefit of ovarian ablation/suppression in premenopausal women who have received adjuvant chemotherapy is uncertain.
[q] See Adjuvant Endocrine Therapy (BINV-I).
[r] Chemotherapy and endocrine therapy used as adjuvant therapy should be given sequentially with endocrine therapy following chemotherapy. The benefits of chemotherapy and of endocrine therapy are additive. However, the absolute benefit from chemotherapy may be small. The decision to add chemotherapy to endocrine therapy should be individualized, especially in those with a favorable prognosis and in women age ≥ 60 y where the incremental benefit of chemotherapy may be smaller. Available data suggest sequential or concurrent endocrine therapy with radiation therapy is acceptable.
[s] There are insufficient data to make chemotherapy recommendations for those over 70 y old. Treatment should be individualized with consideration of comorbid conditions.

> **Note:** All recommendations are category 2A unless otherwise indicated.
> **Clinical Trials:** NCCN believes that the best management of any cancer patient is in a clinical trial. Participation in clinical trials is especially encouraged.

BINV-5

FIGURE 82-1 Algorithm of NCCN guidelines for the treatment of hormone receptor–positive, HER-2-positive breast cancer. *[Reproduced with permission from The NCCN (2.2008) Invasive Breast Cancer. Clinical Practice Guidelines in Oncology. © National Comprehensive Cancer Network, 2008. Available at: http://www.nccn.org. To view the most recent and complete version of the guideline, go online to www.nccn.org.]*

mortality at 15 years.[2] Comparison of CMF (cyclophosphamide, methotrexate, and 5-fluorouracil) with anthracycline-containing regimens demonstrated that the use of anthracycline-based therapies resulted in a breast cancer mortality rate ratio of 0.84 (p < 0.00001) when compared to CMF. Thus, the NCCN recommends that anthracycline containing therapies be the preferred regimen for node-positive patients. However, the EBCTCG did not analyze the effect of HER-2 status upon the efficacy of anthracycline-based treatment. Retrospective evaluation has shown that the benefit of anthracycline-based chemotherapy may be closely linked to its effect on HER-2-positive tumors.[8-12] In addition, several trials have found that anthracycline-based therapies may have greater benefit in patients with HER-2-positive breast cancer, leading the NCCN to note this relationship in its guidelines.[11-14]

Randomized trials comparing AC (doxorubicin and cyclophosphamide) to CMF have shown no significant differences in relapse-free and overall survival.[15-17] However, 2 trials involving node-positive patients that randomized patients to CEF (cyclophosphamide, epirubicin, and 5-fluorouracil) versus CMF (cyclophosphamide, methotrexate, and 5-fluorouracil) demonstrated that the use of CEF resulted in a statistically significant improvement in relapse-free survival, with one trial demonstrating a significant increase in overall survival.[18,19]

The addition of a sequential taxane-based regimen became accepted after the NSABP B-28 and the Cancer and Leukemia Group B (CALGB) Intergroup trials demonstrated that the sequential addition of paclitaxel to AC (Adriamycin [doxorubicin] and Cytoxan [cyclophosphamide]) resulted in a significant improvement in DFS, with the CALGB Intergroup trial showing that the addition of sequential paclitaxel therapy to AC resulted in an absolute benefit of 3% in overall survival at 5 years.[20,21] Retrospective analysis of the CALGB Intergroup study demonstrated that the absolute benefits in DFS and OS due to chemotherapy were greater for patients with ER-negative, compared with ER-positive, tumors.[22]

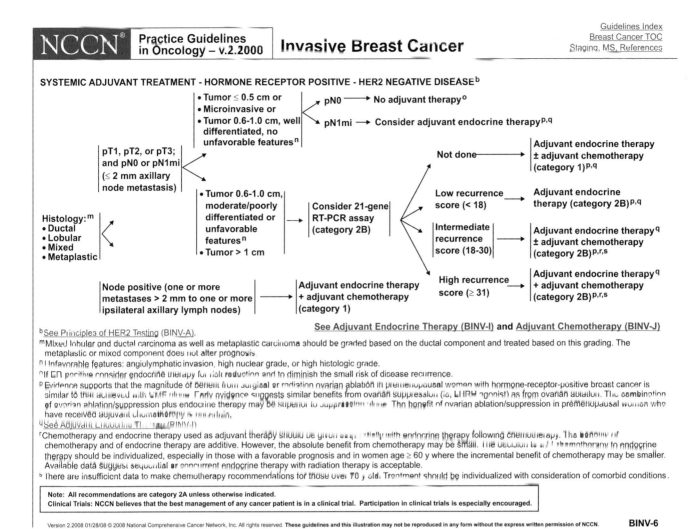

NCCN Practice Guidelines in Oncology – v.2.2000 **Invasive Breast Cancer**

SYSTEMIC ADJUVANT TREATMENT - HORMONE RECEPTOR POSITIVE - HER2 NEGATIVE DISEASE[b]

See Adjuvant Endocrine Therapy (BINV-I) and Adjuvant Chemotherapy (BINV-J)

[b] See Principles of HER2 Testing (BINV-A).

[m] Mixed lobular and ductal carcinoma as well as metaplastic carcinoma should be graded based on the ductal component and treated based on this grading. The metaplastic or mixed component does not alter prognosis.

[n] Unfavorable features: angiolymphatic invasion, high nuclear grade, or high histologic grade.

[o] If ER positive consider endocrine therapy for risk reduction and to diminish the small risk of disease recurrence.

[p] Evidence supports that the magnitude of benefit from surgical or radiation ovarian ablation in premenopausal women with hormone-receptor-positive breast cancer is similar to that achieved with CMF alone. Early evidence suggests similar benefits from ovarian suppression (ie, LHRH agonist) as from ovarian ablation. The combination of ovarian ablation/suppression plus endocrine therapy may be superior to suppression alone. The benefit of ovarian ablation/suppression in premenopausal women who have received adjuvant chemotherapy is uncertain.

[q] See Adjuvant Endocrine Therapy (BINV-I).

[r] Chemotherapy and endocrine therapy used as adjuvant therapy should be given sequentially with endocrine therapy following chemotherapy. The benefit of chemotherapy and of endocrine therapy are additive. However, the absolute benefit from chemotherapy may be small. The decision to add chemotherapy to endocrine therapy should be individualized, especially in those with a favorable prognosis and in women age ≥ 60 y where the incremental benefit of chemotherapy may be smaller. Available data suggest sequential or concurrent endocrine therapy with radiation therapy is acceptable.

[s] There are insufficient data to make chemotherapy recommendations for those over 70 y old. Treatment should be individualized with consideration of comorbid conditions.

> **Note:** All recommendations are category 2A unless otherwise indicated.
> **Clinical Trials:** NCCN believes that the best management of any cancer patient is in a clinical trial. Participation in clinical trials is especially encouraged.

FIGURE 82-2 Algorithm of NCCN guidelines for the treatment of hormone receptor–positive, HER-2-negative breast cancer. *[Reproduced with permission from The NCCN (2.2008) Invasive Breast Cancer. Clinical Practice Guidelines in Oncology. © National Comprehensive Cancer Network, 2008. Available at: http://www.nccn.org. To view the most recent and complete version of the guideline, go online to www.nccn.org.]*

Given the efficacy of taxanes, as well as their lack of cross-resistance with anthracyclines, a multicenter, randomized trial compared the effect of adjuvant TAC (docetaxel, doxorubicin, and cyclophosphamide) with FAC (5-fluorouracil, doxorubicin, and cyclophosphamide) upon DFS in patients with node-positive breast cancer.[23] Investigators found that TAC resulted in an improvement in DFS at 5 years (75% vs 68%, $p = 0.001$). Treatment with TAC, in comparison to FAC, was associated with a 30% lower risk of death (HR 0.70, $p = 0.008$). However, the incidence of grade 3 or greater nonhematologic adverse events, grade 3 or greater neutropenia, and grade 3 or greater infections was higher in the TAC group.

To determine the optimal choice and schedule of taxane, the Eastern Cooperative Oncology Group E1199 randomized patients to treatment with paclitaxel or docetaxel given at 3-week intervals for 4 cycles or 1-week intervals for 12 doses; taxane therapy followed 4 cycles of AC therapy.[24] The trial found that, when compared with patients receiving paclitaxel every 3 weeks, the odds ratio for DFS was 1.27 among those receiving weekly paclitaxel ($p = 0.006$), 1.23 among those receiving docetaxel every 3 weeks ($p = 0.02$), and 1.09 among those receiving weekly docetaxel ($p = 0.29$). The weekly administration of paclitaxel also resulted in an improved overall survival (odds ratio, 1.32; $p = 0.01$) over the 3-week interval regimen.

Taxane-based regimens were further studied in a phase III trial, which randomized patients with operable breast cancer to adjuvant therapy with either AC (doxorubicin and cyclophosphamide) or TC (docetaxel and cyclophosphamide).[25] At 5 years, TC was associated with a significant improvement in DFS rate (HR 0.67, $p = 0.015$), with a trend toward an improvement in OS (HR 0.76, $p = 0.13$). These findings support consideration of TC as a regimen in the treatment of early breast cancer, but further studies are necessary to evaluate whether the exclusion of anthracyclines altogether is warranted in this setting.

SYSTEMIC ADJUVANT TREATMENT - HORMONE RECEPTOR NEGATIVE - HER2 POSITIVE DISEASE[b]

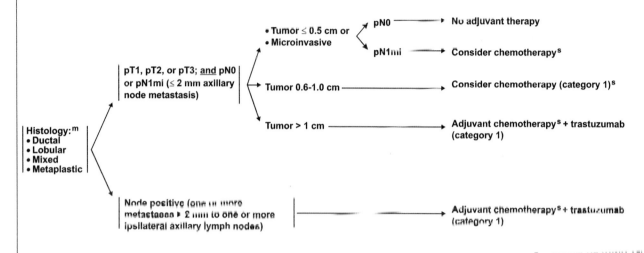

[b] See Principles of HER2 Testing (BINV-A).

[m] Mixed lobular and ductal carcinoma as well as metaplastic carcinoma should be graded based on the ductal component and treated based on this grading. The metaplastic or mixed component does not alter prognosis.

[s] There are insufficient data to make chemotherapy recommendations for those over 70 y old. Treatment should be individualized with consideration of comorbid conditions.

Note: All recommendations are category 2A unless otherwise indicated.
Clinical Trials: NCCN believes that the best management of any cancer patient is in a clinical trial. Participation in clinical trials is especially encouraged.

FIGURE 82-3 Algorithm of NCCN guidelines for the treatment of hormone receptor–negative, HER-2-positive breast cancer. *[Reproduced with permission from The NCCN (2.2008) Invasive Breast Cancer. Clinical Practice Guidelines in Oncology. © National Comprehensive Cancer Network, 2008. Available at: http://www.nccn.org. To view the most recent and complete version of the guideline, go online to www.nccn.org.]*

Dose density has been evaluated in 5 trials; only 2 of these studies have demonstrated a benefit in the reduction in interval between treatments.[26-30] Of these trials, the only trial to include taxanes and to evaluate the benefit of dose density in the absence of dose alterations was the CALGB Intergroup trial 9741, which compared the effects of concurrent versus sequential chemotherapy (doxorubicin followed by paclitaxel followed by cyclophosphamide, vs doxorubicin plus cyclophosphamide followed by paclitaxel) given either every 2 weeks (with filgrastim support) versus every 3 weeks.[27] While there was no difference between the concurrent and sequential scheduling of these regimens, dose-dense therapy resulted in a 26% improvement in DFS (*p* = 0.01) and a 31% improvement in OS (*p* = 0.013).

Adjuvant Endocrine Therapy

The real first generation of targeted therapy was endocrine therapy, blocking the binding of the estrogen and/or progesterone

receptors (ER). Targeting of the estrogen and/or progesterone receptors enabled clinicians to treat patients with therapies that demonstrated both significant efficacy and decreased toxicity in comparison to traditional cytotoxic regimens.

Premenopausal Women

The EBCTCG overview found that the use of tamoxifen for 5 years in ER-positive premenopausal breast cancer patients was associated with a reduction in the annual rate of recurrence by approximately 40%, as well as a decrease in breast cancer-related deaths by 34%.[2] Randomized trials have found that the optimal duration of tamoxifen is 5 years.[31,32] However, tamoxifen has known potential side effects, including uterine cancer, thromboembolic disease, and cataracts.

For patients who are unable to take or tolerate tamoxifen, ovarian suppression, in the form of surgical oophorectomy or luteinizing hormone-releasing hormone (LHRH) agonists, is another viable option. The EBCTCG analysis showed that

SYSTEMIC ADJUVANT TREATMENT - HORMONE RECEPTOR NEGATIVE - HER2 NEGATIVE DISEASE[b]

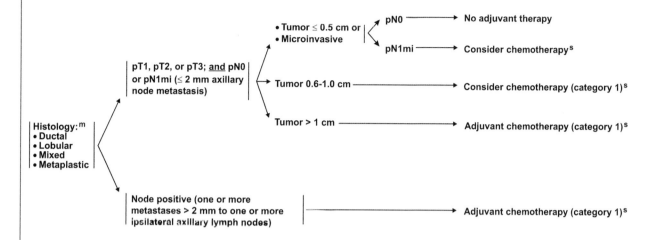

See Follow-Up (BINV-15)
See Adjuvant Endocrine Therapy (BINV-I) and Adjuvant Chemotherapy (BINV-J)

[b]See Principles of HER2 Testing (BINV-A).

[m]Mixed lobular and ductal carcinoma as well as metaplastic carcinoma should be graded based on the ductal component and treated based on this grading. The metaplastic or mixed component does not alter prognosis.

[s] There are insufficient data to make chemotherapy recommendations for those over 70 y old. Treatment should be individualized with consideration of comorbid conditions.

> **Note:** All recommendations are category 2A unless otherwise indicated.
> **Clinical Trials:** NCCN believes that the best management of any cancer patient is in a clinical trial. Participation in clinical trials is especially encouraged.

FIGURE 82-4 Algorithm of NCCN guidelines for the treatment of hormone receptor–negative, HER-2-negative breast cancer. *[Reproduced with permission from The NCCN (2.2008) Invasive Breast Cancer. Clinical Practice Guidelines in Oncology. © National Comprehensive Cancer Network, 2008. Available at: http://www.nccn.org. To view the most recent and complete version of the guideline, go online to www.nccn.org.]*

ovarian ablation or suppression resulted in a statistically significant decrease in recurrence ($p < 0.00001$) and breast cancer mortality ($p = 0.004$), but this difference appeared to occur only in the absence of other systemic therapies.[33] A subsequent meta-analysis of 16 randomized trials demonstrated that, when used as the only systemic adjuvant treatment, LHRH agonists did not significantly reduce recurrence (28.4% relative reduction, $p = 0.08$); however, the addition of LHRH agonists to tamoxifen, chemotherapy, or both reduced recurrence by 12.7% ($p = 0.02$).[34]

Postmenopausal Women

In postmenopausal women, studies have demonstrated the efficacy of aromatase inhibitors in the treatment of early-stage breast cancer. Aromatase inhibitors have been studied as initial, sequential (following tamoxifen), and extended therapy.

Initial use of an aromatase inhibitor, in comparison to tamoxifen monotherapy, was studied in the ATAC (Arimidex, Tamoxifen, Alone or in Combination) trial, which randomized

patients to initial treatment with tamoxifen alone, anastrozole alone, or the combination of tamoxifen and anastrozole. The study demonstrated that, compared to tamoxifen, anastrozole significantly prolonged DFS (HR 0.87, $p = 0.01$) and time-to-recurrence (HR 0.79, $p = 0.0005$).[35] No additional benefit was found from the combination of tamoxifen and anastrozole therapy.

The Breast International Group (BIG) 1-98 trial randomized patients to 1 of 4 treatment arms: tamoxifen alone for 5 years, letrozole alone for 5 years, tamoxifen for 2 years followed by letrozole for 3 years, or letrozole for 2 years followed by tamoxifen for 3 years. An updated interim analysis of this trial compared the tamoxifen and letrozole monotherapy arms; it demonstrated that DFS was significantly improved in the letrozole arm (0.82, $p = 0.007$).[36] Four other trials have evaluated the use of tamoxifen for 2 to 3 years followed sequentially by a third-generation aromatase inhibitor. The Italian Tamoxifen Anastrozole (ITA) trial, the Intergroup Exemestane Study (IES), the Austrian Breast and Colorectal

Cancer Study Group (ABCSG) trial, and the Arimidex Nolvadex trial have demonstrated that sequential therapy with tamoxifen and an aromatase inhibitor is associated with a significant improvement in DFS when compared to tamoxifen therapy alone.[37-39]

Furthermore, extended endocrine therapy was evaluated through the MA-17 trial, which initially randomized patients who had completed 4.5 to 6 years of adjuvant tamoxifen to treatment with placebo or letrozole. After a median follow-up of 30 months (range, 1.5-61.4 months), women in the letrozole arm exhibited an improved DFS (HR 0.58, $p < 0.001$) and distant DFS (HR 0.60, $p = 0.002$) when compared to those in the placebo arm.[40]

Differences in patient population and trial design prevent cross-trial comparison; thus, the optimal sequencing (initial treatment, sequential treatment, or extended use) and duration of aromatase inhibitor therapy are not presently known. However, these studies have consistently shown the benefit of aromatase inhibitor treatment over tamoxifen monotherapy. Thus, due to these encouraging findings, it is recommended that postmenopausal women who exhibit no contraindication or intolerance to an aromatase inhibitor be treated with a third-generation aromatase inhibitor as initial therapy, sequentially after tamoxifen, or as extended therapy following tamoxifen. There appear to be no significant differences among the 3 aromatase inhibitors that would lead to a recommendation of one agent over another.

Adjuvant Trastuzumab-Based Therapy

The treatment of HER-2-positive breast cancer has undergone significant advances since the cloning of the HER-2 oncogene in 1984.[41] In 2005, the interim results of the NSABP B-31 trial, the North Central Cancer Treatment Group (NCCTG) N9831 study, and the Herceptin Adjuvant (HERA) Breast International Group (BIG) 01-01 trial, were presented. The combined results of the NSABP B-31 and NCCTG N9831 trials demonstrated that, at 3 years, the addition of trastuzumab to adjuvant chemotherapy resulted in an absolute improvement in DFS of 12%, as well as a 33% reduction in the risk of death ($p = 0.015$).[42] The HERA trial confirmed these findings, as it demonstrated that the addition of trastuzumab to neoadjuvant or adjuvant chemotherapy resulted in an 8.4% improvement in DFS at 2 years.[43]

Shortly after the presentation of these initial findings, the NCCN revised its practice guidelines to incorporate trastuzumab in its guidelines for systemic adjuvant therapy. Thus, patients with HR-positive, HER-2-positive invasive breast tumors that are less than or equal to 0.5 cm, microinvasive, or well differentiated (but measure 0.6-1 cm) should receive consideration for adjuvant endocrine therapy alone if they are node negative or have micrometastatic nodal disease.[44] In the case of node negative (or pN1mi) tumors that measure 0.6 to 1 cm, are moderately differentiated, or have unfavorable features (ie, lymphovascular invasion, high nuclear grade, or high histologic grade), adjuvant chemotherapy followed by endocrine therapy should be considered. However, HR-positive, HER-2-positive breast tumors that are greater than 1 cm and/or are node positive should receive an adjuvant trastuzumab-based chemotherapy, followed by endocrine therapy.

For the adjuvant treatment of HR-negative, HER-2-positive breast cancer, chemotherapy is more highly considered due to the absence of endocrine therapy options. Thus, only patients with tumors that are microinvasive or measure less than 0.5 cm should receive no adjuvant therapy. The remainder of the patients in this group should receive consideration for chemotherapy and trastuzumab.

FUTURE DIRECTIONS

As translational research in the field of breast cancer continues, the goals of breast cancer treatment expand to encompass not only the successful eradication of disease, but also to render fewer side effects and enable improved quality of life during and after therapy. In addition, current research focuses on the ability to expand on the previous success of endocrine and chemotherapeutic agents through novel combinations and sequencing.

Microarray technology has led to the development of prognostic signatures that contribute to the prediction of the risk of recurrence for lymph node negative, HR-positive operable breast cancers. Among these indicators, 2 genetic profiles are widely used and are currently involved in prospective validation trials: the Amsterdam 70-gene profile (Mammaprint) and the Recurrence Score (Oncotype Dx). The Mammaprint assay utilizes fresh frozen breast tumor tissue to differentiate good-prognosis from poor-prognosis tumors.[45] External validation of this profile through 2 retrospective studies led to the approval of Mammaprint by the Food and Drug Administration (FDA).[46,47] The MINDACT (Microarray In Node negative Disease may Avoid ChemoTherapy) trial is currently enrolling patients in order to prospectively compare the 70-gene prognostic signature to traditional clinical-pathologic methods for assessing the risk of recurrence in women with lymph-node-negative disease. Pending these results, the Mammaprint assay is not recommended by the NCCN guidelines.

Unlike the Mammaprint assay, the Recurrence Score (Oncotype Dx) analyzes 21 genes within paraffin-embedded tumor tissue in order to develop a Recurrence Score.[48] External validation of the Recurrence Score occurred through the comparison of its predictions (low, intermediate, or high risk) to the outcomes of the patients in the tamoxifen-only arm of the National Surgical Adjuvant Breast and Bowel Project (NSABP), which demonstrated that the rates of distant recurrence at 10 years in the low-risk, intermediate-risk, and high-risk groups were 6.8%, 14.3%, and 30.5%, respectively. The TAILORx (Trial Assigning IndividuaLized Options for Treatment) study, which is currently accruing patients, will aim to prospectively validate this assay. Pending the results of the MINDACT and TAILORx trials, the Oncotype DX test may be considered an option to assist in the risk stratification of patients with node-negative, HR-positive, HER-2-negative breast cancers measuring 0.1 to 1 cm (with unfavorable features) or greater than 1 cm.[44]

Optimal endocrine therapy continues to be evaluated through clinical trials. The SOFT (Suppression of Ovarian Function Trial) will randomize premenopausal women who have completed chemotherapy or surgery (if chemotherapy is not planned) to 1 of 3 arms: tamoxifen monotherapy, tamoxifen in combination with triptorelin, or exemestane in combination with triptorelin. In addition, the TEXT (Tamoxifen and Exemestane) trial will compare the efficacy of tamoxifen versus exemestane in women undergoing ovarian suppression, and the PERCHE (Premenopausal Endocrine Responsive Chemotherapy) study will evaluate the benefit of chemotherapy for patients who are receiving ovarian suppression in combination with either tamoxifen or exemestane. For postmenopausal women, the MA-17 trial is currently evaluating the optimal duration of adjuvant aromatase inhibitor therapy; it will do so by randomizing women who have completed 5 years of letrozole therapy to treatment with either placebo or letrozole.

In the field of HER-2-positive breast cancer, current trials are evaluating the effect of dual inhibition of important targets, in combination with chemotherapy, upon DFS. For example, the BETH (Bevacizumab with Trastuzumab Adjuvant Therapy for HER-2-positive Breast Cancer) trial will evaluate the effect of adding bevacizumab to chemotherapy plus trastuzumab in patients with resected node-positive or high risk node-negative, HER-2-positive breast cancer. In addition, the ALTTO (Adjuvant Lapatinib And/Or Trastuzumab Treatment Optimisation) study will randomize patients to adjuvant therapy involving 1 of 4 arms: lapatinib monotherapy, trastuzumab alone, trastuzumab followed by lapatinib, or lapatinib concomitantly with trastuzumab.

While it is not possible to list all of the ongoing trials in the field of breast cancer, it is important to note a continued surge of research in one direction—toward more effective, tolerable, safe, and targeted therapies.

SUMMARY

The treatment of primary invasive breast cancer has undergone significant advances over the past decades. Endocrine therapy has established itself as a cornerstone in the treatment of HR-positive breast cancer. However, the optimal duration and sequence of this therapy continues to require further study. For patients with HR-negative breast cancer, trials have established the benefits (or lack of benefit) of dose escalation, dose density, and sequencing of agents. While no single regimen has been established as optimal, encouraging studies have established additional regimens (such as the combination of docetaxel and cyclophosphamide) that may be effective in this diverse population of patients. Finally, recent trials have demonstrated the effect of trastuzumab upon survival in HER-2-positive patients, giving hope to a population that once suffered from an aggressive and relentless disease.

REFERENCES

1. Jemal A, Siegel R, Ward E, et al. Cancer statistics, 2008. *CA Cancer J Clin.* 2008;58:71-96. Available from http://www.ncbi.nlm.nih.gov/entrez/query.fcgi?cmd=Retrieve&db=PubMed&dopt=Citation&list_uids=18287387.

2. Clarke M. Meta-analyses of adjuvant therapies for women with early breast cancer: the Early Breast Cancer Trialists' Collaborative Group overview. *Ann Oncol.* 2006;17(suppl 10):59-62. Available from http://www.ncbi.nlm.nih.gov/entrez/query.fcgi?cmd=Retrieve&db=PubMed&dopt=Citation&list_uids=17018753.

3. Olivotto IA, Bajdik CD, Ravdin PM, et al. Population-based validation of the prognostic model ADJUVANT! for early breast cancer. *J Clin Oncol.* 2005;23:2716-2725. Available from http://www.ncbi.nlm.nih.gov/entrez/query.fcgi?cmd=Retrieve&db=PubMed&dopt=Citation&list_uids=15837986.

4. Ravdin PM, Siminoff LA, Davis GJ, et al. Computer program to assist in making decisions about adjuvant therapy for women with early breast cancer. *J Clin Oncol.* 2001;19:980-991. Available from http://www.ncbi.nlm.nih.gov/entrez/query.fcgi?cmd=Retrieve&db=PubMed&dopt=Citation&list_uids=11181660.

5. Wolmark N, Wang J, Mamounas E, et al. Preoperative chemotherapy in patients with operable breast cancer: nine-year results from National Surgical Adjuvant Breast and Bowel Project B-18. *J Natl Cancer Inst Monogr.* 2001;30:96-102. Available from http://www.ncbi.nlm.nih.gov/entrez/query.fcgi?cmd=Retrieve&db=PubMed&dopt=Citation&list_uids=11773300.

6. Kuerer HM, Newman LA, Smith TL, et al. Clinical course of breast cancer patients with complete pathologic primary tumor and axillary lymph node response to doxorubicin-based neoadjuvant chemotherapy. *J Clin Oncol.* 1999;17:460-469. Available from http://www.ncbi.nlm.nih.gov/entrez/query.fcgi?cmd=Retrieve&db=PubMed&dopt=Citation&list_uids=10080586.

7. Bear HD, Anderson S, Smith RE, et al. Sequential preoperative or postoperative docetaxel added to preoperative doxorubicin plus cyclophosphamide for operable breast cancer:National Surgical Adjuvant Breast and Bowel Project Protocol B-27. *J Clin Oncol.* 2006;24:2019-2027. Available from http://www.ncbi.nlm.nih.gov/entrez/query.fcgi?cmd=Retrieve&db=PubMed&dopt=Citation&list_uids=16606972.

8. Mass R. The role of HER-2 expression in predicting response to therapy in breast cancer. *Semin Oncol.* 2000;27(suppl 11):46-52; discussion 92-100. Available from http://www.ncbi.nlm.nih.gov/entrez/query.fcgi?cmd=Retrieve&db=PubMed&dopt=Citation&list_uids=11236028.

9. Menard S, Valagussa P, Pilotti S, et al. Response to cyclophosphamide, methotrexate, and fluorouracil in lymph node-positive breast cancer according to HER2 overexpression and other tumor biologic variables. *J Clin Oncol.* 2001;19:329-335. Available from http://www.ncbi.nlm.nih.gov/entrez/query.fcgi?cmd=Retrieve&db=PubMed&dopt=Citation&list_uids=11208823.

10. Muss HB, Thor AD, Berry DA, et al. c-erbB-2 expression and response to adjuvant therapy in women with node-positive early breast cancer. *N Engl J Med.* 1994;330:1260-1266. Available from http://www.ncbi.nlm.nih.gov/entrez/query.fcgi?cmd=Retrieve&db=PubMed&dopt=Citation&list_uids=7908410.

11. Paik S, Bryant J, Tan-Chiu E, et al. HER2 and choice of adjuvant chemotherapy for invasive breast cancer: National Surgical Adjuvant Breast and Bowel Project Protocol B-15. *J Natl Cancer Inst.* 2000;92:1991-1998. Available from http://www.ncbi.nlm.nih.gov/entrez/query.fcgi?cmd=Retrieve&db=PubMed&dopt=Citation&list_uids=11121461.

12. Thor AD, Berry DA, Budman DR, et al. erbB-2, p53, and efficacy of adjuvant therapy in lymph node-positive breast cancer. *J Natl Cancer Inst.* 1998;90:1346-1360. Available from http://www.ncbi.nlm.nih.gov/entrez/query.fcgi?cmd=Retrieve&db=PubMed&dopt=Citation&list_uids=9747866.

13. Paik S, Bryant J, Park C, et al. erbB-2 and response to doxorubicin in patients with axillary lymph node-positive, hormone receptor-negative breast cancer. *J Natl Cancer Inst.* 1998;90:1361-1370. Available from http://www.ncbi.nlm.nih.gov/entrez/query.fcgi?cmd=Retrieve&db=PubMed&dopt=Citation&list_uids=9747867.

14. Pritchard KI, Shepherd LE, O'Malley FP, et al. HER2 and responsiveness of breast cancer to adjuvant chemotherapy. *N Engl J Med.* 2006;354:2103-2111. Available from http://www.ncbi.nlm.nih.gov/entrez/query.fcgi?cmd=Retrieve&db=PubMed&dopt=Citation&list_uids=16707747.

15. Bang SM, Heo DS, Lee KH, et al. Adjuvant doxorubicin and cyclophosphamide versus cyclophosphamide, methotrexate, and 5-fluorouracil chemotherapy in premenopausal women with axillary lymph node positive breast carcinoma. *Cancer.* 2000;89:2521-2526. Available from http://www.ncbi.nlm.nih.gov/entrez/query.fcgi?cmd=Retrieve&db=PubMed&dopt=Citation&list_uids=11135211.

16. Fisher B, Anderson S, Tan-Chiu E, et al. Tamoxifen and chemotherapy for axillary node-negative, estrogen receptor-negative breast cancer: findings from National Surgical Adjuvant Breast and Bowel Project B-23. *J Clin Oncol.* 2001;19:931-942. Available from http://www.ncbi.nlm.nih.gov/entrez/query.fcgi?cmd=Retrieve&db=PubMed&dopt=Citation&list_uids=11181655.

17. Fisher B, Brown AM, Dimitrov NV, et al. Two months of doxorubicin-cyclophosphamide with and without interval reinduction therapy compared with 6 months of cyclophosphamide, methotrexate, and fluorouracil in positive-node breast cancer patients with tamoxifen-nonresponsive tumors: results from the National Surgical Adjuvant Breast and Bowel

Project B-15. *J Clin Oncol*. 1990;8:1483-1496. Available from http://www.ncbi.nlm.nih.gov/entrez/query.fcgi?cmd=Retrieve&db=PubMed&dopt=Citation&list_uids=2202791.

18. Benefit of a high-dose epirubicin regimen in adjuvant chemotherapy for node-positive breast cancer patients with poor prognostic factors: 5-year follow-up results of French Adjuvant Study Group 05 randomized trial. *J Clin Oncol*. 2001;19:602-611. Available from http://www.ncbi.nlm.nih.gov/entrez/query.fcgi?cmd=Retrieve&db=PubMed&dopt=Citation&list_uids=11157009.

19. Levine MN, Pritchard KI, Bramwell VH, et al. Randomized trial comparing cyclophosphamide, epirubicin, and fluorouracil with cyclophosphamide, methotrexate, and fluorouracil in premenopausal women with node-positive breast cancer: update of National Cancer Institute of Canada Clinical Trials Group Trial MA5. *J Clin Oncol*. 2005;23:5166-5170. Available from http://www.ncbi.nlm.nih.gov/entrez/query.fcgi?cmd=Retrieve&db=PubMed&dopt=Citation&list_uids=16051958.

20. Henderson IC, Berry DA, Demetri GD, et al. Improved outcomes from adding sequential Paclitaxel but not from escalating Doxorubicin dose in an adjuvant chemotherapy regimen for patients with node-positive primary breast cancer. *J Clin Oncol*. 2003;21:976-983. Available from http://www.ncbi.nlm.nih.gov/entrez/query.fcgi?cmd=Retrieve&db=PubMed&dopt=Citation&list_uids=12637460.

21. Mamounas EP, Bryant J, Lembersky B, et al. Paclitaxel after doxorubicin plus cyclophosphamide as adjuvant chemotherapy for node positive breast cancer: results from NSABP B-28. *J Clin Oncol*. 2005;23:3686-3696. Available from http://www.ncbi.nlm.nih.gov/entrez/query.fcgi?cmd=Retrieve&db=PubMed&dopt=Citation&list_uids=15897552.

22. Berry DA, Cirrincione C, Henderson IC, et al. Estrogen-receptor status and outcomes of modern chemotherapy for patients with node positive breast cancer. *JAMA*. 2006;295:1658-1667. Available from http://www.ncbi.nlm.nih.gov/entrez/query.fcgi?cmd=Retrieve&db=PubMed&dopt=Citation&list_uids=16609087.

23. Martin M, Pienkowski T, Mackey J, et al. Adjuvant docetaxel for node-positive breast cancer. *N Engl J Med*. 2005;352:2302-2313. Available from http://www.ncbi.nlm.nih.gov/entrez/query.fcgi?cmd=Retrieve&db=PubMed&dopt=Citation&list_uids=15930421.

24. Sparano JA, Wang M, Martino S, et al. Weekly paclitaxel in the adjuvant treatment of breast cancer. *N Engl J Med*. 2008;358:1663-1671. Available from http://www.ncbi.nlm.nih.gov/entrez/query.fcgi?cmd=Retrieve&db=PubMed&dopt=Citation&list_uids=18420499.

25. Jones SE, Savin MA, Holmes FA, et al. Phase III trial comparing doxorubicin plus cyclophosphamide with docetaxel plus cyclophosphamide as adjuvant therapy for operable breast cancer. *J Clin Oncol*. 2006;24:5381-5387. Available from http://www.ncbi.nlm.nih.gov/entrez/query.fcgi?cmd=Retrieve&db=PubMed&dopt=Citation&list_uids=17135639.

26. Bonadonna G, Zambetti M, Moliterni A, et al. Clinical relevance of different sequencing of doxorubicin and cyclophosphamide, methotrexate, and Fluorouracil in operable breast cancer. *J Clin Oncol*. 2004;22:1614-1620. Available from http://www.ncbi.nlm.nih.gov/entrez/query.fcgi?cmd=Retrieve&db=PubMed&dopt=Citation&list_uids=15117983.

27. Citron ML, Berry DA, Cirrincione C, et al. Randomized trial of dose-dense versus conventionally scheduled and sequential versus concurrent combination chemotherapy as postoperative adjuvant treatment of node-positive primary breast cancer: first report of Intergroup Trial C9741/Cancer and Leukemia Group B Trial 9741. *J Clin Oncol*. 2003;21:1431-1439. Available from http://www.ncbi.nlm.nih.gov/entrez/query.fcgi?cmd=Retrieve&db=PubMed&dopt=Citation&list_uids=12668651.

28. Fisher B, Anderson S, Tan-Chiu E, et al. Tamoxifen and chemotherapy for lymph node-negative, estrogen receptor-negative breast cancer: findings from National Surgical Adjuvant Breast and Bowel Project B-23. *J Clin Oncol*. 1998;16:2382-2391. Available from http://www.ncbi.nlm.nih.gov/entrez/query.fcgi?cmd=Retrieve&db=PubMed&dopt=Citation&list_uids=9667255.

29. Linden HM, Haskell CM, Green SJ, et al. Sequenced compared with simultaneous anthracycline and cyclophosphamide in high-risk stage I and II breast cancer: final analysis from INT-0137 (S9313). *J Clin Oncol*. 2007;25:656-661. Available from http://www.ncbi.nlm.nih.gov/entrez/query.fcgi?cmd=Retrieve&db=PubMed&dopt=Citation&list_uids=17308269.

30. Nitz UA, Mohrmann S, Fischer J, et al. Comparison of rapidly cycled tandem high-dose chemotherapy plus peripheral-blood stem-cell support versus dose-dense conventional chemotherapy for adjuvant treatment of high-risk breast cancer: results of a multicentre phase III trial. *Lancet*. 2005;366:1935-1944. Available from http://www.ncbi.nlm.nih.gov/entrez/query.fcgi?cmd=Retrieve&db=PubMed&dopt=Citation&list_uids=16325695.

31. Fisher B, Dignam J, Bryant J, Wolmark N. Five versus more than five years of tamoxifen for lymph node-negative breast cancer: updated findings

from the National Surgical Adjuvant Breast and Bowel Project B-14 randomized trial. *J Natl Cancer Inst*. 2001;93:684-690. Available from http://www.ncbi.nlm.nih.gov/entrez/query.fcgi?cmd=Retrieve&db=PubMed&dopt=Citation&list_uids=11333290.

32. Stewart HJ, Forrest AP, Everington D, et al. Randomised comparison of 5 years of adjuvant tamoxifen with continuous therapy for operable breast cancer. The Scottish Cancer Trials Breast Group. *Br J Cancer*. 1996;74:297-299. Available from http://www.ncbi.nlm.nih.gov/entrez/query.fcgi?cmd=Retrieve&db=PubMed&dopt=Citation&list_uids=8688340.

33. Effects of chemotherapy and hormonal therapy for early breast cancer on recurrence and 15-year survival: an overview of the randomised trials. *Lancet*. 2005;365:1687-1717. Available from http://www.ncbi.nlm.nih.gov/entrez/query.fcgi?cmd=Retrieve&db=PubMed&dopt=Citation&list_uids=15894097.

34. Cuzick J, Ambroisine L, Davidson N, et al. Use of luteinising-hormone-releasing hormone agonists as adjuvant treatment in premenopausal patients with hormone-receptor-positive breast cancer: a meta-analysis of individual patient data from randomised adjuvant trials. *Lancet*. 2007;369:1711-1723. Available from http://www.ncbi.nlm.nih.gov/entrez/query.fcgi?cmd=Retrieve&db=PubMed&dopt=Citation&list_uids=17512856.

35. Howell A, Cuzick J, Baum M, et al. Results of the ATAC (Arimidex, Tamoxifen, Alone or in Combination) trial after completion of 5 years' adjuvant treatment for breast cancer. *Lancet*. 2005;365:60-62. Available from http://www.ncbi.nlm.nih.gov/entrez/query.fcgi?cmd=Retrieve&db=PubMed&dopt=Citation&list_uids=15639680.

36. Coates AS, Keshaviah A, Thurlimann B, et al. Five years of letrozole compared with tamoxifen as initial adjuvant therapy for postmenopausal women with endocrine-responsive early breast cancer: update of study BIG 1-98. *J Clin Oncol*. 2007;25:486-492. Available from http://www.ncbi.nlm.nih.gov/entrez/query.fcgi?cmd=Retrieve&db=PubMed&dopt=Citation&list_uids=17200148.

37. Boccardo F, Rubagotti A, Guglielmini P, et al. Switching to anastrozole versus continued tamoxifen treatment of early breast cancer. Updated results of the Italian tamoxifen anastrozole (ITA) trial. *Ann Oncol*. 2006;17(suppl 7):10-14. Available from http://www.ncbi.nlm.nih.gov/entrez/query.fcgi?cmd=Retrieve&db=PubMed&dopt=Citation&list_uids=16760270.

38. Coombes RC, Kilburn LS, Snowdon CF, et al. Survival and safety of exemestane versus tamoxifen after 2-3 years' tamoxifen treatment (Intergroup Exemestane Study): a randomised controlled trial. *Lancet*. 2007;369:559-570. Available from http://www.ncbi.nlm.nih.gov/entrez/query.fcgi?cmd=Retrieve&db=PubMed&dopt=Citation&list_uids=17307102.

39. Jakesz R, Jonat W, Gnant M, et al. Switching of postmenopausal women with endocrine-responsive early breast cancer to anastrozole after 2 years' adjuvant tamoxifen: combined results of ABCSG trial 8 and ARNO 95 trial. *Lancet*. 2005;366:455-462. Available from http://www.ncbi.nlm.nih.gov/entrez/query.fcgi?cmd=Retrieve&db=PubMed&dopt=Citation&list_uids=16084253.

40. Goss PE, Ingle JN, Martino S, et al. Randomized trial of letrozole following tamoxifen as extended adjuvant therapy in receptor positive breast cancer: updated findings from NCIC CTG MA.17. *J Natl Cancer Inst*. 2005;97:1262-1271. Available from http://www.ncbi.nlm.nih.gov/entrez/query.fcgi?cmd=Retrieve&db=PubMed&dopt=Citation&list_uids=16145047.

41. Schechter AL, Stern DF, Vaidyanathan L, et al. The neu oncogene: an erb-B-related gene encoding a 185,000-Mr tumour antigen. *Nature*. 1984;312:513-516. Available from http://www.ncbi.nlm.nih.gov/entrez/query.fcgi?cmd=Retrieve&db=PubMed&dopt=Citation&list_uids=6095109.

42. Romond EH, Perez EA, Bryant J, et al. Trastuzumab plus adjuvant chemotherapy for operable HER2-positive breast cancer. *N Engl J Med*. 2005;353:1673-1684. Available from http://www.ncbi.nlm.nih.gov/entrez/query.fcgi?cmd=Retrieve&db=PubMed&dopt=Citation&list_uids=16236738.

43. Piccart-Gebhart MJ, Procter M, Leyland-Jones B, et al. Trastuzumab after adjuvant chemotherapy in HER2-positive breast cancer. *N Engl J Med*. 2005;353:1659-1672. Available from http://www.ncbi.nlm.nih.gov/entrez/query.fcgi?cmd=Retrieve&db=PubMed&dopt=Citation&list_uids=16236737.

44. *The NCCN Clinical Practice Guidelines in Oncology™ Breast Cancer (Version 1.2009). © 2009 National Comprehensive Cancer Network, Inc. Available at: NCCN.org*. Accessed January 28, 2009.

45. van 't Veer LJ, Dai H, van de Vijver MJ, et al. Gene expression profiling predicts clinical outcome of breast cancer. *Nature*. 2002;415:530-536. Available from http://www.ncbi.nlm.nih.gov/entrez/query.fcgi?cmd=Retrieve&db=PubMed&dopt=Citation&list_uids=11823860.

46. van de Vijver MJ, He YD, van't Veer LJ, et al. A gene-expression signature as a predictor of survival in breast cancer. *N Engl J Med.* 2002;347:1999-2009. Available from http://www.ncbi.nlm.nih.gov/entrez/query.fcgi?cmd=Retrieve&db=PubMed&dopt=Citation&list_uids=12490681

47. Buyse M, Loi S, van't Veer L, et al. Validation and clinical utility of a 70-gene prognostic signature for women with node-negative breast cancer. *J Natl Cancer Inst.* 2006;98:1183-1192. Available from http://www.ncbi.nlm.nih.gov/entrez/query.fcgi?cmd=Retrieve&db=PubMed&dopt=Citation&list_uids=16954471.

48. Paik S, Shak S, Tang G, et al. A multigene assay to predict recurrence of tamoxifen-treated, node-negative breast cancer. *N Engl J Med.* 2004;351:2817-2826. Available from http://www.ncbi.nlm.nih.gov/entrez/query.fcgi?cmd=Retrieve&db=PubMed&dopt=Citation&list_uids=15591335.

CHAPTER 83

Selection of Patients for Therapy

William Irvin, Jr
Keith Amos

Initial observational studies of the natural history of breast cancer (untreated) viewed all breast cancers as the same, causing death a median of 2.7 years after presentation.[1] Similarly, initial treatment trials[2-4] viewed breast cancer as a homogeneous disease with no consideration of possible biological differences. Fortunately, in the 1960s, breast cancer heterogeneity was beginning to be recognized and included such factors as tumor size, the number of tumor-involved lymph nodes,[5-7] and later the influence of estrogen receptor (ER) and progesterone receptor (PR).[8-10]

This progress in understanding the heterogeneity of breast cancer has accelerated in the past 2 decades. Another example of this heterogeneity is the human epidermal growth receptor 2 (HER-2) and its correlation with relapse and survival.[11,12] Approximately 20% of tumors have high levels of HER-2 expression (3+ by immunohistochemical staining or an amplified HER-2 gene number copy by fluorescence in situ hybridization). HER-2 represents an important prognostic factor because it identifies patients who may benefit from HER-2-directed therapy.[13-15] Most recently, gene expression studies have identified several major subtypes of breast cancer[16]: the luminal subtypes, which typically express hormone receptor (HR)-related genes, and 2 HR-negative subtypes, the HER-2+/ER- subtype and the basal-like subtype. Prognosis varies by subtype, with worse outcomes traditionally seen with the 2 HR-negative subgroups compared to the luminal subgroups.[17-19] "Triple-negative" breast cancer (phenotypically ER, PR, and HER-2 negative) have an early aggressive clinical course when compared with other forms of breast cancer, but the effect appears transient.

This chapter reviews selection of therapy (especially preoperative therapy) in regard to molecular and genetic profiling and the use of genomic testing and Internet mathematical tools (Adjuvant!) for risk stratification.

MOLECULAR AND GENETIC PROFILING OF BREAST CANCER

Gene Expression Arrays

Initially, the heterogeneity of breast cancer was defined by light microscopy histologic differences with hematoxylin and eosin (H&E) stains and then specific immunostains. Moving beyond conventional light microscopy and basic histology, gene expression microarrays attempt to identify which genes are overexpressed or underexpressed in a given breast cancer specimen as compared with normal controls.

From breast cancer specimens, sets of DNA sequences are immobilized on solid substrates. Genes of interest are labeled and hybridization to the array occurs. After a period of time, an image of the array is obtained showing the individual nucleic acid species based on the amount of hybridization to complementary DNAs in known positions on the array. Different fluorescent dyes are used to quantify the relative abundance of a particular gene; the ratio of the intensities of 2 fluorescent dyes provides this answer. This allows researchers to examine and compare genes under varying conditions, that is, to know when and where a gene is expressed.[20,21]

Clustering of breast cancers according to their intrinsic gene expression patterns by gene expression array profiling studies on breast tumors reveal at least 5 intrinsic subtypes: [16-19] luminal A and B, HER-2+/ER-negative, normal breast-like, basal-like, and potentially a "claudin-low" subtype (low expression of luminal and cell-cell junction proteins)[22] (Fig. 83-1). This technology has illustrated that "breast cancer" represents a group of biologically distinct diseases. The "luminal" subtypes are named because of their similarity in gene expression pattern to the luminal epithelial component of the breast. Luminal A and B

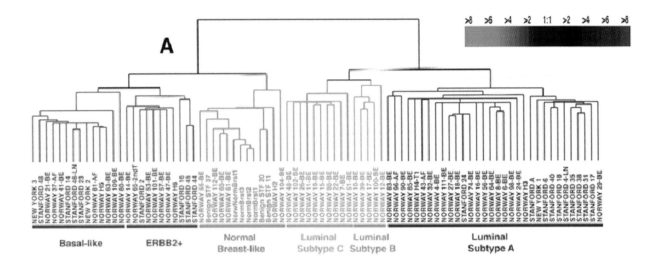

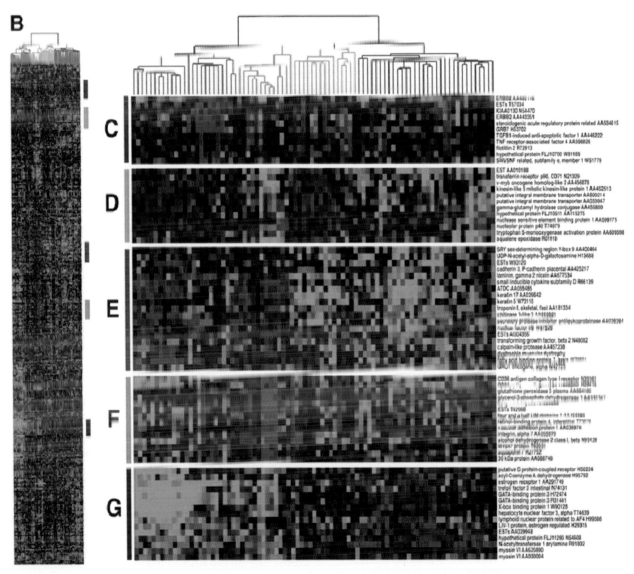

FIGURE 83-1 Gene expression patterns of 85 experimental samples representing 78 carcinomas, 3 benign tumors, and 4 normal tissues, analyzed by hierarchical clustering using the 476cDNA intrinsic clone set. (*Reproduced, with permission, from Sørlie T, Perou CM, Tibshirani R, et al. Proc Natl Acad Sci USA. 2001;98:10869-10874.*)

are both ER and PR positive, but luminal A tumors are more likely to be lower grade, have lower proliferative indices, higher expression of ER genes, and a lower chance of HER-2 overexpression. The HER-2+/ER-negative subtype is characterized by the overexpression of HER-2 and the lack of ER genes. The basal subtype typically is "triple negative," or ER, PR, and HER-2 negative, but these terms are not complete synonyms because 20% of basal tumors are not triple negative (although 91% of triple-negative cancers have basal-like gene expressions).[23] These breast cancer subtypes are highly reproducible,[17-19] are concordant between the primary tumor and the metastasis,[24] are found in the preneoplastic lesion ductal carcinoma in situ,[25] and persist before and after therapy.

Although they are the gold standard to identify breast cancer subgroups, RNA-based microarrays are not suitable for routine use in clinical environments for both technical reasons and the need for frozen tumors. However, these gene expression analyses have helped explain the genetic heterogeneity of breast cancer and have caused a shift in planning treatment trials for breast cancer for specific subtypes.

One of the most important contributions seen from this molecular breast cancer classification system is identifying the poor prognostic basal subtype. The initial studies examining outcome by intrinsic subtype uniformly found a poor prognosis in basal breast cancer.[17,19] In population-based studies such as the Carolina Breast Cancer Study, the triple-negative phenotype demonstrated reduced breast cancer–specific survival compared with luminal phenotypes as predicted by the early translational studies.[26] In a single institution cohort study involving more than 1600 patients, triple-negative breast cancer had an increased likelihood of distant recurrence (hazard ratio 2.6, 95% confidence interval [CI], 2-3.5) and death (hazard ratio 3.2, 95% CI 2.3-4.5) within 5 years of diagnosis, but not after 5 years because the peak of distance recurrence peaked at 3 years.[27] Another study also showed a difference in overall survival between triple-negative and non-triple-negative cancers that was most obvious at 3 years and decreased to no difference at 10 years.[28]

21-Gene Assay (Oncotype DX)

Oncotype DX Recurrence Score (Genomic Health, Inc; Redwood City, California) is a 21-gene breast cancer assay that predicts the 10-year distant recurrence risk and benefit to adjuvant chemotherapy in node-negative/HR-positive disease treated with tamoxifen. In 2001, the Genomic Health Company developed a reverse transcriptase polymerase chain reaction method for paraffin block tissues. Model-building studies using data from 447 breast cancer cases, including 233 cases from NSABP B-20, were used to select the 21-gene assay. The 21-gene assay has been validated for women with early stage, lymph node–negative, ER-positive breast cancers using available paraffin blocks from the National Surgical Adjuvant Breast and Bowel Project (NSABP) B-14 and the Kaiser Permanente Study.[29]

To determine an individual patient's risk for recurrence, a fixed paraffin-embedded tumor block or six 10-μm sections and 1 H&E slide are submitted to Genomic Health for analysis. The 21-gene assay is performed. Results are reported using

TABLE 83-1 21-Gene Assay Clinical Validation Results from NSABP B-14 Disease Relapse-Free Survival

Risk Category	Recurrence Score	Patients, %	10-yr Rate of Distant Recurrence (95% CI)
Low	<18	51	7%* (4.0–10)
Intermediate	18–30	22	14% (8–20)
High	≥31	27	31%* (24–37)

*$p < 0.00001$
CI = confidence interval.
Adapted from Paik S, Shak S, Tang G, et al. A multigene assay to predict recurrence of tamoxifen-treated, node-negative breast cancer. *N Engl J Med*. 2004;351(27):2817-2826.

a numeric recurrence score (RS) from 0 to 100. The RS is used to predict the average rate of distant recurrence at 10 years. Recurrence Scores are subdivided into low-, intermediate-, and high-risk groups (Table 83-1).[29]

The recurrence score also has a correlation with magnitude of chemotherapy benefit. For patients with high-risk recurrence scores (RS ≥ 31), there was 28% absolute benefit from a combination of tamoxifen and chemotherapy (relative risk: 0.26; 95% CI, 0.13-0.53).[30] In the low recurrence score group, there was no clear reduction in distant recurrence at 10 years (relative risk: 1.31; 95% CI, 0.46-3.78; increase of 1% in absolute risk). The benefit of chemotherapy in the intermediate recurrence score group was less clear (relative risk: 0.61; 95% CI, 0.24-1.59; increase of 2% in absolute risk).[30]

Because of this uncertainty, this group is the subject of further study. The TAILORx (Trial Assigning Individualized Options for Treatment) breast cancer trial is designed to determine whether adjuvant hormonal therapy alone is as effective as adjuvant hormonal therapy in combination with chemotherapy for certain women with breast cancer. Eligibility criteria include women with ER-positive and/or PR-positive, HER-2/neu negative breast cancer who are lymph node negative. The primary study group is women with recurrence scores between 11 and 25. These patients are randomized to receive adjuvant hormonal therapy alone or adjuvant chemotherapy in combination with hormonal therapy. This study was activated in 2006, and the accrual goal is approximately 10,000 patients.[31]

70-Gene Assay (MammaPrint)

MammaPrint is a 70-gene assay that uses molecular technology to determine the likelihood of distant recurrence within 5 to 10 years after initial diagnosis for node-negative disease in women 60 years of age or less. MammaPrint was developed by the Agendia Company located in Amsterdam, Netherlands. Investigators from the Netherlands Cancer Institute in Amsterdam (NKI) studied a core set of 70 genes that were found to be significantly associated with distant metastasis at

10 years.[32] The 70-gene assay has been on the market in Europe since 2005 and was cleared by the Food and Drug Administration for use in the United States in 2007. It has been independently validated for breast cancer patients with the following criteria: age less than 61 years, tumor size smaller than 5.0 cm, lymph node negative, and ER-positive status. This test should be limited to lymph node negative stage 1 or stage 2 patients.[33]

To perform a test, a MammaPrint Specimen Collection and Transportation Kit should be obtained. The 3-mm punch biopsy device from the kit is used to a fresh specimen for analysis from the surgical specimen within 1 hour of surgery. The tumor biopsy is placed in preservative solution to avoid RNA degradation. The biopsy specimen is then shipped to an Agendia laboratory for analysis. Upon receipt, each specimen is reviewed for histology and RNA quality. A specimen is rejected if there are less than 30% tumor cells histologically. The expression of 70 preselected genes is determined using DNA microarray technology. The data is analyzed using a specific algorithm that determines the MammaPrint Index and the expression profile of the sample as low risk or high risk for distant metastasis.

Tumor samples with a MammaPrint Index above a threshold of 0.4 are low risk. Tumor samples with a MammaPrint Index equal to or smaller than this threshold are classified as high risk. A low-risk patient has a 95% chance of being metastasis-free within the following 5 years (90% within the following 10 years), whereas a high-risk patient has a 78% chance of being metastasis-free within the following 5 years (71% within the following 10 years).[32]

The Microarray for Node Negative Disease May Avoid Chemotherapy Trial (MINDACT) is a multicenter, prospective, randomized phase III trial with planned accrual of nearly 6000 European breast cancer patients. The primary objective of MINDACT is to expand the 70-gene indication through identification and validation of novel gene expression signatures that can predict clinical response to chemotherapy and endocrine therapy.

76-Gene Prognostic Signature and Two-Gene Expression Ratio

Two other prognostic profiles have been studied in the literature but are not currently recommended for clinical use. The 76-gene prognostic profile for node-negative disease risk-stratifies patients into a good or poor profile group for risk of early distant metastasis. It has been validated in several studies and has shown similar prognostic performance to the 70-gene assay.[34-36] A 2-gene ratio has been validated in node-negative, ER-positive patients treated with adjuvant tamoxifen monotherapy.[37-39] Homeobox gene 13 (HOXB13) and interleukin 17B receptor (IL17BR) were analyzed as a ratio HOXB13:IL17BR (marketed as H/I; AvariaDx; Carlsbad, California), and the studies have shown that the higher the ratio, the worse the relapse-free survival, disease-free survival, and overall survival.[37-40]

PROGNOSTIC MODELS TO DETERMINE INDIVIDUAL PATIENT RISK

Several clinically useful prognostic indices incorporating relevant clinical information have been developed. These include the Nottingham Prognostic Index, the St. Gallen's risk categories,

and a Web-based model, Adjuvant! online. Currently, neither the National Comprehensive Cancer Network (NCCN) nor the American Society of Clinical Oncology (ASCO) have guidelines regarding the use of these prognostic indices.

Nottingham Prognostic Index

The Nottingham Prognostic Index (NPI) is calculated using tumor grade (1-3) plus lymph node stage (1-3) plus maximum tumor diameter (centimeters multiplied by 0.2) giving a range from 2.08 (no lymph nodes, grade 1, size 0.4 cm) to 6.8 (nodal stage 3, grade 3, size 4.9 cm).[41] It has been prospectively validated and is applicable to all operable breast cancers.[42-47] The NPI can be divided into 6 groups: excellent (2.08-2.4), good (2.42-≤3.4), moderate I (3.42-≤4.4), moderate II (4.42-≤5.4), poor (5.42-≤6.4), and very poor (6.5-6.8), with the 10-year breast cancer specific survivals 96%, 93%, 81%, 74%, 50%, and 38%, respectively.[48]

St. Gallen's

The St. Gallen's consensus meeting updated its risk stratification criteria in 2005, continuing to place patients into low-, intermediate-, or high-risk categories. Low-risk includes node negative and the tumor 2 cm or larger, grade 1, no peritumoral vascular invasion, HER-2 negative, and patient 35 years or more. Intermediate-risk includes node negative and the tumor larger than 2 cm, or grade 2 to 3, or peritumoral vascular invasion, or HER-2+, or age less than 35 years, or node positive (1-3) and HER-2 negative. High-risk includes 1 to 3 positive nodes and HER-2+ or 4 or more positive nodes.[49] In an independent retrospective validation, this risk categorization had high prognostic value. The 5-year distant disease-free survivals for the low-, intermediate-, and high-risk groups were 100%, 92%, and 72%, respectively ($p < 0.00005$).[50]

Adjuvant!

To help physicians and their patients make treatment decisions and understand prognosis, Adjuvant! (www.adjuvantonline.com) was designed to estimate objectively the benefit of adjuvant systemic therapy for individual breast cancer patients.[51] Adjuvant! includes patient age, comorbid conditions, tumor grade, HR status, tumor size, and the number of involved lymph nodes. The estimates of benefit on Adjuvant! were derived from estimating a patient's risk of a negative event (death or relapse) and then multiplying that by the proportion of negative events that a given adjuvant therapy will prevent. The Surveillance, Epidemiology, and End Results (SEER) registry estimates of outcome for breast cancer in the United States were used for estimates of prognosis. Efficacy estimates of adjuvant tamoxifen and chemotherapy were initially derived from the Early Breast Cancer Trialists' Collaborative Group 1998 meta-analysis data and then updated with the 2000 Overview Analysis of Randomized Adjuvant Tamoxifen and Chemotherapy Breast Cancer Trials.[53-55] The efficacy of combined endocrine and chemotherapy was developed from the product of the individual risk reductions from endocrine therapy and chemotherapy alone.[52]

On the main screen of Adjuvant! the physician enters patient information: age, comorbidity status, ER status, histologic grade, tumor size, positive nodes, and adjuvant therapy option. An option exists for adjustments to a "prognostic factor impact calculator" where the user enters the relative risk of the high-risk group versus the low-risk group and the percentage of patients in the high-risk group. Adjuvant! does not make projections based on HER-2 status or the use of trastuzumab. The physician is able to print for the patient the 10-year risk of recurrence and overall survival graphs with risk reduction estimates with endocrine therapy, chemotherapy, and combined therapy.

Adjuvant! has been validated based on comparison of predicted overall survival (OS), breast cancer–specific survival (BCSS), and event-free survival (EFS) estimates with observed outcomes for 4083 British Columbian women with stage I or II breast cancer. The 10-year predicted and observed outcomes were within 1% for OS, BCSS, and EFS ($p > 0.05$) across all patients. In subgroup analysis, Adjuvant! overestimated OS, BCSS, and EFS in women less than 35 years of age or with lymphatic or vascular invasion (LVI), for these 2 factors are not automatically incorporated into the Adjuvant! calculation. When the prognostic factor impact calculator was adjusted for the distribution of LVI, the predicted and observed outcomes were not significantly different.[56] Adjuvant! is an important tool for physician-patient communication regarding probability.

PRACTICE GUIDELINES FOR GENOMIC TESTING

The breast cancer practice guidelines for both NCCN and ASCO include the use of genomic testing of tumors for treatment. The NCCN breast cancer guidelines (www.nccn.org) include the consideration of 21-gene testing for tumors larger than 1.0 cm or tumors measuring 6 mm to 1.0 cm that are moderately/poorly differentiated or with unfavorable features including angiolymphatic invasion, high nuclear grade, or high histologic grade. The ASCO guidelines support the use of the 21-gene assay in node-negative, ER-positive breast cancer to help identify patients who are predicted to obtain the most benefit from adjuvant tamoxifen and may not require the use of adjuvant chemotherapy.[57] The use of genomic testing in these well-known clinical practice guidelines has solidified the role of molecular tumor diagnostics in breast cancer treatment planning.

PREOPERATIVE THERAPY

Historically, definitive surgical therapy for the primary tumor has been the initial treatment for patients presenting with breast cancer. Neoadjuvant therapy was first used in patients with unresectable, advanced, or inflammatory breast cancer with the goal of treating and shrinking the primary tumor. Increasingly, neoadjuvant therapy is used as a strategy for breast-conservation therapy for patients who present with locally advanced disease; it may also be used in any patient with an indication for adjuvant systemic cytotoxic treatment. The main goals of neoadjuvant therapy are to reduce mortality from breast cancer with reduced toxicity, to improve surgical options,

and to acquire early information on response of the tumor.[58] A multidisciplinary approach between medical, surgical, and radiation oncology should be taken with all patients for whom neoadjuvant therapy is considered.

There are a number of advantages to a chemotherapy first approach. Biologically, groups have shown that the proliferation rate of metastatic foci increases after resection of the primary tumor in animal models.[59,60] The cosmetic result of breast-conservation therapy is improved if less of the breast is resected after receiving neoadjuvant chemotherapy. Resistance to chemotherapy can be identified, and ineffective chemotherapy regimens can be discontinued to avoid toxicity. A pathologic complete response (pCR) can be seen in the primary tumor and lymph nodes in 15% to 30% of patients.[61]

The NSABP B-18 trial was a phase III trial to evaluate differences in neoadjuvant and adjuvant chemotherapy. Patients with operable breast cancer were randomized to receive either neoadjuvant versus adjuvant Adriamycin and cyclophosphamide (AC) in 4 cycles. The overall response rate was 80% in the preoperative group. Among the cohort of patients with tumors larger than 5 cm, 22% underwent breast conservation compared with 8% in the adjuvant therapy group. Patients who received neoadjuvant chemotherapy were more likely to have axillary downstaging (59% vs 42%). Eighty-seven percent of patients with a complete clinical response had pathologically negative axillary nodes versus 50% with stable disease. However, there was no difference in the disease-free survival and overall survival between the 2 groups.[62] With a median follow-up of 9 years, the overall survival was 69% in the neoadjuvant therapy arm and 70% in the adjuvant therapy arm (not statistically different).[63] The European Organization for Research and Treatment of Cancer (EORTC) conducted a trial of similar design confirming the results of NSABP B-18.[61]

Hormonal therapy has also been used in the neoadjuvant setting. In a double-blind phase III randomized trial, 4 months of neoadjuvant letrozole, 2.5 mg daily, was compared with tamoxifen, 20 mg daily, in postmenopausal women with ER- and/or PR-positive breast cancer. For the letrozole patients, 60% responded and 48% underwent successful breast-conserving surgery compared with 41% ($p = 0.004$) and 36% ($p = 0.036$) for tamoxifen patients.[64] Phase II data exist comparing neoadjuvant anastrozole or exemestane for 3 months compared with neoadjuvant doxorubicin and paclitaxel in ER-/PR-positive patients with similar overall objective response rates between the endocrine and the chemotherapy groups; however, this topic needs to be further studied before these data can be universally applied.[65] Neoadjuvant therapy with endocrine agents should only be employed in HR-positive patients for whom cytotoxic chemotherapy is contraindicated and if breast-conserving therapy is not possible first.[58]

BREAST-CONSERVING THERAPY AFTER NEOADJUVANT THERAPY

The surgical assessment of patients both before and after neoadjuvant therapy is often driven by a goal of breast conservation. A metallic tissue marking clip should be percutaneously placed at the tumor site prior to initiation of neoadjuvant therapy. This clip can be useful in facilitating prior tumor location in patients who have a complete clinical response with neoadjuvant therapy. In patients with a complete clinical response, approximately 50% will have no residual invasive disease on pathologic analysis.[66] Some patients will have ductal carcinoma in situ in the absence of invasive disease. The pathologic response pattern to neoadjuvant therapy is variable. Some tumors regress in a concentric pattern, and others regress with scattered tumor satellites. Despite clinical response, if a large area of calcifications remains on mammogram, a mastectomy should be considered. Negative margins should be achieved with a lumpectomy. The management of patients with a large burden of disease at surgery following neoadjuvant treatment is a topic of ongoing research.

STAGING

Pathologic staging after treatment is determined using the revised American Joint Committee on Cancer (yAJCC) staging, adopted in January 2003 (y designation if pathologic staging occurs after neoadjuvant therapy; a detailed discussion on staging was presented earlier in this text).[67] Other

than the yAJCC staging, the residual cancer burden (RCB) has been shown to be a significant predictor of distant relapse-free survival. RCB is calculated as a continuous index combining pathologic measurements (size and cellularity) and nodal metastasis (number and size). RCB-0 identifies patients with pCR. Cutoff points were assigned to define the other 3 categories: RCB-I (minimal residual disease), RCB-II (moderate residual disease), and RCB-III (extensive residual disease). The cutoff between RCB-III and II was defined as the 87th percentile (RCB 3.28) and the cutoff between RCB-II and I was the 40th percentile (RCB 1.36). The difference between RCB-0 (best) and III (worst) in terms of 5-year rates of distant relapse was 48.2% (95% CI, 28 to 66). RCB adds prognostic power at least to stage II/III yAJCC tumors.[68]

FUTURE DIRECTIONS

Table 83-2 lists the current ongoing trials for the molecular and genetic profiling and genetic testing of tumors found on www.clinicaltrials.gov.[69,70] Table 83-3 lists therapeutic agents being studied for selection of therapy in the neoadjuvant setting.[71] As described in Table 83-3, there is no lack of a shortage of agents being tested in this setting, and the number will only grow as new agents are developed.

TABLE 83-2 Ongoing Trials: Molecular and Genetic Profiling and Genetic Testing of Tumors

Description	Purpose
Randomized clinical trial to evaluate the predictive accuracy of a gene expression profile-based test to select patients for preoperative taxane/anthracycline chemotherapy for stage I–III breast cancer	To prospectively evaluate the predictive accuracy of a gene expression profile-based test to foretell pathologic complete response (pCR) to preoperative paclitaxel/5-fluorouracil, doxorubicin, cyclophosphamide (FAC)
Procurement of normal breast tissue and metastatic breast cancer tissue for molecular profiling	To define the molecular profile for normal breast tissue, primary breast tumors, and metastatic tumors
A pilot study to establish a standardized protocol for gene microarray analysis in patients receiving neoadjuvant chemotherapy for breast cancer: Identifying factors predictive of a response to paclitaxel	To determine the feasibility of accruing women to a trial with serial breast biopsies and to determine a standard protocol template for gene microarray analysis
Genetic factors affecting breast cancer progression	To correlate variations in genes with breast cancer progression and survival
A randomized phase II trial evaluating the performance of genomic expression profiles to direct the use of preoperative chemotherapy for early stage breast cancer	To determine whether genomic profiling for drug sensitivity can improve the pCR rate as compared with random assignment of patients to therapy
Serum protein profiling as a predictor of gemcitabine sensitivity in breast cancer with prior exposure to anthracyclines and taxanes	To identify a serum protein profile that predicts gemcitabine/carboplatin sensitivity or resistance
Predicting response and toxicity in patients receiving chemotherapy for breast cancer: A multicenter genomic, proteomic, and pharmacogenomic correlative study	To correlate tumor gene expression and serum and tumor proteomic profiles with response to commonly used chemotherapies
Evaluating the role of genotype in tamoxifen therapy	To evaluate whether endoxifen levels can be increased in intermediate metabolizers by increasing the dose of tamoxifen from 20 mg daily to 40 mg daily

TABLE 83-3 Therapeutic Agents Being Evaluated Preoperatively

Everolimus and letrozole
Cisplatin
Bevacizumab in combination with standard therapy
Cisplatin and bevacizumab
Trastuzumab plus everolimus
Trastuzumab plus vinorelbine
Zoledronic acid plus standard chemotherapy
Capecitabine plus docetaxel
Bevacizumab plus letrozole
Trastuzumab plus albumin-bound nanoparticle paclitaxel
Sunitinib
Trastuzumab plus bevacizumab
Capecitabine
Sorafenib
Cetuximab and capecitabine
Vorinostat
Lapatinib plus trastuzumab
Gemcitabine plus paclitaxel and trastuzumab

NECESSARY FUTURE STUDIES TO ADVANCE THE FIELD

Future studies will not only need to continue to evaluate heterogeneity in the tumor but will also need to consider another possibility for outcome differences: heterogeneity in the patient. For example, the cytochrome P450 (CYP450) metabolic enzyme CYP2D6 has a major role in tamoxifen metabolism, breaking tamoxifen down to its active metabolites N-desmethyl tamoxifen, 4-hydroxy-tamoxifen, and endoxifen (4-hydroxy-N-desmythltamoxifen).[74,75] Endoxifen is 100 times more potent in antiestrogen effect than tamoxifen (equivalent to 4-hydroxy-tamoxifen), but it is present in plasma at least 6 times more than 4-hydroxy-tamoxifen.[74-76] The CYP2D6 gene is polymorphic; thus variant gene sequences that result in proteins with absent or reduced enzyme function produce lower plasma levels of the tamoxifen metabolites, including endoxifen.[74] Goetz et al shows that women who were homozygous for the null-activity CYP2D6 alleles tended to have worse relapse-free survival.[77] Furthermore, an analysis in Korean women suggested that the time to progression in women with metastatic breast cancer on tamoxifen was shorter in women with lower steady-state plasma concentrations of endoxifen.[78] These studies, in part, have prompted debate on guidelines for dosing tamoxifen; however, at this time, insufficient evidence is available to point to a clear solution.

Table 83-4 summarizes topics of research of unanswered questions in the specific areas covered in this chapter. In the area of molecular and genetic profiling of breast cancer, correlative studies showing the effects of downstream inhibition of molecular pathways (ie, inhibition of epidermal growth factor receptor [EGFR] in responders and nonresponders in triple-negative disease) is needed to better understand how to treat resistant disease and to speed up new drug development. Along with this, further correlative studies with DNA microarray analysis of the effect of treatment on breast cancer subtype are also needed. Establishing the connection between CYP2D6 genotype, endoxifen levels, and outcomes in patients treated with tamoxifen will allow for more precise selection of the most effective hormonal therapy. Also, the future of pharmacogenomics will provide studies for establishing individual patient and tumor susceptibility to specific chemotherapeutic agents.

TABLE 83-4 Necessary Future Studies

Molecular and genetic profiling of breast cancer	1. Correlative studies showing the effects of downstream inhibition of molecular pathways (ie, inhibition of EGFR in responders and non-responders in triple-negative disease) 2. Further DNA microarray analysis of the effect of treatment on breast cancer subtype 3. Establishing the connection, if any, between CYP2D6 genotype, endoxifen levels, and outcomes in patients treated with tamoxifen
Genomic testing of tumors	1. Establish specific testing to determine tumor susceptibility to specific chemotherapeutic agents 2. Establish specific criteria to determine to whom chemotherapy is likely to do harm rather than benefit
Adjuvant!	1. Establish inclusion and validation for HER-2 and treatment with trastuzumab
Preoperative therapy	1. Further "residual disease trials" for patients with significant disease after neoadjuvant therapy and local treatment 2. Continued evaluation of incorporating targeted therapy (against VEGF, EGFR, and HER-2) preoperatively

EGFR, epidermal growth factor receptor; HER-2, human epidermal growth receptor 2; VEGF, vascular endothelial growth factor.

Clinically needed are further "residual disease trials" (trials for patients with significant disease at surgery after neoadjuvant chemotherapy) to provide possibly risk-lowering treatment to patients with high-risk disease. Also necessary for advancing treatment is further analysis of preoperative targeted therapy against vascular endothelial growth factor, EGFR, or HER-2, for example.

SUMMARY

Our increasing understanding of the molecular and genetic profile of breast cancer and the use of prognostic indices such as Adjuvant! and genomic tests such as the 70-gene prognostic signature and the 21-gene panel has changed the selection of patients for therapy (and the selection of therapy for patients). Much room is present though for improvement in this selection for efficacy and safety, and studies are ongoing and being developed to address these issues, especially as novel diagnostic, prognostic, and therapeutic interventions come available. Newer staging tools, such as the RCB, are being integrated with yAJCC staging to help clinicians more accurately provide prognostic information to their patients. Future studies are focusing on novel combinations of neoadjuvant treatment and whether treating residual disease with chemotherapy is beneficial.

REFERENCES

1. Bloom HJ, Richardson WW, Harries EJ. Natural history of untreated breast cancer (1805–1933). Comparison of untreated and treated cases according to histological grade of malignancy. *Br Med J.* 1962;2(5299):213-221.
2. Harrington SW. Results of surgical treatment of unilateral carcinoma of breast in women. *J Am Med Assoc.* 1952;148(12):1007-1011.
3. Lewis D, Rienhoff WF. Results of operations at the Johns Hopkins Hospital for cancer of the breast: performed at the Johns Hopkins Hospital from 1889 to 1931. *Ann Surg.* 1932;95(3):336-400.
4. Bonadonna G, Brusamolino E, Valagussa P, et al. Combination chemotherapy as an adjuvant treatment in operable breast cancer. *N Engl J Med.* 1976;294(8):405-410.
5. Fisher B, Ravdin RG, Ausman RK, et al. Surgical adjuvant chemotherapy in cancer of the breast: results of a decade of cooperative investigation. *Ann Surg.* 1968;168(3):337-356.
6. Fisher B, Slack NH. Number of lymph nodes examined and the prognosis of breast carcinoma. *Surg Gynecol Obstet.* 1970;131(1):79-88.
7. Fisher B. The surgical dilemma in the primary therapy of invasive breast cancer: a critical appraisal. *Curr Probl Surg.* 1970:1-53.
8. Fisher B, Redmond C, Brown A, et al. Influence of tumor estrogen and progesterone receptor levels on the response to tamoxifen and chemotherapy in primary breast cancer. *J Clin Oncol.* 1983;1(4):227-241.
9. Fisher B, Wickerham DL, Brown A, Redmond CK. Breast cancer estrogen and progesterone receptor values: their distribution, degree of concordance, and relation to number of positive axillary nodes. *J Clin Oncol.* 1983;1(6):349-358.
10. Fisher B, Redmond CK, Wickerham DL, et al. Relation of estrogen and/or progesterone receptor content of breast cancer to patient outcome following adjuvant chemotherapy. *Breast Cancer Res Treat.* 1983;3(4):355-364.
11. Slamon DJ, Clark GM, Wong SG, et al. Human breast cancer: correlation of relapse and survival with amplification of the HER-2/neu oncogene. *Science.* 1987;235(4785):177-182.
12. Owens MA, Horten BC, Da Silva MM. HER2 amplification ratios by fluorescence in situ hybridization and correlation with immunohistochemistry in a cohort of 6556 breast cancer tissues. *Clin Breast Cancer.* 2004;5(1):63-69.
13. Romond EH, Perez EA, Bryant J, et al. Trastuzumab plus adjuvant chemotherapy for operable HER2-positive breast cancer. *N Engl J Med.* 2005;353(16):1673-1684.
14. Piccart-Gebhart MJ, Procter M, Leyland-Jones B, et al. Trastuzumab after adjuvant chemotherapy in HER2-positive breast cancer. *N Engl J Med.* 2005;353(16):1659-1672.
15. Joensuu H, Kellokumpu-Lehtinen PL, Bono P, et al. Adjuvant docetaxel or vinorelbine with or without trastuzumab for breast cancer. *N Engl J Med.* 2006;354(8):809-820.
16. Perou CM, Sorlie T, Eisen MB, et al. Molecular portraits of human breast tumours. *Nature.* 2000;406(6797):747-752.
17. Sorlie T, Perou CM, Tibshirani R, et al. Gene expression patterns of breast carcinomas distinguish tumor subclasses with clinical implications. *Proc Natl Acad Sci USA.* 2001;98(19):10869-10874.
18. Sorlie T, Tibshirani R, Parker J, et al. Repeated observation of breast tumor subtypes in independent gene expression data sets. *Proc Natl Acad Sci USA.* 2003;100(14):8418-8423.
19. Sotiriou C, Neo SY, McShane LM, et al. Breast cancer classification and prognosis based on gene expression profiles from a population-based study. *Proc Natl Acad Sci USA.* 2003;100(18):10393-10398.
20. Eisen MB, Brown PO. DNA arrays for analysis of gene expression. *Methods Enzymol.* 1999;303:179-205.
21. DeRisi JL, Iyer VR, Brown PO. Exploring the metabolic and genetic control of gene expression on a genomic scale. *Science.* 1997;278(5338):680-686.
22. Herschkowitz JI, Simin K, Weigman VJ, et al. Identification of conserved gene expression features between murine mammary carcinoma models and human breast tumors. *Genome Biol.* 2007;8(5):R76.
23. Kreike B, van Kouwenhove M, Horlings H, et al. Gene expression profiling and histopathological characterization of triple-negative/basal-like breast carcinomas. *Breast Cancer Res.* 2007;9(5):R65.
24. Weigelt B, Hu Z, He X, et al. Molecular portraits and 70-gene prognosis signature are preserved throughout the metastatic process of breast cancer. *Cancer Res.* 2005;65(20):9155-9158.
25. Livasy CA, Perou CM, Karaca G, et al. Identification of a basal-like subtype of breast ductal carcinoma in situ. *Hum Pathol.* 2007;38(2):197-204.
26. Carey LA, Perou CM, Livasy CA, et al. Race, breast cancer subtypes, and survival in the Carolina Breast Cancer Study. *JAMA.* 2006;295(21):2492-2502.
27. Dent R, Trudeau M, Pritchard KI, et al. Triple-negative breast cancer: clinical features and patterns of recurrence. *Clin Cancer Res.* 2007;13(15 Pt 1):4429-4434.
28. Tischkowitz M, Brunet JS, Begin LR, et al. Use of immunohistochemical markers can refine prognosis in triple negative breast cancer. *BMC Cancer.* 2007;7:134.
29. Paik S, Shak S, Tang G, et al. A multigene assay to predict recurrence of tamoxifen-treated, node-negative breast cancer. *N Engl J Med.* 2004;351(27):2817-2826.
30. Paik S, Tang G, Shak S, et al. Gene expression and benefit of chemotherapy in women with node-negative, estrogen receptor-positive breast cancer. *J Clin Oncol.* 2006;24(23):3726-3734.
31. Sparano JA. TAILORx: trial assigning individualized options for treatment (Rx). *Clin Breast Cancer.* 2006;7(4):347-350.
32. van de Vijver MJ, He YD, van't Veer LJ, et al. A gene-expression signature as a predictor of survival in breast cancer. *N Engl J Med.* 2002;347(25):1999-2009.
33. Buyse M, Loi S, van't Veer L, et al. Validation and clinical utility of a 70-gene prognostic signature for women with node-negative breast cancer. *J Natl Cancer Inst.* 2006;98(17):1183-1192.
34. Foekens JA, Atkins D, Zhang Y, et al. Multicenter validation of a gene expression-based prognostic signature in lymph node-negative primary breast cancer. *J Clin Oncol.* 2006;24(11):1665-1671.
35. Desmedt C, Piette F, Loi S, et al. Strong time dependence of the 76-gene prognostic signature for node-negative breast cancer patients in the TRANSBIG multicenter independent validation series. *Clin Cancer Res.* 2007;13(11):3207-3214.
36. Haibe-Kains B, Desmedt C, Piette F, et al. Comparison of prognostic gene expression signatures for breast cancer. *BMC Genomics.* 2008;9:394.
37. Ma XJ, Hilsenbeck SG, Wang W, et al. The HOXB13:IL17BR expression index is a prognostic factor in early-stage breast cancer. *J Clin Oncol.* 2006;24(28):4611-4619.
38. Jansen MP, Sieuwerts AM, Look MP, et al. HOXB13-to-IL17BR expression ratio is related with tumor aggressiveness and response to tamoxifen of recurrent breast cancer: a retrospective study. *J Clin Oncol.* 2007;25(6):662-668.
39. Goetz MP, Suman VJ, Ingle JN, et al. A two-gene expression ratio of homeobox 13 and interleukin-17B receptor for prediction of recurrence and survival in women receiving adjuvant tamoxifen. *Clin Cancer Res.* 2006;12(7 Pt 1):2080-2087.
40. Ma XJ, Wang Z, Ryan PD, et al. A two-gene expression ratio predicts clinical outcome in breast cancer patients treated with tamoxifen. *Cancer Cell.* 2004;5(6):607-616.
41. Haybittle JL, Blamey RW, Elston CW, et al. A prognostic index in primary breast cancer. *Br J Cancer.* 1982;45(3):361-366.

42. Todd JH, Dowle C, Williams MR, et al. Confirmation of a prognostic index in primary breast cancer. *Br J Cancer.* 1987;56(4):489-492.
43. D'Eredita G, Giardina C, Martellotta M, Natale T, Ferrarese F. Prognostic factors in breast cancer: the predictive value of the Nottingham Prognostic Index in patients with a long-term follow-up that were treated in a single institution. *Eur J Cancer.* 2001;37(5):591-596.
44. Sundquist M, Thorstenson S, Brudin L, Wingren S, Nordenskjold B. Incidence and prognosis in early onset breast cancer. *Breast.* 2002;11(1):30-35.
45. Balslev I, Axelsson CK, Zedeler K, et al. The Nottingham Prognostic Index applied to 9,149 patients from the studies of the Danish Breast Cancer Cooperative Group (DBCG). *Breast Cancer Res Treat.* 1994;32(3):281-290.
46. Kollias J, Murphy CA, Elston CW, et al. The prognosis of small primary breast cancers. *Eur J Cancer.* 1999;35(6):908-912.
47. Kollias J, Elston CW, Ellis IO, Robertson JF, Blamey RW. Early-onset breast cancer—histopathological and prognostic considerations. *Br J Cancer.* 1997;75(9):1318-1323.
48. Blamey RW, Ellis IO, Pinder SE, et al. Survival of invasive breast cancer according to the Nottingham Prognostic Index in cases diagnosed in 1990–1999. *Eur J Cancer.* 2007;43(10):1548-1555.
49. Goldhirsch A, Glick JH, Gelber RD, et al. Meeting highlights: international expert consensus on the primary therapy of early breast cancer 2005. *Ann Oncol.* 2005;16(10):1569-1583.
50. Yau TK, Soong IS, Chan K, et al. Evaluation of the prognostic value of 2005 St Gallen risk categories for operated breast cancers in Hong Kong. *Breast.* 2008;17(1):58-63.
51. Ravdin PM. A computer program to assist in making breast cancer adjuvant therapy decisions. *Semin Oncol.* 1996;23(1 suppl 2):43-50.
52. Ravdin PM, Siminoff LA, Davis GJ, et al. Computer program to assist in making decisions about adjuvant therapy for women with early breast cancer. *J Clin Oncol.* 2001;19(4):980-991.
53. Early Breast Cancer Trialists' Collaborative Group (EBCTCG). Tamoxifen for early breast cancer: an overview of the randomised trials. *Lancet.* 1998; 351(9114):1451-1467.
54. Early Breast Cancer Trialists' Collaborative Group (EBCTCG). Polychemotherapy for early breast cancer: an overview of the randomised trials. *Lancet.* 1998; 352(9132):930-942.
55. Early Breast Cancer Trialists' Collaborative Group (EBCTCG). Effects of chemotherapy and hormonal therapy for early breast cancer on recurrence and 15-year survival: an overview of the randomised trials. *Lancet.* 2005;365(9472):1687-1717.
56. Olivotto IA, Bajdik CD, Ravdin PM, et al. Population-based validation of the prognostic model ADJUVANT! for early breast cancer. *J Clin Oncol.* 2005;23(12):2716-2725.
57. Harris L, Fritsche H, Mennel R, et al. American Society of Clinical Oncology 2007 update of recommendations for the use of tumor markers in breast cancer. *J Clin Oncol.* 2007;25(33):5287-5312.
58. Kaufmann M, von Minckwitz G, Bear HD, et al. Recommendations from an international expert panel on the use of neoadjuvant (primary) systemic treatment of operable breast cancer: new perspectives 2006. *Ann Oncol.* 2007;18(12):1927-1934.
59. Kaplan HS, Murphy ED. The effect of local roentgen irradiation on the biological behavior of a transplantable mouse carcinoma; increased frequency of pulmonary metastasis. *J Natl Cancer Inst.* 1949;9(5-6):407-413.
60. Fisher B, Gunduz N, Saffer EA. Influence of the interval between primary tumor removal and chemotherapy on kinetics and growth of metastases. *Cancer Res.* 1983;43(4):1488-1492.
61. van der Hage JA, van de Velde CJ, Julien JP, Tubiana-Hulin M, Vandervelden C, Duchateau L. Preoperative chemotherapy in primary operable breast cancer: results from the European Organization for Research and Treatment of Cancer trial 10902. *J Clin Oncol.* 2001;19(22):4224-4237.
62. Fisher B, Bryant J, Wolmark N, et al. Effect of preoperative chemotherapy on the outcome of women with operable breast cancer. *J Clin Oncol.* 1998;16(8):2672-2685.
63. Wolmark N, Wang J, Mamounas E, Bryant J, Fisher B. Preoperative chemotherapy in patients with operable breast cancer: nine-year results from National Surgical Adjuvant Breast and Bowel Project B-18. *J Natl Cancer Inst Monogr.* 2001(30):96-102.
64. Ellis MJ, Coop A, Singh B, et al. Letrozole is more effective neoadjuvant endocrine therapy than tamoxifen for ErbB-1- and/or ErbB-2-positive, estrogen receptor-positive primary breast cancer: evidence from a phase III randomized trial. *J Clin Oncol.* 2001;19(18):3808-3816.
65. Semiglazov VF, Semiglazov VV, Dashyan GA, et al. Phase 2 randomized trial of primary endocrine therapy versus chemotherapy in postmenopausal patients with estrogen receptor-positive breast cancer. *Cancer.* 2007;110(2):244-254.
66. Kuerer HM, Newman LA, Buzdar AU, et al. Pathologic tumor response in the breast following neoadjuvant chemotherapy predicts axillary lymph node status. *Cancer J Sci Am.* 1998;4(4):230-236.
67. Singletary SE, Allred C, Ashley P, et al. Revision of the American Joint Committee on Cancer staging system for breast cancer. *J Clin Oncol.* 2002;20(17):3628-3636.
68. Symmans WF, Peintinger F, Hatzis C, et al. Measurement of residual breast cancer burden to predict survival after neoadjuvant chemotherapy. *J Clin Oncol.* 2007;25(28):4414-4422.
69. U.S. National Institute of Health; clinicaltrials.gov. Molecular profiling breast cancer. Available at: http://www.clinicaltrials.gov/ct2/results?term=molecular+profiling+breast+cancer.
70. U.S. National Institute of Health; clinicaltrials.gov. Genomic testing breast cancer. Available at: http://www.clinicaltrials.gov/ct2/results?term=genomic+testing+breast+cancer.
71. U.S. National Institute of Health; clinicaltrials.gov. Breast cancer preoperative therapy. Available at: http://www.clinicaltrials.gov/ct2/results?term=breast+cancer+preoperative+therapy&pg=1.
72. Crewe HK, Ellis SW, Lennard MS, Tucker GT. Variable contribution of cytochromes P450 2D6, 2C9 and 3A4 to the 4-hydroxylation of tamoxifen by human liver microsomes. *Biochem Pharmacol.* 1997;53(2):171-178.
73. Desta Z, Ward BA, Soukhova NV, Flockhart DA. Comprehensive evaluation of tamoxifen sequential biotransformation by the human cytochrome P450 system in vitro: prominent roles for CYP3A and CYP2D6. *J Pharmacol Exp Ther.* 2004;310(3):1062-1075.
74. Jin Y, Desta Z, Stearns V, et al. CYP2D6 genotype, antidepressant use, and tamoxifen metabolism during adjuvant breast cancer treatment. *J Natl Cancer Inst.* 2005;97(1):30-39.
75. Lim YC, Li L, Desta Z, et al. Endoxifen, a secondary metabolite of tamoxifen, and 4-OH-tamoxifen induce similar changes in global gene expression patterns in MCF-7 breast cancer cells. *J Pharmacol Exp Ther.* 2006;318(2):503-512.
76. Stearns V, Johnson MD, Rae JM, et al. Active tamoxifen metabolite plasma concentrations after coadministration of tamoxifen and the selective serotonin reuptake inhibitor paroxetine. *J Natl Cancer Inst.* 2003;95(23):1758-1764.
77. Goetz MP, Rae JM, Suman VJ, et al. Pharmacogenetics of tamoxifen biotransformation is associated with clinical outcomes of efficacy and hot flashes. *J Clin Oncol.* 2005;23(36):9312-9318.
78. Lim HS, Ju Lee H, Seok Lee K, et al. Clinical implications of CYP2D6 genotypes predictive of tamoxifen pharmacokinetics in metastatic breast cancer. *J Clin Oncol.* 2007;25(25):3837-3845.

CHAPTER 84

Neoadjuvant Endocrine Therapy

E. Jane Macaskill
J. Michael Dixon

Traditionally, neoadjuvant chemotherapy has been used to downstage locally advanced and unresectable primary breast tumors to make them operable.[1,2] Endocrine therapy has emerged as an attractive alternative in the neoadjuvant setting for postmenopausal women with estrogen receptor–positive (ER+) breast cancer, with comparatively less toxicity. Direct comparison between neoadjuvant chemotherapy and endocrine therapy has not been addressed in large randomized studies as the selection of patients for either treatment has to date been based upon menopausal status and ER status of the tumor. One Russian study randomized 121 postmenopausal women with T2-4 ER+ and/or progesterone–receptor-positive (PR+) breast cancer to receive either neoadjuvant doxorubicin and paclitaxel chemotherapy (n = 62) or neoadjuvant endocrine treatment with anastrozole (n = 30) or exemestane (n = 29) for 3 months prior to surgery.[3] Clinical and mammographic objective response rates (ORR) were similar for endocrine therapy and chemotherapy, and there was a trend for greater rates of breast-conserving surgery with endocrine therapy with no significant differences in local recurrence rates at 34 months. Grade 3/4 alopecia, neutropenia, cardiotoxicity, and neuropathy were experienced by significant numbers of women in the chemotherapy group. Neoadjuvant endocrine therapy was better tolerated, the most common adverse events being hot flushes, fatigue, vaginal bleeding, and arthralgia. These data support the view that endocrine therapy is a safe alternative to chemotherapy, with similar response rates but less toxicity. In ER+ breast cancer there is also some evidence to suggest that neoadjuvant chemotherapy is less effective than in ER– breast cancer. A recent retrospective study of 1731 patients who had primary chemotherapy showed a significantly lower rate of pathologic complete response to chemotherapy in patients with hormone receptor–positive tumors compared with those with hormone receptor–negative tumors (8% vs 24%; $p < .0001$).[4] These data

are consistent with the observation that patients with hormone receptor–positive disease are less chemosensitive and respond better to endocrine therapy. There is also evidence to suggest that the histological response to chemotherapy and endocrine therapy differ, with higher rates of central scarring in tumors treated with neoadjuvant letrozole (58.5% vs 2%, $p = .035$).[5] Central scarring correlates with clinical response and explains why, following endocrine therapy, excising the residual mass results in complete excision more often than after neoadjuvant chemotherapy where scattered widespread foci of disease are significantly more common.[5] In this study, complete pathological response rate, as expected, was seen significantly more frequently after neoadjuvant chemotherapy, although this was not seen in the randomized study by Semiglazov.[3]

WHICH PATIENTS WILL BENEFIT FROM NEOADJUVANT THERAPY OVER PRIMARY SURGERY?

With careful selection there are benefits of neoadjuvant therapy compared with primary surgery. The most significant benefits are in postmenopausal patients with large operable or locally advanced inoperable ER+ tumors, which can be downstaged to become operable or to be suitable for less extensive surgery, such as breast conservation in those originally thought to require mastectomy. It is widely accepted that breast conservation followed by radiotherapy provides improved quality of life, better cosmetic outcomes, and comparable disease control compared with mastectomy, although this has yet to be proven in any long-term study following neoadjuvant therapy. The majority of patients who are spared mastectomy are elderly but studies have shown that older women are no more likely to choose mastectomy than younger women if given a choice.

For patients who are unfit for surgery due to significant comorbidities, neoadjuvant treatment can allow downstaging prior to resection under local anesthesia, or for a select group of patients with short life expectancy, neoadjuvant endocrine therapy alone can provide long-term disease control.

SELECTION OF PATIENTS FOR NEOADJUVANT ENDOCRINE THERAPY

In early studies with tamoxifen patients were not selected on the basis of ER or PR status. It has since been shown that ER positivity is an important predictor for response to tamoxifen and aromatase inhibitors.[6] Selection of patients for neoadjuvant endocrine therapy in patients with ER+ tumors needs to be based upon the likely benefit that can be obtained from such treatment. Patients who are likely to benefit are those with locally advanced breast cancer who may, after response, become operable; those with large operable tumors that have the potential for conversion from mastectomy to breast-conserving surgery if the tumor volume can be reduced; and those with a large cancer suitable for breast-conserving surgery whose cosmetic outcome may be improved by allowing a less extensive local excision with tumor shrinkage. Patients who are unlikely to benefit are (1) those who have operable disease that is multifocal that usually requires mastectomy regardless of response with treatment and (2) patients with certain tumor types that have been shown to respond slowly or indiscernibly to treatment such as invasive lobular carcinomas (ILCs) and mucinous carcinomas. Response in such patients can be difficult to assess. There is a need in patients with ILC to assess extent of disease accurately prior to treatment, and in mucinous cancers to consider longer durations of treatment, which are often necessary to see shrinkage in such cancers.

SELECTION OF ENDOCRINE AGENT FOR NEOADJUVANT THERAPY

Tamoxifen was the first widely used neoadjuvant endocrine therapy, but there have been a number of studies published recently investigating the role of aromatase inhibitors in this setting. The results and outcomes of these studies are discussed below and provide evidence upon which treatment decisions can be based.

Studies with Tamoxifen

Most of the studies using tamoxifen as a primary treatment have compared surgery with or without tamoxifen to the use of tamoxifen alone, and thus were not designed to assess tamoxifen in the true neoadjuvant setting. These studies do, however, show the effect of tamoxifen as a primary treatment. There have been 3 large randomized trials of tamoxifen alone versus surgery alone. While 1 trial found no difference between the 2 treatments at 6 years,[7] a Nottingham study found a significant increase in local progression in the tamoxifen-alone group at a median follow-up of 145 months.[8] This was confirmed in a multicenter European study that also reported a shorter time to

progression and shorter disease-free survival, as well as poorer locoregional control in the tamoxifen-alone group at a median 120 months follow-up.[9]

Three randomized trials have compared tamoxifen alone with surgery followed by tamoxifen. In an Italian study, 474 patients were randomized to surgery followed by 5 years tamoxifen or to 5 years tamoxifen alone.[10] No difference was found in overall survival or breast-cancer-specific survival at 80 months, but there was a significantly higher local progression rate in the tamoxifen-only arm (106 vs 27; $p = .0001$). In the 2 studies that have reported follow-up to 12 years there was a significant increase in the rate of local recurrence in the tamoxifen-alone group, and a significantly higher overall mortality and mortality from breast cancer in the tamoxifen-only groups, although in 1 of these 2 studies the increase in mortality was observed only after 3 years.[11,12] In none of the randomized trials were patients selected on the basis of ER status, and this will have influenced outcome as ER negative patients will have gained no benefit from tamoxifen. One conclusion from these studies was that using long-term tamoxifen treatment without surgery should be reserved for patients in whom life expectancy is short (2-3 years maximum).[11]

These studies did not clarify how long tamoxifen is effective when given as the sole therapy to women with hormone-sensitive cancer. One study did report long-term follow-up data for 113 patients over the age of 70 who had been treated with tamoxifen as the sole therapy.[13] The median time to failure of local control was 2.5 to 3 years, with more than half of the responders relapsing by 5 years. In Edinburgh, a series of 100 women more than 70 years of age, with ER+ tumors, were treated to investigate the time course of response with neoadjuvant tamoxifen.[14] Modified World Health Organization (WHO) criteria were used to evaluate tumor response in the neoadjuvant setting as follows:

- Partial response (PR): reduction in tumor size 50% or more from pretreatment size
- Minor response (MR): reduction in tumor size 25% or more and less than 50% from pretreatment size
- No change (NC): less than 25% decrease or less than 25% increase in tumor size from pretreatment size
- Complete response (CR): no measurable tumor
- Progressive disease (PD): 25% or more increase in tumor size from pretreatment size

After 3 months of tamoxifen, 72 patients had responded (CR, PR, or MR) and 1 patient had progressive disease (PD). The remaining 27 patients continued on tamoxifen for a further 3 months, during which time 4 responded and 5 progressed (Fig. 84-1). The observation drawn from these data is that it is unlikely that patients who do not have a response by 3 months will have a response with prolonged further treatment, and so if patients do not respond to hormonal therapy within this time period alternative treatments need to be considered.

The first studies using neoadjuvant aromatase inhibitors were performed in Edinburgh and produced promising results,[15-17] and have since led to large randomized studies comparing tamoxifen with aromatase inhibitors, the results of which are discussed below.

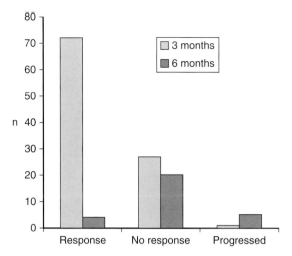

FIGURE 84-1 Response rates to neoadjuvant tamoxifen over time in Edinburgh study.[14]

Studies with Letrozole

Tamoxifen has been compared with letrozole in the neoadjuvant setting in a study referred to as the PO24 study, in which 337 postmenopausal women with large ER+ or PR+ breast cancers that required mastectomy or were locally advanced and inoperable were randomized to receive letrozole or tamoxifen for 4 months as primary treatment.[18] Objective response rates by palpation, mammography, and ultrasound were assessed, showing a significantly higher clinical response rate in letrozole-treated patients (55% vs 36%; $p < .001$), and significant results in favor of letrozole on ultrasound and mammograms. There was a significantly higher rate of breast-conserving surgery in the letrozole group than in the tamoxifen group, even in those patients with locally advanced cancer (Fig. 84-2). When these results

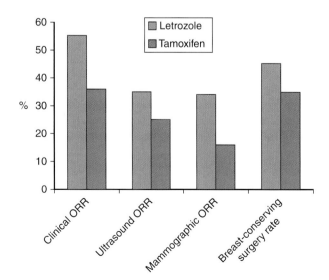

FIGURE 84-2 Outcomes from PO24 trial of neoadjuvant letrozole (L) versus tamoxifen (T) for 4 months.[18] (L versus T clinical ORR $p \leq .001$; ultrasound ORR $p = .042$; mammographic ORR $p < .001$; breast-conserving surgery rate $p = .022$.)

were analyzed with respect to ER Allred scores, it was evident that not only were response rates to letrozole higher in the high ER score categories (6-8), but they were also higher in patients who had lower ER scores (3-5); among these patients responses were achieved only with letrozole.[6,19] This has significant implications for the treatment of patients with tumors with low ER scores who may still benefit from neoadjuvant letrozole treatment if required, whereas tamoxifen may not be as effective in tumors with low levels of ER expression.

Studies with Anastrozole

There have been 2 large randomized studies comparing anastrozole with tamoxifen in postmenopausal women with hormone receptor–positive breast cancer.

In the IMPACT (IMmediate Preoperative Arimidex, Tamoxifen or Combined with Tamoxifen), 330 patients from the UK and Germany were randomized to receive anastrozole or tamoxifen or both in combination for 3 months prior to surgery.[20] The primary end point was objective clinical response measured by calipers, with ultrasound measurement as a secondary end point. This study found that there was no significant difference in objective response between the 3 treatments as measured by calipers and ultrasound. Among patients with HER-2-positive tumors, anastrozole had a numerically higher clinical response rate than tamoxifen ($p = .18$). At 3 months, among those patients initially assessed as requiring mastectomy, significantly more were deemed suitable for breast-conserving surgery in the anastrozole arm than tamoxifen arm ("feasible surgery," 46% vs 22%; $p = .03$). Not all patients accepted this recommendation, and there was no significant difference in numbers actually undergoing breast conservation ("actual surgery") between anastrozole and tamoxifen groups at 3 months (44% vs 31%; $p = .23$).

In the PROACT (PReOperative Arimidex Compared with Tamoxifen) trial the entry criteria were similar to the IMPACT trial, but also included patients whose tumors were inoperable and those on concurrent chemotherapy.[21] Patients were randomized to receive either anastrozole (n = 202) or tamoxifen (n = 201), both with placebo, for 3 months. The primary end point was objective tumor response measured by ultrasound scan. Caliper measurement was included as a secondary end point, alongside surgical assessment at baseline and 3 months. No significant difference in ORR was seen between treatment arms in all patients, although a trend was noted in favor of anastrozole in those patients who had hormonal therapy alone. There was, however, a significantly higher ORR in favor of anastrozole in those patients initially assessed as requiring mastectomy (36.6% vs 24.2% on ultrasound, $p = .03$; and 48.6% vs 35.8% with calipers, $p = .04$). This also translated into a significant improvement for those initially requiring mastectomy with 43.0% of those treated by anastrozole being treatable by breast-conserving surgery versus 30.8% with tamoxifen ($p = .04$), and greater numbers of those with initially inoperable tumors having a surgical procedure performed with anastrozole ($p = NS$).

A combined analysis of these 2 studies with a total combined population of 535 patients compared ORR and improvement

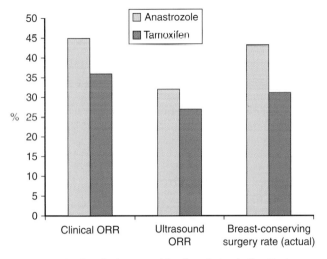

FIGURE 84-3 Results from combined analysis of all patients from IMPACT and PROACT trials of neoadjuvant anastrozole versus tamoxifen for 3 months.[22] (A versus T clinical ORR p = .052, ultrasound ORR p = .191; breast-conserving surgery (actual) p = .019.)

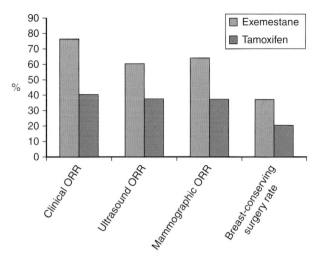

FIGURE 84-4 Results from Russian study of neoadjuvant exemestane versus tamoxifen for 3 months.[26] (E versus T clinical ORR p = .05, ultrasound ORR p = .092; mammographic p = .082; breast-conserving surgery rate p = .05.)

in surgery, and failed to show any significant difference between tamoxifen and anastrozole in the whole group (Fig. 84-3).[22] There was, however, a significant improvement in ORR in favor of anastrozole in the subgroup of patients who were considered to require mastectomy or be inoperable at the outset (47% vs 35% p = .026) and on ultrasound response (36% vs 26%; p = .048). There was a significant change in feasible (anastrozole 47% vs tamoxifen 35%; p = .021) and actual surgery (anastrozole 43% vs tamoxifen 31%; p = .019) in those patients whose tumors were thought to require a mastectomy or were inoperable at initial assessment. These data suggest anastrozole is superior to tamoxifen in tumors that are large and require mastectomy or are inoperable or locally advanced at diagnosis.

Studies with Exemestane

Four studies have reported the use of exemestane in the neoadjuvant setting—the first from Edinburgh, in which 10 of 12 patients with large operable or locally advanced primary breast cancer treated for 12 weeks with exemestane had more than 50% reduction in tumor size. Ten patients initially required mastectomy, but only 2 required mastectomy after 3 months of exemestane.[16]

The German Neoadjuvant Aromasin® Initiative (GENARI) trial randomized 27 patients to 16 weeks exemestane, of which 10 had a partial response and 17 stable disease, and 14 underwent breast-conserving surgery.[23]

In a French study 38 postmenopausal women were given 4 to 5 months of exemestane prior to surgery.[24] Clinical response as measured on ultrasound confirmed complete response in 5.9%, partial response in 64.7%, and stable disease in 23.5%. Breast-conserving surgery was achieved in 45.2%. These studies all have small numbers and assess exemestane only, but show promising results for the role of exemestane in neoadjuvant treatment.

A Japanese study has reported results of 4 months neoadjuvant exemestane in ER+ and/or PR+ large breast cancers.[25] Evidence of a pathological response was observed in 13 (43%)

of 30 patients who underwent surgery at 4 months, and a clinical response was seen in 27 (66%) of 41 evaluable patients. Breast-conserving surgery was performed in 27 (90%) of 30 patients who underwent surgery at 4 months.

Exemestane has been compared with tamoxifen in 1 study in which 151 postmenopausal women were randomized to either exemestane or tamoxifen for 3 months preoperatively.[26] Clinical ORR assessed by palpation was the primary end point. Secondary end points were response measured on mammogram and ultrasound, and number of patients undergoing breast-conserving surgery. Clinical objective response on palpation was superior in the exemestane group (76.3%) compared to tamoxifen (40.0%; p = .05) (Fig. 84-4). There was no significant difference in objective response on ultrasound (E 60.5% vs T 37.3%; p = .092) or on mammogram (E 64.0% vs T 37.3%; p = .082). Exemestane treatment resulted in a higher rate of breast-conserving surgery than tamoxifen (36.8% vs 20.0%, p = .05). Exemestane had a similar rate of reported adverse events to tamoxifen. These data are not yet published and thus the data supporting the use of exemestane in the neoadjuvant setting are less robust than for those for letrozole and anastrozole.

A recent meta-analysis of aromatase inhibitors versus tamoxifen for neoadjuvant treatment included the PO24, IMPACT, PROACT, and the Semiglazov exemestane trials and pooled results from these 4 trials.[27] Combined results showed superior rates for aromatase inhibitors compared with tamoxifen for clinical ORR (RR, 1.29; 95% CI, 1.14-1.47; p < .001), ultrasound ORR (RR, 1.29; 95% CI, 1.10-1.51; p = .002), and breast-conserving surgery rate (RR, 1.36; 95% CI, 1.16-1.59; p < .001).

OPTIMUM DURATION OF NEOADJUVANT TREATMENT

Randomized studies of aromatase inhibitors and tamoxifen have assessed response over 3 to 4 months. Studies using tamoxifen alone were not designed to assess the optimum duration of tamoxifen in the neoadjuvant setting but compare it to surgery. None of these studies have addressed the optimum duration of neoadjuvant endocrine treatment, the 3 to 4 months duration for the randomized studies being largely based on experience with neoadjuvant chemotherapy. More recent studies with longer durations of neoadjuvant chemotherapy have, however, suggested that prolonging treatment duration increases the overall response rate.[28]

One prospective study published recently from Edinburgh included 184 women with large operable or locally advanced ER+ breast cancers who were treated with neoadjuvant letrozole.[29] Patients were reviewed initially after 2, 6, and 12 weeks of treatment to assess tolerance and to measure response by clinical measurement with calipers and imaging (ultrasound and clinical measurements at 0, 6, and 12 weeks and mammography at 0 and 12 weeks). At 3 months all patients were reviewed by a single surgeon and a treatment decision taken. The decision was either to perform surgery, to continue letrozole or, following discussion at a multidisciplinary meeting, to switch to another therapy. This decision was based on an assessment of response, operability, fitness for operation, and willingness of the patient to proceed to surgery. Patients who continued letrozole beyond 3 months were reviewed at 6, 9, 12, 18, and 24 months and yearly thereafter.

One hundred and twenty-seven patients (69.8%) had a complete or partial response by 3 months and only 4 patients had disease progression (>25% increase in tumour volume). Of the 119 patients who had surgery at 3 months, 99 had breast-conserving surgery and 19 had mastectomy. The 19 undergoing mastectomy included 15 patients who had locally advanced breast cancer that was not initially considered suitable for surgery, but these patients became operable following 3 months of letrozole. Sixty-three patients continued on letrozole beyond 3 months. The mean reduction in clinical volume in the first 3 months in these 63 patients was 46.7%, with a median of 52%. There was a sustained response with continued treatment with further reductions in volume between 3 and 6 months (mean 46.6%, median 50%), between 6 and 12 months (mean 47.8%, median 37%), and 12 to 24 months (mean 35.8%, median 33%) (Fig. 84-5). Prolonged treatment with neoadjuvant letrozole treatment resulted in an increase in the number of patients who were converted from requiring a mastectomy or who were inoperable to be suitable for breast-conserving surgery from 81 of 134 (60%) at 3 months with 96 (72%) eventually being treated with breast conservation. At the time of publication the median follow-up was 3 years, and the median time to treatment failure had not yet been reached with 70% of those on prolonged letrozole treatment having disease control on letrozole alone. These data show that in selected patients prolonged treatment with letrozole can result in sustained response with tumor shrinkage. It remains our view that surgery followed by radiotherapy in patients undergoing breast-conserving surgery should be carried out after a satisfactory response to neoadjuvant letrozole has been achieved. In patients who are not suitable for or who refuse surgery, neoadjuvant letrozole given for prolonged periods appears safe and appears to provide this group of women with long-term disease control.

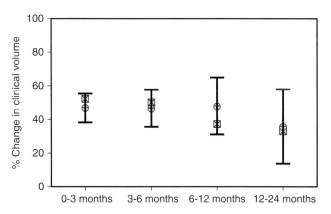

FIGURE 84-5 Results from Edinburgh study of prolonged treatment with letrozole showing sustained response with duration of treatment.[29] Mean (circles) and median (squares) values with 95% CI of the mean for change in clinical volume between 0 and 3 months, 3 and 6 months, 6 and 12 months, and 12 and 24 months.

PREDICTING RESPONSE TO NEOADJUVANT THERAPY

ER and PR Status

Selection of patients who will benefit from neoadjuvant therapy is based upon clinical criteria and on tumor factors. Estrogen receptor status has been shown in tamoxifen trials to be the most important predictor of response to treatment, and this has been confirmed in studies with the aromatase inhibitors. In the PO24 study comparing letrozole with tamoxifen, both agents achieved significantly more responses in patients with ER rich (Allred 6-8) tumors than those with ER poor (Allred 2-5) tumors.[6] Responses to letrozole were significantly better for PR+ tumors than for PR– tumors, and a similar but weaker trend was also seen with tamoxifen (Fig. 84-6). There was a close direct correlation between the degree of ER positivity and likelihood of response to letrozole in this study. Response rates were still more than 30% in cancers with Allred scores of 3 to 5 with letrozole, but there were no tamoxifen-induced responses seen in patients with these scores, although the numbers in these subgroups were too small to draw definitive conclusions.

In the IMPACT study of anastrozole versus tamoxifen, ER scores were measured by histoscore, and analyzed by quartiles, with significantly more responders having cancers in the highest ER quartile ($p = .02$) in the intention-to-treat (ITT) population.[20]

HER-2 Status

A study from Edinburgh of 3 months neoadjuvant anastrozole has shown no significant difference in response to anastrozole between HER-2-positive and HER-2-negative tumors.[30] In an Edinburgh study of 172 postmenopausal women receiving neoadjuvant letrozole, at 3 months assessment the clinical responses were similar in HER-2-positive and HER-2-negative tumors (61% vs 69%; $p = .506$).[31]

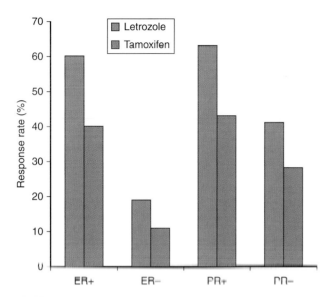

FIGURE 84-6 Response rates assessed by clinical measurement from PO24 trial of neoadjuvant letrozole versus tamoxifen according to tumor ER and PR status.[6]

In the PO24 study, tumors that were both ER+ and overexpressed HER-1 or HER-2 had an 88% response rate to letrozole compared with a 21% response rate to tamoxifen (*p* = .0004).[6] In HER-1/2-negative tumors, there was also superiority of letrozole in response rates, although the difference was less dramatic than that in HER-1/2-positive cancers (54% for letrozole vs 41% for tamoxifen). These data indicate that letrozole is effective in both HER-1/2-positive and HER-1/2-negative tumors, whereas tamoxifen appears comparatively less effective in HER-1/2-positive tumors.

A combined analysis of tumor samples from 503 patients treated in either the PO24 trial or the Edinburgh neoadjuvant audit of letrozole has reported similar findings.[32] In the letrozole-treated patients from PO24 and Edinburgh, there was no significant difference in clinical response between HER-1 positive and HER-1 negative tumors. In the HER-2-positive tumors, letrozole had a significantly better clinical response rate than tamoxifen. In the HER-2-positive tumors there was a trend toward improved clinical efficacy for letrozole compared with tamoxifen for clinical and mammographic response rates.

In the IMPACT study, 34 of the 239 tumors assessable were HER-2 positive. Of these tumors, objective response was seen in 58% with anastrozole, 22% with tamoxifen, and 31% with the combination (anastrozole vs tamoxifen HR 4.9; 95% CI 0.53-63.22; *p* = .18).[20] These results did not reach significance, but the analysis was underpowered due to the small sample size of this subgroup of tumors. These results suggest that anastrozole is effective in both HER-2-positive and HER negative tumors, with tamoxifen being somewhat less effective in HER-2 tumors.

▪ Proliferation

Results are also available from neoadjuvant trials on the effects of aromatase inhibitors and tamoxifen on the proliferation rate

of breast cancers as measured by Ki67. In the PO24 study, there was a significantly greater reduction in proliferation with letrozole than with tamoxifen (reduction in geometric mean Ki67 of 87% with letrozole compared with 75% for tamoxifen; *p* = .0009).[19] As part of the IMPACT trial, immunohistochemical analysis was assessed after 2 weeks of treatment and at surgery (12 weeks after commencement of hormonal treatment). There was a significantly greater reduction in Ki67 in the anastrozole group compared with both tamoxifen alone or the combination at 2 weeks (*p* = .004) and 12 weeks (*p* < .001). There was no significant relationship between Ki67 changes and clinical response. Recent results from the IMPACT study have shown a statistically significant correlation between the level of Ki67 at 2 weeks and relapse-free survival after a median 37 months follow-up (HR 2.01; *p* = .002).[33] The implication of these findings is that there is a predictive value in the residual rate of proliferation after 2 weeks of treatment and that measuring the 2 week Ki67 could be a valuable tool for predicting long-term outcome. This is now being tested in a randomized study (Perioperative Endocrine Therapy—Individualized Care [POETIC]).

Neoadjuvant therapy has the advantage to the clinician of allowing direct assessment of response to treatment of a tumor, in comparison to the adjuvant setting where lack of response or resistance to treatment is only discovered at the point of tumor recurrence. By clinical observation such as that described in the Edinburgh letrozole study, it can be determined whether a tumor is responsive to a particular endocrine agent, allowing the use of the same agent of known efficacy in the adjuvant setting following surgery.

A further benefit of neoadjuvant therapy is the potential to allow access to the cancer during treatment to allow investigation of mechanisms of response and resistance as well as allowing identification of potential predictors of response. By correlating response to an agent with biological changes that occur within the cancer over a relatively short neoadjuvant period of 3 to 4 months, it should be possible to better understand how drugs work and, more importantly, why they sometimes do not work.

FUTURE DIRECTIONS

The comparative benefits seen with aromatase inhibitors over tamoxifen in neoadjuvant studies to date have led to their increased use in the clinical setting. Good response to treatment in the neoadjuvant setting allows the clinician confidence of the efficacy of the drug, and where a response is evident the same drug can be given in the adjuvant setting after surgery and/or radiotherapy. Patients with low ER tumors are less responsive to tamoxifen, and in such patients aromatase inhibitors or immediate surgery, if appropriate, is a more pertinent choice of treatment.

There remains the issue of development of resistance to treatment with aromatase inhibitors. Ongoing studies assessing the role of aromatase inhibitors in combination with signal transduction inhibitors to prevent resistance are ongoing. There have been promising results in this area with the combination of letrozole and everolimus, a mammalian target of rapamycin (mTOR) inhibitor in the neoadjuvant setting.[34] In this study, 270 patients with newly diagnosed ER+ breast cancer larger than 2 cm were randomized to receive either letrozole 2.5 mg and everolimus 10 mg once daily or letrozole 2.5 mg and placebo for 16 weeks prior to surgery. There was a higher response rate in the group who received letrozole and RAD001 on ultrasound scan (58% with everolimus and letrozole and 47% with letrozole alone, $p = .035$) and on clinical examination (66.7% everolimus and letrozole vs 54.5% letrozole alone, $p = .021$). The problem was that less than 50% of patients were able to tolerate the 2 drugs together so this combination of these doses is unlikely to be used outside of this trial. This study does show, however, that combination of endocrine and the newer biologically targeted agents can improve response rates, so further studies with different agents are ongoing.

NECESSARY FUTURE STUDIES

While studies to date have shown benefits of neoadjuvant therapy in terms of tumor shrinkage and resulting improvement in cosmetic outcomes, the longer-term benefits have yet to be clarified. Neoadjuvant endocrine therapy needs to be compared with neoadjuvant chemotherapy in a larger study. Also, neoadjuvant endocrine therapy needs to be compared with adjuvant endocrine therapy. Even if there is no improvement in disease-free and overall survival with neoadjuvant endocrine therapy, the benefits of limiting surgery in elderly patients are obvious and merits its continued use in individual patients.

SUMMARY

Neoadjuvant endocrine therapy is a safe alternative to neoadjuvant chemotherapy in postmenopausal patients with ER+ tumors. Initial studies with tamoxifen and aromatase inhibitors have shown that ER is an important predictor of response, with tamoxifen only being effective in ER rich tumors, but with responses seen in patients with all levels of ER with aromatase inhibitors. Aromatase inhibitors appear equally effective in both HER-2-positive and HER-2-negative tumors, whereas tamoxifen appears somewhat less effective in HER-2-positive tumors. Letrozole, anastrozole, and exemestane have all been shown to have better rates of breast conservation, and in patients with large inoperable tumors improved response rates are seen with the aromatase inhibitors compared with tamoxifen. The optimum duration of neoadjuvant treatment has yet to be identified, but in selected patients prolonged treatment with letrozole has been shown to result in sustained tumor shrinkage.

REFERENCES

1. Perloff M, Lesnick GJ. Chemotherapy before and after mastectomy in stage III breast cancer. *Arch Surg.* 1982;117(7):879-881.
2. Schick P, Goodstein J, Moor J, Butler J, Senter KL. Preoperative chemotherapy followed by mastectomy for locally advanced breast cancer. *J Surg Oncol.* 1983;22(4):278-282.
3. Semiglazov VF, Semiglazov V, Ivanov V, et al. The relative efficacy of neoadjuvant endocrine therapy vs chemotherapy in postmenopausal women with ER positive breast cancer. *Proc Am Soc Clin Oncol.* 2004; 22(14s):519.
4. Guarneri V, Broglio K, Kau SW, et al. Prognostic value of pathologic complete response after primary chemotherapy in relation to hormone receptor status and other factors. *J Clin Oncol.* 2006;24:1037-1044.
5. Julian H, Dixon JM, Thomas JS. Central scarring is a common pattern of tumour response to neoadjuvant letrozole therapy for breast cancer but not neoadjuvant chemotherapy and correlates with tumour shrinkage and suitability for conservation surgery. *Breast Cancer Res Treat.* 2006;100(suppl 1): S188; abs 4050.
6. Ellis MJ, Coop A, Singh B, et al. Letrozole is more effective neoadjuvant endocrine therapy than tamoxifen for ErbB-1- and/or ErbB-2-positive, estrogen receptor-positive primary breast cancer: evidence from a phase III randomized trial. *J Clin Oncol.* 2001;19(18):3808-3816.
7. Gazet JC, Ford HT, Coombes RC, et al. Prospective randomized trial of tamoxifen vs surgery in elderly patients with breast cancer. *Eur J Surg Oncol.* 1994;20(3):207-214.
8. Kenny FS, Robertson JFR, Ellis IO, et al. Long-term follow-up of elderly patients randomised to primary tamoxifen or wedge mastectomy as initial therapy for operable breast cancer. *Breast.* 1998;7:335-339.
9. Fentiman IS, Christiaens MR, Paridaens R, et al. Treatment of operable breast cancer in the elderly: a randomised clinical trial EORTC 10851 comparing tamoxifen alone with modified radical mastectomy. *Eur J Cancer.* 2003;39(3):309-316.
10. Mustacchi G, Ceccherini R, Milani S, et al. Tamoxifen alone versus adjuvant tamoxifen for operable breast cancer of the elderly: long-term results of the phase III randomized controlled multicenter GRETA trial. *Ann Oncol.* 2003;14(3):414-420.
11. Fennessy M, Bates T, Macrae DG, on behalf of the Closed Trials Working Party of the Cancer Research UK Breast Cancer Trials Group. Late follow-up of a randomized trial of surgery plus tamoxifen versus tamoxifen alone in women aged over 70 years with operable breast cancer. *Br J Surg.* 2004;91(6):699-704.
12. Bates T, Fennessy M, Riley DL, on behalf of the CRC Breast Cancer Trials Group UK. Breast cancer in the elderly: surgery improves survival. The results of a Cancer Research Campaign Trial. *Eur J Cancer.* 2001; 37(5s):7.
13. Horobin JM, Preece PE, Dewar JA, et al. Long-term follow-up of elderly patients with locoregional breast cancer treated with tamoxifen only. *Br J Surg.* 1991;78:213-217.
14. Dixon JM. Neoadjuvant therapy: surgical perspectives. In: Miller WR, Ingle JN. *Endocrine Therapy in Breast Cancer.* New York: Marcel Dekker: 2002:197-212.
15. Dixon JM, Love CDB, Bellamy COC, et al. Letrozole as primary medical therapy for locally advanced and large operable breast cancer. *Breast Cancer Res Treat.* 2001;66(3):191-199.
16. Miller WR, Dixon JM. Endocrine and clinical endpoints of exemestane as neoadjuvant therapy. *Cancer Control.* 2002;9(2s):9-15.
17. Dixon JM, Renshaw L, Bellamy C, et al. The effects of neoadjuvant anastrozole (Arimidex) on tumor volume in postmenopausal women with breast cancer: a randomized, double-blind, single-center study. *Clin Cancer Res.* 2000;6(6):2229-2235.
18. Eiermann W, Paepke S, Appelstaedt J, et al. Preoperative treatment of postmenopausal breast cancer patients with letrozole: a randomized double-blind multicenter study. *Ann Oncol.* 2001;12:1527-1532.
19. Ellis MJ, Coop A, Singh B, et al. Letrozole inhibits tumor proliferation more effectively than tamoxifen independent of HER1/2 expression status. *Cancer Res.* 2003;63:6253-6231.
20. Smith I, Dowsett M, Ebbs SR, et al. Neoadjuvant treatment of postmenopausal breast cancer with anastrozole, tamoxifen, or both in combination: the immediate preoperative anastrozole, tamoxifen, or combined with tamoxifen (IMPACT) multicenter double-blind randomized trial. *J Clin Oncol.* 2005;23(22):5108-5116.
21. Cataliotti L, Buzdar AU, Noguchi S, et al. Comparison of anastrozole versus tamoxifen as preoperative therapy in postmenopausal women with hormone receptor-positive breast cancer: the Pre-Operative "Arimidex" Compared to Tamoxifen (PROACT) trial. *Cancer.* 2006;106(10):2095-2103.
22. Smith I. Anastrozole versus tamoxifen as preoperative therapy for oestrogen receptor-positive breast cancer in postmenopausal women: combined analysis of the IMPACT and PROACT trials. Presented at 4th European Breast Cancer Conference, Hamburg, Germany, 17 March 2004.
23. Krainick U, Astner A, Jonat W, et al. Phase II study to define safety and efficacy of exemestane as preoperative therapy for postmenopausal patients with primary breast cancer—final results of the German Neoadjuvant Aromasin Initiative (GENARI). *Breast Cancer Res Treat.* 2003;82(1s):S55; abs 239.
24. Tubiana-Hulin M, Spyratos F, Becette V, et al. Phase II study of neo-adjuvant exemestane in postmenopausal patients with operable breast cancer. *Breast Cancer Res Treat.* 2003;82(1s):S106; abs 443.

25. Takei H, Suemasu K, Inoue K, et al. Multicenter phase II trial of neoadjuvant exemestane for postmenopausal patients with hormone receptor-positive operable breast cancer: Saitama Breast Cancer Clinical Study Group (SBCCSG-03). *Breast Cancer Res Treat.* 2008;107:87-94.

26. Semiglazov VF, Semiglazov VV, Ivanov VG, et al. Neoadjuvant endocrine therapy: exemestane vs tamoxifen in postmenopausal ER+ breast cancer patients (T1-4, N1-2, M0). *Proc Am Soc Clin Oncol.* 2005;23(16s):abs 530.

27. Seo JH, Kim YH, Kim JS. Meta-analysis of pre-operative aromatase inhibitor versus tamoxifen in postmenopausal woman with hormone receptor-positive breast cancer. *Cancer Chemother Pharmacol.* 2009;63: 261-266.

28. Bear HD, Anderson S, Brown A, et al. The effect on tumor response of adding sequential preoperative docetaxel to preoperative doxorubicin and cyclophosphamide: preliminary results from national surgical adjuvant breast and bowel project protocol B-27. *J Clin Oncol.* 2003;21:4165-4174.

29. Dixon JM, Renshaw L, Macaskill EJ, et al. Increase in response rate by prolonged treatment with neoadjuvant letrozole. *Breast Cancer Res Treat.* 2009;113(1):145-151.

30. Dixon JM, Jackson J, Hills M, et al. Anastrozole demonstrates clinical and biological effectiveness in oestrogen-receptor-positive positive breast cancers, irrespective of the erbB2 status. *Eur J Cancer.* 2004;40:2742-2747.

31. Young O, Murray J, Renshaw L, et al. Neoadjuvant letrozole is equally effective in HER2 positive and negative breast cancers. *Breast Cancer Res Treat.* 2004;88(1s):S36; abs 411.

32. Ellis MJ, Tao Y, Young O, et al. Estrogen-independent proliferation is present in estrogen-dependent HER2-positive primary breast cancer after neoadjuvant letrozole. *J Clin Oncol.* 2006;24:3019-3025.

33. Dowsett M, A'Hern R, Smith I, on behalf of the IMPACT Trialists. Ki67 after 2 weeks' endocrine treatment predicts relapse-free survival (RFS) in the IMPACT trial. *Breast Cancer Res Treat.* 2005;94(s1):abs 45.

34. Baselga J, Semiglazov V, van Dam P, et al. Phase II double-blind randomized trial of daily oral RAD001 (everolimus) plus letrozole (LET) or placebo (P) plus LET as neoadjuvant therapy for ER+ breast cancer. *Breast Cancer Res Treat.* 2007;106:S107; abs 2066.

CHAPTER 85

Neoadjuvant Chemotherapy

Funda Meric-Bernstam

NEOADJUVANT CHEMOTHERAPY: ADVANTAGES AND DISADVANTAGES

Neoadjuvant (or preoperative) chemotherapy is being increasingly used for the treatment of breast cancer. Response to neoadjuvant chemotherapy may convert an inoperable breast cancer to an operable tumor. By downsizing the tumor, neoadjuvant chemotherapy also increases the possibility of breast-conserving surgery in a larger number of patients[1,2] (Fig. 85-1A). In addition, in patients who have operable breast cancer at the onset, the delivery of neoadjuvant chemotherapy allows for excisions of smaller volumes of breast tissue. Indeed, this was shown in a study by Boughey et al[3] in which patients treated with neoadjuvant therapy were compared with patients who underwent adjuvant chemotherapy. For patients who had an initial tumor size greater than 2 cm, neoadjuvant chemotherapy was found to allow for significantly smaller volumes of breast tissue to be excised (113 cm³ vs 213 cm³, $p = 0.004$). In this study, the delivery of neoadjuvant chemotherapy did not alter the reexcision rate or the number of operations performed in the 2 groups.

Another rationale for neoadjuvant systemic therapy is that this allows for the immediate treatment of micrometastases; however, this has not been associated with an increase in survival in most trials to date (Figs. 85-1B and 85-1C). In contrast, a major advantage is that tumor response to chemotherapy is a strong predictor of outcome. Thus neoadjuvant systemic therapy can be used as an in vivo assay of systemic therapy efficacy. This, in theory, can allow for testing of new therapy regimens in the neoadjuvant setting, allowing for shorter and smaller trials to be conducted using chemotherapy response as the primary end point. In addition, the neoadjuvant setting allows the opportunity to identify biomarkers that can predict response as well as identify pharmacodynamic markers of response, that is

to say, markers that can change within the primary tumor with the administration of chemotherapy, which can be an early molecular signal of therapy activity. Although the standard of care at this point has been to not deliver any further therapy in patients who have received a full course of neoadjuvant chemotherapy even if they have significant residual disease, there is now increasing interest in clinical trials of further therapy based on the residual cancer burden, as well as the molecular phenotype of the residual disease for subsequent treatment planning.

Neoadjuvant chemotherapy does, however, have potential disadvantages, including loss of pretherapy pathologic staging (tumor size and lymph node status). This raises the potential for both over- and undertreatment with chemotherapy and radiation therapy. Furthermore, neoadjuvant chemotherapy does lead to a delay in local and regional therapy and is associated with a small risk of tumor progression. These disadvantages need to be weighed against the advantages to select the appropriate sequence for surgery and chemotherapy for each patient.

PATIENT SELECTION

In general, appropriate neoadjuvant regimens mirror the chemotherapy regimens administered in the adjuvant setting. For this reason, the choice of neoadjuvant regimen depends upon the nature of the tumor and patient-centered factors such as comorbidity. Specific regimens are described at length in Chapter 87.

Predictors of Response to Neoadjuvant Chemotherapy

Neoadjuvant chemotherapy is the standard of care for patients with inflammatory and locally advanced breast cancers. Neoadjuvant chemotherapy is indeed necessary before local

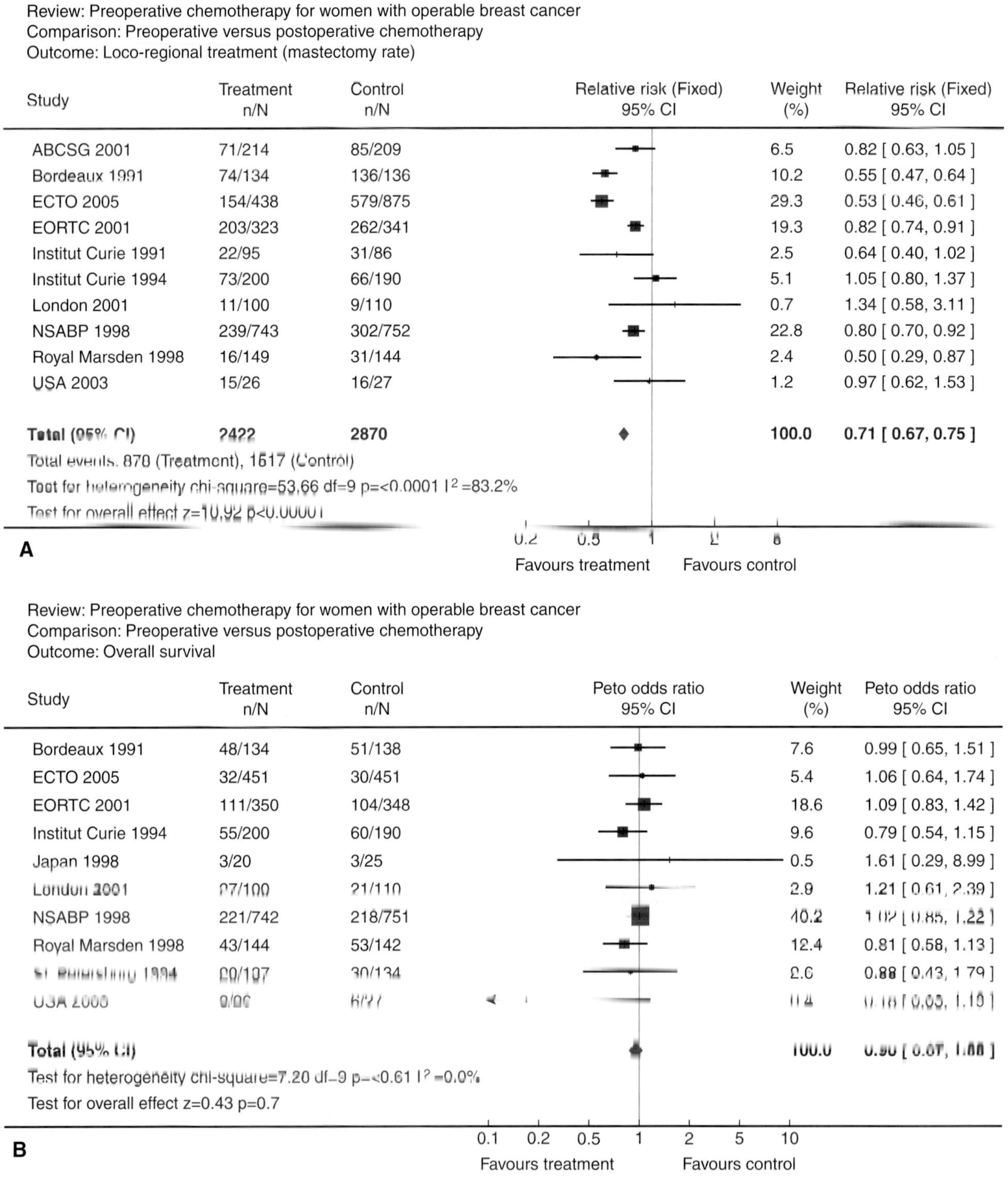

Review: Preoperative chemotherapy for women with operable breast cancer
Comparison: Preoperative versus postoperative chemotherapy
Outcome: Loco-regional treatment (mastectomy rate)

Study	Treatment n/N	Control n/N	Relative risk (Fixed) 95% CI	Weight (%)	Relative risk (Fixed) 95% CI
ABCSG 2001	71/214	85/209		6.5	0.82 [0.63, 1.05]
Bordeaux 1991	74/134	136/136		10.2	0.55 [0.47, 0.64]
ECTO 2005	154/438	579/875		29.3	0.53 [0.46, 0.61]
EORTC 2001	203/323	262/341		19.3	0.82 [0.74, 0.91]
Institut Curie 1991	22/95	31/86		2.5	0.64 [0.40, 1.02]
Institut Curie 1994	73/200	66/190		5.1	1.05 [0.80, 1.37]
London 2001	11/100	9/110		0.7	1.34 [0.58, 3.11]
NSABP 1998	239/743	302/752		22.8	0.80 [0.70, 0.92]
Royal Marsden 1998	16/149	31/144		2.4	0.50 [0.29, 0.87]
USA 2003	15/26	16/27		1.2	0.97 [0.62, 1.53]
Total (95% CI)	**2422**	**2870**		**100.0**	**0.71 [0.67, 0.75]**

Total events: 878 (Treatment), 1517 (Control)
Test for heterogeneity chi-square=53.66 df=9 p=<0.0001 I^2=83.2%
Test for overall effect z=10.92 p<0.00001

A

0.2   0.5   1   2   5
Favours treatment   Favours control

Review: Preoperative chemotherapy for women with operable breast cancer
Comparison: Preoperative versus postoperative chemotherapy
Outcome: Overall survival

Study	Treatment n/N	Control n/N	Peto odds ratio 95% CI	Weight (%)	Peto odds ratio 95% CI
Bordeaux 1991	48/134	51/138		7.6	0.99 [0.65, 1.51]
ECTO 2005	32/451	30/451		5.4	1.06 [0.64, 1.74]
EORTC 2001	111/350	104/348		18.6	1.09 [0.83, 1.42]
Institut Curie 1994	55/200	60/190		9.6	0.79 [0.54, 1.15]
Japan 1998	3/20	3/25		0.5	1.61 [0.29, 8.99]
London 2001	27/100	21/110		2.9	1.21 [0.61, 2.39]
NSABP 1998	221/742	218/751		40.2	1.02 [0.85, 1.22]
Royal Marsden 1998	43/144	53/142		12.4	0.81 [0.58, 1.13]
St Petersburg 1994	28/107	30/134		2.6	0.88 [0.43, 1.79]
USA 2003	9/26	8/27		0.4	0.18 [0.03, 1.16]
Total (95% CI)				**100.0**	**0.90 [0.87, 1.08]**

Test for heterogeneity chi-square=7.20 df=9 p=<0.61 I^2=0.0%
Test for overall effect z=0.43 p=0.7

B

0.1   0.2   0.5   1   2   5   10
Favours treatment   Favours control

FIGURE 85-1 Neoadjuvant chemotherapy for women with operable breast cancer. Comparison of preoperative versus postoperative chemotherapy. **A.** Locoregional treatment (mastectomy rate). **B.** Overall survival. **C.** Disease-free survival. *(Reproduced, with permission, from Mieog JS, van der Hage JA, van de Velde CJ. Preoperative chemotherapy for women with operable breast cancer.* Cochrane Database Syst Rev. *2007:CD005002.)*

intervention for inflammatory breast cancer. Locally advanced breast cancer can be further subdivided into several groups. Patients who have internal mammary lymph node involvement (N3B), supraclavicular lymph node involvement (N3C), or chest wall invasion (T4A)[4] in general require neoadjuvant chemotherapy to assist in surgical therapy. In contrast, other patients with locally advanced breast cancer may be technically operable at the onset, but neoadjuvant preoperative chemotherapy is still preferred; patients with limited skin involvement (selected T4B), patients with nonfixed matted nodes (selected N2), and patients with limited involvement of infraclavicular lymph nodes (N3A). Patients who have a large tumor compared

Review: Preoperative chemotherapy for women with operable breast cancer
Comparison: Preoperative versus postoperative chemotherapy
Outcome: Disease-free survival

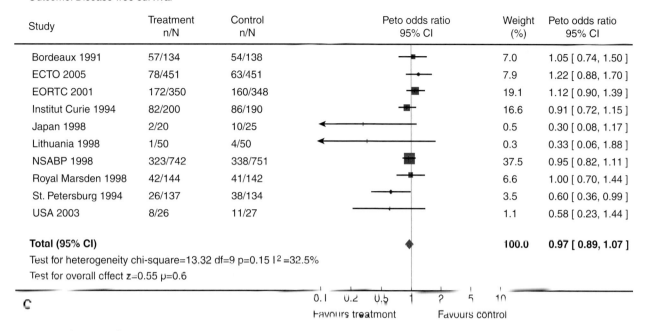

Study	Treatment n/N	Control n/N	Peto odds ratio 95% CI	Weight (%)	Peto odds ratio 95% CI
Bordeaux 1991	57/134	54/138		7.0	1.05 [0.74, 1.50]
ECTO 2005	78/451	63/451		7.9	1.22 [0.88, 1.70]
EORTC 2001	172/350	160/348		19.1	1.12 [0.90, 1.39]
Institut Curie 1994	82/200	86/190		16.6	0.91 [0.72, 1.15]
Japan 1998	2/20	10/25		0.5	0.30 [0.08, 1.17]
Lithuania 1998	1/50	4/50		0.3	0.33 [0.06, 1.88]
NSABP 1998	323/742	338/751		37.5	0.95 [0.82, 1.11]
Royal Marsden 1998	42/144	41/142		6.6	1.00 [0.70, 1.44]
St. Petersburg 1994	26/137	38/134		3.5	0.60 [0.36, 0.99]
USA 2003	8/26	11/27		1.1	0.58 [0.23, 1.44]
Total (95% CI)				100.0	**0.97 [0.89, 1.07]**

Test for heterogeneity chi-square=13.32 df=9 p=0.15 I^2=32.5%
Test for overall effect z=0.55 p=0.6

0.1 0.2 0.5 1 2 5 10
Favours treatment   Favours control

C

FIGURE 85-1 *(Continued)*

with their breast size that desire breast-conserving surgery would also benefit from preoperative therapy followed by breast-conserving surgery (Fig. 85-2). An alternative to this approach would be the use of a large wide local excision of the breast with oncoplastic breast remodeling in patients in whom the breast anatomy would allow this approach or breast-conserving surgery with latissimus flap closure to reachieve breast contour. However, neoadjuvant chemotherapy allowing downsizing is usually the initially preferred approach, with consideration of the other 2 surgical techniques to assist in patients in whom chemotherapy does not achieve enough tumor downsizing to allow for breast conservation.

In contrast, there are patients in whom preoperative therapy is undesirable. Patients undergoing preoperative therapy need to have a definitive diagnosis of invasive cancer. Therefore, if a patient has a breast mass, a core biopsy is needed to demonstrate the invasive nature of this tumor rather than a fine-needle aspirate before initiation of chemotherapy. Furthermore, markers for therapeutic planning, including estrogen receptor (ER), progesterone receptor (PR), and HER-2, need to be obtained on the tumor for proper therapeutic management. In addition, patients in whom the tumor extent is not clear are not good candidates for neoadjuvant therapy. Examples include patients with ill-defined tumor extent on imaging or patients in whom the extent of invasive versus noninvasive cancer is unclear. These scenarios have systemic therapy implications, as chemotherapy may be overtreatment for these patients, and furthermore, it may affect radiation therapy planning. For example, the invasive tumor size (T3 vs not) may affect the ultimate recommendations regarding the need for radiation therapy. If there is no definite need for chemotherapy, surgery first is preferred.

As studies to date have demonstrated that neoadjuvant chemotherapy confers neither better nor worse overall survival compared with postoperative therapy (Fig. 85-1B), neoadjuvant chemotherapy is an acceptable alternative to postoperative therapy in any patient who definitely requires chemotherapy. However, this necessitates that there is an experienced multidisciplinary team available, that the tumor response can be closely monitored, and that the patient is compliant. This is preferably done on a clinical trial.

In pretreatment planning, one needs to consider the clinical predictors of response to neoadjuvant chemotherapy. These include treatment regimen–related features, such as the drugs administered, number of cycles delivered, and the therapy schedule. They also include clinicopathologic features, such as tumor size, grade, histologic type, and ER/PR status. Special scenarios to consider include patients with invasive lobular carcinoma histology. Invasive lobular carcinoma is associated with a very low pathologic complete response (pCR) rate (3% for invasive lobular carcinoma vs 15% for invasive ductal carcinoma).[5] Also of note, patients who do not have pCR but have lobular histology have a significantly better outcome compared with patients who have residual disease but ductal histology, suggesting that while looking at residual disease for prognostic prediction, one also needs to take histology into consideration. Furthermore, delivery of neoadjuvant chemotherapy for invasive lobular carcinoma has also been shown not to significantly improve the ability to do breast-conserving surgery.[6] Taken together, the relative benefit of neoadjuvant therapy with standard chemotherapy seems quite limited for patients with invasive lobular carcinoma.

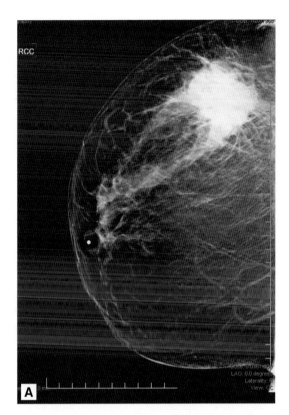
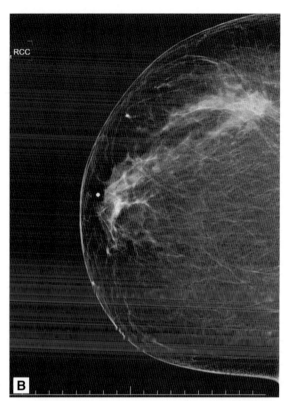

FIGURE 85-2 Downsizing of a T3 tumor with neoadjuvant chemotherapy. The prechemotherapy **(A)** and postchemotherapy **(B)** mammograms are demonstrated. Final pathology demonstrated concentric shrinkage of the tumor with residual T1 tumor excised with widely negative margins on breast-conserving surgery.

For ER-positive cancer, there are also relatively low pathologic response rates. Indeed, in the University of Texas MD Anderson Cancer Center series, the pCR rate was 8% for hormone receptor–positive tumors versus 24% in hormone receptor–negative tumors ($p > 0.001$).[7] However, patients with hormone receptor–positive disease who did have pCR had a significant survival benefit compared with those who did not. In spite of the relatively low pCR rates obtained in hormone receptor–positive tumors, neoadjuvant chemotherapy is reasonable for patients with large hormone receptor–positive tumors who desire breast-conserving surgery. However, surgery first is preferred for node-negative patients for whom the need for chemotherapy is unclear. Surgery first would allow for definitive pathology size and nodal status assessment and will allow the patient to participate in the adjuvant therapy trials, such as the Trial Assigning IndividuaLized Options for Treatment (Rx) or the TAILORx trial. Alternative therapy options for these patients include preoperative aromatase inhibitors for postmenopausal patients.

Because of their relatively poor prognosis, patients with triple-negative breast cancer have been of significant interest. Interestingly, patients with triple-negative breast cancer have higher pCR rates than non–triple-negative breast cancer patients (22% vs 11%, $p = 0.0034$). If pCR is achieved, patients with triple-negative breast cancer have similar overall survival rates as patients with non–triple-negative breast cancer.[8] However, if residual disease remains after chemotherapy, triple-negative breast cancer has a worse overall survival rate compared with non–triple-negative breast cancer with residual disease. Thus patients with triple-negative breast cancer may indeed benefit from neoadjuvant chemotherapy, as they have a significant likelihood of achieving tumor downsizing and pCR. Furthermore, neoadjuvant chemotherapy allows us to identify patients at highest risk for relapse, and these patients may be targeted for clinical trials assessing the role of additional adjuvant therapy for chemoresistant tumors.

The treatment of patients with HER-2-positive disease has recently evolved with the introduction of HER-2-targeted therapies. There have been dozens of clinical trials looking at HER-2-targeted agents in the neoadjuvant setting, with variable responses. One of the most striking responses was seen in a clinical trial conducted by Buzdar et al.[9] In this single-institution study conducted at MD Anderson Cancer Center, patients with HER-2-positive disease (amplified by fluorescent in situ hybridization or 3+ by immunohistochemistry) were enrolled to receive either paclitaxel followed by fluorouracil, epirubicin, and cyclophosphamide (FEC) or paclitaxel and FEC in combination with the trastuzumab. The clinical trial had a planned sample size of 164 patients but was stopped early after the enrollment of 42 patients based on the clear superiority of the investigational arm. Indeed, the pCR rate was 65.2% in the trastuzumab arm, compared with 26% in the standard chemotherapy arm. This study demonstrated the definitive benefit of anti-HER-2 strategies in achieving pCR. Clearly, this makes the case for anti-HER-2 targeted therapies in the neoadjuvant setting to achieve significant tumor downsizing in this patient population. This also raises the exciting possibility that the multiple evolving targeted therapies can further improve tumor downsizing and pCR rates for other breast cancer subtypes, further improving breast conservation rates.

Breast Conservation after Neoadjuvant Chemotherapy

For successful breast-conserving surgery after neoadjuvant chemotherapy, appropriate patient selection is critical. Large residual tumor size versus breast size, multicentric disease, persistent skin edema, contraindications or unwillingness to receive radiation therapy, and inflammatory breast cancer are considered contraindications for breast-conserving surgery.[10] Overall, the indications for breast-conserving surgery are fairly similar to the criteria for breast-conserving surgery de novo.

THERAPY PLANNING

Prechemotherapy Work-Up

A prerequisite for successful breast-conserving surgery after neoadjuvant chemotherapy is adequate determination of tumor extent before chemotherapy. Imaging usually includes a bilateral mammography and ultrasonography of the breast, axilla, and infraclavicular, supraclavicular, and internal mammary nodes to identify regional disease. Fine-needle aspiration of any suspicious axillary or supraclavicular lymph nodes is performed for documentation of nodal involvement. There are also evolving data suggesting a role for magnetic resonance imaging (MRI) for both prediction of response to chemotherapy as well as assessment of tumor response and determination of tumor extent after neoadjuvant therapy. It is important at the onset to biopsy any suspicious lesions in the ipsilateral breast to rule out multicentric disease and in the contralateral breast to rule out bilateral disease before the initiation of systemic therapy.

Response Monitoring On-Therapy

It is important for patients receiving neoadjuvant therapy to be monitored by a multidisciplinary team while on therapy to document response and to rule out any tumor progression. Usually, tumor response is monitored by a combination of physical exam and imaging. Marker placement is performed for future tumor localization if the tumor is less than 2 cm in size up front or if the tumor shrinks by 50% or more after the first cycle of chemotherapy or if the tumor shrinks to 2 cm or less in size after the second course of chemotherapy. If the patient has multifocal disease, either all lesions can be marked with separate markers or lesions that are furthest apart can be marked to assist in surgical planning.

Preoperative Work-Up and Surgical Technique

Preoperative work-up should include reassessment of tumor extent, which may include mammography and/or ultrasonography and possibly MRI. The imaging study that demonstrates

the most extensive residual disease should be used for localization. The goal is to remove all remaining evidence of tumor. For example, if a tumor mass originally seen had decreased in size but there are extensive surrounding suspicious calcifications, in general, the calcifications felt to be associated with the malignant process would be targeted for complete excision. In patients with extensive calcifications or multifocal disease, bracketing with 2 or more wires can be used to excise the tumor en bloc with a rim of normal breast tissue (Fig. 85-3). In patients in whom there is no residual tumor, surgery is still necessary, because at least half of the patients with complete clinical response (physical exam, mammogram, ultrasound) still have residual carcinoma on pathology. Needle localization for breast conservation can be done with mammographic or ultrasonographic guidance. Usually ultrasound is preferred for lesions that are easily detectable by ultrasound. Mammographic localization is preferred for patients who have calcifications extending outside of the tumor mass. Mammographic localization of metallic markers is performed for those patients with no residual disease on imaging of the primary site or for those who have satellite nodules. Mammograms after localization are invaluable for assisting in 3-dimensional visualization of the localization; surgical planning can be further assisted by intraoperative ultrasound. Also, for mammographic localization, good communication with the surgeon and radiologist is also of great value. The surgical approach is to target the residual disease with 1-cm margins of normal surrounding breast parenchyma rather than the original volume of involvement. Breast-conserving surgery in the setting of neoadjuvant chemotherapy is made somewhat challenging, as physical exam, mammography, and ultrasound findings have all been shown to have relatively poor correlation with post–neoadjuvant chemotherapy tumor volumes.[11] With all breast-conserving surgery, important aspects include orientation of the specimen and inking of the margins. Intraoperative margin analysis may assist in identification of close margins and allow for directed intraoperative reexcisions. Although multiple approaches have been used for this, 1 approach is assessment of gross pathology, along with specimen radiographs of sections and selective frozen section analysis as described for breast-conserving surgery de novo.[12] Intraoperative assessment with specimen mammography can be especially invaluable in patients who have extensive calcifications or multifocal disease (Fig. 85-4). Positive margins on final pathology necessitate reexcision or completion mastectomy. Close margins are controversial; however, margins less than 2 mm have been associated with higher local recurrence rates in some studies.[13] Patients who have close margins in the setting of scattered islands of residual disease may especially benefit from reexcision or consideration of completion mastectomy.

NODAL STAGING WITH NEOADJUVANT THERAPY

Prognostic Implications of Nodal Status after Neoadjuvant Chemotherapy

The goal of axillary surgery is to obtain accurate staging, including the presence or absence of axillary metastases and the number of nodes involved, while simultaneously achieving

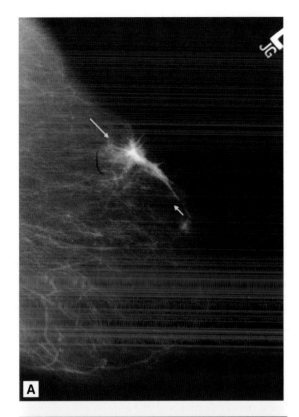

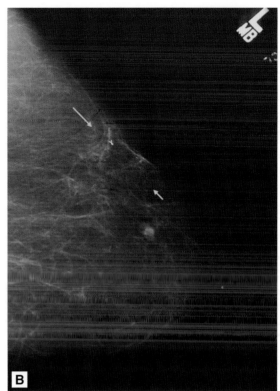

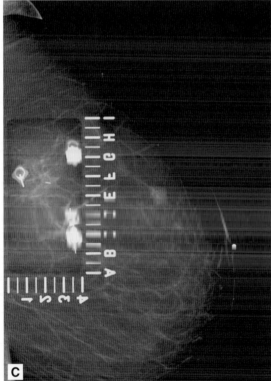

FIGURE 85.3 **A.** Preoperative mammogram, with extent of the calcifications designated by arrows. The primary tumor was localized with a metallic clip. **B.** At the completion of chemotherapy, mammography demonstrates complete resolution of the tumor mass, however, with extent of residual calcifications unchanged, again demonstrated by arrows. **C.** Localization of a postchemotherapy tumor with bracketing as demonstrated with the postlocalization mammogram.

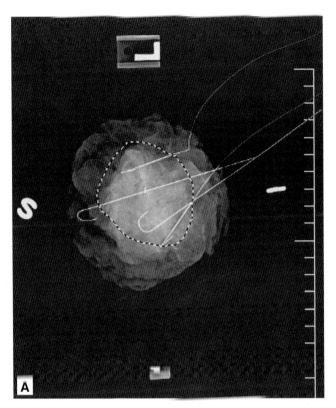
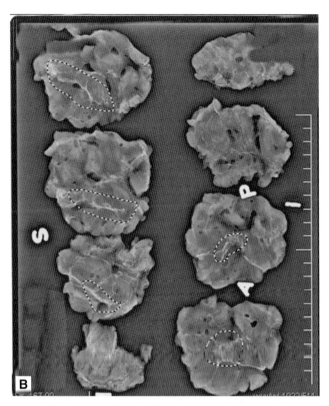

FIGURE 85-4   A. Gross specimen mammogram demonstrating removal of targeted lesion that has been bracketed. **B.** Radiographs of sections of the specimen allow for assessment of extent of calcifications and demonstrate that radiographically clear margins have been obtained.

regional control, with the potential of impacting survival. Although neoadjuvant chemotherapy has multiple recognized advantages, it also has a disadvantage—it may interfere with staging information gained from axillary dissection or sentinel node biopsy. Concern is that patients who have axillary lymph node metastasis before therapy indeed may have eradication of their axillary lymph node metastasis and therefore may be node-negative upon surgical staging after neoadjuvant chemotherapy. This was demonstrated in a series from MD Anderson when patients with locally advanced breast cancer who had cytologically documented axillary lymph node metastasis were treated on 1 of 2 prospective trials of doxorubicin-based neoadjuvant chemotherapy. Of 191 patients who were cytologically documented to be node-positive at the outset, 43 patients (20%) had histologically negative nodes at the time of surgery. Ten percent of these "node-negative" patients were found to have occult nodal metastasis when the lymph nodes were investigated with more scrutiny using immunohistochemistry.[14] However, the rest of the patients demonstrate that neoadjuvant chemotherapy can indeed eradicate disease in the lymph nodes, thus altering the staging.

The prognostic value of lymph node status after neoadjuvant chemotherapy has been assessed in some studies. A series from McCready et al[15] looked at 136 patients with locally advanced breast cancer treated with neoadjuvant chemotherapy with fluorouracil, doxorubicin, and cyclophosphamide. Univariate analysis revealed that the number of positive lymph nodes was significantly associated with disease-free and overall

survival. However, subsequent studies demonstrated that although the nodal status is indeed prognostic after neoadjuvant chemotherapy, it may not confer the same prognosis as the same pathologic lymph node status before chemotherapy.[16] For example, patients who are lymph node negative after neoadjuvant chemotherapy consist of patients who were node negative up front, as well as patients who had nodal involvement and had chemotherapy-induced eradication of their nodal metastasis. These groups do not necessarily have the same outcome. Furthermore, the finding of 1 to 3 lymph nodes or 4 to 9 lymph nodes after preoperative chemotherapy appears to be associated with a worse outcome than having the same nodal status when surgery is performed initially.[16] Thus although axillary lymph node status remains prognostic after preoperative neoadjuvant chemotherapy, pathologically positive lymph nodes after chemotherapy appear to be associated with a worse prognosis than the same nodal status before chemotherapy. These patients may have had larger initial tumor burden in their nodes, and thus this represents a chemotherapy-resistant population. These patients may benefit from clinical trials with cross-over chemotherapy regimens and novel therapies.

Sentinel Node Biopsy after Neoadjuvant Chemotherapy

Whether sentinel node biopsy should be performed before or after neoadjuvant chemotherapy has been an area of significant controversy. One concern about sentinel node biopsy after neoadjuvant chemotherapy has been regarding the identification rate. It has been argued that chemotherapy-associated changes in the breast may lead to changes in the lymphatic drainage pattern, interfering with identification of a sentinel node, or worse, with identification of an alternate lymph node compared with the sentinel node that would have been identified if the procedure was done up front, before chemotherapy. This could potentially lead to a false-negative finding. Furthermore, it has also been hypothesized that involved lymph nodes may have differential responses to chemotherapy, and although metastasis in the sentinel node could be potentially eradicated, additional non-sentinel nodes in the axilla may still contain lymph node metastasis, again leading to a false-negative result. These hypotheses were originally fueled by a small retrospective series from the University of Washington where 53 patients who underwent sentinel node biopsy up front had a false-negative rate of 9% while 13 patients who underwent neoadjuvant chemotherapy had a false-negative rate of 33%.[17] The authors concluded that neoadjuvant chemotherapy is associated with an unacceptably high false-negative rate. This has led to the proposal that sentinel node biopsy be performed before chemotherapy, and for patients who have a positive sentinel node after chemotherapy, axillary lymph node dissection can be performed after the completion of chemotherapy. Patients for whom sentinel node biopsy is negative can proceed to chemotherapy as planned with no further axillary surgery.[18,19] In contrast, several subsequent single-institution studies have suggested that sentinel node biopsy after neoadjuvant chemotherapy does, in fact, have an acceptable false-negative rate (eg, Breslin et al[20]), except in the setting of inflammatory breast cancer.[21] In the National Surgical Adjuvant Breast and Bowel Project (NSABP) B27 clinical trial, in which patients were randomized with neoadjuvant chemotherapy with doxorubicin and cyclophosphamide (AC) or AC followed by docetaxel, of 2411 patients, 420 (18%) had sentinel node biopsy in addition to axillary lymph node dissection off protocol. This study showed a false-negative rate of 10.7% for sentinel node biopsy after neoadjuvant chemotherapy. No significant difference was identified among false-negative rates by tumor response or other patient and tumor characteristics.[22] Subsequently, a meta-analysis was performed of sentinel node biopsy after neoadjuvant chemotherapy. A total of 1273 patients were reported in 21 studies with a pooled identification rate of 90% and a pooled false-negative rate of 12% (95% confidence interval of 10%-15%).[23] This false-negative rate for sentinel node biopsy is not that different from what has been reported in multicenter trials of sentinel node biopsy de novo, in the absence of neoadjuvant chemotherapy. Thus sentinel node biopsy after neoadjuvant chemotherapy based on current data may be an acceptable approach. However, patients who have cytologically proven lymph node involvement before chemotherapy have been reported to have higher false-negative rates.[24] At this time, axillary lymph dissection is recommended for patients with cytologically proven positive nodes before chemotherapy. However, with the increasing efficacy of chemotherapy regimens, the role of sentinel node mapping in this group may need to be reassessed in the future. There is an American College of Surgeons Oncology Group clinical trial that will be addressing this specific question.

LOCAL CONTROL WITH BREAST CONSERVATION AFTER NEOADJUVANT CHEMOTHERAPY

There have been concerns about the local control that would be achieved with breast conservation after neoadjuvant chemotherapy. Although some tumors concentrically shrink, allowing for the residual tumor to be more easily identified and margins to be easily assessed, other tumors can have a residual scattered island viable tumor, often referred to as "cookie crumble" pattern or multifocal residual disease. Concerns about breast conservation in patients with this kind of response pattern have been raised, because in theory, margins may appear negative on analysis, but there may be multifocal residual disease outside of the margins in this scenario.

Long-term results of local control with breast-conserving surgery have yet to be reported in the setting of neoadjuvant chemotherapy. One of the largest single-institution series has been reported from MD Anderson Cancer Center.[25] In 340 patients who were treated with anthracycline-based neoadjuvant chemotherapy, breast-conserving surgery was performed directed at the postchemotherapy residual disease, and all patients received radiation therapy with a boost. This study reported a 5-year ipsilateral breast tumor recurrence-free survival rate of 95%, demonstrating that adequate local control could be obtained in carefully selected patients, treated by a dedicated multidisciplinary team. In this study, ipsilateral breast tumor recurrence-free survival did not significantly differ based on presenting T-stage (between T1, T2, T3, T4 tumors); however, patients with T3 and T4 tumors who received breast-conserving surgery in this study were likely offered this option based on their responsiveness to neoadjuvant chemotherapy. It was noted, however, that patients who had T3 or T4 tumors and had multifocal residual disease did have lower ipsilateral breast tumor 5-year recurrence-free survival rates (80% for T3/T4 multifocal positive vs 97% for T3 multifocal negative, 95% for T1/T2 multifocal positive, and 96% for T1/T2 multifocal negative, $p = 0.0008$.) Determinants of ipsilateral breast tumor recurrence in this study included clinical nodal stage (N2/3 vs N0/1), residual tumor size greater than 2 cm, and multifocal residual disease or presence of lymphovascular invasion demonstrated a trend toward higher rate of ipsilateral breast tumor recurrence. Assigning each of these factors 1 point, a prognostic score was created to predict ipsilateral breast tumor recurrence. Patients having a prognostic index score of 0, 1, 2, and 3 had corresponding 5-year ipsilateral breast tumor recurrence rates of 99%, 94%, 88%, and 82%, respectively.[26] It is interesting to note that the same prognostic factors also are prognostic for locoregional control after mastectomy. Of concern, the small cohort of patients who had a prognostic index of 3 to 4 who underwent mastectomy were found to have a higher likelihood of being locoregional recurrence-free compared with those patients who underwent breast-conserving surgery (81% for mastectomy vs 39% for breast-conserving surgery, $p = 0.009$).[27] This finding does suggest that it may be possible to identify clinical and pathologic features that can help identify patients who are at higher risk of locoregional recurrence with breast-conserving surgery after neoadjuvant chemotherapy. However, this model has yet to be validated in larger prospective series.

FUTURE DIRECTIONS

Neoadjuvant Therapy as a Discovery Tool for Markers of Response

Neoadjuvant therapy is expanding with the evolving understanding of molecular oncology and the availability of high-throughput tools for rapid assessment of molecular phenotype. The ability to assess the prognosis of tumors and the ability to predict response to therapies are rapidly evolving. Neoadjuvant therapy is an ideal setting for which markers of response can be identified. Biopsies of tumors while in vivo can be coupled with standard chemotherapy or novel therapeutics, allowing for predictors of response that can determine outcome prospectively to be identified. Furthermore, the neoadjuvant setting can allow for biopsies of the tumors on-therapy to see if novel targeted therapies are indeed inhibiting presumed targets and whether target inhibition affects clinical and pathologic response. Other alterations in the tumor, such as apoptosis or inhibition of proliferation (eg, as measured with Ki-67) can be followed as another surrogate of response. Finally, assessment of residual disease with high-throughput strategies may allow for changes in the tumor characteristics, and this may allow for identification of mechanisms of resistance. This also may allow for selection of therapies that will target the chemoresistant clones. Biomarker assessments are critical to the development of new agents in the clinic; therefore, consideration should be given to incorporation of correlative studies in all neoadjuvant therapy trials.

Neoadjuvant-Targeted Therapy Trials

With standard chemotherapy achieving pCR in only 10% to 30% of patients, there is a need for more personalized medicine—in other words, to tailor the therapies delivered and to treat the breast cancer more effectively and potentially with the least toxicity. Molecular targeted therapies can exploit differences in gene expression as well as growth and survival signaling between cancer cells and normal cells. There are numerous oncogenic pathways identified in breast cancer that are potentially "druggable." These include the ERB2 receptor family, insulin-like growth factor receptors, src inhibitors, angiogenesis inhibitors, inhibitors of PI3K/Akt/mTOR pathway, histone deacetylase (HDAC) inhibitors, and proteosomal pathway inhibitors.[28] It is critical to determine which targets are best and which combinations of targeted therapies can enhance the efficacy of standard therapy. Neoadjuvant therapy trials allow for rapid assessment of in vivo efficacy looking at clinical and pathologic response.

The remarkable success of trastuzumab in the neoadjuvant setting in enhancing pCR rates for HER-2-positive tumors[9] emphasizes the value of targeted therapies in the neoadjuvant therapy setting. Additional ongoing clinical trials looking at HER-2-targeted therapies include the American College of Surgeons Oncology Group Z1041 trial, which examines the optimal chemotherapy combination with trastuzumab. Other ongoing HER-2-targeted trials compare lapatinib or combination lapatinib plus trastuzumab with trastuzumab alone in combination with chemotherapy, such as NSABP-41, GeparQuattro, Cancer and Leukemia Group B (CALGB) 40601, and Neo-ALTTO (NeoAdjuvant Lapatinib and/or Trastuzumab Treatment Optimization). The last 2 trials are intriguing due to preplanned cross-validation of predictive biomarkers, which may allow determination of resistance and sensitivity patterns. There are also several ongoing trials assessing other targets, including the use of the antiangiogenesis agent bevacizumab. These include the NSABP-40 HER-2-negative trial, the CALGB 40603 trial, which is limited to triple-negative disease only and examines both an antiangiogenic question and the question of platinum sensitivity in triple-negative disease, and the GeparQuattro trial. Many other targeted therapies that are earlier in development are also being examined in the neoadjuvant setting, allowing both identification of clinical activity and simultaneous study of biologic factors related to this activity.

Necessary Future Studies

Whether neoadjuvant chemotherapy or neoadjuvant endocrine therapy is preferable in postmenopausal women with ER-positive tumors remains an area of controversy that needs to be addressed in future studies. Whether patients who do not have significant response to standard neoadjuvant chemotherapy would derive survival benefit from additional therapy also needs to be determined.

Importantly, neoadjuvant therapy studies can be used to prospectively test any predictive markers that have been generated for standard chemotherapy as well as individual chemotherapy regimens and separate combination therapies. It is likely that predictive markers will need to be generated for each combination being given. Thought needs to be given regarding how to best bring novel therapies into clinical trials, especially in the neoadjuvant therapy setting. One option is to treat patients with a standard of care and if they achieve no response, to consider novel targeted therapies. Another approach is to use molecular markers to identify benefits for patients unlikely to benefit from standard therapy and offer these patients targeted therapies trials. Yet another option is to select patients likely to respond based on preclinically generated predictive markers of response and test these markers for their ability to enrich for responders in the clinical setting. Successful incorporation of correlative studies into neoadjuvant therapy trials is most likely to enhance the efficacy of neoadjuvant therapies, and introduction of biomarker evaluation for patient selection is likely to lead to higher success in achieving pCR in the neoadjuvant setting, facilitate selection of combination therapies, and potentially assist in identifying patients who do not respond to standard therapies and may benefit from additional targeted postoperative adjuvant therapies.

SUMMARY

Neoadjuvant therapy is the standard of care for inflammatory breast cancer and locally advanced breast cancer. Neoadjuvant chemotherapy should also be considered for patients with large breast tumors who desire breast conservation. In patients who definitely need chemotherapy, neoadjuvant chemotherapy can be offered in the presence of a dedicated multidisciplinary team and close follow-up, and preferably on a clinical trial.

Neoadjuvant chemotherapy leads to tumor downsizing in most patients, thus improving the ability to perform breast conservation, with acceptable local control in appropriately selected patients. With improving personalized therapies, neoadjuvant treatment is likely to lead to increasing numbers of patients eligible for breast conservation in the future.

REFERENCES

1. Fisher B, Bryant J, Wolmark N, et al. Effect of preoperative chemotherapy on the outcome of women with operable breast cancer. *J Clin Oncol.* 1998;16:2672-2685.
2. Wolmark N, Wang J, Mamounas E, Bryant J, Fisher B. Preoperative chemotherapy in patients with operable breast cancer: nine-year results from National Surgical Adjuvant Breast and Bowel Project B-18. *J Natl Cancer Inst Monogr.* 2001:96-102.
3. Boughey JC, Peintinger F, Meric-Bernstam F, et al. Impact of preoperative versus postoperative chemotherapy on the extent and number of surgical procedures in patients treated in randomized clinical trials for breast cancer. *Ann Surg.* 2006;244:464-470.
4. Greene FL, Page DL, Fleming ID, et al. *AJCC Cancer Staging Manual.* 6th ed. New York, NY: Springer; 2002.
5. Cristofanilli M, Gonzalez-Angulo A, Sneige N, et al. Invasive lobular carcinoma classic type: response to primary chemotherapy and survival outcomes. *J Clin Oncol.* 2005;23:41-48.
6. Boughey JC, Wagner J, Garrett BJ, et al. Neoadjuvant chemotherapy in invasive lobular carcinoma may not improve rates of breast conservation. *Ann Surg Oncol.* 2009;16:1606-1611.
7. Guarneri V, Broglio K, Kau SW, et al. Prognostic value of pathologic complete response after primary chemotherapy in relation to hormone receptor status and other factors. *J Clin Oncol.* 2006;24:1037-1044.
8. Liedtke C, Mazouni C, Hess KR, et al. Response to neoadjuvant therapy and long-term survival in patients with triple-negative breast cancer. *J Clin Oncol.* 2008;26:1275-1281.
9. Buzdar AU, Valero V, Ibrahim NK, et al. Neoadjuvant therapy with paclitaxel followed by 5-fluorouracil, epirubicin, and cyclophosphamide chemotherapy and concurrent trastuzumab in human epidermal growth factor receptor 2-positive operable breast cancer: an update of the initial randomized study population and data of additional patients treated with the same regimen. *Clin Cancer Res.* 2007;13:228-233.
10. Singletary SE, McNeese MD, Hortobagyi GN. Feasibility of breast-conservation surgery after induction chemotherapy for locally advanced breast carcinoma. *Cancer* 1992;69:2849-2852.
11. Chagpar AB, Middleton LP, Sahin AA, et al. Accuracy of physical examination, ultrasonography, and mammography in predicting residual pathologic tumor size in patients treated with neoadjuvant chemotherapy. *Ann Surg.* 2006;243:257-264.
12. Cabioglu N, Hunt KK, Sahin AA, et al. Role for intraoperative margin assessment in patients undergoing breast-conserving surgery. *Ann Surg Oncol.* 2007;14:1458-1471.
13. Rouzier R, Extra JM, Carton M, et al. Primary chemotherapy for operable breast cancer: incidence and prognostic significance of ipsilateral breast tumor recurrence after breast-conserving surgery. *J Clin Oncol.* 2001;19:3828-3835.
14. Kuerer HM, Sahin AA, Hunt KK, et al. Incidence and impact of documented eradication of breast cancer axillary lymph node metastases before surgery in patients treated with neoadjuvant chemotherapy. *Ann Surg.* 1999;230:72-78.
15. McCready DR, Hortobagyi GN, Kau SW, et al. The prognostic significance of lymph node metastases after preoperative chemotherapy for locally advanced breast cancer. *Arch Surg.* 1989;124:21-25.
16. Meric F, Mirza NQ, Buzdar AU, et al. Prognostic implications of pathological lymph node status after preoperative chemotherapy for operable T3N0M0 breast cancer. *Ann Surg Oncol.* 2000;7:435-440.
17. Nason KS, Anderson BO, Byrd DR, et al. Increased false negative sentinel node biopsy rates after preoperative chemotherapy for invasive breast carcinoma. *Cancer.* 2000;89:2187-2194.
18. Schrenk P, Hochreiner G, Fridrik M, Wayand W. Sentinel node biopsy performed before preoperative chemotherapy for axillary lymph node staging in breast cancer. *Breast J.* 2003;9:282-287.
19. Sabel MS, Schott AF, Kleer CG, et al. Sentinel node biopsy prior to neoadjuvant chemotherapy. *Am J Surg.* 2003;186:102-105.
20. Breslin TM, Cohen L, Sahin A, et al. Sentinel lymph node biopsy is accurate after neoadjuvant chemotherapy for breast cancer. *J Clin Oncol.* 2000;18:3480-3486.
21. Stearns V, Ewing CA, Slack R, et al. Sentinel lymphadenectomy after neoadjuvant chemotherapy for breast cancer may reliably represent the axilla except for inflammatory breast cancer. *Ann Surg Oncol.* 2002;9:235-242.
22. Mamounas EP. Sentinel lymph node biopsy after neoadjuvant systemic therapy. *Surg Clin North Am.* 2003;83:931-942.
23. Xing Y, Foy M, Cox DD, et al. Meta-analysis of sentinel lymph node biopsy after preoperative chemotherapy in patients with breast cancer. *Br J Surg.* 2006;93:539-546.
24. Shen J, Gilcrease MZ, Babiera GV, et al. Feasibility and accuracy of sentinel lymph node biopsy after preoperative chemotherapy in breast cancer patients with documented axillary metastases. *Cancer.* 2007;109:1255-1263.
25. Chen AM, Meric-Bernstam F, Hunt KK, et al. Breast conservation after neoadjuvant chemotherapy: the MD Anderson cancer center experience. *J Clin Oncol.* 2004;22:2303-2312.
26. Chen AM, Meric-Bernstam F, Hunt KK, et al. Breast conservation after neoadjuvant chemotherapy. *Cancer.* 2005;103:689-695.
27. Huang EH, Strom EA, Perkins GH, et al. Comparison of risk of local-regional recurrence after mastectomy or breast conservation therapy for patients treated with neoadjuvant chemotherapy and radiation stratified according to a prognostic index score. *Int J Radiat Oncol Biol Phys.* 2006;66:352-357.
28. Ocana A, Pandiella A. Identifying breast cancer druggable oncogenic alterations: lessons learned and future targeted options. *Clin Cancer Res.* 2008;14:961-970.

CHAPTER 86

Endocrine Therapy

Prudence A. Francis

Among postoperative therapies for early breast cancer, endocrine therapy is responsible for the greatest reduction in the risk of recurrence and death. Following resection of hormone receptor–positive breast cancer, adjuvant endocrine therapy reduces the risk of local recurrence, distant metastasis, and contralateral breast cancer. Currently new medical oncology treatments described as targeted therapies are improving outcomes in a variety of malignancies. Tamoxifen treatment for breast cancer represents the first successful application of a targeted therapy, where the drug targets the estrogen receptor (ER) on any residual tumor cells. Tamoxifen is described as a selective estrogen receptor modulator (SERM) because of its varying effects in different tissues, where it may act as an antagonist (eg, breast) or an agonist (eg, uterus).

The most recent Early Breast Cancer Trialists' Collaborative Group (EBCTCG) Oxford overview analysis was published in 2005. This analysis found that among women with ER-positive tumors who were randomized to receive 5 years of adjuvant tamoxifen, the annual breast cancer recurrence rate was almost halved (41% proportional risk reduction) and the breast cancer mortality rate was reduced by one-third (34% proportional risk reduction) compared with those who did not receive tamoxifen.[1] These benefits were observed across all age groups, regardless of the use of chemotherapy, and in both node-negative and node-positive disease. While the relative (proportional) risk reduction is similar for these different patient groups with ER-positive tumors, the absolute benefit from treatment with tamoxifen is greater for women at higher risk for relapse (Table 86-1).

The EBCTCG overview analysis also shows that for women who were randomized to receive adjuvant tamoxifen for 5 years, there is evidence of a protective carry-over effect with continued divergence of the risk of recurrence curves after tamoxifen treatment has been ceased during years 6 to 10. The mortality curves for patients treated with and without tamoxifen continue to diverge with 15 years of follow-up, indicating that the benefits are substantial and persistent. In women with ER-positive disease, adjuvant tamoxifen also reduces the risk of contralateral breast cancer by about one-third.

Recurrences after surgery for early breast cancer are not confined to the first 5 years, and this is particularly true for hormone receptor–positive breast cancer. For hormone receptor–negative breast cancer, recurrences occur predominantly during the first 5 years after surgery, whereas for hormone receptor–positive breast cancer there remains a significant ongoing risk of recurrence during years 6 to 15 after surgery, in addition to the risk of a second primary breast cancer. The EBCTCG overview data show that for women with ER-positive tumors who receive adjuvant tamoxifen, there are as many recurrences in years 6 to 15 as there are during the first 5 years after surgery.[1] Appreciation of the prolonged time course after surgery in which recurrences of hormone receptor–positive breast cancer occur, has led to more research on the role of extended endocrine therapy.

PATIENT SELECTION

To achieve optimal outcomes in early breast cancer, accurate assessment of tumor hormone receptor status is crucial, so that all patients who may benefit from endocrine therapy are identified. One recent study has suggested that when immunohistochemical methods are used, assaying core biopsies may provide more reliable ER and PR (progesterone receptor) estimations than assaying the excised tumor.[2] To optimize the likelihood of detecting the presence of hormone receptors, it may be preferable to routinely assay core biopsies of invasive breast cancer for hormone receptors. However when significant hormone receptor staining is not detected in the initial core biopsy, it may still be reasonable to assay the resected tumor for hormone receptors,

TABLE 86-1 Benefit from 5 Years of Adjuvant Tamoxifen in ER-Positive (or Unknown) Breast Cancer

	Absolute Difference in Recurrence at 10 Years[*]	Absolute Difference in Mortality at 10 Years[*]
Node-positive breast cancer	~15%	~12%
Node-negative breast cancer	~12%	~5%

[*]The benefits may be slightly larger for women with ER-positive tumors, as this analysis included some tumors with unknown ER status.
Data from the Early Breast Cancer Trialists' Collaborative Group.

in case of a false-negative result with the prior testing or heterogeneity of the tumor.

Adjuvant endocrine therapy should be considered for all women with tumors that show *any* level of expression of ER or PR. Approximately 75% of breast cancers fall into this category. In endocrine therapy trials, hormone receptor–positive breast cancer is generally defined as tumors with 10% or more cells staining positively by immunohistochemistry for ER and/or PR. However, patients with tumors that show occasional cells (ie, 1%-9% cells) staining positively for ER or PR may derive benefit from endocrine therapy.[3] Therefore while endocrine therapy should not be relied upon as the sole systemic therapy for these tumors, it should be included as part of the therapy. Endocrine therapy is not recommended for women with tumors with completely absent ER and PR hormone receptor staining (0% cells positive), with the exception of possible prophylaxis against second tumors in BRCA1 or BRAC2 gene carriers.[4]

PREMENOPAUSAL WOMEN

Tamoxifen

Hormonal therapy with tamoxifen 20 mg orally daily, is considered a standard component of adjuvant systemic therapy for premenopausal women with tumors expressing ER or PR hormone receptors, regardless of age or nodal status. Other than tamoxifen, there are no data on the use of other SERMs such as raloxifene or toremifene in the adjuvant setting in premenopausal women. In women with tumors with completely absent hormone receptor staining (0% cells positive) for ER and PR, adjuvant tamoxifen may be detrimental.[5] The EBCTCG overview shows that 5 years of therapy is significantly more effective than 1 to 2 years of tamoxifen.[1] Currently, 5 years of adjuvant tamoxifen is considered standard therapy for premenopausal women, however the optimal duration for adjuvant tamoxifen remains uncertain.

The large randomized ATLAS (Adjuvant Tamoxifen Longer Against Shorter) trial tested a longer duration of adjuvant therapy with tamoxifen and a preliminary presentation of the trial results reported a reduction in breast cancer recurrences with 10 years of tamoxifen compared with 5 years but with no

significant effect on mortality.[6] Results specific for premenopausal women were not presented, although the effect was expected to be similar across age groups. The aTTom (adjuvant Tamoxifen To offer more?) trial similarly randomized women to an additional 5 years of tamoxifen versus ceasing hormonal therapy after at least 4 years of adjuvant tamoxifen. A preliminary presentation of the aTTom trial results showed a nonsignificant reduction in recurrence rates for women randomized to continue tamoxifen in years 5 to 10.[7] Detailed publication of the aTTom and ATLAS trial results and/or longer follow-up may clarify the clinical relevance of these results for women who remain premenopausal after 5 years of tamoxifen. Given the survival advantage observed in postmenopausal women with node-positive tumors who receive extended hormonal therapy during years 6 to 10,[8] duration of endocrine therapy is an important question for younger women.

Tamoxifen is effective regardless of menstrual status, while aromatase inhibitors are only effective in postmenopausal women. Tamoxifen may result in infrequent menses or prolonged amenorrhea in women who biochemically remain premenopausal. In women under 50 years of age, prolonged amenorrhea on tamoxifen may lead to the false conclusion that a woman is postmenopausal if confirmatory biochemical verification of the estradiol level is not undertaken. Tamoxifen was initially used as a fertility treatment and women of childbearing potential receiving tamoxifen should be informed that they may become pregnant, even if not menstruating. As tamoxifen may harm a developing fetus, women receiving tamoxifen should be advised to utilize nonhormonal methods to avoid pregnancy. In some clinical situations, women may elect to cease tamoxifen prior to completing 5 years because of a desire for pregnancy.

HER-2 overexpression in breast tumors is associated with an adverse prognosis and an increased risk for early relapse. There are data from preclinical studies, metastatic disease, and the adjuvant setting[9-11] to indicate that the presence of HER-2 overexpression may be associated with tamoxifen resistance in hormone receptor–positive breast cancer. Currently it is recommended that tamoxifen be included in the adjuvant therapy for premenopausal women with hormone receptor–positive tumors with associated HER-2 overexpression, although additional adjuvant therapies such as chemotherapy and trastuzumab (Herceptin) may be more important in this patient subset.

Ovarian Suppression or Ablation

Ovarian function suppression refers to the reversible induction of menopause with temporary cessation of ovarian estrogen production in premenopausal women by regular injections of gonadotropin-releasing hormone (GnRH) agonists, also known as luteinizing hormone-releasing hormone (LHRH) agonists. Generally GnRH injections are administered on a 4 weekly (monthly) schedule. Depot GnRH agonist preparations administered every 3 months are available, although there has been some uncertainty about the adequacy of suppression in women with the less frequent administration schedule. Even with the monthly injection schedule, GnRH agonists may not achieve complete ovarian function suppression in some patients,[12] and pregnancy has occasionally been reported in women receiving GnRH therapy. The possibility of incomplete ovarian function suppression in premenopausal women with GnRH agonists is particularly relevant if an aromatase inhibitor is given in combination and the efficacy of this adjuvant therapeutic approach in premenopausal women is currently being tested in clinical trials. The Austrian Breast and Colorectal Cancer Study Group adjuvant ABCSG-12 trial randomized premenopausal women with hormone-responsive breast cancer to receive 3 years of ovarian suppression (by GnRH) plus either tamoxifen or anastrozole. The women in ABCSG-12 were additionally randomized to either receive zolendronic acid (a bisphosphonate) or not. In a preliminary presentation of the results there was no significant difference in outcome between patients receiving tamoxifen or anastrozole.[13] The ABCSG-12 trial was possibly underpowered to definitively answer this question, which is also being studied in the larger ongoing Tamoxifen and Exemestane Trial (TEXT) and Suppression of Ovarian Function Trial (SOFT) randomized adjuvant trials.[14]

Ovarian ablation refers to the permanent induction of menopause with permanent cessation of ovarian estrogen production in premenopausal women by either surgical oophorectomy or ovarian irradiation. Surgical oophorectomy may be performed by laparoscopic surgery or laparotomy. Ovarian irradiation is not generally favored as a method of ovarian ablation due to the quick recovery from laparoscopic oophorectomy, potential for unsuccessful ovarian ablation with irradiation, and the concern that radiation of healthy tissues may result in long-term or late toxicity. If ovarian irradiation is performed as a method of ovarian ablation, hormone levels should be subsequently checked, to ensure that estradiol has fallen to a postmenopausal level.

In premenopausal women with hormone receptor–positive breast cancer, ovarian suppression (by GnRH agonists) and ovarian ablation are effective adjuvant endocrine treatments.[1] There is no evidence that ovarian suppression or ablation is more effective than tamoxifen. Adjuvant endocrine therapy by means of ovarian suppression or ablation has been shown to provide a similar benefit to adjuvant chemotherapy with the CMF (cyclophosphamide, methotrexate, and 5-fluorouracil) first-generation chemotherapy regimen.[15] Ovarian suppression or ablation is considered a valid alternative to chemotherapy in premenopausal women with early breast cancer who are appropriately selected for endocrine responsiveness and without

other high-risk features.[16] Tumors most suited to this therapeutic approach (1) exhibit strong staining for both ER and PR in the majority of cells, (2) are HER-2 negative, and (3) have no or limited nodal involvement. For women over 40 years of age, when reversibility of menopause is not desired, surgical ovarian ablation may be a better alternative to ovarian suppression by GnRH agonists. In younger women, ovarian suppression by GnRH agonists is more commonly favored, as temporary induction of menopause may reduce the long-term effects associated with permanent premature menopause. The optimal duration of ovarian function suppression adjuvant therapy is uncertain, although 2 years of therapy could be considered as a minimum duration. Trials have generally utilized between 2 and 5 years of GnRH therapy. Given that longer durations of oral hormonal adjuvant therapy are more effective than 2 years, it seems plausible that longer durations of ovarian function suppression may also be more effective.

When ovarian suppression or ablation therapy is chosen as an alternative to adjuvant chemotherapy in premenopausal women, it is ordinarily combined with tamoxifen. There is evidence that adding 5 years of tamoxifen to GnRH agonist therapy provides additional benefit.[17] By contrast, for premenopausal women who receive 5 years of adjuvant tamoxifen either with or without prior adjuvant chemotherapy, there is no clear evidence that adding ovarian suppression or ablation provides significant additional risk reduction, over and above that achieved by tamoxifen. This question is currently being studied in the randomized Suppression of Ovarian Function Trial (SOFT). As many premenopausal women become postmenopausal after adjuvant chemotherapy, any potential additive effect of ovarian ablation is likely to be observed predominantly in younger women or those who retain ovarian function. While there are concerns regarding the potential for resistance to tamoxifen in the subset with hormone receptor–positive breast cancer plus HER-2 overexpression, a combined endocrine approach with ovarian ablation plus tamoxifen was found to be an effective adjuvant strategy in this patient subset in a premenopausal trial.[18]

Endocrine Effects of Chemotherapy

In premenopausal women with hormone receptor–positive breast cancer, chemotherapy reduces the risk of recurrence through direct cytotoxic effects but may also have indirect endocrine effects. Chemotherapy may result in transient ovarian function suppression clinically manifested by temporary amenorrhea or permanent ovarian function suppression with menopause. Premenopausal women with hormone receptor–positive breast cancer who experience amenorrhea for at least 3 months following adjuvant chemotherapy have been found to have a reduced risk of recurrence compared to those who continue to menstruate.[5,19] Women with chemotherapy-induced amenorrhea and experiencing menopausal symptoms may find this information encouraging. The likelihood of undergoing permanent menopause following adjuvant chemotherapy is both age and regimen dependent, with virtually no women under the age of 30 years experiencing permanent amenorrhea and a minority in their 30s.[20] Shorter adjuvant chemotherapy regimens completed within 3 months are associated with a lower probability of amenorrhea than 6 to 8 cycle regimens administered over 4 to 6 months.

Women who experience chemotherapy-induced amenorrhea should not receive adjuvant endocrine therapy with an aromatase inhibitor alone as the likelihood of ovarian recovery is significant, particularly among those under 40 years old. Even for women in their 40s who have chemotherapy-induced amenorrhea with biochemical confirmation of postmenopausal estradiol, caution should be taken with commencement of an aromatase inhibitor. In one study, among 45 such women with a median age of 47 (range, 39-52 years), 12 women (27%) had recovery of ovarian function on the aromatase inhibitor.[21] It is feasible that the ovarian function recovery was actually stimulated by the aromatase inhibitor in these women, given that aromatase inhibitors are currently being utilized to induce ovulation for in vitro fertilization (IVF) programs. It should be noted that in a previously premenopausal woman, a single measurement of hormone (estradiol, FSH, and LH) levels showing postmenopausal levels after chemotherapy does not predict the potential for recovery of ovarian function. The potential for recovery of ovarian function is greater with shorter adjuvant chemotherapy regimens, compared with 6-month regimens that include oral cyclophosphamide. Tamoxifen is a more reliable option for women with chemotherapy-induced amenorrhea, unless serial monitoring of hormone levels is planned.

POSTMENOPAUSAL WOMEN

Tamoxifen

Current American Society of Clinical Oncology (ASCO) guidelines recommend that an aromatase inhibitor should be included as a component of adjuvant endocrine therapy for postmenopausal women, either initially or after a course of tamoxifen.[22] However tamoxifen remains an effective adjuvant therapy for postmenopausal women. Five years of adjuvant endocrine therapy with tamoxifen is the gold standard against which newer endocrine therapies have been compared. Therapy with tamoxifen alone may be an appropriate choice for women in whom aromatase inhibitors are poorly tolerated, contraindicated, or for women with low-risk tumors when the toxicity profile of tamoxifen is deemed preferable to the toxicity profile of aromatase inhibitors for that individual. Currently for most postmenopausal patients who are commenced on tamoxifen, consideration may be given to a switch to an aromatase inhibitor after an initial ~2 years of tamoxifen. In postmenopausal women who receive initial tamoxifen, if this hormonal therapy is poorly tolerated, then an earlier switch to an aromatase inhibitor should be considered.

It should be noted that the increased risk for the serious toxicities associated with tamoxifen such as endometrial tumors and thromboembolism predominantly occurs in postmenopausal women. In postmenopausal women with a prior history of thrombosis, initial treatment with an aromatase inhibitor may be a safer option. For women considered at higher risk for early recurrence, an aromatase inhibitor is generally chosen instead of tamoxifen for the commencement of endocrine therapy. In the Breast International Group (BIG) 1-98 trial, factors associated with an increased risk of early recurrence include nodal positivity (particularly 4 or more positive nodes), HER-2 overexpression, only 1 hormone receptor-positive, high-grade tumor, large tumor size, and vascular invasion.[23]

The International Breast Cancer Study Group conducted 2 randomized trials (IBCSG 12 and 14) in node-positive postmenopausal women comparing 5 years of adjuvant endocrine therapy with tamoxifen 20 mg orally daily with toremifene 60 mg orally daily. Analysis of these trials showed that toremifene resulted in similar outcomes to tamoxifen (ie, not significantly different) as an adjuvant endocrine therapy for this patient population and was an acceptable alternative.[24] The 5-year disease-free survival was 72% and 69% for toremifene and tamoxifen, respectively. The 5-year overall survival rates were 85% and 81%, respectively.

Aromatase Inhibitors

Prior to menopause, estrogen is predominantly produced by the ovaries, but after menopause estrogen is predominantly produced in adipose tissue by the enzyme aromatase. Aromatase inhibitors act to reduce the already low estrogen levels in postmenopausal women by blocking the conversion of precursor hormones to estrogen in adipose tissue. If a patient is receiving an aromatase inhibitor, then hormone-replacement therapy is contraindicated. There are currently 3 third-generation aromatase inhibitors (AIs) in clinical practice that have been shown to improve outcomes compared with 5 years of tamoxifen for postmenopausal women with hormone receptor-positive breast cancer. These agents are anastrozole (Arimidex), letrozole (Femara), and exemestane (Aromasin). There are 3 ways of utilizing aromatase inhibitors that have been shown to be effective in adjuvant endocrine therapy for postmenopausal women (Table 86-2).

Early Use of Aromatase Inhibitors

The ATAC and BIG 1-98 randomized trials have shown that 5 years of adjuvant therapy with anastrozole or letrozole will significantly reduce the risk of recurrence compared with 5 years of tamoxifen.[25,26] The absolute differences in disease-free survival for women in these trials at 5 years are 2.4% and 2.9%, respectively.[27,28] The ATAC trial has the longest follow-up and shows that the benefit of anastrozole therapy over tamoxifen has continued to increase over time, with an absolute difference in disease-free survival of 4.1% at 9 years. However, no significant differences in overall survival have emerged in either of these trials, with follow-up of 100 months in the ATAC trial and 51 months in the BIG 1-98.[27,28]

Sequential Use of Aromatase Inhibitors

Several randomized trials have shown that the sequential use of an aromatase inhibitor during years 3 to 5 after an initial ~2 years of adjuvant tamoxifen reduces recurrences compared with 5 years of adjuvant tamoxifen.[29-32] While the initial analyses of these trials did not show a significant survival advantage, modest survival advantages have emerged with longer follow-up[33] or by performing a combined analysis of trials with similar designs.[34]

TABLE 86-2 Effective Adjuvant Endocrine Therapy Strategies Utilizing Aromatase Inhibitors in Postmenopausal Women

Timing of Aromatase Inhibitor (AI)	AI Shown to Be Effective	Trial Acronyms
Early use of an AI for 5 y instead of tamoxifen	Anastrozole	ATAC
	Letrozole	BIG 1-98
Sequential use of an AI in 3-5 y after an initial ~2 y of tamoxifen	Anastrozole	ABCSG 8, ARNO 95, ITA
	Exemestane	IES
Extended use of an AI for 5 y after ~5 y of tamoxifen	Letrozole (Exemestane*)	MA.17 (NSABP-B33*)

*Trial closed prematurely due to MA.17 trial results.

The optimal timing for commencement of an aromatase inhibitor in adjuvant therapy for postmenopausal women is currently uncertain. The strategies of early use versus sequential use of an aromatase inhibitor for adjuvant therapy have been compared in the BIG 1-98 trial, with results of this comparison not yet available.

The toxicity profiles of tamoxifen and aromatase inhibitors show differences that may be a factor in treatment selection or treatment changes for individual patients. While both medications result in vasomotor symptoms, on average these are somewhat more frequent with tamoxifen. Tamoxifen is more frequently associated with vaginal discharge and pruritus while aromatase inhibitors are associated with more vaginal dryness and dyspareunia. Tamoxifen tends to be somewhat protective of bone density in the postmenopausal setting, while aromatase inhibitors are associated with an increased risk for osteoporosis and fracture and monitoring of bone density is recommended. Tamoxifen is associated with an increase risk for thromboembolism compared with the aromatase inhibitors. Aromatase inhibitors appear to be associated with a less favorable profile than tamoxifen with regard to cholesterol and cardiac events. Tamoxifen is associated with an increased risk of benign and malignant gynecologic pathology and hysterectomy rates compared with aromatase inhibitors. Aromatase inhibitors may be associated with arthralgias, arthritis, and myalgias, which for some patients are sufficiently debilitating to limit therapy. Leg cramps are more frequent with tamoxifen, while carpal tunnel syndrome is more frequent with aromatase inhibitors.

Extended Use of Aromatase Inhibitors

The MA.17 trial randomized postmenopausal women with hormone receptor–positive breast cancer who had received ~5 years of adjuvant tamoxifen to either no additional therapy or to commence 5 years of extended hormonal therapy with letrozole during years 6 to 10. The MA.17 trial showed a significant reduction in the risk of breast cancer recurrence in postmenopausal women receiving extended adjuvant hormonal therapy with letrozole in years 6 to 10 after prior tamoxifen.[35] The estimated 4-year disease-free survival rates were 93% with letrozole therapy compared with 87% in the group with no additional therapy. A subsequent analysis of the MA.17 trial revealed a significant improvement in overall survival for patients with lymph node–positive tumors who received extended hormonal therapy with letrozole after 5 years of tamoxifen.[8]

PATIENT CARE ISSUES

When chemotherapy is also given, a randomized trial has shown that tamoxifen should be given sequentially following completion of the chemotherapy and not concurrently with chemotherapy.[36] Tamoxifen may be given concurrently with other therapies such as radiation and trastuzumab. Women who receive adjuvant chemotherapy followed by tamoxifen frequently report weight gain that they attribute to tamoxifen; however, in placebo-controlled breast cancer prevention trials, tamoxifen does not result in significant weight gain.

Tamoxifen is associated with an increased risk from thromboembolism. Women who are taking tamoxifen should be advised to consider temporary cessation of tamoxifen in the perioperative period, if surgery is planned.[37] The increased risk from thromboembolism and cerebrovascular events (stroke) associated with adjuvant tamoxifen therapy appears to be counterbalanced by a reduced risk of cardiovascular disease including myocardial infarction,[1,38] possibly as a result of favorable lipid changes. In a meta-analysis of randomized trials comparing aromatase inhibitors with tamoxifen in postmenopausal women, there was a significantly increased risk of grade 3 or 4 cardiovascular events, with the current generation of aromatase inhibitors compared to tamoxifen, with a relative risk ratio of 1.34 ($p = 0.004$).[39] It is uncertain whether aromatase inhibitors directly increase the risk for cardiovascular events, or whether they simply lack the protective effects of tamoxifen.

While tamoxifen is associated with an increased risk for both benign and malignant uterine pathology, there is no evidence that performing uterine ultrasound screening in asymptomatic women receiving tamoxifen is beneficial and it may result in unecessary anxiety and gynecologic procedures. Patients thought to be postmenopausal receiving either tamoxifen or an aromatase inhibitor should be encouraged to report any vaginal bleeding. In younger postmenopausal patients, initial assessment of bleeding requires ascertainment of their current hormonal status (estradiol level), and if they are confirmed as postmenopausal, gynecologic investigation is warranted.

Metabolism of tamoxifen to its active metabolite endoxifen is influenced by genetic variation and also certain medications. Medications that are potent inhibitors of tamoxifen metabolism include the antidepressants paroxetine and fluoxetine, while other antidepressants in this category such as venlafaxine are weaker inhibitors with less potential for interaction. Antidepressants may be prescribed to ameliorate vasomotor symptoms associated with tamoxifen in addition to treatment of depression. Genetic variations in cytochrome P450 2D6 (CYP2D6) may influence the response to tamoxifen and the toxicity (ie, vasomotor symptoms). Women with 2 null variant alleles of the CYP2D6 gene, which occurs in up to 10% of European and North American populations, are described as poor metabolizers. Retrospective data in postmenopausal women treated with tamoxifen suggest that poor metabolizers by virtue of either genetic variation or prescription of potent CYP2D6 inhibitors have a higher risk of breast cancer recurrence.[40]

While patient compliance with adjuvant chemotherapy is usually good, compliance is a significant issue for women recommended adjuvant hormonal therapy over several years.[41] At follow-up visits it is important to assess endocrine therapy side effects and compliance. A significant proportion of women do not complete the planned course of hormonal therapy for a variety of reasons, often related to side effects. However, some women may have poor compliance due to erroneous views on the likelihood of serious toxicities, while others may have the mistaken belief that the adjuvant hormonal therapy is less important than the chemotherapy that they completed, not fully understanding the additive benefits.

BONES AND BISPHOSPHONATES

In premenopausal women, ovarian suppression, ovarian ablation, tamoxifen, and chemotherapy have all been associated with reduced bone mineral density. If a patient is receiving adjuvant tamoxifen, then concurrent therapy with another SERM, such as raloxifene, for osteoporosis should be avoided because of potential for interactions. In postmenopausal women, tamoxifen is partially protective of bone density, while aromatase inhibitors are associated with an increased risk for osteoporosis and fracture. It is recommended that women who receive an aromatase inhibitor have a baseline DEXA (bone mineral density) scan with subsequent monitoring of bone density during therapy. Other routine measures that may be helpful in patients at risk for loss of bone density are calcium and vitamin D supplementation, regular weight-bearing exercises, and avoidance of smoking. The American Society of Clinical Oncology has developed guidelines in relation to bone health in women with breast cancer.[42]

Numerous studies have shown that both oral and intravenous bisphosphonates can mitigate treatment induced loss of bone density women with early breast cancer. However, bisphosphonates are also being studied in the adjuvant setting to determine if they can reduce the risk of recurrence/metastasis. The Austrian Breast and Colorectal Cancer Study Group ABCSG-12 trial randomized premenopausal women with hormone-responsive early breast cancer to receive 3 years of ovarian suppression (by GnRH) combined with either tamoxifen or anastrozole. Trial participants were additionally randomized to receive intravenous zolendronic acid (a bisphosphonate) twice yearly or no bisphosphonate. In a preliminary presentation of the ABCSG-12 trial results, while there were no significant differences in outcome according to the oral hormonal therapy, women who were randomized to receive zolendronic acid had

fewer relapses[13] and better bone density.[43] Other bisphosphonate trials (Z-FAST and ZO-FAST) randomized postmenopausal women receiving adjuvant endocrine therapy with an aromatase inhibitor (letrozole) to either initial zolendronic acid administered twice yearly or (delayed) zolendronic acid administered if osteoporosis developed during adjuvant hormonal therapy. These trials were designed to assess the impact bisphosphonate therapy on bones and were not powered to assess for reduction in breast cancer recurrences. However, in a joint analysis of these trials and consistent with the preliminary results of ABCSG-12 trial, there were numerically fewer recurrences observed in the patient group randomized to initial zolendronic acid.[44] Upcoming studies may shed additional light on this topic; the AZURE randomized trial tested a more frequent dosing schedule of zolendronic acid versus no zolendronic acid in women of all ages planned to receive adjuvant chemotherapy for early breast cancer, and the National Surgical Adjuvant Breast and Bowel Project (NSABP) B-34 study examined 3 years of oral clodronate versus placebo in a similar population. Results of these trials are expected shortly and may provide further evidence regarding the potential for bisphosphonate therapy to influence breast cancer recurrence rates. A randomized trial conducted by SWOG (S0307) is comparing different bisphosphonates (zolendronic acid, clodronate, and ibandronate) in the adjuvant setting.

FUTURE DIRECTIONS

There are several large randomized clinical trials of adjuvant endocrine therapy that are currently accruing or have completed accrual with final results not yet reported (Table 86-3). For premenopausal women with hormone receptor–positive breast cancer, the Tamoxifen and Exemestane Trial (TEXT) and the Suppression of Ovarian Function Trial (SOFT) are pivotal trials.[14] TEXT is comparing the efficacy of tamoxifen versus exemestane (an aromatase inhibitor) in women receiving ovarian function suppression by GnRH for 5 years. It is hoped that the improvement in outcome observed in postmenopausal women with aromatase inhibitors compared with tamoxifen can be replicated in premenopausal women who undergo ovarian function suppression (Fig. 86-1). SOFT is comparing ovarian function suppression plus tamoxifen or ovarian function suppression plus exemestane to standard endocrine therapy with tamoxifen for 5 years. Only patients who have a confirmed premenopausal estradiol level (after chemotherapy if given) are eligible for SOFT (Fig. 86-2). The Prevention of Early Menopause Study (POEMS) is enrolling premenopausal women with hormone receptor–negative breast cancer and testing if the administration of a GnRH agonist with adjuvant chemotherapy can protect against chemotherapy-induced premature ovarian failure. Because chemotherapy-induced amenorrhea is associated with a reduced risk of recurrence in women with hormone receptor–positive breast cancer,[19] the POEMS study is restricted to women with hormone receptor–negative breast cancer in whom cessation of ovarian estradiol production should theoretically provide no benefit.

In postmenopausal women, the results of the BIG 1-98 trial will be crucial in assessing the optimal way to utilize aromatase

TABLE 86-3 Adjuvant Endocrine Therapy Randomized Trials

Trial Acronym	Patient Population	Trial Treatment Arms	No. Patients
TEXT IBCSG 25-02	Premenopausal ER and/or PR positive	GnRH + tamoxifen 5 y GnRH + exemestane 5 y	2600
SOFT IBCSG 24-02	Premenopausal after chemotherapy if given ER and/or PR positive	Tamoxifen 5 y OFS + tamoxifen 5 y OFS + exemestane 5 y	3000
POEMS* SWOG 0230	Premenopausal ER and PR negative	Chemotherapy Chemotherapy + GnRH	416
BIG 1-98 IBCSG 18-98	Postmenopausal ER and/or PR positive	Tamoxifen 5 y Letrozole 5 y Tamoxifen 2 y → letrozole 3 y Letrozole 2 y → tamoxifen 3 y	8000
TEAM (amended)	Postmenopausal ER and/or PR positive	Exemestane 5 y Tamoxifen 2 y → exemestane 3 y	4400
NCIC-CTG MA.27	Postmenopausal ER and/or PR positive	Anastrozole 5 y Exemestane 5 y	6840
FACE	Postmenopausal Node positive ER and/or PR positive	Anastrozole 5 y Letrozole 5 y	4000

ER, estrogen receptor; GnRH, gonadotropin-releasing hormone agonist (triptorelin); OFS, ovarian function suppression (by GnRH or ovarian ablation); PR, progesterone receptor.
*Trial testing prevention of premature menopause.

inhibitors in clinical practice. In the BIG 1-98 trial, the comparison of 5 years of therapy with letrozole versus tamoxifen has shown that letrozole results in a reduced risk of recurrence.[26] However, the results of the BIG 1-98 trial complete 4-arm comparison that includes the sequential therapy arms are awaited and should delineate the optimal treatment strategy for postmenopausal women during the first 5 years of endocrine therapy (Fig. 86-3). The TEAM trial design was amended following trial data on aromatase inhibitor efficacy, and is now comparing exemestane monotherapy to a sequential strategy of tamoxifen followed by exemestane. The NCIC CTG MA.27 and FACE trials are performing head-to-head comparisons of different aromatase inhibitors to assess for possible differences in efficacy and/or toxicity.

The MA.17 randomized trial showed an improved outcome in postmenopausal women receiving extended adjuvant hormonal

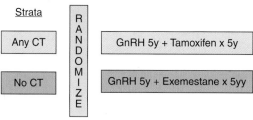

FIGURE 86-1 Schema, Tamoxifen and Exemestane Trial (TEXT) CT, chemotherapy.

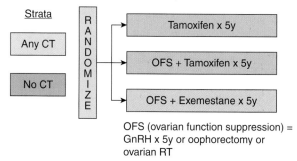

FIGURE 86-2 Schema, Suppression of Ovarian Function Trial (SOFT).

BIG 1-98 Postmenopausal trial

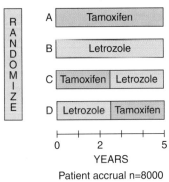

FIGURE 86-3 Breast International Group (BIG) 1-98 trial.

therapy with letrozole in years 6 to 10 after prior tamoxifen.[35] A number of other trials are testing extended adjuvant endocrine therapy in patients who have previously received approximately 5 years of adjuvant endocrine therapy (Table 86-4). The ATLAS trial randomized women to longer versus standard duration of adjuvant tamoxifen therapy with 11,500 women randomized to 10 years versus 5 years of therapy. Preliminary presentation of results described a reduction in recurrences with 10 years of therapy.[6] The aTTom trial studied a similar question and preliminary results reported a nonsignificant

decrease in recurrence with 10 years of tamoxifen.[7] Full publication of the ATLAS and aTTOM trial results is awaited. The SOLE (Study of Letrozole Extension) trial is testing the efficacy of intermittent versus continuous endocrine therapy with letrozole during years 6 to 10 in postmenopausal women who have already received ~5 years of adjuvant endocrine therapy. It is postulated that the increase in estrogen levels that occurs with the intermittent schedule may induce apoptosis in residual tumor cells that have become resistant to the prolonged aromatase inhibitor therapy low-estrogen environment. The LATER trial will test prevention of late relapses and new (second) primary breast cancers that are known to occur at increased frequency in women with a prior history of breast cancer. The NSABP B-42 and the MA.17 R (MA.17 Re-randomization) trials are studying the optimal duration of aromatase inhibitor therapy in postmenopausal women.

Necessary Future Studies

Randomized clinical trials have provided a wealth of data on adjuvant endocrine therapy that have shaped current clinical practice. However, there are adjuvant endocrine therapy questions that remain unanswered. While one randomized trial showed that sequential chemotherapy followed by tamoxifen is a superior strategy to concurrent chemo-hormonal therapy,[36] there are no data applicable to estrogen-lowering treatments such as GnRH agonists in premenopausal women and aromatase

TABLE 86-4 Trials Testing Extended Adjuvant Endocrine Therapy 5 Years or More After Initial Endocrine Therapy for Hormone Receptor–Positive Breast Cancer

Trial Acronym	Patient Population	Trial Treatment Arms	No. Patients
ATLAS	All ages ER positive/unknown Prior tamoxifen 5 y	Tamoxifen 5 more y Cease tamoxifen	11,500*
aTTOM	All ages ER positive/unknown Prior tamoxifen >4 y	Tamoxifen 5 more y Cease tamoxifen	7000
SOLE IBCSG 35-07	Postmenopausal Node positive Prior hormone Rx 4-6 y	Continuous letrozole 5 y Intermittent letrozole 5 y	4000
LATER ANZ 0501	Postmenopausal >1 y since completed 5 y of endocrine Rx	Letrozole 5 y Placebo 5 y	2500
NSABP B-42	Postmenopausal 5 y of prior endocrine Rx with either AI or tamoxifen → AI	Letrozole 5 y Placebo 5 y	3840
MA.17R	MA.17 participant or prior tamoxifen for 5 y followed by letrozole 5 y	Letrozole 5 y Placebo 5 y	4700

AI, aromatase inhibitor; ER, estrogen receptor.
*Additional patients were randomized to other durations.

inhibitors in postmenopausal women. Currently, in the absence of evidence regarding optimal scheduling for these therapies, adjuvant aromatase inhibitors are typically given after chemotherapy. Both sequential and concurrent strategies for GnRH agonists and chemotherapy have been utilized in clinical trials that were studying other questions and there is no evidence as to the optimal strategy. In addition, when GnRH therapy is utilized as an adjuvant therapy in premenopausal women, there are no trials addressing the optimal duration of therapy.

Adjuvant therapy trials are now increasingly done separately for different tumor phenotypes such as HER-2-positive and HER-2-negative breast cancer. Yet all the randomized adjuvant endocrine therapy trials thus far have been done across a broad population of hormone receptor–positive patients, which includes a minority of patients who also have HER-2-positive tumors. It is possible that the optimal endocrine strategies for patients with tumors that are HER-2 positive may differ from the optimal strategies for HER-2-negative patients. For example, the value of combining therapy with tamoxifen and ovarian suppression in this subset in premenopausal women may be different to that in the HER-2-negative subset. There remains some uncertainty regarding the benefit of 5 years of tamoxifen in premenopausal women with this tumor phenotype.

Fulvestrant (Faslodex) is an ER antagonist administered by monthly injection, and unlike tamoxifen does not exert any agonist effects. Fulvestrant has similar efficacy to anastrozole in postmenopausal women with advanced hormone-receptor-positive breast cancer. A randomized trial has been conducted in advanced breast cancer to assess if the combination of anastrozole plus fulvestrant provides better tumor control than anastrozole alone. If the trial suggests the combination is superior in advanced disease, then an adjuvant trial testing anastrozole with or without fulvestrant in postmenopausal hormone receptor–positive breast cancer will be the next step.

Further research is required into the role of genetic variations in enzymes responsible for tamoxifen metabolism and genetic variations in the enzyme (aromatase) responsible for production of estrogen in postmenopausal women. There are data to suggest increased recurrence rates among postmenopausal women who are poor metabolizers of tamoxifen due to genetic variant alleles of CYP2D6.[40] However, not all results are consistent with this finding and there is no information pertinent to premenopausal women. Genetic variations in tamoxifen-metabolizing enzymes may also be associated with variations in degree of toxicity experienced by patients (eg, vasomotor symptoms), and this area requires more detailed study for both tamoxifen and the aromatase inhibitors.

Resistance to endocrine therapy is a major problem in the treatment of hormone receptor–positive breast cancer. Methods to identify hormone receptor–positive tumors that are resistant to a particular endocrine therapy are needed. Gene microarray research that correlates variations in tumor gene expression with differences in patient outcomes may assist our future ability to predict responsiveness to specific endocrine therapies. Some progress has been made in identifying patients with hormone receptor–positive breast cancer at risk for early recurrence, but identification of patients who are destined to experience a late relapse should also be the focus of research.

Ultimately therapy tailored to specific patient and tumor features will lead to optimal adjuvant therapy.

SUMMARY

Adjuvant endocrine therapy should be considered for women with resected breast tumors that show any expression of either ER and/or PR. In patients with hormone receptor–positive breast cancer, adjuvant therapy with tamoxifen for 5 years results in significant reductions in the risk of local recurrence, distant metastases, contralateral breast cancer, and overall deaths. Benefits from tamoxifen are observed in all age groups and regardless of chemotherapy or nodal status. The benefits continue in the years after tamoxifen therapy has been ceased. Hormone receptor–positive breast cancers may relapse over a prolonged time course of up to 15 years after surgery, which suggests a role for extended endocrine therapy beyond 5 years.

For premenopausal women, tamoxifen for 5 years is the current standard of care regardless of age, menstrual status, or chemotherapy. Ovarian function suppression or ablation may be used as an alternative to chemotherapy in premenopausal women with tumors selected for endocrine responsiveness and lacking high-risk features. In premenopausal women who receive tamoxifen with or without chemotherapy, the role of adding ovarian suppression or ablation is under investigation. Aromatase inhibitors are also being investigated in premenopausal women. Chemotherapy frequently has indirect endocrine effects through suppression of ovarian function. For postmenopausal women, aromatase inhibitors are now recommended to be included as part of the adjuvant endocrine therapy, although the optimal time to commence this therapy (initially or after prior tamoxifen) and duration remain uncertain. Bisphosphonates protect against therapy-induced loss of bone density and may play a role in reducing recurrences.

REFERENCES

1. Early Breast Cancer Trialists' Collaborative Group (EBCTCG). Effects of chemotherapy and hormonal therapy for early breast cancer on recurrence and 15-year survival: an overview of the randomized trials. *Lancet.* 2005;365:1687-1717.
2. Mann GB, Fahey VD, Feleppa F, et al. Reliance on hormone receptor assays of surgical specimens may compromise outcomes in patients with breast cancer. *J Clin Oncol.* 2005;23:5148-5154.
3. Eifel P, Axelson JA, Costa J, et al. National Institutes of Health Consensus Development Conference Statement: adjuvant therapy for breast cancer, November 1-3, 2000. *J Natl Cancer Inst.* 2001;93:979-989.
4. Reebeck TR, Lynch HT, Neuhausen SL, et al. Prophylactic oophorectomy in carriers of BRCA1 or BRCA2 mutations. *N Engl J Med.* 2002;346:1616-1622.
5. International Breast Cancer Study Group. Tamoxifen after adjuvant chemotherapy for premenopausal women with lymph node-positive breast cancer: International Breast Cancer Study Group Trial 13-93. *J Clin Oncol.* 2006;24:1332-1341.
6. Peto R, Davies C, on behalf of the ATLAS Collaboration. Atlas (Adjuvant Tamoxifen, Longer Against Shorter): International randomized trial of 10 versus 5 years of adjuvant tamoxifen among 11500 women-preliminary results. San Antonio Breast Cancer Symposium, December 2007, Late Breaking Abstract # 48.
7. Gray RG, Rea DW, Handley K, et al. aTTOM (adjuvant Tamoxifen—To Offer More?): randomized trial of 10 versus 5 years of adjuvant tamoxifen among 6,934 women with estrogen receptor-positive (ER+) or ER untested breast cancer: preliminary results. *J Clin Oncol.* 2008;26 (suppl):abstract 513,105.

8. Goss PE, Ingle JN, Martino S, et al. Randomized trial of letrozole following tamoxifen as extended adjuvant therapy in receptor-positive breast cancer: updated findings from NCIC CTG MA.17. *J Natl Cancer Inst.* 2005;97:1262-1271.

9. Tetu B, Brisson J. Prognostic significance of the pattern of immunostaining and adjuvant therapy. *Cancer.* 1994;73:2358-2365.

10. Borg A, Baldetorp B, Ferno M, et al. ERBB2 amplification is assoicated with tamoxifen resistance in steroid-receptor positive breast cancer. *Cancer Lett.* 1994;81:137-144.

11. Carlomagno C, Perrone F, Gall C, et al. C-erbB2 overexpression decreases the benefit of adjuvant tamoxifen in early stage breast cancer without axillary node metastases. *J Clin Oncol.* 1996;14:2702-2708.

12. Jimenez-Gordo AM, de las Heras B, Zamora P, et al. Failure of goserelin ovarian ablation in premenopausal women with breast cancer: two case reports. *Gynecol Oncol.* 2000;76:126-127.

13. Gnant M, Mlincritsch B, Schippinger W, et al. Adjuvant ovarian suppression combined with tamoxifen or anastrozole, alone or in combination with zolendronic acid, in premenopausal women with endocrine-responsive, stage I and II breast cancer: first efficacy results from ABCSG-12. *J Clin Oncol.* 2008;26:1006s.

14. Price KN, Goldhirsch A. Clinical trials update: International Breast Cancer Study Group. *Breast Cancer Res.* 2005;7:252-254.

15. LHRH-agonists in Early Breast Cancer Overview group. Use of luteinizing-hormone-releasing hormone agonists as adjuvant treatment in premenopausal patients with hormone receptor positive breast cancer: a meta-analysis of individual patient data from randomized adjuvant trials. *Lancet.* 2007;369:1711-1723.

16. Goldhirsch A, Wood WC, Gelber RD, et al. Progress and promise: highlights of the international expert consensus on the primary therapy of early breast cancer 2007. *Ann Oncol.* 2007;18:1133-1144.

17. Davidson NE, O'Neill AM, Vukov AM, et al. Chemoendocrine therapy for premenopausal women with axillary lymph node-positive, steroid hormone receptor-positive breast cancer: results from INT 0101 (E5188). *J Clin Oncol.* 2005;23:5973-5982.

18. Love RR, Duc NB, Havighurst TC, et al. HER-2/neu overexpression and response to oophorectomy plus tamoxifen adjuvant therapy in estrogen receptor positive premenopausal women with operable breast cancer. *J Clin Oncol.* 2003; 21:453-457.

19. Pagani O, O'Neill A, Castiglione M, et al. Prognostic impact of amenorrhea after adjuvant chemotherapy in premenopausal breast cancer patients with axillary node involvement: results of International Breast Cancer Study Group (IBCSG) trial VI. *Eur J Cancer.* 1998;34:632-640.

20. Bines J, Oleske DM, Cobleigh MA. Ovarian function in premenopausal women treated with adjuvant chemotherapy for breast cancer. *J Clin Oncol.* 1996;14:1718-1729.

21. Smith IE, Dowsett M, Yap YS, et al. Adjuvant aromatase inhibitors for early breast cancer after chemotherapy-induced amenorrhea: caution and suggested guidelines. *J Clin Oncol.* 2006;24:2444-2447.

22. Winer EP, Hudis C, Burstein HJ, et al. American Society of Clinical Oncology technology assessment on the use of aromatase inhibitors as adjuvant therapy for postmenopausal women with hormone receptor-positive breast cancer: status report 2004. *J Clin Oncol.* 2005;23:619-629.

23. Mauriac L, Keshaviah A, Debled M, et al. Predictors of early relapse in postmenopausal women with hormone receptor-positive breast cancer in the BIG 1-98 trial. *Ann Oncol.* 2007;18:859-867.

24. International Breast Cancer Study Group. Toremifene and tamoxifen are equally effective for early stage breast cancer; first results of International Breast Cancer Study Group trials 12-93 and 14-93. *Ann Oncol.* 2004;15:1749-1759.

25. The ATAC (Arimidex, Tamoxifen Alone of in Combination) Trialists' Group. Anastrozole alone or in combination with tamoxifen versus tamoxifen alone for adjuvant treatment of postmenopausal women with early breast cancer: first results of the ATAC randomized trial. *Lancet.* 2002;359:2131-2139.

26. The Breast International Group (BIG) 1-98 Collaborative Group. A comparison of letrozole and tamoxifen in postmenopausal women with early breast cancer. *N Engl J Med.* 2005;353:2747-2757.

27. ATAC Trialists' Group. Effect of anastrozole and tamoxifen as adjuvant treatment for early stage breast cancer: 100-month analysis of the ATAC trial. *Lancet Oncol.* 2008;9:45-53.

28. Coates AS, Keshaviah A, Thurlimann B, et al. Five years of letrozole compared with tamoxifen as initial adjuvant therapy for postmenopausal women with enodcrine-responsive early breast cancer: update of study BIG 1-98. *J Clin Oncol.* 2007;25:486-492.

29. Kaufmann M, Jonat W, Hilfrich J, et al. on behalf of the German Adjuvant Breast Cancer Group. Survival benefit of switching to anastrozole after 2 years treatment with tamoxifen versus continued tamoxifen therapy: the ARNA 95 study. *J Clin Oncol.* 2006;24:14S; Abstract 547.

30. Coombes RC, Hall E, Gibson LJ, et al. on behalf of the Intergroup Exemestane Study. A randomized trial of exemestane after two to three years of tamoxifen therapy in postmenopausal women with primary breast cancer. *N Engl J Med.* 2004;350:1081-1092.

31. Jakesz R, Jonat W, Gnant M, et al. on behalf of the ABCSG, the GABG. Switching of postmenopausal women with endocrine responsive early breast cancer to anastrozole after 2 years adjuvant tamoxifen: combined results of ABCSG trial 8 and ARNO 95 trial. *Lancet.* 2005;366:455-462.

32. Boccardo F, Rubagotti A, Puntoni M, et al. Switching to anastrozole versus continued tamoxifen treatment of early breast cancer: preliminary results of the Italian Tamoxifen Anastrozole Trial. *J Clin Oncol.* 2005;23: 5148-5147.

33. Coombes RC, Kilburn LS, Snowdon CF, et al. Survival and safety of exemestane versus tamoxifen after 2-3 years of tamoxifen treatment (Intergroup Exemestane Study): a randomised controlled trial. *Lancet.* 2007;369:559-570. Erratum in *Lancet.* 2007;369:906.

34. Jonat W, Gnant M, Boccardo F, et al. Effectiveness of switching from adjuvant tamoxifen to anastrozole in postmenopausal women with hormone-sensitive early-stage breast cancer: a meta analysis. *Lancet Oncol.* 2006;7:991-996.

35. Goss PE, Ingle JN, Martine S, et al. A randomized trial of letrozole in postmenopausal women after 5 years of tamoxifen for early stage breast cancer. *N Engl J Med.* 2003;349;1793-1802.

36. Albain KS, Green SJ, Ravdin PM, et al. Adjuvant chemohormonal therapy for primary breast cancer should be sequential instead of concurrent: initial results from intergroup trial 0100 (SWOG-8814). *Proc Am Soc Clin Oncol.* 2002;21:37a.

37. IBIS Investigators. First results from the International Breast Cancer Intervention Study (IBIS-1): a randomized prevention trial. *Lancet.* 2002;360: 817-824.

38. Braithwaite RS, Chlebowski RT, Lau J, et al. Meta-analysis of vascular and neoplastic events associated with tamoxifen. *J Gen Intern Med.* 2003;18: 937-947.

39. Cuppone F, Bria E, Verma S, et al. Do adjuvant aromatase inhibitors increase the cardiovascular risk in postmenopausal women with early breast cancer? *Cancer.* 2008;112:260-267.

40. Goetz MP, Knox SK, Suman VJ, et al. The impact of cytochrome P450 2D6 metabolism in women receiving adjuvant tamoxifen. *Breast Cancer Res Treat.* 2007;101:113-121.

41. Partridge AH, Wang PS, Winer E, et al. Nonadherence to adjuvant tamoxifen therapy in women with primary breast cancer. *J Clin Oncol.* 2003;81:602-606.

42. Hillner BE, Ingle JN, Chlebowski RT, et al. American Society of Clinical Oncology 2003 update on the role of bisphosphonates and bone health issues in women with breast cancer. *J Clin Oncol.* 2003;21:4042-4057.

43. Gnant MF, Mlineritsch B, Luschin-Ebengreuth G, et al. Zoledronic acid prevents cancer treatment induced bone loss in premenopausal women receiving adjuvant endocrine therapy for hormone-responsive breast cancer: a report from the Austrian Breast and Colorectal Study Group. *J Clin Oncol.* 2007;25:820-828.

44. Brufsky A, Bundred N, Coleman R, et al. An Integrated analysis of zoledronic acid for prevention of aromatase inhibitor-associated bone loss in postmenopausal women with early breast cancer receiving adjuvant letrozole. *Oncologist.* 2008;13:503-514.

CHAPTER 87

Adjuvant Chemotherapy

Sara M. Tolaney
Ian E. Krop

The goal of adjuvant systemic therapy for early-stage breast cancer is to eliminate micrometastatic disease, thus preventing future recurrences. Adjuvant systemic therapy, chemotherapy, targeted therapy, and/or endocrine therapy, has led to a substantial decline in breast cancer mortality in women with operable breast cancer. Although chemotherapy can be effective in preventing distant failure, not all patients benefit. Many patients would remain disease free without therapy, and others would relapse despite treatment. The decision to use adjuvant chemotherapy involves a careful assessment of its benefits and potential risks. New insights into the biology of breast cancer have provided improved tools to predict more accurately the benefits of chemotherapy in a given patient, thus allowing chemotherapy to be used in patients who most likely will benefit and sparing those who are less likely to benefit. This chapter focuses on adjuvant systemic chemotherapy; the benefit of targeted therapy and endocrine therapy are detailed elsewhere in this text.

THE IMPACT OF CHEMOTHERAPY

The Early Breast Cancer Trialists' Collaborative Group (EBCTCG) has provided key insights about the benefits of adjuvant chemotherapy. The EBCTCG was formed to perform meta-analyses of randomized trials in the adjuvant setting and has been updated approximately every 5 years. The 2000 Overview Analysis (published in 2005) reaffirms the role of adjuvant chemotherapy in the treatment of early-stage breast cancer.[1] This analysis involved 28,764 women treated in 60 trials that randomized patients to combination chemotherapy versus no chemotherapy and demonstrated a significant improvement in both the rate of recurrence (relative risk [RR]: 0.77) and breast cancer mortality (RR: 0.83). The relative and absolute risk reductions for both recurrence and death from

adjuvant chemotherapy were similar in women with node-negative or node-positive disease, although the absolute benefits were greater in women with node-positive disease. The reduction in risk of recurrence with chemotherapy is seen within the first 5 years after randomization and is maintained at the 10- and 15-year time points.

The absolute benefit of adjuvant chemotherapy in a given patient requires knowledge of that patient's baseline risk of recurrence as well as the expected relative risk reduction from chemotherapy. A patient's baseline recurrence risk is a function of both the anatomic extent of disease (ie, tumor size and lymph node status) and the molecular characteristics of the tumor (ie, tumor grade and hormone receptor [HR] and human epidermal growth receptor 2 [HER-2] status). The RR reduction from chemotherapy (ie, a tumor's sensitivity to chemotherapy) appears to be largely based on the molecular characteristics of the tumor, independent of anatomic features, as discussed later.

Considering a patient's baseline risk and the relative benefit from chemotherapy identifies groups of patients with markedly different benefits from chemotherapy. Patients who have high baseline risk and chemo-sensitive cancers receive the greatest absolute benefit from chemotherapy, whereas those with low baseline risk and relatively chemo-insensitive cancers receive the least benefit from chemotherapy. Those patients with high baseline risk and relatively chemo-insensitive cancers and those with low baseline risk and chemo-sensitive cancers are likely to derive a modest benefit.

IMPACT OF CHEMOTHERAPY ON SPECIFIC BREAST CANCER PHENOTYPES

It is now clear that the different subtypes of breast cancer, defined by HR (estrogen and progesterone receptor [ER and PR]) expression and HER-2 status, have differing sensitivity to adjuvant chemotherapy. A recent retrospective analysis suggested that women with HR-positive breast cancer derive significantly less benefit from adjuvant chemotherapy compared with those with HR-negative breast cancer.[2] This analysis included 3 randomized trials conducted by the Cancer and Leukemia Group B (CALGB) involving 6644 women with node-positive breast cancer. Results from this study demonstrated 23% more ER-negative patients survived to 5 years without a recurrence if they received more intensive adjuvant chemotherapy compared with only 7% of patients with ER-positive tumors. The results of the Overview Analysis also support this finding, suggesting that absolute survival benefit from adjuvant chemotherapy is greater in ER-negative disease compared with ER-positive disease.[1]

A subsequent analysis of CALGB 9344 that included HER-2 status provided even more precise delineation of chemosensitivity by tumor subtype. This study evaluated the addition of paclitaxel to 4 cycles of doxorubicin and cyclophosphamide (AC) in patients with node-positive disease.[3] HER-2 positivity was associated with benefit from the addition of paclitaxel after adjuvant treatment with AC independent of ER status.[4] In contrast, cancers that were HER-2 negative and ER-positive derived little benefit from the addition of paclitaxel.

It is worth noting that data from the overview meta-analysis initially suggested patient age predicted benefit from chemotherapy. For women less than 50 years of age, adjuvant chemotherapy reduced the risk of recurrence and death from breast cancer by 37% and 30%, respectively.[1] For women 50 to 69 years of age, the risk of recurrence and death from breast cancer was decreased by 19% and 12%, respectively. However, in an updated analysis, focusing only on patients with HR-negative cancers, benefits from chemotherapy were similar in older and younger women.[5] This finding suggests that the earlier analysis may have been influenced by the fact that HR-negative breast cancer is much more common in younger women then in older women and that if controlled for tumor biology, the impact of age on chemotherapy benefit is uncertain.

SELECTION OF PATIENTS FOR THERAPY

Although receptor status can be helpful in making decisions about chemotherapy as described earlier, baseline risk factors such tumor size, lymph node status, and tumor grade must also be taken into consideration. A Web-based program, Adjuvant! Online, is available to help in estimating the risk of disease recurrence and death for patients with and without adjuvant chemotherapy.[6] This tool uses information derived from SEER databases, meta-analyses, and individual studies. Population-based validation studies have confirmed the value of this program.[7]

In addition to computerized modeling, genomic assays of tumor samples may also help in the selection of the optimal adjuvant treatment approach. The Oncotype DX assay is a 21-gene panel performed on paraffin-embedded tumor tissue using reverse transcriptase-polymerase chain reaction analysis. This assay uses the expression pattern of 16 breast cancer–associated genes to derive a recurrence score (RS) based on their expression profile relative to 5 reference genes. RS were initially obtained in 668 tumor blocks from patients with node-negative breast cancer who were treated with tamoxifen on NSABP B-14.[8,9] RS was

divided into low- (RS <18), intermediate-(18-30), or high-risk (≥31), and Kaplan-Meier estimates of 10-year recurrence rates were 7%, 14%, and 31%, respectively. In addition, they were able to demonstrate a significant relationship between RS and overall survival. Further analysis was done using 651 patients enrolled in NSABP B-20.[10] This trial randomized patients with node-negative ER-positive breast cancer to tamoxifen alone or tamoxifen with chemotherapy. Distant recurrence-free survival (DRFS) rates were not significantly different in patients with low RS treated with tamoxifen with or without chemotherapy; however, DRFS was significantly worse in patients with high RS who received tamoxifen alone without chemotherapy. This suggests that chemotherapy is not beneficial for patients with node-negative ER-positive breast cancer receiving tamoxifen with a low RS, but it does provides significant benefit to those with a high RS. The benefits of adjuvant chemotherapy in individuals with intermediate RS are unclear. To better define the benefits of adjuvant treatment for those with intermediate scores, the TAILORx study is randomizing these patients to hormonal therapy alone or chemotherapy followed by hormonal therapy.[11] Of note is the fact that the RS criteria for an intermediate score were changed from 11 to 25 for the trial. The study plans to enroll at least 10,000 women with HR-positive, HER-2-negative, node-negative breast cancer. However the trial results will likely not be available until 2013. Although data from the NSABP B-14 and B-20 indicate that the Oncotype DX test can be used to help determine if adjuvant chemotherapy may be beneficial in women with ER-positive node-negative tumors, there are now recent studies suggesting that this test may also be helpful in node-positive patients.[12,13]

Other genomic tests are available in addition to Oncotype DX, however, these tests require fresh-frozen tissue, making their applicability more limited.[14] The Mammoprint assay is a 70-gene assay that is offered as a prognostic test for women less than 61 years of age with either ER-positive or ER negative breast cancer.[15] The test results are dichotomous and report either a high or low risk of recurrence. It has not yet been studied if the assay can also predict sensitivity to adjuvant therapies. The Microarray In Node Negative Disease May Avoid Chemotherapy (MINDACT) trial is a prospective trial of primarily lymph node-negative breast cancer that opened in August 2007.[16] All patients are assessed by prognostic factors included in Adjuvant! Online and by the 70-gene Mammoprint assay. If both assays predict a high-risk status, the patient receives adjuvant cytotoxic chemotherapy and also hormonal therapy if ER positive. If both assays indicate a low risk, no chemotherapy is given, and ER-positive patients are given hormonal therapy only. When there is discordance between the prediction of risk as assessed by Adjuvant! Online and the Mammoprint assay, patients are randomized to receive treatment based on either the Mammoprint or Adjuvant! Online results.

In addition to these tools to help clinicians predict risk of recurrence and possible benefit from adjuvant therapies, practice guidelines are put together by 2 major groups: the National Comprehensive Cancer Network (NCCN) and the St. Gallen Consensus.[17] The NCCN guidelines suggest consideration of chemotherapy for women whose breast cancers are 1 cm or more or node positive, regardless of receptor status. These guidelines recommend taking into consideration tumor grade and the presence of lymphovascular invasion for patients with tumors between 0.6 to 1.0 cm to determine if adjuvant chemotherapy should be administered. Trastuzumab is recommended, in addition to adjuvant chemotherapy for women with HER-2-positive tumors 1 cm or more or node positive.

TIMING OF THERAPY

Chemotherapy may be administered prior to surgery or after surgical resection. Although neoadjuvant chemotherapy was initially used for locally advanced breast cancer, it has become more common to use in patients with operable breast cancer. This approach allows more individuals to undergo breast-conserving therapy (BCT) and also allows the observation of responses to systemic treatment within the breast. The foundation for the use of preoperative chemotherapy in operable breast cancer came from the National Surgical Adjuvant Breast and Bowel Project (NSABP) B-18 trial, which randomized women to 4 cycles of AC either before or after surgery and found no statistically significant differences in disease-free survival (DFS) and overall survival (OS) between the 2 groups.[18,19] Preoperative therapy reduced tumor size in about 80% of women, and significantly more were able to undergo BCT (68% vs 60%; *p* = 0.001). These findings have been confirmed in other preoperative studies, including NSABP B-27.[19,20] Although it is true that preoperative treatment allows tumor response in the breast to be monitored during treatment, it should be noted that there are no clear data to indicate how that information can be used to influence further treatment in that individual.

If chemotherapy is administered postoperatively, therapy is generally administered 4 to 6 weeks after surgery. A retrospective analysis found there was no statistically significant benefit to DFS or OS to starting chemotherapy less than 3 weeks compared with more than 3 weeks after surgery.[21] There is, however, data to suggest that a delay to chemotherapy of more than 12 weeks reduces both DFS and OS.[22]

Many women who receive adjuvant chemotherapy also require radiation therapy. Concurrent administration of chemotherapy and radiation therapy is not recommended due to concerns for increased toxicity. There is some theoretical concern that delaying radiation until after chemotherapy may lead to a higher incidence of local recurrence, particularly with the use of more prolonged chemotherapy regimens. A prospective randomized trial was conducted that randomized women to postoperative radiation either before or after chemotherapy, and it found no significant difference in rates of locoregional or distant recurrence, or death.[23,24] Given these data, radiation therapy is generally not initiated until completion of adjuvant chemotherapy.

Just as radiation therapy should be delayed until completion of chemotherapy, hormonal therapy also should not be initiated until after completion of chemotherapy for patients with HR-positive breast cancer. The Southwest Oncology Group (SWOG) 8814 study of postmenopausal women with node-positive, ER-positive breast cancer randomized 1477 women to 1 of 3 arms: tamoxifen alone for 5 years; 6 cycles of cyclophosphamide, doxorubicin, and 5-fluorouracil (CAF) with concurrent

tamoxifen; or 6 cycles of CAF followed by tamoxifen. This study demonstrated that the 10-year DFS (60% vs 53%) and OS (68 vs 62%) were superior in patients given sequential chemotherapy and tamoxifen compared with those given concurrent therapy. As a result of these data, sequential rather than concurrent therapy has been adopted as the standard of care when both chemotherapy and hormonal therapy are administered.[25]

OPTIMAL CHEMOTHERAPY REGIMENS

The benefits of combination chemotherapy for the adjuvant treatment of early-stage breast cancer were initially established in the 1970s by Bonadonna and colleagues.[26] They randomized lymph node-positive patients after mastectomy to 12 monthly cycles of cyclophosphamide, methotrexate, and 5-fluorouracil (CMF) or to observation and found that CMF results in a significant improvement in DFS and OS. A subsequent study evaluated the possibility of reducing the duration of CMF and found that 6 cycles of CMF yielded identical results to those obtained with 12 cycles.[27] A long-term analysis with a median follow-up of 25 years confirmed that longer duration of treatment did not improve treatment outcome, with an estimated DFS of 39% after 12 cycles and 38% after 6 cycles.[28]

Over the next several years, multiple randomized trials evaluated the benefit of anthracyclines in adjuvant therapy. The National Surgical Adjuvant Breast and Bowel Project (NSABP) B-15 and B-23 studies found that 4 cycles of AC was equivalent to 6 cycles of CMF with regard to DFS and OS.[29,30] The 2000 Overview Analysis compared CMF-based and anthracycline-based polychemotherapy and found that among the 14,000 women they examined, there was a small but significant improvement in DFS and OS favoring anthracycline-containing regimens.[1] Although 4 cycles of AC has not directly been shown to be superior to CMF, AC chemotherapy has become a commonly used regimen, likely in part due to the shorter duration of this regimen.

Multiple randomized trials have examined the benefit of adding a taxane (either paclitaxel or docetaxel) to anthracycline-based adjuvant chemotherapy (Table 87-1). Two large randomized trials have examined the use of paclitaxel in addition to anthracycline-based chemotherapy, and both of these studies suggest a survival benefit for the addition of paclitaxel. CALGB 9344 found that the addition of paclitaxel to AC was associated with an improvement in 5-year DFS (70% vs 65%) and OS (80% vs 77%).[3] An unplanned subgroup analysis suggested that the benefit may be restricted to ER-negative breast cancer. NSABP B-28 was a similar study that randomized 3060 node-positive patients to 4 cycles of AC with or without sequential paclitaxel, and demonstrated an improvement in 5-year DFS (76% vs 72%) but no difference in OS.[31] As opposed to CALGB 9344, this study did not demonstrate a difference in benefit based on ER status.

Four large studies have evaluated the benefit of adding docetaxel to an anthracycline-based regimen. Two of these 4 trials demonstrated an improvement in survival with the addition of docetaxel; 2 did not. The first of these studies, PACS 01, randomized 1999 patients to 6 cycles of fluorouracil,

TABLE 87-1 Adjuvant Taxane Trials

Trial	Arms	DFS, %	p Value	OS, %	p Value
CALGB 9344*	AC	65	0.002	77	0.006
	AC → P	70		80	
NSABP B-28	AC	72	0.008	85	0.46
	AC → P	76		85	
PACS 01	FEC × 6	73	0.041	87	0.05
	FEC × 3 → D × 3	78		91	
BCIRG 001 (TAX 316)	TAC × 6	75	0.001	87	0.008
	FAC × 6	68		81	
NSABP B-27	AC	67	—	81	—
	AC → D	72	0.22	83	0.82
	AC → Surgery → D	70	0.24	81	0.51
ECOG 2197	AC	85	0.78	91	0.62
	AT	85		92	
US Oncology	AC	80	0.015	87	0.13
	TC	86		90	

AC, doxorubicin and cyclophosphamide; AT, doxorubicin and docetaxel; D, docetaxel; DFS, disease-free survival; FAC, 5-fluorouracil, doxorubicin, and cyclophosphamide; FEC, fluorouracil, epirubicin, and cyclophosphamide; OS, overall survival; P, paclitaxel; TAC, docetaxel, doxorubicin, and cyclophosphamide; TC, docetaxel and cyclophosphamide.
*Trial was actually a 3 × 2 design; patients were randomized to 1 of 3 doses of doxorubicin (60 mg/m^2, 75 mg/m^2, or 90 mg/m^2) that was administered with cyclophosphamide, 600 mg/m^2; after treatment with AC, patients were randomized to paclitaxel or no paclitaxel.

epirubicin, and cyclophosphamide (FEC) or to 3 cycles of FEC followed by 3 cycles of docetaxel (FEC-D) as adjuvant therapy for node-positive breast cancer,[32] and demonstrated FEC-D resulted in an improvement in DFS (73.2% vs 78.4%) and OS (90.7% vs 86.7%). The Breast Cancer International Research Group (BCIRG) study 001 (TAX 316) randomly assigned 1491 patients with node-positive breast cancer to docetaxel plus doxorubicin and cyclophosphamide (TAC) for 6 cycles or 5-fluorouracil plus doxorubicin and cyclophosphamide (FAC) for 6 cycles and demonstrated an improvement in DFS (75% vs 68%) and OS (87% vs 81%) for those receiving TAC.[33] Two other trials, however, failed to demonstrate an improvement with the addition of docetaxel. NSABP B-27 randomized 2411 women to 4 cycles of AC followed by surgery, 4 cycles of AC followed by docetaxel and then surgery, or 4 cycles of AC followed by surgery and then docetaxel for 4 cycles.[34] The addition of preoperative or postoperative docetaxel after preoperative AC did not significantly improve DFS or OS. The ECOG 2197 trial randomized patients to 4 cycles of AC versus 4 cycles of doxorubicin plus docetaxel (AT) every 3 weeks and found no difference in DFS (85% in both arms) or OS (91% vs 92%), but did find that AT was associated with more toxicity.[35]

There has also been an interest in evaluating whether a taxane can replace an anthracycline. The US Oncology trial randomized 1016 women with node-negative and node-positive breast cancer to 4 cycles of AC or to 4 cycles of docetaxel plus cyclophosphamide (TC) administered every 3 weeks. This study demonstrated an improvement in both DFS (86% vs 80%) and OS (90% vs 87%) favoring TC over AC.[36] There was a higher incidence of myalgia, arthralgia, edema, and febrile neutropenia in patients receiving TC, whereas there was more nausea and vomiting in those receiving AC. Based on this data, many physicians have started administering TC to patients with underlying cardiac disease instead of AC. However it is still unclear as to how TC will compare to more prolonged chemotherapy regimens, such as dose-dense AC followed by paclitaxel.

The schedule of administration of taxane after adjuvant anthracycline therapy also appears to be important. The ECOG 1199 trial enrolled 4950 women, all of whom were initially treated with 4 cycles of AC administered every 3 weeks, and were then randomized to 4 cycles of paclitaxel or docetaxel given every 3 weeks for 4 cycles or the same agents weekly for 12 weeks.[37] Both the weekly paclitaxel and the every 3 week docetaxel demonstrated a statistically significant improvement in DFS compared with every 3 week paclitaxel. Overall survival was improved for weekly paclitaxel compared with every 3 week paclitaxel. This study also found that neuropathy was more frequent with the weekly paclitaxel than with the every 3 week paclitaxel. Although this study demonstrates that 4 cycles of AC administered every 3 weeks followed by 12 weekly doses of paclitaxel is the preferred approach, this regimen has not yet been compared with dose-dense AC followed by paclitaxel (discussed later).

DOSE INTENSITY AND DOSE DENSITY

In vitro data provided initial support for the idea that a higher dose of chemotherapy per cycle administered may not only provide additional benefit from the chemotherapy agent but might also provide the ability to overcome drug resistance. This concept was tested in CALGB 8541, which randomized 1550 women with node-positive breast cancer to 1 of 3 dose levels of CAF. Both DFS and OS were superior for patients on the moderate-dose and high-dose arms, compared with those on the low-dose arms. The dose administered on the high-dose arm is now considered the standard CAF regimen. NSABP B22 and B25 evaluated escalating doses of cyclophosphamide with a set dose of doxorubicin and found no benefit for the higher dose cyclophosphamide in terms of DFS or OS.[38,39] In addition, higher cyclophosphamide doses are associated with a higher incidence of acute myelogenous leukemia and myelodysplastic syndrome. CALGB 9344 examined the benefit of escalating doses of doxorubicin in addition to a standard dose of cyclophosphamide and found that higher doses of doxorubicin were not associated with an improvement in DFS or OS.[3] Given the data just cited, escalating doses of anthracycline or alkylator therapy have not led to an improvement in outcome, and therefore standard doses of these agents are what are currently being administered in clinical practice.

Although dose escalation of chemotherapy has not been demonstrated to improve outcomes in breast cancer, there does appear to be a benefit to increasing the density of chemotherapy. The concept of dose-dense chemotherapy is based on the Norton-Simon model, which predicts that shortening the dosing interval without increasing the dose will minimize tumor cell regrowth between cycles.[40] Dose density has been tested in a large phase III trial in node-positive breast cancer in CALGB 9741. This study compared sequential doxorubicin, 60 mg/m^2, paclitaxel, 175 mg/m^2, and cyclophosphamide, 600 mg/m^2, against concurrent Adriamycin and cyclophosphamide for 4 cycles followed by paclitaxel for 4 cycles, at the same dose levels. A separate randomization compared every 2 week with every 3 week dosing. The every 2-week chemotherapy was given with granulocyte colony-stimulating factor (G-CSF). Dose-dense chemotherapy given every 2 weeks was associated with a significant improvement in DFS and OS compared with the standard every 3-week regimen.[41] Furthermore, the use of G-CSF in the every 2-week schedule resulted in a significant decrease in the incidence of grade IV neutropenia and fewer treatment delays due to hematologic toxicity.[42] Dose-dense chemotherapy has become a standard adjuvant chemotherapy regimen for patients with node-positive early-stage breast cancer.

TOXICITY OF TREATMENT

Both acute and potential long-term toxicities from adjuvant chemotherapy may occur. Since the development of more effective antiemetic therapies and growth factor support, chemotherapy has become more tolerable to patients. Potential acute side effects from treatment include alopecia, nausea, emesis, fatigue, mucositis, myelosuppression, and anemia. Specific toxicities depend on the chemotherapy agent administered. Taxane-based therapy may be associated with neuropathy, myalgias, and hypersensitivity reactions, whereas anthracycline-based therapy is associated with more nausea, mucositis, and gastrointestinal disturbances.

In addition to these acute toxicities, long-term side effects from treatment may occur. Potential long-term sequelae include weight gain,[43,44] ovarian failure with associated menopausal symptoms,[45] osteoporosis, neuropathy,[46] cognitive dysfunction,[47,48] fatigue,[49] and sexual difficulties.[50] The most serious long-term complications from chemotherapy include cardiac dysfunction and leukemia. Congestive heart failure develops in 0.5 to 1.0% of patients receiving an anthracycline-based regimen, and in approximately 0.5% to 4% of patients receiving trastuzumab-based therapy.[51,52] Leukemia is a rare complication and occurs in less than 0.5% of women after anthracycline-based treatment.[53] Because of these potential long-term toxicities, follow-up care for breast cancer survivors is an integral part of their therapy.[54] In general, patients should have follow-up visits every 6 months for 2 to 5 years, and then annually thereafter.[55]

FUTURE DIRECTIONS

The development of new targeted therapies has revolutionized the treatment of breast cancer. Although it is clear that trastuzumab has resulted in dramatic improvements for women with HER-2-positive breast cancer, approximately 15% of patients treated with trastuzumab-based therapy in the adjuvant setting still relapse (Table 87-2).[56] In an effort to decrease recurrence

TABLE 87-2 Adjuvant Trastuzumab Trials

Trial	Treatment Arm	Control Arm	No. of Patients	Hazard Ratio for DFS	p Value
NSABP B-31/NCCTG 9831	AC → PH	AC → P	3969	0.49	<0.0001
HERA	Chemotherapy → H	Chemotherapy	3387	0.54	<0.0001
BCIRG-006	AC → DH	AC → D	3222	0.49	<0.0001
	DCH			0.61	0.00015
FinHer	DH → CEF	D → CEF	232	0.46	0.0078
	VH → CEF	V → CEF			

AC, doxorubicin and cyclophosphamide; CEF, cyclophosphamide, epirubicin, and 5-fluorouracil; D, docetaxel; DCH, docetaxel, carboplatin, and trastuzumab; DFS, disease-free survival; H, trastuzumab; P, paclitaxel; V, vinorelbine.

rates further, investigators are evaluating whether new HER-2-targeted agents such as lapatinib may provide benefit when administered either with, or instead of, trastuzumab. Lapatinib is an oral small molecule dual kinase inhibitor of epidermal growth factor receptor and HER-2. Lapatinib has demonstrated activity as a single agent in HER-2-positive metastatic breast cancer in phase II trials,[57] and evidence from a phase III study in 2006 demonstrated that lapatinib in combination with capecitabine is active in patients who progressed on prior trastuzumab-containing regimens.[58] There are also recent data to suggest that the combination of trastuzumab and lapatinib may be superior to lapatinib alone based on data in the metastatic setting.[59] The ALTTO trial is a 4-arm study, with a goal accrual of 8000 patients, evaluating standard adjuvant chemotherapy followed by trastuzumab versus lapatinib versus the combination versus the sequence. This trial will help answer the question as to whether the combination of trastuzumab and lapatinib is superior to either single agent when administered in the adjuvant setting (Table 87-3).

Bevacizumab is a humanized monoclonal antibody against vascular endothelial growth factor that has demonstrated efficacy in the metastatic setting.[60] A pilot study was conducted looking at the combination of dose-dense chemotherapy with bevacizumab and demonstrated feasibility of this regimen. This has led to a large adjuvant trial, ECOG 5103, a double-blind randomized trial that will enroll approximately 5000 patients with node-positive or high-risk node-negative breast cancer. Patients will be randomized to 1 of 3 arms: AC followed by weekly paclitaxel, AC with bevacizumab followed by weekly paclitaxel with bevacizumab, or AC with bevacizumab followed by weekly paclitaxel with bevacizumab followed by bevacizumab

monotherapy. This trial will not only help establish whether bevacizumab adds to standard adjuvant chemotherapy for breast cancer but will also address whether increasing the duration of exposure to bevacizumab is beneficial. There is also interest in exploring whether adding bevacizumab to trastuzumab-based therapy will be beneficial for HER-2-positive patients, and several trials are ongoing investing this combination.

The use of platinum-based chemotherapy for patients with triple-negative (HR- and HER-2-negative) breast cancer is also being explored. Evidence indicates that BRCA tumors may be less capable of repairing specific types of DNA errors, and in vitro data suggest that these tumors are particularly sensitive to the DNA damage induced by cisplatin chemotherapy.[61] It therefore seems reasonable to believe that tumors with a similar phenotype to BRCA tumors, the triple-negative tumors, may also demonstrate sensitivity to cisplatin. There are currently studies investigating the use of cisplatin in both the neoadjuvant and adjuvant setting for these triple-negative tumors.

The inherent DNA repair defect in BRCA-deficient cells has also provided a rationale for the approach of inhibiting the DNA repair protein PARP (polyadenosine 5' diphosphoribose polymerase) to generate lesions that require BRCA for repair, resulting in synthetic lethality.[62] PARP inhibitors, with and without the use of cisplatin, are currently being tested in clinical trials.

NECESSARY FUTURE STUDIES

There have been several exciting developments for the treatment of breast cancer over the past several years, including the development of trastuzumab, which has revolutionized the

TABLE 87-3 Future Directions: Ongoing and Planned Studies

Trial	Treatment Arms	No. of Patients	Status of Trial
ECOG 5103	AC → P AC + B → P + B AC + B → P + B → B	4950	Open
BCIRG 006 (BCIRG)	DCH (or DH → FEC) + H DCHB or (DHB → FEC) → HB	3500	Open
ALTTO	Completion anthracycline-based chemotherapy, administered with or without concurrent paclitaxel: H × 52 wk L × 52 wk H → L (total 52 wk) H + L × 52 wk	8000	Open
TAILORx	OncotypeDX <11: hormonal therapy OncotypeDX 11–25: randomized to hormonal therapy or chemotherapy OncotypeDx >25: chemotherapy	10,000	Open
US Oncology	TC vs TAC	2000	Open
CALGB 40101	AC × 4 vs P × 4 vs AC × 6 vs P × 6	4646	Open

AC, doxorubicin and cyclophosphamide; B, bevacizumab; D, docetaxel; DCH, docetaxel, carboplatin, and trastuzumab; H, trastuzumab; P, paclitaxel; TAC, docetaxel, doxorubicin, and cyclophosphamide; TC, docetaxel, cyclophosphamide.

treatment of patients with HER-2-positive disease. In addition, there are several new biological agents, including bevacizumab and lapatinib, which may enhance the efficacy of standard chemotherapy. With increasing awareness that breast cancer is not just one disease but many distinct subtypes, the treatment of breast cancer will continue to evolve. The goal will be to further tailor treatment to the biology of the individual's tumor, and this will come about through adjuvant and neoadjuvant trials that include robust correlative assays to identify biomarkers that predict responsiveness and resistance to therapy. These studies will not only help us predict response to chemotherapy but will likely help lead to the development of additional targeted therapies. It will also be important to develop methods to predict who will develop specific toxicities to individual therapies, in order to help prevent adverse effects from treatment. Focusing on a more individualized approach to breast cancer treatment will allow for continued improvements in efficacy while minimizing toxicity.

SUMMARY

Adjuvant chemotherapy for the treatment of breast cancer is an important part of therapy for many patients with operable breast cancer, and its use has contributed to the overall decline in mortality from this disease. Not all patients will benefit, however, and the decision to use chemotherapy in an individual requires an understanding of the absolute risk reduction the patient can expect from chemotherapy. To calculate this risk reduction requires knowledge of the patient's baseline risk of recurrence and the relative benefit of chemotherapy based on the molecular subtype of their tumor. Anatomic features, such as tumor size and lymph node involvement, as well as the cancer's biological characteristics, such as grade and receptor status, factor into this calculation. More recently, genomic tests such as the Oncotype DX recurrence score can provide additional accuracy in calculating the benefits of chemotherapy. Once the absolute risk reduction associated with chemotherapy is known, it must be balanced against the toxicity of the treatment. A patient's preferences are also an important factor in the decision whether to include chemotherapy in an individual's treatment program.

When deciding on the particular chemotherapy regimen to use, in general, for patients with lower risk disease, AC for 4 cycles or docetaxel and cyclophosphamide (TC) for 4 cycles may be considered. If patients have higher risk tumors, dose-dense chemotherapy with AC followed by paclitaxel or docetaxel plus doxorubicin, and cyclophosphamide (TAC) can be administered. At this point, there are no clear data indicating that HR status should be used to select a specific type of chemotherapy. For patients with node-positive, HER-2-positive breast cancer, AC followed by paclitaxel and trastuzumab (ACTH) or docetaxel, carboplatin, and trastuzumab (TCH) should be considered. Several biological agents are also being investigated in clinical trials that may change the future of adjuvant chemotherapy. Patients should be followed carefully during and after completion of chemotherapy to monitor for any potential toxicity.

REFERENCES

1. Effects of chemotherapy and hormonal therapy for early breast cancer on recurrence and 15-year survival: an overview of the randomised trials. *Lancet.* 2005;365(9472):1687-1717.
2. Berry DA, Cirrincione C, Henderson IC, et al. Estrogen-receptor status and outcomes of modern chemotherapy for patients with node-positive breast cancer. *JAMA.* 2006;295(14):1658-1667.
3. Henderson IC, Berry DA, Demetri GD, et al. Improved outcomes from adding sequential Paclitaxel but not from escalating Doxorubicin dose in an adjuvant chemotherapy regimen for patients with node-positive primary breast cancer. *J Clin Oncol.* 2003;21(6):976-983.
4. Hayes DF, Thor AD, Dressler LG, et al. HER2 and response to paclitaxel in node-positive breast cancer. *N Engl J Med.* 2007;357(15):1496-1506.
5. Adjuvant chemotherapy in oestrogen-receptor-poor breast cancer: patient-level meta-analysis of randomised trials. *Lancet.* 2008;371(9606):29-40.
6. Ravdin PM, Siminoff LA, Davis GJ, et al. Computer program to assist in making decisions about adjuvant therapy for women with early breast cancer. *J Clin Oncol.* 2001;19(4):980-991.
7. Olivotto IA, Bajdik CD, Ravdin PM, et al. Population-based validation of the prognostic model ADJUVANT! for early breast cancer. *J Clin Oncol.* 2005;23(12):2716-2725.
8. Fisher B, Dignam J, Bryant J, Wolmark N. Five versus more than five years of tamoxifen for lymph node-negative breast cancer: updated findings from the National Surgical Adjuvant Breast and Bowel Project B-14 randomized trial. *J Natl Cancer Inst.* 2001;93(9):684-690.
9. Paik S, Shak S, Tang G, et al. A multigene assay to predict recurrence of tamoxifen-treated, node-negative breast cancer. *N Engl J Med.* 2004; 351(27):2817-2826.
10. Paik S, Tang G, Shak S, et al. Gene expression and benefit of chemotherapy in women with node-negative, estrogen receptor-positive breast cancer. *J Clin Oncol.* 2006;24(23):3726-3734.
11. Sparano JA. TAILORx: trial assigning individualized options for treatment (Rx). *Clin Breast Cancer.* 2006;7(4):347-350.
12. Albain K, Barlow W, Shak S, et al. Prognostic and predictive value of the 21 gene recurrence score assay in postmenopausal, node-positive, ER-positive breast cancer (S8814, INT0100). *Breast Cancer Res Treat.* 2007;106(S1):A10.
13. Loldstein L, Ravdin P, Gray R, et al. Prognostic utility of the 21-gene assay compared with Adjuvant! in hormone receptor (HR) positive operable breast cancer with 0-3 positive axillary nodes treated with adjuvant chemo-hormonal therapy (CHT): an analysis of intergroup trail E2197. *Breast Cancer Res Treat.* 2007;106 (S1):A63.
14. Ross JS, Hatzis C, Symmans WF, Pusztai L, Hortobagyi GN. Commercialized multigene predictors of clinical outcome for breast cancer. *Oncologist.* 2008;13(5):477-493.
15. van de Vijver MJ, He YD, van't Veer LJ, et al. A gene-expression signature as a predictor of survival in breast cancer. *N Engl J Med.* 2002;347(25):1999-2009.
16. Bogaerts J, Cardoso F, Buyse M, et al. Gene signature evaluation as a prognostic tool: challenges in the design of the MINDACT trial. *Nat Clin Pract Oncol.* 2006;3(10):540-551.
17. National Comprehensive Cancer Network (NCCN) guidelines. Available at: www.ncn.org/professionals/physician_gls/default.asp. Accessed 10.30.09.
18. Fisher B, Bryant J, Wolmark N, et al. Effect of preoperative chemotherapy on the outcome of women with operable breast cancer. *J Clin Oncol.* 1998;16(8):2672-2685.
19. Rastogi P, Anderson SJ, Bear HD, et al. Preoperative chemotherapy: updates of National Surgical Adjuvant Breast and Bowel Project Protocols B-18 and B-27. *J Clin Oncol.* 2008;26(5):778-785.
20. Bear HD, Anderson S, Brown A, et al. The effect on tumor response of adding sequential preoperative docetaxel to preoperative doxorubicin and cyclophosphamide: preliminary results from National Surgical Adjuvant Breast and Bowel Project Protocol B-27. *J Clin Oncol.* 2003;21(22):4165-4174.
21. Shannon C, Ashley S, Smith IE. Does timing of adjuvant chemotherapy for early breast cancer influence survival? *J Clin Oncol.* 2003;21(20):3792-3797.
22. Lohrisch C, Paltiel C, Gelmon K, et al. Impact on survival of time from definitive surgery to initiation of adjuvant chemotherapy for early-stage breast cancer. *J Clin Oncol.* 2006;24(30):4888-4894.
23. Recht A, Come SE, Henderson IC, et al. The sequencing of chemotherapy and radiation therapy after conservative surgery for early-stage breast cancer. *N Engl J Med.* 1996;334(21):1356-1361.
24. Bellon JR, Come SE, Gelman RS, et al. Sequencing of chemotherapy and radiation therapy in early-stage breast cancer: updated results of a prospective randomized trial. *J Clin Oncol.* 2005;23(9):1934-1940.

25. Albain KS BW, O'Malley F, et al. Concurrent (CAFT) versus sequential (CAF-T) chemohormonal therapy (cyclophosphamide, doxorubicin, 5-fluorouracil, tamoxifen) versus T alone for postmenopausal, node-positive, estrogen (ER) and/or progesterone (PgR) receptor-positive breast cancer: mature outcomes and new biologic correlates on phase III intergroup trial 0100 (SWOG-8814). San Antonio Breast Cancer Symposium 2004. Abstract 37.

26. Bonadonna G, Brusamolino E, Valagussa P, et al. Combination chemotherapy as an adjuvant treatment in operable breast cancer. *N Engl J Med.* 1976;294(8):405-410.

27. Tancini G, Bonadonna G, Valagussa P, Marchini S, Veronesi U. Adjuvant CMF in breast cancer: comparative 5-year results of 12 versus 6 cycles. *J Clin Oncol.* 1983;1(1):2-10.

28. Bonadonna G, Moliterni A, Zambetti M, et al. 30 years' follow up of randomised studies of adjuvant CMF in operable breast cancer: cohort study. *BMJ.* 2005;330(7485):217.

29. Fisher B, Brown AM, Dimitrov NV, et al. Two months of doxorubicin-cyclophosphamide with and without interval reinduction therapy compared with 6 months of cyclophosphamide, methotrexate, and fluorouracil in positive-node breast cancer patients with tamoxifen-nonresponsive tumors: results from the National Surgical Adjuvant Breast and Bowel Project B-15. *J Clin Oncol.* 1990;8(9):1483-1496.

30. Fisher B, Anderson S, Tan-Chiu E, et al. Tamoxifen and chemotherapy for axillary node-negative, estrogen receptor-negative breast cancer: findings from National Surgical Adjuvant Breast and Bowel Project B-23. *J Clin Oncol.* 2001;19(4):931-942.

31. Mamounas EP, Bryant J, Lembersky B, et al. Paclitaxel after doxorubicin plus cyclophosphamide as adjuvant chemotherapy for node-positive breast cancer: results from NSABP B-28. *J Clin Oncol.* 2005;23(16):3686-3696.

32. Roche H, Fumoleau P, Spielmann M, et al. Sequential adjuvant epirubicin-based and docetaxel chemotherapy for node-positive breast cancer patients: the FNCLCC PACS 01 Trial. *J Clin Oncol.* 2006;24(36):5664-5671.

33. Martin M, Pienkowski T, Mackey J, et al. Adjuvant docetaxel for node-positive breast cancer. *N Engl J Med.* 2005;352(22):2302-2313.

34. Bear HD, Anderson S, Smith RE, et al. Sequential preoperative or postoperative docetaxel added to preoperative doxorubicin plus cyclophosphamide for operable breast cancer: National Surgical Adjuvant Breast and Bowel Project Protocol B-27. *J Clin Oncol.* 2006;24(13):2019-2027.

35. Goldstein LJ, O'Neill A, Sparano JA, et al. Concurrent doxorubicin plus docetaxel is not more effective than concurrent doxorubicin plus cyclophosphamide in operable breast cancer with 0 to 3 positive axillary nodes: North American Breast Cancer Intergroup Trial E 2197. *J Clin Oncol.* 2008;26(25):4092-4099.

36. Jones SE, Savin MA, Holmes FA, et al. Phase III trial comparing doxorubicin plus cyclophosphamide with docetaxel plus cyclophosphamide as adjuvant therapy for operable breast cancer. *J Clin Oncol.* 2006;24(34):5381-5387.

37. Sparano JA, Wang M, Martino S, et al. Weekly paclitaxel in the adjuvant treatment of breast cancer. *N Engl J Med.* 2008;358(16):1663-1671.

38. Fisher B, Anderson S, Wickerham DL, et al. Increased intensification and total dose of cyclophosphamide in a doxorubicin-cyclophosphamide regimen for the treatment of primary breast cancer: findings from National Surgical Adjuvant Breast and Bowel Project B-22. *J Clin Oncol.* 1997;15(5):1858-1869.

39. Fisher B, Anderson S, DeCillis A, et al. Further evaluation of intensified and increased total dose of cyclophosphamide for the treatment of primary breast cancer: findings from National Surgical Adjuvant Breast and Bowel Project B-25. *J Clin Oncol.* 1999;17(11):3374-3388.

40. Fornier M, Norton L. Dose-dense adjuvant chemotherapy for primary breast cancer. *Breast Cancer Res.* 2005;7(2):64-69.

41. Citron ML, Berry DA, Cirrincione C, et al. Randomized trial of dose-dense versus conventionally scheduled and sequential versus concurrent chemotherapy as postoperative treatment of node-positive primary breast cancer: first report of intergroup trial C9741/cancer and leukemia group B trial 9741. *J Clin Oncol.* 2003;21:1431-1439.

42. Norton L. Conceptual and practical implications of breast tissue geometry: toward a more effective, less toxic therapy. *Oncologist.* 2005;10(6):370-381.

43. Makari-Judson G, Judson CH, Mertens WC. Longitudinal patterns of weight gain after breast cancer diagnosis: observations beyond the first year. *Breast J.* 2007;13(3):258-265.

44. Levine EG, Raczynski JM, Carpenter JT. Weight gain with breast cancer adjuvant treatment. *Cancer.* 1991;67(7):1954-1959.

45. Walshe JM, Denduluri N, Swain SM. Amenorrhea in premenopausal women after adjuvant chemotherapy for breast cancer. *J Clin Oncol.* 2006;24(36):5769-5779.

46. Postma TJ, Vermorken JB, Liefting AJ, Pinedo HM, Heimans JJ. Paclitaxel-induced neuropathy. *Ann Oncol.* 1995;6(5):489-494.

47. Hurria A, Lachs M. Is cognitive dysfunction a complication of adjuvant chemotherapy in the older patient with breast cancer? *Breast Cancer Res Treat.* 2007;103(3):259-268.

48. Vardy J, Rourke S, Tannock IF. Evaluation of cognitive function associated with chemotherapy: a review of published studies and recommendations for future research. *J Clin Oncol.* 2007;25(17):2455-2463.

49. Ganz PA, Bower JE. Cancer related fatigue: a focus on breast cancer and Hodgkin's disease survivors. *Acta Oncol.* 2007;46(4):474-479.

50. Broeckel JA, Thors CL, Jacobsen PB, Small M, Cox CE. Sexual functioning in long-term breast cancer survivors treated with adjuvant chemotherapy. *Breast Cancer Res Treat.* 2002;75(3):241-248.

51. Zambetti M, Moliterni A, Materazzo C, et al. Long-term cardiac sequelae in operable breast cancer patients given adjuvant chemotherapy with or without doxorubicin and breast irradiation. *J Clin Oncol.* 2001;19(1):37-43.

52. Smith I, Procter M, Gelber RD, et al. 2-year follow-up of trastuzumab after adjuvant chemotherapy in HER2-positive breast cancer: a randomised controlled trial. *Lancet.* 2007;369(9555):29-36.

53. Chaplain G, Milan C, Sgro C, Carli PM, Bonithon-Kopp C. Increased risk of acute leukemia after adjuvant chemotherapy for breast cancer: a population-based study. *J Clin Oncol.* 2000;18(15):2836-2842.

54. Tolaney SM, Winer EP. Follow-up care of patients with breast cancer. *Breast.* 2007;16(suppl 2):S45-50.

55. Khatcheressian JL, Wolff AC, Smith TJ, et al. American Society of Clinical Oncology 2006 update of the breast cancer follow-up and management guidelines in the adjuvant setting. *J Clin Oncol.* 2006;24(31):5091-5097.

56. Romond EH, Perez EA, Bryant J, et al. Trastuzumab plus adjuvant chemotherapy for operable HER2-positive breast cancer. *N Engl J Med.* 2005;353(16):1673-1684.

57. Blackwell KL, Kaplan EH, Franco SX, Marcom PK, Maleski JE, Sorensen MJ, Berger MS. A phase II, open-label, multicenter study of GW572016 in patients with trastuzumab-refractory metastatic breast cancer. *J Clin Oncol.* 2004;22(14S). ASCO Annual Meeting Proceedings. Abstract 3006.

58. Geyer CE, Forster J, Lindquist D, et al. A phase III randomized, open-label, international study comparing lapatinib and capecitabine vs capecitabine in women with refractory advanced or metastatic breast cancer (EGF100151). Paper presented at: American Society of Clinical Oncology, Atlanta, GA, 2006.

59. O'Shaughnessy J, Blackwell KL, Burstein H, Storniolo AM, et al. A randomized study of lapatinib alone or in combination with trastuzumab in heavily pretreated HER2+ metastatic breast cancer progressing on trastuzumab therapy. *J Clin Oncol.* 2008;26:1015.

60. Miller K, Wang M, Gralow J, et al. Paclitaxel plus bevacizumab versus paclitaxel alone for metastatic breast cancer. *N Engl J Med.* 2007;357(26):2666-2676.

61. Ince TA, Richardson AL, Bell GW, et al. Transformation of different human breast epithelial cell types leads to distinct tumor phenotypes. *Cancer Cell.* 2007;12(2):160-170.

62. De Soto JA, Deng CX. PARP-1 inhibitors: are they the long-sought genetically specific drugs for BRCA1/2-associated breast cancers? *Int J Med Sci.* 2006;3(4):117-123.

CHAPTER 88

Biologic Therapy

Janet K. Horton
E. Claire Dees
Nancy Klauber-DeMore

Biologic therapy involves the delivery of a systemic agent that can be specifically targeted toward a unique cellular feature, often a component of a cell surface receptor. Over the last decade, the approach to systemic therapy in breast cancer has been revolutionized by the development and efficacious application of biologic agents. Rapid translation of laboratory data to the clinic has resulted in meaningful differences in patient outcomes.

Three biologic therapies—trastuzumab, lapatinib, and bevacizumab—are now approved for use in patients with breast cancer. Preclinical and clinical data supporting the use of these agents are the focus of this chapter.

TRASTUZUMAB (HERCEPTIN)

Biology

Human epidermal growth factor receptor 2 (ErbB2/HER-2) is a 185-kd transmembrane protein overexpressed in 20% to 25% of breast cancer patients and correlated with adverse survival outcomes.[1-3] Trastuzumab, a humanized monoclonal antibody to HER-2, was developed to antagonize the role of HER-2 in the progression of breast tumors. After preclinical studies demonstrated growth inhibition in breast cancer cell lines and xenograft models,[4,5] phase I data revealed a favorable safety profile.[6,7] Efficacy trials were subsequently initiated.

Use in Patients with Metastatic Disease

In 1996, Baselga et al[6] reported the results of a phase II study assessing the efficacy of trastuzumab as a single agent in the treatment of HER-2-overexpressing metastatic breast cancer. Forty-six patients received a loading dose of trastuzumab followed by 10 weekly doses. One complete remission and 4 partial remissions were seen (11.6%) in this heavily pretreated group.[6] Pegram et al[7] subsequently reported the results of a similar phase II clinical trial evaluating the combination of trastuzumab and cisplatin. Thirty-nine patients with HER-2 overexpression (2+ or 3+ by immunohistochemistry [IHC]) and progressive metastatic disease on standard therapy received a loading dose followed by 8 weekly doses of trastuzumab. Those without disease progression could continue treatment with maintenance cisplatin and trastuzumab until disease progression or unacceptable toxicity. The toxicity profile seen in this trial was comparable to historical controls treated with cisplatin alone. Almost half of the patients did not progress during the study period, and a quarter had a partial response lasting a median of 5.1 months. As in the first trial, no immunologic adverse events were noted, and pharmacokinetic analysis showed no drug interaction.[7] Two hundred and twenty-two patients from multiple continents were accrued to another trial evaluating response rates to weekly trastuzumab (until disease progression) in HER-2-overexpressing metastatic breast cancer patients. The overall response rate was 22% (8 complete responses) and median time to progression was 9.1 months, despite the fact that greater than 60% of the patients had received prior chemotherapy for metastatic disease. Patients with higher levels of HER-2 overexpression (3+ vs 2+) were noted to have more favorable responses to trastuzumab. Only 14% (n = 29) of patients experienced severe adverse events thought to possibly be related to study drug, several occurring in more than 1 patient as follows: pain (9), chills (5), dyspnea (2), and abdominal pain (2).[8]

With encouraging preliminary results, randomized trials enrolling larger numbers of patients were designed to definitively assess the efficacy of trastuzumab. One hundred and fourteen patients with HER-2-overexpressing (2+ or 3+ by IHC) metastatic breast cancer who declined first-line cytotoxic chemotherapy were randomized to 2 mg/kg of trastuzumab versus 4 mg/kg weekly. Twenty-six percent of the patients had an objective response. No clear relationship to dose level was detected.[9]

In a landmark trial, Slamon et al[10], randomized 469 women with progressive HER-2-overexpressing (2+ or 3+ by IHC) metastatic breast cancer to chemotherapy alone (doxorubicin or epirubicin/ cyclophosphamide or paclitaxel if they had received prior adjuvant anthracycline) or chemotherapy combined with trastuzumab. Although patients had not received prior chemotherapy for metastatic disease, many had received adjuvant chemotherapy and the study regimen was chosen accordingly. The addition of trastuzumab to chemotherapy resulted in an improved median time to disease progression (7.4 vs 4.6 months), higher rate of overall response (50% vs 32%), longer duration of response (9.1 vs 6.1 months), and a significantly longer median survival (25.1 to 20.3 months). This improvement in survival was seen despite a trial design that allowed patients progressing on chemotherapy alone to receive open-label trastuzumab.[10]

Unexpectedly high cardiac dysfunction was seen in 27% of patients receiving an anthracycline in combination with trastuzumab, but only 13% of patients receiving trastuzumab combined with paclitaxel (16% vs 2% with class III/IV New York Heart Association [NYHA] dysfunction). Seventy-five percent of those requiring treatment for cardiac dysfunction improved with standard medical care.[10] Subsequent elegant preclinical studies confirmed the importance of HER-2 in maintenance of cardiac myocytes.[11] Current recommendations for use of trastuzumab suggest avoiding concurrent use with anthracyclines and monitoring cardiac function during use. For metastatic breast cancer patients with normal cardiac function and HER-2-overexpressing disease, combination therapy with trastuzumab and chemotherapy is now standard of care.

Use in the Adjuvant Setting

Promising data in the metastatic setting led to the evaluation of adjuvant trastuzumab. In 2005, combined results of the National Surgical Adjuvant Breast and Bowel Project (NSABP) B-31 and North Central Cancer Treatment Group (NCCTG N9831) were reported. After definitive resection of HER-2 positive (IHC 3+ or amplified by fluorescence in situ hybridization [FISH]), node-positive, or high-risk node-negative (5.7% of cases) breast cancer, women received adjuvant doxorubicin/cyclophosphamide (AC) followed by paclitaxel with or without weekly trastuzumab (begun during paclitaxel) and followed by trastuzumab alone for a total of 52 weeks of HER-2 targeted therapy. Data was reported on over 3000 women with a median follow-up of 2 years. Disease-free survival was significantly improved from 67.1% in the control group to 85.3% in those receiving trastuzumab (hazard ratio [HR] 0.48); overall survival at 3 years was similarly significantly improved from 91.7% in the control group to 94.3% in the trastuzumab group (HR = 0.67). Eligibility was limited to women with normal ejection fraction after AC; 4.1% of women treated with trastuzumab experienced a cardiac event compared with 0.8% with chemotherapy alone.[12]

At the same time, Piccart-Gebhart et al[13] reported results of the 1-year randomization arm of the Herceptin Adjuvant (HERA) trial, which included women with HER-2-positive (IHC 3+ or amplified by FISH) breast cancer randomized after completion of investigators'-discretion adjuvant chemotherapy (several regimens were permitted) to 1 or 2 years of trastuzumab versus no further infusional therapy (the 2-year randomization results have not been reported). This study included node-negative women at a much higher rate (32%-33%) than in the NSABP and NCCTG trials. Women received 1 year of trastuzumab therapy, 6 mg/kg every 3 weeks. An ejection fraction of 55% or greater and no prior cardiac history was required for entry onto the trial. At a median follow-up of 1 year, the HR of relapse for the trastuzumab arm was 0.54, representing an 8.4% absolute improvement in 2-year disease-free survival.[13] In a subsequent report at a median of 2 years of follow-up, improved survival was seen (HR 0.66; 95% CI 0.47-0.91).[14] In spite of more rigorous cardiac eligibility criteria, decreased ejection fraction occurred in 7.1% of the trastuzumab group compared with 2.2% of the observation group, and the clinical cardiotoxicity was 1.7% versus 0.06%. Finally, Breast Cancer International Research Group (BCIRG) 006, which enrolled over 3000 women with node-positive or high-risk node-negative, HER-2 positive (by FISH) breast cancer, compared chemotherapy only (AC followed by docetaxel [AC-T]) with the same chemotherapy with 1 year of trastuzumab beginning during docetaxel (AC-TH) or a novel nonanthracycline regimen of docetaxel plus carboplatin with 1 year of trastuzumab during and after chemotherapy (TCH). This study has been reported at a median of 36 months revealing a significant improvement in disease-free survival with either trastuzumab-based regimen compared with chemotherapy alone (HR 0.61 for AC-TH; HR 0.67 for TCH), and significantly less cardiotoxicity with the nonanthracycline trastuzumab regimen (0.004% TCH vs 1.8% AC-TH), suggesting that much of the benefit may be accrued without the anthracycline and toxicity can be minimized in appropriate patients.[15] A very small but intriguing study, FinHER, included patients with HER-2-positive (by FISH) tumors among a larger trial examining adjuvant vinorelbine versus docetaxel followed by fluorouracil/epirubicin/cyclophosphamide (FEC). The 232 patients with HER-2-positive tumors were randomized to receive or not receive 9 weeks of trastuzumab during the chemotherapy. Results from this subgroup revealed a significantly improved 3-year recurrence-free survival in those who received trastuzumab (HR 0.42), and no significant increase in cardiac events.[16] While too small to be definitive, this study raises the question of whether far shorter durations of adjuvant trastuzumab may be possible, a concept which is being tested in the AOUMODENA trial.

Together these trials brought about the widespread use of trastuzumab in the adjuvant therapy of HER-2+, node-positive, and high-risk node-negative women with breast cancer. Outstanding questions that remain include determining the optimal duration of therapy, the necessity of concurrent chemotherapy, the optimal chemotherapy backbone, and the potential utility of adding other targeted agents such as lapatinib.

Concurrent with Radiotherapy

Preclinical studies link HER-2 overexpression in breast cancer with radioresistance.[17] When HER-2 is exogenously overexpressed in normal breast cancer cell lines, the HER-2-overexpressing cells

TABLE 88-1 Selected Active Phase III Trials in HER-2-Positive Breast Cancer

Trial	Eligibility	Setting/Primary End Point	Randomization
NSABP B-41	Stage II-III	Neoadjuvant/pCR	AC-paclitaxel ± H, L, or HL
CALGB 40601	Stage II-III	Neoadjuvant/pCR	Paclitaxel ± H, L, or HL
Geparquinto (setting III)	Stage I-III	Neoadjuvant/pCR	EC-docetaxel ± H vs L
ALTTO/BIG 2-06/N063D	Stage I-III	Adjuvant/DFS	Chemotherapy with or followed by H, L, H→L, or LH→L
Neo-ALTTO	Stage II-III	Neoadjuvant/pCR	Paclitaxel ± H, L, or HL (with lead-in phase single-agent biologic)
TEACH	Stage I-III	Adjuvant/DFS	Chemotherapy → L vs placebo
BETH/NSABP B-44	Stage II-III	Adjuvant/invasive DFS	Chemotherapy/trastuzumab ± B
ECOG 1105	Chest wall recurrence—1st-line stage IV	PFS	Paclitaxel/trastuzumab ± carboplatin ± B
NCIC MA.31	1st-line stage IV	PFS	Taxane ± H vs L
CLEOPATRA	1st-line stage IV	PFS	Docetaxel/trastuzumab ± pertuzumab

AC, adriamycin/cyclophosphamide; B, bevacizumab; C, carboplatin; D, docetaxel; ddAC, dose dense doxorubicin and cyclophosphamide every 2 weeks × 4; EC: epirubicin, cyclophosphamide H, trastuzumab; L, lapatinib; T, paclitaxel; pCR; pathologic complete response; DFS, disease-free survival; PFS, progression free survival.

acquire radioresistance compared with their parental counterparts, a phenomenon that can be reversed with exposure to trastuzumab.[17,18] These results suggest that trastuzumab may be a radiosensitizer.

The most robust clinical data combining radiotherapy and trastuzumab stems from the combined NSABP/NCCTG analysis where radiation was given concurrently with trastuzumab. Regional nodal irradiation was permitted or required with the exception of internal mammary node irradiation, which was specifically prohibited in both trials. In addition to its distant effects, trastuzumab reduced local recurrence by half in treated patients.[12] Whether this is an effect of the trastuzumab alone on local control, or a sensitizing interaction between the radiation and trastuzumab is unclear. Prospective studies should help to clarify the role of HER-2 in clinical radiation response.

Ongoing Trials

Multiple ongoing phase III trials are evaluating a wide range of potential trastuzumab applications from new drug combinations in the metastatic setting to the role of trastuzumab in the neoadjuvant setting (Table 88-1).

LAPATINIB (TYKERB)

Biology

In addition to HER-2, other members of the ErbB family are known to promote tumor growth. ErbB1 (EGFR), in particular, has been linked to the growth of several solid tumor types. EGFR family members form hetero- or homodimer pairs after

ligand binding that result in activation of downstream signaling pathways. Thus, targeting of multiple receptors with 1 drug is appealing. Lapatinib, a small molecule tyrosine kinase inhibitor, is a reversible inhibitor of ErbB1 (EGFR) and ErbB2 (HER-2).

Use in the Locally Advanced/Metastatic Setting

Early phase data demonstrated that lapatinib was well tolerated[19,20] with diarrhea and rash the most frequent adverse events. As a result, multiple phase II/III studies were initiated to assess the clinical efficacy of lapatinib. In the first phase II evaluation of lapatinib as monotherapy, 229 women with refractory advanced or metastatic breast cancer were given 1500 mg of lapatinib once daily until disease progression. Despite the fact that more than 3 quarters of patients had received 4 or more prior treatment regimens, a clinical benefit (progression-free for at least 6 months) was seen in approximately 6% of HER-2 + patients. No correlation was seen with the level of EGFR expression. No tumor response was seen in patients who did not overexpress HER-2. The most common adverse events were diarrhea (59%), nausea (37%), and rash (32%). Nine patients experienced a decline in left ventricular ejection fraction and one was symptomatic.[21]

Another randomized, multicenter study examined the feasibility of lapatinib as first-line therapy. Patients with stage IIIB, IIIC, and IV HER-2-overexpressing (by FISH; confirmed centrally) breast cancer were randomized to 500 mg or 1500 mg twice daily lapatinib prior to receiving any other chemotherapy, immunotherapy, or biologic therapy. One hundred thirty-eight patients were recruited worldwide. Twenty-four percent experienced a complete or partial response with no significant dose response noted. Median duration of response was 28.4 weeks. No unexpected toxicity was noted.[22] Interestingly, a recently reported phase III trial in women with progression on trastuzumab randomized patients to lapatinib or lapatinib plus ongoing trastuzumab and found that progression-free survival was improved in those with dual biologic therapy despite progression on one.[23]

Women with HER-2+ (IHC 3+ or amplification by FISH) locally advanced or metastatic breast cancer having experienced progression on anthracycline, taxane, and trastuzumab containing regimens were eligible for the pivotal randomized trial evaluating lapatinib (1250 mg daily) plus capecitabine (2000 mg/m^2 in divided doses days 1-14 of a 21-day cycle) versus capecitabine (2500 mg/m^2) alone. Three hundred ninety-nine women were accrued and an improvement in response rate from 14% to 24% as well as a trend toward improved survival was seen with the addition of lapatinib. Grade 4 adverse events were equivalent between the 2 groups. Four asymptomatic decreases in left ventricular ejection fraction were noted, all of which recovered without discontinuation of therapy.[24] Based upon these data, lapatinib was FDA-approved for use with capecitabine in trastuzumab-refractory HER-2-positive disease. Other relevant studies include a phase III trial evaluating the combination of paclitaxel (175 mg/m^2 every 3 weeks) with or without lapatinib (1500 mg per day) in patients with incurable stage III/IV breast cancer[25] where a significant improvement in response rate, time to progression, and event-free survival was seen largely in the HER-2+ subset.

Current studies focus on the use of this drug earlier in therapy and for special populations such as inflammatory breast cancer and central nervous system (CNS) metastasis. A phase II evaluation of single-agent lapatinib in women with inflammatory breast cancer refractory to anthracycline-containing regimens has also been completed. Patients in cohort A (2+ or 3+ by IHC or amplified by FISH) and B (expression of EGFR without HER-2) received 1500 mg daily. Forty-five heavily pretreated patients were enrolled. Two complete responses and 13 partial responses were seen in the HER-2-overexpressing group (50%). Median duration of response was 16.9 weeks. Only 1 patient in the EGFR+ cohort experienced a partial response, thus closing accrual to that group[26] and lending further credence to other studies suggesting that HER-2-positivity is required for lapatinib activity.

Approximately 30% of women with advanced HER-2+ disease will develop brain metastasis despite treatment with trastuzumab. In fact, the efficacy of trastuzumab in controlling systemic parenchymal disease seems to have changed patterns of failure in HER-2+ patients leading to increased CNS involvement.[27] Although trastuzumab does not appear to cross the blood-brain barrier,[28] small molecules such as lapatinib may be able to penetrate and either prevent or treat CNS metastasis. Exploratory analysis in the phase III trial comparing capecitabine/lapatinib with capecitabine alone noted a decrease in symptomatic CNS progression as a first site in the combination group (11 vs 4 women).[24] In a recent phase II trial, Lin et al[29] evaluated response to lapatinib in patients with HER-2-overexpressing breast cancer and measurable CNS involvement. Patients had received trastuzumab and progressed after whole brain or stereotactic irradiation. Lapatinib 750 mg was delivered twice

a day. Although the drug was well tolerated and produced a partial response in 25% of patients with measurable disease outside the CNS, only 1 patient achieved a partial response (PR) in the CNS[29] using traditional criteria. However, CNS disease is poorly suited for conventional response assessment, and volumetric studies were more suggestive of activity (3/34 with volumetric reductions of at least 30%; 7/34 with reductions of 10-30%). For this reason, further studies evaluating the combination of lapatinib and cytotoxic agents in patients with HER-2+ brain metastasis are under way.

Concurrent with Radiotherapy

Like HER-2, EGFR has been shown to play a role in radiation resistance. In 2 EGFR-overexpressing breast cancer cell lines, lapatinib has been shown to sensitize cells to radiation.[30] A phase I trial designed to determine the maximum tolerated dose of lapatinib given concurrently with radiation and the impact of this pairing on downstream signaling pathways is ongoing.[31]

Ongoing Trials

Multiple phase III trials are in progress evaluating the role of lapatinib in the neoadjuvant, adjuvant, and metastatic settings (Table 88-1).

BEVACIZUMAB (AVASTIN)

Biology

Angiogenesis, the process of new capillary formation from pre-existing vessels, is necessary for tumor growth and metastasis. The initiation of the angiogenic program, the angiogenic switch, requires the acquisition of the angiogenic phenotype through a series of molecular events leading to increased expression of angiogenic factors and/or downregulation of naturally occurring inhibitors. Vascular endothelial growth factor (VEGF) is thought to play a pivotal, rate limiting role in tumor angiogenesis. VEGF is an endothelial cell mitogen and inducer of angiogenesis in vivo.[32] Proof of the role of VEGF in tumor angiogenesis was accomplished in a preclinical model where treatment of tumors in nude mice with a monoclonal antibody to VEGF inhibited tumor growth. Presently, the only FDA approved angiogenesis inhibitor for the treatment of breast cancer is bevacizumab, a monoclonal antibody against VEGF.

Use in Metastatic Disease

Bevacizumab is a recombinant human monoclonal antibody against VEGFA that prevents VEGF from binding to its receptor, and has been studied in phase I-III clinical trials in patients with metastatic breast cancer. As a single agent in heavily pretreated metastatic breast cancer, it produces either objective response or prolonged (>22 weeks) disease stabilization in 15% to 20% of patients.[33] Although generally well tolerated, notable toxicities include hypertension, proteinuria, and thromboembolic or wound complications. Bevacizumab combined with conventional chemotherapies such as docetaxel[34] and vinorelbine[35] also demonstrates activity in patients with pretreated metastatic breast cancer. These data supported the initiation of a randomized phase III trial that combined bevacizumab and capecitabine in breast cancer patients previously treated with an anthracycline and a taxane.[36] Although the addition of bevacizumab to capecitabine resulted in a significant increase in response rate (19.8% vs 9.1%) and was well tolerated, it did not significantly improve the primary end point, progression-free survival (4.86 months vs 4.17 months), or overall survival (15.1 months vs 14.5 months).

By contrast, in an open label, randomized phase III first-line trial[37] for patients with locally recurrent or metastatic breast cancer comparing paclitaxel plus bevacizumab with paclitaxel alone, bevacizumab significantly prolonged the median progression-free survival (11.8 months vs 5.9 months) and increased the response rate in all patients (28.2% vs 14.2%, $p < .0001$). It did not improve overall survival (26.7 months vs 25.2 months) as compared with paclitaxel alone. Another study combining bevacizumab with docetaxel confirmed this improvement in progression-free survival, albeit to a far less impressive extent.[38] Based on these data, the FDA approved bevacizumab in combination with paclitaxel for the first-line treatment of patients with metastatic HER-2-negative breast cancer in 2008.

Neoadjuvant Studies

There is only limited data on the use of bevacizumab in the neoadjuvant setting, but the initial data support enthusiasm. In a first study, 34 patients with nonmetastatic and metastatic unresectable breast tumors were treated with docetaxel with or without bevacizumab. There were 5 complete clinical responses and 24 partial responses.[39] In another neoadjuvant trial,[40] patients with inflammatory and locally advanced breast cancer received bevacizumab alone for the first cycle followed by 6 cycles of bevacizumab with doxorubicin and docetaxel. After completion

of neoadjuvant chemotherapy, 8 out of 13 patients had confirmed partial responses, with evidence of a decrease in vascular permeability on dynamic contrast magnetic resonance imaging (MRI).[40]

One concern regarding the use of bevacizumab in the neoadjuvant setting is problems with wound healing. Wound healing requires angiogenesis, and impaired surgical wound healing in patients who undergo surgery during treatment with bevacizumab is a known complication.[41] Because of this, patients should not undergo major surgery until 4 to 6 weeks after discontinuation of bevacizumab. Further studies are needed with bevacizumab in the neoadjuvant setting prior to instituting this therapy outside of a clinical trial.

Ongoing Trials with Bevacizumab in Breast Cancer

There are 59 active clinical trials of bevacizumab for patients with breast cancer in the neoadjuvant, adjuvant, and metastatic settings, in combination with chemotherapy or biologic therapy. Of these, 14 are phase III trials (Table 88-2). A complete listing of trials can be accessed at http://www.cancer.gov/clinicaltrials.

FUTURE DIRECTIONS

Examination of the optimal HER-2 targeting in the adjuvant setting and determining the role of antiangiogenic therapy in early breast cancer is the subject of multiple ongoing and planned studies as detailed in Table 88-1. Angiogenesis remains a target of interest and there are a number of VEGF- and VEGF receptor-targeted compounds and antibodies in development beyond bevacizumab. Further, there are a number of multitargeted oral tyrosine kinase inhibitors in development.

TABLE 88-2 Selected Active or Recently Closed Phase III Trials in Breast Cancer Patients Using Bevacizumab

Trial	Eligibility	Setting/Primary End Point	Randomization
NSABP B-40	HER-2-negative stage I-IIIA	Neoadj/pCR	Chemotherapy ± B
GeparQuinto (setting I)	HER-2-negative stage I-III	Neoadj/pCR	EC-docetaxel ± B
ECOG 5103	HER-2-negative node + or high risk N–	Adjuvant/DFS	AC-paclitaxel ± B
CALGB 40603	Triple-negative stage II-III	Neoadj/pCR	(Paclitaxel ± carboplatin → dd AC) ± B (not yet open)
BEATRICE	Triple-negative stage I-III	Adjuvant/invasive DFS	Chemotherapy ± B
RIBBON 1	Stage IV	PFS	Chemotherapy ± B (closed to accrual)
RIBBON 2	Pretreated stage IV	PFS	Chemotherapy ± B (closed to accrual)
CALGB 40503	ER+ stage IV	PFS	Tamoxifen or aromatase inhibitor ± B
GEICAM/2006-11	Postmenopausal Hormone receptor+ 1st line stage IV	PFS	Letrozole ± B

AC, adriamycin/cyclophosphamide; B, bevacizumab; DFS, disease-free survival; dd, dose dense; EC, epirubicin, cyclophosphamide; ER, estrogen receptor; N, node; pCR, pathologic complete response; PFS, progression-free survival.

For example, the phase II evaluation of sunitinib (which targets VEGF and platelet-derived growth factor [PDGF] among others) in metastatic breast cancer was recently published.[42] Another oral small molecule kinase inhibitor, dasatinib, is currently being evaluated in phase II trials. Other signal transduction inhibitors being evaluated in breast cancer trials include those that target PI3 kinase, AKT, mammalian target of rapamycin (mTOR) and other kinases important in pathways of cell growth, transformation and survival.

HER-2 remains an important target, and there are multiple trials comparing or combining trastuzumab and lapatinib; moreover, there are a number of new HER-2-targeted drugs such as pertuzumab and T-DM1 that are promising. Another member of the HER family, EGFR, has emerged as a target for breast cancer therapy. There are a number of anti-EGFR antibodies and small molecules currently used in the therapy of other tumor types (eg, cetuximab and panatumumab in colorectal cancer and erlotinib in lung cancer). In the breast cancer field, single-agent therapy with EGFR inhibitors in unselected breast cancer has largely been disappointing. However, there are 2 recent trials of interest adding EGFR inhibitors to anti-estrogen therapy. In the first, Kent Osborne et al[43] presented a randomized phase II trial of tamoxifen with or without gefitinib in metastatic breast cancer. In a group of 200 patients with newly diagnosed breast cancer, the addition of gefitinib improved progression-free survival (PFS) by 2 months but also increased toxicity. These results are consistent with the concept that the HER pathway may play a role in acquired resistance to tamoxifen in some patients.[43] The second recent study addressing this question randomly assigned patients to anastrozole plus gefitinib or placebo. Again, the addition of the EGFR inhibitor markedly improved PFS in this small study.[44] In contrast, a similar study in the neoadjuvant setting was negative[45]; thus, this remains an area of ongoing research. Finally, preclinical studies have suggested that basal-like breast cancer may be EGFR dependent and therefore EGFR-directed therapy has been incorporated into 2 recent trials of therapy for the ER-, PR-, and HER-2-negative (triple negative) subtype with evidence of activity.[46,47] A large, ongoing European trial that randomized nearly 200 women with metastatic triple negative breast cancer to cisplatin alone or with cetuximab will further define the role of EGFR targeting in this selected population.

Apoptosis also remains a target of anticancer drug development with compounds targeting Bcl-2 and the IAPs, for example. The insulin-like growth factor 1 (IGF1) receptor is an active target in breast cancer drug development because of its role in cell survival, EGFR cross talk, and vascularization. There are over 25 new compounds and antibodies targeting this receptor tyrosine kinase in development. Inhibitors of PARP, which is critical for DNA repair, are being actively investigated, particularly in patients who are BRCA mutation carriers or possess triple negative tumors, which have been suggested to have aberrant DNA repair due to dysfunction of the BRCA1 pathway. Finally, cell cycle control and check points are another group of targets being exploited. Early phase trials of aurora kinases, which are critical in cell cycle control and chromosome segregation, are ongoing.

Beyond the already approved agents, it is too early to tell which of these targets or agents will make the most meaningful contributions in the treatment of breast cancer and how they will best be combined with other biologic therapies or cytotoxic chemotherapy. Further, it is not yet clear what biomarkers or gene expression profiles may best predict response to each class of agents. For this reason enrollment of patients on these clinical trials with correlative science end points is critical, not only because it offers them the best novel approaches, but also to move forward our understanding of how best to treat this complex disease.

NECESSARY FUTURE STUDIES

In addition to the biologic therapies discussed above, there are a variety of new, targeted agents on the horizon. Recent advances in our understanding of angiogenesis, cell cycle control, apoptosis, and important signal transduction pathways have prompted an explosion of new drug development, with numerous compounds in development targeting critical biologic pathways, and numerous early phase trials ongoing that are beyond the scope of this review. It is not yet clear which of these compounds or targets will be most relevant in the treatment of breast cancer; another issue that must be addressed is how to appropriately select tumors for a biologic approach. It is well established that even biomarkers such as ER and HER-2 often fail, and for many of our current approaches such as anti-angiogenic therapy we have no biomarker at all. Part of the complication arises from the complexity of signaling pathways and the redundancy that is normal in human cancer.[48] If we are to move to truly individualized therapy, we must develop the means to profile tumors and combine targeted strategies, which means that we must merge tissue-based studies with clinical trials, making the role of the surgeon even more important.

SUMMARY

Breast cancer management has become progressively more complex, requiring the assimilation of data not only from the patient's clinical presentation but also from specific tumor biomarkers. Targeted and biologic therapies in breast cancer continue to progress rapidly, and the field of molecular targeted therapy has emerged. During the past decade there has been an improvement in the options available for patients with metastatic breast cancer with the successful translation into the clinic of biologic therapy for breast cancer with trastuzumab, lapatinib, and bevacizumab. Of these 3 agents, only trastuzumab is presently approved for use in the adjuvant setting, but ongoing clinical trials may lead to the adjuvant use of lapatinib and bevacizumab in the near future.

REFERENCES

1. Ravdin PM, Chamness GC. The c-erbB-2 proto-oncogene as a prognostic and predictive marker in breast cancer: a paradigm for the development of other macromolecular markers—a review. *Gene.* 1995;159(1):19-27.
2. Seshadri R, Firgaira FA, Horsfall DJ, et al. Clinical significance of HER-2/neu oncogene amplification in primary breast cancer. The South Australian Breast Cancer Study Group. *J Clin Oncol.* 1993;11(10):1936-1942.
3. Slamon DJ, Clark GM, Wong SG, et al. Human breast cancer: correlation of relapse and survival with amplification of the HER-2/neu oncogene. *Science.* 1987;235(4785):177-182.

4. Baselga J, Mendelsohn J. The epidermal growth factor receptor as a target for therapy in breast carcinoma. *Breast Cancer Res Treat.* 1994;29(1):127-138.

5. Carter P, Presta L, Gorman CM, et al. Humanization of an anti-p185HER2 antibody for human cancer therapy. *Proc Natl Acad Sci USA.* 1992;89(10):4285-4289.

6. Baselga J, Tripathy D, Mendelsohn J, et al. Phase II study of weekly intravenous recombinant humanized anti-p185HER2 monoclonal antibody in patients with HER2/neu-overexpressing metastatic breast cancer. *J Clin Oncol.* 1996;14(3):737-744.

7. Pegram MD, Lipton A, Hayes DF, et al. Phase II study of receptor-enhanced chemosensitivity using recombinant humanized anti-p185HER2/neu monoclonal antibody plus cisplatin in patients with HER2/neu-overexpressing metastatic breast cancer refractory to chemotherapy treatment. *J Clin Oncol.* 1998;16(8):2659-2671.

8. Cobleigh MA, Vogel CL, Tripathy D, et al. Multinational study of the efficacy and safety of humanized anti-HER2 monoclonal antibody in women who have HER2-overexpressing metastatic breast cancer that has progressed after chemotherapy for metastatic disease. *J Clin Oncol.* 1999;17(9):2639-2648.

9. Vogel CL, Cobleigh MA, Tripathy D, et al. Efficacy and safety of trastuzumab as a single agent in first-line treatment of HER2-overexpressing metastatic breast cancer. *J Clin Oncol.* 2002;20(3):719-726.

10. Slamon DJ, Leyland-Jones B, Shak S, et al. Use of chemotherapy plus a monoclonal antibody against HER2 for metastatic breast cancer that over-expresses HER2. *N Engl J Med.* 15 2001;344(11):783-792.

11. Crone SA, Zhao YY, Fan L, et al. ErbB2 is essential in the prevention of dilated cardiomyopathy. *Nature Med.* 2002;8(5):459-465.

12. Romond EH, Perez EA, Bryant J, et al. Trastuzumab plus adjuvant chemotherapy for operable HER2-positive breast cancer. *N Engl J Med.* 2005;353(16):1673-1684.

13. Piccart-Gebhart MJ, Procter M, Leyland-Jones B, et al. Trastuzumab after adjuvant chemotherapy in HER2-positive breast cancer. *N Engl J Med.* 2005;353(16):1659-1672.

14. Smith I, Procter M, Gelber RD, et al. 2-year follow-up of trastuzumab after adjuvant chemotherapy in HER2-positive breast cancer: a randomised controlled trial. *Lancet.* 2007;369(9555):29-36.

15. Slamon D, Eiermann W, Robert N, et al. BCIRG 006: 2nd interim analysis phase III randomized trial comparing doxorubicin and cyclophosphamide followed by docetaxel (AC->T) with doxorubicin and cyclophosphamide followed by docetaxel and trastuzumab (AC->TH) with docetaxel, carboplatin and trastuzumab (TCH) in Her2neu positive early breast cancer patients. *San Antonio Breast Cancer Symposium.* San Antonio, TX; 2006.

16. Joensuu H, Kellokumpu-Lehtinen PL, Bono P, et al. Adjuvant docetaxel or vinorelbine with or without trastuzumab for breast cancer. *N Engl J Med.* 2006;354(8):809-820.

17. Pietras RJ, Poen JC, Gallardo D, et al. Monoclonal antibody to HER-2/neureceptor modulates repair of radiation-induced DNA damage and enhances radiosensitivity of human breast cancer cells overexpressing this oncogene. *Cancer Res.* 1999;59(6):1347-1355.

18. Liang K, Lu Y, Jin W, et al. Sensitization of breast cancer cells to radiation by trastuzumab. *Mol Cancer Ther.* 2003;2(11):1113-1120.

19. Moy B, Goss PE. Lapatinib: current status and future directions in breast cancer. *Oncologist.* 2006;11(10):1047-1057.

20. Burris HA 3rd, Hurwitz HI, Dees EC, et al. Phase I safety, pharmacokinetics, and clinical activity study of lapatinib (GW572016), a reversible dual inhibitor of epidermal growth factor receptor tyrosine kinases, in heavily pretreated patients with metastatic carcinomas. *J Clin Oncol.* 2005;23(23):5305-5313.

21. Burstein HJ, Storniolo AM, Franco S, et al. A phase II study of lapatinib monotherapy in chemotherapy-refractory HER2-positive and HER2-negative advanced or metastatic breast cancer. *Ann Oncol.* 2008;19(6):1068-1074.

22. Gomez HL, Doval DC, Chavez MA, et al. Efficacy and safety of lapatinib as first-line therapy for ErbB2-amplified locally advanced or metastatic breast cancer. *J Clin Oncol.* 2008;26(18):2999-3005.

23. O'Shaughnessy J, Blackwell KL, Burstein H, et al. A randomized study of lapatinib alone or in combination with trastuzumab in heavily pretreated HER2+ metastatic breast cancer progressing on trastuzumab therapy. American Society of Clinical Oncology. *J Clin Oncol.* 2008;26.

24. Geyer CE, Forster J, Lindquist D, et al. Lapatinib plus capecitabine for HER2-positive advanced breast cancer. *New Engl J Med.* 2006;355(26):2733-2743.

25. Di Leo A, Gomez H, Aziz Z, et al. Lapatinib (L) with paclitaxel compared to paclitaxel as first-line treatment for patients with metastatic breast cancer: A phase III randomized, double-blind study of 580 patients. American Society of Clinical Oncology. *J Clin Oncol.* 2007;25:1011.

26. Johnston S, Trudeau M, Kaufman B, et al. Phase II study of predictive biomarker profiles for response targeting human epidermal growth factor receptor 2 (HER-2) in advanced inflammatory breast cancer with lapatinib monotherapy. *J Clin Oncol.* 2008;26(7):1066-1072.

27. Bendell JC, Domchek SM, Burstein HJ, et al. Central nervous system metastases in women who receive trastuzumab-based therapy for metastatic breast carcinoma. *Cancer.* 2003;97(12):2972-2977.

28. Pestalozzi BC, Brignoli S. Trastuzumab in CSF. *J Clin Oncol.* 2000;18(11):2349-2351.

29. Lin NU, Carey LA, Liu MC, et al. Phase II trial of lapatinib for brain metastases in patients with human epidermal growth factor receptor 2-positive breast cancer. *J Clin Oncol.* 2008;26(12):1993-1999.

30. Zhou H, Kim YS, Peletier A, et al. Effects of the EGFR/HER2 kinase inhibitor GW572016 on EGFR- and HER2-overexpressing breast cancer cell line proliferation, radiosensitization, and resistance. *Int J Radiat Oncol Biol Phys.* 2004;58(2):344-352.

31. Horton JK, Kimple RJ, Sartor CI, et al. Radiosensitization of locally recurrent or chemotherapy-refractory locally advanced breast cancer with lapatinib: a phase I trial. *2008 ASTRO Translational Advances in Radiation Oncology and Cancer Imaging Symposium.* Arlington, VA; 2008.

32. Ferrara N. Vascular endothelial growth factor: basic science and clinical progress. *Endocr Rev.* 2004;25(4):581-611.

33. Sledge GW, Miller K, Novotny WF, et al. A phase II trial of single-agent rhumab VEGF (recombinant humanized monoclonal antibody to vascular endothelial cell growth factor) in patients with relapsed metastatic breast cancer. American Society of Clinical Oncology. *Proc Am Soc Clin Oncol.* 2000;19.

34. Ramaswamy B, Elias AD, Kelbick NT, et al. Phase II trial of bevacizumab in combination with weekly docetaxel in metastatic breast cancer patients. *Clin Cancer Res.* 2006;12(10):3124-3129.

35. Burstein HJ, Parker LM, Savoie J, et al. Phase II trial of the anti-VEGF antibody bevacizumab in combination with HER1 for refractory advanced breast cancer. *Breast Cancer Res Treat.* 2002;76(suppl 1):115.

36. Miller KD, Chap LI, Holmes FA, et al. Randomized phase III trial of capecitabine compared with bevacizumab plus capecitabine in patients with previously treated metastatic breast cancer. *J Clin Oncol.* 2005;23(4):792-799.

37. Miller K, Wang M, Gralow J, et al. Paclitaxel plus bevacizumab versus paclitaxel alone for metastatic breast cancer. *N Engl J Med.* 2007;357(26):2666-2676.

38. Miles D, Chan A, Romieu G, et al. Randomized, double-blind, placebo-controlled, phase III study of bevacizumab with docetaxel or docetaxel with placebo as first-line therapy for patients with locally recurrent or metastatic breast cancer (mBC): AVADO. American Society of Clinical Oncology. *J Clin Oncol.* 2008;26.

39. Overmoyer B, Silverman P, Leeming R, et al. Phase II trial of neoadjuvant docetaxel with or without bevacizumab in patients with locally advanced breast cancer. American Society of Clinical Oncology. *J Clin Oncol.* 2004;22.

40. Wedam SB, Low JA, Yang SX, et al. Antiangiogenic and antitumor effects of bevacizumab in patients with inflammatory and locally advanced breast cancer. *J Clin Oncol.* 2006;24(5):769-777.

41. Hurwitz H, Saini S. Bevacizumab in the treatment of metastatic colorectal cancer: safety profile and management of adverse events. *Semin Oncol.* 2006;33(5 Suppl 10):S26-34.

42. Burstein HJ, Elias AD, Rugo HS, et al. Phase II study of sunitinib malate, an oral multitargeted tyrosine kinase inhibitor, in patients with metastatic breast cancer previously treated with an anthracycline and a taxane. *J Clin Oncol.* 2008;26(11):1810-1816.

43. Osborne K, Neven P, Dirix L, et al. A randomized phase II study of gefitinib (IRESSA) or placebo in combination with tamoxifen in patients with hormone receptor positive metastatic breast cancer. *San Antonio Breast Cancer Symposium.* San Antonio, TX; 2007.

44. Cristofanilli M, Valero V, Mangalik A, et al. A phase II multicenter, double-blind, randomized trial to compare anastrazole plus gefitinib with anastrazole plus placebo in postmenopausal women with hormone receptor-positive (HR+) metastatic breast cancer (MBC). American Society of Clinical Oncology. *J Clin Oncol.* 2008;26.

45. Smith IE, Welsh G, Skene A, et al. A phase II placebo-controlled trial of neoadjuvant anastrozole alone or with gefitinib in early breast cancer. *J Clin Oncol.* 2007;25:3816-3822.

46. Carey LA, Rugo HS, Marcom PK, et al. TBCRC 001: EGFR inhibition with cetuximab added to carboplatin in metastatic triple-negative (basal-like) breast cancer. American Society of Clinical Oncology. *J Clin Oncol.* 2008;26.

47. O'Shaughnessy J, Weckstein DJ, Vukelja SJ, et al. Preliminary results of a randomized phase II study of weekly irinotecan/carboplatin with or without cetuximab in patients with metastatic breast cancer. *San Antonio Breast Cancer Symposium.* San Antonio, TX; 2007.

48. Citri A, Yarden Y. EGF-ERBB signalling: towards the systems level. *Nat Rev Mol Cell Biol.* 2006;7(7):505-516.

CHAPTER 89

Pregnancy and Breast Cancer

David W. Ollila
Susan McKenney

INTRODUCTION AND EPIDEMIOLOGY

Treating a pregnant woman diagnosed with breast cancer is a difficult clinical scenario facing a variety of clinicians, obstetricians, radiologists, surgeons, medical oncologists, and radiation oncologists, just to name a few. Unfortunately, there is a paucity of randomized, clinical trial data to guide the treating physicians.[1,2] Thus the clinicians must rely on retrospective data and clinical experience to determine an individual patient's treatment plan. This chapter will summarize the best currently available evidence for treating a pregnant woman with breast cancer.

The traditional definition of pregnancy-associated breast cancer (PABC) is that the diagnosis of breast cancer is made during pregnancy or within 1 year afterwards. Using this definition, epidemiologic data demonstrate that a breast cancer is diagnosed once in every 3000 pregnancies.[3] The median age of pregnant women affected with breast cancer is 33 years (range, 23-47 years).[2,4] As more and more women are delaying motherhood until their 30s or even 40s,[5] PABCs should be increasing, but convincing epidemiologic data are not yet available.

PROGNOSIS

Historically, PABC patients had a dismal prognosis. Kilgore and Bloodgood[6] reported no survivors, whereas Haagensen and Stout[7] reported an 8.6% overall 5-year survival rate, and White[8] reported a 17% 5-year survival rate.

Harrington[9] is credited with reviving at least a bit of optimism for these patients in 1937 by demonstrating a 61% 5-year survival rate among patients with negative lymph nodes. However, the majority of PABC patients present with metastatic disease in the regional nodal basin.[10] When compared with age-matched, nonpregnant peers, the node-negative and node-positive 5-year survival is quite similar.[11] Petrek et al[11] reported that patients with PABC with tumor-free lymph nodes had an 82% 5-year survival rate, compared with an 82% rate for their nonpregnant counterparts. The pregnant patients with tumor-involved lymph nodes had a 47% 5-year survival rate compared with a 59% rate in the control patients; the difference was not statistically significant. This similar survival rate between pregnant breast cancer patients and their nonpregnant peers has been confirmed by others[12-15] (Table 89-1).

DIAGNOSIS

The homogeneously dense breast tissue in pregnant and lactating women makes routine screening methods almost useless because little information is gained owing to the increased water content and loss of fat in the breast during pregnancy.[16] If a dominant breast mass is detected on self-exam or clinician exam, then diagnostic mammograms can be performed with minimal risk to the fetus with the use of abdominal shielding and might yield important information regarding suspicious microcalcifications or masses. Ultimately though, sonography is probably the imaging method of choice for imaging the breasts of pregnant women. Breast sonography provides a rapid and accurate method of differentiating cystic lesions from solid masses during pregnancy and poses no risk to the developing fetus.[17] Gadolinium-enhanced breast magnetic resonance imaging (MRI) is increasingly used for staging and treatment decisions in breast cancer,[18] but gadolinium is contraindicated during pregnancy because it crosses the placenta. Thus a noncontrast MRI does not improve the diagnostic accuracy for the breast radiologist.

In pregnant women with breast abnormalities noted on clinical or radiologic examinations, the goal is to make an accurate

TABLE 89-1 Percentage of Pregnancy-Associated Breast Cancer Patients Surviving 5 Years According to Lymph Node Status

| Investigators | Institution | n | 5-YEAR SURVIVAL RATE (%) | |
			Negative Lymph Nodes	Positive Lymph Nodes
Haagensen and Stout, 1943[7]	Columbia-Presbyterian Medical Center	20	0	0
White, 1954[8]	University of Washington School of Medicine	40	72	6
Holleb, 1962[57]	Memorial Sloan-Kettering Cancer Institute	45	58	21
Applewhite et al, 1973[58]	Louisiana State University	48	56	18
Deemarsky and Neishtadt, 1980[59]		32	73	43
King et al, 1985[60]	Mayo Clinic	38	82	36
Ribiero et al, 1986[61]	The Christie Hospital and Holt Radium Institute	28	79	45
Petrek et al, 1991[11]	Memorial Sloan-Kettering Cancer Center	39	82	47
Kuerer et al, 1996[14]	Mount Sinai School of Medicine	26	60	45
Bonnier et al, 1997[15]	Multicenter study, France	154	63	31

pathologic diagnosis of the abnormality with the least invasive method. There is controversy surrounding each diagnostic method. The least invasive diagnostic method would be a fine-needle aspiration (FNA), but this may be associated with both increased false-positive[19] and increased false-negative rates. Also, when the breast is markedly engorged, as it is during pregnancy or lactation, FNA is technically more difficult to perform because of the small-caliber needle. Others[20] have demonstrated that FNA in the diagnosis of breast lesions in pregnant women can be highly accurate with no false positives. The literature is divided on the utility of FNA in pregnant women with breast masses.

Another minimally invasive option to obtain a pathologic diagnosis in the pregnant women would be a core-needle biopsy of the breast abnormality. Most clinicians are wary of this technique in the postpartum lactating breast because of the possible complication of a milk fistula.[21] However, in the pregnant breast, milk fistula formation is not an issue. For nonpregnant women, the literature suggests that image-guided core biopsy has the highest yield for a cancer diagnosis and minimizes false negatives.[22] For patients with a high level of suspicion for breast cancer, when the core-needle biopsy does not yield a cancer diagnosis, an incisional or excisional biopsy must be performed to establish the diagnosis.

TREATMENT

Decision Making in the Treatment of Gestational Breast Cancer

When pregnant women are diagnosed with breast cancer, it is an extremely complex and overwhelming time for them, their family, and often the medical team treating them. Treatment decisions are best made with the guidance of a multidisciplinary team and include discussions about specific approaches to managing the breast cancer and protecting the fetus during the treatment. It is important to clarify that the goals of treatment do not force a woman to choose between keeping a pregnancy or treating the cancer—both be accomplished safely, in the vast majority of cases, with the thoughtful planning of a multidisciplinary team.

The focus of the treatment portion of this chapter will be on gestational breast cancer, and not those who are diagnosed postpartum. The treatment algorithms for most postpartum breast cancer patients are very similar to those used in nonpregnant women. The surgical management of gestational breast cancer represents a unique challenge, both in the breast and in the axilla. To properly plan a patient's treatment, 3 fundamental questions need to be answered: (1) How far along is the patient in her pregnancy? (2) What is the estimated radiologic size of the patient's breast cancer? (3) Is there axillary nodal disease?

Surgery in the Treatment of Gestational Breast Cancer

Surgery during Pregnancy

Accurately calculating weeks of gestation allows the clinicians to avoid any possible, even if theoretical, drug-induced fetal defect, particularly in the first trimester. As will be detailed in the following paragraphs, the currently available evidence suggests that no commonly used anesthetic drug is a teratogen, but one cannot assume that some potential for teratogenicity does not exist. Therefore, surgical procedures during the first trimester should be avoided to allow the initial phase of fetal organogenesis to be completed.

Surgical procedures in the third trimester increase the risk of preterm labor. To avoid this possibility, most obstetricians will try to deliver the baby at 37 weeks, because these babies are classified as term infants.[23] Sometimes, a specific patient's case necessitates delivery before 37 weeks. However, these late preterm infants, those delivered between 34 and 36 6/7 weeks, have a well-documented increase in medical complications than their term counterparts, including temperature instability, hypoglycemia, respiratory distress, jaundice, apnea, seizures, and feeding problems.[24]

Anesthetic Issues

General anesthesia is necessary for a mastectomy or axillary dissection, and either general anesthesia or heavy conscious sedation is necessary for a partial mastectomy or sentinel node procedure. The surgeon caring for the pregnant breast cancer patient needs to be aware of a few basic principles.

Anesthetic issues in the pregnant patient can be divided into 2 major concerns: teratogenicity of the anesthetic agents and maternal physiologic changes as a result of anesthetic agents.[25] The teratogenicity of anesthetic agents, defined as the potential effect in chromosomal damage or in carcinogenesis in the fetus, is minimal. Studies that have specifically evaluated the effects of anesthetic agents on the fetus have concluded that the morbidity to the fetus is primarily from the underlying disease, not from the anesthetic agents.[26] In an excellent, comprehensive review article, no anesthetic agents were listed as definitively causative of fetal malformations.[27] Paralytics do not cross the placenta. Inhalational and local anesthetics, muscle relaxants, narcotic analgesics, and benzodiazepines have all been shown, with reasonable certainty, to be safe in pregnancy.[26-28]

Multiple cardiovascular and pulmonary physiologic changes occur in the mother during pregnancy. Both the surgeon and anesthesiologist should be aware of these alterations to prevent fetal hypoxia and hypotension. The cardiovascular system of the pregnant patient is hyperdynamic, with an increased cardiac output and an increased heart rate. Total blood volume increases up to 40%, whereas red blood cell volume rises by approximately 25%. This results in a relative anemia of pregnancy, with a drop in hematocrit by approximately 30%. The enlarging uterus pushes both diaphragms cephalad, causing a decreased functional reserve capacity by approximately 20%. Hyperventilation should be avoided, as maternal respiratory alkalosis is easy to produce because resting CO_2 is already reduced to 32 mm Hg. Respiratory alkalosis shifts the oxyhemoglobin dissociation curve to the left and thus may impair transfer of oxygen across the placenta. Umbilical blood flow is also decreased with alkalosis. End-tidal CO_2 monitoring may help avoid both over- and underventilation.[29] Communication between the anesthesia and surgical teams throughout the preoperative, intraoperative, and recovery room phases is critically important to both the mother and the fetus.

Axillary Procedure during Pregnancy

Historically, the patient's surgical option during pregnancy has been a complete level I and II axillary dissection as part of a modified radical mastectomy. In a gestational breast cancer patient, knowledge of the regional axilla histologic status may strongly influence the patient's treatment paradigm. For instance, a patient with histologically proven axillary disease may receive a more aggressive chemotherapy regimen as opposed to a patient with tumor-free axillary nodes. For patients with palpable adenopathy, an image-guided FNA or core biopsy should be performed to establish the histologic axillary nodal status.

In patients with no palpable axillary adenopathy, the pregnant patient should be able to derive the same benefit as her nonpregnant peer and avoid a completion axillary dissection if the sentinel node (SN) is tumor-free. The SN technology has allowed clinicians to accurately stage the regional nodal basin in nonpregnant patients with T1, T2, or T3 breast carcinomas.[30-37] For pregnant patients who present with breast cancer, the ideal timing of the SN procedure becomes very difficult.

Most pregnant patients present with tumors 1 cm or larger and therefore will likely receive systemic chemotherapy as part of their treatment regimen.[37] Thus these women become possible candidates for neoadjuvant chemotherapy. We strongly advocate for a prospective, randomized trial in nonpregnant breast cancer patients to answer this very important clinical question. We could then extrapolate the results to the gestational breast cancer patient.

Two retrospective studies have demonstrated in a small number of pregnant patients the safety of the SN procedure. In one study, 3 academic medical centers in North Carolina formed an institutional review board-approved collaborative registry and identified 10 pregnant patients who had an SN procedure. They reported that, within this small data set, the SN procedure performed with technetium-labeled sulfur colloid and/or isosulfan blue dye (Lymphazurin US Surgical Corporation, Norwalk, Conn) appeared safe to the fetus[38] and accurately determined the histologic status of the regional nodal basin. The other, a retrospective review of a prospectively generated database at the Moffitt Cancer Center identified 10 pregnant patients who had undergone an SN procedure. They also demonstrated that the SN procedure with technetium-labeled sulfur colloid and/or isosulfan blue dye did not have any adverse outcomes on the fetus[39] and was accurate in a limited data set.

However, there are 2 caveats to using the lymphatic mapping agents most widely in use. First, there are numerous data to support the safety of the technetium-labeled sulfur colloid in pregnant patients[12,40,41] (Fig. 89-1). However, there are no studies documenting the safety of isosulfan blue dye in pregnant women.[42,43] Therefore, we would conclude that if the SN procedure is going to be undertaken in patients with gestational breast cancer, it should be performed with technetium-labeled sulfur colloid alone. Even combined, the small sample size of these 2 trials is insufficient to conclude that isosulfan blue dye can be safely used in the pregnant patient.

Breast Surgical Options

Breast Preservation during Pregnancy with Delayed Breast Radiation

As mentioned previously, the historical surgical option during pregnancy has been a modified radical mastectomy. However, there are convincing data from Petrek et al[11] and Berry et al[12] that pregnant breast patients can safely undergo breast preservation. This is another example in critical timing decisions for the patient, the surgeon, and the anesthesia team. The pregnant

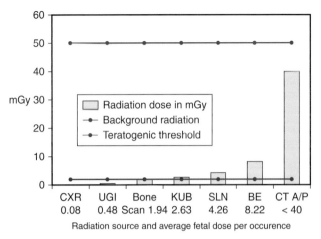

mGy–milligray, unit of kinetic energy transferred to matter; CXR–chest x-ray; UGI - upper gastrointestinal fluoroscopy; KUB–abdominal x-ray; BE–barium enema; CT A/P–computed tomography of abdomen and pelvis

FIGURE 89-1 Absorbed fetal radiation doses (in mGy) for common diagnostic x-ray tests and SN mapping in relation to average annual environmental background radiation exposure and the threshold for adverse fetal effect. (*Reproduced with permission from Mondi MM, Cuenca RL, Ullila DW, et al. Sentinel lymph node biopsy during pregnancy: initial clinical experience. Ann Surg Oncol. 2007;14:218-221.*)

patient can undergo a partial mastectomy and SN procedure and/or axillary dissection, depending on the clinical scenario, from the beginning of the second trimester until usually between 34 and 37 weeks' gestation. The patient then can commence with their systemic adjuvant chemotherapy during the second and third trimester of pregnancy or after delivery of subsequent radiation if indicated.

After the systemic therapy is completed, the patient is then ready to complete her standard whole-breast radiotherapy.[44] Because there are no published breast-preservation trials including gestational breast cancer patients, one must extrapolate from the data obtained in nonpregnant women. Investigators[45] have hypothesized that the pregnant patient's endogenous hormones change the breast's anatomic structure and may result in increased local recurrence rates. A pregnant woman's breast, however, with the large inter-anastomosing network of ducts and sizable lymph and blood vessels, is not anatomically and physiologically similar to the less active breast of a premenopausal woman. It is not certain that the same results after lumpectomy and irradiation will occur with lumpectomy during pregnancy and delayed postpartum radiation. This remains conjecture. There are no published series to suggest that the local recurrence rate after breast conservation in pregnant women is greater than that of their nonpregnant peers.

Breast Preservation during Pregnancy with Gestational Breast Radiotherapy

Completing breast preservation during pregnancy by delivering standard whole-breast radiotherapy unnecessarily exposes the fetus to teratogenic doses of radiation. The actual dose reaching the fetus can be estimated by thermoluminescent dosimeters placed in an anatomic phantom shielding. The developing fetus

receives a biologically significant percent of the total breast dose. The radiation leakage from the radiation unit should not exceed 0.1% of the direct beam exposure rate, as measured from a meter from the radiation source.[46] A larger amount of radiation, however, reaches the fetus from internal scatter by the mother's tissues (which cannot be reduced by external shielding). Thus the standard breast radiation therapy course of approximately 5000 cGy exposes the fetus to from 10 cGy early in pregnancy to 200 cGy or more late in pregnancy and so should be rejected as a treatment option.

Systemic Therapy for Gestational Breast Cancer

The clinicopathologic parameters used to choose between a neoadjuvant or adjuvant chemotherapy approach have been thoroughly discussed elsewhere in this section of the textbook. For the pregnant patient diagnosed with breast cancer, the fetus must be considered. In order to avoid administering chemotherapy during crucial periods of organogenesis, it is avoided during the first trimester whenever possible. Fetal exposure to chemotherapy at this time may cause spontaneous abortion or congenital malformation. The data supporting chemotherapy and its safety to the fetus during the second and third trimesters are for the most part based on retrospective reviews and case reports.[47] The use of endocrine therapy, if the tumor's hormone receptors are positive, is not recommended until after delivery secondary to reports of birth defects.[48]

The drugs most commonly used in treating nonpregnant breast cancer patients are the anthracycline doxorubicin, usually given with cyclophosphamide in the "AC" regimen, and often fluorouracil in regimens such as CAF. The most extensive literature has been with the CAF regimen. Small case series are limited, but suggest no apparent defects in children born after chemotherapy exposure.[12] The use of methotrexate is contraindicated due to its high teratogenic properties.[49] More recently, the taxanes have established efficacy in the treatment of nonpregnant breast cancer patients; however, evidence of safety in the setting of pregnancy are less clear.[50] Newer agents such as the monoclonal antibodies (eg, trastuzumab) also have little to no data on safety during pregnancy.[47]

Delivering chemotherapy during pregnancy poses unique challenges because of the physiological changes that occur in the woman. These changes include increases in fluid and blood volumes, cardiac output, pulmonary vascular resistance, and renal and hepatic metabolism, all together making calculating doses difficult in predicting for toxicities.[51] Many of the side effects of chemotherapy are also seen in a normal pregnancy, not complicated by a cancer treatment. Symptoms such as nausea, vomiting, fatigue, anemia, and deep vein thrombosis can be managed carefully using practice guidelines.[52] Managing more complex events such as infection and pulmonary or cardiac compromise requires careful integration between medical oncology and high-risk maternal fetal medicine. Timing of delivery of the fetus is critical for women on chemotherapy. The recommended delivery timeframe should be should be 3 to 4 weeks after the last dose of chemotherapy to allow for the mother's and newborn's blood counts to recover.[53,54]

Obstetrical Outcomes after Chemotherapy

One of the main obstetrical outcomes after chemotherapy is low birth weight infants, reported in up to 40% of cases. It is unclear whether the stunted growth is caused by the chemotherapy or as a result of early labor.[55] The long-term effects of exposure to chemotherapy in utero are not well studied. One study[56] has followed 84 children whose mothers received chemotherapy for hematologic malignancies for a median of 19 years, and no child demonstrated any physical, psychological, or neurologic abnormality, nor was there evidence of increase in malignancies. Twelve second-generation children in that same group are alive and without sequelae.[56]

COORDINATED HIGH-RISK OBSTETRIC AND ONCOLOGY NURSING MANAGEMENT

For the nonpregnant patient, the multidisciplinary team consists of a medical, surgical, and radiation oncologists, along with radiology and pathology colleagues. For the gestational breast cancer patient, it is essential that a dedicated high risk physician from maternal fetal medicine be integrated in helping with timing of decisions during the treatment path. Psychosocial concerns are paramount, and nursing provides the coordination and orchestration of care between these disciplines. Social work can assist with finances and resources for the woman and her family. Because pregnancy can have many meanings for the woman, it is important not to overlook what spiritual significance this pregnancy may represent. Having access to bringing a hospital chaplain into the group could be invaluable.

In many academic institutions or large community hospitals, nurses are designated as clinical specialists providing and coordinating care within specific disease programs. For a gestational breast cancer patient, coordinated care is essential. At small academic centers or small community hospitals, there may not be such a dedicated nurse specialist to assist in this effort. For example, at the University of Texas MD Anderson Cancer Center, they have a model of care whereby a nurse liaison coordinates between the institution and the outside hospital, which will be providing the patient's obstetric care.[54] At the University of North Carolina, Chapel Hill, we use nurse navigators, functioning in much the same way, ensuring that the cancer care and the obstetric care is coordinated. We are fortunate that within our health care system we have forged paths with our high-risk obstetrics colleagues to streamline care in these situations.

The coordination of care incorporates obtaining pertinent data on the woman's pathologic diagnosis and stage, as well as her full medical and obstetrical history, both present and past. This includes last menstrual period and estimated date of conception. Ensuring that medical records are shared with all members of the multidisciplinary team is important for treatment decision making and timing of the delivery. This type of case would be best discussed at a multidisciplinary conference, where all members can actually discuss the treatment plan and relevant issues.

The nurse specialist in breast cancer is instrumental in providing educational resources to the gestational breast cancer patient and her family. Whether they be pre- or postoperative care plans, chemotherapy side effects, or whole-breast radiotherapy side effects, the nurse has an obligation to assess the woman's understanding of her treatment plan and to this end will provide and ensure safety for her and the fetus.

There are many resources available for patient education on treatment paths as well as psychosocial support for treating women with breast cancer who are pregnant. The National Cancer Institute, American College of Surgeons, American Society of Clinical Oncology, and National Comprehensive Cancer Network are all such organizations. These organizations also provide practice guidelines reflecting best practices. In the circumstance of gestational breast cancer, there are very little data driven from clinical trials supporting those paths. There is consensus on best medical practice based on retrospective case reviews.

FUTURE DIRECTIONS AND NECESSARY FUTURE STUDIES

Of course, the prospective, randomized trial remains the gold standard for establishing paradigm-changing treatments. However, in this specialized niche population, a prospective, randomized trial will never be performed. Thus we are left with a single institution or registry data to help determine the best treatment course for these patients. Several are ongoing, both in the United States and Europe. For example, the MD Anderson Cancer Center prospective trial will enroll 50 pregnant women requiring chemotherapy, treat with a uniform CAF regimen, and follow both mother's and child's outcome, and the German Breast Group includes a registry with similar outcomes. Given the concern both to mother and child of chemotherapy given to the pregnant patient, a great resource would be provided by a nationwide registry and longitudinal studies of both early and late outcomes for both the patient and the children.

SUMMARY

In summary, patients diagnosed with gestational breast cancer need a highly skilled and coordinated team of clinicians to develop a strategy for treating their breast cancer. No longer is a modified radical mastectomy the only option for patients who have breast cancer diagnosed during their pregnancy. The collaborative and team effort ensures that the patient maximizes her oncologic outcome while also maximizing the term delivery of a healthy newborn infant.

REFERENCES

1. Navrozoglou I, Vrekoussis T, Kontostolis E, et al. Breast cancer during pregnancy: a mini-review. *Eur J Surg Oncol.* 2008;34:837-843.
2. Molckovsky A, Madarnas Y. Breast cancer in pregnancy: a literature review. *Breast Cancer Res Treat.* 2008;108:333-338.
3. Anderson JM. Mammary cancers and pregnancy. *Br Med J.* 1979;1:1124-1127.
4. Wallack MK, Wolf JA Jr, Bedwinek J, et al. Gestational carcinoma of the female breast. *Curr Probl Cancer.* 1983;7:1-58.
5. Ventura SJ, Mosher WD, Curtin SC, et al. Trends in pregnancies and pregnancy rates by outcome: estimates for the United States, 1976-96. *Vital Health Stat 21.* 2000:1-47.

6. Kilgore R, Bloodgood J. Tumors and tumor-like lesions of the breast in association with pregnancy. *Arch Surg.* 1929;10.2079.

7. Haagensen C, Stout A. Carcinoma of the breast: criteria of operability. *Ann Surg.* 1943;118:859-870, 1032-1051.

8. White T. Carcinoma of the breast and pregnancy. *Ann Surg.* 1954;139:9.

9. Harrington S. Carcinoma of the breast: results of surgical treatment when the carcinoma occurred in course of pregnancy or lactation and when pregnancy occurred subsequent to operation, 1910-1933. *Ann Surg.* 1937;106:690.

10. Gentilini O, Masullo M, Rotmensz N, et al. Breast cancer diagnosed during pregnancy and lactation: biological features and treatment options. *Eur J Surg Oncol.* 2005;31:232-236.

11. Petrek JA, Dukoff R, Rogatko A. Prognosis of pregnancy-associated breast cancer. *Cancer.* 1991;67:869-872.

12. Berry DL, Theriault RL, Holmes FA, et al. Management of breast cancer during pregnancy using a standardized protocol. *J Clin Oncol.* 1999;17:855-861.

13. Zemlickis D, Lishner M, Degendorfer P, et al. Maternal and fetal outcome after breast cancer in pregnancy. *Am J Obstet Gynecol.* 1992;166:781-787.

14. Kuerer HM, Cunningham JD, Brower ST, Tartter PI. Breast carcinoma associated with pregnancy and lactation. *Surg Oncol.* 1997;6:93-98.

15. Bonnier P, Romain S, Dilhuydy JM, et al. Influence of pregnancy on the outcome of breast cancer: a case-control study Societe Française de Senologie et de Pathologie Mammaire Study Group. *Int J Cancer.* 1997;72:720-727.

16. Liberman L, Giess CS, Dershaw DD, et al. Imaging of pregnancy-associated breast cancer. *Radiology.* 1994;191.245-248.

17. Scott-Conner CE, Schorr SJ. The diagnosis and management of breast problems during pregnancy and lactation. *Am J Surg.* 1995;170:401-405.

18. Schelfout K, Van Goethem M, Kersschot E, et al. Contrast-enhanced MR imaging of breast lesions and effect on treatment. *Eur J Surg Oncol.* 2004;30:501-507.

19. Finley JL, Silverman JF, Lannin DR. Fine-needle aspiration cytology of breast masses in pregnant and lactating women. *Diagn Cytopathol.* 1989;5:255-259.

20. Gupta RK. The diagnostic impact of aspiration cytodiagnosis of breast masses in association with pregnancy and lactation with an emphasis on clinical decision making. *Breast J.* 1997;3:131-134.

21. Schackmuth EM, Harlow CL, Norton LW. Milk fistula: a complication after core breast biopsy. *AJR Am J Roentgenol.* 1993;161:961-962.

22. Hylton N, Carey LA, DeMichele A, et al. Characterizing the biology and response of locally advanced breast cancer in women undergoing neoadjuvant therapy: preliminary results from the I-SPY trial. Presented at the San Antonio Breast Cancer Symposium, San Antonio, TX, December 13-16, 2007.

23. Bastek JA, Sammel MD, Paré E, et al. Adverse neonatal outcome examining the risks between preterm, late preterm, and term infants. *American Journal of Obstetrics and Gynecology.* 2008;199:367.e361-367.e368.

24. Raju TN, Higgins RD, Stark AR, Leveno KJ. Optimizing care and outcome for late-preterm (near-term) infants: a summary of the workshop sponsored by the National Institute of Child Health and Human Development. *Pediatrics.* 2006;118:1207-1214.

25. Malangoni MA, Wagh M. Tumor vs management of general surgical problems in the pregnant patient. *Am J Surg.* 2004;187:170-180.

26. Rosen MA. Management of anesthesia for the pregnant surgical patient. *Anesthesiology.* 1999;91:1159-1163.

27. Koren G, Pastuszak A, Ito S. Drugs in pregnancy. *N Engl J Med.* 1998;338:1128-1137.

28. Cohen SE. Nonobstetric surgery during pregnancy. In: Chestnut DH, ed. *Obstetric Anesthesia, Principles and Practice.* St. Louis, MO: CV Mosby; 1999:279-302.

29. Nuevo FR. Anesthesia for nonobstetric surgery in the pregnant patient. In: Birnbach DJ, Gatt SP, Datta S, eds. *Textbook of Obstetric Anesthesia.* New York, NY: Churchill Livingstone; 2000:289-298.

30. Giuliano AE, Dale PS, Turner RR, et al. Improved axillary staging of breast cancer with sentinel lymphadenectomy. *Ann Surg.* 1995;222:394-399; discussion 399-401.

31. Giuliano AE, Kirgan DM, Guenther JM, Morton DL. Lymphatic mapping and sentinel lymphadenectomy for breast cancer. *Ann Surg.* 1994;220:391-398; discussion 398-401.

32. Krag DN, Weaver DL, Alex JC, Fairbank JT. Surgical resection and radiolocalization of the sentinel lymph node in breast cancer using a gamma probe. *Surgical Oncology.* 1993;2:335-339; discussion 340.

33. Albertini JJ, Lyman GH, Cox C, et al. Lymphatic mapping and sentinel node biopsy in the patient with breast cancer. *JAMA.* 1996;276:1818-1822.

34. Schrenk P, Hochreiner G, Fridrik M, Wayand W. Sentinel node biopsy performed before preoperative chemotherapy for axillary lymph node staging in breast cancer. *Breast J.* 2003;9:282-287.

35. Sabel MS, Schott AF, Kleer CG, et al. Sentinel node biopsy prior to neoadjuvant chemotherapy. *Am J Surg.* 2003;186:102-105.

36. Ollila DW, Neuman HB, Sartor C, et al. Lymphatic mapping and sentinel lymphadenectomy prior to neoadjuvant chemotherapy in patients with large breast cancers. *Am J Surg.* 2005;190:371-375.

37. Krag DN, Anderson SJ, Julian TB, et al. Technical outcomes of sentinel-lymph-node resection and conventional axillary-lymph-node dissection in patients with clinically node-negative breast cancer: results from the NSABP B-32 randomised phase III trial. *Lancet Oncol.* 2007;8:881-888.

38. Mondi MM, Cuenca RE, Ollila DW, et al. Sentinel lymph node biopsy during pregnancy: initial clinical experience. *Ann Surg Oncol.* 2007;14:218-221.

39. Khera SY, Kiluk JV, Hasson DM, et al. Pregnancy-associated breast cancer patients can safely undergo lymphatic mapping. *Breast J.* 2008;14:250-254.

40. Keleher A, Wendt R 3rd, Delpassand E, et al. The safety of lymphatic mapping in pregnant breast cancer patients using Tc-99m sulfur colloid. *Breast J.* 2004;10:492-495.

41. Hale J. X-ray protection. In: Taveras JM, Ferrucci JT, eds. *Radiology.* 15th ed. Philadephia, PA: Lippincott Williams & Wilkins; 2001:2-3.

42. Loibl S, von Minckwitz G, Gwyn K, et al. Breast carcinoma during pregnancy. International recommendations from an expert meeting. *Cancer.* 2006;106:237-246.

43. Schwartz GF, Giuliano AE, Veronesi U. Proceedings of the consensus conference on the role of sentinel lymph node biopsy in carcinoma of the breast, April 19-22, 2001, Philadelphia, PA. *Cancer.* 2002;94:2542-2551.

44. Schnitt SJ, Harris JR. Evolution of breast-conserving therapy for localized breast cancer. *J Clin Oncol.* 2008;26:1395-1396.

45. Veronesi U, Luini A, Del Vecchio M, et al. Radiotherapy after breast-preserving surgery in women with localized cancer of the breast. *N Engl J Med.* 1993;328:1587-1591.

46. National Council on Radiation Protection and Measurements. *Report #39: Basic Radiation Protection Criteria.* Washington, DC: NCRP; 1971.

47. Kelly HL, Collichio FA, Dees EC. Concomitant pregnancy and breast cancer: options for systemic therapy. *Breast Dis.* 2005;23:95-101.

48. Cullins SL, Pridjian G, Sutherland CM. Goldenhar's syndrome associated with tamoxifen given to the mother during gestation. *JAMA.* 1994;271:1905-1906.

49. Cardonick E, Iacobucci A. Use of chemotherapy during human pregnancy. *Lancet Oncol.* 2004;5:283-291.

50. Gadducci A, Cosio S, Fanucchi A, et al. Chemotherapy with epirubicin and paclitaxel for breast cancer during pregnancy: case report and review of the literature. *Anticancer Res.* 2003;23:5225-5229.

51. Redmond GP. Physiological changes during pregnancy and their implications for pharmacological treatment. *Clin Invest Med.* 1985;8:317-322.

52. Rimes S, Gano J, Hahn K, et al. Caring for pregnant patients with breast cancer. *Oncol Nurs Forum.* 2006;33:1065-1069.

53. Williams SF, Schilsky RL. Antineoplastic drugs administered during pregnancy. *Semin Oncol.* 2000;27:618-622.

54. Rimes S, Gano J, Milbourne A. Care of the pregnant patient with cancer. *Oncology Nurse.* 2008;22:13-22.

55. Pavlidis N, Pentheroudakis G. The pregnant mother with breast cancer: diagnostic and therapeutic management. *Cancer Treat Rev.* 2005;31:439-447.

56. Aviles A, Neri N. Hematological malignancies and pregnancy: a final report of 84 children who received chemotherapy in utero. *Clin Lymphoma.* 2001;2:173-177.

57. Holleb AI, Farrow JH. The relation of carcinoma of the breast and pregnancy in 283 patients. *Surg Gynecol Obstet.* 1962;115:65-71.

58. Applewhite RR, Smith LR, DiVincenti F. Carcinoma of the breast associated with pregnancy and lactation. *Am Surg.* 1973;39:101-104.

59. Deemarsky L, Neishtadt E. Breast cancer and pregnancy. *Breast.* 1980;7:17.

60. King RM, Welch JS, Martin JK Jr, Coulam CB. Carcinoma of the breast associated with pregnancy. *Surg Gynecol Obstet.* 1985;160:228-232.

61. Ribeiro G, Jones DA, Jones M. Carcinoma of the breast associated with pregnancy. *Br J Surg.* 1986;73:607-609.

CHAPTER 90

Inflammatory Breast Cancer

Viviana Negrón González
Julia L. Oh
Massimo Cristofanilli
Gildy V. Babiera

Inflammatory breast cancer (IBC) is one of the rarest and most aggressive forms of breast cancer, having relatively distinct clinicopathological features and the lowest survival rates. Its presentation was first described in 1814 by Bell as "a purple color on the skin over the tumor accompanied by shooting pains," which he identified as "a very unpropitious beginning."[1] In 1889, Bryant noted the role of cancer cells obstructing the lymphatics in the development of inflammatory signs.[2] The term "inflammatory carcinoma of the breast" was coined by Lee and Tannebaum in 1924. Currently, based on the American Joint Committee on Cancer (AJCC) Staging System, IBC is classified as T4d and described as a "clinicopathological entity that is characterized by diffuse erythema and edema (peau d'orange), often without an underlying mass. These clinical findings should involve the majority of the breast . . . "[3] It should be stressed that IBC is primarily a clinical diagnosis and thus, in the absence of clinical findings, involvement of the dermal lymphatics alone does not indicate the diagnosis of IBC. In this chapter, we review the epidemiology, clinical presentation, diagnostic modalities, and treatment, and discuss the current controversies of IBC.

EPIDEMIOLOGY

The incidence of IBC is 1% to 6% in the United States. However, results from the 2005 Surveillance, Epidemiology, and End Results program revealed that the IBC incidence rate increased from 2.0/100,000 woman-years for 1988 to 1990 to 2.5/100,000 woman-years for 1997 to 1999. This is a marked contrast with the incidence rates for other types of invasive breast cancers, which decreased during the same time.[4]

Before 1990, it was believed that IBC was particularly prevalent in North Africa, specifically in Tunisia, because pre-1990 reports revealed a higher than 50% incidence of IBC in those areas.[5] However, a review of 419 cases diagnosed as T4d between 1975 and 1996 at a single Tunisian institution revealed the incidence of IBC in Tunisia to be approximately 7%.[5] This decrease in IBC incidence was attributed to the fact that prior studies had included not only T4d breast cancers, but also ulcerated breast cancers (T4b), which clearly exemplifies the complexities in the diagnosis of IBC.

Studies done using breast biopsy tissue from Tunisian patients with IBC revealed an increased incidence in the detection of viral sequences and antigens that resemble mouse mammary tumor virus.[6] This relationship is currently under investigation in several institutions in the United States to confirm the etiopathogenetic role of mouse mammary tumor virus in IBC. Currently, various molecular factors associated with IBC have been identified, but the causative agent remains to be isolated.

CLINICAL CHARACTERISTICS

IBC has a characteristic clinical presentation of skin changes and breast enlargement that occurs rapidly, typically within 3 months (Fig. 90-1).[7] Although the AJCC definition calls for clinical findings to involve the majority of the breast, some researchers are calling for the disease to be diagnosed when there is less skin involvement so that an earlier diagnosis and possibly a better outcome might be obtained.[8] IBC is often considered to have

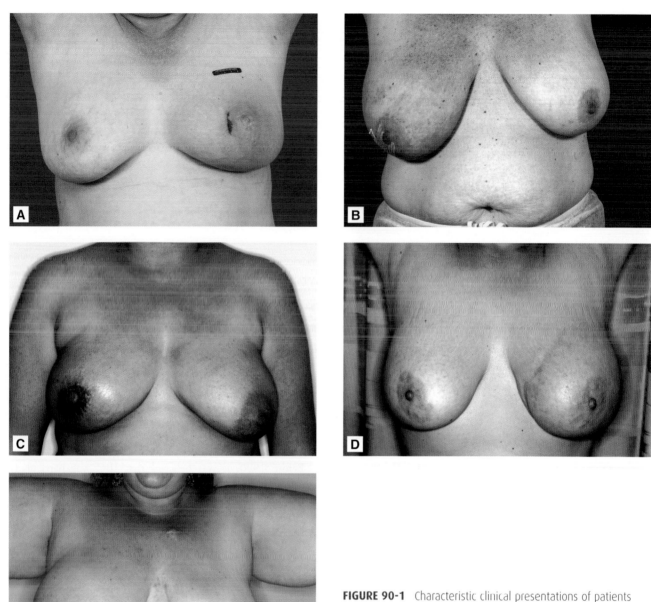

FIGURE 90-1 Characteristic clinical presentations of patients with IBC. **A.** Patient with left breast IBC; note erythema and peau d'orange. **B.** Patient with right breast IBC; note erythema and marked breast edema. **C.** Patient with right breast IBC; note skin changes and edema. **D.** Patient with left breast IBC; note breast edema and erythema. **E.** Patient with right breast IBC; note erythema and peau de orange.

3 clinical variants: primary, secondary, and occult (Table 90-1).[2] The occult variant has a better prognosis.

Although IBC is most commonly associated with ductal carcinoma, lobular and medullary carcinomas may also be associated with an IBC diagnosis. The mean age at diagnosis is 58 years, and black women appear to be more affected with this disease than are other women.[4] IBC is often estrogen receptor (ER) negative (up to 83% of cases), and it is associated with a higher nuclear grade tumor and a higher incidence of lymph node involvement compared with other types of breast cancer.[9] As reported in the literature, the incidence of involved axillary lymph nodes can reach 72.3% (range, 60%-85%), with supra-clavicular lymph node involvement seen in 11.6% of cases.[10] Further, IBC is associated with a higher incidence (~20%) of distant metastasis at the time of diagnosis than are other breast cancers. It has also been reported that a high body mass index in breast cancer patients is associated with a poor overall survival rate.[11] However, Chang et al[11] found no statistical survival difference between obese and nonobese patients with IBC. They also found that premenopausal women with IBC had a worse survival rate than did postmenopausal women with IBC.[11]

TABLE 90-1 Variants of Inflammatory Breast Cancer (IBC)

Variant	Characteristics
Primary	Signs of inflammation
	No palpable breast mass
	Enlarged ipsilateral axillary lymph node
	Presence of clinically, radiologically, and pathologically indistinct invasive carcinoma
Secondary	Skin manifestation in breast that previously contained cancer
	After mastectomy, skin manifestation in opposite breast or distant cutaneous recurrence
	Clinical course and behavior similar to primary IBC
Occult	No clinical evidence of inflammation
	Tumor emboli present in dermal lymphatics on histological exams
	Has a better prognosis

In general, the diagnosis of IBC is an independent predictor of a poor prognosis, with death from this disease occurring nearly twice as often as in other breast cancers.[8,12,13] In their institutional review of 398 patients treated for IBC at the University of Texas MD Anderson Cancer Center between 1974 and 2005, Gonzalez-Angulo et al[13] revealed a median overall survival duration of 4.2 years and a mean time to disease recurrence of 2.3 years. These findings demonstrate a marked contrast with those for stage I breast cancer, which has a 5-year overall survival rate of 90% or more.[14] Finally, both "estrogen (ER)/progesterone (PR)-negative receptor status" and high nuclear grade are associated with a poorer overall survival rate for patients diagnosed with IBC.

DIFFERENTIAL DIAGNOSIS

IBC has characteristic clinical findings, but may be confused with locally advanced breast cancer (LABC), which can present with the same physical findings. Thus, a thorough medical history is crucial to distinguish between the 2 as treatment and prognosis can differ significantly. LABC and IBC were previously thought to represent different points on the same disease spectrum, but it has since been well established that they are distinct entities, each with distinct clinical behaviors and outcomes (Table 90-2).[12,15] For example, in IBC the physical signs are secondary to the characteristic dermal lymphatic invasion by tumor cells, whereas in LABC the physical signs typically are believed to represent tumor that has progressed as a result of delayed diagnosis or neglect.[16] A critical difference between the 2 is the time frame during which the signs of disease develop. IBC arises quickly (<3 months), while LABC often develops slowly. IBC is usually detected by the patient because of the rapid progression of changes to the skin, and fewer than 50% of IBC patients present with a well-defined mass.[7] In contrast, LABC is usually detected by the patient because of the presence of a mass over a long period of time, which is sometimes neglected.

The treatment strategy for both IBC and LABC includes neoadjuvant chemotherapy, surgery, and radiotherapy. However, 2 of the most important reasons for distinguishing between them are the differences in the actual local treatment prescribed and the survival outcomes. The outcome for patients with IBC

TABLE 90-2 Comparison between Locally Advanced Breast Cancer (LABC) and Inflammatory Breast Cancer (IBC)

LABC	IBC
Arises over a longer period of time (>3 months)	Arises quickly (<3 months)
No dermal lymphatic involvement[16]	Probable dermal lymphatic involvement[16]
Palpable mass usually detected by patient	Rapid, progressive changes to skin usually detected by patient
Older patients	Younger patients
Positive ER/PR common*,[12]	Negative ER/PR common*,[12]
	Positive node involvement common†,[12]
	High tumor grade common[12]
No micrometastasis	Possible micrometastasis
Possible increase in angiogenesis and lymphangiogenesis	Probable increase in angiogenesis and lymphangiogenesis
Possible overexpression of HER-2/neu, RhoC GTPase, and NF-κB[15]	Probable overexpression of HER-2/neu, RhoC GTPase, and NF-κB[15]
Incidence increases with age‡,[12]	Incidence plateaus after age 50 years[12]
Overall survival rate of 44%-79% at 5 years[7]	Overall survival rate of 41% at 5 years[7]

*Patients with ER-negative LABC have a poorer overall survival rate than patients with ER-positive IBC.[12]
†Data for positive node involvement in IBC was too incomplete for assessment.[12]
‡The incidence of LABC increases rapidly until age 50 years and then increases slowly; the incidence of IBC increases until age 50 years and then flattens.[12]

is less favorable than that for patients with LABC, with IBC patients being at twice the risk of death from disease as LABC patients.[12] A series studied by Hortobagyi et al[7] revealed 5-year overall survival rates for patients with stage IIIA or IIIB LABC to be 79% and 44%, respectively, while the overall 5-year survival rate for patients with IBC was 41%.

Mastitis is another condition that must be differentiated from IBC. Mastitis usually occurs during lactation, and the skin changes are accompanied by the flu-like symptoms of fatigue, fever, chills, and leukocytosis.[2] An abscess may also be present. A mammogram may be normal or show increased tissue density, while a sonogram may show increased vasculature, skin thickening, or an abscess in the breast.[17] Mastitis responds well to antibiotics; therefore, any suspected mastitis that persists for longer than 2 weeks or that does not respond to antibiotics warrants a biopsy to exclude IBC.

Radiation dermatitis must also be distinguished from IBC. It is usually limited to areas within the radiation field and often resembles a sun burn. Moist desquamation can occur, but typically these changes resolve within 2 to 3 weeks. Edema is not typically observed.[2]

Other conditions to be considered in the differential diagnosis of IBC include breast lymphoma, Paget disease, erysipelas, tuberculosis, metastatic gastric or ovarian cancer,[18] and calciphylaxis.[19] With so many conditions to be excluded, it is imperative to obtain a thorough medical history and to perform a complete physical exam, as well as radiological studies and biopsies, to distinguish all these conditions from IBC. A heightened awareness of IBC is extremely important to its early diagnosis because the longer it goes undiagnosed the worse it is for a patient who has an already poor survival outcome.

DIAGNOSTIC MODALITIES

Radiological Studies

Although IBC is a clinical diagnosis, imaging studies play an important role in the complete assessment of patients because they provide characterization and delineation of the disease in the breast and enable the evaluation of the contralateral breast, regional lymph node basin, distant metastasis, and response to therapy. The standard imaging modalities used in IBC are mammography and ultrasonography, both of which provide better imaging than in previous years owing to technological advances. Similarly, technological innovations have enabled magnetic resonance imaging (MRI) and positron emission tomography by means of computed tomography (PET/CT) to be used in the early diagnosis and staging of IBC. Because technological advances in radiology have improved the imaging of breast tissue, the idea that IBC is not associated with a breast mass[7] is being challenged by current findings.

Mammography

Despite its standard use, mammography is the least sensitive imaging modality used in the differential diagnosis of IBC. The importance of mammography lies in the early detection of abnormality. The most common mammographic findings for IBC are skin thickening and trabecular distortion, which are seen in 83% and 73% of IBC patients, respectively.[20] On mammograms, skin thickening indicative for IBC is first seen in the inferior areolar region, in contrast with other etiologies in which skin thickening is local or segmental.[21]

Previously, IBC was often diagnosed without an associated breast mass because mammography could not distinguish a mass between variations in the increased density of the diseased breast.[22] A study comparing radiological findings in IBC patients during 1988 to 2000 revealed that a mass was identified on only 16% of the mammograms.[21] However, in a study comparing radiological findings in IBC patients from 2003 to 2007, an associated mass was identified on 32% of the mammograms.[20] This marked difference may be secondary to technological improvements in mammography.

Ultrasonography

The sensitivity to changes in structure and pathology provided by ultrasonography make it a reliable means by which to conduct image-guided biopsy to diagnose IBC, and to assess regional lymph node involvement. In a study comparing radiological findings in 76 patients with IBC, a breast mass, architectural distortion, and skin thickening was seen in 95% of the sonograms.[20] Yang et al[20] reported that a loss of architecture could be ultrasonographically identified by a characteristic "linear infiltrative hypoechogenecity" dissecting the parenchyma. Another study comparing radiological findings in patients with IBC showed that axillary, supraclavicular, and infraclavicular lymph node involvement was seen in 93%, 50%, and 50% of the sonograms, respectively.[22] Such findings demonstrate the reliability of ultrasonography in supporting a diagnosis for IBC and in assessing disease spread to regional lymph nodes.

MRI

Developed for medical use in the 1970s, recent technological innovations have enabled MRI to be applied to breast cancer. Current comparative studies of imaging modalities used in IBC[20,22] indicate that the sensitivity of MRI appears to be superior to that of mammography or ultrasonography in diagnosing IBC. In 99 cases of IBC, MRI revealed a mass and/or architectural distortion in 100% of cases, skin thickening in 97%, multicentric disease in 73%, and axillary lymph node involvement in 88%.[20] Such results appear to make MRI an excellent imaging modality for this disease, and perhaps in the near future it may become the study of choice for IBC. However, disadvantages of MRI exist, including patient discomfort, lack of tolerance, and the single coil size, the latter of which may exclude patients who have bigger or smaller breasts (Fig. 90-2).

PET/CT

Another relatively new imaging modality being investigated for the initial staging of IBC is PET/CT. Yang et al[20] reported that skin thickening and breast parenchymal lesions could be identified in 96% of PET/CT scans from 24 patients with IBC. In their review of radiological studies done in patients with IBC, Le-Petross et al[22] reported that PET/CT revealed multicentricity in 63% of cases, regional nodal disease in 88%, and distant metastasis in 38%. Given all these findings, PET/CT can be

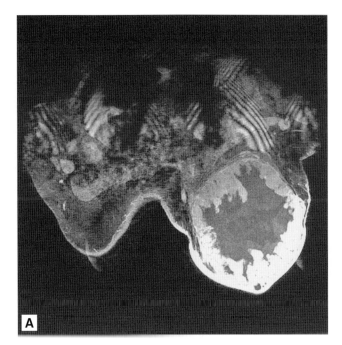
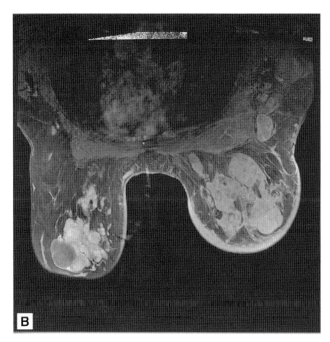

FIGURE 90-3 MRI findings in patients with IBC. **A**, Patient with right IBC; note enhancing mass and skin thickness. **B**, Patient with right IBC; note marked skin thickness.

considered a useful imaging modality for the initial staging of IBC. However, experience in imaging with PET/CT for IBC is still in its early stages and its role remains to be defined (Fig. 90-3).

Biopsy

IBC is a clinicopathological disease and biopsy can certainly help confirm the diagnosis. The presence of dermal lymphatic tumor emboli is considered specific for IBC; however, this finding is not a prerequisite for the diagnosis because it may only be seen in upto 75% of cases.[2] Surgical skin biopsy can be performed for obtaining a diagnosis of IBC, the goal of which is to include part of the area with skin changes in order to detect lymphatic involvement. However, skin punch biopsy can also be considered as it allows various cores to be obtained, making this an adequate biopsy method as well. In cases with a palpable mass or adenopathy, an additional core biopsy of these entities may establish the diagnosis.

The role of fine-needle aspiration is not well established. It has been reported that the difficulty in obtaining an adequate sample, which can require multiple attempts, and the need for an experienced cytopathologist to perform the procedure make this method impractical.[2]

PATHOLOGICAL FINDINGS

As stated previously, the presence of dermal lymphatic invasion is characteristic of IBC (Fig. 90-4). It is this lymphatic obstruction that gives rise to the inflammatory signs. IBC tends to be a ductal malignancy characterized by early lymphatic invasion and lymph node involvement. Studies have revealed that, unlike other types of breast cancer, IBC cells overexpress E-cadherin.[9] IBC cells lose the ability to express E-cadherin when invading

the lymphatic channels, but they regain overexpression once they enter the circulation. The presence of E-cadherin stabilizes the tumor emboli in the lymphatics. The tumor emboli are hypoxic in the center, making them more resistant to both chemotherapy and radiotherapy.[9] Increased angiogenesis in IBC has been correlated with significantly higher microvascular density and increased levels of carbonic anhydrase IX.[9] The expression levels of lymphangiogenic growth factors, such as vascular endothelial growth factors (VEGF) C and D, are also increased.

IBC has a high incidence of HER-2/neu and c-myb overexpression. It is also more commonly associated with p53 mutation than other breast cancers.[9] Other factors commonly overexpressed in IBC are RhoC GTPase, an oncogene involved with cytoskeletal reorganization that contributes to a cancer's metastatic potential and serves as a predictor of poor survival, and NF-κB, a transcription factor that mediates apoptosis, proliferation, and migration in tumor cells.[9] Meanwhile, WISP3, a tumor suppressor gene that inhibits the ability of tumor cells' abilities to invade and grow, is commonly lost in IBC.[9] All these factors combined may contribute to the aggressive characteristics and behavior exhibited by IBC, which makes them ideal candidates for future targeted therapies.

TREATMENT

IBC was originally thought to be a fatal disease, with a 5-year overall survival rate of upto 5% for patients treated with surgery or irradiation alone. However, in the past 4 decades the treatment of IBC has been revolutionized with the addition of chemotherapy to the regimen. Currently, the management of IBC requires a multidisciplinary approach, which combines chemotherapy,

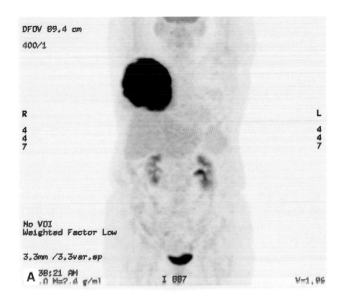

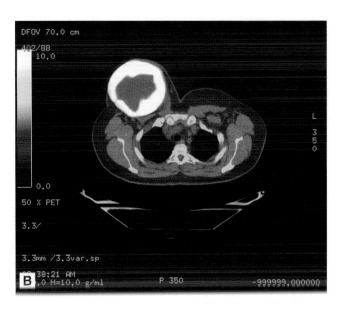

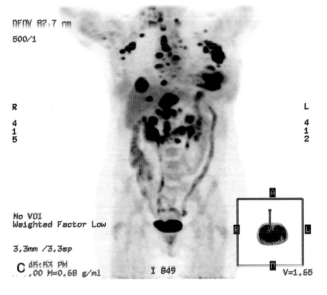

FIGURE 90-3 PET and PET/CT findings in patients with IBC. **A.** Patient with right breast IBC. **B.** PET/CT scan of the same patient as in **(A)**. **C.** Metastatic left breast IBC; note multiple lesions.

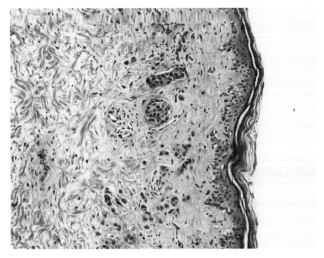

FIGURE 90-4 Dermal lymphatic invasion by tumor emboli in IBC. Note tumor emboli present in the dermal lymphatics.

surgery and radiotherapy. This combination has improved the 3-year overall survival to 50%.[23]

Chemotherapy

Primary chemotherapy is the initial approach in the treatment of IBC (Fig. 90-5). It was originally used only when IBC was deemed inoperable at the time of presentation and there was poor disease control with the other modalities. The standard chemotherapy regimen for IBC is anthracycline based.[24] Typical regimens used are FAC (cyclophosphamide, doxorubicin, and 5-fluorouracil) or FEC (cyclophosphamide, epirubicin, and 5-fluorouracil). The introduction of taxanes (paclitaxel and docetaxel) to the FAC regimen have markedly increased the rate of complete pathological response from 10% to 25%, which has increased overall survival from 41 to 52 months.[25] This improvement in overall survival is more dramatic in patients with ER-negative IBC.

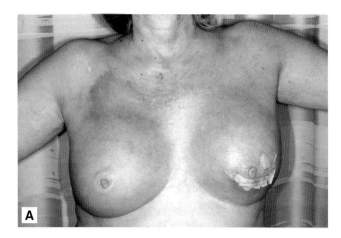
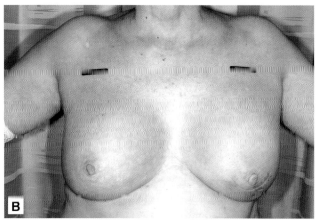

FIGURE 90-5 Clinical response of bilateral IBC to neoadjuvant chemotherapy. **A.** Skin manifestation prior to neoadjuvant chemotherapy. **B.** Marked improvement in skin changes post–neoadjuvant chemotherapy.

IBC patients with HER-2/neu overexpression are candidates for the use of trastuzumab and lapatinib. In a review of 111 patients, Dawood et al[26] found that the use of trastuzumab decreased the hazard of death for HER-2/neu-positive IBC patients compared with that for HER-2/neu-negative patients (hazard ratio, 0.56; 95% CI, 0.34-0.93). The use of lapatinib, a reversible inhibitor of the ErbB1 and ErbB2 tyrosine kinases that induces growth arrest and/or apoptosis in ErbB1/ErbB2 cell lines, was studied by Cristofanilli et al[27] in 21 patients with recurrent HER-2-positive IBC. That study demonstrated a 95% clinical response rate, but data regarding survival are still pending.

Antiangiogenic therapies using bevacizumab (Avastin) have shown limited benefit as neoadjuvant chemotherapy for patients with IBC, although changes in the biological activities of tumors have been noted.[28] Current clinical trails are testing the effects of tyrosine-kinase inhibitors on VEGF and lymphangiogenesis, but results have not yet been reported.

Surgery

The role of mastectomy after chemotherapy in patients with IBC is controversial. In 1 study in which 54 patients received neoadjuvant chemotherapy with radiotherapy only or with surgery and radiotherapy, De Boer et al[29] found that surgery did not appear to have any impact on the frequency of local recurrence. This was demonstrated by both groups having similar rates of local disease recurrence: 34% for those who received surgery and radiotherapy and 42% for those who received radiotherapy only (p value not specified).[29] Nevertheless, a review of the literature done by Kell and Morrow[30] revealed that, although various studies had similar results to those of De Boer et al, other studies have noted benefits of surgical treatment, such as gaining additional clinical information with which to guide future treatment, removing potential chemoresistant foci, and improving local disease control. In a review of 172 patients with IBC, a study performed by Fleming et al[31] found that the combination of chemotherapy, mastectomy, and radiotherapy improved local disease control and decreased local recurrence.

A comparison of all studies to determine the discrepancies in outcomes is difficult to perform because of the selection bias inherent in each. Using the response to neoadjuvant chemotherapy to determine which patients received radiotherapy only versus which received surgery and radiotherapy may play a determining role in the results of comparative studies.[30] The best way to assess the contribution surgical treatment makes to the management of IBC is to conduct a prospective randomized trial.[30] As of today, no randomized trail comparing triple therapy (chemotherapy, surgery, and radiotherapy) with dual therapy (chemotherapy and surgery or chemotherapy and radiotherapy) has been performed.

Currently, the surgical treatment of choice for patients with IBC is a modified radical mastectomy.[30] This should be performed 2 or 3 weeks after the completion of chemotherapy. The operative field should include all skin changes because it has been demonstrated that positive surgical margins are associated with poorer rates for overall survival, disease-free survival, and local control. In their study of IBC patients Curcio et al[1] reported that 3-year overall survival, disease-free survival, and local control rates for patients with a negative margin were 47.4%, 37.5%, and 60.3%, respectively, while the same rates were 0%, 16.7%, and 31.3%, respectively, for patients with a positive margin. Given these findings and the difficulty in judging the extent of residual disease, breast-conserving surgery is ill advised for patients with IBC.[32] Moreover, the standard practice is to perform an axillary dissection in IBC patients because 55% to 85% of patients will have a clinically positive axilla.

The use of sentinel lymph node biopsy is not recommended in IBC patients because it is believed that the tumor cells block the lymphatics, making them unable to carry the tracer necessary to identify the sentinel node. In a study of IBC patients who underwent sentinel lymph node biopsy, Stearns et al[33] noted that the procedure had an identification rate of 75%. The false negative rate also appeared to be high, but the total patients evaluated were too small to make definitive conclusions. Therefore, the low identifcation rate combined with the high probability of axillary inovlvement and the potential for inadequate locoregional control, is why sentinel lymph node biopsy is not routinely recommended for patients with IBC.

Breast reconstruction is feasible in patients with IBC who have no medical contraindications for the procedure. However, the timing of reconstruction is controversial. Arguments against immediate reconstruction include difficulties in delivering adequate doses of radiation to the disease site and surveying the area for recurrence.[34] Radiotherapy decreases wound healing and may cause contraction as well as atrophy and fibrosis, which can affect the cosmetic outcome for reconstructions that used autologous tissue transfer in the immediate setting. A study by Tran et al[35] revealed that the incidence for late complications was significantly higher for patients undergoing immediate versus those undergoing delayed TRAM reconstruction. The complications seen in patients who had immediate TRAM reconstruction included fat necrosis, volume loss, and flap contractures. No difference was seen between the 2 groups in the rate of early complications.[35] In cases where radiotherapy will be given postoperatively, implant-based reconstruction is not recommended because of a large incidence of contracture.[36] A review by Spear and Onyewu[37] revealed a complication rate of 52.5% among 40 patients who underwent immediate reconstruction with implants before receiving radiotherapy, with complications including contractures (32.5%), extrusion (5%), and infection (12.5%). In contrast, a study by Chin et al[34] revealed no difference in outcomes between patients undergoing immediate versus delayed autologous-based reconstructions. They also revealed no differences in the rates for disease-free and overall survival between patients who had undergone reconstruction and those who had not.[34]

Skin-sparing mastectomy, the current modality used when performing immediate reconstruction, is obviously not an option for patients with IBC owing to the amount of skin that may need to be removed to ensure negative margins. In addition, because a significant proportion of skin may need to be removed, implant-based reconstruction often is not recommended. Nevertheless, the option of reconstruction, particularly in the delayed fashion can provide a better quality of life for these patients.

Radiotherapy

Following systemic chemotherapy and mastectomy, radiation therapy is indicated for all patients with nonmetastatic IBC. To date, there have been no randomized trials comparing accelerated hyperfractionation to conventional once daily fractionation. The rapid disease progression seen in IBC supports the rationale for accelerated hyperfractionated radiation treatment. This schedule delivers 51 Gy to the chest wall, supraclavicular fossa, and internal mammary nodes with 1.5 Gy twice a day with a 6-hour interval between fractions. Subsequently, the mastectomy scar and any regional, undissected lymph nodes that were involved are boosted to an additional 15 Gy in the same twice-daily fashion, bringing the total dose to 66 Gy. Investigators from the MD Anderson Cancer Center reported a 5-year local-regional control rate of 84% in a study of 192 patients with IBC.[38] The majority of patients in their study received twice-daily postmastectomy radiation therapy. On multivariate analysis, tumor response to neoadjuvant chemotherapy and negative margins were statistically significant predictors of improved locoregional control. The 5-year locoregional control rates were 95% for patients with a clinical complete response compared to 51% for patients with less than a partial response (less than 50% reduction in tumor volume). These results are particularly promising in a disease where local recurrence is

frequently accompanied by simultaneous distant metastases; therefore, the ability to attain locoregional control is likely to translate into improved survival.

The morbidity associated with achieving such results can be significant. Radiation therapy for IBC is associated with early and late skin toxicity. Depending on the initial extent of skin changes, the area treated may be larger than used for standard, non-IBC postmastectomy cases and a bolus on the chest wall is used to intentionally increase the skin dose. This results in considerable moist desquamation toward the last week of radiation and can be very uncomfortable for the patient. Late toxicity may include fibrosis and telangiectasias at the chest wall as well as lymphedema. Because the skin in IBC patients is at very high risk of dermal recurrence, immediate breast reconstruction is discouraged. Immediate reconstruction would compromise target coverage at the medial chest wall and internal mammary nodes due to the constraints of nearby lung and heart tissue.[39] For any patient in whom postmastectomy radiation therapy is indicated, a flat and smooth chest wall provides the optimal anatomy to deliver dose to the targets with minimum dose to the surrounding normal structures.

Depending on the preferences of the institution, patients are often referred to the radiation oncologist before initiating chemotherapy to allow for a comprehensive assessment of the extent of disease. Photographs are taken to document any skin changes that extend beyond the breast to ensure their inclusion in the radiation field. Generous margins will further prevent a recurrence at the field edge. In addition to treating the chest wall, comprehensive irradiation of all ipsilateral lymphatics is indicated due to the exceedingly high risk of regional metastases. This requires careful attention to the initial staging ultrasound to accurately assess the anatomic location of involved lymph nodes for future targeting. After patients complete their systemic therapy, repeat imaging of the ipsilateral supraclavicular, infraclavicular, and internal mammary lymph nodes will be performed to evaluate disease response to determine the final boost dose. The involved nodes should be contoured on axial computed tomography (CT) images and dosimetry planned with 3-dimensional dose calculation algorithms to ensure that all targets receive the optimal dose. In summary, radiation therapy is critical in the multimodality management of patients with IBC. Future directions to reduce the morbidity while maintaining locoregional control are being investigated.

FUTURE DIRECTIONS

To our knowledge, there are currently few active clinical trials regarding systemic treatment options for patients with IBC. The biological features of IBC make several molecular markers (angiogenic factors, E-cadherin, and RhoC) possible targets for novel therapy. The role of bevacizumab, an antiangiogenic inhibitor, in IBC is still under investigation. Prior studies of anti-VEGF agents with chemotherapy did not have promising results in IBC patients, but other members of the VEGF family may be more active agents. The role of farnesyl transferase inhibitors is also currently being studied, and the impressive results for lapatinib reported by Cristofanilli et al,[27] which will be evaluated in an upcoming phase III clinical trail, will perhaps add another therapeutic agent to the current regimen.

Another future therapy may be the concurrent use of chemotherapy and irradiation. Unpublished data from MD Anderson regarding the use of capecitabine (Xeloda) and radiotherapy in patients with inoperable breast cancer have revealed favorable results, with 91% of patients becoming operable.[40] This may represent another future therapy for patients with IBC.

Finally, public educational campaigns geared toward the community, primary care physicians, and community surgeons may help in the early diagnosis and treatment of patients with this disease, with the hope of improving their survival.

SUMMARY

IBC is the most aggressive variant of breast cancer and has one of the worst outcomes. With the addition of chemotherapy to the treatment regimen of IBC in the 1970s, the 5-year overall survival rate increased to 40%.[13] However, a retrospective review of 398 IBC patients treated from 1974 to 2005 at MD Anderson[13] revealed that no significant improvement in the survival rate by decade of diagnosis has since occurred despite the various advances in systemic and locoregional treatments made in the past 30 years for other breast cancers. This suggests that the addition of chemotherapy was the last major advancement in the fight against IBC and that additional research on the biology of this disease is necessary to develop more targeted and effective therapies.

REFERENCES

1. Curcio LD, Rupp E, Williams WL, et al. Beyond the palliative mastectomy in inflammatory breast cancer—a reassessment of margin status. *Ann Surg Oncol*. 1999;6(3):249-254.
2. Resetkova E. Pathologic aspects of inflammatory breast cancer: part 1. Histomorphology and differential diagnosis. *Semin Oncol*. 2008;35(1):25-32.
3. Greene FL, Page DL, Fleming ID, et al. Breast. In: Greene FL, Page DL, Fleming ID, et al. *AJCC Cancer Staging Manual*. 6th ed. Chicago, IL: Springer; 2002:221-240.
4. Hance KW, Anderson WF, Devesa SS, et al. Trends in inflammatory breast carcinoma incidence and survival: the Surveillance, Epidemiology, and End Results program at the National Cancer Institute. *J Natl Cancer Inst*. 2005;97(13):966-975.
5. Boussen H, Bouzaiene H, Ben H, et al. Inflammatory breast cancer in Tunisia: reassessment of incidence and clinicopathological features. *Semin Oncol*. 2008;35(1):17-24.
6. Levine PH, Mesa-Tejada R, Keydar I, et al. Increased incidence of mouse mammary tumor virus-related antigen in Tunisian patients with breast cancer. *Int J Cancer*. 1984;33(3):305-308.
7. Hortobagyi GN, Singletary SE, Buchholz TA. Locally advanced breast cancer. In: Singletary SE, Robb GL, Hortobagyi GN. *Advanced Therapy of Breast Disease*. 2nd ed. Hamilton, ON: BC Decker; 2004:498-508.
8. Levine PH, Veneroso C. The epidemiology of inflammatory breast cancer. *Semin Oncol*. 2008;35(1):11-16.
9. Gong Y. Pathologic aspects of inflammatory breast cancer: part 2. Biologic insight of its aggressive phenotype. *Semin Oncol*. 2008;35(1):33-40.
10. Amparo RS, Miguel Angel CD, Ana LH, et al. Inflammatory breast carcinoma: pathological or clinical entity? *Breast Cancer Res Treat*. 2000;64(3):269-273.
11. Chang S, Alderfer JR, Asmar L, Buzdar AU. Inflammatory breast cancer survival: the role of obesity and menopausal status at diagnosis. *Breast Cancer Res Treat*. 2000;64(2):157-163.
12. Anderson WF, Chu KC, Chang S. Inflammatory breast carcinoma and noninflammatory locally advanced breast carcinoma: distinct clinicopathologic entities? *J Clin Oncol*. 2003;21(12):2254-2259.
13. Gonzalez-Angulo AM, Hennessy B, Broglio K, et al. Trends for inflammatory breast cancer: is survival improving? *Oncologist*. 2007;12(8):904-912.
14. Schnitt SJ, Guidi AJ. Pathology of invasive breast cancer. In: Harris JR, Lippman ME, Morrow M, et al. *Diseases of the Breast*. 3rd ed. Philadelphia, PA: Lippincott Williams & Wilkins; 2004:541-584.
15. Chia S, Swain SM, Byrd DR, et al. Locally advanced and inflammatory breast Cancer. *J Clin Oncol*. 2008;26(5):786-790.
16. Ahern V, Brennan M, Ung O, et al. Locally advanced and inflammatory breast cancer. *Aust Fam Physician*. 2005;34(12):1027-1032.
17. Cardeñosa G. Stroma. In: Cardeñosa G. *Breast Imaging Companion*. 3rd ed. Philadelphia, PA: 2008:368-423.
18. Sato T, Muto I, Fushiki M, et al. Metastatic breast cancer from gastric and ovarian cancer mimicking inflammatory breast cancer: report of two cases. *Breast Cancer*. 2008;15(4):315-320.
19. Bonilla LA, Dickson-Witmer D, Witmer DR, et al. Calciphylaxis mimicking inflammatory breast cancer. *Breast J*. 2007;13(5):514-516.
20. Yang WT, Le-Petross HT, Macapinlac H, et al. Inflammatory breast cancer: PET/CT, MRI, mammography, and sonography findings. *Breast Cancer Res Treat*. 2008;109(3):417-426.
21. Günhan-Bilgen I, Üstün EE, Memis A. Inflammatory breast carcinoma: mammographic, ultrasonographic, clinical, and pathological findings in 142 cases. *Radiology*. 2002;223(3):829-838.
22. Le-Petross CH, Bidaut L, Yang WT. Evolving role of imaging modalities in inflammatory breast cancer. *Semin Oncol*. 2008;35(1):51-63.
23. McIntyre SB, Sabel MS. Inflammatory breast cancer. In: Harris JR, Lippman ME, Morrow M, et al. *Diseases of the Breast*. 3rd ed. Philadelphia, PA: Lippincott Williams & Wilkins; 2004:971-982.
24. Dawood S, Ueno NT, Cristofanilli M. The medical treatment of inflammatory breast cancer. *Semin Oncol*. 2008;35(1):64-71.
25. Cristofanilli M, Gonzalez-Angulo AM, Buzdar AU, et al. Paclitaxel improves the prognosis in estrogen receptor-negative inflammatory breast cancer: the M. D. Anderson Cancer Center experience. *Clin Breast Cancer*. 2004;4(6):415-419.
26. Dawood S, Broglio K, Gong Y, et al. Prognostic significance of HER-2 status in women with inflammatory breast cancer. *Cancer*. 2008;112(9):1905-1911.
27. Cristofanilli M, Boussen H, Baselga J, et al. A phase II combination study of lapatinib and paclitaxel as a neoadjuvant therapy in patients with newly diagnosed inflammatory breast cancer (IBC) [abstract]. *Breast Cancer Res Treat*. 2006;100(Suppl 1):S5.
28. Bonthala Wedam S, Low JA, Yang SX, et al. Antiangiogenic and antitumor effects of bevacizumab in patients with inflammatory and locally advanced breast cancer. *J Clin Oncol*. 2006;54(5):769-770.
29. De Boer RH, Allum WH, Gui GPH, et al. Multimodality therapy in inflammatory breast cancer: is there a place for surgery? *Ann Oncol*. 2000;11(9):1147-1153.
30. Kell MR, Morrow M. Surgical aspects of inflammatory breast cancer. *Breast Dis*. 2005,2006;22(1):67-73.
31. Fleming RYD, Asmar L, Buzdar AU, et al. Effectiveness of mastectomy by response to induction chemotherapy for control in inflammatory breast carcinoma. *Ann Surg Oncol*. 1997;4(6):452-461.
32. Singletary SE. Surgical management of inflammatory breast cancer. *Semin Oncol*. 2008;35(1):72-77.
33. Stearns V, Ewing CA, Slack R, et al. Sentinel lymphadenectomy after neoadjuvant chemotherapy for breast cancer may reliably represent the axilla except for inflammatory breast cancer. *Ann Surg Oncol*. 2002;9(3):235-242.
34. Chin PL, Andersen JS, Somlo G, et al. Esthetic reconstruction after mastectomy for inflammatory breast cancer: is it worthwhile? *J Am Coll Surg*. 2000;190(3):304-309.
35. Tran NV, Chang DW, Gupta A, Kroll SS. Comparison of immediate and delayed free TRAM flap breast reconstruction in patients receiving postmastectomy radiation therapy. *Plast Reconstr Surg*. 2001;108(1):78-82.
36. Kronowitz SJ, Robb GL. Breast reconstruction and radiation therapy. In: Singletary SE, Robb GL, Hortobagyi GN. *Advanced Therapy of Breast Disease*. 2nd ed. Hamilton, ON: BC Decker; 2004:427-438.
37. Spear SL, Onyewu C. Staged breast reconstruction with saline-filled implants in the irradiated breast: recent trends and therapeutic implications. *Plast Reconstr Surg*. 2000;105(3):930-942.
38. Bristol IJ, Woodward WA, Strom EA, et al. Locoregional treatment outcomes after multimodality management of inflammatory breast cancer. *Int J Radiat Oncol Biol Phys*. 2008;72(2):474-484.
39. Motwani SB, Strom EA, Schechter NR, et al. The impact of immediate breast reconstruction on the technical delivery of postmastectomy radiotherapy. *Int J Radiat Oncol Biol Phys*. 2006;66(1):76-82.
40. Woodward WA, Buchholz TA. The role of locoregional therapy in inflammatory breast cancer. *Semin Oncol*. 2008;35(1):78-86.

CHAPTER 91

Breast Cancer Vaccines

Elizabeth A. Mittendorf
Brian J. Czerniecki
George E. Peoples

Advances in the molecular characterization of human tumors have led to increased interest in the development of targeted therapeutics to include monoclonal antibodies and cancer vaccines. Interest in the development of cancer vaccines has increased since these advances led to the identification of tumor-associated antigens (TAAs).[1-3] TAAs expressed by tumors are able to elicit a specific immune response. In addition to having an antigen that serves as a target for the immune response, a successful tumor vaccine requires a platform to present the antigen to the immune system and an environment that is conducive to immune stimulation. The goal of researchers, therefore, has been to identify TAAs and deliver them to the immune system in the context of a vaccine with the appropriate secondary signals required to prompt a robust, protective immune response.

Breast cancer vaccines are appealing because they represent a nontoxic therapeutic modality with great specificity. Another potential benefit of breast cancer vaccines is that they stimulate an immunologic memory response, potentially allowing for a sustained effect without recurrent therapy. In addition, because vaccines are designed to stimulate the immune system, patients are unlikely to develop resistance to this form of targeted therapy. In this chapter, we will review the basics of the immune system's response to vaccination, discuss vaccine formulations, including the TAAs that serve as targets in breast cancer, and present current strategies for incorporating vaccines into treatment algorithms for patients with breast cancer.

BASIC VACCINE IMMUNOLOGY

The human immune system consists of both innate and adaptive arms. The innate immune system is made up of cells such as mast cells, phagocytes, natural killer cells, basophils, and eosinophils that defend the host in a nonspecific manner. This system provides immediate defense against infection but is unable to confer long-lasting or protective immunity. The major functions of the innate immune system therefore include the recruitment of immune cells to sites of infection or inflammation through release of cytokines, activation of the complement cascade, removal of foreign substances, and activation of the adaptive immune system by antigen presentation. The adaptive immune system then is able to confer long-lasting immunity by mounting 2 types of a response: humoral and cellular. Humoral immunity (the antibody response) involves B cells interacting with a foreign antigen, leading to differentiation into plasma cells or memory cells. Plasma cells are able to secrete specific antibodies against the antigen, while memory cells are longer lasting and function to respond quickly to future exposures of the antigen. Cellular immunity (the T-cell response) involves an interaction between T cells and processed fragments of proteins (peptides) that are present on the surface of other cells in association with major histocompatibility (MHC) molecules.

There are 2 types of MHC molecules: class I and class II (Fig. 91-1). Class I MHC molecules are found on nearly all nucleated cells. They can be loaded with peptides of 8 to 10 amino acids that are generated endogenously within the cytosol of the cell. Peptides associated with class I MHC molecules are translocated to the cell surface, where they can be recognized by specific receptors on CD8+ lymphocytes, also known as cytotoxic T cells (CTLs). CTLs confer cytolytic activity by releasing perforin and cytotoxins that induce apoptosis in the target cell. Historically, the majority of cancer vaccines have been designed to stimulate a CTL response.

Class II MHC molecules are found on a few specialized cell types, including dendritic cells, B cells, and macrophages, all of

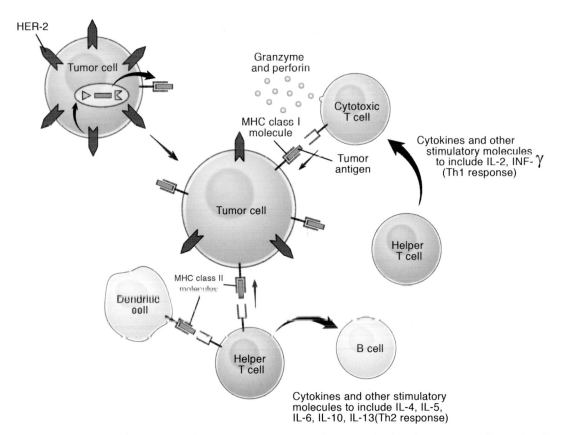

FIGURE 91-1 Basic tumor immunology. Tumor cells express tumor associated antigens (TAA) such as HER-2 on their cell surface. These TAA can be processed by tumor cells such that peptides derived from the TAA are complexed with MHC class I or MHC class II molecules and presented on the cell surface. MHC class I molecules complexed with peptides are recognized by cytotoxic T cells, which when activated, release granzyme and perforin, which induce apoptosis in the target cell. MHC class II molecules complexed with peptides are recognized by helper T cells. Helper T cells release multiple different cytokines including IL-2 and INF-γ, which stimulate CTL and IL-4, IL-5, IL-6, IL-10, and IL-13, which in turn stimulate B cells and the humoral immune response.

which are professional antigen-presenting cells (APC). APCs are efficient at phagocytosis and provide the co-stimulatory molecules needed to activate T cells. An APC is able to engulf a protein, break it apart, and present the peptides on the APC surface during a class II MHC response. Once loaded with the peptide on its cell surface, the APC is then able to stimulate CD4+ lymphocytes, also known as T helper (Th) cells. In addition, there are some tumor cells that express MHC class II molecules including breast, melanoma, and lung cancer.[4] These tumor cells are also able to load peptide associated with MHC class II molecules on their surface therefore they can also stimulate Th cells. Two predominant Th cell subtypes exist, Th1 and Th2, and each of these subtypes has a unique role. Th1 cells are responsible for activating and regulating the development and persistence of cell-mediated immunity.[5] Cytokines produced by Th1 cells include interleukin (IL)-2 and interferon gamma (INF-γ). Using a transgenic mouse model, Park and colleagues demonstrated that Th1 cells are also essential to induce complement fixing antibody and that this resulted in the prevention of breast cancer development.[6] Th2 cells are associated with the humoral immune response and produce several different cytokines, including IL-4, IL-5, IL-6, IL-10, and IL-13, which have roles in B-cell maturation, clonal expansion, and class switching.[7]

Clearly, Th cells mediate an antitumor immune response through multiple mechanisms, and there is increasing evidence that generation of a Th-cell response will be required for a vaccine strategy to be effective.

VACCINE FORMULATION

Vaccine Platform: Selecting a Delivery System

In designing breast cancer vaccines, investigators have employed different platforms for delivering antigens to the immune system. Several of these platforms, their purported benefits, and their potential drawbacks are discussed in the next sections. Additional vaccine formulations, including genetically engineered plasmid DNA vectors, recombinant viral vectors, and recombinant bacteria, which deliver defined TAAs using gene transfer, are in the early stages of development and will not be discussed in detail in this chapter.

Whole Tumor Cell Vaccines

One strategy involves delivering vaccines derived from whole tumor cells, which has the potential advantage of delivering the complete antigen pool of a tumor, theoretically activating a polyclonal immune response. These vaccines can be composed of autologous or allogeneic tumor cells. Autologous tumor cell vaccines are produced by isolating tumor cells from an individual patient and processing these tumor cells into a vaccine in vitro by combining the cells with an immunoadjuvant (described further below) or by genetically modifying the cells. The vaccine is then administered to the patient from whom the tumor cells were initially isolated. One purported benefit of this strategy is that it delivers antigens that may be unique to an individual's tumor.[8] Unfortunately, this strategy is limited by the need to obtain a sufficient quantity of tumor cells from the patient.[8] Allogeneic tumor cells are an alternative that utilize tumor cells isolated from one patient or an established tumor cell line that are subsequently killed and processed, and then administered to another patient. Allogeneic tumor cells can be used as a source of antigen because tumors from various patients have overlapping antigen expression profiles[8-10] and because the tumor antigen-specific immune response can be initiated by cross-priming.[8,11,12] Because tumor cells are not inherently immunogenic, either autologous or allogeneic tumor cells must be delivered in the presence of a strong immune-stimulating adjuvant, such as bacillus Calmette-Guérin (BCG), granulocyte macrophage colony-stimulating factor (GM-CSF), or cytokines known to promote T-cell proliferation. Another disadvantage of a whole tumor cell strategy is that the majority of the tumor cell is made up of normal antigens, and therefore only a small amount of relevant immunogenic antigen is actually delivered.

Peptide-Based Vaccines

Peptide-based vaccines use antigenic peptides derived from TAAs to induce peptide-specific immune regulators, including antibodies, Th cells, and CTLs, that can recognize and lyse tumor cells expressing the immunogenic peptide on their surface. The element of the immune system that is stimulated depends on the peptide utilized and the class of MHC molecule with which the peptide is complexed. Because peptides are only weakly immunogenic, they too must be combined with an immunoadjuvant to stimulate a response.

Peptides can be easily manufactured on a large scale and at a low cost; therefore peptide-based vaccines are simple to construct. One drawback of peptide vaccines is that they are HLA restricted, which limits the number of patients who could benefit from this type of vaccination. For instance, E75, a HER-2-derived peptide discussed in the "HER-2" section later in the chapter, is HLA-A2/A3 restricted.[13] Approximately 50% of patients are HLA-A2+, and an additional 15% are HLA-A3+,[14] suggesting that approximately two-thirds of patients with breast cancer could benefit from an E75 peptide vaccine. To overcome this limitation, investigators have begun identifying peptides for other common HLA types; therefore, it is conceivable that someday every patient could receive an HLA-specific peptide vaccine. A second drawback of vaccination with a single peptide is that the vaccine activates only one arm of the immune system. Using E75 again as an example, because E75 is presented by class I MHC molecules, it stimulates only CTLs. Thus, strategies to incorporate multiple peptides, including those that stimulate CTLs and others that stimulate Th cells, into a single, multi-epitope vaccine, are currently being investigated.[15] Other investigators have utilized longer class II MHC helper peptides that contain class I MHC CTL peptides sequestered completely within their sequence. Patients immunized with the longer peptides mount both a Th cell and CTL response for an enhanced overall immunologic response.[7,16]

Dendritic Cell Vaccines

Dendritic cells (DCs) are the immune system's most effective APCs. When activated, DCs express high levels of both class I and class II MHC molecules for priming CD8+ and CD4+ T cells. In addition, DCs provide potent costimulatory molecules and cytokines required for T-cell activation, suggesting that they may be used to induce a broad, potent, tumor-specific immune response.

Constructing a DC vaccine involves extracting DCs from a patient, using stimulants to mature and expand large quantities of the DCs, exposing these DCs to antigens from the patient's cancer cells, and then injecting the completed vaccine into the patient so the DCs can stimulate an immune response. Although it appears simple, this process is complex, which has limited the clinical development of this vaccination strategy. One issue is with acquiring DCs, which can be obtained from the peripheral blood or derived from peripheral blood precursors, such as monocytes or mobilized CD34+ precursors. The peripheral blood concentration is low and, therefore, obtaining quantities sufficient for repetitive vaccinations is difficult. In addition, peripheral DCs are frequently functionally defective in patients with breast cancer.[8,17] Monocyte-derived DCs can be obtained in large quantities but require a maturation step for immune activation. CD34-derived DCs can be robustly expanded but are expensive to generate. Once obtained, DCs can be loaded with antigen in the form of peptides, proteins, mRNA, or whole tumor cells or their lysates.

Additional challenges exist for an effective DC vaccine strategy. For example, investigators have recognized the importance of secretion of the cytokine IL-12 by DCs in order to enhance the survival and functional avidity of CTLs. CTLs sensitized in the presence of IL-12 are able to recognize the peptide at 10- to 100-fold lower concentrations than CTLs sensitized in its absence.[18] IL-12 also plays a role in Th development. Given the importance of IL-12 in generating an antitumor immune response, the timing of IL-12 secretion must be accounted for when determining the optimal time-point for harvesting in vitro–activated DCs for administration to patients.[19]

Tumor Antigens: Selecting a Target

Identifying antigens that can serve as targets for an immune response is a critical, but challenging, aspect of vaccine development, as tumors arise from tissues normally present in the body; therefore, many of the antigens presented on a tumor's cell surface are normal proteins, or self-antigens. Self-antigens are routinely sampled by the immune system, which may lead to the development of tolerance, limiting the ability of these antigens to stimulate an immune response. There is evidence,

TABLE 91-1 Tumor Antigens Investigated as Potential Targets for Breast Cancer Vaccines

Antigen	Description	Relevance in Breast Cancer	Reference
Carcinoembryonic antigen	Glycoprotein involved with cell adhesion	Expressed in breast cancer as well as carcinoma of the colon, rectum, lung, and pancreas	25
HER-2	Member of the epidermal growth factor family of receptor tyrosine kinases	Overexpressed in up to 30% of breast cancers; associated with a poor prognosis	27,28
hTERT	Catalytic protein component of telomerase that protects telomeric ends of chromosomes from degradation during cell division	Expressed in nearly all human cancer cells including breast cancer cells	23
Mammaglobin A	Glycoprotein of unknown function	Overexpressed in 80% of primary and metastatic breast cancers	29
MUC-1	Membrane-associated glycoprotein expressed in ductal tissues	Upregulated and aberrantly glycosylated in breast cancer	24
p53	Normal p53 contributes to DNA repair and apoptosis	Mutated in approximately 20% of breast cancers	26

however, that the immune system can recognize tumor cells based on the absolute level and/or timing of the expression of certain "normal" proteins.[20,21] Additional factors that determine the suitability of an antigen to serve as a target for immunotherapy include its tissue expression profile; the diversity, scope, and avidity of the antigen-specific T-cell repertoire; and the commonality of the antigen between patients.[8,22] A number of antigens have been tested as potential targets for breast cancer vaccines (Table 91-1).[23-29] Two proteins that have been investigated extensively for use in breast cancer vaccines are mucin-1 (MUC-1) and HER-2.

MUC-1

The MUC-1 gene is a member of the mucin family, which encodes a membrane-bound phosphoprotein expressed on the apical surface by many types of ductal epithelia. It is characterized by heavy glycosylation and a 20 amino acid tandem repeat segment. MUC-1 has multiple functions, including protecting mucous membranes by binding pathogens, signal transduction, and modulating the immune system.[30] In breast cancer, MUC-1 is up-regulated and aberrantly glycosylated. Changes in glycosylation result in shortening of the complex carbohydrate side chains, which in turn results in exposure of peptide and carbohydrate epitopes that can serve as targets for immunotherapy.[31] Several clinical trials of MUC-1–based vaccines, using both peptide and DC platforms, have been reported. One of the earliest clinical trials involved a peptide vaccine consisting of a synthetic MUC-1 peptide mixed with BCG administered to 63 patients with adenocarcinomas of the breast, pancreas, or colon.[32] Overall, the vaccine was well tolerated. Skin biopsies at the injection sites showed delayed-type hypersensitivity (DTH) reactions to MUC-1 peptides, as well as intense T-cell infiltration. Approximately one-third of the

patients demonstrated a 2- to 4-fold increase in MUC-1 specific CTLs.[32] Additional early clinical trials investigating MUC-1 vaccines reported inconsistent results on whether MUC-1 vaccination induced a humoral response or a peptide-specific CTL response.

Subsequently, investigators have explored alternative strategies for targeting the MUC-1 antigen. Sialyl-Tn (STn) is a carbohydrate associated with MUC-1 on a number of human cancer cells that is associated with more aggressive disease. The cancer vaccine Theratope (STn-KLH, where KLH [keyhole limpet hemocyanin] is an immunogenic carrier protein to which antigens can be coupled) was designed by incorporating a synthetic STn antigen that emulates the STn seen in human tumors. Theratope was investigated in the largest breast cancer vaccine trial to date.[33] This phase III trial enrolled 1028 women with metastatic breast cancer who had stable disease or who achieved a response after initial chemotherapy. Patients were randomized to receive either Theratope (STn-KLH) or control (KLH alone). While Theratope was demonstrated to be safe and capable of generating an immune response, no differences were found in time to disease progression or overall survival between the patients who received Theratope and those who received the control.[33] Additional analyses of the data from this trial did show a trend toward improved time to disease progression and overall survival in patients who also received concomitant hormone therapy.[34] In addition, the median overall survival was longer in patients who had an adequate antibody response to STn.[35]

HER-2

HER-2 is a member of the epidermal growth factor receptor family of transmembrane tyrosine kinases. The HER-2 gene is amplified and the encoded protein is overexpressed in a variety of malignancies, including up to 30% of breast cancers.[27,28] This overexpression can result in a 100- to 200-fold increase in the concentration of the HER-2 protein in tumor tissue compared to normal tissue.[36] Because of this differential expression, it was hypothesized that HER-2 may serve as a tumor antigen. Subsequent work demonstrated that HER-2 overexpression leads to higher levels of T-cell precursors and peptides that can activate T cells in vivo and in vitro.[37] Theoretically, processing the overexpressed HER-2 protein results in an increased supply of peptides, which may then occupy a large number of MHC molecules in competition with other peptides, activating or amplifying an immune response against HER-2-expressing tumors.[36,37] In addition, antibodies that react with HER-2 have been detected in the serum of patients with breast cancer.[21] Taken together, these data suggest that HER-2 is an appropriate target for vaccine development.

Since the HER-2 protein's identification as a TAA, several peptides derived from it have been investigated for use in anticancer vaccines. E75 (HER-2/neu, 369-377), originally described by Fisk and colleagues,[36] is the most studied HER-2-derived peptide both in vitro and in vivo. Promising preclinical studies led to 3 clinical trials of E75 for patients with metastatic disease.[16,38,39] In these trials, the E75 peptide was used in combination with an immunoadjuvant (incomplete Freund adjuvant or GM-CSF) and injected intradermally. Though these trials were small, enrolling fewer than 15 patients, they found that the E75 peptide was safe and capable of inducing a peptide-specific immune response. Unfortunately, little has been reported regarding the potential clinical impact of this HER-2 immunity, which is likely because the enrolled patients had late-stage disease and large residual tumor burdens.[15] E75 has also been used as part of a DC vaccine. In a pilot study enrolling 10 patients with advanced breast or ovarian cancer, Brossart and colleagues demonstrated that autologous DCs loaded with the E75 peptide and reinfused back into the patients were successful in inducing a peptide-specific CTL response.[40] However, no data are available regarding the clinical efficacy of this vaccine strategy.

Disis and colleagues, who conducted one of the early E75 trials, have investigated other HER-2 peptide vaccines. In one trial, they administered a HER-2 peptide vaccine containing longer peptides that bind class II MHC molecules and, therefore, stimulate a Th response.[41] Over 90% of patients who received the vaccine developed T-cell immunity to HER-2 peptides, and over 60% developed HER-2 protein–specific immunity, suggesting that the vaccine formulations contained peptides that were naturally processed. Therefore, immunization with the helper peptides resulted in the generation of T cells that could respond to the HER-2 protein processed by APCs.[7,41] Recognizing the importance of Th immunity, this group ran a subsequent trial in patients with stage III or IV breast or ovarian cancer who were administered HER-2-derived class II MHC helper peptides, which contained sequestered class I MHC binding motifs (ie, the helper peptide, p369-384, contained within its sequence the E75 class I MHC peptide, p369-377).[16] Comparing the results of the Disis study to that of a second study[42] that was run concurrently and immunized patients with just the E75 peptide, Knutson and Disis found

that patients immunized with the helper peptide generated greater magnitude and durability of T-cell immunity to the E75 peptide. The higher responses to E75 correlated with higher responses to the longer helper peptide that fully encompassed E75.[7] Despite the fact that the clinical trials have demonstrated these vaccines' ability to generate HER-2-specific immunity, they have yet to demonstrate clinical efficacy.

CURRENT VACCINATION STRATEGIES

Therapeutic Vaccines

The lack of clinical efficacy seen with previous vaccine trials is likely attributable to multiple factors. One factor is that most of the clinical trials investigating vaccines enrolled patients with late-stage disease and were utilizing vaccines as a therapeutic modality. As was previously discussed above, the largest therapeutic breast cancer vaccine trial completed to date administering Theratope was largely disappointing as it failed to demonstrate improved time to disease progression or overall survival in patients who were immunized. This trial and others enrolling patients with later-stage disease point out several concerns that must be addressed when considering vaccines to be used as a therapeutic modality. Patients with late-stage disease likely have heavy tumor burdens, tumor-induced immunosuppression, and immune system dysfunction resulting from prior chemotherapy. In addition, as tumors grow, they develop immune escape mechanisms such as downregulation of HLA expression and the induction of a tolerative tumor microenvironment.[13] As an example of the latter, regulatory T cells (Tregs) are found in increased numbers in the peripheral blood and tumor microenvironment of breast cancer patients.[44]

In an attempt to address some of these challenges and make therapeutic vaccines more effective, some investigators have targeted Tregs. This subpopulation of T cells suppresses activation of the immune system and appears to contribute to tolerance of cancer cell antigens. Recognizing the potential impact of Tregs on a vaccine's effectiveness, researchers have begun to employ both nonspecific and specific strategies aimed at overcoming this immune suppression. Included among the nonspecific strategies is using low-dose cyclophosphamide, which has been demonstrated to inhibit or deplete Tregs. Inhibition of Tregs using a preconditioning dose of cyclophosphamide could enhance the CD8+ T cell response to vaccination.[45] Emens and colleagues at Johns Hopkins University are currently enrolling patients with HER-2-overexpressing metastatic breast cancer on a phase II study of trastuzumab, cyclophosphamide, and an allogeneic GM-CSF-secreting breast cancer vaccine. One objective of the trial is to measure the impact of cyclophosphamide pretreatment on Tregs.[46] Other investigators have begun employing specific strategies to attack Tregs including administering a toxin aimed at a specific receptor identified on the Treg cell surface. ONTAK (denileukin diftitox) is a recombinant DNA-derived cytotoxic protein that is active against cells, including Tregs, that express the IL-2 receptor (IL-2R). A phase one-half single-arm clinical trial in patients with advanced refractory breast cancer is being conducted by Disis and colleagues at the University of Washington to determine if ONTAK will show antitumor activity. One primary objective of this trial is to evaluate the effect of ONTAK administration on peripheral blood Tregs.[47]

Other mechanisms have also been targeted in order to enhance the efficacy of therapeutic vaccines. Cytotoxic T lymphocyte antigen-4 (CTLA-4) is a T-cell inhibitory receptor expressed primarily on CD4+ T cells that is involved with down-regulation of T-cell response. Ipilimumab is a human monoclonal antibody against CTLA-4 that has been used in several clinical trials against a variety of cancers. At doses required to achieve an antitumor effect when used as monotherapy, ipilimumab has resulted in significant side effects to include autoimmune colitis.[48] Using lower doses in a pilot study enrolling 11 patients with a variety of malignancies (3 colon cancer, 4 non-Hodgkin lymphoma, 4 prostate cancer) who had experienced disease progression after administration of a cancer vaccine, O'Mahoney and colleagues showed a reduction in the number of Tregs as well as tumor regression in 2 patients with lymphoma.[49] In another study infusing ipilimumab after vaccination with irradiated, autologous tumor cells engineered to secrete GM-CSF, Hodi and colleagues demonstrated antitumor immunity without grade 3 or 4 toxicity in 11 patients with metastatic melanoma. Eight of 11 patients experienced meaningful antitumor effects defined as tumor regressions or prolonged stable disease.[0] Taken together, these data suggest that there may be a role for targeting CTLA-4 as part of a cancer vaccination strategy.

Vaccines Administered in the Neoadjuvant or Adjuvant Setting: A Preventive Approach

Given the limitations of these previous trials and the complexities of using vaccines as a therapeutic modality, researchers have begun investigating the use of cancer vaccines in a model similar to that used for infectious disease. Conventional vaccines against infections are designed to be protective, not therapeutic (ie, immunity is established before disease onset). The focus in several clinical trials for breast cancer vaccines, therefore, has shifted to immunization during early-stage disease or in the adjuvant disease-free setting to prevent disease recurrence. Two such strategies are discussed in the next sections.

Dendritic Cell Vaccines for Ductal Carcinoma in Situ

Czerniecki and colleagues are investigating a vaccine in HER-2-overexpressing ductal carcinoma in situ (DCIS). They are exploiting the relatively long latency period between the appearance of DCIS and the development of invasive breast cancer as an opportunity for administering novel neoadjuvant interventions. Specifically, Czerniecki and colleagues have used DCs pulsed with HER2 class I and II MHC peptides as a vaccine administered prior to surgery. This strategy may alter the natural history of DCIS lesions, reduce the risk of recurrence, and potentially decrease the amount of other therapy (ie, surgery or radiation) required.[50]

Czerniecki and colleagues have previously done extensive work on DC vaccines, including developing a unique strategy of preconditioning DCs for an IL-12 burst upon encountering the CD40 ligand. IL-12 enhances the functional avidity of CD8+ cells and increases these cells' tumor-recognizing and

killing properties.[18] In addition to secreting IL-12, DCs produce other cytokines involved in anti-tumor CD4+ and CD8+ T-cell activity.[51] In a clinical trial enrolling patients with HER-2-overexpressing DCIS, 4 weekly vaccinations with autologous HER-2 peptide-pulsed DCs were administered into normal groin lymph nodes under ultrasound guidance. Following completion of the inoculation series, patients underwent surgical resection of their disease. Though this trial was small (n = 11 evaluable patients), the early results are encouraging. Vaccinated patients showed high rates of peptide-specific CD4+ and CD8+ T cells, as well as accumulation of T and B lymphocytes in the breast and induction of complement-dependent, tumorilytic antibodies. Seven of the 11 patients had a significant decrease in HER-2 expression in their resected tumors, often with measurable decreases in residual DCIS, suggesting that vaccination altered the tumor phenotype, a process that the authors referred to as "targeted immunoediting."[52] Looking forward, vaccines may play a role as a chemopreventive strategy in patients with DCIS.

Peptide Vaccines to Prevent Disease Recurrence

Other investigators have pursued using peptide vaccines to prevent disease recurrence in breast cancer patients who are disease free after standard therapy. Initial trials involved administering E75 mixed with GM-CSF as a vaccine.[53] Recently, results from 2 concurrent phase II trials have been reported by Peoples and colleagues.[13] The combined trials enrolled over 185 patients, making it the largest trial of a preventive vaccine strategy in breast cancer to date. The vaccine was demonstrated to be safe and effective in raising an immune response, with all patients developing CD8+ T cells that recognized HER-2-expressing tumor cells and DTH reactions to E75 postvaccination. A primary analysis of the clinical response initiated after a median follow-up of 18 months demonstrated a decrease in the rate of recurrence for those who had been vaccinated versus unvaccinated controls (5.6% vs 14.2%, $p = 0.04$).[13] At a later follow-up (median, 26 months), the recurrence rate was 8.3% in the vaccinated group compared to 14.8% in the observation group ($p = 0.17$).[54] Thus, while a trend toward a benefit from vaccination continued, statistical significance had been lost. Interestingly, there was also an alteration in the recurrence pattern with the lack of bone-only metastatic disease in the vaccinated patients.[55] To address this waning immunity, this group is exploring the role of booster inoculations, similar to those used to maintain immunity against infectious disease. In addition, this group is investigating vaccines administering HER-2-derived class II MHC peptides to stimulate the Th-cell response, multi-epitope vaccines designed to stimulate both arms of the adaptive immune system, and combination immunotherapy using peptide vaccines with the HER-2-targeted monoclonal antibody Trastuzumab.[56,57] In addition, a randomized phase III clinical trial for the optimally dosed and boosted E75 peptide is in development.

ONGOING TRIALS

Table 91-2 lists ongoing breast cancer vaccine trials.[58] Review of this table identifies many of the strategies discussed above that are currently being investigated in order to optimize the

TABLE 91-2 Ongoing Breast Cancer Vaccine Trials Registered through the National Cancer Institute

Clinical Trial	Protocol IDs
Phase I/II Study of Vaccinia-CEA-TRICOM Vaccine Before Dose-Intensive Induction Chemotherapy and Fowlpox-CEA-TRICOM Vaccine after Dose-Intensive Induction Chemotherapy and Immune Depletion in Patients with Previously Untreated Metastatic Breast Cancer	NCT00053170
Phase I/II Randomized Study of Vaccination Comprising p53-Infected Autologous Dendritic Cells in Women with p53-Overexpressing Stage III Breast Cancer Undergoing Neoadjuvant or Adjuvant Chemotherapy and Adjuvant Radiotherapy	NCT00082641
Phase I/II Study of Vaccine Comprising a HER2/neu-Positive Allogeneic Tumor Cell Line Transfected with the Sargramostim (GM-CSF) Gene in Combination with Low-Dose Interferon Alfa and Low-Dose Cyclophosphamide in Patients with HER2/neu-Positive Stage IV Breast Cancer	NCT00095862
Histocompatibility Leukocyte Antigen (HLA)-A*0201 Restricted Peptide Vaccine Therapy in Patients with Breast Cancer	NCT00677326
Histocompatibility Leukocyte Antigen (HLA)-A*2402 Restricted Peptide Vaccine Therapy in Patients with Breast Cancer	NCT00678509
Phase II Randomized Pilot Study of Docetaxel with versus without Vaccinia-CEA-MUC-1-TRICOM Vaccine, Fowlpox-CEA-MUC-1-TRICOM Vaccine, and Sargramostim (GM-CSF) in Patients with Metastatic Breast Cancer	NCT00217750
Phase II Study of HER-2/neu Intracellular Domain Peptide-Based Vaccine in Combination with Trastuzumab (Herceptin) in Patients with HER2/neu-Positive Stage IIIB, IIIC, or IV Breast Cancer	NCT00343109
Phase II Study of Trastuzumab (Herceptin), Cyclophosphamide, and Allogeneic GM-CSF-Secreting Breast Tumor Vaccine in Patients with HER2/neu-Overexpressing Metastatic Breast Cancer	NCT00397371
Phase II Study of Multiepitope Autologous Dendritic Cell Vaccine, Trastuzumab (Herceptin), and Vinorelbine Ditartrate in Patients with HER2/neu-Overexpressing Locally Recurrent or Metastatic Breast Cancer	NCT00266110
Phase II Randomized Study of Adjuvant GP2 Peptide/GM-CSF Vaccine or AE37 Peptide/GM-CSF Vaccine versus Sargramostim (GM-CSF) in Patients with Lymph Node-Positive or High-Risk Lymph Node-Negative, HER2/neu-Expressing Breast Cancer	NCT00524277
Phase I Study of Telomerase: 540-548 Peptide Vaccine Emulsified in Montanide ISA-51 and Sargramostim (GM-CSF) in Patients with HLA-A2-Expressing Stage IV Breast Cancer	NCT00079157
Phase I Study of Vaccination Comprising Allogeneic Sargramostim (GM-CSF)-Secreting Breast Cancer Cells with or without Cyclophosphamide and Doxorubicin in Women with Stage IV Breast Cancer	NCT00093834
Phase I Pilot Study of Neoadjuvant Ultrasound-Guided Intranodal Vaccine Therapy Comprising Autologous Dendritic Cells Pulsed with Recombinant HER2/neu Peptides in Patients with Ductal Carcinoma In Situ of the Breast	NCT00107211
Adenovirus Encoding Rat HER-2 in Patients with Metastatic Breast Cancer (AdHER2.1)	NCT00307229
Xenogeneic HER2/Neu DNA Immunization for Patients with Metastatic and High Risk Breast Cancer: A Phase I Study to Assess Safety and Immunogenicity	NCT00393783
Phase I Study of Adjuvant pNGVL3-hICD Vaccine and Sargramostim in Patients with HER2/neu-Overexpressing Stage III or IV Breast or Ovarian Cancer	NCT00436254
A Safety and Immunology Study of a Modified Vaccinia Vaccine for HER-2(+) Metastatic Breast Cancer	NCT00485277
Multipeptide Vaccine for Advanced Breast Cancer	NCT00573495
Study of Cancer Peptides Vaccine Plus GM-CSF as Adjuvant Treatment for High Risk (TXN2-3M0) or Metastatic Breast Cancer with No Evidence of Disease	NCT00674791
Phase I Study of Replication-Incompetent Ad-sig-hMUC-1/ecdCD40L Vaccine in Women with Previously Treated Metastatic Breast Cancer	NCT00706615
Pilot Study of Sialyl Lewis -Keyhole Limpet Hemocyanin Conjugate Vaccine and QS21 in Patients with Metastatic Breast Cancer	NCT00470574
Randomized Study of Vaccine Therapy Comprising MUC1 Antigen, HER-2/neu Peptides, and Sargramostim (GM-CSF)and/or CpG Oligodeoxynucleotide in Patients with Previously Treated Stage II or III Adenocarcinoma of the Breast	NCT00640861

From www.cancer.gov/Search/SearchClinicalTrialsAdvanced.aspx. Accessed November 5, 2008.

immune response generated by vaccines. Completion of these trials will further our understanding of how a vaccine may stimulate a response against TAA as well as provide insight into how vaccines may be incorporated into the algorithm for the clinical management of breast cancer.

FUTURE DIRECTIONS

It is anticipated that the ongoing paradigm shift discussed above will continue; that breast cancer vaccines will be utilized in patients with early-stage disease rather than late-stage disease when large tumor burdens make immunotherapy less effective. It is conceivable that a vaccine that is initially demonstrated effective in the adjuvant setting could ultimately be utilized as a truly preventive vaccine administered to women identified by their genomic signature as being at high risk for developing breast cancer. Clinical trials with appropriate immunologic assays and biomarker surrogates will be necessary to evaluate such an approach given the prolonged clinical end points intrinsic to prevention trials.

SUMMARY

Advances in the molecular characterization of breast cancer have led to increased interest in targeted therapies, including vaccines recognizing TAAs. Cancer vaccines have important potential advantages over other available therapies for breast cancer because they are nontoxic and have great specificity. Early clinical trials demonstrated that breast cancer vaccines have the ability to stimulate an antigen-specific immune response. Unfortunately, early vaccine trials failed to demonstrate clinical efficacy, which is likely attributable to the fact that most of these trials enrolled patients with late-stage disease and used vaccines as a therapeutic modality. In addition, early vaccine formulations primarily targeted a CTL response; more recent studies have demonstrated that a successful vaccine needs to stimulate Th cells as well in order to maximize the vaccine's immunogenicity. Recognizing the limitations of early trials, researchers have begun investigating vaccination strategies designed to stimulate a more robust immune response in early-stage disease or in the adjuvant setting to prevent disease recurrence. Results of early clinical trials employing this strategy are encouraging and suggest that vaccines will have clinical efficacy in this setting.

REFERENCES

1. Boon T, Coulie PG, Van den Eynde B. Tumor antigens recognized by T cells. *Immunol Today.* 1997;18:267-268.
2. Rosenberg SA. Cancer vaccines based on the identification of genes encoding cancer regression antigens. *Immunol Today.* 1997;18:175-182.
3. Van den Eynde B, Brichard VG. New tumor antigens recognized by T cells. *Curr Opin Immunol.* 1995;7:674-681.
4. Altomonte M, Fonsatti E, Visintin A, Maio M. Targeted therapy of solid malignancies via HLA class II antigens: a new biotherapeutic approach? *Oncogene.* 2003;22:6564-6569.
5. Kalams SA, Walker BD. The critical need for CD4 help in maintaining effective cytotoxic T lymphocyte responses. *J Exp Med.* 1998;188:2199-2204.
6. Park JM, Terabe M, Sakai Y, et al. Early role of CD4+ Th1 cells and antibodies in HER-2 adenovirus vaccine protection against autochthonous mammary carcinomas. *J Immunol.* 2005;174:4228-4236.
7. Knutson KL, Disis ML. Augmenting T helper cell immunity in cancer. *Curr Drug Targets.* 2005;5:365-371.
8. Emens LA. Cancer vaccines: on the threshold of success. *Expert Opin Emerg Drugs.* 2008;13:295-308.
9. Cox AL, Skipper J, Chen Y, et al. Identification of a peptide recognized by five melanoma-specific human cytotoxic T cell lines. *Science.* 1994;264:716-719.
10. Van Der Bruggen P, Zhang Y, Chaux P, et al. Tumor-specific shared antigenic peptides recognized by human T cells. *Immunol Rev.* 2002;188:51-64.
11. Huang AY, Bruce AT, Pardoll DM, Levitsky HI. In vivo cross-priming of MHC class I-restricted antigens requires the TAP transporter. *Immunity.* 1996;4:349-355.
12. Thomas AM, Santarsiero LM, Lutz ER, et al. Mesothelin-specific CD8(+) T cell responses provide evidence of in vivo cross-priming by antigen-presenting cells in vaccinated pancreatic cancer patients. *J Exp Med.* 2004;200:297-306.
13. Peoples GE, Holmes JP, Hueman MT, et al. Combined clinical trial results of a HER2/neu (E75) vaccine for the prevention of recurrence in high-risk breast cancer patients: U.S. Military Cancer Institute Clinical Trials Group study I-01 and I-02. *Clin Cancer Res.* 2008;14:797-803.
14. Lee T. In: *Distribution of HLA Antigens in North American Caucasians, North American Blacks and Orientals.* New York, NY: Springer-Verlag; 1990.
15. Mittendorf EA, Peoples GE. HER-2/neu peptide breast cancer vaccines: current status and future directions. *Breast Diseases: A Year Book Quarterly.* 2007;17:318-320.
16. Knutson KL, Schiffman K, Disis ML. Immunization with a HER-2/neu helper peptide vaccine generates HER-2/neu CD8 T-cell immunity in cancer patients. *J Clin Invest.* 2001;107:477-484.
17. Satthaporn S, Robins A, Vassanasiri W, et al. Dendritic cells are dysfunctional in patients with operable breast cancer. *Cancer Immunol Immun.* 2004;53:510-518.
18. Xu S, Koski GK, Faries M, et al. Rapid high efficiency sensitization of CD8+ T cells to tumor antigens by dendritic cells leads to enhanced functional avidity and direct tumor recognition through an IL-12-dependent mechanism. *J Immunol.* 2003;171:2251-2261.
19. Koski GK, Cohen PA, Roses RE, et al. Reengineering dendritic cell-based anti-cancer vaccines. *Immunol Rev.* 2008;222:256-276.
20. Disis ML, Knutson KL, Schiffman K, et al. Pre-existent immunity to the HER-2/neu oncogenic protein in patients with HER-2/neu overexpressing breast and ovarian cancer. *Breast Cancer Res Treat.* 2000;62:245-252.
21. Disis ML, Pupa SM, Gralow JR, et al. High-titer HER-2/neu protein-specific antibody can be detected in patients with early stage breast cancer. *J Clin Oncol.* 1997;15:3363-3367.
22. Gilboa E. The makings of a tumor rejection antigen. *Immunity.* 1999;11:263-270.
23. Bednarek AK, Sahin A, Brenner AJ, et al. Analysis of telomerase activity levels in breast cancer: positive detection at the in situ breast carcinoma stage. *Clin Cancer Res.* 1997;3:11-16.
24. Chung MA, Luo Y, O'Donnell M, et al. Development and preclinical evaluation of a Bacillus Calmette-Guerin-MUC1-based novel breast cancer vaccine. *Cancer Res.* 2003;63:1280-1287.
25. Hodge JW. Carcinoembryonic antigen as a target for cancer vaccines. *Cancer Immunol Immun.* 1996;43:127-134.
26. Runnebaum IB, Nagarajan M, Bowman M, et al. Mutations in p53 as potential molecular markers for human breast cancer. *Proc Natl Acad Sci USA.* 1991;88:10657-10661.
27. Slamon DJ, Clark GM, Wong SG, et al. Human breast cancer: correlation of relapse and survival with amplification of the HER-2/neu oncogene. *Science.* 1987;235:177-182.
28. Slamon DJ, Godolphin W, Jones LA, et al. Studies of the HER-2/neu proto-oncogene in human breast and ovarian cancer. *Science.* 1989;244:707-712.
29. Watson MA, Dintzis S, Darrow CM, et al. Mammaglobin expression in primary, metastatic, and occult breast cancer. *Cancer Res.* 1999;59:3028-3031.
30. Curigliano G, Rescigno M, Goldhirsch A. Immunology and breast cancer: therapeutic cancer vaccines. *Breast.* 2007;16(suppl 2):S20-S26.
31. Miles DW, Taylor-Papadimitriou J. Mucin based breast cancer vaccines. *Expert Opin Invest Drugs.* 1998;7:1865-1877.
32. Goydos JS, Elder E, Whiteside TL, et al. A phase I trial of a synthetic mucin peptide vaccine. Induction of specific immune reactivity in patients with adenocarcinoma. *J Surg Res.* 1996;63:298-304.
33. Miles D, Papazisis K. Rationale for the clinical development of STn-KLH (Theratope) and anti-MUC-1 vaccines in breast cancer. *Clin Breast Cancer.* 2003;3(suppl 4):S134-S138.
34. Mayordomo J, Tres A, Miles D, et al. Long-term follow-up of patients concomitantly treated with hormone therapy in a prospective controlled randomized multicenter clinical study comparing STn-KLH vaccine with KLH control in stage IV breast cancer following first line chemotherapy [abstract]. *Proc Am Soc Clin Oncol.* 2004;23:188.

35. Ibrahim N, Murray J, Parker J, et al. Humoral immune response to naturally occurring STn in metastatic breast cancer patients (MBC pts) treated with STn-KLH vaccine. *Proc Am Soc Clin Oncol.* 2004;23:174. Abstract.

36. Fisk B, Blevins TL, Wharton JT, Ioannides CG. Identification of an immunodominant peptide of HER-2/neu protooncogene recognized by ovarian tumor-specific cytotoxic T lymphocyte lines. *J Exp Med.* 1995;181:2109-2117.

37. Ioannides CG, Ioannides MG, O'Brian CA. T-cell recognition of oncogene products: a new strategy for immunotherapy. *Mol Carcinog.* 1992;6:77-82.

38. Murray JL, Gillogly ME, Przepiorka D, et al. Toxicity, immunogenicity, and induction of E75-specific tumor-lytic CTLs by HER-2 peptide E75 (369-377) combined with granulocyte macrophage colony-stimulating factor in HLA-A2+ patients with metastatic breast and ovarian cancer. *Clin Cancer Res.* 2002;8:3407-3418.

39. Zaks TZ, Rosenberg SA. Immunization with a peptide epitope (p369-377) from HER-2/neu leads to peptide-specific cytotoxic T lymphocytes that fail to recognize HER-2/neu+ tumors. *Cancer Res.* 1998;58:4902-4908.

40. Brossart P, Wirths S, Stuhler G, et al. Induction of cytotoxic T-lymphocyte responses in vivo after vaccinations with peptide-pulsed dendritic cells. *Blood.* 2000;96:3102-3108.

41. Disis ML, Gooley TA, Rinn K, et al. Generation of T-cell immunity to the HER-2/neu protein after active immunization with HER-2/neu peptide-based vaccines. *J Clin Oncol.* 2002;20:2624-2632.

42. Knutson KL, Schiffman K, Cheever MA, Disis ML. Immunization of cancer patients with a HER-2/neu, HLA-A2 peptide, p369-377, results in short-lived peptide-specific immunity. *Clin Cancer Res.* 2002;8:1014-1018.

43. Mittendorf EA, Peoples GE, Singletary SE. Breast cancer vaccines: promise for the future or pipe dream? *Cancer* 2007:110:1677-1686.

44. Liyanage UK, Moore TT, Joo HG, et al. Prevalence of regulatory T cells is increased in peripheral blood and tumor microenvironment of patients with pancreas or breast adenocarcinoma. *J Immunol.* 2002;169:2756-2761.

45. Salem ML, Kadima AN, El-Naggar SA, et al. Defining the ability of cyclophosphamide preconditioning to enhance the antigen-specific CD8+ T-cell response to peptide vaccination: creation of a beneficial host microenvironment involving type I IFNs and myeloid cells. *J Immunother.* 2007;30:40-53.

46. Phase II study of trastuzumab (Herceptin), cyclophophamide, and allogeneic GM-CSF-secreting breast cancer. Available at: http://www.cancer.gov/search/ViewClinicalTrials.aspx?cdrid=510161&version=HealthProfessional&protocolsearchid=5390376. Accessed November 5, 2008.

47. http://www.cancer.gov/search/ViewClinicalTrials.aspx?cdrid=526414&version=HealthProfessional&protocolsearchid=5390702. Accessed November 5, 2008.

48. Hodi FS, Butler M, Oble DA, et al. Immunologic and clinical effects of antibody blockade of cytotoxic T lymphocyte-associated antigen 4 in previously vaccinated cancer patients. *Proc Natl Acad Sci USA.* 2008;105:3005-3010.

49. O'Mahony D, Morris JC, Quinn C, et al. A pilot study of CTLA-4 blockade after cancer vaccine failure in patients with advanced malignancy. *Clin Cancer Res.* 2007;13:958-964.

50. Czerniecki BJ, Roses RE, Koski GK. Development of vaccines for high-risk ductal carcinoma in situ of the breast. *Cancer Res.* 2007;67:6531-6534.

51. Wesa A, Kalinski P, Kirkwood JM, et al. Polarized type-1 dendritic cells (DC1) producing high levels of IL-12 family members rescue patient TH1-type antimelanoma CD4+ T cell responses in vitro. *J Immunother.* 2007;30:75-82.

52. Czerniecki BJ, Koski GK, Koldovsky U, et al. Targeting HER-2/neu in early breast cancer development using dendritic cells with staged interleukin-12 burst secretion. *Cancer Res.* 2007;67:1842-1852.

53. Peoples GE, Gurney JM, Hueman MT, et al. Clinical trial results of a HER-2/neu (E75) vaccine to prevent recurrence in high-risk breast cancer patients. *J Clin Oncol.* 2005;23:7536-7545.

54. Mittendorf EA, Holmes JP, Ponniah S, Peoples GE. The E75 HER2/neu peptide vaccine. *Cancer Immunol Immunother.* 2008;57:1511-1521.

55. Amin A, Benavides LC, Holmes JP, et al. Assessment of immunologic response and recurrence patterns among patients with clinical recurrence after vaccination with a preventive HER2/neu peptide vaccine: from US Military Cancer Institute Clinical Trials Group Study I-01 and I-02. *Cancer Immunol Immunother.* 2008;57:1817-1825.

56. Holmes JP, Benavides LC, Gates JD, et al. Results of the first phase I clinical trial of the novel II-key hybrid preventive HER-2/neu peptide (AE37) vaccine. *J Clin Oncol.* 2008;26:3426-3433.

57. Mittendorf EA, Storrer CE, Shriver CD, et al. Investigating the combination of trastuzumab and HER2/neu peptide vaccines for the treatment of breast cancer. *Ann Surg Oncol.* 2006;13:1085-1098.

58. Search for Clinical Trials: Advanced Search. Available at: http://www.cancer.gov/Search/SearchClinicalTrialsAdvanced.aspx. Accessed November 5, 2008.

CHAPTER 92

Metastatic Breast Cancer

Hope S. Rugo

Although significant advances have been made in the treatment of breast cancer resulting in continued improvement in survival, more than 40,000 women will die of the disease this year.[1] Approximately 30% of women diagnosed with early-stage breast cancer will develop a systemic metastatic recurrence, with only a few of these patients achieving long-term survival with standard chemotherapy.[2] In addition, 5% to 10% of women are diagnosed with metastatic disease at first presentation of breast cancer. Overall survival (OS) for patients with metastatic disease has changed little over the last 50 years, despite a marked increase in the choice of active agents for treatment. The availability of new targeted biological therapies, particularly trastuzumab for HER-2/neu overexpressing disease, as well as new hormonal and chemotherapeutic agents, has clearly improved outcome for patients with certain biological subtypes of this disease. However, the concept of treating metastatic breast cancer as a chronic disease is still largely theoretical because most patients will survive less than 5 years following diagnosis.

The most significant advances in the treatment of metastatic breast cancer are not limited to the inclusion of new targeted biological therapies. Most recently, the introduction of new cytotoxic agents, new formulations of existing drugs, rationally designed combination therapy, and variation of dose and schedule have resulted in improvements in outcome with generally well-tolerated toxicity profiles. The advantage of these studies is not only seen in improved options for patients with metastatic disease, but also in the ability to test more promising treatment approaches in the adjuvant setting. In addition, there are more options for hormonal therapy, as well as a greater understanding of how and when to use treatment directed toward the estrogen receptor (ER). However, treatments invariably fail, and some tumors are initially resistant to therapy. A better understanding of the biology that drives tumor growth and resistance to therapy has helped to identify new potential targets as well as develop new therapies, but clearly additional study is needed.

PRINCIPLES OF THERAPY

The primary goal of treatment for metastatic disease is to control symptoms and to prolong survival in the context of maximizing quality of life. Treatment is palliative, but effective therapy can significantly prolong life. The choice of therapy is based on a variety of factors including biological markers, extent and pattern of disease, prior treatment, patient performance status, and patient preference. Biological markers correlate with the pattern of organ involvement and prognosis; hormone receptor (HR)-positive disease most commonly presents in bone and soft tissues, and visceral involvement is usually limited early in the course of disease. In contrast, visceral involvement dominates in HR-negative and HER-2/neu-positive disease, with risk of pending organ dysfunction. The National Comprehensive Cancer Network provides guidelines for evaluation and treatment of advanced disease that are available online at http://www.nccn.org.

INITIAL EVALUATION OF PATIENTS WITH METASTATIC DISEASE

Extent of metastatic disease is an important determinant of therapy and is determined with baseline studies that are also used for future assessment of treatment effect. In addition, organ dysfunction may preclude certain therapies. Therefore, initial evaluation should begin with complete laboratory studies including complete blood count, liver function, renal function, electrolytes, calcium and albumin, as well as scans. In addition to computed tomography (CT) scanning of the chest, abdomen, and pelvis, a bone scan should be obtained. Positron emission tomography/CT scanning is now often used as a single test to evaluate both visceral organs and bone,[3] although bone scans may be a more sensitive determinant of osteoblastic lesions.[4] One accessible lesion should be biopsied, both to confirm the origin of the metastatic cells[5] and to reassess biological markers including ER, progesterone receptor (PR), and HER-2/neu. With progression to metastatic disease, HR status may occasionally change primarily with loss of receptor expression,[6] and several reports have suggested that the same is true for HER-2/neu,[7] although this remains to be validated. In addition, clinical behavior or a pattern of organ involvement that is inconsistent with marker results should prompt reevaluation because the outcome could have a significant impact on therapeutic decisions.

IMPORTANT TREATMENT CONSIDERATIONS

A variety of factors play a role in determining the most appropriate treatment during the course of metastatic disease. These include biological markers, history and type of adjuvant treatment, disease-free interval, and extent of disease. Cancers are initially divided into 3 major groups: HR positive, HER-2/neu positive, or receptor negative, also referred to as triple negative. Treatment decisions are generally based on these receptors and modified with the factors just listed. Patients with HR-positive disease are usually treated with sequential hormone therapy[8] leaving chemotherapy for the treatment of hormone resistant disease. Chemotherapy is also used to treat HR-negative disease, and in combination with targeted biological agents including trastuzumab or lapatinib for HER-2/neu positive disease and bevacizumab (see Chapter 88). Table 92-1 outlines chemotherapy options for the treatment of advanced breast cancer, and includes both approved indications as well as regimens for which clinical data exists. Radiographic testing and evaluation of symptoms is used to assess the effectiveness of therapy.[9]

HORMONE THERAPY

Hormonal therapy for advanced breast cancer has evolved significantly in the more than 100 years since initial data documenting the effect of ovarian ablation on advanced breast cancer in premenopausal women.[10] ER and PR are now routinely measured, and it is now well understood that expression of these receptors determines response to hormone therapy. The approach to treating HR-positive advanced breast cancer must take into account the type and extent of adjuvant hormonal therapy, time since last hormonal treatment, and the biological aggressiveness of the disease.[8] Options include sequencing of the nonsteroidal aromatase inhibitors (AI) letrozole and anastrozole, the steroidal AI exemestane, fulvestrant (a novel ER antagonist without agonist effects), tamoxifen (a selective ER modulator), and megestrol acetate (a synthetic progestational agent).[11] High doses of estrogen may also be effective; toxicities such as thrombosis, nausea, and bloating may limit therapy.[12] Table 92-2 lists the hormonal options for the treatment of advanced breast cancer.

It does not appear that the exact sequencing of specific agents is important in terms of outcome. Although in 3 randomized trials AIs were found to be superior or equivalent to tamoxifen as first-line treatment for metastatic disease in terms of response and time to progression (TTP), no survival benefit was found. The recent EFFECT trial randomized almost 700 women with advanced disease recurring or progressing after treatment with a nonsteroidal AI to receive either fulvestrant or exemestane.[13] Median TTP was identical at 3.7 months in both groups as was the overall response rate (ORR) and rate of carcinoma of breast (CB). Interestingly, for patients who did respond, the median duration of response was quite long, ranging from 9.8 to 13.5 months, and CB was seen in up to 29% of patients with visceral dominant disease and regardless of prior response to the nonsteroidal AI. Based on these data, it seems that sequential hormonal therapy can continue to provide benefit to patients with hormone responsive disease, despite progression on relatively similar agents. Patients with short response duration in the adjuvant or metastatic setting are less likely to benefit from continued hormonal manipulations.

TABLE 92-1 Chemotherapy for Metastatic Breast Cancer: Active Single Agents and Combinations

Single Agents	Combinations	Biological Combinations
Paclitaxel	Docetaxel/capecitabine	Trastuzumab/chemotherapy
Docetaxel	Gemcitabine/paclitaxel	Lapatinib/capecitabine
Nab-paclitaxel	Carbo/cisplatin combinations	Trastuzumab/lapatinib
Doxorubicin	Ixabepilone/capecitabine	Bevacizumab/taxane
Epirubicin	Vinorelbine/capecitabine	Trastuzumab/bevacizumab
L. doxorubicin*	Gemcitabine/vinorelbine	
Capecitabine		
Gemcitabine		
Vinorelbine		
Ixabepilone		
Carbo or cisplatin		
Irinotecan		
Pemetrexed		

*L. doxorubicin = liposomal pegylated doxorubicin.

TABLE 92-2 Hormonal Treatment for Advanced Breast Cancer

Category	Agent
Selective Estrogen Response Modifiers (SERMs)	Tamoxifen Toremifene
Selective Estrogen Receptor Downregulator (SERD)	Fulvestrant
Estrogens	DES Estradiol
Aromatase inhibitors (nonsteroidal)	Anastrozole Letrozole
Aromatase Inhibitors (steroidal)	Exemestane
GnRH agonists	Goserelin Leuprolide Triptorelin

DES, diethylstilbestrol; GnRH, gonadotropin-releasing hormone.

CHEMOTHERAPY

Sequential Single-Agent Chemotherapy

Given the widespread use of adjuvant chemotherapy, many patients with advanced disease will have received prior treatment with anthracyclines and taxanes. Significant advances in the use of taxanes in the treatment of metastatic disease have improved subsequent options for therapy, as well as the availability of a broad range of active agents.

The taxanes function as inhibitors of the microtubules that are essential for cell division[14,15] and are one of the most effective class of agents available for treating both early- and late-stage breast cancer. Paclitaxel and docetaxel, originally identified as natural products from the yew tree, are considered a standard of care in the treatment of metastatic disease[16,17] with single-agent response rates (RR) of 32% to 68%.[18]

Variations in schedule of administration have been tested in both the metastatic and adjuvant settings for both paclitaxel and docetaxel.[17,19] Weekly paclitaxel, based on mathematical models by Norton[20] that predict superiority for more frequent dosing, appears to offer improved efficacy with reduced hematologic toxicity,[21] as well as a potential antiangiogenic effect.[22] Cancer and Leukemia Group B (CALGB) 9840[23] randomized 577 women with taxane-naive metastatic breast cancer to receive weekly paclitaxel versus every 3 week paclitaxel. Weekly paclitaxel was superior to every 3 week paclitaxel with respect to RR (40% vs 28%; $p = 0.017$) and TTP (9 vs 5 months; $p = 0.0008$), with less granulocytopenia but more sensory neuropathy from weekly dosing. Other studies evaluating a dose relationship for paclitaxel given every 3 weeks documented improved RRs[24] at 175 mg/m^2 compared with 135 mg/m^2, but no differences in response and greater toxicity when higher doses were used.[25] In the treatment of metastatic breast cancer, weekly paclitaxel appears to be superior to every 3 week paclitaxel

and is currently the preferred schedule of administration for this taxane.

In contrast to paclitaxel, weekly dosing of docetaxel[26] is associated with less bone marrow and neurotoxicity as well as stomatitis but significantly more non-life-threatening toxicities including nail changes (onycholysis) and canalicular stenosis (tearing) compared to every 3 week dosing.[27] Thus the standard dosing schedule for docetaxel is every 3 weeks. Increasing every 3 week docetaxel dose to 60, 75, or 100 mg/m^2 has been demonstrated to increase ORR[27] (22.1%, 23.3%, and 36%, respectively) and TTP, but with a significant increase in both hematologic and nonhematologic toxicity and no benefit in terms of survival.

Head-to-Head Comparison of Docetaxel to Paclitaxel

Preclinical studies identified potentially important differences between paclitaxel and docetaxel/[28] Compared with paclitaxel, docetaxel demonstrated a higher intracellular concentration in target cells[29] as well as a greater affinity for the tubulin binding site.[30,31] The toxicity of the 2 taxanes differs, with paclitaxel associated more commonly with neurotoxicity and hypersensitivity and docetaxel with fluid retention, asthenia, as well as nail, eye, and skin changes.

An open-label, randomized phase III trial was designed to directly compare paclitaxel and docetaxel as second-line therapy for metastatic breast cancer.[32] The 449 patients were assigned to either paclitaxel, 175 mg/m^2, or docetaxel, 100 mg/m^2, every 3 weeks until progression or toxicity. Although fewer patients discontinued docetaxel for progression than paclitaxel (47% vs 75%), more patients stopped docetaxel for adverse events (26% vs 8%). TTP was prolonged for patients receiving docetaxel (5.7 vs 3.6 months, hazard ratio [HR]: 1.64, $p < 0.0001$), as was survival, with median overall survival (OS) 15.4 versus 12.7 months (HR: 1.41, $p = 0.03$). Febrile neutropenia was more frequent in patients receiving docetaxel than paclitaxel (14.9% vs 1.8%), as was asthenia, peripheral edema, stomatitis, and neurosensory changes.

Based on this phase III trial, every 3 week docetaxel appears to be superior in efficacy, but more toxic, than every 3 week paclitaxel. Weekly paclitaxel is superior to every 3 week paclitaxel, bringing into question whether difference in optimal schedule of administration could be responsible for the superiority of docetaxel. To improve quality of life and reduce toxicity, higher doses of docetaxel should be given with prophylactic myeloid growth factors.[33]

Newer Microtubule Targeted Agents

New formulations of existing agents have the advantage of potentially modifying the toxicity profile as well as possibly improving tumor penetrance leading to enhanced efficacy. Nab-paclitaxel is an albumin-bound, solvent-free novel formulation of the insoluble drug paclitaxel in the form of albumin-based nanoparticles that eliminates the need for premedications and the risk of hypersensitivity from paclitaxel.[34] Binding of drug to albumin receptors (glycoprotein 60 [gp60]) on the endothelial cell wall of the tumor neovasculature[35] may result in enhanced tumor cell uptake of *nab*-paclitaxel and therefore enhanced antitumor activity.

A phase III trial in patients with metastatic breast cancer compared *nab*-paclitaxel (n-pac), 260 mg/m², to paclitaxel, 175 mg/m², given every 3 weeks.[36] Treatment with n-pac resulted in improved RR (33% vs 19%; $p < 0.001$) and TTP (5.0 vs 3.7 months; $p = 0.030$) compared with paclitaxel, with reduced grade 4 neutropenia (9% vs 22%; $p < 0.001$) despite a 49% higher paclitaxel dose. Grade 3 sensory neuropathy was more common with n-pac than paclitaxel (10% vs 2%; $p < 0.001$) but improved at a median of 22 days. No hypersensitivity reactions occurred with n-pac despite the absence of premedication and shorter administration time.

Two large phase II studies evaluating weekly n-pac demonstrated RRs of 12% to 15% in taxane-resistant metastatic disease,[37,38] with low rates of grade 3 sensory neuropathy and minimal hematologic toxicity. A phase II trial randomized 300 patients with untreated metastatic breast cancer to 4 different arms: A: n-pac, 300 mg/m² every 3 weeks; B: n-pac, 100 mg/m² weekly (3 on, 1 off); C: n-pac, 150 mg/m² weekly (3 on, 1 off); and D: docetaxel, 100 mg/m² every 3 weeks.[39] Weekly n-pac resulted in the best RR (B: 62%, C: 70%, A: 43%, D: 38%), and high dose weekly n-pac was associated with the best progression-free survival (PFS) (arm C vs D, HR: 0.46; $p = 0.002$; arm C vs B, HR: 0.55; $p = 0.009$). The least toxicity was seen with arm B.

A large phase III, randomized trial is planned to open in 2009 and will compare weekly n-pac, 150 mg/m² given weekly for 3 of every 4 weeks, to every 3 week docetaxel, 100 mg/m², in women with metastatic breast cancer. The *nab* platform can be applied to other hydrophobic chemotherapy and biological agents; phase I studies of every 3 week *nab*-docetaxel are ongoing, and other *nab*-based agents are in development.

Epothilones

The epothilones are a novel class of nontaxane microtubule stabilizers with unique properties obtained by fermentation of myxobacteria *Sorangium cellulosum*.[40,41] The cytotoxic activity of epothilones, like those of the taxanes, have been linked to suppression of cell growth by promoting accelerated assembly of stable microtubules, which consequently leads to cell cycle arrest and eventual cell death.[40,42]

The most advanced epothilone in development, and the only epothilone approved for human use, is the semisynthetic analog of epothilone B ixabepilone. The tubulin polymerizing activity of ixabepilone is 2 to 10 times more potent than either paclitaxel or docetaxel,[43,44] and this agent is able to at least in part avoid several mechanisms that lead to drug resistance.[42,45,46] Like the taxanes, ixabepilone is solubilized with Cremophor; however, steroids are generally not necessary, and with minimal premedication, hypersensitivity reactions are not observed.

Phase II trials of ixabepilone, 40 mg/m² by intravenous infusion over 3 hours every 3 weeks, in metastatic breast cancer have demonstrated a partial RR of 42% in anthracycline pretreated tumors,[47] and 12% in anthracycline and taxane refractory heavily pretreated metastatic breast cancer.[48,49] The largest phase II trial treated 113 patients with anthracycline, taxane,

and capecitabine pretreated disease and reported a RR of 11.5% with an overall clinical benefit rate of 25%; PFS was 3.1 months.[50] Grade 3 or 4 sensory neuropathy, seen in 14%, improved in less than 6 weeks. An ongoing phase II trial is comparing every 3 week to weekly dosing of ixabepilone, with a comparator arm of weekly paclitaxel; all patients also receive bevacizumab. A phase III CALGB and North Central Cancer Treatment Group (NCCTG) trial (CALGB 40502) is comparing weekly ixabepilone and weekly nab-paclitaxel to weekly paclitaxel in patients with untreated metastatic breast cancer; all patients will also receive bevacizumab. Correlative studies in this trial will explore mechanisms of resistance and sensitivity to the taxane and epothilone.

Other Agents

A number of single agents have demonstrated efficacy in the treatment of metastatic breast cancer. The most widely used following anthracyclines and taxanes is capecitabine, an oral fluoropyrimidine prodrug that is converted to 5FU. Phase II studies demonstrated ORR of 20% to 28% with median OS of 12.8 to 15.2 months in women with anthracycline and taxane pretreated disease using the standard dose of 1250 mg/m² in 2 divided doses for 14 days followed by 7 days rest.[51,52] Capecitabine is oral, does not cause hair loss, and is relatively well tolerated when delivered at a slightly lower dose of 1000 mg/m² with the primary toxicity being hand-foot syndrome and modest diarrhea.

Other effective single agents used to treat advanced breast cancer include gemcitabine,[53] vinorelbine,[54] irinotecan,[55] and platinum compounds.[56] With the exception of the platinum compounds, phase II trials have demonstrated RRs in the range of 15% to 25% in patients with chemotherapy-resistant disease, with response durations in the 4- to 6-month range. Treatment with platinum compounds in chemotherapy refractory disease results in RRs of less than 10% in unselected metastatic disease. Pegylated liposomal doxorubicin is well tolerated when dosed appropriately.[57] The liposomal preparation does not have typical anthracycline toxicities; there is no alopecia, minimal nausea and bone marrow suppression, and it is dosed once a month. Weekly low-dose anthracyclines,[58] including epirubicin and doxorubicin, are also relatively well tolerated.

Metronomic therapy refers to frequent and often daily administration of low doses of chemotherapy and has been demonstrated in preclinical models to have antiangiogenic properties and to overcome at least some mechanisms of resistance.[59,60] Continuous low-dose oral cyclophosphamide with intermittent methotrexate as treatment for metastatic breast cancer with minimal pretreatment resulted in RR of 19% and stable disease in 32% of women with an associated decrease in circulating levels of vascular endothelial growth factor.[61] This interesting schedule is now being tested in women with residual cancer following neoadjuvant chemotherapy in combination with bevacizumab.

Combination Chemotherapy

It has long been observed that combinations of chemotherapy agents can increase RRs in advanced disease.[62,63] Long-term follow-up of patients treated at MD Anderson Cancer Center suggests that those patients who achieve a complete remission with first-line chemotherapy are the most likely to be long-term survivors of the disease.[2] These data have been used to support the use of more aggressive or combination chemotherapy to improve chances of remission, although it is more likely that biology determines both the quality and duration of response. The subsequent findings of the Eastern Cooperative Group (ECOG) trial 1193,[64] demonstrating an improvement in RR with the combination of doxorubicin and paclitaxel compared with either doxorubicin or paclitaxel alone without a corresponding improvement in survival but an increase in toxicity discouraged the general use of combination therapy. ECOG 1193 incorporated a second-line crossover design for single-agent therapy arm, enabling tracking of response and TTP in patients switching postprogression to either doxorubicin or docetaxel from the alternative agent. Results were again similar between the 2 arms, suggesting that the order of specific agents is less important than access to continued treatment. A recent meta-analysis of 9 randomized trials found treatment with single-agent taxanes or anthracyclines to result in comparable survival compared with taxane combination regimens,[65] although there were differences in PFS and RR. Data such as this is biased not only by subsequent therapy but also by rapidly changing standards in the treatment of early stage disease and the incorporation of biological therapy.

Two recent rationally designed nonanthracycline combinations have demonstrated a significant improvement in outcome compared with single-agent chemotherapy. Based on preclinical data demonstrating synergy, 256 patients with anthracycline pretreated metastatic breast cancer were randomized to receive either docetaxel, 100 mg/m² every 3 weeks, or docetaxel, 75 mg/m² every 3 weeks, combined with capecitabine, 1250 mg/m² twice daily, for 2 of every 3-week cycle.[66] TTP, ORR, and OS (14.5 vs 11.5 months) were improved with the combination; however, toxicity was significantly increased. In addition, only 15% of patients initially treated with docetaxel received capecitabine following progression, bringing into question the potential similar benefit from access to multiple single-agent sequential therapy in comparison to upfront combination therapy without subsequent options.

A second rationally based combination also demonstrated significant benefit in advanced disease. The 529 patients with a history of prior anthracycline-based adjuvant therapy were randomized to receive either paclitaxel, 175 mg/m² every 3 weeks, or the combination of paclitaxel at the same dose with gemcitabine, 1250 mg/m² day 1 and 8 of each 3-week cycle, as first-line therapy for metastatic disease.[67] RR, TTP, and OS (18.6 vs 15.8 months) were improved in the combination arm, but, again, few patients received subsequent chemotherapy. Toxicity with this combination was modestly increased.

A phase III trial compared capecitabine to the combination of capecitabine and ixabepilone in patients with taxane-resistant and anthracycline pretreated metastatic breast cancer.[49] The 752 women were randomized to either ixabepilone, 40 mg/m² every 3 weeks given with capecitabine, 2000 mg/m² in 2 divided doses days 1 to 14 every 3 weeks, or capecitabine alone. PFS was longer in the combination arm compared with treatment

with capecitabine alone (5.8 vs 4.2 months; HR: 0.75; $p = 0.0003$), as was the RR (35% vs 14%; $p < 0.0001$). The combination arm resulted in increased toxicity including grade 3/4 neutropenia, febrile neutropenia, and grade 3/4 peripheral neuropathy.

Taken together, these data demonstrate that modern versions of combination chemotherapy result in improved RR and TTP, even in anthracycline- and taxane-resistant disease. However, the lack of consistent posttrial therapy limits our ability to evaluate any benefit in survival using this approach, and clearly toxicity is enhanced. Keeping the goal of therapy in mind in the metastatic setting, combination regimens should be reserved for patients with a short disease-free interval from adjuvant therapy or for those with a life-threatening visceral crisis.

SPECIAL TOPICS

Targeted Biological Therapy

Combinations of chemotherapy and anti-HER-2-directed or antiangiogenic therapy are covered in Chapter 88. There is great interest in combining hormone therapy with targeted biologics to reverse or delay resistance. Both preclinical and clinical data suggest that HER-2-positive breast cancer is relatively resistant to hormone therapy, leading to the hypothesis that hormone sensitivity might be restored with blockade of the growth factor receptor.[68,69] Both trastuzumab and lapatinib combined with an AI have been shown to improve RR and TTP compared with an AI alone in metastatic disease overexpressing both HER-2/neu and HR,[70,71] and an ongoing trial is evaluating the effect of combining fulvestrant with lapatinib as second-line hormone therapy in both HER-2-positive and normal disease.

Other growth factor receptors have been implicated in resistance to hormone therapy in HR-positive disease. The insulin-like growth factor receptor (IGFR) appears to phosphorylate the ER and may play an important role in receptor cross-talk in the development of hormone resistance.[72] Several IGFR inhibitors are in early clinical trials to investigate this hypothesis. The vascular endothelial growth factor (VEGF) induces proliferation of breast cancer cells, and increased levels of VEGF have been associated with poor response to endocrine therapy.[73] Based on encouraging results from a phase II study,[74] CALGB 40503 is comparing first-line therapy of advanced, HR-positive breast cancer with an AI to the combination of an AI and inhibition of angiogenesis with bevacizumab. The combination of targeted biological therapy and hormone therapy is being tested in many ongoing and planned trials;[68,75] future studies will need to focus on both identifying resistant tumor phenotypes and identifying specific pathways that drive tumor growth in an individual tumor.

Triple-Negative Breast Cancer

Triple-negative breast cancer, defined by low expression of receptors for estrogen, progesterone, and HER-2/neu, is a particularly aggressive subgroup of this disease associated with high proliferative rates, early recurrence, and short survival.[76] In the metastatic setting, patients with triple-negative disease present the biggest therapeutic challenge due to limited and ineffective options.

DNA-damaging agents, such as platinum compounds, could potentially be effective in cancer cells with impaired DNA repair, such as those with BRCA1 or BRCA2 mutations, and they are often used in combination outside of clinical trials. One study randomized patients with advanced triple-negative disease to receive the antibody to epidermal growth factor receptor, cetuximab, or the combination of cetuximab and carboplatin.[77] Patients who progressed on cetuximab alone could cross over to receive the combination therapy. The RR to cetuximab alone was only 6% (2 of 31), but rose to 17% (4 of 24) with the addition of carboplatin, suggesting potential single-agent effectiveness of the platinum salt. Additional studies are evaluating the role of cisplatin and carboplatin in the treatment of triple-negative disease. Several small neoadjuvant studies in triple negative and BRCA1 mutation associated cancers have demonstrated pathologic complete response rates of 72% in a small BRCA1 mutation carrier trial[78], and upto 22% in unselected women with triple negative disease followed treatment with cisplatin alone.[79] A planned cooperative group neoadjuvant trial will evaluate the role of carboplatin combined with paclitaxel and bevacizumab in patients with triple negative disease.

Other targeted biological therapies are being evaluated in the treatment of triple-negative metastatic breast cancer and include antiangiogenic agents in combination with chemotherapy, and poly(ADP-ribose) polymerase 1 (PARP1) inhibitors.[80] PARP1 is a nuclear protein involved in critical pathways of DNA repair. Germ-line mutations in BRCA are associated with a defect in homologous recombination, another DNA repair pathway, and a high lifetime risk of breast and ovarian cancers. Preclinical studies indicate that PARP1 inhibitors target BRCA-deficient cell lines and tumors with high specificity.[81] Several PARP1 inhibitors are being evaluated in the clinical setting in both BRCA-associated metastatic breast cancer as well as in triple negative disease in combination with chemotherapy. Two doses of the oral PARP1 inhibitor olaparib (100 or 400 mg BID given continuously) were tested in a small phase II study in patients with BRCA1 and 2 associated metastatic breast cancer.[82] Interestingly, both patients with BRCA1 (usually triple negative) and BRCA2 (usually hormone receptor positive) associated cancers had evidence of tumor response, suggesting that the critical factor in sensitivity to these agents is a defect in the DNA repair pathway, rather than the triple negative phenotype. Twenty seven patients were treated on each arm; the response rate was higher in patients receiving the higher dose of oleparib (41% vs 22%), as was PFS (5.7 months vs 3.8 months) with the only toxicity being modest fatigue, nausea, and vomiting. A phase III trial is planned.

Triple negative cancers have been found to upregulate PARP1, and may also have acquired mutations in the BRCA gene. The most exciting data with PARP inhibitors was presented at ASCO in 2009.[83] In this randomized phase II trial, 116 patients with metastatic triple negative breast cancer were randomized to receive weekly gemcitabine and carboplatin, with or without the intravenous PARP1 inhibitor BSI-201

given in 4 IV infusions over two weeks. Remarkably, in this initial analysis of 86 patients, response rates (16% vs 48 %, $p < .01$), PFS (3.3 vs 6.9 mos., $p < .0001$, HR 0.34) and OS (5.7 months vs 9.2 months, $p = .0005$, HR 0.34) were all significantly improved in patients received the PARP inhibitor, despite the ability for patients on the control arm to cross over to the PARP inhibitor on disease progression. Toxicity was not increased with the addition of BSI-201 to the chemotherapy combination. This data is still preliminary, but the final results should be available in the near future, and a phase III registration study of the same design is rapidly accruing patients. A number of other oral PARP inhibitors are in phase I trials, and there are at least two ongoing neoadjuvant trials incorporating PARP inhibitors in platinum based regimens. It will remain to be seen whether there are any long-term toxicities to inhibition of this critical component of DNA repair.

FUTURE DIRECTIONS

A number of ongoing or planned clinical trials are investigating different schedules and new combinations of chemotherapy agents in an attempt to improve response and TTP without increasing toxicity. Many new studies are directed toward specific disease subtypes, such as triple-negative disease, and are combining new targeted biologics with chemotherapy or hormone therapy based on preclinical models of improved activity. Gene expression profiles are under evaluation to predict response or resistance to specific therapies and to identify breast cancer subtypes. The majority of trials are measuring blood markers that could enable early identification of futility and allow identification of cell surface markers. The best studied to date are circulating tumor cells[84]; circulating endothelial cells and proteins are also under evaluation.

NECESSARY FUTURE STUDIES

New hormone and chemotherapy agents have significantly improved the options for treatment of metastatic breast cancer. Nonetheless, this remains an incurable disease with a relatively short survival. In addition, specific subtypes are associated with poor response to available therapies. The most important future studies include understanding the biology of metastatic disease to allow prediction of response to specific agents. To achieve this goal, it is critical that tumor tissue be obtained to allow correlation of biological factors and clinical end points. New technologies should allow assessment of specific targets with modest amounts of tissue. Ideally, tissue would be obtained before and during treatment. Practically, most studies struggle to obtain material from initial diagnosis that may miss changes that occur in the transition to metastatic disease and the acquisition of resistance. In any case, ongoing and future studies will hopefully result in the identification of gene signatures or specific markers that will allow individualization of treatment.

As our understanding of biology improves, treatment will be increasingly directed toward rational combinations to improve response and reverse or delay resistance. This includes combinations with hormone therapy as well as chemotherapy. In addition, combinations of targeted biological agents to block multiple pathways or more than part of a specific pathway may prove particularly effective. To this end, new studies should be directed toward biological subtypes, rather than to metastatic breast cancer as a single entity. The ultimate goal of improving therapy in the metastatic setting is to apply the most effective treatments to early-stage disease, eventually eliminating the risk of recurrence.

SUMMARY

Many new treatments are available for the treatment of metastatic breast cancer that have improved both survival and tolerability. However, advanced disease remains incurable with subgroups of highly resistant tumors. Treatment goals include palliation of symptoms and prolonging survival. Sequential hormone therapy has proven to be effective in hormone-sensitive disease; progress has been made in partially reversing hormone resistance in HER-2/neu-positive disease with the addition of HER 2 directed therapy. Ongoing studies are also evaluating combinations of hormone agents with antiangiogenic therapy. New chemotherapy agents may be able to overcome some mechanisms of drug resistance or are associated with improved toxicity profiles; schedule and dosage is important. Sequential single agent chemotherapy is usually associated with a better toxicity profile than combination regimens, although combinations often result in improved RR and TTP. For patients with rapidly progressive and resistant disease, combination therapy may be the most appropriate approach. Triple-negative disease represents a heterogeneous subgroup of difficult to treat metastatic breast cancers for which there is intense study to find more effective agents.

REFERENCES

1. Jemal A, Siegel R, Ward E, et al. Cancer statistics, 2008. *CA Cancer J Clin.* 2008;58(2):71-96.
2. Greenberg PA, Hortobagyi GN, Smith TL, et al. Long-term follow-up of patients with complete remission following combination chemotherapy for metastatic breast cancer. *J Clin Oncol.* 1996;14(8):2197-2205.
3. Shie P, Cardarelli R, Brandon D, Erdman W, Abdulrahim N. Meta-analysis: comparison of F-18 fluorodeoxyglucose-positron emission tomography and bone scintigraphy in the detection of bone metastases in patients with breast cancer. *Clin Nucl Med.* 2008;33(2):97-101.
4. Abe K, Sasaki M, Kuwabara Y, et al. Comparison of 18FDG-PET with 99mTc-HMDP scintigraphy for the detection of bone metastases in patients with breast cancer. *Ann Nucl Med.* 2005;19(7):573-579.
5. Chang EY, Johnson W, Karamlou K, et al. The evaluation and treatment implications of isolated pulmonary nodules in patients with a recent history of breast cancer. *Am J Surg.* 2006;191(5):641-645.
6. Lower EE, Glass EL, Bradley DA, Blau R, Heffelfinger S. Impact of metastatic estrogen receptor and progesterone receptor status on survival. *Breast Cancer Res Treat.* 2005;90(1):65-70.
7. Meng S, Tripathy D, Shete S, et al. HER-2 gene amplification can be acquired as breast cancer progresses. *Proc Natl Acad Sci USA.* 2004;101(25):9393-9398.
8. Rugo HS. Hormonal therapy for advanced breast cancer. *Hematol Oncol Clin North Am.* 2007;21(2):273-291.
9. Harris L, Fritsche H, Mennel R, et al. American Society of Clinical Oncology 2007 update of recommendations for the use of tumor markers in breast cancer. *J Clin Oncol.* 2007;25(33):5287-5312.
10. Beatson GT. On the treatment of inoperable cases of carcinoma of the mamma: suggestions for a new method of treatment with illustrative cases. *Lancet.* 1869;2:104-107.
11. Bertelli G, Paridaens R. Optimal sequence of hormonotherapy in advanced breast cancer. *Curr Opin Oncol.* 2006;18(6):572-577.
12. Ellis MJ, Dehdahti F, Kommareddy A, et al. A randomized phase 2 trial of low dose (6 mg daily) versus high dose (30 mg daily) estradiol for patients with estrogen receptor positive aromatase inhibitor resistant advanced breast cancer. *Breast Cancer Res Treat.* 2008;106(S1):16.
13. Gradishar W, Chia SK, Piccart M. Fulvestrant versus exemestane following prior non-steroidal aromatase inhibitor therapy: first results from EFECT, a randomized, phase III trial in postmenopausal women with advanced breast cancer. *Breast Cancer Res Treat.* 2006;100(S1):12.
14. Zhou J, Giannakakou P. Targeting microtubules for cancer chemotherapy. *Curr Med Chem Anticancer Agents.* 2005;5(1):65-71.
15. Jordan MA, Wilson L. Microtubules as a target for anticancer drugs. *Nat Rev Cancer.* 2004;4:253-265.
16. Eisenhauer EA, Vermorken JB. The taxoids. Comparative clinical pharmacology and therapeutic potential. *Drugs.* 1998;55(1):5-30.
17. Sparano JA. Taxanes for breast cancer: an evidence-based review of randomized phase II and phase III trials. *Clin Breast Cancer.* 2000;1(1):32-40; discussion 41-32.
18. Seidman AD. Systemic treatment of breast cancer. Two decades of progress. *Oncology (Williston Park).* 2006;20(9):983-990; discussion 991-982, 997-988.
19. Eniu A, Palmieri FM, Perez EA. Weekly administration of docetaxel and paclitaxel in metastatic or advanced breast cancer. *Oncologist.* 2005;10(9):665-685.
20. Norton L. Kinetic concepts in the systemic drug therapy of breast cancer. *Semin Oncol.* 1999;26(1 suppl 2):11-20.
21. Seidman AD, Hudis CA, Albanell J, et al. Dose-dense therapy with weekly 1-hour paclitaxel infusions in the treatment of metastatic breast cancer. *J Clin Oncol.* 1998;16(10):3353-3361.
22. Kerbel RS, Viloria-Petit A, Klement G, Rak J. "Accidental" anti-angiogenic drugs. anti-oncogene directed signal transduction inhibitors and conventional chemotherapeutic agents as examples. *Eur J Cancer.* 2000;36(10):1248-1257.
23. Seidman AD, Berry D, Cirrincione C, et al. Randomized phase III trial of weekly compared with every-3-weeks paclitaxel for metastatic breast cancer, with trastuzumab for all HER 2 overexpressors and random assignment to trastuzumab or not in HER-2 nonoverexpressors: final results of Cancer and Leukemia Group B protocol 9840. *J Clin Oncol.* 2008;26(10):1642-1649.
24. Nabholtz JM, Gelmon K, Bontenbal M, et al. Multicenter, randomized comparative study of two doses of paclitaxel in patients with metastatic breast cancer. *J Clin Oncol.* 1996;14(6):1858-1867.
25. Winer EP, Berry DA, Woolf S, et al. Failure of higher-dose paclitaxel to improve outcome in patients with metastatic breast cancer: cancer and leukemia group B trial 9342. *J Clin Oncol.* 2004;22(11):2061-2068.
26. Hainsworth JD, Burris HA III, Greco FA. Weekly administration of docetaxel (Taxotere): summary of clinical data. *Semin Oncol.* 1999;26 (3 suppl 10):19-24.
27. Tabernero J, Climent MA, Lluch A, et al. A multicentre, randomised phase II study of weekly or 3-weekly docetaxel in patients with metastatic breast cancer. *Ann Oncol.* 2004;15(9):1358-1365.
28. Ringel I, Horwitz SB. Studies with RP 56976 (Taxotere): a semisynthetic analogue of Taxol. *J Natl Cancer Inst.* 1991;83:288-291.
29. Riou J-F, Petitgenet O, Combeau C, et al. Cellular uptake and efflux of docetaxel (Taxotere) and paclitaxel (Taxol) in P388 cell line. *Proc Am Soc Clin Oncol.* 1994;35:385.
30. Diaz JF, Andreu JM. Assembly of purified GDP-tubulin into microtubules induced by Taxol and Taxotere: reversibility, ligand stoichiometry, and competition. *Biochemistry.* 1993;32:2747-2755.
31. Lavelle F, Bissery MC, Combeau C, et al. Preclinical evaluation of docetaxel (Taxotere). *Semin Oncol.* 1995;22(2 suppl 4):3-16.
32. Jones SE, Erban J, Overmoyer B, et al. Randomized phase III study of docetaxel compared with paclitaxel in metastatic breast cancer. *J Clin Oncol.* 2005;23(24):5542-5551.
33. Crawford J, Althaus B, Armitage J, et al. Myeloid growth factors. Clinical practice guidelines in oncology. *J Natl Compr Canc Netw.* 2007;5(2):188-202.
34. Gradishar WJ. Albumin-bound paclitaxel: a next-generation taxane. *Expert Opin Pharmacother.* 2006;7(8):1041-1053.
35. Desai N, Trieu V, Yao R, Labao E, Soon-Shiong P. Increased endothelial transcytosis of nanoparticle albumin-bound paclitaxel (ABI-007) by gp60-receptors: a pathway inhibited by Taxol. *Breast Cancer Res Treat.* 2004;88(S1):1071.
36. Gradishar WJ, Tjulandin S, Davidson N, et al. Phase III trial of nanoparticle albumin-bound paclitaxel compared with polyethylated castor oil-based paclitaxel in women with breast cancer. *J Clin Oncol.* 2005;23(31):7794-7803.

37. Blum JL, Savin MA, Edelman G, et al. Long term disease control in taxane-refractory metastatic breast cancer treated with nab paclitaxel. *Proc Am Soc Clin Oncol.* 2004;22(14S):543.

38. O'Shaughnessy JA, Blum JL, Sandbach JF, et al. Weekly nanoparticle albumin paclitaxel (Abraxane) results in long-term disease control in patients with taxane-refractory metastatic breast cancer. *Breast Cancer Res Treat.* 2004;88(S1):1070.

39. Gradishar W, Krasnojon D, Cheporov S, et al. Randomized comparison of weekly or every-3-week (q3w) nab-paclitaxel compared to q3w docetaxel as first-line therapy in patients (pts) with metastatic breast cancer (MBC). *Proc Am Soc Clin Oncol.* 2007;25(18S):1032.

40. Bollag DM, McQueney PA, Zhu J, et al. Epothilones, a new class of microtubule-stabilizing agents with a Taxol-like mechanism of action. *Cancer Res.* 1995;55(11):2325-2333.

41. Cortes J, Baselga J. Targeting the microtubules in breast cancer beyond taxanes: the epothilones. *Oncologist.* 2007;12(3):271-280.

42. Kavallaris M, Verrills NM, Hill BT. Anticancer therapy with novel tubulin-interacting drugs. *Drug Resist Updat.* 2001;4(6):392-401.

43. Wartmann M, Altmann KH. The biology and medicinal chemistry of epothilones. *Curr Med Chem Anticancer Agents.* 2002;2(1):123-148.

44. Altmann KH. Recent developments in the chemical biology of epothilones. *Curr Pharm Des.* 2005;11(13):1595-1613.

45. Fojo AT, Menefee M. Microtubule targeting agents: basic mechanisms of multidrug resistance (MDR). *Semin Oncol.* 2005;32(6 suppl 7):S3-8.

46. Kavallaris M, Kuo DY, Burkhart CA, et al. Taxol-resistant epithelial ovarian tumors are associated with altered expression of specific b-tubulin isotypes. *J Clin Invest.* 1997;100:1282-1293.

47. Roche H, Yelle L, Cognetti F, et al. Phase II clinical trial of ixabepilone (BMS 247550), an epothilone B analog, as first-line therapy in patients with metastatic breast cancer previously treated with anthracycline chemotherapy. *J Clin Oncol.* 2007;25(23):3415-3420.

48. Conte P, Thomas E, Martin M, Klimovsky J, Tabernero J. Phase II study of ixabepilone in patients (pts) with taxane-resistant metastatic breast cancer (MBC): final report. *J Clin Oncol.* 2006;24(S18):10505.

49. Thomas ES, Gomez HL, Li RK, et al. Ixabepilone plus capecitabine for metastatic breast cancer progressing after anthracycline and taxane treatment. *J Clin Oncol.* 2007;25(33):5210-5217.

50. Perez EA, Lerzo G, Pivot X, et al. Efficacy and safety of ixabepilone (BMS-247550) in a phase II study of patients with advanced breast cancer resistant to an anthracycline, a taxane, and capecitabine. *J Clin Oncol.* 2007;25(23):3407-3414.

51. Blum JL, Jones SE, Buzdar AU, et al. Multicenter phase II study of capecitabine in paclitaxel-refractory metastatic breast cancer. *J Clin Oncol.* 1999;17(2):485-493.

52. Fumoleau P, Largillier R, Clippe C, et al. Multicentre, phase II study evaluating capecitabine monotherapy in patients with anthracycline- and taxane-pretreated metastatic breast cancer. *Eur J Cancer.* 2004;40(4):536-542.

53. Dent S, Messersmith H, Trudeau M. Gemcitabine in the management of metastatic breast cancer: a systematic review. *Breast Cancer Res Treat.* 2008;108(3):319-331.

54. Zelek L, Barthier S, Riofrio M, et al. Weekly vinorelbine is an effective palliative regimen after failure with anthracyclines and taxanes in metastatic breast carcinoma. *Cancer.* 2001;92(9):2267-2272.

55. Perez EA, Hillman DW, Mailliard JA, et al. Randomized phase II study of two irinotecan schedules for patients with metastatic breast cancer refractory to an anthracycline, a taxane, or both. *J Clin Oncol.* 2004;22(14):2849-2855.

56. Carrick S, Ghersi D, Wilcken N, Simes J. Platinum containing regimens for metastatic breast cancer. *Cochrane Database Syst Rev.* 2004(3):CD003374.

57. Coleman RE, Biganzoli L, Canney P, et al. A randomised phase II study of two different schedules of pegylated liposomal doxorubicin in metastatic breast cancer (EORTC-10993). *Eur J Cancer.* 2006;42(7):882-887.

58. Barni S, Archili C, Lissoni P, et al. A weekly schedule of epirubicin in pretreated advanced breast cancer. *Tumori.* 1993;79(1):45-48.

59. Kerbel RS, Klement G, Pritchard KI, Kamen B. Continuous low-dose anti-angiogenic/metronomic chemotherapy: from the research laboratory into the oncology clinic. *Ann Oncol.* 2002;13(1):12-15.

60. Kerbel RS, Kamen BA. The anti-angiogenic basis of metronomic chemotherapy. *Nat Rev Cancer.* 2004;4(6):423-436.

61. Colleoni M, Rocca A, Sandri MT, et al. Low-dose oral methotrexate and cyclophosphamide in metastatic breast cancer: antitumor activity and correlation with vascular endothelial growth factor levels. *Ann Oncol.* 2002;13(1):73-80.

62. Miles D, von Minckwitz G, Seidman AD. Combination versus sequential single-agent therapy in metastatic breast cancer. *Oncologist.* 2002;7(suppl 6):13-19.

63. Nabholtz JM, Riva A. Taxane/anthracycline combinations: setting a new standard in breast cancer? *Oncologist.* 2001;6(suppl 3):5-12.

64. Sledge GW, Neuberg D, Bernardo P, et al. Phase III trial of doxorubicin, paclitaxel, and the combination of doxorubicin and paclitaxel as front-line chemotherapy for metastatic breast cancer: an intergroup trial (E1193). *J Clin Oncol.* 2003;21(4):588-592.

65. Piccart-Gebhart MJ, Burzykowski T, Buyse M, et al. Taxanes alone or in combination with anthracyclines as first-line therapy of patients with metastatic breast cancer. *J Clin Oncol.* 2008;26(12):1980-1986.

66. O'Shaughnessy J, Miles D, Vukelja S, et al. Superior survival with capecitabine plus docetaxel combination therapy in anthracycline-pretreated patients with advanced breast cancer: phase III trial results. *J Clin Oncol.* 2002;20(12):2812-2823.

67. Albain KS, Nag S, Calderillo-Ruiz G, et al. Global phase III study of gemcitabine plus paclitaxel (GT) vs. paclitaxel (T) as frontline therapy for metastatic breast cancer (MBC): First report of overall survival. *Proc Am Soc Clin Oncol.* 2004;22(14S):510.

68. Ellis M. Overcoming endocrine therapy resistance by signal transduction inhibition. *Oncologist.* 2004;9(suppl 3):20-26.

69. Osborne CK, Shou J, Massarweh S, Schiff R, Crosstalk between estrogen receptor and growth factor receptor pathways as a cause for endocrine therapy resistance in breast cancer. *Clin Cancer Res* 2005;11(2 Pt 2):865s-870s.

70. Mackey JR, Kaufman B, Clemens M, et al. Trastuzumab prolongs progression free survival in hormone dependent and HER2 positive metastatic breast cancer. *Breast Cancer Res Treat.* 2006;100(S1):3.

71. Johnston S, Pegram M, Press M, et al. Lapatinib combined with letrozole vs. letrozole alone for front line postmenopausal hormone receptor positive (HR+) metastatic breast cancer (MBC): first results from the EGF30008 Trial. *Breast Cancer Res Treat.* 2008;106(S1):46.

72. Juncker-Jensen A, Lykkesfeldt AE, Worm J, et al. Insulin-like growth factor binding protein 2 is a marker for antiestrogen resistant human breast cancer cell lines but is not a major growth regulator. *Growth Horm IGF Res.* 2006;16(4):224-239.

73. Liang Y, Brekken RA, Hyder SM. Vascular endothelial growth factor induces proliferation of breast cancer cells and inhibits the anti-proliferative activity of anti-hormones. *Endocr Relat Cancer.* 2006;13(3):905-919.

74. Traina TA, Rugo H, Caravelli J, et al. Letrozole with bevacizumab is feasible in patients with hormone receptor-positive metastatic breast cancer. *Proc Am Soc Clin Oncol.* 2006;24:133.

75. Johnston SR. Clinical trials of intracellular signal transductions inhibitors for breast cancer—a strategy to overcome endocrine resistance. *Endocr Relat Cancer.* 2005;12(suppl 1):S145-157.

76. Schneider BP, Winer EP, Foulkes WD, et al. Triple-negative breast cancer: risk factors to potential targets. *Clin Cancer Res.* 2008;14(24):8010-8018.

77. Carey L, Rugo HS, Markam PK, et al. TBCRC 001: EGFR inhibition with cetuximab added to carboplatin in metastatic triple-negative (basal-like) breast cancer. *J Clin Oncol.* 2008;26:1009.

78. Gronwald J, Byrski T, Huzarski T, et al. Neoadjuvant therapy with cisplatin in BRCA1-positive breast cancer patients. *J Clin Oncol.* 27:15s, 2009 (suppl; abstr 502)

79. Garber JE, Richardson A, Harris LN, et al. Neo adjuvant cisplatin (CDDP) in triple-negative breast cancer (BC). San Antonio Breast Cancer Symposium 2006, abstr 3074.

80. Lord CJ, Ashworth A. Targeted therapy for cancer using PARP inhibitors. *Curr Opin Pharmacol.* 2008;8(4):363-369.

81. Martin SA, Lord CJ, Ashworth A. DNA repair deficiency as a therapeutic target in cancer. *Curr Opin Genet Dev.* 2008;18(1):80-86.

82. Tutt J, Robson M, Garber JE, et al. Phase II trial of the oral PARP inhibitor olaparib in BRCA-deficient advanced breast cancer. *Clin Oncol.* 27:18s, 2009 (suppl; abstr CRA501).

83. O'Shaughnessy J, Osborne C, Pippen J, et al. Efficacy of BSI-201, a poly (ADP-ribose) polymerase-1 (PARP1) inhibitor, in combination with gemcitabine/carboplatin (G/C) in patients with metastatic triple-negative breast cancer (TNBC): results of a randomized phase II trial. *J Clin Oncol.* 27:18s, 2009 (suppl; abstr 3).

84. Cristofanilli M, Hayes DF, Budd GT, et al. Circulating tumor cells: a novel prognostic factor for newly diagnosed metastatic breast cancer. *J Clin Oncol.* 2005;23:1420-1430.

RADIATION

Bruce G. Haffty

CHAPTER 93

Conceptual Basis and Principles of Radiation Oncology

Bruce G. Haffty
Venkat Narra
Ning J. Yue

OVERVIEW

As a discipline, radiation oncology primarily deals with the use of ionizing radiation in the treatment of malignant diseases. Occasionally therapeutic doses of radiation may be used to treat benign processes, such as heterotopic bone formation, meningiomas, and other benign proliferative diseases. Radiation has a very prominent role in the management of breast cancer after lumpectomy, as adjuvant therapy after mastectomy, in the management of locoregional relapse of disease, and in the palliation of metastatic disease. Management of breast cancers can typically cover up to 20% to 25% of a general radiation oncology practice. The next few chapters will cover in more detail the role of radiation therapy after breast conserving therapy, the rapidly evolving role of partial breast irradiation, postmastectomy radiation, and the role of radiation in palliation and metastatic disease.

A basic review of the underlying principles of the physics, radiation biology, and radiation planning is essential to understanding the role of radiation therapy in the management of breast cancer. It is beyond the scope of this text to comprehensively review the underlying principles of radiation physics and biology, and the reader is referred to more comprehensive textbooks for more detailed information.[1-5] However, in this chapter we will highlight some of the basic principles of physics and radiation biology and outline some of the basics of radiation planning to give the reader an appreciation of the underlying principles, rationale, and process of radiation in the management of breast cancer.

BASIC PHYSICS OF RADIATION THERAPY

Radiation therapy uses a form of electromagnetic radiation, commonly referred to as ionizing radiation, generated from x-rays, gamma rays, electrons, and other forms of particles. *Ionizing radiation* consists of highly energetic particles that can eject at least 1 electron from an atom. Ionizing ability depends on the energy of individual particles or waves. Although x-rays or gamma rays are the principle form of ionizing radiation used in conventional radiation therapy, other forms of ionizing radiation include protons, beta particles, neutrons, alpha particles, and heavy ions. The ability of photons to ionize an atom or molecule varies across the electromagnetic spectrum. Although x-rays and gamma rays have high enough energy to ionize almost any molecule or atom, near ultraviolet and visible light are ionizing to very few molecules, and microwaves and radiowaves are nonionizing radiation within the electromagnetic spectrum.[3,4]

Ionizing radiation ejects electrons from atoms. These fast electrons continue on to produce additional ionizations, amplifying the effect of the initial photon interactions. One of the more critical and essential interactions of x-rays is the creation of ion pairs from interactions with the abundant water in cells and tissues that lead to the formation of free radicals. This process represents the primary mechanism through which damage is created in irradiated cells. Certain substances, such as antioxidants or high doses of certain vitamins, theoretically can absorb some of these free radicals, thereby counteracting the effects of radiation.[6,7]

Although radiation interaction in human tissues can damage a variety of cellular components, DNA remains the essential and primary target of radiation in the management of malignant disease. DNA double-strand breaks, caused by ionizing radiation interaction in cells, likely represent the most critical lesions. As discussed below, lack of repair of double-strand breaks, or misrepair, results in cell death and other biologic effects of radiation. The chemical and biological changes in tissue result from exposure to ionizing radiation, caused by the deposition of energy from the radiation into the tissue. The *absorbed dose* is the energy actually absorbed per unit mass in the irradiated volume. The unit of absorbed dose is the Gray (Gy), defined as 1 J/kg of irradiated medium.[3-5]

Production of X-Rays and External Photon Beam Radiation

The practice of radiation therapy began very soon after Roentgen's discovery of x-rays in the 1890s. Within just a few years of the discovery of x-rays, reports of altering the course of malignant disease and palliation of malignancy with the use of therapeutic doses of radiation appeared in the early literature.[3] External-beam radiation units are commonly categorized by the energy range of the beam: contact units (40-50 kV), superficial (50-150 kV), orthovoltage (150-500 kV), supervoltage (500-1000 kV), and megavoltage (> 1000 kV or > 1 MV). In general, the higher the energy, the more penetrating the beam will be. Although higher-energy beams have advantages with respect to sparing skin and treating more deeply seated tumors, in the earlier years of therapy, most radiation therapy was delivered with x-rays generated at relatively low-energy units below approximately 300 kV, due to the limitations of the available technology of the time.

It was not until the 1950s and the availability of high-activity sources of cobalt 60 (^{60}Co) that megavoltage units came into widespread use. Cobalt units contain a source of ^{60}Co, which emits gamma rays of 1.17 and 1.33 MV, and were therefore more suitable for treating more deeply seated tumors while providing some sparing of the skin, as compared with the lower-energy orthovoltage units. Although linear accelerators have replaced cobalt units in the majority of facilities in the United States, cobalt units continue to be used in many facilities throughout the world. Because the cobalt source is always active and cannot be turned on or off, the radiation beam is turned on and off by moving the source from a shielded position to an exposed position. Although linear accelerators have predominantly replaced cobalt units in the majority of external-beam facilities, cobalt sources are still routinely used in the "gamma knife" stereotactic radiation device commonly used to deliver stereotactic radiosurgical treatments in a variety of brain applications.

When the megavoltage cobalt units were being developed, many were manufactured with isocentric gantries. The gantry of an isocentric unit rotates about a horizontal axis, so that the source remains in a plane perpendicular to this axis, and the radiation beam always passes through a single point on the axis in space, known as the *isocenter*, around which both treatment table and collimator also rotate, as shown in Figures 93-1A through C. This is the fundamental design of current modern linear accelerators as well.

Modern linear accelerators (also known as *linacs*) are now found in virtually all radiation therapy departments and have replaced most low-energy x-rays units and isotope teletherapy units. Most medical linacs accelerate electrons and the resulting electron beam strikes a target, producing x-rays that are collimated and directed to the patient. Modern linear accelerators generate x-ray beams generally ranging from 4 to 18 MV, with the use of 6-MV photons being most commonly used for external-beam whole-breast irradiation. Many of the current machines have 2 energies to choose from, as more deeply seated tumors, such as prostate or pelvic tumors, may be better treated by more penetrating beams of 10 MV or more. Figures 93-2A through C show a modern linear accelerator with a patient under treatment for breast cancer.

Electron Beams

Although linear accelerators most commonly operate in the photon or x-ray mode, the accelerated electron beam can be focused directly at the patient in the electron mode. Here, the target and flattening filter are moved out of the electron field, and the electron beam is directed through a scattering foil and then directly to the patient for electron beam therapy. The direct electron beam is not as penetrating as x-rays, and the dose falls off fairly rapidly from the surface of the patient. The penetration of an electron beam compared with that of a photon beam in tissue is shown in Figure 93-3, where the dose in tissue is near maximum at the surface for an electron beam, then rapidly falls off. For a photon beam, the skin is spared because the dose starts to buildup just below the skin surface, reaches its maximum at a certain depth, then gradually falls off. Therefore, electrons are useful in treating the skin and near the surface of the patient, while sparing deeper underlying tissues and as such are ideally suited to boost the tumor bed after whole-breast irradiation, to boost the scar after mastectomy, and by some, to treat the chest wall after mastectomy.

Linear Accelerator Machines

Most electron accelerators consist of a microwave power source (magnetron), a linear accelerator guide to accelerate the electrons, a bending magnet, an x-ray target which the electrons hit to produce the x-rays; a flattening filter, which filters and flattens the beam for uniform clinical use; an ionization chamber to monitor dose delivered; and a collimator to delineate the final dimensions of the field. Fields could be further shaped and customized to the specific clinical situation with blocks, generally made from cerrobend, which were placed between the collimator and the patient, to achieve a final customized, shaped field based on the specific clinical case. When treating directly with electrons, the target and flattening filter are moved out of the electron beam, and a scattering foil is used for direct electron beam treatment. When shaping the electron field, the final stage of collimation of an electron beam must be close to the skin surface. Therefore, a cone or electron applicator is commonly used to shape electron beams.

Although custom cerrobend blocks were used routinely in the past to allow custom shaping of the field for each clinical

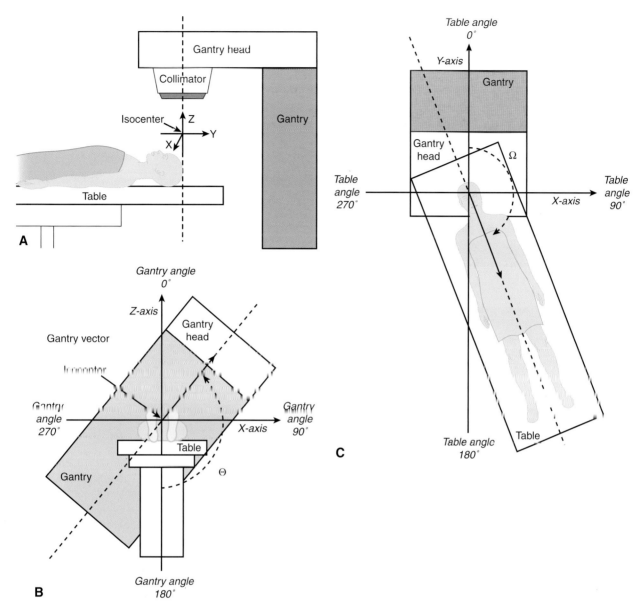

FIGURE 93-1 **A.** Isocenter and its relative location to machine gantry, treatment table, and collimator. **B.** Gantry rotates around an axis, passing the isocenter. **C.** Treatment table rotates around an axis, passing the isocenter.

case, most modern linear accelerators incorporate a multileaf collimator (MLC) within the head of the linear accelerator. These devices effectively allow custom shaping of the field within the linear accelerator itself and can be used to further shape and refine the beam. MLCs were originally envisioned as a field-shaping device to eliminate the hazards and tedious work of creating custom cerrobend blocks to shape the field. With advances in computer technology and treatment planning, the leaves of the MLC can be moved in and out of the field rapidly during treatment, effectively resulting in the ability to modulate the intensity of portions of the beam during treatment. Effectively, portions of the beam can be blocked during a specific treatment, attenuating the intensity of a given portion of the beam for part of the treatment. This results in a

radiation beam that cannot only be shaped, but intensity-modulated during treatment to improve either the homogeneity of radiation distribution or radiation conformity during treatment. This is discussed in detail later, under radiation treatment planning.

Brachytherapy

Although the majority of radiation treatment is delivered by external-beam radiation generated from linear accelerators, radiation can also be delivered from radioactive sources placed directly in or adjacent to the target tissue. The short distance between the source of radiation and the tumor or target tissue relates directly to the root of the

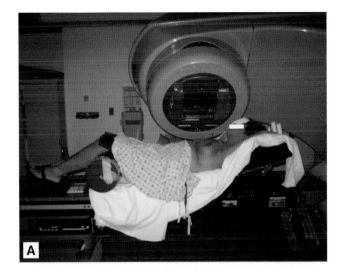

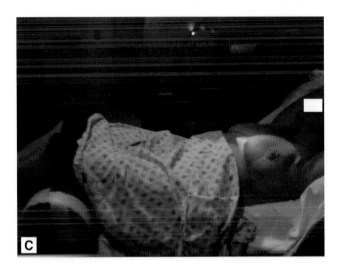

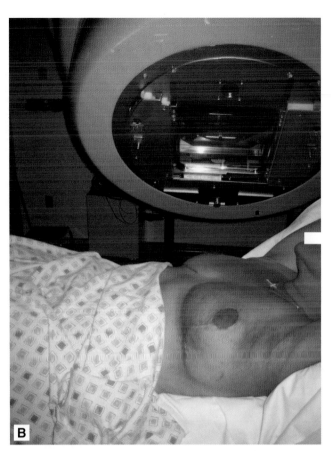

FIGURE 93-2 **A.** A breast cancer patient is receiving external-beam radiation treatment on a modern linac. **B.** Close-up of a patient under external-beam radiation treatment on a modern linac. **C.** Close-up of a patient under external-beam radiation treatment on a modern linac, showing 1 of the treatment light fields.

term brachytherapy which is derived from the Greek word *brachios*, meaning short distance. It has been most commonly used in the treatment of prostate and gynecologic tumors, but more recently it has been used with increasing frequency in patients treated with accelerated partial-breast irradiation, with devices such as the MammoSite[8] (Hologic; Bedford, Massachusetts). A potential advantage of brachytherapy is that a high dose can be delivered directly to the target, because the absorbed dose falls off very rapidly with increasing distance from the source.

The physics of brachytherapy is fundamentally based on the phenomenon of radioactive decay. More detailed discussion of the physics of brachytherapy can be found elsewhere, but some general concepts are introduced here.[3,5] Most atoms are stable and not radioactive. However, in some atoms, the ratio of the number of neutrons to protons leads to instability, and these nuclei undergo changes that lead to a more stable configuration. These reactions are accompanied by the emission of particles and electromagnetic radiation as the nucleus releases

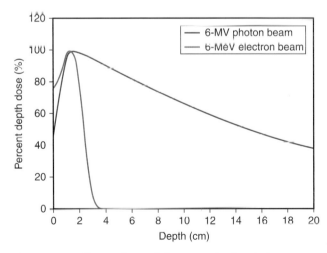

FIGURE 93-3 Comparison of dose penetration between 6-MV photon and 6-MeV electron beams.

energy. These changes are referred to as *radioactive decay*, and the process of emission of radiation is described as *radioactivity*. The rate of decay of a radionuclide is directly proportional to the number of atoms of a radionuclide present in a given sample. As the number of atoms of the radionuclide decreases (as they change into the progeny nuclide), the rate of decay, or *radioactivity*, of the sample decreases. The rate of radioactivity change of different radionuclides is most likely different and is normally quantified with half-life, which is defined as the time required for the activity to decay to half the initial value.

In general radiation oncology practice, most commonly used radionuclides are photon emitters in the energy range of 20 keV to 1.0 MeV, although brachytherapy can be performed by using photon emitters, beta, or other particle emitters. Photons with energy lower than 20 keV and beta rays with energy lower than 500 keV can be easily attenuated in superficial layers of tissue and are of limited clinical value. In clinical practice, the radionuclide is normally made into sealed source, encapsulated with an inert metal. This metallic encapsulation may filter out low-energy photons and beta particles, leading to a possible different energy spectrum of sealed source from its corresponding pure radionuclide. It is common that for low-energy photon emitters, such as iodine-125 (^{125}I) and palladium 103 (^{103}Pd), different models of sealed source manufactured by different vendors possess different photon spectra because of different design of the source encapsulation. A useful physical quantity to describe the photon energy of sealed source is half-value layer in lead, which is the thickness of lead that would reduce the photon intensity to half the initial value.[3]

In Table 93-1, the properties of several commonly used brachytherapy sources are listed. Their range of dominant photon energies is as follows: iridium 192 (^{192}Ir) (0.06-0.88 MeV), cesium 137 (^{137}Cs) (0.662 MeV), ^{125}I (Model 6711-OncoSeed) (0.022-0.035 MeV), ^{103}Pd (Model 200) (0.020-0.023 MeV), ^{131}Cs (Model Cs-1) (0.017-0.034 MeV), gold 198 (0.071-1.09 MeV, primarily 0.412 MeV), and radium 226 (^{226}Ra) (0.047-2.45 MeV). ^{125}I, ^{103}Pd, and ^{131}Cs sources offer low-energy photons and have relatively short half-lives (in days), which make them desirable choices for permanent implants, in which the sources are placed and left inside the patient permanently. These are commonly used in the treatment of prostate cancer with permanent iodine or palladium seeds. Longer-lived sources, such as ^{192}Ir, ^{137}Cs, and ^{226}Ra, are more suitable for both low dose rate

(LDR) and high dose rate (HDR) temporary implants, in which the sources are placed inside or near the target volume to deliver the desired dose and then are removed from the patient after. Compared with other clinically available sources, ^{192}Ir source has much higher specific radioactivity (radioactivity per unit mass). This unique characteristic of ^{192}Ir makes it possible to manufacture a source with high radioactivity but small size and makes ^{192}Ir a natural choice for the HDR brachytherapy treatment, in which the source is often transported to inside the patient via fairly narrow catheters or tubes. The HDR units are often used as sources to introduce into balloon-based brachytherapy, such as the MammoSite device, discussed in more detail in Chapter 95.

The clinical brachytherapy sources are available in different forms. ^{192}Ir is available as solid wire, individual seeds, or ribbons. ^{125}I, ^{103}Pd, and ^{131}Cs are available as individual seeds and may also be available in absorbable ribbons. ^{226}Ra and ^{137}Cs are available as tubes or needles. As mentioned above, the encapsulations of the radionuclides are manufacturer dependent in terms of material and construction design. Even the distribution of radionuclide inside source is also manufacturer dependent. Because of these differences, each source design requires its own dose rate distribution determination because the amount of attenuation depends on the geometry of the design, especially for low-energy particle emitters, such as ^{125}I, ^{103}Pd, and ^{131}Cs.

Brachytherapy can be delivered by a number of techniques, including interstitial implants, where radioactive sources are generally placed in multiple catheters implanted directly into the tumor bed; intracavitary implants, where radioactive sources can be placed in a body cavity adjacent to the target tissue; intraluminal implants, where sources are placed in the lumen of a vessel, duct, or airway; or molds, where the sources are placed in a mold or plaque and placed on the skin or mucosal surface to treat a lesion on the surface. Though theoretically the above-mentioned sources can be used in any technique, due to the differences in source design, size, and dosimetry characteristics, ^{226}Ra and ^{137}Cs sources are mostly used in intracavitary implants; ^{125}I, ^{103}Pd, and ^{131}Cs are mostly used in interstitial and plaque implants; and ^{192}Ir is used in both interstitial and intracavitary implants.

Brachytherapy procedures can be further categorized as temporary or permanent implants. Temporary implants can be delivered on an outpatient basis or can require that the patient be hospitalized for the duration of the treatment, which generally

TABLE 93-1 Properties of Sealed Photon-Emitting Sources in Clinical Use

Isotope	Half-Life	Dominant Photon Energy Range (MeV)	Average Energy (MeV)	First Half-Value Layer (mm Pb)
Iridium 192	73.83 days	0.06-0.88	0.35	2.2
Cesium 137	30 years	0.662	0.662	5.6
Palladium 103 (Model 200)	17.0 days	0.020-0.023	0.021	0.008
Iodine 125 (6711- OncoSeed)	59.4 days	0.022-0.035	0.027	0.016
Gold 198	2.7 days	0.071-1.09	0.412	2.5
Cesium 131 (Model Cs-1)	9.7 days	0.017-0.034	0.030	0.021
Radium 226	1600 years	0.047-2.45	0.83	12.0

lasts no more than a few days. Permanent implants, which are practical only for interstitial treatments, require that the sources remain in the tissue permanently. For these treatments, sources with relatively short half-lives are used, so that the majority of the dose is delivered within a few weeks or months. Permanent implants must use sources with low-energy emissions so that the dose rate at the patient's external surface does not present a significant risk of radiation exposure to others. These patients frequently can be released from the hospital as soon as their medical condition permits.

Temporary implants are further classified as HDR or LDR. HDR temporary implants normally deliver radiation to the target volume at a rate higher than 1200 cGy/h and may require only a few minutes of irradiation for 1 fraction of treatment, whereas LDR temporary implants deliver radiation at a rate between 4 and 200 cGy/h and usually require a few days of irradiation. HDR brachytherapy treatment is almost always delivered using a remotely controlled afterloading system. The system is controlled with a computer, which is stationed outside the treatment room. Most of the systems use a tiny ^{192}Ir source with a radioactivity of about 10 Ci, which is welded onto the end of a motor-driven cable. The source, along with the cable, is housed in a shielded safe within the unit. Figure 93-4 shows one such kind of unit. The treatment is preceded by first placing catheters or applicators into or near the target volume. Based on the dose prescription, a specialized treatment planning system uses optimization algorithms to determine the source dwell positions and corresponding dwell times in each of the catheters or applicators. The dose distribution can be further improved by manually adjusting either the dose distribution itself or dwell positions and times on the planning computer. Right before the treatment, the catheters or applicators are connected with guide tubes to the ports of the system. Verifications are conducted with imaging devices to further confirm the positioning accuracy of the catheters or applicators. During the treatment, the source is sequentially sent from the safe to the dwell positions in the applicators by a command from a remote-control console, after medical staffs exit the treatment room. The source can be retracted back into the safe anytime if needed. After the treatment is completed, the source is always remotely retracted back into the safe, and catheters or applicators can be either removed or temporarily left in place for additional treatments.

Brachytherapy was used frequently in the earlier years of breast-conserving therapy as a method of boosting the lumpectomy site. With the widespread availability of external electron beam units, brachytherapy gradually fell out of favor for the boost to the tumor bed. However, over the past 10 years, brachytherapy has been used increasingly for partial breast irradiation in the form of multi-catheter interstitial implants and single-catheter techniques such as the MammoSite device. The multi-catheter interstitial implants are normally performed with ^{192}Ir sources in ribbons and are temporary LDR brachy treatment, whereas the single-catheter techniques are normally conducted with an HDR unit. These are discussed more extensively in Chapter 95.

BASICS OF RADIATION BIOLOGY

As noted above, DNA remains the primary target of ionizing radiation, where breaks that cannot be repaired by the rapidly dividing and proliferating cancer cell ultimately result in cell death. These breaks may either restitute, fail to rejoin, and result in deletion of a portion of the chromosome, or the broken ends may reassort and give rise to a chromosomal aberration. The phase of the cell cycle in which the cell is located at the time of irradiation is critical to the type of aberration produced. Chromosome-type aberrations result if the cell is irradiated before DNA replication, whereas chromatid-type aberrations are produced by irradiation of cells that have completed DNA synthesis.

In addition to direct damage from radiation to the DNA within a cell, it appears that cells not directly exposed to radiation may also exhibit effects resulting from the irradiation (bystander effect of radiation).[9]

Models of Cell Survival

The radiation cell survival curve is a fundamental basic radiation biology tool used to determine radiation sensitivity of cell lines in vitro and to gain insight regarding the effectiveness of radiation under different conditions. These curves are commonly used to determine the radiation sensitivity for a particular cell type; estimate the additive, synergistic, or protective value of agents administered in combination with radiation; or determine the effectiveness of specific fractionation schemes.

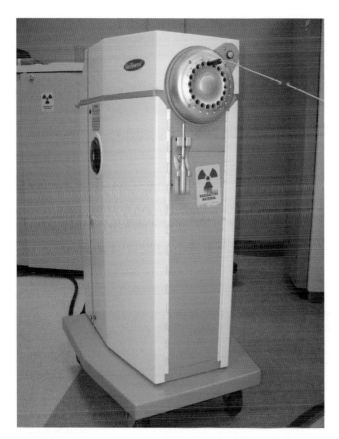

FIGURE 93-4 VariSource HDR remote afterloader (Varian Medical Systems, Palo Alto, California).

Radiosensitivity and Cell Cycle Phase

The cell cycle is classically categorized into 4 distinct phases: G_1 phase, S phase, G_2 phase (collectively known as interphase), and M phase. The first phase within interphase, from the end of the previous M phase until the beginning of DNA synthesis, is called G_1 (G indicating *gap* or *growth*). During this phase, the biosynthetic activities of the cell, which had been considerably slowed down during M phase, resume at a high rate. This phase is marked by synthesis of various enzymes that are required in S phase, mainly those needed for DNA replication. Duration of G_1 is highly variable. The subsequent S phase starts when DNA synthesis commences; when it is complete, all of the chromosomes have been replicated and converted to sister chromatids. Thus during this phase, the amount of DNA in the cell has effectively doubled. The duration of S phase is relatively constant among cells. The cell then enters G_2, where significant protein synthesis occurs, which lasts until the cell enters mitosis. Inhibition of protein synthesis during G_2 phase prevents the cell from undergoing mitosis. After mitosis, cells may be in a quiescent or senescent state (G_0). Nonproliferative cells enter the quiescent G_0 state from G_1 and may remain quiescent for long periods of time. Cellular senescence is a state that occurs in response to DNA damage or degradation that would make the progeny of a cell nonviable. Alternatively damaged cells can undergo self-destruction by apoptosis. The M phase is composed of 2 processes: mitosis, in which the chromosomes are divided, and cytokinesis, in which the cytoplasm divides, forming separate distinct cells. Cells that have stopped dividing are said to have entered the G_0 or quiescent phase.

The sensitivity of cells to radiation differs depending upon their position in the cell cycle at the time of irradiation. Cells are generally most sensitive during G_2 and in M, whereas resistance is usually greatest in the latter part of S. Early S and G_1 cells exhibit intermediate radiosensitivity, although a resistant period may be evident early in G_1.[4]

This differential cell cycle phase radiosensitivity represents an important factor in radiotherapy because surviving cells that were in a resistant phase at the time of an initial irradiation may continue through the cell cycle. Therefore, at the time of a second irradiation, a cell that may have been in a relatively resistant portion of the cell cycle could have progressed into a more sensitive phase and sustain radiation damage that will result in lethality.

Reassortment sensitization occurs primarily in more actively dividing cell populations, which may be found in certain types of cancers, and is largely absent in late-responding normal tissue. This represents a fundamental basis for fractionated radiotherapy, because without cell cycle reassortment, a substantially higher radiation dose may be necessary to eradicate a tumor.

Time, Dose, and Fractionation

The key factors in determining the effect of radiation on tumors and normal tissues are the total dose, the fraction size, and the time over which the dose is delivered. Extending the time over which a specific radiation dose is delivered lessens its toxicity because tissues and tumors have a means of counteracting the lethal effects of radiation by repair between fractions and over

the course of therapy. Theoretically, if the time to deliver a series of radiation doses is extended, a higher total dose may be necessary to provide a particular level of tumor control. Thus even though treatment prolongation may diminish the severity of acute effects, this may lead to a loss of tumor control. Depending on the circumstances, some clinicians may extend treatments for patients who have had prolonged breaks. Fraction size also plays a critical role in radiation response. The dose to achieve a particular level of tumor control or the tolerance dose for normal tissues generally decreases with increasing fraction size.

It is often useful to have a means to compare with a numerical score the theoretical biological impact of different treatment regimens. This can be accomplished using the linear-quadratic (LQ) model to calculate the biologically effective dose (BED),[10-12] which is used to compare different fractionation regimens. The LQ model is based on the radiation cell survival curves. Most of radiation survival curves can be mathematically described with an equation

$$\ln S_{ext} = -\alpha N D \left(1 + \frac{D}{\alpha/\beta}\right),$$

where S_{ext} is cells surviving fraction after radiation, N is number of fractions, D is daily fractional dose, α and β are constant coefficients for a certain type of cells, and the quantity

$$N D \left(1 + \frac{D}{\alpha/\beta}\right)$$

is termed the BED. Although this relatively simple equation does not take repair, repopulation, reassortment, and reoxygenation into account, it is a quick and convenient way to establish approximate equivalence among different fractional schemes. The equivalence between 2 different fractional schemes can be mathematically expressed as

$$\ln S_{ext,1} = \ln S_{ext,2},$$

which leads to

$$-\alpha N_1 D_1 \left(1 + \frac{D_1}{\alpha/\beta}\right) \approx -\alpha N_2 D_2 \left(1 + \frac{D_2}{\alpha/\beta}\right).$$

Based on this equation, a new fractional scheme can be designed from an established fractional scheme as

$$N_{new} D_{new} \left(1 + \frac{D_{new}}{\alpha/\beta}\right) \approx N_{estab} D_{estab} \left(1 + \frac{D_{estab}}{\alpha/\beta}\right).$$

One has to keep in mind that the above equation is only an estimate. Many other factors need to be taken into account, including both early and late normal tissue toxicity effects.

FRACTIONATION IN BREAST CANCER

The treatment of breast cancer, as with most solid tumors, uses standard fractionation of 180 to 200 cGy daily, delivered over 5 to 6 weeks to a total dose of 4500 to 5000 cGy. This dose is generally delivered to areas thought to be at risk for subclinical microscopic disease, which would include the breast or chest wall and, in selected patients, the regional lymphatics, depending on the clinical situation. This standard dose of approximately 50 Gy with standard fractionation has been shown in many disease sites to be adequate to control subclinical microscopic disease. Areas at higher risk (eg, the lumpectomy cavity after breast-conserving therapy or in some cases the chest wall scar after mastectomy, or sites of positive or close margins) will require a boost, which typically would be an additional 1000 to 1600 cGy in 200-cGy per day fractions.

Using a variety of formulas, including the BED method described earlier, a number of alternative fractionation schedules have been developed and evaluated and are currently in use for the treatment of breast cancer. One of the more common alternate schemes was tested in a randomized trial in Canada and established equivalent toxicity and local control comparing 50 Gy in 25 fractions over 5 weeks with 4250 Gy of 16 fractions in 3.5 weeks.[13] A number of other fractionation schemes have been evaluated or are under investigation, and these are summarized in Table 93-2.

As will be discussed in Chapter 95 on partial breast irradiation, the smaller volumes allow for larger fraction sizes to be treated over a shorter time. It has been established that the current fractionation scheme of 3.4 to 3.85 Gy, delivered twice daily to a total of 34 to 38.5 Gy over 5 days is biologically equivalent to approximately 50 Gy delivered over 5 weeks.

Over the next several years, the results of ongoing randomized trials may help to further define acceptable fractionation schedules that result in similar rates of local control and cosmetic outcomes achieved with conventional fractionation.

THE PROCESS OF RADIATION THERAPY

The process of radiation therapy begins with the consult with the radiation oncologist. Oftentimes in collaboration with the surgeon and medical oncologist, the radiation oncologist will do a formal consultation with the patient, which includes a complete history and physical examination, review of diagnostic studies and pertinent laboratory results, and review of the pathology, and will order any additional diagnostic studies required to render a final recommendation. Breast cancer patients are often seen by multiple physicians in a single multidisciplinary setting, or will be presented at multidisciplinary tumor boards where a full discussion of treatment options, sequencing, and optimal management is discussed.

If recommendations regarding the need for radiation are made, the radiation oncologists will coordinate the timing and integration of radiation with the surgeons, oncologists, and other physicians involved in the care and management of the patient. The specific role of radiation treatment in the management of breast cancer after lumpectomy and mastectomy and in the palliative setting is discussed in the following 3 chapters.

Patients requiring radiation proceed to simulation, treatment planning, and treatment as described below.

Simulation

Simulation in radiotherapy is a process of defining radiation beams, including beam directions, portals, type of radiation, and so on, to encompass the target volume while sparing normal tissues to achieve the desired treatment goals. In addition, the simulation process includes patient immobilization device selection and reference marker placement for reliable day-to-day treatment

TABLE 93-2 Common Fractionation Schedules in Breast Cancer

Volume	Fraction Size (cGy)	Number of Fractions/Time	Total Dose (cGy)	Notes/Reference
Whole breast	180-200	25-30 (Delivered over 5-6 weeks)	4500-5000	Most common fractionation scheme, usually followed by a boost of 200 × 5[15]
Whole breast	266	16 (Delivered over 3.5 weeks)	4250	Equivalent in toxicity and local control to standard treatment in randomized trial[13]
Whole breast	320	13 (Delivered over 5 weeks)	4160	Equivalent local control in randomized trial to 200 × 25[16]
Whole breast	300	13 (Delivered over 5 weeks)	3900	Slightly lower local control than 320 × 13[16]
Partial breast	340-385	10 (Delivered twice daily over 1 week)	3400-3850	Being tested in randomized trial to whole breast[17]

positioning reproducibility. The defined beams and patient positioning information will be subsequently used in treatment. One of the prerequisites for a successful simulation is precise and accurate knowledge of geometric locations of the target volume and critical normal structures of the patient, based on the information gained from a variety of diagnostic, physical, and pathologic examinations. Patient comfort and feasibility of the beam placement should also be taken into consideration.

Before CT scanners became available in a radiation oncology department, the simulation had been primarily conducted with a radiotherapy simulator that resembled a treatment machine or directly on a treatment machine. During the simulation, the patient is positioned on the machine table, commonly with an immobilization device (e.g., a breast board is often used for a breast cancer patient), and reference landmarks are placed on the patient's skin for future reference. The simulator beam is aimed at the target volume from different angles, and patient images are acquired. The image acquisition can be done with films or electronic imaging devices, depending on the availability of imaging technology. On the acquired images, beam portals are further defined and outlined to optimize the encompassment of the target volume and sparing of critical structures. This conventional simulation process is apparently suboptimal because the images are 2-dimensional and the beam angles and portals are more based on experience rather than dosimetric evaluation.

The introduction of CT simulator into radiotherapy represents a revolutionary advancement of the simulation process. The simulation using a CT simulator is termed virtual simulation. The CT simulator by itself is very similar to a conventional diagnostic CT scanner, except for a flat tabletop and possible larger opening. Similar to the conventional simulation, the CT-based simulation starts with the patient positioned on the CT table with a suitable immobilization device and reference landmarks properly placed. CT images are then obtained over a range of volume of interest. The CT images provide 3-dimensional anatomic information and make more accurate delineation of the target volume and normal structures. These images are transferred to a computer on which a specially designed software package is used to simulate the treatment machine and the patient using the 3-dimentional digital information contained in the CT images. A typical CT treatment plan of a patient receiving radiation therapy to the breast is shown in Figure 93-5. Normally, the target volumes and a variety of anatomic structures are delineated with tools in the software package and are presented in a 3-dimensional space that is closely correlated to the simulated treatment machine via the reference landmarks. Beam angles, portals, and

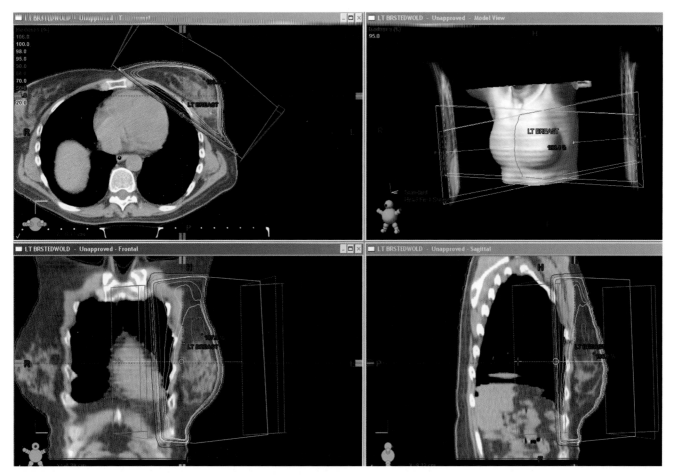

FIGURE 93-5 Radiation treatment plan for tangential breast irradiation.

other beam-limiting devices are selected and evaluated to achieve the optimal coverage of the target volume and the sparing of critical structures. The later part of process is closely associated with the treatment planning process. As a matter of fact, it is becoming more and more a part of the treatment planning process instead of the simulation process, because the goal of treatment is optimal dose coverage of the target volume and radiation sparing of critical structures, instead of simple geometric portal coverage of beams over the target volume and beam portal avoidance of critical structures.

CT-based virtual simulation is becoming a standard in breast cancer radiation management. Though breast cancer patients are normally simulated and treated in supine position, some patients, particular those with large chest diameters or pendulous breasts, may benefit from a prone position simulation and treatment in terms of dose homogeneity and lung sparing.[14] For treatment with the patient in a supine position, the most common immobilization device is the breast board, on which the patient can be positioned at different angles with the arm extending above the head and held in a reproducible and relatively comfortable position (see Fig. 93-2).

Treatment Planning

The treatment planning process is to derive a treatment strategy to achieve treatment objectives based on the evaluations of the calculated dose distributions. This process is usually performed on a treatment planning computer with sophisticated planning and dose-calculation software. The treatment strategy includes the choice of beam energy, type, numbers, orientations, beam-limiting devices, and so on.

In breast cancer radiation treatment, the primary objective is to provide homogeneous dose coverage to the target volume and to minimize radiation to lung and heart (especially in left breast treatment). The target volume may include the entire or partial breast, chest wall, and involved lymph nodes.

For whole-breast treatment, the most commonly used irradiation technique is 2 tangential photon field technique, in which 1 medial tangential field and 1 lateral tangential field are aimed to cover the entire breast, chest wall, and lower axilla. A third anterior-posterior (AP) field may be used to irradiate the supraclavicular nodes if needed, as shown in Figure 93-6. In the boost treatment of surgical scars, or to boost the lumpectomy bed, electron beams are commonly used to treat the superficially located tissues. An electron beam boost to a tumor bed is shown in Figure 93-7. Because breasts often present slopes relative to the tangential fields, wedges are almost always used as tissue compensators to improve the uniformity inside the breast. Modern beam delivery technologies, such as dynamic wedge and electronic compensator, have been used to replace the conventional hard wedges and to further improve the dose homogeneity in the treatment fields. Another consideration is tissue inhomogeneity correction. Because the tangential beams pass through a certain amount of lung and lung density is much lower than that of regular breast

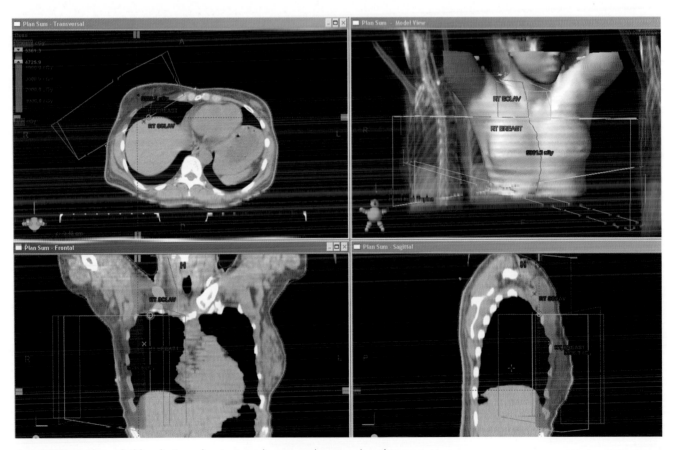

FIGURE 93-6   Three-field radiation plan to treat breast and regional nodes.

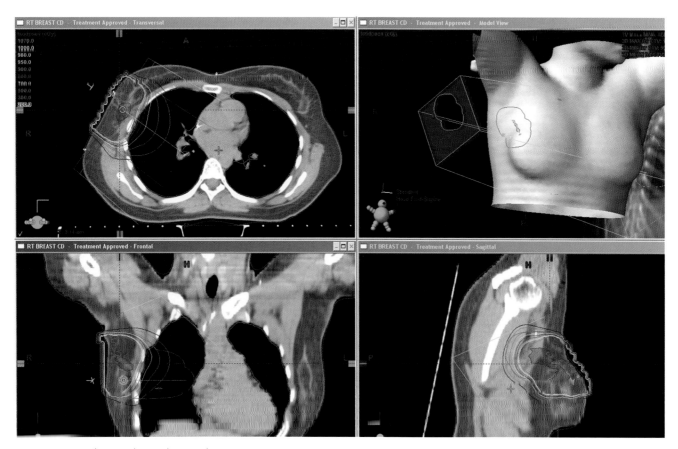

FIGURE 93-7 Electron beam boost plan.

tissue, this density inhomogeneity may lead to discrepancy between calculated dose distribution and actual delivered dose if the inhomogeneity is not properly taken into account during the dose-calculation process. Traditionally, this density inhomogeneity is not taken into account during breast radiation dose calculation because of the limitations of dose-calculation algorithms. The clinical significance of the discrepancy and the degree of importance of the inhomogeneity correction remain to be investigated for breast cancer radiation treatment.

Treatment planning for partial-breast irradiation is more complicated. The surgical cavity and planning target volumes need to be delineated on the CT simulation images. A total of 3 to 5 beams are needed and are aimed from different angles to achieve desired dose coverage. Avoiding excessive radiation to lung and heart is 1 of the major considerations in the partial-breast irradiation treatment planning process. Partial-breast irradiation is discussed in detail in Chapter 95.

Treatment

Radiation treatment is carried out on the linear accelerator treatment machine according to the strategy derived in the treatment planning process. One of the most important considerations in the treatment is to reproduce the patient position (relative to the treatment beams) as in the plan. This requires treatment setup using an identical immobilization device in the simulation and

other devices to prevent patient movement during treatment. The initial setup is rigorously verified with the most appropriate imaging technologies available to the department. The verification includes imaging the beam portals and patient anatomies and comparing the gained images to the corresponding images in the plan. Periodic physics quality assurance is conducted to ensure that the characteristics of the treatment machine remain as expected. Because most of radiation treatment involves multiple fractions, patient treatment positioning is periodically verified and confirmed before further treatment is delivered.

Treatment information, including both delivered dose and beam parameters, is recorded in the patient's chart and computer-controlled record and verify (RV) system. This information is also periodically checked and reported to avoid any potential mistreatments and dose inaccuracy.

FUTURE STUDIES

There are many new developments in the principles behind radiation oncology that will advance the field in the next few years. These include

- Technological developments: Further refinements in external-beam equipment, planning techniques, and technologies will enhance our ability to deliver the optimal dose to the target tissues and minimize dose to normal structures.

- Fractionation studies: A variety of ongoing randomized trials are evaluating different fractionation schedules, which will result in equivalent local control and minimal normal tissue damage.
- Partial-breast irradiation: Randomized trials throughout the world are investigating the effectiveness of partial-breast irradiation compared with whole-breast irradiation in selected women with breast cancer.
- Biological studies: Methods of combining radiation with chemotherapy, hormonal therapy, and other biological agents are currently under investigation and will likely result in combination treatment strategies to optimize local control with acceptable toxicity.

SUMMARY

The appropriate delivery of radiation treatment for patients with breast cancer is highly dependent on detailed input from physicists, dosimetrists, basic scientists, nurses, and radiation oncologists from the radiation team, working collaboratively with colleagues from medical oncology and surgical oncology and other members of the multidisciplinary breast team. The technological advancements in the past few years have had a tremendous impact on our ability to refine radiation treatments, minimize dose to normal tissues, and deliver the most homogenous dose possible to the target tissues. Combining radiation with chemotherapy, hormonal therapy, and novel biological therapies remains an active area of investigation.

Alternate methods of delivering radiation, including novel techniques for partial-breast irradiation, continue to undergo rigorous evaluation. Only through prospective randomized trials will we continue to move the field forward. The following chapters are devoted to the specific topics of breast-conserving therapy with radiation, partial-breast irradiation, postmastectomy radiation, and the palliative use of radiation in patients with breast cancer.

REFERENCES

1. Steel GG. *Basic Clinical Radiobiology for Radiation Oncologists.* London, UK: Edward Arnold; 1993.
2. Hall FJ. *Radiobiology for the Radiologist.* 4th ed. Philadelphia, PA: Lippincott; 1993.
3. Khan FM. *The Physics of Radiation Therapy.* 2nd ed. Baltimore, MD. Williams & Wilkins; 1994.
4. Hall EJ, Giaccia AJ. *Radiobiology for the Radiologist.* 6th ed. Philadelphia, PA: Lippincott Williams & Wilkins; 2006.
5. Haffty BG, Wilson L. *Handbook of Radiation Oncology.* 1st ed. Sudbury, MA: Jones and Bartlett; 2009.
6. Prasad KN. Rationale for using multiple antioxidants in protecting humans against low doses of ionizing radiation. *Br J Radiol.* 2005;78:485-492.
7. Prasad NR, Menon VP, Vasudev V, et al. Radioprotective effect of sesamol on gamma-radiation induced DNA damage, lipid peroxidation and anti-oxidants levels in cultured human lymphocytes. *Toxicology.* 2005;209: 225-235.
8. Vicini FA, Beitsch PD, Quiet CA, et al. First analysis of patient demographics, technical reproducibility, cosmesis, and early toxicity: results of the American Society of Breast Surgeons MammoSite breast brachytherapy trial. *Cancer.* 2005;104:1138-1148.
9. Morgan WF, Sowa MB. Non-targeted bystander effects induced by ionizing radiation. *Mutat Res.* 2007;616:159-164.
10. Fowler JF. The linear-quadratic formula and progress in fractionated radiotherapy. *Br J Radiol.* 1989;62:679-694.
11. Barendsen GW, Dose fractionation, dose rate and iso-effect relationships for normal tissue responses. *Int J Radiat Oncol Biol Phys.* 1982;8:1981-1997.
12. Thames HD Jr, Withers HR, Peters LJ, et al. Changes in early and late radiation responses with altered dose fractionation: implications for dose-survival relationships. *Int J Radiat Oncol Biol Phys.* 1982;8:219-226.
13. Whelan T, MacKenzie R, Julian J, et al. Randomized trial of breast irradiation schedules after lumpectomy for women with lymph node-negative breast cancer. *J Natl Cancer Inst.* 94:1143-1150, 2002.
14. Stegman LD, Beal KP, Hunt MA, et al. Long-term clinical outcomes of whole-breast irradiation delivered in the prone position. *Int J Radiat Oncol Biol Phys.* 2007;68:73-81.
15. Fisher B, Anderson S, Bryant J, et al. Twenty-year follow-up of a randomized trial comparing total mastectomy, lumpectomy, and lumpectomy plus irradiation for the treatment of invasive breast cancer. *N Engl J Med.* 2002;347:1233-1241.
16. Owen JR, Ashton A, Bliss JM, et al. Effect of radiotherapy fraction size on tumour control in patients with early-stage breast cancer after local tumour excision: long-term results of a randomised trial. *Lancet Oncol.* 2006;7:467-471
17. Arthur DW, Vicini FA. Accelerated partial breast irradiation as a part of breast conservation therapy. *J Clin Oncol.* 2005;23:1726-1735.

CHAPTER 94

Whole-Breast Radiation Following Breast-Conserving Therapy for Noninvasive and Invasive Cancers

Meena S. Moran

Breast-conserving therapy (BCT), consisting of surgical removal of the primary tumor followed by radiation therapy to the intact breast, is now considered a standard treatment approach for early-stage breast cancer. Increasing numbers of patients are becoming eligible for breast conservation after the diagnosis of breast cancer, due to improvements in early detection and patient awareness. In addition, patients presenting with larger tumors that previously would have required mastectomy may now be eligible for BCT using neoadjuvant chemotherapy to downsize the tumor, followed by local excision and radiation. Data from multiple randomized prospective studies have demonstrated equivalent long-term survival outcomes for BCT compared to mastectomy and the benefit of adding adjuvant radiation therapy after conservative surgery. Furthermore, there are numerous retrospective single-institutional series that support the use of conservative surgery and radiation therapy in early-stage breast cancer. This chapter will discuss the indications and validity of postoperative, whole-breast radiation therapy for noninvasive and invasive cancer, and will address special considerations and future directions for radiation therapy as a component of breast conservation therapy for early-stage breast cancer.

LOBULAR CARCINOMA IN SITU

Lobular carcinoma in situ (LCIS) is generally considered a risk indicator for the development of invasive carcinoma, and not a malignancy in and of itself. Although the overall management of pure LCIS remains somewhat controversial, patients are often treated with conservative surgery alone or sometimes mastectomy. In addition, there are substantial data to support the use of tamoxifen for LCIS, to reduce the risk of future invasive breast cancer,[1] In patients who undergo surgical excision with pure LCIS histology, the literature on the use of radiotherapy postoperatively is very limited.[2,3] After a recent workshop on LCIS conducted by EUSOMA members in London, the group concluded that "there is little data to recommend radiation therapy in the clinical management of LCIS."[4] Therefore, based on insufficient data to support its usage, radiation therapy after local excision is not typically utilized in the management of pure LCIS.

For patients who have LCIS as a component of their invasive breast cancer, the decision for BCT should be based on the evaluation of the invasive component alone. If LCIS is present at the surgical margin of an invasive carcinoma, no further re-excision is required so long as the invasive component is completely excised. Despite some conflicting data from single-institutional series,[5-7] it is generally accepted that local control does not appear to be compromised with LCIS as a component of invasive cancer. Therefore, BCT is a reasonable treatment option for patients with invasive cancers with associated LCIS, and further excision for margins involved with LCIS alone is not warranted.

WHOLE-BREAST RADIATION FOR DUCTAL CARCINOMA IN SITU

Although ductal carcinoma in situ (DCIS) is a noninvasive breast malignancy with an overall good to excellent prognosis, the biological diversity correlates with the variable malignant potential and therefore the risk of local recurrence can be relatively high with surgery alone. In addition, the natural history of recurrent disease can be significantly different from the primary DCIS, with a risk of approximately 50% of the recurrences being invasive disease, with a higher potential for nodal and distant metastasis. For these reasons, preventing recurrence for DCIS is of paramount importance. The local treatment approaches for DCIS include the following: (1) simple mastectomy, (2) breast-conserving surgery and radiation therapy, and (3) breast-conserving surgery alone. The rationale for treatment with breast-conserving surgery and radiation over conservative surgery alone (without radiation) has been substantiated by several large, randomized trails. The diversity in histologic features and differences in malignant potential of DCIS suggests that a proportion of patients may be candidates for surgical excision alone with omission of radiation, yet at this juncture, no prospective studies have been able to identify subgroups of patients who may be potential candidates for observation after surgery. The current standard of care, based on the results of these large randomized, prospective studies, indicates that radiation therapy after breast-conserving surgery significantly reduces the local relapse rates in all subsets of patients with DCIS, decreasing the risk of both invasive and noninvasive recurrences.

Randomized, Prospective Data for DCIS

The prospective study with the longest follow-up comes from the National Surgical Breast and Bowel Project (NSABP). The NSABP B-17 addressed the issue of radiation for DCIS by randomizing 818 patients to lumpectomy alone versus lumpectomy plus radiation therapy.[8] Patients were randomized postoperatively to a standard dose of 50 Gy in 25 fractions over 5 week to the whole breast versus observation. All patients were required to have negative margins. After a median follow-up of 10.75 years, the patients randomized to lumpectomy alone had a relapse rate of 32% versus 16% in patients treated with adjuvant radiation. Approximately 50% of the recurrences in both cohorts were invasive cancers; thus, radiation significantly reduced the risk of invasive and in situ recurrences. There were no differences observed in overall survival with the addition of radiation.

The European Organization for Research and Treatment of Cancer (EORTC) also conducted a landmark study addressing the role of radiation therapy for DCIS less than 5 cm in size resected with negative surgical margins,[9] similarly randomizing patients to observation versus postoperative radiation therapy. Their findings were consistent with the NSABP B-17 trial, resulting in a

statistically significant benefit in local control for DCIS treated with radiation therapy at 10.5 years in all subgroups of patients.

A similarly conducted randomized study of postoperative radiation for DCIS from Sweden (the SweDCIS Trial) found a cumulative incidence of recurrence of 0.07 (95% CI 0.050-0.10) in the radiation arm compared with 0.22 (95% CI 0.18-0.26) in the observation arm at a median follow-up of 5.2 years.[10] This corresponded to an overall hazard ratio of 0.33 (95% CI 0.24-0.47, $p < 0.0001$). Although their findings were consistent with the studies mentioned earlier, this study differed from those trials in that the protocol did *not* require microscopically negative margins prior to radiation; 10% of the patients had positive surgical margins in this study.

The fourth landmark study was conducted in the United Kingdom, Australia, and New Zealand (UK/ANZ DCIS trial), and randomized DCIS patients to 1 of 4 arms after surgery: postoperative radiation, postoperative tamoxifen, a combination of radiation and tamoxifen, or observation.[11] The findings of this study also favored the use of radiation therapy for DCIS, with local recurrences of 8% and 6% for the radiation arms, and 22% and 18% for the nonradiation arms, at a median follow-up of 4.4 years. Again, adjuvant radiation was associated with a statistically significant reduction of in-breast recurrences (HR = 0.38, $p < 0.0001$), with a significant reduction in both invasive and noninvasive cancers. There was no apparent benefit to tamoxifen for DCIS in this study. The findings of these 4 randomized studies are detailed in Table 94-1.

More recently, a meta-analysis of the 4 randomized trials was conducted, pooling the 3665 patients together to determine the cumulative benefit of adjuvant radiation therapy for DCIS.[12] Their findings showed a significant reduction of invasive and in-situ ipsilateral breast cancer, with an odds ratio (OR) of 0.40 (95% CI 0.33-0.60, $p < 0.00001$) and 0.40 (95% CI 0.31-0.53, $p < 0.00001$), respectively. As expected, distant metastases and death rates between the 2 arms did not differ. Interestingly, there were more contralateral breast cancers after adjuvant RT in comparison to the observation arm, with a 1.53-fold higher likelihood of contralateral breast cancer (95% CI 1.05-2.24, $p = 0.03$). Subset analysis did not isolate any DCIS patient groups in whom radiation could be omitted.

All of randomized trails discussed in this section treated patients to 50 Gy in 2-Gy fractions without a boost. Based on

TABLE 94-1 Randomized Prospective Studies of Radiation Therapy for DCIS

Trial	Trail Design	No. Patients	Med F/U (y)	LC Outcomes
NSABP B-17	RT vs Observ.	818	12	16% vs 32%[*]
EORTC	RT vs Observ.	1010	10.5	15% vs 26%[a]
SweDISH	RT vs Observ.	1067	5.2	7% vs 22%[b]
UK/ANZ	RT vs RT + Tam vs. Tam vs Observ.	1701	4.4	8% vs 6% vs. 18% vs 22%[*]

F/U, median follow-up in years; LC, local control; no. patients, total number of patients randomized in study; RT, radiation therapy.
[*]Indicates statistically significant difference.

these data, radiation therapy after local excision for DCIS has been shown to decrease ipsilateral breast tumor recurrences by approximately 60%; this decrease includes both in situ and invasive relapse. No difference in overall survival has been demonstrated with the addition of radiation therapy. At this juncture, this benefit in local control appears to apply broadly to all subsets of patients with DCIS.

Observation after Conservative Surgery for DCIS

There is a clinically relevant need to identify subsets of DCIS patients in whom postoperative radiation may be omitted; thus, the issue of subjecting all DCIS patients to radiation remains an area of controversy, particularly because no survival benefit has been noted. Some institutions continue to stratify patients according the Van Nuys Prognostic Index,[13] a system in which patients are given a score based on margin status, histologic subtype, tumor size, and patient age (Table 94-2). Based on the retrospective analysis of the a cohort of DCIS patients from 2 institutions, the authors of this scoring system recommend breast-conserving surgery alone (postoperative observation) for scores of 4 to 6, surgery plus radiation for scores of 7 to 9 (radiation decreased local recurrence by a statistically significant difference of 15%-12%), and mastectomy for scores of 10 to 12 (because the recurrence rate with breast-conserving surgery and

radiation were unacceptably high at 50% at 5 years in this subgroup). From a clinical standpoint, though the basis for utilizing a "scoring system" for DCIS makes sense, it is important to note that none of the randomized data, either alone or pooled, have been able to isolate pathologic or patient criteria for omission of radiation for DCIS for DCIS. Furthermore, a recent, single-arm prospective study of observation after breast-conserving surgery for DCIS (wide excision alone with larger than 1-cm margins for small, low-grade tumors) was closed early to accrual because of the high number of local recurrences with observation alone.[14]

The topic of excision alone for DCIS will need to continue to be studied in a prospective fashion. Radiation Therapy Oncology Group (RTOG) trial 98-04 was designed to address this question by randomizing low-risk DCIS patients to lumpectomy alone versus lumpectomy plus radiation. Unfortunately, the trial closed due to poor patient accrual. The European Cooperative Oncology Group (ECOG) E-5194 is a prospective study of approximately 1000 DCIS patients (< 2.5 cm low to intermediate grade, or < 1 cm high grade) treated with excision and negative margins larger than 3 mm, with the end points of local recurrence at 5 and 10 years. The result of this study should provide useful information on the efficiency of lumpectomy alone for low-risk DCIS. Currently, it remains unclear how to identify patients with DCIS who can be treated with excision alone. Although future studies may identify patients with DCIS who can be treated with observation after breast-conserving surgery the existing prospective data suggest a significant benefit for radiation therapy for low-, intermediate-, and high-risk groups, based on our current classifications. Future molecular profiling studies may help to stratify patients into risk categories to identify subsets of patients in whom radiation may be omitted.

WHOLE-BREAST RADIATION FOR INVASIVE, EARLY-STAGE BREAST CANCER

The surgical management of early-stage, invasive breast cancer has significantly evolved over the last several decades. Historically, local control of the primary tumor was achieved by removal of the entire breast. We now know that, in appropriately selected patients, removing the primary tumor with a rim of surrounding normal tissue (breast-conserving surgery), followed by radiation therapy to the whole breast, provides equivalent long-term outcomes to mastectomy and offers the patient the opportunity to preserve the breast. Long-term data from large, randomized prospective studies have validated the use of breast-conservation therapy as a standard treatment option for early-stage breast cancer. These studies have demonstrated that less extensive surgery does not compromise breast cancer outcomes when the tumor is completely removed with negative margins and followed by postoperative radiation therapy to the intact breast. Over the last decade, BCT has gained acceptance as a comparable alternative to mastectomy for early-stage breast cancer; in 1991, the National Cancer Institute (NCI) issued a consensus statement stating that "BCT is an appropriate method of primary therapy for the majority of women with stage I and II breast cancer and is preferable because it provides survival

TABLE 94-2 Van Nuys Prognostic Index[*]

Score		Parameter
	Margins	
1		≥ 10 mm
2		1-9 mm
3		< 1 mm
	Histologic Type	
1		G1-2, no necrosis
2		G1-2, + necrosis
3		G3
	Size	
1		< 1.5 cm
2		1.6-4 cm
3		> 4 cm
	Age of Patient	
1		> 60
2		40-60
3		< 40

[*]Scores range from 4 to 12 based on the 4 parameters.

Recommendations

Score 4-6: Breast-conserving surgery alone
Score 7-9: Breast-conserving surgery + radiation
Score 10-12: Mastectomy
Adapted from Silverstein MJ. The University of Southern California/Van Nuys prognostic index for ductal carcinoma in situ of the breast. *Am J Surg.* 2003;186:337-343.

TABLE 94-3 Randomized Prospective Trials Comparing Breast Conservation Therapy to Mastectomy

Trial	Follow-up (y)	No. Patients	OS
NSABP-B06[17]	20	1219	NS
Milan[18]	20	701	NS
Institute Gustave-Roussy[19]	15	179	NS
National Cancer Institute[20]	10	237	NS
Danish Breast Cancer Group[21]	6	905	NS
EORTC[22]	10	868	NS

no. patients, number of patients enrolled in study; NS, difference not significant; OS, overall survival.

equivalent to total mastectomy and axillary dissection."[15] As the efficacy of BCT becomes better understood by both physicians and patients, the rates of BCT in the United States continue to rise.

The goal of BCT should be to achieve local recurrence of upto 1% per year, based on the recommendations of the Consensus Conference of Breast Conservation.[16] While defining the appropriate selection of patients for BCT remains controversial, established criteria are based on the ability to (1) achieve an acceptable cosmetic result (ie, tumor size with respect to breast size), (2) obtain negative margins at surgery, and (3) safely deliver radiation therapy and minimize potential for side effects. Meticulous patient selection, surgical techniques, and radiation delivery are therefore required to optimize local control.

Randomized Prospective Data for BCT In Early-Stage Breast Cancer

There are numerous prospective studies that have been conducted worldwide addressing the role of BCT in early-stage breast cancer. There are 6 modern prospective randomized trials[17-22] comparing mastectomy to conservative surgery plus radiation therapy (Table 94-3). All of these trials have demonstrated that there is no significant difference in distant metastasis, cause-specific survival, or overall survival between mastectomy and BCT. In addition, none of these studies found a difference in contralateral breast cancers or second malignancies between the 2 cohorts.

Given that the efficacy of BCT compared to mastectomy has been proven, it follows that the value of adding radiation to lumpectomy alone needs establishment. Multiple randomized prospective studies[17,23-29] have assessed the role of radiation therapy after breast-conserving surgery (Table 94-4). These studies randomized patients to surgical excision alone versus excision followed by radiation (± adjuvant systemic therapy or tamoxifen). Overall, each of these studies has demonstrated a statistically significant improvement in local control when adding adjuvant radiation therapy to breast-conserving surgery, with an approximately two-thirds reduction in local recurrence. None of the studies have shown that the addition of radiation therapy has resulted in an improvement in survival. Based on the current available data from these randomized prospective trials, radiation therapy after local excision is the standard of care for the majority of patients who choose to conserve their breast. The benefit in local control with the addition of radiation therapy after conservative surgery from the NSABP B-06 20-year

TABLE 94-4 Selected Randomized Prospective Trials of Breast-Conserving Surgery with and without Radiation

Trial	No. Patients	Local CS (%)	Relapse CS + RT (%)	F/U (y)
NSABP B-06[17]	1265	41	12	10
NSABP B-21[23]	1006	17	3	8
Ontario COG[27]	837	35	11	7.6
Milan III[28]	579	24	6	10
Scottish[24]	556			5
ER+		25	3	
ER−		44	14	
British[29]	399	35	13	5
Swedish[24]	585	24	6	6
Uppsala[25]	381	18	2	5
West Midlands, UK[26]	707	18	8	4.2

CS, conservative surgery; CS + RT, conservative surgery and radiation therapy; F/U (y), followup as reported.

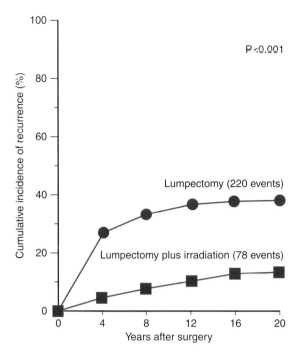

FIGURE 94-1 Twenty-year follow-up from NSABP B-06 trial showing cumulative incidence of a first recurrence of cancer the ipsilateral breast in patients treated with lumpectomy alone versus lumpectomy plus radiation therapy. (Reproduced with permission from Fisher B, Anderson S, Margolese RG, et al. Twenty year follow-up of a randomized trial comparing total mastectomy, lumpectomy, and lumpectomy plus irradiation for the treatment of invasive breast cancer. N Engl J Med. 2002;347:1233-1241.)

follow-up is shown in Figure 94-1. The guidelines by the American College of Radiology (ARS) for BCT in stage I and II patients currently state that "whole breast radiation with or without boost is the standard of care after lumpectomy."[30]

In 2004, a pivotal meta-analysis was published of 15 randomized studies evaluated lumpectomy plus radiation versus lumpectomy alone.[31] Although none of the individual studies assessing the role of radiation after lumpectomy suggested a benefit in survival, this analysis found a small but statistically significant benefit in overall survival with the addition of radiation. In this pooled analysis, 9422 patients were evaluated and as expected, the relative risk of developing an ipsilateral breast tumor recurrence without radiation compared to with radiation was 3.00 (95% CI 2.65-3.40). Furthermore, the relative risk of mortality was 1.086 (95% CI 1.003-1.175), corresponding to an estimated 8.6% (95% CI 0.3-17.5) relative excess mortality if radiotherapy was omitted.

Another landmark meta-analysis performed by the Early Breast Cancer Trialist's Cooperative Group combined data from 42,080 patients from prospective randomized trials addressing the role of radiation for breast cancer.[32] For the subset of patients who had undergone BCT (7311 patients from 10 trials), postoperative radiation therapy was associated with a statistically significant absolute reduction in local recurrence of 19% at 5 years (decrease in local relapse from 26% to 7%). When pooling the data collectively, this translated into an absolute reduction in

breast-cancer-specific mortality of 5.4% at 15 years (Fig. 94-2). Radiation produced similar proportional reduction in local relapse in all women, regardless of age or pathologic characteristics. It was notable that these data demonstrated a 1.8% increase in second malignancies (contralateral breast and lung cancers) and a 1.3% increase in deaths from causes other than breast cancer (particularly heart disease and lung cancer), drawing attention to the toxicities of radiation and the necessity to carefully plan and deliver radiation to minimize the dose to surrounding normal tissue. Despite these additional risks from radiotherapy, the absolute reduction in 15-year overall mortality was similar to the 15-year breast-cancer-specific mortality. The authors concluded that for every 4 local recurrences avoided by optimizing local control, 1 breast cancer death would be avoided. This very important study highlights the relationship between local recurrence and survival, suggesting that despite the increased death from other causes for patients who received radiation, there is an association between improved local control with the addition of radiation therapy and improvement in overall mortality.

OMITTING RADIATION AFTER LOCAL EXCISION IN SPECIFIC SUBSETS OF PATIENTS

Several well designed trials have addressed the role of omitting radiation after breast-conserving surgery for subsets of patients with good prognostic features in whom the absolute benefit of radiation may not be clinically apparent. A trial from Canada attempted to omit radiation in patients over the age of 50 with node-negative, estrogen receptor (ER)-positive tumors less than 5 cm.[33] Patients were randomized to tamoxifen alone versus radiation plus tamoxifen. The rate of local relapse at 5 years was 7.7% in the tamoxifen group and 0.6% in the tamoxifen plus irradiation group ($p < 0.001$), with a corresponding difference in 5-year disease-free survival rates of 84% and 91% ($p = 0.004$). In addition, the axillary relapse rate was significantly higher in patients not receiving radiation. Even with subset analysis of the smaller tumors (< 2 cm), the relapse rates were unacceptably high with the omission of radiation, with 5-year local relapse of 0.4% in the tamoxifen plus radiotherapy arm and 5.9% in the tamoxifen alone arm ($p < 0.001$). Based on these data, there is no justification for omission of radiation therapy in this subset of patients more than 50 years of age.

Another study was performed by the CALGB for patients aged 70 and older with 2 cm or less, ER-positive, node-negative invasive tumors randomized similarly, to tamoxifen alone versus radiation plus tamoxifen after surgical excision.[34] An 8-year update of this study has shown that the risk of relapse with and without radiation was 1% versus 6.3%.[35] Although this difference achieved statistical significance, the relapse rate without radiation was within acceptable levels (< 1% per year). The EBCTCG reported a 5-year absolute reduction in local recurrence of 11% for women aged 70 and older with node-negative disease, which falls into the category of a 10% to 20% absolute reduction in 5-year risk of local recurrence and which, according to the overall analysis, should correspond to an absolute reduction in breast cancer mortality of 4.5% (SE = 0.8),[32] although it is important to note the number of patients 70 or more in the overview were small. Based on these data, the absolute benefit of

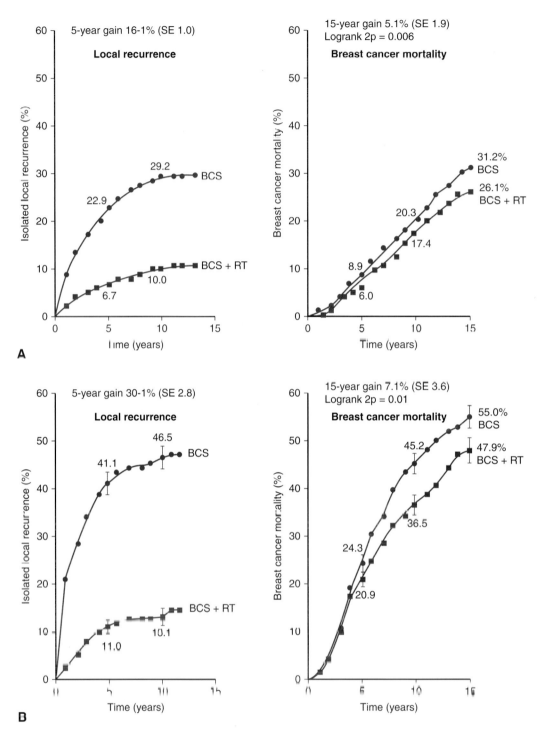

FIGURE 94-2 A. Local recurrence and breast cancer mortality improvements with the addition of radiation therapy to breast-conserving surgery in node-negative patients. **B.** Local recurrence and breast cancer mortality improvements with the addition of radiation therapy to breast-conserving surgery in node-positive patients. *(Reproduced with permission from Effects of radiotherapy and of differences in the extent of surgery for early breast cancer on local recurrence and 15-year survival: an overview of the randomised trials. Lancet. 2005;366:2087-2106.)*

radiation in this specific patient population (> 70) appears to be less compared with younger patients. For elderly patients with small, ER-positive invasive cancers, the advantage of radiation should be weighed against other comorbidities, and the decision to treat with radiation should be individualized. Results of ongoing investigations such as the PRIME II trial (Postoperative Radiation

in Minimal Risk Elderly Patients) will hopefully further define the role of radiation (omission) in low-risk elderly patients.

The NSABP B-21 was a 3-arm study conducted on women with less than 1 cm clinically node-negative invasive cancers.[23] There was no age cutoff in this study. Women were randomized after surgery to tamoxifen alone, radiation alone, or radiation and tamoxifen. The cumulative incidence of ipsilateral breast recurrences was 16.5% in the tamoxifen alone arm, 9.3% in the radiation alone arm, and 2.8% in the combination arm at 8 years. This study suggests that even in low-risk tumors, tamoxifen cannot replace radiation to attain local control, and that the combination of both radiation and tamoxifen has an additive effect in further reducing local relapses.

THE ROLE OF A RADIATION "BOOST"

A radiation "boost" or "cone-down" is an additional 10 to 16 Gy delivered to the tumor bed with a margin after whole-breast radiation therapy. Randomized prospective clinical trials from Lyon, France and the EORTC have assessed the benefit of "boost" versus no "boost" and have found a statistically significant improvement in local control with the addition of a boost in all patient populations with invasive cancer.[36-38] While planning the boost field, it is important to be aware that there are data suggesting that the lumpectomy cavity is inadequately localized with clinically designed boost fields.[39] It is therefore important to identify and carefully plan the treatment of the surgical cavity plus margin with the assistance of radiographic imaging (ie, CT, ultrasound, fluoroscopy) when designing the boost cavity. Although utilization of a boost after whole breast radiation has now been substantiated by randomized data demonstrating the further decrease in ipsilateral breast recurrences with its use, the routine use of boost in all patients remains somewhat controversial due to concerns about the long-term toxicity and the effects on cosmesis.

THE ROLE OF RADIATION THERAPY IN REGIONAL NODAL MANAGEMENT

Radiation therapy directed to the lymphatic nodal basins can achieve excellent regional control of microscopic disease. The efficacy of radiation to the axilla compared with surgical dissection of the axilla was prospectively studied in the NSABP B-04.[40] Now with over 25 years of follow-up, this 3-arm study randomized patients with clinically negative axilla to radical mastectomy (surgical treatment to the axilla), simple mastectomy (no treatment to the axilla), or simple mastectomy plus radiation to the chest wall and regional nodes (radiation to the axilla). No significant differences were observed among the 3 groups of women with clinically negative nodes with respect to disease-free survival, relapse-free survival, distant-disease-free survival, or overall survival. Axillary relapses in patients treated with nodal dissection versus radiation did not differ significantly, suggesting that regional control can be achieved with either of these treatment modalities.

Based on the NSABP B-04 and other studies,[41,42] patients who do not undergo axillary nodal dissection who are at risk for nodal involvement, such as patients who have an involved sentinel node but did not undergo completion dissection, can receive radiation to the axilla with acceptable and durable long-term regional control. In addition, one may choose to omit surgical evaluation and treat the axilla with radiation for patients in whom information regarding the status of lymph nodes will not influence the management with systemic therapy (ie, the elderly patient who will not receive chemotherapy).

For patients who have undergone axillary dissection, the benefit of postoperative radiation to the axilla remains unclear. Due to the significantly higher risk of lymphedema with the combination of dissection and radiation to the axilla, and lack of consistent data to support adjuvant radiation in this setting, postoperative radiation to a dissected axilla should be used judiciously for selected patients with a suspected high risk of residual disease, such as those with extensive nodal involvement, a large number of involved lymph nodes, or an inadequately dissected axilla.

Unfortunately, there is generally a lack of consensus regarding the indications for adjuvant radiation therapy to the regional lymphatics after breast-conserving surgery. For pathologically node-negative patients undergoing BCT, treatment of the whole breast with tangential fields without additional nodal fields is generally the standard practice. Although the axilla is not intentionally targeted, the level 1 and 2 axillary nodes are often encompassed in the typical tangential fields.[43] Axillary regional relapses in pathologically node-negative patients are therefore relatively uncommon.

For pathologically node-positive patients undergoing BCT, the role of radiation to the regional lymphatics is less clear. For patients with 4 or more positive lymph nodes, supraclavicular ± internal mammary (IM) radiation fields are often employed at most centers, with the rationale that these patients are at higher risk of regional nodal relapse. For patients with 1 to 3 positive lymph nodes undergoing BCT, there is increased variability in practices, with some institutions routinely utilizing supraclavicular ± IM fields, while others do not. The EORTC and the NCI Canada (MA-20) are both independently accruing patients onto trials in Europe and North America/Australia, attempting to address the benefit of regional radiation for conservatively treated breast cancer patients. In both of these trials, patients are being randomized to tangential whole-breast radiation versus radiation to the whole breast and regional lymphatics. The results of these trials should better characterize which patients require regional nodal radiation with whole-breast radiation after breast-conserving surgery.

SEQUENCING OF RADIATION WITH SYSTEMIC THERAPY

It is generally accepted that for patients who will not be receiving chemotherapy, radiation should be within 3 to 12 weeks of surgery, to allow for sufficient wound healing and patient recovery from surgery. For patients receiving chemotherapy, the integration with radiation poses an important management issue. With the increase in the use of systemic therapy for early-stage breast cancer, delays in radiation therapy have lead to concerns of increased local failure, particularly in patients with close or positive margins. Several completed randomized studies have addressed the role of sequencing postoperative chemotherapy with radiation therapy. The first of these studies was conducted by the Harvard group, randomizing clinical stage I or II patients after BCT to 4 cycles of cyclophosphamide, doxorubicin, methotrexate with leucovorin rescue, 5-fluorouracil, and prednisone at 3-week intervals, given either before or after radiation therapy. In the most recent update with a median follow-up time of 135 months,[44] there were no significant differences between the CT-first and RT-first arms in time to any event, distant metastasis, or death. In addition, sites of first failure were also not significantly different. Toxicity was higher in the RT-first arm, mainly due to increased rates of neutropenia and pneumonitis. The authors concluded that among breast cancer patients treated with conservative surgery, there was no advantage to giving RT before adjuvant chemotherapy. The risk of local failure was substantial in patients with positive margins, regardless of treatment sequence (20% vs 23% in the 2 arms, respectively). Based on the Consensus Conference on Breast Conservation,[16] there are no current data that strongly support which should be undertaken first, radiation or chemotherapy. Patient choice and institutional traditions should influence the sequencing of chemotherapy and radiation.

The general trend has been to move away from delivering radiation therapy concurrently with chemotherapy due to the potential increase in toxicity, particularly for patients receiving taxanes and anthracyclines. Concurrent treatment with these agents is being evaluated in ongoing studies; at this juncture, concurrent chemotherapy and radiation should only be administered when a patient is enrolled on a protocol and should not be utilized in the routine clinical setting. Based on the ACR guidelines for early-stage breast cancer,[30] sequential therapy is considered the standard of care.

On the other hand, in HER-2/neu-positive patients, trastuzumab is routinely delivered concurrently with radiation therapy. In the randomized trials that have demonstrated the efficacy of trastuzumab, the protocols mandated that the radiation was delivered concomitantly. Of note, IM nodes were not allowed to be included in the radiation portals in these protocols. A recent study from France addressed acute toxicity in patients receiving concurrent trastuzumab and radiation[45]; in this trial, where IM radiation was allowed (71% of the patients had IM radiation), the left ventricular ejection fraction was decreased in 9% of the patients with IM radiation and 5% of those who did not receive IM radiation. Although these numbers did not achieve statistical significance, this study highlights that particular care must be taken to minimize cardiac volume due to the potential increased risk of cardiac toxicity in these patients. IM nodal radiation should be utilized with caution in patients receiving concomitant trastuzumab due to the increase in cardiac volume it inevitably confers. Longer follow-up and additional prospective data on the concomitant use of trastuzumab and radiation are warranted.

The use of hormone therapy (selective ER modulators and aromatase inhibitors) has become common clinical practice in recent years for receptor-positive breast cancer. The optimal timing of when to initiate the hormonal therapy is yet to be determined. Historically, there have been concerns for increased toxicity and radiation resistance with concurrent administration of tamoxifen and radiation. Although large, randomized studies have demonstrated the efficacy of hormone therapy, the integration with radiation was not a point of focus for these studies. Neither the FEMTABIG study (letrozole vs tamoxifen vs sequential treatment) nor the ATAC study (anastrozole vs tamoxifen vs combination of both) specified the sequence of radiation and hormonal treatment. The TEAM study compared exemestane (Aromasine) and tamoxifen, but detailed in the protocol that hormonal treatment had to follow the completion of radiation therapy. Single-institutional retrospective series suggest that there is no difference in whether tamoxifen is administered concurrently or sequentially with radiation.[46-48] Based on the currently available data, there do not appear to be any adverse effects with concurrent hormone and radiation treatment. Further investigation of the effects of sequencing chemotherapy and radiation (concomitantly and sequentially) is necessary.

THE ROLE OF NEOADJUVANT CHEMOTHERAPY FOR BREAST PRESERVATION

Historically, there have been concerns that for a large primary tumor, downsizing with systemic therapy may leave satellite nodules; therefore, breast conservation was not traditionally advocated in these patients. In an initial feasibility study conducted by the MD Anderson group, 143 locally advanced breast cancer patients were given induction chemotherapy followed by mastectomy.[49] Careful pathology review of the specimens demonstrated that almost one-fourth of these patients had significant regression of their tumor to be eligible for breast conservation therapy, with residual tumors smaller than 4 cm in size, no satellite nodules, and complete resolution of skin changes. Of the patients who would have been eligible for BCT with significant regression of their tumor after neoadjuvant chemotherapy, 42% had no residual tumor in the mastectomy specimen. Since that time, several large randomized prospective studies have been conducted speaking to the issue of neoadjuvant chemotherapy and breast conservation. Patients in these studies were both early stage and locally advanced. The largest of these prospective randomized studies was conducted by the NSABP (B-18), in which over 1500 women with stage I to IIIA were randomized to Adriamycin and Cytoxan delivered either neoadjuvantly or adjuvantly.[50] The initial findings of the study were reported at 5 years; more recently, in the 9-year follow-up publication, there continued to be no difference in overall survival or disease-free survival in the pre- or postoperative arms (Fig. 94-3). The breast conservation rate was 68% for the neoadjuvant arm and 60% for the adjuvant arm. Although there was an increase in the rate of ipsilateral breast recurrence in the preoperative chemotherapy group of 10.7% versus 7.6% in the postoperative chemotherapy group, this difference did not achieve statistical significance.

Based on these and other data, there is an approximately 20% to 25% relative increase in eligibility for breast preservation and no overall difference in survival with neoadjuvant compared with adjuvant chemotherapy. Induction chemotherapy followed by breast-conserving surgery and radiation therapy is now considered a reasonable treatment option for patients wishing to conserve their breasts who are not initially candidates for BCT. The available data suggest that this treatment approach is safe and will increase the eligibility for breast preservation in approximately one-fourth of patients with large tumors relative to breast size, and that this approach can even be considered for locally advanced (noninflammatory) breast cancers. Proper patient selection and a meticulous multidisciplinary approach must be applied to these patients.

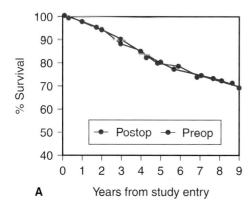

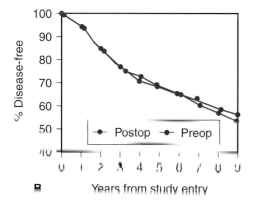

FIGURE 94-3 Results from the 9-year follow-up of the NSABP B-18, preoperative versus postoperative chemotherapy. **A.** Overall survival. **B.** Disease-free survival. *(Reproduced with permission from Wolmark N, Wang J, Mamounas E, et al. Preoperative chemotherapy in patients with operable breast cancer: nine-year results from National Surgical Adjuvant Breast and Bowel Project B-18. J Natl Cancer Inst Monogr. 2001;30:96-102.)*

From a technical standpoint, when the neoadjuvant approach is being considered, it is important to insert radioopaque markers percutaneously into the tumor, in order to localize the surgical site after partial or complete regression of tumor. It is also important to recognize that the clinical assessment of response to chemotherapy tends to overestimate the pathologic extent of disease by approximately 3-fold. Therefore, in a patient who has had a complete *clinical* response to induction chemotherapy, surgical excision of the primary tumor site should not be omitted (chemotherapy followed by radiation, no surgery) in any instances; the risk of *pathologic* residual disease still remains relatively high. Several series have shown higher local relapse rates in patients in whom surgery was omitted after neoadjuvant chemotherapy and followed by radiation alone.[51,52]

SPECIAL CONSIDERATIONS

Previously Radiated Patients

Multiple studies have documented the higher risk of breast cancer in women successfully radiated for the treatment of Hodgkin disease at a young age.[53,54] Very small series have addressed

breast conservation and re-irradiation after Hodgkin disease.[55] Therefore, due to the concerns regarding exceeding normal tissue tolerances and causing significant complications (eg, brachial plexopathy, soft-tissue necrosis), a history of prior radiation therapy is an absolute contraindication for breast-conserving surgery in patients who would require retreatment with an excessively high total radiation dose to a previously radiated breast.[30]

Preganancy

Pregnancy, unless terminated, is an absolute contraindication to treatment with radiation based on ACR guidelines.[30] For women in the first and second trimester of their pregnancy, internal radiation scatter from the radiation to the breast can reach teratogenic and potentially lethal levels. If the patient is in the third trimester and wishes to preserve her breast, conservative surgery can be performed, and radiation treatment given after the patient has delivered. Patients should be counseled accordingly.

Collagen Vascular Disease

A history of collagen vascular disease is thought to be a relative contraindication for BCT due to the potential for increased tissue toxicity in this patient population. Published studies evaluating long-term toxicities in patients with collagen vascular disease suggest that the increased toxicity is predominantly in patients with active systemic lupus erythematosus (SLE) and scleroderma.[56-59] In comparison, patients with rheumatoid arthritis do not appear to have increased late toxicity from radiation and therefore can be considered for breast conservation. The potential for increase in acute and latent toxicities should be relayed to patients wishing to pursue BCT.

Young Age

Younger patients, in comparison to older patients, have a higher risk of local relapse, distant recurrences, and breast-cancer-specific survival after BCT.[60-63] This increased risk may be related to the worse prognostic features such as more estrogen-/progesterone-negative tumors in younger women. Based on the existing data, it is not clear that the risk of recurrence is greater in young patients treated with a breast-conserving approach than with mastectomy.[30] The American College of Surgeons Consensus Recommendation therefore states that young age should not preclude the use of BCT, but that the increased risk of local recurrence should be discussed with patients during the decision-making process.[16]

BRCA Carriers

Of all the newly diagnosed breast cancer cases in the United States, approximately 10% will be secondary to inherited germline mutations, mainly BRCA1 and BRCA2. Affected breast cancer patients who are germline mutation carriers are at high risk for contralateral breast cancer and ovarian cancer. In addition, there is a higher risk of late ipsilateral breast relapse in these patients, thought to be second primaries in the treated breast and not recurrence of the primary tumor, due to the prolonged time to detection (median 8 years), different histology, and location remote to the primary.[64] Patients can potentially decrease their risk of second primary tumors by using adjuvant hormonal therapy or by undergoing bilateral prophylactic oophoretomy.[65] Although additional studies of germline mutation carriers and BCT are warranted, the available data suggest that BRCA mutations carriers can be considered for breast conservation. Patients should be advised regarding the increased risks of ipsilateral and contralateral breast recurrences during the treatment counseling process, and should be offered all potential management options to decrease recurrences, such as tamoxifen and prophylactic oorphorectomy.

Positive and Close Margins

Positive margins are defined as cancer cells at the inked rim of the lumpectomy specimen. It is well documented that positive margins increase the risk of local recurrence after BCT,[66-68] and that the extent of positive margin correlates with the increased risk of relapse,[69] although the magnitude of the recurrence varies greatly in different studies. Furthermore, positive margins are an independent predictor of decreased breast-cancer-specific survival after BCT.[70] Patients presenting to the radiation oncologist with positive margins should therefore be sent back for reexcision. Unfortunately, there is significant controversy regarding the definition of "negative" margin and "close" margin. In general, a margin of normal cells larger than 2 mm results in consistently low local recurrence rates, and is considered acceptable by most radiation oncologists. Although the NSABP defines a negative margin as absence of malignant cells at the inked margins, others suggest that 1- to 2-mm margins should be considered "close," with conflicting local outcomes in this pathologic subgroup.[71,72] At this juncture, the management of close margins remains controversial, with numerous conflicting studies.[73] Every attempt should be made to achieve widely negative margins without compromising cosmetic outcome at the time of initial surgery. For patients with close margins, a more cautious approach with reexcision should be considered.

Extensive Intraductal Component

Extensive intraductal component (EIC) is commonly defined as invasive tumors with 23% or more DCIS within the primary lesion and DCIS present in adjacent breast tissue. Early studies suggested that EIC was a predictor of local relapse, raising concerns about treating EIC-positive patients with BCT.[74,75] More contemporary evidence suggests that breast preservation is safe with acceptable local control in patients with EIC so long as negative margins are achieved.[76] Therefore, meticulous assessment of the margin status in patients with EIC is necessary prior to initiating radiation therapy.

Multifocal/Multicentric Disease

Multifocal disease is defined as multiple tumors within the same quadrant of the breast, whereas multicentric refers to tumors in separate quadrants. For patients with multifocal disease, BCT can be considered so long as the lesions can be completely excised with a negative margin and acceptable cosmetic result.

The data suggest that local relapse after BCT for multifocal disease is not compromised so long as negative margins are obtained. Multicentric disease generally precludes breast conservation, due to the poor cosmetic result with surgical excisions in multiple quadrants followed by radiation therapy and the risk for additional foci of disease. Based on the ACR guidelines, multicentricity is a contraindication for BCT.[30]

Histologic Subtypes

Due to the increased risk of multicentricity, multifocality, and contralateral breast cancers with invasive lobular carcinoma, the role of BCT for early-stage invasive lobular carcinoma has been questioned. Although there are some conflicting data from retrospective data, 2 of the 3 largest studies of invasive lobular carcinoma treated with BCT (compared to invasive ductal) show no significant difference in local relapse after conservative surgery and radiation therapy for lobular versus ductal patients.[77-79] Based on the available data, it is generally accepted that no histologic subtypes are considered at higher risk for breast relapse after BCT.

FUTURE DIRECTIONS

Future directions in early-stage breast cancer management should have the goal of personalizing treatment to the individual patients. Although the overall benefits and contraindications to radiation therapy and BCT with supporting data have been reviewed in this chapter, there remain significant variations of subgroups of patients in these studies, suggesting that some patients are either being undertreated or overtreated. With the identification of molecular markers and gene sequencing, one hopes that the risk of local relapse can be assessed for the individual patient, and the decision of breast-conservation surgery and the addition of radiation therapy can be scientifically based on quantitative estimation of risk of relapse. Additional research endeavors to further define prognostic markers such as serum-based/tissue-based markers and predictive multigene signatures, to identify risk of local relapse, responsiveness to radiation therapy, and increased risk for long-term toxicity, are warranted for patients with early-stage breast cancer.

SUMMARY

Currently the role for postoperative radiation for pure LCIS remains undefined and requires further investigation. For DCIS, local control is significantly improved in all subsets of patients with the addition of radiation compared with breast-conserving surgery alone.

For early-stage, invasive breast cancer, conservative surgery plus radiation therapy produces long-term survival outcomes equivalent to mastectomy. For early-stage, invasive breast cancer, radiation therapy after breast-conserving surgery significantly decreases local relapse in all subsets of patients.

Meta-analysis suggests that with the addition of radiation, improvements in local control may confer a long-term survival benefit.

For early-stage, invasive breast cancer, local control is improved with the addition of a radiation "boost" to the lumpectomy cavity compared with no boost. Radiation to the axillary area offers long-term regional control comparable to axillary nodal dissection

There are no strong data to support the use of chemotherapy or radiotherapy first when sequencing adjuvant treatment for patients undergoing BCT. Currently the usual standard is to deliver chemotherapy prior to radiation. There is no significant difference in long-term survival outcomes if chemotherapy is delivered neoadjuvantly or adjuvantly. There is a greater potential for breast conservation with the neoadjuvant approach.

Relative contraindications for BCT include pregnancy, previously radiated breast (eg, Hodgkin disease), positive margins, multicentric disease, active schleroderma, and lupus.

REFERENCES

1. Wolmark N, Dunn BK. The role of tamoxifen in breast cancer prevention: issues sparked by the NSABP Breast Cancer Prevention Trial (P-1). *Ann NY Acad Sci.* 2001;949:99-108.
2. Cutuli B, de Lafontan B, Quetin P, Mery E. Breast-conserving surgery and radiotherapy: a possible treatment for lobular carcinoma in situ? *Eur J Cancer.* 2005;41:380-385.
3. Cutuli B, Jaeck D, Renaud R, Rodier JF. Lobular carcinoma in situ of the breast: results of a radiosurgical conservative treatment. *Oncol Rep.* 1998;5:1531-1533.
4. Fournier S, Audretsch W, Clemm-Jenssen A, et al. The management of lobular carcinoma in situ (LCIS) the same as ductal carcinoma in situ (DCIS)? *Eur J Cancer.* 2006;42:2205-2211.
5. Moran M, Haffty BG. Lobular carcinoma in situ as a component of breast cancer: the long-term outcome in patients treated with breast-conservation therapy. *Int J Radiat Oncol Biol Phys.* 1998;40:353-358.
6. Abner AL, Connolly JL, Recht A, et al. The relation between the presence and extent of lobular carcinoma in situ and the risk of local recurrence for patients with infiltrating carcinoma of the breast treated with conservative surgery and radiation therapy. *Cancer.* 2000;88:1072-1077.
7. Jolly S, Kestin LL, Goldstein NS, Vicini FA. The impact of lobular carcinoma in situ in association with invasive breast cancer on the rate of local recurrence in patients with early-stage breast cancer treated with breast-conserving therapy. *Int J Radiat Oncol Biol Phys.* 2006;66:365-371.
8. Fisher B, Land S, Mamounas E, et al. Prevention of invasive breast cancer in women with ductal carcinoma in situ: an update of the national surgical adjuvant breast and bowel project experience. *Semin Oncol.* 2001;28: 400-418.
9. Bijker N, Peterse JL, Duchateau L, et al. Risk factors for recurrence and metastasis after breast-conserving therapy for ductal carcinoma-in-situ: analysis of European Organization for Research and Treatment of Cancer Trial 10853. *J Clin Oncol.* 2001;19:2263-2271.
10. Emdin S, Granstrand B, Ringberg A, et al. SweDCIS: Radiotherapy after sector resection for ductal carcinoma in situ of the breast. Results of a randomised trial in a population offered mammography screening. *Acta Oncologica.* 2006;45:536-543.
11. Houghton J. Radiotherapy and tamoxifen in women with completely excised ductal carcinoma in situ of the breast in the UK, Australia, and New Zealand: randomized controlled trial. *Lancet.* 2003;362:95-102.
12. Viani G, Stefano E, Afonso S, et al. Breast-conserving surgery with or without radiotherapy in women with ductal carcinoma in situ: a meta-analysis of randomized trials. *Radiat Oncol.* 2007;2:28.
13. Silverstein MJ. The University of Southern California/Van Nuys prognostic index for ductal carcinoma in situ of the breast. *Am J Surg.* 2003;186:337-343.
14. Wong JS, Kaelin CM, Troyan SL, et al. Prospective study of wide excision alone for ductal carcinoma in situ of the breast. *J Clin Oncol.* 2006;24:1031-1036.
15. NIH Consensus Conference. Treatment of early-stage breast cancer. *JAMA.* 1991;265:391-395.
16. Schwartz GF, Veronesi U, Clough KB, et al. Consensus conference on breast conservation. *J Am Coll Surg.* 2006;203:198-207.
17. Fisher B, Bryant J, Margolese RG, et al. Twenty-year follow-up of a randomized trial comparing total mastectomy, lumpectomy, and lumpectomy

plus irradiation for the treatment of invasive breast cancer. *N Engl J Med.* 2002;347:1233-1241.
18. Veronesi U, Cascinelli N, Mariani L, et al. Twenty-year follow-up of a randomized study comparing breast-conserving surgery with radical mastectomy for early breast cancer. *N Engl J Med.* 2002;347:1227-1232.
19. Arriagada R, Le MG, Rochard F, Contesso G. Conservative treatment versus mastectomy in early breast cancer: patterns of failure with 15 years of follow-up data. Institut Gustave-Roussy Breast Cancer Group. *J Clin Oncol.* 1996;14:1558-1564.
20. Jacobson JA, Danforth DN, Cowan KH, et al. Ten-year results of a comparison of conservation with mastectomy in the treatment of stage I and II breast cancer. *N Engl J Med.* 1995;332:907-911.
21. Blichert-Toft M, Rose C, Andersen JA, et al. Danish randomized trial comparing breast conservation therapy with mastectomy: six years of life-table analysis. Danish Breast Cancer Cooperative Group. *J Natl Cancer Inst Monogr.* 1992;11:19-25.
22. van Dongen JA, Voogd AC, Fentiman IS, et al. Long-term results of a randomized trial comparing breast-conserving therapy with mastectomy: European Organization for Research and Treatment of Cancer 10801 trial. *J Natl Cancer Inst.* 2000;92:1143-1150.
23. Fisher B, Bryant J, Dignam JJ, et al. Tamoxifen, radiation therapy, or both for prevention of ipsilateral breast tumor recurrence after lumpectomy in women with invasive breast cancers of one centimeter or less. *J Clin Oncol.* 2002;20:4141-4149.
24. Forrest AP, Stewart HJ, Everington D, et al. Randomised controlled trial of conservation therapy for breast cancer: 6-year analysis of the Scottish trial. Scottish Cancer Trials Breast Group. *Lancet.* 1996;348:708-713.
25. Liljegren G, Holmberg L, Adami HO, et al. Sector resection with or without postoperative radiotherapy for stage I breast cancer: five year results of a randomized trial. Uppsala-Orebro Breast Cancer Study Group. *J Natl Cancer Inst.* 1994;86:717-722.
26. Spooner D, Morrison JM, Oates GD, et al. The role of radiotherapy in early breast cancer (stage I). A West Midlands Breast Group prospective randomized collaborative study (BR 3002). *Breast* 1995;4:231-232.
27. Clark RM, Whelan T, Levine M, et al. Randomized clinical trial of breast irradiation following lumpectomy and axillary dissection for node-negative breast cancer: an update. Ontario Clinical Oncology Group. *J Natl Cancer Inst.* 1996;88:1659-1664.
28. Veronesi U, Marubini E, Mariani L, et al. Radiotherapy after breast-conserving surgery in small breast carcinoma: long-term results of a randomized trial. *Ann Oncol.* 2001;12:997-1003.
29. Renton SC, Gazet JC, Ford HT, et al. The importance of the resection margin in conservative surgery for breast cancer. *Eur J Surg Oncol.* 1996;22:17-22.
30. White JR, Halberg FE, Rabinovitch R, et al. American College of Radiology appropriateness criteria on conservative surgery and radiation: stages I and II breast carcinoma. *J Am Coll Radiol.* 2008;5:701-713.
31. Vinh-Hung V, Verschraegen C. Breast-conserving surgery with or without radiotherapy: pooled-analysis for risks of ipsilateral breast tumor recurrence and mortality. *J Natl Cancer Inst.* 2004;96:115-121.
32. Effects of radiotherapy and of differences in the extent of surgery for early breast cancer on local recurrence and 15-year survival: an overview of the randomised trials. *Lancet.* 366:2087-2106.
33. Fyles AW, McCready DR, Manchul LA, et al. Tamoxifen with or without breast irradiation in women 50 years of age or older with early breast cancer. *N Engl J Med.* 2004;351:963-970.
34. Hughes KS, Schnaper LA, Berry D, et al. Lumpectomy plus tamoxifen with or without irradiation in women 70 years of age or older with early breast cancer. *N Engl J Med.* 2004;351:971-977.
35. Hughes KS, Schnaper LA, Berry D, et al. Lumpectomy plus tamoxifen with or without irradiation in women 70 years of age or older with early breast cancer: a report of further follow-up. San Antonio Breast Cancer Symposium, 2006. Abstract 11.
36. Bartelink H, Horiot JC, Poortmans P, et al. Recurrence rates after treatment of breast cancer with standard radiotherapy with or without additional radiation. *N Engl J Med.* 2001;345:1378-1387.
37. Poortmans P, Bartelink H, Horiot JC, et al. The influence of the boost technique on local control in breast conserving treatment in the EORTC "boost versus no boost" randomised trial. *Radiother Oncol.* 2004;72:25-33.
38. Romestaing P, Lehingue Y, Carrie C, et al. Role of a 10-Gy boost in the conservative treatment of early breast cancer: results of a randomized clinical trial in Lyon, France. *J Clin Oncol.* 1997;15:963-968.
39. Landis DM, Luo W, Song J, et al. Variability among breast radiation oncologists in delineation of the postsurgical lumpectomy cavity. *Int J Radiat Oncol Biol Phys.* 2007;67:1299-1308.
40. Fisher B, Jeong JH, Anderson S, et al. Twenty-five-year follow-up of a randomized trial comparing radical mastectomy, total mastectomy, and total mastectomy followed by irradiation. *N Engl J Med.* 2002;347:567-575.

41. Galper S, Recht A, Silver B, et al. Is radiation alone adequate treatment to the axilla for patients with limited axillary surgery? Implications for treatment after a positive sentinel node biopsy. *Int J Radiat Oncol Biol Phys.* 2000;48:125-132.

42. Pejavar S, Wilson LD, Haffty BG. Regional nodal recurrence in breast cancer patients treated with conservative surgery and radiation therapy (BCS+RT). *Int J Radiat Oncol Biol Phys.* 2006;66.1320-1327.

43. Schlembach PJ, Buchholz TA, Ross MI, et al. Relationship of sentinel and axillary level I-II lymph nodes to tangential fields used in breast irradiation. *Int J Radiat Oncol Biol Phys.* 2001;51:671-678.

44. Bellon JR, Come SE, Gelman RS, et al. Sequencing of chemotherapy and radiation therapy in early-stage breast cancer: updated results of a prospective randomized trial. *J Clin Oncol.* 2005;23:1934-1940.

45. Belkacemi Y, Gligorov J, Ozsahin M, et al. Concurrent trastuzumab with adjuvant radiotherapy in HER2-positive breast cancer patients: acute toxicity analyses from the French multicentric study. *Ann Oncol.* 2008;19:1110-1116.

46. Ahn PH, Vu HT, Lannin D, et al. Sequence of radiotherapy with tamoxifen in conservatively managed breast cancer does not affect local relapse rates. *J Clin Oncol.* 2005;23:17-23.

47. Pierce LJ, Hutchins LF, Green SR, et al. Sequencing of tamoxifen and radiotherapy after breast-conserving surgery in early-stage breast cancer. *J Clin Oncol.* 2005;23:24-29.

48. Harris EE, Christensen VJ, Hwang WT, et al. Impact of concurrent versus sequential tamoxifen with radiation therapy in early-stage breast cancer patients undergoing breast conservation treatment. *J Clin Oncol.* 2005;23:11-16.

49. Singletary SE, McNeese MD, Hortobagyi GN. Feasibility of breast conservation surgery after induction chemotherapy for locally advanced breast carcinoma. *Cancer.* 1992;69:2849-2852.

50. Wolmark N, Wang J, Mamounas E, et al. Preoperative chemotherapy in patients with operable breast cancer: nine-year results from National Surgical Adjuvant Breast and Bowel Project B-18. *J Natl Cancer Inst Monogr.* 2001;30:96-102.

51. Mauriac L, Durand M, Avril A, Dilhuydy JM. Effects of primary chemotherapy in conservative treatment of breast cancer patients with operable tumors larger than 3 cm. Results of a randomized trial in a single centre. *Ann Oncol.* 1991;2:347-354.

52. Mauriac L, MacGrogan G, Avril A, et al. Neoadjuvant chemotherapy for operable breast carcinoma larger than 3 cm: a unicentre randomized trial with a 124-month median follow-up. Institut Bergonie Bordeaux Groupe Sein (IBBGS). *Ann Oncol.* 1999;10:47-52.

53. Hodgson DC, Koh ES, Tran TH, et al. Individualized estimates of second cancer risks after contemporary radiation therapy for Hodgkin lymphoma. *Cancer.* 2007;110:2576-2586.

54. Mandrell BN. Secondary breast cancer in a woman treated for Hodgkin lymphoma as a child. *Oncology (Williston Park).* 2007;21(suppl):27-29.

55. Deutsch M, Gerszten K, Bloomer WD, Avisar E. Lumpectomy and breast irradiation for breast cancer arising after previous radiotherapy for Hodgkin's disease or lymphoma. *Am J Clin Oncol.* 2001;24:33-34.

56. Chen AM, Obedian E, Haffty BG. Breast-conserving therapy in the setting of collagen vascular disease. *Cancer J.* 2001;7:480-491.

57. De Naeyer B, De Meerleer G, Braems S, et al. Collagen vascular diseases and radiation therapy: a critical review. *Int J Radiat Oncol Biol Phys.* 1999;44:975-980.

58. Morris MM, Powell SN. Irradiation in the setting of collagen vascular disease: acute and late complications. *J Clin Oncol.* 1997;15:2728-2735.

59. Fleck R, McNeese MD, Ellerbroek NA, et al. Consequences of breast irradiation in patients with pre-existing collagen vascular diseases. *Int J Radiat Oncol Biol Phys.* 1989;17:829-833.

60. Fowble BL, Schultz DJ, Overmoyer B, et al. The influence of young age on outcome in early stage breast cancer. *Int J Radiat Oncol Biol Phys.* 1994;30:23-33.

61. Vicini FA, Kestin LL, Goldstein NS, et al. Impact of young age on outcome in patients with ductal carcinoma-in-situ treated with breast-conserving therapy. *J Clin Oncol.* 2000;18:296-306.

62. Vanlemmens L, Hebbar M, Peyrat JP, Bonneterre J. Age as a prognostic factor in breast cancer. *Anticancer Res.* 1998;18:1891-1896.

63. de la Rochefordiere A, Asselain B, Campana F, et al. Age as prognostic factor in premenopausal breast carcinoma. *Lancet.* 1993;341:1039-1043.

64. Haffty BG, Harrold E, Khan AJ, et al. Outcome of conservatively managed early-onset breast cancer by BRCA1/2 status. *Lancet.* 2002;359:1471-1477.

65. Pierce LJ, Levin AM, Rebbeck TR, et al. Ten-year multi-institutional results of breast-conserving surgery and radiotherapy in BRCA1/2-associated stage I/II breast cancer. *J Clin Oncol.* 2006;24:2437-2443.

66. Gage I, Schnitt SJ, Nixon AJ, et al. Pathologic margin involvement and the risk of recurrence in patients treated with breast-conserving therapy. *Cancer.* 1996;78:1921-1928.

67. Solin LJ, Fowble BL, Schultz DJ, Goodman RL. The significance of the pathology margins of the tumor excision on the outcome of patients treated with definitive irradiation for early stage breast cancer. *Int J Radiat Oncol Biol Phys.* 1991;21:279-287.

68. Spivack B, Khanna MM, Tafra L, et al. Margin status and local recurrence after breast-conserving surgery. *Arch Surg.* 1994;129:952-956; discussion 956-957.

69. Wazer DE, Jabro G, Ruthazer R, et al. Extent of margin positivity as a predictor for local recurrence after breast conserving irradiation. *Radiat Oncol Invest.* 1999;7:111-117.

70. Meric F, Mirza NQ, Vlastos G, et al. Positive surgical margins and ipsilateral breast tumor recurrence predict disease-specific survival after breast-conserving therapy. *Cancer.* 2003;97:926-933.

71. Obedian E, Haffty BG. Negative margin status improves local control in conservatively managed breast cancer patients. *Cancer J Sci Am.* 2000;6:28-33.

72. Neuschatz AC, DiPetrillo T, Safaii H, et al. Margin width as a determinant of local control with and without radiation therapy for ductal carcinoma in situ (DCIS) of the breast. *Int J Cancer.* 2001;96(suppl):97-104.

73. Singletary SE. Surgical margins in patients with early-stage breast cancer treated with breast conservation therapy. *Am J Surg.* 2002;184:383-393.

74. Schnitt SJ, Connolly JL, Harris JR, et al. Pathologic predictors of early local recurrence in Stage I and II breast cancer treated by primary radiation therapy. *Cancer.* 1984;53:1049-1057.

75. Schnitt SJ, Connolly JL, Khettry U, et al. Pathologic findings on re-excision of the primary site in breast cancer patients considered for treatment by primary radiation therapy. *Cancer.* 1987;59:675-681.

76. Schnitt SJ, Abner A, Gelman R, et al. The relationship between microscopic margins of resection and the risk of local recurrence in patients with breast cancer treated with breast-conserving surgery and radiation therapy. *Cancer.* 1994;74:1746-1751.

77. Salvadori B, Biganzoli E, Veronesi P, et al. Conservative surgery for infiltrating lobular breast carcinoma. *Br J Surg.* 1997;84:106-109.

78. du Toit RS, Locker AP, Ellis IO, et al. An evaluation of differences in prognosis, recurrence patterns and receptor status between invasive lobular and other invasive carcinomas of the breast. *Eur J Surg Oncol.* 1991,17:251-257.

79. Moran MS, Yang Q, Haffty BG. The Yale University experience of early stage invasive lobular carcinoma (ILC) and invasive ductal carcinoma (IDC) treated with breast conservation treatment (BCT), analysis of clinical-pathologic features, long-term outcomes, and molecular expression of COX-2, Bcl-2 and p53 as a function of histology. *Breast J.* In press.

CHAPTER 95

Accelerated Partial Breast Irradiation

Sharad Goyal
Victor Zannis

The treatment of breast cancer was dominated by radical mastectomy or modified radical mastectomy of the affected breast prior to the 1970s. This included en bloc removal of the breast, muscles of the chest wall, and contents of the axilla, and at the time they were advocated as the most appropriate local therapy for women with early-stage breast cancers. However, the results of the National Surgical Adjuvant Breast and Bowel Project (NSABP) B-06 and other studies found equivalent survival and local control rates among women treated with either mastectomy or lumpectomy followed by whole-breast irradiation (WBI).[1,2] The NSABP B-06, which compared mastectomy to lumpectomy with and without radiotherapy in women with invasive carcinoma, found a 39% local recurrence rate at 20 years with lumpectomy alone, which was decreased to 14% with the addition of radiotherapy.[1] Several other randomized studies demonstrated equivalent long-term survival and disease-free survival rates in patients treated by breast-conserving therapy (BCT) compared to mastectomy.[2-5] Additional randomized studies comparing lumpectomy alone to lumpectomy and radiation clearly demonstrate a 3-fold reduction in local relapse with the use of radiation following breast-conserving surgery.[6-10] More recent meta-analyses of trials comparing lumpectomy alone to lumpectomy and radiation demonstrated not only a 3-fold reduction in local relapse, but a small but statistically significant compromise in overall survival with the omission of radiation following lumpectomy.[11,12] For patients with ductal carcinoma in situ (DCIS), randomized studies conducted by the NSABP and European Organization for Research and Treatment in Cancer (EORTC) comparing lumpectomy alone to lumpectomy and radiation found a 55% and 43% respective reduction in ipsilateral breast cancer events with the addition of radiotherapy.[13,14] From these data, breast-conservation surgery followed by WBI (BCS+RT) became the standard of care for women with stage 0, I, and II breast cancer. BCS+RT involves

the surgical removal of the primary tumor, evaluation of the axillary nodes, and local breast irradiation; this treatment is extremely well tolerated with minimal long-term toxicity and favorable cosmetic outcomes.[15,16] Despite the obvious cosmetic and potential emotional advantages of BCS+RT, 15% to 30% of patients who undergo lumpectomy do not receive postoperative radiotherapy.[17-20] Many patients may choose mastectomy or lumpectomy alone over BCS+RT due to the protracted course of daily treatment involved with WBI, which consists of daily radiotherapy to the whole breast for 25 treatments usually followed by a 5 fraction boost to the tumor bed, all delivered over the course of 6 to 6.5 weeks. Other reasons that steer women away from BCS+RT are physician bias, patient age, fear of radiation treatments, distance from a radiation treatment facility, and socioeconomic factors.[18,21-24]

Based on the numerous randomized studies noted above, it is standard of care for all women, regardless of age or tumor size, to receive radiotherapy in the setting of BCT to reduce local recurrence. However, in recent years investigators have tried to identify subsets of women who may not benefit from the addition of radiotherapy to lumpectomy for early-stage breast cancer. A prospective study from the Cancer and Leukemia Group B (CALGB) randomized women 70 years of age or older whose tumors were less than 2 cm and estrogen receptor–positive to tamoxifen ± radiotherapy.[25] Even though radiotherapy significantly reduced the rate of local recurrence (from 4% to 1%), there was no difference in overall survival, and the investigators concluded that "tamoxifen alone is a reasonable choice for adjuvant treatment in such women." A Canadian trial, published simultaneously, showed that women over age 50 with early-stage breast cancer demonstrated a local relapse rate of 7.7% with lumpectomy and tamoxifen compared to 0.6% with lumpectomy, tamoxifen, and radiation. Although there was no compromise in survival with the omission of radiation, the study was not sufficiently powered to demonstrate small benefits in survival.

Smith et al, using the Surveillance, Epidemiology, and End Results (SEER)-Medicare database, identified 8724 women over age 70 years who met the eligibility criteria for CALGB 9343, and found that radiotherapy not only reduced local recurrence but also reduced the rate of any second breast cancer event and subsequent mastectomy.[26] They further identified subgroups, such as women between 70 and 79 years with low comorbidities and those with lobular histology, that derived the greatest benefit from radiotherapy. Of note, in the SEER-Medicare database of women age 70 or greater, only 59% of patients treated with breast-conserving surgery received radiation. Collectively, these data suggest that some older women may safely avoid radiation but that it is also rational for elderly women with long life expectancies and low comorbidities to receive radiotherapy after lumpectomy. Many fail to do so, however, given the prolonged course of therapy, resources needed in travel, and distance to a radiotherapy center.

In response, accelerated partial breast irradiation (APBI) has been increasingly studied over the past 15 years as a viable alternative to WBI. In general, APBI involves treating the surgical cavity with a 1 to 2 cm margin, thus reducing the volume of breast tissue irradiated by up to 50% using various radiotherapeutic methods. Technical approaches of partial breast irradiation include multicatheter interstitial brachytherapy, single lumen balloon catheter brachytherapy, intracavitary multiple lumen catheter brachytherapy, external 3-dimensional conformal external beam radiotherapy (3D-CRT) and intraoperative radiotherapy (IORT). Treatment is typically delivered postoperatively, over a short period of time, using large fraction sizes. Advocates of APBI state that it is a safe and well-tolerated therapy that allows for equivalent cosmetic outcomes while significantly increasing quality of life and allowing for an effective treatment of breast cancer. To date, pilot studies of various APBI techniques have been studied, and large, multicenter randomized and controlled studies are under way comparing APBI to WBI.

RATIONALE

In standard BCT, radiotherapy is delivered to the whole breast to eliminate areas of occult multicentric in situ or invasive carcinoma. Additional radiotherapy may be delivered to the tumor bed using a "boost" to eliminate the higher burden of microscopic disease that may have been left in close proximity to the tumor bed after lumpectomy.

Following BCS and WBI, the majority of local relapses occur in close proximity to the tumor bed. When discussing a tumor recurrence in the ipsilateral breast, it is important to note the difference between a true recurrence and the development of a second primary in the irradiated breast. A study from Yale defined a second primary as a recurrence distinctly different from the primary tumor with respect to the histologic subtype, location, or ploidy. In patients treated with BCT with 15-year follow-up data,[27,28] patients developed both true recurrences and second primaries at similar rates until approximately 8 years, when true recurrence rates stabilized but second primary

rates continued to rise. Recht et al also found that the majority of true recurrences occurred in the first 5 to 10 years but with increasing follow-up, there was a higher incidence of second primary tumors that developed in other quadrants of the breast.[29] The 20-year update from Veronesi et al comparing mastectomy to BCT showed a nonsignificant difference between the development of true recurrences or second primaries in the ipsilateral breast (0.63 per 100 woman-years of observation) treated with second compared with the contralateral breast (0.66 per 100 woman-years of observation).[2]

Several retrospective as well as prospective, randomized studies comparing lumpectomy ± WBI have shown that the majority of tumor recurrences occurred at or near the original tumor bed.[30,31] Another study by Veronesi found that failures beyond the lumpectomy cavity occurred in 2.9% of patients, consistent with previously published data of 1.5% and 3.5%.[9,32,33] These data suggest that the true benefit of radiotherapy may be to decrease the recurrence of tumor at or near the tumor bed, but may not prevent the development of new, second primary breast cancers that may occur in the irradiated breast.

Given that the majority of true local relapses occur adjacent to the tumor bed, along with available pathologic data demonstrating only minimal microscopic tumor burden more than 1 to 2 cm beyond the primary tumor, a rationale now exists for more localized treatment in selected patients. With APBI, a conformal dose of radiation is delivered to a limited volume of breast in a short period of time. Unfortunately, the majority of data regarding APBI involves single institution, nonrandomized studies with small patient populations. To assess the efficacy of APBI, a large, prospective randomized study is needed. Currently, an intergroup trial (National Surgical Adjuvant Breast and Bowel Project B and Radiation Therapy Oncology Group) is randomizing patients with early-stage breast cancer to WBI versus APBI. Accrual has been brisk and is currently enrolling "high-risk" patients including women less than 50 years of age with DCIS or invasive disease or any patient with node-positive or hormone negative invasive cancer.

PATIENT SELECTION

Accurate patient selection for APBI is crucial to prevent locoregional failures. To date, the American Brachytherapy Society and the American Society of Breast Surgeons (ASBS) have released similar versions of patient selection criteria for APBI, based mainly on both retrospective and prospective studies (Table 95-1). The American Brachytherapy Society criteria for patient selection include age 50 years or more, tumor upto 3 cm in greatest dimension, invasive ductal histology, negative lymph node status, negative marginal status (defined as "no tumor at ink"), applicator placement within 10 weeks of final lumpectomy procedure, and a postlumpectomy cavity with 1 dimension of at least 3.0 cm.[34] Very similar to the American Brachytherapy Society recommendations, the ASBS recommendations include age 45 years or older, tumor upto 3 cm in greatest dimension, in-situ or invasive ductal histology, negative lymph node status, and negative marginal status.

TABLE 95-1 Recommendations for Patient Selection

Series	Age	Tumor Size	Histology	Lymph Nodes	Margins
American Brachytherapy Society	>50	≤3 cm	Invasive ductal carcinoma	Negative (ALND or SLN recommended)	Negative (no tumor at inked margin)
American Society of Breast Surgeons	≥45	≤3 cm	Invasive ductal or in situ carcinoma	Negative (ALND or SLN recommended)	Negative

ALND, axillary lymph node dissection; SLN, sentinel lymph node.

The NSABP B-39/Radiation Therapy Oncology Group (RTOG) 0413 trial randomizing patients to WBI versus APBI uses the following criteria: age 18 years or more, in situ or invasive ductal or lobular histology, tumor size ≤3 cm, negative margins, a target lumpectomy cavity upto 30% of the breast volume, and if invasive histology, 0 to 3 positive axillary nodes with a minimum of 6 sampled nodes in patients with positive nodes. Given the survival benefit from irradiation of the chest wall and regional nodal groups in patients with positive nodes, the wisdom of including patients with positive nodes as candidates for APBI has been debated.[35,36] Other clinicopathologic features such as extensive intraductal component, invasive lobular histology, and lymphovascular invasion also still need to be investigated. The results of the NSABP/RTOG randomized trial, which includes patients with the above noted features, may help to refine selection criteria for patients considering APBI as an alternative to WBI. Until more data are available, it appears that the use of APBI per American Brachytherapy Society or ASBS recommendations represents a reasonable cohort of patients to consider for partial breast irradiation. However, we advise the enrollment of patients for APBI on clinical trials, to help establish selection criteria, document patterns of recurrence, identify acute and long-term toxicities, and develop alternative technical approaches and fractionation strategies.

CURRENT TECHNIQUES AND EXPERIENCE IN ACCELERATED PARTIAL BREAST IRRADIATION

The goal in APBI is to deliver a homogeneous dose of radiation in a short period of time to the tumor bed with additional margin. This may be achieved using several distinct radiotherapy techniques and include multicatheter interstitial brachytherapy, single lumen balloon catheter brachytherapy, intracavitary multiple lumen catheter brachytherapy, 3D-CRT, and IORT. Each technique is vastly different from the others in terms of degree of invasiveness, radiation delivery, operator proficiency, acceptance among radiation oncologists, and length of treatment. However, each technique is able to deliver a homogeneous dose of radiation to the target area, which in theory is radiobiologically equivalent to conventional protracted WBI with respect to local tumor control, as well as acute and long-term toxicity.

There is a considerable amount of phase I and II data available investigating APBI with similar local control rates as compared to WBI at 5 years. However, most of these data evolved from patients who received multicatheter interstitial breast brachytherapy, which is an intricate, labor-intensive procedure that requires skill on the part of the radiation oncologist. More recently, the intracavitary catheters, such as the MammoSite balloon catheter, external beam radiotherapy, and IORT, have been investigated as alternative methods of APBI.

Multicatheter Interstitial Brachytherapy

Multicatheter interstitial brachytherapy has been the longest-used APBI technique that originated as a technique for delivering a tumor bed boost following WBI (Table 95-2). Through this approach, flexible afterloading catheters are placed through the breast tissue in several planes, to ensure adequate coverage of the lumpectomy cavity with margin (Fig. 95-1). Generally, these catheters are placed at 1 to 1.5 cm intervals, in several planes, for a total of 10 to 20 catheters to ensure a homogeneous dose covering the target area. Low-activity sources with dose rates in the range of 0.4 to 2 Gy/h are used in low dose rate (LDR) brachytherapy, while high-activity sources with dose rates greater than 12 Gy/h are used in high dose rate (HDR) brachytherapy. Medium dose rate (MDR) and pulsed dose rate (PDR) brachytherapy have also been investigated as alternative methods. With respect to APBI, LDR sources are implanted for approximately 2 to 5 days while the patient is admitted as an inpatient, while HDR brachytherapy allows for an outpatient treatment, fractionated over the course of a week, with a treatment time on the order of seconds to minutes. Implants are carried out using iridium 192 (^{192}Ir) sources of uniform or varying source activities. Remote afterloading with HDR brachytherapy allows for flexibility in treatment planning, given programmable dwell times for each catheter.

The Oschner Clinic in New Orleans, Louisiana, first investigated the use of LDR and HDR interstitial implants following lumpectomy in patients with DCIS or invasive ductal histology, with a tumor size less than 4 cm, negative margins, and 0 to 3 positive axillary nodes.[37] They randomized 50 patients in block fashion to either LDR (45 Gy over 3.5-6 days) or HDR (32 Gy over 4 days in 8 fractions). The target volume included

TABLE 95-2 Multicatheter Interstitial Brachytherapy Accelerated Partial Breast Irradiation Studies

Series	No. of Patients	Dose Rate	APBI Scheme (Dose [Gy] × Fraction No.)	Median FU (mo)	TR/MM (%)	Regional Nodal Failure (%)	Good/ Excellent Cosmesis (%)
Oschner Clinic [37,38] New Orleans, LA	84	HDR LDR	4.0 × 8 45 × 1	84	2.5	6	75
William Beaumont Hospital [39] Royal Oaks, MI	199	HDR LDR	4.0 × 8 or 3.4 × 10 50 × 1	65	2	4	99
RTOG 95-17 [40]	99	HDR LDR	3.4 × 10 45 × 1	45	3	2	NR
NIO I [45,46] Budapest, Hungary	45	HDR	4.33 × 7 or 5.2 × 7	84	0	NR	84
NIO II [47] Budapest, Hungary	126	HDR	5.2 × 7	36	1.2	NR	86

FU, follow-up; HDR, high dose rate; LDR, low dose rate; NIO, National Institute of Oncology; NR, not reported; TR/MM, true recurrence/marginal miss.

the lumpectomy cavity with 2 cm of circumferential breast tissue. In their original report with a median follow-up of 75 months, there was only 1 breast recurrence (2%) and 3 regional nodal failures (6%), with only 1 nodal failure among the 9 patients with positive nodes upon study entry.

In a retrospective, case-control study, King et al identified patients who met the eligibility criteria for the brachytherapy trial but who received WBI.[38] They matched these patients to brachytherapy-treated patients according to characteristics based on tumor size, breast size, and pathologic stage. Using

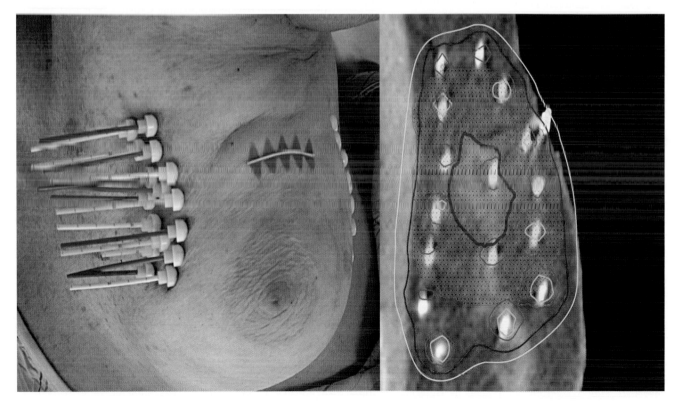

FIGURE 95-1 Multicatheter interstitial implant. *(Courtesy of Douglas Arthur. Reprinted with permission. ©2008 American Society of Clinical Oncology. All rights reserved.)*

this case-control cohort, they found no difference in breast recurrences (2% vs 5%) and locoregional recurrences (8% vs 5%) in patients treated with APBI and WBI, respectively. There was also a nonsignificant difference in cosmesis rated as good or excellent at 20 months between the APBI and WBI groups (75% and 85%, respectively).

The William Beaumont Hospital group has the largest experience using interstitial brachytherapy with the longest reported follow-up of 199 patients with early-stage breast cancer (JNCI).[39] Eighty percent of these patients were treated on institutional protocols with the following criteria: invasive ductal histology, tumor size less than 3.0 cm, negative margins (2 mm or more), age more than 40 years, and negative lymph nodes. The other 20% were treated with APBI for "compassionate" reasons and included patients with close margins, DCIS, participation in other studies, and timing of radiotherapy after lumpectomy. The median age was 65 years and 12% of patients had 1 to 3 positive lymph nodes. One hundred twenty patients were treated with LDR brachytherapy, receiving 50 Gy over 96 hours, while the rest of the cohort underwent HDR brachytherapy, receiving either 32 Gy in 8 fractions or 34 Gy over 10 fractions. The target volume included the lumpectomy cavity with a 1 to 2 cm margin for all patients. The group also included a matched pair analysis to compare the rate of local recurrence between APBI and WBI. At 60 months they reported a low local recurrence rate in both the APBI and WBI groups. There was also no difference in distant metastases, disease free survival, cause-specific survival, or overall survival between the 2 groups. Furthermore, in patients with 60-month follow-up, 99% of patients reported their cosmesis to be good or excellent.

The RTOG conducted the first multi-institutional trial (RTOG 95-17) consisting of interstitial brachytherapy to treat early-stage breast cancer patients.[40] This was a phase I/II trial to determine the feasibility, reproducibility, toxicity, cosmesis, local control, and survival of patients treated with lumpectomy and axillary lymph node evaluation followed by APBI using interstitial brachytherapy. One hundred women were enrolled and 99 were found to be eligible. Eighty-seven patients were T1 and 20 patients had 1 to 3 positive lymph nodes. Thirty-three patients were treated using LDR (45 Gy over 4.5 days) and 66 using HDR (34 Gy over 10 fractions in 5 days). With a median follow-up of 3.7 years, 3 patients developed an in-breast recurrence and 3 patients experienced a nodal failure. In a recent update presented at the American Society of Therapeutic Radiation Oncology in November 2006 with a median follow-up of 6 years, 3% and 6% of patients treated with HDR and LDR experienced an in-breast failure, with the majority of failures being classified as a true recurrence/marginal miss.[41] The authors concluded that "multicatheter partial breast brachytherapy on this trial experienced excellent in-breast control rates."

There have been several European groups that have investigated the efficacy of multicatheter interstitial brachytherapy to deliver APBI. Many of the early studies were fraught with poor patient selection and outdated treatment planning modalities.[42-44] For the purpose of this discussion, we will focus on the more recent European studies, including 1 prospective, randomized controlled study comparing WBI to APBI using interstitial brachytherapy. The National Institute of Oncology (NIO) in Budapest, Hungary, has much experience in the use of HDR interstitial implants to provide APBI.[45,46] They treated women of any age with pathologic T1 tumors (in situ carcinoma and invasive lobular carcinoma were excluded) with negative margins and lymph nodes that were pathologically negative (or <2 mm micrometastases). Forty-five patients were treated to a total of 30.3 Gy (n = 8) or 36.4 Gy (n = 37) in 7 fractions over 4 days. The authors included a control group of patients who met the eligibility criteria during the same time period and were treated with WBI. With a median follow-up of 7 years, the actuarial ipsilateral failure rate was reported as 9% (n = 3) in the APBI group and 12% in the WBI group. All patients treated with APBI who experienced a recurrence were subsequently treated with lumpectomy followed by 46 to 50 Gy WBI, providing a 100% mastectomy-free recurrence rate. The NIO then conducted a single institution randomized study between 1998 and 2004 of patients more than 40 years with the same eligibility criteria as described above.[47] Two hundred fifty-five patients were randomized to 50 Gy WBI (n = 129) or APBI (n = 126) using HDR multicatheter interstitial brachytherapy (36.4 Gy in 7 fractions over 4 days). Patients who were not suitable for implantation received EBRT using an enface electron field of 50 Gy prescribed to the 80% isodose. With a median follow-up of 3 years, the local recurrence rate was reported as 1.3% and 1.9% for APBI and WBI, respectively (p = .99). There was no difference in cause-specific survival, disease-free survival, and distant metastases-free survival. However, they reported fewer grade 2 to 3 skin side effects in patients treated with APBI as compared to WBI (3% vs 17%, p < .001). At 5 years, the actuarial rate of ipsilateral breast failure was 5.5% and 4.4% in PBI and WBI arms, respectively (p = .65). The long-term cosmetic results being rated as good/excellent were 79% and 59% in the PBI and WBI arms, respectively (p = .001).

Single Lumen Balloon Catheter Brachytherapy

The MammoSite balloon brachytherapy device (MammoSite Radiation Therapy System [RTS]; Hologic, Bedford, Massachusetts) was introduced in 2002 and is a form of intracavitary brachytherapy that is simpler in its technique and treatment planning as compared to interstitial brachytherapy (Fig. 95-2). The apparatus consists of a double lumen catheter that is 15 cm in length and 6 mm in diameter. The catheter contains a central lumen that allows for a HDR ^{192}Ir source, and a small adjacent lumen for filling the distally located balloon. This spherical MammoSite balloon catheter is available in 2 sizes when inflated, either 4 to 5 cm or 5 to 6 cm in diameter, for variability in the dimensions of a lumpectomy cavity. An elliptically shaped MammoSite balloon catheter is also available that is a fixed 4 × 6 cm in diameter ellipsoid when inflated.

The MammoSite catheter is implanted after lumpectomy, at the time of surgery directly into the cavity; after surgery under ultrasound guidance through a small, separate incision; or after surgery directly into the cavity through the healing lumpectomy wound. The manufacturer of the MammoSite catheter has also produced a simpler and less expensive balloon catheter called the Cavity Evaluation Device (CED). This allows the

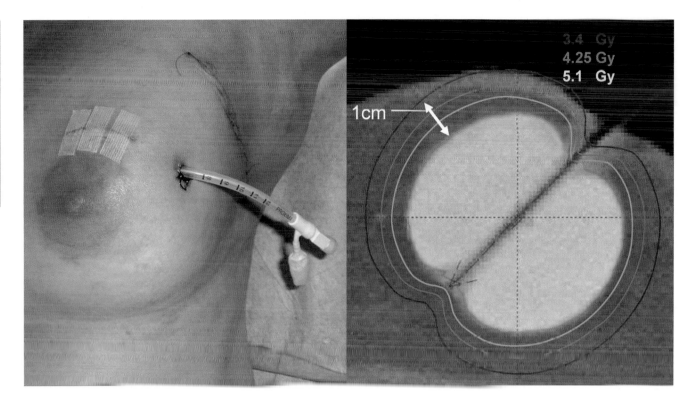

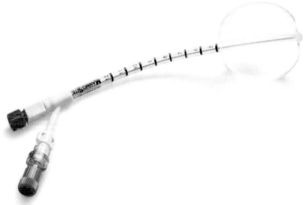

FIGURE 95-2 MammoSite balloon brachytherapy. (Courtesy of Douglas Arthur. Reprinted with permission. ©2008 American Society of Clinical Oncology. All rights reserved.)

surgeon, without wasting a MammoSite device because of poor conformance or inadequate balloon-to-skin distance, to check balloon-cavity conformance and to ensure adequate skin-to-balloon distance while in the operating room. Also, to preclude wasting a MammoSite catheter from disqualifying final nodal and margin histology, the CED may be left in the breast for a few days until the final pathology is reported. If the patient remains a candidate for brachytherapy, the CED may then be exchanged for a MammoSite catheter in the surgeon's office or outpatient clinic under local anesthesia.

After catheter placement, computed tomography (CT) of the breast is performed prior to initiation of treatment to determine that the balloon-to-skin distance is 5 mm or more, the conformity of the balloon to the walls of the lumpectomy cavity is more than 90%, and there is symmetry between the balloon and

the center shaft of the catheter (Fig. 95-2). These guidelines were developed by the ASBS to ensure proper patient selection for this technique.

The ASBS published the outcomes of insertion techniques of a registry trial of 1403 patients who received MammoSite breast brachytherapy.[48] The trial, initiated in May 2002 by the manufacturer who relinquished control of the trial in November 2003, accrued patients from 87 institutions over 30 months. Patients were enrolled per the American Brachytherapy Society eligibility criteria listed earlier in this review. A total of 1237 (87%) patients received APBI via MammoSite, 43 (3%) patients received a boost via MammoSite, and 123 (9%) patients underwent catheter explantation. Explantation was performed for poor skin spacing (35%), irregular cavity (28%), positive margins (9%), and balloon failure (9%). Recently published 3-year data on 1440 early-stage breast cancer patients (1449 cases) treated with MammoSite in the ASBS registry trial with a median follow-up of 30.1 months revealed a 1.6% rate of ipsilateral breast tumor recurrence (IBTR) for a 2-year actuarial rate of 1.04% (1.11% for invasive breast cancer and 0.59% for DCIS).[49] The percentages of breasts with good to excellent cosmetic results at 12 (n = 980), 24 (n = 752), 36 (n = 403), and 48 months (n = 67 cases) were 95%, 94%, 93%, and 93%, respectively.

Cuttino et al presented a pooled analysis of 9 institutions of patients with stage 0, I, and II breast carcinoma with MammoSite between 2000 and 2004 at the American Society of Therapeutic Radiation Oncology annual meeting in November 2006.[50] All 483 patients received 34 Gy in 10 fractions over 5 days. The median follow-up was 2 years, and all patients had a minimum follow-up of 1 year. They found a 1.2% (n = 6) in-breast failure rate; however, only 0.4% of all patients experienced a failure that was characterized as a true recurrence or marginal miss. Cosmetic results were reported as good/excellent in 91% of patients. Administration of prophylactic antibiotics, skin spacing more than 5 mm, and use of multiple dwell positions contributed to less dermatologic toxicity in terms of severe acute skin reactions, severe hyperpigmentation, and grade 3/4 acute skin reactions.

A multi-institutional phase II clinical trial was conducted from May 2003 to January 2006 to evaluate the utility of MammoSite in patients with DCIS.[51] Eligibility criteria included the following: age 45 years or more, unicentric pure DCIS, 1 mm or more margins, tumor size up to 5 cm, clinically node negative, and a postlumpectomy mammogram showing complete resolution of any suspicious microcalcifications. One hundred and thirty three patients were enrolled, with 117 patients receiving the MammoSite implant. Seventeen patients underwent removal of the implant for various reasons, including suboptimal skin distance, positive margins, and irregular cavity. Thus, 100 patients completed treatment with a median follow-up period of 9 months. Two patients experienced an ipsilateral breast recurrence, with 1 being a true recurrent/marginal miss. Ninety-eight percent of patients reported a good/excellent cosmetic result and there was a 4% infection rate, consistent with the other series. Details of these studies can be found in Table 95-3.

Intracavitary Multiple Lumen Catheter Brachytherapy

Given the limitations of single lumen balloon catheters in shaping the radiation dose in the treatment region, many patients with inadequate skin spacing (less than 5-7 mm) or deep-set lesions near the chest wall are often found not to be candidates for this procedure. Given these considerations, intracavitary multiple lumen catheters were developed to allow for greater flexibility in treatment planning, thereby increasing the number of patients eligible for intracavitary brachytherapy. Two devices are currently available: (1) the Strut-Adjusted Volume Implant (SAVI) breast brachytherapy device (Cianna Medical; Aliso Viejo, California), which has 6, 8, or 10 peripheral source channels (Fig. 95-3); and (2) the Contura multi-lumen balloon applicator (SenoRx Inc; Irvine, California), which has 5 fixed lumens in the shaft: 1 centered and 4 offset by 5 mm (Fig. 95-3).

Like the MammoSite catheter, the SAVI and Contura devices are implanted after lumpectomy, either at the time of surgery directly into the cavity or after surgery under ultrasound guidance through a small, separate incision (Fig. 95-4). However, if placement at the time of surgery is preferred, use of the temporary CED catheter described previously allows exchange for the SAVI or Contura device in the office or clinic after brachytherapy eligibility is confirmed by viewing the final pathology report.

Clinical studies evaluating toxicity and local control rate involving both devices are in the beginning phases. However, dosimetric studies have shown that the flexibility of treatment planning with intracavitary multiple lumen catheters create a greater potential for optimization of dose delivery, thereby reducing toxicity in patients with lesions close to skin or rib.[52,53] This flexibility benefits patients who are unable to meet dosimetric requirements using a single lumen catheter (Fig. 95-5).

3D Conformal External Beam Radiotherapy

This technique, although the most widely used form of radiation therapy to treat carcinomas of all types, has the least amount of data supporting its role in APBI. 3D-CRT is a noninvasive method of delivering APBI that provides increased dose

TABLE 95-3 Mammosite Brachytherapy Accelerated Partial Breast Irradiation Studies

Series	No. of Patients	Dose Rate	APBI Scheme (Dose [Gy] × Fraction No.)	Median FU (mo)	TR/MM (%)	Infection Rate (%)	Explantation Rate (%)	Good/Excellent Cosmesis (%)
ASBS Registry Trial[48,71]	1403	HDR	3.4 × 10	15	0.1	8	9	98
Cuttino et al[50]	483	HDR	3.4 × 10	12	0.4	NR	NR	91
Benitez et al[51]	100	HDR	3.4 × 10	9.5	2	4	14.5	98

ASBS, American Society of Breast Surgeons; FU, follow-up; HDR, high dose rate; LDR, low dose rate; NR, not reported; TR/MM, true recurrence/marginal miss.

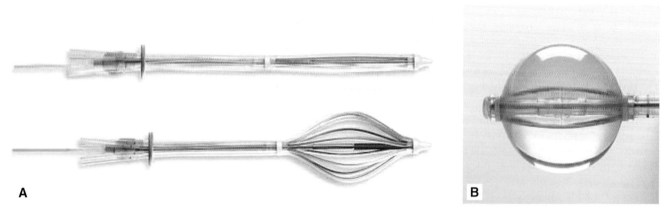

A

B

FIGURE 95-3 **A.** Strut-Adjusted Volume Implant (SAVI) breast brachytherapy device. *(Courtesy of the Texas Cancer Clinic and Cianna Medical, Aliso Viejo, California.)* **B.** Contura multi-lumen balloon applicator. *(Courtesy of SenoRx.)*

homogeneity leading to theoretical potential for better cosmetic outcomes compared with the other techniques (Figs. 95-6 through 95-9). Furthermore, 3D-CRT is a technique that is less operator dependent than interstitial brachytherapy techniques and may include patients who do not meet eligibility criteria for intracavitary devices like MammoSite. In addition, cost analysis studies have indicated that 3D-CRT may be cheaper than brachytherapy techniques that do not require an extra surgical procedure or inpatient hospitalization.[54,55] With the emergence of CT-based simulation, easier identification of the tumor bed and calculation of doses to critical normal structures has also led to an interest in delivering APBI using 3D-CRT.

Vicini et al at the William Beaumont Hospital first used 3D-CRT to deliver APBI in a select group of patients using active breathing control to account for movement of the breast secondary to respiration.[56] They found this technique to be feasible and initiated a phase I/II trial further investigating the role of 3D-CRT in patients who met the eligibility criteria for RTOG 95-17.[57] Thirty-one patients were enrolled and underwent

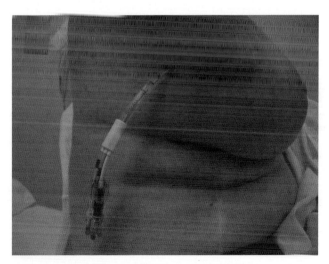

FIGURE 95-4 Contura multi-lumen balloon applicator. *(Courtesy of the Texas Cancer Clinic.)*

CT-based planning. The clinical target volume (CTV) was defined as the lumpectomy cavity plus a 1 to 1.5 cm margin, limited by the skin surface and chest wall. A 1-cm margin was added to form the planning target volume (PTV). The first 5 patients received 34 Gy over 10 twice-daily fractions, while the remainder of the patients received 38.5 Gy over 10 twice daily fractions. With a median follow-up of 10 months, there were no recurrences and a 100% rating of good/excellent cosmesis. The technical aspects of this study were found to be feasible and easily reproducible.

The RTOG conducted a phase I/II trial to evaluate the feasibility and reproducibility of 3D-CRT in delivering APBI.[58] They enrolled 58 patients with stage I or II invasive ductal carcinoma with lesions upto 3 cm and negative surgical margins. After lumpectomy, the surgical cavity was defined on CT scan and this was denoted as the gross tumor volume (GTV). An expansion of 1.0 to 1.5 cm was added to form the CTV. The CTV was restricted to within 5 mm of the skin surface and lung–chest wall interface. An additional margin of more than 1.0 cm was provided to form the PTV, to account for penumbra. However, a separate PTV structure was formed to exclude this volume to within 5 mm of the skin surface and lung–chest wall interface, and was used for the dose volume histogram (DVH) analysis. A total of 38.5 Gy was delivered in 10 fractions over 5 days. Patients were not treated using active breathing control. Port films and orthogonal pair films were taken 4 times during the course of therapy. The dose volume constraints were as follows: less than 50% of the ipsilateral breast should receive less than 50% of the prescribed dose and 25% of the ipsilateral whole breast should receive the prescribed dose; the contralateral breast received less than 3% of the prescribed dose; less than 10% of the ipsilateral lung could receive 30% of the prescribed dose; less than 10% of the contralateral lung could receive 5% of the prescribed dose; less than 5% of the heart could receive a maximum of 5% of the prescribed dose for right-sided lesions, and for left-sided lesions the volume of lung receiving 5% of the dose should be less than conventional WBI; finally, the maximum dose to the thyroid could be 3% of the prescribed dose. The primary end point of the study was to

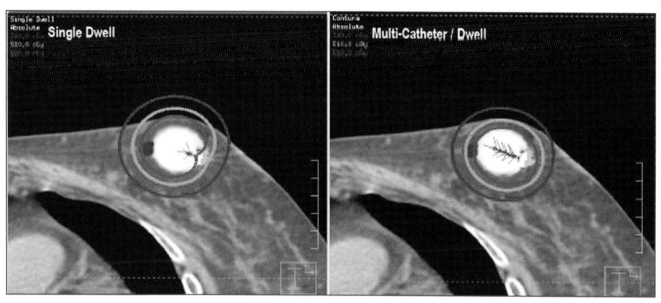

FIGURE 95-5 Isodose comparison between a single-dwell *(left)* and a multicatheter/dwell plan *(right)*. The minimum balloon-to-skin distance is 3 mm. The PTV is shown in light purple. Using multiple catheters and dwell positions reduces the maximum skin dose from 195% to 135% (blue). Per the NSABP B-39 protocol, the maximum allowable skin dose is 145%. *(Courtesy of Frank Vicini.)*

determine if 3D-CRT was reproducible, which was confirmed by the authors, as there were only 4 cases with major variations in the first 42 evaluable plans. All 4 of these major variations arose from the strict DVH constraints on the ipsilateral lung. The results of this study served as the foundation for the NSABP B-39/RTOG 0413 clinical trial that opened in 2005.

Formenti et al at the New York University designed a phase I/II study in 2000 evaluating the role of APBI delivered using 3D-CRT to patients lying in the prone position. Advocates of the prone position state that it reduces normal tissue motion secondary to respiration and cardiac systole, and further allows for the removal of the heart and lungs from the treatment field. This group treated 78 patients with a median follow-up of 28 months, which is the longest published follow-up of APBI using 3D-CRT.[59] There were no recurrences to date, and cosmesis was rated as good/excellent in 92% of patients. Details on the experience with 3D-CRT are listed in Table 95-4.

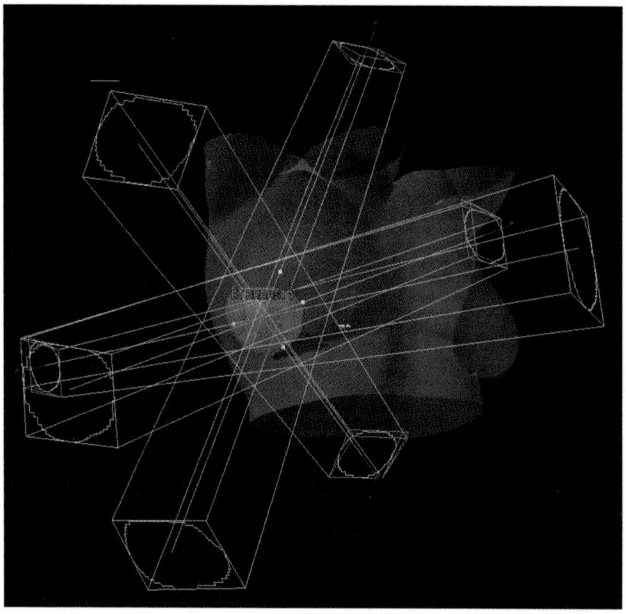

INTRAOPERATIVE RADIOTHERAPY

Intraoperative radiotherapy is a method of delivering a single dose of radiation directly to the tumor bed or to the exposed tumor at the time of surgery. For most tumor sites, it can be used adjuvantly after surgery or as a boost, to be followed by fractionated external beam radiotherapy for either palliative or curative intent. The objective of IORT is to deliver a high single dose of electrons or low-energy photons to the exposed target volume while displacing critical, dose-limiting structures. Traditionally, patients were transported from the operating room to the radiotherapy suite during surgery, or surgery was performed in the radiotherapy suite. However, there are several devices now available that function as mobile IORT machines such as the Intrabeam (Carl Zeiss AG; Oberkochen, Germany), which produces 50 kVp x-rays; and the Mobetron System (Oncology Care Systems Group of Siemens Medical Systems, Intraop Medical Inc; Santa Clara, California) and Novac 7 System (Hitesys spA; Aprilia, Italy), both of which produce electrons between 4 and 12 MeV. While the use of IORT has mainly been studied in depth treating abdominal, genitourinary, and gynecologic malignancies and sarcomas, the experience in breast cancer is limited. Recently, it was actively explored in Europe as part of BCT due to longer treatment delays secondary to rising costs and poor access to health care. Advocates of IORT

FIGURE 95-6 Three-dimensional conformal radiation therapy plan using a 4-field external beam technique using different beam angles to deliver a conformal dose of radiation to the tumor bed.

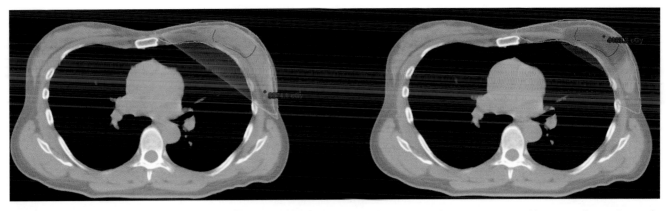

FIGURE 95-7 Amount of normal tissue receiving 90% of prescribed dose: whole-breast irradiation versus partial breast irradiation (3D-CRT).

affirm that a geographical miss, which may occur with standard external beam radiotherapy, are avoided by this technique, where the surgical bed is visualized at the time of radiation therapy. Importantly, before radiotherapy is limited solely to the tumor bed using IORT, obtaining negative margins, which is dependent on histology, accurate patient selection, and the skill of the surgeon, is crucial to the success of IORT.

The theoretical benefit of IORT is the delivery of a large single dose of radiation, either with x-rays or electrons. Large single doses of radiation are thought to be more effective on "late-responding" tissues such as lung and spinal cord, which have a low α/β ratio (2.0-6.3 and 1.7-4.9, respectively).[60] Breast tissue and tumors are thought to have an α/β ratio of 10. The linear-quadratic model, which uses values of α and β to

determine relative effectiveness of a fractionation scheme on early- and late-responding tissues, may not be reliable to use with single fraction sizes greater than 6 to 8 Gy.[61] Given this, estimates of single fraction sizes comparable to the standard 60 Gy delivered over 30 fractions are thought to be 20 to 22 Gy.[61,64] However, the late effect on breast tissue using large single fraction sizes is unknown.

There are several prospective series of patients where IORT was used to deliver radiotherapy as a part of BCT. A study by Veronesi et al at the European Institute of Oncology examined 237 patients with tumors less than 2 cm who received quadrantectomy followed by immediate IORT using the Novac 7, with 222 patients receiving 21 Gy using 3- to 9-MeV electrons.[62] With a mean follow-up of 19 months, 2.5% of patients developed

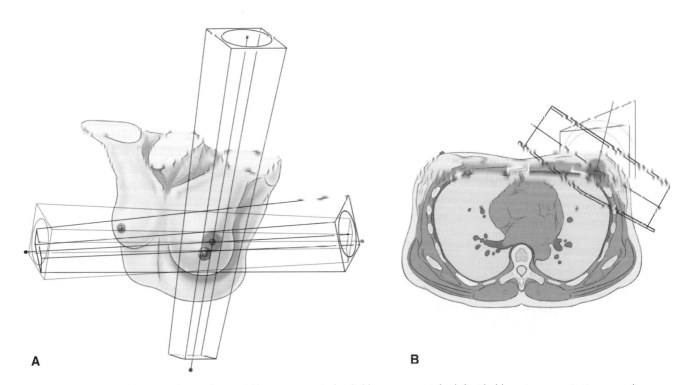

A

B

FIGURE 95-8 External beam radiation for partial breast. **A.** Typical 4-field arrangement for left-sided breast cancer. **B.** Corresponding transverse CT image through center of treatment area of breast.

TABLE 95-4 3D Conformal Radiation Therapy Accelerated Partial Breast Irradiation Studies

Series	No. of Patients	APBI Scheme (Dose [Gy] × Fraction No.)	Position	Median FU (mo)	TR/MM (%)	Mean % of Breast Receiving 100% Dose	Good/ Excellent Cosmesis (%)
RTOG 03-19[58]	46	3.85 × 10	Supine	NR	NR	NR	NR
William Beaumont Hospital[56,57] Royal Oaks, MI	31 31	3.4 × 10 or 3.85 × 10	Supine	10	0	23	100
NYU[59] New York, NY	78	6.0 × 5	Prone	28	0	26	92

FU, follow-up; NR, not reported; RTOG, Radiation Therapy Oncology Group; TR/MM, true recurrence/marginal miss.

adverse effects secondary to IORT and only 1.3% patients developed a recurrence in the ipsilateral breast, all of which were outside of the treatment field. The European Institute of Oncology has met its goal of accruing 824 patients randomized to either WBI plus boost or a single dose of 21 Gy using IORT. The results from this trial are eagerly awaited. Another study conducted by the University College of London examined 105 patients with early-stage breast cancer who received IORT using the Intrabeam system.[61,63] The prescribed dose was one 5 to 20 Gy fraction at a depth of 1 and 0.2 cm, respectively. Twenty-two patients received IORT alone, while 163 patients received it as a boost prior to WBI. Their data has not been reported in full, but preliminarily only 2 recurrences were noted and cosmetic outcomes were described as being good. This group is also accruing 1600 patients to a randomized study designed to test equivalence comparing WBI plus boost to single fraction IORT.

SEQUENCING WITH CHEMOTHERAPY

Systemic therapy has been shown to have a favorable impact on local control in combination with radiotherapy following breast-conservation surgery. Several randomized and retrospective studies have shown a significant decrease in local recurrence in patients treated with lumpectomy followed by a course of systemic therapy and radiotherapy. Even though the positive impact of systemic therapy on local control has been proven, how best to implement systemic therapy with respect to radiation therapy is divisive. With the currently used chemotherapeutic regimens for treating invasive breast cancer, the use of concurrent radiotherapy is discouraged as side effects are significantly increased. A meta-analysis investigating the sequencing of adjuvant radiotherapy and chemotherapy in breast cancer revealed a significant decrease in 5-year locoregional recurrence rates in patients treated with radiotherapy within 8 weeks of surgery (5.8%) compared with treatment between 9 to 16 weeks after surgery (9.1%).[64] Several studies investigating the role of concurrent chemotherapy and radiation therapy showed significant reductions in locoregional recurrence; however, these studies used older chemotherapeutic regimens.[65,66]

With APBI, radiotherapy may be delivered earlier in the course of treatment. Given the short course of treatment, APBI may be sandwiched between surgery and chemotherapy, essentially dissolving the debate of sequencing of radiotherapy with chemotherapy. The NSABP/RTOG study investigating APBI in early-stage breast cancer patients mandates that patients randomized to APBI receive their radiotherapy prior to any recommended chemotherapy administration.

The toxicity results from sequencing APBI between surgery and chemotherapy in a single institution experience from 2 different groups found that patients who received HDR interstitial brachytherapy followed by anthracycline-based regimens experienced increased complications of varying types. A group led by David Wazer found that 50% of these patients experienced fat necrosis as compared with 19% of those patients who did not receive chemotherapy.[67] There was a higher incidence of greater than or equal to grade 2 subcutaneous toxicity and a lower rate of having an excellent cosmetic result. In a study by Arthur et al, there was a striking increase of radiation recall in those patients treated with doxorubicin that continued with varying intensity during each subsequent cycle of chemotherapy.[68] Interestingly, however, their group concluded that LDR brachytherapy was not associated with cosmetic failure when preceding doxorubicin.

With regard to concurrent chemoradiotherapy with APBI, a pilot study presented at the American Society of Therapeutic Radiation Oncology annual meeting in November 2006 by Johns Hopkins University investigated APBI concurrent with dose dense doxorubicin and cyclophosphamide (ddAC).[69] They enrolled women with T1-2, N0-1 invasive breast carcinoma who underwent lumpectomy with negative margins and received ddAC (60 and 600 mg/m^2, respectively) every 14 days with growth factor support concurrently with APBI using 3D-CRT. The radiation was delivered to the tumor bed plus margin in 2.7 Gy fractions over 15 fractions to a total dose of 40.5 Gy. Radiotherapy started within 2 days of the first chemotherapy dose. With 13 patients treated and a median follow-up of 9 months, they reported no radiation recall and no radiation dermatitis greater than grade 1. They reported no signs of late skin or soft tissue toxicity. Even though these results are preliminary and encouraging, it does raise the question in determining the optimal timing and dose fractionation schema of APBI in relation to chemotherapy.

In an analysis of the ASBS MammoSite registry trial, Haffty et al reported that cosmetic outcome appeared to be superior in those patients whose chemotherapy was initiated more than 3 weeks after the last MammoSite brachytherapy treatment. Cosmetic outcome was good to excellent in 94% of women receiving chemotherapy later than 3 weeks after the last fraction, compared with 72.2% good to excellent cosmesis in women receiving chemotherapy within 3 weeks of the last MammoSite fraction ($p = .01$).[70] The cosmetic outcome in women receiving chemotherapy after 3 weeks following the fraction was similar to the cosmetic outcome of the overall population not receiving chemotherapy. Of note, the incidence of radiation recall was 18% in patients receiving chemotherapy within 3 weeks of the last MammoSite fraction compared with 7% for those receiving chemotherapy greater than 3 weeks after the last fraction. Longer follow-up and additional data will be required to determine the optimal timing of chemotherapy following APBI with the various techniques employed.

ONGOING TRIALS AND FUTURE DIRECTIONS

Accelerated partial breast irradiation is an exciting development in the treatment of early-stage breast cancer patients. However, more data are needed to determine its efficacy and equivalence in the treatment paradigm of these patients. The phase III trial being conducted by the NSABP/RTOG randomizing patients to WBI or APBI is of much interest given the large scope of the trial. Unfortunately, early data from this trial are several years from being reported and meaningful results are more than 10 years away. Fortunately, there are several trials being conducted worldwide investigating WBI versus APBI using the various techniques described in this chapter. A randomized trial is being conducted by the Breast Cancer Working Group of the Groupe Européen de Curiethérapie–European Society for Therapeutic Radiology and Oncology to determine equivalence between WBI and APBI using multicatheter brachytherapy. A complete list of ongoing phase III trials is listed in Table 95-5. Determining which patients are best suited to receive APBI in lieu of WBI and vice versa are expectations that should be addressed by the ongoing phase III trials. Research is still needed to help determine the optimal dose per fraction, timing with chemotherapy, and treatment of patients with adverse risk factors. To date, results from the phase I/II studies discussed above are encouraging and may lead to a shift in the treatment paradigm in early-stage breast cancer patients. Only through enrollment of patients in these ongoing randomized clinical trials, and through development of novel phase I/II programs evaluating other issues related to fractionation, positioning, and techniques, can we continue to move forward in this rapidly evolving field of accelerated partial breast irradiation.

SUMMARY

Partial-breast irradiation has emerged as a common method of treatment for patients with early-stage breast cancer. It has the advantage over conventional WBI of allowing treatment to be

TABLE 95-5 Ongoing Phase III Clinical Trials

Series	No. of Patients	Trial Design	Control Arm	Experimental Arm
NSABP B-39 RTOG 0413	3000	Equivalence	50-50.4 Gy WB ± 10-16 Gy Boost	1. Interstitial brachytherapy, or 2. MammoSite, or 3. 3D conformal EBRT
European Brachytherapy Breast Cancer GEC-ESTRO Working Group	1170	Noninferiority	50-50.4 Gy WB + 10 Gy Boost	Brachytherapy only 7.0 Gy × fractions HDR 30.3 Gy 7 fractions HDR 50 Gy PDR 50 Gy PDR
European Institute of Oncology	824	Equivalence	50 Gy WB + 10 Gy Boost	Intraoperative Single fraction EBRT 21 Gy × 1
University College of London	1600	Equivalence	WB (per center) + Boost	Intraoperative Single fraction EBRT 5 Gy × 1
NIO Budapest, Hungary	570	Noninferiority	50 Gy WB	1. Interstitial brachytherapy (5.2 Gy × 7) or 2. Electrons (50 Gy)

EBRT, external beam radiation therapy; GEC-ESTRO, Groupe Européen de Curiethérapie–European Society for Therapeutic Radiology and Oncology; Gy, gray; HDR, high dose rate; NIO, National Institute of Oncology; NSABP, National Surgical Adjuvant Breast and Bowel Project; PDR, pulsed dose rate; RTOG, Radiation Therapy Oncology Group; WB, whole breast.

delivered in an accelerated fashion, over 1 to 2 weeks. Ongoing trials will help to further refine which patient populations are most suitable for this approach, and novel technologies are rapidly evolving that will help to further refine and improve the delivery of accelerated partial breast irradiation.

REFERENCES

1. Fisher B, Anderson S, Bryant J, et al. Twenty-year follow-up of a randomized trial comparing total mastectomy, lumpectomy, and lumpectomy plus irradiation for the treatment of invasive breast cancer. *N Engl J Med.* 2002;347:1233-1241.

2. Veronesi U, Cascinelli N, Mariani L, et al. Twenty-year follow-up of a randomized study comparing breast-conserving surgery with radical mastectomy for early breast cancer. *N Engl J Med.* 2002;347:1227-1232.

3. Blichert-Toft M, Rose C, Andersen JA, et al. Danish randomized trial comparing breast conservation therapy with mastectomy: six years of life-table analysis. Danish Breast Cancer Cooperative Group. *J Natl Cancer Inst Monogr.* 1992:19-25.

4. Poggi MM, Danforth DN, Sciuto LC, et al. Eighteen-year results in the treatment of early breast carcinoma with mastectomy versus breast conservation therapy: the National Cancer Institute Randomized Trial. *Cancer.* 2003;98:697-702.

5. van Dongen JA, Voogd AC, Fentiman IS, et al. Long-term results of a randomized trial comparing breast-conserving therapy with mastectomy: European Organization for Research and Treatment of Cancer 10801 trial. *J Natl Cancer Inst.* 2000;92:1143-1150.

6. Clark RM, Whelan T, Levine M, et al. Randomized clinical trial of breast irradiation following lumpectomy and axillary dissection for node-negative breast cancer: an update. Ontario Clinical Oncology Group. *J Natl Cancer Inst.* 1996;88:1659-1664.

7. Fisher B, Bryant J, Dignam JJ, et al. Tamoxifen, radiation therapy, or both for prevention of ipsilateral breast tumor recurrence after lumpectomy in women with invasive breast cancers of one centimeter or less. *J Clin Oncol.* 2002;20:4141-4149.

8. Liljegren G, Holmberg L, Bergh J, et al. 10-year results after sector resection with or without postoperative radiotherapy for stage I breast cancer: a randomized trial. *J Clin Oncol.* 1999;17:2326-2333.

9. Veronesi U, Marubini E, Mariani L, et al. Radiotherapy after breast-conserving surgery in small breast carcinoma: long-term results of a randomized trial. *Ann Oncol.* 2001;12:997-1003.

10. Winzer KJ, Sauer R, Sauerbrei W, et al. Radiation therapy after breast-conserving surgery; first results of a randomised clinical trial in patients with low risk of recurrence. *Eur J Cancer.* 2004;40:998-1005.

11. Clarke M, Collins R, Darby S, et al. Effects of radiotherapy and of differences in the extent of surgery for early breast cancer on local recurrence and 15-year survival: an overview of the randomised trials. *Lancet.* 2005;366:2087-2106.

12. Vinh-Hung V, Verschraegen C. Breast-conserving surgery with or without radiotherapy: pooled-analysis for risks of ipsilateral breast tumor recurrence and mortality. *J Natl Cancer Inst.* 2004;96:115-121.

13. Fisher B, Dignam J, Wolmark N, et al. Lumpectomy and radiation therapy for the treatment of intraductal breast cancer: findings from National Surgical Adjuvant Breast and Bowel Project B-17. *J Clin Oncol.* 1998;16:441-452.

14. Julien JP, Bijker N, Fentiman IS, et al. Radiotherapy in breast-conserving treatment for ductal carcinoma in situ: first results of the EORTC randomised phase III trial 10853. EORTC Breast Cancer Cooperative Group and EORTC Radiotherapy Group. *Lancet.* 2000;355:528-533.

15. Vrieling C, Collette L, Fourquet A, et al. The influence of the boost in breast-conserving therapy on cosmetic outcome in the EORTC "boost versus no boost" trial. EORTC Radiotherapy and Breast Cancer Cooperative Groups. European Organization for Research and Treatment of Cancer. *Int J Radiat Oncol Biol Phys.* 1999;45:677-685.

16. Vrieling C, Collette L, Fourquet A, et al. The influence of patient, tumor and treatment factors on the cosmetic results after breast-conserving therapy in the EORTC 'boost vs. no boost' trial. EORTC Radiotherapy and Breast Cancer Cooperative Groups. *Radiother Oncol.* 2000;55:219-232.

17. Farrow DC, Hunt WC, Samet JM. Geographic variation in the treatment of localized breast cancer. *N Engl J Med.* 1992;326:1097-1101.

18. Lazovich DA, White E, Thomas DB, et al. Underutilization of breast-conserving surgery and radiation therapy among women with stage I or II breast cancer. *JAMA.* 1991;266:3433-3438.

19. Mann BA, Samet JM, Hunt WC, et al. Changing treatment of breast cancer in New Mexico from 1969 through 1985. *JAMA.* 1988;259:3413-3417.

20. Ballard-Barbash R, Potosky AL, Harlan LC, et al. Factors associated with surgical and radiation therapy for early stage breast cancer in older women. *J Natl Cancer Inst.* 1996;88:716-726.

21. Athas WF, Adams-Cameron M, Hunt WC, et al. Travel distance to radiation therapy and receipt of radiotherapy following breast-conserving surgery. *J Natl Cancer Inst.* 2000;92:269-271.

22. Kelemen JJ 3rd, Poulton T, Swartz MT, et al. Surgical treatment of early-stage breast cancer in the Department of Defense Healthcare System. *J Am Coll Surg.* 2001;192:293-297.

23. Schroen AT, Brenin DR, Kelly MD, et al. Impact of patient distance to radiation therapy on mastectomy use in early-stage breast cancer patients. *J Clin Oncol.* 2005;23:7074-7080.

24. Whelan T, Levine M, Gafni A, et al. Mastectomy or lumpectomy? Helping women make informed choices. *J Clin Oncol.* 1999;17:1727-1735.

25. Hughes KS, Schnaper LA, Berry D, et al. Lumpectomy plus tamoxifen with or without irradiation in women 70 years of age or older with early breast cancer. *N Engl J Med.* 2004;351:971-977.

26. Smith BD, Gross CP, Smith GL, et al. Effectiveness of radiation therapy for older women with early breast cancer. *J Natl Cancer Inst.* 2006;98:681-690.

27. Obedian E, Fischer DB, Haffty BG. Second malignancies after treatment of early-stage breast cancer: lumpectomy and radiation therapy versus mastectomy. *J Clin Oncol.* 2000;18:2406-2412.

28. Smith TE, Lee D, Turner BC, et al. True recurrence vs. new primary ipsilateral breast tumor relapse: an analysis of clinical and pathologic differences and their implications in natural history, prognoses, and therapeutic management. *Int J Radiat Oncol Biol Phys.* 2000;48:1281-1289.

29. Recht A, Come, SE, Troyan, S, et al. Local-regional recurrence after mastectomy or breast-conserving therapy. In: Harris JR LM, Morrow M, et al., eds. *Diseases of the Breast.* 2nd ed. Philadelphia, PA: Lippincott Williams & Wilkins; 2000:731-748.

30. Fisher B, Anderson S. Conservative surgery for the management of invasive and noninvasive carcinoma of the breast: NSABP trials. National Surgical Adjuvant Breast and Bowel Project. *World J Surg.* 1994;18:63-69.

31. Holli K, Saaristo R, Isola J, et al. Lumpectomy with or without postoperative radiotherapy for breast cancer with favourable prognostic features: results of a randomized study. *Br J Cancer.* 2001;84:164-169.

32. Uppsala Orebro Breast Cancer Study Group. Sector resection with or without postoperative radiotherapy for stage I breast cancer: a randomized trial. *J Natl Cancer Inst.* 1990;82:1851.

33. Clark RM, McCulloch PB, Levine MN, et al. Randomized clinical trial to assess the effectiveness of breast irradiation following lumpectomy and axillary dissection for node-negative breast cancer. *J Natl Cancer Inst.* 1992;84:683-689.

34. Arthur DW, Vicini FA, Kuske RR, et al. Accelerated partial breast irradiation: an updated report from the American Brachytherapy Society. *Brachytherapy.* 2003;2:124-130.

35. Overgaard M, Jensen MB, Overgaard J, et al. Postoperative radiotherapy in high-risk postmenopausal breast-cancer patients given adjuvant tamoxifen: Danish Breast Cancer Cooperative Group DBCG 82c randomised trial. *Lancet.* 1999;353:1641-1648.

36. Ragaz J, Olivotto IA, Spinelli JJ, et al. Locoregional radiation therapy in patients with high-risk breast cancer receiving adjuvant chemotherapy: 20-year results of the British Columbia randomized trial. *J Natl Cancer Inst.* 2005;97:116-126.

37. Kuske RR BJ, Wilenzick RM, et al. Brachytherapy as the sole method of breast irradiation in Tis, T1, T2, N0-1 breast cancer. *Int J Radiat Oncol Biol Phys.* 1994;30:245.

38. King TA, Bolton JS, Kuske RR, et al. Long-term results of wide-field brachytherapy as the sole method of radiation therapy after segmental mastectomy for T(is,1,2) breast cancer. *Am J Surg.* 2000;180:299-304.

39. Vicini FA, Kestin L, Chen P, et al. Limited-field radiation therapy in the management of early-stage breast cancer. *J Natl Cancer Inst.* 2003;95:1205-1210.

40. Kuske RR, Winter K, Arthur D, et al. A phase I/II trial of brachytherapy alone following lumpectomy for select breast cancer: toxicity analysis of Radiation Therapy Oncology Group 95-17. *Int J Radiat Oncol Biol Phys.* 2002;54:87.

41. Kuske RR, Winter K, Arthur D, et al. A phase II trial of brachytherapy alone following lumpectomy for select breast cancer: tumor control and survival outcomes of RTOG 95-17. *Int J Radiat Oncol Biol Phys.* 2006;66:S29-30.

42. Fentiman IS, Deshmane V, Tong D, et al. Caesium(137) implant as sole radiation therapy for operable breast cancer: a phase II trial. *Radiother Oncol.* 2004;71:281-285.

43. Fentiman IS, Poole C, Tong D, et al. Iridium implant treatment without external radiotherapy for operable breast cancer: a pilot study. *Eur J Cancer.* 1991;27:447-450.

44. Poti Z, Nemeskeri C, Fekeshazy A, et al. Partial breast irradiation with interstitial 60CO brachytherapy results in frequent grade 3 or 4 toxicity. Evidence based on a 12-year follow-up of 70 patients. *Int J Radiat Oncol Biol Phys.* 2004;58:1022-1033.

45. Polgar C, Fodor J, Major T, et al. Radiotherapy confined to the tumor bed following breast conserving surgery current status, controversies, and future projects. *Strahlenther Onkol.* 2002;178:597-606.

46. Polgar C, Major T, Somogyi A, et al. Sole brachytherapy of the tumor bed after breast conserving surgery: a new radiotherapeutic strategy for patients at low risk of local relapse. *Neoplasma.* 1999;46:182-189.

47. Polgar C, Major T, Fodor J, et al. High-dose-rate brachytherapy alone versus whole breast radiotherapy with or without tumor bed boost after breast-conserving surgery: seven-year results of a comparative study. *Int J Radiat Oncol Biol Phys.* 2004;60:1173-1181.

48. Zannis V, Beitsch P, Vicini F, et al. Descriptions and outcomes of insertion techniques of a breast brachytherapy balloon catheter in 1403 patients enrolled in the American Society of Breast Surgeons MammoSite breast brachytherapy registry trial. *Am J Surg.* 2005;190:530-538.

49. Vicini F, Beitsch PD, Quiet CA, et al. Three-year analysis of treatment efficacy, cosmesis, and toxicity by the American Society of Breast Surgeons MammoSite Breast Brachytherapy Registry Trial in patients treated with accelerated partial breast irradiation (APBI). *Cancer.* 2008;112:758-766.

50. Cuttino LW, Keisch M, Jenrette JM, et al. Multi-institutional experience using the MammoSite radiation therapy system (RTS) in the treatment of early-stage breast cancer: 2 year results. *Int J Radiat Oncol Biol Phys.* 2006;66:S30-31.

51. Benitez PR, Streeter O, Vicini F, et al. Preliminary results and evaluation of MammoSite balloon brachytherapy for partial breast irradiation for pure ductal carcinoma in situ: a phase II clinical study. *Am J Surg.* 2006;192:427-433.

52. Kim L, Sebastian L, Gholizan M et al. Initial dosimetric experience with the contura multi-lumen balloon applicator. American Society for Therapeutic Radiology and Oncology (ASTRO) Annual Meeting; 2008; Boston, MA.

53. Yashar CM, Quiet C, Scanderberg V, et al. Use of the breast brachytherapy device (SAVI) to obtain flexible dose modulation for normal structures in close proximity to device. American Society of Clinical Oncology (ASCO) Breast Cancer Symposium; 2008; Washington, DC.

54. Ellerin BE, Seidenfeld J, Formenti SC. A systematic review of post-lumpectomy radiation therapy regimens. *Proc Am Soc Clin Oncol.* 2004;23:683.

55. Suh WW, Pierce LJ, Vicini FA, et al. A cost comparison analysis of partial versus whole-breast irradiation after breast-conserving surgery for early-stage breast cancer. *Int J Radiat Oncol Biol Phys.* 2005;62:790-796.

56. Baglan KL, Sharpe MB, Jaffray D, et al. Accelerated partial breast irradiation using 3D conformal radiation therapy (3D-CRT). *Int J Radiat Oncol Biol Phys.* 2003;55:302-311.

57. Vicini FA, Remouchamps V, Wallace M, et al. Ongoing clinical experience utilizing 3D conformal external beam radiotherapy to deliver partial breast irradiation in patients with early-stage breast cancer treated with breast-conserving therapy. *Int J Radiat Oncol Biol Phys.* 2003;57:1247-1253.

58. Vicini F, Winter K, Straube W, et al. A phase I/II trial to evaluate three-dimensional conformal radiation therapy confined to the region of the lumpectomy cavity for stage I/II breast carcinoma: initial report of feasibility and reproducibility of Radiation Therapy Oncology Group (RTOG) Study 0319. *Int J Radiat Oncol Biol Phys.* 2005;63:1531-1537.

59. Wernicke AG, Gideaa-Addeo D, Magnolfi C, et al. External beam partial breast irradiation following breast-conserving surgery: preliminary results of cosmetic outcome of NYU 00-23. *Int J Radiat Oncol Biol Phys.* 2006;66:S32.

60. Hall E. *Radiobiology for the Radiologist.* 5th ed. Philadelphia, PA: Lippincott Williams & Wilkins: 2000

61. Vaidya JS, Tobias JS, Baum M, et al. Intraoperative radiotherapy for breast cancer. *Lancet Oncol.* 2004;5:165-173.

62. Veronesi U, Gatti G, Luini A, et al. Full-dose intraoperative radiotherapy with electrons during breast-conserving surgery. *Arch Surg.* 2003;138:1253-1256.

63. Tobias JS, Vaidya JS, Keshtgar M, et al. Reducing radiotherapy dose in early breast cancer: the concept of conformal intraoperative brachytherapy. *Br J Radiol.* 2004;77:279-284.

64. Huang J, Barbera L, Brouwers M, et al. Does delay in starting treatment affect the outcomes of radiotherapy? A systematic review. *J Clin Oncol.* 2003;21:555-563.

65. Obedian E, Haffty BG. Negative margin status improves local control in conservatively managed breast cancer patients. *Cancer J Sci Am.* 2000;6:28-33.

66. Park CC, Mitsumori M, Nixon A, et al. Outcome at 8 years after breast-conserving surgery and radiation therapy for invasive breast cancer: influence of margin status and systemic therapy on local recurrence. *J Clin Oncol.* 2000;18:1668-1675.

67. Berle L, Wazer DE, Graham R, et al. Toxicity, local control and cosmesis after interstitial partial breast HDR brachytherapy alone for T1/T2 breast cancer. *Radiother Oncol.* 2004;71.

68. Arthur DW, Koo D, Zwicker RD, et al. Partial breast brachytherapy after lumpectomy: low-dose-rate and high-dose-rate experience. *Int J Radiat Oncol Biol Phys.* 2003;56:681-689.

69. Zellars RC, Stearns V, Asrari F, et al. Feasibility trial of partial breast irradiation with concurrent dose-dense doxorubicin and cyclophosphamide in early-stage breast cancer. *J Clin Oncol.* 2009 Jun 10;27(17):2816-2822.

70. Haffty BG, Vicini FA, Beitsch P, et al. Timing of chemotherapy after MammoSite radiation therapy system breast brachytherapy: analysis of the American Society of Breast Surgeons MammoSite Breast Brachytherapy Registry Trial. *Int J Radiat Oncol Biol Phys.* 2008.

71. Keisch ME, Vicini F, Beitsch P, et al. Two-year actuarial analysis of 198 patients with DCIS treated with accelerated partial breast irradiation (APBI): efficacy, cosmesis and toxicity in patients on the American Society of Breast Surgeons (ASBS) MammoSite Breast Brachytherapy Registry Trial. *Int J Radiat Oncol Biol Phys.* 2006;66:s213.

CHAPTER 96

Postmastectomy Radiation Therapy

Atif J. Khan
Bruce G. Haffty

It is indeed paradoxical that the use postmastectomy radiation therapy (PMRT) continues to cause considerable debate and controversy despite having been the subject of over 20 randomized prospective trials spanning 5 decades of research activity. In fact, some of the first prospective randomized trials ever conducted attempted to define the role of PMRT.[1] Nonetheless, several important questions still await definitive answers.

Historically, PMRT was offered to the majority of women with breast cancer in the early and mid-20th century.[2] Many of these women had locally advanced breast cancer, and oncologists of the time intuitively understood that additional locoregional therapy was needed for these women with a high burden of locoregional disease. Clinicians became cognizant of the potential risks of PMRT at the same time that surgical techniques improved and systemic therapy was developed. Consequently, the role of PMRT in the nascent therapeutic strategy for women with breast cancer came under rigorous scrutiny.

This chapter will focus exclusively on the topic of PMRT and is divided into 4 themes. First, the rationale for PMRT will be considered, by reviewing data supporting the efficacy of PMRT. Because the rationale for any intervention is contingent on the risks of the intervention, the risks and sequelae of PMRT will also be reviewed in this section. Second, data that attempt to shed light on the often vexing problem of appropriate patient selection will be reviewed. Third, breast reconstruction after mastectomy and its relevance to PMRT will be reviewed. Finally, the technique for PMRT will be discussed as well as the related issues of treatment volume and dose.

RATIONALE

Efficacy of PMRT

The efficacy of irradiating the chest wall and draining lymph nodes after mastectomy in improving locoregional control has been firmly established by multiple older trials comparing mastectomy alone to mastectomy with postoperative radiation.[3-9] These trials typically used outdated radiation techniques and equipment that produced orthovoltage x-rays. Orthovoltage x-rays produce suboptimal dose distributions that would never be used for therapy in the modern context. Because of these reasons, the relevance of these older trials is limited in the context of modern radiation therapy, but they adequately demonstrated 2 important facts: (1) PMRT can effectively reduce the burden of residual locoregional disease; and (2) in terms of treatment volume, radiation therapy is more comprehensive and more "radical" than even the most radical surgery. Notably, these trials did not demonstrate improvements in survival end points.

The locoregional effects of adjuvant systemic therapy alone (without radiation) can be studied through those trials of systemic therapy versus nil that have reported patterns of failure.[10-24] In summary, data demonstrating an improvement in locoregional control with systemic cytotoxic chemotherapy are somewhat inconsistent. However, the most recent Early Breast Cancer Trialists Collaborative Group (EBCTCG) meta-analysis of systemic therapy trials reported statistically fewer isolated local relapses in patients receiving polychemotherapy (recurrence rate ratio of 0.63 and 0.70 for women <50 and 50-69, respectively).[25] However, it appears that increasing the intensity or agents of chemotherapy does not improve locoregional control over standard chemotherapy.[26-31] In contrast, adjuvant tamoxifen seems to improve locoregional control rather consistently, reducing the likelihood of recurrence on average by about one-half.[10,12-14,23] This was also demonstrated in the most recent EBCTCG meta analysis just mentioned, which showed an isolated local recurrence rate ratio of 0.47 with tamoxifen versus without.[25] These observations, along with the demonstrable improvement in survival with systemic agents, call into question the relative benefit of PMRT in improving locoregional and survival end points in patients who have received or will receive systemic therapy.

Several trials have studied the efficacy and added benefit of PMRT in the presence of systemic therapy.[32-44] The most definitive of these have come from the Danish Breast Cancer Cooperative Group[40,41] and the British Columbia Cancer Agency.[42] In addition to these, the updated findings of EBCTCG meta-analysis of postoperative radiation trials, which will be discussed later,[45] have decisively altered practice and reaffirmed the role of PMRT in modern breast oncology.

The Danish Breast Cancer Cooperative Group's protocol 82b randomized premenopausal women with high-risk breast cancer after modified radical mastectomy (total mastectomy and level 1 and 2 axillary dissection) to either 9 cycles of CMF chemotherapy or to 8 cycles of CMF chemotherapy and radiation therapy to the chest wall and regional nodes between the first and second cycles of chemotherapy.[40] High-risk status was defined as positive lymph nodes, tumor size greater than 5 cm, or invasion of the skin or pectoralis fascia. Radiation therapy was delivered to a total dose of 50 Gy in 25 fractions or 48 Gy in 22 fractions using an anterior electron field to treat the chest wall and internal mammary nodes (IMNs) and a matched anterior photon field to treat the supraclavicular, infraclavicular and axilla lymph nodes. A posterior axillary photon field was used in patients with a large anterior-posterior separation. Over 92% of all patients were treated with megavoltage equipment. The study enrolled 1708 patients from 1982 to 1989. With a median follow-up of 114 months, the irradiated group demonstrated statistically significant improvements in locoregional recurrence (32% vs 9%), disease-free survival (35% vs 48% at 10 years), and overall survival (45% vs 54% at 10 years). Notably, over half of all locoregional recurrences were on the chest wall.

In the companion 82c protocol,[41] postmenopausal women younger than 70 with high-risk breast cancer (defined as in 82b) were randomized after modified radical mastectomy to receive either 30 mg of tamoxifen daily for 1 year beginning 2 to 4 weeks after surgery alone or with concurrent radiation therapy delivered to the chest wall and draining lymph nodes. Radiotherapy details were identical to the 82b trial. Similar to the 82b trial, over 90% of women were treated with megavoltage equipment. Between 1982 and 1990, a total of 1375 patients were recruited and followed for a median time of 10 years. As in the 82b study, the irradiated group demonstrated statistically significant improvements in locoregional recurrence (35% vs 8%), disease-free survival (24% vs 36%), and overall survival (36% vs 45%). Again, the majority of locoregional recurrences were on the chest wall, but the proportion of recurrences at all locoregional subsites was lower with PMRT than without. The Danish investigators deserve much praise for

these well-designed efforts, which although not without flaw (as will be discussed later), clearly demonstrated that in certain patient subsets, aggressive locoregional control could translate into improved survival—independent of systemic therapy.

The British Columbia trial enrolled 318 node-positive premenopausal breast cancer patients and randomized them after modified radical mastectomy to either radiation therapy or no additional locoregional therapy.[42] Both groups received adjuvant CMF chemotherapy for 12 months (first 80 patients) or 6 months. Radiation therapy was delivered to the chest wall to a dose of 37.5 Gy in 16 daily fractions through opposed tangential photon fields. The supraclavicular and axilla nodes were treated with an AP field and a posterior axillary field, as is conventionally done, with a target midaxilla dose of 35 Gy. Bilateral IMNs were treated with an additional anterior field to a dose of 37.5 Gy in 16 fractions. All treatments were delivered with cobalt machines, between cycle 4 and 5 of chemotherapy. After a median follow-up of 20 years, the 20-year survival free of locoregional disease developing before systemic disease was 61% in the chemotherapy alone arm and 87% in the irradiated group. The irradiated group had significantly higher 20-year event-free survival (25% vs 38%), systemic disease-free survival (31% vs 48%), breast-cancer-specific survival (38% vs 53%), and overall survival (37% vs 47%). There were slightly more non-breast-cancer deaths in the irradiated group (9% vs 4%, $p = 0.11$). There were 3 cardiac deaths (2%) in the irradiated group versus 1 (0.6%) in the control group ($p = 0.62$), and 9% of patients in the irradiated group developed arm edema compared with 3% in the control group ($p = 0.035$).

The EBCTCG has collected primary data from every randomized trial of adjuvant radiotherapy in breast cancer, and periodically reports the ongoing analyses on the benefits and risks of radiation therapy in these patients. The most recent report from 2005 reviewed data on 9933 patients enrolled on 25 trials of PMRT, all of which were unconfounded by the use of systemic therapy.[45] Node-positive patients who had axillary clearance and received radiation therapy after mastectomy had a 5-year locoregional recurrence rate of 6%, compared to 23% for unirradiated controls (15 year rates were 8% vs 29%). In every large trial of PMRT in node-positive women, radiation therapy produced comparable proportional reductions in local recurrence in all women irrespective of age or tumor characteristics and regardless of time period—indeed a powerful demonstration of the efficacy of radiation therapy in reducing local recurrence.

Because the proportional reductions in local failures were similar across heterogeneous patient groups, the absolute reductions in local recurrence were variable and dependent on the *control risk*, that is, larger reductions were seen in subsets with greater risk and smaller reductions were noted in women with lower risk. For patients with a control risk of local recurrence that exceeded 10%, the addition of RT improved local recurrence irrespective of systemic therapy (chemotherapy and/or hormonal therapy). Importantly, the overall 17% absolute improvement in *5-year* local control translated into a 5.4% absolute improvement in *15-year* breast cancer mortality (60.1% vs 54.7%, $2p = 0.0002$).[45] In terms of absolute effects, a 4:1 ratio of benefit was seen, whereby a 20% absolute reduction in 5-year local recurrence resulted in a 5% absolute reduction in 15-year breast cancer mortality. Furthermore, women with node-positive disease who were irradiated after mastectomy and axillary clearance experienced a 4.4% absolute improvement in all-cause mortality over controls ($2p = 0.0009$), a difference not detected in the prior EBCTCG report published in 2000.[46]

In their review of the EBCTCG data, Punglia and associates note that treatments that had little or no effect on decreasing the 5-year local recurrence rate produced no benefit in 15-year breast cancer mortality.[47] They also draw attention to a subgroup analysis in the report that showed that the use of radiation therapy after mastectomy in node-positive patients improved 15-year survival only in patients who also received adjuvant systemic therapy and not in patients who were treated with mastectomy alone. This lends credence to the concept of an independent yet cooperative effect of adjuvant locoregional therapy and adjuvant systemic therapy.

Updated data from the EBCTCG was presented at the 2007 annual meeting of the American Society of Clinical Oncology.[48] In contrast to prior reports, the subgroup of patients with 1 to 3 positive lymph nodes demonstrated statistically significant improvements in 15-year breast cancer mortality (50.9% vs 43.3%, $2p = 0.002$) and all-cause mortality (56.1% vs 50.9%, $2p = 0.05$) with PMRT. In addition, a study of prognostic factors for 5-year local recurrence risks identified tumor grade as a highly significant factor, even when controlling for other known risk factors. These findings will undoubtedly be expounded upon in the next full report from the EBCTCG trialists.

The value of the EBCTCG overview cannot be overstated. However, the relevance of its findings may be limited by the inclusion of trials that used fractionation schemes, treatment machines, and treatment volumes that are antiquated by today's standards, as well as by the other limitations inherent to all meta-analyses. Attempts to correct for these limitations suggest that the EBCTCG results may actually *underestimate* the benefit of PMRT. For example, Van de Steene and coworkers conducted a similar meta-analysis and demonstrated improved odds ratios for survival with PMRT by excluding trials that began before 1970, trials with small sample sizes (< 600 patients), trials with poor survival rates (crude survival less than 80%), and trials that used outdated fractionation schemes.[49] Similarly, Whelan and associates performed a meta-analysis of PMRT trials that specifically included systemic therapy in both the control and experimental groups.[50] As with the EBCTCG study, the addition of RT led to reductions in the risk of any recurrence (odds ratio = 0.69) and death (odds ratio = 0.83). Finally, Gebski and colleagues performed a meta-analysis in which they carefully attempted to control for the quality of radiation delivery in PMRT trials. The authors defined optimal dose as 40 to 60 Gy delivered in 2-Gy fractions (nonconventional fractionation schemes were converted to 2-Gy equivalents using bioeffective dose calculations) and appropriate treatment volumes as both chest wall and regional lymphatics (but not necessarily inclusive of the IMNs).[51] The data from the EBCTCG meta-analyses were then reanalyzed applying these criteria. Locoregional control was greater for trials with optimal dose and volume (80%), compared to those with suboptimal dose (70%) or volume (64%). An improvement in breast

cancer mortality was limited to those trials that used appropriate doses and fields for irradiation (6.4% absolute increase in survival, $p < 0.001$).

It is worth noting that the survival improvements demonstrated in the collective Danish and British Columbia experiments are among the most remarkable improvements in survival ever reported for any adjuvant therapy in a randomized trial. Taken together, these studies show that certain patient cohorts have a high risk for locoregional recurrence that cannot be addressed by systemic therapy alone. Reducing the rates of locoregional failure can result in improved survival, perhaps because persistent or recurrent locoregional disease serves as a source of distant metastases and subsequent death. The collective PMRT data seems to indicate that adjuvant locoregional therapy and adjuvant systemic therapy independently benefit patients on the principle of spatial cooperation, with the former addressing microscopic locoregional residual disease and the latter addressing systemic micrometastases.

Risks of PMRT

Perhaps the most concerning risk of PMRT for treating physicians is the risk of radiation-induced cardiac morbidity. As described earlier, the EBCTCG meta-analysis as well as other registry data have detected increased risks of cardiac mortality in irradiated patients.[45,46,52] An older meta-analysis by Cuzick and colleagues contributed significantly to the PMRT discourse.[53,54] First published in 1987 and then updated in 1994, the meta-analysis pooled data from 10 early trials (all initiated before 1975 and all without chemotherapy) of mastectomy with or without PMRT, and, in the second report, attempted to define cause-specific mortality in over 4000 patients who died at least 10 years after enrolling on study.[53,54] The time period during which these trial were conducted saw an important shift of surgical technique away from radical mastectomy to less radical surgery. In women who had a radical mastectomy, an 18% deficit in all-cause mortality was found in women who received radiation therapy compared to controls who were observed. However, there was no difference in the group that had either simple or modified radical mastectomy followed by RT versus those who were observed. There was a nonsignificant 7% decrement in survival reported for all patients who received radiation therapy ($p = 0.21$). Older, node-negative women treated on the earlier trials with radical mastectomy contributed most to this observed decrement. Cause-specific mortality analysis revealed an excess of cardiac mortality in patients who received radiation therapy, and was greatest in the 3 trials in which the largest doses were given. The standardized mortality ratio (SMR) for cardiac mortality for left- versus right-sided irradiation was 1.34 ($p = 0.09$). Breast-cancer mortality was improved with PMRT and tended to balance cardiac-related mortality at 10 years. Nonetheless, the meta-analysis by Cuzick and associates raised significant concerns in the oncology community about the safety of PMRT, although it was clearly burdened by all the usual limitations of a meta-analysis of older trials.

There was excess mortality from heart disease and lung cancer in women studied on the updated EBCTCG report (including women treated with an intact breast), as well as and excess cancer incidence mainly in the contralateral breast and lung. The averaged detrimental effects of irradiation were minor, with 15-year absolute loss of 1.8% for contralateral breast cancer and 1.3% for non-breast-cancer mortality. Importantly, the proportional excess of non-breast-cancer deaths was greatest 5 to 14 years and >15 years after randomization, and the mean dates of randomization for these 2 groups were 1975 and 1970, respectively. The authors of the EBCTCG correctly note that the late hazards evident in their report could well be substantially lower for modern radiation therapy technique and regimens.

An analysis of the Danish postmastectomy trial patients by Hojris and associates found equal rates of ischemic heart disease and acute myocardial infarction (MI) in the irradiated and unirradiated group.[55] Approximately 3% of patients in both groups had ischemia-related morbidity at a median follow-up of 117 months, and less than 1% of patients in both arms had death due to cardiac causes, with no notable differences when comparing left- versus right-sided irradiation. It should be mentioned that the Danish investigators deserve praise for their careful technique aimed at minimizing cardiac irradiation; the authors used customized blocks and all patients had a chest wall ultrasound to measure chest wall thickness so the correct electron energy could be selected for the IM field. On the one hand, these numbers can be interpreted to mean that, with good technique, the cardiac risks are minimal; on the other, these numbers may underestimate the true burden of radiation-related cardiac morbidity due to the competing risk of breast-cancer death in this high-risk population, and also because this study was an unplanned retrospective report on a prospectively studied patient cohort.

In their review of 960 patients treated on the first Stockholm Breast Cancer Trial (modified radical mastectomy alone vs preoperative vs postoperative RT accrued 1971-1976), Gyenes and associates reported 58 acute MI in the study population for a crude rate of 6%.[56] There were no differences in acute MI or death due to cardiovascular disease (n = 63/960) between irradiated and unirradiated patients. In addition, only patients in the high-dose-volume group had an excess hazard of cardiovascular death (HR 2, 95% CI 1.0-3.9, $p = 0.04$). A retrospective study by Harris and coworkers examined cardiac events in a series of 961 women irradiated to the intact breast and reported no interaction between left- versus right-sided RT on cardiac mortality or congestive heart disease.[57] However, a significant association was noted between left-sided irradiation and the subsequent development of coronary artery disease (20-year actuarial risk 25% vs 10% for right-sided, $p < 0.001$) and MI (15% vs 5%, $p < 0.002$). In their experience, coexistent hypertension was an independent hazard for the development of coronary artery disease.

A study of the SEER database conducted by Giordano and colleagues compared 15-year cardiac mortality rates in left- versus right-sided breast cancer as a function of the year of diagnosis in patients who received RT.[58] As in other studies, the presumption was that patients with left-sided lesions received more heart irradiation than those with right-sided lesions. Although the authors demonstrated excess cardiac mortality in left-sided breast cancer patients diagnosed from 1973 to 1979 (13% vs 10%,

$p = 0.02$), they found no significant difference in patients irradiated in the most recent time periods (approximately 9% for both groups in the 1980-1984 cohort, and 5-6% in the 1985-1989 cohort). Beginning in 1979, the hazard of death from ischemic heart disease in left-sided breast cancer patients (vs right-sided) declined by an average of 6% per year. Taken together, these data are certainly reassuring and imply that improvements in image-based treatment delivery should further reduce cardiac morbidity associated with radiation therapy.

Additional non-life-threatening late risks of postmastectomy radiation can include arm edema, fibrosis, shoulder stiffness, and brachial plexopathy. In a valuable report from the Danish postmastectomy trialists, patients irradiated at Aarhus University Hospital who were alive and without evidence of disease were invited to participate in a study of the late effects of PMRT.[59] Eighty-four patients accepted the invitation and were eligible for analysis, and these patients were carefully assessed for late toxicity based primarily on LENT-SOMA criteria. More women in the irradiated group had lymphedema (17% vs 9%) and impaired shoulder movement (16% vs 2%) that interfered with work or daily activities. Irradiated patients also had more arm paresthesias (21% vs 7%) and more arm weakness (14% vs 3%). Perhaps because this analysis was limited by small numbers, only the decline in shoulder function reached statistical significance. Symptomatic pulmonary complications and cardiac events were equal in irradiated and unirradiated patients. In a separate report of 161 patients with neurologic follow-up who were irradiated on the Danish 82 protocols, 5% of patients had disabling and 8% had mild radiation-induced brachial plexopathies.[60] Finally, Kunht and associates reported acute and chronic reactions in 194 patients receiving PMRT. Twenty-two percent of patients had any incidence of chronic effects, mostly from arm edema (28/43).[61] Five patients had telangiectasia and 1 patient had plexopathy.

In summary, randomized trials as well as data from meta-analyses provide a strong rationale for PMRT in patients at high risk for residual locoregional disease, regardless of the use of systemic therapy in these patients. Additional locoregional therapy in the form of RT reduces LR recurrence rates by a factor of approximately two-thirds, and 1 breast-cancer death is averted for every 4 LR recurrences prevented by RT. The risks of PMRT are modest but demonstrable, and cardiac effects may largely be attributable to radiotherapy techniques and schedules no longer in use. The cardiac detriment of modern-day PMRT is unknown.

PATIENT SELECTION

Node-Positive Patients

Axillary node-positivity is the most significant predictor of locoregional recurrence after mastectomy. It should be remembered, however, that approximately two-thirds of locoregional recurrences occur on the chest wall, and that axillary failures are far less common.[62-65] Therefore the degree of node positivity should be viewed as a nonspecific surrogate for locoregional recurrence risk (ie, risk not limited to axillary failure).

The Danish and Canadian PMRT trials demonstrated stable relative risk reductions for all events in all groups of node-positive patients. However, there are 2 general criticisms of these studies that limit the translation of these findings to all node-positive patients: (1) the adequacy of the systemic therapy in the control arms of these studies and (2) the issue of the "background risk" in the study populations.

The EBCTCG meta-analysis of systemic therapy revealed a modest but statistically significant improvement for anthracycline-containing polychemotherapy regimens over CMF-based regimens.[25] How this small incremental benefit affects locoregional control is unknown, but a significant benefit in patients with high risk for locoregional microscopic residual seems unlikely. For example, we do know that neither the addition of taxanes nor increases in the intensity or density of chemotherapy demonstrably improve locoregional control in node-positive patients, although they do improve survival end points, presumably by addressing micrometastases.[26-31] Given these data it is probably safe to conclude that present-day chemotherapy regimens would not significantly alter the findings of the postmastectomy trials. However, the Danish 82c trial treated the postmenopausal patients (untested for ER/PR status) with only 1 year of tamoxifen[41] and it is unknown how a longer duration of hormonal therapy in an exclusively hormone-receptor-positive population would modulate the risk of locoregional recurrence and, in turn, the benefit of PMRT.

The second and more significant issue that limits interpretation of the Danish and British Columbia trials is that node-positive patients on the control arms of these trials had higher locoregional recurrence rates than commonly reported for patients treated in the United States and elsewhere.[40-42,62] This difference is even more apparent in the subgroup of patients with 1 to 3 positive lymph nodes, who comprised about 60% of patients on

these studies. The 18-year probability of locoregional recurrence (as first site of failure) was 59% for patients with 4 or more positive nodes, and 37% for those with 1 to 3 positive nodes in the control arms of the Danish trials.[66] Similarly, the 20-year *isolated* locoregional recurrence rate was 41% for patients with 4 or more positive nodes, and 21% for patients with 1 to 3 positive nodes on the control arm of the Canadian trial.[42] Locoregional recurrence developing any time before distant failure (ie, cumulative LRR as first failure) was 39% for the entire unirradiated group, but was not reported by number of positive nodes.

In contrast to this, several large series of patients treated in the United States and elsewhere have reported locoregional recurrence rates in the range of 6% to 13% for patients with 1 to 3 positive nodes (Table 96-1).[63,64,67,68] For example, Recht and associates reviewed the ECOG experience of over 2000 node-positive patients treated with adjuvant systemic therapy but without RT. The 10-year rate of LRR (with or without distant failure) was 13% for patients with 1 to 3 positive nodes, and 29% for patients with 4 or more involved nodes.[64] The MD Anderson Cancer Center (MDACC) reviewed recurrence data for postmastectomy patients treated on studies of doxorubicin-based chemotherapy without RT. The 10-year actuarial total LRR was 13% for patients with 1 to 3 positive nodes and 26% for patients with more than 3 positive nodes.[63] This seems to indicate that the background risk for locoregional recurrence in the Danish and BC trials was higher than average, and this may have exaggerated the benefit of PMRT in this population.

Differences in axillary surgical evaluation may account for these differences: a median of 7 lymph nodes were removed in the Danish studies and a median of 11 lymph nodes were examined in patients on the Canadian trial.[40-42] These differences in axillary evaluation may have shifted the entire spectrum of risk; patients scored as having 1 to 3 positive lymph nodes may actually have

TABLE 96-1 Locoregional Recurrence Rates in Patients Not Treated with Radiation after Mastectomy in Randomized Clinical Trials

Patterns-of-Failure Studies	No. Patients	Locoregional Recurrence Rates at 10 Years (%)
NSABP[67]		
1-3 + LN	2957	6-11
≥ 4 + LN	2784	14-25
IBCSG[70]		
1-3 + LN	2408	14-27
≥ 4 + LN	1659	24-35
ECOG[64]		
1-3 + LN	1018	13
≥ 4 + LN	998	29
MD Anderson[63]		
1-3 + LN	466	13
≥ 4 + LN	419	26

ECOG, Eastern Cooperative Oncology Group; IBCSG, International Breast Cancer Study Group; NSABP, National Surgical Adjuvant Breast and Bowel Project.

had 4 or more positive nodes on full dissection. This in turn could have magnified the benefits of PMRT. Tellingly, failure in the axilla either alone or as a component of LRR represented 43% of all LRR in the Danish studies,[62] compared to 14% in the MDACC study cited in the preceding paragraph.[63]

Although the differences in the extent of axillary evaluation may account for the differences in the control risk observed between the PMRT trial population and the other reported populations, it should be noted that the studies in Table 96-1 have reported results typically at a median of 10 years of follow-up. In contrast, the Danish studies report 18-year recurrence rates, and also document a consistent LRR of about 1% per year between follow-up years 10 and 25.[62] Similarly, in the BC trial, which has reported 20-year recurrence rates, approximately 20% of LRRs occurred after follow-up year 10.[42] Other identified and unidentified risk factors, such as T4 tumors and/or pectoral fascia invasion, may have been over-represented in the postmastectomy trials,[62] increasing the background risk for locoregional failure. For example, in a combined report of patients with 1 to 3 positive axillary nodes treated on the control arm of the British Columbia postmastectomy trial (n = 82) and similar patients treated on prospective systemic therapy trials at the MDACC (n = 462), statistically significant differences were detected in patients on the BC trial who were younger (median age 43 vs 48) and had more lympovascular invasion (52% vs 33%), in addition to fewer examined nodes (median 10 vs 16).[69] The resultant 10-year Kaplan–Meier estimates of LRR were 21.5% and 12.6% for the BC and MDACC patients, respectively.

Still, several reports have demonstrated the prognostic impact of total dissected nodes, nodal ratio (number of involved to uninvolved nodes), and number of total uninvolved nodes on LRR and even overall survival.[63,64,67-72] Indeed, in the combined BC/MDACC study described above, nodal ratio greater than 0.20 was reliably associated with a 10-year LRR > 20% across both groups of patients.[69] Attempts by Danish investigators to reanalyze their patients to include only those with adequate dissections are limited by the fact that these patients were not stratified by this important risk factor at randomization.[73] This issue remains unclear and contested and will perhaps be settled by ongoing randomized trials (see "Future Directions" later in the chapter). The American Society of Therapeutic Radiology and Oncology (ASTRO), the American Society of Clinical Oncology (ASCO), and other advisory organizations have endorsed the routine use of PMRT in women with 4 or more involved nodes and node-positive women with tumors greater than 5 cm; these groups have a high (> 20-25%) risk of locoregional recurrence without RT.[74-77] Both societies recognize the uncertain benefit of PMRT in patients with T1/T2 primaries with 1 to 3 positive nodes (stage II) in whom the risk of LRR is intermediate (around 10-20%).[75,76]

Given this uncertainty in intermediate risk patients, several groups have attempted to identify patients within the 1 to 3 positive lymph node group who may benefit from PMRT (Table 96-2). This group of patients is heterogenous in terms of various potential clinicopathologic factors that may allow differentiation into low- and high-risk cohorts. An important

TABLE 96-2 Variables Associated with 10-year Locoregional Recurrence Risk Exceeding 15% after Mastectomy and Chemotherapy in Patients with 1-3 Positive Lymph Nodes

Study	No. Patients	Variables
Wallgren et al[68]	2404	Premenopausal, G2 or G3, LVSI Postmenopausal, G3 Postmenopausal, G2, T2 disease
Taghian et al[67]	2403	Age < 50, T2 disease
Recht et al[64]	1018	Premenopausal, T1 disease
Truong et al[72]	821	Age < 45* 25% of lymph nodes involved* ER-negative disease* G3 disease T2 disease LVSI Medial tumor location*
Katz et al[78]	466	Tumor size > 4 cm Invasion of skin/nipple Invasion of pectoralis fascia Close or positive margins

DF, distant failure; ER, estrogen receptor; G2 or 3, grade 2 or 3; LRF, local-regional failure, LVSI, lymphovascular space invasion.
*Retain significance on multivariate analysis.

effort came from the Ludwig investigators who reviewed data on over 5300 patients enrolled on the first 7 trials of the International Breast Cancer Study Group (IBCSG).[68] These trials of systemic therapy required a minimum of 8 dissected lymph nodes and negative margins. In the node-positive patients, multivariate analysis revealed that 4 or more positive nodes and high grade were independent predictors of increased LRR, and LVI and tumor size larger than 2 cm were additional risk factors in premenopausal and postmenopausal patients, respectively. In patients with 1 to 3 involved lymph nodes, premenopausal patients with LVI and grade 3 tumors had cumulative incidence functions (CIFs) exceeding 20% for any LRR. Postmenopausal women with grade 3 tumors and tumors larger than 2 cm also had high risk. In a later report, the same group reported results from IBCSG trials 1 to 9 and demonstrated the significant independent impact, in a multivariate model, of the number of uninvolved lymph nodes.[70] In the group of patients with 1 to 3 lymph nodes (n = 2402), factors that independently predicted a CIF for LRR exceeding 20% included age younger than 40, fewer than 10 uninvolved lymph nodes, and LVI.

The MDACC has reported results from their cohort of 1031 patients treated on 5 prospective trials between 1975 and 1994 with mostly cyclophosphamide- and doxorubicin-based chemotherapy without subsequent radiation therapy.[63,71,78] Katz and associates reported 3 factors significant for isolated and total LRR on multivariate analysis of the entire group: T stage, number of involved nodes, and extranodal extension ≥ 2 mm. Restricting the analysis to patients with T1/T2 disease and 1 to 3 axillary nodes (n = 404, overall isolated 10-year LRR risk of 10%), multivariate predictors of LRR were fewer examined nodes, higher T stage, and extracapsular extension (ECE), with isolated 10-year LRR in excess of 25% for patients with ECE (33%) and tumor size greater than 4 cm (26%).[63] In a study of pathologic factors predictive of LRR, Katz and associates reported that close or positive margins and gross multicentric disease were also predictive of LRR on multivariable analysis.[78] Other predictors for higher LRR in the subgroup of patients with 1 to 3 positive nodes included invasion of skin and nipple, pectoral fascia invasion, and close or positive margins, but not multicentricity. This experience is corroborated by Fowble and associates, who reported that patients with multicentric disease had a 5-year actuarial risk of an isolated LRR of only 8% in the absence of other risk factors for postmastectomy chest wall relapse.[79]

The MDACC group also performed an RPA analysis on all patients (including those with 4 or more nodes) to assign relative weights to the various prognostic factors, focusing especially on nodal ratio and pathologic tumor size.[71] In the 913 patients with available data, a nodal ratio of greater than 0.20 was the most significant predictor of LRR, and patients with higher nodal ratios and tumor sizes 3.5 cm or more had LRR rates of 40% at 8 years, while those with nodal ratios less than 0.20 and tumor size less than 5 cm had a low risk of LRR (10% at 8 years).

Truong and coworkers reported on 821 women with T1 and T2 primary lesions with 1 to 3 positive lymph nodes treated with mastectomy and systemic therapy (in 94%) within the British Columbia Cancer Agency.[72] Twelve candidate clinicopathologic factors were tested in a multivariate model for their effect on LRR. Age less than 45, nodal ratio greater than 25%, ER-negative status, and medial location independently predicted for isolated and any LRR, with age having the greatest effect (hazard ratio 3.44). The authors suggested using age and nodal ratio as first-line discriminants of risk, and medial location and ER-negative status as secondary factors.

Recht and colleagues reported on the outcomes of over 2016 patients enrolled on 4 randomized ECOG studies of systemic therapy with a median follow-up of 12 years. A total of 983 patients had tumors 5 cm or less and 1 to 3 positive lymph nodes. In a multivariate analysis of all patients, increasing tumor size, increasing number of positive nodes, ER-negative status, and decreasing number of examined nodes were significant independent predictors of LRR.[64] Cheng and colleagues identified 110 patients with 1 to 3 positive axillary nodes treated at their institution with modified radical mastectomy and systemic therapy but without radiation (median number of nodes examined, 17).[80] Sixty-nine patients received adjuvant chemotherapy and 84 received adjuvant hormonal therapy with tamoxifen. The 4 most significant factors on univariate analysis (age < 40 years, tumor ≥ 3 cm, ER-negative disease, and lymphovascular invasion) could segregate patients into high-risk (with 3 or 4 factors) and low-risk groups (with 2 or fewer factors). On multivariate analysis, only tumor size (< 3 cm vs > 3 cm) was significant for LRR. In a similar Hungarian study of 249 patients with T1 and T2 tumors with 1 to 3 positive axillary nodes, half of whom were treated with PMRT,[81] only age (≤ 45 years) and size (T2) emerged as independent predictors of LRR on multivariate analysis.

Node-Negative Patients

The most recent EBCTCG overview demonstrated a modest 5-year local recurrence rate of 6% after mastectomy and axillary clearance in node-negative patients. The addition of PMRT reduced this rate to 2% ($2p = 0.0002$), producing a small absolute 5-year gain of 4%.[45] Given the low overall risk of LRR in node-negative patients, PMRT is not routinely indicated. Nonetheless, several investigators have attempted to identify subsets within the node-negative group who have LRR risks high enough to warrant PMRT.

In a multivariate analysis of the IBCSG trial patients (discussed earlier in the "Node-Positive Patients" section), vessel invasion was a significant risk factor of LRR in node-negative patients, as was size larger than 2 cm in premenopausal node-negative patients.[68] Jagsi and associates reported a retrospective analysis of a cohort of 870 node-negative patients (excluding T4 patients) treated with modified radical mastectomy without RT at the Massachusetts General Hospital between 1980 and 2000.[82] A multivariate analysis of several potential risk factors for total LRR revealed 4 significant independent predictors: margin status (< 2 mm), premenopausal status, size (> 2 cm), and LVI. Of these, premenopausal status and LVI had the greatest hazard ratios (3.8 and 3.2, respectively). The 10-year total LRR rates were approximately 20% with 2 adverse factors and 40% with 3 adverse factors; however, approximately two-thirds of the patients in this cohort did not receive systemic therapy.

Floyd and associates published a study on 70 patients with pathologic T3N0 disease treated at multiple centers with mastectomy and systemic therapy, but without radiation, and reported a 5-year locoregional recurrence of only 8%[83] Those who had LVSI had a 21% locoregional recurrence compared to a 4% rate for those without LVSI. Taghian and coworkers reported results on 313 patients with pathologic stage T3N0 disease who were treated with mastectomy, systemic treatment, and no radiation on NSABP clinical trials.[84] The 10-year LRR for this series was only 7%, with 24 of the 28 locoregional recurrences developing only on the chest wall.

Truong and colleagues focused exclusively on patients with T1/T2 node-negative breast cancer treated within the British Columbia Cancer Agency and examined clinicopathologic data on this patient cohort from their Outcome Database.[85] The actuarial 10-year LRR risk was 8% in 1505 such women treated with mastectomy without RT. Grade, LVI, T stage, and systemic therapy use were all statistically significant independent predictors of LRR. Recursive partitioning analysis revealed the first split at presence of histologic grade 3 (actuarial 10-year rate of LRR 12% vs 6%). The simultaneous presence of LVI increased the Kaplan–Meier estimate for 10-year LRR to 21%. In patients with grade 3 disease without LVI, patients with T2 tumors and no systemic therapy had a 10-year LRR in excess of 20%. On a similar note, Yildirim and associates reported on 502 patients treated with modified radical mastectomy for T1/T2 node-negative disease in a retrospective study from Ankara Oncology Hospital in Turkey.[86] With a median follow-up of 77 months, only 3% of patients had LRR. Although the numbers were small, multivariate analysis identified tumor size larger than 2 cm and LVI as predictors for high LRR risk in women upto 40 years and tumor size larger than 3 cm, LVI, grade, and HER-2 status as risk factors in the older women. The 10-year risk of LRR exceeded 30% for younger women with both risk factors, and older women with at least 3 risk factors. Finally, Cheng and coworkers have reported on gene expression profiles that are predictive of LRR after mastectomy, although the number of locoregional events in their patients with 1 to 3 positive nodes was very small.[87] Tissue and gene expression markers hold promise as valuable predictors of clinical behavior in postmastectomy patients.

Margin Status

Margin status is a risk factor for local failure in multiple solid tumor types. However, information documenting and quantifying the risk of LRR in postmastectomy patients is scarce because margin issues are decidedly uncommon after mastectomy. Furthermore, interpreting the available data is complicated by the variable definitions of close or positive margins and the small denominators in the handful of existing reports. In what is probably the most extensive experience, the British Columbia Cancer Agency group identified 94 women with tumor at the inked margin of resection after mastectomy in their Outcomes Database.[88] Forty-one of these patients received PMRT, while 53 did not; the cumulative crude LRR was 11.3% versus 4.9% in observed and irradiated groups, respectively, with no significant difference between the 2 groups. Factors that resulted in a cumulative crude LRR of

approximately 20% (17%-23%) in the unirradiated group were aged upto ≤ 50 years, T2 tumor size, grade III histology, and LVI. The corresponding rates with RT were in the single digits (0-9%), but all comparisons were limited by small numbers and were nonsignificant. Notably, none of the 22 women with positive margins without these associated features had LRR. Freedman and associates reviewed 34 patients with close or positive margins (tumor margin ≤ 10 mm; n = 2 for tumor at margin) after mastectomy whose primary tumor was smaller than 5 cm with 0 to 3 positive axillary nodes and who received no postoperative radiation.[89] Five chest wall recurrences appeared at a median interval of 26 months (range, 7-127 months), resulting in an 8-year cumulative incidence of a chest wall recurrence of 18%. The risk of local relapse was confined to younger women (age 50 or younger) compared to older women (28% vs 0 at 8 years, p = 0.04). In a multivariate analysis by Katz and associates of factors predictive of LRR in patients treated with mastectomy and chemotherapy without irradiation, close or positive margins were a significant independent predictor of LRR.[78] Although only 29 patients were available for the margin analysis, the 10-year LRR was 45%; interestingly, the risk was 33% for those with pectoralis fascia invasion even when negative margins were achieved.

POST-INDUCTION CHEMOTHERAPY

With the widespread use of neoadjuvant chemotherapy, new questions regarding the indications for PMRT have emerged. As discussed above, risk stratification after mastectomy is based largely on pathologic findings in the mastectomy specimens. However, induction chemotherapy changes the extent of pathologic disease in most patients, and almost certainly affects the risk discriminants traditionally used to select patients for PMRT. Bucholz and coworkers addressed this issue in a comparative study of 150 postmastectomy patients treated with neoadjuvant and 1031 postmastectomy patients treated with adjuvant chemotherapy.[90] The locoregional recurrence rate associated with a particular pathologic extent of disease after surgery was higher among patients treated with induction chemotherapy compared to those who had up-front surgery. This makes intuitive sense in that this was a comparison between the extent of residual disease after chemotherapy and original, untreated disease. These findings suggest that both pretreatment disease factors and the extent of pathologic residual disease after chemotherapy should be considered in assessing risk for LRR.

A subsequent report by Huang and colleagues established the efficacy of PMRT after neoadjuvant chemotherapy and also attempted to identify features that would predict for higher LRR rates if RT was omitted.[91] The authors studied a cohort of 676 patients treated on institutional protocols of doxorubicin-based neoadjuvant chemotherapy followed by mastectomy. One-hundred and thirty-four of these patients had PMRT while the remainder (n = 542) did not. Because patients were offered RT at the discretion of the treating radiation oncologist, the irradiated cohort had significant overrepresentation of adverse prognostic factors such as higher T-stage and N-stage, residual after chemotherapy, number of positive nodes, and close/involved margins. Nonetheless, the locoregional recurrence rate was significantly lower in the group treated with PMRT (10-year actuarial locoregional recurrence rates were 11% and 22%, respectively, $p = 0.0001$). RT significantly reduced the risk of developing LRR in patients with 4 or more positive nodes and residual tumor larger than 2 cm after chemotherapy (10-year rates 16% vs 59% and 14% vs 31%). Patients presenting with stage I and II disease with a pathologic complete response (pathCR) and patients who had stage II disease with 1 to 3 positive nodes after chemotherapy did not have improvements in LRR with RT. Multivariate analysis revealed 6 factors as independently predictive of LRR: (1) radiation use (HR 4.7, 95% CI 2.7-8.1), (2) nodal ratio > 0.20, (3) stage IIIB or IV disease, (4) no tamoxifen use, (5) ER-negative disease, and (6) poor response to induction chemotherapy. RT use was also an independent factor improving cause-specific survival (HR 2.0, 95% CI 1.4-2.9). Notably, attainment of clinical or pathCR was not an independent factor on multivariate analysis for either locoregional control or cause-specific survival.

Garg and collaborators tried to address which patients given neoadjuvant chemotherapy for clinical stage I and II breast cancer should receive radiation therapy.[92] They reviewed 132 such patients treated with doxorubicin-based induction chemotherapy followed by mastectomy but without postoperative radiation therapy. Although limited by small numbers, initial clinical T3N0 disease ($n = 19$) and 4 or more positive lymph nodes after chemotherapy ($n = 6$) correlated significantly with higher rates of locoregional recurrence (29% and 67%, respectively). Age 40 or younger and the absence of tamoxifen therapy also predicted for higher LRR. In contrast, 42 patients with clinical stage II disease who had 1 to 3 positive lymph nodes after neoadjuvant chemotherapy had a relatively low rate of locoregional recurrence (5-year rate of 5%).

RECONSTRUCTION AND POSTMASTECTOMY RADIATION THERAPY

Many women desire breast reconstruction after mastectomy, and this poses several challenges in the management of these women should they also require radiation therapy. A multidisciplinary collaboration is warranted in partnership with the patient to ensure an optimal aesthetic outcome without compromising the proven benefits of timely PMRT. Although a detailed discussion is beyond the scope of this chapter, breast reconstruction efforts can generally be categorized as either implant-based or autologous tissue reconstructions. In addition, reconstructions can be performed at the time of the mastectomy (immediate reconstructions) or at some time after mastectomy, usually after the completion of radiotherapy (delayed reconstructions). Implant-based approaches are technically less challenging, avoid the potential morbidities associated with the donor site, and can be offered to women who may not have adequate autologous tissue in potential donor sites. Typically, implant-based reconstructions occur immediately after mastectomy because tissue expansion after RT can be

problematic. Autologous reconstructions can be immediate or delayed and can be performed using a transverse rectus abdominus myocutaneous (TRAM) flap, a latissimus dorsi flap, or a flap based on the deep inferior epigastric artery (DIEP flap) or gluteal arteries.

Immediate reconstructions are often paired with a skin-sparing mastectomy. This allows the important advantage of preserving sensate skin and the natural tissue and skin folds for reconstruction. However, these advantages are offset by the possible adverse effects of radiation therapy on an immediate reconstruction. In addition, the reconstruction may potentially compromise the design and delivery of PMRT.

High rates of contracture, fibrosis, and poor cosmesis have been reported in patients who have immediate implant-based reconstructions. These changes can develop late but are usually progressive. Spear and associates reviewed the data on 40 consecutive patients who had undergone a 2-stage saline implant reconstruction followed by RT and compared their outcomes to 40 controls.[93] Fifty-three percent of irradiated reconstructions had complications compared to 10% in controls, including a 33% capsular contracture rate in the irradiated patients compared to none in the controls ($p < 0.00005$). Krueger and associates reviewed data on 19 patients who had expander/implant reconstruction and radiation therapy and found that 13 (68%) had complications, compared to 19/62 (31%) in unirradiated controls ($p = 0.006$).[94] Implant failure rates were 37% and 8% ($p = 0.005$), respectively. In contrast, complication rates seem to be lower for patients who have immediate *autologous* reconstructions.[95,96]

The effects of PMRT on immediate versus delayed TRAM reconstructions have been reported by Tran and coworkers.[97] Twenty-four of 32 patients in the immediate reconstruction group had contracture, compared to 0/70 in the delayed reconstruction group ($p < 0.0001$). Furthermore, 28% of the patients with immediate reconstruction required an additional flap or prosthesis to improve cosmesis. Kronowitz and associates have reported on a novel treatment algorithm to reconcile the benefits of immediate reconstruction and the uncertainty of eventual pathologic indications for PMRT; in the "delayed-immediate" breast reconstruction, patients have a skin-sparing mastectomy, with preservation of sensate skin, and subpectoral placement of a tissue expander.[98] After final pathology is reviewed, those patients who do not require PMRT proceed to an "immediate" (within 2 weeks) autologous reconstruction, while the remainder have a delayed autologous reconstruction after PMRT. The expander is kept inflated throughout chemotherapy and then deflated before the radiation simulation.

The contour of the chest wall after reconstruction can create challenges in the design and delivery of radiation to the necessary target volume. In a recent report, Motwani and coworkers reviewed 112 radiation plans designed to treat postmastectomy breast reconstructions and found that 52% of these required compromises in field design due to geometrical constraints imposed by the reconstruction. Of these, 33% were scored as moderate compromises and 19% major compromises.[99] Only 7% of similar plans in matched controls without reconstructions had compromises due to patient anatomy ($p < 0.0001$).

Technique

Treatment Volume, Dose, and Prescription

The target volumes at greatest risk for recurrence, the chest wall and the supraclavicular lymph nodes, should be included. The entire mastectomy flaps, inclusive of the mastectomy scar and the drain sites, should be irradiated. In the rare case of a high-risk node-negative breast cancer being treated with PMRT, the supraclavicular field may be omitted due to the low risk of regional failure reported in these patients.[82,84] An exhaustive discussion of field design is beyond the scope of the present discussion, and only salient features will be described. Most commonly, a monoisocentric photon technique in which opposed photon fields that are tangent to the chest wall are matched at isocenter to a superior AP (anterior-posterior) supraclavicular field. The medial border of the chest wall fields is typically at midsternum and the lateral border is at the mid- or posterior axillary line as clinically indicated. The inferior edge is 2 cm inferior to the level of where the inframammary fold existed. The superior border of the chest wall fields is set at the palpable inferior edge of the clavicular limb. This occurs in the match plane between the tangent fields and the third (or fourth) field. In general, 2 to 3 cm of lung in the tangents is required for adequate coverage of the chest wall.

All of the steps of a conventional fluoroscopic simulation can be reproduced virtually on image data acquired at the time of a CT simulation, and fields designed as described above. Alternatively, the entire chest wall can be treated with electrons, but variations in patient thickness and slope can make optimal dosimetry difficult with this technique. The target dose to the chest wall is 45 to 50 Gy in conventional 1.8- to 2-Gy fractions. Ideally, the treatment volume should be homogenous for dose, with acceptable ranges within 95% to 107% of prescription dose. Contributions from 15-mV photons should be minimized and bolus placement should be considered to ensure superficial coverage. Advances beyond the conventional techniques such as forward-planned intensity-modulated radiation therapy (IMRT), electronic compensation, and inverse-planned IMRT (Fig. 96-1) can be considered by the radiation oncologist to meet treatment objectives.

The supraclavicular field is typically an AP photon field with the upper border above the AC joint (or just flashing the skin), medial border at the vertebral pedicles, and lateral border at the coracoid process in patients who have had complete axillary dissections. In the case of an undissected or inadequately dissected axilla, the lateral border can be placed to include the medial two-thirds of the humeral head. A posterior axillary boost (PAB) can be designed to supplement dose to the axillary apex if the contribution from the AP supraclavicular field to the midplane is inadequate. Often, 50 Gy prescribed to the supraclavicular volume will result in 40 to 45 Gy to the axillary apex without need for a PAB.

No consensus exists on the inclusion of the IMN chains. Advocates of IMN irradiation correctly point out that the postmastectomy radiation trials discussed earlier did include the IMNs and that microscopic involvement of these nodes can be high. However, IMN failures are exceedingly unusual (0.1% in the ECOG experience).[64] This issue will not likely be settled at least until the results of ongoing randomized trials of regional nodal irradiation are mature. If the IMNs are to be included, several techniques are available. The partially wide tangents technique in which the tangent fields are altered to deepen coverage in the upper 3 intercostal spaces, is commonly used (Fig. 96-2). Another popular technique is the use of a 5- to 6-cm wide electron patch matched to the entry point of the medial tangent and tilted to a gantry angle 5 to 10 degrees less than the medial tangent. Nine- or 12-MeV electrons can be employed to treat at the requisite CT-defined depth. At 80% to 90% of prescribed dose, acute skin reactions may necessitate substituting the electron field with a photon field in the same geometry to allow skin sparing. The target dose is 45 to 50 Gy.

The area around the scar is commonly boosted with an additional 8 to 12 Gy with electrons. An electron "cut-out" can be created to treat a 2- to 3-cm margin around the mastectomy scar and/or drain sites. An elegant and creative way to avoid matching electron fields in patients with complex scar geometry or extensive chest wall curvature (especially after reconstruction) has been described in which a customized surface applicator

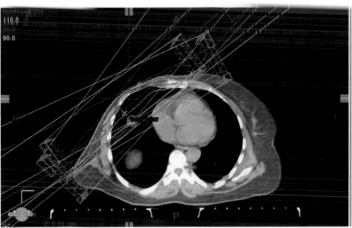
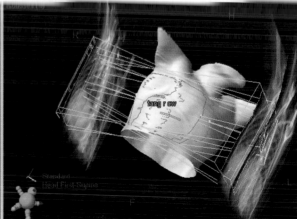

FIGURE 96-1 Illustration of an inversely planned IMRT plan for chest-wall irradiation.

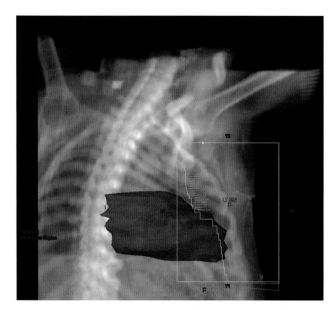

FIGURE 96-2 Digitally reconstructed beams eye view of a partially wide tangent field.

with embedded high dose rate (HDR) afterloading catheters is used for delivery of dose (Fig. 96-3).[100]

FUTURE DIRECTIONS

The results of 3 ongoing randomized trials will shed crucial light on currently unanswered question regarding the use of radiation therapy after mastectomy. The European SUPREMO (Selective Use of Postoperative Radiotherapy after Mastectomy) trial is currently open and will attempt to answer the critical question of appropriate patient selection criteria. This trial randomizes "intermediate-risk" operable breast cancer (node-positive stage II tumors and node-negative tumors larger than 2 cm with adverse features [high grade or LVI]) to chest wall

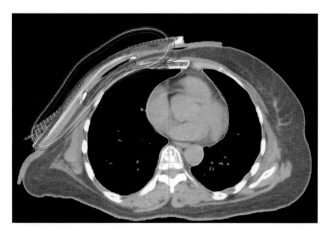

FIGURE 96-3 Customized brachytherapy surface applicator for delivery of chest wall boost.

irradiation or observation after mastectomy. A biological sub-study of the SUPREMO trial will develop tissue microarrays from the projected study population of 3700 patients to determine if immunohistochemical signatures are associated with relapse patterns.

The value of regional nodal irradiation is being tested in the National Cancer Institute-Canada's MA.20 and the EORTC 22922 studies, which, however, are studying this issue in the context of breast-conservation therapy. The MA.20 study randomized women with positive axillary nodes, women with T3N0 disease, and node-negative women with tumors larger than 2 cm and fewer than 10 nodes examined and 1 of the following risk factors: (1) negative ER, (2) high-grade disease, and (3) LVI to either breast irradiation alone or breast and regional nodal irradiation. The EORTC study is examining the benefit of irradiating the IMNs and medial supraclavicular nodes in node-positive women and in women with central or medial tumor location. The information that will become available when these trials are mature may help guide radiotherapy target volume definitions in the PMRT setting.

Necessary Future Studies

The development of molecular signatures predictive for locoregional recurrence may revolutionize how we select patients for PMRT. Significant progress has been made in this area with regards to systemic therapy, with rapid translation of these predictive assays into clinical practice. Similar work is needed with regard to locoregional therapies.

The sequencing of PMRT and cytotoxic chemotherapy can perhaps be revisited. Although data addressing this issue exist in the setting of early-stage disease with breast-conservation therapy, the results are not applicable to the PMRT setting where locoregional risks are higher. It is indeed possible that earlier locoregional therapy may improve outcome

SUMMARY

PMRT improves locoregional control, breast cancer-mortality and all-cause mortality in appropriately selected patients, and should be considered for all patients who have a projected locoregional recurrence rate of 20%. Node-positive patients with 4 or more involved nodes should routinely be offered PMRT, as should patients with 1 to 3 involved nodes and primary tumors larger than 5 cm (T3 disease). Patients with T4 disease, skin involvement, and/or involvement of the chest wall should routinely be offered PMRT.

Patients with T1/T2 disease and 1 to 3 involved nodes have an intermediate risk of recurrence (10%-20%) and should be considered for PMRT if they have fewer than 10 nodes removed, nodal ratio greater than 0.20, high tumor grade, LVI, age less than 45, positive margins, or hormone-receptor negativity.

Node-negative patients generally have low rates of locoregional recurrence, including those with T3N0 disease. PMRT can be considered in patients who have at least 3 of these additional adverse features: young age, histologic grade 3, LVI, T2 size, and absence of systemic therapy.

Patients who are clinical stage III, T3/T4, and have 4 or more nodes positive, or residual tumor larger than 2 cm after induction chemotherapy, should be offered PMRT. Pathologic complete response rates are an unreliable marker for locoregional recurrence risk.

Successful postmastectomy reconstruction requires a carefully planned multidisciplinary treatment program.

REFERENCES

1. Cole M. The place of radiotherapy in the management of early breast cancer. Br J Cancer. 1964;51:216-20.
2. Lichter A. Cancer of the Breast. 2nd ed. Philadelphia, PA: Elsevier; 2004.
3. EBCTCG. Treatment of Early Breast Cancer. Vol 1. Worldwide Evidence, 1985-1990. Oxford: Oxford University Press;1990:111.
4. Haybittle J, Brinkley D, Houghton J, et al. Postoperative radiotherapy and late mortality: Evidence from the Cancer Research Campaign Trial for early breast cancer. BMJ. 1989;298:1611 1614.
5. Höst H, Brennhovd M, Loeb M. Postoperative radiotherapy in breast cancer—Long term results from the Oslo study. Int J Radiat Oncol Biol Phys. 1986;12:727-732.
6. Jones J, Ribeiro G. Mortality patterns over 34 years of breast cancer patients in a clinical trial of postoperative radiotherapy. Clin Radiol. 1989;40:204-208.
7. Lythgoe J, Palmer M. Manchester Regional Breast Study—5 and 10 year results. Br J Surg. 1982;69:693-696.
8. Rutqvist L, Lax I, Fornander M, et al. Cardiovascular mortality in a randomized trial of adjuvant radiation therapy versus surgery alone in primary breast cancer. Int J Radiat Oncol Biol Phys. 1992;22:887-896.
9. Stewart H, Jack W, Everington D, et al. South-east Scottish trial of local therapy in node negative breast cancer. Breast. 1994;3:31-39.
10. Ingle J, Everson L, Wieand S, et al. Randomized trial of observation versus adjuvant therapy with cyclophosphamide, fluorouracil, prednisone with or without tamoxifen following mastectomy in postmenopausal women with node-positive breast cancer. J Clin Oncol. 1988;6:1388-1396.
11. Bonadonna G, Valagussa P, Moliterni A, et al. Adjuvant cyclophosphamide, methotrexate, and fluorouracil in node-positive breast cancer. N Engl J Med. 1995;332:901 906.
12. Castiglione-Gersch M, Johnsen C, Goldhirsh A, et al. The International (Ludwig) Breast Cancer Study Group trials I-IV: 5 years follow-up. Ann Oncol. 1994;5:717 724.
13. Crivellari D, Price K, Gelber R, et al. Adjuvant endocrine therapy compared with no systemic therapy for elderly women with early breast cancer: 21 year results of International Breast Cancer Study Group trial IV. J Clin Oncol. 2003;21:4517-4523.
14. Fisher B, Dignam J, Bryant J, et al. Five versus more than five years of tamoxifen therapy for breast cancer patients with negative lymph nodes and estrogen receptor-positive tumors. J Natl Cancer Inst. 1996;88:1529-1542.
15. Fisher B, Dignam J, Eleftherios P, et al. Sequential methotrexate and fluorouracil for the treatment of node-negative breast cancer patients with estrogen receptor-negative tumors: eight-year results of from National Surgical Adjuvant breast and bowel project (NSABP) B-13 and first report of findings from NSABP-B-19 comparing methotrexate and fluorouracil with conventional cyclophosphamide, methotrexate, and fluorouracil. J Clin Oncol. 1996;14:1982-1992.
16. Fisher B, Fisher E, Redmond C, et al. Ten-year results from the national surgical adjuvant breast and bowel project (NSABP) clinical trial evaluating L-phenylalanine mustard (L-PAM) in the management of primary breast cancer. J Clin Oncol. 1985;4:929-941.
17. Goldhirsh A, Castiglione M, Gelber R, et al. A single perioperative adjuvant chemotherapy course for node-negative breast cancer: five-year results of trial V. International Breast Cancer Study Group (formerly Ludwig Group) J Natl Cancer Inst Monogr. 1992:89-96.
18. Mansour E, Eudey L, Tormey D, et al. Chemotherapy versus observation in high-risk node-negative breast cancer patients. J Natl Cancer Inst Monogr. 1992:97-104.
19. Morrison J, Howell A, Kelly K, et al. West Midlands Oncology Association trials of adjuvant chemtherapy in operable breast cancer: results after a median follow-up of 7 years. I. Patients with involved axillary lymph nodes. Br J Cancer. 1989;60:911 918.

20. Morrison J, Kelly K, Howell A, et al. West Midlands Oncology Association trial of adjuvant chemotherapy in node-negative breast cancer. J Natl Cancer Inst Monogr. 1992:85-88.
21. Richards M, O'Reilly S, Howell A, et al. Adjuvant cyclophosphamide, methotrexate, and fluorouracil in patients with axillary node-positive breast cancer: an update of the Guy's Manchester trial. J Clin Oncol. 1990;8:2032-2039.
22. Rubens R, Knight R, Fentiman I, et al. Controlled trial of adjuvant chemotherapy with melphalan for breast cancer. Lancet. 1983;1:839-843.
23. Taylor S, Knuiman W, Sleeper L, et al. Six-year results of the Eastern Cooperative Oncology Group Trial of observation versus CMFP versus CMFPT in postmenopausal patients with node-positive breast cancer. J Clin Oncol. 1989;7(7):879-889.
24. Zambetti M, Valagussa P, Bonadonna G, et al. Adjuvant cyclophosphamide, methotrexate and fluorouracil in node-negative and estrogen receptor negative breast cancer. Ann Oncol. 1996;7:481-485.
25. EBCTCG. Effects of chemotherapy and hormonal therapy for early breast cancer on recurrence and 15-year survival: an overview of the randomized trials. Lancet. 2005;365:1687-1717.
26. Marks L, Halperin E, Prosnitz L, et al. Postmastectomy radiotherapy following adjuvant chemotherapy and autologous bone marrow transplantation for breast cancer patients with > 10 positive axillary lymph nodes. Int J Radiat Oncol Biol Phys. 1992;23:1021 6.
27. Citron M, Berry D, Cirrincione C, et al. Randomized trial of dose dense versus conventionally scheduled and sequential versus concurrent combination chemotherapy as postoperative adjuvant treatment of node-positive primary breast cancer: first report of Intergroup trial C 9741/Cancer and Leukemia Group B trial 9741. J Clin Oncol. 2003;21:1431-1439.
28. Fisher B, Anderson S, Wickerham D, et al. Increased intensification and total dose of cyclophosphamide in a doxorubicin-cyclophosphamide regimen for the treatment of primary breast cancer: findings of the National and Surgical Adjuvant Breast and Bowel Project B-22. J Clin Oncol. 1997;15:1858-1869.
29. Hoeller U, Heide J, Kroeger N, et al. Radiotherapy after high-dose chemotherapy and peripheral blood stem-cell support in high-risk breast cancer. Int J Radiat Oncol Biol Phys. 2002;53:1234-9.
30. Sartor C, Peterson B, Woolf S, et al. Effect of addition of adjuvant paclitaxel on radiotherapy delivery and locoregional control of node positive breast cancer: Cancer and Leukemia Group B 9344. J Clin Oncol. 2005;23:30-40.
31. Wood W, Budman D, Korzun A, et al. Dose and dose intensity of adjuvant chemotherapy for stage II, node-positive breast carcinoma. N Engl J Med. 1994;330:1253-1259.
32. Blomqvist C, Tiusanen K, Elomaa I, et al. The combination of radiotherapy, adjuvant chemotherapy (cyclophosphamide-doxorubicin-ftorafur) and tamoxifen in stage II breast cancer. Long-term follow-up results of a randomized trial. Br J Cancer. 1992;66:1171-1176.
33. Buzdar A, Hortobagyi G, Kau S, et al. Breast cancer adjuvant therapy at the MD Anderson Cancer Center—results of four prospective studies. In: Salmon S, ed. Adjuvant therapy of Cancer. Philadelphia, PA: Lippincott, 1993:220-231.
34. Griem K, Henderson I, Gelman R, et al. The 5-year results of a randomized trial of adjuvant radiation therapy after chemotherapy in breast cancer patients treated with mastectomy. J Clin Oncol. 1987;5:1546-1555.
35. Klefstrom P, Grohn P, Heinonen E, et al. Adjuvant postoperative radiotherapy, chemotherapy, and immunotherapy in stage III breast cancer. Cancer. 1987;60:936-942.
36. Martinez A, Ahmann D, O'Fallow J, et al. An interim analysis of the randomized surgical adjuvant trial for patients with unfavorable breast cancer. Int J Radiat Oncol Biol Phys. 1984;10(suppl 2):106.
37. McArdle C, Crawford D, Dykes E, et al. Adjuvant radiotherapy and chemotherapy in breast cancer. Br J Surg. 1986;73:264-266.
38. Muss H, Cooper M, Brockschmidt, et al. A randomized trial of chemotherapy (L-PAM vs CMF) and irradiation for node-positive breast cancer. Eleven year follow-up of Piedmont Oncology Association trial. Breast Cancer Res Treat. 1991;18:77-84.
39. Olson J, Neuberg D, Pandya K, et al. The role of radiotherapy in the management of operable locally advanced breast cancer: results of a randomized trial by the Eastern Cooperative Oncology Group. Cancer. 1997;79:1138-1149.
40. Overgaard M, Hansen P, Overgaard J, et al. Postoperative radiotherapy in high-risk premenopausal women with breast cancer who receive adjuvant chemotherapy. N Engl J Med. 1997;337:949-955.
41. Overgaard M, Jensen M, Overgaard J, et al. Postoperative radiotherapy in high-risk postmenopausal breast-cancer patients given adjuvant tamoxifen: Danish Breast Cancer Cooperative Group DBCG 82c randomized trial. Lancet. 1999;353:1641-1648.

42. Ragaz J, Olivotto I, Spinelli J, et al. Locoregional radiation therapy in patients with high-risk breast cancer receiving adjuvant chemotherapy: 20 year results of the British Columbia randomized trial. *J Natl Cancer Inst.* 2005;97:116-126.

43. Tennvall-Nittby L, Tengrup I, Landberg T, et al. The total incidence of loco-regional recurrence in a randomized trial of breast cancer TNM stage II. The South Sweden Breast Cancer Trial. *Acta Oncol.* 1993;32:641-646.

44. Velez-Garcia E, Carpenter J, Jr, Moore M, et al. Postsurgical adjuvant chemotherapy with or without radiotherapy in women with breast cancer and positive axillary nodes: a Southeastern Cancer Study Group (SEG) trial. *Eur J Cancer.* 1992;28:1833-1837.

45. EBCTCG. Effects of radiotherapy and of differences in the extent of surgery for early breast cancer on local recurrence and 15-year survival: an overview of the randomised trials. *Lancet.* 2005;366:2087-2106.

46. EBCTCG. Favourable and unfavourable effects on long-term survival of radiotherapy for early breast cancer: an overview of the randomised trials. *Lancet.* 2000;355:1757-1770.

47. Punglia R, Morrow M, Winer E, Harris J. Local therapy and survival in breast cancer. *N Engl J Med.* 2007;356:2399-2405.

48. Darby S. New results from the worldwide overview of individual patient data from the randomised trials of radiotherapy. 2007 Annual ASCO meeting. Available at http://www.asco.org/ASCO/Abstracts+%26+Virtual+Meeting/Virtual+Meeting?&vmview=vm_session_presentations_view&confID=47&trackID=1&sessionID=431. Accessed on November 4, 2009.

49. Van de Steene J, Soete G, Storme G. Adjuvant radiotherapy for breast cancer significantly improves overall survival: the missing link. *Radiother Oncol.* 2000;55:263-272.

50. Whelan TJ, Julian J, Wright J, et al. Does locoregional radiation therapy improve survival in breast cancer? A meta-analysis. *J Clin Oncol.* 2000;18:1220-1229.

51. Gebski V, Lagvela M, Keech A, et al. Survival effects of postmastectomy adjuvant radiation therapy using biologically equivalent doses: a clinical perspective. *J Natl Cancer Inst.* 2006;98:26-38.

52. Rutqvist L, Johansson H. Mortality by laterality of the primary tumor among 55,000 breast cancer patients from the Swedish Cancer Registry. *Br J Cancer.* 1990;61:866-868.

53. Cuzick J, Stewart H, Peto R, et al. Overview of randomized trials of postoperative adjuvant radiotherapy in breast cancer. *Cancer Treat Rep.* 1987;71:15-29.

54. Cuzick J, Stewart H, Rutqvist L, et al. Cause-specific mortality in long-term survivors of breast cancer who participated in trials of radiotherapy. *J Clin Oncol.* 1994;12:447-453.

55. Hojris I, Overgaard M, Christensen J, et al. Morbidity and mortality of ischaemic heart disease in high-risk breast-cancer patients after adjuvant postmastectomy systemic treatment with or without radiotherapy: analysis of DBCG 82b and 82c randomised trial. *Lancet.* 1999;354:1425-1430.

56. Gyenes G, Rutqvist L, Liedberg A, Fornander T. Long-term cardiac morbidity and mortality in a randomized trial of pre- and postoperative radiation therapy versus surgery alone in primary breast cancer. *Radiother Oncol.* 1998;48:185-190.

57. Harris E, Correa C, Hwang W, et al. Late cardiac mortality and morbidity in early-stage breast cancer patients after breast-conservation treatment. *J Clin Oncol.* 2006;24:4100-4106.

58. Giordano S, Kuo Y, Freeman J, et al. Risk of cardiac death after adjuvant radiotherapy for breast cancer. *J Natl Cancer Inst.* 2005;97:419-424.

59. Hojris I, Andersen J, Overgaard M, Overgaard J. Late treatment-related morbidity in breast cancer patients randomized to postmastectomy radiotherapy and systemic treatment versus systemic treatment alone. *Acta Oncol.* 2000;39:355-372.

60. Olsen N, Pfeiffer P, Johanssen L, et al. Radiation-induced brachial plexopathy: neurological follow-up in 161 recurrence-free breast cancer patients. *Int J Radiat Oncol Biol Phys.* 1993;26:43-49.

61. Kuhnt T, Richter C, Enke H, et al. Acute radiation reaction and local control in breast cancer patients treated with postmastectomy radiotherapy. *Strahlenther Onkol.* 1998;174:257-261.

62. Nielsen H, Overgaard M, Grau C, et al. Study of failure pattern among high-risk breast cancer patients with or without postmastectomy radiotherapy in addition to adjuvant systemic therapy: Long-term results from the Danish Breast Cancer Cooperative Group (DBCG) 82b and 82c randomized studies. *J Clin Oncol.* 2006;24:2268-2275.

63. Katz A, Strom EA, Buchholz TA, et al. Locoregional recurrence patterns after mastectomy and doxorubicin-based chemotherapy: implications for postoperative irradiation. *J Clin Oncol.* 2000;18:2817-2827.

64. Recht A, Gray R, Davidson NE, et al. Locoregional failure 10 years after mastectomy and adjuvant chemotherapy with or without tamoxifen

65. without irradiation: experience of the Eastern Cooperative Oncology Group. *J Clin Oncol.* 1999;17:1689-1700.

65. Woodward W, Strom E, Tucker S, et al. Locoregional recurrence after doxorubicin-based chemotherapy and postmastectomy: implications for breast cancer patients with early-stage disease and predictors for recurrence after postmastectomy radiation. *Int J Radiat Oncol Biol Phys.* 2003;57:336-344.

66. Nielsen H, Overgaard M, Grau C, et al. Locoregional recurrence after mastectomy in high-risk breast cancer—risk and prognosis. An analysis of patients from the DBCG 82 b& c randomization trials. *Radiother Oncol.* 2006;79:147-155.

67. Taghian A, Jeong JH, Mamounas E, et al. Patterns of locoregional failure in patients with operable breast cancer treated by mastectomy and adjuvant chemotherapy with or without tamoxifen and without radiotherapy: results from five National Surgical Adjuvant Breast and Bowel Project randomized clinical trials. *J Clin Oncol.* 2004;22:4247-4254.

68. Wallgren A, Bonetti M, Gelber R, et al. Risk factors for locoregional recurrence among breast cancer patients: results from International Breast Cancer Study Group Trial I-VII. *J Clin Oncol.* 2003;21:1205-1213.

69. Truong P, Woodward W, Thames H, et al. The ratio of positive to excised nodes identifies high-risk subsets and reduces inter-institutional differences in locoregional recurrence risk estimates in breast cancer patients with 1-3 positive nodes: an analysis of prospective data from British Columbia and the MD Anderson Cancer Center. *Int J Radiat Oncol Biol Phys.* 2007;68:59-65.

70. Karlsson P, Cole B, Price K, et al. The role of number of uninvolved lymph nodes in predicting locoregional recurrence in breast cancer. *J Clin Oncol.* 2007;25:2019-2026.

71. Katz A, Buchholz TA, Thames H, et al. Recursive partitioning analysis of locoregional recurrence patterns following mastectomy: implications for adjuvant irradiation. *Int J Radiat Oncol Biol Phys.* 2001;50:397-403.

72. Truong P, Olivotto I, Kader H, et al. Selecting breast cancer patients with T1-T2 tumors and one to three positive axillary nodes at high postmastectomy locoregional recurrence risk for adjuvant radiotherapy. *Int J Radiat Oncol Biol Phys.* 2005;61:1337-1347.

73. Overgaard M, Nielsen H, Overgaard J. Is the benefit of postmastectomy irradiation limited to patients with four or more positive nodes, as recommended in the international consensus reports? A subgroup analysis of the DBCG 82 b&c randomized trials. *Radiother Oncol.* 2007;82:247-253.

74. Eifel P, Axelson JA, Costa J, et al. National Institutes of Health Consensus Development Conference Statement: adjuvant therapy for breast cancer, November 1-3, 2000. *J Natl Cancer Inst.* 2001;93:979-989.

75. Harris J, Halpin-Murphy P, Mcneese M, et al. Consensus statement on postmastectomy radiation therapy. *Int J Radiat Oncol Biol Phys.* 1999;44:989-990.

76. Recht A, Edge SB, Solin LJ, et al. Postmastectomy radiotherapy: clinical practice guidelines of the American Society of Clinical Oncology. *J Clin Oncol.* 2001;19:1539-1569.

77. Taylor ME, Haffty BG, Shank BM, et al. Postmastectomy radiotherapy. American College of Radiology. ACR Appropriateness Criteria. *Radiology.* 2000;215(suppl):1153-1170.

78. Katz A, Strom EA, Buchholz TA, et al. The influence of pathologic tumor characteristics on locoregional recurrence rates following mastectomy. *Int J Radiat Oncol Biol Phys.* 2001;50:735-742.

79. Fowble B, Yeh IT, Schultz DJ, et al. The role of mastectomy in patients with stage I-II breast cancer presenting with gross multifocal or multicentric disease or diffuse microcalcifications. *Int J Radiat Oncol Biol Phys.* 1993;27:567-573.

80. Cheng J, Chen C, Liu M, et al. Locoregional failure of postmastectomy patients with 1-3 positive axillary lymph nodes without adjuvant radiotherapy. *Int J Radiat Oncol Biol Phys.* 2002;52:980-988.

81. Fodor J, Polgar C, Major T, Nemeth G. Locoregional failure 15 years after mastectomy in women with one to three positive axillary nodes with or without irradiation. *Strahlenther Onkol.* 2003;179:197-202.

82. Jagsi R, Abi Raad R, Goldberg S, et al. Locoregional recurrence rates and prognostic factors for failure in node-negative patients treated with mastectomy: implications for postmastectomy radiation. *Int J Radiat Oncol Biol Phys.* 2005;62:1035-1039.

83. Floyd S, Buchholz T, Haffty B, et al. Low local recurrence rate without postmastectomy radiation in node-negative breast cancer patients with tumors 5 cm and larger. *Int J Radiat Oncol Biol Phys.* 2006;66:358-364.

84. Taghian A, Jeong J, Mamounas E, et al. Low locoregional recurrence rate among node-negative breast cancer patients with tumors 5 cm or larger treated by mastectomy, with or without adjuvant systemic therapy and without radiotherapy: results from five National Surgical Adjuvant Breast and Bowel Project randomized clinical trials. *J Clin Oncol.* 2006;24:3927-2932.

85. Truong P, Lesperance M, Culhaci A, et al. Patient subsets with T1-T2, node-negative breast cancer at high locoregional recurrence risk after mastectomy. *Int J Radiat Oncol Biol Phys.* 2005;62:175-182.

86. Yildirim E, Berberoglu U. Can a subgroup of node-negative breast carcinoma patients with T1-T2 tumor who may benefit from postmastectomy radiotherapy be identified? *Int J Radiat Oncol Biol Phys.* 2007;68:1024-1029.

87. Cheng S, Horng C, West M, et al. Genomic prediction of locoregional recurrence after mastectomy in breast cancer. *J Clin Oncol.* 2006;24:4594-4602.

88. Truong P, Olivotto I, Speers C, et al. A positive margin is not always an indication for radiotherapy after mastectomy in early breast cancer. *Int J Radiat Oncol Biol Phys.* 2004;58:797-804.

89. Freedman GM, Fowble BL, Hanlon AL, et al. A close or positive margin after mastectomy is not an indication for chest wall irradiation except in women aged fifty or younger. *Int J Radiat Oncol Biol Phys.* 1998;41:599-605.

90. Buchholz T, Katz A, Strom E, et al. Pathological tumor size and lymph node status predict for different rates of locoregional recurrence after mastectomy for breast cancer patients treated with neoadjuvant versus adjuvant chemotherapy. *Int J Radiat Oncol Biol Phys.* 2002;53:880-888.

91. Huang E, Tucker S, Strom E, et al. Postmastectomy radiation improves local-regional control and survival for selected patients with locally advanced breast cancer treated with neoadjuvant chemotherapy and mastectomy. *J Clin Oncol.* 2004;22:4691-4699.

92. Garg A, Strom E, McNeese M, et al. T3 disease at presentation or pathological involvement of four or more lymph nodes predict for locoregional recurrence in stage II breast cancer treated with neoadjuvant chemotherapy

93. Spear S, Onyewu C. Staged breast reconstruction with saline-filled implants in the irradiated breast: recent trends and therapeutic implications. *Plast Reconstr Surg.* 2000 Mar;105(3):930-942.

94. Krueger E, Wilkins E, Strawderman M, et al. Complications and patient satisfaction following expander/implant breast reconstruction with and without radiotherapy. *Int J Radiat Oncol Biol Phys.* 2001;49:713-721.

95. Soong I, Yau T, Ho C, et al. Post-mastectomy radiotherapy after immediate autologous breast reconstruction in primary treatment of breast cancers. *Clin Oncol (R Coll Radiol).* 2004;16:283-289.

96. Chawla A, Kachnic L, Taghian A, et al. Radiotherapy and breast reconstruction: complications and cosmesis with TRAM versus tissue expander/implant. *Int J Radiat Oncol Biol Phys.* 2002;54:520-526.

97. Tran N, Chang D, Gupta A, et al. Comparison of immediate and delayed free TRAM flap breast reconstruction in patients receiving postmastectomy radiation therapy. *Plast Reconstr Surg.* 2001;108:78-82.

98. Kronowitz S, Hunt K, Kuerer H, et al. Delayed-immediate breast reconstruction. *Plast Reconstr Surg.* 2004;113:1617-1628.

99. Motwani S, Strom E, Schechter N, et al. The impact of immediate breast reconstruction on the technical delivery of postmastectomy radiotherapy. *Int J Radiat Oncol Biol Phys.* 2006;66:76-82.

100. Stewart A, O'Farrell D, Bellon J, et al. CT computer-optimized high-dose-rate brachytherapy with surface applicator technique for scar boost radiation after breast reconstruction surgery. *Brachytherapy.* 2005;4:224-229.

and mastectomy without radiotherapy. *Int J Radiat Oncol Biol Phys.* 2004;59:138-145.

CHAPTER 97

Radiation Therapy in Metastatic Disease

Kathleen C. Horst

BRAIN METASTASES

Incidence

Brain metastases are the most common intracranial neoplasm in adults. It is estimated that approximately 10% to 16% of patients with metastatic breast cancer will develop clinically evident brain metastases,[1] while up to 30% of patients will have brain metastases identified at autopsy.[2] Intraparenchymal metastases occur via hematogenous spread to the watershed area of the brain at the junction of the gray and white matter.[3] The presence of metastases in the supratentorial and infratentorial compartments is in proportion to the relative weight and blood supply of these areas, with 85% occurring in the cerebral hemispheres, 10% to 15% in the cerebellum, and 1% to 3% in the brainstem.[4] Leptomeningcal metastases are less common than intraparenchymal metastases and are found in 5% to 16% of patients at autopsy.[1,2]

Young age,[5] estrogen receptor (ER)–negative status,[6-8] the presence of pulmonary metastases,[7] and HER-2 overexpression[6,9] have all been described as risk factors for the development of brain metastases in patients with metastatic breast cancer. With improvements in systemic therapies and overall survival of patients with metastatic disease, the incidence of brain metastases appears to have increased over the last several years.[10] In particular, with the introduction of trastuzumab, a humanized monoclonal antibody that binds to the extracellular segment of the HER-2/neu (erbB2) receptor and does not penetrate the blood-brain barrier,[11] a higher incidence of central nervous system (CNS) metastases has been observed in patients receiving trastuzumab for metastatic breast cancer, ranging from 28% to 43%.[9] This observation suggests that the incidence of CNS metastases may be higher in patients with HER-2-positive metastatic breast cancer whose systemic disease is well controlled with this newer agent.

Clinical Presentation

While some patients may be asymptomatic, the most common presenting symptom is headache, which can occur in 24% to 48% of patients.[12,13] Other presenting signs and symptoms include nausea/vomiting (4%), gait ataxia (7%), focal weakness (20%), seizures (12%), speech difficulty and/or visual changes (5%), or impaired cognitive function (14% to 34%).[12,14,15] Symptoms can be a result of the metastatic tumor itself, depending on the location, or from surrounding vasogenic edema. Cranial neuropathies suggest leptomeningeal involvement or invasion into the cavernous sinus.

Although the clinical suspicion of new onset brain metastases is higher in patients with known metastatic breast cancer, any patient with a history of breast cancer who presents with such signs or symptoms should undergo additional evaluation with a thorough neurologic examination and diagnostic imaging.

Diagnostic Imaging

Gadolinium-enhanced brain magnetic resonance imaging (MRI) is the best diagnostic test for brain metastases as it has been shown to be more sensitive than contrast-enhanced computed tomography (CT), particularly with respect to identifying lesions less than 10 mm and lesions in the posterior fossa.[16] Most brain metastases appear hypointense to isointense with respect to gray matter on T1-weighted images and enhance in a solid or ring-like pattern following administration of intravenous gadolinium contrast. On T2-weighted images, metastatic lesions may appear relatively hypointense to normal brain while cystic or necrotic areas or surrounding vasogenic edema are hyperintense (Fig. 97-1).[17]

A diagnosis of breast cancer metastatic to the brain cannot be made solely on the acquired imaging studies, although the diagnosis is likelier in the setting of known metastatic breast cancer or if there are multiple enhancing lesions.[18] In a patient

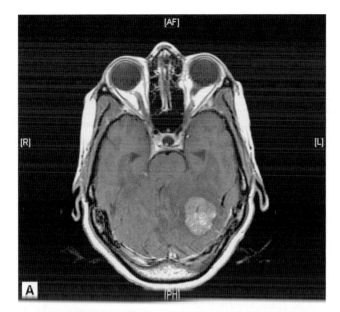

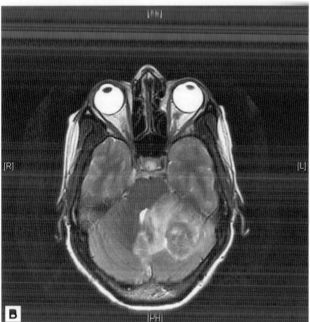

FIGURE 97-1 **A.** Axial T1-weighted MRI showing a heterogeneously enhancing left cerebellar hemisphere mass, which exerts significant mass effect with downward tonsillar herniation and obstructive hydrocephalus. **B.** Axial T2-weighted MRI showing surrounding vasogenic edema. This patient underwent surgical resection followed by postoperative radiotherapy.

with a history of breast cancer and no evidence of distant metastatic disease, a neurosurgical biopsy would be appropriate to establish the diagnosis.

Prognosis

Investigators from the Radiation Therapy Oncology Group (RTOG) have defined 3 prognostic groups based on a recursive partitioning analysis of various prognostic factors.[19] Of 1200 patients with brain metastases from a variety of solid tumors, patients less than 65 years of age with a Karnofsky Performance Status (KPS) greater than 70 who have controlled primary

tumor without evidence of extracranial disease had a median survival of 7.1 months after whole-brain radiotherapy. Patients with a KPS less than 70 had a median survival of only 2.3 months. All other patients had a median survival of 4.2 months. This prognostic index was validated using a phase III trial, confirming that age, performance status, status of the primary tumor, and the extent of metastatic disease are valid prognostic factors that can help guide treatment decisions.[20]

With more recent data demonstrating that the number of brain metastases is prognostic, a new index, the Graded Prognostic Assessment (GPA), has been developed to reflect age, KPS, the presence or absence of extracranial metastases, and the number of brain metastases.[21] Additional predictors of survival in patients with brain metastases include longer disease-free interval[22] and HER-2 amplification.[23]

Management

Symptomatic Treatment

Corticosteroids An initial bolus of corticosteroids followed by a maintenance dose of 4 mg every 6 hours can help mitigate symptoms within several hours, particularly if there is a significant component of vasogenic edema as noted on the T2-weighted images. Because of significant side effects associated with corticosteroids, such as mood changes, insomnia, elevated blood sugar, weight gain, gastrointestinal bleeding, and increased susceptibility to infections,[24] tapering of the steroid dose is often recommended during definitive treatment.

Antiepileptic Drugs The incidence of seizure is influenced by the location of the metastatic lesion, with patients having a higher incidence when lesions are located in the parietal, frontal, or temporal lobes and lowest in the occipital lobe.[25] Patients who present with seizure have an approximately 70% chance of having recurrent seizures, and antiepileptic drugs (AEDs) are often prescribed.[25] The choice of AED in patients who will be undergoing radiotherapy is important, as there have been several reports of patients developing Stevens-Johnson syndrome while on phenytoin during whole-brain radiotherapy.[26] In patients with metastatic brain lesions who have not experienced a seizure, AEDs are not effective in preventing first seizures. The prophylactic use of AEDs, therefore, should not be used routinely in such patients given the lack of efficacy and potential side effects.[27]

Definitive Treatment

Surgery For patients with a single metastasis, complete surgical resection followed by whole-brain radiotherapy (WBRT) has been shown in a randomized trial to improve local control and overall survival compared to a needle biopsy plus radiotherapy.[28] Randomized trials have also shown that combined modality therapy, complete surgical resection followed by whole-brain radiotherapy, improves local control compared to surgery alone (local recurrence of 10% vs 46%, $p < .001$)[29] and improves survival compared to WBRT alone for patients with a single brain metastasis (median survival of 10 months vs 6 months, *p* = .04).[30] It is therefore important to obtain a brain MRI for complete evaluation to determine whether or not a patient has a single metastasis or multiple metastases, as small lesions may otherwise be missed on a contrast-enhanced CT. The current accepted standard of care for patients with a single metastasis who are deemed appropriate surgical candidates with a good performance status and controlled extracranial disease is complete surgical resection followed by WBRT.

The role of surgery in patients with multiple brain metastases is not well established. While retrospective studies suggest improvement in outcome with surgery in patients with multiple metastases,[31] there are no randomized data supporting combined modality therapy with surgery and WBRT over WBRT alone in these patients. Surgical resection is therefore limited to those patients with large lesions causing neurologic compromise secondary to mass effect or significant edema, or if a pathologic diagnosis is required.

Whole-Brain Radiotherapy Most chemotherapeutic agents have limited efficacy in the treatment of brain metastases because of the blood-brain barrier and resulting low CNS levels for agents delivered intravenously.[32] As such, whole-brain radiotherapy is used to palliate symptoms and improve quality of life in patients with multiple brain metastases and, as previously mentioned, has been shown to decrease the rate of local recurrence in patients with a single brain metastasis after surgical resection.[29] Multiple randomized trials have evaluated various treatment schedules, ranging from 10 gray (Gy) in a single fraction to 50 Gy in 20 fractions.[33,34] While no study has demonstrated superior outcomes with one schedule over another, most patients in the United States receive 30 Gy in 10 daily fractions over 2 weeks, or 37.5 Gy in 15 daily fractions over 3 weeks.

Acute toxicities related to WBRT include skin erythema, hair loss, fatigue, nausea, and anorexia. Approximately 75% to 85% of patients with headaches or seizure activity will achieve some palliation of symptoms either during the treatment course or within 3 to 4 weeks posttreatment. Unfortunately, only 50% of patients with more severe neurologic signs or symptoms such as motor dysfunction will have a partial or complete response. Long-term toxicities of WBRT may include memory loss, lethargy, dementia, personality changes, and endocrine dysfunction.[35]

Stereotactic Radiosurgery Stereotactic radiosurgery (SRS) refers to highly conformal, high-dose radiation that is delivered to a relatively small target using multiple beams with minimal exposure to normal tissues. This treatment was originally developed by a Swedish neurosurgeron, Lars Leksell, as a potential substitute for surgical resection.[36] Several techniques are currently available for SRS: the Gamma Knife system (cobalt 60 source), linac (linear accelerator)-based radiosurgery, or the CyberKnife® Robotic Radiosurgery System (linear accelerator with an image-guided robotic system).

Although there are no randomized data comparing surgical resection of a single brain metastasis with SRS, the addition of SRS to WBRT had been shown to improve local control in patients with a single metastasis compared with WBRT alone.[37,38] Given the concern about long-term neurocognitive dysfunction with the use of whole-brain radiotherapy, questions remain as to whether a focal therapy such as SRS could provide adequate initial treatment in patients with limited CNS disease and whether WBRT can be deferred without compromising outcomes. Several retrospective series found no difference in survival between patients treated with SRS alone and those treated with WBRT plus SRS,[39,40] yet approximately 50% of patients treated with SRS alone developed additional brain metastases. The only published phase III trial investigating SRS plus WBRT versus SRS alone in 132 patients with limited (≤4) brain metastases reported no difference in overall survival between the 2 treatment groups (median survival of 7.5 months vs 8.0 months in the WBRT + SRS and SRS alone groups, respectively; *p* = .42).[41] The 12-month rate of brain tumor recurrence, however, was significantly higher in the SRS-alone group (76.4%) compared with the WBRT + SRS group (46.8%; *p* < .001). Although intracranial relapse is more common when WBRT is omitted from the initial treatment in patients with ≤4 brain metastases, the use of up-front WBRT with SRS did not improve overall survival, suggesting that early detection of recurrence and early salvage with WBRT may prevent neurologic complications and neurologic death. The use of SRS alone without up-front WBRT is currently controversial, with some advocating that patients with multiple metastases should receive WBRT up front with SRS reserved for recurrences.[42] Future studies are required before SRS alone is considered the standard of care in patients with limited brain metastases.

In patients with a single metastasis treated with surgical resection, some retrospective studies suggest that SRS alone to the postoperative bed without WBRT can provide local control in up to 79% of patients at 1 year posttreatment, and that WBRT can be reserved for salvage treatment.[43]

Side effects of SRS depend on the location of the treated metastasis but can include headaches, nausea, exacerbation of existing neurologic deficits, or seizures, particularly in patients with temporal lobe lesions. Doses usually range between 15 and 24 Gy, depending on the size of the lesion, with SRS limited to tumors less than 3 cm.[44] With larger tumors, the risk of radiation necrosis with high-dose radiosurgery increases significantly and fractionated treatment should be considered.

Future areas of research for breast cancer patients will need to address possible CNS prophylactic strategies with perhaps new agents that have improved penetration into the CNS, particularly for patients with HER-2-positive breast cancer who appear to have a higher incidence of brain metastases since the introduction of trastuzumab.

In summary, breast cancer patients who present with persistent headaches or neurologic compromise should undergo brain MRI. If there is a single brain lesion that appears suspicious for metastatic disease, surgical resection should be considered if the patient is an appropriate surgical candidate with a good performance status and controlled systemic disease. Whole-brain radiotherapy should be administered adjuvantly based on phase III data demonstrating a reduction of local recurrence from 46% to 10% (*p* < .001) without a difference in median survival (43 weeks vs 48 weeks, *p* = .39).[29] Some retrospective series support using SRS alone to the postoperative bed,[43] but frequent monitoring would be necessary to detect recurrences early for salvage treatment. If a patient with a single metastasis is not deemed to be a good surgical candidate or the lesion is considered unresectable given its location in eloquent areas of the brain that may result in significant postoperative neurologic sequelae, WBRT should be used with consideration of an SRS boost. SRS alone in patients with a single metastasis is used in some institutions but is still considered an area of investigation.

In patients with multiple brain metastases, surgical resection is reserved for those situations in which a confirmation of diagnosis is required, such as the first presentation of metastatic disease, or for those patients who may have a dominant lesion causing significant neurologic dysfunction, midline shift, or herniation. WBRT should otherwise be given with consideration of an SRS boost if there are upto 4 lesions or larger lesions that may not be well controlled with WBRT alone. SRS alone in patients with upto 4 metastatic lesions is controversial. Although it is not currently considered standard treatment, it is used in some situations with the expectation that close follow-up is necessary and WBRT may need to be given as salvage therapy.

CHOROIDAL METASTASES

Incidence

Due to its high vascularity, the choroid is the most common location of ocular metastases from breast cancer, followed by the orbit, iris, ciliary body, optic nerve, and eyelid.[45] Autopsy studies estimate a 9% to 37% incidence of choroidal metastases from breast cancer upon death.[46,47] A prospective screening program of 120 patients with known disseminated breast cancer found that 5% had asymptomatic choroidal disease.[48] The incidence of symptomatic metastases, however, is lower (1% to 2%).[49] Breast cancer patients with metastatic disease to more than 1 organ and involvement of lung and brain are at higher risk of developing choroidal metastases.[48] Although most patients presenting with choroidal lesions have known metastatic cancer, it has been reported to be the initial manifestation of breast cancer in 4% to 46% of patients or the initial site of metastatic disease in 12% to 31% of patients.[40,50]

Clinical Presentation

The most common symptom is blurred vision, occurring in 75% to 91% of patients. Other presenting symptoms include visual field defects (22%), photopsia (15%), floaters (6%), or pain (1%).[45,51] Choroidal metastases are often unilateral with an equal distribution between the right and left eyes, but can be bilateral in 30% to 40% of patients with multifocality noted in 32% to 50%.[48,51]

Diagnostic Workup

Patients with a history of breast cancer or known metastatic cancer who develop visual symptoms should be referred for a thorough ophthalmologic examination. Based on a screening program that detected asymptomatic lesions in 5% of patients with disseminated breast cancer, some clinicians recommend screening for high-risk patients.[48] A-scan ultrasonography will reveal medium to medium-high internal reflectivity while B-scan

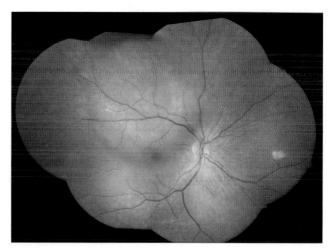

FIGURE 97-2 Choroidal metastasis from breast cancer.

ultrasonography will show acoustic solidity. Choroidal metastases usually appear as yellow, spotted subretinal lesions often with secondary retinal detachment (Fig. 97-2).[40,51] A biopsy is considered only in patients with no detectable primary or other sites of metastatic cancer.[52] Because the incidence of CNS disease increases after the development of ocular metastasis,[45] a brain MRI should be obtained to determine whether there is any evidence of CNS involvement.

Management

Patients who have choroidal metastases may be treated with chemotherapy and/or hormonal therapy with stabilization or regression of the lesions; however, results are often delayed.[53] Because choroidal metastases are usually radiosensitive, external beam radiotherapy is the most commonly used treatment and has been shown to stabilize or improve vision, control lesions, and prevent secondary retinal detachment.[54-56] Several retrospective series have shown tumor responses in 70% to 90% of patients,[57,58] with stabilization or improvement of vision in approximately 60% to 80%.[51,57,58] Patients who subsequently receive chemotherapy have higher response rates compared to those who receive radiotherapy alone.[58] Factors that are predictive of response include age less than 55, excellent preradiotherapy vision, smaller tumors with a tumor base diameter less than 15 mm, and no evidence of retinal detachment at the time of treatment.[55,59] Radiation dose has also been shown to be predictive of outcome, with 72% of patients treated with doses greater than 35.5 Gy having a complete response compared to 33% of patients treated with less than 35.5 Gy.[51] Although higher doses can result in improved tumor responses and improved visual acuity, increased late effects are associated with doses greater than 40 Gy.[58] In order to balance optimal response with toxicity, radiation treatment doses of 35.5 to 40 Gy are often recommended.

Acute side effects of external beam radiotherapy to the choroid include dry eye, hair loss, skin erythema, and conjunctival irritation.[52] Long-term side effects are not well described since many patients do not survive to experience such late toxicities, but potentially include increased risk of cataract formation

(5%), neovascular glaucoma (<1%), and radiation retinopathy (2%).[45,51] Lens-sparing treatment techniques can potentially minimize the risk of cataract formation.

In patients who present with bilateral synchronous disease, bilateral irradiation is recommended. In patients with unilateral disease, the question remains as to whether the contralateral choroids should be treated. In one series of 36 patients with unilateral choroid disease, 3 of 26 (11.5%) patients developed new contralateral metastases if only unilateral radiotherapy was given compared with 0 of 10 patients (0%) who had bilateral irradiation.[51] A second series reported a lower risk of developing metachronous metastases in nonirradiated contralateral eyes (2 of 41 patients, 4.8%) but similar results in the prophylactically irradiated eyes (0 of 8 metastases, 0%).[60] German investigators found that none of the patients with unilateral metastases treated with unilateral radiotherapy developed contralateral choroidal metastases during follow-up, suggesting that a unilateral field without sparing of the contralateral choroid will result in 50% to 70% of the prescribed dose being delivered to the contralateral choroid, a dose that may be sufficient to treat micrometastatic disease in the contralateral eye.[58] Most treatment recommendations therefore are for bilateral irradiation in patients with bilateral metastases, but unilateral treatment for those with unilateral disease in order to minimize any toxicity to the uninvolved eye.

Prognosis

Patients diagnosed with choroidal metastases have a poor prognosis, with a median survival after diagnosis and treatment ranging from 7 to 31 months and 1-year survivals of 59% to 65%.[45,51,61]

BONE METASTASES AND SPINAL CORD COMPRESSION

Incidence

Approximately three-quarters of patients with metastatic breast cancer will develop metastatic disease to the bone.[62] Isolated bone metastases appear to be more common in patients with ER-positive breast cancer,[63] while patients with triple-negative breast cancers (defined as ER-negative, progesterone receptor [PR]-negative, and HER-2/neu- negative) are more likely to develop visceral disease as the site of first distant recurrence and have a poorer prognosis.[64]

Clinical Presentation

Patients with metastatic disease to the bone can be asymptomatic, with disease identified only on routine imaging, or will often present with localized pain as the initial symptom. Pain related to bone metastases can be persistent and often requires increasing doses of pain medication. Bone metastases can lead to pathological fractures, hypercalcemia, neurologic complications, or spinal cord compression.[63,65] Common sites of symptomatic metastases include the axial skeleton, pelvic bones, and humeral or femoral heads. Areas that can be symptomatic but are less commonly reported by patients as problematic are the skull, ribs, and the diaphysis of the long bones. Bony disease to the clivus or base of the skull can result in neurologic symptoms or cranial nerve deficits if not treated.

Spinal Cord Compression

Pain is usually the first symptom of spinal cord compression and often precedes other neurologic symptoms by approximately 2 to 3 months.[66] Persistent back pain in patients with a history of breast cancer or with known metastatic disease should therefore be promptly evaluated for early diagnosis. Once disease progresses, patients may present with upper or lower extremity weakness, numbness in a radicular distribution or with a spinal sensory level, or bladder or bowel incontinence. These patients should be evaluated urgently as their functional and neurologic outcome is improved if there is minimal delay in diagnosis and treatment occurs prior to any significant spinal cord damage.[67] If there is clinical and radiographic evidence of spinal cord compression or cauda equina syndrome, corticosteroids should be administered immediately and the patient should be referred for urgent evaluation by a neurosurgeon and radiation oncologist.

Diagnostic Imaging

Metastatic bone lesions from breast cancer can be osteolytic, causing destruction of bone; osteoblastic, causing new bone formation; or mixed-pattern. Approximately 80% of patients with bone metastases have predominantly osteolytic lesions.[65,68] Plain radiographs are the simplest and most cost-effective imaging technique to identify bone metastases and pathologic fractures. Although the specificity is high, plain radiography has only approximately 60% sensitivity for identifying malignant lesions.[69]

Bone scintigraphy with technetium 99m–labeled diphosphonates is widely used for the detection of bone metastases given its high sensitivity compared with plain spinal radiographs and its ability to evaluate the entire skeleton at a relatively low cost.[70] Because abnormalities on a bone scan simply reflect the presence of an osteoblastic response, its specificity for detecting malignancy is lowered by benign processes such as osteoarthritis and inflammation. It is also difficult to interpret when following response to treatment, as the osteoblastic reaction may persist and the bone scan may remain positive even if there was a good clinical response to treatment.

Computed tomography is often used for routine staging of breast cancer and can help identify disruption of the bony cortex, which may suggest epidural tumor extension.[71] Disadvantages of CT, however, include the use of ionizing radiation and its limited ability to clearly identify the spinal cord and epidural space. Although one series found that CT of the thorax, abdomen, and pelvis identified 98% of metastatic bone lesions compared with 100% identified on bone scan, CT has not yet replaced bone scan for detection of bone metastases but is still commonly used to follow patients.[72]

The role of fluorodeoxyglucose positron emission tomography (FDG-PET) has increasingly been used in the staging and restaging of various malignancies, including breast cancer. In comparison to bone scan for detection of bone metastases, [F-18]FDG-PET appears to have a higher specificity (98% vs 87%) but a lower sensitivity (69% vs 88%)[73] Although it has a high specificity, the sensitivity of [F-18]FDG-PET in detecting bone metastases has been reported to range anywhere from 56.5% to 100%.[70,74] In particular, [F-18]FDG-PET has been found to be superior to bone scan in detecting osteolytic metastases, but is significantly less sensitive in detecting osteoblastic lesions.[75] One advantage of using PET is in following responses, with one study reporting that 76.4% of [F-18]FDG-avid lesions became negative after treatment while most remained abnormal on CT and positive on bone scan.[68] Despite the high specificity and the potential to detect osseous metastases at an earlier stage, it is still inconclusive as to whether FDG-PET should replace bone scan in metastatic breast cancer.[73] Since FDG-PET is more sensitive for osteolytic lesions and bone scintigraphy is more sensitive for osteoblastic lesions, both studies should be considered complementary until results of ongoing studies are available.[76]

Magnetic resonance imaging has been shown to be superior to CT and bone scan in detecting epidural involvement by tumor and can offer better visualization of paravertebral soft tissue involvement by tumor.[77] In patients with neurologic symptoms or suspicion of spinal cord compression, MRI can help facilitate management strategies by identifying the extent of epidural or paravertebral disease and determining whether there is any evidence of compression fracture and subsequent bony retropulsion into the spinal canal (Fig. 97-3). If a patient presents with clinical signs and symptoms concerning for spinal cord compression or cauda equina syndrome, an MRI with intravenous gadolinium contrast should be obtained to optimize management decisions.

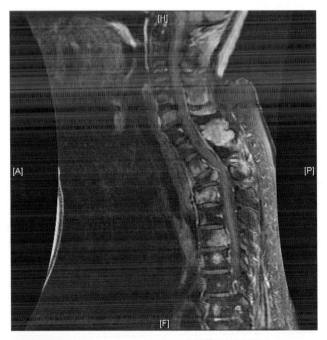

FIGURE 97-3 Multiple areas of metastatic disease with multiple compression fractures, particularly at T3 where there is flattening of the vertebral body and retropulsion resulting in cord compression.

Management

The goals of treating metastatic disease to the bone are to improve pain and decrease pain medication requirements; to prevent pathologic fractures, particularly in weight-bearing bones; and to preserve function and mobility.

Surgery

The role of surgery for metastatic disease to the bone is primarily limited to those bony areas that are at risk of or have already sustained a pathologic fracture, such as the femoral neck and shaft or the humerus. Surgical fixation can stabilize the long bones and provide improved mobility and function.

Patients with metastatic disease to the spine, on the other hand, do not usually undergo surgical resection unless there is evidence of spinal cord compression or bony retropulsion into the spinal canal. These patients have improved outcomes if they are initially treated with surgical decompression. A phase III randomized trial demonstrated that 84% of patients treated with surgical decompression followed by radiotherapy were able to walk after treatment compared with only 57% of patients treated with radiotherapy alone (*p* = .001). In addition, patients in the surgical group compared with the radiotherapy-alone group had a significant reduction in the use of corticosteroids (*p* = .0093) and opiates (*p* = .002) for management of symptoms.[78] Based on these results, patients who present with spinal cord compression who are surgical candidates should undergo surgical decompression prior to radiotherapy for optimal recovery of neurologic function.

Radiotherapy

In addition to postoperative treatment after surgical decompression or bone stabilization, external beam radiotherapy is commonly used to treat painful, metastatic bone lesions in which the pain is not well controlled with medication. Although 10% of patients may experience a temporary pain flare, or worsening of symptoms, shortly after initiating treatment,[79] radiotherapy can provide pain relief in approximately 76% of breast cancer patients with bony metastases and complete pain relief in up to 65% of patients.[80] Radiotherapy is also used to treat spinal metastases where there may be early involvement into the spinal canal or neural foramina in order to prevent neurologic compromise, and to prevent pathologic fractures, particularly in weight-bearing bones such as the femur.

Many different radiation fractionation schedules have been studied, ranging from a single fraction of 8 Gy to a total dose of 30 to 40 Gy delivered in multiple daily fractions over the course of 2 to 4 weeks. Clinical trials have shown that single treatments and shorter fractionation schedules provide equivalent pain control compared with longer treatment schedules, thus providing adequate palliation with improved patient convenience and cost-effectiveness.[81-83] Patients treated with a single fraction or shorter fractionation schedules, however, are twice as likely to require retreatment for long-term pain control compared with those who receive longer treatment courses initially.[83,84]

Stereotactic Body Radiotherapy

While external beam radiotherapy is still considered the standard treatment for metastatic disease to the spine, stereotactic body radiotherapy (SBRT) is emerging as a treatment option for patients with limited disease. This technique is often employed in patients who have previously been irradiated to the spine in an attempt to minimize any additional dose and toxicity to the spinal cord. Treatments often consist of 10 to 25 Gy in 1 to 5 fractions delivered using a linac-based technique or the CyberKnife.[85,86] Early investigations support that image-guided radiosurgery for spinal tumors is relatively safe and can offer long-term pain control in 65% to 86% of patients,[86,87] but patient selection is important. Patients with spinal cord compression should not be treated with radiosurgery.[85]

RADIATION THERAPY FOR LOCAL CONTROL IN PATIENTS WITH METASTATIC DISEASE

Although goals shift from cure to palliation in the setting of metastatic breast cancer, there is a subset of patients with metastatic disease who may have limited disease burden and/or more indolent disease, such as those with bone-only metastases. In these patients management decisions regarding local control of the primary lesion are unclear. Surgical series have suggested that patients with metastatic disease who undergo complete surgical resection of the primary lesion have a significantly better prognosis compared with those not treated surgically.[88] These results have been criticized for having significant selection bias; however, in patients with a good performance status and stable systemic disease, treatment of the primary lesion can certainly impact their overall quality of life. In such patients, local radiotherapy, either postoperatively or as definitive treatment of the breast, can help palliate symptoms such as pain or discomfort, skin ulceration, and lymphedema in patients with bulky nodal disease.

FUTURE DIRECTIONS

Patients with breast cancer are surviving longer with advances in systemic therapy. As these patients are living longer with their disease, palliative therapy for symptomatic disease plays an increasingly important role. How best to integrate localized radiation treatment with systemic therapy, including cytotoxic chemotherapy, endocrine therapy, and novel biological therapies, will continue to be an active area of investigation for patients with metastatic breast cancer.

SUMMARY

Radiation therapy has an important role in the management of patients with metastatic breast cancer. Patients with metastatic disease to the brain, orbits, or bone should be referred for consideration of radiotherapy. Radiotherapy to the primary lesion even in the setting of metastatic disease may benefit patients in terms of symptom management and quality of life.

REFERENCES

1. Tsukada Y, Fouad A, Pickren JW, Lane WW. Central nervous system metastasis from breast carcinoma. Autopsy study. *Cancer.* 1983;52(12):2349-2354.
2. Lee YT. Breast carcinoma: pattern of metastasis at autopsy. *J Surg Oncol.* 1983;23(3):175-180.
3. Hwang TL, Close TP, Grego JM, Brannon WL, Gonzales F. Predilection of brain metastasis in gray and white matter junction and vascular border zones. *Cancer.* 1996;77(8):1551-1555.
4. Delattre JY, Krol G, Thaler HT, Posner JB. Distribution of brain metastases. *Arch Neurol.* 1988;45(7):741-744.
5. Evans AJ, James JJ, Cornford EJ, et al. Brain metastases from breast cancer: identification of a high-risk group. *Clin Oncol (R Coll Radiol).* 2004;16(5):345-349.
6. Hicks DG, Short SM, Prescott NL, et al. Breast cancers with brain metastases are more likely to be estrogen receptor negative, express the basal cytokeratin CK5/6, and overexpress HER2 or EGFR. *Am J Surg Pathol.* 2006;30(9):1097-1104.
7. Slimane K, Andre F, Delaloge S, et al. Risk factors for brain relapse in patients with metastatic breast cancer. *Ann Oncol.* 2004;15(11):1640-1644.
8. Maki DD, Grossman RI. Patterns of disease spread in metastatic breast carcinoma: influence of estrogen and progesterone receptor status. *AJNR Am J Neuroradiol.* 2000;21(6):1064-1066.
9. Bendell JC, Domchek SM, Burstein HJ, et al. Central nervous system metastases in women who receive trastuzumab-based therapy for metastatic breast carcinoma. *Cancer.* 2003;97(12):2972-2977.
10. Weil RJ. Does trastuzumab increase the risk of isolated central nervous system metastases in patients with breast cancer? *Nat Clin Pract Oncol.* 2006;3(5):236-237.
11. Pestalozzi BC, Brignoli S. Trastuzumab in CSF. *J Clin Oncol.* 2000;18(11):2349-2351.
12. Posner JB. Brain metastases: 1995. A brief review. *J Neurooncol.* 1996;27(3):287-293.
13. Forsyth PA, Posner JB. Headaches in patients with brain tumors: a study of 111 patients. *Neurology.* 1993;43(9):1678-1683.
14. Zimm S, Wampler GL, Stablein D, Hazra T, Young HF. Intracerebral metastases in solid-tumor patients: natural history and results of treatment. *Cancer.* 1981;48(2):384-394.
15. Nussbaum ES, Djalilian HR, Cho KH, Hall WA. Brain metastases. Histology, multiplicity, surgery, and survival. *Cancer.* 1996;78(8):1781-1788.
16. Davis PC, Hudgins PA, Peterman SB, Hoffman JC Jr. Diagnosis of cerebral metastases: double-dose delayed CT vs contrast-enhanced MR imaging. *AJNR Am J Neuroradiol.* 1991;12(2):293-300.
17. Arastoo Vossough M, Gilberto Gonzalez R, Henson JW. Imaging neurologic manifestations of oncologic disease. In: Schiff D, Wen PY, eds. *Current Clinical Oncology: Cancer Neurology in Clinical Practice.* Totowa, NJ: Humana Press; 2002:15-30.
18. Friedman WA, Sceats DJ Jr, Nestok BR, Ballinger WE Jr. The incidence of unexpected pathological findings in an image-guided biopsy series: a review of 100 consecutive cases. *Neurosurgery.* 1989;25(2):180-184.
19. Gaspar L, Scott C, Rotman M, et al. Recursive partitioning analysis (RPA) of prognostic factors in three Radiation Therapy Oncology Group (RTOG) brain metastases trials. *Int J Radiat Oncol Biol Phys.* 1997;37(4):745-751.
20. Gaspar LE, Scott C, Murray K, Curran W. Validation of the RTOG recursive partitioning analysis (RPA) classification for brain metastases. *Int J Radiat Oncol Biol Phys.* 2000;47(4):1001-1006.
21. Sperduto PW, Berkey B, Gaspar LE, Mehta M, Curran W. A new prognostic index and comparison to three other indices for patients with brain metastases: an analysis of 1,960 patients in the RTOG database. *Int J Radiat Oncol Biol Phys.* 2008;70(2):510-514.
22. Lagerwaard FJ, Levendag PC, Nowak PJ, et al. Identification of prognostic factors in patients with brain metastases: a review of 1292 patients. *Int J Radiat Oncol Biol Phys.* 1999;43(4):795-803.
23. Wolstenholme V, Hawkins M, Ashley S, Tait D, Ross G. HER2 significance and treatment outcomes after radiotherapy for brain metastases in breast cancer patients. *Breast.* 2008;17(6):661-665.
24. Wen PY, Schiff D, Kesari S, et al. Medical management of patients with brain tumors. *J Neurooncol.* 2006;80(3):313-332.
25. Sperling MR, Ko J. Seizures and brain tumors. *Semin Oncol.* 2006;33(3):333-341.
26. Delattre JY, Safai B, Posner JB. Erythema multiforme and Stevens-Johnson syndrome in patients receiving cranial irradiation and phenytoin. *Neurology.* 1988;38(2):194-198.
27. Glantz MJ, Cole BF, Forsyth PA, et al. Practice parameter: anticonvulsant prophylaxis in patients with newly diagnosed brain tumors. Report of the Quality Standards Subcommittee of the American Academy of Neurology. *Neurology.* 2000;54(10):1886-1893.
28. Patchell RA, Tibbs PA, Walsh JW, et al. A randomized trial of surgery in the treatment of single metastases to the brain. *N Engl J Med.* 1990;322(8):494-500.

29. Patchell RA, Tibbs PA, Regine WF, et al. Postoperative radiotherapy in the treatment of single metastases to the brain: a randomized trial. *JAMA.* 1998;280(17):1485-1489.

30. Noordijk EM, Vecht CJ, Haaxma-Reiche H, et al. The choice of treatment of single brain metastasis should be based on extracranial tumor activity and age. *Int J Radiat Oncol Biol Phys.* 1994;29(4):711-717.

31. Bindal RK, Sawaya R, Leavens ME, Lee JJ. Surgical treatment of multiple brain metastases. *J Neurosurg.* 1993;79(2):210-216.

32. Lin NU, Bellon JR, Winer EP. CNS metastases in breast cancer. *J Clin Oncol.* 2004;22(17):3608-3617.

33. Borgelt B, Gelber R, Kramer S, et al. The palliation of brain metastases: final results of the first two studies by the Radiation Therapy Oncology Group. *Int J Radiat Oncol Biol Phys.* 1980;6(1):1-9.

34. Borgelt B, Gelber R, Larson M, et al. Ultra-rapid high dose irradiation schedules for the palliation of brain metastases: final results of the first two studies by the Radiation Therapy Oncology Group. *Int J Radiat Oncol Biol Phys.* 1981;7(12):1633-1638.

35. DeAngelis LM, Delattre JY, Posner JB. Radiation-induced dementia in patients cured of brain metastases. *Neurology.* 1989;39(6):789-796.

36. Leksell L. The stereotaxic method and radiosurgery of the brain. *Acta Chir Scand.* 1951;102(4):316-319.

37. Andrews DW, Scott CB, Sperduto PW, et al. Whole brain radiation therapy with or without stereotactic radiosurgery boost for patients with one to three brain metastases: phase III results of the RTOG 9508 randomised trial. *Lancet.* 2004;363(9422):1665-1672.

38. Kondziolka D, Patel A, Lunsford LD, Kassam A, Flickinger JC. Stereotactic radiosurgery plus whole brain radiotherapy versus radiotherapy alone for patients with multiple brain metastases. *Int J Radiat Oncol Biol Phys.* 1999;45(2):427-434.

39. Shirato H, Takamura A, Tomita M, et al. Stereotactic irradiation without whole-brain irradiation for single brain metastasis. *Int J Radiat Oncol Biol Phys.* 1997;37(2):385-391.

40. Sneed PK, Lamborn KR, Forstner JM, et al. Radiosurgery for brain metastases: is whole brain radiotherapy necessary? *Int J Radiat Oncol Biol Phys.* 1999;43(3):549-558.

41. Aoyama H, Shirato H, Tago M, et al. Stereotactic radiosurgery plus whole-brain radiation therapy vs stereotactic radiosurgery alone for treatment of brain metastases: a randomized controlled trial. *JAMA.* 2006;295(21):2483-2491.

42. Patchell RA, Regine WF, Renschler M, et al. Comments about the prospective randomized trial by Aoyama et al. *Surg Neurol.* 2006;66(5):459-460.

43. Soltys SG, Adler JR, Lipani JD, et al. Stereotactic radiosurgery of the postoperative resection cavity for brain metastases. *Int J Radiat Oncol Biol Phys.* 2008;70(1):187-193.

44. Shaw E, Scott C, Souhami L, et al. Single dose radiosurgical treatment of recurrent previously irradiated primary brain tumors and brain metastases: final report of RTOG protocol 90-05. *Int J Radiat Oncol Biol Phys.* 2000;47(2):291-298.

45. Demirci H, Vine AK, Elner VM. Choroidal metastasis from submandibular salivary gland adenoid cystic carcinoma. *Ophthalmic Surg Lasers Imaging.* 2008;39(1):57-59.

46. Bloch RS, Gartner S. The incidence of ocular metastatic carcinoma. *Arch Ophthalmol.* 1971;85(6):673-675.

47. Nelson CC, Hertzberg BS, Klintworth GK. A histopathologic study of 716 unselected eyes in patients with cancer at the time of death. *Am J Ophthalmol.* 1983;95(6):788-793.

48. Wiegel T, Kreusel KM, Bornfeld N, et al. Frequency of asymptomatic choroidal metastasis in patients with disseminated breast cancer: results of a prospective screening programme. *Br J Ophthalmol.* 1998;82(10):1159-1161.

49. Albert DM, Rubenstein RA, Scheie HG. Tumor metastasis to the eye. I. Incidence in 213 adult patients with generalized malignancy. *Am J Ophthalmol.* 1967;63(4):723-726.

50. Merrill CF, Kaufman DI, Dimitrov NV. Breast cancer metastatic to the eye is a common entity. *Cancer.* 1991;68(3):623-627.

51. Rosset A, Zografos L, Coucke P, Monney M, Mirimanoff RO. Radiotherapy of choroidal metastases. *Radiother Oncol.* 1998;46(3):263-268.

52. Chong JT, Mick A. Choroidal metastasis: case reports and review of the literature. *Optometry.* 2005;76(5):293-301.

53. Letson AD, Davidorf FH, Bruce RA Jr. Chemotherapy for treatment of choroidal metastases from breast carcinoma. *Am J Ophthalmol.* 1982;93(1):102-106.

54. Chu FC, Huh SH, Nisce LZ, Simpson LD. Radiation therapy of choroid metastasis from breast cancer. *Int J Radiat Oncol Biol Phys.* 1977;2(3-4):273-279.

55. Rudoler SB, Corn BW, Shields CL, et al. External beam irradiation for choroid metastases: identification of factors predisposing to long-term sequelae. *Int J Radiat Oncol Biol Phys.* 1997;38(2):251-256.

56. Thatcher N, Thomas PR. Choroidal metastases from breast carcinoma: a survey of 42 patients and the use of radiation therapy. *Clin Radiol.* 1975;26(4):549-553.

57. Rudoler SB, Shields CL, Corn BW, et al. Functional vision is improved in the majority of patients treated with external-beam radiotherapy for choroid metastases: a multivariate analysis of 188 patients. *J Clin Oncol.* 1997;15(3):1244-1251.

58. Wiegel T, Bottke D, Kreusel KM, et al. External beam radiotherapy of choroidal metastases—final results of a prospective study of the German Cancer Society (ARO 95-08). *Radiother Oncol.* 2002;64(1):13-18.

59. Mewis L, Young SE. Breast carcinoma metastatic to the choroid. Analysis of 67 patients. *Ophthalmology.* 1982;89(2):147-151.

60. Amichetti M, Caffo O, Minatel E, et al. Ocular metastases from breast carcinoma: a multicentric retrospective study. *Oncol Rep.* 2000;7(4):761-765.

61. Shields CL, Shields JA, Gross NE, Schwartz GP, Lally SE. Survey of 520 eyes with uveal metastases. *Ophthalmology.* 1997;104(8):1265-1276.

62. Coleman RE. Skeletal complications of malignancy. *Cancer.* 1997;80(8 suppl):1588-1594.

63. Coleman RE, Rubens RD. The clinical course of bone metastases from breast cancer. *Br J Cancer.* 1987;55(1):61-66.

64. Dent R, Hanna WM, Trudeau M, et al. Pattern of metastatic spread in triple-negative breast cancer. *Breast Cancer Res Treat.* 2009;115(2):423-428.

65. Akhtari M, Mansuri J, Newman KA, Guise TM, Seth P. Biology of breast cancer bone metastasis. *Cancer Biol Ther.* 2008;7(1):3-9.

66. Helweg-Larsen S, Sorensen PS. Symptoms and signs in metastatic spinal cord compression: a study of progression from first symptom until diagnosis in 153 patients. *Eur J Cancer.* 1994;30A(3):396-398.

67. Husband DJ. Malignant spinal cord compression: prospective study of delays in referral and treatment. *BMJ.* 1998;317(7150):18-21.

68. Du Y, Cullum I, Illidge TM, Ell PJ. Fusion of metabolic function and morphology: sequential [18F]fluorodeoxyglucose positron-emission tomography/computed tomography studies yield new insights into the natural history of bone metastases in breast cancer. *J Clin Oncol.* 2007;25(23):3440-3447.

69. Jarvik JG, Deyo RA. Diagnostic evaluation of low back pain with emphasis on imaging. *Ann Intern Med.* 2002;137(7):586-597.

70. Hamaoka T, Madewell JE, Podoloff DA, Hortobagyi GN, Ueno NT. Bone imaging in metastatic breast cancer. *J Clin Oncol.* 2004;22(14):2942-2953.

71. Weissman DE, Gilbert M, Wang H, Grossman SA. The use of computed tomography of the spine to identify patients at high risk for epidural metastases. *J Clin Oncol.* 1985;3(11):1541-1544.

72. Bristow AR, Agrawal A, Evans AJ, et al. Can computerised tomography replace bone scintigraphy in detecting bone metastases from breast cancer? A prospective study. *Breast.* 2008;17(1):98-103.

73. Shie P, Cardarelli R, Brandon D, Erdman W, Abdulrahim N. Meta-analysis: comparison of F-18 Fluorodeoxyglucose-positron emission tomography and bone scintigraphy in the detection of bone metastases in patients with breast cancer. *Clin Nucl Med.* 2008;33(2):97-101.

74. Fogelman I, Cook G, Israel O, Van der Wall H. Positron emission tomography and bone metastases. *Semin Nucl Med.* 2005;35(2):135-142.

75. Cook GJ, Houston S, Rubens R, Maisey MN, Fogelman I. Detection of bone metastases in breast cancer by 18FDG PET: differing metabolic activity in osteoblastic and osteolytic lesions. *J Clin Oncol.* 1998;16(10):3375-3379.

76. Schirrmeister H. Detection of bone metastases in breast cancer by positron emission tomography. *Radiol Clin North Am.* 2007;45(4):669-676; vi.

77. Godersky JC, Smoker WR, Knutzon R. Use of magnetic resonance imaging in the evaluation of metastatic spinal disease. *Neurosurgery.* 1987;21(5):676-680.

78. Patchell RA, Tibbs PA, Regine WF, et al. Direct decompressive surgical resection in the treatment of spinal cord compression caused by metastatic cancer: a randomised trial. *Lancet.* 2005;366(9486):643-648.

79. Roos DE, O'Brien PC, Smith JG, et al. A role for radiotherapy in neuropathic bone pain: preliminary response rates from a prospective trial (Trans-tasman radiation oncology group, TROG 96.05). *Int J Radiat Oncol Biol Phys.* 2000;46(4):975-981.

80. Arcangeli G, Giovinazzo G, Saracino B, et al. Radiation therapy in the management of symptomatic bone metastases: the effect of total dose and histology on pain relief and response duration. *Int J Radiat Oncol Biol Phys.* 1998;42(5):1119-1126.

81. Chow E, Hoskin PJ, Wu J, et al. A phase III international randomised trial comparing single with multiple fractions for re-irradiation of painful bone metastases: National Cancer Institute of Canada Clinical Trials Group (NCIC CTG) SC 20. *Clin Oncol (R Coll Radiol).* 2006;18(2):125-128.

82. Hartsell WF, Scott CB, Bruner DW, et al. Randomized trial of short- versus long-course radiotherapy for palliation of painful bone metastases. *J Natl Cancer Inst.* 2005;97(11):798-804.

83. Steenland E, Leer JW, van Houwelingen H, et al. The effect of a single fraction compared to multiple fractions on painful bone metastases: a global analysis of the Dutch Bone Metastasis Study. *Radiother Oncol.* 1999;52(2):101-109.

84. Bone Pain Trial Working Party. 8 Gy single fraction radiotherapy for the treatment of metastatic skeletal pain: randomised comparison with a multifraction schedule over 12 months of patient follow-up. *Radiother Oncol.* 1999;52(2):111-121.

85. Gibbs IC, Chang SD. Radiosurgery and radiotherapy for sacral tumors. *Neurosurg Focus.* 2003;15(2):E8.

86. Ryu S, Jin R, Jin JY, et al. Pain control by image-guided radiosurgery for solitary spinal metastasis. *J Pain Symptom Manage.* 2000;35(3):292-290.

87. Gerszten PC, Burton SA, Ozhasoglu C, Welch WC. Radiosurgery for spinal metastases: clinical experience in 500 cases from a single institution. *Spine.* 2007;32(2):193-199.

88. Khan SA, Stewart AK, Morrow M. Does aggressive local therapy improve survival in metastatic breast cancer? *Surgery.* 2002;132(4):620-626; discussion 626-627.

SECTION 9

FOLLOW-UP AND COMPLICATIONS FOLLOWING DIAGNOSIS AND THERAPY

Tara Breslin
Mehra Golshan

CHAPTER 98

Guidelines for Follow-Up

Alicia Growney
Jennifer J. Griggs

Breast cancer survivors number more than 2,000,000 in the United States alone.[1] Improvements in screening technology, increased uptake of screening, and advances in adjuvant therapy[2] as well as the aging of the population are bound to lead to even greater numbers of breast cancer survivors over time. The Institute of Medicine report entitled *From Cancer Patient to Cancer Survivor: Lost in Transition* reported on the health, psychosocial, family, employment, and financial needs of survivors of cancer and provided recommendations for improving the quality of care and health outcomes of cancer survivors.[3] Follow-up of the breast cancer survivor is one important aspect of survivorship care.

As described in preceding chapters, multimodality therapy of breast cancer is associated with acute side effects such as postoperative pain, skin toxicity from radiation, fatigue, alopecia, and anemia related to chemotherapy. As people recover from these effects, new issues requiring attention may arise (Table 98-1). The long-term and late effects of cancer and its treatment are addressed in other chapters of this section.

Physicians who care for survivors of breast cancer—including surgeons, medical oncologists, radiation oncologists, primary care physicians, gynecologists, and mental health professionals—have the opportunity to address the concerns of breast cancer survivors and to intervene to improve functional status and quality of life. In addition, physical therapists, dieticians, sexual health therapists, and social work professionals provide care to survivors as described in earlier chapters. Coordinating the care of breast cancer survivors among multiple providers can itself become a challenge for patients. In addition, patients are often not clear about the purpose of follow-up care.[4] Finally, the medical costs of breast cancer follow-up are substantial.[5,6] In one study of 391 women, the average estimated costs per year per patient were $1800.[6]

PURPOSE OF FOLLOW-UP

There are several goals of scheduled follow-up care in breast cancer survivors[7]: detection and management of second primary breast cancers and locoregional breast cancer recurrences, detection and management of late and long-term effects of treatment, management of adjuvant endocrine therapy, recognition of genetic cancer syndromes, and promotion of healthy behaviors. Provision of information to survivors on the treatments they received and what they should expect during the months and years after treatment is important to achieve and preserve optimal health in survivors and their families.

There is no evidence that follow-up with cancer care providers improves the likelihood or duration of *survival* in patients after breast cancer. In addition, specialized cancer care does not appear to decrease the risk of catastrophic events such as spinal cord compression, pathologic fractures, hypercalcemia, or decline in functional status attributable to cancer recurrence.[8] In contrast, prompt evaluation of symptoms that may reflect metastatic recurrence is critical to avoid and treat such events and other symptoms of metastatic disease. The risk of recurrent disease even 5 years after completion of therapy ranges from 2% (for women with stage I disease) to nearly 15% (for women with stage III disease) over the following 5 years.[9] The evaluation of women suspected of having metastatic recurrence is described earlier in the textbook.

Primary care physicians may assume the care of breast cancer patients if familiar with the issues faced by breast cancer survivors and if experienced in examining women after breast surgery and radiation therapy.[8] In a randomized study of primary care follow-up compared with cancer specialist follow-up, 968 (58%) of 1760 patients invited to participate agreed to be randomized. Enrolled patients were followed by either their family

TABLE 98-1 Examples of Long-Term and Late Issues Among Breast Cancer Survivors

Issues related to physical health after breast cancer and its treatment
  Fatigue
  Premature menopause
  Bone health
  Side effects of endocrine therapy
  Sexual health
  Cardiac dysfunction
  Risk of secondary cancers
  Pregnancy after breast cancer
  Lymphedema
  Disruption of cognitive function
Psychological and social aspects of survivorship
  Concerns about recurrence
  Impact of cancer on the family
  Sexual health
  Impact of cancer on employment and financial health

physician, who was provided a 1-page information sheet about recommended follow-up care, or their treating cancer providers. There were no differences in the occurrence or detection of serious clinical events between the 2 groups of patients. Prompt referral of patients with metastasis will allow the newly diagnosed patient with stage IV disease to receive optimal management of her disease in a timely fashion.

Shared follow-up between cancer specialists and primary care physicians represents another model for the care of an increasing number of cancer survivors. Patients cared for in a shared care model see both their primary care physicians and their oncologists in a well-coordinated schedule of follow-up. This model requires frequent and high quality communication between providers and clear expectations about the role of each provider.[10] Shared care with a primary care provider increases the likelihood that appropriate screening for other medical problems, such as hyperlipidemia, and preventive services, such as influenza vaccination.[11] Nurse practitioners familiar with the principles of follow-up may provide care to well patients after completion of breast cancer treatment.[12]

RECOMMENDATIONS FOR FOLLOW-UP

Recommendations for follow-up in breast cancer include a history and physical, breast imaging, appropriate referral for genetic counseling, and regular pelvic examinations. Patients should also be informed about symptoms of recurrence. Guideline-concordant follow-up care has been shown to minimize costs of care while maximizing health outcomes, including quality of life.[13,14] Recommended follow up of women who have completed multimodality therapy of breast cancer is summarized in Table 98-2.

Medical History

A careful history for symptoms of recurrence or of long-term and late effects of treatment is important in caring for the cancer survivor.[15] The recommended frequency of a medical history is every 3 to 6 months for the first 3 years after completion of multimodality therapy. Thereafter, the frequency of follow-up visits can decrease to every 6 months in the fourth and fifth years followed by annual visits thereafter.[16,17] Symptom assessment should determine the presence of symptoms that may suggest metastatic recurrence of cancer or the development of long-term adverse effects of treatment, such as cardiomyopathy related to anthracycline use. Neurologic symptoms or deficits should similarly prompt further investigation of possible distant metastases, although neuropathy is a known side effect of some chemotherapy agents, such as the taxanes. Any bone pain should be thoroughly investigated and evaluated with plain films and bone scan to evaluate for metastatic disease. It is important to distinguish between bone pain and joint symptoms that may occur in patients experiencing menopause or in and with adjuvant endocrine therapy in avoid overuse of imaging studies. Postmenopausal women on tamoxifen should be asked if they have had any vaginal bleeding, as such bleeding may indicate the presence of endometrial cancer, an uncommon but important adverse effect of tamoxifen.

Patients who are on tamoxifen should not take medications that inhibit CYP2D6, such as the selective serotonin receptor antagonists fluoxetine and paroxetine, because these drugs inhibit conversion of tamoxifen to its active metabolite, endoxifen, and may reduce the effectiveness of tamoxifen.[18]

Physical Examination

A physical examination should be performed during follow-up visits.[16] A careful examination of bilateral nodal basins, including cervical, supraclavicular, and axillary nodes, should be performed at every encounter, in addition to examination of the breasts in the upright and supine position for changing asymmetry, skin changes, new dominant masses, nodularity, or skin thickening. Cardiovascular and pulmonary examinations should be performed to evaluate for the presence of pleural or pericardial effusions or cardiac dysfunction. An examination of the abdomen should be done to evaluate for evidence of hepatomegaly or right upper quadrant tenderness. In the patient with upper extremity lymphedema, early referral to an experienced physical therapist may reduce the severity of long-term lymphedema and decrease the functional impairment associated with lymphedema.

Breast Imaging

In addition to the physical examination, the patient should undergo annual mammography to be completed 1 year from the previous screening mammogram. For patients treated with breast-conserving therapy, initial postradiation mammograms are generally performed 6 months after the completion of treatment, with subsequent annual mammograms performed 12 months from the previous screening exam.[17] Despite clear and consistent guidelines about the use of surveillance breast

TABLE 98-2 Follow-Up of Breast Cancer Survivors after Completion of Multimodality Therapy

History and physical examination	Every 3 to 6 months for the first 3 years of follow-up; every 6 months for years 4 and 5; annually after 5 years Visits should include provision of information about symptoms of recurrence Women should be counseled to perform breast self-examination monthly, although there is no clear evidence that breast self-examination improves outcome
Mammography	Annually Women who had breast-conserving therapy should have a mammogram of the treated breast approximately 6 months after completion of radiation therapy
Referral for genetic counseling	Indicated for patients with a compelling personal or family history (see also Chapter 8)
Pelvic examination	Regular gynecologic care is recommended. Women on tamoxifen should be told to report any postmenopausal bleeding
Monitoring of bone health	Indicated for women who are at risk of loss of bone mineral density (for example, women who have premature menopause due to chemotherapy or women on aromatase inhibitors)
Lifestyle counseling	Patients should be informed of screening recommendations for other cancers, importance of strategies for weight loss, smoking cessation resources
Referral to appropriate specialists	Patients should be offered referral to specialty services, such as physical therapy for the management of lymphedema, registered dieticians, supportive psychotherapists, sex therapists, financial counselors, and employment attorneys

imaging, several studies have demonstrated underuse of mammography among survivors of breast cancer.[6,19] For example, in one study, only 61.9% of women with stages I or II disease received mammography in the first year of follow up.[6] In another study of patients in the combined Surveillance, Epidemiology, and End Results–Medicare data set, only 56.7% had mammography yearly over a 3-year period. Nonclinical factors, such as black race and being unmarried, have been associated with underuse of surveillance mammography,[6,19] suggesting that high-quality surveillance care is not applied equally to all women.

Magnetic resonance imaging (MRI) should be offered to women who are at particularly high risk of a second primary breast cancer, such as women with an inherited susceptibility to breast cancer by virtue of having a BRCA1 or BRCA2 mutation. The role of surveillance MRI in women not deemed to be at high risk of a second primary cancer has not been established.

Additional Tests

Analyses of multiple randomized controlled trials designed to assess the effectiveness of different follow-up strategies on morbidity, mortality, and quality of life in breast cancer patients have concluded there was no survival benefit or difference in disease-free survival in patients who were subjected to more intensive monitoring with laboratory and radiographic tests compared with regular examinations and mammography.[20] Routine laboratory studies in asymptomatic patients, including hepatic transaminases, alkaline phosphatase, tumor markers, and bone scans, have not been shown to improve disease-free survival, overall survival, or quality of life and are thus not recommended.[16,21] Such testing often leads to additional imaging and invasive procedures and thus increases patient and family anxiety and costs of care with no proven benefit.[7]

Despite the increase in risk of endometrial cancer in women treated with tamoxifen, endometrial ultrasound and biopsies are not indicated in asymptomatic patients on tamoxifen.[22] Population-based research has shown that many patients receive imaging (eg, computerized tomographic scans of the chest and abdomen and bone scans) and blood tests without clear indications. It does appear that the use of nonrecommended testing is decreasing in frequency, perhaps as a result of dissemination of guidelines.[23]

Referral for Genetic Counseling

Revisiting the patient's family history of cancer is important as the patient can become aware of relevant cancers in her family only after multimodality treatment is complete and because new cancers can obviously develop in family members in the years after a patient's diagnosis and treatment. A familiarity with the genetic cancer syndromes described in Chapter 8 will help providers identify patients who should be referred for genetic counseling. Patients often have misconceptions about genetic counseling and testing that can be addressed by a knowledgeable clinician. Primary care physicians may require information support from oncology specialists in knowing for whom genetic counseling is indicated. For example, in a survey of a national sample of physicians conducted in 1999 through 2000, oncologists were significantly more likely than primary care physicians to recognize that mutations in BRCA1 and BRCA2 can be transmitted through paternal inheritance.[24]

Lifestyle Counseling

In addition to the above, breast cancer follow-up provides the opportunity to counsel patients on healthy behaviors.[25] Having completed treatment for breast cancer, survivors may be motivated to start exercise and weight reduction programs. Opportunities to counsel patients about smoking cessation and alcohol intake should be taken advantage of in the follow-up period. Referral to appropriate services can be offered to patients desiring additional support with smoking cessation and problem alcohol use.

Raising patient and family awareness of screening guidelines for other cancers, such as colorectal cancer, is appropriate in the breast cancer survivor, and such recommendations can be reinforced during follow-up visits. Lifestyle measures may reduce the risk of loss of bone mineral density in women at risk of osteopenia and osteoporosis as described next.

Monitoring of Bone Health

Bone health is often affected by systemic therapy of breast cancer. Chemotherapy, premature menopause caused by chemotherapy and luteinizing hormone–releasing hormone analogs, and aromatase inhibitors can all decrease bone mineral density.[26,27] Although protective against loss of bone mineral density in postmenopausal women, tamoxifen causes loss of bone mineral density in premenopausal women.

Current recommendations for patients on aromatase inhibitors include routine monitoring of bone health with dual x-ray absorptiometry (DXA).[26] The frequency with which DXA testing should be performed will depend on the baseline bone mineral density and the presence of other risk factors as well as the intended duration of aromatase inhibitor use.

Premenopausal women who experience chemotherapy-induced menopause are also at risk of osteopenia and osteoporosis and should be advised to follow the lifestyle measures described below and to have monitoring of bone density with DXA at periodic intervals (depending on severity of bone mineral loss and other risk factors).

Patients who are found to have osteopenia or osteoporosis should be evaluated for other possible causes of bone loss, such as vitamin D deficiency, hypercalciuria, and hyperparathyroidism given the prevalence of these conditions among breast cancer survivors with osteopenia and osteoporosis.[28]

Protective strategies for minimizing the risk of skeletal complications of systemic therapy include adequate intake of calcium and vitamin D, regular weight-bearing exercise, smoking cessation, reduction of alcohol consumption, and the addition of bisphosphonates in patients with osteoporosis.[26,29]

Information Support

After completion of surgery, chemotherapy, and radiation therapy, the intensity of visits to medical providers decreases at the same time patients face new information needs. Follow-up visits with cancer providers tend to be brief and in general do not provide adequate time or opportunity to address the information needs of breast cancer survivors.[30]

Studies that have evaluated the adequacy of survivorship information have shown that most patients are dissatisfied with the quantity and quality of information.[31-34] The tendency of health care providers to underestimate the importance of information to patients[35,36] is likely to contribute to such frustration and to the limited time available in the typical follow-up visit. Issues such as sexual health and problems with fertility after treatment (see Chapter 101) are often left unaddressed in the course of a busy outpatient practice.

From Cancer Patient to Cancer Survivor: Lost in Transition from the Institute of Medicine offered a number of recommendations to address the information needs of cancer survivors.[3] One such recommendation is that patients be provided a treatment summary and survivor care plan at the conclusion of multimodality therapy.[3,37,38] Treatment summaries and survivor care plans may serve as a vehicle for the delivery of both general and tailored information to patients and their medical providers, including their primary care providers. Preparing a treatment summary and survivor care plan requires communication between cancer providers in order to reflect accurately the treatments received and recommendations for follow-up.[37,38] In addition, the survivor care plan serves as a discussion tool for patients and their doctors and can help raise issues previously not addressed. Recommended elements of treatment summaries and survivor care plans are listed in Table 98-3.

FUTURE DIRECTIONS AND NECESSARY STUDIES TO ADVANCE THE FIELD

The groundswell of interest in cancer survivorship, spurred on by advocacy groups, professionals caring for and learning from their patients, and the Institute of Medicine report, has identified areas for further research. As the number of breast cancer survivors grows and the workforce shortages in medicine increase, providing high-quality care of survivors will become more challenging. Thus novel ways of delivering follow-up care need to be investigated. Particularly challenging is the care of people who do not have access to specialized follow-up care, such as people living in rural areas with a lower concentration of providers, people with limited health literacy, and other vulnerable populations, such as the medically uninsured. Web-based interfaces to provide some aspects of follow-up care may increase access to high-quality care, and research addressing Web-based and other follow-up strategies is ongoing.

TABLE 98-3 Suggested Elements of a Breast Cancer Treatment Summary and Care Plan

Treatment Summary

Date of diagnosis
Age at diagnosis
Affected breast(s)
Menopausal status at diagnosis

Tumor characteristics

Stage
Histologic subtype
Hormone receptor status
Histologic grade
HER2 status
Angiolymphatic invasion

Treatments

Locoregional therapy
Surgery
Date(s) of surgery
Surgery performed
Sentinel lymph node/axillary lymph node dissection
Type of reconstruction if applicable
Complications
Radiation therapy
Dates of radiation
Radiation field
Radiation dose; boost dose (if applicable); total dose
Unplanned treatment interruptions and any complications
Systemic therapy
Chemotherapy
Dates of chemotherapy
Drugs given
Schedule
Number of cycles
Total cumulative dose of anthracyclines (if applicable)
Complications
Trastuzumab and dates
Endocrine therapy
Name of drug and dates
Planned duration of endocrine therapy

Names and contact information of cancer care providers

Survivorship Care Plan

Recommended frequency and type of follow-up
Symptoms that should prompt a call to providers
Information about recommended lifestyle modifications to improve long-term health and quality-of-life outcomes
Information about possible long-term effects of treatment and expected course of recovery
Information about possible effects of cancer and its treatment on relationships, employment
Information about professional resources available for addressing the above issues

Also acknowledged is the lack of data supporting the recommendation for treatment summaries and survivor care plans. Although policymakers, advocates, and health care professionals all endorse the use of such documents, research to define the best ways to create, tailor, implement, and maintain updated data treatment summaries and care plans is needed.

Finally, follow-up recommendations, specifically recommendations against routine imaging and blood tests, are based on studies that used chest x-rays, bone scans, and blood tests that are nonspecific and were conducted in an era of limited treatment options. Detection of preclinical recurrence at the point of minimal disease burden and tailored treatment with well-tolerated therapies may improve survival amongst survivors of breast cancer. Such a strategy is being proposed as part of cancer control efforts within the cooperative group setting. With the number of breast cancer survivors and the costs of such therapies, study design of the utmost rigor will be required to change recommendations about follow-up care in breast cancer survivors.

SUMMARY

Just as the care of the breast cancer patient involves multiple specialists during initial treatment, follow-up strategies require coordination of care to provide high-quality, patient-centered care that meets patients' needs without excessive and unnecessary use of medical care resources. Appropriate follow-up involves coordinated care between medical providers, prompt evaluation of symptoms that may indicate metastatic recurrence, avoidance of tests not indicated by available evidence, and anticipatory management of long-term possible complications, such as loss of bone mineral density. In addition, counseling patients about resources available to them will allow them to access the services of other health care and nonmedical professionals.

REFERENCES

1. Stat bite: Number of cancer survivors by site, 2003. *J Natl Cancer Inst.* 2006;98:1514.
2. Berry DA, Cronin KA, Plevritis SK, et al. Effect of screening and adjuvant therapy on mortality from breast cancer. *N Engl J Med.* 2005;353:1784-1792.
3. Hewitt M, Greenfield S, Stovall E. *From Cancer Patient to Cancer Survivor: Lost in Transition.* Washington, DC: Institute of Medicine and National Research Council, The National Academies Press; 2005.
4. Loprinzi CL, Hayes D, Smith T. Doc, shouldn't we be getting some tests? *J Clin Oncol.* 2000;18:2345-2348.
5. Hensley ML, Dowell J, Herndon JE 2nd, et al. Economic outcomes of breast cancer survivorship: CALGB study 79804. *Breast Cancer Res Treat.* 2005;91:153-161.
6. Mandelblatt JS, Lawrence WF, Cullen J, et al. Patterns of care in early-stage breast cancer survivors in the first year after cessation of active treatment. *J Clin Oncol.* 2006;24:77-84.
7. Hayes DF. Clinical practice. Follow-up of patients with early breast cancer. *N Engl J Med.* 2007;356:2505-2513.
8. Grunfeld E, Levine MN, Julian JA, et al. Randomized trial of long-term follow-up for early-stage breast cancer: a comparison of family physician versus specialist care. *J Clin Oncol.* 2006;24:848-855.
9. Brewster AM, Hortobagyi GN, Broglio KR, et al. Residual risk of breast cancer recurrence 5 years after adjuvant therapy. *J Natl Cancer Inst.* 2008;100:1179-1183.
10. Oeffinger KC, McCabe MS. Models for delivering survivorship care. *J Clin Oncol.* 2006;24:5117-5124.

11. Earle CC, Burstein HJ, Winer EP, Weeks JC. Quality of non-breast cancer health maintenance among elderly breast cancer survivors. *J Clin Oncol.* 2003;21:1447-1451.

12. Koinberg IL, Fridlund B, Engholm GB, Holmberg L. Nurse-led follow-up on demand or by a physician after breast cancer surgery: A randomised study. *Eur J Oncol Nurs.* 2004;8:109-117; discussion 118-120.

13. Mille D, Roy T, Carrere MO, et al. Economic impact of harmonizing medical practices: Compliance with clinical practice guidelines in the follow-up of breast cancer in a French Comprehensive Cancer Center. *J Clin Oncol.* 2000;18:1718-1724.

14. Lash TL, Clough-Gorr K, Silliman RA. Reduced rates of cancer-related worries and mortality associated with guideline surveillance after breast cancer therapy. *Breast Cancer Res Treat.* 2005;89:61-67.

15. Ganz PA. Monitoring the physical health of cancer survivors: A survivorship-focused medical history. *J Clin Oncol.* 2006;24:5105-5111.

16. Khatcheressian JL, Wolff AC, Smith TJ, et al. American Society of Clinical Oncology 2006 update of the breast cancer follow-up and management guidelines in the adjuvant setting. *J Clin Oncol.* 2006;24:5091-5097.

17. National Comprehensive Cancer Network. *NCCN Practice Guidelines in Oncology: v.2.2009 Breast Cancer.* Fort Washington, PA: NCCN; 2008.

18. Jin Y, Desta Z, Stearns V, et al. CYP2D6 genotype, antidepressant use, and tamoxifen metabolism during adjuvant breast cancer treatment. *J Natl Cancer Inst.* 2005;97:30-39.

19. Keating NL, Landrum MB, Guadagnoli E, Winer EP, Ayanian JZ. Factors related to underuse of surveillance mammography among breast cancer survivors. *J Clin Oncol.* 2006;24:85-94.

20. Rojas MP, Telaro E, Russo A, et al. Follow-up strategies for women treated for early breast cancer. *Cochrane Database Syst Rev.* 2005;CD001768.

21. Harris L, Fritsche H, Mennel R, et al. American Society of Clinical Oncology 2007 update of recommendations for the use of tumor markers in breast cancer. *J Clin Oncol.* 2007;25:5287-5312.

22. Fung MF, Reid A, Faught W, et al. Prospective longitudinal study of ultrasound screening for endometrial abnormalities in women with breast cancer receiving tamoxifen. *Gynecol Oncol.* 2003;91:154-159.

23. Keating NL, Landrum MB, Guadagnoli E, Winer EP, Ayanian JZ. Surveillance testing among survivors of early-stage breast cancer. *J Clin Oncol.* 2007;25:1074-1081.

24. Wideroff L, Vadaparampil ST, Greene MH, et al. Hereditary breast/ovarian and colorectal cancer genetics knowledge in a national sample of US physicians. *J Med Genet.* 2005;42:749-755.

25. Demark-Wahnfried W, Aziz NM, Rowland JH, Pinto BM. Riding the crest of the teachable moment: Promoting long-term health after the diagnosis of cancer. *J Clin Oncol.* 2005;23:5814-5830.

26. Theriault RL, Biermann JS, Brown E, et al. NCCN Task Force Report: Bone Health and Cancer Care. *J Natl Compr Canc Netw.* 2006;4(suppl 2):S1-20; quiz S21-22.

27. Saad F, Adachi JD, Brown JP, et al. Cancer treatment-induced bone loss in breast and prostate cancer. *J Clin Oncol.* 2008;26:5465-5476.

28. Camacho PM, Dayal AS, Diaz JL, et al. Prevalence of secondary causes of bone loss among breast cancer patients with osteopenia and osteoporosis. *J Clin Oncol.* 2008;26:5380-5385.

29. Ravdin PM. Managing the risk of osteoporosis in women with a history of early breast cancer. *Oncology (Williston Park).* 2004;18(11):1385-1390, 1393; discussion 1394.

30. Beaver K, Luker KA. Follow-up in breast cancer clinics: Reassuring for patients rather than detecting recurrence. *Psychooncology.* 2005;14:94-101.

31. Janz NK, Mujahid MS, Hawley ST, et al. Racial/ethnic differences in adequacy of information and support for women with breast cancer. *Cancer.* 2008;113:1058-1067.

32. Griggs JJ, Sorbero ME, Mallinger JB, et al. Vitality, mental health, and satisfaction with information after breast cancer. *Patient Educ Couns.* 2007;66:58-66.

33. Rozmovits L, Ziebland S. What do patients with prostate or breast cancer want from an internet site? A qualitative study of information needs. *Patient Educ Couns.* 2004;53:57-64.

34. Salminen E, Vire J, Poussa T, Knifsund S. Unmet needs in information flow between breast cancer patients, their spouses, and physicians. *Support Care Cancer.* 2004;12:663-668.

35. Laine C, Davidoff F, Lewis CE, et al. Important elements of outpatient care: a comparison of patients' and physicians' opinions. *Ann Intern Med.* 1996;125:640-645.

36. Waitzkin H. Information giving in medical care. *J Health Soc Behav.* 1985;26:81-101.

37. Earle CC. Failing to plan is planning to fail: Improving the quality of care with survivorship care plans. *J Clin Oncol.* 2006;24:5112-5116.

38. Ganz PA, Hahn EE. Implementing a survivorship care plan for patients with breast cancer. *J Clin Oncol.* 2008;26:759-767.

CHAPTER 99

Tumor Registry

Luke M. Funk
Caprice C. Greenberg

High quality cancer registries are critical for any modern health care system. They provide organizations and governments with vital data for allocating public health resources in an efficient manner. They enable investigators to study cancer at both patient and population-based levels, and allow clinicians to develop optimal methods for the prevention, diagnosis, and treatment of disease. Tumor registries facilitate important comparisons between different regions, races, genders, and age groups. When a registry has been operating for many years, survival and other prognostic data become available. Trends can also be followed, which allows public health experts to project future incidence rates and predict the need for screening programs, treatment programs, and new facilities.

In the United States and elsewhere, there are 2 main types of tumor registries. Population-based registries include national, regional, or state databases that provide data on the general population. Their purpose is to capture incidence, prevalence, survival, and mortality data for all new cancer cases in a defined population.[1] Hospital-based registries, on the other hand, provide data that characterize cancer care at the institutional level. This allows researchers to study specific treatment protocols and provides insight into the practice patterns at different hospitals.

HISTORY OF TUMOR REGISTRIES

One of the first organized attempts to systematically collect cancer data occurred in 1900 when the Prussian Ministry of Culture sent questionnaires to every physician in Germany. The goal of the survey was to document the total number of cancer cases, but due to a poor response rate it was regarded as a failure.[1] A similar problem was also experienced in Massachusetts in the 1920s after surveys aimed at identifying cancer cases were largely disregarded by practitioners.[2] In 1935, the Connecticut State Department of

Health established one of the first cancer research divisions in the United States. Six years later, the Connecticut Tumor Registry was created, which subsequently became one of the first successful American tumor registries.[3] To date, over 400 reports have been published with information from this state database.[4]

In 1942, Denmark established the first national cancer registry, the Danish Cancer Registry. In this system, Danish physicians reported cases on a volunteer basis and were given access to mortality and death certificate data.[5] The World Health Organization followed Denmark's lead in 1950 with the development of the first set of cancer registration guidelines.[6] The International Union Against Cancer also created the Committee on Geographic Pathology, which emphasized the importance of recording all new cancer cases within a defined geographic population.[7] With the information obtained from these initial efforts, the first volume of *Cancer Incidence in Five Continents* was published in 1966. The International Association of Cancer Registries (IACR) was founded later that year.[8] The IACR currently serves as the membership organization for population-based registries worldwide and has set the standards for cancer registration and training for over 40 years.[9]

US TUMOR REGISTRIES

Surveillance, Epidemiology, and End Results Database

Background

With the passage of the National Cancer Act of 1971, Congress initiated the first comprehensive, national effort to systematically collect cancer data in the United States. Citing cancer as a leading cause of death with an increasing incidence, Congress mandated that the National Cancer Institute (NCI) lead an effort to "collect, analyze and disseminate all data useful in the prevention, diagnosis and treatment of cancer, including the establishment of an international cancer research data bank."[10] In 1973, the NCI established the Surveillance, Epidemiology, and End Results (SEER) database, which has since become a leading source of information on cancer incidence and survival in the United States.[11] Since its inception, the SEER program has grown substantially. Currently, it covers 26% of the US population and includes 18 different registry sites in 12 states and 6 metropolitan areas.[12]

To identify cancer cases, information from hospital records, nursing homes, radiotherapy units, private laboratories, and death certificates is monitored by each registry.[13] Data regarding all cancer cases within a geographic area are collected by the appropriate registry and submitted to the NCI. Patient demographics, date of diagnosis, primary cancer site/type, stage at diagnosis, first course of treatment, and type of surgical treatment or radiotherapy recommended within 4 months of diagnosis are among the key pieces of information that are gathered.[14]

SEER Applications

In its annual report titled the SEER Cancer Statistics Review (CSR), the NCI publishes data on the incidence, mortality, survival, and lifetime risks for specific types of cancer. For example, according to the SEER CSR, the breast cancer incidence rate from 2001 to 2005 was 68.5 per 100,000 person-years while the mortality rate was 14.1 per 100,000 person-years. Five-year survival was 88.7%, which contrasted sharply with the 60% survival rate during the early 1950s. Data regarding race are also available. For example, from 2001 to 2005, the age-adjusted death rate for white breast-cancer patients was 13.7% compared with 19.9% for African Americans.[15]

The NCI, the American Cancer Society, and the Centers for Disease Control and Prevention (CDC) also collaborate to publish the Annual Report to the Nation on the Status of Cancer. In the 2007 report, which included 82% of the US population, breast cancer incidence rates had decreased 3.5% per year from 2001 to 2004. This was the first consistent decrease in breast cancer incidence in nearly 2 decades.[16]

Independent researchers can also use SEER data. Racial and ethnic disparities in breast cancer are among the areas that have been explored. One study published in May of 2008 revealed that the age-adjusted mortality rate for African American women under 40 years of age was 2 times higher than for white women. African American women were also more likely to be diagnosed with regional or distant disease.[17] Another report showed that although breast cancer incidence dropped significantly in the United States between 2001 and 2004, white women experienced a 14% decline while African American rates were essentially unchanged.[18] Additional areas of investigation have included the prognostic importance of breast cancer micrometastases,[19] breast cancer mortality trends according to estrogen receptor status and age,[20] and outcomes following surgical resection of breast tumors in patients with metastatic disease.[21]

To obtain the SEER data, researchers can either query the database online using SEER*Stat software or obtain a CD or DVD. A limited-use data agreement form must be completed.[22,23] There is no fee associated with accessing SEER data.

Limitations

While the SEER population is comparable to the US population, there are significantly more urban and foreign-born individuals represented in SEER registries (88.2% vs 79% and 17.3% vs 11.1%, respectively).[24] Individuals residing within SEER regions are also more affluent, have a higher rate of employment, and have more cancer specialists within their geographic areas.[25] Additionally, the SEER data do not capture information about cancer screening, cancer detection, comorbidities, or treatment provided more than 4 months after diagnosis. To study these variables, SEER data must be linked with outside resources, such as the Medicare system.

SEER-Medicare Linked Database

Background

Recognizing the limitations of the SEER data, the federal government established the SEER-Medicare database in 1991. As the primary health insurer for 97% of the US population aged 65 and older, Medicare adds a number of informative variables to the SEER dataset. Medicare files contain information regarding dates of service, diagnostic codes, procedure codes, charges for services, and reimbursement, as well as identifying data for hospitals and physicians.[26] Researchers can also analyze outpatient, home health care, and hospice claims data.

SEER-Medicare Applications

SEER-Medicare data allow investigators to study cancer care along its entire spectrum. Medicare claims prior to diagnosis, such as mammography, can be used to examine cancer screening and detection methods.[27,28] While SEER only reports initial treatments, Medicare claims data capture most major cancer-related procedures.[29] Medicare files also contain information on the use of adjuvant chemotherapy.[30,31] Disparities in diagnostic or therapeutic interventions as they relate to age, race, sex, income, location, or provider can also be measured.[32,33] SEER-Medicare can also be linked with the American Medical Association Masterfile and the Unique Physician Identification Number Registry to study how provider characteristics affect the delivery of care.[34]

Cost is another important area that has been studied. One recent publication characterized over 300,000 patients aged 65 and older who were diagnosed with breast, lung, colorectal, or prostate cancer between 1991 and 2002. During this 11-year period, the average cost for the initial care of a breast cancer patient increased from $4,189 to $20,964. In 2002, Medicare payments for the initial care of these 4 cancers exceeded $6.7 billion.[35] Survivorship,[36] cancer recurrence,[37,38] and end-of-life care[39,40] have also been evaluated using SEER-Medicare data. Additionally, investigators have studied treatment and survival differences between Medicare beneficiaries enrolled in health maintenance organizations compared to fee-for-service plans.[41,42]

Limitations

Since the SEER-Medicare database only includes information on individuals aged 65 and older, investigators must be careful when generalizing results to the rest of the population. These concerns are especially relevant when considering practice patterns, utilization rates, and outcomes for certain types of breast cancer care. For example, older patients are less likely to undergo breast reconstruction after mastectomy[43] or receive axillary dissections for stage I or II breast cancers.[44] Surgeons are also less likely to refer older breast cancer patients to medical oncologists.[45] Additionally, while breast-conservation therapy plus irradiation is the standard of care for younger patients with early breast cancers, recent literature suggests that lumpectomy plus tamoxifen without irradiation may be sufficient for women 70 years of age or older.[46]

The SEER-Medicare database also lacks claims data for oral prescription drugs. This is particularly pertinent for breast cancer research since hormone replacement therapy plays a prominent role. This may change with inclusion of Part D Medicare claims data. Claims for HMO enrollees, who comprised 14% of the Medicare population in 2001, are missing in the SEER-Medicare database as well.[26]

Accessing SEER-Medicare Data

Given the sensitivity of the information contained in the SEER-Medicare database, the files are not available for public use. Investigators who wish to pursue research projects must sign data-use agreements with both the Centers for Medicare and Medicaid Services (CMS) and SEER. Each research proposal must be approved prior to obtaining the data. Costs vary depending on the type of data file requested. Due to the complexity of the data files, both SEER and CMS offer assistance with data analysis.[47]

National Program of Cancer Registries

Background

State cancer registries are another important source of population-based cancer data. Prior to 1992, few states had tumor registries and those that did often lacked adequate resources and legislative support.[48] To address this need, the US Congress passed the Cancer Registries Amendment Act in 1992.[49] This gave the CDC authority to establish and fund the National Program of Cancer Registries (NPCR). The NPCR has since provided grant money and technical assistance to state health departments for the development of statewide cancer registries. Today, the NPCR assists registries in 45 states. These data cover 96% of the US population and represent the entire US population when combined with the SEER database.[50-52]

The primary goals of the NPCR are to provide data for health care resource allocation, determine cancer patterns in different populations, study cancer prevention programs, and provide data to investigators. To receive funding, state registries are required to submit basic demographic information, clinical information including the date and modality of the first treatment course, and pathologic data such as tumor site and morphology. Each registry must also submit an annual statewide report to the CDC.[53]

Evaluating NPCR Data

Together with the North American Association of Central Cancer Registries and the NCI, the CDC publishes an annual report titled United States Cancer Statistics: Incidence and Mortality (USCS). This report summarizes invasive cancer incidence and mortality rates, which are categorized by primary site, sex, race, age, state, and region. According to the USCS, breast cancer was the most common malignancy among women (117.7 cases per 100,000 persons) and the second most common cause of death (24.4 cases per 100,000 persons) in 2004.[54] The NPCR also disseminates a public use data set of cancer incidence rates hosted on a CDC website named WONDER (Wide-Ranging Online Data for Epidemiologic Research).[55] A US County Cancer Incidence Dataset is also available online.[56]

In 2007, the CDC conducted a literature review of studies that used NPCR data and identified nearly 300 publications.[57] Twenty-three percent of these studies were specific to breast cancer. Among them were an epidemiologic study on differences between ductal and lobular carcinoma in situ in California,[58] an examination of the carcinogenic potential of breast implants in Connecticut,[59] and an analysis of mammography screening in Hawaii.[60] A study from Illinois assessed urban and rural differences in the management of breast cancer,[61] while another from New Jersey focused on the relationship between health insurance coverage and clinical outcomes.[62] Long-term hormone-replacement therapy and the risk of breast cancer was the topic of another publication from the Wisconsin breast cancer registry.[63] These examples illustrate the capabilities of state cancer registries and the NPCR.

National Cancer Data Base

Background and Participation

Established in 1989 through a joint program between the American College of Surgeon's Commission on Cancer (CoC) and the American Cancer Society, the National Cancer Data Base (NCDB) is the largest clinical registry in the world with data from over 20 million cancer patients.[64] More than 1400 US hospitals contribute to the NCDB[65,66] and 75% of newly diagnosed cancer cases are identified.[64]

As opposed to SEER and NPCR, the NCDB is a compilation of hospital-based registries. To participate in the NCDB program, hospitals must be accredited by the CoC, which requires participating hospitals to provide basic diagnostic and treatment services and monitor quality improvement by establishing cancer committees and the cancer registry.[67,68] Data collected for the NCDB are similar to those collected for the SEER and NPCR databases and include basic demographic, clinical (staging, type of first treatment, disease recurrence, survival), and pathologic information. Each hospital is asked to provide annual follow-up data on at least 90% of its registry patients. The accuracy of the data is evaluated each year by both automated systems and site surveyors from the CoC.[66]

Evaluating NCDB Data

Perhaps the strongest feature of the NCDB is its ability to provide data about individual institutions. This allows important comparisons in the quality of care provided by hospitals throughout the country, including lower volume hospitals that provide the majority of cancer care in the United States.[69]

The NCDB also has the ability to benchmark hospitals, which allows for quality improvement analysis at each institution.

In 2007, the National Quality Forum endorsed 5 quality measures regarding cancer treatment. Three of these were specific to breast cancer—administration of radiation therapy within 1 year of diagnosis for women under age 70 receiving breast-conserving surgery, consideration of combination chemotherapy within 4 months of diagnosis for women under 70 with stage II or III hormone receptor–negative breast cancer, and consideration of tamoxifen or a third generation aromatase inhibitor within 1 year of diagnosis for women with stage II or III hormone receptor–positive breast cancer.[70]

Hospitals with CoC-approved cancer programs are now benchmarked according to their adherence to these parameters. Though these data are not publicly available, hospitals can examine their performances on these measures and compare their results to other participating hospitals.

Public benchmark reports are also available. Though they do not identify specific hospitals, these reports provide information on 11 common types of cancer. Information regarding each state, hospital type, gender, race, stage, histology, first treatment, and surgical procedure is publicly available.[71] Surgical and adjuvant therapy treatment trends can also be evaluated with NCDB data.[72,73]

Limitations

Since not all hospitals participate in the NCDB program, the database is not a true population-based registry. Thus despite its large size, investigators must be careful when generalizing results to the population. Additionally, though public benchmarks are available online, the majority of the database is not accessible unless an investigator is affiliated with a participating CoC hospital.

Individual Hospital Databases

Single institutional databases are also important sources of data. Linkages with banked tissue have been particularly important for breast cancer research. For example, much of the early BRCA1/BRCA2 research originated from hospital-based registry data, which identified Ashkenazi Jewish patients who had undergone surgery and had tissue available for study.[74] Hospital-based tumor registries have also been important for HER-2/neu[75] and estrogen and progesterone receptor[76] genetic analysis.

Quality improvement programs can also be initiated with hospital-based registry data. The National Comprehensive Cancer Network (NCCN) is one example. Functioning as a coalition of 20 cancer centers in the United States, the NCCN collects data from each institution using both data abstracting and patient surveys. These data are subsequently used for research and for development of evidence-based breast cancer quality measures.[77] The NCCN Breast Cancer Outcomes Database includes patient information from each institution including comorbidities, menopausal status, trial participation and follow-up, and standard demographic and pathologic information. Each year, NCCN provides institutional leaders and clinicians with a report outlining compliance with the standard of care.[78,79] Each institution can subsequently use these data to improve care at their respective institutions.

FUTURE DIRECTION OF TUMOR REGISTRIES

United States

The NCI is currently expanding its cancer surveillance activities in an effort to explore patterns and trends in cancer rates. One area under active research involves the use of Geographic Information Systems (GIS) to display spatial data as layered maps. Using newly developed software, researchers can create maps that identify cancer clusters and present statistical data that are more interpretable. One example is the Long Island Geographic Information System, which examines relationships between breast cancer and the environment in 4 counties in Connecticut and New York.[80] Advanced statistical models are also being used to predict the geographical distribution of new cancer cases by creating associations between risk factors, demographics, and mortality rates in the SEER database. The NCI believes that the application of these methods will lead to more accurate projections of new cancer cases each year.[81]

Tumor registries will also advance the field of genetic epidemiology. For example, researchers within the Genetic Epidemiology Branch at the NCI are using tissue microarrays from invasive breast tumors obtained from a population-based breast cancer registry. Their goal is to identify molecular markers involved in key pathways of breast tumor development.[82] The NCI has also established the Breast and Colon Cancer Family Registries, which include information and tissue specimens from over 12,500 families. Identification of cancer susceptibility genes and other risk factors in cancer development are primary focuses of this project.[83]

The NCDB has plans to strengthen its quality improvement initiatives over the next several years. The NCDB plans on releasing de-identified data to CoC-hospital investigators that will include data on surgical margin status, chemotherapy, hormonal therapy, and radiation therapy.[66] Making NCDB data available for public use is also being considered.

Globally

The systematic collection of cancer data on a worldwide basis will require significant time, effort, and financing over the next several decades. Many developing countries still consider cancer registration a luxury, not a priority. Poor health care infrastructure, inaccurate clinical records and population estimates, and limited death certificate availability are among the most important barriers to establishing population-based registries in the developing world.[84] As a result, while 99% of the North American population was covered by cancer registries in 2006, only 11% of the African population was followed.[9]

Over half of the world's annual cancer cases arise in developing countries. This accounts for at least 5 million new cancer cases each year. Parkin and colleagues have estimated that 23% of all female cancers in the world are breast cancers.[85] As the chronic disease burden increases over the next 10 to 20 years because of improvements in infectious disease and malnutrition management, these numbers will continue to rise. Tumor registry data will become vital sources of information for these nations. Fortunately, the developed world has begun to mobilize its resources.

One program, known as the Pediatric Oncology Networked Database (POND), uses the Internet as a clinical research data collection tool.[86] Established in 2004, this online tumor registry allows investigators to study the epidemiologic patterns of malignancies in low-income countries.[87] Providers from around the world can enter and share de-identified patient data including standard tumor registry information. Nutritional, psychosocial, socioeconomic, and chemotherapy information can also be analyzed. As of 2007, 7 countries in Central America were using POND resources to establish hospital-based tumor registries.[88]

The Breast Health Global Initiative (BHGI) was founded in 2002 and consists of an international group of providers dedicated to establishing evidence-based, affordable clinical practice guidelines for limited resource countries. Creating individual and facility-based medical records are 2 of the program's initial goals.[89] Currently, the BHGI is focused on implementing these data collection systems along with diagnostic and treatment plans in low-income countries. Implementation guidelines for International Breast Health and Cancer Control were published in October 2008.[90,91]

SUMMARY

Tumor registries have been important in the care of cancer patients for over 100 years. They began as handwritten logs kept by individual practitioners, but have subsequently transformed into powerful data sets capable of maintaining massive amounts of information. Governments, hospitals, providers, researchers, and patients depend on them for accurate and timely analysis of cancer data. Over the next several decades, they will continue to play an important role as technology improves and fields such as GIS and genetic epidemiology continue to grow. As life expectancies around the world continue to increase, organized and efficient cancer care will be critical for ensuring the health of the global population. Cancer registries will be a vital part of this process.

REFERENCES

1. Jensen OM, Parkin DM, MacLennan R, et al., eds. *Cancer Registration: Principles and Methods.* IARC Scientific Publication No. 95. Lyon, France: International Agency for Research on Cancer; 1991.
2. Hoffman FL. Discussion to the paper of FC Wood. *Am J Public Health.* 1930;20:19-20.
3. Griswold MH, Wilder CS, Cutler SJ, Pollack ES. *Cancer in Connecticut 1935-51.* Hartford, CT: Connecticut State Department of Health: 1955.
4. Connecticut Department of Public Health. Connecticut Tumor Registry, bibliography. Available at: http://www.ct.gov/dph/LIB/dph/ctr/pdf/CTR_Bibliography.PDF. Accessed August 1, 2008.
5. Clemmesen J. Statistical studies in the aetiology of malignant neoplasms. *Acta Pathol Microbiol Scand.* 1965;4(suppl 174).
6. Stocks P. Cancer registration and studies of incidence by surveys. *Bull World Health Organ.* 1959;20:697-715.
7. Clemmesen J. *Symposium on the Geographic Pathology and Demography of Cancer.* Paris: Council for the Coordination of International Congresses of Medical Statistics: 1951.
8. Union Internationale Contre le Cancer. *Cancer Incidence in Five Continents, Vol. 1.* Doll R, Payne P, Waterhouse JAH, eds. Geneva, Switzerland: Union Internationale Contre le Cancer: 1966.
9. Parkin D. The evolution of the population-based cancer registry. *Nat Rev Cancer.* 2005;6(8):603-612.
10. The National Cancer Act of 1971 (PL 92-218). Available at: http://legislative.cancer.gov/history/phsa/1971. Accessed July 7, 2008.
11. Hankey BF, Ries LA, Edwards BK. The Surveillance, Epidemiology, and End Results program: a national resource. *Cancer Epidemiol Biomarkers Prev.* 1999;8:1117-1121.
12. SEER Registries. Available at: http://www.seer.cancer.gov/registries. Accessed June 27, 2008.
13. SEER Cancer Statistics Review 1975-2005. Available at: http://www.seer.cancer.gov/csr/1975_2005/results_single/sect_01_intro.28pgs.pdf. Accessed June 28, 2008.
14. Gloeckler Ries LA, Reichman ME, Lewis DR, et al. Cancer survival and incidence from the Surveillance, Epidemiology, and End Results (SEER) program. *Oncologist.* 2003;8(6):541-552.
15. SEER Cancer Statistics Review, 1975-2005. Available at: http://seer.cancer.gov/csr/1975_2005. Accessed August 18, 2008.
16. Espey DK, Wu XC, Swan J, et al. Annual report to the nation on the status of cancer, 1975-2004, featuring cancer in American Indians and Alaska Natives. *Cancer.* 2007;110(10):2119-2152.
17. Baquet CR, Mishra SI, Commiskey P, et al. Breast cancer epidemiology in blacks and whites: disparities in incidence, mortality, survival rates and histology. *J Natl Med Assoc.* 2008;100(5):480-488.
18. Hausauer AK, Keegan TH, Chang ET, Clark CA. Recent breast cancer trends among Asian/Pacific Islander, Hispanic, and African-American women in the US: changes by tumor subtype. *Breast Cancer Res.* 2007;9(6):R90.
19. Chen SL, Hoehne FM, Giuliano AE. The prognostic significance of micrometastases in breast cancer: a SEER population-based analysis. *Ann Surg Oncol.* 2007;14(12):3378-3384.
20. Jemal A, Ward E, Thun MJ. Recent trends in breast cancer incidence rates by age and tumor characteristics among U.S. women. *Breast Cancer Res.* 2007;9(3):R28.
21. Gnerlich J, Jeffe DB, Deshpande AD, Beers C. Surgical removal of the primary tumor increases overall survival in patients with metastatic breast cancer: analysis of the 1988-2003 SEER data. *Ann Surg Oncol.* 2007;14(8):2187-2194.
22. SEER Publications. Available at: http://www.seer.cancer.gov/publications. Accessed June 29, 2008.
23. SEER. 1973-2005 SEER Data. Available at: http://seer.cancer.gov/data/access.html. Accessed July 24, 2008.
24. Characteristics of the SEER Population Compared with the Total United States Population. Available at: http://www.seer.cancer.gov/registries/characteristics.html. Accessed June 29, 2008.
25. Nattinger AB, McAuliffe TL, Shapira MM. Generalizability of the surveillance, epidemiology, and end results registry population: factors relevant to epidemiologic and health care research. *J Clin Epidemiol.* 1997;50:939-945.
26. Warren JL, Klabunde CN, Schrag D, et al. Overview of the SEER-Medicare data: content, research applications, and generalizability to the United States elderly population. *Med Care.* 2002;40(8 suppl):IV-3-18.
27. Freeman JL, Klabunde CN, Schussler N, et al. Measuring breast, colorectal, and prostate cancer screening with Medicare claims data. *Med Care.* 2002;40(8 suppl):IV-36-42.
28. McCarthy EP, Burns RB, Coughlin SS, et al. Mammography use helps to explain differences in breast cancer stage at diagnosis between black and white women. *Ann Intern Med.* 1998;128(9):729-736.
29. Cooper GS, Virnig B, Klabunde CN, et al. Use of SEER-Medicare data for measuring cancer surgery. *Med Care.* 2002;40(8 suppl):IV-43-48.
30. Warren JL, Harlan LC, Fahey A, et al. Utility of the SEER-Medicare data to identify chemotherapy use. *Med Care.* 2002;40(8 suppl):IV-55-61.
31. Du X, Goodwin JS. Patterns of use of chemotherapy for breast cancer in older women: findings from Medicare claims data. *J Clin Oncol.* 2001;19:1455-1461.
32. Gross CP, Smith BD, Wolf E, Anderson M. Racial disparities in cancer therapy: did the gap narrow between 1992 and 2002? *Cancer.* 2008;112(4):900-908.
33. Hershman DL, Buono D, McBride RB, et al. Surgeon characteristics and receipt of adjuvant radiotherapy in women with breast cancer. *J Natl Cancer Inst.* 2008;100(3):199-206.
34. Baldwin LM, Adamache W, Klabunde CN, et al. Linking physician characteristics and Medicare claims data: issues in data availability, quality and measurement. *Med Care.* 2002;40(8 suppl):IV-82-95.
35. Warren JL, Yabroff KR, Meekins A, et al. Evaluation of trends in the cost of initial cancer treatment. *J Natl Cancer Inst.* 2008;100(12):888-897.
36. Field TS, Doubeni C, Fox MP, et al. Under utilization of surveillance mammography among older breast cancer survivors. *J Gen Intern Med.* 2008;23(2):158-163.
37. Stokes ME, Thompson D, Montoya EL, et al. Ten-year survival and cost following breast cancer recurrence: estimates from SEER-Medicare data. *Value Health.* 2008;11(2):213-220.
38. Earle CC, Nattinger AB, Potosky AL, et al. Identifying cancer relapse using SEER-Medicare data. *Med Care.* 2002;40(8 suppl):IV-75-81.

39. Lackan NA, Ostir GV, Freeman JL, et al. Decreasing variation in the use of hospice among older adults with breast, colorectal, lung and prostate cancer. *Med Care.* 2004;42(2):116-122.

40. Lackan NA, Freeman JL, Goodwin JS. Hospice use by older women dying with breast cancer between 1991-1996. *J Palliat Care.* 2003;19(1):49-53.

41. Potosky AL, Merrill RM, Riley GF, et al. Breast cancer survival and treatment in HMO and fee-for-service settings. *J Natl Cancer Inst.* 1997;89:1683-1691.

42. Riley GF, Potosky AL, Klabunde CN, et al. Stage at diagnosis and treatment patterns among older women with breast cancer: an HMO and fee-for-service comparison. *JAMA.* 1999;281(8):720-726.

43. Greenberg CC, Schneider EC, Lipsitz SR, et al. Do variations in provider discussions explain socioeconomic disparities in postmastectomy breast reconstruction? *J Am Coll Surg.* 2008;206(4):605-615.

44. Edge SB, Gold K, Berg CD, et al. Patient and provider characteristics that affect the use of axillary dissection in older women with stage I-II breast carcinoma. *Cancer.* 2002;94(10):2534-2541.

45. Thwin SS, Fink AK, Lash TL, Silliman RA. Predictors and outcomes of surgeons' referral of older breast cancer patients to medical oncologists. *Cancer.* 2005;104(5):936-942.

46. Hughes KS, Schnaper LA, Berry D, et al. Lumpectomy plus tamoxifen with or without irradiation in women 70 years of age or older with early breast cancer. *N Engl J Med.* 2004;351(10):971-977.

47. SEER Medicare Linked Database. Available at http://healthservices.cancer.gov/seermedicare. Accessed June 30, 2008.

48. National Program of Cancer Registries, About the Program. Available at: http://www.cdc.gov/cancer/npcr/about.htm. Accessed July 5, 2008.

49. Cancer Registries Amendment Act (PL 102-515). Available at: http://www.cdc.gov/cancer/NPCR/npcrpdfs/publaw.pdf. Accessed July 7, 2008.

50. Centers for Disease Control and Prevention. State cancer registries: status of authorizing legislation and enabling regulations—United States, October 1993. *Morb Mortal Wkly Rep.* 1994;43(4):71, 74-75.

51. Weir HK, Berg GD, Manley EC, Belloni KA. The National Program of Cancer Registries: explaining state variations in average cost per case reported. *Prev Chronic Dis.* 2005;2(3):1-10.

52. Wingo PA, Jamison PM, Hiatt RA, et al. Building the infrastructure for nationwide cancer surveillance and control—a comparison between the National Program of Cancer Registries (NPCR) and the Surveillance, Epidemiology, and End Results (SEER) program (United States). *Cancer Causes Control.* 2003;14(2):175-193.

53. National Program of Cancer Registries, Data Release Activities. Available at: http://www.cdc.gov/cancer/npcr/datarelease.htm. Accessed July 6, 2008.

54. US Cancer Statistics Working Group. *United States Cancer Statistics: 2004 Incidence and Mortality.* Atlanta: US Department of Health and Human Services, Centers for Disease Control and Prevention and National Cancer Institute: 2007.

55. CDC Wonder. Available at: http://wonder.cdc.gov. Accessed July 11, 2008.

56. National Cancer Institute, State Cancer Profiles. Available at: http://www.statecancerprofiles.cancer.gov. Accessed July 11, 2008.

57. National Program of Cancer Registries, Literature Review of Data from Statewide Cancer Registries in the U.S. Available at: http://www.cdc.gov/cancer/npcr/review.htm. Accessed July 12, 2008.

58. Baldwin UL. An epidemiologic study of differences between mammary ductal and lobular carcinoma in situ: analysis of 11,436 cases from the California Cancer Registry. *Anat Pathol.* 1996;1:193-203.

59. Kern KA, Flannery JT, Kuehn PG. Carcinogenic potential of silicone breast implants: a Connecticut statewide study. *Plast Reconstr Surg.* 1997;100(3):737-747; discussion 748-749.

60. Maskarinec G, Wilkens L, Meng L. Mammography screening and the increase in breast cancer incidence in Hawaii. *Cancer Epidemiol Biomarkers Prev.* 1997;6(3):201-208.

61. Howe HL, Katterhagen JG, Yates J, Lehnherr M. Urban-rural differences in the management of breast cancer. *Cancer Causes Control.* 1992;3(6):533-539.

62. Ayanian JZ, Kohler BA, Abe T, Epstein AM. The relation between health insurance coverage and clinical outcomes among women with breast cancer. *N Engl J Med.* 1993;329(5):326-331.

63. Newcomb PA, Longnecker MP, Storer BE, et al. Long-term hormone replacement therapy and risk of breast cancer in postmenopausal women. *Am J Epidemiol.* 1995;142(8):788-795.

64. US Census Bureau, General medical and surgical hospitals. Available at: http://factfinder.census.gov. Accessed August 1, 2008.

65. National Cancer Data Base. Available at: http://www.facs.org/cancer/ncdb. Accessed July 10, 2008.

66. Bilimoria KY, Stewart AK, Winchester DP, Ko CY. The National Cancer Data Base: a powerful initiative to improve cancer care in the United States. *Ann Surg Oncol.* 2008;15(3):683-690.

67. Commission on Cancer. Available at: http://www.facs.org/cancer/public about.html. Accessed August 1, 2008.

68. Commission on Cancer. Cancer Program Approval. Available at: http://www.facs.org/cancer/coc/whatis.html. Accessed July 10, 2008.

69. Reid-Lombardo KM, Gay G, Patel-Parekh L, et al. Treatment of gastric adenocarcinoma may differ among hospital types in the United States, a report from the National Cancer Data Base. *J Gastrointest Surg.* 2007;11:410-9; discussion 419-420.

70. National Cancer Database, National Quality Forum Endorsed Commission on Cancer Measures for Quality of Cancer Care for Breast and Colorectal Cancers. Available at: http://www.facs.org/cancer/qualitymeasures.html. Accessed July 12, 2008.

71. National Cancer Data Base, Patterns of Diagnosis and Treatment for Selected Cancers Diagnosed 1998-2005. Available at: http://cromwell.facs.org/BMarks/BMPub/Ver9/DxRx/BMPub_DxRx9.cfm. Accessed August 1, 2008.

72. Kennedy T, Stewart AK, Bilimoria KY, et al. Treatment trends and factors associated with survival in T1aN0 and T1bN0 breast cancer patients. *Ann Surg Oncol.* 2007;14:2918-2927.

73. Singletary SE, Patel-Parekh L, Bland KI. Treatment trends in early-stage invasive lobular carcinoma: a report from the National Cancer Data Base. *Ann Surg.* 2005;242(2):281-289.

74. Foulkes WD, Wong N, Brunet JS, et al. Germ-line BRCA1 mutation is an adverse prognostic factor in Ashkenazi Jewish women with breast cancer. *Clin Cancer Res.* 1997;3:2465-2469.

75. Rosen PP, Lesser ML, Arroyo CD, et al. Immunohistochemical detection of HER2/neu in patients with axillary lymph node negative breast carcinoma. A study of epidemiologic risk factors, histologic features, and prognosis. *Cancer.* 1995;75(6):1320-1326.

76. Ihemelandu CU, Leffall LD Jr, Dewitty RL, et al. Molecular breast cancer subtypes in premenopausal African-American women, tumor biologic factors and clinical outcome. *Ann Surg Oncol.* 2007;14(10):2994-3003.

77. *NCCN: NCCN Clinical Practice Guidelines in Oncology.* 1st ed. Jenkintown, PA: The National Comprehensive Cancer Network: 2006. Available at: www.nccn.org. Accessed August 2, 2008.

78. Weeks J, Niland J, Hughes ME, et al. *Institutional Variation in Concordance with Guidelines for Breast Cancer Care in the National Comprehensive Cancer Network: Implications for Choice of Quality Indicators.* Seattle, WA: Academy Health Annual Research Meeting: 2006.

79. Hassett MJ, Hughes ME, Niland JC. Selecting high priority quality measures for breast cancer quality improvement. *Med Care.* 2008;46(8):762-770.

80. National Cancer Institute, Long Island Geographic Information System (LGIS). Available at: http://li-gis.cancer.gov/overview/overviewLIBCSP.html. Accessed August 20, 2008.

81. National Cancer Institute, Geographic Information Systems. Available at: http://gis.cancer.gov. Accessed August 2, 2008.

82. National Cancer Institute, Division of Cancer Epidemiology and Genetics. Available at: http://dceg.cancer.gov/gch/research/population. Accessed August 2, 2008.

83. National Cancer Institute, Breast and Colon Cancer Family Registries. Available at: http://epi.grants.cancer.gov/CFR/about_breast.html. Accessed August 24, 2008.

84. Valsecchi ML, Steliarova-Foucher E. Cancer registration in developing countries: luxury or necessity? *Lancet Oncol.* 2008;9(2):159-167.

85. Parkin DM, Bray F, Ferlay J, Pisani P. Global cancer statistics, 2002. *CA Cancer J Clin.* 2005;55(2):74-108.

86. Pediatric Oncology Networked Database (POND). Available at: https://www.pond4kids.org/pond/home. Accessed July 25, 2008.

87. Ayoub L, Fu L, Pena A, et al. Implementation of a data management program in a pediatric cancer unit in a low income country. *Pediatr Blood Cancer.* 2007;49(1):23-27.

88. Howard SC, Metzger ML, Wilimas JA, et al. Childhood cancer epidemiology in low-income countries. *Cancer.* 2008;112(3):461-472.

89. Anderson BO, Jakesz R. Breast cancer issues in developing countries: an overview of the breast health global initiative. *World J Surg.* 2008;32(12):2578-2585.

90. Report from the Breast Health Global Initiative. Available at: http://www.fhcrc.org/science/phs/bhgi/news/2008/BHGI_Report_2008.pdf. Accessed August 2, 2008.

91. Guidelines for International Breast Health and Cancer Control Implementation. *Cancer.* 2008;113(S8):2215-2371.

CHAPTER 100

Psychosocial

Michelle B. Riba
Prachi Agarwala

HISTORICAL OVERVIEW

In 1952, Renneker and Cutler published the results of a distinguished group of surgeons and psychoanalysts. In examining the psychosomatic aspects of breast cancer, they found a typical postmastectomy depression in most patients.[1] Sutherland and Orbach reported that a majority of women who had undergone a radical mastectomy experienced significant depression, anxiety, and low self-esteem, along with extended impairments in physical and sexual functioning.[2] Follow-up studies have affirmed that approximately 25% of women who undergo radical or modified radical mastectomies experience significant psychological distress in the year following surgery[3,4] In the last half century, considerable clinical and research attention has been placed on the psychosocial effects of breast cancer and the various and evolving surgical treatments, reconstruction options, and combination therapies.[5,6]

There have been numerous studies that have addressed the psychosocial aspects of mastectomy from the woman's perspective,[7] the man's viewpoint,[8] and the impact on the family.[9] Issues such as loss, changes in self-esteem, sexuality, body image and fears of disfigurement, mood and anxiety, suicidal ideation, sleep disturbances, and quality of life have been studied in the context of the treatments offered at the time.[10,11] Wellisch and associates noted that in their sample of 31 men that sexuality and intimacy were "severely stressed and often negatively altered after mastectomy." Men were also polarized about the surgeon—some viewing the surgeon as an adversary, some as an ally.[8]

Jamison and associates called attention to depression and suicidal thoughts after a mastectomy. In their study, one-fourth of women had considered suicide for reasons they associated with their mastectomies or to depression.[7] This same group of patients had previously rated their pre-mastectomy sexual satisfaction significantly higher than the other women. Klein wrote

of the adverse psychological effects of mastectomy on the family—the husband's feelings of inadequacy to protect his wife and children's worries about their mother's survival transforming into depression and anxiety.[9]

The role of the surgeon has been noted to be central to a patient's psychosocial journey. Surgeons' attributes in this process have included the importance of honesty, providing appropriate hope and involvement of the patient's partner, and timely referral for counseling and rehabilitation.[12] Baile and colleagues noted that training physicians in giving bad news and improving communication techniques was an important component of medical education and was helpful to patients' recovery.[13] The doctor–patient relationship and the trust the patient puts in the surgeon remain core values in cancer care. Physician suggestions and preferences; how the surgeon communicates with the patient, partner, and family; and treatment team dynamics are of consummate importance. In a busy practice, with complicated and complex issues and a high level of stress for patients, attending to the psychosocial needs of patients and families can take a significant amount of time and effort, often without reimbursement. Melding medical and psychosocial treatment to meet the needs of the patient remains an important and difficult challenge.[14]

Throughout this historical period, surgical procedures and techniques have improved, allowing for less invasive measures and increased sparing of the breast (breast-conserving therapy); there are enhanced options for reconstruction and more successful, targeted use of adjuvant chemotherapeutic treatments and radiation therapy. The recognition of the importance of genetic testing has impacted the types of prophylactic surgeries recommended. Better screening techniques have allowed earlier detection of breast cancers in women and men of all ages. Cultural factors are now integrated into decision-making and treatment.[15] These improvements have spurred the need for

TABLE 100-1 Risk Factors for Developing a Psychiatric Disorder Related to Breast Cancer Surgery

Past history of psychiatric illness
Family history of psychiatric illness
Younger age
Substance use
Single status
Cognitive impairment
Pain
Physical disability
Adjuvant chemotherapy
Family coherence
Young children
Limited access to medical care
Financial strain

TABLE 100-2 Factors That May Increase Psychosocial Distress Related to Breast Cancer Surgery

Body image
Physical functioning
Premature menopause
Infertility
Sexuality/Intimacy
Sleep disturbance
Pain
Fear of recurrence or death
Survivorship
New diagnosis
Change in treatment modality
Treatment failure
Effects of radiation/chemotherapy
Numerous medical appointments

better understanding of the psychosocial impact of the surgical procedures and combination of modalities in breast surgical cancer treatment (Table 100-1).

Since so much has changed and continues to evolve in the evaluation and treatment of breast cancer, it is difficult to simply focus on the psychosocial aspects of the surgical procedures per se. Patients are often treated in a multidisciplinary approach, over a long period of time. Further, the types of surgeries are multiple, including biopsy, sentinel node assessment, lumpectomy or mastectomy and reconstruction, with possible revisions. A patient may be in several different radiology or surgical suites, with a number of physicians and other clinicians and physician extenders, all of whom may have different communication styles and important roles in the patient's overall treatment plan. For a particular patient, it might be difficult to sort out the impact of a particular treatment or clinician in the overall care; sometimes the diagnoses change once the patient is evaluated in an academic multidisciplinary setting.[16]

As treatments have evolved, psychosocial distress has also been better defined and the scope understood. We have learned, for example, that groups of patients, whether having lumpectomy or mastectomy, have similar difficulties in emotional well-being and sexual functioning in the months after surgery (Table 100-2).[5,17,18] While we may think that we are delivering good news by telling a patient that she is a good candidate for breast-conserving therapy, the patient may experience this as bad news, worrying the surgeon may be leaving behind cancerous cells. Patients who are not adequately screened for depression, or such psychiatric illnesses as body dysmorphic disorder, may seek reconstruction options and not be pleased with the results, increasing their ongoing psychosocial distress. When we do not screen for psychological distress or psychiatric problems prior to reconstruction or prophylactic mastectomy, certain patients might suffer from further loss, self-doubt, or second guessing of their decision.[19] Nutrition, exercise, and complementary therapies may also be useful adjuncts in helping patients to retain psychosocial health and fitness and need to be explored with

patients as to their interest and willingness to engage in these types of treatments.

Breast cancer surgery for women, as well as for men, has traditionally been seen as a symbolic representation of disease and mortality. Strain and Grossman performed some of the groundbreaking work in describing common psychological issues in impending surgery. Concerns included threat to the sense of personal invulnerability, concern that one's life is being entrusted largely to strangers, separation from the familiar environment of home and family members, fears of loss of control or death while under anesthesia, fears of being partially awake during surgery, and worry of damage to the body.[20] In breast cancer surgery, factors that are associated with more severe psychological reactions include history of psychiatric disorder, problems with body image, a history of unsatisfying or negative sexual experiences, and difficulty discussing personal, especially sexual, problems.[11,21]

Cancer is no longer as stigmatizing a disease as it was 50 years ago. The focus is now on survivorship, rather than just on the proximate event, which promises to be a more beneficial approach in the long-term care of the patient and family. The Institute of Medicine, in its 2007 report on "Cancer Care for the Whole Patient" (p. 1), noted that attention to psychosocial concerns is often "the exception rather than the rule in oncology practice today."[22] While advances in treatment are transforming cancer, the Institute of Medicine emphasized the importance of a biopsychosocial approach to cancer care in its 2006 report (p. 1): "Today, it is not possible to deliver good quality cancer care without using existing approaches, tools, and resources to address patients' psychosocial health needs. All patients with cancer, and their families, should expect and receive cancer care that ensures the provision of appropriate psychosocial health services."[22]

This chapter will review some of the more common psychosocial problems and issues in the surgical treatment of breast cancer, as well as options for screening and treatment of these psychiatric disorders. Suggestions for future directions, both in clinical care and research, will be provided.

PREVALENT PSYCHIATRIC DISORDERS

Depressive Disorders

Twenty percent to 40% of patients with breast cancer are likely to suffer from a depressive disorder.[23] Stanton found that women with breast cancer were more vulnerable to depressive disorders than healthy women.[24] Disorders include adjustment disorder, major depressive disorder, and a mood disorder related to a general medical condition. Patients are most likely to suffer from a depressive disorder in the 6 months after initial diagnosis and treatment.[25]

Patients often demonstrate a constellation of symptoms. Sleep is frequently disturbed, with difficulty falling and staying asleep. Compared to the general population, women with breast cancer have about twice the rate of insomnia.[26] Patients can experience appetite and energy changes. They may have a decreased ability to concentrate. Guilt may also be a significant component. Patients often experience guilt regarding surviving the disease, as well as the perceived burden on the family. Friedman and associates studied 123 women with breast cancer. Women blamed themselves for a variety of reasons, notably poor coping skills, anxiety, problems with expression of emotions, and delay in seeking medical consultation. Patients with a higher level of self-blame were found to have higher levels of depression and a decreased quality of life.[27] Suicidal thoughts may also be present and should be assessed.

Surgical treatments may affect the development of a depressive disorder. Waljee and associates studied 714 patients who underwent breast-conserving surgery over a 4-year period. They determined that breast asymmetry, common after this surgical treatment, increased stigma and fear of recurrence. Women with pronounced asymmetry had a higher incidence of depressive symptoms.[28] Conversely, Brandberg and colleagues found that in 90 patients undergoing bilateral prophylactic mastectomy, the rate of depression had not changed 1 year after the procedure.[29]

Depression often negatively impacts a patient's perception of symptoms, side effects, and treatment. Fann and associates reviewed 20 years of literature related to breast cancer and depression.[25] They noted that patients diagnosed with depression suffered from an increased number of side effects and the experience of these symptoms was intensified. Side effects included fatigue, hot flashes, cognitive impairment, and sexual dysfunction. Depression also amplified the subjective experience of pain. The somatic symptoms associated with depression may be exacerbated by side effects of a treatment modality or confused as simply effects of the treatment. Opportunities for treatment can often be overlooked.[30]

Symptoms of depression may lead to the impression that a patient is not compliant with medically advised treatment. As mentioned, poor concentration is often a component of depression. Patients can have difficulty understanding treatment recommendations or remembering to follow through on daily treatment goals.[25] Depression itself is also known to be a significant risk factor for poor adherence to treatment and a cause for inability to make a decision for surgery. In 2000, DiMatteo and associates performed a quantitative review of

studies that correlated depression and treatment noncompliance. Depressed patients were 3 times more likely to be nonadherent to treatment.[31]

Anxiety Disorders

Anxiety disorders range from anxiety related to a general medical condition to generalized anxiety disorder (GAD), panic disorder, and posttraumatic stress disorder (PTSD). Patients with GAD experience excessive worry for greater than 6 months, with associated tension, fatigue, irritability, and sleep disturbance. Recurrent panic attacks and fear of experiencing additional attacks are the hallmarks of panic disorder. Bilateral prophylactic mastectomy has been demonstrated to decrease the incidence of anxiety 1 year after the surgical procedure.[29]

Posttraumatic stress disorder may develop after a traumatic event, such as learning the prognosis of the illness or a treatment modality. Patients reexperience the event in some manner, avoid stimuli that are reminders of the trauma, and have increased arousal states (eg, hypervigilance, sleep disturbance). Shelby and colleagues studied 74 women treated with either breast-conserving surgery or modified radical mastectomy and found 12 were diagnosed with PTSD.[32] These patients were more likely to have a history of an anxiety or mood disorder, substance use, or a past trauma. Eighty-three percent of the patients diagnosed with PTSD had undergone a modified radical mastectomy. Fifteen patients met criteria for subsyndromal PTSD, diagnosed if patients met only 1 or 2 of the 3 criteria. These patients were more likely to have had a history of a mood disorder. There was no difference in the percentage of patients who underwent a modified radical mastectomy versus breast-conserving surgery. They were shown to have mild impairment in overall functioning and did benefit from treatment of the subsyndromal symptoms.[32]

METHODS OF SCREENING AND EVALUATION

There are a number of screening measures available for clinical use. The key to successful monitoring is to assess symptoms in a routine fashion over several visits, and preferably over the course of care, into survivorship. Screening may be viewed as trying to determine the patients with the most severe psychopathology and referring those patients for treatment. More promising would be screening that helps us better understand distress at the particular point in time of the patient's surgical and medical treatment, and then helping to improve the patient's emotional and physical well-being.[33]

The National Comprehensive Cancer Network (NCCN) practice guidelines state that patients should be screened during the initial visit and at other relevant times, such as with change in disease status or treatment.[34] Clinicians may benefit from gaining experience and comfort with a systemized method of assessment for psychosocial distress as a part of regular follow-up appointments.

The Handbook of Psychiatric Measures contains a wide range of assessment methods, from measures for general psychiatric symptoms and health to measures for specific diagnoses. Each measure is accompanied by a description, the psychometric

NCCN® Practice Guidelines in Oncology – v.1.2008 | **Distress Management**

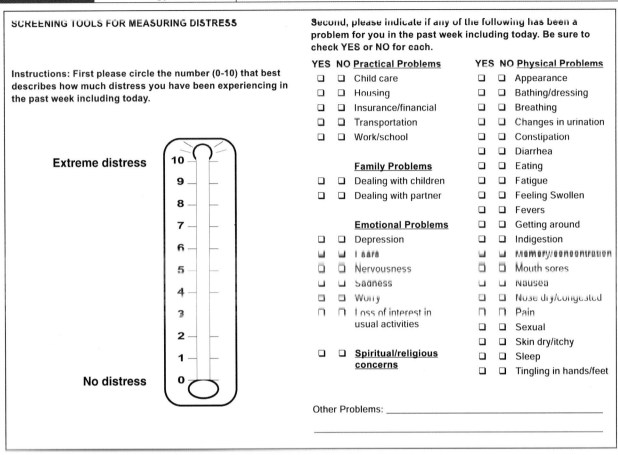

FIGURE 100-1 Screening tool for management of distress. *(Reproduced with permission from the NCCN 1.2008 Distress Management Clinical Practice Guidelines in Oncology. National Comprehensive Cancer Network, 2007. Available at: http://www.nccn.org.)*

properties, and references.[35] A brief description of 3 available measures is given in the next sections.

National Comprehensive Cancer Network Distress Thermometer

Patients are instructed to rate their overall level of distress on a scale from 0 to 10 as a visual analog (Fig. 100-1). They are then asked more specifically about several problems areas, including finances, emotions, and physical and spiritual concerns. The thermometer measures symptomology over the past week. The distress thermometer has been studied and validated for different cancer populations and in different parts of the world. Decision points on the scale, regarding which patients should be provided with educational materials or referred to mental health providers, continue to be fine-tuned.[36]

Profile of Mood States Questionnaire

The Profile of Mood States (POMS) questionnaire is a 65-item questionnaire that is frequently used in studies of mood

disturbance and breast cancer. It has been demonstrated to be both reliable and valid.[37] There are 6 scales: depression, tension, anger, confusion, vigor, and fatigue. Patients in ahil in rate their symptoms over the past week on a 5-point Likert scale. There is also a shortened version of this scale (the SF form)

Impact of Event Scale

The Impact of Event Scale (IES) is a 15-item scale used to assess a patient's perception of stress related to a specific trauma.[38] There are 2 subscales: intrusion (ideas, images, feelings) and avoidance (ideas, images, situations). Symptoms are rated on a 4-point Likert scale, not true to often true.

Psychiatric Consultation

Evaluation by a psychiatrist can be helpful in determining treatment options. A mental health assessment is indicated for patients with worsening psychiatric symptoms and suicidal thoughts. Psychiatrists may perform portions of the Structured Clinical Interview for the Diagnostic and Statistical Manual

(SCID) to help clarify a diagnosis and better understand treatment needs.[39]

TREATMENT OPTIONS

Psychotherapy

Psychological interventions have been demonstrated to be effective forms of treatment for psychiatric disorders in patients with cancer. In 2002, Barsevick and associates examined scientific studies, systematic reviews, and practice guidelines related to the clinical management of depression in cancer patients. They found that behavioral therapies, as well as psychoeducation, were beneficial and effective in reducing depressive symptoms.[40] Group interventions have been shown to be valuable. Cohesion within the group, a high feeling of connectedness between members, and an increased number of sessions were correlated with a decreased level of distress and number of side effects.[41]

Cognitive behavioral therapy (CBT) is an effective treatment for both depressive and anxiety disorders. Hunter and associates demonstrated significant decreases in both depression and anxiety after group CBT in patients after surgical and radiation/chemotherapeutic treatments. This reduction in symptoms continued for 3 months after treatment.[42] CBT can be administered both individually and in group settings. The goal of CBT is to address both cognitive distortions and behaviors that may be contributing to the illness. For depressive disorders, therapists may address isolative behaviors, sleep disturbances, and the patient's perception of support and illness. Avoidance behaviors, exposure, and relaxation techniques are likely to be tackled in patients with anxiety disorders. CBT can also be used for insomnia. Epstein and Dirksen studied 72 women, after primary treatment for breast cancer, with insomnia. They found that short-term cognitive behavioral interventions were effective in treating insomnia in this cohort.[26]

Supportive-expressive therapy (SET) is a treatment modality shown to reduce mood disturbances and improve coping strategies. It is based on a treatment manual. The goals of SET are to build social support, enhance communication between the patient and treatment staff, and improve symptom control. The expression of a high level of emotions points the therapist to specific issues that should be addressed. SET allows patient to examine existential concerns about life, death, isolation, and identity.[43] Kissane and coworkers studied 227 women with metastatic breast cancer to determine if SET, in a group setting, could improve survival rates. They found no difference in survival rates; however, patients experienced a significant reduction in depressive and trauma symptoms, as well as hopelessness. In addition, there was a marked increase in social functioning.[44]

Psychotropic Medications

Selective serotonin reuptake inhibitors (SSRIs) are most commonly used as first-line agents. A consensus of experts in depression in women, including peri-menopausal women, stated that SSRIs should be used as first-line pharmacologic agents in depressive disorders.[45] Roscoe and associates studied 94 breast cancer patients undergoing chemotherapy who were

suffering from depression. Paroxetine was found to be superior to placebo in decreasing depressive symptoms.[46] Fluoxetine has been shown to decrease depressive symptoms, increase quality of life, and increase the patient's completion of adjuvant treatments.[47] Sertraline was demonstrated to decrease hot flashes associated with adjuvant treatments.[48] SSRIs are also indicated for anxiety disorders. Hoffman and coworkers performed a comprehensive review of anxiety disorder pharmacotherapies. They determined that SSRIs should be as first-line agents for anxiety disorders. The dose of SSRI needed for treatment of anxiety symptoms is typically higher than is used for depressive disorders.[49] The decision of which SSRI to prescribe is most often made based on targeted concerns, such as mood disorders, sleep disturbances, side effects, and medication interactions.

A growing area of concern, however, is the interactions of SSRIs and other antidepressants with chemotherapy agents. Tamoxifen has been shown to decrease the rate of death from breast cancer in hormone receptor-positive breast cancers.[50] Tamoxifen is metabolized to endoxifen via CYP2D6; endoxifen is a potent anti-estrogen. Patients with poor or inhibited metabolism of CYP2D6 were found to have increased rates of breast cancer recurrence.[51] SSRIs are known to be inhibitors of CYP2D6, at varying strengths. Stearns and coworkers studied breast cancer patients taking tamoxifen. After paroxetine was initiated, the concentration of endoxifen significantly decreased.[52] In a subsequent study, Borges and associates found that treatment with strong inhibitors of CYP2D6, such as paroxetine and fluoxetine, caused low levels of endoxifen. Treatment with weak inhibitors, including sertraline and citalopram, led to intermediate levels of endoxifen.[53] Further studies examining the effects of antidepressants that do not inhibit CYP2D6, notably escitalopram and venlafaxine, are needed.

Tricyclic antidepressants (TCAs) have also been demonstrated to be effective in breast cancer patients. Their side effects, however, limit their use. Pezzella and associates compared the effectiveness of paroxetine and amitriptyline in breast cancer patients. Both paroxetine and amitriptyline were shown to decrease depressive symptoms effectively. However, amitriptyline led to higher rates of anticholinergic side effects.[54] Serotonin and norepinephrine reuptake inhibitors (SNRIs) are also indicated for both depressive and anxiety disorders.[49] Venlafaxine can also be used as a treatment for hot flashes. Loibl and associates demonstrated that venlafaxine was more effective than clonidine in reducing the frequency of hot flashes in breast cancer patients on adjuvant treatments.[55] Benzodiazepines are also commonly used for short-term anxiolysis. The addictive potential, however, limits their use. The benzodiazepines can be helpful while an SSRI is being titrated to an effective dose. The choice of which benzodiazepine is often based on the half-life and route of metabolism, as well as past history of use and history of substance abuse or dependence.[49]

Postmastectomy pain syndrome has been described in the literature and in common clinical practice. Vadivelu and colleagues reviewed recent literature on this syndrome and found that about one-half of patients undergoing mastectomy or beast reconstruction experienced postoperative pain syndromes.[56] The syndrome typically consists of burning, stabbing pain in the axilla, arm, and chest wall of the affected side, worsened by movement and poorly responsive to opioid medications.[57] Amitriptyline[58] and venlafaxine[59] have been demonstrated to improve neuropathic pain in small samples of breast cancer patients, compared to placebo. Rueben and associates studied 100 patients with breast cancer scheduled for either a partial or radical mastectomy with axillary dissection to determine if venlafaxine could prevent the pain syndrome. There was no difference in opioid usage between the groups. In patients started on venlafaxine prior to surgery, pain scores with movement were decreased, as was the incidence of chest wall, arm, and axillary pain.[60]

FUTURE DIRECTIONS

Future directions in psychosocial research and clinical care include finding screening tools that are easy for clinicians to use and that patients find helpful. While tools such as the NCCN Distress Thermometer are readily accessible, we must better understand the obstacles and difficulties of integrating such screening and evaluation methods in standard clinical practice.[61] Patients and families must come to expect such evaluation as a standard of care. As our understanding of breast cancer genetics increases, we must appreciate the impact of individualized medical and psychosocial treatment approaches for each patient. This includes the interaction of psychotropic medications and chemotherapeutic agents. In addition to medication and psychotherapy, new psychosocial interventions continue to be studied. Several papers have been published examining the role of exercise on quality of life following breast cancer diagnosis and treatment. Randomized control trials are needed to establish the efficacy of exercise and physical activity. The long-term benefits are not yet known. Evolving technology has provided breast cancer patients and their families with new coping strategies. Online support groups, Web sites, and blogs are now available tools to express emotions, seek support, and learn about others' experiences.[62] The effects of these tools are just now being examined to determine the impact on mood, functionality, and quality of life. As we learn more about the impact of exercise,[63] stress, acupuncture, and evidence for complementary treatments, we will be better able to understand and perhaps prevent depression, anxiety, and other comorbidities in patients with breast cancer. Finally, the impact of breast cancer on partners, family, and children should continue to be evaluated as technology, early detection, prognoses, and treatments progress.

SUMMARY

The psychosocial aspects of breast cancer surgery are very important for the patient, family, and surgeon. Understanding patients' normal and abnormal reactions allows clinicians to better understand treatment adherence, adjustment to family, work and other social aspects, quality of life, and overall rehabilitation. As surgical techniques and options change and improve, and new combinations of treatment and protocols develop, it is all the more important to evaluate how patients may improve with such treatments, medically, surgically, and psychosocially. The Institute of Medicine has given us a mandate to include such psychosocial care in the overall treatment of patients regularly and routinely. How to accomplish this for patients, from the beginning of care, into survivorship, is a challenge and opportunity.

REFERENCES

1. Renneker R, Cutler M. Psychosocial problems of adjustment to cancer of the breast. *JAMA*. 1952;148:833-839.
2. Sutherland AM, Orbach CE. Psychological impact of cancer and cancer surgery: II. Depressive reactions associated with surgery for cancer. *Cancer*. 1953;6:958-962.
3. Morris T, Greer HS, White P. Psychological and social adjustment to mastectomy. *Cancer*. 1977;40:2381-2387.
4. Maguire GP, Lee EG, Bevington DJ, et al. Psychiatric problems in the first year after mastectomy. *Br Med J*. 1978;1:1963-1965.
5. Steinberg MD, Juliano MA, Wise L. Psychological outcome of lumpectomy versus mastectomy in the treatment of breast cancer. *Am J Psychiatry*. 1985;142:1.
6. Monteiro-Grillo I, Marques-Vidal P, Marilia J. Psychosocial effect of mastectomy versus conservative surgery in patients with early breast cancer. *Clin Transl Oncol*. 2005;11:499-503.
7. Jamison KR, Wellisch DK, Pasnau RO. Psychosocial aspects of mastectomy: I. The woman's perspective. *Am J Psychiatry*. 1978;135:432-436.
8. Wellisch DK, Jamison KR, Pasnau RO. Psychosocial aspects of mastectomy: II. The man's perspective. *Am J Psychiatry*. 1978;135:543-546.
9. Klein R. A crisis to grow on. *Cancer*. 1971;28:1660-1665.
10. Ganz PA, Schag AC, Lee JJ, et al. Breast conservation versus mastectomy: is there a difference in psychological adjustment or quality of life in the year after surgery? *Cancer*. 1992;69:1729-1738.
11. Jacobsen PB, Roth AJ, Holland JC. Surgery. In: Holland JC, ed. *Psychooncology*. Oxford, UK: Oxford University Press; 1998;257-268.
12. Anstice E. The emotional operation. *Nurs Times*. 1970;66:837-838.
13. Baile WF, Buckman R, Lenzi R, et al. SPIKES—a six-step protocol for delivering bad news: application to the patient with cancer. *Oncologist*. 2005;5:302-311.
14. Butow PN, Maclean M, Dunn SM et al. The dynamics of change: cancer patients' preferences for information, involvement and support. *Ann Oncol*. 1997;64:181-182.
15. Ho SMY, Saltel P, Machavoine JL, et al. Cross-cultural aspects of cancer care. In: Moore RJ, Spiegel D, eds. *Cancer, Culture and Communication*. New York: Springer; 2004:157-183.
16. Newman EA, Guest AB, Helvie MA, et al. Changes in surgical management resulting from case review at a breast cancer multidisciplinary tumor board. *Cancer* 2006;107:2346-2351.
17. Fallowfield LJ, Baum M, Maguire GP. Effects of breast conservation on psychological morbidity associated with diagnosis and treatment of early breast cancer. *Br Med J*. 1986;293:1331-1334.
18. Schain WS, d'Angelo TM, Dunn ME, et al. Mastectomy versus conservative surgery and radiation therapy: psychosocial consequences. *Cancer*. 1994;73:1221-1228.
19. Rowland JH, Holland JC, Chaglassian T, Kinne D. Psychological response to breast reconstruction: expectations for and impact on postmastectomy functioning. *Psychosomatics*. 1993;34:241-250.
20. Strain JJ, Grossman S. *Psychological Care of the Medically Ill*. New York, NY: Appleton-Century-Crofts; 1975.
21. Holland JC, Rowland JH. Psychological reactions to breast cancer and its treatment. In: Harris JR, Hellman S, Henderson IC, Kinne DW, eds. *Breast Diseases*. Philadelphia, PA: Lippincott Williams & Wilkins; 1987: 632-647.
22. *Cancer Care for the Whole Patient: Meeting Psychosocial Health Needs*. Institute of Medicine, National Academy of Sciences; 2007:1.
23. Von Ah D, Kang DH. Correlates of mood disturbance in women with breast cancer: patterns over time. *J Adv Nurs*. 2008;61:676-689.
24. Stanton AL. Psychosocial concerns and interventions for cancer survivors. *J Clin Oncol*. 2006;24:5132-5137.
25. Fann JR, Thomas-Rich AM, Katon WJ, et al. Major depression after breast cancer: a review of epidemiology and treatment. *Gen Hosp Psychiatry*. 2008;30:112-126.
26. Epstein DR, Dirksen SR. Randomized trial of a cognitive-behavioral intervention for insomnia in breast cancer survivors. *Oncol Nurs Forum*. 2007;34:E51-E59.
27. Friedman LC, Romero C, Elledge R, et al. Attribution of blame, self-forgiving attitude and psychological adjustment in women with breast cancer. *J Behav Med*. 2007;30:351-357.

28. Waljee JF, Hu ES, Ubel PA, et al. Effect of esthetic outcome after breast-conserving surgery on psychosocial functioning and quality of life. *J Clin Oncol*. 2008;26:3331-3337.

29. Brandberg Y, Sandelin K, Erikson S, et al. Psychological reactions, quality of life, and body image after bilateral prophylactic mastectomy in women at high risk for breast cancer: a prospective 1-year follow-up study. *J Clin Oncol*. 2008;26:3943-3949.

30. Spiegel D, Riba M. Psychological aspects of cancer. In: DeVita VT, Lawrence TS, Rosenberg SA, eds. *Principles and Practice of Oncology*. 8th ed. Philadelphia, PA: Lippincott Williams & Wilkins; 2008:2817-2826.

31. DiMatteo MR, Lepper HS, Croghan TW. Depression is a risk factor for non-compliance with medical treatment. *Arch Intern Med*. 2000;160:2101-2107.

32. Shelby RA, Golden-Kreutz DM, Andersen BL. PTSD diagnoses, subsyndromal symptoms and comorbidities contribute to impairments for breast cancer survivors. *J Traumatic Stress*. 2008;21:165-172.

33. Garssen B, de Kok E. How useful is a screening instrument? *Psychooncology*. 2008;17:726-728.

34. National Comprehensive Cancer Network. Practice Guidelines in Oncology—Distress Management v.1.2008. Retrieved on August 28, 2008, from www.nccn.org.

35. Rush AJ, First MB, Blacker D, eds. *Handbook of Psychiatric Measures*. 2nd ed. Washington, DC: American Psychiatric Publishing; 2008.

36. Hoffman BM, Zevon MA, D'Arrigo MC, et al. Screening for distress in cancer patient: the NCCN rapid-screening measure. *Psychooncology*. 2004;13:792-799.

37. Cella DF, Tulsky DS, Gray G, et al. The functional assessment of cancer therapy scale: development and validation of the general measure. *J Clin Oncol*. 1993;11:570-579.

38. Horowitz M, Wilner N, Alvarez W. Impact of event scale: a measure of subjective stress. *Psychosom Med*. 1979;41:209-218.

39. Spitzer RL, Williams JB, Gibbon M, First MB. The structured clinical interview for DSM-III-R (SCID). I. History, rationale, and description. *Arch Gen Psychiatry*. 1992;49:624-629.

40. Barsevick AM, Sweeney C, Haney E, Chung E. A systematic qualitative analysis of psychoeducational interventions for depression in patients with cancer. *Oncol Nurs Forum*. 2002;29:73-84; quiz 85-87.

41. Andersen BL, Shelby RA, Golden-Kreutz DM. RCT of a psychological intervention for patients with cancer: I. Mechanisms of change. *J Consult Clin Psychol*. 2007;75:927-938.

42. Hunter MS, Coventry S, Hamed H, et al. Evaluation of a group cognitive behavioural intervention for women suffering from menopausal symptoms following breast cancer treatment. *Psychooncology*. 2009;18(5):560-563.

43. Classen CC, Kraemer HC, Blasey C, et al. Supportive-expressive group therapy for primary breast cancer patients: a randomized prospective multicenter trial. *Psychooncology*. 2008;17:438-447.

44. Kissane DW, Grabsch B, Clarke DM, et al. Supportive-expressive group therapy for women with metastatic breast cancer: survival and psychosocial outcome from a randomized control trial. *Psychooncology*. 2007;16:277-286.

45. Altshuler LL, Cohen LS, Moline ML, et al. Treatment of depression in women: a summary of expert consensus guidelines. *J Psychiatr Pract*. 2001;7:185-208.

46. Roscoe JA, Morrow GR, Hickok JT, et al. Effect of paroxetine hydrochloride on fatigue and depression in breast cancer patients receiving chemotherapy. *Breast Cancer Res Treat*. 2005;89:243-249.

47. Navari RM, Brenner MC, Wilson MN. Treatment of depressive symptoms in patients with early stage breast cancer undergoing adjuvant therapy. *Breast Cancer Res Treat*. 2008;112(1):197-201.

48. Kimmick GG, Lorato J, McQuellon R, et al. Randomized, double blind, placebo controlled crossover study of sertraline for treatment of hot flashes in women with early stage breast cancer taking tamoxifen. *Breast J*. 2006;12:114-122.

49. Hoffman EJ, Mathew SJ. Anxiety disorders: a comprehensive review of pharmacotherapies. *Mt Sinai J Med*. 2008;75:248-268.

50. Effects of chemotherapy and hormonal therapy for early breast cancer on recurrence and 15-year survival: an overview of the randomised trials. *Lancet*. 2005;365:1687-1717.

51. Goetz MP, Knox SK, Suman VJ, et al. The impact of cytochrome P450 2D6 metabolism in women receiving adjuvant tamoxifen. *Breast Cancer Res Treat*. 2007;101:113-121.

52. Stearns V, Johnson MD, Rae JM, et al. Active tamoxifen metabolite plasma concentrations after coadministration of tamoxifen and the selective serotonin reuptake inhibitor paroxetine. *J Natl Cancer Inst*. 2003;95:1758-1764.

53. Borges S, Desta Z, Li L, et al. Quantitative effect of CYP2D6 genotype and inhibitors on tamoxifen metabolism: implication for optimization of breast cancer treatment. *Clin Pharmacol Ther*. 2006;80:61-74.

54. Pezzella G, Moslinger-Gehmayr R, Contu A. Treatment of depression in patients with breast cancer: a comparison between paroxetine and amitriptyline. *Breast Cancer Res Treat*. 2001;70:1-10.

55. Loibl S, Schwedler K, von Minckwitz G, et al. Venlafaxine is superior to clonidine as treatment of hot flashes in breast cancer patients—a double blind, randomized study. *Ann Oncol*. 2007;18:689-693.

56. Vadivelu N, Schreck M, Lopez J, et al. Pain after mastectomy and breast reconstruction. *Am Surg*. 2008;74:285-296.

57. Stevens PE, Dibble SL, Miaskowski C. Prevalence, characteristics and impact of post-mastectomy pain syndrome: an investigation of women's experiences. *Pain*. 1995;61:61-68.

58. Kalso ET, Tasmuth T, Neuvonen PJ. Amitriptyline effectively relieves neuropathic pain following treatment of breast cancer. *Pain*. 1995;64:293-302.

59. Tasmuth T, Hartel B, Kalso ET. Venlafaxine in neuropathic pain following treatment of breast cancer. *Eur J Pain*. 2002;6:17-24.

60. Reuben SS, Makari-Judson G, Lurie SD. Evaluation of efficacy of the perioperative administration of venlafaxine XR in the prevention of post-mastectomy pain syndrome. *J Pain Sympt Manage*. 2004;27:133-139.

61. Mitchell AJ. Pooled results from 38 analyses of the accuracy of distress thermometer and other ultra-short methods of detecting cancer-related mood disorders. *J Clin Oncol*. 2007;25:4670-4681.

62. Shaw BR, Jeong Yeob Han, Hawkins RP, et al. Communicating about self and others within an online support group for women with breast cancer and subsequent outcomes. *J Health Psychol*. 2008;13:930-939.

63. Kolden GG, Strauman TJ, Ward A, et al. A pilot study of group exercise training (GET) for women with primary breast cancer: feasibility and health benefits. *Psychooncology*. 2002;11:447-456.

CHAPTER 101

Fertility, Sexuality, and Menopausal Symptom Management

Kathryn J. Ruddy
Ann H. Partridge

Improvements in the detection and treatment of breast cancer have resulted in a growing number of breast cancer survivors. It has been estimated that there are now more than 2 million breast cancer survivors in the United States alone, and many more worldwide.[1] As these women go on to live healthy and productive lives, many will experience burdensome menopausal symptoms, such as hot flashes and vaginal dryness, and impairments in sexual functioning. Couzi et al[2] reported that, of women previously diagnosed with early-stage breast cancer, 65% suffered hot flashes, 44% night sweats, 48% vaginal dryness, 26% dyspareunia, 44% difficulty sleeping, and 44% feeling depressed. Physical and emotional problems arising from the diagnosis and treatment of breast cancer may compound each other, creating a complex interplay of symptoms. Sexual problems may result from a combination of the psychosocial trauma associated with the diagnosis of breast cancer, changes in body image, and treatment side effects. Atrophic vaginitis, a constellation of symptoms including vaginal dryness and associated urogenital inflammation, atrophy, stenosis, pruritus, and dyspareunia, is particularly problematic for sexual functioning.[3] Without treatment, these symptoms can be lasting and severe. Speer et al[4] found that breast cancer survivors an average of 4.4 years after treatment had reduced sexual functioning in all domains except desire when compared with previously published data on women without a history of cancer. In a direct comparison with age-matched control women, Broeckels et al[3] found that women who had been treated for breast cancer at least 5 years previously reported worse sexual functioning including greater lack of sexual interest, inability to relax and enjoy sex, difficulty becoming aroused, and difficulty achieving an orgasm.

Menopausal symptoms may have a substantial impact on quality of life, body image, sexual function, and self-esteem.[5,6] These symptoms also impact adherence to hormonal therapies.[7] For the approximately 25% of breast cancer patients who are premenopausal at diagnosis, treatment may result in amenorrhea and potential infertility. Menopausal status and fertility potential after breast cancer is an area of great concern for young cancer survivors and may impact treatment decisions.[8] Understanding the factors contributing to these symptoms and long-term effects and implementing strategies to avoid or ameliorate them is likely to improve symptoms and quality of life for breast cancer survivors.

Several factors contribute to the development or worsening of menopausal symptoms, sexual dysfunction, and amenorrhea and infertility in breast cancer survivors. Peri- and postmenopausal women generally are recommended to discontinue symptom-relieving hormone-replacement therapy when they are diagnosed with breast cancer. Abrupt withdrawal often precipitates severe hot flashes and vaginal dryness, which weaning more slowly may lessen.[9] Surgery and radiation therapy can impair function locally, and systemic therapy including chemotherapy and hormonal therapy may precipitate menopausal symptoms and changes in ovarian function through a number of mechanisms.

EFFECTS OF LOCAL THERAPY

Surgical treatments for breast cancer including mastectomy or partial mastectomy and lymph node surgery directly alter a woman's body contour, which may affect body image adversely. Lasting changes in sensation often occur postoperatively, particularly in the setting of mastectomy. Chronic pain syndromes due to nerve damage in the breast and axillary area as well as impaired upper-extremity range of motion and lymphedema can also interfere with sexual functioning. Local irradiation may compound these upper body changes. Bukovic et al[10] reported that rates of satisfaction with sexual life in breast cancer patients treated with mastectomy (plus radiation for more advanced tumors) and in those treated with lumpectomy plus radiation (for early-stage tumors) both dropped from 70% and 73%, respectively, before treatment to 57% and 50%, respectively, after treatment. In contrast, Monteiro-Grillo et al[11] found that mastectomy had a more negative impact than lumpectomy. Surveying 61 women who had undergone breast-conserving therapy and 64 who had undergone modified radical mastectomy, these authors found that mastectomy was associated with more negative body image, more change in social behaviors, and poorer quality of life. Reconstructive surgery may be an important contributor to healthy sexuality for women who undergo mastectomy. Several studies suggest that immediate reconstruction is more protective of sexual functioning than delayed reconstruction.[12,13]

EFFECTS OF SYSTEMIC THERAPY

Systemic therapy, including chemotherapy and hormonal therapy, may affect a woman's sexual and reproductive functioning both directly and indirectly. In the short term, chemotherapy causes physical losses, including hair loss, nausea and vomiting, and skin and nail changes, all potentially altering body image and libido. Chemotherapy is fatiguing emotionally and physically, and fatigue may be of long duration. In pre- and perimenopausal women, chemotherapy can be directly toxic to the ovaries, resulting in amenorrhea and depletion in systemic estrogen levels, which may be temporary or permanent. This abrupt decrease in estrogen levels may cause severe menopausal symptoms, including hot flashes and vaginal dryness. Regardless of menopausal status, tamoxifen is associated with hot flashes due to its antiestrogenic effects, although it acts in a proestrogenic manner in the vagina with an associated increased incidence of vaginal discharge and rare but significant risk of uterine cancer. Aromatase inhibitors (AIs) lack this estrogenic action in the vagina and endometrium and therefore cause more vaginal dryness compared with tamoxifen (approximately 18% compared with approximately 8%).[16,17] With the increasing use of AIs, the absolute number of breast cancer patients affected by symptomatic atrophic vaginitis is likely to increase. In contrast to hot flashes, vaginal atrophy usually increases over time, so treatments are likely to be required as long as the patient remains estrogen-deficient. In the Arimidex, Tamoxifen, Alone or in Combination (ATAC) trial comparing these treatments in postmenopausal women with early breast cancer, women receiving the AI were more likely to report vaginal dryness (18.5% vs 9.1%), diminished libido (34.0% vs 26.1%), and dyspareunia (17.3% vs 8.1%) as compared with women receiving tamoxifen.[18] In premenopausal women, ovarian suppression or bilateral oophorectomy induces a sudden menopause that often is associated with severe symptoms. A study comparing different systemic regimens for breast cancer in premenopausal women

found that ovarian suppression with goserelin acetate increased temporary sexual dysfunction during treatment, but adjuvant chemotherapy increased sexual dysfunction even 3 years afterwards, likely because of more lasting damage to the ovaries from the chemotherapy.[19]

Sexual dysfunction, including lack of lubrication, dyspareunia, decreased libido, and difficulty with orgasm, affects at least 50% of women after breast cancer.[20] Risk factors for sexual dysfunction include younger age, premature menopause, and the use of chemotherapy.[21] In younger women, Burwell et al[20] found that negative body image is linked with mastectomy, hair loss from chemotherapy, concern with weight gain or loss, poorer mental health, lower self-esteem, and poor communication with a partner. Fobair et al[22] found that young women's sexual difficulties are exacerbated by vaginal dryness, poor mental health, being married, and negative body image. In postmenopausal women with a history of breast cancer, Greendale et al[23] found that sexual impairment was associated with older age, less time since diagnosis, poor relationship quality, vaginal discomfort, higher education, fewer hot flashes, urinary incontinence, history of mastectomy, and poorer perceived health and body image. Impaired sleep due to nocturnal hot flashes and night sweats in cancer survivors may impact sexual functioning, libido, and quality of life. Anxiety and depression after treatment for breast cancer may be compounded by hormonal changes and may add to sexual dysfunction.

Premenopausal women may become infertile due to direct gonadotoxicity of chemotherapy. Although hormonal therapy effects on ovarian function and menopausal symptoms appear to be reversible with discontinuation of the medication, fertility declines naturally over the time it takes to receive optimal hormonal treatment.

ASSESSMENT AND MANAGEMENT OF MENOPAUSAL SYMPTOMS AND SEXUAL DYSFUNCTION

Assessment of menopausal symptoms should include documentation of the frequency and severity of vasomotor symptoms (hot flashes and night sweats), symptoms of atrophic vaginitis (vaginal dryness, dyspareunia, urinary urgency, and frequency), reduced libido, and sleep disturbance.[24] The decision whether to treat menopausal symptoms pharmacologically will depend on their severity, impact on activities of daily living, and patient preferences. Measuring quality of life may facilitate treatment decisions using menopause-specific instruments such as the MENQOL (Menopause-Specific Quality of Life Questionnaire) or breast cancer-specific instruments such as the FACT-ES (Functional Assessment of Cancer Therapy–Endocrine Symptoms).[25,26] Sexual functioning after breast cancer can be assessed with standardized, validated instruments such as the Sexual Activity Questionnaire or the Greene Scale, although these measures are most commonly used in a research setting.[27,28] Ganz et al[5] proved that a comprehensive menopausal intervention program, in which pharmacologic and behavioral interventions are recommended if appropriate, can improve menopausal symptoms and sexual functioning as compared with usual care. For many women, a multifaceted approach may be warranted to improve

TABLE 101-1 Side Effects of Breast Cancer Therapies and Management Strategies

	Symptom	Management Strategy
Physical	Hot flashes/night sweats	Medications including SSRIs and SNRIs
		Cooling pillows and/or layered clothing
	Vaginal dryness/dyspareunia	Vaginal moisturizers and lubricants, ideally nonhormonal
	Anorgasmia/poor arousal	Lubricants, vibrators, counseling for patient and partner
	Sleep deprivation	Sleep hygiene strategies, hypnotic medications
		Treatment of hot flashes, depression
	Changes in body contour	Breast reconstruction
	Weight gain	Exercise, nutrition
Emotional	Anxiety	Medications including SSRIs and SNRIs
	Depression	Medications including SSRIs and SNRIs
	Relationship Strain	Counseling for patient and partner
	Lack of libido	Counseling for patient and partner, cognitive restructuring

SNRI, serotonin and norepinephrine reuptake inhibitor; SSRI, selective serotonin reuptake inhibitor.

these symptoms and related problems. Table 101-1 provides a synopsis of suggested management strategies for a variety of physical and emotional symptoms that may result from treatment for breast cancer.

Combined estrogen and progesterone hormone-replacement therapy is a very effective mechanism for alleviation of menopausal symptoms in women without breast cancer.[29-31] However, it carries cardiovascular risks even in women without a history of cancer,[32] and due to potential stimulation of cancer cells, it is likely not safe to use after breast cancer. Two Swedish randomized controlled trials, the Stockholm trial and the hormonal replacement therapy after breastcancer diagnosis—is it safe? (HABITS) trial, were both stopped early because the HABITS trial (but never the Stockholm trial) revealed increased recurrences in those receiving hormone-replacement therapy after treatment for breast cancer. In the HABITS trial of 442 breast cancer survivors in Scandinavia, women randomized to hormone-replacement therapy and followed for a median of 4 years had 3.5-fold more cancer recurrences than those randomized to placebo.[33] The absence of increased risk in the Stockholm trial may result from lower-risk patients and more participants concomitantly receiving tamoxifen (which should at least blunt the stimulatory impact of estrogen on the breast cancer cells). For women on tamoxifen, hormone-replacement therapy appears to have limited efficacy in alleviating hot flashes.[34] Therefore, for most breast cancer survivors, nonhormonal treatments are recommended.[35] Nevertheless, for women with low-risk disease and severe symptoms, short-term hormone-replacement therapy may be appropriate.[36]

Management of Hot Flashes

The natural history of vasomotor symptoms after breast cancer is not well-studied, but in spontaneous menopause, vasomotor symptoms are known to decrease in frequency and severity after 12 months of amenorrhea.[37,38] Therefore, it is reasonable to take a watch-and-wait approach for some women or to try to discontinue treatments for hot flashes on an intermittent basis in order to assess whether symptoms recur. Little is known about factors regulating hot flashes arising from endocrine therapy for breast cancer. In women without cancer who are experiencing natural menopause, hot flashes are thought to be caused by the loss of estrogen's modulating effect on the hypothalamic thermoregulating mechanism.[39] After spontaneous menopause, hot flashes may be triggered by stimuli such as spicy food, hairdryers, or anxiety. For individual breast cancer survivors, recording triggers in a diary may help women to avoid triggers and prevent hot flashes. Some women find it helpful to wear natural fibers and to dress in layers so that clothes can easily be removed during hot flashes. Use of a cold pack may also lessen symptoms when they occur. Acupuncture, paced breathing, and hypnosis are promising treatment methods, but their benefit over sham procedures remains unproven.

Evidence is conflicting regarding whether hot flashes are reduced by lifestyle modifications such as weight loss (for overweight women), regular exercise, and cessation of smoking.[24] In 1 study, hot flashes were found to be more severe in overweight women and in smokers.[40] There is also some preliminary data suggesting that exercise reduces the risk of or ameliorates hot flashes.[41]

Routine nonhormonal strategies for management of hot flashes include relaxation techniques, cooling pillows, selective serotonin reuptake inhibitors (SSRIs), serotonin and norepinephrine reuptake inhibitors (SNRIs), gabapentin, and clonidine. Details of pharmacologic therapies are provided in Table 101-2. A meta-analysis of 10 randomized controlled trials involving 1581 women in total and 14 pilot trials with 325 total participants suggested that therapeutic efficacy of treatments for hot flashes is similar in women with and without a history of breast cancer and with or without tamoxifen treatment.[42] This meta-analysis found evidence that hot flashes are moderately decreased by venlafaxine, mildly to moderately decreased by fluoxetine, mildly decreased by clonidine, and not substantially decreased

TABLE 101-2 Oral Pharmacologic Interventions for Menopausal Symptoms

	Clonidine	SSRI/SNRI	Gabapentin
Efficacy: Mean difference in daily number of hot flashes vs placebo per meta-analysis (95% CI)[47]	−0.95(−1.44 to −0.47)	−1.13(−1.70 to 0.57)	−2.05 (−2.80 to −1.30)
Proven duration of action	Up to 8 weeks	Up to 6 weeks	Up to 12 weeks
Discontinuation due to side effects in clinical trials for hot flashes	40%[60]	10%-20%[92]	10%[93]
Common side effects	Dry mouth and insomnia or drowsiness	Dry mouth, blurred vision, sexual dysfunction	Dizziness, drowsiness, unsteadiness

SNRI, serotonin-norepinephrine reuptake inhibitor; SSRI, selective serotonin reuptake inhibitor.

by vitamin E or black cohosh.[42] Alternative therapies such as dong quai, evening primrose oil, and ginseng have not appeared promising in studies to date.[43] Evidence for the efficacy of soy products in reducing hot flashes is contradictory.[44] Furthermore, it is not clear how safe soy is for breast cancer survivors due to potential stimulation of breast cancers by the phytoestrogens it contains. Therefore, given that black cohosh has been occasionally linked to liver failure and high-dose vitamin E was shown to increase all-cause mortality in other settings, most providers favor SSRI/SNRI, gabapentin, or clonidine therapy, all of which have been studied and demonstrated some efficacy in the treatment of hot flashes in breast cancer survivors.[45,46]

There are few head-to-head studies of different drugs, with most research comparing an agent with placebo in a small population of women who average more than 14 hot flashes per week, and conclusions are complicated by the significant placebo effect seen in many studies.[47] Comparing venlafaxine with placebo in postmenopausal women without cancer, Evans et al[48] did not find a significant benefit, but Loprinzi et al[49] did find a reduction in number of daily hot flashes using 37.5 or 75 mg of venlafaxine in a larger study. Two studies by Stearns et al,[50,51] each with approximately 150 participants, both showed a significant reduction with paroxetine (10-20 mg daily or 12.5-25 mg of controlled release). Kalay et al[52] found that citalopram effectively improved scores on 2 scales of menopausal symptoms, but Suvanto-Luukonen et al[53] did not find a significant impact of citalopram or fluoxetine over placebo. A cross-over design comparing placebo with 50 mg of sertraline on women receiving tamoxifen revealed decreased hot flashes in those taking sertraline. In those who are taking tamoxifen, medications that inhibit CYP2D6 (eg, paroxetine and fluoxetine) should be avoided because they prevent effective breakdown of tamoxifen into its most active metabolite, endoxifen.[54,55] Venlafaxine and citalopram are not strong CYP2D6 inhibitors, so their use is thought to be safe even in those taking tamoxifen.[56] Although the side effects of SSRIs and SNRIs can include weight gain, insomnia, and decreased libido, patients may still feel better on these medications if hot flashes are very problematic. SSRIs and SNRIs are generally contraindicated in women taking monoamine oxidase inhibitors and should be used cautiously or preferably avoided in women with bipolar disorder because of the risk of inducing mania.

If there is no response in 4 weeks, then the treatment is unlikely to be effective, and it is reasonable to consider trying a different SSRI, SNRI, or another class of drugs. Gabapentin appears be an effective alternative and may be used as an alternative first-line treatment or instead of SSRI/SNRIs or in women with sexual dysfunction or who do not respond to or cannot take SSRI/SNRIs.[57,58] There does not appear to be a benefit of adding gabapentin to SSRI/SNRIs.[58] In tamoxifen users with a history of breast cancer, a reduced frequency and severity of hot flashes has been seen with clonidine, a centrally acting α-adrenergic agonist that reduces vascular reactivity, at either 0.1 mg/day transdermally or 0.1 mg/day orally.[59,60] However, side effects with this agent, including dizziness and hypotension, may be problematic.

Management of Vaginal Dryness and Atrophic Vaginitis

Nonhormonal vaginal lubricants are appropriate first-line therapies for vaginal dryness and atrophic vaginitis. Replens is a vaginal moisturizer that can be applied vaginally every 2 to 3 days to prevent itching, burning, and pain. This can cause some vaginal discharge, so some women prefer to use genital lubricants externally and/or internally as needed for sexual activity. Water-based or silicone-based products are preferable to glycerine-based products, which can promote yeast infection. Astroglide, Liquid Silk (Bodywise Limited), and Sensua Organics are effective personal lubricants that can be used to reduce dyspareunia on their own or in combination with Replens. All are safe to use with latex condoms and can be applied directly to a condom if desired. For symptoms that do not respond to nonhormonal therapy, vaginal estrogen preparations can be considered. Options for topical vaginal estrogen include an estradiol-releasing vaginal ring, estrogen-based vaginal creams, pessaries containing estriol, and a slow-release 17β-estradiol tablet. There is controversy regarding the use of topical intravaginal estrogens because of concern that systemic absorption may stimulate breast cancer recurrences.

Small retrospective studies suggest that vaginal estrogens do not adversely affect outcome in breast cancer patients,[61] but an estradiol vaginal tablet, Vagifem (Novo Nordisk Femcare AG; Princeton, New Jersey), increased serum estradiol levels in an evaluation of 7 postmenopausal women on AIs.[62] Therefore, vaginal estradiol could reduce the efficacy of an AI, but vaginal estriol, a less potent estrogen, may be safe. More research is needed regarding the safety of vaginal estrogens after breast cancer. Nevertheless, judicious use of vaginal preparations may be necessary for some women with severe vaginal symptoms. In women whose atrophic vaginitis is refractory to treatment, vaginal stenosis can develop, and vaginal dilators may be needed to relieve symptoms and allow intercourse.

Management of Libido and Orgasm Problems

Given the multifactorial etiology of sexual dysfunction in breast cancer survivors, a comprehensive approach to treatment is often necessary. Ameliorating symptoms described previously including fatigue and vaginal dryness may improve desire and orgasm potential. The differentiation between poor desire and poor arousal is difficult and usually requires direct questioning. For problems with arousal and orgasm, vibrators, pubococcygeus muscle exercises, and pelvic physical therapy can be helpful. Using an integrative approach, behavioral strategies such as sensate focus and focused breathing can improve both desire and arousal.

Treatment of libido disorders in this setting is challenging. Although several randomized controlled trials have shown that the combination of transdermal testosterone with estradiol improves sexual functioning in noncancer patients who have undergone surgical menopause or who have hypoactive sexual desire disorder,[63-67] a placebo-controlled cross-over study of transdermal testosterone in postmenopausal women with a history of cancer showed no difference in libido change between testosterone and placebo.[68] The authors attribute this lack of benefit to estrogen depletion.

Counseling for the individual patient can build coping skills and improve sexual functioning via cognitive restructuring. When anxiety or depression is present, psychotherapy or medications to improve mood and reduce anxiety may be helpful in ameliorating libido. Even in women not suffering from anxiety and depression, nonhormonal options for improving sexual function may include antidepressants. A noncontrolled study by Mathias et al[69] found that bupropion 150 mg daily for 8 weeks was associated with better sexual function. Furthermore, couples counseling can also be important for enhancing communication and understanding between the patient and her partner.

MANAGEMENT OF FERTILITY CONCERNS AND INFERTILITY

Of the approximately 180,000 women diagnosed with breast cancer each year in the United States, more than 40,000 are premenopausal, and many of these women may not yet have finished their child-bearing at diagnosis.[70] Some of these women are interested in having a biological child after breast cancer. Because nulliparity and late first pregnancy increase risk for breast cancer, a disproportionate number of breast cancer

patients may be nulliparous or may not yet have finished their child-bearing at diagnosis. Although there is theoretic concern that pregnancy after breast cancer could stimulate recurrence, many studies have actually found better outcomes in women who become pregnant after breast cancer.[71] This may reflect a "healthy mother bias," as women who are healthier may be more likely to conceive, but regardless, there is no evidence that pregnancy should be avoided after breast cancer, although optimal breast cancer treatment (often 5 years of hormonal therapy) and avoidance of pregnancy during the period of highest risk of recurrence are often recommended.

The American Society of Clinical Oncology has recommended that all cancer patients receive the following care related to fertility: (1) assessment for and communication regarding risk of infertility; (2) for those who are at risk of infertility and interested in fertility preservation, referral to a specialist with expertise in fertility preservation method. In order to manage these patients, a thorough understanding of the risk of infertility after treatment for breast cancer is necessary. Women who are older and who receive more gonadotoxic chemotherapy regimens are more likely to experience menopause after treatment for breast cancer and therefore are at higher risk of losing the ability to have a biological child. In one study, rates of menstrual bleeding 6 months after completion of chemotherapy were approximately 85% in those less than 35 years of age, 61% in those 35 to 40 years, and less than 25% in those more than 40 years, with higher rates after the regimens that contained less total cyclophosphamide.[72] Whether amenorrhea adds to the risk of infertility after chemotherapy is uncertain. Because the decision to attempt pregnancy after breast cancer is complex and relatively rare, there are little to no data comparing actual conception rates between different regimens. In fact, studies suggest that only 5% to 15% of young women with breast cancer will later become pregnant.[73-75] Those who do should be referred to a high-risk obstetrician for medical care during the pregnancy given the risk of disease recurrence during pregnancy and complications related to the history of breast cancer treatment.

Rates of amenorrhea have been collected in studies of various chemotherapies, but not for all regimens and not using identical definitions for amenorrhea. The most significant limitation of these data is that it is unknown how closely amenorrhea (temporary, in some cases) reflects fertility impairment.[71] Data are limited, but estimations of rates of amenorrhea with common regimens are presented in Table 101-3.

Although breast cancer treatments including chemotherapy and hormonal therapy may result in ovarian dysfunction and associated infertility, many young breast cancer survivors remain premenopausal after therapy is complete. However, even in women who regain menses after chemotherapy, fertility may be compromised by premature menopause or decreased ovarian reserve. For a 32-year-old woman who receives doxorubicin and cyclophosphamide as adjuvant therapy, the likelihood that menses will return is high. However, her risk of menopause in the next 5 years may be higher than other nontreated women her age. Even someone only 25 at diagnosis and menstruating 2 years later was shown in one study to have a 16% risk of menopause at 5 years after cyclophosphamide, methotrexate, and fluorouracil, but a 75% risk at 10 years (at only age 35 years).[76] Concern about

TABLE 101-3 Risk of Amenorrhea with Common Treatment Regimens[72,94-98]

Regimen	Age < 30 Years	Age 30-40 Years	Age > 40 Years
None	~0	< 5	20-25
AC × 4	–	13	57-63
CMF × 6	19	31-38	76-96
CAF/CEF × 6	23-47		80-89
TAC × 6		62	
AC × 4, T × 4		38 (15% age < 40)	

AC, doxorubicin and cyclophosphamide; CAF, cyclophosphamide, doxorubicin, and fluorouracil; CEF, cyclophosphamide, epirubicin, and fluorouracil; CMF, cyclophosphamide, methotrexate, and fluorouracil; T, paclitaxel; TAC, docetaxel, doxorubicin, and cyclophosphamide.
Adapted from Partridge and Ruddy (2007).[71]

menopause occurring earlier in breast cancer survivors who remain premenopausal immediately after chemotherapy may impact the time frame in which pregnancies will be planned. Though tamoxifen and/or ovarian suppression do not appear to directly damage the ovaries, women are all less fertile after 5 years of hormonal therapy due to the natural decline of ovarian function over time. Increasing attention is focusing on how best to measure ovarian reserve at the time of diagnosis and in follow-up in order to determine fertility potential after treatment.[77,78] Serum levels of hormones and ultrasound measurement of antral follicle count may inform decisions about whether the chance of future fertility will be low.

Fertility preservation strategies should be considered as early as possible in the course of a woman's breast cancer care if she desires a future pregnancy, and fertility is likely to be impaired for her after treatment. Assessment of fertility concerns can be difficult in the setting of a new cancer diagnosis because of the inevitable stress relating to prognosis and treatment. However, it is important that these concerns be elicited early, as most fertility preservation techniques (listed in Table 101-4) are generally considered before systemic therapy is begun. Options for fertility preservation all have limitations. The most tested option for fertility preservation at the time of diagnosis is embryo cryopreservation.[8] This requires that a woman have a partner or use

TABLE 101-4 Strategies for Fertility Preservation in Women with Breast Cancer

Method	Risks	Efficacy
GNRH agonists	Menopausal symptoms and bone thinning	Efficacy unknown, studies ongoing
Embryo cryopreservation	Requires sperm source Requires delay in initiation of systemic therapy Concern that hormonal stimulation may adversely impact prognosis Ethically problematic if patient dies	20%-30% pregnancy rate per transfer of 2-3 embryos
Oocyte cryopreservation	Requires delay in initiation of systemic therapy Concern that hormonal stimulation may adversely impact prognosis	Approximately 2% pregnancy rate per thawed oocyte
Ovarian tissue cryopreservation	Invasive May increase risk of infertility in low-risk situation Potential for reintroduction of malignant cells at reimplantation	Case report level evidence (few babies born to date)

GNRH, gonadotropin-releasing hormone.

a sperm donor and also that she undergo ovarian stimulation and ultrasound-guided egg retrieval, requiring at least 2 weeks of delay of breast cancer therapy.[79] Fertilization and storage of embryos occurs, so after treatments are completed, a woman can have these embryos implanted and can sustain a pregnancy even if her ovaries are no longer functioning. Pregnancy rates of 20% to 30% per transfer of 2 of 3 embryos have been reported.[80] Novel regimens of ovarian stimulation are using letrozole and tamoxifen to attempt to reduce potential stimulation of breast cancer cell growth in the setting of the supraphysiologic estradiol levels that result from conventional regimens. Preliminary data from these strategies suggest safety in the short term, although concerns remain.[8,81,82] However, the control groups in these studies may be less than ideal, as women who are at lower baseline risk may be more likely to want to delay therapy for 2 weeks in order to freeze eggs. Thus the safety of embryo cryopreservation remains controversial, particularly in women with hormone receptor–positive tumors.

There are also experimental techniques such as oocyte and ovarian tissue preservation, which are usually only offered if a woman does not have a desirable sperm source with which to create embryos (which store better). These techniques are not as well studied or effective as embryo cryopreservation. A recent meta-analysis revealed that approximately 2% of frozen oocytes produced live births as of 2006, though techniques continue to improve.[83] At 1 center, when 200 women aged 11 to 39 underwent ovarian tissue preservation before cancer treatment (55% for breast cancer), 2 of the 4 who underwent re-implantation by the time of publication had resumed ovarian cycling within approximately 6 months.[84] Ongoing studies are evaluating the use of gonadotropin-releasing hormone agonists (GNRH-a) to attempt to protect the ovaries of women with hormone receptor–negative tumors from cycling (and being damaged) during chemotherapy. The efficacy of this strategy is unproven to date, though there is some promising evidence in other cancers as well as in breast cancer.[73,85-88] However, at least 1 small trial found that GNRH-a during chemotherapy did not prevent amenorrhea after cyclophosphamide,[89] another found that GNRH-a did not improve measures of ovarian reserve after chemotherapy for Hodgkin lymphoma,[90] and a third showed no improvement in follicle-stimulating hormone levels or resumption of menstruation after chemotherapy for breast cancer.[91]

SUMMARY

It is important that clinicians educate and support patients through menopausal and sexual consequences of breast cancer treatment and that fertility concerns are evaluated before initiating therapy in premenopausal women. Continued progress in identifying and treating the long-lasting side effects of breast cancer treatment will help optimize the quality of life of breast cancer survivors. The American Society of Clinical Oncology has recommended that all cancer patients receive the following care related to fertility: (1) assessment for and communication regarding risk of infertility; (2) for those who are at risk of infertility and interested in fertility preservation, referral to a specialist with expertise in fertility preservation method. Advances in reproductive technologies will help women who do

experience infertility after cancer treatment. Additional research is needed to enhance understanding of how currently used chemotherapeutic regimens impact ovarian function at different ages and to develop measures of ovarian reserve to help women make decisions regarding treatment that may affect fertility. Further studies are also needed to investigate strategies for improving menopausal symptoms and sexual side effects without impairing efficacy of cancer treatment. There is a particular need for strategies to help women who are diagnosed in the premenopausal period, as most research to date has been focused on a postmenopausal population.

REFERENCES

1. Ries LG, Melbert D, Krapcho M, et al. SEER Cancer Statistics Review, 1975-2005. Bethesda, MD: National Cancer Institute; 2008.
2. Couzi RJ, Helzlsouer KJ, Fetting JH. Prevalence of menopausal symptoms among women with a history of breast cancer and attitudes toward estrogen replacement therapy. *J Clin Oncol.* 1995;13:2737-2744.
3. Broeckel JA, Thors CL, Jacobsen PB, et al. Sexual functioning in long-term breast cancer survivors treated with adjuvant chemotherapy. *Breast Cancer Res Treat.* 2002;75:241-248.
4. Speer JJ, Hillenberg B, Sugrue DP, et al. Study of sexual functioning determinants in breast cancer survivors. *Breast J.* 2005;11:440-447.
5. Ganz PA, Greendale GA, Petersen L, et al. Managing menopausal symptoms in breast cancer survivors: results of a randomized controlled trial. *J Natl Cancer Inst.* 2000;92:1054-1064.
6. Gupta P, Sturdee DW, Palin SL, et al. Menopausal symptoms in women treated for breast cancer: the prevalence and severity of symptoms and their perceived effects on quality of life. *Climacteric.* 2006;9:49-58.
7. Partridge AH. Non-adherence to endocrine therapy for breast cancer. *Ann Oncol.* 2006;17:183-184.
8. Partridge AH. Fertility preservation: a vital survivorship issue for young women with breast cancer. *J Clin Oncol.* 2008;26:2612-2613.
9. Schover LR. The impact of breast cancer on sexuality, body image, and intimate relationships. *CA Cancer J Clin.* 1991;41:112-120.
10. Bukovic D, Fajdic J, Hrgovic Z, et al. Sexual dysfunction in breast cancer survivors. *Onkologie.* 2005;28:29-34.
11. Monteiro-Grillo I, Marques-Vidal P, Jorge M. Psychosocial effect of mastectomy versus conservative surgery in patients with early breast cancer. *Clin Transl Oncol.* 2005;7:499-503.
12. Stevens LA, McGrath MH, Druss RG, et al. The psychological impact of immediate breast reconstruction for women with early breast cancer. *Plast Reconstr Surg.* 1984;73:619-628.
13. Al-Ghazal SK, Sully L, Fallowfield L, et al. The psychological impact of immediate rather than delayed breast reconstruction. *Eur J Surg Oncol.* 2000;26:17-19.
14. Franchelli S, Leone MS, Berrino P, et al. Psychological evaluation of patients undergoing breast reconstruction using two different methods: autologous tissues versus prostheses. *Plast Reconstr Surg.* 1995;95:1213-1218; discussion 1219-1220.
15. Schain WS, Wellisch DK, Pasnau RO, et al. The sooner the better: a study of psychological factors in women undergoing immediate versus delayed breast reconstruction. *Am J Psychiatry.* 1985;142:40-46.
16. Howell A, Cuzick J, Baum M, et al. Results of the ATAC (Arimidex, Tamoxifen, Alone or in Combination) trial after completion of 5 years' adjuvant treatment for breast cancer. *Lancet.* 2005;365:60-62.
17. Cella D, Fallowfield LJ. Recognition and management of treatment-related side effects for breast cancer patients receiving adjuvant endocrine therapy. *Breast Cancer Res Treat.* 2008;107:167-180.
18. Cella D, Fallowfield L, Barker P, et al. Quality of life of postmenopausal women in the ATAC ("Arimidex," tamoxifen, alone or in combination) trial after completion of 5 years' adjuvant treatment for early breast cancer. *Breast Cancer Res Treat.* 2006;100:273-284.
19. Berglund G, Nystedt M, Bolund C, et al. Effect of endocrine treatment on sexuality in premenopausal breast cancer patients: a prospective randomized study. *J Clin Oncol.* 2001;19:2788-2796.
20. Burwell SR, Case LD, Kaelin C, et al. Sexual problems in younger women after breast cancer surgery. *J Clin Oncol.* 2006;24:2815-2821.
21. Schover LR. Premature ovarian failure and its consequences: vasomotor symptoms, sexuality, and fertility. *J Clin Oncol.* 2008;26:753-758.

22. Fobair P, Stewart SL, Chang S, et al. Body image and sexual problems in young women with breast cancer. *Psychooncology*. 2006;15:579-594.

23. Greendale GA, Petersen L, Zibecchi L, et al. Factors related to sexual function in postmenopausal women with a history of breast cancer. *Menopause*. 2001;8:111-119.

24. Hickey M, Saunders CM, Stuckey BG. Management of menopausal symptoms in patients with breast cancer: an evidence-based approach. *Lancet Oncol*. 2005;6:687-695.

25. Hilditch JR, Lewis J, Peter A, et al. A menopause-specific quality of life questionnaire: development and psychometric properties. *Maturitas*. 1996;24:161-175.

26. Fallowfield LJ, Leaity SK, Howell A, et al. Assessment of quality of life in women undergoing hormonal therapy for breast cancer: validation of an endocrine symptom subscale for the FACT-B. *Breast Cancer Res Treat*. 1999;55:189-199.

27. Thirlaway K, Fallowfield L, Cuzick J. The Sexual Activity Questionnaire: a measure of women's sexual functioning. *Qual Life Res*. 1996;5:81-90.

28. Greene JG. Constructing a standard climacteric scale. *Maturitas*. 1998;29:25-31.

29. Vestergaard P, Hermann AP, Stilgren L, et al. Effects of 5 years of hormonal replacement therapy on menopausal symptoms and blood pressure-a randomised controlled study. *Maturitas*. 2003;46:123-132.

30. Madalinska JB, van Beurden M, Bleiker EM, et al. The impact of hormone replacement therapy on menopausal symptoms in younger high-risk women after prophylactic salpingo-oophorectomy. *J Clin Oncol*. 2006;24:3576-3582.

31. Peeyananjarassri K, Baber R. Effects of low-dose hormone therapy on menopausal symptoms, bone mineral density, endometrium, and the cardiovascular system: a review of randomized clinical trials. *Climacteric*. 2005;8:13-23.

32. Farquhar CM, Marjoribanks J, Lethaby A, et al. Long term hormone therapy for perimenopausal and postmenopausal women. *Cochrane Database Syst Rev*. 2005;CD004143.

33. Holmberg L, Iversen OE, Rudenstam CM, et al. Increased risk of recurrence after hormone replacement therapy in breast cancer survivors. *J Natl Cancer Inst*. 2008;100:475-482.

34. Sestak I, Kealy R, Edwards R, et al. Influence of hormone replacement therapy on tamoxifen-induced vasomotor symptoms. *J Clin Oncol*. 2006;24:3991-3996.

35. Gainford MC, Simmons C, Nguyen H, et al. A practical guide to the management of menopausal symptoms in breast cancer patients. *Support Care Cancer*. 2005;13:573-578.

36. Trinh XB, Peeters F, Tjalma WA. The thoughts of breast cancer survivors regarding the need for starting hormone replacement therapy. *Eur J Obstet Gynecol Reprod Biol*. 2006;124:250-253.

37. Einbond LS, Shimizu M, Xiao D, et al. Growth inhibitory activity of extracts and purified components of black cohosh on human breast cancer cells. *Breast Cancer Res Treat*. 2004;83:221-231.

38. McKinlay SM. The normal menopause transition: an overview. *Maturitas*. 1996;23:137-145.

39. Shaw CR. The perimenopausal hot flash: epidemiology, physiology, and treatment. *Nurse Pract*. 1997;22:55-56, 61-66.

40. Whiteman MK, Staropoli CA, Langenberg PW, et al. Smoking, body mass, and hot flashes in midlife women. *Obstet Gynecol*. 2003;101:264-272.

41. Thurston RC, Joffe H, Soares CN, et al. Physical activity and risk of vasomotor symptoms in women with and without a history of depression: results from the Harvard Study of Moods and Cycles. *Menopause*. 2006;13:553-560.

42. Loprinzi CL, Barton DL, Sloan JA, et al. Mayo Clinic and North Central Cancer Treatment Group hot flash studies: a 20-year experience. *Menopause*. 2008;15:655-660.

43. Kronenberg F, Fugh-Berman A. Complementary and alternative medicine for menopausal symptoms: a review of randomized, controlled trials. *Ann Intern Med*. 2002;137:805-813.

44. MacGregor CA, Canney PA, Patterson G, et al. A randomised double-blind controlled trial of oral soy supplements versus placebo for treatment of menopausal symptoms in patients with early breast cancer. *Eur J Cancer*. 2005;41:708-714.

45. Antoine C, Liebens F, Carly B, et al. Safety of alternative treatments for menopausal symptoms after breast cancer: a qualitative systematic review. *Climacteric*. 2007;10:23-26.

46. Miller ER 3rd, Pastor-Barriuso R, Dalal D, et al. Meta-analysis: high-dosage vitamin E supplementation may increase all-cause mortality. *Ann Intern Med*. 2005;142:37-46.

47. Nelson HD, Vesco KK, Haney E, et al. Nonhormonal therapies for menopausal hot flashes, systematic review and meta analysis. *JAMA*. 2006;295:2057-2071.

48. Evans ML, Pritts E, Vittinghoff E, et al. Management of postmenopausal hot flushes with venlafaxine hydrochloride: a randomized, controlled trial. *Obstet Gynecol*. 2005;105:161-166.

49. Loprinzi CL, Kugler JW, Sloan JA, et al. Venlafaxine in management of hot flashes in survivors of breast cancer: a randomised controlled trial. *Lancet* 2000;356:2059-2063.

50. Stearns V, Slack R, Greep N, et al. Paroxetine is an effective treatment for hot flashes: results from a prospective randomized clinical trial. *J Clin Oncol*. 2005;23:6919-6930.

51. Stearns V, Beebe KL, Iyengar M, et al. Paroxetine controlled release in the treatment of menopausal hot flashes: a randomized controlled trial. *JAMA*. 2003;289:2827-2834.

52. Kalay AE, Demir B, Haberal A, et al. Efficacy of citalopram on climacteric symptoms. *Menopause*. 2007;14:223-229.

53. Suvanto-Luukkonen E, Koivunen R, Sundstrom H, et al. Citalopram and fluoxetine in the treatment of postmenopausal symptoms: a prospective, randomized, 9-month, placebo-controlled, double-blind study. *Menopause*. 2005;12:18-26.

54. Stearns V, Johnson MD, Rae JM, et al. Active tamoxifen metabolite plasma concentrations after coadministration of tamoxifen and the selective serotonin reuptake inhibitor paroxetine. *J Natl Cancer Inst*. 2003;95:1758-1764.

55. Jin Y, Desta Z, Stearns V, et al. CYP2D6 genotype, antidepressant use, and tamoxifen metabolism during adjuvant breast cancer treatment. *J Natl Cancer Inst*. 2005;97:30-39.

56. Lash TL, Pedersen L, Cronin-Fenton D, et al. Tamoxifen's protection against breast cancer recurrence is not reduced by concurrent use of the SSRI citalopram. *Br J Cancer* 2008;99:616-621.

57. Pandya KJ, Thummala AR, Griggs JJ, et al. Pilot study using gabapentin for tamoxifen-induced hot flashes in women with breast cancer. *Breast Cancer Res Treat*. 2004;83:87-89.

58. Loprinzi CL, Kugler JW, Barton DL, et al. Phase III trial of gabapentin alone or in conjunction with an antidepressant in the management of hot flashes in women who have inadequate control with an antidepressant alone: NCCTG N03C5. *J Clin Oncol*. 2007;25:308-312.

59. Goldberg RM, Loprinzi CL, O'Fallon JR, et al. Transdermal clonidine for ameliorating tamoxifen-induced hot flashes. *J Clin Oncol*. 1994;12:155-158.

60. Pandya KJ, Raubertas RF, Flynn PJ, et al. Oral clonidine in postmenopausal patients with breast cancer experiencing tamoxifen-induced hot flashes: a University of Rochester Cancer Center Community Clinical Oncology Program study. *Ann Intern Med*. 2000;132:788-793.

61. Dew JE, Wren BG, Eden JA. A cohort study of topical vaginal estrogen therapy in women previously treated for breast cancer. *Climacteric*. 2003;6:45-52.

62. Kendall A, Dowsett M, Folkerd E, et al. Caution: vaginal estradiol appears to be contraindicated in postmenopausal women on adjuvant aromatase inhibitors. *Ann Oncol*. 2006;17:584-587.

63. Shifren JL, Braunstein GD, Simon JA, et al. Transdermal testosterone treatment in women with impaired sexual function after oophorectomy. *N Engl J Med*. 2000;343:682-688.

64. Goldstat R, Briganti E, Tran J, et al. Transdermal testosterone therapy improves well-being, mood, and sexual function in premenopausal women. *Menopause*. 2003;10:390-398.

65. Braunstein GD, Sundwall DA, Katz M, et al. Safety and efficacy of a testosterone patch for the treatment of hypoactive sexual desire disorder in surgically menopausal women: a randomized, placebo-controlled trial. *Arch Intern Med*. 2005;165:1582-1589.

66. Buster JE, Kingsberg SA, Aguirre O, et al. Testosterone patch for low sexual desire in surgically menopausal women: a randomized trial. *Obstet Gynecol*. 2005;105:944-952.

67. Nathorst-Boos J, Floter A, Jarkander Rolff M, et al. Treatment with percutaneous testosterone gel in postmenopausal women with decreased libido: effects on sexuality and psychological general well-being. *Maturitas*. 2006;53:11-18.

68. Barton DL, Wender DB, Sloan JA, et al. Randomized controlled trial to evaluate transdermal testosterone in female cancer survivors with decreased libido; North Central Cancer Treatment Group protocol N02C3. *J Natl Cancer Inst*. 2007;99:672-679.

69. Mathias C, Cardeal Mendes CM, Ponde de Sena E, et al. An open-label, fixed-dose study of bupropion effect on sexual function scores in women treated for breast cancer. *Ann Oncol*. 2006;17:1792-1796.

70. Jemal A, Siegel R, Ward E, et al. Cancer statistics, 2007. *CA Cancer J Clin*. 2007;57:43-66.

71. Partridge AH, Ruddy KJ. Fertility and adjuvant treatment in young women with breast cancer. *Breast*. 2007;16(suppl 2):S175-S181.

72. Petrek JA, Naughton MJ, Case LD, et al. Incidence, time course, and determinants of menstrual bleeding after breast cancer treatment: a prospective study. *J Clin Oncol*. 2006;24:1045-1051.

73. Fox KR, Scialla J, Moore H. Preventing chemotherapy-related amenorrhea using leuprolide during adjuvant chemotherapy for early-stage breast cancer. *Proc Am Soc Clin Oncol*. 2003;22:13. Abstract 50.

74. Partridge A, Gelber S, Peppercorn J, et al. Fertility outcomes in young women with breast cancer: A web-based survey. *Proc Am Soc Clin Oncol.* 2004;23:538. Abstract 6085.

75. Ives A, Saunders C, Bulsara M, et al. Pregnancy after breast cancer: population based study. *BMJ.* 2007;334:194.

76. Partridge A, Gelber S, Gelber RD, et al. Age of menopause among women who remain premenopausal following treatment for early breast cancer: long-term results from International Breast Cancer Study Group Trials V and VI. *Eur J Cancer.* 2007;43:1646-1653.

77. Ruddy K, Partridge A, Gelber S, et al. Ovarian reserve in women who remain premenopausal after chemotherapy for early stage breast cancer. Presented at the Annual Meeting of the American Society of Clinical Oncology, Chicago, IL, May 30-June 3, 2008.

78. Lutchman Singh K, Muttukrishna S, Stein RC, et al. Predictors of ovarian reserve in young women with breast cancer. *Br J Cancer.* 2007;96:1808-1816.

79. Sonmezer M, Atabekoglu C. Assisted reproduction and breast cancer. *Minerva Ginecol.* 2007;59:403-414.

80. Lobo RA. Potential options for preservation of fertility in women. *N Engl J Med.* 2005;353:64-73.

81. Oktay K, Buyuk E, Libertella N, et al. Fertility preservation in breast cancer patients: a prospective controlled comparison of ovarian stimulation with tamoxifen and letrozole for embryo cryopreservation. *J Clin Oncol.* 23:4347-53, 2005

82. Azim AA, Costantini Ferrando M, Oktay K. Safety of fertility preservation by ovarian stimulation with letrozole and gonadotropins in patients with breast cancer: a prospective controlled study. *J Clin Oncol* 2008:26:2630-2635.

83. Oktay K, Gil AP, Bang H. Efficiency of oocyte cryopreservation: a meta-analysis *Fertil Steril.* 2006;06:70 00.

84. Sanchez M, Novella-Maestre E, Teruel J, et al. The ovarian transplant for Fertility Preservation. *Clin Transl Oncol.* 2008;10:495-498.

85. Recchia F, Saggio G, Amiconi G, et al. Gonadotropin releasing hormone analogues added to adjuvant chemotherapy protect ovarian function and improve clinical outcomes in young women with early breast carcinoma. *Cancer.* 2006;106:514-23.

86. Blumenfeld Z, Eckman A. Preservation of fertility and ovarian function and minimization of chemotherapy-induced gonadotoxicity in young women by GnRH-a. *J Natl Cancer Inst Monogr.* 2005;40-43.

87. Castelo-Branco C, Nomdedeu B, Camus A, et al. Use of gonadotropin-releasing hormone agonists in patients with Hodgkin's disease for preservation of ovarian function and reduction of gonadotoxicity related to chemotherapy. *Fertil Steril.* 2007;87:702-705.

88. Pereyra Pacheco B, Mendez Ribas JM, Milone G, et al. Use of GnRH analogs for functional protection of the ovary and preservation of fertility during cancer treatment in adolescents: a preliminary report. *Gynecol Oncol.* 2001;81:391-397.

89. Waxman JH, Ahmed R, Smith D, et al. Failure to preserve fertility in patients with Hodgkin's disease. *Cancer Chemother Pharmacol.* 1987;19:159-162.

90. Giuseppe L, Attilio G, Edoardo DN, et al. Ovarian function after cancer treatment in young women affected by Hodgkin disease (HD). *Hematology.* 2007;12:141-147.

91. Ismail-Khan R, Minton S, Cox C, et al. Preservation of ovarian function in young women treated with neoadjuvant chemotherapy for breast cancer: A randomized trial using the GnRH agonist (triptorelin) during chemotherapy. Presented at the Annual Meeting of the American Society of Clinical Oncology Annual Meeting, Chicago, IL, May 30-June 3, 2008.

92. Stearns V. Serotonergic agents as an alternative to hormonal therapy for the treatment of menopausal vasomotor symptoms. *Treat Endocrinol.* 2006;5:83-87.

93. Butt DA, Lock M, Lewis JE, et al. Gabapentin for the treatment of menopausal hot flashes: a randomized controlled trial. *Menopause.* 2008;15:310-318.

94. Goodwin PJ, Ennis M, Pritchard KI, et al. Risk of menopause during the first year after breast cancer diagnosis. *J Clin Oncol.* 1999;17:2365-2370.

95. Burstein HJ, Winer EP. Primary care for survivors of breast cancer. *N Engl J Med.* 2000;343:1086-1094

96. Martin M, Pienkowski T, Mackey J, et al. Adjuvant docetaxel for node-positive breast cancer. *N Engl J Med* 2005;352:2302-2313.

97. Parulekar WR, Day AG, Ottaway JA, et al. Incidence and prognostic impact of amenorrhea during adjuvant therapy in high-risk premenopausal breast cancer: analysis of a National Cancer Institute of Canada Clinical Trials Group Study: NCIC CTG MA.5. *J Clin Oncol.* 2005;23:6002-6008.

98. Fornier MN, Modi S, Panageas KS, et al. Incidence of chemotherapy-induced, long-term amenorrhea in patients with breast carcinoma age 40 years and younger after adjuvant anthracycline and taxane. *Cancer.* 2005;104:1575-1579.

CHAPTER 102

Disparities in Breast Cancer

Nicholas Osborne
Lisa Newman

Breast cancer is the most common female malignancy in the United States and worldwide. The World Health Organization estimates that more than 1 million cases of breast cancer occur annually. In 2000, the last year in which worldwide data was available, more than 400,000 women died of breast cancer.[1] Over the last several decades, a growing literature has described disparities in the incidence, treatment, and survival from breast cancer between populations delineated by socioeconomic, racial/ethnic, and cultural characteristics. Despite a growing recognition that disparities exist, the underlying causes of these disparities are not well understood. Factors affecting the incidence of and survival from breast cancer are no doubt multifactorial, including biological and genetic factors, environmental factors, reproductive factors, and dietary factors. Despite significant advances in the detection and treatment of breast cancer, these disparities have persisted. This review will focus primarily on disparities in breast cancer incidence, treatment, and outcome between African American and white women, as this represents the best established literature.

DISPARITIES IN BREAST CANCER EPIDEMIOLOGY AND MORTALITY

Evidence of the racial and socioeconomic differences in the incidence and mortality from breast cancer is compelling. The best population-based evidence of these disparities comes from the Surveillance, Epidemiology, and End Results (SEER) Program. This program was started in the United States in 1973 to describe the incidence and outcomes from cancers. Initially, 9 sites were involved, including 5 states (Connecticut, Hawaii, Iowa, New Mexico, and Utah) and 4 major cities (Detroit, Atlanta, San Francisco, and Seattle); however, the program has now grown to include 16 sites. In 2001, sites were added in Louisiana, Kentucky, New Jersey, and California to further improve the representation of minorities. This database now represents the largest collection of cancer registries in the United States. The SEER program is estimated to include 26% of the US population. SEER coverage includes 23% of African Americans, 40% of Hispanics, 42% of American Indians and Alaska Natives, 53% of Asians, and 70% of Hawaiian/Pacific Islanders.[2] Although race is documented in the SEER database, the racial and ethnic heterogeneity of the US population presents a challenge to correctly accounting for these complex relationships. Despite this limitation, the SEER database has provided researchers and clinicians with robust population-based estimates of the cancer incidence and survival.

Disparities in Breast Cancer Epidemiology

The incidence of breast cancer has significant racial variation. Using the most recent SEER data, African American women have a lower age-adjusted incidence of breast cancer as compared with white women (117.5 vs 130.6 per 100,000 respectively) (Fig 102-1). Similarly, Asian/Pacific Islander, Hispanic, and American Indian/Alaskan Native women all have lower incidence of breast cancer as compared with white women (89.6, 90.1, and 75.0 per 100,000 women, respectively).[2]

Although African American women have a lower cumulative incidence of breast cancer as compared with white women, young African American women have higher incidence of breast cancer as compared with similarly aged white women. In women younger than 45 years, African American women have a higher incidence of breast cancer as compared with white women, and this incidence equalizes in the fifth decade. After age 50, white women have a significantly higher incidence of breast cancer. As a consequence, African American women have a lower median age at diagnosis as compared with white women (57 vs 62 years, respectively).[3]

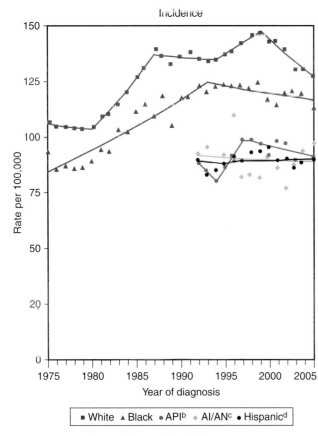

Incidence

FIGURE 102-1 The incidence of female breast cancer using SEER data (1975-2005). [Data from Ries LAG, Melbert D, Krapcho M, et al (eds). SEER Cancer Statistics Review, 1975-2005. Bethesda, MD: National Cancer Institute, 2008. Available at: http://seer.cancer.gov/csr/1975_2005/.]

Legend: ■ White ▲ Black ● API[b] ◆ AI/AN[c] ● Hispanic[d]

Disparities in Histopathology and Tumor Stage

Overall, nearly three-quarters of all women diagnosed with breast cancer have infiltrating ductal carcinoma. The histologic type, grade, and stage of breast cancer varies significantly with race. In particular, African American women had a significantly higher risk of presenting with inflammatory breast cancer as compared with white women (relative risk [RR] = 1.4; 95% confidence interval [CI], 1.3-1.5).[4] Similarly, several studies have shown that African American women have a higher risk of medullary breast cancer.[5,6] Some have suggested that the higher incidence of medullary tumors may in fact be a reflection of a higher frequency of misdiagnosed high-grade infiltrating ductal carcinoma lesions, which can often be confused with medullary cancer.[3] Regardless, it appears that African American women are more likely to present with more aggressive tumor types.

As well as presenting with more aggressive histology, African American women are also more likely to present with locally advanced disease (RR = 1.8; 95% CI, 1.7-2.0).[4] In this analysis, African American women were more likely to present at a younger age and generally had worse survival.

African American women have consistently been shown to present with more advanced disease and hormone receptor–negative

disease. The results of several of these studies are shown in Table 102-1. In 2002, Anderson and colleagues reported that African American women were more likely to present with estrogen receptor–negative disease; these findings have been confirmed by multiple studies.[7-10] Several studies have also noted that African American women are more likely to present with tumors expressing multiple abnormal proteins, including p53, p16, and cyclins D1 and E.[11,12] Although African American women are more likely to present with estrogen receptor–negative tumors, it appears that there is no racial difference in the rate of HER-2/neu overexpression.[13,14]

In summary, African American women are more likely to present with more advanced breast cancer, at a younger age, and they are more likely to present with estrogen receptor–negative tumors. These characteristics may in part explain differences in breast cancer outcomes, but as will be detailed throughout the chapter, significant evidence exists that even after controlling for the more advanced disease burden, African Americans continue to fair worse than their white counterparts.

DISPARITIES IN BREAST CANCER MORTALITY

Despite a lower cumulative incidence of breast cancer, African American women have a paradoxically higher mortality from breast cancer.[2] African American women diagnosed with breast cancer between 1996 and 2004 had a significantly lower 5-year survival as compared with white women (77.8 vs 90.5, respectively).[2] Figure 102-2 shows the trend in breast cancer mortality stratified by race. The mortality rates from breast cancer have decreased for white women and remained relatively stable among all other racial/ethnic groups. As discussed earlier, African American women are more likely to present with more advanced disease as compared with white women. Even when accounting for more advanced presentations, African American women continue to have a lower survival from breast cancer.[2]

DISPARITIES IN BREAST CANCER SCREENING

African American women present with more advanced disease as compared with white American women. These differences in presentation may be partially explained by differential utilization of breast cancer screening. The widespread adoption of mammography after age 40 has been credited as a significant factor in improving breast cancer outcomes.[15] This improvement in outcomes has largely been a consequence of identifying breast cancer at an earlier stage. In the period from 1985 to 2005, the incidence of breast cancer diagnosed as in situ nearly tripled.[2] Despite these improvements, African American women continue to present with more advanced disease. The existing data regarding the racial differences in the utilization of screening mammography is conflicting. Several studies using survey data from the National Health Interview Survey have reported similar rates of mammography between African American and white American women.[16,17] Similarly, in an analysis of survey data from the Behavioral Risk Factor Surveillance System combined from registry data, African American women had a lower rate of screening mammography;

TABLE 102-1 Differences In Presentation of African American and White American Women with Breast Cancer: Results of Multiple Recent Studies

Study	Dataset	Features	White Americans	African Americans
Chlebowski et al, 2005	WHI Postmenopausal	N	3455	242
		Mean tumor size (cm)	1.56	1.6
		High-grade tumors (%)	25	43
		ER-negative (%)	13	29
		PR-negative (%)	24	41
		Mortality hazard (95% CI)	1.0 (ref)	1.79 (1.05-3.05)
Li et al, 2003	SEER	N	97,999	10,560
		Stage (%)		
		I	50.4	35.4
		III/IV	11.3	18.9
		High-grade tumors (%)	32.1	43.2
		Tumor 5 cm (%)	8	15
		Node negative (%)	53.9	42.6
		ER-negative (%)	22	39.2
		PR-negative (%)	31.7	46.6
		Mortality hazard (95% CI)	1.0 (ref)	1.5 (1.4-1.6)
Li et al 18, 2002	SEER	N	75978	6915
	Age ≥ 50 years	Stage (%)		
		I	53.2	39.1
		III/IV	11.1	19.1
		High-grade tumors (%)	29	37.6
		Tumor 5 cm (%)	7.4	11.1
		Node negative (%)	51.3	43.2
		ER-negative (%)	15.2	24.1
		PR-negative (%)	23.8	30.4
Newman et al, 2002	Detroit SEER	N	1378	507
	Age ≥ 40 years	Localized Stage (%)	52.1	42.4
		Median tumor size (cm)	2.6	3.4
		Node-negative (%)	45.7	33.3
		ER-negative (%)	44.4	61.9
		PR-negative (%)	48.8	59.7
		Mean survival (months)	50	45
Shavers et al, 2003	SEER	N	2638	724
	Age ≥ 35 years	Stage (%)		
		I	26.7	16.4
		III/IV	12.3	16.7
		High-grade tumors (%)	43.3	54.8
		Median tumor size (cm)	2.5	2.8
		Node negative (%)	44.6	36.5
		ER-negative (%)	33.1	34.4
		PR-negative (%)	35.4	35.6
		5-year disease-specific survival	76.5	66.6
		Mortality hazard (95% CI)	1.0 (ref)	1.3 (1.0-1.6)
Elledge et al, 1994	San Antonio database	N	4885	1016
		Age ≥ 50 Years	76.1	62.6
		P53-pos (%)	50.9	54.9
		Tumor 5 cm (%)	10.9	27.7
		Node-negative (%)	57.9	48.8
		Tumor-5 cm (%)	10.9	27.7
		Node-negative (%)	57.9	48.8
		ER-negative (%)	22.1	37.9
		PR-negative (%)	44	59.2
		HER-2/neu-positive (%)	16.1	13.8
		5-year overall survival (%)	75	65
		Median survival (months)	166	117

Adapted from Newman and Martin.[3]

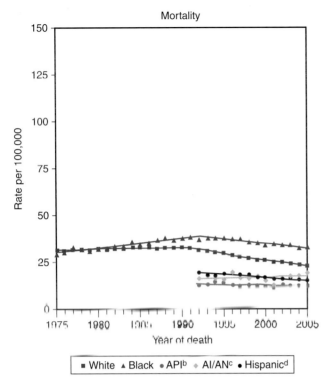

FIGURE 102-2 The mortality of female breast cancer using SEER data (1975–2005). [Data from Ries LAG, Melbert D, Krapcho M, et al (eds). SEER Cancer Statistics Review, 1975-2005. Bethesda, MD: National Cancer Institute; 2008.Available at: http://seer.cancer.gov/csr/1975_2005/.]

however, this difference was not significant.[18] Despite similar rates of screening mammography, African American women continued to have a lower odds of presenting with early stage disease. In contrast, in an analysis of mammography registry data from the National Cancer Institute–funded Breast Cancer Surveillance Consortium, African American women were more likely to receive inadequate screening mammography as compared with white American women (RR = 1.2; 95% CI, 1.2-1.2). This analysis also noted that African American women were more likely to present with large, advanced stage, lymph node–positive tumors regardless of screening interval as compared with white American women.[19] In an earlier analysis of Medicare claims data for mammography was linked to the SEER registry, McCarthy et al[20] estimated that 30% of the delayed presentation of African American women can be explained by disparate use of screening mammography.

The true utilization of screening mammography among African American women remains unclear. It is evident from both the survey data and registry data, however, that African American women are more likely to present with more advanced disease as compared with white women, even among patients with similar screening patterns.

DISPARITIES IN BREAST CANCER TREATMENT

Although the disparities in breast cancer outcomes between African American and white American women may be partially explained by differences in presentation as noted above, treatment related differences could potentially explain why

African American women with equal stage cancers continue to fair worse than their white counterparts.

Breast-Conserving Surgery

As noted above, African American women present with more advanced breast disease and they have a higher mortality from breast cancer as compared with white American women at all stages of disease. The equivalent treatment of invasive breast cancer with either breast-conserving surgery or mastectomy relies upon the multidisciplinary approach to breast cancer. Despite nearly equivalent rates of breast-conserving surgery, African American women are less likely to receive appropriate adjuvant locoregional therapy (radiation therapy). In an analysis of early-stage breast cancer patients using the SEER registry from 1992 to 2002, African American women had equivalent rates of lumpectomy, but they were 24% less likely to receive the requisite radiation therapy in combination with lumpectomy.[21] This disparity remained significant after controlling for the earlier age of diagnosis, more advanced disease and tumor biology, and geographic variation. Similarly, in a recent analysis of SEER data from the Atlanta site, African American women were again noted to have lower rates of postoperative radiation therapy after breast-conserving surgery.[22]

Sentinel Lymph Node Biopsy Versus Axillary Lymph Node Dissection

Until recently, the axillary lymph node dissection has been the standard-of-care for staging breast cancer. Given the significant morbidity associated with the axillary lymph node dissection, the use of less-invasive methods has been pursued. The sentinel lymph node biopsy has become an accepted alternative to the axillary lymph node dissection in patients with nonpalpable axillary nodes. Although this technique has been shown to decrease the morbidity associated with breast surgery, it appears that racial differences in the utilization of sentinel node biopsy exist. In an analysis of SEER data, African American women were 36% less likely to receive lymphatic mapping and sentinel node biopsy as compared with white American women.[23] These findings were supported in a subsequent analysis by Bickell et al,[24] who found that among early-stage breast cancer patients in New York, African American women were significantly less likely to receive a sentinel node biopsy as compared with white American women.

Adjuvant Systemic Treatment

Just as African American women are less likely to receive post-operative radiation after lumpectomy, researchers have noted that African American women may be less likely to receive and complete adjuvant chemotherapy. In a 2003 study of cancer registrars, White and colleagues[25] noted that African American and Hispanic women received indicated adjuvant chemotherapy for node-positive disease less frequently than white American women (78.7% vs 85.3%, respectively). Similarly, in a cross sectional study of breast cancer patients in New York, Bickell et al reported that African American women were twice as likely to be inadequately treated with either radiation therapy, chemotherapy, or endocrine therapy as compared with white women.[24] Importantly, African American women are not only less likely to receive chemotherapy, they are also less likely to complete a full course of chemotherapy. Hershman and colleagues[26] demonstrated that among women diagnosed with early-stage breast cancer, one-third of African American women did not receive a full course of chemotherapy, as compared with one-fifth of white American women. In a separate analysis, Hershman and colleagues[27] noted that African American women are more likely to have their chemotherapy delayed or terminated early due to neutropenia.

Breast Reconstruction

After mastectomy, the reconstruction of the breast can be accomplished immediately or in a delayed fashion. In both instances, African American women have lower rates of reconstruction. Using the National Cancer Database, Morrow et al[28] reported that African American women were less likely to order breast reconstruction as compared with white American women. In a similar analysis from The University of Texas MD Anderson Cancer Center, African American women were significantly less likely to receive reconstruction, regardless of race, as compared with white American women (20% vs 40%, respectively).[29] Of note, African American women were not only less likely to receive a reconstruction referral, they were also less likely to be offered reconstruction when they met with a plastic surgeon. In an analysis of the SEER registry, Alderman and colleagues[30] noted that national rates of immediate and delayed reconstruction are low, and that in particular, African American women are about 50% less likely to receive an early reconstruction as compared with white American women. Of those women who did receive a reconstruction, African American women are more likely to receive complex tissue grafts as compared with white American women.[30] In a more recent analysis using the National Comprehensive Cancer Network Outcomes Project, reconstruction rates were significantly higher (42%) for all women; however, Medicaid and Medicare patients were significantly less likely to receive reconstruction. In this analysis, African American women trended toward less frequent reconstruction; however, this trend was not significant.[31]

In summary, African American women experience significant disparities in the treatment of breast cancer. These differences in treatment are no doubt partially responsible for the worse outcomes experienced by African American women. In the next section, we will explore the potential causes for these disparities.

MECHANISMS FOR DISPARITIES

The Institute of Medicine highlighted disparities in health care in the landmark publication "Unequal Treatment" in 2003. As outlined in their discussion of the causes of racial disparities, they identified several key sources: patient-specific (genetic differences, disease biology), social, economic, and cultural influences; and provider and system-level prejudices and stereotyping.[32] This model allows for researchers and policymakers to identify 3 key participants in patient care: the patient, the provider, and the system. Unequal Treatment focused much energy on understanding differences in patient preferences that could explain these disparities. In the remaining sections of this chapter, we will focus on attention on understanding the potential causes of these disparities, including biological factors, socioeconomic factors, clinical comorbidities, environmental exposures, cultural beliefs, and racial discrimination. For the purpose of this chapter, we will focus on the existing literature regarding biological factors, socioeconomic factors, and clinical comorbidities.

Biological Factors

As noted earlier, African American women are more likely to present at a younger age with breast cancer as compared with their white counterparts. Similarly, African American women are more likely to present with tumors with more aggressive characteristics, including later stage, positive lymph nodes, and hormone receptor negativity. Some of these disparities in presentation may be due to inherent genetic differences between African American and white American women. Other biological factors that have been observed include differences in the reproductive history of African American patients and differences in hormone replacement.

The relatively higher frequency of multiparous women among African American women may explain their lower lifetime risk of developing breast cancer (as compared with white Americans). Multiple pregnancies are thought to decrease the lifetime exposure to estrogen and thus decrease the risk of developing breast cancer. In contrast, there is a slightly increased risk of breast cancer in the early postpartum period. Because younger pregnancies are more common among African American women, researchers speculate that this early postpartum risk of breast cancer may be responsible for the higher frequency of early cancers among African American women. This hypothesis has been supported by several studies.[33,34] In a case-control study based upon patients from the SEER registry, Ursin and colleagues[35] found that for every level of parity, African American women had a smaller decrease in their overall risk of developing breast cancer as compared with white American women. Interestingly, in this study, there was no observed increase in the risk of breast cancer immediately after birth. Given the conflicting evidence regarding the interaction of race and parity on breast cancer risk, further research will be necessary.

The growing understanding of molecular biology and the aberrant cell signaling that can lead to cancer offers hope to further explain differences in cancer presentation and outcomes. It is estimated that hereditary breast cancer accounts for between 3% and 8% of all breast cancer.[36,37] The most studied mutations associated with breast and ovarian cancer are the BRCA1 and BRCA2 mutations. To date, most studies have focused on high-risk white American women. Several case series have reported mutations in the BRCA1 and BRCA2 genes in African American women. In a comparative analysis of high-risk families from multiple ethnic and racial groups, Nanda et al[38] demonstrated that African American women had a lower rate of deleterious BRCA1 and BRCA2 mutations and, conversely, had a higher rate of sequence variations as compared with non-Hispanic, non-Jewish white women. Overall, rates of BRCA1 or BRCA2 mutations were lower among African American families as compared with Ashkenazi Jewish families. Of note, the mean number of breast cancer cases in families with BRCA1 or BRCA2 mutations was lower for African American families as compared with non–African American families (3.4 vs 4.4, $p = 0.01$).[38] In a case-control study from North Carolina, white American women had a 3 times higher frequency of BRCA2 mutations as compared with African American women.[39] In a study of international families with breast cancer, researchers failed to identify any deleterious mutations in the BRCA2 gene among African American or African families.[40] In contrast, several studies of American families have reported mutations in both the BRCA1 and BRCA2 genes found in families whose ancestry can be traced back to West Africa.[41,42] Of note, the majority of the slave trade during the 18th and 19th centuries was focused along the West African coast. In a review of the literature in 2003, Olopade and colleagues[43] identified 26 distinct mutations in the BRCA1 and 18 deleterious mutations in the BRCA2 genes in African American or African families. More than 50% of these mutations were unique to the group studied, suggesting that BRCA gene mutations may be under-recognized among African American women. Although BRCA1 and BRCA2 mutations are the most recognized inherited germline mutations responsible for breast and ovarian cancer, there are no doubt undetermined genetic mutations that may also confer a higher risk of aggressive tumor biology to African American women.

In collaboration with Ghanaian physicians, Newman and colleagues[44] have begun to analyze breast cancer specimens from native Ghanaian women with breast cancer. These researchers hypothesize that if African American women have genetic predispositions toward more advanced and aggressive disease, these should be present in their ancestral populations as well. African women have a younger peak incidence of breast cancer, approximately 10 to 15 years earlier than that of Western nations.[44] In a study of HER-2/neu polymorphism among 200 Ghanaian, 257 white American, and 90 African American healthy women, researchers found that the Val-allele (associated with younger onset breast cancer) was absent in Ghanaian women whereas it was present in 20% of white American and 24% of African American women.[45] In a study of Nigerian breast cancer patients younger than 40 years, BRCA1 or BRCA2 sequence variations were detected in 29 of 39 patients (74%).[46]

Hereditary causes of breast cancer are an important factor in mitigating the disparities in tumor presentation and outcomes. There is a paucity of population-based data regarding the genetic polymorphisms and genetic mutations that may contribute to the younger onset of disease and more aggressive characteristics of tumors among African American women. Further research will be instrumental in understanding the role of hereditary factors in these disparities.

Socioeconomic Factors

Socioeconomic status is a commonly used term in the disparities literature. The definition of socioeconomic status unfortunately is not constant in the health services literature. Socioeconomic status is a multidimensional construct, which can be broken down into 3 core domains: income/wealth, education, and occupation.[47] Unfortunately, these variables are often poorly measured in administrative databases and are incompletely answered in survey data. Nevertheless, socioeconomic factors are an important determinant of health status and may play a key role in the relationship between race and health outcomes from breast cancer.

Although multiple studies have treated socioeconomic status as a confounder in the relationship between race and health outcomes from breast cancer, few studies have focused on using socioeconomic status to explain these disparities. In addition, studies using multi-institutional registries, SEER database or Medicare data, rely upon census level measures of socioeconomic status, including area-based poverty level, educational attainment, and employment levels. The average values are assigned to all inhabitants of that area (census tract, zip code). These area based methods assume that individuals who live within those census tracts or zip codes all have the same socioeconomic characteristics, thus underestimating neighborhood heterogeneity. Studies have suggested that the misclassification of individuals appears random and that this introduces a null bias and that these area-based estimates are likely conservative estimates of the individual's socioeconomic status.[48] In contrast, these area-based methods may offer the advantage of accounting for neighborhood level factors that are unmeasured in individual socioeconomic variables, such as access to hospitals, pharmacies, and transportation.[49]

Despite these limitations to the existing data, lower socioeconomic status is associated with less aggressive treatment and worse outcomes from breast cancer. In many studies, the use of socioeconomic status variables attenuates the relationship between African American race and breast cancer mortality[50]. Using data from the Metropolitan Detroit Cancer Surveillance System (MDCSS) linking SEER data to the Medicaid claims data files, Bradley et al[51] found that low socioeconomic status (defined by receiving Medicaid insurance and poverty level) is associated with later stage of diagnosis, inadequate treatment, and mortality. In a multivariate model accounting for race, age, cancer stage, insurance status, and poverty level, African American women who underwent breast surgery were less likely to receive breast-conserving therapy.[51] Similarly, Albano and colleagues[52] noted that individual educational attainment was inversely correlated with cancer mortality. Interestingly, African American women had a higher mortality from breast cancer at each level of educational attainment as compared with white American women, except for less than 9 years of education. In a meta-analysis of 20 studies that provided both socioeconomic and race measures, Newman et al[50] noted that even after controlling for studies that explain socioeconomic status, race continued to remain a significant predictor of mortality from breast cancer.

Although the measurement of socioeconomic status is problematic, it appears that low socioeconomic status is a negative predictor of outcome from breast cancer. Continued research is necessary to further interaction of socioeconomic status and race on breast cancer outcomes.

Comorbidities

Patients with more severe clinical comorbidities are less likely to receive aggressive treatment. Numerous studies have noted that comorbidities are correlated with worse outcomes from breast cancer.[53-55] The presence of multiple clinical comorbidities increases the mortality independent of the effect of age or race.[55] In an early analysis, Eley et al[56] noted that increasing clinical comorbidity burden explained 25% of the racial disparity of all-cause mortality, but not breast cancer–specific mortality. In a more recent analysis, Tammemagi and colleagues[57] demonstrated that more than 77 comorbidities were associated with worse outcomes from breast cancer. In particular, the more comorbidities that a patient carried, the higher the all-cause mortality for that patient. Of note, African American women were more likely to be diagnosed with multiple comorbidities (odds ratio = 3.20; 95% CI, 2.17-4.72). After adjusting for comorbidities, the racial disparity in all-cause mortality was attenuated by nearly half.[57] This finding suggests that aggressive treatment of comorbidities may lead to improved outcomes for all breast cancer patients and in particular African American women, who have a disproportionately higher comorbidity index.

SUMMARY

Racial and ethnic disparities exist in breast cancer epidemiology, treatment, and outcome. This chapter has focused on the disparities between African American and white American women. In reality, disparities exist for multiple ethnicities and disadvantaged groups. Further research is requisite to understanding the underlying causes of these disparities and intervening to diminish these disparities. The causes are no doubt multifactorial, including biological factors, socioeconomic factors, clinical comorbidities, environmental exposures, cultural beliefs, and provider-level prejudices or racial discrimination. The increasing data available from large, prospectively collected registries will be instrumental in understanding the patient-level, provider-level, and system-level variation. In addition, the increasing availability of molecular and genetic markers will help to explain the possible genetic predisposition toward more severe breast cancer. This marriage of both health services research and molecular biology offers the best opportunity to eliminate existing disparities.

REFERENCES

1. Stewart BW, Kleihues P. *World Cancer Report*. Geneva, Switzerland: International Agency for Research on Cancer, World Health Organization; 2003.
2. Ries LAG, Melbert D, Krapcho M, et al (eds). SEER Cancer Statistics Review, 1975-2005. Bethesda, MD: National Cancer Institute; 2008. Available at: http://seer.cancer.gov/csr/1975_2005/.
3. Newman LA, Martin IK. Disparities in breast cancer. *Curr Probl Cancer*. 2007;31:134-156.
4. Hance KW, Anderson WF, Devesa SS, Young HA, Levine PH. Trends in inflammatory breast carcinoma incidence and survival: The Surveillance, Epidemiology, and End Results Program at the National Cancer Institute. *J Natl Cancer Inst*. 2005;97:966-975.
5. Kovi J, Mohla S, Norris HJ, Sampson CC, Heshmat MY. Breast lesions in black women. *Pathol Annu*. 1989;24:199-218.
6. Trock BJ. Breast cancer in African American women: epidemiology and tumor biology. *Breast Cancer Res Treat*. 1996;40:11-24.
7. Anderson WF, Chatterjee N, Ershler WB, Brawley OW. Estrogen receptor breast cancer phenotypes in the Surveillance, Epidemiology, and End Results database. *Breast Cancer Res Treat*. 2002;76:27-36.
8. Li CI, Malone KE, Daling JR. Differences in breast cancer hormone receptor status and histology by race and ethnicity among women 50 years of age and older. *Cancer Epidemiol Biomarkers Prev*. 2002;11:601-607.
9. Li CI, Malone KE, Daling JR. Differences in breast cancer stage, treatment, and survival by race and ethnicity. *Arch Intern Med*. 2003;163:49-56.
10. Shavers VL, Harlan LC, Stevens JL. Racial/ethnic variation in clinical presentation, treatment, and survival among breast cancer patients under age 35. *Cancer*. 2003;97:134-147.
11. Jones BA, Kasl SV, Howe CL, et al. African-American/White differences in breast carcinoma: p53 alterations and other tumor characteristics. *Cancer*. 2004;101:1293-1301.
12. Porter PL, Lund MJ, Lin MG, et al. Racial differences in the expression of cell cycle-regulatory proteins in breast carcinoma. *Cancer*. 2004;100:2533-2542.
13. Elledge RM, Clark GM, Chamness GC, Osborne CK. Tumor biologic factors and breast cancer prognosis among white, Hispanic, and black women in the United States. *J Natl Cancer Inst*. 1994;86:705-712.
14. Stark AT, Claud S, Kapke A, et al. Race modifies the association between breast carcinoma pathologic prognostic indicators and the positive status for HER-2/neu. *Cancer*. 2005;104:2189-2196.
15. Feig SA. Effect of service screening mammography on population mortality from breast carcinoma. *Cancer*. 2002;95:451-457.
16. National Healthcare Disparities Report, 2005. Agency for Healthcare Research and Quality, Rockville, MD. Available at: http://www.ahrq.gov/qual/nhdr05/nhdr05.htm. Accessed August 28, 2008.
17. Sabatino SA, Coates RJ, Uhler RJ, et al. Disparities in Mammography use among US women aged 40-64 years, by Race, Ethnicity, Income, Health Insurance Status 1993 and 2005. *Med Care*. 2008;46:692-700.
18. Jasset P, Luo FY, Cunningham L. Factoring racial/ethnic disparities in female breast cancer: screening rates and stage at diagnosis. *Am J Public Health*. 2006;96:2165-2172.
19. Smith-Bindman R, Miglioretti DL, Lurie N, et al. Does utilization of screening mammography explain racial and ethnic differences in breast cancer? *Ann Intern Med*. 2006;144:541-553.
20. McCarthy EP, Burns RB, Coughlin SS, et al. Mammography use helps to explain differences in breast cancer stage at diagnosis between older black and white women. *Ann Intern Med*. 1998;128:729-736.
21. Du XL, Gor BJ. Racial disparities and trends in radiation therapy after breast-conserving surgery for early-stage breast cancer in women, 1992 to 2002. *Ethn Dis*. 2007;17:122-128.
22. Lund MJ, Brawley OP, Ward KC, et al. Parity and disparity in first course treatment of invasive breast cancer. *Breast Cancer Res Treat*. 2008;109:545-557.
23. Maggard MA, Lane KE, O'Connell JB, Nanyakkara DD, Ko CY. Beyond the clinical trials: how often is sentinel lymph node dissection performed for breast cancer? *Ann Surg Oncol*. 2005;12:41-47.
24. Bickell NA, Wang JJ, Oluwole S, et al. Missed opportunities: racial disparities in adjuvant breast cancer treatment. *J Clin Oncol*. 2006;24:1357-1362.
25. White J, Morrow M, Moughan J, et al. Compliance with breast-conservation standards for patients with early-stage breast carcinoma. *Cancer*. 2003;97:893-904.
26. Hershman D, McBride R, Jacobson JS, et al. Racial disparities in treatment and survival among women with early-stage breast cancer. *J Clin Oncol*. 2005;23:6639-6646.
27. Hershman D, Weinberg M, Rosner Z, et al. Ethnic neutropenia and treatment delay in African American women undergoing chemo-therapy for early-stage breast cancer. *J Natl Cancer Inst*. 2003;95:1545-1548.
28. Morrow M, Scott SK, Menck HR, Mustoe TA, Winchester DP. Factors influencing the use of breast reconstruction postmastectomy: a National Cancer Database study. *J Am Coll Surg*. 2001;192:1-8.
29. Tseng JF, Kronowitz SJ, Sun CC, et al. The effect of ethnicity on immediate reconstruction rates after mastectomy for breast cancer. *Cancer*. 2004;101:1514-1523.
30. Alderman AK, McMahon L Jr, Wilkins EG. The national utilization of immediate and early delayed breast reconstruction and the effect of sociodemographic factors. *Plast Reconstr Surg*. 2003;111:695-703.
31. Christian CK, Niland J, Edge SB, et al. A multi-institutional analysis of the socioeconomic determinants of breast reconstruction. *Ann Surg*. 2006;243:241-249.
32. Smedley BD, StithAY, Nelson AR, eds. *Unequal Treatment: Confronting Racial and Ethnic Disparities in Health Care*. Washington, DC: National Academy Press; 2002.
33. Palmer JR, Wise LA, Horton NJ, Adams-Campbell LL, Rosenberg L. Dual effect of parity on breast cancer risk in African-American women. *J Natl Cancer Inst*. 2003;95:478-483.

34. Pathak DR, Osuch JR, He J. Breast carcinoma etiology: current knowledge and new insights into the effects of reproductive and hormonal risk factors in black and white populations. *Cancer.* 2000;80:1230-1238.

35. Ursin G, Bernstein L, Wang Y, et al. Reproductive factors and risk of breast carcinoma in a study of white and African-American women. *Cancer.* 2004;101:353-362.

36. Easton DF. The inherited component of cancer. *Br Med Bull.* 1994;50:527-535.

37. Eeles RA, Stratton MR, Goldgar DE, Easton DF. The genetics of familial breast cancer and their practical implications. *Eur J Cancer.* 1994;30A:1383-1390.

38. Nanda R, Schumm LP, Cummings S, et al. Genetic testing in an ethnically diverse cohort of high-risk women: a comparative analysis of BRCA1 and BRCA2 mutations in American families of European and African ancestry. *JAMA.* 2005;294:1925-1933.

39. Mu H, Newman B, Rousseau C, et al. Frequency of breast cancer attributable to BRCA1 and BRCA2 in a population-based series of Caucasian and African American women. *Am J Hum Genet.* 1999;63(suppl):A21.

40. Wagner TM, Hirtenlchner K, Shen P, et al. Global sequence diversity of BRCA2: analysis of 71 breast cancer families and 95 control individuals of worldwide populations. *Hum Mol Genet.* 1999;8:413-423.

41. Mefford HC, Baumbach L, Panguluri RC, et al. Evidence for a BRCA1 founder mutation in families of West African ancestry [letter]. *Am J Hum Genet.* 1999;65:575-578.

42. Stoppa-Lyonnet D, Laurent-Puig P, Essioux L, et al. BRCA1 sequence variations in 160 individuals referred to a breast/ovarian family cancer clinic. *Am J Hum Genet.* 1997;60:1021-1030.

43. Olopade OI, Fackenthal JD, Dunston G, et al. Breast cancer genetics in African Americans. *Cancer.* 2003;97(suppl):236-245.

44. Fregene A, Newman LA. Breast cancer in sub-Saharan Africa: how does it relate to breast cancer in African-American women? *Cancer.* 2005;103:1540-1550.

45. Ameyaw M, Thornton N, McLeod H. Re: Population-based, case-control study of HER2 genetic polymorphism and breast cancer risk. *J Natl Cancer Inst.* 2000;92:1947.

46. Fackenthal JD, Sveen L, Gao Q, et al. Complete allelic analysis of BRCA1 and BRCA2 variants in young Nigerian breast cancer patients. *J Med Genet.* 2005;42:276-281.

47. Braveman PA, Cubbin C, Egerter S, et al. Socioeconomic status in health research: one size does not fit all. *JAMA.* 2005;294:2879-2888.

48. Subramanian S, Chen J, Rehkopf D, et al. Comparing individual- and area-based socioeconomic disparities: a multilevel analysis of Massachusetts births, 1989–1991. *Am J Epidemiol.* 2006;164:823-834.

49. Krieger N, Chen J, Waterman P, et al. Painting a truer picture of US socioeconomic and racial/ethnic health inequalities: the public health disparities geocoding project. *Am J Public Health.* 2005;95:312-323.

50. Newman LA, Griffith KA, Jatoi I, et al. Meta-analysis of survival in African American and white American patients with breast cancer: ethnicity compared with socioeconomic status. *J Clin Oncol.* 2006;24:1342-1349.

51. Bradley CJ, Given CW, Roberts C. Race, socioeconomic status, and breast cancer treatment and survival. *J Natl Cancer Inst.* 2002;94:490-496.

52. Albano JD, Ward E, Jemal A, et al. Cancer mortality in the United States by education level and race. *J Natl Cancer Inst.* 2007;99:1384-1394.

53. Satariano WA, Ragland DR. The effect of comorbidity on 3-year survival of women with primary breast cancer. *Ann Intern Med.* 1994;120:104-110.

54. West DW, Satariano WA, Ragland DR, Hiatt RA. Comorbidity and breast cancer survival: a comparison between black and white women. *Ann Epidemiol.* 1996;6:413-419.

55. Yancik R, Wesley MN, Ries LA, et al. Effect of age and comorbidity in postmenopausal breast cancer patients aged 55 years and older. *JAMA.* 2001;285:885-892.

56. Eley JW, Hill HA, Chen VW, et al. Racial differences in survival from breast cancer: results of the National Cancer Institute Black/White Cancer Survival Study. *JAMA.* 1994;272:947-954.

57. Tammemagi CM, Nerenz D, Neslund-Dudas C, Feldkamp C, Nathanson D. Comorbidity and survival disparities among black and white patients with breast cancer. *JAMA.* 2005;294:1765-1772.

CHAPTER 103

Surgical Complications and Management

Kandice E. Kilbride

The complication rates following surgery of the breast and axilla are considered low. The mortality after these procedures is less than 1%; most complications are wound related (ie, surgical site infections and seroma). These complications may lead to cosmetic compromise and psychological distress to the patient; result in increased costs, prolonged hospital stays, and frequent outpatient visits; and potentially delay important adjuvant therapies. In this chapter, the following topics are addressed:

- Early systemic complications (ie, cardiovascular complications, thromboembolic events, and allergic reactions)
- Early wound-related complications, including hematomas, wound infections, and seromas
- Long-term complications such as chronic breast cellulitis, lymphedema, and chronic pain
- Future directions for scientific study

EARLY SYSTEMIC COMPLICATIONS

In a prospective review of 3107 patients using National Surgical Quality Improvement Program (NSQIP) data, El-Tamer et al reported a 30-day mortality rate of 0.128% after surgery for breast cancer. The mortality rate was significantly increased in patients after mastectomy when compared with lumpectomy (0.24% vs 0.0%), but death remained a rare postoperative event. Breast cancer operations are commonly performed on an elective basis, enabling thorough preoperative evaluation and potential optimization of patients deemed to be high risk. In addition, patients with breast cancer are relatively healthy overall, as most (>85%) patients are classified as ASA 1 or 2.[1]

Furthermore, breast and axillary procedures are classified as clean, soft tissue operations, with no violation of the thoracic or abdominal cavity. As a result, serious infections are rare. As most patients are considered low risk, the incidence of cardiac

complications after breast surgery is also low; the incidence of cardiovascular complications is 0.06% in mastectomy patients. The incidence of stroke is 0.1%. Pulmonary complications are also rare, even with the use of general anesthesia.[1]

Thromboembolic Events

It is well established that patients with a diagnosis of cancer are at an increased risk of thrombotic events. The estimated annual incidence of thrombotic events in the general population is 0.117%; cancer patients have a 4-fold increase in risk.[2] The pathogenesis of the hypercoagulable state in cancer is multifactorial: activation of the coagulation and fibrinolytic cascades, change in the vascular endothelium, generation of acute phase reactants, and hemodynamic compromise.[3]

Patients undergoing surgery for breast cancer often exhibit multiple factors that put them at increased risk of thrombotic events: advanced age, diagnosis of malignancy, use of previous chemotherapy or hormonal therapy, and indwelling central venous catheters.[4] The risk of thrombosis is patients with breast cancer is somewhat lower when compared with other malignancies (brain, pancreas, primary liver). The MD Anderson Cancer Center reported their results in a series of 3898 patients who underwent 4416 breast surgical procedures. Seven women developed venous thrombosis within 60 days of surgery, for a rate of 0.16% per procedure.[2]

There is little consensus regarding the optimal strategy for thromboembolic prophylaxis in the breast cancer population. Randomized trials in the general surgical, orthopedic, and gynecologic literature have demonstrated a substantial reduction in risk of thrombosis with use of prophylactic measures, with only a minimal increase in bleeding complications.[5] However, little data exist on the use of prophylactic measures in those patients undergoing surgery for breast cancer. Breast surgical procedures are increasingly performed on an ambulatory, outpatient basis and tend not to be prolonged cases, questioning the need for prophylaxis.[6] Surgeons are fearful that bleeding complications may result from preoperative anticoagulation.

A survey of 137 breast surgeons in the United Kingdom demonstrated wide variation both in the perceived risk of deep venous thrombosis (DVT) in the patient population and prophylaxis practices. Thirty percent of surgeons surveyed did not routinely prescribe thromboprophylaxis. In those who did, 9 different regimens were reported; the most common was subcutaneous heparin alone, followed by subcutaneous heparin with compressive stockings. Sixty-three percent of the surgeons who did not use routine prophylaxis considered their patient population "low risk" for venous thrombosis; 75.7% of the surgeons who frequently prescribed prophylaxis considered their patients "high risk."[7]

Friis et al compared the use of low-molecular-weight heparin (LMWH) to compression hose in their series of 425 Danish women undergoing breast cancer surgery. No patient developed clinical evidence of DVT. The incidence of hematoma in women who received LMWH was 18.7%, compared with 6.0% in those treated with hose alone. In both groups, almost half of patients with hematoma required reoperation. In multivariate analysis, LMWH prophylaxis was independently associated with postoperative hematoma formation when compared with compressive stockings (OR 3.13, 95% CI 1.38-7.13).[5] Additionally, in a recent series published in the *British Journal of Surgery*, Hardy et al found the use of LMWH to be associated with a 4-fold increase in hemorrhagic complications when compared with unfractionated heparin. No patient in either group developed a clinically evident DVT or pulmonary embolism (PE) within 30 days of surgery; the overall incidence of hematoma requiring reoperation was less than 2% in both groups.[8] The incidence of DVT in these studies may be underrepresented, as up to 25% of patients may have no clinical manifestations.[5]

The National Comprehensive Cancer Network has attempted to address the issue of venous thrombosis in the cancer population. According to the most recent guidelines released in 2008, it is recommended that all hospitalized patients with cancer should undergo mechanical prophylaxis with pneumatic compression devices. Prophylactic anticoagulation with LMWH or unfractionated heparins should be considered in conjunction with pneumatic compression devices for those patients with multiple risk factors and no contraindications to anticoagulation.[9] There is no consensus as to whether or not women with early stage breast cancer should routinely receive anticoagulants prior to outpatient or ambulatory breast surgery.

▪ Allergic Reactions Associated With Lymphatic Mapping

Lymphatic mapping with sentinel lymph node biopsy (SLNB) has become the standard of care for staging the axillary lymph nodes in women undergoing primary surgery for early stage breast cancer. Most surgeons use a combination of radiolabeled sulfur colloid and blue dye, with overall identification rates ranging from 65.5% to 94%.[10] Adverse reactions have been reported in 1% to 4% of cases, most of which were minor in severity, including interference with pulse oximetry, discoloration of body fluids, and skin rashes.[11] With widespread clinical adaptation of SLNB, isosulfan blue has been shown to be associated with life-threatening reactions.

Multiple authors have reported their experience with isosulfan blue dye in lymphatic mapping for breast cancer. In the largest series of 2392 patients who underwent SLNB for breast cancer at Memorial Sloan-Kettering Cancer Center using isosulfan blue dye, 1.6% patients had an allergic reaction. Sixty-nine percent presented with urticaria, pruritus, or skin reaction. Only 0.5% patients developed a severe episode of hypotension; the mean interval from injection to development of reaction was 44 minutes.[12] Similar findings were reported by the authors at MD Anderson Cancer Center in their review of 1835 patients who had SLNB procedures for various types of cancer. The overall incidence of adverse events that could be attributed to isosulfan blue dye was 1.5%. In the subset of 583 patients undergoing breast surgical procedures, incidence was 2.0%. Most of these reactions (75%) were skin reactions, but half were associated with hypotensive episodes.[13]

Risk factors for the development of adverse reactions to isosulfan blue are unknown. Isosulfan blue is a triphenylmethane dye that is present in medications, cosmetics, and textiles; common use of these dyes may lead to sensitization by the general population.[9] Patient allergies to other medications and environmental factors have not been associated with development of adverse reactions.[13] Isosulfan blue contains 2 sulfur atoms, but no correlation has been made between a history of sulfa allergy and adverse events. Montgomery et al noted a 2.6% incidence of allergic reactions to isosulfan blue in patients with sulfa allergy, but this was not statistically different from those without.[12] Chronic use of beta blockade and corticosteroids are unrelated to adverse events. Daley et al found the only significant risk factor for the development of an adverse reaction was chronic use of angiotensin-converting enzyme (ACE) inhibitor and angiotensin receptor blocker medications prior to surgery. The exact mechanism of this relationship is unknown; those patients may be more susceptible to hypotension, but skin reactions were also noted, suggesting other factors.[13]

Concern regarding incidence of life-threatening anaphylaxis and a recent national shortage has prompted use of methylene blue as a substitute for isosulfan blue. Methylene blue has been shown to have equivalent identification rates (99.1% vs 98.9%) and lower cost profiles ($31 per patient vs $191 per patient), without the associated risk of severe adverse reactions.[14] However, methylene blue, especially when injected in the intradermal plane, may be associated with severe skin reactions in up to 21% of patients. In a series of 24 patients who received methylene blue injections during SLNB for breast cancer, 5 presented with skin lesions ranging from superficial ulceration to necrosis. Skin toxicity is thought to result from oxidizing properties of methylene blue leading to local inflammatory reactions and vasospasm.[15] Therefore, intraparenchymal injection is the preferred route when using methylene blue.[9]

Regardless of the type of blue dye used, intradermal injection can lead to prolonged staining of the skin. In a cohort of 33 patients who underwent SLNB with intradermal injection of 1 mL isosulfan blue, 64% reported blue staining of the skin at the injection site after 6 months, and 41% reported persistent staining after 1 year. None of the women considered it to be a psychological or cosmetic issue; however, it is important to warn patients of this finding.[16]

EARLY WOUND-RELATED COMPLICATIONS

Bleeding

The common use of electrocautery in breast surgical procedures has reduced the risk of bleeding complications, but the incidence of hematoma has been reported in up to 11% of patients.[17] Mastectomy patients have a wide surface area of dissection; lumpectomy often requires fracture of breast parenchyma without dissection of avascular planes. Postoperative bleeding complications are associated with increased risk of postoperative wound infection[18] and can lead to poor cosmesis and discomfort for the patient. Small hematomas will be absorbed over time, but larger hematomas can expand quickly and may require reoperation for evacuation, irrigation, and closure.[6]

Use of medications with antiplatelet activity such as aspirin, other nonsteroidal anti-inflammatories, and herbal medications, in the perioperative period can increase the risk of bleeding complications.[6] Intravenous ketorolac has been increasingly used as an adjunct for the acute management of surgical pain; it provides effective pain relief in the postoperative period while reducing the need for narcotics.[19] Some surgeons have expressed concern with the use of ketorolac, as it inhibits platelet aggregation and can increase bleeding time. The only data evaluating bleeding complications with the use of ketorolac after breast surgical procedures were reported by Sharma et al, who published a series of 215 patients who underwent transverse rectus abdominis musculocutaneous (TRAM) flap flap reconstruction. The incidence of hematoma in those patients who received ketorolac was 1.5%; this was statistically similar to those who did not.[20]

Wound Infections

Surgical site infections are the third most common nosocomial infections and the most common infection in surgical patients.[21] Overall wound infection rates after breast surgery vary between reports, from 3% to 19%. Most wound infections are superficial, occur as a result of skin flora (most commonly *Staphylococcus aureus* and *Streptococcus epidermidis*), and can be managed with a short course of antibiotics.[6]

Patient-related risk factors for the development of wound infections have been widely studied. Age is consistently identified as a risk factor, with older patients more likely to develop postoperative wound infections.[18] Obesity has also been associated with increased morbidity and risk of wound infection in patients undergoing breast surgery.[1] Patients on chronic steroids preoperatively are at 1.4 times higher risk of surgical site infections (95% CI 1.18-1.63); smokers and diabetic patients are also at higher risk.[18] Smoking causes a reduction in tissue blood flow and oxygen tension, and as shown by Sorensen et al, smokers have a 3-fold increased risk of wound infections and 9-fold increase in skin flap necrosis after breast surgery.[22,23] A recent review of 260 mastectomy patients showed that any blood

glucose value over 150 mg/dL during the perioperative period increased the risk of postoperative wound infection 3-fold (95% CI 1.2-6.2).[24] In a review of 425 patients undergoing breast cancer surgery, diabetes was the single most significant factor for the development of wound infection (multivariate OR 4.22, 95% CI 1.10-16.2).[22] El-Tamer et al also found the preoperative albumin and hematocrit to be independent predictors of postoperative wound infection, likely related to overall nutritional state and immunologic defense.[1]

Treatment-related factors have also been correlated with the risk of wound infections in this patient population. As reported by NSQIP data, patients undergoing mastectomy are more likely to have postoperative wound infections when compared with lumpectomy (2.8% vs 1.4%, *p* = .007); however, other studies have been somewhat inconsistent.[1] In patients undergoing SLNB for staging of their breast cancer, wound infection rate was 1.0%, as shown by data from the American College of Surgeons Oncology Group (ACOSOG) Z0010 trial. This is significantly lower than the accepted rates of infection (6%-19%) after axillary dissection (ALND).[25] Furthermore, patients who undergo chemotherapy prior to their definitive breast surgery have a 2.8 times higher risk of surgical site infection (95% CI 1.4-5.8).[24]

The use of preoperative antibiotic coverage has been evaluated in multiple randomized trials. A meta-analysis by Platt et al noted a 38% reduction in wound infection rates with the use of antimicrobial prophylaxis.[26] Other studies have reported equivocal results.[27,28] As a result, some clinicians have chosen to limit preoperative antibiotics to those patients at high risk for postoperative wound infection and those involving foreign bodies, such as guidewire placement or implant reconstruction.[6] Weber et al concluded that the timing of antimicrobial prophylaxis was also a significant risk factor for surgical site infection; lowest rates were seen when antibiotics were administered 30 to 74 minutes before surgery.[23]

Seromas

Seromas are accumulations of fluid under the skin resulting from transected lymphatic channels that occur during surgical dissection. They may occur in the dead spaces of lumpectomy cavities, axillary wounds, and the anterior chest wall.[6] Histologic evaluation of the fluid shows that it also contains components associated with an acute inflammatory exudate (ie, immune globulins, granulocytes, and leukocytes).[29] Seromas are commonly reported complications after breast and axillary surgery, and may be considered side effects rather than complications. The incidence varies significantly throughout the literature (2.5%-72%). Seromas can be managed with percutaneous aspiration, which is required in 10% to 80% of patients, as reported by Pogson et al.[30] Aspiration is fairly well tolerated, as the axillary and mastectomy incisions tend to be insensate. Persistent seromas can be a source of significant physical and psychological morbidity for patients, with increased costs, frequent visits, and potential delay of wound healing and initiation of adjuvant therapies.

The data are inconclusive regarding patient factors associated with seroma formation. Lumachi et al reported a higher incidence of seroma in older patients after ALND (60.0 vs 53.8 years, *p* = .02); however, others found no association.[31,32]

Increased body mass index (BMI) is also a risk factor for seroma formation, as shown in the same study.[31]

It has been suggested that more extensive surgical dissection is associated with risk of seroma formation. As reported by Kuroi et al in a systematic review, 6 studies comparing breast-conserving therapy with mastectomy have shown equivocal data regarding seroma formation. Immediate reconstruction at time of mastectomy is associated with lower incidence of seroma, while extended radical mastectomy is associated with higher rates of seroma when compared with simple mastectomy.[32] Regarding ALND, 4 studies have shown no association with the number of nodes removed and seroma formation.[31] However, it has been demonstrated that the use of SLNB has significantly reduced seroma rates when compared with ALND. Guiliano et al reported the presence of a seroma in 1.5% of patients after SLNB, compared with 15% in women who underwent SLNB followed by ALND, despite external drainage in ALND patients.[33]

It has been hypothesized that the use of electrocautery for dissection leads to damage of adjacent lymphatics, leading to leakage of lymph fluid into surgical cavities.[14] Studies evaluating surgical technique have suggested an increase in seroma formation with use of electrocautery, but results are inconsistent. A randomized study of 160 patients undergoing breast-conserving therapy or modified radical mastectomy showed that the rate of seroma formation is independent of method of dissection (electrocautery vs cold knife dissection).[34] In contrast, Porter et al reported a significant increase in seroma formation with use of electrocautery in mastectomy patients.[35] Some authors have expected a reduction in seroma rates with the use of ultrasonic scissors (harmonic scalpel), as it occludes vascular and lymphatic channels without extensive thermal injury.[36] The data evaluating the use of ultrasonic scissors in patients undergoing mastectomy showed no reduction in overall drainage and no advantage regarding incidence of seroma formation.[29] Lumachi et al prospectively studied the use of ultrasonic scissors in 92 women undergoing ALND. The incidence of seroma was decreased when compared with electrocautery (20% vs 40.4%), but this difference did not reach statistical significance.[31] Another study by Irshad and Campbell noted a significant reduction in seroma rates with the use of ultrasonic scissors for ALND.[37]

Some authors have reported the use of external compression or suture fixation in order to facilitate adherence of the skin flaps to the chest wall, thereby closing the dead space and inhibiting seroma formation. Based on data from a meta analysis that reviewed the effect of dead space closure on seroma rates, 2 randomized controlled trials failed to show a reduction in postoperative drainage with the use of external compressive dressings when compared with a loosely fitting surgical bra.[31,38,39] In contrast, the authors of the meta-analysis concluded that multiple studies suggest there was a significant decrease in the incidence of seroma and reduction in drainage time with suture fixation of the skin flaps, without sacrificing shoulder mobility.[31] However, this method was associated with a significant increase in operating time.[30]

As shown by Lotze et al, patients who receive early physiotherapy experience higher volumes and longer time of drainage.[40]

In an attempt to reduce the shearing forces that may contribute to seroma formation, authors have limited shoulder mobilization in patients undergoing mastectomy. Placement of bandages and slings to prevent early use showed little benefit.[30] Limitation of physiotherapy until after the drains have been removed may reduce seroma formation; Schultz et al reported a significant reduction in patients who started physiotherapy on the first postoperative day (38%) compared with the seventh postoperative day (22%). There was no significant difference in outcome of shoulder function at 4 to 6 month follow-up.[41]

Chemical maneuvers such as sclerosing agents and topical coagulants have also been investigated in attempt to decrease seroma. Fibrin sealants have been used in a variety of surgical settings; animal models have suggested a decrease in seroma formation after mastectomy.[42] A meta-analysis of 11 randomized controlled trials evaluating the use of fibrin glue was published by Carless and Henry; they noted an overall seroma rate of 1.7% to 53.1%, and concluded that fibrin sealant was not effective in preventing seroma formation or reducing volume of postoperative drainage.[44]

The use of external drainage tubes is a common practice following both mastectomy and ALND; drainage of lymphatic fluid closes dead space and allows for adherence of skin flaps to the chest wall. Patients are discharged with the drains in situ, and they are removed when the output decreases, usually within 7 to 10 days. These drains are often cumbersome to patients, require maintenance upon discharge, and may be associated with increased discomfort and infection.[43] In addition, it has been suggested that continuous closed suction drainage prevents closure of transected lymphatics, leading to prolonged fluid accumulation.[44] A systematic review by Kuroi et al reported that the incidence of seroma was not influenced by the number of drains placed or intensity of negative suction pressure. Furthermore, evidence regarding the optimal timing of drain removal is inconclusive in randomized controlled trials.[32]

CHRONIC COMPLICATIONS AFTER BREAST AND AXILLARY SURGERY

Chronic Breast Cellulitis

Chronic or delayed breast cellulitis has been described in the literature to occur in a minority (1%-12%) of patients after breast-conserving therapy. Patients with this condition present with diffuse breast erythema, edema, warmth, and tenderness; this is distinct from acute cellulitis, as it lacks systemic manifestations and has a more indolent course.[45] It is speculated to result from bacterial infection of tissues with impaired lymphatic drainage as a result of surgery and radiation.[46] This condition can cause significant concern as it may present with findings similar to an inflammatory recurrence.[6] Once imaging is obtained to rule out recurrence, a short course of oral antibiotics is recommended, reserving intravenous therapy for the most severe of cases.[45]

Indelicato et al reported a series of 50 patients with delayed breast cellulitis, noting an independent association with history of postoperative hematoma, seroma, or lymphedema. In addition, as confirmed by other series, violation of soft tissue with seroma aspiration or hematoma evacuation also increases the risk of long-term breast cellulitis.[45,46]

Lymphedema

Lymphedema resulting from breast cancer treatment is one of the most dreaded and problematic sources of morbidity for patients. The incidence is generally accepted at approximately 30%, although reported rates vary. The wide variation of data in the literature is likely a result of differing definitions of what constitutes lymphedema, use of indirect methods of measurement, and inconsistent duration of follow-up. A longitudinal study by Hayes et al reported that at any given point in the 18 months following treatment, at least 1 in 10 women experienced symptoms of lymphedema (point prevalence 8.0%-14.9%). Most cases present early, but some patients may present as late as 18 months to 3 years after treatment.[47]

It has become accepted that more extensive treatment (extent of surgery, use of radiotherapy) increases risk of lymphedema. Those patients who undergo mastectomy are 6 times more likely to experience lymphedema when compared with patients after breast-conserving therapy (OR 6.21 1.4-27.6).[47] In addition, multiple randomized trials have shown a decreased incidence of lymphedema after SLNB when compared with ALND. In 2904 patients who underwent SLNB as part of the ACOSOG Z0010 trial, 7% were found to have lymphedema at 6-months follow-up. This is compared with the accepted incidence of 7% to 20% with ALND by recent reports. Using multivariate analysis, increasing age and increasing BMI were independent predictors for the development of lymphedema after SLNB.[25]

Lymphedema may be associated with long-term sequelae. Hayes et al showed that women with lymphedema were twice as likely to complain of upper-body impairment when compared with those without.[47] Additionally, patients may develop *Stewart-Treves syndrome*, which consists of angiosarcoma occurring in a lymphedematous upper extremity. These lesions are bluish-reddish macules or nodules on the skin, which appear approximately 10 years after treatment; patients with history of nodal irradiation and ALND are at highest risk. This syndrome is one of the most feared complications of lymphedema, as patients often present with metastatic disease. Median survival is approximately 2 years.[6]

Neurologic Complications

Limitation in arm and shoulder mobility has been thoroughly described as a complication of both breast and axillary surgery. The pathophysiology of "frozen shoulder" is similar to other soft tissue contractures that occur in conditions with reduced mobility. In a recent series, Nesvold et al evaluated 263 patients to compare arm and shoulder mobility after breast cancer surgery. They noted that patients after mastectomy were 2.3 times more likely to experience impaired flexion and abduction of the shoulder when compared with patients after breast-conserving therapy. They also found that women were less likely to complain of moderate and severe symptoms of impaired arm function, shoulder stiffness, and pain after breast-conserving therapy then after mastectomy.[48]

Ideally, mobilization of the shoulder should begin as soon as possible after surgery. Early mobilization exercises may consist of wall walking and pendulum exercises. In patients with frozen shoulder and limited arm abduction, aggressive treatment with physical therapy may be warranted prior to initiation of radiotherapy to prevent progressive fibrosis and worsening contracture.[49]

Axillary web syndrome is characterized by axillary pain radiating down the ipsilateral arm and limitation of shoulder mobility in the presence of fibrotic bands that extend from the axilla distally down the arm. This clinical syndrome was first described by Moskovitz et al in 44 of 750 patients who developed axillary web syndrome after ALND. In this cohort, 43% of patients had preservation of the intercostobrachial nerve at the time of ALND, suggesting that ligation of this nerve does not contribute to axillary web syndrome.[50] Sentinel lymph node biopsy is associated with a lower incidence of this syndrome; Leidenius et al reported an incidence of 20% after SLNB, as compared with 72% after ALND ($p < .01$).[51] Use of SLNB is also associated with decreased severity of impaired shoulder mobility; the median deficiency in shoulder abduction in patients after SLNB was 2 degrees, compared with 61 degrees after ALND ($p = .0003$).[51] Depending on the severity of pain and limitation of motion, treatment consists of a combination of nonsteroidal anti-inflammatories and analgesics with physical therapy, manual fibrous release, and range of motion exercises.[48] However, this syndrome is often self-limited, and likely to resolve without sequelae within 3 months.[50,51] Axillary web syndrome has been described as an axillary variant of *Mondor disease*, a thrombophlebitis of the superficial veins of the breast that presents with painful subcutaneous cords on the chest wall. This is also self-limited, resolving spontaneously within 2 to 10 weeks after presentation.[50]

Patients may also experience paresthesias after axillary surgical procedures; the incidence and outcomes vary between authors. As shown in the ACOSOG Z0010 clinical trial, the incidence of axillary paresthesia 6 months after SLNB was 8.6%. Ninety-two percent of patients described the symptoms as "mild." Younger women may be more susceptible to these symptoms, as shown by multivariate analysis (OR 0.79, 95% CI 0.71-0.87).[25]

Less extensive surgical dissection is associated with lower incidence of paresthesias, as patients after SLNB are 50% less likely to report symptoms when compared with ALND.[52] In a randomized trial comparing SLNB with ALND, Veronesi et al reported a 2% incidence of axillary paresthesias after SLNB, compared to 85% with ALND.[53] In addition, in node-positive patients who often require both procedures, questions arise about whether delaying the completion of ALND may contribute to the high incidence of complications. A recent update of the ACOSOG Z0010 and Z0011 trials reviewed this issue, comparing the complication rates between immediate and delayed ALND in women undergoing breast-conserving therapy. Immediate ALND was associated with greater frequency of postoperative complications, including axillary paresthesias (50% vs 42%, $p = .02$), seromas (18% vs 12%, $p = .01$), and limited shoulder mobility (49% vs 36%, $p < .01$).[54]

Persistent pain after breast surgery was first described by Wood in 1978 in a case series of 5 women with intercostobrachial entrapment syndrome after mastectomy.[55] The incidence of persistent pain after breast surgery is estimated to reach approximately 50%, but definitions vary. The exact etiology of pain after breast surgery is unclear; it is thought to be neuropathic in nature, resulting from (1) dissection of neurovascular structures leading to focal injuries from traction and/or scarring, (2) chronic nerve compression from ischemia, scarring, and fibrosis, or (3) neuroma formation causing spontaneous pain from trapped axons.[56,57] Jung et al have classified neuropathic pain after breast surgery into 4 categories: intercostobrachial neuralgia, phantom breast pain, neuroma pain, and others.[58] This pain may be localized to the upper chest wall, axilla, arm, or shoulder regions, and has been described as stabbing, shooting, gnawing, and aching.[56] Women who experience pain after breast surgery are at greater risk of psychological distress, leading to difficulty performing activities of daily living, alteration of body image, and decreased sexual interest and function.[59]

The sensation of persistence of the breast after its removal by mastectomy has been characterized as *phantom breast syndrome.* The presence of phantom sensations is a known complication in patients after limb amputation, and has been reported in patients after removal of other organs. In breast surgery patients, studies report the incidence to range from 17% to 64%. As noted by Kroner in a review of 120 Danish women after mastectomy, phantom breast syndrome was experienced in 25.8% patients, and often persists at 1-year follow-up. Fifty-two percent of patients reported this sensation to be painful.[60]

The preponderance of data exists in the postmastectomy population, but the presence of pain after breast surgery is not limited to those patients with cancer. Barton et al reported pain to be the most common complication in 269 women after bilateral prophylactic mastectomy using data from the Cancer Research Network.[61] Chronic pain was also noted in 22% of patients after reduction mammoplasty, and 40% of patients after augmentation.[56]

Little is known about the risk factors for the development of chronic pain after breast surgery. Due to the low prevalence of breast cancer in men, studies are limited to female participants.[56] Increased BMI may be a factor in chronic pain after breast surgery.[57] The frequency of pain after breast surgery is associated with younger age, as shown by multiple authors. In a cohort of 69 breast reduction patients, Wallace et al found a significant correlation with longer from time to pain and younger age (34 years vs 48 years, $p < .05$).[56] Caffo et al also reported lower median age in patients with pain after breast cancer surgery (57 years vs 61 years, $p = .01$).[62] In their series, Macdonald et al. noted a reduction in chronic pain after mastectomy with advancing age: 91% in women aged 30 to 49 versus 55% in women aged 50 to 69, and 29% in women over 70.[57] Furthermore, the presence of pain before surgery has been shown to be a risk factor for development of phantom breast pain after mastectomy.[60] Some suggest that patients with increased pain intensity in the acute postoperative period are more likely to develop chronic pain.[63]

Treatment-related factors may also have an impact on the development of chronic pain. A higher incidence of pain has been reported in patients treated with breast-conserving therapy when compared with mastectomy,[62] supporting the hypothesis that use of radiation may increase the risk of postsurgical pain. This may also be secondary to neuroma formation within the lumpectomy

incision, resulting in spontaneous pain from trapped axons.[58] In patients treated with mastectomy, addition of reconstruction is associated with an increased incidence of chronic pain syndrome (31% after mastectomy alone vs 49% with reconstruction).[56] Furthermore, the type and timing of reconstruction may impact development of chronic pain, with increased pain reported after implant versus native tissue reconstructions and delayed versus immediate reconstructions.[56] Patients who undergo SLNB are 50% less likely to experience sensory morbidity when compared with ALND.[52] The use of chemotherapy has not been shown to correlate with chronic pain.[56,62]

Treatment of chronic pain symptoms after breast cancer surgery poses a management challenge to clinicians. Few randomized controlled trials exist concerning treatment modalities in this population. Amitriptyline has been examined in a trial of neuropathic pain after breast surgery, and was shown to significantly improve pain relief compared with placebo; however, 5 of 8 patients who experienced relief stopped the medication due to side effects.[64] Another trial evaluating efficacy of venlafaxine showed greater overall relief when compared with placebo, but little benefit in measurement of daily pain ratings, the primary end point of the study.[62,63] Data suggest that neuropathic pain syndromes in other areas of the body share symptoms and characteristics with chronic pain after breast surgery; therefore, attempts are being made to use other efficacious modalities and treatments in this population.[58]

There have been few studies reporting long-term outcome in patients with pain after breast surgery. Studies evaluating chronic breast pain are difficult to interpret, as they are frequently based on patient surveys, often relying on pain or recollection without clinical correlation regarding presurgical quality of life, presence of presurgical pain, and documented narcotic use. An epidemiological study from Scotland evaluated 408 women after mastectomy with mean postoperative interval of 3.0 years, and noted an incidence of pain in 43% patients. When reevaluating quality of life and outcome 6 years later, the authors noted persistence of pain in 52% and complete resolution in 38% of the 113 responders. Women reported still suffering with activities of daily of living, but overall quality of life was improved. This suggests that the intensity of pain may decrease over time, or women may develop better adaptive mechanisms.[60]

FUTURE DIRECTIONS

As the complications mentioned in this chapter are a source of significant morbidity, multiple trials are in progress in attempt to lower complication rates after breast and axillary surgery, thereby improving quality of life. Areas of active research include the following:

- Institutional comparisons of complication rates using information from sources such as the NSQIP database to determine national benchmarks and standards of care
- Multiple trials sanctioned by the National Cancer Institute to better identify risk factors for infection, seromas, lymphedema, and chronic pain[65]

- Trials evaluating reduction of symptoms of lymphedema with use of decongestive lymphatic massage therapy, kinesiobandages, strength training, and selenium therapy[65]
- Studies using lidocaine patches, acupuncture therapy, and pentoxifylline therapy to improve symptoms and quality of life for patients with chronic pain[65]

In addition, we are awaiting results from 3 trials that have closed to accrual. Final follow-up of the ACOSOG Z0010, ACOSOG Z0011, and NSABP B-32 trials may clarify the long-term benefits and complications of SLNB when compared with ALND.[65,66] Ideas for further study include a randomized trial comparing the use of heparin/LMWH as thromboprophylaxis for breast surgical patients, a randomized trial comparing the use of ketorolac as an adjunct pain reliever and its impact on bleeding risk, and more studies evaluating neuropathic pain treatments in the breast cancer population.

SUMMARY

Breast surgical procedures are routinely performed in an ambulatory elective setting and most patients are healthy; as a result, perioperative mortality is less than 1%, and complication rates are low in this population. Most commonly patients will experience a wound-related complication such as wound infection, postoperative bleeding, or seroma. While minor, these complications can be a significant source of morbidity to patients and result in delayed healing, increased cost, and potential delay of adjuvant therapies. Patients with breast cancer are also at risk of venous thrombosis, but data are inconclusive regarding the need for prophylaxis with risk of bleeding. Long-term complications such as cellulitis, lymphedema, limited shoulder motion, and chronic pain syndromes can lead to decreased functional capacity and quality of life; the optimal management strategy is to identify factors that increase the risk of developing these complications and prevent them if possible.

REFERENCES

1. El-Tamer MB, Ward BM, Schifftner T, et al. Morbidity and mortality following breast cancer surgery in women: national benchmarks for standards of care. *Ann Surg.* 2007;245(5):665-671.
2. Andtbacka RH, Babiera G, Singletary SE, et al. Incidence and prevention of venous thromboembolism in patients undergoing breast cancer surgery and treated according to clinical pathways. *Ann Surg.* 2006;243(1):96-101.
3. Caine GJ, Stonelake PS, Rea D, Lip GYH. Coagulopathic complications in breast cancer. *Cancer.* 2003;98(8):1578-1586.
4. Geerts WH, Heit JA, Clagett GP, et al. Prevention of venous thromboembolism. *Chest.* 2001;119(suppl):132-175.
5. Friis E, Horby J, Sorensen LT, et al. Thromboembolic prophylaxis as a riDsk factor for postoperative complications after breast cancer surgery. *World J Surg.* 2004;28:540-543.
6. Vitug AF, Newman LA. Complications in breast surgery. *Surg Clin N Am.* 2007;87:431-451.
7. Cameron IC, Azmy IAF. Thromboprophylaxis in patients undergoing surgery for breast cancer. *Breast.* 2001;10:535-537.
8. Hardy RG, Williams L, Dixon JL. Use of enoxaparin results in more haemorrhagic complications after breast surgery than unfractionated heparin. *Brit J Surg.* 2008;95:834-836.
9. National Comprehensive Cancer Network Practice Guidelines in Oncology. Available at: http://www.nccn.org/professionals/physician_gls/PDF/vte.pdf. Accessed October 5, 2008.
10. Thevarajah S, Huston TL, Simmons RM. A comparison of the adverse reactions associated with isosulfan blue versus methylene blue dye in sentinel lymph node biopsy for breast cancer. *Amer J Surg.* 2005;189:236-239.
11. Masannat Y, Shenoy H, Speirs V, Hanby A, Horgan K. Properties and characteristics of the dyes injected to assist axillary sentinel node localization in breast surgery. *Eur J Surg Onc.* 2006;32:381-384.
12. Montgomery LL, Thorne AC, Van Zee KJ, et al. Isosulfan blue dye reactions during sentinel lymph node mapping for breast cancer. *Anesth Analg.* 2002;95:385-388.
13. Daley MD, Norman PH, Leak JA, et al. Adverse events associated with the intraoperative injection of isosulfan blue. *J Clin Anesth.* 2004;16:332-341.
14. Blessing WD, Stolier AJ, Teng SC, Bolton JS, Fuhrman GM. A comparison of methylene blue and lymphazurin in breast cancer sentinel node mapping. *Amer J Surg.* 2002;184:341-345.
15. Stradling B, Aranha G, Gabram S. Adverse skin lesions after methylene blue injections for sentinel lymph node localization. *Amer J Surg.* 2002;184:350-352.
16. Govaert GAM, Oostenbroek RJ, Plaisier PW. Prolonged skin staining after intradermal use of patent blue in sentinel lymph node biopsy for breast cancer. *Eur J Surg Onc.* 2005;31:373-375.
17. Bakker X, Roumen RM. Bleeding after excision of breast lumps. *Eur J Surg.* 2002;168:401-403.
18. Neumayer L, Schifftner TL, Henderson WG, Khuri SF, El-Tamer M. Breast cancer surgery in Veterans Affairs and selected university medical centers: Results of the Patient Safety in Surgery Study. *JACS.* 2007;204(6):1235-1241.
19. Severino FB, Sinatra RS, Paige D, Silverman DG. Intravenous ketorolac as an adjunct to patient-controlled analgesia (PCA) for management of postgynecologic surgical pain. *J Clin Anesth.* 1994;6:23-27.
20. Sharma S, Chang DW, Koutz C, et al. Incidence of hematoma associated with ketorolac after TRAM flap breast reconstruction. *Plast Recon Surg.* 2001;107(2):352-355.
21. Neumayer L, Hosokawa P, Itani K, et al. Multivariable predictors of postoperative surgical site infection after general and vascular surgery: results from the Patient Safety in Surgery Study. *JACS.* 2007;204(6):1178-1186.
22. Sorensen LT, Horby J, Friis E, Pilsgaard B, Jorgensen T. Smoking as a risk factor for wound healing and infection in breast cancer surgery. *Eur J Surg Onc.* 2002;28:815-820.
23. Weber WP, Marti WR, Zwahlen M, et al. The timing of surgical antimicrobial prophylaxis. *Ann Surg.* 2008;247(6):918-926.
24. Villar-Compte D, Alvarez de Iturbe I, Martin-Onraet A, et al. Hyperglycemia as a risk factor for surgical site infections in patients undergoing mastectomy. *Amer J Infect Control.* 2008;36(3):192-198.
25. Wilke LG, McCall LM, Posther KE, et al. Surgical complications associated with sentinel lymph node biopsy: results from prospective international cooperative group trial. *Ann Surg Onc.* 2006;13(4):491-500.
26. Platt R, Zaleznik DF, Hopkins CC, et al. Perioperative antibiotic prophylaxis for herniorrhapy and breast surgery. *N Engl J Med.* 1990;322(3):153-160.
27. Wagman LD, Tegtmeier B, Beatty JD. A prospective, randomized double-blind study of the use of antibiotics at the time of mastectomy. *Surg Gynecol Obstet.* 1990;170(1):12-16.
28. Gupta R, Sinnett D, Carpenter R, et al. Antibiotic prophylaxis for postoperative wound infection in clean elective breast surgery. *Eur J Surg Onc.* 2000;26(4):363-366.
29. Galatius H, Okholm M, Hoffmann J. Mastectomy using ultrasonic dissection: effect on seroma formation. *Breast.* 2003;12:338-341.
30. Pogson CJ, Adwani A, Ebbs SR. Seroma following breast cancer surgery. *Eur J Surg Onc.* 2003;29:711-717.
31. Lumachi F, Brandes AA, Burelli P, et al. Seroma prevention following axillary dissection in patients with breast cancer using ultrasound scissors: a prospective clinical study. *J Cancer Surg.* 2004;30:526-530.
32. Kuroi K, Shimozuma K, Taguchi T, et al. Evidence-based risk factors for seroma formation in breast surgery. *Jap J Clin Onc.* 2006;36(4):197-206.
33. Guiliano AE, Haigh PI, Breannan MB, et al. Prospective observational study of sentinel lymphadenectomy without further axillary dissection in patients with sentinel node negative breast cancer. *J Clin Oncol.* 2000;18:2553-2559.
34. Nadkarni M, Rangole A, Sharma R, et al. Influence of surgical technique on axillary seroma formation: a randomized study. *Anz J Surg.* 2007;77:385-389.
35. Porter KA, O'Connor S, Rimm E, Lopez M. Electrocautery as a risk factor in seroma formation following mastectomy. *Amer J Surg.* 1998;176:8-11.
36. Deo SVS, Shukla N. Modified radical mastectomy using harmonic scalpel. *J Surg Onc.* 2000;74:204-207.
37. Irshad K, Campbell H. Use of harmonic scalpel in mastectomy and axillary dissection for breast cancer. *Eur J Cancer.* 2002;38(suppl 3):104.
38. Chen SC, Chen MF. Timing of shoulder exercise after modified radical mastectomy: a prospective study. *Chang Keng I Hsueh Tsa Chih.* 1999;22:37-43.

39. O'Hea BJ, Ho MN, Petrek JA. External compression dressing versus standard dressing after axillary lymphadenectomy. *Amer J Surg.* 1999;177:450-453.

40. Lotze MT, Duncan MA, Gerber LH, Wolrering EA, Rosenburg SA. Early versus delayed shoulder motion following axillary dissection. *Ann Surg.* 1981;193:288-295.

41. Schultz I, Barholm M, Grondal S. Delayed shoulder exercises in reducing seroma frequency after modified radical mastectomy. a prospective randomized study. *Ann Surg Oncol.* 1997;4(4):293-297.

42. Carless PA, Henry DA. Systematic review and meta-analysis of the use of fibrin sealant to prevent seroma formation after breast cancer surgery. *Brit J Surg.* 2006;93:810-819.

43. Soon PSH, Clark J, Magarey CJ. Seroma formation after axillary lymphadenectomy with and without use of drains. *Breast.* 2005;14:103-107.

44. Chintamani, Singhal V, Singh J, Vansal A, Saxena S. Half versus full vacuum suction drainage after modified radical mastectomy for breast cancer—a prospective randomized trial. *BMC Cancer.* 2005;5(11).

45. Indelicato DJ, Grobmyer SR, Newlin H, et al. Delayed breast cellulitis: an evolving complication of breast conservation. *Int J Rad Onc Biol Phys.* 2006;66(5):1339-1346.

46. Brewer VH, Hahn KA, Rohrbach BW, Bell JL, Baddour LM. Risk factor analysis for breast cellulitis complicating breast conservation therapy. *Clin Infect Dis.* 2000;31:654-659.

47. Hayes SC, Janda M, Cornish B, Battistutta D, Newman B. Lymphedema after breast cancer: incidence, risk factors and effect on upper body function. *J Clin Onc.* 2008;26(21):3536-3542.

48. Nesvold IL, Dahl AA, Lokkevik E, Mengshoel AM, Fossa SD. Arm and shoulder morbidity in breast cancer patients after breast conserving therapy versus mastectomy. *Acta Oncologica.* 2008;47:835-842.

49. Cheville AL, Tchou J. Barriers to rehabilitation following surgery for primary breast cancer. *J Surg Onc.* 2007;95:409-418.

50. Moskovitz, AH, Anderson BO, Yeung RS, et al. Axillary web syndrome after axillary dissection. *Amer J Surg.* 2001;181:434-439.

51. Leidenius M, Leppanen E, Krogerus L, von Smitten K. Motion restriction and axillary web syndrome after sentinel node biopsy and axillary clearance in breast cancer. *Amer J Surg.* 2003;185:127-130.

52. Temple LK, Baron R, Cody HS, et al. Sensory morbidity after sentinel lymph node biopsy and axillary dissection: a prospective study of 233 women. *Ann Surg Onc.* 2002;9(7):654-662.

53. Veronesi U, Paganelli G, Viale G, et al. A randomized comparison of sentinel-node biopsy with routine axillary dissection in breast cancer. *N Engl J Med.* 2003;349:546-553.

54. Olson JA, McCall LM, Beitsch P, et al. Impact of immediate versus delayed axillary node dissection on surgical outcomes in breast cancer patients with positive sentinel nodes: results from American College of Surgeons Oncology Group Trials Z0010 and Z0011. *J Clin Onc.* 2008;26(21):3530-3535.

55. Wood KM. Intercostobrachial nerve entrapment syndrome. *South Med J.* 1978;71(6):662-663.

56. Wallace MS, Wallace AM, Lee J, Dobke MK. Pain after breast surgery: a survey of 282 women. *Pain.* 1996;66:195-205.

57. Macdonald L, Bruce J, Scott NW, Smith WCS, Chambers WA. Long-term follow-up of breast cancer survivors with post-mastectomy pain syndrome. *Brit J Cancer.* 2005;92:225-230.

58. Jung BF, Herrmann D, Griggs J, Oaklander AL, Dworkin RH. Neuropathic pain associated with non-surgical treatment of breast cancer. *Pain.* 2005;118:10-14.

59. Kudel I, Edwards RR, Kozachik S, et al. Predictors and consequences of multiple persistent postmastectomy pains. *J Pain Symptom Mgmt.* 2007;34(6):619-627.

60. Kroner K, Krebs B, Skov J, Jorgensen HS. Immediate and long term phantom breast syndrome after mastectomy: incidence, clinical characteristics, and relationship to pre-mastectomy breast pain. *Pain.* 1989;36:327-334.

61. Barton MB, West CN, Liu IA, et al. Complications following bilateral prophylactic mastectomy. *JNCI Monographs.* 2005;35:61-66.

62. Caffo O, Amichetti M, Ferro A, et al. Pain and quality of life after surgery for breast cancer. *Breast Cancer Res Treat.* 2003;80:39-48.

63. Tasmuth T, Hartel B, Kalso E. Venlaxafine in neuropathic pain following treatment of breast cancer. *Eur J Pain.* 2002;6:17-24.

64. Kalso E, Tasmuth T, Neuvonen PJ. Amitripytline effectively relieves neuropathic pain following treatment of breast cancer. *Pain.* 1995;64:293-302.

65. National Cancer Institute Clinical Trials Search Results. Available at: http://www.cancer.gov/search/ResultsClinicalTrials.aspx?protocolsearchid=5136133. Bethesda, MD. Accessed September 15, 2008.

66. National Surgical Adjuvant Breast and Bowel Project: Clinical Trials Information. Pittsburgh, PA. Available at: http://www.nsabp.pitt.edu/. Accessed September 15, 2008.

CHAPTER 104

Lymphedema

Steve Norton

PATHOGENESIS

Lymphedema is caused when protein-rich fluid accumulates in the interstitium due to impaired function of lymphatic tissues. Proteins and other macromolecular wastes with water constitute lymphatic functional loads; these wastes rely upon specially structured absorptive and transport structures in regional anatomy for their return to the central circulation. When lymph stasis prevails, inflammatory processes and fibrosis (lymphostatic fibrosis) trigger changes in tissue density, further entrapping superficial vessels and accelerating the mechanical insufficiency.[1]

PRIMARY AND SECONDARY LYMPHEDEMA

A brief description of primary lymphedema highlights the genetic variability of lymphatic constitution and may explain why seemingly similar patients receiving the same surgical protocol will have different risks for lymphedema over time (Table 104-1). In primary lymphatic diseases and syndromes (eg, Turner syndrome, Noonan syndrome), which include lymphatic dysplasias, these structural malformations involve the mechanisms for uptake, transport, and filtration of lymph. Inherited traits are found in Nonne–Milroy disease, Meige disease, and Distichiasis syndrome.[2] The majority of these developmental insufficiencies (87%)[1,3] manifest before the age of 35 and cause hypoplasia of vessels and nodes. Syndromes involving hyperplasia, node fibrosis, or aplasia also occur with much less frequency (Fig. 104-1).[2] As a result, dysplasia predisposes regions of drainage to inadequate lymph collection, resulting in edema and secondary tissue changes such as chronic inflammation and reactive fibrosis. Since there is no method currently available to image lymphatic vessels safely, it remains a mystery how robust the constitution

of lymphatic anatomy is in each patient. Of interest are variations in upper limb drainage that circumvent the axillary nodes to empty at supraclavicular sites. Anatomists theorize that these particular anomalies create advantageous collateral pathways to prevent lymphedema in those fortunate enough to possess these variations.[4]

The focus of this chapter's discussion is secondary lymphedema, the type caused by a known, significant insult to lymphatic tissues (Table 104-2). It is well documented that lymphedema occurs with great frequency when direct trauma is rendered to regional nodes and/or vessel structures. Degradation of lymphatic health is also noted when adjacent tissues such as superficial and deep veins become diseased, when cellulitis occurs, or when accumulations of adipose or radiation fibrosis mechanically disrupt drainage of skin lymphatics.[1,3,5] The following discussion is aimed at assisting with differential diagnosis, since all edemas do not occur in pure form.

PATHOPHYSIOLOGY AND LYMPHATIC INSUFFICIENCIES

Lymphedema always involves a compromised mechanical function within the lymphatic tissues leading to inadequate uptake of tissue loads and protein-rich fluid accumulation. The unique function of lymphatic vessels as compared to blood vessels involves peristaltic pulsation (intrinsic contractions) of lymphangion segments, resulting in continual transport of fluid regardless of activity level or limb position.[4,6] At the level of the lymph capillary plexus, inelastic collagen-anchoring filaments tethered to overlapping inter-endothelial junctions ("swinging tips")[4] passively respond to increases in interstitial fluid pressure by opening under tension, allowing fluid to be pulled into the lumen to form lymph. Once this heightened interstitial pressure

TABLE 104-1 Causes of Primary Lymphedema
Hypoplasia
Hyperplasia
Aplasia
Node Fibrosis

TABLE 104-2 Common Causes of Secondary Lymphedema
Lymphadenectomy
Radiation therapy
Trauma
Infection
Malignancy
Obesity
Chronic Venous Insufficiency

has been alleviated, the junction closes as the anchoring filament relaxes.[4,7] Because lymph uptake relies upon continual, uninterrupted emptying of proximal vessels and nodes, disruption of afferent vessels at the node results in lymph vessel hypertension, valvular incompetence with reflux, vessel fatigue/failure, and lack of new lymph formation at the capillary level.[4] Further mechanical compromises occur when surrounding tissues form lymphostatic fibrosis, which acts to entrap vessels and capillary plexuses, limiting free function.

Reactive Fibrosis (Lymphostatic Fibrosis)

During lymph stasis, activated macrophages respond to accumulations of lipoperoxides caused by free radicals not absorbed by compromised lymphatics. In the interstitium these macrophages release interleukin 1, causing fibroblast migration and fibrocyte or adipocyte accumulations.[4] These inflammatory processes and cells responding to protein accumulation populate the interstitium, creating additional lymphatic loads (LLs) on already mechanically insufficient lymphatic tissues.[4,6,8] Furthermore, hypertensive lymph collectors themselves become obstructed by clot formations, and vessel walls sclerose (mural insufficiency) if treatment is not administered to interrupt and reverse disease progression.[4,9] Additionally, although lymph collectors and capillaries are not as radiation sensitive as the nodes, microvascular retreat within radiation tissues further accelerates fibrotic tissue formation, leading to regional vessel entrapment. Interestingly, as undifferentiated cells, fibroblast morphology seems to depend upon host body type, resulting in a hardened (fibrosclerosis) tissue formation in thin individuals or "spongy" swelling of the subcutis in heavier patients.

Healthy Lymphatic Function

Transport capacity (TC) is generally estimated to be 10 times the level of daily-required LL.[3,4,9] Lymph time volume (LTV) directly reflects the current LL by adjusting with an increase in contractile amplitude and frequency in tissues local to the newly formed fluids. Systemically LL is approximately 2 L/d; if required LTV adjusts (lymphatic safety factor)[4] when necessary to a level of approximately 20 L/d without failure for extended periods. Therefore, TC equals maximum LTV (TC = MLTV) and functional reserve (FR) represents the difference between TC and LL at any moment in time (Fig. 104-2).[4]

Mechanical Insufficiency

In secondary lymphedema, mechanical insufficiency results when TC is reduced from an assumed robust and normal level due to external trauma. FR is therefore decreased and LL approaches or exceeds the diminished TC, resulting in accumulations of macromolecular debris.[4,5,9,10] Because FR is determined by ill-defined, inherited lymphatic constitution minus the relative amount of lymphatic trauma suffered, a timeline to the expression of lymphedema symptoms remains an unpredictable and highly variable phenomenon (Fig. 104-3).

Dynamic Insufficiency

With its adjustable LTV (lymphatic safety factor) and considerable FR, the lymphatic system both regionally and systemically has an

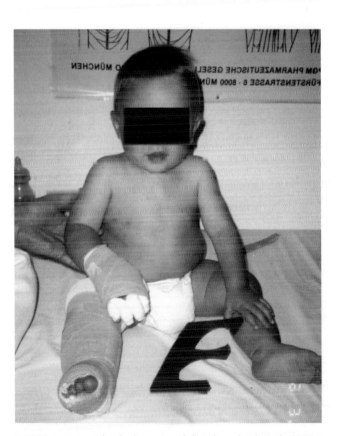

FIGURE 104-1 Milroy's disease with bandage (pediatric).

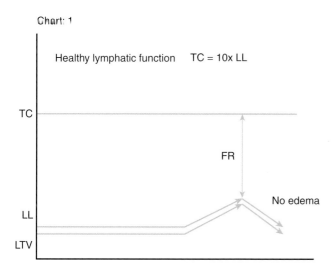

Chart: 1

Healthy lymphatic function   TC = 10x LL

FIGURE 104-2 Healthy lymphatic function.

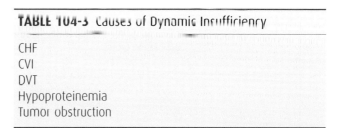

TABLE 104-3 Causes of Dynamic Insufficiency
CHF
CVI
DVT
Hypoproteinemia
Tumor obstruction

the lymphatic system's adaptive function fatigues and then fails (Table 104-3, Fig. 104-4).

Combined Insufficiency

Based upon the former described pathologies it is possible to encounter a combination of mechanical and dynamic insufficiencies. With a lower than normal TC and a higher than normal LL, the gap between demand and capacity yields more of a burden on the lymphatic and venous systems. Postmastectomy-related lymphedema with concomitant congestive heart failure, CHF, is a local failure compounded with the need for extremely high water loads with greatly limited uptake from surrounding veins and lymphatics (Fig. 104-5).

STAGES OF DISEASE PROGRESSION

Lymphedema progression can be best described by clinical impression rather by calculation of limb volume or girth change. Lymphedema progression is most accurately described by clinical impression rather than limb volume calculation or girth measurement. As such, the clinical findings of limb enlargement represent both fluid retention as well as tissue metaplasia accompanied by palpable changes in density and texture (induration) at the epidermal and subcutaneous tissue layers.[3,4,9] Since mechanically insufficient lymphatic response leads to increased population of interstitial proteins, extravascular oncotic pressure draws water away from the microcirculation, feeding the swelling.

Impressive capacity to absorb and transport fluid loads. When the neighboring venous system is patent, the net ultrafiltrate (UF) at the level of the microcirculation is approximately 10%. This net UF represents a LL, with the remaining 90% of tissue fluids returning directly through the venous limb of the capillary loop.[4,5,9,10] When venous health is degraded, hypertension and resultant passive hyperemia cause an increased blood capillary pressure (BCP), resulting in high levels of UF from the venous limb, cancelling venous resorptive capacity.[5] These excessively high LLs represent a potential pathologic demand, taxing the lymphatic system if not therapeutically countered. Such "dynamic" forces may consume much of the FRs, but if not exceeding maximum LTV, tissues will not show clinically evident edema. In this scenario, once the venous water loads exceed the TC of the still healthy lymphatic system, excesses will substantiate a low-protein, clinically apparent venous edema.[3,4,9] It is important to note that this physiologic imbalance leads to secondary lymphedema as

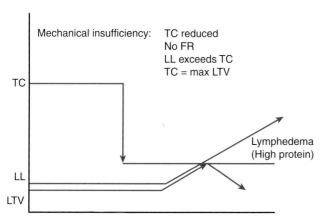

Mechanical insufficiency: TC reduced
No FR
LL exceeds TC
TC = max LTV

Lymphedema
(High protein)

FIGURE 104-3 Mechanical insufficiency.

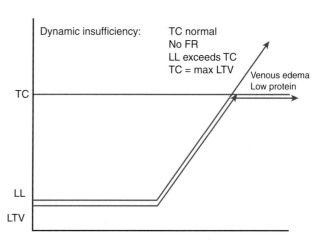

Dynamic insufficiency: TC normal
No FR
LL exceeds TC
TC = max LTV

Venous edema
Low protein

FIGURE 104-4 Dynamic insufficiency.

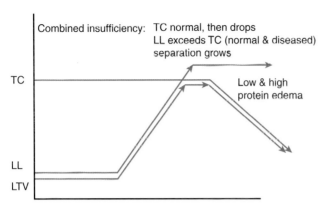

Combined insufficiency: TC normal, then drops
LL exceeds TC (normal & diseased)
separation grows

Low & high
protein edema

FIGURE 104-5   Combined insufficiency.

TABLE 104-4 Stage 0: Subjective Complaints
Achiness
Pain
Heaviness
Waterlogged sensation
Tightness

The resulting lymphedema does not resolve with limb positioning or elevation, as this osmotic pressure holds fluid firmly against the forces of gravity (Table 104-5).[4]

Clinical Impression

The stages of lymphedema progression involve secondary connective tissue disease combined with disturbed uptake and transport of fluid and reflect these attributes in a universal and classic clinical picture. Four distinct stages exist.

Stage 0 (Latency Stage)

Much evidence exists to support the relevance of stage 0 regarding disease progression. Clinical expression is not yet evident unless highly sensitive measurement devices are employed. In this stage patients verbalize a classic list of complaints since there is sound cause to validate the imbalance within the regional lymphatic system. Typical descriptors, such as limb heaviness, achiness, pain, "waterlogged," or tightness, are universal and quite common.[11-15] Until recently, such subjective utterances were dismissed as inconsequential or baseless; however, when not addressed with therapeutic suggestions, stage 0 lymphedema always progresses to stage 1.

As lymph load approaches TC, patient sensitivity to these subtle changes can be reflected in limb volume changes of between 3% and 5% above baseline.[14] While clinical examination is not sensitive enough to detect such subtle imbalances, lymphedema specialists have learned to regard these complaints as highly relevant (Table 104-4).

Stage 1 (Reversible)

In the natural progression of ever-increasing macromolecular waste, the diminished TC is more easily reached or exceeded, creating a transient swelling state. During stage 1, limb elevation, decreased activity level, or self-administered manual therapy resolves the condition as the lymphatic system catches up with the workload placed upon it. Swelling is too recent to have triggered an inflammatory response, so the term "reversible" has been coined to describe its fully remitting characteristics.[1,3,4]

Stage 2 (Spontaneously Irreversible)

In this stage the swelling is ever-present, although it may appear minimal. The fact that a clinically measureable, and visibly apparent swelling is unremitting, indicates onset. LLs that cannot be handled even when the limb is elevated or when activity levels are lessened (and so cannot spontaneously reverse).[3,4] In stage 2 the first indications of fibrosis are apparent, as pitting is subtly more difficult to achieve and skin texture is palpably harder when compressed. Stage 2 is generally characterized as being free of papilloma formations and hyperkeratosis, which are only associated with stage 3.[1,3,4,16] If neglected, stage 2 can advance, becoming massively swollen and pitting resistant even in the absence of such extreme external skin changes. As such, stage 2 may be a lifelong stage for many patients with upper extremity lymphedema.

Stage 3 (Lymphostatic Elephantiasis)

This stage indicates the presence of extreme lymphostatic fibrosis and is usually associated with limb contour distortions and massive girth (Fig. 104-6). Although subcutaneous fibrosis impregnates the tissues throughout the natural course of progression, an additional rough, warty keratin layer (hyperkeratosis) appears with or within papilloma formation (papillomatosis). These severe tissue changes characterize the term elephantiasis, and are unique to lymphedema as a disease process.[1,3,4,9,16] Stage 3 is not uncommon in lower-extremity cases due to neglect, gravity, dependency, and masking or hiding the problem under clothing. Additionally, legs experience a higher incidence of primary lymphedema, which follows a more protracted timeline without an appropriate, accurate diagnosis. Fortunately in the breast cancer population it is uncommon to see prolonged lymphostasis leading to such severe disease expression. This is likely attributable to the vast educational resources available to breast cancer patients, which prompt recognition and earlier diagnosis and treatment. Additionally, patient self-consciousness and the inability to hide a hand swelling attract more attention, prompting therapeutic interventions earlier in the disease progression (Fig. 104-7).

TABLE 104-5 Stages of Lymphedema

Stage 0: Latency stage	Reduced transport capacity and functional reserve No visible, palpable edema, subjective complaints
Stage 1: Reversible	Reduces with elevation, pitting when present, no fibrosis
Stage 2: Spontaneously irreversible	No resolution, may fluctuate, pitting more difficult, fibrosis present
Stage 3: Lymphostatic Elephantiasis	Dermal hardening, non-pitting, papillomas, hyperkeratosis, extreme girth in some

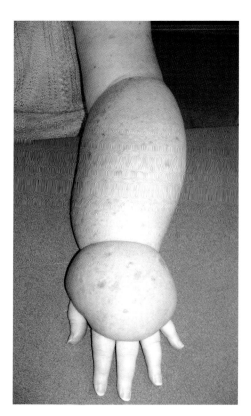

FIGURE 104-6 Stage 3 arm.

SYMPTOMS AND CHARACTERISTICS

Typical/Classic

Lymphedema results in regional immune suppression and leads to an increase in opportunistic infections such as *cellulitis*. As skin integrity suffers, scaling and dryness allow resident skin pathogens (strep and staph) to gain access through the skin barrier. Protein-rich interstitial fluid creates a favorable medium for bacterial colonization. Lymphocyte migration is reduced, and dissected AP nodal sites are slow to detect invaders. Furthermore, stagnant lymph fosters a further delay in immune response.[3,4,9]

Pain is not directly associated with lymphedema in the majority of cases, since the skin accommodates a gradual and insidious accumulation of fluids.[3,4,9,18] Secondary discomfort at the shoulder, elbow, or wrist may be explained by the increased weight of the limb,[4,18] deconditioning, or decreased range of motion. Since the progression is strikingly slow in most cases, gravity and centrifugal forces pull fluids towards distal limb areas, causing an entrenched and stubborn pitting quality. As lymph vessels congest, valvular incompetence feeds the *distal worsening* to include fingers, toes, and dorsal hand/foot regions. Prominent upper extremity structures such as the styloids, epicondyles, and olecranon become progressively less distinct, creating a *columnar* limb appearance. As distinct lymphatic failure is not taxing to the venous system, *skin color remains normal* and blood supply patent, warding off the development of secondary *ulcerations* (Table 104-6).[3,4]

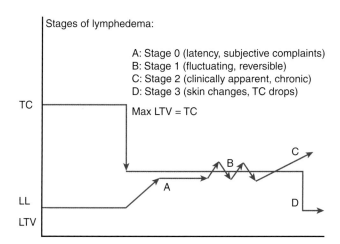

Stages of lymphedema:

A: Stage 0 (latency, subjective complaints)
B: Stage 1 (fluctuating, reversible)
C: Stage 2 (clinically apparent, chronic)
D: Stage 3 (skin changes, TC drops)

Max LTV = TC

TC

LL
LTV

FIGURE 104-7 Stages of lymphedema.

TABLE 104-6 Symptoms and Characteristics of Lymphedema

Slow, gradual progression
Pitting in early stages
Distal to proximal advancement (may spare hand)
Loss of bony contours (columnar)
Dorsal "buffalo hump" if hand involved
Normal skin color (accept stage 3)
History of infection common
Ulcerations rare (pure lymphedema)
Rarely painful (discomfort common)
Asymmetric if bilateral (lower extremities)

Atypical Characteristics

In upper extremity presentations the most notable departures from the norm involve *hand-sparing* and *proximally pronounced* lymphedema. When encountered, these presentations suggest a proximal traumatic disturbance, which has not yet resulted in distal vessel fatigue. In time forearm and hand regions will likely show signs of fluid accumulations as tendonous features and superficial veins become immersed. Rarely, fluid tends to *pool* in one limb region (hand, mid-arm, forearm only) without progressing to involve more tissue. Another atypical characteristic involves a markedly *accelerated progression through the stages* of severity leading to extreme fibrotic tissue changes with or without massive limb girth expressions.

Severity

The severity of breast cancer related lymphedema can be directly correlated to factors such as timeline since initial expression and extent of cancer therapy (number of nodes resected, number of positive nodes, and use of radiotherapy).[11,19-21] Additionally, common exacerbators such as the number of episodes of infection,[4,9,18] weight gain, injury,[13,22] diuretics,[18,22] disuse, pneumatic compression therapy[4,23] and ill-fitting compression sleeves/gloves, contribute to worsening in most cases. The single most important contributor to increasing severity is lack of patient education leading to lack of treatment and/or improper attempts at therapy, which cause further harm.

Postoperative Edema

Immediately following axillary intervention, an increase in upper limb edema of 10% can be expected in 35% of patients.[24] Interestingly, bilateral limb girth increases also occur (32%) in unilateral axillary interventions.[24] These bilateral changes are postulated as reinforcement that the interaxillary anastomosis shares workload when the ipsilateral quadrant is disabled.[24,25] In many cases edema reduces to normal or slightly above in weeks[14,24] and does not return. When edema returns following full healing, it is considered evidence of permanent lymphatic failure and can be accurately classified as secondary lymphedema. The time to secondary onset has been shown to be approximately 6.9 months postoperatively[14] but may not express for many years into the future. Volume changes of 150 mL are not clinically detectable yet support patient complaints (latency stage), and at 200 mL approximately 10% become clinically detectable.[26] As such, a narrow window exists where clinical intervention can more effectively reverse this already burgeoning disequilibrium.

Post-Radiation

Radiation therapy increases the risk of developing lymphedema.[28-30] Radiation fibrosis of the skin and node beds causes symptom expression by challenging the lymphatic systems efforts to adapt to flow disruption. Since this process can be slow it helps explain the delays in diagnosis that lead to advanced stages so commonly encountered in specialized lymphedema clinics. Immediately following radiation, most cases of true secondary lymphedema have not yet expressed, so lymphedema therapist exposure to pronounced swelling is usually limited. Physical therapy focuses on restoration of full range of motion, supple skin, and soft tissue to lessen the mechanical interruption of skin lymphatics and collateral drainage.[31] Should there be a need for lymphedema therapy at the time of radiotherapy, therapists strategize to encourage remote sites of collateral drainage and stay clear of desquamation areas.

Malignant Lymphedema

Primary tumors or recurrent malignancy may provoke swelling due to obstruction of local lymph vessels and regional nodes. Furthermore, local impingement inhibits venous return, arterial perfusion, nerve conduction, and joint function, leading to a distinct constellation of clinical symptoms.[3,4] Malignant lymphedema can be described as proximally pronounced, painful, and rapidly progressing, and is associated with cyanosis, shiny, tight skin, loss of shoulder joint function (with brachial or supraclavicular involvement), and shortening of the neck to acromion distance secondary to guarding against pain.[3,4] Even without many of these phenomena, early detection of recurrence has been clinically evidenced during lymphedema therapy sessions whereby a formerly compliant swelling suddenly becomes treatment resistant. Lymphedema therapists are trained to detect these changes so that medical oncology interventions can be adjusted in a timely fashion.

DIAGNOSIS

Clinical

Lymphedema can be accurately diagnosed using history and physical examination (palpation, inspection).[3,4,9,31] Since axillary trauma has occurred, ipsilateral upper quadrant TC is expectedly reduced. Using the universal characteristics as a guide, while ruling out recurrence, renders sufficient information to arrive at a diagnosis. Breast conservation techniques spare tissue but subject the flaccid breast to potential accumulations, especially when pendulous. Breast and trunk lymphedema are becoming more prevalent solely or in combination with arm swelling so evaluation must include trunk inspection.

Imaging

Lymphography involves a subcutaneous injection of lymphotropic dye (Patent Blue V) followed by x-ray[3,4,9] and provides highly resolute images of lymphatic structures. Lymphography is invasive, painful, damaging to lymphatics, and potentially lethal (1 in 1800), and is therefore no longer recommended.[4] *Lymphangioscintigraphy* (LAS) employs interdigital subcutaneous injection of protein-labeled radioisotopes followed by imaging at time intervals to gather information about uptake and transport time to support a diagnosis. Since images are hazy and false negatives common, well-trained radiotherapists familiar with lymphology and lymphedema specifically can best administer this test. Furthermore, standard criteria for LAS administration are not agreed upon, so measures may not be similarly conclusive.

Limb Measuring Instruments and Methods

The diagnosis of lymphedema can be supported by measurement technologies sensitive to changes in limb volume. One such device is known as the Perometer, which uses a method known as opto-electronic volumetry (Fig. 104-8). By scanning the limb with infrared beams circumferentially, an accurate recording of girth can be measured at 4-mm intervals along the limb length and transmitted to a computer program.[32] This device is used primarily in the research setting and is not typically afforded by outpatient clinics where most patients access care. Preoperative and postoperative measurements at intervals lead to early detection. Therefore wider dissemination of this tool will allow clinicians and surgeons to better assess breast cancer therapy outcomes guiding intervention for lymphedema at the mildest presentation. Studies vary as to assigning the diagnosis of lymphedema to percentage increases of limb volume (3%, 5%, 10%).[14,24,26] Most often, subjective complaints are associated with subtle fluid increases and bolster the diagnosis.

Another device, the *Impedimed XCA* (introduced in 2007) uses *bioelectrical impedance* (Fig. 104-9) to calculate ratios between intracellular and extracellular fluids by passing a weak electrical current through the involved and uninvolved limbs and comparing results. Edematous tissue renders less impedance supporting an accurate diagnosis. Results are compared to average measurements gained from vast population studies measuring impedance levels and then scaling results.[33] Bioelectrical impedance is an emerging, affordable, and portable technology, which will be widely available in clinical settings to support lymphedema diagnosis. Serial measurement of circumference using a standard garment *tape measure* is still the most widely accessible approach. Intra-rater reliability is comparable to any currently used tool but cannot compare when employed for early detection or screening purposes or when various raters are used to assess the same patient.[34] *Water displacement* techniques for limb volume

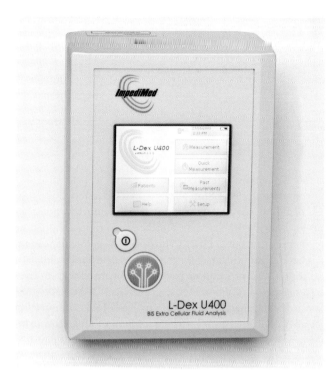

FIGURE 104-9 Extracellular fluid analysis (ImpediMed). *(Reproduced with permission from ImpediMed, San Diego, California.)*

calculation, although accurate, prove impractical in most clinical settings and are therefore rarely used (Table 104-7).

TREATMENT

Historical Approaches and Failed Therapies

Classically lymphedema has been approached without a clear appreciation for, or understanding of, the underlying structure and function of the lymphatic tissues (Table 104-8).

Elevation as sole therapy provides short-lived results since the ever-increasing macromolecular wastes retain water against the effects of gravity. This increase in interstitial colloid osmotic pressure must be addressed with interventions targeted at improving lymphatic function; otherwise disease progression will predictably result. Furthermore, the suggestion of elevation alone is impractical, promotes deconditioning, alters lifestyle if for prolonged periods, and only serves to delay disease progression.[4]

Elastic garments prove inadequate since they attempt to treat this complex condition with compression alone. Medically correct garments are engineered with thoughtful attention to quality textiles and offer gradient support, which facilitates proximal flow. However, without precise tissue stimulation leading to improved lymphangioactivity, macromolecular wastes

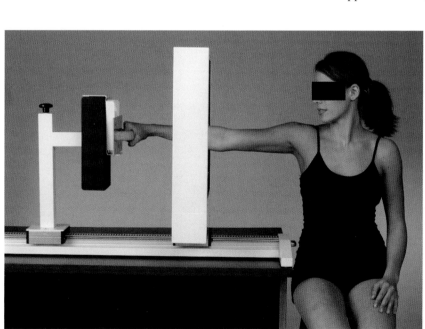

FIGURE 104-8 Arm perometer. *(Reproduced with permission Julius Zorn, Inc. Cuyahoga Falls, Ohio.)*

TABLE 104-7 Limb Measuring Instruments

Optoelectronic volumetry
Bioelectrical impedance
Tape measure (classic)
• Water displacement

cannot be removed. Increases in interstitial pressure provided by compression sleeves and gloves only serve to retard the process of further fluid accumulations. When removed, spontaneous girth increases render an imprecise fit, and in a short time a countertherapeutic effect. Furthermore, garments cannot combat the osmotic forces generated by ever-increasing interstitial wastes. Except for those patients fortunate enough to have been diagnosed in the latency stage or stage 1, disease progression involving metaplasia will ensue. The elastic compression garment is a cornerstone in the continuum of long-term management, but must not be used as a stand-alone treatment.[4]

Until the introduction of complete decongestive therapy, *pneumatic compression pumps* were considered the standard of care. Without an appreciation for the unique structure and function of lymph capillaries and vessels as well as the architecture of skin territories (root areas), the pump cannot provide more than a temporary girth reduction.

Results rendered by the pump can be universally described as involving proximal congestion, accelerated fibrosis development, and a rapid refilling of tissues when removed.[4,35-37] Pneumatic pumps disregard the ipsilateral territory of the excised regional nodes, effectively dumping fluid from the arm into the trunk. Since chest and back vessels drain toward the axilla, fluid cannot drain from within this quadrant. While compression forces generated by the pump are caused by a static inflation–deflation pressure cycle, which does not stimulate lymphangio-activity, pumped fluids contain mostly water, leaving the proteins and other large wastes behind.[37] This action effectively dehydrates the limb as would a diuretic, accelerating lymphostatic fibrosis and leading to a permanently enlarged limb that is no longer fluid filled. Although appropriately prescribed to address water-rich edemas of venous origin, *diuretics* as treatment for lymphedema similarly disregard the fact that lymphedema is a protein-rich edema. Long-term, high-dose diuretic administration leads to treatment-resistant

TABLE 104-8 Historic Approaches: Failed Therapies

Elevation
Elastic garments
Diuretics
Surgery
Pneumatic pumps
Benzopyrones (Coumarin)

limbs similar to those that have received intensive pneumatic compression.[4] *Benzopyrones* such as coumarin promote proteolysis by stimulating macrophage migration into the interstitium. Although some benefits have been noted including limb softening, hepatotoxic reactions and death have been attributed to the drug. Since bioflavonoid are naturally occurring benzopyrones, rutin (vitamin P) has been recommended as a safe alternative; however, no formal studies have been conducted to support its efficacy and dosage.[38,39] *Surgical treatment approaches* for lymphedema utilize either excisional (debulking) or microsurgical techniques. The most extensive technique, the "radical Charles procedure," completely debulks all involved tissue down to the level of the muscle fascia.[4,17] Split-thickness grafts are then harvested from excised skin and donor sites, applied, and limb reduction is achieved (Fig. 104-10). Most of these procedures have been applied to lower extremity lymphedema, offering an alarming cosmetic result. Less radical surgeries championed by Thompson and Homan favor long incisions, preserving the skin but excising subcutaneous edematous portions to achieve girth reductions. In any case the superficial lymphatic system is removed, leading to a further mechanical insufficiency. Microsurgical approaches may involve any number of procedures including autologous transplantation of vessels to bridge defects at regional node beds, lymphovenous anastomosis (LVA), lymph-nodo-venous anastomosis (LNVA) liposuction, and vein bypass grafts.[40-44] Since venous pressures generally exceed intralymphatic pressures, regurgitation and clot formations occlude the vessel lumen.

Current Approaches

The current "international gold standard" for the treatment of lymphedema is *complete decongestive therapy (CDT)*. The originators of the method, Michael and Etelka Foeldi, discovered a unique symbiotic relationship between 4 distinct modalities that addressed the various challenges inherent to the disease process.[23] In 1989 the system was imported to the United States by Robert Lerner and has since become the mainstay domestically.

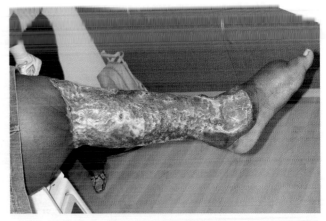

FIGURE 104-10 Radical Charles procedure for lymphedema debulking.

Complete decongestive therapy (2 phase)

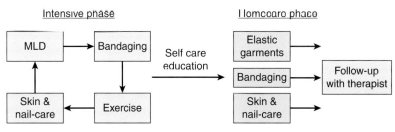

FIGURE 104-11 Complete decongestive therapy (CDT): gold-standard lymphedema management.

approaches the patient with intensive daily treatment sessions to strengthen this collateral flow as a pathway to circumvent the surgical disruption. Since similar collateral anastomoses exist between the ipsilateral upper and lower trunk quadrants at the region of the waist laterally, MLD can again be used to reinforce drainage to inguinal nodes.[46] Treatment strategies further recruit deeper-situated lymphatics such as the thoracic duct, and subclavian trunks that empty at the juncture of the internal jugular and subclavian veins (venous angles) to improve global uptake.[45]

CDT is a *2-phase approach* involving an intensive clinical effort, followed by a semi-intensive home care program geared towards autonomous management, stabilization, and continual improvement. CDT is comprised of manual lymph drainage (MLD), compression bandaging, exercise, skin and nail hygiene, and self-care education. The fifth element, self-care education, is a domestic addition, since access to services and reimbursement took years to develop, leading patients to rely upon honed self-care skills.

The next sections illuminate the beneficial attributes of each modality to the program whole (Fig. 104-11).

Manual Lymph Drainage

Manual lymph drainage is a form of soft-tissue mobilization that provides traction to the skin, causing favorable stimulation to superficial lymph vessels and nodes. As stated in the "Pathophysiology and Lymphatic Insufficiencies" section earlier in the chapter, lymph capillaries contain large inter-endothelial inlets called "swinging tips" akin to overlapping shingles. Each overlapping cell is tethered to the interstitial matrix by anchoring filaments so that increases in fluid cause immediate distension and inflow of lymph. Manual traction of the skin using MLD promotes more uptake of lymph fluid by stretching these filamentous structures, opening swinging tips.[4,45] Deeper-situated lymph collectors have been proven to respond to intraluminal stretch and pull stimulation caused by fluid engorgement and respond with reflexive intrinsic contractions of each lymphangion segment, promoting proximal flow. Similarly application of MLD provides extrinsic stimulation of the lymphangion towards the same end, drawing fluid into the system at the level of the capillaries and promoting flow at the level of the vessels toward regional lymph nodes. With a contraction frequency of 6/min, MLD has been shown to triple this output (18-20/min), greatly enhancing systemic transport.[4,7] MLD applied to breast-cancer-related lymphedema approaches the patient as if the entire upper quadrant (territory of ipsilateral axillary nodes) is involved even if evidence of swelling exists only in the arm. Since interaxillary anastomotic collaterals exist at the sternum anteriorly and between the scapulae posteriorly, MLD can be applied to the contralateral axillary nodes and territory to create a siphon, drawing fluid from an area of high pressure to one of lower pressure. MLD

Compression Bandaging

Compression bandaging provides tissue support following MLD to prevent reflux, retard the formation of new fluid, and mechanically soften areas of fibrosis. Lymphedema bandaging techniques provide a high working pressure[4] (inelastic containment property) to harness the muscle and joint pumps as a propellant for lymph while resisting retrograde flow created by gravity and centrifugal forces during movement. Pure cotton materials coupled with specialized padding create a soft cast-like environment, which confines the swollen tissues without constriction. By relying upon high working and conversely low resting pressures[4] (constitution property) to decrease limb swelling, great control over intensity can be achieved with little to no soft-tissue injury or discomfort. This bulky, inelastic complex is worn following each MLD treatment until the following day's session to intensively control the reduction process without fluctuations. Once a plateau is reached, tissue stabilization and self-care education become the goals of additional sessions. Coupled with continued MLD, a thoroughly decongested limb and trunk quadrant can be maintained or even improved upon in time. In home care, self-management relies heavily upon compression in the form of daytime elastic sleeves (with or without gloves) followed by nighttime compression bandaging to decongest any fluid that may have accumulated in the less supportive sleeve environment. Skin care highlighting hygiene and dermal integrity coupled with activity or specialized exercises performed within the bandage round out the long-term program.

Exercise

Exercise is always performed with adequate support to counteract fluid formation. During the intensive phase, limbs are bandaged to provide complete containment round the clock. Gentle exercises encourage blood flow into the muscle, which when contracted creates a favorable internal pressure (working pressure), effectively squeezing the subcutaneous space between the wall of the bandage and muscle.[3,4] Since every bandage strives to provide a gradient of support, fluid is encouraged towards proximal. Padding layers within the bandage complex thoughtfully imbed themselves, mechanically softening fibrosis while further stimulating lymphangioactivity. During the home care phase patients may continue to coordinate exercise programs so that bandages are still worn, or may graduate to wearing elastic sleeves during exercise if the limb has achieved adequate stability.

Skin and Nail Hygiene

Skin and nail hygiene constitute another major cornerstone of effective lymphedema management. Without well-hydrated, intact skin, cellulitic infections will occur with regularity in many individuals whose immune response has been diminished by regional lymphadenectomy.[3,4,9,31,47] CDT strives to protect the skin from all forms of injury, highlighting the health of the superficial vessel network. Additionally, constriction of any kind along the limb or at the trunk where territories share collateral flow is contraindicated. Patients receive clear guidelines to educate and reinforce appropriate behavior to prevent infection secondary to avoidable external events. Since most cellulitis is caused by resident skin pathogens (*Streptococcus* and *Staphylococcus*), a low skin pH is sought to control colonization. Special lotions provide support for the skin's "acid mantle," while other strategies involve using silver-impregnated textiles to control skin bacteria within fabrics of elastic sleeves and some bandage materials.[3,4,47]

Self-Care Education

Self-care education highlights the unfortunate reality of lymphedema as a chronic condition. Without daily management, lymphedema will destabilize and begin to saturate tissues, causing the expected skin changes. As such, it is of paramount importance for each therapist to equip his or her patient with the necessary self-care tools and knowledge to maintain and even maximize the clinically achieved results. The ability of patients to don/doff compression garments and bandages, exercise safely, preserve skin integrity, monitor for infection, and respond appropriately is the mainstay of autonomous function.

FUTURE DIRECTIONS

Although CDT provides the current benchmark by which other therapies are measured, future interventions for lymphedema sufferers will likely involve strategies that minimize the impact of cancer therapy, identify lymphatic insufficiency as early as possible, and preserve, repair or replace lymphatic tissues directly.

Gene therapy currently seeks to manipulate vascular endothelial growth factors VEGF-C and VEGF-D and their receptors (VEGFR-2 and VEGFR-3) to permit lymphangiogenesis. In the primary lymphedema patient, hypoplasia has been traced to 3 genes: VEGFR-3, FOXC-2, and SOX-18.[4,17] Since these genes are responsible for embryologic formation of both blood and lymph vessels, further specificity is required to identify precise lymphangiogenic factors to avoid overgrowth and tumor formations. Future therapy will focus on tissue engineering towards repair or replacement of lymphatics and will target applications for both primary and secondary lymphedema.

Hyperbaric therapy seeks to disrupt the formation of radiation fibrosis, which entraps skin lymphatics as the subcutaneous tissue becomes impregnated with inflammatory elements while microcirculation retreats. Few studies have been conducted and evidence does not yet exist to support this hypothesis, but current research is forthcoming.

Pharmacologic therapy geared toward proteolysis as has been explored by benzopyrone therapy will continue to receive attention. Drugs that improve lymphangioactivity, such as Daflon, have been shown to decrease limb volumes by 6.8%[4,46] and lead to functional improvement of lymphatics as verified by LAS. Topical application of 8-epi-prostaglandin F2 (PGF2) to lymphedema sufferers decreased lymph capillary pressure markedly, but is yet untested as a treatment for lymphedema.[4] Many other chemicals such as serotonin, histamine, acetylcholine, dopamine, leukotrienes, and noradrenalin increase the activity of the lymph pumps but have only been studied in animals.[4] The horizon for new therapies is wide open as lymphedema becomes better recognized as a disease deserving of pharmacologic intervention.

Surgical therapy to improve drainage consists of myriad forms, which have all proven ineffective. Although microsurgical interventions continue to be explored, no radically new techniques are currently emerging.

PREVENTION AND AVOIDANCE BEHAVIORS

With a known decrease in regional and/or systemic TC, 2 main categories of concern must be noted regarding prevention: (1) insults that increase LL and (2) those that would challenge skin integrity, setting the stage for infection. Active or passive hyperemia within the microcirculation unmitigated by a counteracting increase in interstitial pressure will fluid load tissues and further tax the already diminished lymphatic absorption and transport functions. As such, known stressors triggering arterial limb dilation such as heat, inflammation, excessive strain, overuse (unmonitored exercise), injury, friction, and infection must be avoided. Venous limb stressors such as constriction, dependency, disuse, venipuncture, and even weight gain must also be avoided and monitored, since a resulting passive hyperemia will again fluid load the interstitium.[4] With local immune function depressed, skin preservation education is essential. Avoiding excessively dry skin, minor skin injury, burns, and insect bites constitutes a reasonable lifestyle adjustment that is easily made by most patients. The 3 most common triggers for development of lymphedema are weight gain, injury, and infection,[12,47] and these are largely controllable situations (Table 104.9).

Early Detection

Historically a clinical presentation of edema was the only trusted indicator used to generate an accurate diagnosis. However, it must be noted that once lymphedema has progressed to this stage of clinical presentation (stage 2), albeit mild, a treatment-resistant quality emerges requiring a full spectrum of modalities. As discussion illuminates the "gold standard of care," CDT,[23] which necessarily employs multiple modalities, it becomes apparent that single-modality approaches in comparison prove impotent in reversing, stabilizing, and maintaining lymphedema and its sequelae. In this regard, early detection of lymphedema promises to interrupt the processes contributing to chronic progression and further supports more efficient utilization of health care services and patient resources.

TABLE 104-2 Avoidance Behaviors

Decrease Lymphatic Load
Heat excesses
Overuse
Inflammation
Strain
Injury
Infection
Constriction
Venipuncture
Dependency
Disuse
Weight gain
Preserve Skin Integrity
Hydrate skin
Avoid burns, bites
Minor skin injury
- Rashes, allergies

Detection Tools

Limb volume increase is clinically undetectable up to approximately 150 mL.[14] Only the most astute and well-versed clinician can detect such low levels of edema through palpation or tape-measure methods, so diagnosis is difficult to verify in this earliest time frame. With tools such as bioelectrical impedance (Impedimed XCA) and optoelectronic volumetry (Perometry), subtle increases can be easily calculated. Levels as low as 3%, 5%, and 10% of edema increase above baseline have been used to support lymphedema as a diagnosis toward immediate intervention.[4,24,26] Since perometry can also detect bilateral postoperative fluid, uniform increases cannot be factored into these calculations. Postoperative fluid increases temporarily return to normal in many and those who progress to ≥ 3%, average onset 6.9 months, can be considered to have lymphedema.[14] In 77% of breast-cancer-related lymphedema, onset occurs in the first 3 years following axillary treatments, with a rate of further occurrence at 1% per year following.[12] Screening should therefore prove valuable for the majority of new-onset cases if available at the time of cancer intervention and extended through ongoing oncologic management.

Avoiding Progression (Early Staging)

With new technologies for detection of subtle limb volume increases, clinicians can intervene at the earliest levels in the progression timeline. The diagnosis of lymphedema can be assigned at this earliest preclinical stage, where subjective compliant is coupled with known local lymphatic disruption. Since Axillary Lymph Node Dissection (ALND) and Radiotherapy (XRT) breast-cancer-related lymphedema ranges from 33% to 49%, and 4% to 17% following Sentinel Lymph Node Dissection (SLND) and XRT, a growing evidence base supports this intervention via early detection.[14,48] The form that intervention should take will be debated as outcome measures reflect; however, compression

therapy with elastic sleeves has been shown to restore swelling to baseline within 4 weeks followed by self-administered compression as necessary long-term.[14]

Early Intervention Strategies

To combat edema formation associated with a lowered lymphatic TC, several approaches are being studied, which are described in the next sections.

Compression

Evidence supports the use of elastic sleeves, gauntlets, and gloves to counteract early lymph formation in stage 0 patients by increasing interstitial pressure.[14] Unfortunately, compression offers little stimulation to lymph vessels to improve transport of lymph loads. As such, universal clinical impression verifies the inadequacy of elastic support as sole therapy once lymphedema has triggered secondary inflammation, whereby protein loads have increased to significantly influence a counteracting interstitial oncotic pressure.

Manual Lymph Drainage

Our current understanding of lymphatic anatomy and physiology suggests that when disabled or distressed, the lymphatic vessel function will respond by

- Recruiting intact collateral vessels of the affected territory
- Utilizing intact anastomoses between lymphatic territories
- Increasing LTV[4]

When clinically apparent lymphedema is treated with MLD, the intervention strategy seeks to enhance these processes and facilitate improved lymphatic function (efficiency of absorption and transport) toward neighboring lymph node beds and territories. With earlier diagnosis supported by detection devices such as perometry and bioimpedance, MLD is being utilized to prevent disease progression. Studies are currently underway to examine the relationship between self-applied preventative MLD and onset of lymphedema. Since lymphatic distress is expected following axillary trauma, preventative clinical intervention providing skilled application of MLD may become standard of care once all breast cancer patients are routed through preoperative limb measurement pathways. With the inclusion of basic lymphedema education and ongoing postoperative screening, most patients will be the beneficiaries of less intensive and shorter courses of therapy, utilizing a fraction of the resources usually required to correct such a chronic condition.

Exercise

Although a pure physiologic model of the microcirculation suggests that exercise-related hyperemia further loads the interstitium, taxing subnormal lymphatic response, several studies suggest that moderate, controlled exercise in the predisposed patient cannot be considered a definitive trigger for lymphedema.[30] Research also supports the clinical observation that exercise without compression causes exacerbation in clinically involved limbs.[30] When exercise is employed and a limb is supported with appropriately prescribed compression, swelling will not be exacerbated.[30] Clinical guidelines routinely caution against exercise following axillary intervention but several known benefits may be unachievable such as protection against chronic disease, improved strength, and improved function and range of motion and as well as enhanced feelings of physical and psychological empowerment after cancer therapy.[30,49,50] Additionally, exercise increases lymph flow and the uptake of interstitial proteins, and further enhances lymph transport via the thoracic duct due to intrathoracic pressure changes associated with the breathing cycle.[51] Since venous hypertension may also result from axillary cancer therapy, flexibility (stretching) routines may facilitate fewer contractures, improving venous and lymphatic return.[30] As such, current approaches towards preventing lymphedema must include exercise as a core component.

Complete Decongestive Therapy

In almost every case where early detection devices have not been accessible, lymphedema will have progressed to a chronic yet mild presentation. In such instances, which substantiate the majority of case presentations, intervention requires a multimodality approach such as complete decongestive therapy (CDT) to reverse, stabilize, and mechanically soften lymphostatic fibrosis. A short course of consecutive therapy sessions is generally required to gain control, tailor the approach, and educate the patient adequately for autonomous care. When a course of CDT is administered in this early stage of severity, limb swellings may be completely reversed, requiring far less long-term diligent attention.

CLINICAL ADVICE TO PRACTICING SURGEONS

Perhaps the most critical factor responsible for the high incidence of lymphedema is the absence of understanding regarding lymphedema pathogenesis on the part of the physician. Without an appreciation for lymphedema as a chronic condition of highly variable and delayed onset, breast surgeons often lose sight of the direct connection to former cancer therapy, discounting the need to educate all patients. Lymphedema may express immediately following surgery or delay expression for several decades. Regardless, the underlying damage predisposing the quadrant cannot be mistaken. Also, it must be assumed that FR in lymphatic transport vary widely in the population leading to inabilities that remit incomplete or skewed comprehension. Incidence of occurrence is clearly associated with extent of axillary surgery and administration of adjuvant radiation therapy. However, until further refinements in surgical and radiation technique emerge, lymphedema cannot be avoided, nor can blame be placed on therapeutic approaches targeted at lymphatic tissues.

Decreasing Morbidity

With a greater appreciation for lymphedema as a distinct disease process with its signature traits, physicians can assist patients immeasurably with early education about the risk as well as the pathways for management currently available. It is widely agreed upon that lymphedema cannot be prevented with current cancer management strategies; however, *early education and detection* leading to immediate therapeutic intervention can interrupt lymphedema progression and reverse and control severity, leading to significant quality-of-life improvement. As has been explored, lymphedema becomes rapidly chronic, requiring extensive therapy, while abbreviated approaches have proven inadequate in the majority of this population, leading to mistreatment, self-care failures, hopelessness, and further dread of the condition. As the ranks of well-trained therapists providing CDT grows, lymphedema care is becoming widely accessible, welcoming physician support as a comprehensive team effort to avoid neglect.

Identify Risk Levels

Following sentinel lymph node biopsy the risk of developing lymphedema is quite low but increases with each additional node dissected. Radiation therapy alone, regardless of extent of surgery, further increases risk; and since breast conservation techniques are always preferable, inclusion of radiation therapy supports comprehensive treatment. The most thoughtful approach to counseling involves acknowledging the very real odds of developing lymphedema based upon the most current statistics. As has been stated, incidence may be as high as 49% or more based upon current sound data. Discussion can then lead patients to well-trained therapists so that specific education and detection services can construct a current clinical picture to further tailor an intervention.

Patient Information

With instant access to the Internet, patients quickly become frightened about lymphedema and are easily disillusioned regarding treatment options. It is of paramount importance that patients receive early advice aimed at protecting them from radical or experimental treatments. Basic clarification of the signs and symptoms of latency stage lymphedema, as well as the known triggers, will support the information provided by a referred lymphedema therapist.

RESOURCES, REFERRALS, AND SERVICES

Since lymphedema therapy specialists are not available in all medical centers, a list of regional resources should be compiled to streamline a search to those who possess training in CDT. It should also be noted that a further level of certification is possible once CDT training is completed. Following 1 year of clinical practice, therapists can differentiate themselves as specialists by completing an examination offered by the *Lymphology Association of North America (LANA)*. This organization does not accredit educational bodies but serves to reinforce the body of knowledge, which represents our most current understanding of the disease and its safe and effective treatment.

The *National Lymphedema Network (NLN)*, established in 1988, is a highly regarded resource for patients and clinicians. With its Medical Advisory Committee comprised of leading national experts, responsible current perspectives and tools are provided via website and quarterly newsletter. Other resources include the *Lymphatic Research Foundation (LRF)*, an organization which focuses efforts on finding a cure for lymphatic diseases. The LRF funds research fellowships to help further our specific understanding of the genetics of lymphology, via first-of-their-kind lymphatic tissue banking efforts and patient registries. The *International Society of Lymphology (ISL)* brings together research scientists and clinicians from around the world and publishes a quarterly peer-reviewed journal. Established in 1966, the ISL remains a leading resource for strengthening the field of lymphology as a unique area of specialization. An indispensable English-translated textbook, *Textbook of Lymphology*,[4] is unmatched in scope and has recently become available in the United States, so is highly recommended for all physicians.

SUMMARY

Lymphedema is an increasingly common and recognized comorbidity of cancer therapy affecting nearly half (49%) of all patient who self-report symptoms following ALND and XRT,[11-13] with incidence ranging from 4% to 17% following SLNB and ARL.[16-19] Subjective complaints routinely precede the onset of clinically apparent swelling, implying a need to screen all surgical candidates before and after surgical intervention to detect changes, assess risk levels, and develop a strategy for early intervention when indicated. Although breast surgeons cannot prevent lymphedema with current cancer management techniques, understanding the risk levels, early signs, and availability of specialized resources can lead to interruption of this chronic, dreaded disease process. The pathophysiology of lymphedema has not been widely accessible in English-translated medical textbooks until very recently, which has stunted the American physicians' appreciation for this distinct disease.

REFERENCES

1. Lerner R. Chronic Lymphedema. *Textbook of Angiology.* Springer; 2000.
2. Northrup KA, Witte MH, Witte CL. Syndromic classification of hereditary lymphedema. *Lymphology.* New York, NY. 2003;36:162-189.
3. Weissleder H, Schuchhardt C. *Lymphedema Diagnosis and Therapy.* 3rd ed. Cologne, Germany. 2001.
4. Foeldi M, Foeldi E, Kubik S. *Textbook of Lymphology.* Urban & Fischer; Munich, Germany. 2003.
5. Foeldi M. The role of the lymphatic system in post-thrombotic syndrome. *Lymphology.*
6. Szuba A, Rockson S. Lymphedema: anatomy, physiology and pathogenesis. *Vasc Med.*1997;2:321-326.
7. Kubik S, Manestar M. Anatomy of the lymph capillaries and precollectors of the skin. In: Bollinger A, Partsch H, Wolfe JHN, eds. *The Initial Lymphatics.* Stuttgart, Germany. Thieme-Verlag; 1985:66-74.
8. Piller NB. Macrophage and tissue changes in the developmental phases of secondary lymphedema and during conservative therapy with benzopyrone. *Arch Histol Cytol.* 1990:53:209-218.
9. Olszewski W. *Lymphstasis: Pathophysiology, Diagnosis and Treatment.* CRC Press, Boca Raton, Florida. 1991:330.
10. Foeldi E, Foeldi M, Clodius L. The lymphedema chaos: a lancet. *Ann Plast Surg.* 1989;22:505.
11. Petrek JA, Pressman PI, Smith RA. Lymphedema: current issues in research and management. *CA Cancer J Clin.* 2000;50:292-307.
12. Petrek JA, Senie RT, Peters M, et al. Lymphedema in a cohort of breast carcinoma survivors 20 years after diagnosis. *Cancer.* 2001;92:1386-1377.
13. Armer JM, Radina ME, Culbertson SD. Predicting breast cancer-related lymphedema using self-reporting symptoms. *Nurs Res.* 2003;52:370-379.
14. Stout N, Pfalzer A, McGarvey C, et al. Preoperative assessment enables the early diagnosis and successful treatment of lymphedema. *Cancer.* 2008;112: 2809-2810.
15. Armer J, Fu MR, Wainstock JM, et al. Lymphedema following breast cancer treatment, including sentinel lymph node biopsy. *Lymphology.* 2004;37:73-91.
16. Casely-Smith JR. Alterations of untreated lymphedema and its grades over time. *Lymphology.* 1995;28:174-185.
17. Browse N, Burnand K, Mortimer P. *Diseases of the Lymphatics.* Arnold; London, UK. 2003.
18. Casely-Smith JR. *Modern Treatment for Lymphedema.* Lymphedema Association of Australia; Adelaide, Australia. 1997.
19. Clark B, Sitzia J, Harlow W. Incidence and risk of arm oedema following treatment for breast cancer: a three year follow up study. *QJM.* 2005;98:343-348.
20. Soran a, D'Angelo G. Breast cancer related lymphedema—what are the significant predictors and how they affect the severity of lymphedema? *Breast J.* 2006;12:536-543.
21. Larson D, Weinstein M, Goldberg I. Edema of the arm as a function of extent of axillary surgery in patients with stage I-II carcinoma of the breast treated with primary radiotherapy. *Int J Radiat Oncol Biol Phys.* 1986;12:1575-1582.
22. Werner RS, McCormick B, Petrek J. Arm edema in conservatively managed breast cancer: obesity is a major predictive factor. *Radiology.* 1991;180:177-184.
23. Consensus Document of the International Society of Lymphology Executive Committee. *Lymphology.* 2003;36:84-91.
24. Haines TP, Sinnamon P. Early arm swelling after breast surgery: changes on both sides. *Breast Cancer Res Treat.* 2007;101:105-112.
25. Wolfgang R, Leduc O, Leduc A. Imaging techniques in the management and prevention of posttherapeutic upper limb edemas. *Cancer.* 1998;83:2805-2813.
26. Armer J. The problem of post-breast cancer lymphedema: impact and measurement issues. *Cancer Invest.* 2005;23:76-83.
27. Ryttov N, Holm NV. Influence of adjuvant irradiation on the development of the late arm lymphedema and impaired shoulder mobility after mastectomy for carcinoma of the breast. *Acta Oncol.* 1988;27:667-670.
28. Perre CI, Hoefnagel CA, Kroon BB. Altered lymphatic drainage after lymphadenectomy or radiotherapy of the axilla in patients with breast cancer. *Br J Surg.* 1996;83:1258.
29. Christensen S, Lundgren E. Sequelae of axillary dissection vs. axillary sampling with or without irradiation for breast cancer. A randomized trial. *Acta Chir Scand.* 1989;155:515-519.
30. Ahmed R, Thomas W, Schmitz K. Randomized controlled trial of weight training and Lymphedema in Breast Cancer Survivors. *J Clin Oncol.* 2006;24:1-8.
31. Lerner R, Petrek J. *Diseases of the Breast.* Lippincott-Raven. Philadelphia, PA; 1998:896-903.
32. Stanton AW, Northfield JW, Mortimer PS. Validation of an optoelectronic volumeter (Perometer). *Lymphology.* 1997;30:77-97.
33. Cornish BH, Chapman M, Hirst C. Early diagnosis of lymphedema using multiple frequency bioimpedance. *Lymphology.* 2001;34:2-11.
34. Karges JR, Mark BE, Stikeleather SJ. Concurrent validity of upper extremity volume estimates: comparison of calculated volume derived from girth measurements and water displacement volume. *Phys Ther.* 2003;83:134-145.
35. Pappas CJ, O'Donnell TF. Long-term results of compression treatment of lymphedema. *J Vasc Surg.* 1992;16:555-562.
36. Yamazaki Z, Idezuk Y. Clinical experiences using pneumatic massage therapy for edematous limbs over the last ten years. *Angiology.* 1981;39:154-163.
37. Leduc A, Bastin R, Bourgeois P. Lymphatic reabsorption of proteins and pressotherapies. *Prog Lympol.* 1988;11: 591-592.
38. Casely-Smith JR. Treatment of lymphedema of the arm and legs with 5.6 benzo-a-pyrone. *N Engl J Med.* 1993;329:1158-1163.
39. Loprinzi C. Lack of effect of Coumarin in women with lymphedema after treatment of breast cancer. *N Engl J Med.* 1999;340:346-350.
40. Campisi C. Peripheral lymphedema: new advances in microsurgical treatment and long term outcome. *Microsurgery.* 2003;23:522-525.
41. Gloviczki P. Principles of surgical treatment of chronic lymphedema. *Int Angiol.* 1999;18:42-46.
42. Vignes S. Role of surgery in the treatment of lymphedema. *Rev Med Intern.* 2002;23:426-430.
43. Kim D. Excisional surgery for chronic advanced lymphedema. *Surg Today.* 2004;34:134-137.
44. Brorson H. Liposuction in arm lymphedema treatment. *Scand J Surg.* 2003;92:287-295.
45. Whittlinger H. *Textbook of Dr. Vodder's Manual Lymphatic Drainage.* Heidelberg, Germany: Haug; 1982.

46. Leduc A, Caplan I, Leduc O. Lymphatic drainage of the upper limb. *Lymphology.* 1993 4;13:13-19.
47. National Lymphedema Network Medical Advisory Committee. *Postion Statement Topic: Lymphedema Risk Reduction Practices.* National Lymphedema Network, Oakland, CA. 2005.
48. Petrek J, Heelan M. Incidence of breast carcinoma related lymphedema. *Cancer.* 1998;83(suppl A):2776-2781.
49. Freidenreich CM. physical activity and cancer prevention: From observational to intervention research. *Cancer Epidemiol Biomarkers Prev.* 2001;10:287-301.
50. Pinto BM, Maruyama NC. Exercise in the rehab of breast cancer survivors. *Psychooncology.* 1999;8:191-206.
51. Brennan MJ, Miller LY. Overview of treatment options and the review of the current role and use of compression garments, intermittent pumps, and exercise in the management of lymphedema. *Cancer.* 1998,83:2821-2827.

CHAPTER 105

Diet and Exercise in Breast Cancer Survivorship

Jennifer Ligibel

Accumulating evidence suggests that lifestyle behaviors such as physical activity and dietary patterns may impact breast cancer prognosis. Observational data suggest that patients who are overweight and inactive have higher rates of breast cancer recurrence and overall mortality as compared to patients who are leaner and more active.[1-4] Interventional studies in breast cancer survivors have demonstrated that changes in diet and physical activity patterns are feasible and are associated with improvements in quality of life, less treatment-related weight gain, and fewer disease- and treatment-related side effects.[5] Some preliminary evidence suggests that lifestyle change may also improve prognosis in breast cancer,[6] but much work still needs to be done to validate this and determine which types of lifestyle change are most important. This chapter provides an overview of the observational and interventional work in this area, as well as clinical recommendations for breast cancer survivors.

PHYSICAL ACTIVITY AND BREAST CANCER PROGNOSIS

Four recent prospective observational studies have demonstrated that women who are physically active after breast cancer diagnosis have a better prognosis than sedentary women (Table 105-1). The Nurses' Health Study investigators looked at the relationship between physical activity and rates of breast cancer recurrence and death in a cohort of 2987 women diagnosed with stage I-IIIa breast cancer and demonstrated that patients who engaged in more than 9 metabolic equivalent task (MET) hours/week of physical activity, equivalent to walking at an average pace for 3 h/wk, had a 50% lower risk of breast cancer recurrence, breast cancer death, and all-cause mortality than women who were inactive.[3] The decreased risk of recurrence and death associated with exercise was seen in both pre- and postmenopausal patients and was independent of body mass

index (BMI). Similar results were seen the Collaborative Women's Longevity Study, which collected information regarding physical activity behaviors from 4482 women who had been diagnosed with early-stage breast cancer at least 5 years previously.[4] Women expending more than 2.8 MET h/wk had lower breast cancer mortality when compared to women with lower levels of activity (hazard ratio [HR] 0.65, 95% CI 0.39-1.08 for 2.8-7.9 MET h/wk; and HR 0.59, 95% CI 0.35-1.01 for 8.0-20.9 MET h/wk). Results were again independent of patient age or BMI.

The Health, Eating, Activity and Lifestyle (HEAL) study also prospectively evaluated the relationship between physical activity and breast cancer outcomes.[7] The study collected information regarding activity 3 years after diagnosis from 668 women with early-stage breast cancer. After 6 years median follow-up and 164 deaths, the study demonstrated that women who engaged in at least 9 MET h/wk of activity had a HR for total death of 0.33 (95% CI 0.15-0.73). Although the relatively small number of events limited the power, the study also suggested that women who decreased activity after diagnosis had an increased risk of death (HR 3.95, 95% CI 1.45-10.50) and those who increased activity had a decreased risk of death (HR 0.55, 95% CI 0.22-1.38) as compared to those who maintained a constant level of activity.

The Women's Healthy Eating and Living (WHEL) study assessed the impact of physical activity, body weight, and dietary patterns upon survival in 1490 patients diagnosed with early-stage breast cancer.[8] The study demonstrated a linear trend between mortality and physical activity, with participants who engaged in more than 1320 MET min/wk having a 42% lower risk of death as compared to inactive participants (p for trend = 0.02). There was also a significant relationship between fruit and vegetable intake and mortality ($p = 0.02$), but no trend toward decreasing mortality with increasing fruit and vegetable intake ($p = 0.08$). A composite measurement looking

TABLE 105-1 Prospective Observational Studies of Physical Activity after Diagnosis and Breast Cancer Outcome

Study	N	Menopausal Status	Median Follow-Up (mo)	Timing of Exercise Assessment	Results
Nurses' Health Study (NHS)[3]	2987	Pre and Post	96	At least 2 years post-diagnosis	At least 9 MET h/wk had significant reduction in recurrence, breast cancer death, and overall death: HR 0.57 (0.38-0.85)
Women's Healthy Eating and Living Study (WHEL)[8]	1490	Pre and Post	80	At study enrollment (within 4 years of diagnosis)	Patients who consumed ≥ 5 vegetable/fruit servings/d plus 9 MET h/wk of activity had significant reduction in mortality: HR 0.56 (0.31-0.98)
Collaborative Women's Longevity Study (CWLS)[4]	4482	Pre and post	66	More than 5 years post-diagnosis	Patients who exercised at least 2.8 MET h/wk had significant reduction in breast cancer death: HR 0.58 (0.45-0.75)
Health, Eating, Activity and Lifestyle Study (HEAL)[7]	688	Pre and post	77	3 years after diagnosis	Patients who exercised at least 9 MET h/wk had significant reduction in breast cancer death: HR 0.33 (0.15-0.73)

at fruit and vegetable intake and physical activity showed that participants who both consumed 5 or more servings of fruits and vegetables per day and completed at least 540 MET min/wk of physical activity week (equivalent to walking at a moderate pace for 3 h/wk) had a mortality of 4.8%, compared to 10.4% to 10.7% in participants who had either (but not both) high physical activity or high fruit/vegetable intake, and 11.5% in participants who had low physical activity and low fruit and vegetable intake. The impact of increased physical activity and fruit/vegetable intake was most significant in women whose tumors were estrogen receptor (ER) positive, although there were fewer events in the ER negative subset.

One study has also examined the relationship between physical activity before breast cancer diagnosis and breast cancer outcomes. Abrahamson and colleagues collected information regarding physical activity behaviors from 1264 premenopausal women with newly diagnosed early-stage breast cancer.[9] Participants were asked to recall the average frequency of moderate and vigorous activity that they engaged in at age 13, age 20, and in the year prior to breast cancer diagnosis. The study demonstrated a modest improvement in overall survival in women who engaged in the highest quartile of activity in the year prior to diagnosis as compared to the lowest (HR 0.78, 95% CI 0.56-1.08). The relationship was stronger in women who were overweight or obese at the time of breast cancer diagnosis (HR 0.70, 95% CI 0.49-0.99). There was no relationship

seen between physical activity at ages 13 and 20 and breast cancer prognosis.

In aggregate, these studies encompass more than 10,000 breast cancer patients. Despite the fact that each trial has looked at exercise at a different point in time, all 5 studies demonstrate that breast cancer patients who engage in moderate amounts of physical activity have better disease-free and overall survival as compared to inactive patients. However, despite this evidence, studies have suggested that many women become less active after breast cancer diagnosis. The Health, Eating, Activity, and Lifestyle (HEAL) study evaluated changes in physical activity in the year after diagnosis in a population-based cohort of 812 patients with newly diagnosed early-stage breast cancer.[10] Patients were asked to specify the frequency and duration of participation in a number of different household and recreational activities in the year prior to diagnosis and in the month prior to the interview. Patients were found to decrease total physical activity levels by approximately 2.0 h/wk (11% of total activity) from pre-diagnosis to post diagnosis. Obese patients demonstrated greater decreases in recreational physical activity than overweight or normal-weight patients. The greatest decreases in activity were observed in women undergoing both radiation and chemotherapy, but activity was found to decrease even in women treated with surgery alone. A follow-up questionnaire administered 3 years post-diagnosis to cohort members who remained free of disease demonstrated that less than

50% of patients had resumed pre-diagnosis levels of physical activity even 3 years after their diagnosis, demonstrating that declines in physical activity after diagnosis can be long-lasting in a significant proportion of breast cancer patients.[11]

Physical Activity Intervention Studies

To date, no randomized trial has evaluated the impact of increased physical activity after diagnosis on breast cancer outcomes. However, dozens of interventional studies have looked at the feasibility and potential benefits of exercise both in patients undergoing adjuvant treatment and in breast cancer survivors.[5,12-14] Most of these trials have been small and enrolled patients at a single institution, although 3 recent trials enrolled patients across multiple institutions to distance-based exercise interventions, with or without a dietary component.[15-17] A full review of these studies is beyond the scope of this chapter, but several recent reviews and a meta-analysis have demonstrated that exercise interventions may safely be implemented in breast cancer patients both during and after therapy.[5,12-14] Although results are not completely consistent, studies have also demonstrated that patients who participate in exercise programs experience improvements in quality of life, cancer-related fatigue, and side effects of treatment. Some trials also demonstrated improvements in biomarkers associated with breast cancer risk and prognosis, but again, results were not consistent across trials.[18-20]

DIET AND BREAST CANCER PROGNOSIS

Breast cancer incidence has historically varied widely across the world, with Western countries such as the United States and Europe experiencing relatively high rates of the disease and Eastern countries such as China and Japan experiencing lower rates. Migration studies demonstrate that immigrants from low-risk areas of the world experience higher rates of breast cancer after moving to countries such as the United States, leading investigators to postulate that environmental or behavioral differences must be responsible for these differences in breast cancer risk.[21,22] As a result, more than 1400 studies have been done to evaluate the relationship between dietary intake of fat, fruits and vegetables, supplements, and other nutrients and breast cancer risk.[23,24]

Investigators have also been interested in the relationship between dietary intake and cancer prognosis. Dozens of studies have looked at dietary intakes and breast cancer outcomes.[24-26] Investigators have been especially interested in studying the relationship between dietary fat intake and breast cancer prognosis, given the huge differences in fat intake across the world and the large body of work examining the relationship between dietary fat intake and breast cancer risk. A recent review looked at 13 studies evaluating the relationships between fat consumption and breast cancer outcomes,[25] and demonstrated that 6 of these studies showed an inverse relationship between fat intake and breast cancer outcomes. However, dietary fat intake is often strongly correlated with body weight, which is a known prognostic factor in early stage breast cancer. Four of the 6 studies showing a relationship between dietary fat intake and breast cancer prognosis thus became nonsignificant when analyses were adjusted for BMI and total caloric intake.

Studies have also looked at prognosis in relation to intake of fruits and vegetables, protein, carbohydrates and moderate amounts of alcohol.[25,26] Although several individual studies have shown a relationship between intake of a specific dietary nutrient and breast cancer prognosis, there have generally been no consistent relationships between diet and breast cancer prognosis. One recent paper has suggested that there may be nonlinear relationships between intake of some nutrients and breast cancer prognosis, with patients with either higher or lower than average intake of protein, fat, and other nutrients experiencing a worse prognosis as compared to individuals with more average diets, but these findings require further confirmation.[26]

Dietary Intervention Studies

Two large-scale, randomized trials have examined the impact of dietary modification on disease outcomes in early-stage breast cancer (Table 105-2). The Women's Interventional Nutrition Study (WINS) randomized 2437 women with stage I-IIIa breast cancer to a low-fat dietary intervention or usual care control group.[27] Eligibility included breast cancer diagnosis within 12 months and a baseline diet including at least 20% of daily calories from fat. Participants randomized to the dietary intervention decreased dietary fat intake modestly, and had lower body weight at the end of the study as compared to controls. After a median follow-up of 5.6 years and 227 relapse events, disease-free survival was significantly better in patients randomized to the dietary intervention as compared to the controls (HR 0.76, 95% CI 0.60-0.98). With further follow-up, this difference was no longer statistically significant, but an exploratory subgroup analysis at that time demonstrated a significant improvement in survival in ER-negative patients randomized to the intervention group (HR 0.41, $p = 0.003$).[28]

The Women's Healthy Eating and Living (WHEL) study looked at the impact of a low-fat, high fruit and vegetable diet on disease-free survival in 3088 women with stage I-IIIa breast cancer.[29] Eligibility criteria included breast cancer diagnosis within 4 years. There were no restrictions on baseline diet. Participants randomized to the dietary intervention significantly increased intake of fruits and vegetables, and decreased percentage of dietary calories from fat. The study was designed so that patients did not reduce calories, so as to avoid any confounding effect of weight loss on dietary change. There were no changes in body weight. After a median follow-up of 7.3 years and 518 relapse events, there was no difference in recurrence rates in the diet and control groups (16.7 vs 16.9%, $p = 0.63$).

Thus evidence regarding the impact of dietary change on breast cancer outcomes is inconsistent. WINS suggests that a low-fat diet and/or modest weight loss may lead to improvements in prognosis for patients with early-stage breast cancer, perhaps especially for patients with hormone-receptor-negative breast cancer.[27] However, the WHEL study[29] did not show even a suggestion of improvement in breast cancer outcome in patients participating in an intensive, long-term dietary intervention, and observational evidence has not suggested a link between diet and breast cancer outcomes.[25] Further work is needed before evidence-based dietary guidelines can be developed for breast cancer survivors.

TABLE 105-2 Dietary Intervention Studies

	Women's Intervention Nutrition Study (WINS)[6]	Women's Healthy Eating and Living Study (WHEL)[29]
N	2437	3088
Time since diagnosis	Within 12 months	Within 4 years
Baseline diet	≥20% calories from fat	No restrictions
Stage	I-IIIa	I-IIIa
Average age	58.5	53
Primary end point	Relapse-free survival	Invasive breast cancer event, overall survival
Dietary intervention	Low fat	Low fat; high fruits, vegetables, fiber; isocaloric
Weight loss	Yes, 6 lb	No
Median follow-up	60 mo	7.3 years
Number of events	277	518 recurrences 315 deaths
Results	HR 0.76 (95% CI 0.60-0.98)	Recurrence: HR 0.96 (95% CI 0.80-1.14) Death: HR 0.91 (95% CI 0.72-1.15)

WEIGHT AND BREAST CANCER PROGNOSIS

Abe and colleagues reported the first study looking at the relationship between body weight and breast cancer recurrence in 1976.[30] The study demonstrated that women who were overweight or obese had a 55.6% 5-year survival rate, as compared to 79.9% in leaner women. The study also demonstrated that obese women were more likely to have larger tumors, with higher rates of lymphatic invasion and nodal involvement. Since the initial report by Abe and associates, there have been more than 50 studies examining the relationship between body weight and prognosis.[1,2,31] Studies have looked at weight in a variety of different ways. Older studies generally picked a weight cut point without regard to patient height, whereas more recent studies divided patients based on Quetelet score (weight/height) or BMI (kg/m^2). Regardless of the method used to categorize excess body weight, the majority of these studies demonstrated a strong association between baseline weight and breast cancer outcomes. Several of these studies demonstrate a quadratic or J-shaped relationship between body weight and prognosis,[32,33] suggesting that the risk of adverse prognosis increases exponentially with increasing weight.

A recent review of trials published through 2004 demonstrates that 36 of 51 published trials showed an association between some measure of excess adiposity and poor prognosis, in most cases after adjustment for known prognostic factors such as tumor size, nodal involvement, and tumor grade.[1,2,31] A meta-analysis combining data from several of these trials demonstrated a hazard ratio for recurrence at 5 years of 1.78 (95% CI 1.5-2.11) and for death at 10 years of 1.36 (95% CI 1.19-1.55) for women in higher-weight categories. When the meta-analysis was restricted to trials utilizing BMI to categorize patient weight, the hazard ratio for recurrence at 5 years was 1.91 (95% CI 1.52-2.40) and for death at 10 years was 1.6 (95% CI 1.38-1.76) for women in the highest category of BMI as compared to those in the lowest.[2,31]

Weight Change after Breast Cancer Diagnosis

A few trials have also evaluated the association between weight gain after diagnosis and rates of recurrence (Table 105-3), but results have not been consistent. Three studies looked at recurrences in small groups of patients treated with older chemotherapy regimens, which often incorporated significant doses of steroids and were thus associated with more weight gain than is typically seen with modern chemotherapy regimens.[34-36] One study reported no association between weight gain and recurrence risk.[36] Another study reported an increased risk of death in 5 women who gained more than 10 kg,[34] and the third reported that women who gained a significant percentage of their body weight had an increased risk of recurrence.[35] One additional older study looked at breast cancer outcomes in 545 women treated with a year-long chemotherapy regimen.[37] Premenopausal women gained an average of 5.9 kg and postmenopausal women 3.6 kg. After 6.6 years median follow-up, premenopausal women who gained more than the average amount of weight had a significantly increased risk of death (HR 1.6, p = 0.04), but not of recurrence (HR 1.5, p = 0.15) as compared to women who gained less than the average amount of weight. There was no association between weight gain and recurrence or death in postmenopausal women.

Two more recent trials have looked at the association between weight gain and breast cancer outcomes in larger groups of breast cancer patients. In a study of more than 5000 women treated for early breast cancer, the Nurses' Health Study Investigators demonstrated a significant increase in the risk of recurrence in nonsmoking women who gained more than 2 kg/m^2 (RR 1.64, 1.07-2.51) compared to women who lost or maintained weight.[38] In contrast, Caan and colleagues reported no relationship between either moderate (5%-10% body weight) or more significant (more than 10% body weight) weight gain after diagnosis and breast cancer outcomes in 3215 women with early-stage breast cancer taking part in 2 large cohort studies (HR 0.8, 95% CI 0.6-1.1 and HR 0.9, 95% CI 0.7-1.2, respectively).[39] The group also reported an increased risk of breast cancer recurrence and death in women who lost more than 10% of their body weight in the 4 years following breast cancer diagnosis (HR 1.7, 95% CI 1.0-2.6 and HR 2.1, 95% CI 1.3-3.4, respectively),[40] but this finding has not been corroborated in other studies. Thus although there is consistent evidence that increased weight at the time of breast cancer diagnosis is associated with poor prognosis, more work is needed to determine whether weight gain and weight loss after breast cancer diagnosis are related to breast cancer outcome.

Weight Loss Intervention Studies

Despite the large number of observational studies demonstrating an association between increased weight at diagnosis and poor prognosis in patients with early breast cancer, there is currently no direct evidence that weight loss decreases risk of breast cancer recurrence, and to date, only a few small pilot trials have reported results of weight loss interventions in breast cancer survivors. Goodwin and colleagues reported that 70% of participants met weight goals in a trial looking at the ability of a multidisciplinary weight management intervention, comprised of support groups providing diet and exercise counseling, to help patients lose weight or avoid weight gain during adjuvant chemotherapy.[41] Mefferd and colleagues also performed a randomized trial of a cognitive behavioral therapy weight loss intervention in 85 overweight breast cancer survivors and demonstrated significant reductions in body weight, body fat, and lipids following the 16-week intervention ($p = 0.05$).[42] Shaw and colleagues performed a randomized pilot study in 64 obese women with early-stage breast cancer and demonstrated that participants randomized to a low-fat or a low-calorie diet experienced significant weight loss and reduction in body fat as compared to controls ($p = 0.006$ and 0.008, respectively).[43] Finally, Djuric and colleagues randomized 48 obese breast cancer survivors to 1 of 3 dietary intervention arms (Weight Watchers program, individualized dietary counseling, or a combination of the two), or to a control group.[44] Women assigned to the combination group lost a significant amount of weight as compared to the controls by 3 months, and maintained this through the 12-month study. Women assigned to the individualized counseling group lost a significant amount of weight by the end of the study, but the Weight Watchers-alone group did not experience significant weight loss.

One ongoing randomized trial will look at the impact of weight loss after diagnosis on breast cancer outcomes. The Lifestyle Intervention Study for Adjuvant Treatment of Early Breast Cancer (LISA) will randomize more than 2000 postmenopausal women with hormone-receptor-positive, stage I-IIIa breast cancer to an educational control group or to a 2-year, telephone-based weight loss intervention, modeled on the Diabetes Prevention Project.[45] The primary objective of the trial is to determine the impact of participation in a telephone-based weight loss intervention upon disease-free survival in women with hormone-receptor-positive breast cancer. Secondary objectives include assessing the impact of the intervention upon survival, distant disease-free survival, weight, quality of life, and the incidence of arthritis and diabetes.

POTENTIAL BIOLOGICAL MEDIATORS OF RELATIONSHIP BETWEEN ENERGY BALANCE AND BREAST CANCER PROGNOSIS

The biological mechanisms underlying the relationship between lifestyle factors and breast cancer are not well understood. In postmenopausal women, obesity is associated with higher levels of estrone and estradiol due to increased peripheral aromatization of adrenal androgens in adipose tissue and decreased binding to sex-hormone-binding globulin.[46] Observational studies performed prior to the widespread use of the aromatase inhibitors as adjuvant therapy for early-stage breast cancer have demonstrated that higher levels of sex steroids are a poor prognostic factor. Rock and colleagues performed a nested case-control study looking at the relationship between levels of estradiol, testosterone, and sex-hormone-binding globulin (measured an average of 23 months from diagnosis) and risk of breast cancer recurrence in 153 matched pairs of peri- and postmenopausal women from the control arm of the WHEL study.[47] The investigators demonstrated a significant increase in the risk of recurrence with increasing levels of estradiol (HR 1.41 for each unit increase in log concentration of estradiol), but did not see any relationship between levels of testosterone or sex-hormone-binding globulin. Micheli and colleagues looked at the relationship between testosterone levels (measured an average of 3 months after diagnosis) and recurrence in 194 postmenopausal women with stage I and IIa breast cancers not treated with hormonal therapy.[48] Patients with testosterone levels above the median of 4.0 ng/mL were found to have significantly lower event-free survival as compared to women with testosterone levels below the median (HR 2.05, 95% CI 1.28-3.27).

Although variations in levels of sex steroids may explain, at least in part, the relationship between energy balance and breast cancer in postmenopausal women, obesity and inactivity are also associated with poor prognosis in premenopausal women.[1-3] In premenopausal women, sex steroids derive primarily from the ovaries and are thus not as affected by excess weight. Additionally, preoperative estradiol levels in premenopausal women are not related to risk of breast cancer recurrence or death,[49] suggesting that obesity must affect prognosis through some mechanism other than sex-steroid levels in this population.

Studies have demonstrated that obesity and inactivity are associated with higher levels of insulin and other metabolic hormones in both pre- and postmenopausal women.[50,51] Insulin promotes proliferation of malignant breast cells in vitro[52] and is a structural homologue of insulinlike growth factor 1 (IGF-1), which has been demonstrated to have mitogenic properties in vitro and is associated with an increased risk of premenopausal breast cancer.[53] Two recent observational studies have also suggested that elevated insulin levels are associated with poor prognosis in early-stage breast cancer. Goodwin and colleagues measured fasting insulin levels shortly after diagnosis in 512 women with early-stage breast cancer. After a 50-month median follow-up,

TABLE 105-3 Selected Observational Studies of Weight Gain and Breast Cancer Outcome

Study	N	Years of Enrollment	Events	Average Weight Gain	Follow-up (y)	Results
Camoriano et al[37]	545	1979-1985	Not reported	5.9 kg premenopausal 3.6 kg postmenopausal	6.6	Significant increase in risk of death in premenopausal women who gained weight (RR 1.6, $p < 0.05$). No significant increase in recurrence risk in premenopausal women, or in risk of recurrence or death in postmenopausal women who gained weight
Kroenke et al (Nurses' Health Study)[38]	5204	1976-2000	860 deaths, 681 recurrences	33% of women gained between 0.5 and 2 kg/m² (average 6 lb) 14% of women gained more than kg/m² (average 17 lb)	9	Women who gained 0.5-2.0 kg/m² had RR for recurrence of 1.35 (95% CI 0.93-1.95), and those who gained > 2.0 kg/m² had RR of 1.64 (95% CI 1.07-2.51)
Caan et al[39]	3215	1995-2002	333 breast cancer events	3.17 kg WHEL cohort 1.81 LACE cohort	6.2	No relationship between either moderate (5%-10% body weight) or more significant weight gain (> 10%) and cancer recurrence

women in the highest quartile of insulin levels were found to have twice the risk of distant recurrence and 3.1 times the risk of death as women with the lowest insulin levels.[32] Another recent study demonstrated that women with high levels of c-peptide, a breakdown product of insulin production, at the time of breast cancer diagnosis were found to have a lower event-free survival as compared to women with lower levels of c-peptide.[54] Finally, a third recent study has demonstrated that breast cancer patients with "metabolic syndrome," a condition including elevated fasting glucose levels and increased abdominal adiposity, had a 3-fold increase in the risk of cancer recurrence as compared to patients without these features.[55]

In addition to insulin, other substances have been implicated in the relationship between obesity and breast cancer. Epidemiologic studies have shown that high plasma levels of IGF-1 are associated with increased risk of breast cancer, especially in premenopausal women.[53,56] In vitro data also suggest that IGF-1 signaling plays a central role in the development and progression of breast cancer.[57,58] Additionally, adipose cells produce several other hormones and biologically active substances, such as leptin, adiponectin, and hepatocyte growth factor (HGF). In vitro studies have suggested that these adipose-related hormones can impact growth of breast cancer cells lines,[59,60] and recent work has demonstrated adiponectin receptor expression in breast tumors, as well as over-expression of adiponectin in adipose tissue adjacent to malignant breast tissue.[61] Case control studies have demonstrated lower levels of

adiponectin and higher levels of leptin in women who develop breast cancer as compared to controls,[61-63] and one recent cohort study has shown a trend toward decreased breast cancer risk in postmenopausal women with adiponectin levels in the highest quartile.[64]

Numerous studies in non-breast-cancer populations have demonstrated that lifestyle interventions can decrease visceral body fat, improve insulin sensitivity, and lead to alterations in other metabolic hormones in both diabetic and nondiabetic populations.[65-67] One study has recently demonstrated that participation in a mixed-strength and aerobic exercise intervention led to a 28% decrease in fasting insulin levels in a group of overweight breast cancer survivors.[19] However, other groups have failed to show exercise-induced changes in levels of insulin and other metabolic hormones in breast cancer survivors.[18,20] Further work is needed to evaluate the biological mechanisms through which physical activity, weight, and diet may impact breast cancer prognosis.

FUTURE DIRECTIONS

There is currently a large body of observational data suggesting that physical activity, body weight, and possibly diet may influence breast cancer prognosis. However, other than the WINS and WHEL randomized dietary intervention trials, there have been few randomized studies evaluating the impact of lifestyle change after diagnosis upon breast cancer outcomes. Additionally,

TABLE 105-4 Clinical Recommendations for Breast Cancer Survivors

	Recommendation	Level of Evidence
Diet	Balanced diet important for weight maintenance, consider low-fat diet	WINS study[27] suggested that low-fat diet may lead to better prognosis, but WHEL did not show improvement with similar diet[29]
Physical activity	At least 3-5 h/wk of moderate exercise such as walking at a 2.5-3 mile/h pace	Observational evidence showing better prognosis in women who exercise moderately + interventional studies showing better quality of life, fatigue, and symptoms[3,4,7]
Weight	Avoid weight gain, consider modest weight loss (5%-10% body weight) for women who have a BMI > 25 kg/m²	Observational evidence suggesting poor prognosis in women who are overweight at the time of diagnosis, WINS possibly showing that weight loss improves prognosis[27]

the biological mechanisms through which lifestyle factors may impact breast cancer are currently poorly understood.

The ongoing LISA will provide the first information from a randomized trial regarding the impact of a weight loss intervention upon breast cancer recurrence in postmenopausal women with hormone-receptor-positive breast cancer. Additional randomized studies are needed to evaluate the impact of weight loss upon breast cancer outcomes in other groups of patients, such as premenopausal women and those with hormone-receptor-negative disease, whom the WINS study suggested may derive significant benefit from behavioral change after diagnosis. Further work is also needed to confirm the impact of dietary change upon this group of women with hormone-receptor-negative breast cancer.

Additionally, given the strong observational data suggesting a relationship between physical activity and breast cancer prognosis, randomized trials are needed to test whether increasing activity after breast cancer diagnosis leads to improvements in prognosis. Finally, more work needs to be done to determine the biological mechanisms through which these lifestyle changes may impact breast cancer prognosis, in order to provide insight into metabolic and other factors that impact breast cancer development and progression, and also to help identify patient populations who may especially benefit from lifestyle modifications after breast cancer diagnosis.

SUMMARY

Observational studies have suggested that breast cancer patients who engage in modest levels of physical activity,[3,4,7] and perhaps those who maintain a BMI between 19 and 25,[1,2] have a better prognosis than do patients who are inactive or heavier. Interventional studies have also demonstrated that women who increase physical activity, lose weight, and change dietary patterns after breast cancer diagnosis have a better quality of life, less fatigue, and fewer cancer- and treatment-related symptoms.[5,13,14] Although there is currently little randomized evidence that changes in diet and exercise behaviors after breast cancer diagnosis will decrease the risk of breast cancer recurrence, one randomized trial suggested that decreasing dietary fat might

lead to better outcomes. Further randomized trials will be needed to evaluate the impact of increased physical activity, weight loss, and dietary change upon breast cancer prognosis. Given the evidence currently available, it is reasonable to suggest the lifestyle recommendations for breast cancer survivors given in Table 105-4.

REFERENCES

1. Chlebowski R, Aiello E, McTiernan A. Weight loss in breast cancer patient management. *J Clin Oncol.* 2002;20:1128-1143.
2. Goodwin P. Energy balance and cancer prognosis: breast cancer. In: McTiernan A, ed. *Cancer Prevention and Management Through Exercise and Weight Control.* Taylor and Francis Group; 2006:405-435.
3. Holmes M, Chen W, Feskanich D, et al. Physical activity and survival after breast cancer diagnosis. *JAMA.* 2005;293:2479-2486.
4. Holick C, Newcomb P, Trentham-Dietz A, et al. Physical activity and survival after diagnosis of invasive breast cancer. *Cancer Epidemiol Biomarkers Prev.* 2008;17:379-386.
5. Galvao D, Newton R. Review of exercise interventions studies in cancer patients. *J Clin Oncol.* 2005;23:899-909.
6. Chlebowski R, Blackburn G, Thomson C, et al. Dietary fat reduction and breast cancer outcome: interim efficacy results from the Women's Intervention Nutrition Study. *J Natl Cancer Inst.* 2006;98:1767-1776.
7. Irwin M, Smith A, McTiernan A, et al. Influence of pre- and postdiagnosis physical activity on mortality in breast cancer survivors: the health, eating, activity, and lifestyle study. *J Clin Oncol.* 2008;26:3958-3964.
8. Pierce J, Stefanick M, Flatt S, et al. Greater survival after breast cancer in physically active women with high vegetable-fruit intake regardless of obesity. *Clin Oncol.* 2007;17:2345-2351.
9. Abrahamson P, Gammon M, Lund M, et al. Recreational physical activity and survival among young women with breast cancer. *Cancer.* 2006;107:1777-1785.
10. Irwin M, Crumley D, McTiernan A, et al. Physical activity levels before and after a diagnosis of breast carcinoma. *Cancer.* 2003;97:1746-1757.
11. Irwin M, McTiernan A, Bernstein L, et al. Physical activity levels among breast cancer survivors. *Med Sci Sports Exerc.* 2004;36:1484-1491.
12. Markes M, Brockow T, Resch K. Exercise for women receiving adjuvant therapy for breast cancer. *Cochrane Database Syst Rev.* 2006;4:CD005001. DOI: 10.1002/14651858.CD005001.pub2.
13. Doyle C, Kushi L, Byers T, et al. Nutrition and physical activity during and after cancer treatment: an American Cancer Society guide for informed choices. *CA: Cancer J Clin.* 2006;56:323-353.
14. McNeeley M, Campbell K, Rowe B, et al. Effects of exercise on breast cancer patients and survivors: a systematic review and meta-analysis. *Can Med Assoc J.* 2006;175:34-41.
15. Demark-Wahnefried W, Clipp E, Lipkus I, et al. Main outcomes of the FRESH START trial: a sequentially tailored, diet and exercise mailed print intervention among breast and prostate cancer survivors. *J Clin Oncol.* 2007;25:2709-2718.

16. Demark-Wahnfried W, Clipp E, Morey M, et al. Lifestyle intervention development study to improve physical function in older adults with cancer: outcomes from project LEAD. *J Clin Oncol.* 2006;24:3465-3473.

17. Vallance J, Courneya K, Plotnikoff R, et al. Randomized controlled trial of the effects of print materials and step pedometers on physical activity and quality of life in breast cancer survivors. *J Clin Oncol.* 2007;25:2352-2359.

18. Fairey A, Courneya K, Field C, et al. Effects of exercise training on fasting insulin, insulin resistance, insulin-like growth factors, and insulin-like growth factor binding proteins in postmenopausal breast cancer survivors: a randomized controlled trial. *Cancer Epidemiol Biomarkers Prev.* 2003;12:721-727.

19. Ligibel J, Campbell N, Partridge A, et al. Impact of a mixed strength and endurance exercise intervention on insulin levels in breast cancer survivors. *J Clin Oncol.* 2008;26:907-912.

20. Schmitz K, Ahmed R, Hannan P, Yee D. Safety and efficacy of weight training in recent breast cancer survivors to alter body composition, insulin, and insulin-like growth factors. *Cancer Epidemiol Biomarkers Prev.* 2005;14:1672-1680.

21. Chie W, Chen C, Chen C, et al. Geographic variation of breast cancer in Taiwan: international and migrant comparison. *Anticancer Res* 1995;15:2745-2749.

22. Stanford J, Herrington L, Schwartz S, Weiss N. Breast cancer incidence in Asian migrants to the United States and their descendants. *Epidemiology.* 1995;6:181-183.

23. Michels K, Mohllajee A, Roset-Bahmanyar E, et al. Diet and breast cancer: a review of the prospective observational studies. *Cancer* 2007;109:2712-2749. Available from file:///H./Exercise%20papers/Vit%20D/Fuchs,%20colon.htm

24. Berrino F, Krogh V, Riboli E. Epidemiology studies on diet and cancer. *Tumori.* 2003;89:581-585.

25. Rock C, Demark-Wahnefried W. Nutrition and survival after the diagnosis of breast cancer: a review of the evidence. *J Clin Oncol.* 2002;20:3302-3316.

26. Goodwin P, Ennis M, Pritchard K, et al. Diet and breast cancer: evidence that extremes in diet are associated with poor survival. *J Clin Oncol.* 2003:2500-2507.

27. Chlebowski R, Blackburn G, Elashoff R, et al. Mature analysis from the womens intervention nutrition study (WINS) evaluating dietary fat reduction and breast cancer outcome San Antonio Breast Cancer Symposium, 2006.

28. Chlebowski R, Blackburn G, Hoy M, et al. Survival analyses from the Women's Intervention Nutrition Study (WINS) evaluating dietary fat reduction and breast cancer outcome. *Am Soc Clin Oncol.* 2008;26(suppl). Abstract 522.

29. Pierce J, Natarajan L, Caan B, et al. Influence of a diet very high in vegetables, fruit, and fiber and low in fat on prognosis following treatment for breast cancer: the Women's Healthy Eating and Living (WHEL) randomized trial. *JAMA.* 2007;298:289-298.

30. Abe R, Kumagi G, Kimura M, et al. Biological characteristics of breast cancer in obesity. *Tohoku J Exp Med.* 1976;120:351-359.

31. Goodwin P, Boyd N. Body size and breast cancer prognosis: a critical review of the evidence. *Breast Cancer Res Treat.* 1990;16:205-214.

32. Goodwin P, Ennis M, Pritchard K, Trudeau M. Fasting Insulin and outcome in early-stage breast cancer: results of a prospective cohort study. *J Clin Oncol.* 2002;20:42-51.

33. Suissa C, Pollak M, Spitzer W, Margolese R. Body size and breast cancer prognosis: a statistical explanation of the discrepancies. *Cancer Res* 1989;49:0111-3111.

34. Chlebowski R, Weiner J, Reynolds R, et al. Long-term survival following relapse after 5-FU but not CMF adjuvant breast cancer therapy. *Breast Cancer Res Treat.* 1986;7:23-29.

35. Bonomi P, Bunting N, Fishman D, et al. Weight gain during adjuvant chemotherapy or hormono-chemotherapy for stage II breast cancer in relation to disease free survival. *Breast Cancer Res Treat.* 1984;4:339. Abstract.

36. Levine E, Raczynski J, Carpenter J, et al. Weight gain with breast cancer adjuvant treatment. *Cancer.* 1991;67:1954-1959.

37. Camoriano J, Loprinzi C, Ingle J, et al. Weight change in women treated with adjuvant therapy or observed following mastectomy for node-positive breast cancer. *J Clin Oncol.* 1990;8:1327-1334.

38. Kroenke C, Chen W, Rosner B, Holmes M. Weight, weight gain, and survival after breast cancer diagnosis. *J Clin Oncol.* 2005;23:1370-1378.

39. Caan B, Emond J, Natarajan L, et al. Post-diagnosis weight gain and breast cancer recurrence in women with early stage breast cancer. *Breast Cancer Res Treat.* 2006;99:47-57.

40. Caan B, Kwan M, Hartzell G, et al. Pre-diagnosis body mass index, post-diagnosis weight change, and prognosis among women with early stage breast cancer. *Cancer Causes Control* 2008 Published online August 20, 2008.

41. Goodwin P, Esplen M, Butler K, et al. Multidisciplinary weight management in locoregional breast cancer: results of a phase II study. *Breast Cancer Res Treat.* 1998;48:53-64.

42. Mefferd K, Nichols J, Pakiz B, Rock C. A cognitive behavioral therapy intervention to promote weight loss improves body composition and blood lipid profiles among overweight breast cancer survivors. *Breast Cancer Res Treat.* 2007;104:145-152.

43. Shaw C, Mortimer P, Judd P. Randomized controlled trial comparing a low-fat diet with a weight-reduction diet in breast cancer lymphedema. *Cancer.* 2007;109:1949-1956.

44. Djuric Z, DuLaura N, Jenkins I, et al. Combining weight-loss counseling with the Weight Watchers plan for obese breast cancer survivors. *Obesity Res.* 2002;10:657-665.

45. Group DPPR. Reduction in the incidence of type 2 diabetes with lifestyle intervention or metformin. *N Engl J Med.* 2002;346:393-403.

46. Kaye S, Folsom A, Soler J, et al. Associations of body mass and fat distribution with sex hormone concentrations in postmenopausal women. *Int J Epidemiol.* 1991;20:151-156.

47. Rock C, Flatt S, Laughlin G, et al. Reproductive steroid hormones and recurrence-free survival in women with a history of breast cancer. *Cancer Epidemiol Biomarkers Prev.* 2008;17:614-620.

48. Micheli A, Meneghini E, Secreto G, et al. Plasma testosterone and prognosis of postmenopausal breast cancer patients. *J Clin Oncol.* 2007;25:2685-2690.

49. Pujol P, Daures J, Brouillet J, et al. A prospective prognostic study of the hormonal milieu at the time of surgery in premenopausal breast carcinoma. *Cancer.* 2001;91:1854-1861.

50. Soler J, Folsom A, Kaye S, Prineas R. Associations of abdominal adiposity, fasting insulin, sex hormone binding globulin, and estrone with lipids and lipoproteins in post-menopausal women. *Atherosclerosis.* 1989;79:21-27.

51. Peiris A, Sothman M, Hennes M, et al. Relative contributions of obesity and body fat distribution to alterations in glucose insulin homeostasis: predictive values of selected indices in premenopausal women. *Am J Clin Nutr.* 1989;49:758-764.

52. Belfiore A, Frittitta L, Constantino A, et al. Insulin receptors in breast cancer. *J Endocrinol Invest.* 1996;784:173-188.

53. Hankinson S, Willett W, Colditz G, et al. Circulating concentrations of insulin-like growth factor-1 and risk of breast cancer. *Lancet.* 1998;351:1393-1396.

54. Pollak M, Chapman J, Shepherd L, et al. Insulin resistance, estimated by serum C-peptide level, is associated with reduced event-free survival for postmenopausal women in NCIC CTG MA.14 adjuvant breast cancer trial. *J Clin Oncol.* 2006;24:524.

55. Pasanisi P, Berrino F, De Petris M, et al. Metabolic syndrome as a prognostic factor for breast cancer recurrences. *Int J Cancer.* 2006;119:236-238.

56. Li B, Khosravi M, Berkel H. Free IGF-1 and breast cancer risk. *Int J Cancer.* 2001;91:736-739.

57. Bradley L, Gierthy J, Pentecost B. Role of the insulin-like growth factor system on an estrogen-dependent cancer phenotype in the MCF-7 human breast cancer cell line. *J Steroid Biochem Mol Biol.* 2008;109:185-196.

58. Creighton C, Casa A, Lazard Z, et al. Insulin-like growth factor-I activates gene transcription programs strongly associated with poor breast cancer prognosis. *J Clin Oncol.* 2008;26:4078-4085.

59. Garofalo C. Obesity hormone leptin: a new target in breast cancer? *Breast Cancer Res.* 2007;9:301-302.

60. Rose D, Komninou D, et al. Obesity, adipocytokines, and insulin resistance in breast cancer. *Obesity Rev.* 2004;5:153-165.

61. Korner A, Pazaitou-Panayiotou K, Kelesidis T, et al. Total and high molecular weight adiponectin in breast cancer: in vitro and in vivo studies. *J Clin Endocrinol Metab.* 2007;92:1041-1048.

62. Mantzoros C, Petridou E, Dessypris N, et al. Adiponectin and breast cancer risk. *J Clin Endocrinol Metab.* 2004;89:1102-1107.

63. Chen D, Chung Y, Yeh Y, et al. Serum adiponectin and leptin levels in Taiwanese breast cancer patients. *Cancer Lett.* 2006;237:109-114.

64. Tworoger S, Eliassen A, Kelesidis T, et al. Plasma adiponectin concentrations and risk of incident breast cancer. *J Clin Endocrinol Metab.* 2007;92:1510-1516.

65. Hawley J. Exercise as a therapeutic intervention for the prevention and treatment of insulin resistance. *Diabetes Metab Res Rev.* 2004;20:383-393.

66. Frank L, Sorensen B, Yasui Y, et al. Effects of exercise on metabolic risk variables in overweight postmenopausal women. A randomized clinical trial. *Obesity Res.* 2005;13:615-625.

67. Braith R, Stewart K. Resistance exercise training: its role in the prevention of cardiovascular disease. *Circulation.* 2006;113:2642-2650.

INDEX

Note: Page numbers followed by *f* or *t* refer to figures or tables, respectively.